Non-Neoplastic Disorders of the Lower Respiratory Tract

ATLAS OF NONTUMOR PATHOLOGY

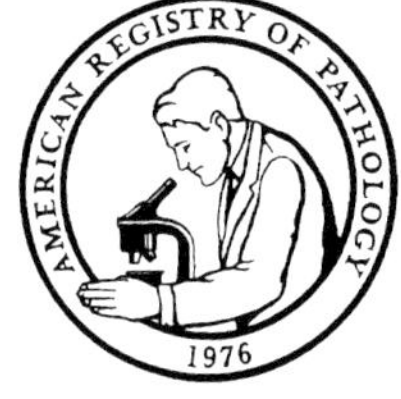

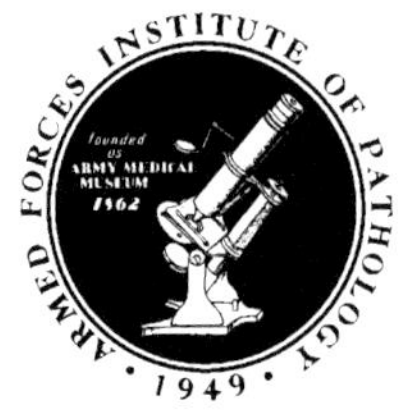

ATLAS OF NONTUMOR PATHOLOGY

First Series
Fascicle 2

Non-Neoplastic Disorders of the Lower Respiratory Tract

William D. Travis, MD
Thomas V. Colby, MD
Michael N. Koss, MD
Melissa L. Rosado-de-Christenson, Col, USAF, MC, FACR
Nestor Luiz Müller, MD, PhD
Talmadge E. King Jr., MD

Published by the
American Registry of Pathology
and the
Armed Forces Institute of Pathology
Washington, DC

In Collaboration with
Universities Associated for Research
and Education in Pathology, Inc.
Bethesda, Maryland

2002

ATLAS OF NONTUMOR PATHOLOGY

Manuscript Reviewed by:
Andrew G. Nicholson, DM, FRCPath
Victor L. Roggli, MD

Accepted for Publication
2001

Available from the American Registry of Pathology
Armed Forces Institute of Pathology
Washington, DC 20306-6000
www.afip.org
ISBN: 1-881041-79-4

INTRODUCTION TO SERIES

This is the second Fascicle of the Atlas of Nontumor Pathology, a complementary series to the Armed Forces Institute of Pathology (AFIP) Atlas of Tumor Pathology, first published in 1949.

For several years, various individuals in the pathology community have suggested the formation of a new series of monographs concentrating on this particular area. In 1998, an Editorial Board was appointed and outstanding authors chosen shortly thereafter.

The purpose of the Atlas is to provide surgical pathologists with ready expert reference material most helpful in their daily practice. The lesions described relate principally to medical non-neoplastic conditions as exemplified by our first three Fascicles on endocrine, pulmonary, and skin diseases. Many of these lesions represent complex entities and, when appropriate, we have included contributions from internists, radiologists, and surgeons. This has led to some increase in the size of the monographs but the emphasis remains on diagnosis by the surgical pathologist.

Previously, the Fascicles have been available on CD-ROM format as well as in print. In order to provide the widest possible advantages of both modalities, we have formatted the print Fascicle on the World Wide Web. Use of the Internet allows cross-indexing within the Fascicles as well as linkage to MedLine.

Our goal is to continue to provide expert information at the lowest possible cost. Therefore, marked reductions in pricing are available to residents and fellows as well as to staff purchasing on a subscription basis.

We believe that the Atlas of Nontumor Pathology will serve as an outstanding reference for surgical pathologists as well as an important contribution to the literature of other medical specialties.

Donald West King, MD
Leslie H. Sobin, MD
J. Thomas Stocker, MD
Bernard Wagner, MD

PREFACE

This book is the second in a series of Fascicles on the pathology of non-neoplastic diseases and is devoted to a very challenging organ system: the lower respiratory tract. As this subject is inherently multidisciplinary, we have included two radiologists and a pulmonologist as authors to supplement the pathology authors' contributions. The advent of high-resolution computed tomography has transformed the field of interstitial lung disease and provides an outstanding representation of the gross pathology. Its inclusion in this volume provides many radiologic as well as pathologic images. Hopefully, this has resulted in a text that will help clinicians and radiologists, as well as pathologists, in better understanding this difficult subject.

This series of non-neoplastic Fascicles is the inspiration of the editor, Dr. Donald West King, and the associate editors, Drs. Leslie H. Sobin, J. Thomas Stocker, and Bernard Wagner. We are grateful to them for allowing us to publish this work in this series. The success of this series of publications will be a tribute to their vision and leadership.

William D. Travis, MD
Department of Pulmonary and Mediastinal Pathology
Armed Forces Institute of Pathology

Thomas V. Colby, MD
Department of Pathology and Laboratory Medicine
Mayo Clinic Scottsdale

Michael N. Koss, MD
Department of Pathology
Keck School of Medicine
University of Southern California, Los Angeles

Melissa L. Rosado-de-Christenson, Col, USAF, MC, FACR
Department of Radiologic Pathology
Armed Forces Institute of Pathology
Department of Radiology and Nuclear Medicine
Uniformed Services University of the Health Sciences

Nestor Luiz Müller, MD, PhD
Department of Radiology
Vancouver Hospital & Health Sciences Centre

Talmadge E. King Jr., MD
Department of Medicine
University of California, San Francisco

ACKNOWLEDGMENTS

Many thanks to Lois B. Travis, MD, ScD, for all her love and encouragement and to Dr. David M. and Jeanne D. Travis for teaching me the value of hard work and education.

Thank you to each of the co-authors of this textbook for your hard work, excellent contributions, and friendship. Special thanks are extended to Drs. Victor Roggli and Andrew Nicholson for their excellent reviews and constructive comments.

In addition, thanks to the many individuals who contributed case material or illustrations that have been acknowledged in the legends for the respective figures. Without your generosity, the educational value of this textbook would have been greatly diminished. We also greatly appreciate the constructive comments on chapter 12 from the Department of Infectious and Tropical Disease Pathology of the AFIP by Ronald C. Neafie, MS, Chief, Parasitic Disease Pathology Branch; Mary K. Klassen-Fischer, Maj, USAF, MC, Chief, Fungal Diseases Pathology; and Peter L. McEvoy, Col, MC, Chief, Infectious and Tropical Disease Pathology Division.

Thanks to Veronica Ferris, MFS, Lead Medical Photographer for her excellent photography and to Tammie Winters, Administrator, Department of Pulmonary and Mediastinal Pathology for outstanding administrative support through this project.

William D. Travis, MD

To my family, the source of my strength.

Thomas V. Colby, MD

I would like to acknowledge the unending support of my wife, Dr. Linda Koss Kelly in this and other academic efforts. In addition, two people have provided encouragement over the years: Dr. Donald West King, formerly Executive Director of the American Registry of Pathology, and Dr. Liselotte Hochholzer, formerly Chairperson of the Department of Pulmonary and Mediastinal Pathology. Finally, Drs. Charles C. Marboe and Glauco Frizzera, both from New York, NY, and Dr. Susan Abbondanzo of the Department of Hematopathologic Pathology at the AFIP provided micrographs or other material support.

Michael N. Koss, MD

I thank my husband Dr. Paul J. Christenson and my children Jennifer and Heather for their loving support during my work on this book. I thank my colleagues in the Departments of Radiologic Pathology and Pulmonary and Mediastinal Pathology at the AFIP for their input and assistance towards the completion of the project. I am particularly grateful to the countless radiology residents who attended the AFIP's Radiologic Pathology Courses over the years and to those who continue to participate. Their case contributions enrich the Radiologic Pathology Archives and the entire Institute. Teaching these young physicians has been my greatest privilege. Their insightful questions and comments enhanced my understanding of radiologic-pathologic correlation and helped me develop as an educator, a radiologist, and a medical officer.

Melissa L. Rosado-de-Christenson, Col, USAF, MC, FACR

To my wife Ruth for your love and encouragement, and to our children for their understanding.

Nestor L. Müller MD, PhD

I would like to express my gratitude to Mozelle D. King for her support and encouragement.

Talmadge E. King Jr., MD

Permission to use copyrighted illustrations has been granted by:

American College of Chest Physicians
Chest 1994;106:1209–14. For table 18-2.

American Medical Association
Arch Pathol 1970;90:577–82. For figure 17-28.

American Thoracic Society
Am Rev Respir Dis 1992;146:1615–22. For figure 10-17.
Am J Respir Crit Care Med 2000;161:1300–5. For figure 9-28.
Am J Respir Crit Care Med 2002. For table 3-2 and figures 3-1 and 3-2.

Appleton & Lange
Pathol Annu 1968;3:367–98. For figures 10-6 and 10-7.

Butterworth Heinemann
Occupational Lung Disorders, 1994. For figure 16-5.

Copenhagen Munksgaard International Publishers
Am J Reprod Immunol 1992;28:247–50. For tables 5-2 and 13-4.

The Gordon Museum, London, England
For figures 10-12, 10-26, 12-1, 12-46, 12-53, 12-55, 15-24, and 16-47.

Kinpodo Publishing
Lymphatic System of the Human Lung, 1989. For figures 1-11 and 1-12

Lippincott Williams & Wilkins
Am J Surg Pathol 1999;23:1288–93. For figure 3-118.
Am J Surg Pathol 2000;24:19–33. For figure 3-22.
Am J Surg Pathol 2001;25:479–84. For figure 3-121.
Lab Invest 1984;50:711–25. For figure 3-141.

Massachusetts Medical Society
N Engl J Med 1983;308:1469. For figure 16-41.
N Engl J Med 1990;323:1681. For figure 9-25, left.
N Engl J Med 2000;342:1334–49. For figures 3-41 and 3-42.
N Engl J Med 2000;343:269–80. For figures 10-1, 10-3, 10-4, and 10-5.
N Engl J Med 2001;344:350–62. For figures 10-38 and 10-39.

Mayo Clinic Proceedings
Mayo Clin Proc 1985;60:531–7. For figure 12-134.

McGraw-Hill
Pulmonary Diseases and Disorders, vol 1, 1988. For figures 1-5 and 1-13.

Mosby Yearbook
Essentials of Human Embryology, 1988. For figure 1-1.

Radiological Society of North America
Radiographics 1995;15:255–70. For figures 12-69, 12-71, and 12-91.
Radiographics 1995;15:271–86. For figure 12-80.

Raven Press
Fungal Diseases of the Lung, 2nd ed., 1993. For table 12-12.

Urban & Schwarzenberg
Cell and Tissue Biology: A Textbook of Histology, 1988. For figure 1-14.

WB Saunders
Ann Diagn Pathol 1998;2:321–34. For figures 14-15, 14-17, and 14-18.
Chronic Airflow Obstruction in Lung Disease, 1976. For figures 10-8 and 10-9.
Hum Pathol 1992;23:529–41. For table 13-3.
Katzenstein and Askin's Surgical Pathology of Non-Neoplastic Lung Disease, 1997. For figure 3-31.
Textbook of Respiratory Medicine, 1994. For table 12-3 and figure 10-37.

Contents

NON-NEOPLASTIC DISORDERS OF THE LOWER RESPIRATORY TRACT

1

EMBRYOLOGY AND ANATOMY

EMBRYOLOGY

The stages of lung development (1–9) are summarized in Table 1-1 and figure 1-1. In the embryo, the developing lower respiratory tract is first seen as a groove in the floor of the primitive pharynx, caudal to the pharyngeal pouches. The groove evaginates into a distinct laryngotracheal diverticulum, which elongates caudally into the primitive mesenchyme as the primordial lung bud. Bronchial buds arise by progressive dichotomous division, and the segmental, subsegmental, and more distal airways are formed. Orderly branching is influenced by the surrounding mesodermal component and its extracellular matrix in which soluble growth factors activate proliferation genes at the points of branching (2). Bronchial cartilage, muscle, and connective tissue are derived from the mesenchyme surrounding the bronchial buds. The development of the major airways, termed the embryonic phase, occurs between 3 and 6 weeks' gestation.

From the 6th to 16th week of gestation, the small airways, up to the terminal bronchioles, are formed; 16 weeks after conception, the formation of the conducting airways is complete. This is termed the pseudoglandular phase (fig. 1-2).

The next stage of development, the canalicular phase, occurs between 16 and 28 weeks. The acinus and its accompanying vascular supply develop and terminal bronchioles give rise to respiratory bronchioles, with terminal sacs representing primitive alveoli (fig. 1-3). Some respiratory function may be possible toward the end of this phase because of the presence of vascularized terminal sacs.

The saccular phase is identifiable by the 28th week and extends to the 36th week of gestation. Saccules form and are lined by flattened type 1 alveolar lining cells. The alveolar capillary network develops in the surrounding mesenchyme, and lymphatics are formed.

The alveolus is distinguished by the following features: it arises from an alveolar duct, it is lined almost exclusively by alveolar lining cells, and the capillaries in the alveolar wall are exposed to at least two contiguous alveoli (1). The alveolar phase begins at approximately 36 weeks' gestation and extends to as late as 8 years of age. Vascularized alveoli become fully formed and are lined by attenuated type 1 alveolar lining cells (fig. 1-4). Although the alveolar stage begins at about 36 weeks of gestation, mature

Table 1-1

PHASES OF LUNG DEVELOPMENT[a]

Phase	Gestation	Major Events
Embryonic	26 days to 6 weeks	Development of major airways
Pseudoglandular	6 to 16 weeks	Development of airways to terminal bronchioles
Canalicular	16 to 28 weeks	Development of the acinus and its vascularization
Saccular	28 to 36 weeks	Subdivision of saccules by secondary crests
Alveolar	36 weeks to term (and up to 4 years of age)	Acquisition of alveoli

[a]Modified from reference 5.

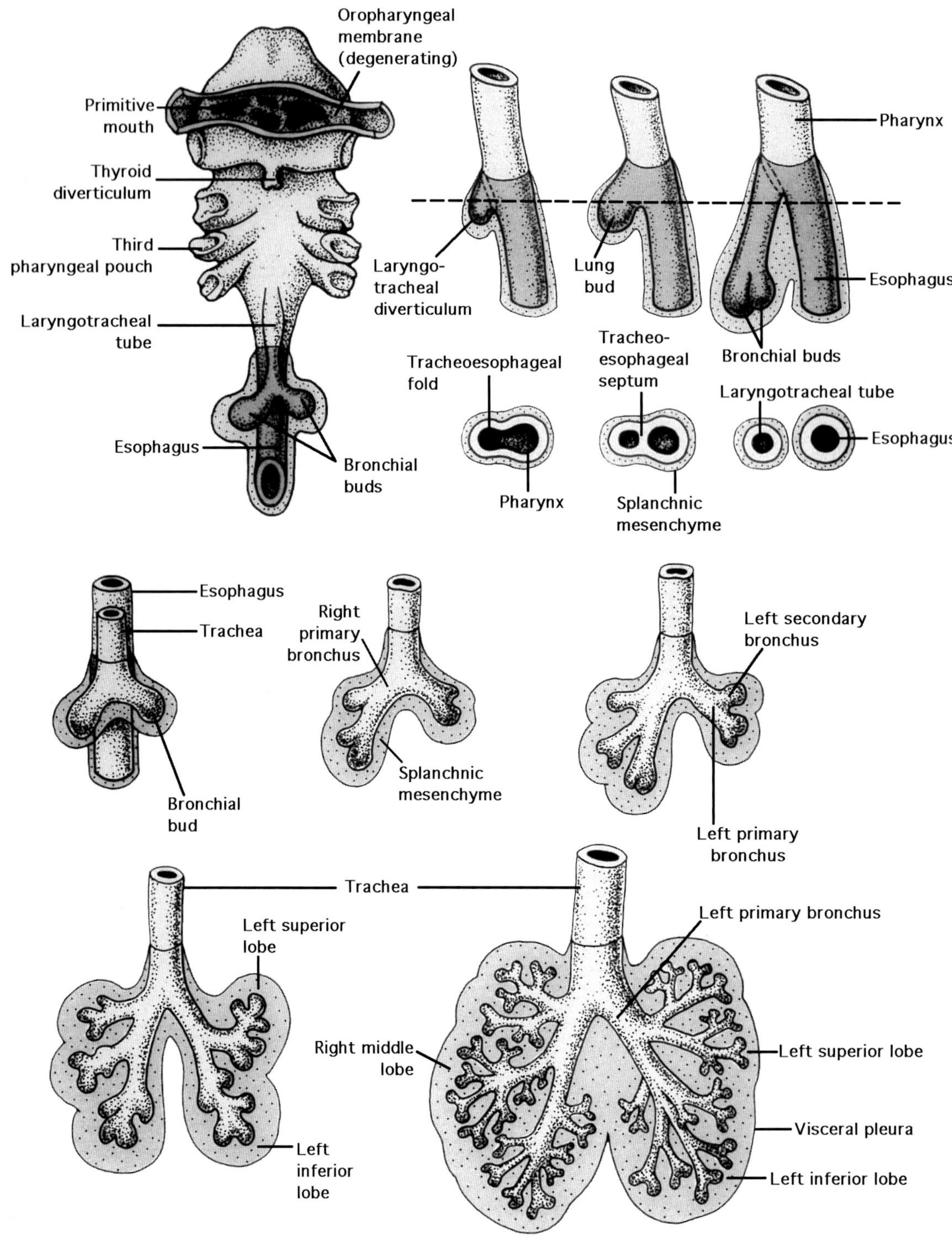

Figure 1-1

EARLY EMBRYOLOGIC DEVELOPMENT OF THE LUNG

The embryonic lungs first arise as the laryngotracheal diverticulum in the primitive gut. This elongates and forms bronchial buds which progressively divide dichotomously within the splanchnic mesenchyme. (Figures 10-1 and 10-4 from Moore KL, Herbst M, Thompson M. Essentials of human embryology. St. Louis: Mosby Yearbook; 1988.)

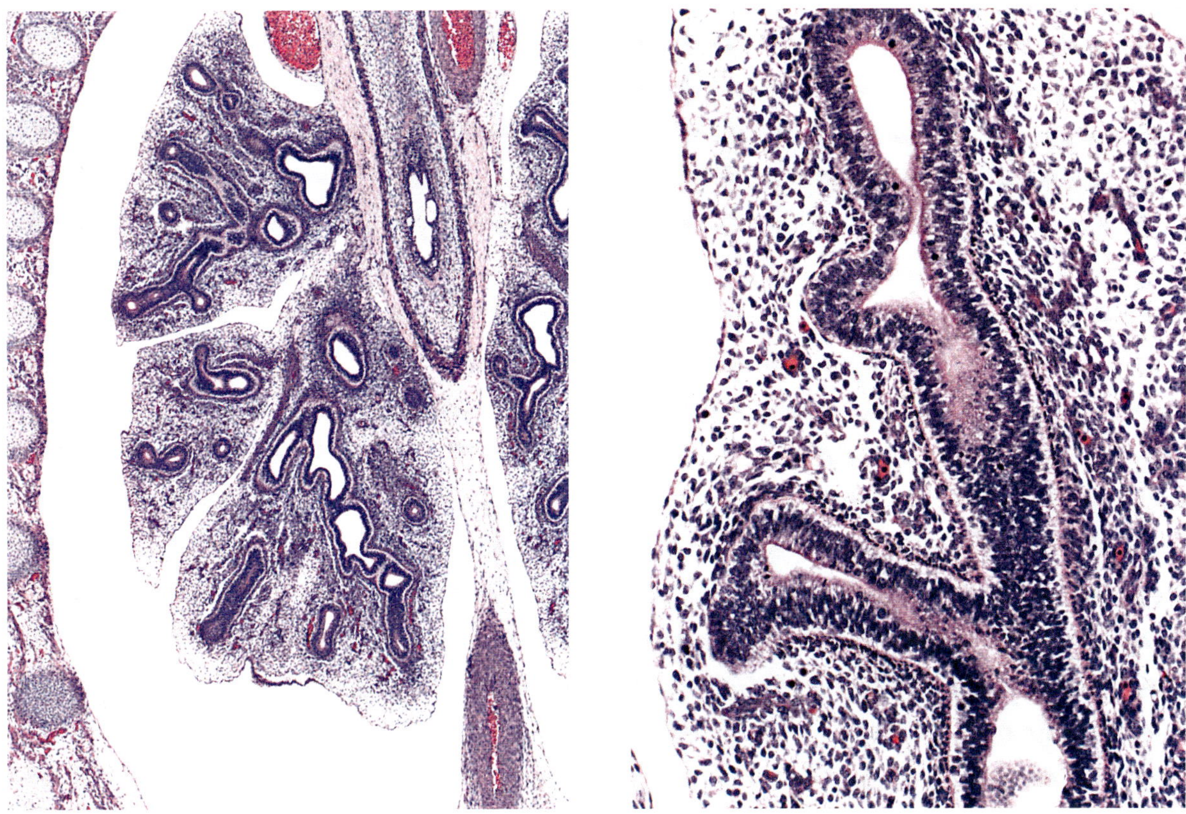

Figure 1-2

PSEUDOGLANDULAR PHASE OF LUNG DEVELOPMENT

The primitive right lung is seen in the chest cavity of this 7-week-old fetus (left). Three lobes covered by mesothelium are apparent. Simple tubular structures divide within a primitive mesenchymal matrix (right). The epithelium is reminiscent of endometrial epithelium.

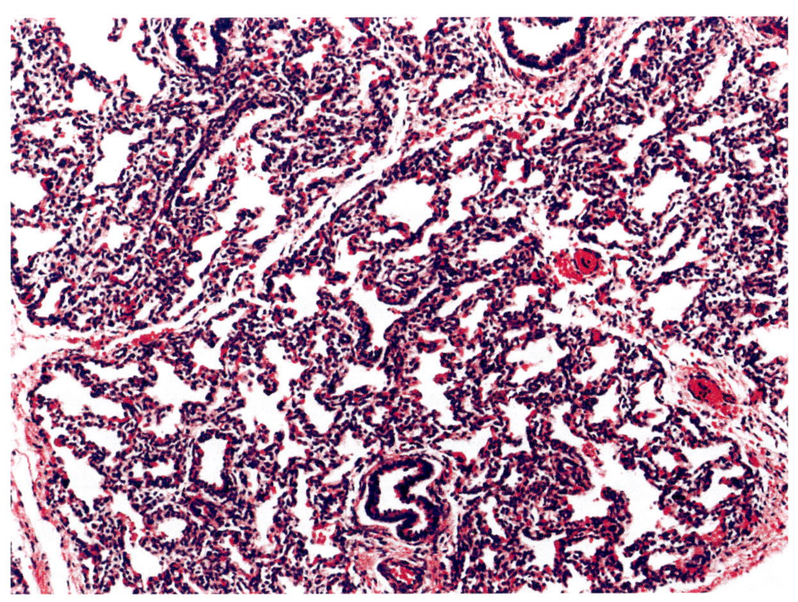

Figure 1-3

CANALICULAR PHASE OF LUNG DEVELOPMENT (26-WEEK FETUS)

Early vascularized air sacs are lined by cuboidal epithelium. There is marked interstitial thickening. Note the relatively small pulmonary artery compared to the bronchiole.

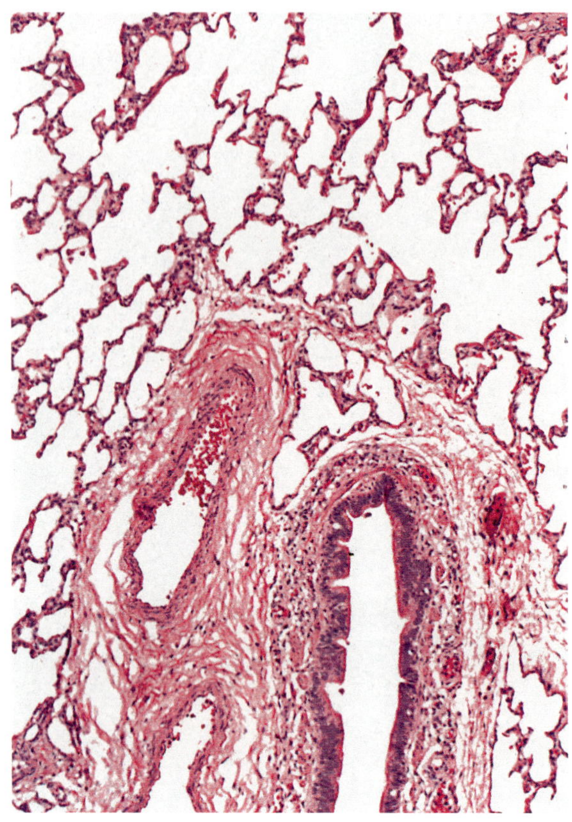

Figure 1-4

ALVEOLAR PHASE OF LUNG DEVELOPMENT

Well-inflated sections from a 1-month-old full-term infant show recognizable alveoli with only slight thickening of the alveolar walls. The pulmonary artery approaches the size of the bronchiole and its wall thickness is less than that of a systemic artery.

alveoli are not found until approximately 5 weeks after birth.

The pulmonary artery is formed from the 6th branchial arch which first appears at approximately 32 days of gestation. Branches arise from this arch and extend into the mesenchyme along the lung buds. Thereafter, the pulmonary arterial system forms in tandem with the branching bronchial buds. Arteries that follow the airways are termed conventional pulmonary arteries. Supernumerary arteries are also recognized; they come off at right angles to supply airspaces adjacent to bronchovascular bundles. Muscularization of the arteries does not keep up with the pace of appearance of new bronchioles. Muscularization of pulmonary arteries beyond the level of the terminal bronchiole begins only in the first year of life and progresses to early adulthood, when it is seen all the way to the alveolar wall. In the fetus and neonate, the walls of pulmonary arteries appear thick in histologic sections, since until birth the pulmonary circulation is a high pressure system similar to the systemic circulation. After birth, there is progressive decrease in the proportion of the arterial media as the pulmonary system becomes a low pressure system (fig. 1-4).

The pulmonary venous system develops from an evagination in the wall of the atrium in the sino-atrial region. The primitive pulmonary vein grows toward the lung buds, and ultimately, following fusions and further divisions, four major pulmonary veins are formed which enter the left atrium. Branches of the veins grow into the mesenchyme around the lung buds and into interlobular septa.

The visceral and parietal pleurae arise within the primordial mesenchyme surrounding the developing lung (fig. 1-2).

The development of the lung can be divided into lung growth, corresponding to cell multiplication, and lung maturation, referring to attainment of normal distensibility and compliance (1). Lung growth can be assessed by: lung weight and/or volume and its ratio to total fetal weight/volume; DNA amount or concentration in the lung; total alveolar surface area; and total alveolar number. Lung growth is affected by the available intrathoracic space and by the volume of liquid in the fetal lung (3). Disruption of lung liquid dynamics is associated with abnormalities in lung growth: oligohydramnios (decreased lung liquid) leads to lung hypoplasia, whereas experimental tracheal ligation (which increases lung liquid) is associated with increased lung growth (hyperplasia).

Normal lung maturation leads to a stable, distensible and compliant lung, and is affected by many physical and hormonal factors (1). Lung maturation requires normal synthesis, storage, and secretion of surfactant, and this can be affected by hormones (including steroid hormones, insulin, and epinephrine), growth factors, and many other agents (8). At birth, the lung is a liquid-filled organ that must quickly adapt to being an air-filled organ, probably by decreased secretion and increased reabsorption of lung liquid.

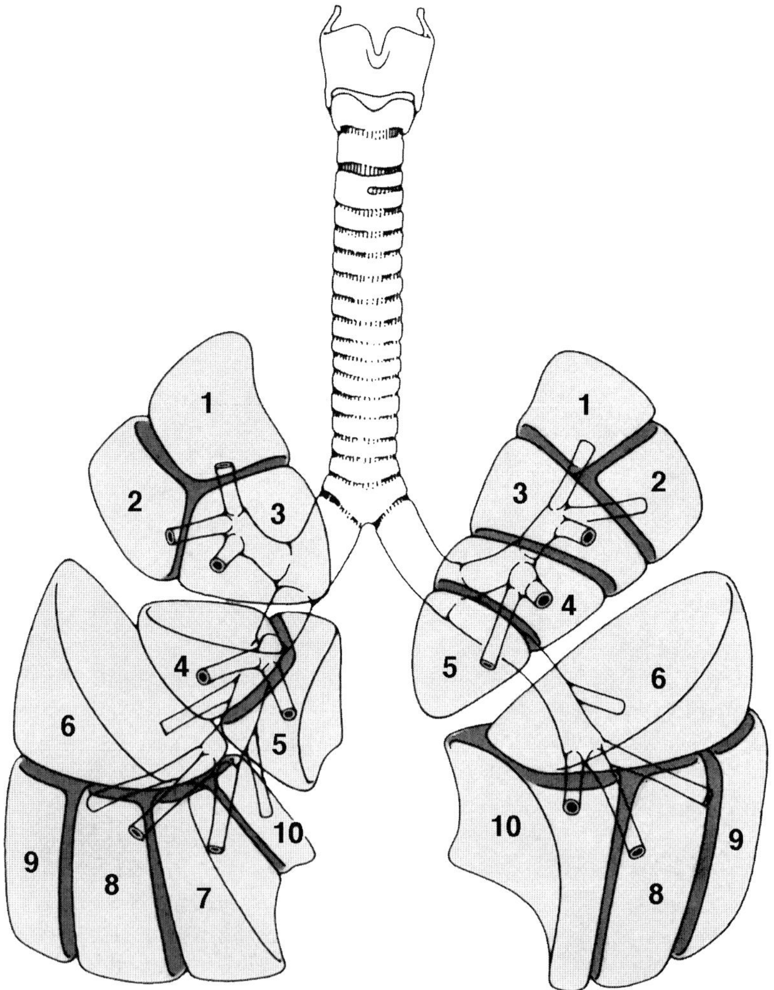

Figure 1-5

BRONCHOPULMONARY SEGMENTS OF THE HUMAN LUNG

Left upper and right upper lobes: 1, apical; 2, posterior; 3, anterior; 4, superior lingular; 5, inferior lingular segments. Right middle lobe: 4, lateral; 5, medial segments. Lower lobes: 6, superior apical; 7, medial basal; 8, anterior basal; 9, lateral basal; 10, posterior basal segments. The medial basal segment (7) is absent in the left lung. (Figure 2-2 from Weibel ER, Taylor CR. Design and structure of the human lung. In: Fishman AP, ed. Pulmonary diseases and disorders, vol. 1, 2nd ed. New York: McGraw-Hill; 1988.)

ANATOMY AND HISTOLOGY

The anatomy and histology of the lung are well described (10–36). The average weight of both lungs for men is approximately 850 g and for women, 750 g. The lungs are divided into five lobes: the right upper, right middle, and right lower lobes and the left upper and left lower lobes. The proximal bronchial branches define 10 bronchopulmonary segments within these lobes (fig. 1-5). A lobule is the smallest anatomic compartment of the lung that is grossly apparent. Lobules are 1 to 2 cm in diameter, polygonal, and bound by complete or incomplete connective tissue interlobular septa. Lobules and their demarcating septa are best appreciated grossly in the periphery of the lung, particularly in cigarette smokers, where the septa are highlighted by accumulations of anthracotic pigment in the septal lymphatics (fig. 1-6). Lobules have centrally located bronchoarterial bundles. Identification of lobules has become important for correlating radiologic studies of the lung, particularly high-resolution computed tomography (HRCT), with the gross and histologic findings.

The functional unit of the lung is the pulmonary acinus, where gas transfer takes place. A lobule may contain from 3 to 30 acini. An acinus is defined as "the complex of all airways that are distal to terminal bronchioles and thus are served by a first order respiratory bronchiole," which is termed a "transitional bronchiole" (17). Acini include multiple respiratory bronchioles and their supplied alveolar ducts

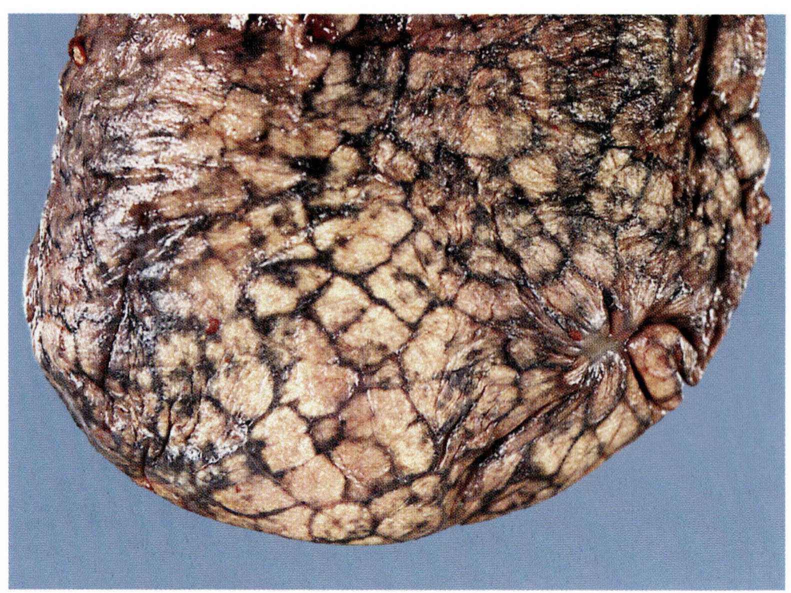

Figure 1-6

PULMONARY LOBULES

This collapsed lobectomy specimen from a smoker shows anthracotic pigment highlighting the interlobular septa which surround the lobules. In a normally inflated specimen, the lobules would be approximately 2 cm in diameter. The carcinoma for which this resection was done is seen as a puckered region at 4 o'clock.

and alveoli. Acinar volume averages 187 mm^3 (17), and acini may be up to 9 mm in greatest dimension (average, 7.5 mm) (17,29). Assuming an average diameter of 7.5 mm, there are approximately 25,000 acini in normal adult male lungs, with a volume of 5.25 L (29).

The airways undergo up to about 23 generations of dichotomous branching beyond the carina, 20 proximal to the level of the respiratory bronchioles. The trachea and bronchi have cartilage in their walls. Tracheal cartilage is U-shaped, with a posterior band of smooth muscle. The bronchi have circumferential cartilaginous rings. The bronchi and the bronchioles are the conducting airways of the lung. The smallest bronchi (cartilaginous airways) are approximately 1 mm in diameter; airways smaller than 1 mm are bronchioles (membranous airways). Bronchioles lack cartilaginous rings and have a smooth muscle investment in their walls. Respiratory bronchioles have functional alveoli in their walls and are part of the pulmonary acinus. The term "small airways" has been used for airways 2 mm in diameter and smaller, and refers to both small bronchi as well as bronchioles.

Within the acinus (respiratory bronchioles, alveolar ducts, alveoli) (fig. 1-7), gas transfer takes place across a very thin membrane between the air-blood interface. This membrane is comprised of cytoplasm of a type 1 alveolar lining cell, fused basement membranes of the type 1 alveolar lining cell and the adjacent endothelial cell, and the attenuated endothelial cell cytoplasm of the alveolar capillary. Adjacent alveoli communicate by the pores of Kohn. These develop after birth. They average 13 to 21 per alveolus and are thought to be involved in collateral ventilation (18).

Lambert's canals communicate directly between airways and adjacent alveoli. These are rarely observed morphologically, but their functional effects in collateral ventilation are apparent to physiologists. Healing inflammatory changes in the bronchioles may be associated with peribronchiolar metaplasia, with growth of bronchiolar epithelium through Lambert's canals (fig. 1-8).

The lung has a dual vascular supply. The pulmonary arteries accompany airways into the lung periphery where they progressively divide into a ramifying capillary network in the alveolar wall. The rich alveolar capillary network is interanastomosing and wraps around the axis of the alveolar wall to provide a maximum surface area for blood-gas exchange (fig. 1-9). Bronchial arteries are systemic, arising from the aorta or intercostal arteries; they form a plexus in the bronchial wall which extends peripherally as far as the respiratory bronchioles. Proximally, bronchial arteries anastomose with those that supply the trachea, which derive from branches

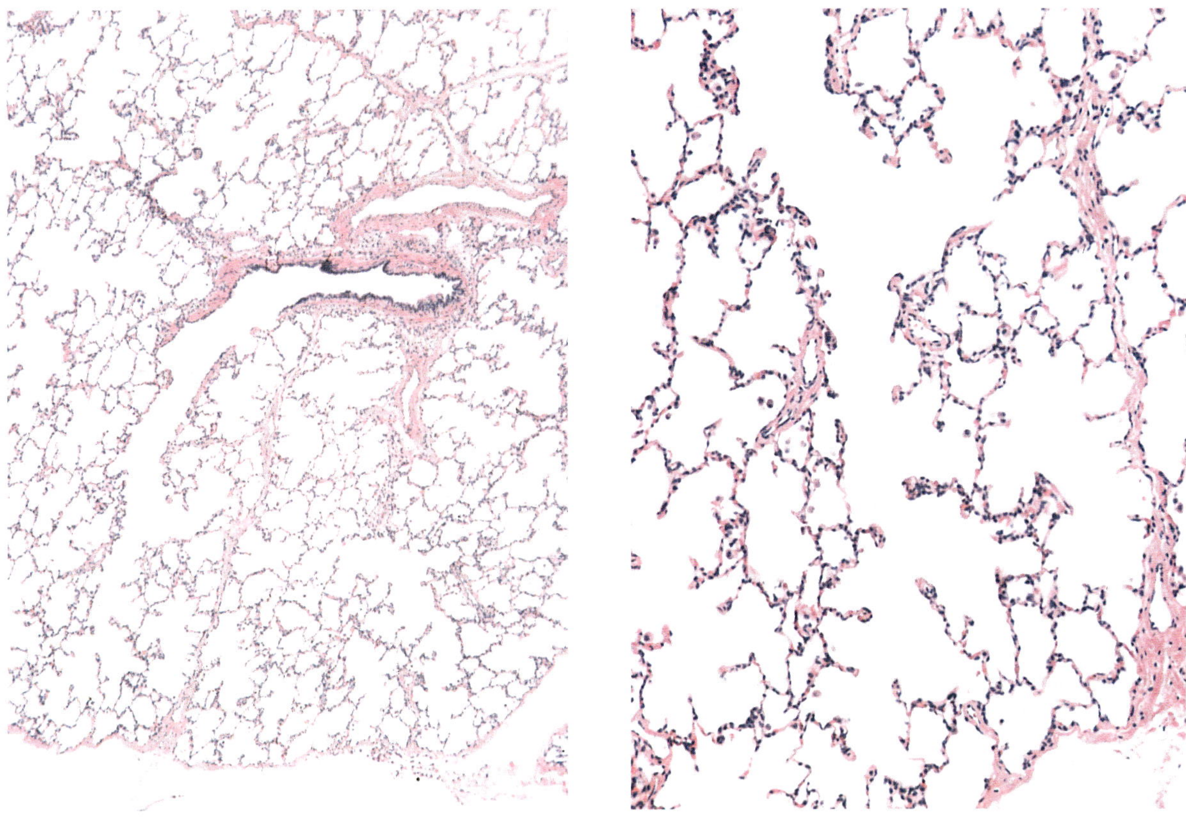

Figure 1-7

PULMONARY ACINUS

A membranous bronchiole connects with a respiratory bronchiole (left), which is continuous with alveolar ducts and alveoli adjacent to the septum and pleura. The alveolar walls are delicate and thin (right), and allow maximum surface area for gas exchange.

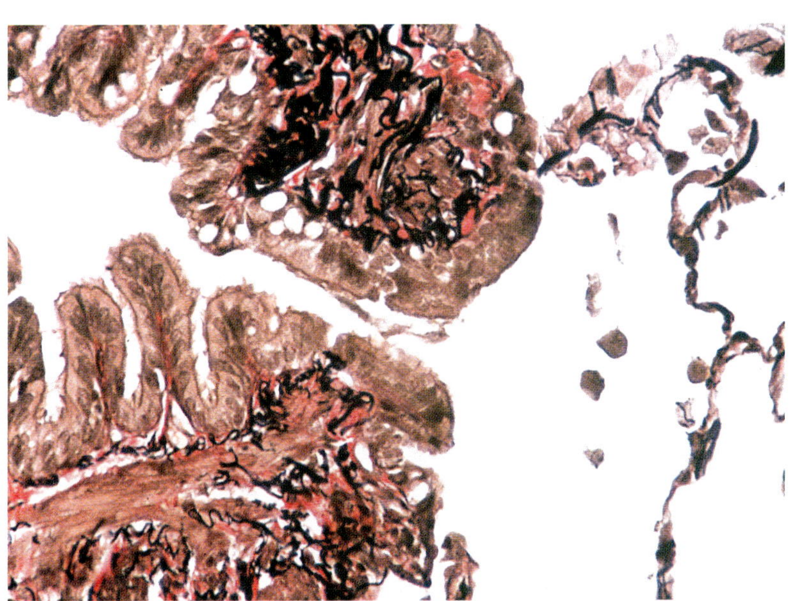

Figure 1-8

CANAL OF LAMBERT

This histologic section of a normal bronchiole shows a direct communication between the bronchiolar lumen and an adjacent alveolus.

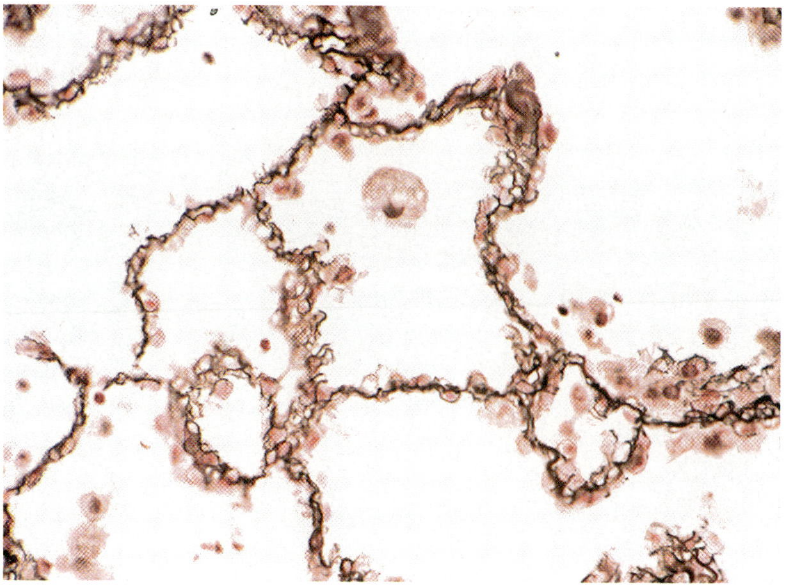

Figure 1-9

NORMAL ALVEOLAR WALL

This reticulin stain highlights the rich capillary network of the delicate alveolar septum.

of the inferior thyroid artery. Branches of the bronchial arteries also supply the visceral pleura and some of the interstitial connective tissue.

The pulmonary venous system arises from the efferent blood flow through the alveolar capillary network of the periphery of the lobules, where small veins can be seen entering pulmonary septa. Bronchopulmonary segments are often drained by more than one pulmonary vein.

In histologic sections, pulmonary arteries have an internal and external elastic membrane, whereas veins have a single external elastica (fig. 1-10). In pathologic states, especially those with fibrosis or pulmonary hypertension, distinction between arteries and veins may be difficult, even with elastic tissue stains. This is because veins may be "arterialized," and their elastica may be reduplicated. In such instances, anatomic location is extremely important, since arteries accompany airways and veins can be identified within interlobular septa. In histologic sections of adult lungs, the pulmonary artery and its accompanying bronchiole should be about the same size; in pathologic conditions a discrepancy can be seen in the size of either of these structures (36).

The lymphatic drainage of the lung is quite complex (fig. 1-11). In general, the lymphatics follow the bronchovascular structures and are found in the pleura and septa. They can be identified along pulmonary arteries, airways to the level of respiratory bronchioles, venules in the periphery of lobules, and veins in the septa. A rich lymphatic network is also found in the visceral pleura. Lymphatics are generally inapparent in histologic sections but become more obvious in pathologic states such as pulmonary edema and lymphangitic carcinoma. Pulmonary lymphatics contain valves (in contrast to pulmonary veins).

Lymphoid tissue, including clusters of histiocytes, can be found along lymphatic vessels, particularly at sites of branching of larger airways where inhaled particulate antigens are likely to settle and where there is respiratory epithelium specialized for absorption. This lymphoid tissue is termed bronchus-associated lymphoid tissue (BALT) and is generally not apparent histologically in the absence of antigenic stimulation (30). It is organized into discrete lymph nodes around the larger bronchi (intrapulmonary peribronchial lymph nodes) and in the hilum. Lymph nodes are occasionally found in the periphery of the lung, usually in the pleura or in the septa (19). Lymphatic drainage from the pulmonary lymphatics is primarily cephalad to lymph node groups in the chest, but also to lymph nodes in the abdomen (fig. 1-12).

BALT is part of the generalized mucosa-associated lymphoid tissue (MALT) found in a number of organs in the body, most notably the gastrointestinal tract (10,11,16,30). Technically,

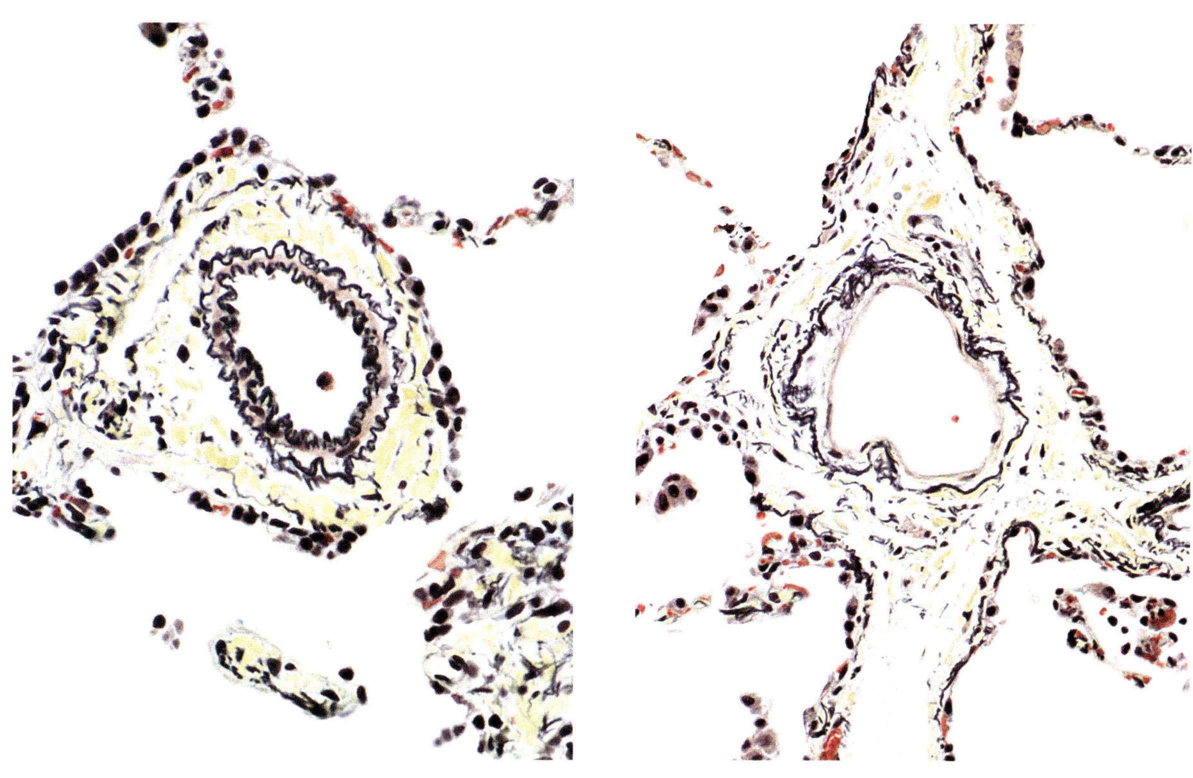

Figure 1-10

NORMAL PULMONARY ARTERY AND VEIN

The artery has a dual elastica (left) and a vein (right) in a single external elastic lamina, which is highlighted with elastic tissue staining.

the term BALT is used for lymphoid tissue along the airways, but hyperplasia of this tissue is commonly accompanied by hyperplastic lymphoid tissue along all of the lymphatic routes in the lung, including the septa and pleura. Lymphoid hyperplasia along airways shows a close apposition of lymphoid follicles to the overlying airway epithelium, which may be somewhat flattened and infiltrated by lymphocytes.

The major cell types found in the lower respiratory tract are summarized in Tables 1-2 and 1-3. The cells lining the airways and alveoli are endodermally derived and have a number of specialized modifications. The respiratory tract is organized to produce and to propel mucus proximally, and to facilitate gas transfer distally (figs. 1-13, 1-14). In the large airways, the goblet cells (and the submucosal glands [see below]) produce mucus, which forms a coat lining the airways. This mucus coat is propelled proximally by the ciliated cells of the airways. It is composed of glycoprotein (which includes mucins), lipids, proteoglycans, immunoglobulins (secretory IgA), lysozyme, lactoferrin, peroxidase, actin, DNA, and other substances which together form a potent defense mechanism (33). The mucus also traps particulate debris. Normal function of the mucociliary escalator depends on normal maintenance of the airway epithelium. Inflammatory and irritative states may change the cellular composition of the mucosa of the airways (for example, increased goblet cells and increased mucus production, squamous metaplasia with loss of ciliated cells), and alter normal function and produce or contribute to pathologic states. Basal cells in the airway epithelium are precursors to goblet and ciliated cells. Scattered neuroendocrine cells, some of which have dendritic processes, are present in the basal layer of the airway epithelium but not the alveoli. They represent 0.17 percent of all airway epithelial cells (12). Small clusters of neuroendocrine cells

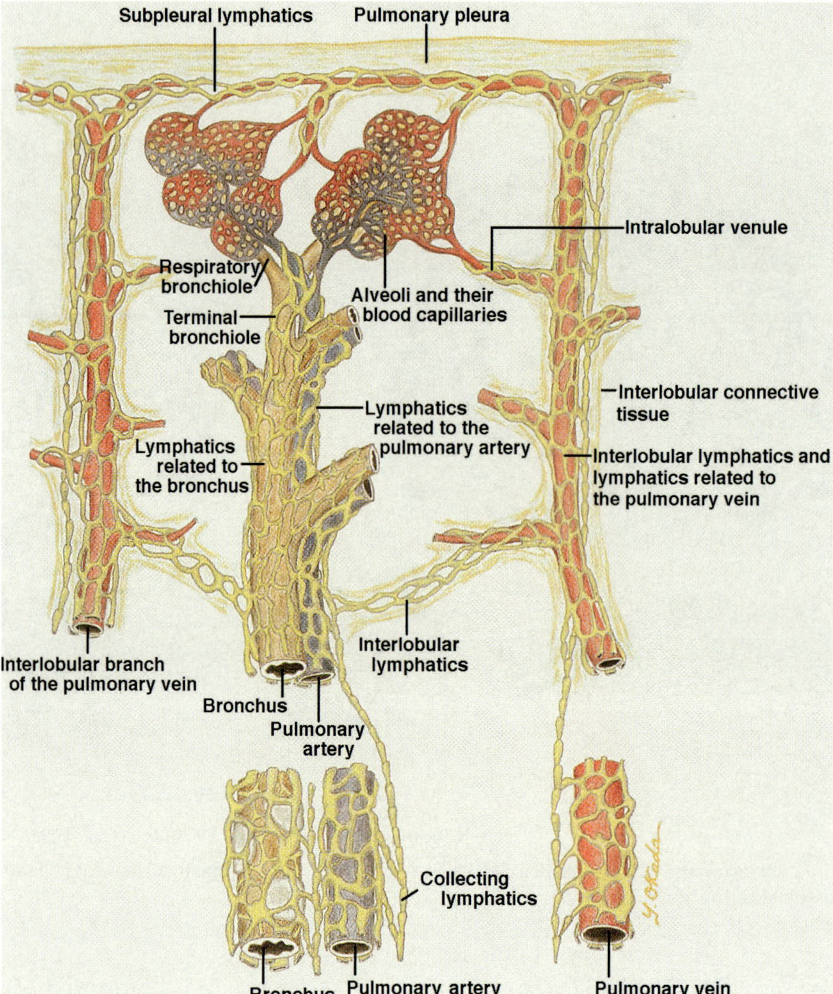

Figure 1-11

HISTOLOGIC DIAGRAM OF THE PULMONARY LYMPHATICS

Pulmonary lymphatics are found along bronchovascular structures, pulmonary veins, and within the septa and pleura. (Figure 1 from Okada Y. Lymphatic system of the human lung. Kyoto, Japan: Kinpodo Publishing; 1989.)

(neuroepithelial bodies) can be identified at airway branch points. The ultrastructural features of the ciliated cells are well described (20,21), and in syndromes associated with abnormal ciliary function, ultrastructural abnormalities may be identified (see chapter 9).

In small airways, there is a progressive decrease in number of goblet cells and ciliated cells and a concomitant increase in Clara cells. The mucosa assumes a cuboidal appearance in contrast to the pseudostratified columnar pattern seen in large airways (fig. 1-13).

The major cells found in the alveoli include type 1 (squamous) alveolar lining cells, which cover over 90 percent of the alveolar surface area; type 2 alveolar lining cells (granular pneumocytes); and alveolar macrophages. Ultrastructurally, type 2 alveolar lining cells contain lamellar inclusions which represent precursors of surfactant. Type 2 alveolar lining cells represent precursor cells to type 1 cells and proliferate following injury and during chronic inflammatory states. Scavenger alveolar macrophages are present within the alveoli (and increase in chronic inflammatory and irritative states); they are involved in phagocytosis of foreign material and are a major component of the inflammatory and immune response. Type 1 alveolar lining cells have thin, very attenuated cytoplasm, inapparent in routine hematoxylin and eosin–stained sections but easily appreciated with immunohistochemical stains for epithelia

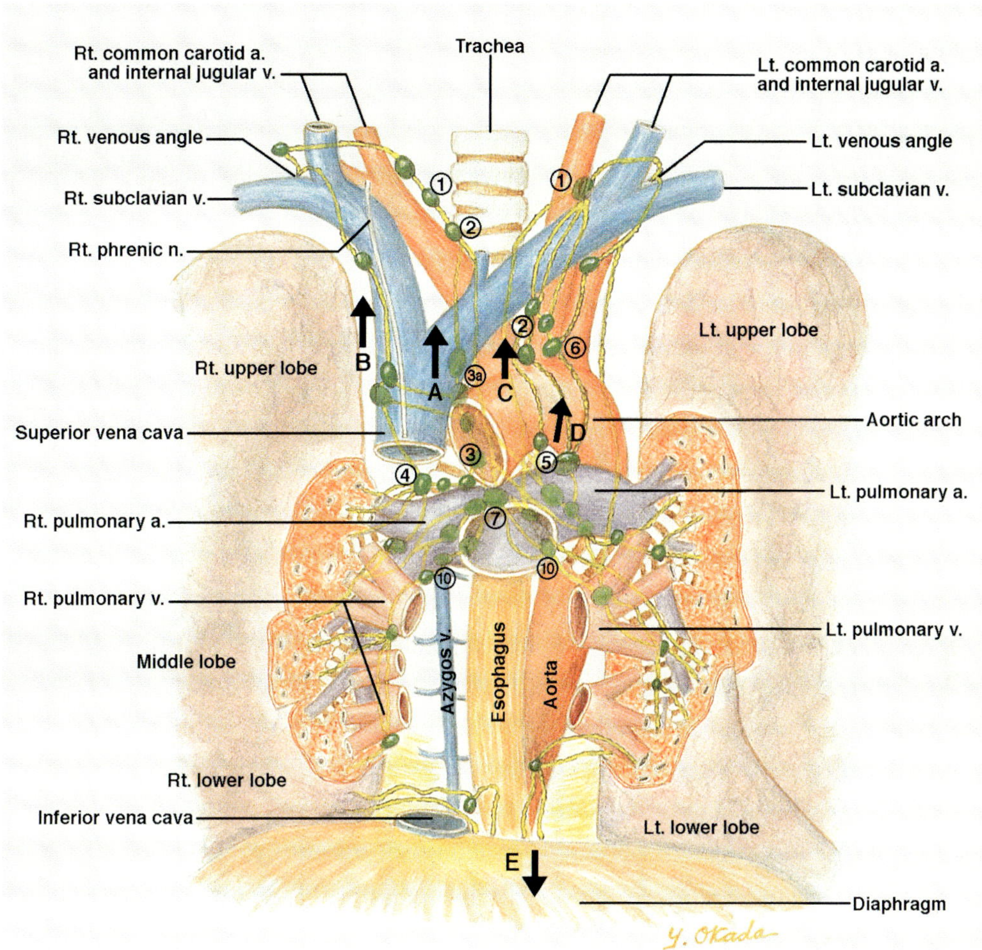

Figure 1-12

LYMPHATIC DRAINAGE OF THE LUNG

The drainage is primarily cephalad along the right paratracheal route (A), right brachiocephalic route (B), left paratracheal route (C), and para-aortic route (D). Some deep drainage into the abdomen (E) takes place from the inferior thoracic cavity. (Figure 4 from Okaha Y. Lymphatic system of the human lung. Kyoto, Japan: Kinpodo Publishing; 1989.)

(such as cytokeratin or epithelial membrane antigen), whereas type 2 alveolar lining cells are easily appreciated in routine sections.

Glands of minor salivary type are found in the submucosa of the trachea and bronchi (but not the bronchioles). Anatomically, three regions are recognized in these glands: the ciliated duct, the connecting duct, and the secretory tubules lined by serous and mucous cells. These seromucous glands are invested by a myoepithelial cell layer which probably functions in secretion. Particularly in older individuals, oncocytes (oncocytic metaplasia) may be found in the connecting duct, or replacing serous or mucous cells in the secretory tubules.

The lung contains an interstitial compartment which provides its connective tissue framework. The interstitium is generally inconspicuous but can be recognized along bronchovascular bundles, around veins, and where it forms interlobular septa. Within the interstitium, there are collagen fibers, elastic fibers, mesenchymal cells, and a few inflammatory cells. In the pediatric lung, the interstitial space is more apparent, usually manifesting as a thickening of the alveolar walls; this pattern is present up to about 4 years of age.

Table 1-2

MAJOR CELLS OF THE LOWER RESPIRATORY TRACT

Cell Type	Main Features	Functions	Location	Comments
Ciliated	Columnar, cuboidal, ciliated bronchial lining cells; each cell has approximately 250 cilia at the apical surface and each cilium is approximately 6 μm long	Proximal transport of mucus stream (mucociliary escalator)	Bronchi and bronchioles	Decreased number and morphologic abnormalities seen with chronic irritation
Goblet	Columnar mucus-secreting cells; contain mucus or glycoprotein which discharges apically	Contribute to airway mucus	Bronchi, more numerous proximally; small numbers in bronchioles	Increased number in chronic airway irritation
Basal	Short cells with relatively little cytoplasm oriented along the membrane; do not reach the luminal surface of the epithelium	Precursor cell of ciliated and goblet cells	Bronchi; rare in bronchioles	---
Neuroendocrine	Basal-oriented cells with numerous dense-core (neurosecretory) granules single or in groups (neuroepithelial bodies); the latter near the airway bifurcation	Specific functions not known in detail; considered part of the diffuse neuroendocrine system	Bronchi and bronchioles	---
Oncocytic	Eosinophilic mitochondrial-rich cells in submucosal gland ducts	Ion secretory functions	Submucosal glands	Increasing number with aging
Squamous (metaplasia)	Stratified squamous epithelium is an abnormal reaction, replacing normal pseudostratified respiratory epithelium	Protective, reparative	Bronchi and bronchioles; scarred alveoli	Metaplastic response to irritation or repair
Clara	Columnar nonciliated bronchiolar cells; protuberant apical cytoplasm with large ovoid electron-dense granules; comprise the majority of nonciliated bronchial cells	Secretory functions contributing to the mucus pool and maintaining extracellular lining fluid; progenitor of other bronchiolar cells; role in surfactant and protease inhibitor production	Predominantly in bronchioles	---
Type 1 alveolar pneumocyte	Large, flat, squamous alveolar lining cells; cover approximately 93% of alveolar surface area; incapable of division	Provide a thin air-blood interface for gas transfer	Alveoli	---
Type 2 alveolar pneumocyte	Columnar alveolar lining cells comprising 16% of the lung parenchyma; microvillous surface; synthesize and secrete surfactant (lamellar ultrastructural inclusions); capable of division	Maintain alveolar stability and produce surfactant; stem cell alveoli acting as progenitor type 1 pneumocytes	Alveoli	Increased in reparative states and as a response to chronic injury
Alveolar macrophages	Marrow-derived phagocytic cells	Involved in alveolar defense, cytokine production, and inflammatory and immune processes	Alveoli, airway, submucosa, lymphatic, and lymphoid tissue	---

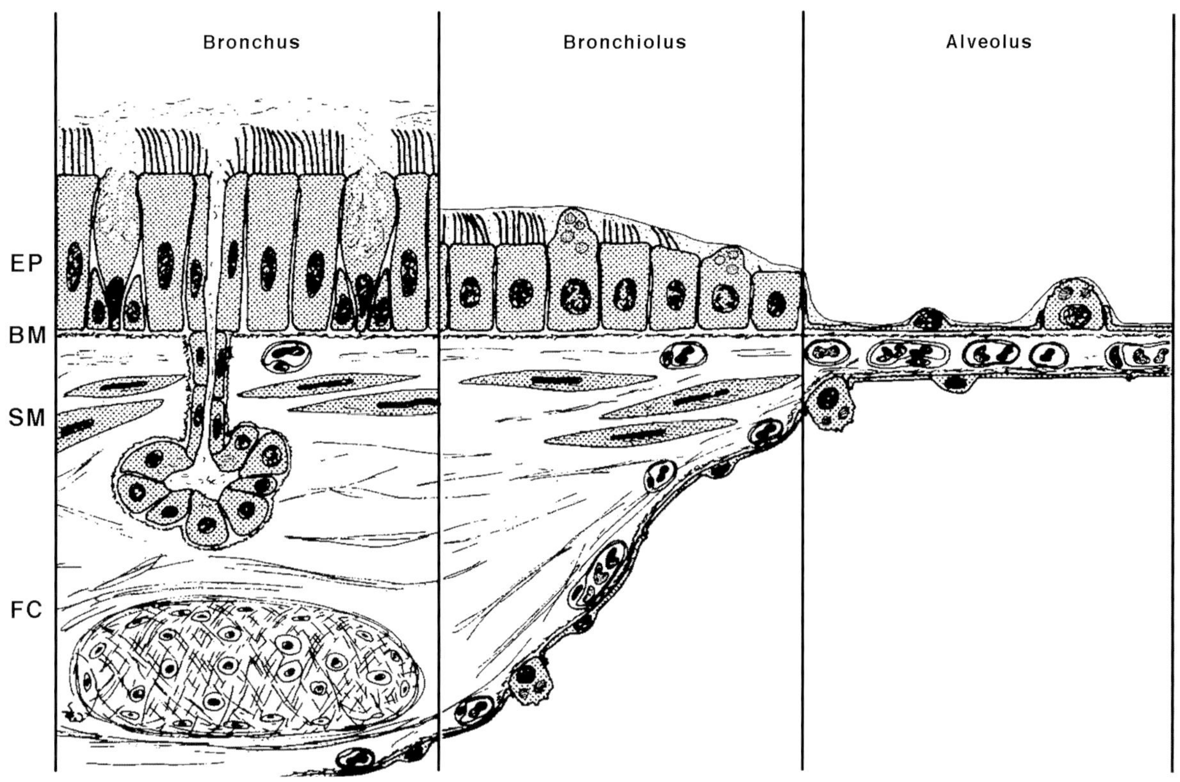

Figure 1-13

SCHEMATIC REPRESENTATION OF THE SURFACE EPITHELIUM OF THE RESPIRATORY TRACT

Columnar ciliated cells are most prominent in the bronchus, whereas cuboidal-shaped cells and Clara cells with apical protrusions containing granules are more prominent in the bronchiole. The alveolus contains primarily type 1 (membranous) alveolar lining cells to facilitate gas transfer, interspersed with type 2 cells that protrude into the alveolar lumen. (Figure 2-6 from Weibel ER, Taylor CR. Design and structure of the human lung. In: Fishman AP, ed. Pulmonary diseases and disorders, vol. 1, 2nd ed. New York: McGraw-Hill; 1988.)

Table 1-3

OTHER CELLS OF THE LOWER RESPIRATORY TRACT

Endothelial cells and pericytes	Mesothelial pleural lining
Interstitial fibrocytes, fibroblasts, and myofibroblasts	Cartilage and bone
Lymphocytes (intravascular and interstitial)	Smooth muscle
Langerhans type histiocytes (in airway mucosa)	Peripheral nerve and small ganglia
Intravascular megakaryocytes	Myoepithelial cells
Mast cells	

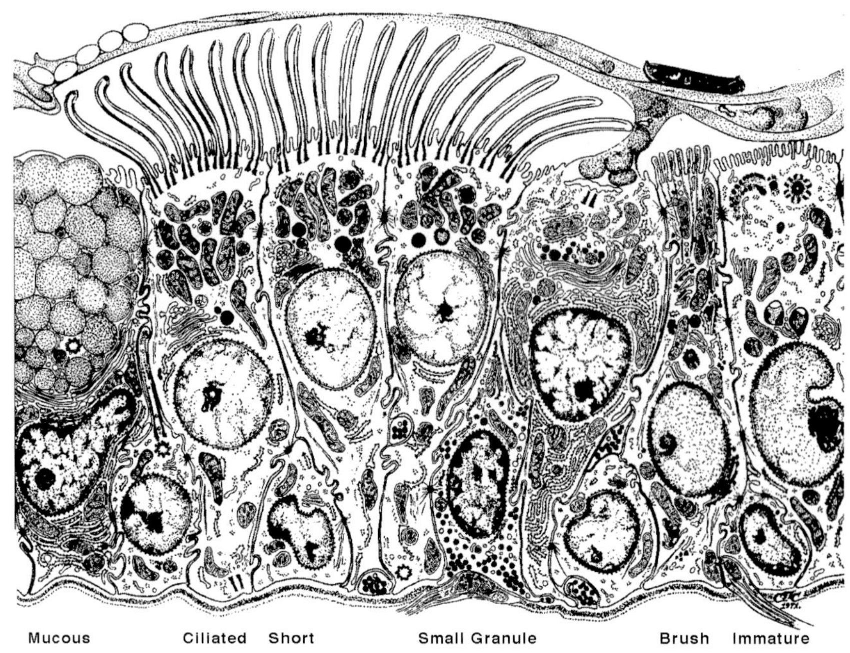

Figure 1-14

ULTRASTRUCTURAL SCHEMATIC REPRESENTATION OF RESPIRATORY TRACT EPITHELIUM IN A BRONCHUS

The various cell types comprising this epithelium are illustrated along with their ultrastructural features. Brush cells had been primarily recognized in animals. (Figure 25-11 from Sorokin SP. The respiratory system. In: Weiss L, ed. Cell and tissue biology: a textbook of histology. Baltimore: Erban & Schwarzenberg; 1988).

REFERENCES

Embryology

1. DiFiore JW, Wilson JM. Lung development. Semin Pediatr Surg 1994:3:221–32.
2. Hilfer SR. Morphogenesis of the lung: control of embryonic and fetal branching. Annu Rev Physiol 1996;58:93–113.
3. Hooper SB, Harding R. Fetal lung liquid: a major determinant of the growth and functional development of the fetal lung. Clin Exp Pharmacol Physiol 1995;22:235–47.
4. Inselman LS, Mellins RB. Growth and development of the lung. J Pediatr 1981;98:1–15.
5. Langston C, Kida K, Reed M, Thurlbeck WN. Human lung growth in late gestation and in the neonate. Am Rev Respir Dis 1984;129:607–13.
6. Moore KL. The developing human, 3rd ed. Philadelphia: WB Saunders; 1982.
7. Moore KL. Essential of human embryology. Philadelphia: BC Decker; 1988.
8. Price WA, Stiles AD. New insights into lung growth and development. Curr Opinion Pediatr 1996;8:202–8.
9. Thurlbeck WM. Lung growth and development. In: Thurlbeck WM, Churg AM, eds. Pathology of the lung, 2nd ed. New York: Thieme; 1995:37–87.

Anatomy and Histology

10. Bienenstock J. Bronchus-associated lymphoid tissue. Int Arch Allergy Appl Immun 1985;76:62–9.
11. Bienenstock J, Befus AD. Gut- and bronchus-associated lymphoid tissue. Am J Anat 1984; 170:437–45.
12. Boers JE, den Brok JL, Koudstaal J, Arends JW, Thunissen FB. Number and proliferation of neuroendocrine cells in normal human airway epithelium. Am J Respir Crit Care Med 1996; 154:758–63.
13. Breeze RG, Wheeldon EB. The cells of the pulmonary airways. Am Rev Respir Dis 1977; 116:705–7.
14. Colby TV, Yousem SA. Lungs. In: Sternberg SS, ed. Histology for pathologists, 2nd ed. New York: Lippincott-Raven; 1997.
15. Gail DB, Lenfant CJ. Cells of the lung: biology and clinical implications. Am Rev Respir Dis 1983;127:366–87.
16. Gould SJ, Isaacson PG. Bronchus-associated lymphoid tissue (BALT) in human fetal and infant lung. J Pathol 1993;169:229–34.
17. Haefleli-Bleuer B, Weibel E. Morphometry of the human pulmonary acinus. Anat Record 1988;220:401–14.

18. Hasleton PS, Curry A. Anatomy of the lung. In: Hasleton PS, ed. Spencer's pathology the lung, 5th ed. New York: McGraw-Hill; 1996:1–44.
19. Kradin RL, Spirn PW, Mark EJ. Intrapulmonary lymph nodes. Clinical, radiological, and pathologic features. Chest 1985;87:662–7.
20. Kuhn C III. Normal anatomy and histology. In: Thurlbeck WM, Churg AM, eds. Pathology of the lung, 2nd ed. New York: Thieme; 1995:1–36.
21. Kuhn C III. Ultrastructure and cellular function in the distal lung. In: Thurlbeck WM, Abell MR, eds. The lung. Baltimore: Williams & Wilkins; 1978.
22. Langston C, Kida K, Reed M, Thurlbeck WM. Human lung growth in late gestation and in the neonate. Am Rev Respir Dis 1984;129:607–13.
23. Lehnert BE. Pulmonary and thoracic macrophage subpopulations and clearance of particles from the lung. Environ Health Perspect 1992;97:17–46.
24. Nagaishi C. Functional anatomy and histology of the lung. Baltimore: University Park Press, 1972.
25. Okada Y. Lymphatic system of the human lung. Kyoto-shi: Kinpodo, 1989.
26. Pabst R, Tschernig T. Lymphocytes in the lung: an often neglected cell. Numbers, characterization and compartmentalization. Anat Embryol 1995;192:293–9.
27. Richmond I, Pritchard GE, Ashcroft T, Avery A, Corris PA, Walters EH. Bronchus associated lymphoid tissue (BALT) in human lung: its distribution in smokers and non-smokers. Thorax 1993;48:1130–4.
28. Sorokin SP. The respiratory system. In: Weiss L, ed. Cell and tissue biology, 6th ed. Baltimore: Urban & Schwarzenberg; 1988:753–814.
29. Thurlbeck WM. Quantitative anatomy of the lung. In: Thurlbeck WM, Churg AM, eds. Pathology of the lung, 2nd ed. New York: Thieme; 1995:89–98.
30. Tschernig T, Kleemann WJ, Pabst R. Bronchus-associated lymphoid tissue (BALT) in the lungs of children who had died from sudden infant death syndrome and other causes. Thorax 1995;50:658–60.
31. Wagenvoort CA, Wagenvoort N. Pathology of pulmonary hypertension. New York: Wiley; 1977.
32. Wang NS. Anatomy. In: Dail DH, Hammar SP, eds. Pulmonary pathology, 2nd ed. New York: Springer; 1994:21–44.
33. Wanner A, Salathe M, O'Riordan TG. Mucociliary clearance in the airways. Am J Respir Crit Care Med 1996;154:1868–902.
34. Weibel ER. Design and structure of the human lung. In: Fishman AP, ed. Pulmonary diseases and disorders, 2nd ed. New York: McGraw Hill; 1988:11–60.
35. Weibel ER. Lung cell biology. In: Fishman AP, Fisher AB, eds. Handbook of physiology. Bethesda, MD: American Physiological Society; 1985:47–91.
36. Yaegashi H, Takahashi T. The airway dimension in ordinary human lung. Arch Pathol Lab Med 1994;118:969–74.

2
HANDLING AND ANALYSIS OF BRONCHOALVEOLAR LAVAGE AND LUNG BIOPSY SPECIMENS WITH APPROACH TO PATTERNS OF LUNG INJURY

The assessment of patients with non-neoplastic lung diseases requires a multidisciplinary approach with evaluation of clinical, radiologic, and pathologic parameters. This chapter will review general principles for the evaluation of lung biopsies from such patients.

The interpretation of lung biopsies from patients with non-neoplastic lung diseases is often difficult for surgical pathologists for a variety of reasons. First, in most cases the diagnosis is not purely pathologic and requires correlation with clinical and radiologic findings. Second, the terminology is confusing, with many abbreviations for various entities. Of these various terms there tends to be an overuse of the diagnoses of usual interstitial pneumonia (UIP), desquamative interstitial pneumonia (DIP), and bronchiolitis obliterans organizing pneumonia (BOOP). Most interstitial lung diseases are relatively uncommon, so few pathologists have substantial experience or training in studying large numbers of cases. It is important to systematically examine lung biopsies, looking for possible lesions at all major anatomic locations such as the pleura, septa, airways, vessels, and alveolar spaces. Lesions of the blood vessels and airways, such as veno-occlusive disease and obliterative bronchiolitis, respectively, are often overlooked. In addition, large numbers of lung biopsies show a variety of nonspecific histologic patterns. If the biopsy is too small, if it shows marked crush artifact, or if it is obtained from the wrong site the tissue sample may be inadequate. There is a tendency to overinterpret some of these inadequate samples to suggest a specific diagnosis when the findings are nonspecific.

Another potential problem is encountering an unsuspected immunosuppressed patient. This can happen because of an occult condition or if the pathologist has not been given an adequate history. Occasionally, patients with opportunistic infections present with interstitial lung diseases prior to recognition of an underlying immunosuppressed condition, such as infection with human immunodeficiency virus (HIV). If special stains for microorganisms are not performed in such cases, infectious agents such as *Pneumocystis carinii* may be initially overlooked (66). This is discussed in more detail in chapters 12 and 13.

CLINICAL AND RADIOLOGIC CORRELATION

Accurate diagnosis of most non-neoplastic pulmonary conditions requires careful correlation with clinical and radiologic features. Ideally, this information should be provided at the time that the specimen is delivered to the pathology department. Unfortunately, in a busy practice, this information is often not available or is inaccurate. For this reason, pathologists often need to take the initiative to obtain this critical information. Depending on the morphologic findings, the information shown in Table 2-1 may be extremely helpful in arriving at a final diagnosis. It can be especially important to correlate the clinical and radiologic data when the lung biopsy is small, such as obtained in a bronchoscopic or needle biopsy.

It is very useful for the pulmonologist, radiologist, and pathologist to review all of the data together in a conference where each present their respective findings, especially if there is discordance between the lung biopsy findings and the clinical or radiologic information. While this may not be possible in all cases, if it is done routinely in complicated cases it helps to open lines of communication that carry over to other simpler cases. During prolonged clinical follow-up, it is useful to periodically re-review the lung biopsy in light of the new clinical information that accumulates. Occasionally, new information becomes available that sheds a light on subtle lung biopsy findings that were previously overlooked or thought not to be important. Also, in complex cases consultation with other experienced pathologists may help in pattern recognition and confirmation of the predominant pathologic features.

Table 2-1

CLINICAL AND RADIOLOGIC INFORMATION CRITICAL TO THE PATHOLOGIST

What is the severity of the patient's illness?
  Are they severely ill on a ventilator in an intensive care unit?
  Are they ambulatory with few or moderate symptoms?

What are the symptoms?
  Cough, dyspnea, fever, hemoptysis

What is the type of onset?
  Gradual, acute, or subacute

Does the patient have underlying disease?
  Immunodeficiency, collagen vascular disease, vasculitis

Are there environmental exposures?
  Asbestos, bird antigens, toxic fumes

Is there a history of medication?
  Corticosteroids, cytotoxic agents, antibiotics

Are there laboratory abnormalities?
  Anemia, elevated serum eosinophil counts, antineutrophil cytoplasmic antibodies, serum precipitins against *Aspergillus,* rheumatoid factor

What are the chest radiographic findings?
  Normal, diffuse or localized opacities, nodular or patchy consolidation, airspace or interstitial, upper or lower lobe predominance
  Is there a pleural effusion?

What does the HRCT show?
  Ground-glass opacities, bronchiectasis, evidence of airways disease, lower lobe, subpleural, microcystic, or honeycomb change, bilateral upper lobe cysts and nodules, diffuse cystic changes bilaterally

What are the results of pulmonary function tests?
  Obstructive, restrictive, mixed obstructive or restrictive, normal

BRONCHOALVEOLAR LAVAGE

Bronchoalveolar lavage (BAL), performed during fiberoptic bronchoscopy, is a useful adjunct to lung biopsy in the diagnosis of nonneoplastic lung diseases in a limited number of settings (4). There are no absolute contraindications to the performance of BAL beyond those commonly associated with bronchoscopy. It is beyond the scope of this text to address BAL in any detailed fashion as this has been done in other major references (4,11,19,26,28,35,38,42,52,75,76,102), so only a few comments will be made here.

BAL is a minimally invasive technique that may provide important information about diagnosis and yield insights into immunologic, inflammatory, and infectious processes taking place at the alveolar level (4). There is limited information regarding the optimal site in the lung for BAL (49,50). In localized disease, lavage of the involved segment is likely to yield the best results. In diffuse disease, the right middle lobe or lingula is lavaged most commonly because, when the patient is supine, the anatomy favors maximal recovery of fluid and cells from these sites. Lavage in one site appears adequate, especially if a volume of 100 mL or greater is instilled. Since this volume samples approximately one million alveoli (1.5 to 3.0 percent of the lung), it provides a representative picture of the inflammatory and immune processes in the alveoli regardless of the site of the lavage. Nevertheless, fluid from two or three different areas may yield more specific results when there is marked radiologic heterogeneity in the disease process.

There are a number of steps involved in the optimal processing and examination of BAL samples (49,50). The recovered lavage fluid should be pooled into a single container (siliconized glass or noncell adherent plastic), well mixed, and the total volume measured. Controversy exists about whether to include the first aliquot of fluid recovered with the remainder. The first aliquot is usually a small volume and represents a disproportionate amount of bronchial airway material (epithelial cells and neutrophils) compared to alveolar fluid. BAL fluid generally should be transported to the laboratory on ice but can be stored or transported at room temperature if processing will occur in less than 1 hour. The cells remain viable in BAL fluid for up to 4 hours when stored at 25°C. The lavage fluid frequently contains large amounts of mucus. Filtration of the fluid through sterile cotton gauze or nylon mesh is often performed to prevent the mixing of this material with the cell pellet after centrifugation; filtration also results in the preferential loss of bronchial epithelial cells. An aliquot of the fluid and cells should be stored in case future testing is required, including, when appropriate, fixing approximately 3 million cells in cacodylate buffered glutaraldehyde for electron microscopic studies.

The total number of leukocytes recovered by lavage is determined by examination of a sample of the pooled fluid with a hemocytometer. The cell counts are most accurate when done on the original, pooled sample before any washing procedure has been performed; washing results in a loss of total cells and a decrease in cell viability. The total white cell count is usually expressed both as the total number of cells recovered per lavage and as the concentration of cells per milliliter of recovered fluid. Red blood cells and epithelial cells should be enumerated but are not included in the total white cell count. Differential cell counts are most frequently determined on slides prepared either by cytocentrifugation or filtration. With either technique, the differential counts are performed with a light microscope employing X25 and X40 objectives. At least 8 to 10 slides are prepared. Counts are made from random fields of 200 to 500 cells.

Esterase staining is often employed to distinguish immature macrophages from large lymphocytes. The number of ciliated or squamous epithelial cells should be noted, but they are not included in the differential count. Because this procedure is operator dependent, it should be performed by an experienced and properly trained cytotechnologist. Cytocentrifugation is the more commonly used method. Differential counting is commonly performed on air-dried (15 to 30 minutes), May-Grunwald-Giemsa– or Wright-Giemsa–stained preparations. There is less distortion of cell structure and less cell loss (especially the selective loss of lymphocytes) when the original sample (before centrifugation and resuspension) is used for the cytocentrifuge preparation. Special stains for iron, inorganic dust, malignant cells, and microorganisms may be performed if desired. With the filtration method, differential cell counts are performed after trapping cells on a filter. The cells are then stained with hematoxylin and eosin (H&E) or the modified Papanicolaou technique. Filtration offers two advantages: cell retention by the filter is high, providing a more accurate representation of the cell types and numbers recovered by lavage, and slides can be stored indefinitely without significant loss of cell detail or staining.

No clear criteria exist for determining the adequacy of the BAL specimen (49,50). Unsatisfactory BAL specimens contain fewer than 2 million total cells; have fewer than 10 alveolar macrophages per high-power field; contain excessive numbers of epithelial cells, either showing morphologic degenerative changes or exceeding the number of alveolar macrophages present; contain a mucopurulent exudate of polymorphonuclear cells; contain excessive red blood cells due to trauma during the procedure; and contain degenerative changes or laboratory artifacts obscuring cell identity. The most common method of presenting results is to present cell differential data in the same manner used for peripheral blood, that is, each white cell type is given as a percentage of the total white cells recovered (49,50). The advantage of this method is that it provides the data in a fashion that is familiar. A disadvantage is that the numbers presented are proportions of the total and, as such, changes in the absolute numbers of a single cell line necessarily affect the reported percentages of all cell lines. With the total cell method, the differential is combined with the total cell count to quantify the absolute number of each cell type per volume of fluid recovered. The advantage of this method is that it also gives insight into the total number of effector cells present in the alveolar structures. Unfortunately, such quantification is most meaningful if standardized lavage volumes are instilled and recovered. At present, such standardization is not possible, and the differential percentage count of total BAL cells is the more commonly used approach.

The usefulness of routine measurement of the noncellular components of BAL in clinical practice remains to be determined. It has been extremely difficult to determine what proportion of the fluid recovered by lavage represents alveolar fluid from the distal airways and alveoli, so-called epithelial lining fluid (ELF).

Several approaches have been proposed to determine the volume of epithelial lining fluid recovered by BAL, including quantitation of albumin, total lavage protein, potassium, methylene blue, and urea. Application of immunofluorescent and immunocytochemical techniques to the analysis of cells recovered from BAL has been predominantly confined to research laboratories.

The average number of cells recovered in BAL fluid from normal, healthy, nonsmoking adults ranges from 100 to 150,000/mL of lavage fluid. Smoking increases the number of cells recovered by a factor of four to six, largely due to an increase in the number of macrophages.

BAL is an excellent method of obtaining specimens to rule out infections, particularly opportunistic infections in immunocompromised hosts by pathogenic organisms not known to colonize the lower respiratory tract (see chapters 12 and 13). Combining the BAL findings with cytologic evaluation showing characteristic viral intranuclear or intracytoplasmic inclusion bodies on examination of pulmonary epithelial cells in the lavage fluid may confirm the diagnosis of viral agents such as cytomegalovirus or herpes simplex (1,4,27,55,88). BAL is also useful for detecting other infectious agents, such as bacteria, fungi, and mycobacteria (1,11,27,53,55,81,86,88). Unfortunately, the ability of many potentially pathogenic bacteria to colonize respiratory passages in the absence of invasive disease has made the recovery of these organisms in BAL specimens difficult to interpret (4). Semiquantitative cultures of BAL fluid from patients with bacteria show that the presence of 105 or more colony-forming units/mL of BAL fluid identifies, with reasonable accuracy, patients with bacterial pneumonias (15,44,45). These results may not be applicable to all patients with pneumonia. Isolation of *Candida, Aspergillus,* or nontuberculous mycobacteria species in BAL fluid is not diagnostic of infection since these organisms have been isolated in patients without invasive disease (4).

BAL cellular and fluid components have been widely studied in patients with interstitial lung diseases such as sarcoidosis (13,41,47,87,102), hypersensitivity pneumonitis (5,38,77,78,84), and idiopathic pulmonary fibrosis (3,9,37,54,71,98,100,105). Much of the data focuses on the immunology, pathogenesis, or progression of disease over time since BAL provides a way to evaluate the inflammatory cellular components of the lung multiple times over the course of the patient's disease. However, the BAL findings are not specific for these disorders, and ultimately the diagnosis is based upon clinical, radiographic, and lung biopsy data. In other disorders, such as acute eosinophilic pneumonia, lung biopsies are seldom performed and the diagnosis more often rests upon BAL findings (10,48,73).

BAL provides a relatively noninvasive means of assessing some occupational exposures, for example, asbestos bodies in the lavage fluid indicate exposure to asbestos, while birefringent crystalline particles within the alveolar macrophages on polarized light microscopy indicate exposure to crystalline silicates. Quantitative assessment of the proliferative response of bronchoalveolar mononuclear cells to specific agents is a useful diagnostic test; a well-studied example is chronic beryllium disease (68).

Cytologic examination of cells obtained by BAL has been useful in the diagnosis of malignancy, primary or metastatic (4,75). Protein immunoelectrophoresis of BAL fluid has been helpful in diagnosing lymphoma involving the lung by demonstrating monoclonal gammopathy (4).

HANDLING AND PROCESSING OF SPECIMENS

Types of Lung Biopsy Specimens

A variety of pathologic specimens may be obtained from the lung to evaluate non-neoplastic disorders (Table 2-2). By bronchoscopy one may obtain transbronchial or endobronchial biopsies. Surgical lung biopsies include

Table 2-2

TYPES OF SPECIMENS FOR ASSESSMENT OF NON-NEOPLASTIC LUNG DISEASE

Expectorated material
Broncholith
Mucus plug
Bronchoscopic biopsy
Transbronchial biopsy
Endobronchial biopsy
Needle biopsy
Surgical lung biopsy
Open biopsy by thoracotomy
Reduction surgery for emphysema
Thoracoscopic biopsy
Segmentectomy/lobectomy/pneumonectomy
Explant from transplantation procedure
Pleural biopsy

open wedge biopsies, video-assisted thoracoscopic biopsies, segmentectomies, lobectomies, pneumonectomies, and pleural or mediastinal biopsies. A thoracoscopic approach is useful for obtaining transpleural lung biopsies or pleural biopsies. Thoracoscopic procedures reduce morbidity and the length of hospitalization compared to lung biopsy through open thoracotomy, while providing comparably diagnostic specimens. Percutaneous transthoracic needle biopsies are useful in some conditions.

Transbronchial Biopsies

In virtually all cases the entire transbronchial biopsy specimen should be placed directly into formalin fixative and processed for routine histology. In patients with a high index of suspicion for infection, a piece is submitted for culture. Gently shaking transbronchial biopsy specimens in fixative in the specimen container helps expand the alveolar spaces to avoid the problem of atelectasis. Transbronchial biopsies are useful for the diagnosis of sarcoidosis (56,59, 60,80), infection (12,34,91,106), or tumor. They are especially useful in immunocompromised patients with infections or malignancies that cause diffuse pulmonary infiltrates. In particular, they are useful in transplant and chemotherapy patients (chapters 7, 13, and 14). Details about the interpretation of lung biopsies from immunocompromised patients are found in chapter 13. If diagnostic lesions are sampled, the diagnosis of pulmonary Langerhans' cell histiocytosis (92), lymphangioleiomyomatosis (8, 36), alveolar proteinosis, eosinophilic pneumonia, or amyloidosis can be established.

Step sections can be particularly useful for detecting small lesions, such as granulomas, in patients with sarcoidosis (67). It is common to encounter nondiagnostic histologic findings in bronchoscopic biopsies, and there is a temptation to overinterpret nondiagnostic findings, but if a definitive morphologic lesion cannot be detected, one should be cautious in such cases.

There is a limited role for transbronchial biopsy in the diagnosis of idiopathic interstitial pneumonias. Surgical lung biopsies obtained through thoracotomy or thoracoscopy are needed to establish a diagnosis of most diffuse interstitial lung diseases since a large piece of tissue is necessary to recognize the entire pattern of disorders such as usual interstitial pneumonia (UIP) or nonspecific interstitial pneumonia (NSIP). In addition, many of the idiopathic interstitial pneumonias require the exclusion of lesions that would indicate a specific etiology. With small samples one may not be able to exclude the presence of infectious agents, granulomas, mineral fibers such as asbestos bodies, or tumor cells that might provide a clue to a specific cause. Occasionally, an open biopsy helps to detect a more treatable disorder, such as hypersensitivity pneumonitis. A surgical lung biopsy may allow for evaluation of disease activity: diffuse alveolar damage and, on occasion, organizing pneumonia patterns, can be recognized on transbronchial lung biopsy. However, the organizing pneumonia pattern can be a nonspecific reaction to a wide variety of other lesions. Therefore, the biopsy findings should be carefully correlated with clinical and radiologic findings before suggesting the diagnosis of cryptogenic organizing pneumonia (see chapter 3).

Artifacts or biopsy findings that can cause confusion are discussed in more detail below. These include hemorrhage, specimen atelectasis or crush artifact, pseudolipoid pneumonia, pleural fragments, blue bodies, and entrapped alveoli in the bronchial submucosa with macrophage accumulation.

Surgical Lung Biopsies

Since lung biopsies, particularly surgical biopsies, are usually performed only once during a patient's lifetime, it is critical that they be processed in a manner to maximize diagnostic information. For interstitial lung diseases, it is useful for the surgeon to determine the optimal site of surgical lung biopsy by review of a computed tomography (CT) or high-resolution (HR) CT scan. For diffuse fibrotic disorders it is important not to biopsy the area of worst involvement since this often shows nonspecific endstage fibrosis. It is also valuable to biopsy more than one lobe since fibrotic and inflammatory interstitial diseases often show heterogeneity in the histologic patterns and the additional specimen provides essential diagnostic information. The surgeon should biopsy areas that appear moderately abnormal or in cases of severe disease, relatively normal. Avoiding the tips of the lobes, including the lingula, has been recommended (69), since these sites may show nonspecific fibrotic or inflammatory lesions. There has been some debate in the literature about whether the lingula is a suitable site or whether more than one lobe needs to be biopsied (30,58,69,90,104). If the chest radiographs show localized lesions, the biopsy should be directed to one of these lesions as well as to a transition area between normal and abnormal lung parenchyma.

For the pathologist and surgeon to ensure that the maximum diagnostic information is obtained from lung biopsy specimens, it is important to follow several procedures. A portion of each open lung biopsy specimen should be sent to the microbiology laboratory for cultures and smears. To minimize contamination, it is best to send the specimen directly to the microbiology laboratory from the operating room. However, the pathologist may send culture specimens from the frozen section laboratory if care is taken to avoid contamination.

Inflation of surgical lung biopsies with fixative can help to avoid specimen atelectasis. It can be very difficult to assess interstitial lesions when the alveolar walls are collapsed and compressed together (18). Open or thoracoscopic lung biopsies can be inflated by gently injecting formalin with a syringe and needle or by slicing the specimen into thin sections and shaking them gently in a bottle of fixative. Lobectomy or pneumonectomy specimens can be inflated through a major bronchus. Inflation can creat an artifact by washing out alveolar macrophages.

Frozen sections of open lung biopsy specimens can be invaluable in certain settings. First, they assist in assessing whether adequate tissue has been sampled. In cases where cultures may not have been already obtained, the finding of inflammatory lesions, such as granulomas, on a frozen section should prompt the surgical pathologist to send a small piece of the specimen to the microbiology laboratory for culture. In addition, frozen sections can provide useful diagnostic information in some cases, particularly in patients with acute illnesses. Granulomatous inflammation, diffuse alveolar damage, most tumors, pulmonary hemorrhage, and some infectious agents can be detected. The organisms that are likely to be detected on frozen section analysis are cytomegalovirus (CMV) or numerous fungi. The combination of frozen section analysis and special stains can provide a specific diagnosis for infectious agents in up to 47 percent of cases within 3 hours of an open lung biopsy (105). The results of frozen section biopsies may point to such diagnoses as diffuse pulmonary hemorrhage syndromes or lymphoproliferative disorders where it may be useful to freeze a small piece of tissue for immunofluorescent or molecular studies.

Touch preparations can be performed on both transbronchial and open lung biopsy specimens (29,62). Neoplastic cells and certain infectious agents may be identified in some cases with this method. CMV inclusions may be recognized on routine stains, and rapid methods for the Gomori silver stain or the Gram-Weigert stain can be very useful for identifying *Pneumocystis carinii* (29,79).

Electron microscopy, immunohistochemistry, and nucleic acid hybridization can provide important diagnostic information in certain cases. For electron microscopy, it is important to fix a small piece of tissue in glutaraldehyde at the time of biopsy. For certain immunohistochemistry or nucleic acid hybridization assays, it may be necessary to snap freeze a portion of the specimen in liquid nitrogen and store it in a freezer.

Special Stains

There are a wide variety of ancillary stains and techniques available to the pathologist to assess lung biopsies for the diagnosis of non-neoplastic disorders. While certain stains should be ordered routinely in certain clinical settings, such as stains for infection in the immunocompromised host, in most cases the pathologist must evaluate routine H&E-stained sections to determine whether it is appropriate to obtain special studies, particularly immunohistochemistry or in situ hybridization. These tests should not be ordered without discrimination.

Histochemical Stains. There are a wide variety of special stains that are useful aids in the diagnosis of interstitial lung diseases (2). The most useful connective tissue stains include the Masson trichrome and Movat pentachrome stains. The Masson stain turns dense collagen a deep blue and highlights its fibrillar quality. The Movat stain not only highlights elastic fibers in black, but it also colors loose collagen green and dense collagen yellow. The Congo red stain is helpful in the detection of amyloid. With unpolarized light, a positive Congo red stain gives a deep orange color that turns to apple-green under polarized light. The Prussian blue stain helps to highlight iron. The von Kossa stain highlights calcified inclusions. Elastic van Giesen stains demonstrate elastic fibers in blood vessels or the pleura.

For lung biopsies from immunocompromised patients, special stains for infectious organisms should be performed routinely. For transbronchial biopsies, it is useful to take 10 serial sections from each specimen and stain three sections (cuts 1, 5, and 10) with H&E (96). For a surgical lung biopsy, 5 sections can be cut from each block and cuts 1, 3, and 5 stained with H&E. The remaining unstained slides and any necessary additional sections are used for special stains, which are ordered routinely in immunosuppressed patients. The most important stains for these patients are the Gomori methenamine silver (GMS), and Ziehl-Neelsen stains since these detect *Pneumocystis carinii,* most fungi, and mycobacteria. Periodic acid-Schiff (PAS) is a good fungal stain that can be included in a routine battery of stains for infectious agents since sometimes it is easier to see fungi in the lung with PAS than on the GMS stain. However, the PAS stain does not detect *P. carinii* or *Histoplasma capsulatum* very well. Other stains, such as bacterial stains or immunohistochemistry for viral agents, may be indicated depending on the morphologic findings. For surgical lung biopsies, special stains may initially be performed on one block, but depending on the index of suspicion for infection, additional blocks may be stained. If a questionable focus is seen on the initial H&E-stained sections, additional deeper sections may be requested.

Searching for microorganisms in tissue sections can be a difficult challenge. In immune competent patients, the organisms are usually present within the areas of inflammation or necrosis. Organisms are readily seen on H&E examination including viral inclusions, parasites, or the sulfur granules seen in actinomycosis or botryomycosis. Certain infectious agents are best detected with specific stains (2). Organisms such as *Nocardia* that are weakly acid fast are best detected with the Coate's fite, which reduces the decolorization step. Bacteria are best detected with Brown and Brenn or Brown and Hopps stain. Silver stains such as the Dieterle can be helpful in detecting some bacteria such as *Legionella.* Cultures, serology, and a good exposure or clinical history may be necessary to pinpoint the diagnosis. Rarely, immunosuppressive conditions such as HIV infection may manifest as pulmonary complications in patients who are thought to be immune competent. For this reason, one should perform special stains for organisms, especially *Pneumocystis carinii,* in lung biopsies from patients with unexplained inflammatory infiltrates (see chapter 13).

Special Techniques

For certain disorders special techniques such as immunohistochemistry, in situ hybridization, and other molecular assays using the polymerase chain reaction (PCR) may be diagnostically useful (2). Depending on the antigens in question, immunohistochemistry can be performed on paraffin-embedded or frozen tissue. Immunohistochemistry is a powerful diagnostic tool for malignant lymphomas, certain solid tumors, and undifferentiated malignant neoplasms, but it is also useful for non-neoplastic diseases.

Although most conditions can be diagnosed by light microscopy, immunohistochemistry has several specific uses in non-neoplastic lung diseases. For the diagnosis of Langerhans' cell histiocytosis, Langerhans' cells can be stained with S-100 protein and CD1a antibodies. These work well in formalin-fixed paraffin-embedded sections. For lymphangioleiomyomatosis (LAM), HMB45 and smooth muscle markers may be helpful, particularly in cases where the LAM cell infiltrates are focal, a problem encountered most often in bronchoscopic biopsy specimens. Keratin can highlight epithelial cells to determine the location of an infiltrate. This is important in an atelectatic lung specimen when it is difficult to be sure whether a cellular infiltrate is in the alveolar spaces or the interstitium. KP-1 stains macrophages, which sometimes can be confused with epithelial cells. Immunohistochemistry helps characterize lymphoid infiltrates to determine if the lymphoid cells (lymphocyte common antigen [LCA]/CD45) are T cells (CD3, UCHL-1/CD45RO) or B cells (L26/CD20, CD79a), or if plasma cells are monoclonal (stains for lambda and kappa light chains).

Immunohistochemical methods have recently been applied to the diagnosis of infections caused by mycobacteria (40), *Aspergillus* (27,72), *Histoplasma* (103), *Cryptosporidia* (97), as well as viral agents including cytomegalovirus (43,83), herpesvirus (32), measles (61,82), and respiratory syncytial viruses (31). Immunohistologic methods for detecting fungi in paraffin-embedded tissues include both immunohistochemistry and direct immunofluorescence. Immunohistochemistry can be used to document dual infections in lung biopsies (74). Monoclonal antibodies to *Pneumocystis* have been shown to be of value in the evaluation of sputum and BAL fluid. However, in formalin-fixed, paraffin-embedded tissue sections, immunohistochemistry has not been shown to be of advantage over routine GMS staining. Monoclonal antibody staining may be useful in separating *Pneumocystis carinii* from *Histoplasma capsulatum* (95).

In situ hybridization is useful for identifying viral nucleic acid sequences for herpes simplex, varicella zoster, cytomegalovirus, adenovirus, respiratory syncytial virus, influenza virus, and Epstein-barr virus (2). PCR is effective in detecting infectious agents and determining clonality in lymphoid infiltrates to exclude a lymphoproliferative process.

Electron Microscopy

Electron microscopy is seldom useful for the diagnosis of non-neoplastic lung disorders (16, 70). For diffuse alveolar hemorrhage syndromes and the various manifestations of lupus pneumonitis, the demonstration of electron-dense deposits corresponds to the presence of immune-complex deposits. It can also be used to diagnose viral infections if immunohistochemical stains are inconclusive. In pulmonary Langerhans' cell histiocytosis, Birbeck granules may be demonstrated, however, this diagnosis is usually best established by light microscopy, with occasional use of immunohistochemistry for the detection of CD1a or S-100 protein. One of the situations in which electron microscopy is essential is in evaluating cilia for ciliary dyskinesia syndromes.

General Principles in Lung Biopsy Interpretation

There are several important principles to consider when interpreting lung biopsies for non-neoplastic lung disorders. The low-power scanning impression is critical. From this view one should assess the distribution of the pathology and whether the lung architecture is preserved or lost. All the major structures of the lung should be evaluated: the pleura, airways, vessels, alveoli, and interstitium (Table 2-3). The type of fibrosis should be assessed: is it dense scarring or loose organizing and are there fibroblastic foci present? If there is inflammation, what type is it: acute, chronic, granulomatous, or mixed? Lesions other than interstitial lung disease, such as lymphangitic carcinoma, should be sought.

Systematic scoring methods for evaluating interstitial lung disorders have been published (17,94). These primarily serve as research tools rather than as necessary for routine diagnosis. However, it can be useful to make a general quantitative assessment of these features while evaluating a biopsy for diagnosis, even if these details are not incorporated into a surgical pathology report.

Artifacts and Incidental Lesions. There are a number of artifacts that can be diagnostic pitfalls in lung biopsy interpretation. Awareness of these and the settings in which they occur help avoid common diagnostic errors.

Atelectasis is commonly encountered in lung biopsies in which the airspaces are not properly expanded during processing (fig. 2-1).

Table 2-3

ANATOMIC DISTRIBUTION IN DIFFUSE LUNG DISEASE

Histologic	Radiologic (HRCT)
Broncho/bronchiolocentric	Centrilobular Bronchovascular Nodular (see fig. 2-17)
Angiocentric	Bronchovascular (arterial) Interlobular septal (venous)
Pleural/subpleural	Pleural/subpleural
Lymphatic	Bronchovascular Interlobular septal Pleural/subpleural
Peripheral acinar	Subpleural peripheral (paraseptal)
Septal	Septal
Random nodular	Random nodular
Parenchymal consolidation	Consolidation, ground glass
Diffuse interstitial	Diffuse interstitial, ground glass

This can give the false impression of hypercellularity or interstitial fibrosis. Clues to this artifact include identification of areas of the lung biopsy where the airspaces are either inconspicuous or absent, but the tissue looks very cellular. Evaluation at high magnification demonstrates numerous nuclei of endothelial cells, and alveolar epithelial cells collapsed together. Major structures such as bronchioles and blood vessels also appear compressed together. This artifact is easier to appreciate if there are other areas of the lung biopsy in which the airspaces are well expanded. Hopefully, the pathologic lesion in question will be present in the better expanded areas since it may be very difficult to appreciate subtle interstitial lesions in atelectatic areas of a lung biopsy. Keratin stains may highlight whether such lesions are located in airspaces or the interstitium.

Pseudolipoid pneumonia is another lesion that results from artifactual collapse of airspaces adjacent to airways (fig. 2-2) (24). The collapsed airways create "holes" in the tissue that appear like vacuoles from which lipid may have washed out during processing.

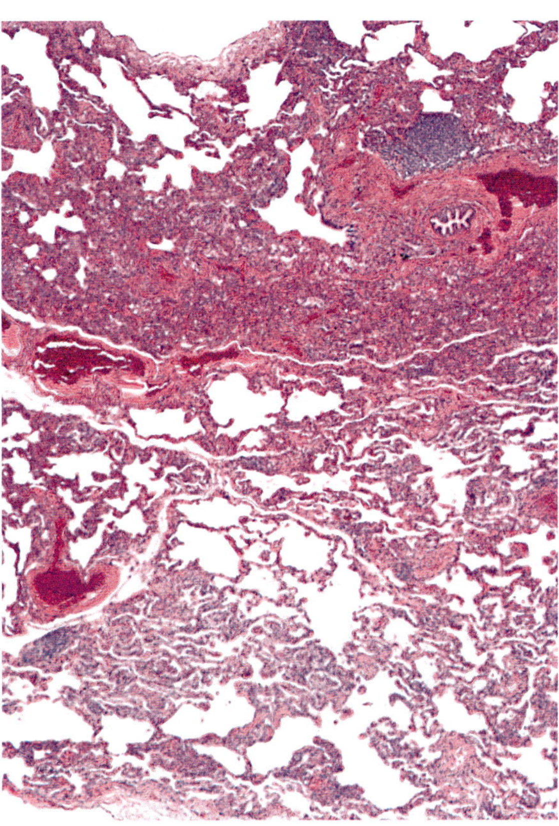

Figure 2-1

SPECIMEN ATELECTASIS

The atelectatic lung (top) appears abnormal at low magnification. However, it represents collapsed alveolar tissue that is difficult to evaluate. The adjacent lung (bottom) is well-expanded and much easier to evaluate, revealing mild interstitial chronic inflammation and alveolar macrophage accumulation.

Submucosal alveolar entrapment may occur in the submucosa of bronchi or bronchioles in bronchoscopic biopsy specimens (fig. 2-3). Occasionally, this can be mistaken for lymphangitic carcinoma. Confusion arises since the alveolar spaces appear above the smooth muscle layer of the airway, probably due to tangential sectioning. Helpful clues are the frequent foamy cytoplasm of the macrophages and the faint brown cytoplasmic pigment that is often present. Awareness of this entrapment phenomenon can avoid a mistaken diagnosis of malignancy. If sufficient concern remains after morphologic assessment, a combination of KP-1 (CD68) and keratin or TTF-1 immunohistochemistry can confirm the

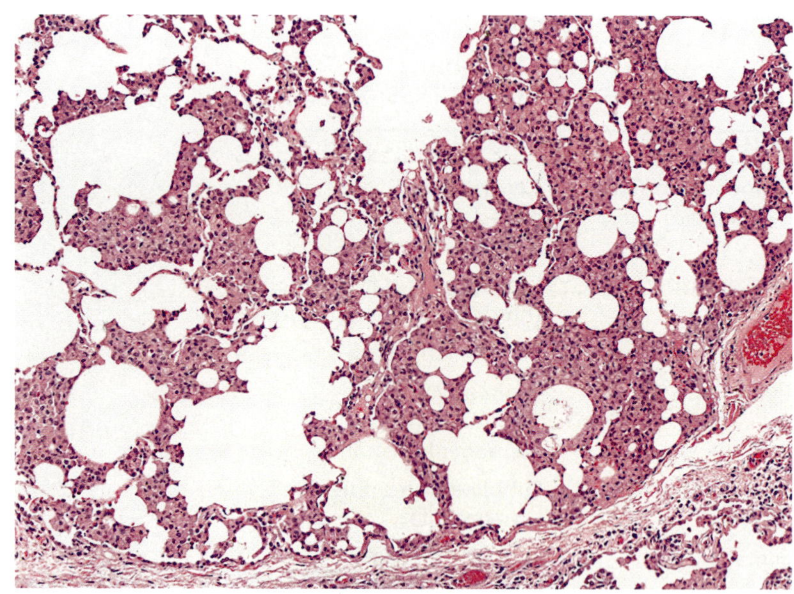

Figure 2-2

PSEUDOLIPOID PNEUMONIA

The vacuolated appearance of these airspaces results from crushed or collapsed airspaces. The lack of vacuolated macrophages shows that the lesion is not due to lipid accumulation.

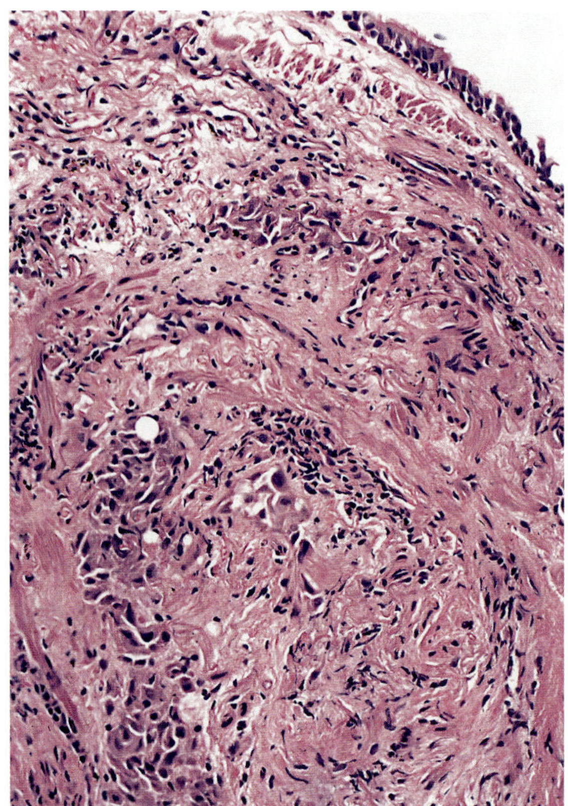

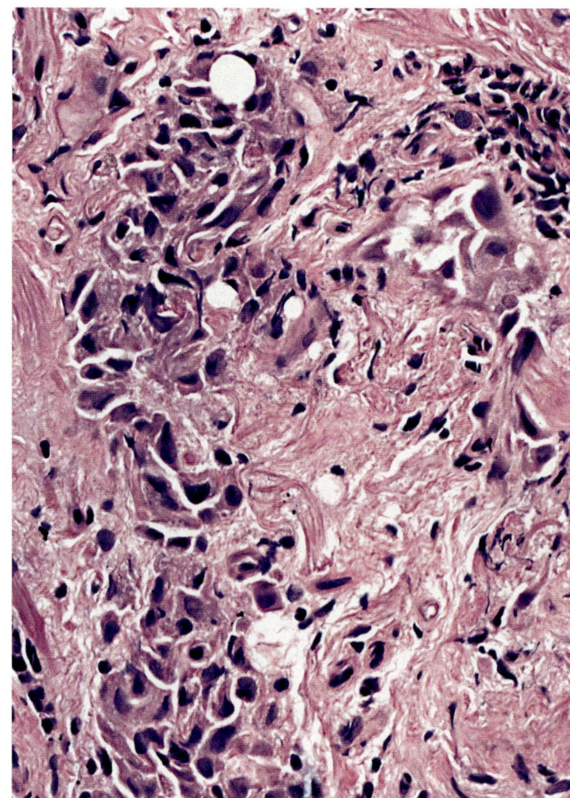

Figure 2-3

SUBMUCOSAL ALVEOLAR ENTRAPMENT

Left: This bronchoscopic specimen shows submucosal alveolar spaces containing macrophages. However, the alveolar spaces appear above the smooth muscle layer of the airway.

Right: Higher power shows alveolar macrophages within compressed alveolar spaces.

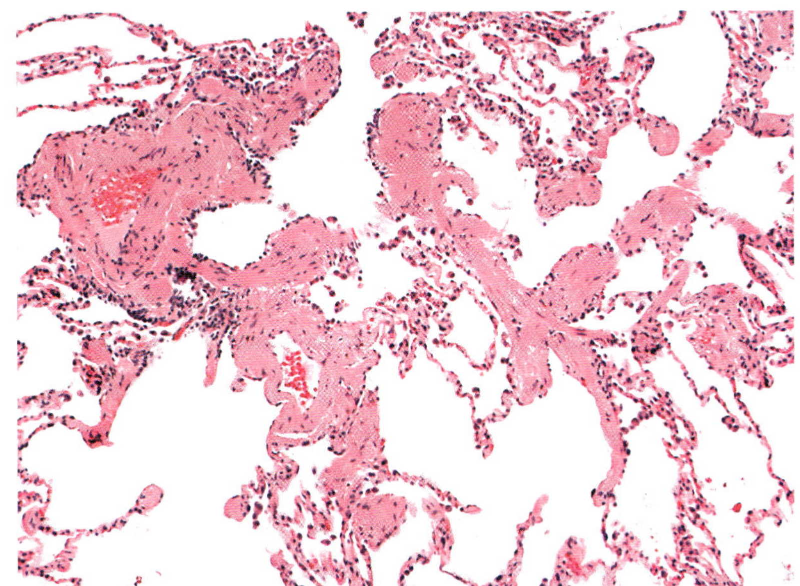

Figure 2-4

ALVEOLAR DUCT SMOOTH MUSCLE

This alveolar duct has prominent smooth muscle, and can be mistaken for hyaline membranes or lymphangioleiomyomatosis.

impression that the cells in question are macrophages and that the spaces are lined by epithelial and not endothelial cells.

Alveolar duct smooth muscle may be mistaken for hyaline membranes, interstitial fibrosis, or lymphangioleiomyomatosis (fig. 2-4). It is important to recognize the anatomic structure of the terminal bronchiole as it transitions into the alveolar ducts. This may be difficult in cases where the specimen shows artifactual atelectasis. In some lung biopsies the alveolar duct smooth muscle is particularly prominent.

Artifactual hemorrhage is a common finding in lung biopsy specimens, particularly transbronchial biopsies (fig. 2-5). It is usually the result of the biopsy procedure and is of no clinical significance. However, it can mistakenly be interpreted as a true pathologic lesion. Usually this is not a difficult problem, but there are cases where it can be a challenge to sort out whether the hemorrhage is truly pathologic or not. Unless there is clinical evidence of acute hemorrhage, such as hemoptysis, one should look for histologic clues to the presence of genuine hemorrhage, such as coarse granules of hemosiderin or erythrophagocytosis, or some tissue reaction such as acute lung injury. Clumps of fibrin sometimes develop within fresh hemorrhage and should not be interpreted as hyaline membranes. In addition, artifactual hemorrhage is often patchy so areas of relatively unaffected lung can be identified. If the lung tissue in the areas with fresh hemorrhage appears the same as in the areas without it, this favors artifactual hemorrhage.

Corpora amylacea are round to oval, intra-alveolar spherical bodies that consist of glycoprotein (fig. 2-6) (7,25,39,57). They are reported in 0.6 to 3.8 percent of autopsies and do not appear to have any specific disease associations (39, 57). They resemble the corpora amylacea seen in the prostate. They measure between 30 and 200 µm, with most being between 60 and 100 µm (7,33,39,57). They have circumferential lines, giving a laminated appearance. They appear pink with H&E, red with Ziehl-Neelsen, blue with Masson trichrome, and magenta with PAS stains (25). Corpora amylacea can be mistaken for alveolar microlithiasis (see chapter 3). Inclusions may be seen within the corpora amylacea and they may appear as black fragments, ring forms, or small polarizable crystals (7,25,33,39,57).

Kuhn's (Mallory's) hyaline consists of dense, waxy, eosinophilic clumps within the cytoplasm of reactive type 2 pneumocytes (fig. 2-7) (51,99). It is derived from cytoplasmic keratin intermediate filaments (51,99). It can be seen in many types of interstitial lung disorders including asbestosis, usual interstitial pneumonia, viral pneumonia, radiation pneumonitis, and bacterial pneumonia (51,99).

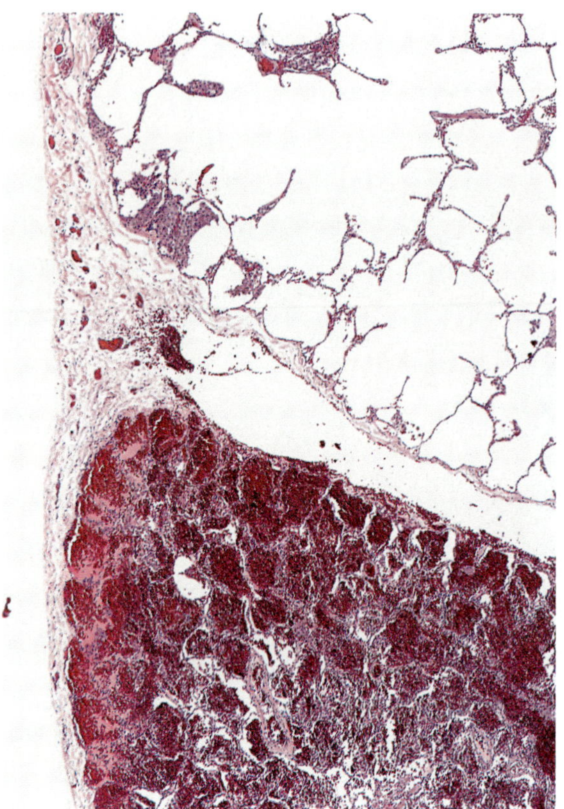

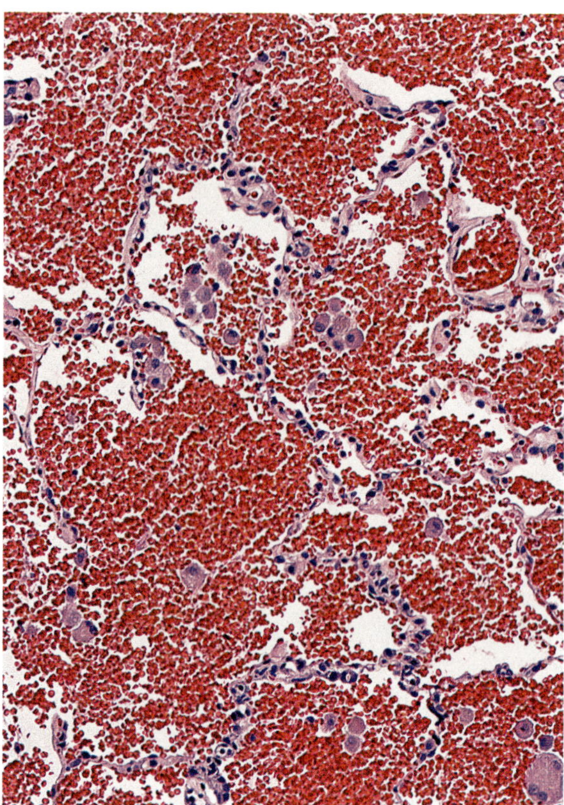

Figure 2-5

ARTIFACTUAL HEMORRHAGE

Left: There is extensive intra-alveolar red blood cell accumulation. The underlying alveolar parenchyma is obscured by the numerous red blood cells, however, the adjacent lung appears relatively normal.

Right: Closer view of the alveolar walls shows normal morphology with no hemosiderin accumulation and no erythrophagocytosis by macrophages.

Megakaryocytes are frequently seen in pulmonary capillaries (fig. 2-8) (46,85). They appear as dark hyperchromatic cells with prominently folded nuclear membranes that are squeezed tightly into the capillary lumens. In contrast to the large rounded appearance and abundant cytoplasm seen in bone marrow specimens, in the pulmonary capillaries the dark nuclear material is often barrel-shaped. Occasionally, multilobulation or branching may be seen (46,85). They can be mistaken for viral inclusions, metastatic malignancy, or embolic trophoblastic tissue. Although megakaryocytes can be stained with factor VIII, usually the morphology is sufficient for recognition.

Vascular encrustation (endogenous pneumoconiosis) occurs in association with chronic hemorrhage due to any cause (fig. 2-9). Hemosiderin deposits on the elastic fibers, resulting in degeneration and fragmentation, frequently elicit a fibrous and giant cell reaction. The elastic fibers are often gray to black and the fragments may appear thicker than normal vascular elastica. These fragmented fibers stain brightly with the Prussian blue stain for iron. The giant cells essentially form a foreign body reaction to the fragmented elastic fibers. They may be mistaken for granulomatous inflammation, and in the context of diffuse pulmonary hemorrhage syndromes they should not be confused with the granulomatous vasculitis of Wegener's granulomatosis. The combination of hemosiderosis and vascular changes also should not be confused with pulmonary veno-occlusive disease.

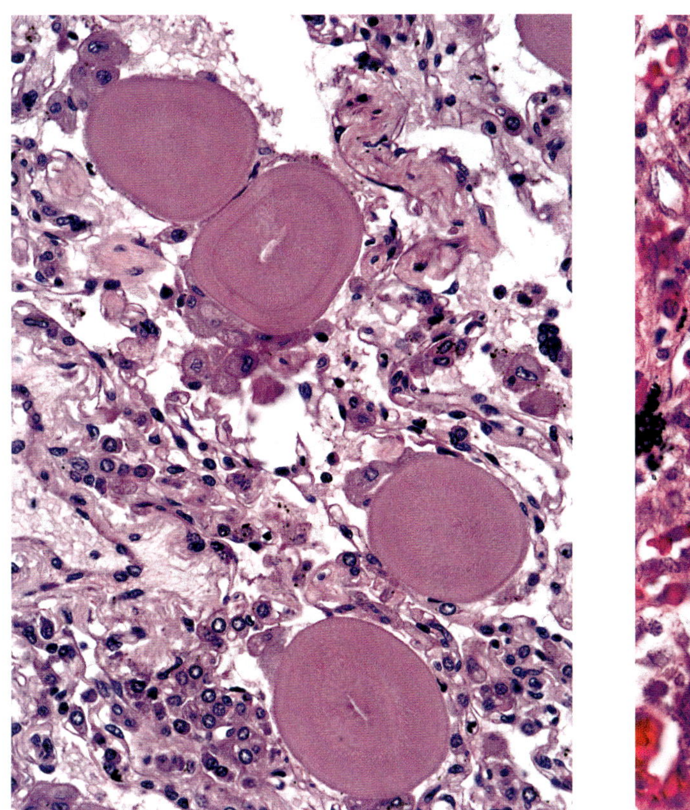

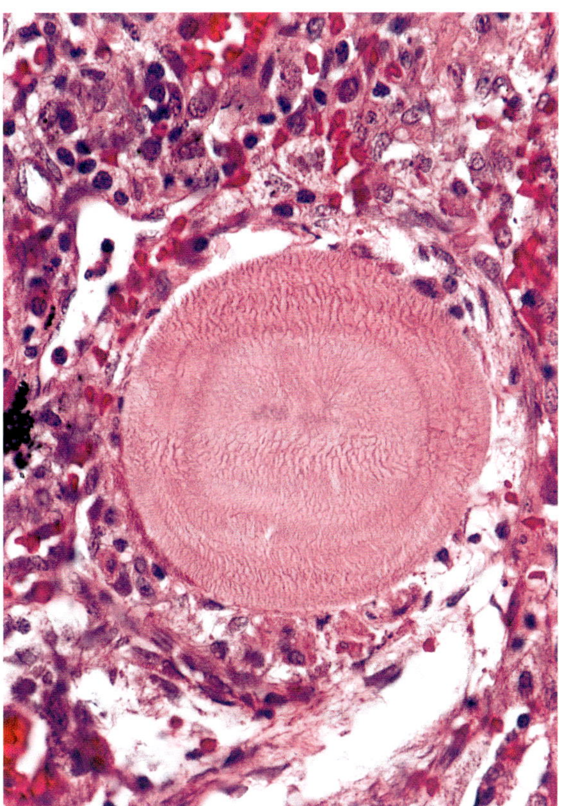

Figure 2-6

CORPORA AMYLACEA

These round to oval eosinophilic bodies consist of proteinaceous material that is concentrically laminated.

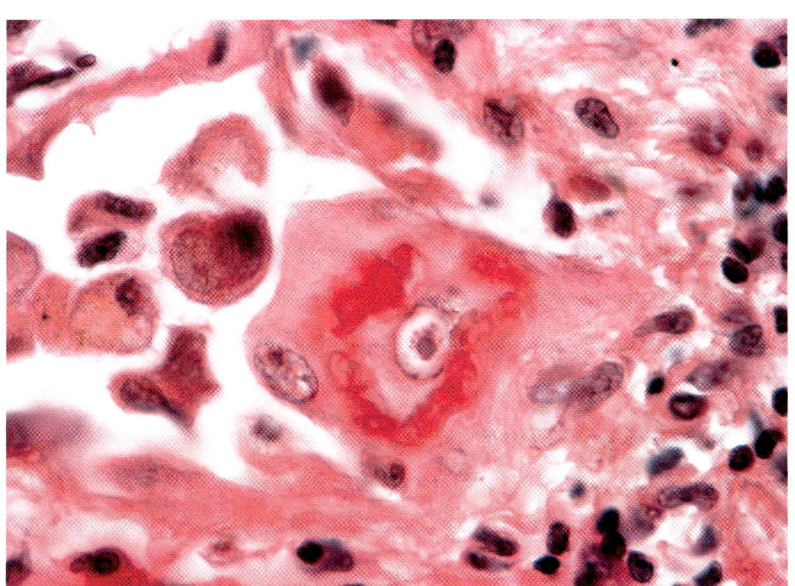

Figure 2-7

KUHN'S (MALLORY'S) HYALINE

The cytoplasm of this hyperplastic pneumocyte contains irregular, rope-like bundles of eosinophilic material. These bundles closely resemble the Mallory's hyaline seen in the liver.

Figure 2-8

INTRACAPILLARY MEGAKARYOCYTE

The hyperchromatic basophilic material that is folded and squeezed into an alveolar wall capillary is a megakaryocyte.

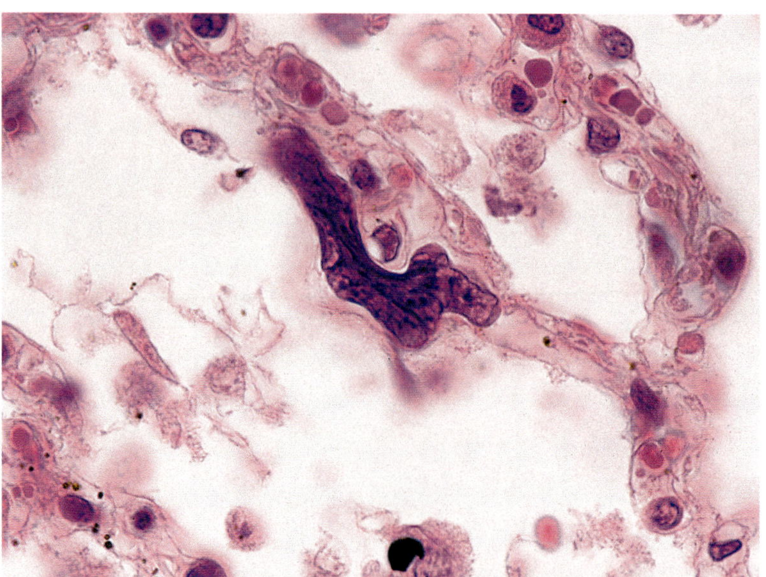

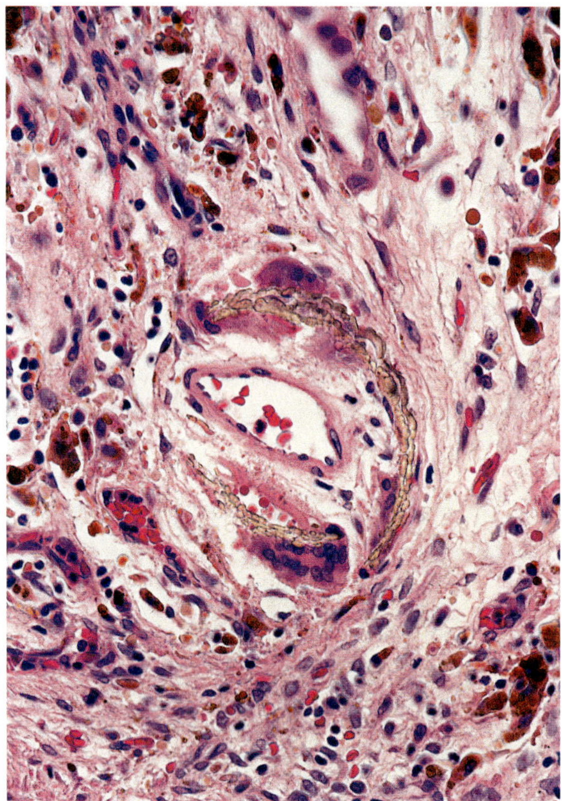

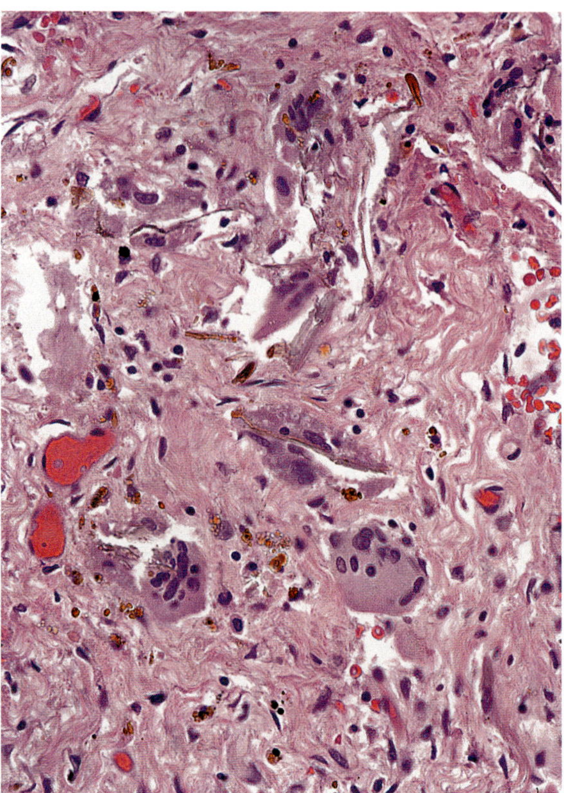

Figure 2-9

VASCULAR ENCRUSTATION

Left: The wall of this blood vessel is thickened by fibrous tissue and fragmented elastic fibers, which are associated with a foreign body giant cell reaction.

Right: The fragmented elastic fibers appear gray or brown when surrounded by an iron protein coat. The latter fibers resemble ferruginous bodies. A giant cell reaction is prominent.

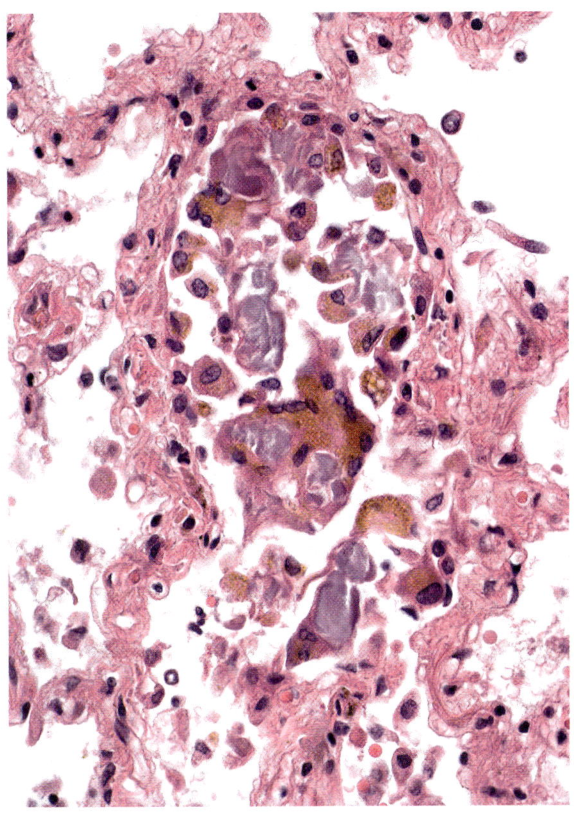

Figure 2-10

BLUE BODIES

These intra-alveolar, laminated, basophilic and calcified bodies are nonspecific, but are often associated with disorders characterized by intra-alveolar macrophage accumulation.

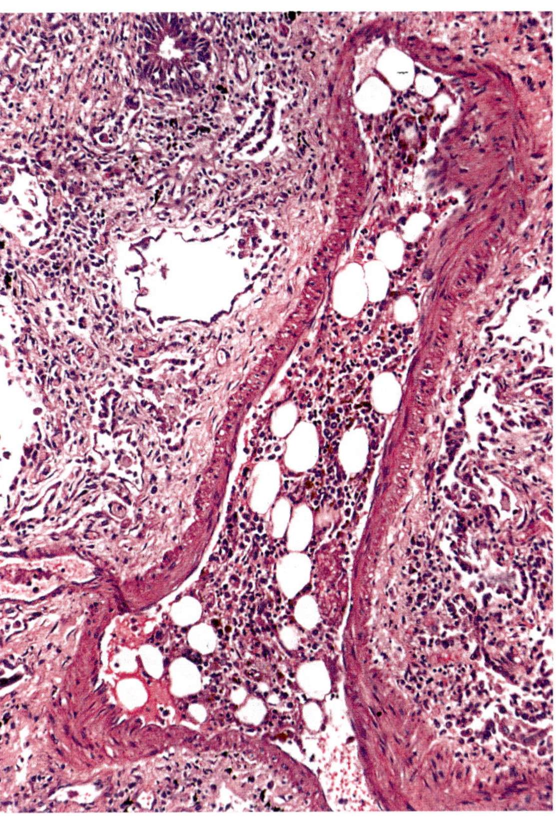

Figure 2-11

BONE MARROW EMBOLI

A fragment of bone marrow with fat and hematopoietic elements is present within the lumen of this blood vessel.

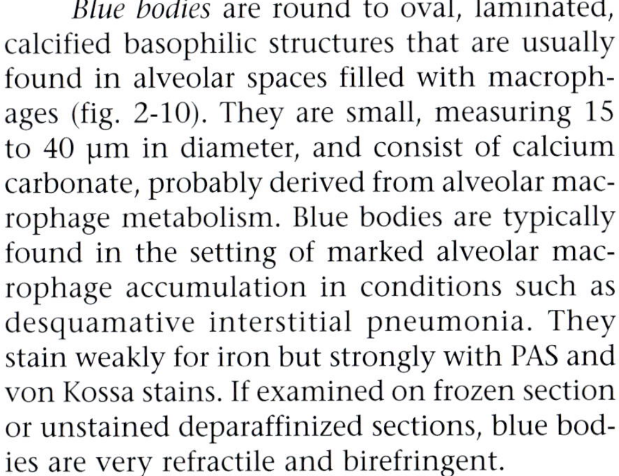

Blue bodies are round to oval, laminated, calcified basophilic structures that are usually found in alveolar spaces filled with macrophages (fig. 2-10). They are small, measuring 15 to 40 µm in diameter, and consist of calcium carbonate, probably derived from alveolar macrophage metabolism. Blue bodies are typically found in the setting of marked alveolar macrophage accumulation in conditions such as desquamative interstitial pneumonia. They stain weakly for iron but strongly with PAS and von Kossa stains. If examined on frozen section or unstained deparaffinized sections, blue bodies are very refractile and birefringent.

Bone marrow emboli are frequent incidental findings in up to 16 percent of autopsy specimens (fig. 2-11). Histologically, they consist of fat admixed with hematopoietic elements, occasionally associated with fragments of bone. However, they are usually of no clinical significance. They are often associated with bone fractures or cardiopulmonary resuscitation, sternal cleavage associated with cardiac surgery, and rarely, metastatic carcinoma to bone or bone infarcts associated with sickle cell anemia.

Minute meningothelioid nodules, or *chemodectomas,* are incidental histologic findings that are commonly encountered in lung biopsies (fig. 2-12). They consist of small perivenular proliferations of round to oval cells which grow in swirling nests that are reminiscent of meningothelial cells. They are usually multiple and can be mistaken for granulomas, interstitial fibrosis, or carcinoid tumorlets. In contrast to

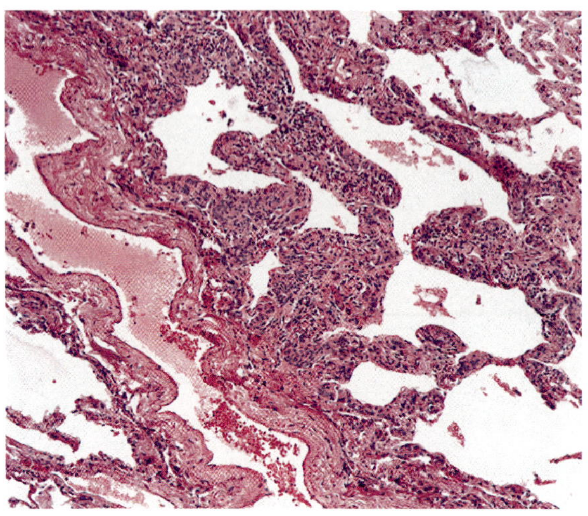

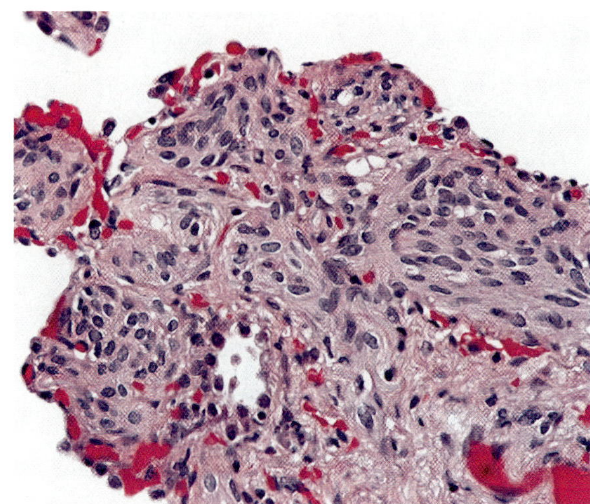

Figure 2-12

MINUTE MENINGOTHELIOID NODULE

Left: The perivenular interstitium is infiltrated by a proliferation of uniform round to oval cells.
Right: These cells have moderate eosinophilic cytoplasm and bland nuclei, and they grow in nests and whorls.

carcinoid tumorlets, they are situated around pulmonary veins rather than airways (21,93).

Occasionally, *pleural fragments* appear in bronchoscopic biopsies and are either overlooked or confused with other lesions (fig. 2-13) (14). The bronchoscope is capable of reaching the periphery of the lung so that the biopsy forceps samples the pleura. In contrast to alveolar parenchyma, the pleura consists of a thin layer of connective tissue lined by mesothelial cells that are either flat or hyperplastic and cuboidal. A layer of elastic fibers can be seen beneath the mesothelial cells. The connective tissue may be mistaken for interstitial fibrosis and the mesothelial cells can be confused with hyperplastic type 2 pneumocytes or atypical cells suspicious for malignancy. Usually this is not a serious diagnostic problem, but if it was deemed necessary, immunohistochemistry for calretinin and TTF-1 could be used to differentiate mesothelial cells and type 2 pneumocytes, respectively.

The "Normal" Lung Biopsy. There are a number of entities that should be considered before suggesting that a lung biopsy is "normal" (Table 2-4). In such specimens the airways and vessels should be carefully examined. Constrictive bronchiolitis may be suspected if the patient has a relatively normal chest radiograph and severe obstructive pulmonary function. Examination of the blood vessels should include evaluation of the arterioles, veins, capillaries, and lymphatics. Lesions such as pulmonary thrombi or emboli, veno-occlusive disease, and plexogenic arteriopathy are easily overlooked. Occasionally, lung biopsies are performed in patients with pulmonary edema, which may be the only pathologic finding. Early diffuse alveolar damage shows only pulmonary edema and focal hyaline membranes. Subtle lesions of Langerhans' cell histiocytosis, lymphangioleiomyomatosis, or alveolar proteinosis can be overlooked. In some cases, even in surgical lung biopsies, the lesion may be completely missed by the surgeon.

PATTERNS OF LUNG INJURY

Many non-neoplastic lung diseases are diffuse, and recognizing patterns of abnormality in such cases is important diagnostically for both the radiologist and the pathologist. In radiologic evaluation, the development of HRCT has allowed much better recognition and characterization of these abnormalities than was possible with conventional chest radiography and has required the radiologist and the pathologist to become familiar with the other's terminology for meaningful clinicopathologic correlation (Tables 2-3, 2-5, 2-6) (6,23,101).

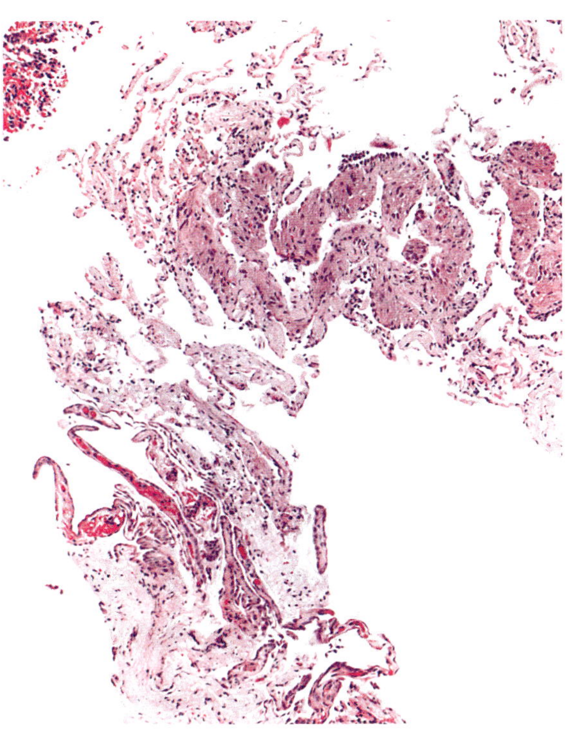

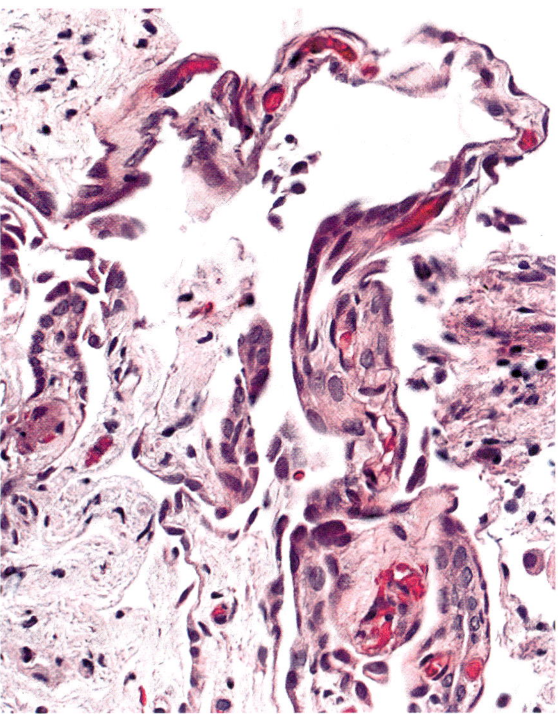

Figure 2-13

PLEURAL FRAGMENTS IN BRONCHOSCOPIC BIOPSIES

Left: These fragments of pleura (bottom) were incidental findings in a bronchoscopic biopsy that also shows lymphangioleiomyomatosis (top).

Right: The pleura consists of a thin layer of fibrous tissue covered by hyperplastic mesothelial cells.

Table 2-4

"NORMAL" BIOPSY IN DIFFUSE LUNG DISEASE

Sampling error (unsampled lesions of Langerhans' cell histiocytosis)
A subtle interstitial infiltrate or early diffuse alveolar damage
Airway disease (especially bronchiolar)
Pulmonary edema
Pulmonary emboli (including fat emboli)
Lymphangioleiomyomatosis with inconspicuous lesions
Pulmonary vascular disease

Table 2-5

USEFULNESS OF HRCT IN THE EVALUATION OF LUNG INJURY[a]

Allows for a specific or nearly specific diagnosis in a small proportion of cases
Narrows considerably the differential diagnosis in many cases
Is an aid in determining the biopsy site for the surgeon or bronchoscopist
Aids the pathologist in narrowing the pathologic differential diagnosis
Allows for a better assessment of the global extent and severity of disease than is possible pathologically based on a (relatively) small sample of lung tissue

[a]Data from references 6,23,63,64,65,89,101.

For the pathologist, pattern recognition is gross or histologic, and there is good correlation between them (20,22,23). For diagnostic surgical pathology, histologic pattern recognition is most useful and is applicable even in small biopsies. Histologically, pattern recognition can be viewed in two ways, each with their own diagnostic usefulness: 1) anatomic distribution

Table 2-6

PATTERN INFORMATION GAINED BY HRCT

Distribution of lesions in the lungs as a whole (upper lobe versus lower lobe, central versus peripheral)
Predilection for a specific anatomic region (centrilobular versus septal)
Qualitative character of the abnormalities identified (ground glass versus consolidation)
Quantitative extent of the abnormalities by visual estimate

Table 2-7

HRCT FINDINGS IN INFILTRATIVE LUNG DISEASE

Predominant Abnormality	Examples of Differential Diagnosis
Septal thickening	Lymphangitic carcinomatosis Lymphoma Sarcoidosis (usually localized)
Irregular linear opacities (reticular pattern)	Usual interstitial pneumonia (idiopathic pulmonary fibrosis) Collagen vascular disease Asbestosis Chronic hypersensitivity pneumonitis
Cystic airspaces	Lymphangioleiomyomatosis Langerhans' cell histiocytosis Honeycomb lung
Nodules	Bronchovascular: sarcoidosis Centrilobular: bronchiolitis, hypersensitivity pneumonitis Miliary: miliary tuberculosis or fungi
Ground-glass attenuation	Hypersensitivity pneumonitis Desquamative interstitial pneumonia Lymphoid interstitial pneumonia Alveolar proteinosis
Consolidation	Chronic eosinophilic pneumonia Bronchiolitis obliterans organizing pneumonia Diffuse alveolar damage Lymphoma

of pathologic lesions according to normal anatomic landmarks in the lung, and 2) reaction patterns of the lung parenchyma.

Anatomic Distribution

Histologic (and gross) recognition of the anatomic distribution of the lesion correlates well with the radiologic distribution as seen with HRCT, and equivalencies can be developed (Tables 2-3, 2-7, figs. 2-14–2-18). Characterization of pathologic lesions according to anatomic distribution rarely leads to a specific diagnosis, but it is helpful in generating and limiting a differential diagnosis, both for the radiologist and the pathologist. For example, histologic identification of granulomatous inflammation that shows a predilection for lymphatic routes is very likely to be sarcoidosis (or berylliosis) in contrast to miliary infections, which do not show such a predilection (figs. 2-15, 2-17). On HRCT, small nodules representing a conglomeration of perilymphatic sarcoid granulomas characteristically are most numerous around the bronchi and vessels in the perihilar regions

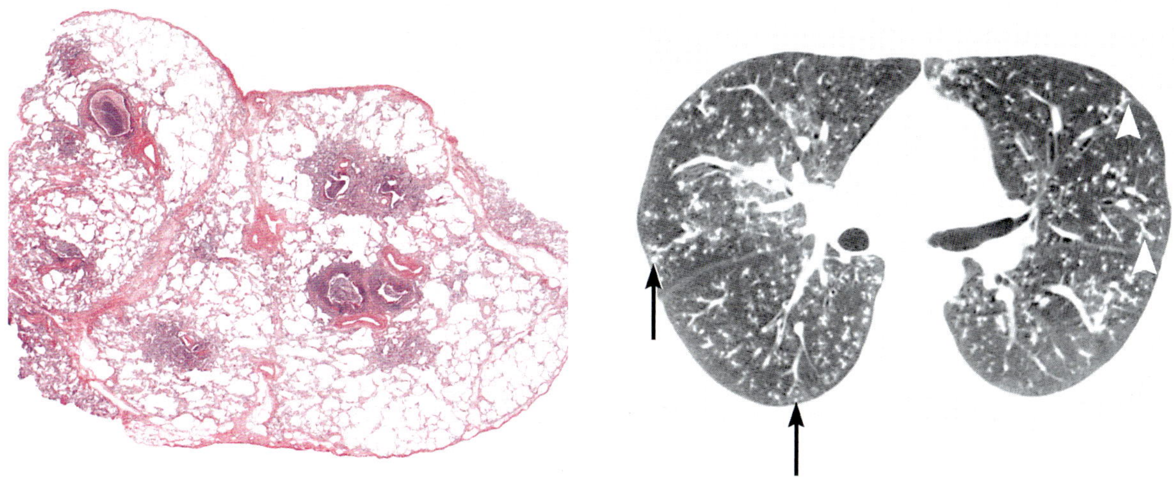

Figure 2-14

BRONCHIOLOCENTRIC DISTRIBUTION

Left: This case of idiopathic chronic bronchiolitis shows ectasia of bronchioles, luminal filling by inflammatory debris, and mural chronic inflammation that is distinctly bronchiolocentric. The remainder of the lung is spared.

Right: HRCT in a patient with bronchiolitis following inhalation of amil nitrate shows the characteristic findings of centrilobular small nodular (arrows) and branching linear (arrowheads) opacities. Centrilobular opacities on HRCT are characteristically a few millimeters away from the pleura, interlobular septa, and large vessels.

of the mid- and upper lung zones. Miliary infections, being hematogenous, have a random distribution but tend to involve mainly the lower lung zones.

Reaction Patterns

Reaction patterns seen histologically in the distal lung parenchyma (Table 2-7) tend to correlate with nonspecific radiologic patterns, specifically, ground-glass attenuation if relatively mild, or consolidation when more severe (figs. 2-19–2-23). Fibrosis can usually be recognized on HRCT by the presence of irregular linear opacities (also known as reticular or interstitial pattern), architectural distortion, dilatation of airways within the areas of fibrosis (known radiologically as traction bronchiectasis and bronchiolectasis), and honeycombing (see chapter 3). While the pattern of distal airspace processes is nonspecific on HRCT, in many cases the diagnosis can be suggested by the distribution of abnormalities. For example, the consolidation in chronic eosinophilic pneumonia characteristically involves the peripheral regions of the upper lobes, while the consolidation in idiopathic bronchiolitis obliterans obstructive pneumonia (BOOP) is often peribronchial in distribution and does not have a propensity to involve mainly the upper lobes (see chapter 3). Examples of HRCT findings (patterns) are shown in Table 2-7; figure 2-24 shows a micronodular pattern.

Recognition of a pathologic reaction pattern is simply a way of looking at a lesion from a different point of view compared to anatomic distribution. Sarcoidosis can be recognized as a granulomatous interstitial pneumonia from the viewpoint of a reaction pattern and as a lesion that follows lymphatic routes from the view of anatomic distribution. It is apparent that in some lesions recognition of both reaction pattern and anatomic distribution may be additive in limiting the differential diagnosis.

The histologic reaction patterns shown in Table 2-8 have many causes, and some of the more common ones are seen in Table 2-9. Examples of lesions showing a given reaction pattern are found throughout the chapters of this Fascicle: for example, diffuse alveolar damage is found with a number of infections, may be caused by a variety of drugs, and may be idiopathic (see chapter 3).

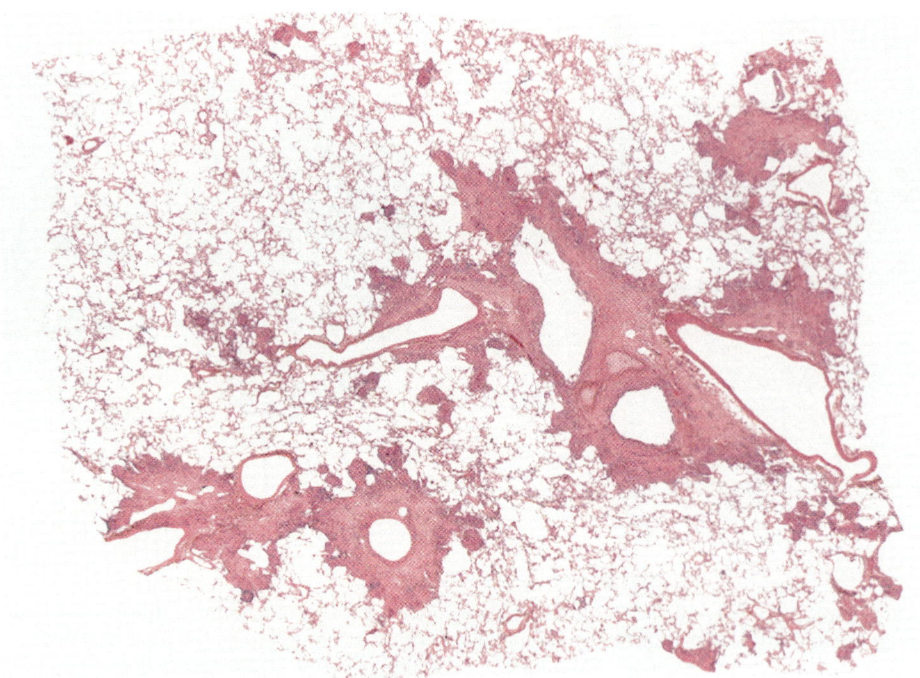

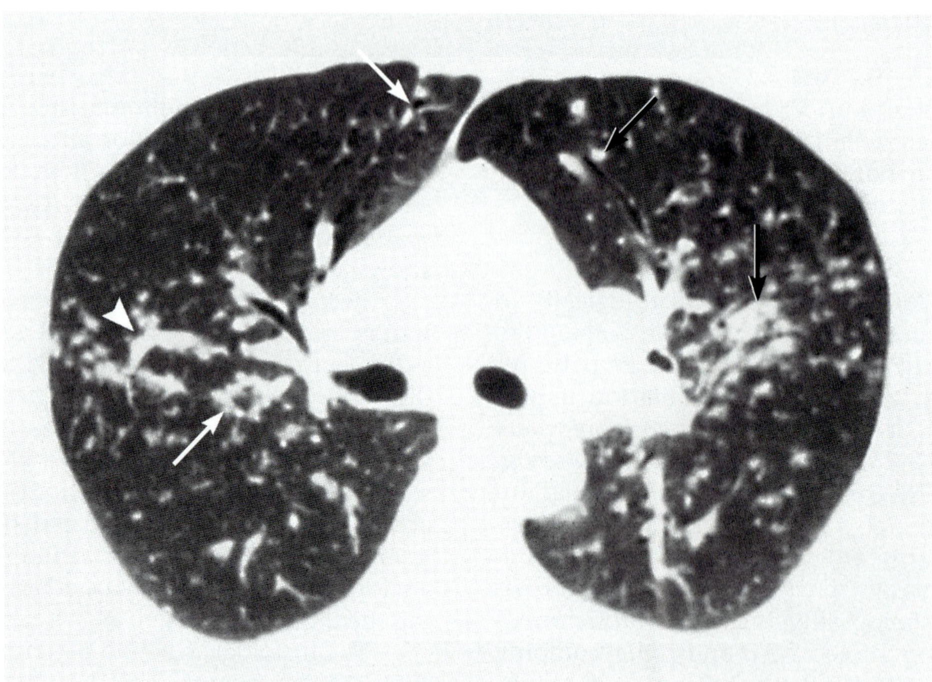

Figure 2-15

LYMPHATIC DISTRIBUTION

Top: The granulomas of sarcoidosis show a predilection to occur along bronchovascular bundles, with relative sparing of the remainder of the lung parenchyma.

Bottom: HRCT in a patient with sarcoidosis demonstrates multiple, bilateral, small nodular opacities. These nodules represent conglomeration of sarcoid granulomas and are located mainly adjacent to bronchi (black arrows), pulmonary vessels (arrowhead), and interlobular septa (white arrows).

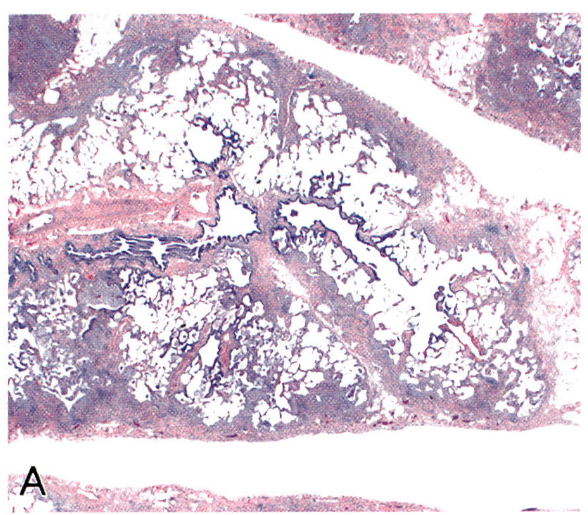

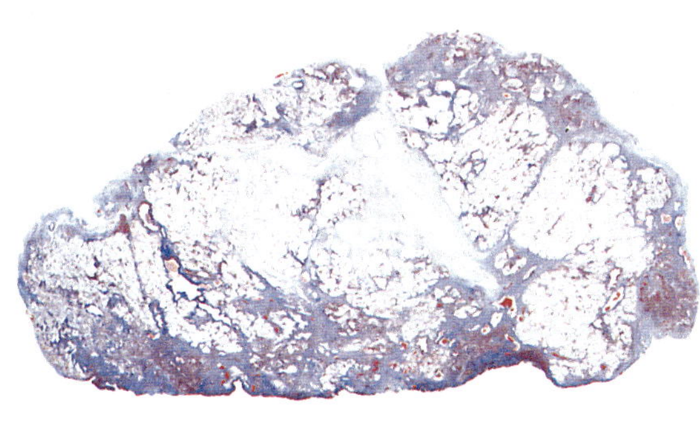

Figure 2-16

PERIPHERAL ACINAR FIBROSIS WITH SUBPLEURAL HONEYCOMBING

A: Early peripheral acinar fibrosis is seen as fibrous thickening in the subpleural and paraseptal zones, with relative sparing of the centrilobular regions.

B: As the severity progresses, dense fibrosis and honeycombing develop in the subpleural regions, as highlighted with a trichrome stain.

C: HRCT in a patient with idiopathic pulmonary fibrosis demonstrates subpleural predominance of the fibrosis and small cystic spaces representing honeycombing.

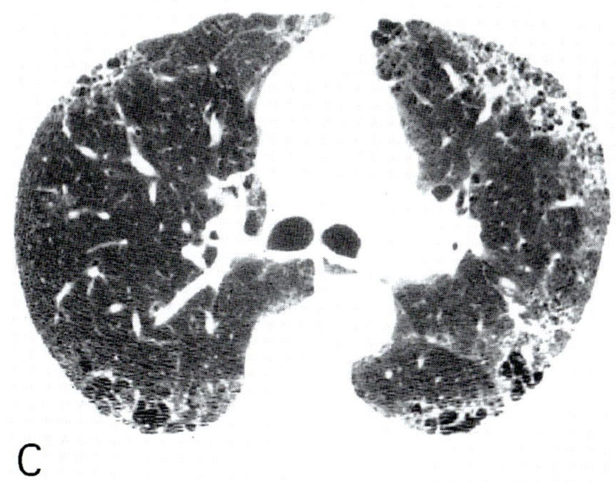

Table 2-8

REACTION PATTERNS OF THE DISTAL LUNG PARENCHYMA

Diffuse alveolar damage
Diffuse alveolar hemorrhage
Organizing pneumonia pattern
Cellular interstitial infiltrates
Desquamative interstitial pneumonia-like pattern
Interstitial fibrosis (usually with honeycombing)
Granulomatous interstitial pneumonia (with or without necrosis)
Lymphocytic interstitial pneumonia/diffuse lymphoid hyperplasia
Bronchiolar injury

Practical Aspects

The characterization of a pathologic finding according to anatomic distribution or reaction pattern is descriptive and not a specific diagnosis. As such, recognition of these patterns are decision points for focusing the differential diagnosis. A pattern can be sought in virtually all histologic specimens from the lung, including transbronchial biopsies.

As with any biologic system, the anatomic distribution and reaction pattern in a given section may be imperfect, involvement of the lung parenchyma may be irregular, and there may be overlap among patterns. For example, sarcoidosis typically follows lymphatic routes, but the involvement may be discontinuous and there may be a predilection for one region over

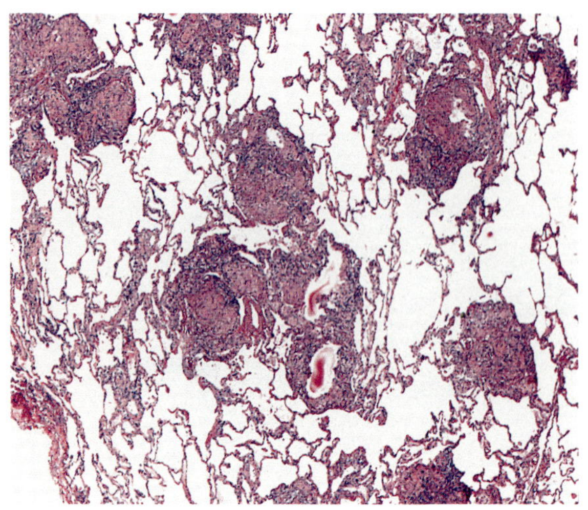

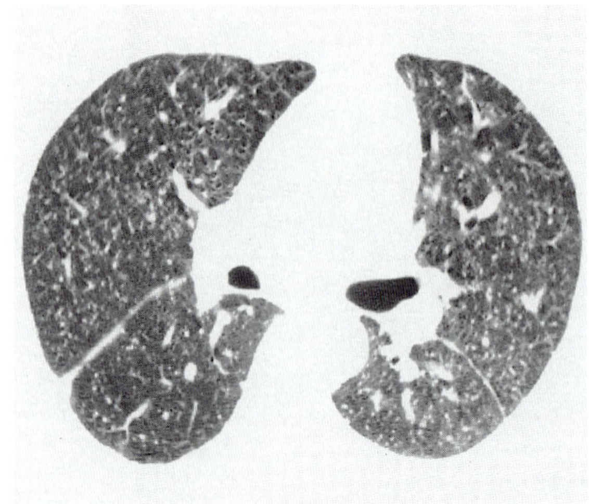

Figure 2-17

RANDOM NODULAR LESIONS

Left: *Mycobacterium avium-intracellulare* manifesting clinically as a diffuse interstitial pneumonia in a nonimmunosuppressed host manifests as randomly scattered, solitary, non-necrotizing granulomas with a cuff of lymphocytes. The lack of lymphatic distribution and lack of coalescence of the granulomas are features that exclude the possibility of sarcoidosis. The relative prominence and size of the granulomas, and lack of chronic inflammatory infiltrate in the alveolar walls, negates a diagnosis of extrinsic allergic alveolitis.

Right: HRCT in a 35-year-old man with miliary tuberculosis demonstrates a random distribution of numerous bilateral nodules measuring approximately 1 to 2 mm.

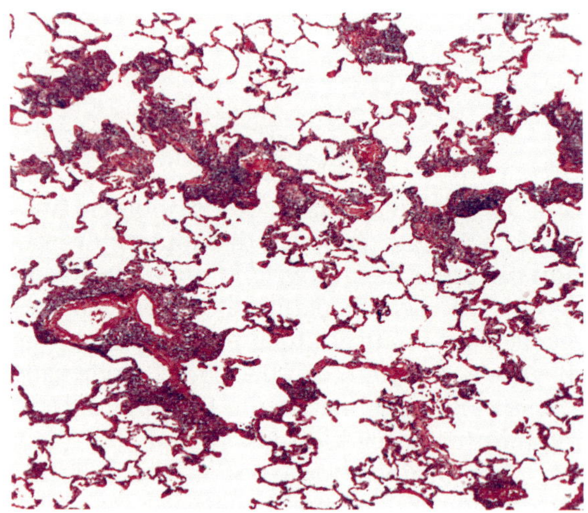

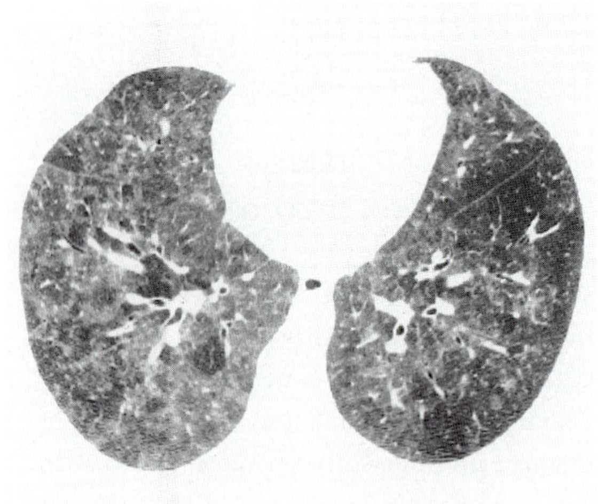

Figure 2-18

INTERSTITIAL INFILTRATES

Left: This case of extrinsic allergic alveolitis shows interstitial inflammation along alveolar ducts (bronchiolocentric distribution). The inflammation is diffuse, lacks nodularity, and manifests radiologically as a ground-glass pattern.

Right: HRCT in a 49-year-old man with extrinsic allergic alveolitis demonstrates extensive bilateral areas of ground-glass attenuation.

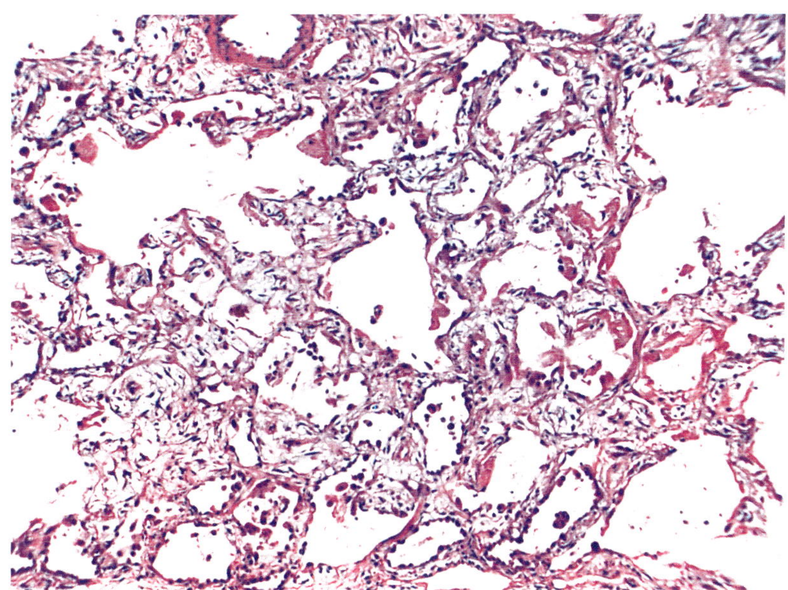

Figure 2-19

DIFFUSE ALVEOLAR DAMAGE

There is uniform edematous change in the alveolar septa and remnants of hyaline membranes lining some airspaces (right center). Other alveolar septa show reparative type 2 pneumocytes (bottom).

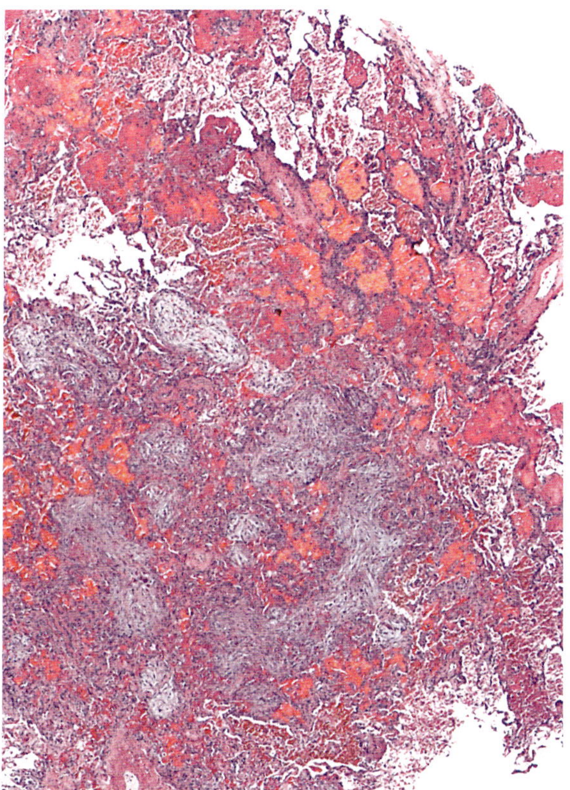

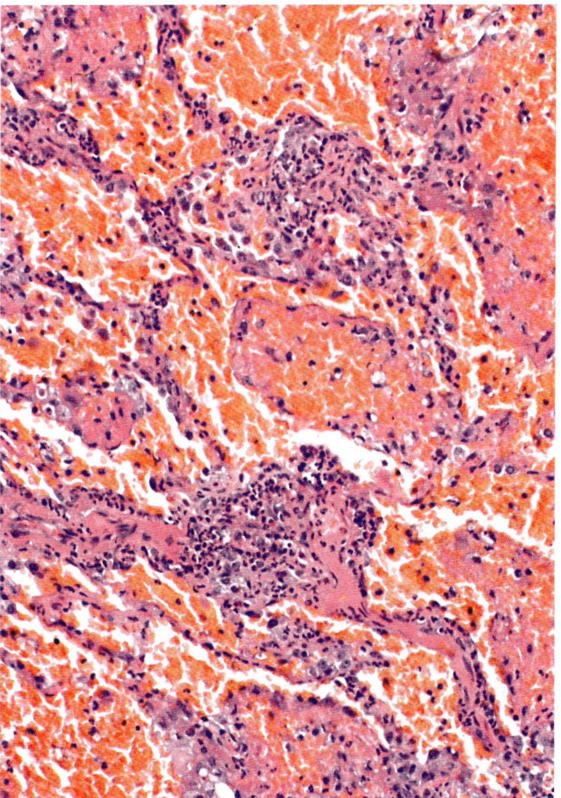

Figure 2-20

ALVEOLAR HEMORRHAGE

Left: There is airspace filling by red blood cells with associated fibrin and occasional hemosiderin-filled macrophages. This case shows some evidence of organization with pale edematous polyps of connective tissue within the airspaces (bottom).

Right: There is also capillaritis (bottom) with neutrophilic infiltrates in alveolar septa.

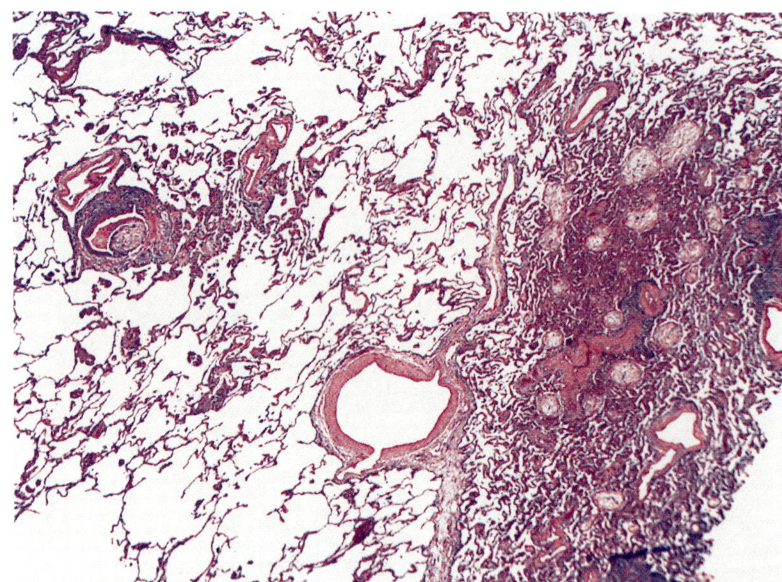

Figure 2-21

ORGANIZING PNEUMONIA PATTERN

This case shows patchy involvement of lung parenchyma by a process that includes organizing polyps of connective tissue within bronchioles (left) and foci of airspace organization with edematous polypoid plugs of connective tissue within the alveolar parenchyma (right).

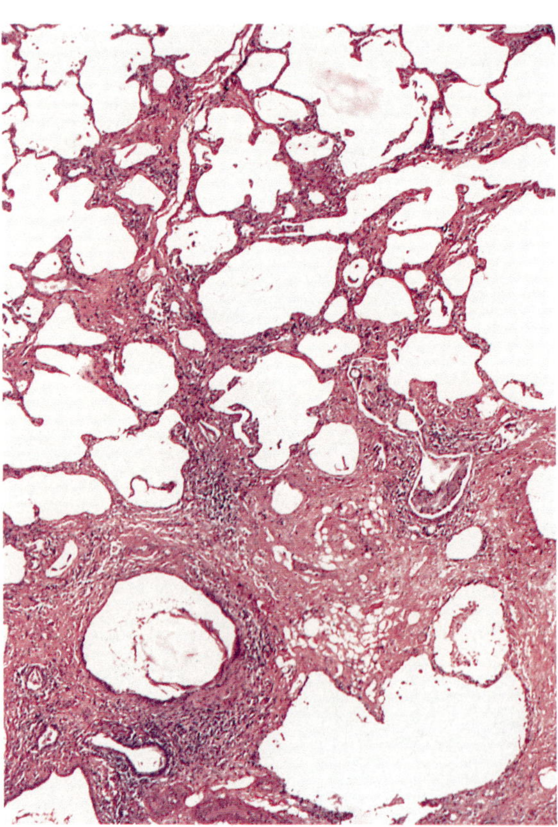

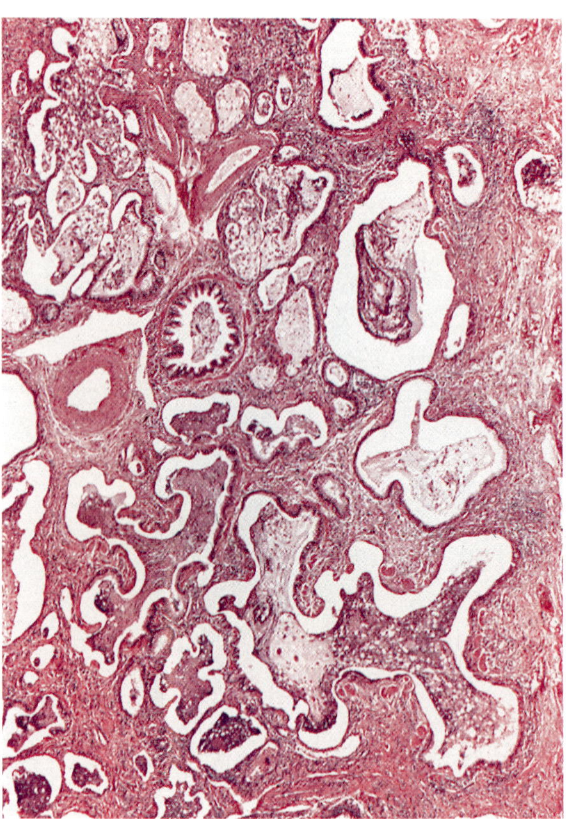

Figure 2-22

INTERSTITIAL FIBROSIS WITH HONEYCOMBING

This pattern typically shows zones of fibrosis with abnormal airspaces (honeycombing) adjacent to foci of less involved lung tissue (left); sometimes large zones of lung tissue are entirely replaced by honeycomb change (right). Typical findings in honeycomb regions include mucostasis, inflammatory cells in the mucus, smooth muscle metaplasia, fibrosis in the septa between the abnormal spaces, and metaplastic, primarily bronchiolar, epithelium lining the spaces.

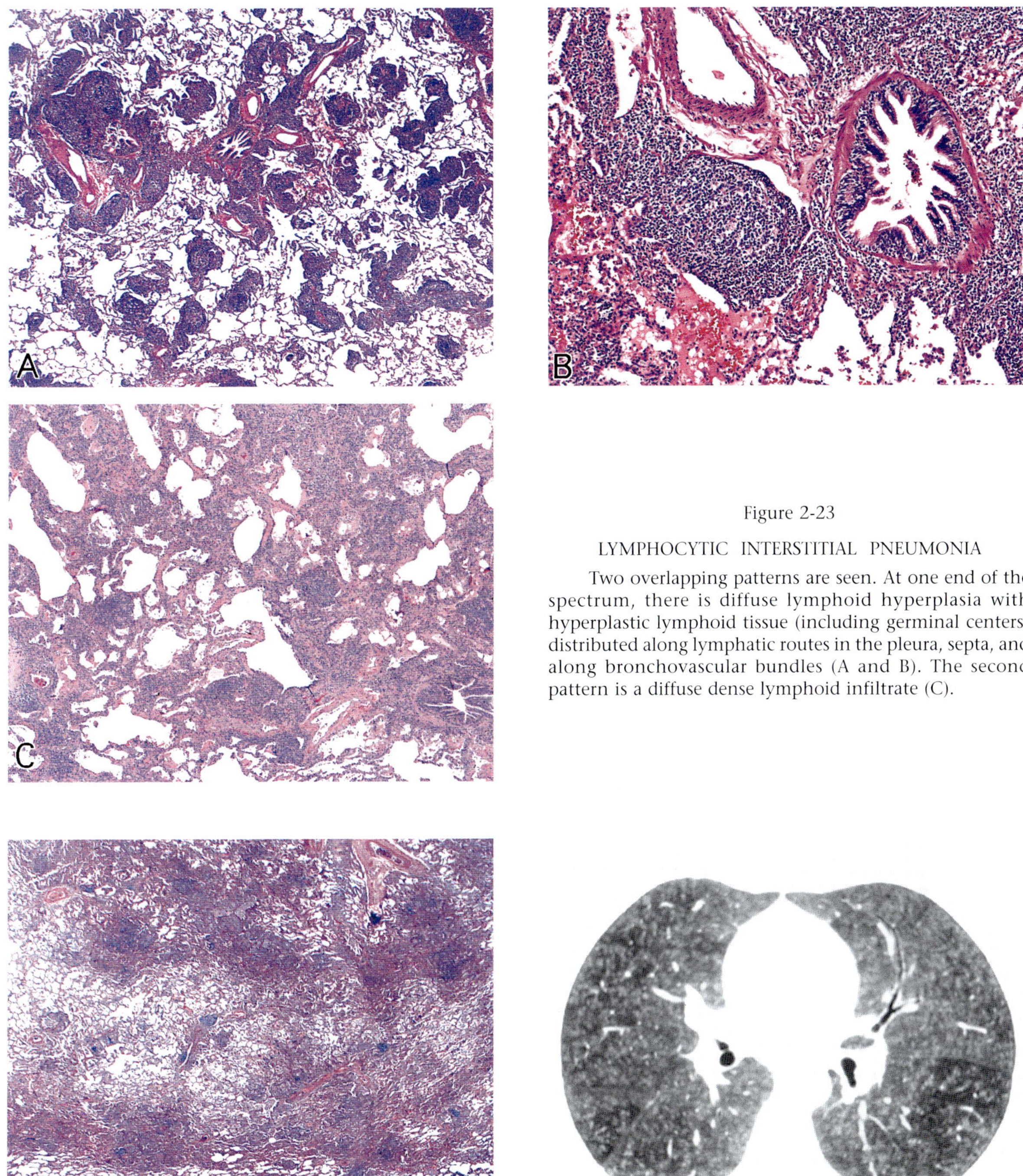

Figure 2-23

LYMPHOCYTIC INTERSTITIAL PNEUMONIA

Two overlapping patterns are seen. At one end of the spectrum, there is diffuse lymphoid hyperplasia with hyperplastic lymphoid tissue (including germinal centers) distributed along lymphatic routes in the pleura, septa, and along bronchovascular bundles (A and B). The second pattern is a diffuse dense lymphoid infiltrate (C).

Figure 2-24

MICRONODULAR PATTERN ON HRCT

Left: One of the more common causes of a micronodular pattern is extrinsic allergic alveolitis. This pattern is apparent histologically by the presence of vague inflammatory nodules distributed along bronchioles with sparing of the pleura. The bronchioles themselves may not be discernible.

Right: HRCT in a 35-year-old woman with extrinsic allergic alveolitis demonstrates numerous, poorly defined, small nodular opacities in a centrilobular distribution.

Table 2-9

REACTION PATTERNS IN DIFFUSE LUNG DISEASE: EXAMPLES OF DIFFERENTIAL DIAGNOSIS

Diffuse Alveolar Damage
- Infections (viral, fungal, bacterial, parasitic)
- Toxic inhalants
- Drugs
- Shock
- Collagen vascular diseases
- Radiation reactions (acute)
- Acute allergic reactions (e.g., hypersensitivity pneumonitis)
- Alveolar hemorrhage syndromes
- Idiopathic (acute interstitial pneumonia/Hamman-Rich syndrome)
- Other miscellaneous conditions

Organizing Pneumonia Pattern (Bronchiolitis Obliterans with Organizing Pneumonia)
- Organizing infections (viral, bacterial, fungal, other)
- Organizing diffuse alveolar damage
- Drug and toxic reactions
- Collagen vascular diseases
- Extrinsic allergic alveolitis (hypersensitivity pneumonitis)
- Chronic eosinophilic pneumonia
- Organizing infectious pneumonias complicating chronic bronchitis and emphysema, bronchiectasis, cystic fibrosis, aspiration
- Location distal to an obstruction
- Part of the peripheral reaction around abscesses, infarcts, Wegener's granulomatosis, others
- Idiopathic (cryptogenic organizing pneumonitis)

Interstitial Fibrosis
- Usual interstitial pneumonia (idiopathic pulmonary fibrosis)
- Lymphocytic interstitial pneumonia
- Collagen vascular diseases
- Drug reactions
- Pneumoconioses (asbestosis, berylliosis, silicosis, hard metal pneumoconiosis, others)
- Sarcoidosis
- Langerhans' cell histiocytosis (eosinophilic granuloma)
- Chronic granulomatous infections
- Chronic aspiration
- Chronic hypersensitivity pneumonitis
- Organized chronic eosinophilic pneumonia
- Organized and organizing diffuse alveolar damage
- Chronic interstitial pulmonary edema/passive congestion
- Radiation (chronic)
- Healed infectious pneumonias

Desquamative Interstitial Pneumonia-Like Pattern
- Desquamative interstitial pneumonia
- Respiratory bronchiolitis associated with interstitial lung disease
- Langerhans' cell histiocytosis
- Drug reactions (especially amiodarone)
- Chronic alveolar hemorrhage
- Eosinophilic pneumonia
- Pneumoconioses (especially talcosis, hard metal, asbestosis)
- Obstructive pneumonias (with foamy macrophages)
- Exogenous lipoid pneumonia and lipid storage diseases
- Infection in immunosuppressed patient ("histiocytic pneumonia")
- As a focal microscopic finding in many conditions

Granulomatous Interstitial Pneumonia (with or without necrosis)
- Sarcoidosis
- Extrinsic allergic alveolitis
- Drug reactions
- Intravenous talcosis (intravenous drug abuse)
- Pneumoconioses (inhalation talcosis, berylliosis)
- Sjögren's syndrome (lymphocytic interstitial pneumonia [LIP] with granulomas)
- Aspiration pneumonia
- Tumors, especially lymphomas
- Bronchocentric granulomatosis
- Allergic granulomatosis
- Necrotizing sarcoid granulomatosis

Lymphocytic Interstitial Pneumonia/Diffuse Lymphoid Hyperplasia
- Infection (especially with *Pneumocystis*)
- Hypersensitivity pneumonitis/extrinsic allergic alveolitis
- Autoimmune disease (especially Sjögren's syndrome)
- Immunodeficiency syndromes
- Drug reactions
- Graft versus host disease
- Miscellaneous

Bronchiolar Injury
- Cellular bronchiolitis[a]
- Constrictive bronchiolitis[a]
- Respiratory bronchiolitis[a]
- Other[a]

[a]See chapter 8 for discussion of bronchiolitis.

another. Most cases of sarcoidosis show a particular predilection for bronchovascular bundles (in a perihilar distribution best identified radiologically) with relative sparing of peripheral septa and pleura (see fig. 3-9). However, occasionally sarcoidosis may show disproportionate pleural involvement.

From a histologic diagnostic point of view, there are many features beyond anatomic distribution and reaction pattern that the pathologist addresses in the evaluation of diffuse lung disease. Necrosis is an example of an additional feature that is extremely helpful diagnostically. In the setting of granulomatous lung disease, necrosis is much more common in infectious than noninfectious processes. Some diffuse lung diseases have distinctive, if not unique, histologic findings that allow for a diagnosis even in the absence of recognition of any anatomic distribution or reaction pattern. For example, the histologic features in Langerhans' cell histiocytosis, lymphangioleiomyomatosis, and pulmonary alveolar microlithiasis (see chapter 3) are unique and specific to those disease entities. Similarly, finding a specific microorganism or malignant cells may lead to a specific diagnosis.

Assuming abnormal lung tissue has been sampled and the initial pathologic interpretation is negative or normal, the pathologist should pay particular attention to the small airways to look for subtle bronchiolar injury; the septa, to seek evidence of pulmonary edema; and the vessels, for evidence of pulmonary vascular disease. Lymphangioleiomyomatosis may be quite subtle and suggest emphysema (see chapter 3), however, the occurrence of emphysema in a relatively young woman (who may very well not be a smoker) should lead one to reconsider the diagnosis.

Sampling error can be addressed in discussions with the surgeon and the radiologist on a case by case basis. Sampling error is, of course, inversely proportional to the size of a sample, and we recommend that traditional open lung biopsies and thoracoscopic lung biopsies be at least 3 cm (preferably 4 cm) in greatest dimension, to minimize sampling error.

REFERENCES

1. Abramson MJ, Stone CA, Holmes PW, Tai EH. The role of bronchoalveolar lavage in the diagnosis of suspected opportunistic pneumonia. Aust N Z J Med 1987;17:407–12.
2. Advanced laboratory methods in histology and pathology, Washington, D.C.: Armed Forces Institute of Pathology; 1994.
3. Agusti C, Xaubet A, Luburich P, Ayuso MC, Roca J, Rodriguez-Roisin R. Computed tomography-guided bronchoalveolar lavage in idiopathic pulmonary fibrosis. Thorax 1996;51:841–5.
4. American Thoracic Society Statement: Clinical role of bronchoalveolar lavage in adults with pulmonary disease. Am Rev Respir Dis 2001;142:481–6.
5. Ando M, Sŭga M. Hypersensitivity pneumonitis. Curr Opin Pulm Med 1997;3:391–5.
6. Austin JH, Müller NL, Friedman PJ, et al. Glossary of terms for CT of the lungs: recommendations of the Nomenclature Committee of the Fleischner Society. Radiology 1996;200:327–31.
7. Barr HS, Ferguson FF. Microlithiasis alveolaris pulmonum: association with diffuse interstitial pulmonary fibrosis. Arch Pathol 1963;76:659–66.
8. Bonetti F, Chiodera PL, Pea M, et al. Transbronchial biopsy in lymphangiomyomatosis of the lung. HMB45 for diagnosis. Am J Surg Pathol 1993;17:1092–102.
9. Boomars KA, Wagenaar SS, Mulder PG, van Velzen-Blad H, van den Bosch JM. Relationship between cells obtained by bronchoalveolar lavage and survival in idiopathic pulmonary fibrosis. Thorax 1995;50:1087–92.
10. Buchheit J, Eid N, Rodgers G Jr, Feger T, Yakoub O. Acute eosinophilic pneumonia with respiratory failure: a new syndrome? Am Rev Respir Dis 1992;145:716–8.
11. Bye MR, Bernstein L, Shah K, Ellaurie M, Rubinstein A. Diagnostic bronchoalveolar lavage in children with AIDS. Pediatr Pulmonol 1987;3:425–8.

12. Cazzadori A, Di Perri G, Todeschini G, et al. Transbronchial biopsy in the diagnosis of pulmonary infiltrates in immunocompromised patients. Chest 1995;107:101–6.
13. Ceuppens JL, Lacquet LM, Marien G, Demedts M, van den Eeckhout A, Stevens E. Alveolar T-cell subsets in pulmonary sarcoidosis. Correlation with disease activity and effect of steroid treatment. Am Rev Respir Dis 1984;129:563–8.
14. Chan JK, Loo KT, Yau BK, Lam SY. Nodular histiocytic/mesothelial hyperplasia: a lesion potentially mistaken for a neoplasm in transbronchial biopsy. Am J Surg Pathol 1997;21:658–63.
15. Chastre J, Fagon JY, Soler P, et al. Diagnosis of nosocomial bacterial pneumonia in intubated patients undergoing ventilation: comparison of the usefulness of bronchoalveolar lavage and the protected specimen brush. Am J Med 1988;85:499–506.
16. Cheah FK, Sheppard MN, Hansell DM. Computed tomography of diffuse pulmonary haemorrhage with pathological correlation. Clin Radiol 1993;48:89–93.
17. Cherniack RM, Colby TV, Flint A, et al. Quantitative assessment of lung pathology in idiopathic pulmonary fibrosis. The BAL Cooperative Group Steering Committee. Am Rev Respir Dis 1991;144:892–900.
18. Churg A. An inflation procedure for open lung biopsies. Am J Surg Pathol 1983;7:69–71.
19. Cobben NA, Jacobs JA, Dieijen-Visser MP, Mulder PG, Wouters EF, Drent M. Diagnostic value of BAL fluid cellular profile and enzymes in infectious pulmonary disorders. Eur Respir J 1999;14:496–502.
20. Colby TV. Atlas of pulmonary surgical pathology. Philadelphia: WB Saunders; 1991.
21. Colby TV, Koss MN, Travis WD. Tumors of the lower respiratory tract. Atlas of Tumor Pathology, 3rd Series, Fascicle 13. Washington, D.C.: Armed Forces Institute of Pathology; 1995.
22. Colby TV, Swensen SJ. Anatomic distribution and histopathologic patterns in diffuse lung disease: correlation with HRCT. J Thorac Imaging 1996;11:1–26.
23. Colby TV, Swensen SJ. Anatomic distribution and histopathologic patterns in interstitial lung disease. In: Schwarz MI, King TE Jr, eds. Interstitial lung disease, 3rd ed. Hamilton: BC Decker; 1998:31–50.
24. Colby TV, Yousem SA. Pulmonary histology for the surgical pathologist. Am J Surg Pathol 1988;12:223–39.
25. Dail DH. Metabolic and other diseases. In: Dail DH, Hammar SP, eds. Pulmonary pathology, 2nd ed. New York: Springer-Verlag; 1994:707–77.
26. de Blic J, Midulla F, Barbato A, et al. Bronchoalveolar lavage in children. ERS Task Force on bronchoalveolar lavage in children. European Respiratory Society. Eur Respir J 2000;15:217–31.
27. Delvenne P, Arrese JE, Thiry A, Borlee-Hermans G, Pierard GE, Boniver J. Detection of cytomegalovirus, Pneumocystis carinii, and aspergillus species in bronchoalveolar lavage fluid. A comparison of techniques. Am J Clin Pathol 1993;100:414–8.
28. Djukanovic R, Wilson JW, Lai CK, Holgate ST, Howarth PH. The safety aspects of fiberoptic bronchoscopy, bronchoalveolar lavage, and endobronchial biopsy in asthma. Am Rev Respir Dis 1991;143:772–7.
29. Domingo J, Waksal HW. Wright's stain in rapid diagnosis of Pneumocystis carinii. Am J Clin Pathol 1984;81:511–4.
30. Flint A, Martinez FJ, Young ML, Whyte RI, Toews GB, Lynch JP III. Influence of sample number and biopsy site on the histologic diagnosis of diffuse lung disease. Ann Thorac Surg 1995;60:1605–7.
31. Fouillard L, Mouthon L, Laporte JP, et al. Severe respiratory syncytial virus pneumonia after autologous bone marrow transplantation: a report of three cases and review. Bone Marrow Transplant 1992;9:97–100.
32. Fraser RS. Catheter-induced pulmonary artery perforation: pathologic and pathogenic features. Hum Pathol 1987;18:1246–51.
33. Friedreich N. Kleinere mittheilungen: I. Corpora amylacea in den lungen. Virchows Arch [Pathol Anat] 1856;9:613–8.
34. Gal AA, Klatt EC, Koss MN, Strigle SM, Boylen CT. The effectiveness of bronchoscopy in the diagnosis of Pneumocystis carinii and cytomegalovirus pulmonary infections in acquired immunodeficiency syndrome. Arch Pathol Lab Med 1987;111:238–41.
35. Goldstein RA, Rohatgi PK, Bergofsky EH, et al. Clinical role of bronchoalveolar lavage in adults with pulmonary disease. Am Rev Respir Dis 1990;142:481–6.
36. Guinee DG Jr, Feuerstein I, Koss MN, Travis WD. Pulmonary lymphangioleiomyomatosis. Diagnosis based on results of transbronchial biopsy and immunohistochemical studies and correlation with high-resolution computed tomography findings. Arch Pathol Lab Med 1994;118:846–9.
37. Haslam PL, Turton CW, Lukoszek A, et al. Bronchoalveolar lavage fluid cell counts in cryptogenic fibrosing alveolitis and their relation to therapy. Thorax 1980;35:328–39.

38. Helmers RA, Hunninghake GW. Bronchoalveolar lavage. In: Wang KP, Mehta AC, eds. Flexible bronchoscopy. Cambridge: Blackwell Science; 1995:160–94.
39. Hollander DH, Hutchins GM. Central spherules in pulmonary corpora amylacea. Arch Pathol Lab Med 1978;102:629–30.
40. Humphrey DM, Weiner MH. Mycobacterial antigen detection by immunohistochemistry in pulmonary tuberculosis. Hum Pathol 1987;18:701–8.
41. Hunninghake GW, Fulmer JD, Young RC Jr, Gadek JE, Crystal RG. Localization of the immune response in sarcoidosis. Am Rev Respir Dis 1979;120:49–57.
42. Hunninghake GW, Gadek JE, Kawanami O, Ferrans VJ, Crystal RG. Inflammatory and immune processes in the human lung in health and disease: evaluation by bronchoalveolar lavage. Am J Pathol 1979;97:149–206.
43. Jiwa M, Steenbergen RD, Zwaan FE, Kluin PM, Raap AK, van der Ploeg M. Three sensitive methods for the detection of cytomegalovirus in lung tissue of patients with interstitial pneumonitis. Am J Clin Pathol 1990;93:491–4.
44. Kahn FW, Jones JM. Analysis of bronchoalveolar lavage specimens from immunocompromised patients with a protocol applicable in the microbiology laboratory. J Clin Microbiol 1988;26:1150–5.
45. Kahn FW, Jones JM. Diagnosing bacterial respiratory infection by bronchoalveolar lavage. J Infect Dis 1987;155:862–9.
46. Kaufman RM, Airo R, Pollack S, Crosby WH, Doberneck R. Origin of pulmonary megakaryocytes. Blood 1965;25:767.
47. Keogh BA, Hunninghake GW, Line BR, Crystal RG. The alveolitis of pulmonary sarcoidosis. Evaluation of natural history and alveolitis-dependent changes in lung function. Am Rev Respir Dis 1983;128:256–65.
48. King MA, Pope-Harman AL, Allen JN, Christoforidis GA, Christoforidis AJ. Acute eosinophilic pneumonia: radiologic and clinical features. Radiology 1997;203:715–9.
49. King TE Jr. Handling and analysis of bronchoalveolar lavage specimens. In: Baughman RP, ed. Bronchoalveolar lavage. St. Louis: Mosby Year Book, 1991:3–25.
50. King TE Jr. Role of bronchoalveolar lavage in the diagnosis of interstitial lung disease. In: Rose BD, ed. Uptodate in medicine. Wellesley: BDR-Uptodate; 2000.
51. Kuhn C, Kuo TT. Cytoplasmic hyalin in asbestosis. A reaction of injured alveolar epithelium. Arch Pathol 1973;95:190–4.
52. Linder J, Rennard S. Bronchoalveolar lavage. Chicago: American Society of Clinical Pathologists; 1988.
53. Linder J, Vaughan WP, Armitage JO, et al. Cytopathology of opportunistic infection in bronchoalveolar lavage. Am J Clin Pathol 1987;88:421–8.
54. Lynch JP, Standiford TJ, Rolfe MW, Kunkel SL, Strieter RM. Neutrophilic alveolitis in idiopathic pulmonary fibrosis. The role of interleukin-8. Am Rev Respir Dis 1992;145:1433–9.
55. Martin WJ, Smith TF, Sanderson DR, Brutinel WM, Cockerill FR, Douglas WW. Role of bronchoalveolar lavage in the assessment of opportunistic pulmonary infections: utility and complications. Mayo Clin Proc 1987;62:549–57.
56. Mayock RL, Bertrand P, Morrison CE, Scott JH. Manifestations of sarcoidosis. Analysis of 145 patients, with a review of nine series selected from the literature. Am J Med 1963;35:67–89.
57. Michaels L, Levene C. Pulmonary corpora amylacea. J Pathol 1957;74:49–56.
58. Miller RR, Nelems B, Müller NL, Evans KG, Ostrow DN. Lingular and right middle lobe biopsy in the assessment of diffuse lung disease. Ann Thorac Surg 1987;44:269–73.
59. Mitchell DM, Emerson CJ, Collins JV, Stableforth DE. Transbronchial lung biopsy with the fibreoptic bronchoscope: analysis of results in 433 patients. Br J Dis Chest 1981;75:258–62.
60. Mitchell DM, Mitchell DN, Collins JV, Emerson CJ. Transbronchial lung biopsy through fibreoptic bronchoscope in diagnosis of sarcoidosis. Br Med J 1980;280:679–81.
61. Moench TR, Griffin DE, Obriecht CR, Vaisberg AJ, Johnson RT. Acute measles in patients with and without neurological involvement: distribution of measles virus antigen and RNA. J Infect Dis 1988;158:433–42.
62. Mones JM, Saldana MJ, Oldham SA. Diagnosis of Pneumocystis carinii pneumonia. Roentgenographic-pathologic correlates based on fiberoptic bronchoscopy specimens from patients with the acquired immunodeficiency syndrome. Chest 1986;89:522–6.
63. Müller NL, Miller RR. Computed tomography of chronic diffuse infiltrative lung disease. Part 1. Am Rev Respir Dis 1990;142:1206–15.
64. Müller NL, Miller RR. Computed tomography of chronic diffuse infiltrative lung disease. Part 2. Am Rev Respir Dis 1990;142:1440–8.
65. Müller NL, Miller RR. Diseases of the bronchioles: CT and histopathologic findings. Radiology 1995;196:3–12.

66. Murphy PM, Fox C, Travis WD, Koenig S, Fauci AS. Acquired immunodeficiency syndrome may present as severe restrictive lung disease. Am J Med 1989;86:237–40.
67. Nagata N, Hirano H, Takayama K, Miyagawa Y, Shigematsu N. Step section preparation of transbronchial lung biopsy. Significance in the diagnosis of diffuse lung disease. Chest 1991;100:959–62.
68. Newman LS, Kreiss K, King TE, Seay S, Campbell PA. Pathologic and immunologic alterations in early stages of beryllium disease. Re-examination of disease definition and natural history. Am Rev Respir Dis 1989;139:1479–86.
69. Newman SL, Michel RP, Wang NS. Lingular lung biopsy: is it representative? Am Rev Respir Dis 1985;132:1084–6.
70. Panchal A, Koss MN. Role of electron microscopy in interstitial lung disease. Curr Opin Pulm Med 1997;3:341–7.
71. Peterson MW, Monick M, Hunninghake GW. Prognostic role of eosinophils in pulmonary fibrosis. Chest 1987;92:51–6.
72. Phillips P, Weiner MH. Invasive aspergillosis diagnosed by immunohistochemistry with monoclonal and polyclonal reagents. Hum Pathol 1987;18:1015–24.
73. Pope-Harman AL, Davis WB, Allen ED, Christoforidis AJ, Allen JN. Acute eosinophilic pneumonia. A summary of 15 cases and review of the literature. Medicine (Baltimore) 1996;75:334–42.
74. Reed JA, Slater LN, Hemann BA, Brigati DJ. Dual organism infection in biopsy specimens from immunocompromised patients: two cases demonstrated by immunocytochemistry. J Clin Lab Anal 1993;7:168–73.
75. Rennard SI. Bronchoalveolar lavage in the assessment of primary and metastatic lung cancer. Respiration 1992;59[Suppl 1]:41–3.
76. Reynolds HY. Bronchoalveolar lavage. Am Rev Respir Dis 1987;135:250–63.
77. Reynolds HY. Hypersensitivity pneumonitis: correlation of cellular and immunologic changes with clinical phases of disease. Lung 1988;166:189–208.
78. Reynolds HY, Fulmer JD, Kazmierowski JA, Roberts WC, Frank MM, Crystal RG. Analysis of cellular and protein content of broncho-alveolar lavage fluid from patients with idiopathic pulmonary fibrosis and chronic hypersensitivity pneumonitis. J Clin Invest 1977;59:165–75.
79. Rosen PP. Frozen section management of a lung biopsy for suspected Pneumocystis pneumonia. Am J Surg Pathol 1977;1:79–82.
80. Rosen Y, Vuletin JC, Pertschuk LP, Silverstein E. Sarcoidosis from the pathologist's vantage point. Pathol Annu 1979;14[Part I]:405–39.
81. Salzman SH. Bronchoscopic techniques for the diagnosis of pulmonary complications of HIV infection. Semin Respir Infect 1999;14:318–26.
82. Sata T, Kurata T, Aoyama Y, Sakaguchi M, Yamanouchi K, Takeda K. Analysis of viral antigens in giant cells of measles pneumonia by immunoperoxidase method. Virchows Arch [A] 1986;410:133–8.
83. Schmidt U, Metz KA, Soukou C, Quabeck K. The association of pulmonary CMV infection with interstitial pneumonia after bone marrow transplantation. Histopathological and immunohistochemical findings in 104 autopsies. Zentralbl Pathol 1993;139:225–30.
84. Semenzato G, Agostini C, Zambello R, et al. Lung T cells in hypersensitivity pneumonitis: phenotypic and functional analyses. J Immunol 1986;137:1164–72.
85. Soares FA. Increased numbers of pulmonary megakaryocytes in patients with arterial pulmonary tumour embolism and with lung metastases seen at necropsy. J Clin Pathol 1992;45:140–2.
86. Sobonya RE, Barbee RA, Wiens J, Trego D. Detection of fungi and other pathogens in immunocompromised patients by bronchoalveolar lavage in an area endemic for coccidioidomycosis. Chest 1990;97:1349–55.
87. Stoller JK, Rankin JA, Reynolds HY. The impact of bronchoalveolar lavage cell analysis on clinicians' diagnostic reasoning about interstitial lung disease. Chest 1987;92:839–43.
88. Stover DE, Zaman MB, Hajdu SI, Lange M, Gold J, Armstrong D. Bronchoalveolar lavage in the diagnosis of diffuse pulmonary infiltrates in the immunosuppressed host. Ann Intern Med 1984;101:1–7.
89. Swensen SJ, Aughenbaugh GL, Douglas WW, Myers JL. High-resolution CT of the lungs: findings in various pulmonary diseases. AJR Am J Roentgenol 1992;158:971–9.
90. Temes RT, Joste NE, Allen NL, Crowell RE, Dox HA, Wernly JA. The lingula is an appropriate site for lung biopsy. Ann Thorac Surg 2000;69:1016–8.
91. Travis WD. Surgical pathology of pulmonary infections. Semin Thorac Cardiovasc Surg 1995;7:62–9.
92. Travis WD, Borok Z, Roum JH, et al. Pulmonary Langerhans cell granulomatosis (histiocytosis X). A clinicopathologic study of 48 cases. Am J Surg Pathol 1993;17:971–86.

93. Travis WD, Colby TV, Corrin B, Shimosato Y, Brambilla E, in collaboration with L.H. Sobin and pathologists from 14 countries. Histological typing of lung and pleural tumors, 3rd ed. Berlin: Springer; 1999.
94. Travis WD, Matsui K, Moss JE, Ferrans VJ. Idiopathic nonspecific interstitial pneumonia: prognostic significance of cellular and fibrosing patterns. Survival comparison with usual interstitial pneumonia and desquamative interstitial pneumonia. Am J Surg Pathol 2000;24:19–33.
95. Travis WD, Pittaluga S, Lipschik GY, et al. Atypical pathologic manifestations of Pneumocystis carinii pneumonia in the acquired immune deficiency syndrome. Review of 123 lung biopsies from 76 patients with emphasis on cysts, vascular invasion, vasculitis, and granulomas. Am J Surg Pathol 1990;14:615–25.
96. Travis WD, Roth DB. Histopathologic evaluation of lung biopsy specimens. In: Shelhamer J, Pizzo PA, Parrillo JE, Masur H, eds. Respiratory disease in the immunosuppressed host. Philadelphia: JB Lippincott; 1991:182–217.
97. Travis WD, Schmidt K, MacLowry JD, Masur H, Condron KS, Fojo AT. Respiratory cryptosporidiosis in a patient with malignant lymphoma. Report of a case and review of the literature. Arch Pathol Lab Med 1990;114:519–22.
98. Turner-Warwick M, Haslam PL. The value of serial bronchoalveolar lavages in assessing the clinical progress of patients with cryptogenic fibrosing alveolitis. Am Rev Respir Dis 1987;135:26–34.
99. Warnock ML, Press M, Churg A. Further observations on cytoplasmic hyaline in the lung. Hum Pathol 1980;11:59–66.
100. Watters LC, Schwarz MI, Cherniack RM, et al. Idiopathic pulmonary fibrosis. Pretreatment bronchoalveolar lavage cellular constituents and their relationships with lung histopathology and clinical response to therapy. Am Rev Respir Dis 1987;135:696–704.
101. Webb WR, Müller NL, Naidich DP. High-resolution CT of the lung. New York: Raven Press; 1992.
102. Weinberger SE, Kelman JA, Elson NA, et al. Bronchoalveolar lavage in interstitial lung disease. Ann Intern Med 1978;89:459–66.
103. Welborn MB Jr, Fahmy A, Gobbel WG Jr. Mucoepidermoid carcinoma of bronchus with chondroid metaplasia and elevated 5-hydroxyindoleacetic acid excretion. J Thorac Cardiovasc Surg 1969;57:618–22.
104. Wetstein L. Sensitivity and specificity of lingular segmental biopsies of the lung. Chest 1986;90:383–6.
105. Wilson WR, Cockerill FR, Rosenow EC. Pulmonary disease in the immunocompromised host (2). Mayo Clin Proc 1985;60:610–31.
106. Zavala DC. Diagnostic fiberoptic bronchoscopy: techniques and results of biopsy in 600 patients. Chest 1975;68:12–9.

3
IDIOPATHIC INTERSTITIAL PNEUMONIA AND OTHER DIFFUSE PARENCHYMAL LUNG DISEASES

GENERAL APPROACH TO DIFFUSE PARENCHYMAL LUNG DISEASES

The diffuse parenchymal lung diseases (DPLD), often collectively referred to as the "interstitial lung diseases," encompass approximately 200 entities in which the lung is altered by a combination of interstitial inflammation, granulomatous inflammation, or fibrosis (1,7,11,15,16,32,42,44,48,49,54,61–64). Most of these diseases affect not only the interstitium of the lung but all anatomic aspects including the pleura, airways, blood vessels, and epithelial cells of the alveoli and bronchioles (8). For this reason, we prefer the term diffuse parenchymal lung diseases (8,19).

This heterogeneous group of disorders is classified together because of similar clinical, radiologic, physiologic, and pathologic manifestations. The DPLDs generally involve both lungs and manifest in an acute, subacute, or chronic manner. The most commonly identifiable causes of DPLD are occupational and environmental exposures or drug reactions. DPLDs include disorders of known cause (e.g., drug or environmental exposures and collagen vascular diseases), granulomatous disorders (e.g., sarcoidosis), and other specific forms of interstitial disease (e.g., lymphangioleiomyomatosis or pulmonary Langerhans' cell histiocytosis) (fig. 3-1). However, the most common and important group of DPLDs is the idiopathic interstitial pneumonias (fig. 3-1) (61).

This chapter provides an overview of the approach to a patient with DPLD, followed by a discussion of the history of the concept of idiopathic interstitial pneumonia (61). The individual causes of DPLD are discussed separately in the following sections of this chapter or in separate chapters in this book as noted in Table 3-1.

Patients with DPLD come to clinical attention in several ways: 1) with symptoms of progressive dyspnea or a persistent, often nonproductive cough; 2) with pulmonary symptoms associated with another disease, such as a connective tissue disease; and 3) for evaluation of an abnormal chest radiograph that was taken for another reason (40).

THE INITIAL EVALUATION OF PATIENTS WITH SUSPECTED DPLD

Clinical Features

Most DPLDs represent clinical-radiologic-pathologic entities, so the final diagnosis requires correlation of information from the clinician, radiologist, and pathologist. The initial evaluation should consist of a complete history and physical examination followed by laboratory

Table 3-1

CLINICAL CLASSIFICATION OF THE DIFFUSE PARENCHYMAL LUNG DISEASES

Drug-Induced Lung Disease (chapter 7)

Environmental and Occupational Exposures
- Pneumoconiosis (chapter 16)
- Hypersensitivity pneumonitis (chapter 3)

Idiopathic Interstitial Pneumonias (chapter 3)
- Idiopathic pulmonary fibrosis/usual interstitial pneumonia (chapter 3)
- Nonspecific interstitial pneumonia (chapter 3)
- Cryptogenic organizing pneumonia (idiopathic bronchiolitis obliterans organizing pneumonia) (chapter 3)
- Acute interstitial pneumonia (chapter 3)
- Respiratory bronchiolitis-interstitial lung disease (chapter 3)
- Desquamative interstitial pneumonia (chapter 3)
- Lymphocytic interstitial pneumonia (chapter 5)

Diffuse Alveolar Damage (chapter 3)

Collagen Vascular Disease and Inflammatory Bowel Disease (chapter 6)

Primary or Unclassified (chapter 3)
- Sarcoidosis (chapter 3)
- Langerhans' cell histiocytosis (histiocytosis X) (chapter 3)
- Lymphangioleiomyomatosis (chapter 3)
- Eosinophilic pneumonia (chapter 3)
- Pulmonary alveolar proteinosis (chapter 3)
- Diffuse alveolar hemorrhage (chapter 3)
- Pulmonary aspiration (chapter 3)
- Alveolar microlithiasis (chapter 3)
- Pulmonary vasculitis (chapter 4)

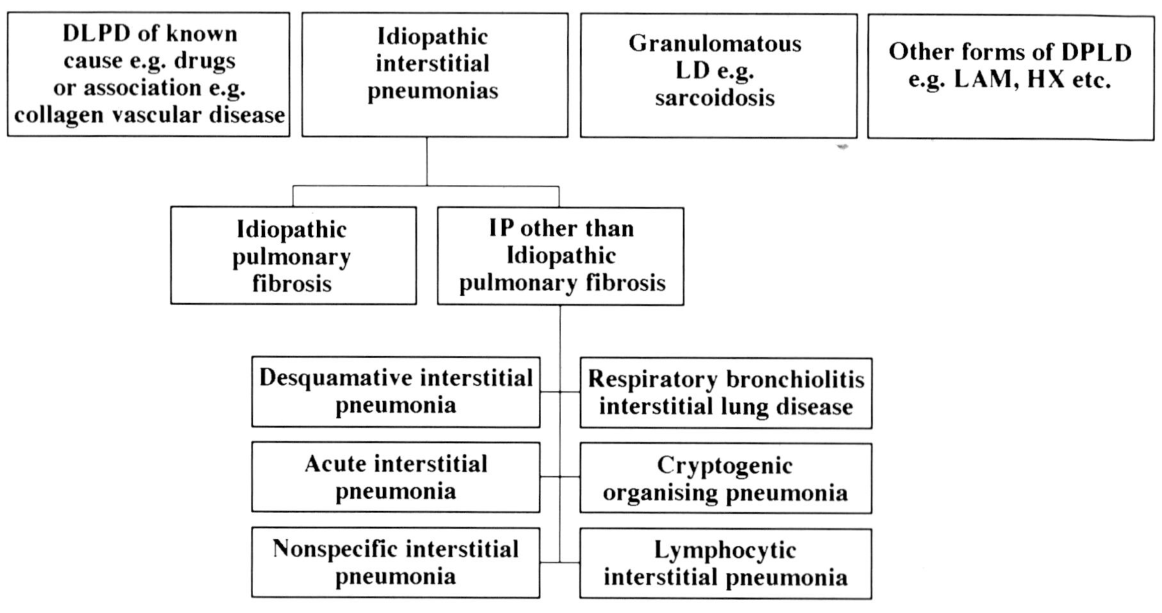

Figure 3-1

DIFFUSE PARENCHYMAL LUNG DISEASES (DPLD)

These consist of disorders of known causes (collagen vascular, environmental, or drug-related disease) as well as disorders of unknown etiology. The latter include idiopathic interstitial pneumonias, granulomatous lung disorders (e.g., sarcoidosis), and other forms of interstitial lung disease including lymphangioleiomyomatosis, pulmonary Langerhans' cell histiocytosis, and eosinophilic pneumonia. The most important distinction among the idiopathic interstitial pneumonias is to distinguish idiopathic pulmonary fibrosis from the other interstitial pneumonias which include nonspecific interstitial pneumonia (a provisional term), desquamative interstitial pneumonia, respiratory bronchiolitis-associated interstitial lung disease, acute interstitial pneumonia, cryptogenic organizing pneumonia, and lymphocytic interstitial pneumonia. (Figure 1 from Travis WD, King TE, Bateman ED, et al. ATS/ERS International Multidisciplinary Consensus Classification of Idiopathic Interstitial Pneumonia. Am J Respir Crit Care Med 2002;165:279.)

testing that includes routine blood tests, serologic studies, pulmonary function tests, arterial blood gas analysis, chest radiograph, high-resolution computed tomography (HRCT), and in many cases, lung biopsy (40,61).

Careful documentation of the past medical, occupational, and environmental history is important in the initial assessment because the cause of the illness is often recognized from the patient's history. The age of the patient may be useful in that some of the DPLDs are more common in patients under the age of 40 years (e.g., sarcoidosis, lymphangioleiomyomatosis, connective tissue disease-associated DPLD, Langerhans' cell histiocytosis, inherited forms of DPLD); others are most often seen in persons over the age of 50 years (e.g., the idiopathic interstitial pneumonias) (27,45,46,56,61). The patient's gender may be helpful in that some processes occur virtually exclusively in women (lymphangioleiomyomatosis and pulmonary involvement in tuberous sclerosis) while others are more common in men (DPLD associated with rheumatoid arthritis or pneumoconiosis). A history of tobacco use is important in the diagnosis of pulmonary Langerhans' cell histiocytosis, desquamative interstitial pneumonia, and respiratory bronchiolitis, however, nonsmokers predominate among patients with sarcoidosis and hypersensitivity pneumonitis (3,5,24,39,65).

The duration of illness before presentation may help narrow the differential diagnosis. The acute or subacute processes are often confused with atypical pneumonias, since many feature diffuse radiographic opacities along with fever and cough (e.g., cryptogenic organizing pneumonia and hypersensitivity pneumonitis). A detailed history of the medications taken by the patient is essential so that drug-induced DPLD can be excluded (69). This should include alternative or over-the-counter medications, oily nose drops or petroleum products, and nutritional supplements. Usually, the patient is taking the drug at presentation; rarely, the presentation with lung disease occurs weeks to years after the drug is discontinued (e.g., carmustine) (69).

The family history is occasionally helpful, since some familial associations have been identified in disorders such as tuberous sclerosis (discussed later), neurofibromatosis, and Hermansky-Pudlak syndrome (see chapter 17) (56).

Signs and Symptoms

Dyspnea is a common complaint in these patients. Importantly, patients with sarcoidosis, silicosis, and pulmonary Langerhans' cell histiocytosis may have extensive parenchymal lung disease on chest radiograph without significant symptoms. This most often occurs early in the course of the disease. A dry cough is common and can be particularly disturbing in conditions that involve the airways such as sarcoidosis, cryptogenic organizing pneumonia, respiratory bronchiolitis, pulmonary Langerhans' cell histiocytosis, and hypersensitivity pneumonitis. Grossly, bloody or blood-streaked sputum occurs in the diffuse alveolar hemorrhage syndromes, lymphangioleiomyomatosis, pulmonary veno-occlusive disease, and granulomatous vasculitides. Wheezing and chest pain is an uncommon manifestation of DPLD. Clinical findings consistent with a connective tissue disease should be carefully recorded (musculoskeletal pain, weakness, fatigue, fever, joint pains or swelling, photosensitivity, Raynaud's phenomenon, pleuritis, dry eyes, and dry mouth). The collagen vascular disorders may be difficult to exclude, since the DPLD occasionally precedes the more typical systemic manifestations by months or years (41).

The physical examination is frequently abnormal, but the findings are nonspecific. Crackles or "velcro rales" are common in most forms of DPLD. The cardiac examination is usually normal except in the middle or late stages of pulmonary fibrosis, when findings of pulmonary hypertension and cor pulmonale (augmented P2, right-sided lift, right-sided gallop) may become evident. Clubbing is a sign of advanced disease and is common in some disorders such as idiopathic pulmonary fibrosis and asbestosis while rare in others such as sarcoidosis, hypersensitivity pneumonitis, and pulmonary Langerhans' cell histiocytosis. Cyanosis occurs as a late manifestation of advanced disease.

Laboratory Tests

The routine laboratory evaluation often is not helpful in narrowing the differential diagnosis. Serologic studies should be obtained if clinically indicated by features suggestive of a connective tissue disease (antinuclear antibodies, rheumatoid factor), environmental exposure (hypersensitivity precipitin panel), or systemic vasculitis (antineutrophil cytoplasmic antibodies, antibasement membrane antibody).

The diagnosis of DPLD is often first suspected after obtaining an abnormal chest radiograph. Importantly, the chest radiograph is normal in as many as 10 percent of patients with some forms of DPLD, particularly those with hypersensitivity pneumonitis. The most common radiographic abnormality on routine chest radiograph is a reticular pattern; however, nodular or mixed patterns (alveolar filling and increased interstitial markings) may often be seen. Although the chest radiograph is useful in suggesting the presence of DPLD, the correlation between the roentgenographic pattern and the stage of disease (clinical or histopathologic) is generally poor. Honeycombing (small cystic spaces) is the only radiologic finding that reliably correlates with the pathologic findings.

HRCT is the most important radiologic method for evaluating patients with DPLDs. Although the accuracy of HRCT in determining the specific etiology has been disappointing, HRCT patterns provide greater diagnostic accuracy than chest radiography. HRCT is particularly useful for detecting disease in patients with a normal chest radiograph or in those who are predisposed to the development of DPLD (58). CT may be useful in selecting the site(s) for lung biopsy. The chest radiographic and HRCT patterns are described for each specific entity.

Complete pulmonary function testing (spirometry, lung volumes, diffusing capacity) and resting room air arterial blood gases should be obtained (21,22). Measurement of lung function is crucial in the assessment of the severity of functional impairment in patients with DPLD. In addition, the pattern of lung function impairment, i.e., an obstructive versus a restrictive pattern, is useful in narrowing the number of possible diagnoses. Most of the interstitial lung disorders have a restrictive defect with reductions in total lung capacity (TLC), functional residual capacity (FRC), and residual volume (RV) (22). Flow rates are decreased (forced expiratory volume [FEV1] and forced volume capacity [FVC]), but the changes are in proportion to the decreased lung volumes; thus, the FEV1/FVC ratio is usually normal or increased. The reduction in lung volumes becomes more pronounced with lung stiffness and worsens with disease progression (21). A pattern of airflow obstruction is suggestive of sarcoidosis, lymphangioleiomyomatosis, hypersensitivity pneumonitis, or chronic obstructive pulmonary disease (COPD) with superimposed interstitial lung disease.

A reduction in the diffusing capacity for carbon monoxide (DLCO) is caused, in part, by effacement of the alveolar capillary units but more importantly results from mismatching of ventilation and perfusion of the alveoli (22). The severity of the DLCO reduction does not correlate well with disease stage. However, severe reductions of DLCO suggest that the patient has DPLD combined with emphysema, pulmonary vascular disease, pulmonary Langerhans' cell histiocytosis, lymphangioleiomyomatosis, or advanced idiopathic interstitial pneumonia.

The resting arterial blood gases may be normal or may reveal hypoxemia (secondary to mismatching of ventilation to perfusion) and respiratory alkalosis (22). Carbon dioxide retention is rare and usually a manifestation of end-stage disease. Because resting hypoxemia is not always evident and because severe exercise-induced hypoxemia may go undetected, it is important to perform exercise testing with serial measurement of arterial blood gases. Arterial oxygen desaturation, a failure to decrease dead space appropriately with exercise (i.e., a high VD/VT ratio), and an excessive increase in respiratory rate with a lower than expected recruitment of tidal volume, provide useful information regarding physiologic abnormalities and the extent of disease. There is evidence that serial assessment of resting and exercise gas exchange is the best method for following disease activity and responsiveness to treatment, especially in patients with interstitial pulmonary fibrosis.

Bronchoalveolar Lavage and Lung Biopsy

The roles of bronchoalveolar lavage and lung biopsy in the assessment of patients with DPLD are discussed in detail in chapter 2. Lung biopsy frequently is required to establish the specific pattern and stage of DPLD. Lung biopsy is especially important to determine the presence or absence of usual interstitial pneumonia. There are several situations in which a lung biopsy should be strongly considered: 1) in a patient with atypical features (age under 50 years, fever, weight loss, hemoptysis, signs of vasculitis); 2) in a patient with a progressive course; 3) when the patient has a normal, atypical, or rapidly changing chest radiograph; 4) in the presence of unexplained extrapulmonary manifestations; or 5) when pulmonary vascular disease of unclear origin is present (see chapter 15) (43). Other indications for lung biopsy are: assess disease activity; exclude neoplastic and infectious processes that occasionally mimic chronic, progressive interstitial disease; identify a more treatable process than originally suspected; and make a definitive diagnosis and predict prognosis before proceeding with therapies which may have serious side effects (43). Relative contraindications to surgical lung biopsy are: 1) radiologic evidence of diffuse end-stage disease, e.g., honeycombing without areas of milder disease activity; 2) serious cardiovascular disease; 3) severe pulmonary dysfunction; 4) advanced age, or other major risks for surgery or general anesthesia; and 5) a high likelihood that adequate-sized biopsies from multiple sites (usually from two lobes) will not be obtained (1,43).

Surgical lung biopsies for DPLD should be obtained from more than one lobe of the lung (10). This is particularly important for the diagnosis of usual interstitial pneumonia (UIP), since heterogeneity exists among different lobes of the lung and areas of a nonspecific interstitial pneumonia (NSIP) pattern can be found in additional lobes of the lung in up to 25 percent of patients (23). If the lung shows severe fibrosis with honeycombing the biopsy specimen should not be taken from the worst-looking areas since these frequently show nonspecific changes. However, if honeycombing is not present, the surgeon should take the biopsy from the abnormal areas of the lung. Correlation with the HRCT may be helpful in directing the surgeon to the most optimal biopsy sites (26).

There needs to be adequate interaction among the clinician, radiologist, surgeon, and pathologist to achieve the maximum benefit from a lung biopsy. The histologic and radiologic abnormalities in the DPLDs are rarely specific and diagnostic in isolation. Most often, the findings are only "characteristic of" or "consistent with" a specific diagnosis or display "nonspecific" reaction patterns common to numerous causes of inflammation and/or fibrosis. Therefore, often it is critical that careful clinical and pathologic correlation is achieved to arrive at a final diagnosis. With such an approach, surgical lung biopsy produces a definitive diagnosis in more than 90 percent of cases of interstitial lung disease occurring in immunocompetent hosts (1). The clinician should provide the radiologist and pathologist with sufficient data to arrive at the most likely diagnosis. This data should include: 1) information regarding the duration of illness, age of patient, and any exposure to occupational or environmental agents; 2) immune status of the patient; 3) any history of drug use (prescribed or illicit); and 4) the clinical impression (1).

CLASSIFICATION OF IDIOPATHIC INTERSTITIAL PNEUMONIAS

In this section the history of classification, the terminology, and the problematic aspects of idiopathic interstitial pneumonias will be discussed.

Liebow Classification

In 1969, Liebow proposed the pathologic classification for interstitial pneumonia listed in Table 3-2 (48). The term "idiopathic" became attached to this group of interstitial pneumonias in subsequent years as it was recognized that these entities occurred in the absence of any detectable cause. In Liebow's original description of these disorders, he emphasized that they represented pathologic patterns and did not focus on their idiopathic aspects (47,48). In fact, much of his initial discussion of usual interstitial pneumonia (UIP) revolved around how this histologic pattern can be caused by viral and mycoplasma pneumonia and toxic exposure, such as to mercury fumes (48). Although diffuse alveolar damage (DAD) was not a specific category in Liebow's classification, he thought that DAD played an important role in the pathogenesis of UIP. Liebow included the term DAD as part of the terminology for the category of bronchiolitis obliterans and DAD. The concept of a group of idiopathic interstitial pneumonias appears to have developed in the late 1970s and early 1980s (17,33,38,68).

During the 1980s, both lymphocytic interstitial pneumonia (LIP) and giant cell interstitial pneumonia (GIP) were no longer included among the idiopathic interstitial pneumonias (Table 3-2). It was shown that many cases classified as LIP actually represented lymphoproliferative disorders (see chapter 5) (12,53). In addition, LIP is associated with collagen vascular disease or human immunodeficiency virus (HIV) infection. It also became known that most cases of GIP were hard metal (cobalt) pneumoconiosis (chapter 16) (2). However, a small number of idiopathic LIP cases remain and these fall into the differential diagnosis with the cellular NSIP pattern.

Katzenstein and Müller/Colby Classifications

Following Liebow's proposal, several new types of idiopathic interstitial pneumonia were described including idiopathic bronchiolitis obliterans organizing pneumonia (BOOP) or cryptogenic organizing pneumonia (COP) (18, 20), acute interstitial pneumonia (AIP) (37), and nonspecific interstitial pneumonia/fibrosis (NSIP) (35). Katzenstein has proposed several revisions of the classification over the past decade. The most recent classification is summarized in Table 3-2 (31,32,34,36).

There is some debate about which entities should be included in the group of idiopathic diffuse lung disorders. Katzenstein includes respiratory bronchiolitis-interstitial lung disease (RB-ILD) since it is probably related to desquamative interstitial pneumonia (DIP) (32,36). However, since virtually all cases of RB-ILD and DIP are related to cigarette smoking, one could argue that they are not really idiopathic. Idiopathic BOOP was not included in Katzenstein's classification

Table 3-2

PREVIOUS CLASSIFICATIONS OF THE IDIOPATHIC INTERSTITIAL PNEUMONIAS[a]

Liebow 1969 (48)	Katzenstein 1997 (30)	Muller & Colby 1997 (49)
Usual interstitial pneumonia	Usual interstitial pneumonia	Usual interstitial pneumonia
Desquamative interstitial pneumonia	Desquamative interstitial pneumonia/respiratory bronchiolitis interstitial lung disease	Desquamative interstitial pneumonia
Bronchiolitis obliterans interstitial pneumonia and diffuse alveolar damage		Bronchiolitis obliterans organizing pneumonia
	Acute interstitial pneumonia	Acute interstitial pneumonia
	Nonspecific interstitial pneumonia	Nonspecific interstitial pneumonia
Lymphocytic interstitial pneumonia		
Giant cell interstitial pneumonia		

[a]Table 1 from Travis WD, King TE, Bateman ED, et al. ATS/ERS International Multidisciplinary Consensus Classification of Idiopathic Interstitial Pneumonia. Am J Respir Crit Care Med 2002;165:281.

based on the argument that most of the connective tissue is within airspaces rather than the interstitium (32,36). Similarly, one could also argue that in RB-ILD and DIP the most conspicuous lesion, the alveolar macrophage accumulation, is within airspaces. Furthermore, none of these disorders is strictly limited to the interstitium since they can be associated with varying degrees of abnormalities of the airspaces, blood vessels, airways, and pleura. In addition to these entities, Müller and Colby included BOOP in their proposed classification (Table 3-2) (49).

American Thoracic Society/European Respiratory Society Classification

Several developments over the past decade have laid the foundation for the recent American Thoracic Society/European Respiratory Society (ATS/ERS) classification project to reevaluate the classification of idiopathic interstitial pneumonias (61). These include the advent of HRCT imaging which improved the detection of disease and the confidence of a specific diagnosis; publication of larger series of reports of patients with these disorders which included more lung biopsies; development of thoracoscopic or noninvasive methods for lung biopsy; and a narrower definition of the histologic criteria for UIP (61). The ATS/ERS classification emphasizes the importance of an integrated approach to diagnosis, requiring careful clinical, radiologic, and pathologic correlation. This approach stresses the importance to the pathologist of knowing as much clinical and radiologic information as possible when handling lung biopsies for the interstitial pneumonias. If this information is not provided by the clinician, the pathologist should make a concerted effort to obtain it in order to assess whether the patient has an idiopathic disorder or not.

The ATS/ERS proposal approaches classification by identifying the pathologic patterns seen on lung biopsy and combining these findings with other clinical information to arrive at a final clinicopathologic diagnosis (Table 3-3). This allows for preservation of existing pathologic and clinical terms while precisely defining the relationship between these terms. In this classification, the separation of UIP from other non-UIP disorders is critical. HRCT plays an important role in the evaluation of these patients (fig. 3-2) since it shows distinctive findings consistent with the presence of the UIP pattern in approximately half of patients with idiopathic pulmonary fibrosis (57).

To clarify the pathologic versus clinical use of the terms for the interstitial pneumonias, when the terms are the same for the pathologic pattern and the clinical diagnosis, it is recommended that the pathologist use the term pattern when referring to the histologic appearance on lung biopsy (Table 3-2) (61). For example, DIP pattern, LIP pattern, or NSIP pattern would be used for the lung biopsy finding and just DIP, LIP, or NSIP for the final clinical diagnosis (61).

Table 3-3 shows the ATS/ERS classification of idiopathic interstitial pneumonias with the

Table 3-3

THE ATS/ERS CLASSIFICATION OF IDIOPATHIC INTERSTITIAL PNEUMONIAS[a]

Histologic Patterns	Clinical-Radiologic-Pathologic Diagnosis
Usual interstitial pneumonia	Idiopathic pulmonary fibrosis/cryptogenic fibrosing alveolitis

Nonspecific interstitial pneumonia
  Cellular pattern[a]
  Fibrosing pattern
	Nonspecific interstitial pneumonia (provisional)[b]

Organizing pneumonia	Cryptogenic organizing pneumonia[c]
Diffuse alveolar damage	Acute interstitial pneumonia
Respiratory bronchiolitis	Respiratory bronchiolitis interstitial lung disease
Desquamative interstitial pneumonia	Desquamative interstitial pneumonia
Lymphocytic interstitial pneumonia	Lymphocytic interstitial pneumonia
Unclassifiable Interstitial Pneumonia	

[a]Modified from reference 61.

[b]This represents a heterogeneous group with poorly characterized clinical and radiologic features that needs further study.

[c]COP is the preferred term, but it is synonymous with idiopathic bronchiolitis obliterans organizing pneumonia.

modification of designating the cellular and fibrosing histologic patterns of NSIP, which we think is important. The panel was reluctant to make this distinction, but now there are four separate series that show no deaths in patients with the cellular pattern and three of these studies show a significantly better survival compared to patients with the fibrosing NSIP pattern (35,51, 52,62). A category of *unclassifiable interstitial pneumonia* was recognized to acknowledge that some interstitial pneumonias defy precise classification for various reasons (see below) (61).

For the purposes of this classification the following terms are regarded as synonymous: idiopathic pulmonary fibrosis (IPF) and cryptogenic fibrosing alveolitis (CFA); pneumonia and pneumonitis; cryptogenic organizing pneumonia (COP) and idiopathic bronchiolitis obliterans and organizing pneumonia (idiopathic BOOP); and idiopathic and cryptogenic.

Commonly Encountered Problems in the Clinical and Pathologic Classification of the Idiopathic Interstitial Pneumonias

Clinical and Pathologic Terminology is Confusing. One of the problems with the nomenclature of idiopathic diffuse lung disorders is the confusion between clinical and pathologic terms. Both Liebow and Katzenstein, as pathologists, made their classifications based primarily on a pathologic approach, although both emphasized the importance of clinicopathologic correlation. When pathologists use the general term "fibrosis" in surgical pathology reports for a descriptive diagnosis, many clinicians assume this represents UIP and often label the patient as having IPF. Thus, it is important for pathologists and clinicians to be as precise as possible with the terms that are used in these cases.

Clinicians have developed their own terminology and clinical approach to classification of idiopathic diffuse lung disorders (17,42). During the 1970s the concept of IPF was proposed by pulmonary clinicians and today it continues to be a widely used diagnostic term (17,42). In the 1970s, the major pathologic subsets recognized in lung biopsies from patients with IPF included UIP and DIP. A major tenet of the concept of IPF was the belief that DIP represented the cellular phase and UIP the fibrotic phase of a single disease (17,42). This contrasted with the concept of Liebow who regarded UIP and DIP as separate entities (48).

Another source of confusion in terminology of the idiopathic diffuse lung disorders is the various clinical terms that have been used. For example, the concept of IPF is primarily used in North America and Asia while in Great Britain

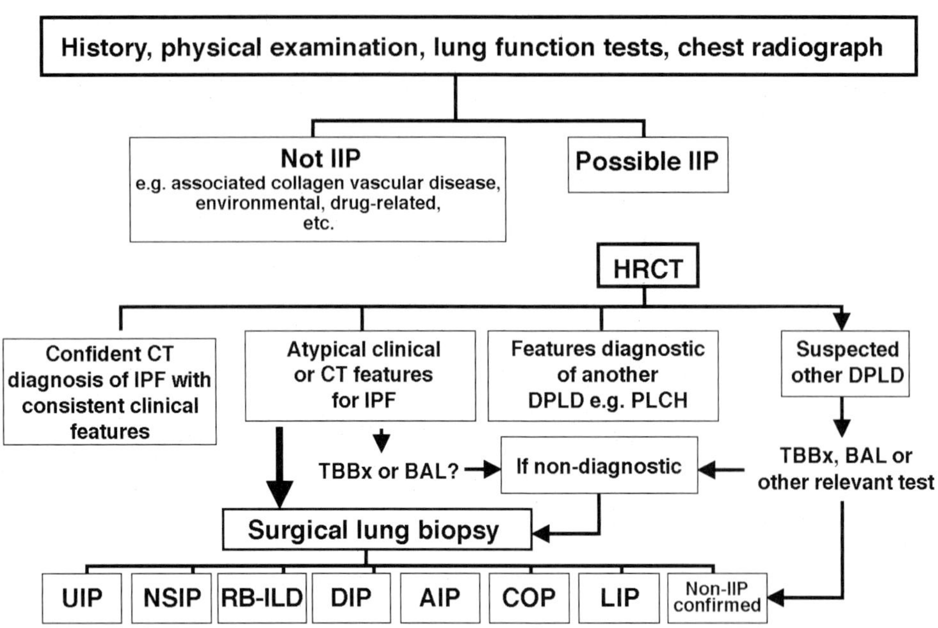

Figure 3-2

THE DIAGNOSTIC PROCESS IN DIFFUSE PARENCHYMAL LUNG DISEASES

The diagnostic process in diffuse pulmonary lung diseases (DPLD) begins with a clinical evaluation which includes a history, physical examination, lung function tests, and a chest radiograph. Based on this information, the patients are divided into two groups: cases that do not represent idiopathic interstitial pneumonia (IIP) due to recognition of associated conditions or underlying exposures and cases that could represent IIP. Patients in the latter category typically receive a high-resolution computed tomograph (HRCT). This generally results in four categories of patients: 1) those with distinctive features that allow for a confident diagnosis of idiopathic pulmonary fibrosis (IPF) in the appropriate clinical setting; 2) those with atypical clinical or CT features of IPF; 3) those with features diagnostic of another DPLD such as pulmonary Langerhans' cell histiocytosis (PLCH); and 4) those with suspected other forms of DPLD. While many patients have surgical lung biopsy, some undergo transbronchial biopsy (TBBX) or bronchoalveolar lavage (BAL). If these findings are nondiagnostic, an open lung biopsy may be necessary to separate the various IIPs from non-IIP DPLD. (Figure 2 from Travis WD, King TE, Bateman ED, et al. ATS/ERS International Multidisciplinary Consensus Classification of Idiopathic Interstitial Pneumonia. Am J Respir Crit Care Med 2002;165:282.)

the term cryptogenic fibrosing alveolitis (CFA) is more popular (4). In the absence of collagen vascular disease, the term "lone" CFA is sometimes used. Other terms that have been used for IPF include Hamman-Rich syndrome, diffuse interstitial fibrosis, "honeycomb lung," Osler-Charcot disease, diffuse pulmonary alveolar fibrosis, and interstitial pneumonias (42). A similar difference in terminology applies to idiopathic BOOP. Idiopathic BOOP is used mostly in North America and Asia, while in Great Britain, the term cryptogenic organizing pneumonia (COP) is more popular.

Furthermore, if one examines how the idiopathic diffuse lung disorders are diagnosed—comparing the perspective of the pathologist with that of the clinician and then the final clinicopathologic diagnosis—it is apparent that there has historically been some inconsistency in how the terms are used and interpreted. For example, considerable confusion has resulted from the use of the term BOOP for a pathologic diagnosis. It is well known that this lesion is a very common and nonspecific histologic reaction seen in many conditions. However, when clinicians see this term in pathologic reports they often assume they are dealing with a case of idiopathic BOOP (discussed later). For this reason, the new ATS/ERS classification recommended using organizing pneumonia as the pathologic term and cryptogenic organizing pneumonia for the clinicopathologic term for the idiopathic syndrome (Table 3-3) (61). In patients with known underlying diseases, such as collagen vascular disease, the term BOOP is appropriate, with mention of the associated condition.

Many pathologists are expected to evaluate lung biopsies with minimal clinical history, especially with the current emphasis on rapid turnaround time. This makes it difficult for a pathologist to make the final clinicopathologic diagnosis. For example, the diagnosis of AIP (idiopathic DAD) requires considerable clinical information. Much of the evaluation to exclude specific causes of the DAD histologic pattern is likely to be completed after the lung biopsy has been evaluated. In fact, the published studies of AIP have been based on a series of patients narrowed from a larger group in which some patients were excluded on the basis of information that was probably not available at the time of biopsy. Even after making a careful diagnosis of AIP, an underlying condition such as a collagen vascular disease may declare itself after the initial pulmonary presentation and the original diagnosis of AIP may need to be revised.

Refinement in the Definition of IPF. Since the mid-1980s, as each new subgroup of pulmonary fibrosis has been recognized, the definition of IPF has become narrower and the group more homogeneous. This has resulted in considerable changes in the natural history and, possibly, treatment of these entities. Bjoraker et al. (6) recently showed how patients with the clinical picture of IPF as defined between 1976 and 1985 had a heterogeneous spectrum of lung biopsy findings, including idiopathic BOOP, DIP, AIP, and NSIP. This study demonstrated that the 2.8-year median survival period of patients with the UIP pattern of interstitial fibrosis was significantly worse than that for patients with the other chronic interstitial pneumonias. Travis et al. (62) recently found that patients with idiopathic UIP had a 5- and 10-year survival rate of 43 and 15 percent, respectively, which was significantly worse than that for DIP and NSIP, both cellular and fibrosing patterns. Nicholson et al. (52) subsequently had a similar finding with a median survival of 24 months for patients with idiopathic UIP, which was also significantly worse than the survival period for those with DIP and NSIP. These data and other studies have supported the separation of DIP from UIP as distinct entities (6,9,25,62). HRCT studies correlated with lung pathology have greatly helped in understanding the importance of separating these disorders (25,28,49,50, 54,55). This has led to a more precise definition of IPF so that for a diagnosis of IPF it is now required to have a radiographic and/or histologic pattern of UIP (1).

It is important to keep this evolution in mind when reading the literature on pulmonary fibrosis since articles published on IPF in the 1970s and 1980s probably included some cases of idiopathic BOOP, DIP, AIP, and NSIP. Thus, the conclusions from these earlier studies may not be comparable with those published using the current criteria. For example, as recently suggested by Costabel and King (59), some of the previously defined prognostic factors may not be relevant for patients with IPF/UIP: cellular histology—more likely DIP or NSIP patients in the older series; younger age—more likely DIP or NSIP; cigarette smoking—likely DIP or RB-ILD; bronchoalveolar lavage (BAL) lymphocytosis—more likely patients with NSIP; and ground-glass opacities—more likely DIP, NSIP, BOOP, or hypersensitivity pneumonitis.

Lack of Experience with Diagnosis of DPLD. Histologic examination is key to the diagnosis, and in many cases determination of the prognosis, of the patients with DPLD (61). However, despite recommendations that histologic examination be routinely performed in these patients, two studies from the United Kingdom have shown that lung biopsies are obtained in only 28 to 33 percent and 8 to 12 percent of patients, respectively (29,30), and in 11 percent of patients in one study from the United States (14). Consequently, most medical centers have limited experience with the histologic evaluation of patients with these disorders. In addition, pathologists commonly rely on experience and gestalt when making a diagnosis based on histologic examination of biopsies from patients with DPLD (13). Therefore, it has been recommended that, whenever possible, biopsy samples from patients with DPLD be examined by a pathologist experienced in respiratory pathology (1,19).

Histologic Patterns are Distinctive but Not Specific. The histologic patterns seen in patients with IPF, DIP, AIP, COP, and NSIP are distinctive but they can be seen not only in an idiopathic setting but also in a variety of other conditions (fig. 3-1). For example, the UIP histologic pattern can be seen in collagen vascular diseases as well as in IPF (see chapter 6). In fact, all of these histologic patterns are seen in patients with associated collagen vascular diseases.

Unclassifiable Cases. There is a subset of patients with interstitial pneumonia that remains unclassifiable after extensive clinical, radiologic, and/or pathologic examination (Table 3-3). Such an unclassifiable category has existed in the World Health Organization (WHO) classification of lung tumors for the past several decades (60,66,67). Although most clinical groups specializing in interstitial lung diseases recognize the existence of such cases, this problem is not addressed in most publications on this subject. For interstitial lung disease, this problem often exists in cases where some critical piece of data is unavailable, for example, there is inadequate clinical information or chest radiologic images or the lung biopsy is inadequate or nondiagnostic due to small size (a bronchoscopic or needle biopsy), poor sampling, or the presence of a nondiagnostic pattern of endstage fibrosis with honeycombing. Some cases may be unclassifiable because there is a major discrepancy between the lung biopsy and radiologic or clinical information. For example, a lung biopsy may show a classical UIP pattern, but the HRCT may show a predominantly upper lobe and airway centered distribution more suggestive of hypersensitivity pneumonitis or some response to an inhaled environmental agent. Even though a UIP pattern may represent the appropriate pathologic diagnosis for such a case, this patient probably does not have IPF or CFA and the case may be unclassifiable.

The ATS/ERS classification of idiopathic interstitial pneumonias proposed that these patients be given the clinicopathologic diagnosis of unclassifiable interstitial pneumonia (Table 3-3) (61). The use of this term varies somewhat from the proposal by Kitaichi et al. (44) since some of those cases may have represented what we now call NSIP (44). Importantly, this category should not be used for cases of clearly defined NSIP or cases where the distinction between the UIP and fibrosing NSIP pattern is difficult (see the differential diagnosis sections of these diseases later in this chapter). The purpose of this concept is not to create a new category to perform clinical studies, but to acknowledge that in some cases it is impossible to make a specific clinicopathologic diagnosis. These cases represent some of the most difficult problems in routine clinical practice.

Differential Diagnosis of Interstitial Pneumonias

Another point of confusion regarding interstitial pneumonias is the differential diagnosis. The differential diagnosis must be approached in two ways: histologically and etiologically. When interpreting lung biopsies, the pathologist must address the differential diagnosis based on the histologic pattern. Sometimes there are histologic clues to an etiology that a pathologist may observe that may or may not have been apparent clinically. Examples include: finding ill-formed granulomas that suggest a hypersensitivity pneumonitis pattern; finding asbestos bodies suggestive of asbestosis; identifying viral inclusions or organisms by examining appropriate special stains in biopsies with unexplained cellular inflammatory infiltrates; and finding a pattern of giant cell interstitial pneumonia suggestive of hard metal pneumoconiosis.

In most cases, though, the pathologist is focused on separating the type of histologic pattern on the lung biopsy, i.e., is it a UIP, organizing pneumonia, or a DAD pattern? The pathologist should always be concerned about potential etiologies when examining a lung biopsy, such as drug reaction, environmental or occupational exposures, or associated connective tissue disease. However, it is primarily the clinicians' responsibility to address most of the etiologic possibilities and in many cases they ultimately determine whether the process is idiopathic or not. After the pathologist has interpreted a lung biopsy, especially if a bronchiolocentric cellular interstitial pneumonia pattern with granulomas is identified, it may be necessary for the clinician to go back to the patient and be more persistent about exposure to inhaled antigens, drugs, or toxic substances. It is crucial that the pathologist and clinician meet regularly to review biopsy samples from patients with DPLD in conjunction with the HRCT and clinical data (61).

USUAL INTERSTITIAL PNEUMONIA (IDIOPATHIC PULMONARY FIBROSIS/ CRYPTOGENIC FIBROSING ALVEOLITIS)

Definition. Usual interstitial pneumonia (UIP) is a histologic pattern seen in the clinical setting of diffuse, bilateral interstitial lung disease. The histologic changes are often distributed along the subpleural and paraseptal regions, and are characterized by patchy, temporally heterogeneous fibrosis with scattered fibroblastic foci at the edges of dense fibrotic scars that cause remodeling of the lung architecture and microscopic honeycombing.

The term UIP has been used in two major ways: as a pathologic pattern and as a clinicopathologic syndrome (165,166). As an idiopathic clinicopathologic syndrome, UIP is synonymous with IPF (73). However, the UIP histologic pattern occurs in a variety of clinical settings including collagen vascular disease. If other known causes of DPLD, such as drug toxicity, environmental exposures, and collagen vascular diseases, have been excluded, the clinicopathologic term IPF (or CFA) is appropriate. Confusion may occur when it is not clearly stated whether one is using the term UIP to describe a clinicopathologic entity or a histologic pattern. Pathologists can work around this problem by using the term UIP pattern when referring only to lung histology.

A variety of other terms have been used for the idiopathic form of UIP. The term classic, usual, or undifferentiated interstitial pneumonia was proposed by Liebow in 1969 (129). Over the past few decades IPF has been used by pulmonary clinicians for a spectrum of pathologic forms of interstitial fibrosis. In Europe, the term CFA is more popular (76) and if there is no underlying collagen vascular disease, the term lone CFA is used (109). For the purposes of this discussion the clinicopathologic term IPF is restricted to cases in which the lung shows a UIP pattern histologically or with HRCT (118). If a patient has DPLD with a UIP pattern in the setting of underlying disease (e.g., rheumatoid arthritis), then the clinicopathologic diagnosis of IPF is inappropriate and the term UIP should be used with mention of the specific associated condition (e.g., UIP with associated rheumatoid arthritis).

Clinical Features. The true incidence and prevalence of IPF are not known. Recent reports on prevalence are 5 to 10 times higher than previously reported: 20.2 cases per 100,000 persons per year for males and 13.2 cases per 100,000 for females (89). The incidence is estimated as 10.7 cases per 100,000 persons per year for males and 7.4 cases per 100,000 for females (89). The incidence of IPF increases with age. More men than women have been reported with IPF. Patients with IPF are often between 50 and 70 years of age; approximately two thirds are over the age of 60 years at the time of presentation (73). It is unclear if a syndrome similar to IPF occurs in children, if so, it is rare. IPF has no distinct geographic distribution and has been reported worldwide in both rural and urban settings, with no predilection by race or ethnicity (73).

The cause of IPF remains unknown. A role for genetic factors is supported by the findings of familial cases (155). Cigarette smoking results in a 1.6- to 2.3-fold excess risk of developing pulmonary fibrosis (78,79,106,161). There is no clear exposure-response pattern with cumulative consumption of cigarettes (79). Long-term exposure to metal dust or wood dust has also been shown to be an independent risk factor for IPF (106). No convincing cultural, serologic, or morphologic evidence supports prior or persistent viral exposure as an etiology (93,124,167).

The typical patient presents with the insidious onset of breathlessness with exertion and a nonproductive cough. Constitutional symptoms are uncommon; however, weight loss, fever, fatigue, myalgias, or arthralgias are occasionally present. The onset may rarely be heralded by a flu-like illness; this type of presentation should suggest another diagnosis. Most patients have these symptoms for months to years (usually around 12 to 18 months) before definitive evaluation (116).

The physical examination is rarely normal. Most patients with IPF are tachypneic, with rapid shallow breaths, probably because of the increased work of breathing. Chest examination shows bibasilar, late inspiratory, fine crackles ("velcro" rales). Clubbing is seen in 40 to 75 percent of patients and is often a late finding in the disease course. Cardiac examination is usually normal except in the middle or late stages of the disease, when findings of pulmonary hypertension (i.e., augmented P_2, right-sided lift, and S_3 gallop) and cor pulmonale may become evident. Similarly, cyanosis is a late manifestation indicative of advanced disease. Spontaneous pneumothorax rarely occurs.

Routine laboratory studies are usually not helpful except to rule out other potential causes of DPLD. An elevated erythrocyte sedimentation rate, hypergammaglobulinemia, low titer–positive antinuclear antibodies and rheumatoid factor, circulating immune complexes, and cryoimmunoglobulins have been identified in these patients (73).

The typical findings of pulmonary function tests are restriction and impairment of gas exchange. Lung function testing is important is assessing the stage of disease at presentation and for following the course of the disease during treatment (94,169,171). The lung volumes (TLC, FRC, and RV) are reduced. Lung volumes may be normal in patients with superimposed chronic obstructive pulmonary disease (101, 160). Lung compliance decreases and lung volumes fall as the disease progresses. Expiratory flow rates, FEV1 and FVC, may be decreased because of the reduction in lung volume, but the FEV1/FVC ratio is maintained. The DLCO is reduced, which may actually precede the loss of lung volume. The resting arterial blood gases reveal hypoxemia and respiratory alkalosis. With exercise, the alveolar-arterial PO_2 difference ([A-a]PO_2) widens, and the arterial PO_2 and oxygen saturation (SO_2) falls. Importantly, the abnormalities identified at rest do not accurately predict the magnitude of the abnormalities that may be seen with exercise. Exercise testing is more sensitive in the detection of abnormalities in oxygen transfer than assessment at rest. In addition, gas exchange during exercise has been demonstrated to be a sensitive parameter for following the clinical course. Pulmonary hypertension develops as the disease progresses.

The pattern of inflammatory cells in the bronchoalveolar lavage (BAL) may be helpful in narrowing the differential diagnosis, but is not diagnostic of IPF (77). Patients with IPF typically have elevations of BAL neutrophils and eosinophils, but these findings are also observed in other fibrosing lung conditions (117). A lone increase in lymphocytes is uncommon in IPF, and when present, another disorder should be excluded (e.g., granulomatous infectious disease, sarcoidosis, hypersensitivity pneumonitis, cryptogenic organizing pneumonia, nonspecific interstitial pneumonia, or lymphocytic interstitial pneumonia) (73).

The diagnosis of IPF requires that a clinical history be carefully taken to eliminate known causes of DPLD, especially those related to occupational and environmental exposures. Unfortunately, several primary DPLDs (sarcoidosis, eosinophilic granuloma, lymphangitic carcinomatosis, hypersensitivity pneumonitis, respiratory bronchiolitis) can often be differentiated only by their histologic appearance; therefore, a lung biopsy is required. In addition, connective tissue diseases may be difficult to exclude because the pulmonary manifestations may precede the more typical systemic manifestations by months or years. The most definitive method of establishing a diagnosis is by surgical lung biopsy (118,153,156,165). Transbronchial biopsy cannot be used to diagnose IPF but is useful in excluding it by showing an alternative specific diagnosis (malignancy, infections, sarcoidosis, hypersensitivity pneumonitis, cryptogenic organizing pneumonia, eosinophilic pneumonia, or Langerhans' cell histiocytosis). Open or thoracoscopic lung biopsy is indicated because it provides an accurate diagnosis; it excludes neoplastic and infectious processes that occasionally mimic chronic, progressive interstitial disease; it occasionally identifies a more treatable process than originally suspected (e.g., chronic extrinsic allergic alveolitis); and it provides a better assessment of disease activity (81, 95,142). It is important that the surgeon obtain an adequate sample from several sites (83,113).

Increasingly, it is recognized that a clinical diagnosis of IPF can be made with a high degree of certainty. For this reason, the ATS recently proposed guidelines for the diagnosis of IPF in the absence of a surgical lung biopsy (Table 3-4) (73). As the definition of IPF has been narrowed to include only cases with the UIP pattern, and with the identification with HRCT of patterns that best correlate with this histologic UIP pattern, it is now recognized that about 50 percent of patients with IPF have a characteristic HRCT pattern (see below) (73,98, 108,150,156,165,172,174). When these specific features are present, radiologists have a high degree of accuracy in predicting the diagnosis of

Table 3-4

ATS CRITERIA FOR DIAGNOSIS OF IDIOPATHIC PULMONARY FIBROSIS IN THE ABSENCE OF A SURGICAL LUNG BIOPSY[a]

Major Criteria[b]

- Exclusion of other known causes of ILD[c] such as certain drug toxicities, environmental exposures, and connective tissue diseases
- Abnormal pulmonary function studies that include evidence of restriction (reduced VC often with an increased FEV1/FVC ratio) and impaired gas exchange (increased $AaPO_2$ with rest or exercise or decreased DLCO)
- Bibasilar reticular abnormalities with minimal ground-glass opacities on HRCT scans
- Transbronchial lung biopsy or BAL showing no features to support an alternate diagnosis

Minor Criteria

- Age > 50 years
- Insidious onset of otherwise unexplained dyspnea on exertion
- Duration of illness ≥ 3 months
- Bibasilar, inspiratory crackles (dry or "velcro" type in quality)

[a]Data from reference 73.

[b]In the immunocompetent adult, the presence of all of the above major diagnostic criteria as well as at least three of the four minor criteria increases the likelihood of a correct clinical diagnosis of IPF.

[c]ILD = interstitial lung disease; VC = vital capacity; FEV = forced expiratory volume; FVC = forced vital capacity; DLCO = diffusion capacity; HRCT = high-resolution computerized tomography; BAL = bronchoalveolar lavage.

UIP. In this setting, bronchoscopic biopsy plays an important role in excluding other specific disorders, as noted above.

Radiologic Findings. Chest radiographs in patients with IPF typically show bilateral, symmetric, irregular linear opacities causing a reticular pattern (fig. 3-3, top) (99,144). Common additional findings include ground-glass opacities, honeycombing, and decreased lung volumes (99,139). The abnormalities may be diffuse but involve mainly the lower lung zones in about 80 percent of cases (86,99,137). Less than 10 percent of patients have a normal chest radiograph at presentation.

The HRCT manifestations of IPF are characteristic and consist of irregular lines (reticular pattern) and honeycombing involving mainly the subpleural lung regions (136,145,150). Honeycombing is evident at presentation on HRCT in 80 to 90 percent of patients with IPF compared to 30 percent of cases on the radiograph (72,163). Early findings of fibrosis on HRCT consist of fine irregular lines within the secondary lobules (intralobular linear opacities), irregular thickening of the interlobular septa, and irregular pleural, vascular, and bronchial interfaces with the lung parenchyma (fig. 3-3, bottom). With progression of fibrosis, the irregular lines become coarser and there is progressive distortion of the lung architecture, dilatation of bronchioles and bronchi (traction bronchiectasis), and honeycombing (fig. 3-4) (72,164). The pattern of abnormalities on HRCT closely reflects the macroscopic pathologic findings (145,146,150). HRCT may demonstrate characteristic findings of IPF in patients who had normal radiographs or radiographs with nonspecific findings (136,151). In approximately 70 percent of patients, areas of ground-glass attenuation are seen on HRCT; these have been shown to correlate with the presence of active alveolitis (127,146).

Patients with HRCT findings of predominant ground-glass attenuation have been shown to be more likely to respond to corticosteroids than patients who have a predominant reticular pattern (126,146,172). However, the majority of patients with IPF have extensive fibrosis at presentation and do not respond to treatment, and areas of ground-glass attenuation often progress to reticulation and honeycombing (102,164).

In the majority of patients, IPF has a slowly progressive course over several years with progressive increase in reticulation and honeycombing on the chest radiograph and HRCT. In a small percentage of patients, IPF progresses

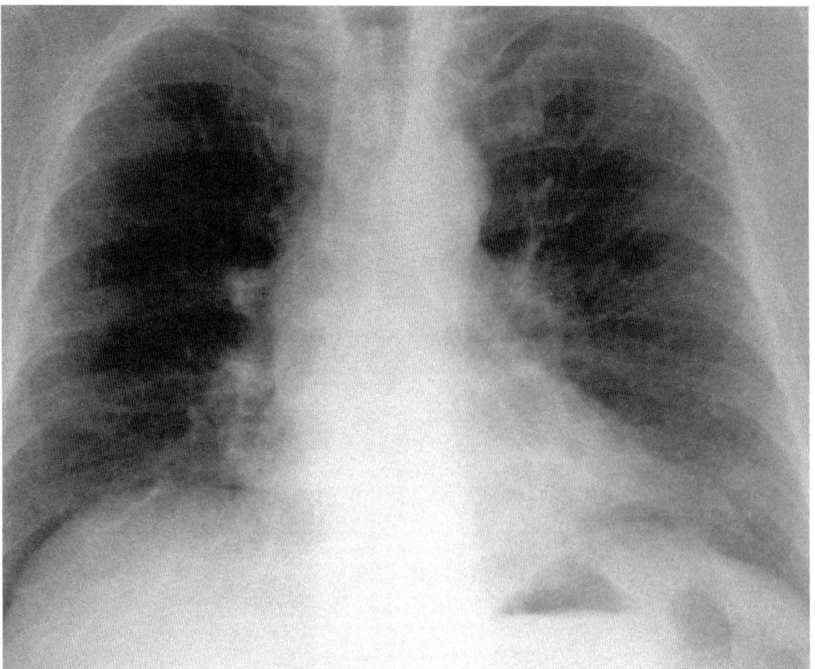

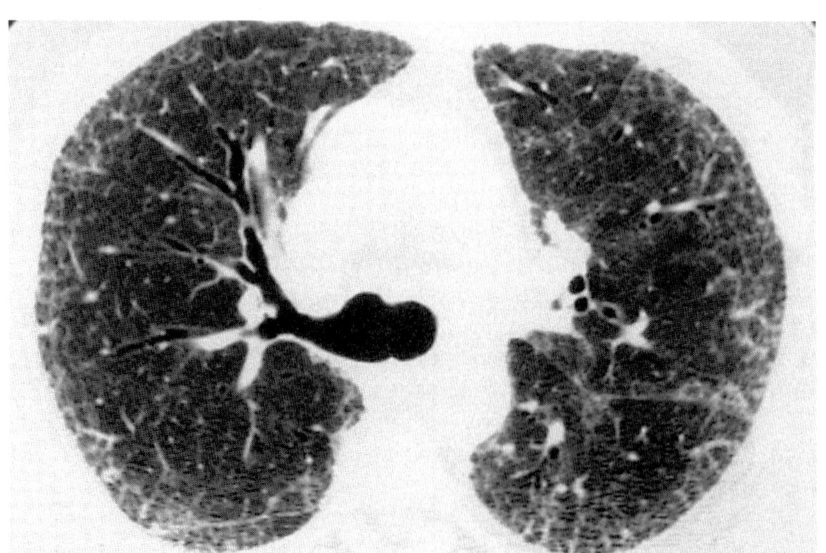

Figure 3-3

USUAL INTERSTITIAL PNEUMONIA PATTERN

Top: PA chest radiograph in a 61-year-old man with IPF shows a fine reticular pattern involving mainly the lower lung zones.

Bottom: HRCT demonstrates predominant subpleural distribution of the abnormalities. The findings include irregular thickening of the interlobular septa, intralobular linear opacities, and subpleural areas of ground-glass attenuation.

rapidly (accelerated deterioration), over 1 month or less. The HRCT in these patients shows extensive areas of ground-glass attenuation, which may be diffuse, multifocal, or peripheral (71,120). Most patients who have accelerated deterioration do not respond to treatment; preliminary results suggest that patients with a predominantly subpleural distribution of ground-glass attenuation are more likely to respond to treatment than patients who have a patchy or diffuse distribution (71,120). Pulmonary carcinoma, which is a potential complication of IPF, may manifest as a focal area of consolidation, as a nodule superimposed on a background of fibrosis, or, less commonly, as massive hilar and mediastinal lymphadenopathy (125).

Pathologic Findings. It is useful to have some historical perspective on the concept of the UIP histologic pattern. As recognized today, classic UIP shows distinctive gross and histologic

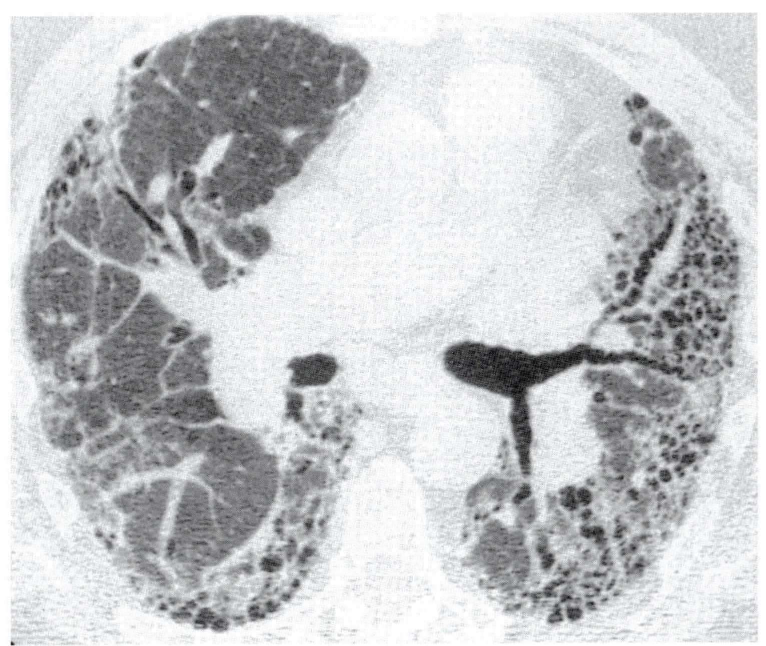

Figure 3-4

USUAL INTERSTITIAL PNEUMONIA: ENDSTAGE

HRCT demonstrates bilateral honeycomb cysts. The honeycombing is more extensive on the left side and is associated with considerable loss of volume of the left lung. A subpleural predominance of the honeycomb cysts is particularly evident on the right side. The patient was a 65-year-old man with longstanding IPF.

features. However, our current histologic criteria for the UIP pattern are substantially different from Liebow's description of this lesion in the late 1960s when the distinction from DAD was not appreciated (129). Since he thought that DAD was an early pattern of UIP, much of Liebow's description of the histology of UIP focused on what we now call DAD. He described UIP as a "highly variegated lesion with evidence of hyaline membrane formation and varying degrees of exudation."

The pathologic criteria for the UIP pattern have been narrowed from Liebow's descriptions in the 1960s and 1970s, due to recognition of additional patterns of pulmonary fibrosis, including DAD, BOOP, and NSIP. The variegated nature and the frequent honeycombing emphasized by Liebow continue to be central criteria of the current pathologic definition of the UIP pattern (128,129).

Gross Findings. The pleural surface of the lungs has a cobble-stoned appearance due to the retraction of scars along the interlobular septa. The overall lung size tends to be small. The cut surface typically shows diffuse fibrosis of the lung parenchyma with lower lobe predominance (fig. 3-5). There is a distinctive distribution in the subpleural regions (fig. 3-5) and along the interlobular septa. The fibrosis is patchy, with areas of fibrotic lung adjacent to relatively

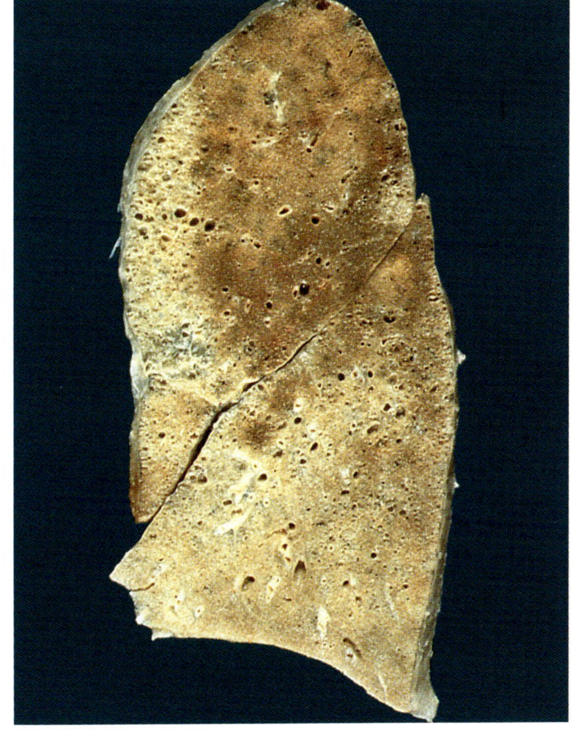

Figure 3-5

USUAL INTERSTITIAL PNEUMONIA PATTERN

There is a predominantly lower lobe, peripheral, subpleural patchy process with fibrotic areas alternating with relatively normal lung. Fibrotic areas are characterized by tan, firm scars causing remodeling of the lung architecture and honeycomb cystic changes.

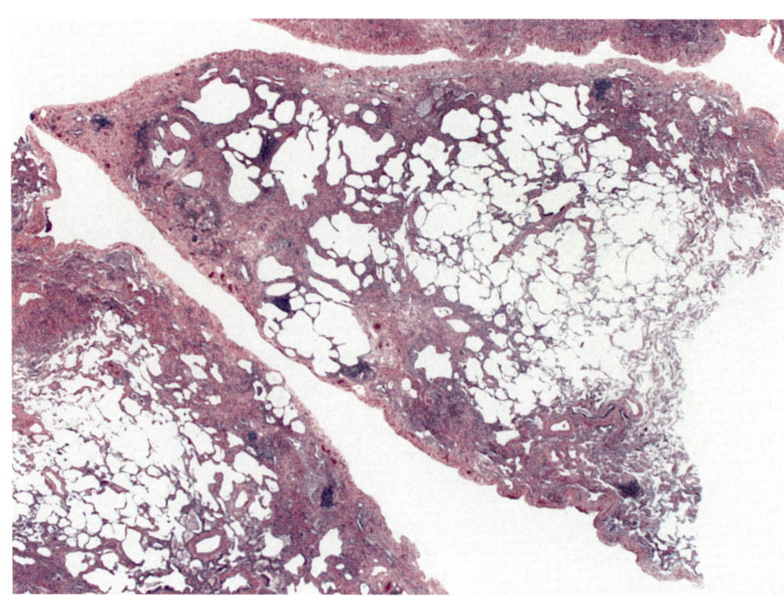

Figure 3-6

USUAL INTERSTITIAL PNEUMONIA PATTERN

Patchy fibrosis with remodeling of the lung architecture shows a striking subpleural distribution.

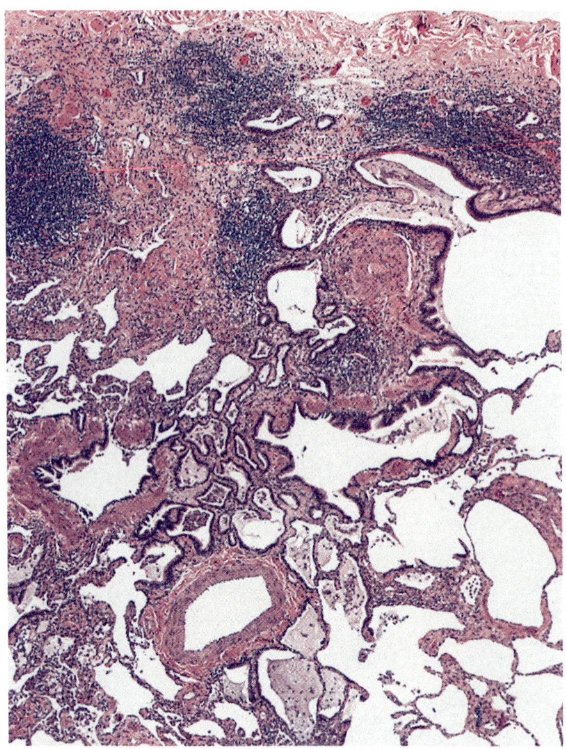

Figure 3-7

USUAL INTERSTITIAL PNEUMONIA PATTERN

Patchy, subpleural fibrosis consists of dense collagenous scarring with remodeling of the lung architecture and small cystic changes. Interstitial chronic inflammation is mild, with a few lymphoid aggregates. Proliferation of bronchiolar epithelium is present on the surface of some of the scarred areas. Areas of "normal" lung lack the active lesions of other interstitial lung disorders.

normal lung. The fibrosis consists of firm, rubbery, white connective tissue frequently associated with honeycomb cystic changes. In cases where an accelerated phase of IPF has occurred, the active areas may show patchy organizing fibrosis with a variegated tan-yellow appearance alternating with areas of relatively preserved lung.

Histologic Findings. The histologic hallmark of the UIP pattern is patchy interstitial fibrosis, often in a subpleural and/or paraseptal distribution, alternating with areas of normal lung (figs. 3-6, 3-7). This feature is best appreciated at low-power magnification (Table 3-5) (88,112, 166). The fibrosis is temporally heterogeneous, with two major types: 1) dense scarring and honeycombing and 2) fibroblastic foci scattered at the edges of the dense scars (fig. 3-8). The dense fibrosis causes remodeling of the lung architecture resulting in collapse of alveolar walls and formation of cystic spaces or honeycombing (fig. 3-9). The dense fibrosis is rich in collagen that stains strongly with a trichrome stain (fig. 3-10, left). The fibroblastic foci consist of a loose type of fibrosis that contains myofibroblasts within a stroma that has few collagen fibers. The Movat stain (fig. 3-10, right) highlights these fibroblastic foci. While connective tissue stains are not necessary for diagnosis, they nicely demonstrate the different types of fibrous connective tissue. Smooth muscle proliferation may be found in areas of dense fibrotic

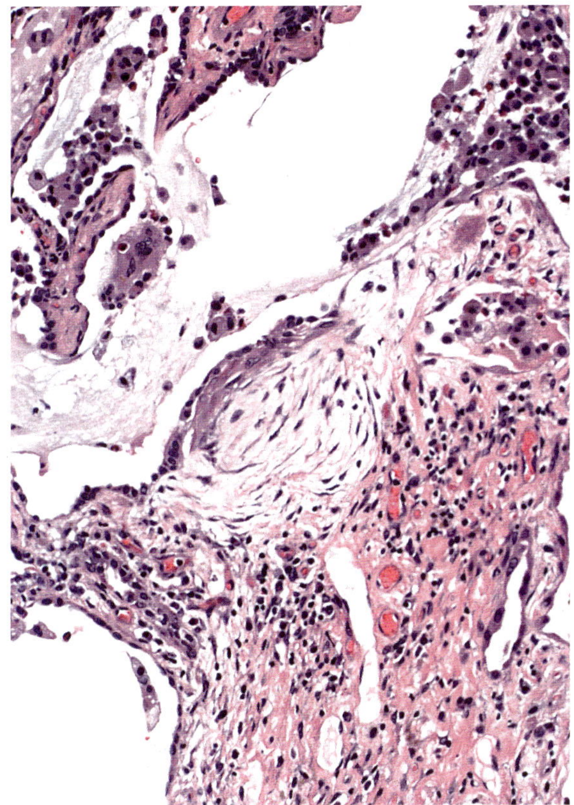

Figure 3-8

USUAL INTERSTITIAL PNEUMONIA PATTERN

The dense collagenous scar is juxtaposed with a fibroblastic focus of loose organizing connective tissue.

Table 3-5

HISTOLOGIC FEATURES OF USUAL INTERSTITIAL PNEUMONIA PATTERN*

Major Features

- Patchy lung involvement
- Frequent subpleural, paraseptal, and/or peribronchiolar distribution
- Dense fibrosis causing remodeling of lung architecture with frequent "honeycomb" fibrosis
- Fibroblastic foci scattered at the edges of the dense scars
- Interstitial inflammation, mild to moderate

Minor Features

- Focal alveolar macrophage accumulation
- Lymphoid aggregates
- Smooth muscle proliferation
- Vascular medial and intimal thickening
- Bronchiolar metaplasia
- Pleuritis, mild/moderate
- Pleural fibrosis, mild/moderate
- Type 2 pneumocyte hyperplasia
- Subpleural fatty metaplasia
- Squamous metaplasia
- Dilated pleural or septal lymphatics
- Alveolar neutrophils
- Cholesterol clefts
- Rare interstitial or alveolar eosinophils
- Metaplastic bone or calcification
- Hyaline cytoplasmic inclusions in pneumocytes
- Focal alveolar fibrin
- Subpleural blebs

Pertinent Negative Findings

- Lack of active lesions of other interstitial diseases (sarcoidosis or Langerhans' histiocytosis)
- Lack of marked interstitial chronic inflammation
- Granulomas: inconspicuous or absent
- Lack of substantial inorganic dust deposits (asbestos bodies [except for carbon black pigment])

*Data from reference 62.

3-11). When severe, the term *muscular cirrhosis of the lung* has been applied (90).

Secondary vascular changes are common and consist of intimal fibrosis and medial thickening (fig. 3-12) (166). The fibrotic thickened alveolar septa tend to be lined by hyperplastic cuboidal epithelial cells or a bronchiolar type of epithelium (fig. 3-13). The epithelial cells overlying the fibroblastic foci are usually attenuated and flat. Occasionally, the pneumocytes lining the alveolar walls are hyperplastic, with abundant cytoplasm, large hyperchromatic nuclei, and prominent nucleoli. Rarely, eosinophilic cytoplasmic inclusions similar to those seen in Mallory's hyaline are present (see fig. 2-7) (168). Bronchiolar or cuboidal epithelium usually lines areas of cystic remodeling or honeycomb fibrosis. Squamous metaplasia may be seen. Interstitial inflammation is usually mild to moderate, consisting mostly of lymphocytes and a few plasma cells. Scattered lymphoid aggregates may be present. Interstitial mast cells, eosinophils, and neutrophils are usually inconspicuous. Occasionally, moderate numbers of interstitial and/or alveolar eosinophils may be seen, but they are typically focal and fall short of eosinophilic pneumonia. Alveolar macrophages are often present, particularly if the patient is a

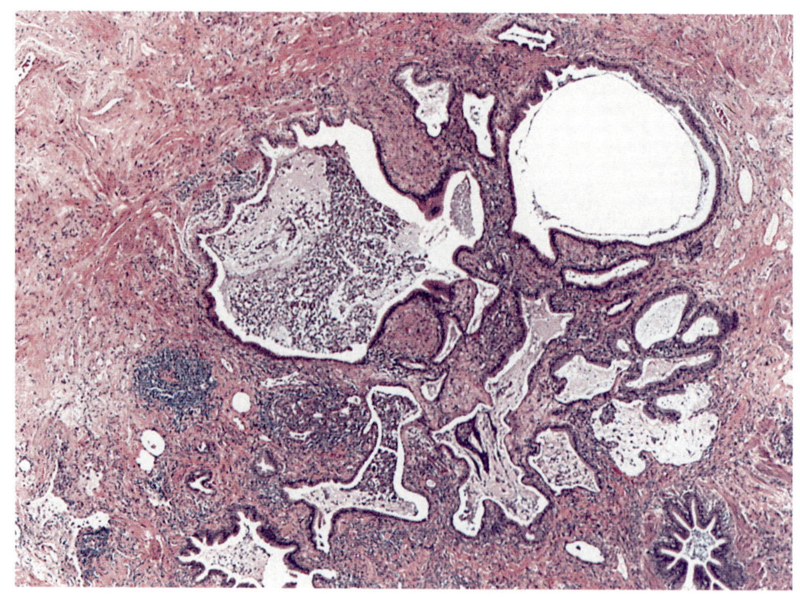

Figure 3-9

USUAL INTERSTITIAL PNEUMONIA PATTERN

Microscopic honeycombing consists of dense fibrosis and complete loss of lung architecture that is replaced by cysts of varying size. The cysts are lined by a metaplastic cuboidal to bronchiolar type of epithelium.

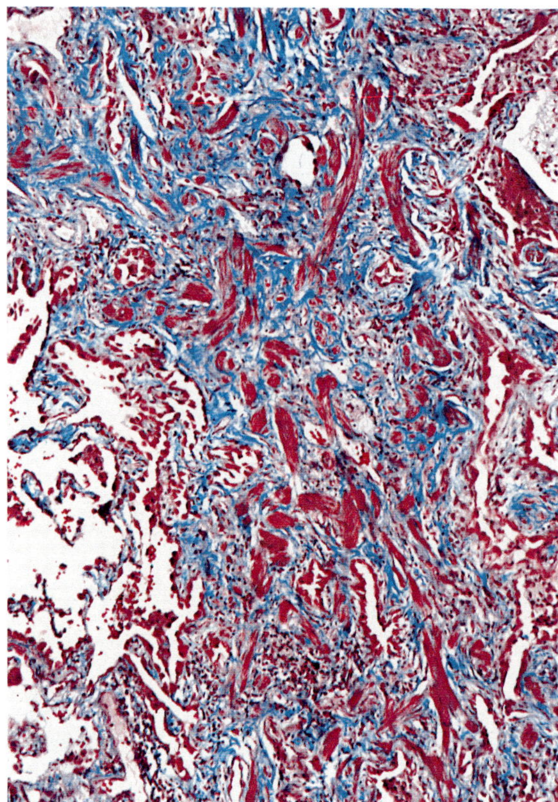

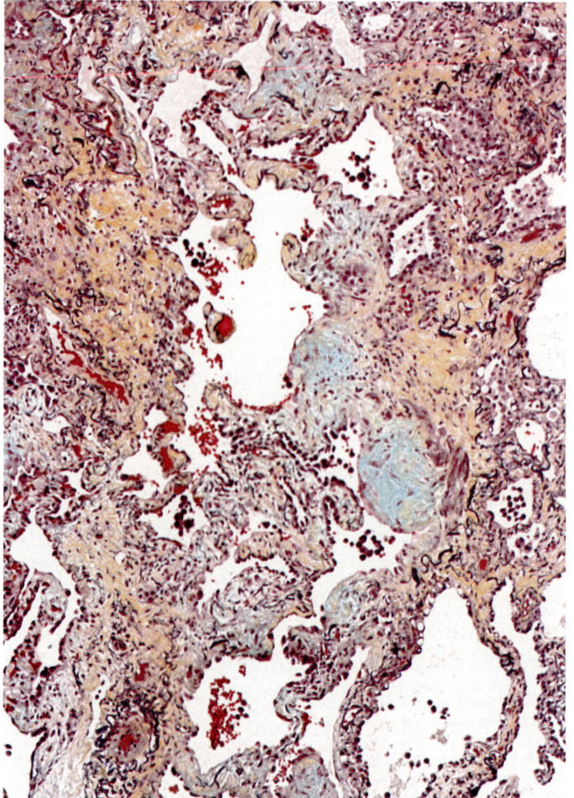

Figure 3-10

USUAL INTERSTITIAL PNEUMONIA PATTERN

Left: The dark blue of the Masson trichrome stain highlights the abundant interstitial dense collagen.
Right: The Movat stain highlights the fibroblastic foci (green) in contrast to the dense fibrosis (yellow).

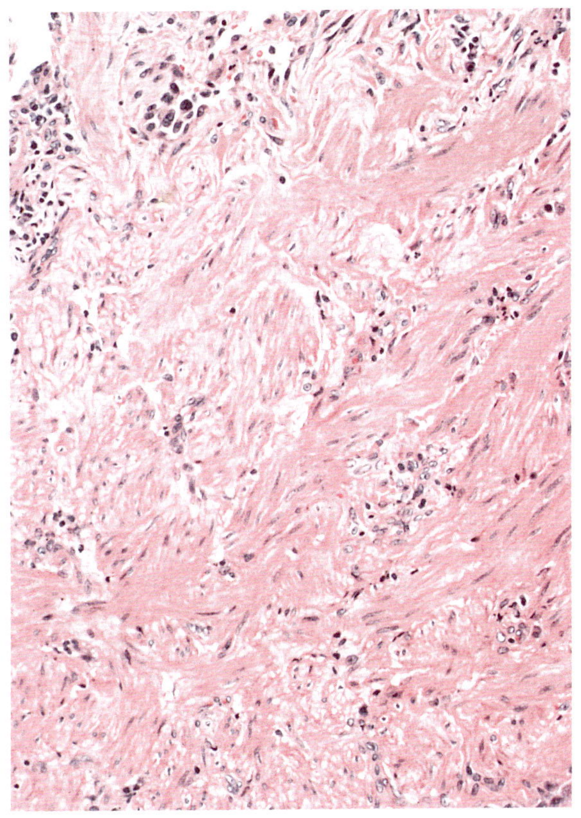

Figure 3-11

USUAL INTERSTITIAL PNEUMONIA PATTERN

Prominent proliferation of smooth muscle is present in this area of scarring.

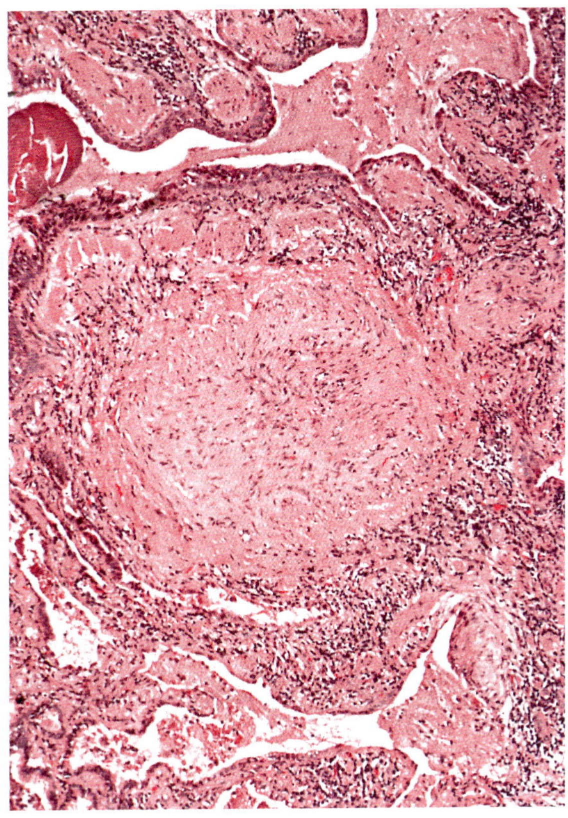

Figure 3-12

USUAL INTERSTITIAL PNEUMONIA PATTERN

Marked medial thickening and intimal proliferation reflect hypertensive vascular changes.

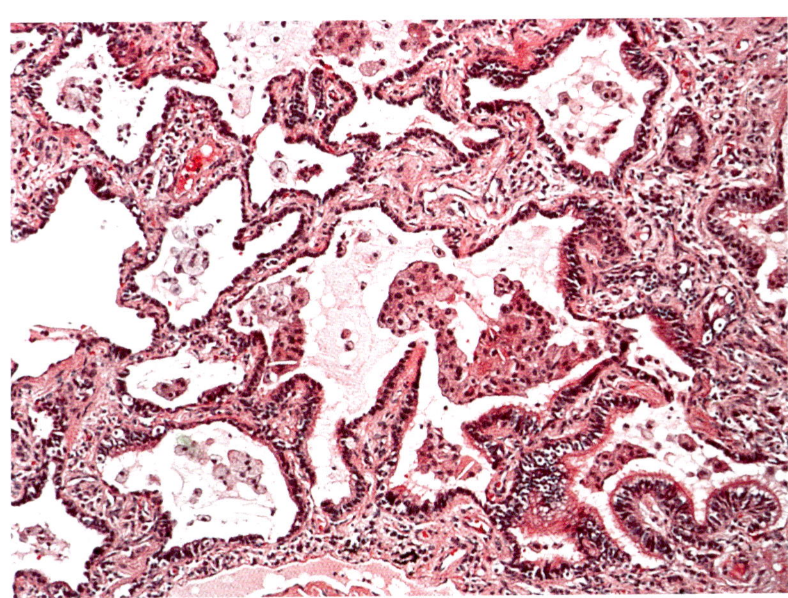

Figure 3-13

USUAL INTERSTITIAL PNEUMONIA PATTERN

There is extensive proliferation of bronchiolar epithelium.

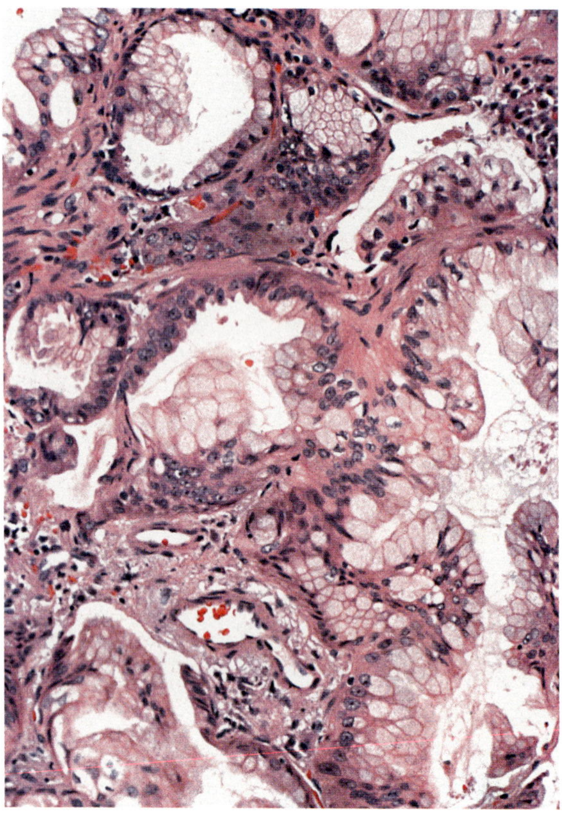

Figure 3-14

USUAL INTERSTITIAL PNEUMONIA PATTERN: WITH ADENOCARCINOMA

In addition to a UIP pattern, this case shows a very exuberant, atypical epithelial proliferation. The glandular proliferation shows micropapillary growth within the lumens of the air-spaces and prominently mucinous epithelial cells with foci of invasion that indicate adenocarcinoma rather than a reactive process.

cigarette smoker. If prominent, the question of DIP or RB-ILD may be raised. An occasional giant cell or a rare, isolated granuloma may be seen, but their presence should raise the possibility of hypersensitivity pneumonitis or collagen vascular disease. In rare cases, lung biopsies show a UIP pattern and many noncaseating granulomas, but the true nature of this disorder and its relationship to conventional UIP versus fibrosing sarcoid, hypersensitivity pneumonitis, or collagen vascular disease remains to be determined. The cysts in areas of microscopic honeycombing may be empty or they may contain mucus and inflammatory cells, particularly macrophages or neutrophils.

There is a spectrum of severity of the fibrosis seen in the UIP pattern (166). When the fibrosis is very extensive and no normal lung is obtained in the lung biopsy, one may only be able to identify the pattern of endstage or honeycomb fibrosis (fig. 3-9). This may reflect a sampling problem if the surgeon took the biopsy from an area of very fibrotic lung. In order to make a definitive pathologic diagnosis of a UIP pattern, areas of normal lung must be present in the biopsy specimen. This is important since a UIP pattern can be seen as the advanced phase of other interstitial disorders. Therefore, areas of relatively normal lung must be examined to exclude the presence of active lesions of other interstitial lung diseases such as sarcoidosis or pulmonary Langerhans' cell histiocytosis. In some patients with a UIP pattern on lung biopsy, specimens from additional lobes of the lung may not meet histologic criteria for UIP and may suggest other patterns such as NSIP. In such a situation, the overall histologic diagnosis should be UIP (95,165).

Lung carcinomas of all histologic types develop in 13 to 31 percent of patients with IPF (125,148). It can be especially difficult to separate prominent reactive epithelial proliferations from well-differentiated adenocarcinomas (fig. 3-14). Exuberant micropapillary proliferation of glandular epithelium, relatively sparse inflammation, prominent mucinous epithelium, invasive growth, and cytologic atypia all favor an adenocarcinoma.

One complication that has received little attention in the pathologic literature is that of acute exacerbation of IPF (71,119,120,176). A small percentage of IPF patients have an accelerated phase of their disease, and after full evaluation and lung biopsy no specific cause, such as an opportunistic infection, is demonstrated. In some cases, patients have had a previous lung biopsy, showing the classic features of a UIP pattern and a second biopsy is performed during the acute illness. In other cases, there is a clinical history consistent with a preexisting UIP pattern and the biopsy is first performed during the acute exacerbation. Usually, lung biopsies show two major patterns: a chronic underlying fibrosis with a UIP pattern and a superimposed acute lesion (fig. 3-15). Several types of acute lesions have been described including

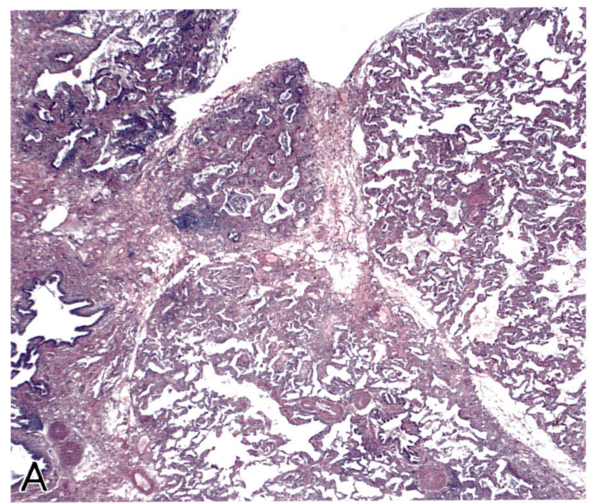

Figure 3-15

USUAL INTERSTITIAL PNEUMONIA PATTERN: ACCELERATED DECLINE

An underlying UIP pattern is present (A), with a superimposed acute lung injury pattern (right), which consists of prominent organizing pneumonia (B), with focal hyaline membranes (C).

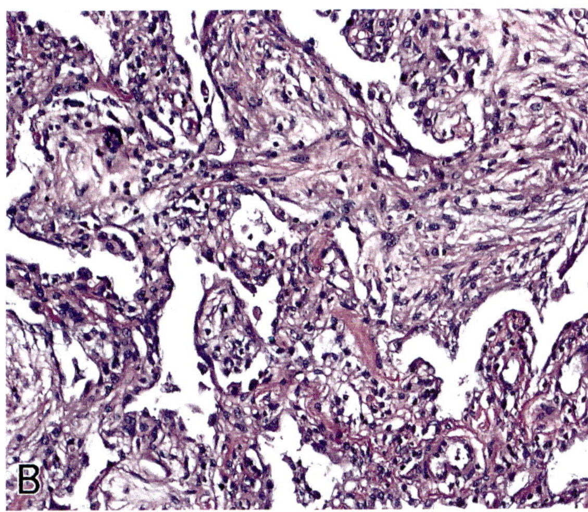

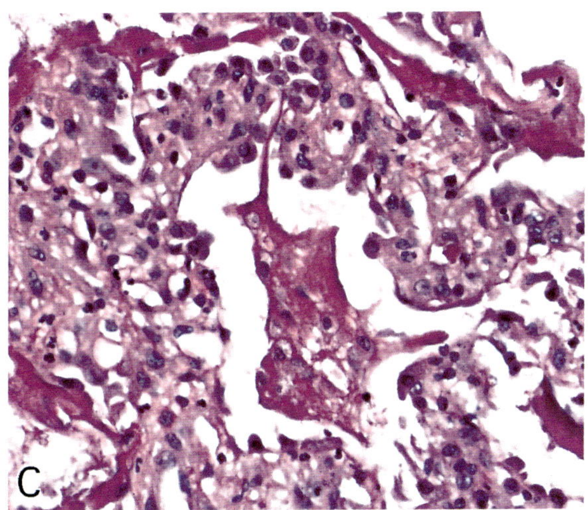

organizing pneumonia (fig. 3-15B), DAD (fig. 3-15C), and hemorrhage with capillaritis (71, 119,176). It may be very difficult to differentiate the chronic from the acute histologic lesions without good clinical correlation.

Histologic Heterogeneity in Different Lobes of Lung. Flaherty et al. (95) recently demonstrated that there is histologic heterogeneity among biopsies from multiple lobes of the lung in patients with IPF. In 26 percent of patients where UIP was found in at least one lobe, a NSIP pattern was found in a separate lobe. Patients with a UIP pattern in all lobes were categorized as having concordant UIP; those with a pattern of UIP in at least one lobe but a NSIP pattern in another lobe were categorized as having discordant UIP. These findings emphasize the importance of taking specimens from more than one lobe of lung at the time of surgical lung biopsy. It also explains some of the difficulty in separating patients with UIP from those with NSIP.

Correlations between Histology and Prognostic or Clinical Parameters. A number of studies have attempted to identify histologic features that predict clinical progression and outcome for patients with IPF (159,169,175). Unfortunately, most of them have not been based on the current concept of IPF which emphasizes the importance of separating the UIP pattern from other DPLDs. Therefore, the suggestion that patients with a cellular pattern on lung biopsy have a better prognosis than those with a fibrotic pattern may reflect differences in survival between patients with a UIP pattern versus a DIP or NSIP pattern. What is needed are studies that examine histologic predictors of survival based on series of patients with careful histopathologic classification of their lung biopsy findings according to current concepts.

A number of correlations have been made between histologic findings on lung biopsy and various clinical parameters. Kanematsu et al. (111) showed a correlation between clubbing and prominent smooth muscle proliferation in the fibrotic portions of the lung in patients with IPF and a UIP pattern of fibrosis ($p<0.01$). Cherniack et al. (87) found DLCO correlated with "desquamation" ($p=0.003$) and total pathology scores ($p=0.0004$) while TLC ($p=0.04$) and FVC ($p=0.0001$) correlated with a cellularity factor score. Watters et al. (169) demonstrated that the total pathology score correlated with a composite clinical-radiographic-physiologic score ($p<0.001$). Gallium-67 citrate scanning was found by Line et al. (130) to correlate with the degree of interstitial cellularity ($p<0.05$) and the degree of alveolar cellularity ($p<0.005$). Travis et al. (166) found that honeycombing ($p=0.049$) or dense interstitial inflammation ($p=0.045$) involving 60 percent or more of the biopsy specimen, and intrapleural fat ($p=0.01$) correlated with a poor prognosis in patients with idiopathic UIP. Multivariate analysis using the Cox method showed that the presence of intrapleural fat ($p=0.0143$) was independent of the other significant histologic factors. Finally, Fulmer et al. (96) showed a high correlation between exercise-induced changes in arterial oxygen pressure per liter of oxygen consumed and the degree of fibrosis ($p<0.001$) as well as the degree of cellularity ($p=0.009$).

In the study by Flaherty et al. (95) on histologic variability among lung biopsies from multiple lobes in IPF patients, patients with concordant UIP were older (63 ± 9 years) than those with discordant UIP (57 ± 12 years), fibrosing NSIP (56 ± 11 years), and cellular NSIP (50 ± 9 years). Similarly, patients with concordant UIP had a lower TLC and DLCO. Survival was better in patients with NSIP compared to both UIP groups ($p<0.001$). Discordant UIP patients had better survival than those with concordant UIP earlier in follow-up ($p=0.09$), although the survival curves converged near the end of the follow-up period. These findings support the conclusion that patients with a histologic pattern of UIP in any lobe should be classified as having UIP.

Pathogenesis. The etiology of IPF/UIP is unknown, but viral, genetic, and immunologic factors are thought to play a role. Evidence that genetic factors are involved include cases of familial IPF (131), reports of human leukocyte antigen (HLA) associations (97,133), and the presence of pulmonary fibrosis in patients with inherited syndromes such as neurofibromatosis (135) and Hermansky-Pudlak syndrome (157). A viral etiology is suggested by presentation with a flu-like illness in a number of patients (115), and reports of associations with hepatitis C (140), Epstein-Barr virus (92), and adenovirus (104,124). The frequency of the UIP histologic pattern in patients with collagen vascular diseases is strong evidence that immunologic factors are important in the pathogenesis. Furthermore, patients with IPF have circulating autoantibodies such as antinuclear antibodies (7 to 25 percent), rheumatoid factor (14 percent), and cryoimmunoglobulins (41 percent) (115).

It has been speculated that after an initial injury, immune complexes activate alveolar macrophages to produce a variety of factors including chemotactic factors that attract neutrophils. Immune complexes can be found in BAL specimens, alveolar epithelial cells, and the luminal side of the capillary walls (115). These events initiate an ongoing fibrogenic process of UIP that is controlled by a variety of growth factors (74), cytokines (70), metalloproteinases, and tissue inhibitors of metalloproteinase (103) that have very complex interactions (138).

Considerable evidence supports the concept that the fibroblastic foci in IPF/UIP represent the leading edges of ongoing microscopic lung injury that are the sites of destruction of the lung architecture, collapse of alveolar walls, and deposition of dense collagen (75,84,85,103, 113,122,123,147). Thus, these countless fibroblastic foci that are diffusely distributed throughout the lungs account for the progressive destruction of the lungs that occurs in UIP. A number of studies have focused on various growth factors, cytokines, integrins, oncogenes, tumor suppressor genes, metalloproteinases, and metalloproteinase inhibitors that participate in the pathogenesis of UIP (70,80,82,103,105,110,114,121, 158). These fibroblastic foci not only reflect the temporal heterogeneity of UIP but they also represent sites of progressive ongoing injury, in contrast to the process that occurs in DAD, NSIP, COP, and DIP, which are thought to follow lung injury at a single point in time resulting in connective tissue of a uniform age (113).

Differential Diagnosis. The differential diagnosis for the UIP pattern includes histologic and etiologic considerations (Table 3-6). This requires a careful clinical as well as pathologic approach. The clinical history should be investigated for drug intake, inhaled antigen exposure, and occupational exposure to minerals such as beryllium, cobalt, asbestos, silicosis, and aluminum. In addition, clinical and serologic manifestations of collagen vascular diseases should be investigated.

The most important issue in assessing lung biopsies for interstitial lung disease is determining whether a UIP or a non-UIP pattern is present. The histologic pattern of UIP must be separated from the patterns of NSIP, DIP, OP, and DAD, since the clinical course and management is so different (Table 3-7). When the classic UIP pattern is present, it is usually not difficult to separate it from the other patterns. The issue of separating the fibrosing NSIP pattern from UIP is often the most challenging, and this is addressed in detail later in this chapter. Due to this difficulty, there are varying levels of certainty in a pathologist's assessment as to whether a UIP pattern is present or not. It can be useful to communicate this level of certainty to clinicians in a comment in the pathology report: 1) Definite UIP pattern, 2) Probable UIP pattern, 3) Possible UIP pattern, 4) Definitely not a UIP pattern. When the pathologic diagnosis is difficult, careful clinical and radiologic correlation is advised.

The separation of the UIP and DIP patterns is usually straightforward, but some UIP cases have prominent alveolar macrophages and some DIP cases may show some focal scarring or honeycomb changes. A marked interstitial inflammatory infiltrate or the presence of granulomatous inflammation should raise the consideration of hypersensitivity pneumonitis, pneumoconiosis, drug-induced pneumonitis, infection, or collagen vascular disease. The pathologist can help in identifying dust deposits such as asbestos bodies or infectious agents. The latter may require special stains for organisms, particularly for *Pneumocystis carinii*. If there is a suspicion of asbestos exposure, iron stains should be performed unless asbestos bodies are seen on hematoxylin and eosin (H&E)–stained sections. Polarization microscopy may help identify birefringent particles that could suggest significant dust deposits; however, a few birefringent particles may be found in lung biopsies from patients with UIP.

Patchy scars with a stellate configuration that are situated on bronchioles should suggest the possibility of a fibrotic phase of Langerhans' cell histiocytosis. The combination of airspace organization and granulomas with peribronchiolar inflammation should suggest hypersensitivity pneumonitis. Prominent giant cell formation in alveolar macrophages should raise concern for giant cell interstitial pneumonia or hard metal pneumoconiosis. Occasionally, honeycomb changes and fibrosis associated with bronchiectasis can be confused with a UIP pattern.

Treatment and Prognosis. The mortality rate for patients with IPF is estimated to be 3.3 in men and 2.5 in women per 100,000 population in Japan (107). Most current studies report that the mean length of survival from the time

Table 3-6

HISTOLOGIC AND ETIOLOGIC DIFFERENTIAL DIAGNOSES FOR USUAL INTERSTITIAL PNEUMONIA PATTERN*

Histologic Patterns
- Nonspecific interstitial pneumonia, fibrosing pattern
- Desquamative interstitial pneumonia pattern
- Fibrotic phases of other interstitial disorders
  - Langerhans' cell histiocytosis
  - Hypersensitivity pneumonitis pattern
  - Diffuse alveolar damage

Etiologic Possibilities
- Collagen vascular disease
- Drug-induced pneumonitis
- Radiation pneumonitis
- Familial idiopathic pulmonary fibrosis
- Hermansky-Pudlak syndrome
- Pneumoconiosis (asbestosis)
- Hypersensitivity pneumonitis
- Idiopathic usual interstitial pneumonia (clinicopathologic term: idiopathic pulmonary fibrosis/cryptogenic fibrosing alveolitis)

*Data from reference 62.

Table 3-7

CLINICAL, RADIOLOGIC, AND HISTOLOGIC DIFFERENTIAL DIAGNOSIS OF IDIOPATHIC PULMONARY FIBROSIS, CRYPTOGENIC ORGANIZING PNEUMONIA, AND ACUTE INTERSTITIAL PNEUMONIA[a]

Feature	IPF/UIP[b]	COP/OP	AIP/DAD
Clinical Presentation			
Age, mean (range)	64 years	56 years	50 years
Duration of symptoms	1–3 years	1–6 months	1–4 weeks
Mechanical ventilation	Rare	Rare	Yes
HRCT			
Main findings	Irregular lines, honeycombing	Consolidation	Consolidation
Predominant distribution	Middle and lower lung zones, subpleural in about 90% of of cases	Patchy, peribronchial, or subpleural in about 60% of cases	Middle and lower lung zones; dependent lung regions
Histology			
Distribution	Patchy, subpleural, paraseptal	Patchy	Diffuse
Hyaline membranes	No	No	Yes
Temporal appearance	Heterogeneous	Uniform	Uniform
Fibroblastic foci	Characteristic, at edge of scars	Absent	Absent
Fibroblastic proliferation	Focal	Patchy, airspace	Diffuse
Interstitial	Focal	No	Yes
Airspace	Minimal	Yes	Sometimes
Type 2 cell proliferation	Focal	Focal	Extensive, diffuse
Dense fibrosis	Characteristic	Absent	Only in late fibrotic phase
Thrombi	No	No	Yes
Clinical Outcome	20–50% 5-year survival	90% 5-year survival	10–50% recovery
Response to steroids	Poor	Excellent	Poor

[a]Compiled and modified from references 112 and 143.
[b]IPF = Idiopathic pulmonary fibrosis/UIP = usual interstitial pneumonia pattern; COP = cryptogenic organizing pneumonia/OP = organizing pneumonia pattern; AIP = acute interstitial pneumonia/DAD = diffuse alveolar damage; HRCT = high-resolution computed tomography.

of diagnosis varies between 3.2 and 5.0 years (73, 83,166). Respiratory failure is the most frequent cause of death in patients with IPF, accounting for approximately 40 percent of the deaths (73, 83,166). However, heart failure, bronchogenic carcinoma, ischemic heart disease, infection, and pulmonary emboli represent other common causes of death in these patients (152).

Conventional management of IPF is primarily based on the concept that suppressing inflammation prevents progression to fibrosis (134,162). However, the use of aggressive immunosuppressive and cytotoxic treatment regimens has largely failed to reduce the death rate in patients with IPF (91,132,134). Only lung transplantation appears beneficial in selected patients (100,141). Future therapies should aim at preventing or inhibiting the fibroproliferative response, and enhancing normal alveolar reepithelialization (162). Novel therapies such as gamma interferon (177) and pirfenidone (149,154) show some promise.

Some IPF patients have an accelerated decline or acute exacerbation of their underlying disease, with a rapid downhill clinical course (71, 120). Typically, the patient develops acute, fulminant respiratory failure, often accompanied by fever, elevation of the erythrocyte sedimentation rate, marked increase in dyspnea, and new opacities that often have an "alveolar" character radiologically. A small percentage of patients may respond to pulse systemic corticosteroid therapy. This condition has a very poor prognosis, and death within 1 week is not unusual.

It is not clear whether patients with UIP associated with collagen vascular disease have a similar or different clinical course. However, it has been shown that the prognosis of patients with progressive systemic sclerosis with lung fibrosis is better than that seen in lone IPF/UIP, even when the patients are controlled for the severity of disease (170,173). This needs to be studied based on current concepts of classification since most of the existing literature predates the updated approach of separating the NSIP from the UIP pattern.

NONSPECIFIC INTERSTITIAL PNEUMONIA, CELLULAR AND FIBROSING PATTERNS

Definition. Nonspecific interstitial pneumonia (NSIP) is an idiopathic interstitial pneumonia with a histologic appearance that does not conform to the characteristic features of UIP, DIP, RB-ILD, DAD, or COP. The main histologic feature of NSIP is the temporally uniform, homogeneous appearance of either inflammation or fibrosis. Most cases of NSIP are of unknown etiology. However, this histologic pattern can be found in association with a number of processes, especially the connective tissue diseases, drug-induced ILD, or chronic hypersensitivity pneumonitis.

It has long been recognized that a substantial proportion of lung biopsies from patients with DPLD of unknown cause show histologic features that do not meet the criteria for one of the major idiopathic interstitial pneumonias, i.e., UIP, DIP, BOOP, AIP, or RB-ILD (190,195). Often, despite the absence of key features, these cases are indiscriminately called UIP and included among the cases of IPF (or CFA). In several IPF studies, many of these cases are identified as the "cellular" phase of UIP, and patients have a better response to corticosteroid therapy and an improved prognosis (183,203,206).

Historical Perspective. The term NSIP was first used to describe noninfectious interstitial pneumonitis in HIV-infected patients (187, 199,202). In 1990, Kitaichi (195) proposed the term "unclassified interstitial pneumonia" for cases of idiopathic interstitial pneumonia that could not be classified as one of the major categories of UIP, DIP, BOOP, or AIP. He suggested that this category be added to the group of idiopathic interstitial pneumonias. In 1994, Katzenstein et al. (190) reported on a series of 64 patients with similar lung biopsy findings and proposed that these cases be called "nonspecific interstitial pneumonia/fibrosis (NSIP)." They showed that the histologic pattern of NSIP occurred in a wide variety of clinical settings and exposures (Table 3-8). Subsequently, the utility of the concept of NSIP gained credence as it was recognized that patients with this pattern had distinctive differences in clinical presentation, HRCT findings, bronchoalveolar cellular profiles, responsiveness to treatment, and prognosis compared to those with IPF/UIP, the lesion with which it was most often confused (178,181,182,185,188,193,194,197,198,201,205).

The term NSIP is problematic in that it implies that the histopathologic findings are "nonspecific." In early descriptions, it was

Table 3-8

UNDERLYING CONDITIONS OR EXPOSURES IN NONSPECIFIC INTERSTITIAL PNEUMONIA[a]

Connective Tissue Disease (n=10, 16%)
- Rheumatoid arthritis (n=4)
- Systemic lupus erythematosus (n=2)
- Polymyositis (n=2)
- Scleroderma (n=1)
- Sjögren's syndrome (n=1)

Other Diseases (n=4, 6%)
- Primary biliary cirrhosis (n=1)
- Hashimoto's thyroiditis (n=1)
- Acute glomerulonephritis (n=1)
- Chronic renal failure (n=1)

Exposures (n=11, 17%)
- Birds (n=2) 1 parrot – proven HP[b]; 1-canary
- Wood stove (n=1)
- Occupational exposures:
  - Grain dust in brewery (n=1), coal and ash in coal handler (n=1), farmer (n=1), veterinarian (n=1), paper factory worker (n=1), garment industry worker (n=2)
- Transfusions for factor IX deficiency (HIV negative) (n=1)
- Symptoms after cleaning jacuzzi (n=1)
- Drug exposure (n=1 each): hydralazine (apresoline), gold, penicillamine

Diffuse Alveolar Damage/Acute Respiratory Distress Syndrome (n=2)

[a]Data from reference 190.
[b]HP = hypersensitivity pneumonitis.

stated that NSIP "should not be considered a specific disease, because it can have a variety of etiologies, including connective tissue diseases, organic dust or other exposures, and prior acute lung injury. Less often, it may reflect a nonrepresentative biopsy of another process"(190). Therefore, there is a lingering tendency to use this term for any interstitial process with atypical features. Also, identification of this pattern may reflect a sampling error as a result of an inadequate lung biopsy and failure to diagnose another process, for example, hypersensitivity pneumonitis. Another problem relates to the description of lung biopsies, especially bronchoscopic biopsies, as "nonspecific." Pathologists must be careful with the use of the term "nonspecific" in a surgical pathology report to avoid confusion with NSIP. A more appropriate term is "nondiagnostic."

Although some investigators argue that NSIP is merely early UIP and not a separate disease, the term NSIP now defines a clinicopathologic subgroup of idiopathic interstitial pneumonias distinct from UIP (178,181,182, 185,188,193,194,197,198,201,205). The ATS/ ERS International Consensus Panel for Classification of Interstitial Lung Disease felt this term was already too ingrained in the literature to change to an alternative term (204). However, due to uncertainty among pulmonologists about this group of patients, the clinical term proposed was *NSIP, provisional.* This implies the need for further evaluation of these patients, realizing that there may be other subsets identified in the future based on clinical, radiologic, and pathologic studies. The varying survival data in currently published studies of patients with NSIP suggest differing interpretation by pathologists of the diagnostic criteria, indicating the need for a better consensus on this issue.

One of the most important aspects of the initial NSIP proposal was the concept of grouping lung biopsies on the basis of the degree of cellularity and fibrosis (190). However, in some of the subsequent papers and reviews of this subject there has been little emphasis on distinguishing between cellular and fibrosing patterns (178,181,189,191,194,201).When using the term NSIP for a clinicopathologic diagnosis, it is important to specify whether it applies to an idiopathic setting (e.g., idiopathic NSIP), or NSIP with underlying disease such as rheumatoid arthritis (e.g., NSIP with associated rheumatoid arthritis).

Clinical Features. The incidence and prevalence of NSIP remain to be defined. However, it appears to be less frequent than UIP but much more common than the other idiopathic interstitial pneumonias (178). The cause of idiopathic NSIP is unknown, but this pattern is becoming well recognized in patients with a variety of systemic diseases, particularly the collagen vascular diseases (181,186). The average duration of illness prior to diagnosis is 8 to 18 months (178,181,182,188,190). The average age ranges from 46 to 57 years (178,181,182,188, 190,201,205), but it can also be found in children (190). It is slightly more common in women. Patients with idiopathic NSIP, cellular pattern, are younger (mean, 39 years, range, 26–50 years) than those with idiopathic UIP ($p=0.006$) and those with idiopathic NSIP, fibrosing pattern (mean, 50 years; range 30 to 71 years; $p = 0.042$) (205). Many of the patients are current or former cigarette smokers (57 to 68 percent) (178,205).

Patients with NSIP present with clinical features that are similar to other idiopathic interstitial pneumonias, especially IPF. The most common symptoms are exertional dyspnea, cough, and fever. Crackles are commonly found on chest examination. Clubbing has been reported in 21 to 40 percent of patients (178,182). Routine laboratory studies are nonspecific. The antinuclear antigen (ANA) and/or rheumatoid factor is positive in a minority of patients (182, 205). BAL shows a modest increase in neutrophils and eosinophils (182). A lymphocytic predominance on BAL examination has been reported and is thought to be helpful in differentiating NSIP from UIP (181,200).

Lung function testing usually reveals a restrictive defect with reduced DLCO (178). Resting arterial blood gases may be normal but exercise gas exchange abnormalities are commonly present (178).

Radiologic Findings. The radiographic and HRCT findings of NSIP are variable and nonspecific. The most common manifestation is areas of consolidation or hazy increased opacity (ground-glass opacities) which may be diffuse but tend to involve mainly the lower lobes (fig.

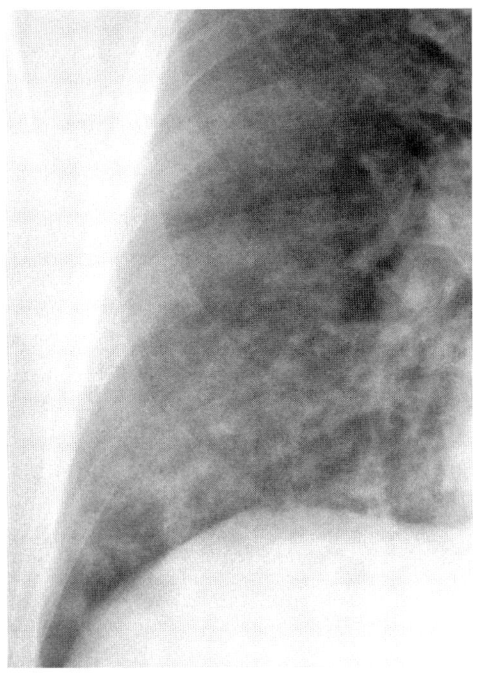

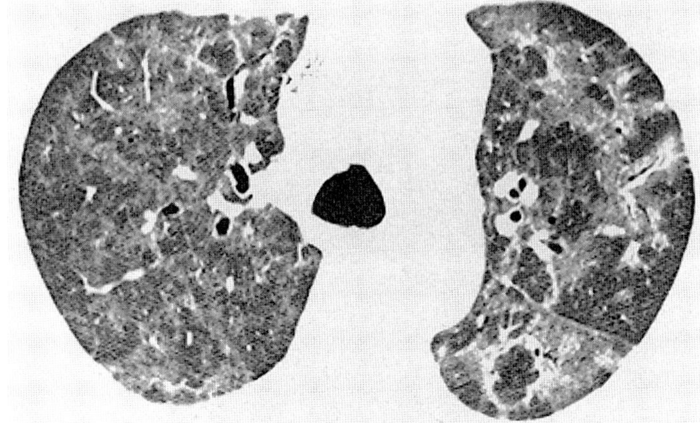

Figure 3-16

NONSPECIFIC INTERSTITIAL PNEUMONIA

Left: Magnified view of the right lower chest in a 61-year-old man with NSIP shows ground-glass opacities and small, poorly defined, patchy areas of consolidation.

Above: HRCT through the upper lobes shows extensive areas of ground-glass attenuation and small areas of consolidation.

3-16, left) (188,193,194,201). Other findings include a reticular pattern or a combination of interstitial and airspace patterns (193,194,201). On HRCT, areas of ground-glass attenuation, which are usually extensive, are seen in virtually all cases (fig. 3-16, above) (188,193,194,201). Although a reticular pattern is commonly present, it is seldom the predominant abnormality (193, 194,201). The radiographic and HRCT findings most commonly mimic those of DIP and hypersensitivity pneumonitis; occasionally, they may resemble those of BOOP or UIP.

Pathologic Findings. NSIP is a diagnosis of exclusion in that the histologic pattern lacks features of UIP, DIP, idiopathic BOOP/COP, and DAD/AIP. It encompasses a broad spectrum of different histologic lesions. Katzenstein et al. (190) described three major subgroups of NSIP based on the lung biopsy findings: cases primarily with interstitial inflammation (group I), those primarily with fibrosis (group III), and those with both inflammation and fibrosis (group II). However, this separation of histologic groups was largely dropped in subsequent writings on NSIP (178,189,191). Nagai et al. (197) separated cellular and fibrosing patterns of NSIP; their cellular cases corresponded to Katzenstein's groups I and II, while their fibrosing cases corresponded to group III. More recently, Travis et al. (205) and Nicholson et al. (198) separated patients with the cellular pattern from those with the fibrosing pattern of NSIP, corresponding to Katzenstein's group I versus groups II and III, respectively (198,205).

The separation of cellular from fibrosing patterns of NSIP is important due to the significantly better prognosis associated with the former pattern (197,198,205). It should be kept in mind that the NSIP, fibrosing pattern, is somewhat of a "wastebasket" and it likely represents a group of miscellaneous non-UIP fibrosing disorders of diverse etiologies.

NSIP, Cellular Pattern. The NSIP, cellular pattern (Table 3-9), consists primarily of mild to moderate, interstitial chronic inflammation, usually with lymphocytes and a few plasma cells (figs. 3-17, 3-18). The lung is usually uniformly involved, but the distribution of the lesions may be patchy. The infiltrate typically involves the alveolar interstitium, but is less severe than the extensive diffuse alveolar septal infiltration observed in LIP. The interstitium around airways, blood vessels, interlobular septa, and pleura may be involved. Intra-alveolar organizing fibrosis (fig. 3-18) may be present, giving a pattern of cellular NSIP and organizing pneumonia. However, there is more interstitial chronic inflammation and more focal organizing pneumonia

Table 3-9

HISTOLOGIC FEATURES OF NONSPECIFIC INTERSTITIAL PNEUMONIA, CELLULAR PATTERN[a]

Major Features
- Mild to moderate interstitial chronic inflammation
- Type 2 pneumocyte hyperplasia in areas of inflammation
- Lung architecture preserved

Minor Features
- Organizing pneumonia
- Lymphoid aggregates
- Alveolar macrophages, focal
- Bronchiolar inflammation
- Bronchiolar fibrosis
- Chronic pleuritis, mild/moderate
- Squamous metaplasia
- Cholesterol clefts
- Thickened arteries

Pertinent Negative Findings
- Dense interstitial fibrosis: inconspicuous or absent
- Honeycomb fibrosis: absent
- Granulomas: inconspicuous or absent
- Eosinophils: inconspicuous or absent
- Lack of viral inclusions and organisms on special stains

[a]Data from reference 205.

than typically seen in the BOOP pattern. Lymphoid aggregates are often present (fig. 3-17).

NSIP, Fibrosing Pattern. The hallmark of the NSIP, fibrosing pattern (Table 3-10), is the presence of dense or loose interstitial fibrosis and the lack of temporal heterogeneity characteristic of UIP (figs. 3-19, 3-20).

Fibroblastic foci, the key lesion that gives the UIP pattern the appearance of temporal heterogeneity, should be absent or inconspicuous. In some cases the pattern of fibrosis is patchy in distribution, causing remodeling of the lung architecture, sometimes with a subpleural distribution. In such cases the lack of fibroblastic foci is especially important in distinguishing fibrosing NSIP from the UIP pattern. Also, the pattern of NSIP shows more diffuse involvement of the lung and greater preservation of alveolar architecture, although the alveolar septal interstitium may be expanded by either dense or loose fibrosis, with or without chronic inflammation. The key feature is that the changes in the affected lung appear to be of the same age or temporally homogeneous (compare with UIP in figures 3-6–3-8). Rare fibroblastic foci may be seen, but they should be inconspicuous and not a part of the intrinsic fibrotic process. Foci of honeycomb fibrosis and

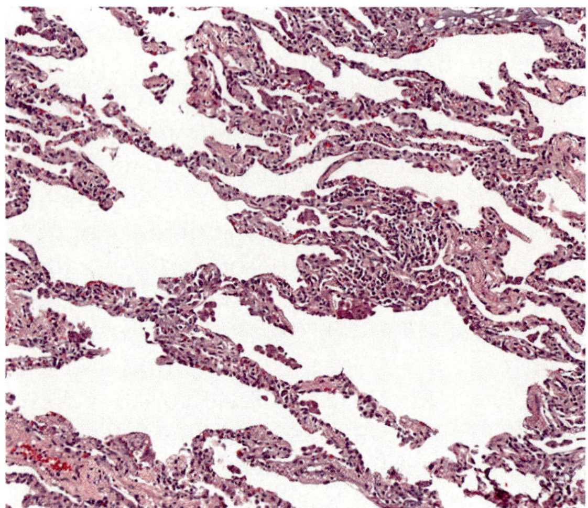

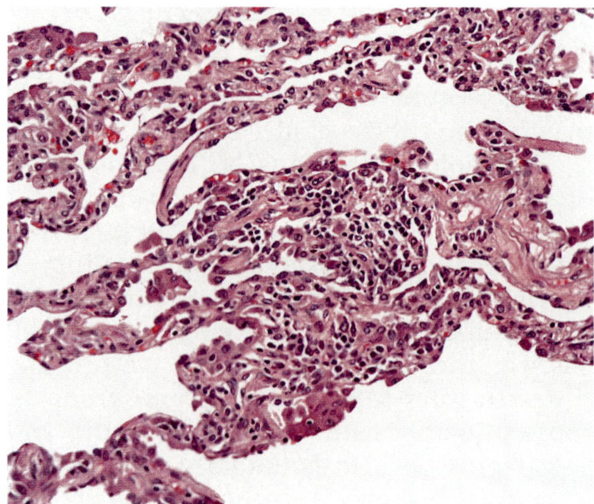

Figure 3-17

NONSPECIFIC INTERSTITIAL PNEUMONIA: CELLULAR PATTERN

Left: Mild to moderate interstitial chronic inflammation causes thickening of the alveolar walls. Some alveolar walls are spared. The architecture of the lung is preserved and there is no increase in dense fibrosis.

Right: The interstitium of the alveolar wall is thickened by inflammation consisting mostly of lymphocytes and plasma cells.

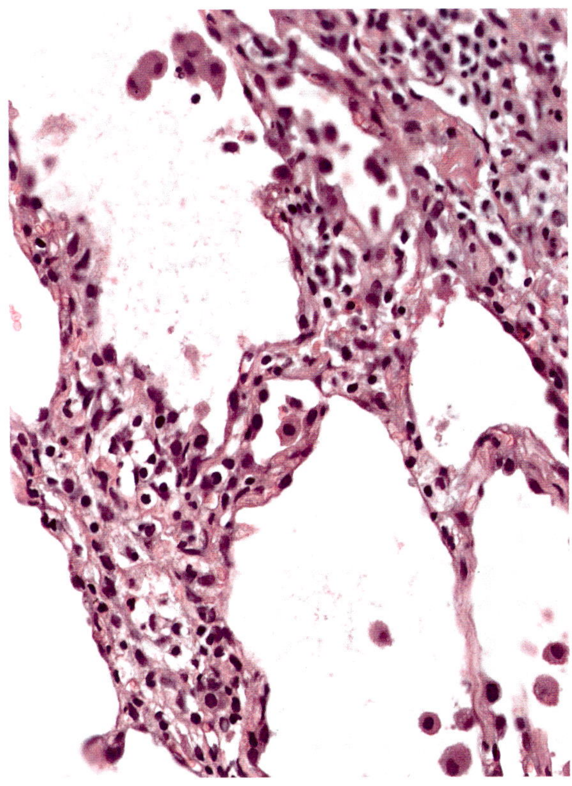

Figure 3-18

NONSPECIFIC INTERSTITIAL PNEUMONIA: CELLULAR PATTERN

There is a mild to moderate interstitial chronic inflammatory infiltrate.

proliferation of interstitial smooth muscle may be seen, but are usually not as prominent and frequent as in UIP. If either fibroblastic foci or honeycomb fibrosis is present, the possibility of a UIP pattern should be carefully excluded. Lymphoid aggregates, chronic pleuritis, and pleural fibrosis are common, and metaplastic bone may be present.

A subset of patients, usually cigarette smokers, may show emphysema, respiratory bronchiolitis, and dense eosinophilic fibrosis causing thickening of alveolar walls. This differs from DIP in that it is patchy and does not show extensive alveolar macrophage accumulation (fig. 3-19C).

Interstitial chronic inflammation is usually mild to moderate and consists mainly of lymphocytes and some plasma cells. Some cases show a fibrosing and cellular pattern with prominent interstitial chronic inflammation

Table 3-10

HISTOLOGIC FEATURES OF NONSPECIFIC INTERSTITIAL PNEUMONIA, FIBROSING PATTERN[a]

Major Features
- Dense or loose interstitial fibrosis lacking the temporal heterogeneity and/or patchy features of UIP
- Lung architecture is often preserved
- Interstitial chronic inflammation: mild or moderate

Minor Features
- Type 2 pneumocyte hyperplasia
- Bronchiolar metaplasia
- Vascular medial and intimal thickening
- Lymphoid aggregates
- Pleural fibrosis or pleuritis
- Bronchiolar fibrosis or bronchiolar inflammation
- Squamous metaplasia
- Intrapleural fatty metaplasia
- Rare eosinophils: alveolar or interstitial
- Alveolar neutrophils
- Atypical pneumocyte hyperplasia
- Organizing pneumonia pattern: focal, inconspicuous, or absent
- Cholesterol clefts
- Metaplastic bone
- Focal alveolar fibrin
- Blue bodies
- Metaplastic calcification

Pertinent Negative Findings
- Fibroblastic foci: inconspicuous or absent—this is especially important in cases with patchy involvement and subpleural or paraseptal distribution
- Lack of airway centricity
- Eosinophils: inconspicuous or absent
- Granulomas: inconspicuous or absent
- Lack of viral inclusions and organisms on special stains

[a]Data from reference 205.

(fig. 3-20). However, due to the many clinical and pathologic similarities between cases showing a fibrosing and cellular or just a fibrosing pattern of NSIP, the single category of NSIP, fibrosing pattern, is used (205).

Differential Diagnosis. *NSIP, Cellular Pattern.* The histologic differential diagnosis for the cellular NSIP pattern includes hypersensitivity pneumonitis, fibrosing NSIP pattern, organizing pneumonia pattern, LIP, and resolving DAD

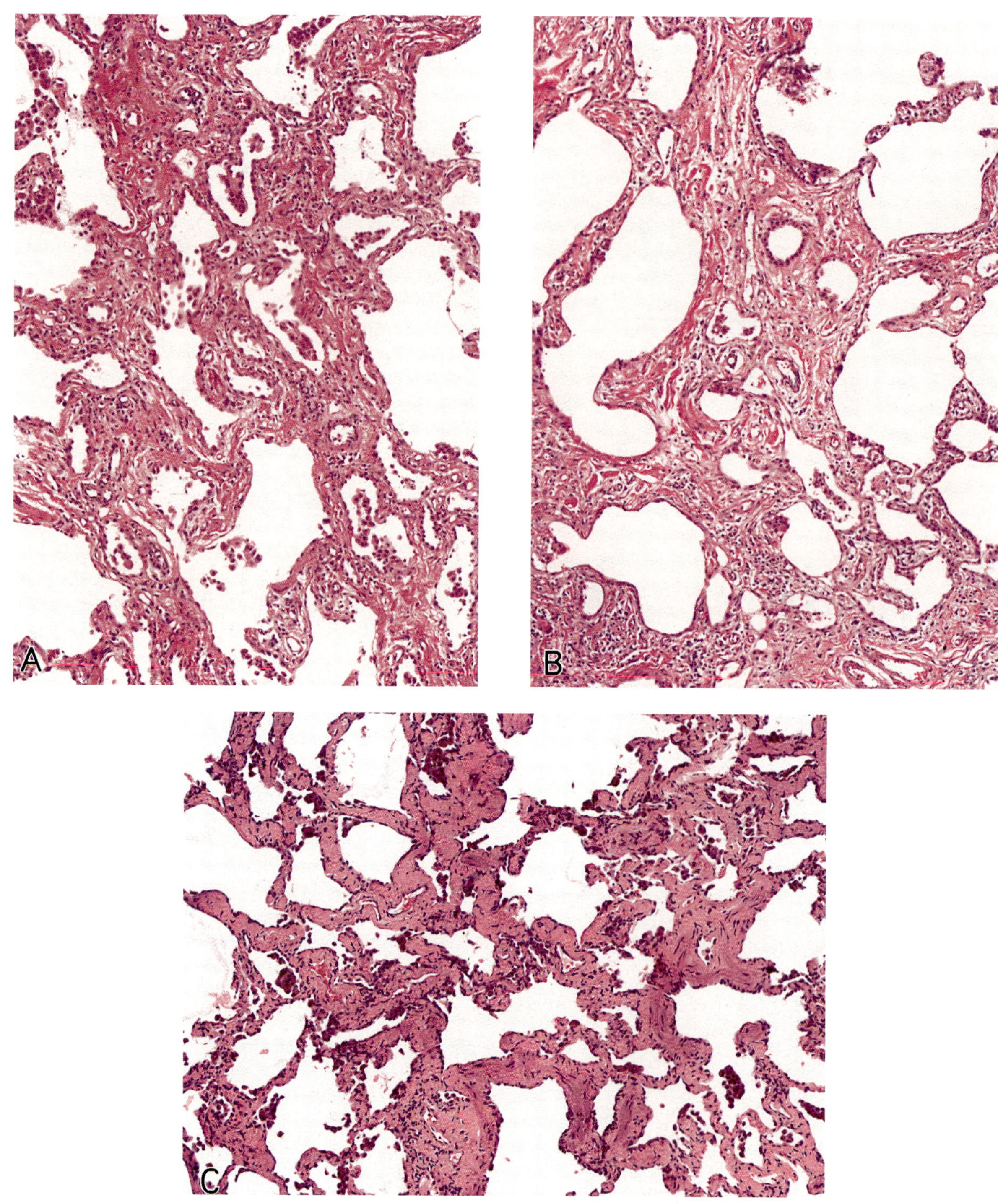

Figure 3-19

NONSPECIFIC INTERSTITIAL PNEUMONIA: FIBROSING PATTERN

A: Marked dense interstitial fibrosis causes thickening of the alveolar walls. However, the architecture of the lung is relatively preserved and the dense fibrosis is approximately the same age, without the presence of fibroblast foci.

B: The alveolar walls are uniformly thickened by dense fibrosis. Fibroblastic foci are absent.

C: The fibrosis shows thickening of the alveolar wall interstitium by dense eosinophilic collagen. Fibroblastic foci are absent.

(Table 3-11; fig. 3-21). Lung biopsies of patients with hypersensitivity pneumonitis typically show scattered, poorly formed granulomas and intraluminal organizing fibrosis (180,192). The presence of loose, poorly formed granulomas in a patient with a cellular NSIP pattern should raise the level of concern to rule out hypersensitivity pneumonitis, infection, collagen vascular disease, or drug-induced pneumonitis. In most cases, the distinction between the cellular NSIP pattern and the fibrosing NSIP pattern with interstitial chronic inflammation is straightforward. In some cases, however, it is difficult to determine whether there is associated dense interstitial fibrosis due to atelectasis or poor specimen processing. Connective tissue stains (e.g., the Masson trichrome stain) help highlight the underlying dense collagen deposits.

The organizing pneumonia pattern is characterized predominantly by intraluminal plugs of loosely organized fibrotic tissue within distal airspaces, including alveoli, alveolar ducts, and bronchioles. The interstitial chronic inflammation is usually relatively mild. In some cases, the cellular NSIP pattern may show occasional foci of intraluminal organizing fibrosis, but this is not the dominant finding and the interstitial chronic inflammation exceeds that seen in COP. Separation of LIP from the cellular NSIP pattern is not well defined, but in LIP there should be extensive alveolar septal infiltration by chronic

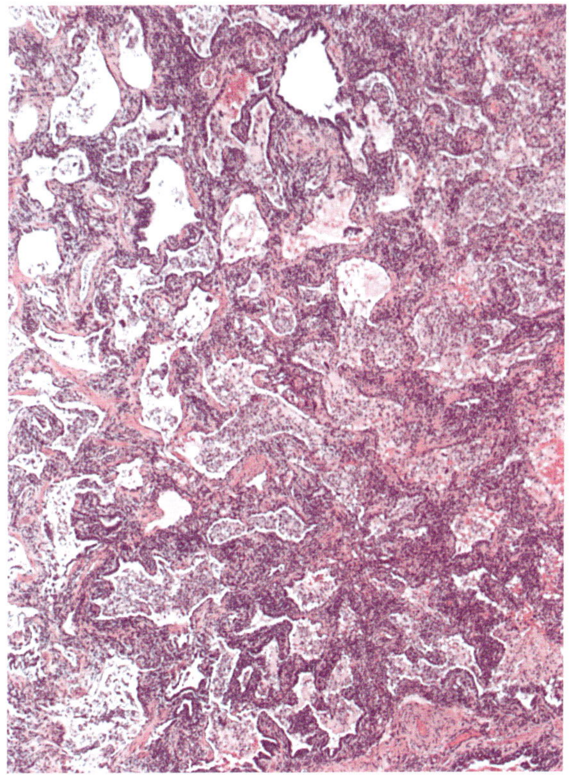

Figure 3-20

NONSPECIFIC INTERSTITIAL PNEUMONIA: CELLULAR AND FIBROSING PATTERN

There is diffuse thickening of the alveolar walls with inconspicuous cystic remodeling of the lung architecture. There is moderate chronic inflammation.

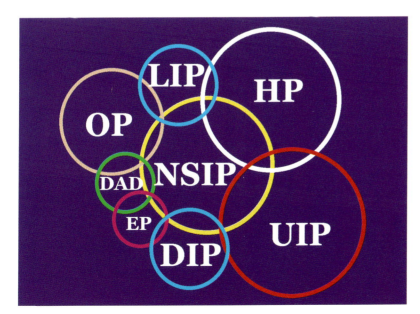

Figure 3-21

NONSPECIFIC INTERSTITIAL PNEUMONIA (NSIP): OVERLAP WITH INTERSTITIAL DISEASES

NSIP has some degree of overlap with a variety of other interstitial diseases. (UIP = usual interstitial pneumonia; HP = hypersensitivity pneumonia; OP = organizing penumonia; DIP = desquamative interstitial pneumonia; EP = eosinophilic pneumonia; LIP = lymphocytic interstitial pneumonia; DAD = diffuse alveolar damage.)

Table 3-11

DIFFERENTIAL DIAGNOSIS OF NONSPECIFIC INTERSTITIAL PNEUMONIA, CELLULAR PATTERN[a]

Histologic Patterns
Nonspecific interstitial pneumonia, fibrosing pattern
Hypersensitivity pneumonitis pattern
Lymphocytic interstitial pneumonitis pattern
Organizing pneumonia pattern
Diffuse alveolar damage, organizing pattern
Possible Etiologies
Collagen vascular disease
Hypersensitivity pneumonitis
Drug-induced pneumonitis
Infection
Immunodeficiency including HIV infection
No detectable cause (idiopathic NSIP, cellular pattern)

[a]Data from reference 205.

Table 3-12

DIFFERENTIAL DIAGNOSIS OF NONSPECIFIC INTERSTITIAL PNEUMONIA, FIBROSING PATTERN[a]

Histologic Patterns
Usual interstitial pneumonia pattern
Nonspecific interstitial pneumonia, cellular pattern
Organizing pneumonia pattern
Fibrotic phase of other interstitial disorders
Hypersensitivity pneumonitis pattern
Langerhans' cell histiocytosis
Desquamative interstitial pneumonia pattern
Diffuse alveolar damage
Possible Etiologies
Collagen vascular disease
Hypersensitivity pneumonitis
Drug-induced pneumonitis
Infection
No detectable cause (idiopathic NSIP, fibrosing pattern)

[a]Data from reference 205.

inflammatory cells, while in the cellular NSIP pattern there is relatively mild and/or patchy interstitial chronic inflammation. The findings in a slowly resolving organizing DAD may be difficult to distinguish from those of the cellular NSIP pattern and require careful correlation with the clinical history. DAD typically shows diffuse involvement of the lung with loosely organizing fibrosis within alveolar septa, and prominent proliferation of type 2 pneumocytes. Infection should be excluded when the cellular NSIP pattern is encountered. The biopsy should be carefully examined for the presence of viral inclusions, granulomas, and organisms using special stains for fungi, *Pneumocystis carinii,* and acid-fast bacilli.

NSIP, Fibrosing Pattern. The etiologic and histologic differential diagnoses for the fibrosing NSIP pattern are listed in Table 3-12. The histologic differential diagnosis includes the UIP pattern and fibrotic forms of other types of interstitial pneumonitis, including hypersensitivity pneumonitis, Langerhans' cell histiocytosis, and DAD, organizing/fibrosing pattern.

The fibrosing pattern of NSIP is the most difficult to separate from the UIP pattern. The UIP pattern frequently shows a subpleural, paraseptal, or peribronchiolar distribution that is seen less often in the fibrosing NSIP pattern. However, the key distinguishing feature of the fibrosing NSIP pattern is the lack of temporal heterogeneity with the prominent fibroblastic foci and dense fibrosis characteristic of the UIP pattern. Fibroblastic foci may be focal or inconspicuous in cases with the NSIP, fibrosing pattern (189–191,197,205). When present, care should be taken to make the distinction from the UIP pattern. It is likely that cases of idiopathic NSIP, fibrosing pattern, were included in previous studies of idiopathic UIP, since only recently have the criteria for the UIP pattern been narrowed to a more precise definition.

The separation of the UIP and fibrosing NSIP patterns is primarily based on histologic examination, but it also requires careful correlation with clinical and radiologic data, especially HRCT scans (Table 3-13). Some lung biopsies interpreted as showing a fibrosing NSIP pattern may represent cases of poorly biopsied UIP. When the quality of the lung biopsy is poor, it should be stated in the pathology report that the distinction between a fibrosing NSIP and UIP pattern cannot be made with certainty. If a lung biopsy from a patient with DPLD shows

Table 3-13

SEPARATION OF NONSPECIFIC INTERSTITIAL PNEUMONIA PATTERN FROM USUAL INTERSTITIAL PNEUMONIA PATTERN[a]

Features	NSIP, Fibrosing Pattern	UIP
Clinical		
Age (range)	49 years (11–78)[b]	51 years (27–70)[c]
Sex (M:F)	28:27[b]	73:37[c]
Duration of symptoms: average (range)	8 mos. (1 week–5 years)	2.5 years
Radiology		
Main findings	Ground-glass attenuation	Irregular lines, honeycombing
Predominant distribution	Diffuse or patchy	Middle and lower lung zones, subpleural in ~90% of cases
Pathology		
Temporal appearance	Uniform	Heterogeneous
Interstitial inflammation	Mild to marked	Mild
Dense interstitial fibrosis	Variable, diffuse or patchy	Patchy
Organizing pneumonia	Not uncommon	Uncommon
Fibroblast foci	Absent or inconspicuous	Characteristic feature
Honeycomb fibrosis	Rare, inconspicuous	Frequent
Alveolar macrophages	Occasional, patchy	Occasional, focal
Prognosis		
5-year survival	90%	20 to 45%
10-year survival	35%	10 to 15%

[a]Summarized from references 179, 190, 196, and 205.
[b]Compiled from references 190 and 205.
[c]Compiled from references 179 and 205.

features that are indeterminate between the UIP and fibrosing NSIP patterns, the term "fibrosing interstitial pneumonia, not further classified" can be used, with an explanation that the pathologist is uncertain about which pattern is present. In some cases it may be possible to favor one pattern versus the other. Such cases may benefit from both intramural and extramural pathologic consultation, and a special attempt should be made to correlate the histologic findings with the HRCT and clinical information.

Biopsies that show a fibrosing NSIP pattern in patients with clinical and radiologic features suggestive of idiopathic UIP (IPF) probably should be diagnosed as idiopathic UIP (IPF). This reflects the problem of histologic heterogeneity or discordant UIP in which biopsies from at least one lobe of the lung show a UIP pattern and biopsies from other lobes show a NSIP pattern (184). In some cases, precise classification may be difficult at the time of lung biopsy and ultimately may be established only after the clinical outcome is clear.

The etiologic possibilities that clinicians must consider in patients with a NSIP pattern on lung biopsy include hypersensitivity pneumonitis, drug-induced pneumonitis, collagen vascular disease, infection, and immunodeficiency syndromes including HIV infection. After receiving a lung biopsy report of a NSIP pattern, clinicians should make a second effort to be certain that all other possibilities have been investigated.

Treatment and Prognosis. NSIP appears to be one of the corticosteroid-responsive lesions, especially if treatment is started during the early phases of the illness. Spontaneous remissions have not been reported. Therefore, untreated patients are expected to experience disease progression and shortened survival times (197,205). Treatment with corticosteroids, with or without immunosuppressive agents, results in improvement or recovery in up to 75 percent of patients with NSIP (182,197).

Travis et al. (205), Nagai et al. (197), and Nicholson et al. (198) found that patients with cellular NSIP had a 100 percent 5-year survival

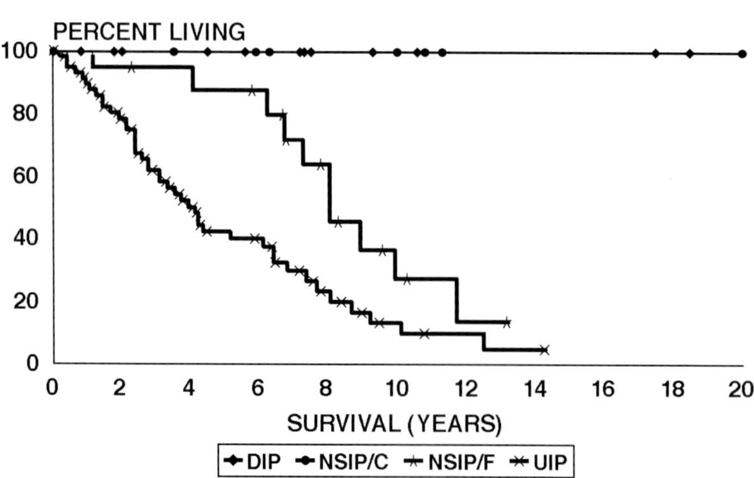

Figure 3-22

KAPLAN-MEIER SURVIVAL CURVES

Kaplan-Meier survival curves for patients with desquamative inter-stitial pneumonia (DIP); nonspecific interstitial pneumonia, cellular pat-tern (NSIP/C); nonspecific inter-stitial pneumonia, fibrosing pattern (NSIP/F); and idiopathic usual inter-stitial pneumonia (UIP). Patients with DIP and cellular NSIP have an excellent survival rate. Patients with idiopathic UIP have the worst rate and those with idiopathic fibrosing NSIP have an intermediate rate (p<0.0001). (Figure 10 from Travis WD, Matsui K, Moss J, Ferrans VJ. Idiopathic nonspecific interstitial pneumonia: prognostic significance of cellular and fibrosing patterns. Survival comparison with usual interstitial pneumonia and desquamative interstitial pneumonia. Am J Surg Pathol 2000;24:19–33.)

rate, significantly better than that for patients with the fibrosing NSIP pattern. The same three studies have shown a statistically more favorable survival rate for patients with the fibrosing NSIP pattern compared to patients with the UIP pattern. In the study by Travis et al., patients with the fibrosing NSIP pattern had a 90 percent 5-year survival rate compared to 43 percent for those with the UIP pattern. At 10 years, the difference in survival rates was far less dramatic (35 versus 15 percent) (fig. 3-22).

Evolving Concept of NSIP

The importance of distinguishing the NSIP pattern from other forms of idiopathic interstitial pneumonia has gained widespread acceptance in the pulmonary community. The clear difference in response to treatment and improved survival for patients with this lesion are useful distinctions from the other idiopathic interstitial pneumonias, particularly UIP/IPF. However, there remains considerable uncertainty regarding its specific clinical, radiologic, and pathologic features. There is a lack of clarity in definition. This partially explains the variable survival data for patients with NSIP in published reports. It is important that the varied pathologic interpretations be resolved, particularly with regard to the differential diagnosis between fibrotic NSIP and other lesions, especially UIP, hypersensitivity pneumonitis, organizing pneumonia, desquamative interstititial pneumonia, bronchiolar fibrosis and rare cases of DAD, eosinophilic pneumonia, and lymphocytic interstitial pneumonia (fig. 3-21). There is currently an ongoing project sponsored by the American Thoracic Society, attempting to resolve some of these differences with the hope of reaching a consensus based on a detailed review of several hundred cases contributed by a panel of expert pathologists, radiologists, and pulmonologists. The report will be published in 2003.

CRYPTOGENIC ORGANIZING PNEUMONIA (BRONCHIOLITIS OBLITERANS ORGANIZING PNEUMONIA)

Definition. Cryptogenic organizing pneumonia (COP) is a distinct clinical entity of unknown etiology with features of a pneumonia. The characteristic histopathologic lesions are excessive proliferations of granulation tissue within small airways and alveolar ducts, associated with chronic inflammation in the surrounding alveoli. COP is also known as idiopathic bronchiolitis obliterans organizing pneumonia.

Table 3-14

TERMS THAT HAVE BEEN USED FOR CRYPTOGENIC ORGANIZING PNEUMONIA/IDIOPATHIC BOOP[a]

Bronchiolitis obliterans with organizing interstitial pneumonia or organizing diffuse alveolar damage (226)
Bronchiolitis obliterans (219)
Organizing pneumonia-like lesion (220)
Unresolved/chronic pneumonia

[a]Modified from reference 211.

In 1985, Epler et al. (218) defined the entity of idiopathic bronchiolitis obliterans organizing pneumonia (BOOP) as a form of interstitial lung disease with distinctive clinical, radiologic, and pathologic characteristics. This entity had been previously recognized under a variety of other terms (Table 3-14) (215,219,220, 226), but the article by Epler et al. had a major influence in drawing attention to it. Davison et al. (215) proposed the alternative term, cryptogenic organizing pneumonia, which is popular in the United Kingdom.

One of the problems with understanding the concept of COP, or idiopathic BOOP, is that the histologic pattern (Table 3-15) is a common nonspecific reaction to a wide variety of types of lung injury (Table 3-16) (227). In the context of DPLD, a secondary cause is usually not found. However, the term BOOP has often been used by pathologists for a nonspecific histologic reaction and clinicians tend to assume a patient has idiopathic BOOP when they hear this term used histologically in a pathology report. As a result, there has been considerable confusion resulting from pathologists using the term BOOP for the histologic pattern without regard for the relatively narrow diagnostic criteria for the clinicopathologic entity of idiopathic BOOP or COP. Consequently, both the pathologist and the clinician must search to rule out an underlying etiology. Infections, collagen vascular diseases, inhalation injuries, hypersensitivity pneumonitis, and lung irradiation are the most frequently associated conditions. Thus, idiopathic BOOP or COP is a diagnosis of exclusion.

Table 3-15

HISTOLOGIC FEATURES OF THE ORGANIZING PNEUMONIA PATTERN[a]

Key Histologic Features
- Organizing pneumonia: intraluminal organizing fibrosis in distal airspaces (bronchioles, alveolar ducts, and alveoli)
- Patchy distribution
- Preservation of lung architecture
- Uniform temporal appearance
- Mild interstitial chronic inflammation

Pertinent Negatives
- Lack of interstitial fibrosis (except for incidental scars or apical fibrosis)
- Absence of granulomas
- Lack of neutrophils or abscesses
- Absence of necrosis
- Lack of hyaline membranes or prominent airspace fibrin
- Lack of prominent infiltration of eosinophils
- Absence of vasculitis

[a]Modified from reference 233.

Table 3-16

CONDITIONS THAT MAY BE ASSOCIATED WITH THE ORGANIZING PNEUMONIA PATTERN[a]

Cryptogenic organizing pneumonia (idiopathic BOOP)
Collagen vascular diseases
Drug reaction
HIV infection
Viral related
Hypersensitivity pneumonitis
Localized organizing pneumonia
Cocaine abuse
Myelodysplastic syndrome
Radiation
Organizing pneumonia distal to obstruction
Vasculitis syndromes (especially Wegener's granulomatosis)
Hemorrhage
Nonspecific reaction adjacent to other lesions (e.g., abscess, infarct, or neoplasm)
Infection (especially *Pneumocystis carinii* pneumonia)

[a]Modified from references 211 and 217.

The ATS/ERS International Consensus Panel for the Classification of Idiopathic Interstitial Pneumonia chose COP as the preferred clinical term over BOOP for idiopathic cases (233). This panel also recommended that pathologists use the term organizing pneumonia rather than BOOP for the histologic pattern seen on lung biopsies since there has been so much confusion over the term BOOP (233). In patients with underlying disease (e.g., rheumatoid arthritis) who have a clinicopathologic condition similar to COP, the clinicopathologic diagnosis of BOOP is appropriate, with mention of the underlying disease (e.g., BOOP associated with rheumatoid arthritis).

Clinical Features. The incidence and prevalence of idiopathic COP are unknown. A prevalence of 6 to 7 cases per 100,000 admissions has been estimated (207). Disease onset is usually in the fifth or sixth decade of life. The clinical presentation mimics that of a community-acquired pneumonia. Three fourths of patients present with less than 2 months' duration of symptoms, and in many it is an acute illness of 1 to 2 weeks' duration (218). Cigarette smoking is not a predisposing factor. A persistent and usually nonproductive cough and shortness of breath are the most common presenting symptoms. A flu-like illness, with fever, malaise, fatigue, and cough, may herald the disease onset. Weight loss (less than 10 pounds) is common. When this condition occurs in a patient with underlying cancer or immunosuppression, it may mimic metastatic malignancy or infection.

Inspiratory crackles are heard on chest examination in most patients. Wheezing is rare and if present is usually heard with crackles. Clubbing is rare. A normal lung examination is seen in 25 percent of patients (218).

Routine laboratory studies are nonspecific. Leukocytosis occurs in 50 percent of patients; the erythrocyte sedimentation rate is commonly elevated, often to 100 mm/hour; and C-reactive protein is positive in 70 to 80 percent of patients (212,221). Autoantibodies are usually negative.

Pulmonary function tests usually show a restrictive defect (223). Lung function is occasionally normal. Gas exchange abnormalities are common. DLCO is reduced in most patients. Hypoxemia at rest and exercise is almost always found.

BAL studies show an increased number of cells recovered with a mixed cellular pattern; i.e., there are increases in the proportion of lymphocytes, neutrophils, and eosinophils (212, 231). Other BAL abnormalities include: presence of foamy macrophages and, occasionally, mast cells (230) and plasma cells; decreased ratio of CD4 to CD8 cells and a normal percentage of CD57+ cells; increased activated T cells, as reflected in human HLA-DR expression (CD3+HLA-DR+ cells [activated T cells); CD8+HLA-DR+ cells [activated suppressor/cytotoxic T cells] CD8+CD57+ cells, and CD8+CD11b- cells [cytotoxic T cells]); and occasionally, interleukin-2 receptor (CD25) expression (214).

Radiologic Findings. The most common radiographic manifestation is unilateral or bilateral areas of airspace consolidation, which have a patchy (fig. 3-23) or predominantly subpleural distribution (218,228). Less common radiographic patterns include ground-glass opacities, nodular opacities, and reticular opacities (210,213,228). The characteristic HRCT finding is bilateral areas of consolidation, which in approximately 60 percent of patients have a predominantly peribronchial or subpleural distribution (fig. 3-24) (225,229). Less common findings include areas of ground-glass attenuation, small nodular opacities which frequently have a centrilobular distribution, and reticular opacities (225,229). Areas of airspace consolidation are seen most commonly in immunocompetent patients who have COP, while atypical findings are seen more commonly in immunocompromised patients and include areas of ground-glass attenuation and nodules. In one study, 91 percent of 32 immunocompetent patients with COP had areas of consolidation, 56 percent had areas of ground-glass attenuation, and 23 percent had small nodules; by comparison, 45 percent of 11 immunocompromised patients had areas of consolidation, 73 percent had areas of ground-glass attenuation, and 55 percent had small nodules (225).

Gross Findings. Since the diagnosis of COP is usually made on open lung biopsy, there are few published gross descriptions of this entity. The lungs show patchy, ill-defined nodular areas of consolidation without scarring or honeycombing. Rarely, patients presenting with a solitary coin lesion (localized organizing

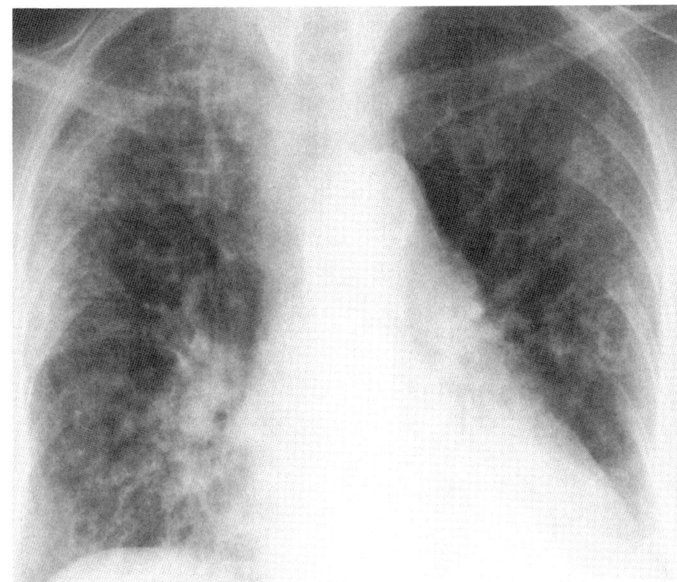

Figure 3-23

CRYPTOGENIC ORGANIZING PNEUMONIA

Posteroanterior chest radiograph demonstrates bilateral areas of consolidation.

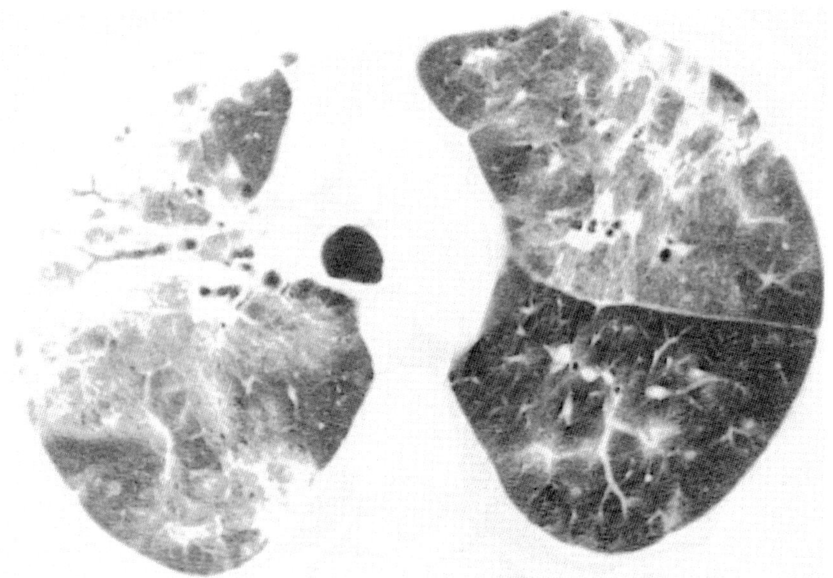

Figure 3-24

CRYPTOGENIC ORGANIZING PNEUMONIA

HRCT shows bilateral areas of consolidation. Although the consolidation has a patchy distribution, it involves predominantly the subpleural and peribronchial regions. There are also patchy areas of ground-glass attenuation.

pneumonia, see below) have histologic findings that are identical to those of COP (216,227).

Histologic Findings. The major histologic features of the organizing pneumonia pattern are summarized in Table 3-15 (211,218,222,224). At low-power microscopy, the process is patchy with relatively normal lung adjacent to zones of organization that may center on a bronchiole (figs. 3-25, 3-26). The organizing fibrosis consists of anastomosing, intraluminal plugs of loose connective tissue that occlude bronchioles (bronchiolitis obliterans), alveolar ducts, and surrounding alveoli (organizing pneumonia) (fig. 3-26). Although bronchioles are frequently involved, the bulk of the connective tissue is situated in the alveolar ducts and alveolar spaces, and bronchiolar involvement is occasionally absent (fig. 3-27). All of the connective tissue appears about the same age and consists of polypoid intraluminal plugs of loose organizing fibrosis (fig. 3-27). The architecture of the lung is preserved, with no remodeling from dense fibrosis or honeycomb changes (Table 3-15). Due to the distal airway

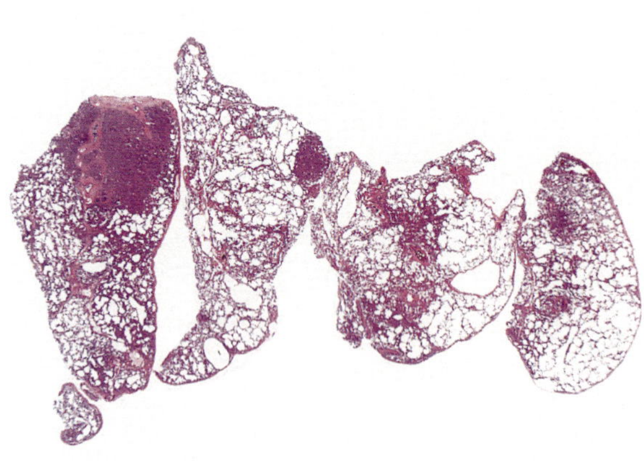

Figure 3-25

ORGANIZING PNEUMONIA PATTERN

The process is patchy with normal lung adjacent to nodular areas of consolidation.

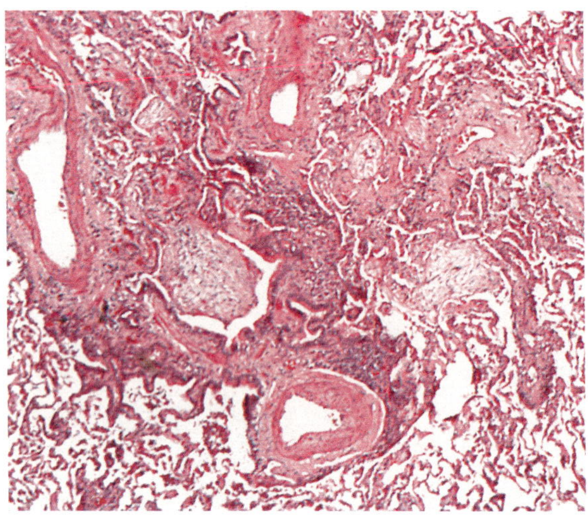

Figure 3-26

ORGANIZING PNEUMONIA PATTERN IN CRYPTOGENIC ORGANIZING PNEUMONIA

Polypoid plugs of loose organizing connective tissue protrude into the lumen of a bronchiole as well as into the surrounding alveolar ducts and spaces.

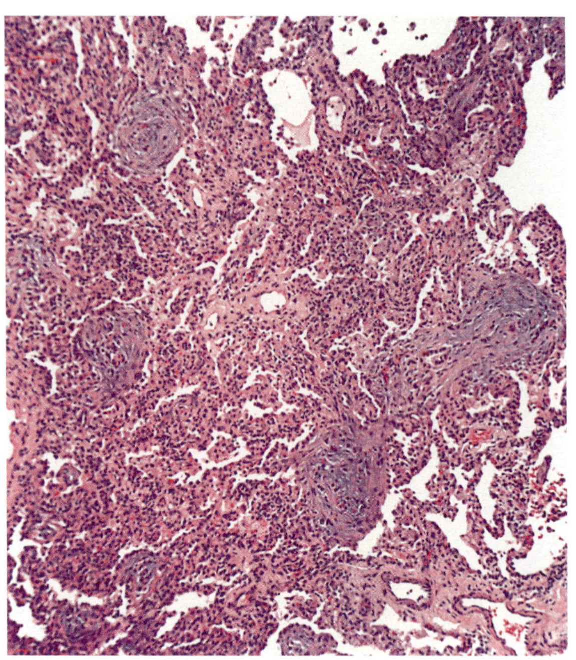

Figure 3-27

ORGANIZING PNEUMONIA PATTERN IN CRYPTOGENIC ORGANIZING PNEUMONIA

The loose organizing connective tissue is evenly spaced and all about the same age. The architecture of the lung is preserved. The connective tissue has a myxoid appearance due to the abundant mucopolysaccharides and paucity of collagen.

occlusion, obstructive or endogenous lipid pneumonia may develop, characterized by the accumulation of foamy, lipid-laden macrophages (fig. 3-28).

The intraluminal polypoid plugs of connective tissue are mucopolysaccharide rich and lack the abundant collagen fibers seen in dense collagen. Therefore, they stain green with the Movat stain in contrast to the yellow staining typically seen with dense fibrosis. Within these intraluminal polypoid plugs there may be small collections of lymphocytes, plasma cells, and histiocytes. Rare alveolar fibrinous exudates may be seen in association with some of the intraluminal fibrosis, but they should not be prominent.

Interstitial inflammation may be mild or moderate and usually consists of lymphocytes and/or plasma cells. A cellular bronchiolitis may be present and scattered germinal centers can be seen. The alveolar walls may be normal or only mildly thickened, and they do not show interstitial fibrosis. Type 2 pneumocyte hyperplasia is usually inconspicuous, but the degree of the epithelial reaction depends on the intensity of the interstitial inflammation. The alveolar parenchyma adjacent to the organizing pneumonia should appear normal. If the lung biopsy

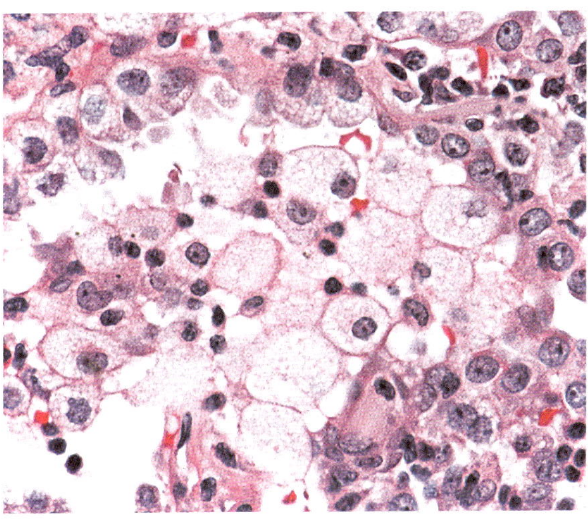

Figure 3-28

ORGANIZING PNEUMONIA PATTERN IN CRYPTOGENIC ORGANIZING PNEUMONIA

Microscopic foci of endogenous lipoid pneumonia are present. The numerous foamy alveolar macrophages are due to the distal airway obstruction.

is not inflated, the tissue around the organizing pneumonia tends to be atelectatic. This should not be mistaken for extensive dense interstitial fibrosis (211). Incidental old fibrotic scars may be present, especially if the biopsy is obtained from the lingula or a lobar tip (211). The scars should not appear to be an intrinsic part of the interstitial pneumonitis and are usually distinct from the lesions of organizing pneumonia.

Diagnosis. The diagnosis of COP requires pathologic, radiologic, and clinical information. When examining a lung biopsy, the pathologist must identify the classic organizing pneumonia pattern and carefully exclude any of the potential histologic lesions listed in Table 3-15 that would indicate an alternative diagnosis. Unless the pathologist has access to a complete clinical history, all imaging information, and the results of all laboratory studies, the best morphologic diagnosis that can be established is *organizing pneumonia, etiology undetermined*. Then the clinician should examine the clinical history, radiologic findings, and results of laboratory studies to see if any of the conditions listed in Table 3-16 are present that could explain the histologic reaction pattern. If there is no underlying disorder that could explain the process and the clinical and radiologic features are appropriate, then the diagnosis of COP can be established.

Although possible, it is difficult to establish a definitive diagnosis of COP based on transbronchial biopsy due to the many different lung processes that can give an organizing pneumonia pattern (Table 3-16). In such cases, one must be especially careful to correlate the biopsy findings with the clinical and radiologic picture, which should be classic for COP (208). If the clinical follow-up does not show the typical prompt response to steroid therapy, a surgical lung biopsy may be indicated.

Differential Diagnosis. The differential diagnosis of COP can be viewed from both a clinical and pathologic perspective. Clinically, COP must be separated from IPF and AIP (see Table 3-7). Patients with COP tend to have a short duration of illness (4 to 6 weeks) while those with IPF have an insidious onset over several years. The radiologic picture of IPF is that of honeycomb fibrosis mostly in the lower lobes, usually in a subpleural distribution. Patients with AIP generally have a relatively fulminant clinical course, with diffuse opacification on chest radiographs, and require management in an intensive care unit with mechanical ventilation. Patients with COP are usually ambulatory and the chest radiographs show patchy nodular opacities. The survival rate for patients with COP is much better than for those with DAD (only about 50 percent survival).

Histologically, the most difficult problem in the diagnosis of the organizing pneumonia pattern is the search for histologic clues that might point to a specific etiology or underlying disease. The organizing pneumonia pattern can also be confused with the UIP, DAD (see Table 3-7), or NSIP patterns. In both the UIP and organizing pneumonia patterns, the lung lesions are patchy, but in the organizing pneumonia pattern all of the connective tissue is the same age, it is intraluminal within conducting airways, there is loose organizing fibrosis, and the architecture of the lung is preserved. This contrasts with the UIP pattern in which the fibrosis shows temporal heterogeneity, with dense scars causing remodeling of the lung architecture and scattered fibroblastic foci at the edges of dense scars. The fibroblastic foci of UIP

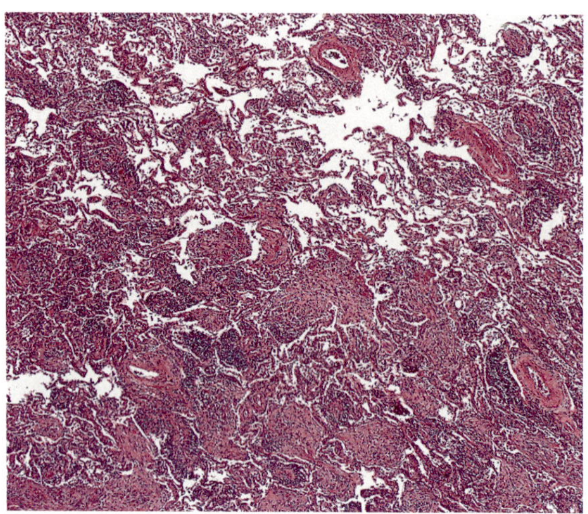
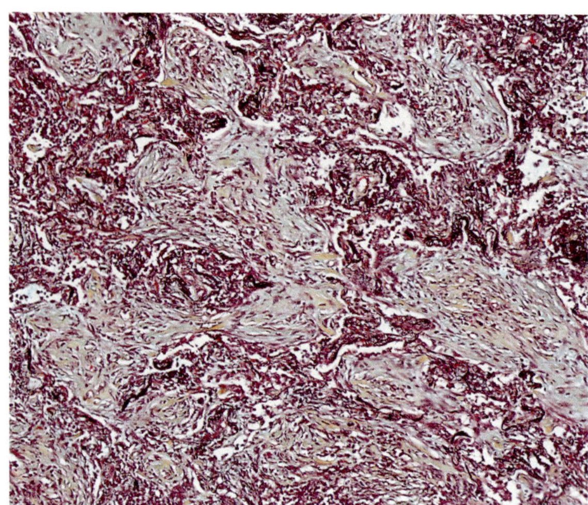

Figure 3-29

LOCALIZED ORGANIZING PNEUMONIA

Left: The patient was found to have a solitary nodule on chest radiography. The nodule consists of organizing pneumonia identical to that in COP, with polypoid plugs of loose connective tissue protruding into the distal airways.

Right: The Movat stain highlights the plugs of loose organizing connective tissue in the alveolar ducts and spaces.

are sometimes prominent and can be confused with the organizing pneumonia pattern. However, in the former, the fibroblastic foci are tightly juxtaposed against dense scars in contrast to the polypoid intraluminal location of the connective tissue in the latter.

The organizing phase of DAD can show focal intraluminal budding fibrosis and resemble the organizing pneumonia pattern. However, DAD can usually be distinguished from organizing pneumonia by the diffuse rather than patchy lung involvement, prominent rather than inconspicuous type 2 pneumocyte hyperplasia, organizing fibrosis causing interstitial thickening rather than purely intraluminal polypoid plugs, hyaline membranes, and foci of acute inflammation and hemorrhage. Vascular fibrin microthrombi are also more likely to be seen in DAD. The cellular pattern of NSIP shows more prominent interstitial chronic inflammation than the organizing pneumonia pattern associated with COP. Foci of organizing pneumonia are often present, but they are not the dominant histologic finding and are only focal (234). If alveolar fibrinous exudates are conspicuous and the process is patchy, the pattern of *acute fibrinous and organizing pneumonia (AFOP)* should be considered (209). Eosinophilic pneumonia comes into the differential diagnosis if eosinophils are prominent, since organizing pneumonia is a common histologic feature in this condition.

Cases that manifest as a solitary pulmonary nodule in asymptomatic patients and show an organizing pneumonia pattern histologically are classified as *localized organizing pneumonia* (fig. 3-29) (232). These lesions have been reported as focal organizing pneumonia (227) and BOOP manifesting as a solitary pulmonary nodule (216). They may be resected with a suspicion of lung cancer, but they require no further treatment and typically do not recur (227). These lesions must be distinguished from inflammatory pseudotumors and focal organizing pneumonia associated with an abscess, acute bronchopneumonia, or necrotizing granulomatous inflammation.

The organizing pneumonia pattern differs from that of constrictive bronchiolitis obliterans (see chapter 8) which shows concentric dense fibrosis causing luminal narrowing rather than polypoid plugs of loose connective tissue in the distal airspaces.

Treatment and Prognosis. Corticosteroid therapy is the most common treatment and leads to complete clinical recovery, physiologic improvement, and normalization of the chest radiograph in two thirds of patients. Approximately one third have persistent disease. Usually, the clinical response is rapid and can be dramatic, within several days or a few weeks. Relapses occur commonly when corticosteroids are withdrawn after 1 to 3 months; they usually respond to corticosteroid treatment. Spontaneous improvement has been reported in a few patients (218,235). The dose of oral corticosteroids needed to treat patients with COP is not known. An oral dose of 30 to 60 mg/day is commonly employed for 3 to 6 months depending on the rate of recovery. High-dose parenteral methylprednisolone, 125 to 250 mg intravenously every 6 hours for 3 to 5 days, has been recommended as initial treatment in patients with progressive COP. For corticosteroid failures, cytotoxic drugs (cyclophosphamide or azathioprine) have been used with limited success.

Patients with predominantly interstitial opacities on the chest radiograph have a poorer prognosis than those with airspace opacities. The overall prognosis for patients with COP is much better than for those with other idiopathic interstitial pneumonias (e.g., IPF). The 5-year survival rate is higher in patients with COP (73 percent) than in those with secondary organizing pneumonia (44 percent) (227). Rapidly fatal COP is uncommon and may actually represent AIP or organizing DAD.

DIFFUSE ALVEOLAR DAMAGE AND ACUTE INTERSTITIAL PNEUMONIA

Definition. Diffuse alveolar damage (DAD) is a form of acute lung injury that progresses through an exudative phase, characterized by pneumocyte and endothelial cell necrosis, edema, and formation of hyaline membranes, to an organizing phase with alveolar septal organizing interstitial fibrosis and prominent type 2 pneumocyte proliferation. In approximately 50 percent of cases this process resolves with restoration of normal lung architecture. In some cases, there is progression to a fibrotic phase in which endstage honeycomb fibrosis develops.

DAD is a histologic pattern of acute lung injury that occurs in a wide variety of clinical settings (Table 3-17) (265,269,270,289,300). It has been compared to a biologic explosion, and causes diffuse, acute damage to both the endothelial and epithelial cells of the alveolar wall (243). Rarely, DAD occurs in the absence of any detectable etiology. Such cases have been called either *idiopathic DAD* or *acute interstitial pneumonia (AIP)* (see below) (267,285).

While this section primarily addresses DAD and AIP, the recently described histologic pattern of *acute fibrinous and organizing pneumonia (AFOP)* will also be mentioned due to its apparent close relationship to DAD.

Clinical Features. The clinical syndrome associated with the histologic finding of DAD is the *acute respiratory distress syndrome (ARDS)*, previously known as the adult respiratory distress syndrome (285). Other synonyms for this syndrome include *acute lung injury, traumatic wet lung, Da Nang lung, noncardiogenic pulmonary edema, congestive atelectasis, Hamman-Rich syndrome,* and *adult hyaline membrane disease* (264). The incidence of ARDS ranges from 1.5 to 8.3 per 100,000 persons per year and represents about 7 percent of all intensive care unit admissions (260,293,299). However, a considerably higher annual incidence is found using the 1994 consensus definition (17.9 per 100,000 for acute lung injury and 13.5 per 100,000 for ARDS) (271). Investigators in the National Institutes of Health (NIH) Acute Respiratory Distress Syndrome Network believe that the actual incidence might approach 75 per 100,000 per year (306). A prospective epidemiologic study using the 1994 consensus definition is under way in Seattle (306).

ARDS is associated with a diverse group of precipitating clinical events. More than 60 causes of ARDS have been identified (Table 3-17) (293). The reason for using the term ARDS is that it denotes a common syndrome despite multiple etiologies or associated illnesses, and implies similar if not identical pathophysiology.

The North American-European Consensus Conference definition for ARDS includes: acute onset of illness, bilateral opacities on chest radiograph, a PaO_2/FIO_2 (fraction of inspired oxygen) ratio of less than 200, a pulmonary arterial wedge pressure less than 18 mm Hg, and no clinical evidence of left heart failure (246, 248,282). In an attempt to define a milder form of injury, the term *acute lung injury (ALI)* was coined with the same criteria as for ARDS except that the PaO_2/FIO_2 ratio is between 200 and 300 (246,248,282).

Table 3-17

CAUSES OF DIFFUSE ALVEOLAR DAMAGE[a]

Shock

Infection
- Bacteremia
- Viral pneumonia (chapter 12)
- Fungal pneumonia (chapter 12)
- *Pneumocystis carinii* pneumonia (chapter 12)
- Severe bacterial pneumonia (chapter 12)

Trauma
- Fat embolism (chapter 15)
- Lung contusion
- Nonthoracic trauma
- Head trauma

Aspiration of Gastric Contents (chapter 3)

Inhalation Injury
- Smoke
- Oxygen
- Corrosive chemical

Drugs (chapter 7)

Metabolic Disorders
- Pancreatitis
- Uremia
- Ingestion of paraquat (chapter 7)

Radiation (chapter 7)

Hematologic Disorders
- Intravascular coagulation
- Transfusion-associated acute lung injury (TRALI)
- Cardiopulmonary bypass

Others
- Burns
- High altitude
- Intravenous administration of contrast material
- Leukemic cell lysis
- Gestational trophoblastic disease
- Near drowning
- Peritoneovenous shunt
- Postlymphangiography
- Collagen vascular disease
- Toxic shock syndrome
- Venous air embolism

Idiopathic
- Acute interstitial pneumonia (Hamman-Rich syndrome)

[a]Modified from references 264 and 285.

The onset of ARDS is commonly quite rapid, occurring most often within 24 to 48 hours of the precipitating event. Tachypnea and dyspnea are the first symptoms, coinciding with arterial hypoxemia and a decreased PaO_2. As ARDS progresses, the dyspnea worsens and the patient develops respiratory failure and noncardiogenic pulmonary edema.

The rapidly progressive respiratory failure is associated with decreased lung compliance but increases in both the shunt fraction and dead space. The hypoxemia is often severe and refractory to oxygen supplementation. The PaO_2 is typically less than 50 to 60 mm Hg despite an inspired oxygen (FIO_2) measurement of more than 60 percent. Total respiratory compliance in patients with ARDS is usually less than 50 mL/cm H_2O (280). BAL cellular and fluid analysis has been widely used to evaluate the inflammatory process in the lungs of patients with ARDS and those at risk for the syndrome. Polymorphonuclear leukocytes and total protein (TP) concentration are increased in the BAL fluid in virtually all patients with ARDS, especially in the early phases of lung injury (260).

Usually it is not difficult to determine the cause of ARDS since the predisposing conditions are often apparent at the onset of the acute lung injury. In the rare instance when none of the common risk factors are present, it is important to use a systematic approach to identify a specific cause of lung injury. Review of the clinical course immediately before the onset of the respiratory failure is the first step. Fiberoptic bronchoscopy for inspection of the airways and for obtaining BAL specimens is often the initial procedure to rule out occult aspiration, diffuse alveolar hemorrhage, infection, and malignancy. Transbronchial and surgical lung biopsies can be performed with reasonable safety, even in severely hypoxemic patients. However, the yield is usually disappointing if the BAL has been nondiagnostic. Surgical lung biopsy is usually performed in patients who are suspected of having disseminated cancer, pulmonary vasculitis, or ARDS superimposed upon another diffuse lung disease, such as interstitial pulmonary fibrosis, sarcoidosis, or connective tissue disease (257).

Radiologic Findings. Chest radiographs performed within the first 12 to 24 hours from the clinical onset of respiratory failure show decreased lung volume but are otherwise normal, unless the ARDS is secondary to an underlying pulmonary process such as aspiration or pneumonia (253,281,294). After 12 to 24 hours, patchy airspace consolidation is present which becomes rapidly confluent and diffuse. The consolidation is often most severe in the peripheral lung regions or, when more widespread, shows small intervening regions of normal parenchyma between the peripheral and more central portions of lung (279). Air bronchograms are frequently seen while septal lines and pleural effusions are uncommon. On CT, the consolidation is often patchy, even when apparently diffuse on the radiograph, and it usually is most marked in the dependent lung regions (fig. 3-30, top) (251,252,273). While pleural effusions are seldom evident on the radiograph unless there are superimposed complications such as heart failure or infection, small unilateral or bilateral effusions are seen on CT in approximately 50 percent of patients with ARDS (296).

With improvement in ARDS the chest radiograph shows a gradually less dense and less heterogeneous consolidation. In patients who remain on mechanical ventilation, after 5 to 7 days the chest radiographs show gradual replacement of consolidation by less dense, ground-glass opacification and the development of small rounded areas of lucency or thin-walled cystic airspaces presumably caused by barotrauma (fig. 3-30, bottom) (250,253,296). After 2 to 3 weeks, reticular opacities become apparent, reflecting the presence of fibrosis (286). In patients who survive, the radiographic abnormalities typically resolve completely (306).

Pathologic Findings. Early pathologic studies defining the morphology of DAD were based on examination of lungs from patients subjected to oxygen therapy and mechanical ventilation (283), shock/trauma (265), or burns (284). Based on these studies, DAD was shown to evolve through several distinct histologic and clinical phases with a fairly consistent sequence of events, listed in Table 3-18 and figure 3-31. The evolution of DAD has been arbitrarily divided into two (265), three (275,300), and five phases (289). The number of phases into which one divides the histologic evolution of DAD is not critical. However, it is useful to be aware that DAD evolves through a sequence of pathologic events that correlate with particular radiologic (fig. 3-30) and clinical changes. It also allows for pathologic assessment of the phase of DAD based on lung biopsy evaluation. While these phases are fairly distinct, they are closely interrelated and overlapping histologic features exist (263,275,300).

The lungs are generally diffusely involved in DAD; however, in some cases the process may appear somewhat patchy, particularly in the early exudative and late resolving phases. Liebow (270a) used the term diffuse to mean the alveoli were diffusely affected, however, one of the most useful histologic features in the recognition of the DAD pattern is that the lung typically shows diffuse rather than patchy involvement. The heterogeneity of the lung alteration in DAD has been appreciated previously by chest CT (273,253) as well as by gross and histologic evaluation of the lungs (300, 307). Yazdy et al. (307) proposed the term *regional alveolar damage* for cases in which the histologic findings of DAD are localized. The term *focal DAD* can also be used for such cases even though the combination of "focal diffuse" is somewhat awkward. In many such cases one can carefully examine the apparently normal lung and see the presence of edema or pneumocyte hyperplasia, indicating that it is not entirely normal. It is not known whether these cases truly represent a completely localized form of acute lung injury or if they simply represent a point in time when a diffuse process is temporarily localized during the initial or resolving stages.

It has been postulated that oxygen therapy and mechanical ventilation play a significant role in causing the development of DAD and ARDS (289,290). It is difficult to separate the effects of oxygen and mechanical ventilation from effects caused by DAD/ARDS itself since both are required to enable these patients to survive. Nevertheless, the histologic picture of DAD and clinical features of ARDS can develop in patients who never received oxygen or mechanical ventilation.

Gross Findings. The lungs affected by DAD are markedly enlarged and heavy. The combined lung weight is often greater than 2,000 g or three to four times the normal weight (289, 297). Lungs examined in the early stages of DAD show congestion and edema (fig. 3-32, left) (289, 297). During the exudative phase the lungs are heavy, the external lung surface distends the overlying pleura, and the cut surface is noncrepitant and dark red to blue (297). As DAD progresses into the proliferative phase, the lungs are

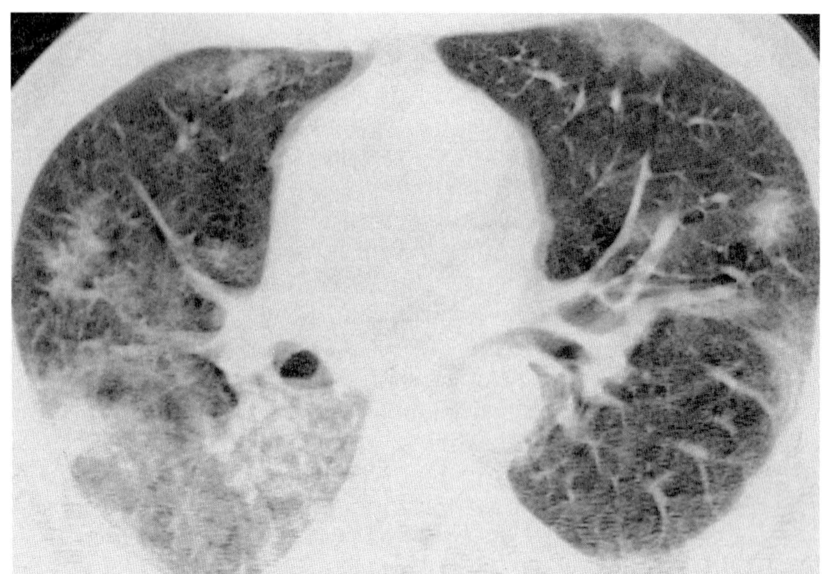

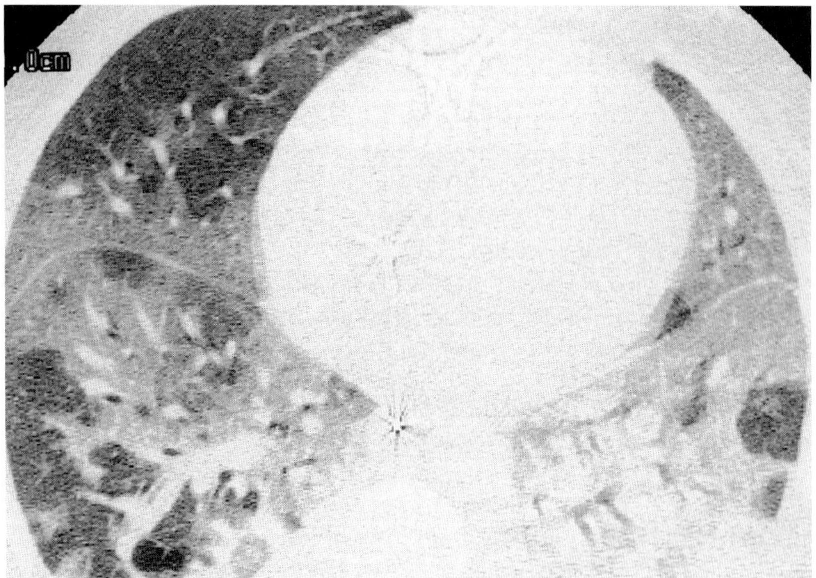

Figure 3-30

ACUTE RESPIRATORY DISTRESS SYNDROME

Top: HRCT in the early stages of ARDS in a 57-year-old man demonstrates patchy bilateral areas of ground-glass attenuation and consolidation. The ARDS was secondary to drug reaction.

Bottom: HRCT performed in the late exudative phase of ARDS in a 45-year-old woman demonstrates areas of consolidation in the dependent lung regions and extensive areas of ground-glass attenuation. Note focal areas of relatively normal parenchyma.

noncrepitant, rubbery, and firm. They may be patchy red-brown or yellow-gray (fig. 3-32, right). A slippery texture has been attributed to the abundant, newly formed connective tissue (300). If progression to the fibrotic phase occurs, the pleural surface shows a coarse, cobblestoned appearance. The cut surface of the lung is pale and spongy, with many fine cysts; airspaces measure 1 to 2 mm in diameter and have thick walls. Irregular areas of dense scarring may be seen. Rarely, honeycomb changes with prominent cysts develop, similar to those seen in bronchopulmonary dysplasia in infants (247).

Histologic Findings. The histologic findings of DAD vary depending on the time at which the tissue sampling occurs (fig. 3-31). These findings fall into three phases: the exudative (acute) phase, the proliferative (organizing) phase, and the fibrotic (chronic) phase (Table 3-18) (265,300). In general, lung biopsies show diffuse histologic changes. Rarely, areas of spared alveolar parenchyma are present. In addition, the connective tissue is usually about the same age, since in most cases of DAD the initial lung injury begins at a single point in time.

Table 3-18

HISTOLOGIC FEATURES OF DIFFUSE ALVEOLAR DAMAGE[a]

Feature	Phase of DAD Exudative	 Proliferative	 Fibrotic
Timing	Edema early (<1 wk)	Organization (repair) intermediate	Fibrosis, late (3 wks)
Macroscopic			
Consistency	Rigid, heavy	Firm, consolidated	Spongy, cystic
Appearance	Hemorrhagic	Pale gray	Pale gray
Microscopic			
Vasculature	Endothelial injury (mild), congestion, neutrophil aggregates, minimal thrombi	Endothelial injury, intimal fibroproliferation, medial hypertrophy, thrombi	Endothelial injury, distortion, compressed, proliferation
Alveoli	Type 1 pneumocyte necrosis, inflammatory, exudate, hyaline membranes, partial collapse	Type 2 pneumocyte proliferation, myofibroblast invasion, increased fibronectin, collagen deposition	Fibrosis, microscopic cysts
Basement membrane	Denuded	Gaps with myofibroblast invasion	Disruption
Alveolar wall	Edema, congestion	Myofibroblast proliferation	Thick collagen
Alveolar duct	Dilated	Myofibroblast proliferation	Fibrosis
Interstitium	Increased volume from edema	Marked increased volume from myofibroblast proliferation	Marked increased volume from dense fibrosis
Pleura	Subpleural ischemic changes	Subpleural necrosis	Subpleural necrosis

[a]Modified from reference 275.

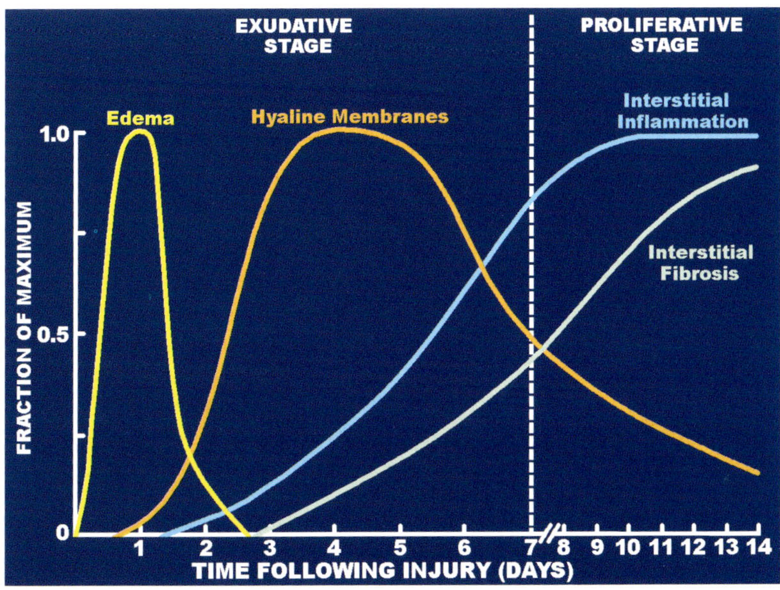

Figure 3-31

DIFFUSE ALVEOLAR DAMAGE

Diagram of the evolution of the histologic patterns of DAD over time. This illustrates the relative rather than absolute times during which various histologic features of DAD occur, emphasizing the overlap between acute and organizing patterns. The times are only estimations and are not intended to be precise. (Figure 2-1 from Katzenstein AL, Askin FB. Katzenstein and Askin's surgical pathology of non-neoplastic lung disease, 3rd ed. Philadelphia: WB Saunders; 1997:17.)

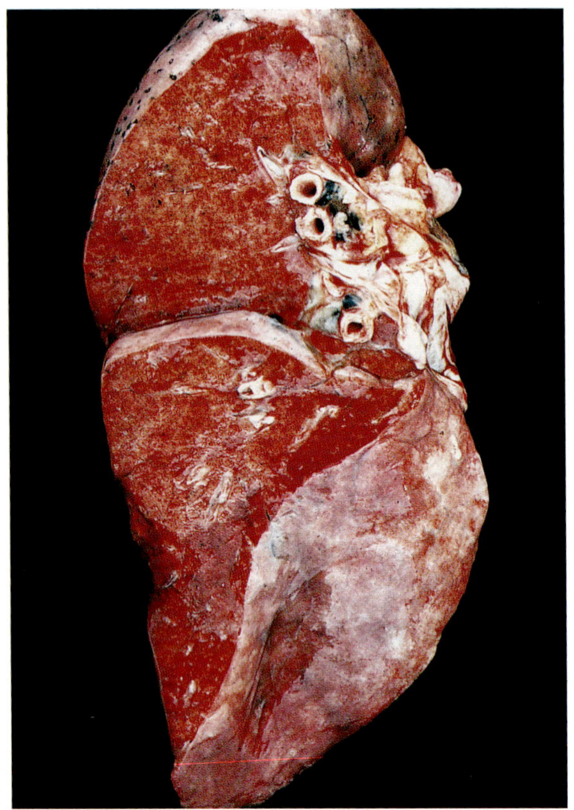

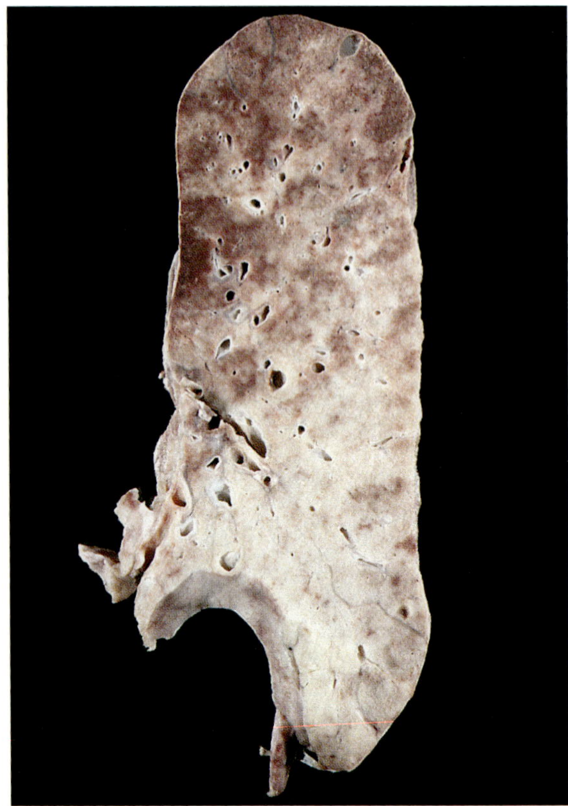

Figure 3-32

DIFFUSE ALVEOLAR DAMAGE: GROSS PATHOLOGY

Acute pattern (left) is characterized by diffuse hemorrhage and edema. Organizing pattern (right) shows extensive tan consolidation.

Exudative (Acute) Phase. The exudative phase of DAD generally takes place the first week following the onset of respiratory failure. The first changes seen by light microscopy are congestion of alveolar capillaries, interstitial and alveolar edema, and intra-alveolar hemorrhage (300). Hyaline membranes are the histologic hallmark of the exudative phase of DAD (figs. 3-33, 3-34).

The earliest changes of DAD are not visible with the light microscope and are appreciated only by electron microscopy (265,284,289, 298). There is injury to type 1 pneumocytes and endothelial cells. This results in edema and exudation of plasma proteins into the alveolar interstitium and spaces. The type 1 pneumocytes undergo extensive necrosis and slough off the alveolar surface (240,265,267,289,298,300). The underlying basement membrane is denuded and becomes the surface of attachment for hyaline membranes and fibrin. Necrosis of type 2 pneumocytes may occur, but these cells are less susceptible to injury than type 1 pneumocytes. Degenerative and necrotic changes are less prominent in endothelial cells than in epithelial cells. The endothelial cells show swelling, widening of intercellular junctions, and increased numbers of pinocytotic vesicles (240,265,267, 289,298,300). In addition, cellular necrosis, disruption and denudation of the basement membrane, and intravascular fibrin accumulation may be seen. The relatively subtle morphologic changes in the endothelial cells may not reflect the extensiveness of the functional damage. This loss of integrity of the alveolar epithelium and endothelium allows for exudation of fluid and fibrin into the interstitium and alveolar spaces.

One or two days following an initial injury, interstitial and alveolar edema as well as alveolar fibrin with hyaline membrane formation can be seen by light microscopy (240,265,

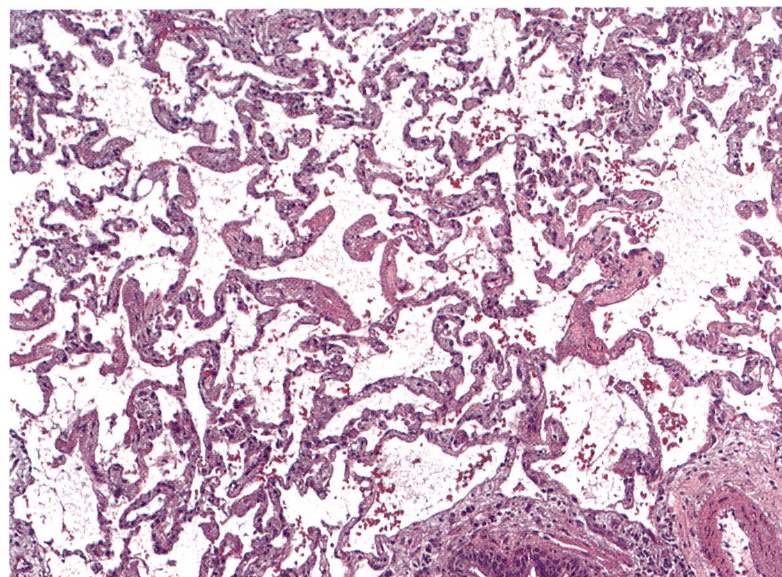

Figure 3-33

DIFFUSE ALVEOLAR DAMAGE: ACUTE PATTERN

The lungs show diffuse involvement by hyaline membranes as well as prominent interstitial and alveolar edema.

267,289,298,300). The degree of interstitial and alveolar edema peaks during the first 1 to 2 days. Hyaline membranes begin to appear by the second day and peak at 4 to 5 days. These eosinophilic "membranes" line the alveolar surfaces and consist of precipitated plasma proteins and the cytoplasmic and nuclear debris from sloughed epithelial cells. The hyaline membranes frequently form in the region of the alveolar ducts (289,290). Intracapillary neutrophil aggregates may be seen, especially after sepsis or trauma. Interstitial inflammation, consisting of lymphocytes, plasma cells, and macrophages, is apparent early and reaches its maximum in about a week. Microvascular thromboemboli are frequently seen and may consist of either hyaline platelet–fibrin thrombi in capillaries and arterioles or laminated fibrin clots in medium-sized and large arterioles (301).

Proliferative (Organizing) Phase. Toward the end of the first week, the proliferative phase of DAD begins. During this phase the exudate within the interstitium and alveolar spaces begins to organize and there is extensive proliferation of type 2 pneumocytes and fibroblasts (figs. 3-35–3-37). Type 2 pneumocytes have a cuboidal morphology as they proliferate along the denuded basement membrane of the damaged alveolar septa (305). Electron microscopy shows that type 2 pneumocytes have lamellar bodies and surface microvilli. They also express

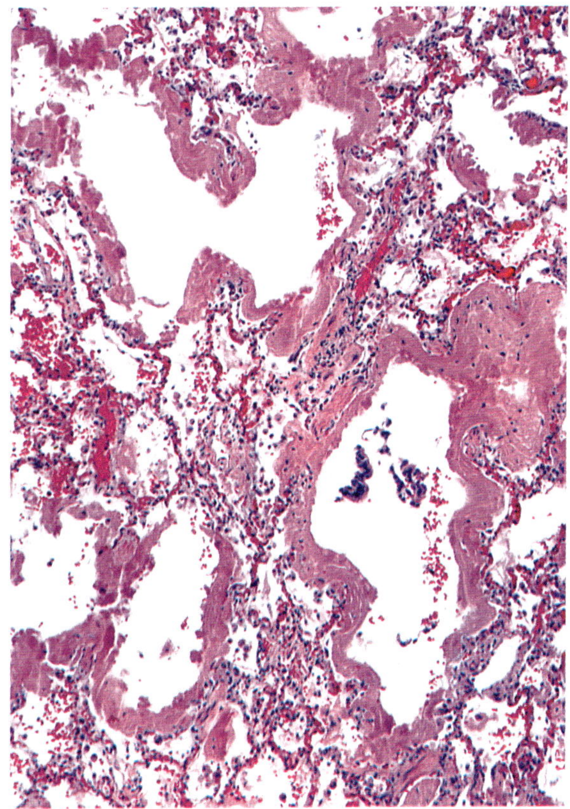

Figure 3-34

DIFFUSE ALVEOLAR DAMAGE: ACUTE PATTERN

The hyaline membranes consist of pink fibrinous material that lines the alveolar ducts.

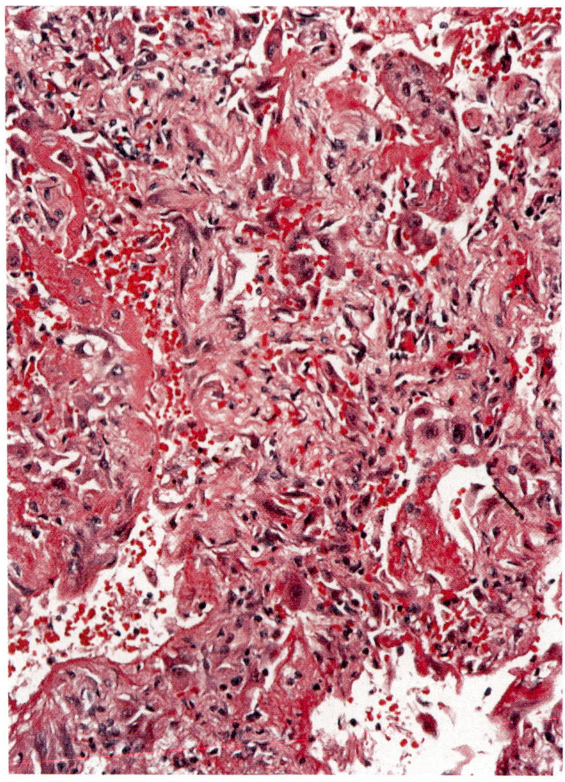

Figure 3-35

DIFFUSE ALVEOLAR DAMAGE: ACUTE AND ORGANIZING PATTERNS

The interstitium of the alveolar walls is markedly thickened by organizing loose connective tissue. Alveolar fibrin and hyaline membranes are also present.

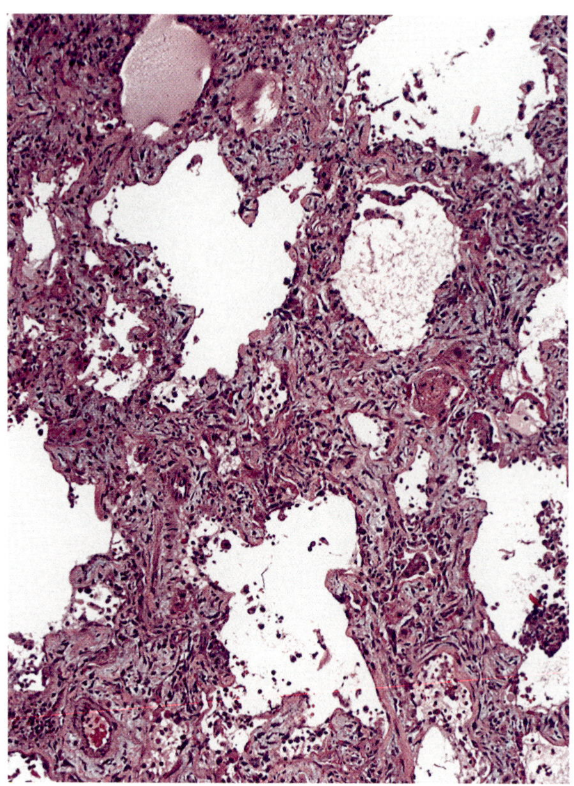

Figure 3-36

DIFFUSE ALVEOLAR DAMAGE: ORGANIZING PATTERN

There is diffuse alveolar septal thickening by proliferation of loose, organizing fibrous connective tissue and prominent type 2 pneumocyte proliferation.

surfactant, which can be detected immunohistochemically. Squamous metaplasia may be seen (fig. 3-38). Some of the proliferating epithelial cells show abundant cytoplasmic hyaline, similar to Mallory's hyaline, which may indicate squamous differentiation (300). The epithelial cells may have large nuclei with prominent nucleoli. Considerable cytologic atypia may be seen, especially in association with viral infections, radiation, or chemotherapy with drugs such as cytoxan or busulfan; however, the atypia can occur in the absence of any known association. As the injured alveolar walls heal, the regenerating type 2 pneumocytes are thought to differentiate into type 1 pneumocytes, allowing restoration of normal alveolar gas exchange.

Fibroblasts and myofibroblasts proliferate within the interstitium and migrate through breaks in the alveolar basement membrane into the intra-alveolar fibrinous exudate (fig. 3-39). This exudate is transformed into granulation tissue that may either undergo resorption as the lung returns to normal or progress to dense fibrosis. Type 2 pneumocytes migrate over the surface of the intra-alveolar granulation tissue, incorporating it into the interstitium.

Pratt et al. (288,289) observed that much of this fibrosis occurs at the level of the alveolar duct and coined the term *alveolar duct fibrosis*. In some cases, the alveolar ducts become obliterated with nodules of organizing fibrosis. In other cases, alveolar duct fibrosis takes the shape of rings of irregular fibrous bands surrounding a central space. If the alveolar duct lumen is filled with an inflammatory exudate, it may be mistaken for a microabscess. If it is filled with hemorrhage, it may be mistaken for a blood vessel.

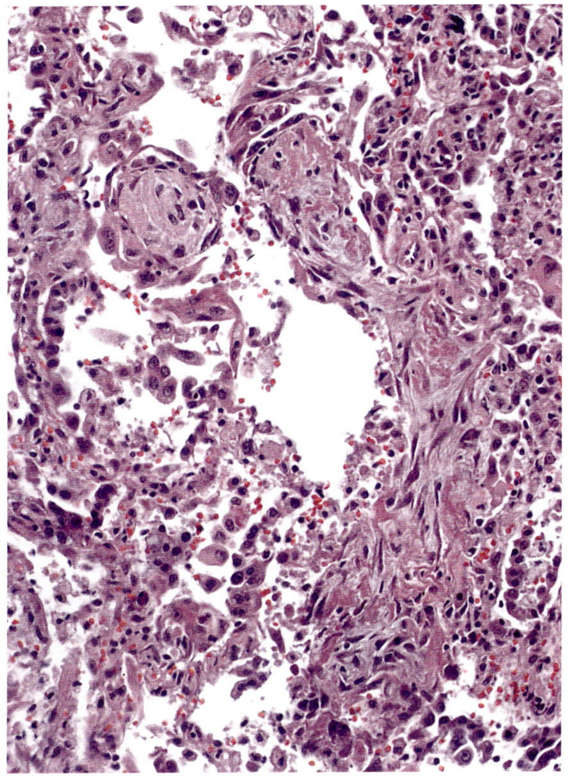

Figure 3-37

DIFFUSE ALVEOLAR DAMAGE: ORGANIZING PATTERN

The fibrosis in the alveolar septal walls consists of a loose organizing type of connective tissue. Prominent hyperplastic type 2 pneumocytes line the alveolar walls.

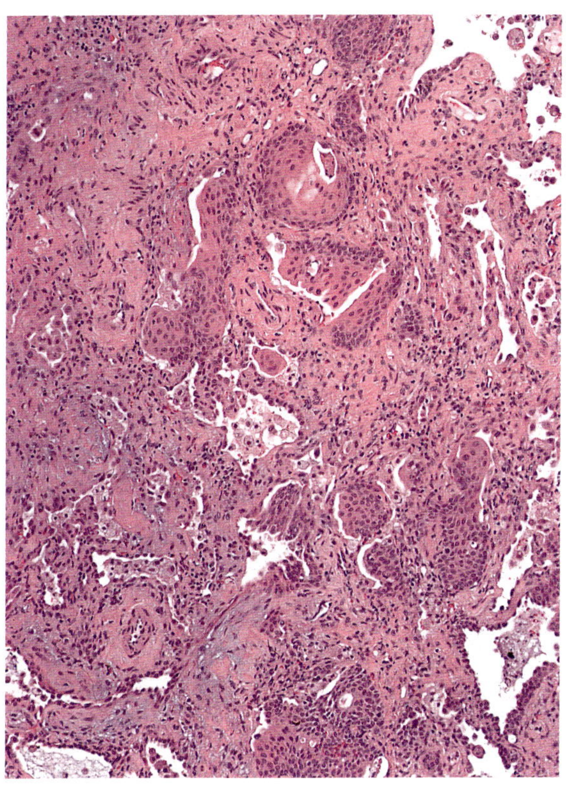

Figure 3-38

DIFFUSE ALVEOLAR DAMAGE: FIBROSING PATTERN

Dense and organizing interstitial fibrosis are accompanied by squamous metaplasia.

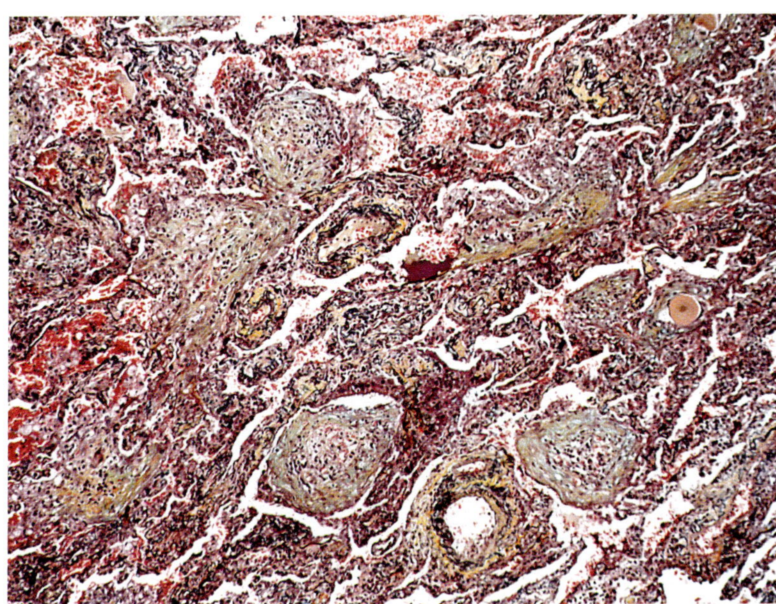

Figure 3-39

DIFFUSE ALVEOLAR DAMAGE: ORGANIZING PATTERN

The intra-alveolar plugs of organizing connective tissue are highlighted by a Movat stain. This gives an appearance resembling an organizing pneumonia pattern. However, in addition, there is thickening of alveolar walls by loose organizing connective tissue, favoring a DAD pattern.

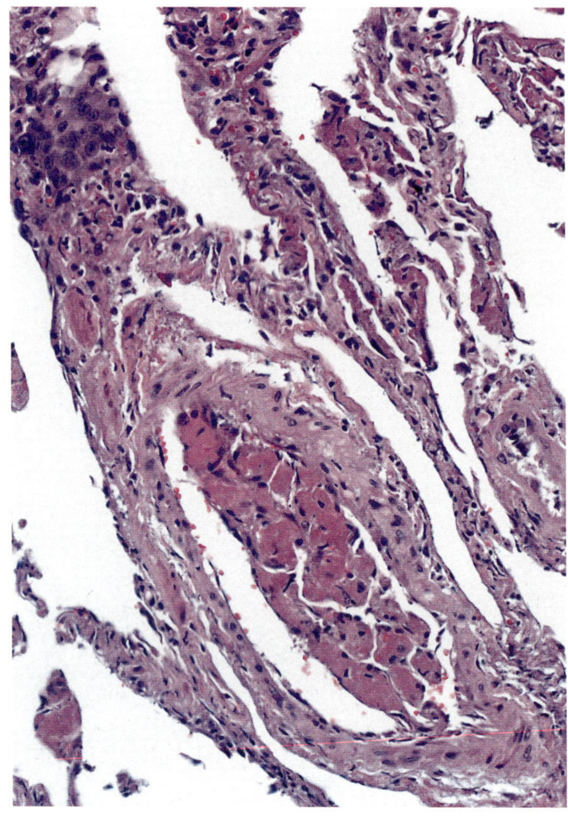

Figure 3-40

DIFFUSE ALVEOLAR DAMAGE: ORGANIZING THROMBUS

Within the lumen of this venule is a fibrin thrombus.

A variety of types of vascular injury are seen in the proliferative phase, each of which contributes to the development of pulmonary hypertension. Vascular thromboemboli are common (fig. 3-40) and peripheral infarcts may be seen (301). The infarcts may be wedge-shaped and subpleural but they may also show unusual patterns such as subpleural, band-like or intermittent lobular necrosis (300,301). Chronic endothelial cell injury can lead to occlusion of capillaries due to hypertrophy of endothelial cells and thickened, reduplicated basement membranes (300,301). Small arteries and veins may be occluded by fibrous intimal proliferation. Lymphatics may be obstructed due to coagulation of proteinaceous edema. Extensive chronic vascular remodeling, increased muscularization, and neomuscularization occur in the proliferative and fibrotic phases of DAD.

Fibrotic (Chronic) Phase. The fibrotic phase of DAD is encountered in patients who survive 3 or 4 weeks on a ventilator. The lungs become extensively remodeled by dense fibrous tissue. The alveolar spaces and bronchioles may be haphazardly enlarged and surrounded by dense fibrosis. Patients who survive more than 2 weeks have a progressive increase in intra-alveolar fibrosis and collagen (249,308). Honeycomb cystic changes may occur in severely fibrotic lungs. Rarely, marked cystic changes occur that resemble the bronchopulmonary dysplasia seen in infants (247).

Histologic Clues to Underlying Cause. Part of the evaluation of lung biopsies showing the pattern of DAD is to look for histologic clues of an etiology. The most important potential cause is infection. Granulomas, viral inclusions, foci of necrosis, and neutrophil collections are all potential clues of infection. Special stains should be performed routinely in such cases for bacteria, mycobacteria, and fungi (especially *Pneumocystis carinii*). Ideally, cultures should be performed on lung biopsy specimens. Other potential histologic clues that suggest an underlying condition include vasculitis, hemorrhage, embolic material such as fat, and the presence of tumor cells.

Pathogenesis. The pathogenesis of DAD is complex, with many cellular events that involve a wide variety of cells such as epithelial cells, endothelial cells, neutrophils, histiocytes, fibroblasts, and smooth muscle cells as well as the extracellular matrix. Many mediators are involved including cytokines, interleukins (240,242,244, 303), tumor necrosis factor-alpha, proteases, oxidants, leukotrienes, oncogenes, suppressor genes, and growth factors (fig. 3-41). It is beyond the scope of this discussion to address these issues in detail, however, several references provide useful reviews of this subject (254,255,258,259,276,287,306).

An important concept in the pathogenesis of DAD is that the intra-alveolar exudates become organized with inflammatory cells, and eventually, fibroblastic connective tissue. This can either resolve to normal lung or become incorporated into the alveolar septa, causing collapse of the alveolar walls and accumulation of dense interstitial fibrosis (fig. 3-42) (240,241,245,249,268).

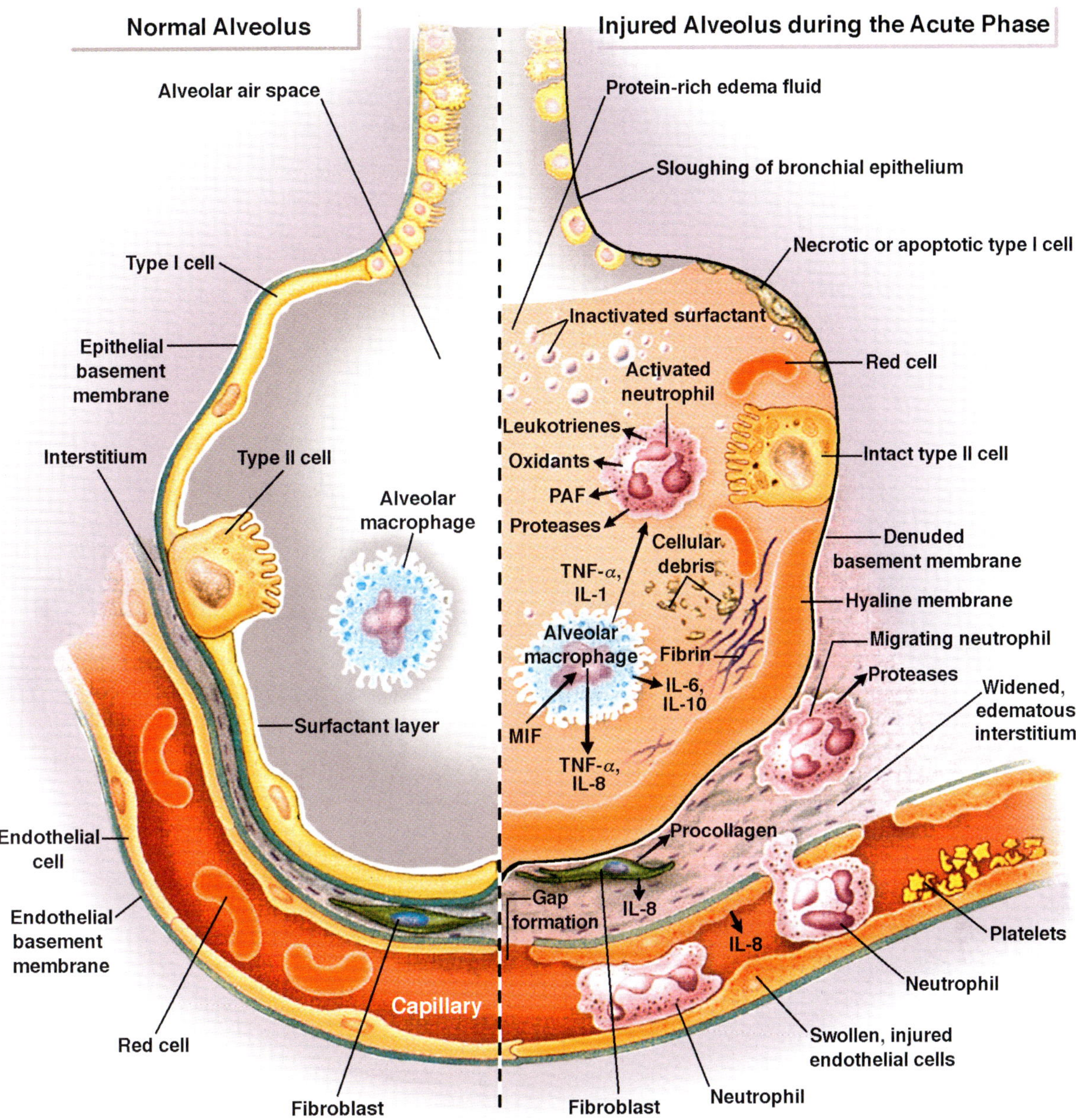

Figure 3-41

PATHOGENESIS OF ACUTE RESPIRATORY DISTRESS SYNDROME: ACUTE PHASE

In contrast to the normal alveolus (left), in the acute phase of the respiratory distress syndrome (right), there is sloughing of both the bronchial and alveolar epithelial cells, with the formation of protein-rich hyaline membranes on the denuded basement membrane. Neutrophils are shown adhering to the injured capillary endothelium and marginating through the interstitium into the airspace, which is filled with protein-rich edema fluid. In the airspace, an alveolar macrophage is secreting cytokines, interleukins (IL) 1,6, 8, and 10, and tumor necrosis factor-alpha (TNF-alpha), which act locally to stimulate chemotaxis and activate neutrophils. Macrophages also secrete other cytokines, including interleukins 1, 6, and 10. Interleukin 1 can stimulate the production of extracellular matrix by fibroblasts. Neutrophils can release oxidants, proteases, leukotrienes, and other proinflammatory molecules, such as platelet-activating factor (PAF). A number of anti-inflammatory molecules are also present in the alveolar milieu, including interleukin 1 receptor antagonist, soluble tumor necrosis factor receptor, autoantibodies against interleukin 8, and cytokines such as interleukins 10 and 11 (not shown). The influx of protein-rich edema fluid into the alveolus has led to the inactivation of surfactant. MIF denotes macrophage inhibitory factor. (Figure 3 from Ware LB, Matthay MA. The acute respiratory distress syndrome. N Engl J Med 2000;342:1339.)

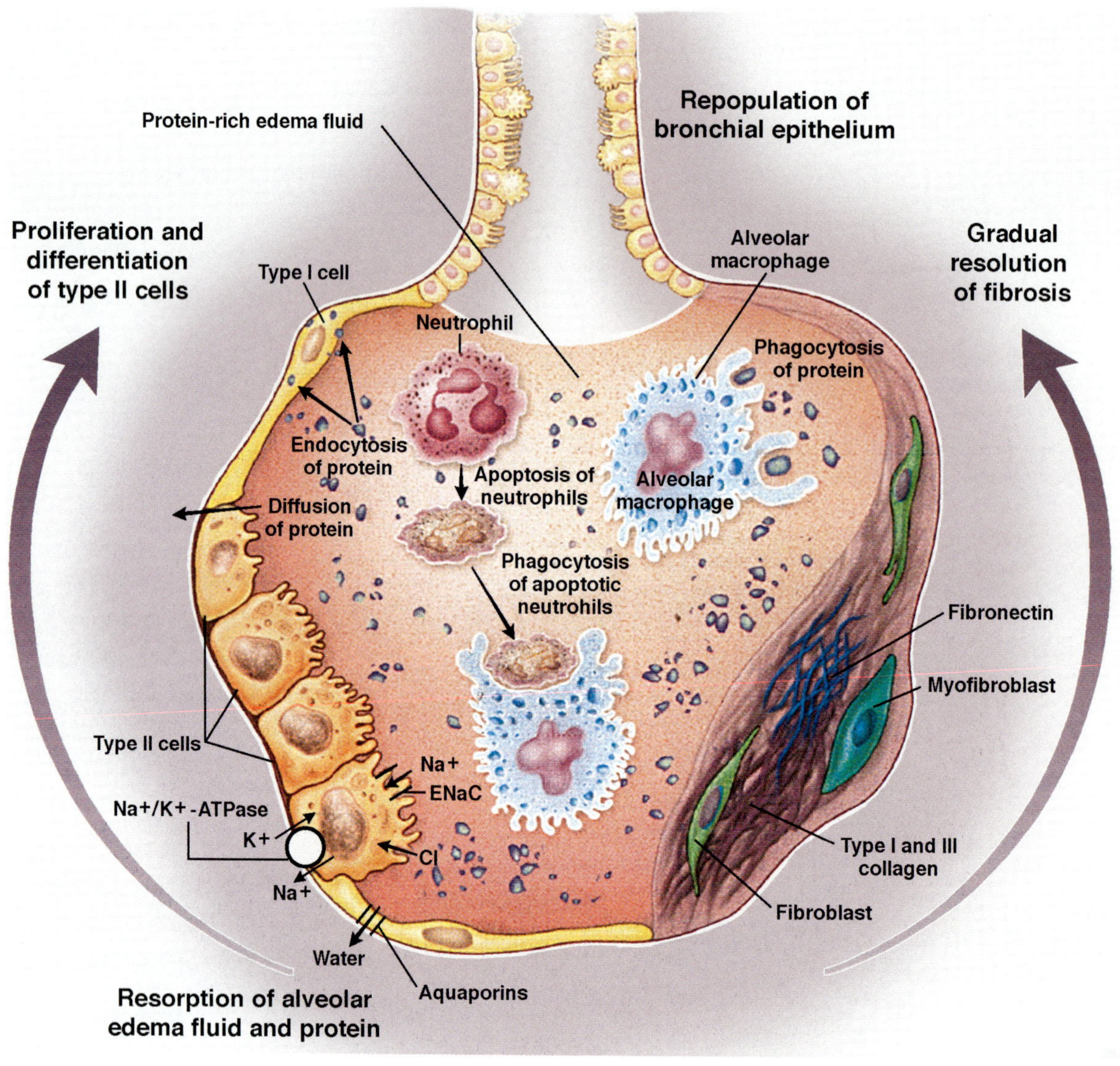

Figure 3-42

PATHOGENESIS OF ACUTE RESPIRATORY DISTRESS SYNDROME: ORGANIZING PHASE AND RESOLUTION

On the left side of the alveolus, the alveolar epithelium is being repopulated by the proliferation and differentiation of alveolar type 2 cells. Resorption of alveolar edema fluid is shown at the base of the alveolus, with sodium and chloride being transported through the apical membrane of type 2 cells. Sodium is taken up by the epithelial sodium channel (ENaC) and through the basolateral membrane of type 2 cells by the sodium pump (Na+/K+ ATPase). The relevant pathways for chloride transport are unclear. Water is shown moving through water channels, the aquaporins, located primarily on type 1 cells. Some water crosses by a paracellular route. Soluble protein is probably cleared by paracellular diffusion and secondarily by endocytosis by alveolar epithelial cells. Macrophages remove insoluble protein and apoptotic neutrophils by phagocytosis. On the right side of the alveolus, the gradual remodeling and resolution of intra-alveolar and interstitial granulation tissue and fibrosis are shown. (Figure 4 from Ware LB, Matthay MA. The acute respiratory distress syndrome. N Engl J Med 2000;342:1342.)

Treatment and Prognosis. Patients with ARDS have an overall mortality rate of approximately 50 percent. Most deaths are due to sepsis or multiorgan dysfunction, however, the therapeutic success of ventilation with low tidal volumes indicates that in some cases death is directly related to lung injury (303,306). Furthermore, it appears that mortality may be decreasing; currently, it is estimated at approximately 35 to 40 percent (236,278,306). Possible explanations for this decrease include more effective treatments for sepsis, changes in the method of mechanical ventilation, and improvement in the supportive care of critically ill patients (306).

In fatal cases, the combination of increasing tachypnea and decreasing tidal volume eventuates in alveolar hypoventilation, progressive hypoxemia, and a rising PCO_2. Patients who survive ARDS may recover normal pulmonary function. However, in severe cases, survivors have interstitial fibrosis (292,304).

Once the diagnosis of ARDS is made, application of certain principles of supportive therapy is warranted regardless of etiology. The therapy for ARDS is primarily supportive and directed at maintaining adequate tissue oxygenation and perfusion, treating hemodynamic instability, and avoiding infectious complications. Recent evidence suggests that traditional approaches to mechanical ventilation can cause or worsen acutely injured lungs. Currently, therapy is directed at the correction of the physiologic abnormalities presenting a threat to organ function while simultaneously minimizing the risk of ventilator-associated lung injury (244,272).

Prognostic Correlations with Lung Biopsy Findings. One would expect that patients with lung biopsies showing extensive fibrosis have a poor clinical outcome. However, several studies by Olson et al. (285) and Suchyta et al. (295) suggest that there is a poor correlation between the severity of lung biopsy findings and clinical outcome. Lamy et al. found that 3 of 13 patients with severe fibrosis survived to regain normal lung function. Olson et al. (285) also saw complete recovery in several patients with AIP who had severe fibrosis on lung biopsy. Suchyta et al. found the severity score for organizing fibrosis correlated with the percent predicted DLCO, however, there was no significant correlation between quantitative scores of histologic abnormalities and predicted lung function more than 1 year after ARDS.

Acute Fibrinous and Organizing Pneumonia

Definition. Acute fibrinous and organizing pneumonia (AFOP) is a histologic pattern that consists of prominent intra-alveolar fibrin and organizing pneumonia, but lacks hyaline membranes or prominent eosinophilia.

AFOP is a histologic pattern that appears to represent a form of lung injury that differs from the histologic patterns of DAD, organizing pneumonia (COP or BOOP), and eosinophilic pneumonia (242). Similar to these patterns of lung injury, the AFOP pattern can occur in an idiopathic setting or with a spectrum of clinical associations. Most patients follow a clinical course similar to that of DAD (304). It is possible some of these cases represent a pre-exudative phase of DAD.

Clinical Features. Beasley et al. (242) recently described 17 patients who had open lung biopsies showing the histologic pattern of AFOP. The patients presented with acute onset of dyspnea, fever, cough, or hemoptysis. The average time from presentation to lung biopsy was 19 days (range, 2 to 60 days). Associations included collagen vascular disease (2 patients), amiodarone therapy (1 patient), positive sputum culture for *Haemophilus influenza* (1 patient), lung culture positive for *Acinetobacter* sp. (1 patient), lymphoma (1 patient), use of hairspray (1 patient), construction work with exposure to wood dusts (1 patient), coal mining (1 patient), and zoological work (1 patient). Six patients had no identifiable etiology or association.

Radiologic Findings. The presence of bilateral basilar opacities is the most common radiologic pattern (242). These opacities appear as diffuse airspace disease or as patchy reticulonodular opacities. Unilateral lung involvement may also occur.

Histologic Findings. The dominant histologic finding is the presence of intra-alveolar fibrin in the form of fibrin "balls" within the alveolar spaces (figs. 3-43, 3-44) (242). The lesion is patchy, with an average airspace involvement of 50 percent (range, 20 to 90 percent). Classic hyaline membranes as seen in DAD are absent. The alveolar fibrin is frequently associated with organizing pneumonia consisting of intraluminal loose connective tissue within the alveolar ducts and bronchioles. The intervening lung parenchyma between the affected areas shows minimal changes, such as a sparse inflammatory infiltrate or minimal interstitial thickening. Vascular thrombi are seen in one third of cases.

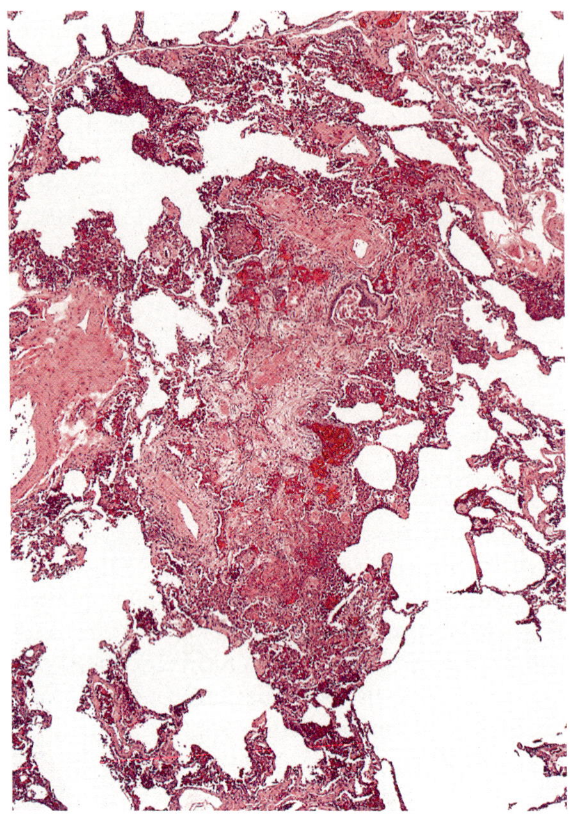

Figure 3-43

ACUTE FIBRINOUS AND ORGANIZING PNEUMONIA

The alveolar spaces are filled with fibrin and organizing loose connective tissue. No hyaline membranes are seen and the process appears patchy rather than diffuse.

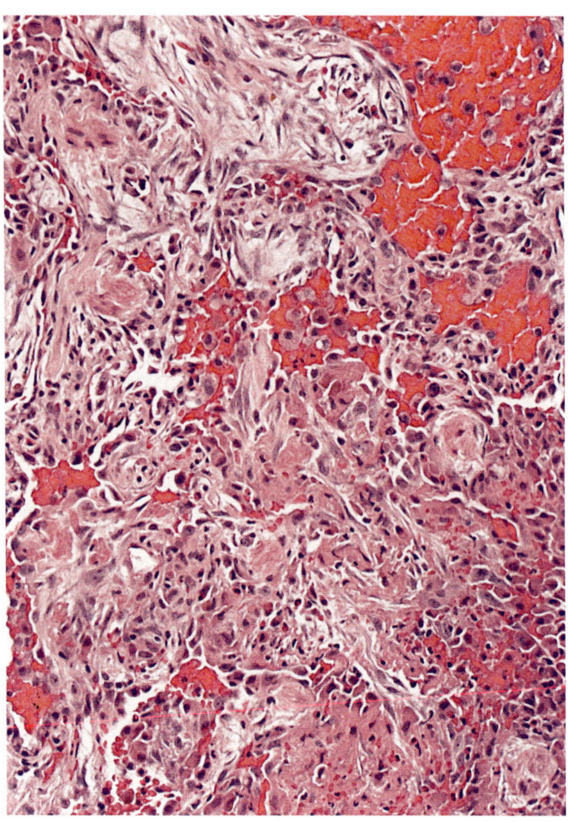

Figure 3-44

ACUTE FIBRINOUS AND ORGANIZING PNEUMONIA

Fibrin and organizing connective tissue fill the alveolar spaces.

Differential Diagnosis. The AFOP histologic pattern must be separated from the patterns of DAD, organizing pneumonia, and eosinophilic pneumonia (242). The lack of hyaline membranes and the patchy nature of the lesion negates DAD and acute eosinophilic pneumonia. The lack of eosinophils negates acute and chronic eosinophilic pneumonia. Focal areas of AFOP are a nonspecific histologic reaction to acute pneumonia and vasculitis such as Wegener's granulomatosis, and are seen adjacent to infarcts and abscesses. In this regard, AFOP shares the same problems with sampling that are encountered with interpreting lung biopsies for the diagnosis of organizing pneumonia.

The etiologic differential diagnosis is similar to that of DAD and includes infection, collagen vascular disease, drug toxicity, and uremia. As with DAD, a careful search must be made for viral inclusions, granulomas, foci of necrosis, and abscesses. Special stains for organisms should also be performed.

Treatment and Prognosis. Follow-up of patients with AFOP in the study by Beasley et al. (242) revealed two clinical patterns of disease progression: one, a fulminant illness with rapid progression to death (in 9 patients, mean survival period of 0.1 year) and two, a more subacute pattern, with recovery (8 patients). Histology and initial symptoms did not correlate with eventual outcome.

The overall mortality rate is similar to that of DAD. In the Beasley study (242), the need for mechanical ventilation was the only parameter that correlated with prognosis in that 5 of 5 patients requiring mechanical ventilation died (p=0.0068). Patients who did not require mechanical ventilation uniformly improved, with normalization of their radiographs and physiologic measurements. There have been no recurrences to date.

Acute Interstitial Pneumonia (Idiopathic Diffuse Alveolar Damage)

Definition. Acute interstitial pneumonia (AIP) is an uncommon, rapidly progressive, fulminant form of lung injury of unknown cause. This clinicopathologic term is synonymous with idiopathic diffuse alveolar damage (DAD). The histologic features are identical with DAD. Lung biopsies are often performed during the organizing phase rather than the exudative phase.

In 1986, Katzenstein et al. (267) defined AIP as the equivalent of idiopathic DAD based on a series of eight patients, and proposed that this entity be added to the group of idiopathic interstitial pneumonias (263). Subsequently, only a few case series and isolated reports have been published on this subject (Table 3-19) (237,238,261,285,291). These cases loosely correspond to cases described by Hamman and Rich (fig. 3-45) (239,256). The ATS/ERS International Consensus Panel for Classification of Idiopathic Interstitial Pneumonias concurred that AIP is the clinical term of choice for patients with idiopathic DAD (302).

Clinical Features. The clinician must have a high index of suspicion to make a diagnosis of AIP. The possibility of AIP should be considered for any patient presenting with a diagnosis of severe community-acquired pneumonia who fails to respond to broad-spectrum antibiotic therapy and in whom no causative agent is identified. AIP differs from ARDS only by the absence of a known precipitating cause or preexisting disease and the lack of a systemic disorder which predisposes to DAD (267,285). The clinical features of AIP are summarized in Table 3-19.

Patients typically present with a prodromal illness resembling an upper respiratory tract viral infection, followed by the onset of acute respiratory failure. Cough and dyspnea are present in 100 and 81 percent of subjects, respectively (304). The duration of symptoms before presentation is usually between 3 and 18 days (291). In fact, most patients with AIP present within 60 days of onset of symptoms, and this is used to differentiate it from other forms of idiopathic interstitial pneumonia

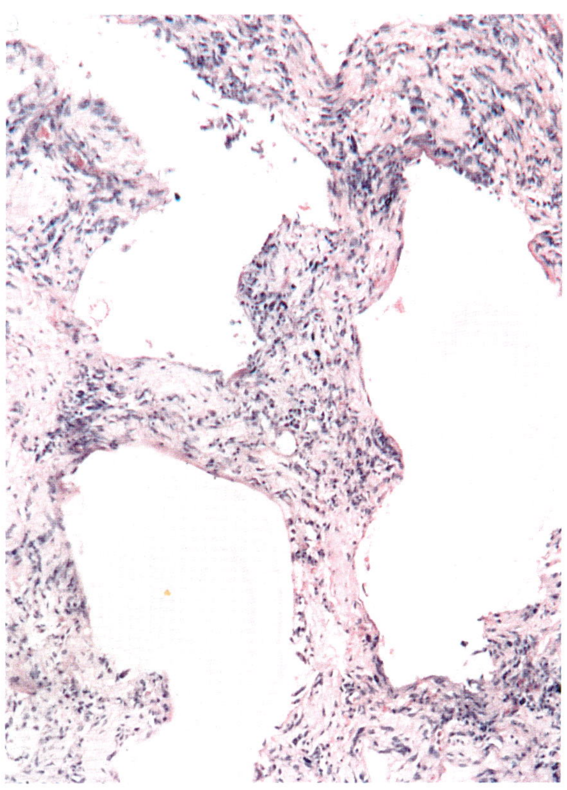

Figure 3-45

ACUTE INTERSTITIAL PNEUMONIA

In a case reported by Hamman and Rich (256), there is prominent type 2 pneumocyte proliferation. These histologic features are virtually identical to those seen in figure 3-36 showing organizing DAD. (Courtesy of Dr. Grover Hutchins, Johns Hopkins University, Baltimore, MD.)

where the symptom duration is often measured in months to years. Except for fever, which occurs in 35 to 50 percent of subjects, there are few systemic symptoms.

Tachypnea is common, and crackles are heard on chest examination in 50 percent of cases. Hypoxemia, often profound, is nearly universal.

Radiologic Findings. The radiologic manifestations of AIP are similar to those of ARDS (262,274,291). The main radiographic finding is rapidly progressive, bilateral airspace consolidation (fig. 3-46, left). HRCT in the exudative and early proliferative stages shows extensive bilateral areas of ground-glass attenuation and areas of consolidation with air bronchograms (fig. 3-46, right) (261,291). The consolidation involves mainly the dependent lung regions. In the late proliferative and fibrotic

Table 3-19

CLINICAL FEATURES OF ACUTE INTERSTITIAL PNEUMONIA

Clinical Feature	Hamman (256) 1944 n=4	Katzenstein (267) 1986 n=8	Olson (285) 1990 n=29	Primack (291) 1993 n=9	Ichikado (261) 1997 n=14	Vourlekis (304) 2000 n=13
Age: yrs, mean (range)	43 (21-68)	28 (13-50)	50 (7-77)	65 (43-83)	53 (40-66)	54 (34-74)
Sex (M:F)	1:3	3:5	14:15	7:2	8:6	6:7
Symptoms/signs (%)				ARI[a] 9 (100)		
URI/flu-like illness	1 (25)	3 (38)	29 (100)		NA	NA
Tachypnea	4 (100)	NA	27 (93)		NA	NA
Dyspnea	4 (100)	2 (25)	27 (93)		NA	9/11 (81%)
Cough	3 (75)	1 (13)	20 (69)		NA	12/12 (100%)
Fever	2 (50)	3 (38)	10 (34)		NA	9/12 (75%)
Cyanosis	2 (50)	NA	3 (10)		NA	NA
Rales	4 (100)	1 (13)	3 (10)		NA	NA
Hypotension	1 (25)	NA	1 (3)		NA	NA
Clinical Outcome						Initial hosp.[d]
Dead (%)	Autopsy series[c]	7/8 (88)	12/24 (50)	8 (88)	Autopsy	4/12 (33%)
Survival (days)[b]				less than 90	series[c]	After recurrence
Mean (range)	58 (31-96)	68 (23-183)	24 (1-136)	days	(14-183)	2/12 (17%)
Recovered (%)	0	1/8	12 (41%)	1 (12)	0	8/12 (67%)
Survival to discharge (days)						1 required HLT[e] 1 died of CHF
Mean (range)	NA	35	48 (11-104); 6 two-year survivors	60	NA	1 O_2 dependent

[a]ARI = acute respiratory tract infection.
[b]Survival = number of survivors divided by number of patients diagnosed by lung biopsy.
[c]Autopsy diagnoses excluded.
[d]hosp. = hospitalization.
[e]HLT = heart-lung transplant; CHF = congestive heart failure.

phase, dilated and distorted bronchi (traction bronchiectasis) can often be seen within the areas of consolidation (261). In the fibrotic phase, there are focal lucencies, cystic spaces representing overinflated regions of lung, and, occasionally, honeycombing (261,291).

Gross Findings. The gross pathologic features of AIP are identical to those of DAD, except underlying causes such as infections or tumors should be absent. Gross findings are more likely to resemble the organizing phase rather than the exudative phase of DAD, since most patients get biopsied or die during the latter phase of AIP.

Histologic Findings. Lung biopsies from patients with AIP show histologic features identical to those of the various exudative, proliferative, and fibrotic phases of DAD. The lung biopsy typically is diffusely involved and the connective tissue appears about the same age (fig. 3-47). Olson et al. (285) found that some lung biopsies vary in severity among different histologic fields. The proliferating type 2 pneumocytes lining the alveolar walls mostly show a low cuboidal or hobnailed morphology, but they often exhibit cytologic atypia with large nuclei and prominent nucleoli (267). Organizing fibrosis is mostly seen within alveolar septa, but it may also be seen within airspaces; this is a prominent feature in over one third of cases (285). Mitotic activity may be seen in the proliferating type 2 pneumocytes and fibroblasts. In 24 to 60 percent of cases, thrombi are seen in small to medium-sized pulmonary arterioles (267,285).

Diagnosis. Since most pathologists review lung biopsies with minimal clinical history, they are seldom in a position to make the ultimate diagnosis of AIP. Usually, the pathologist can only be sure of the diagnosis of "DAD, etiology undetermined." Once the DAD pattern has been established histologically, the biopsy findings need to be correlated with the clinical history and laboratory results to further exclude other

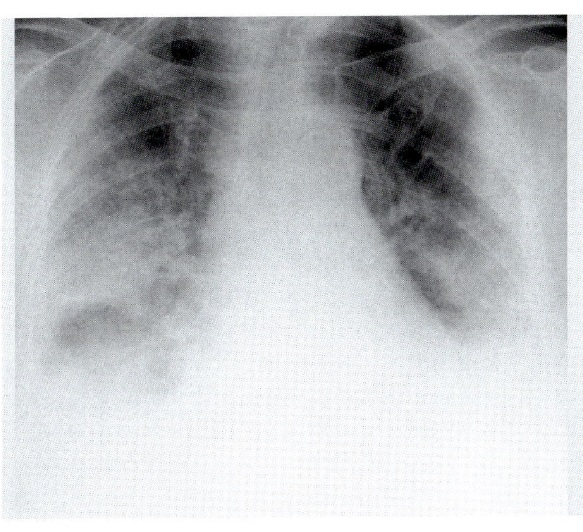

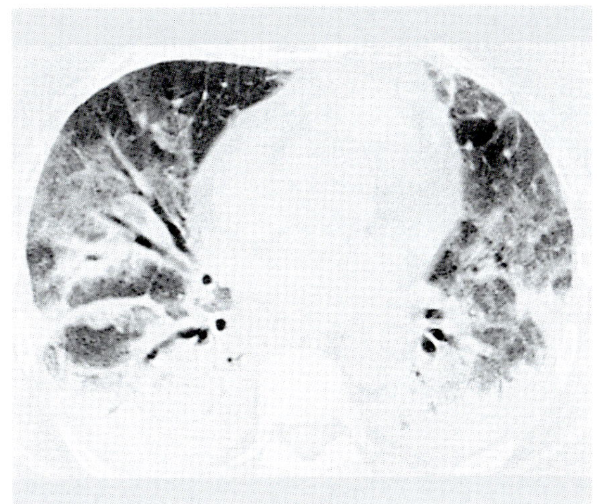

Figure 3-46

ACUTE INTERSTITIAL PNEUMONIA

Left: Anteroposterior chest radiograph demonstrates extensive bilateral areas of consolidation involving mainly the lower lung zones.

Right: HRCT shows that the consolidation involves mainly the dependent lung regions. Areas of ground-glass attenuation are present in the anterior lung. The patient was an 83-year-old woman with AIP.

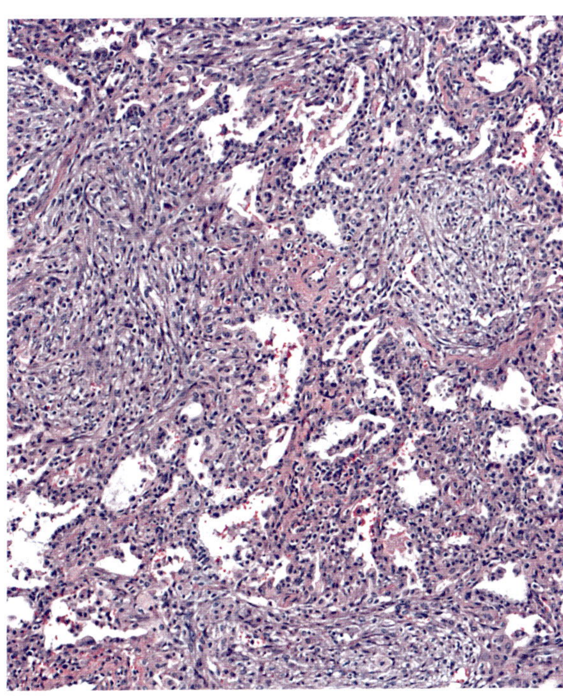

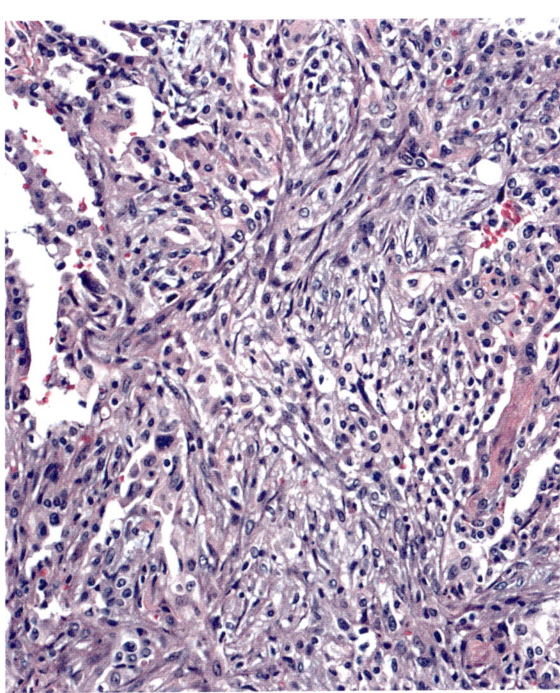

Figure 3-47

ACUTE INTERSTITIAL PNEUMONIA: DIFFUSE ALVEOLAR DAMAGE, ORGANIZING PATTERN

Left: The interstitium is diffusely thickened by uniform, organizing fibrosis. Although the organizing fibrosis has some nodularity, it is situated primarily within the alveolar septal interstitium rather than forming intraluminal polyps as seen in organizing pneumonia.

Right: Closer view shows the alveolar septal location of the organizing fibrosis.

potential etiologies, such as collagen vascular disease. After this clinicopathologic correlation, the diagnosis of AIP may be made (267,285). Therefore, the ultimate diagnosis of AIP is generally made by the clinician after review of the clinical, laboratory, and microbiological data. Since all of these results often are not available until days or weeks after the lung biopsy is performed, it is not possible to be absolutely certain of the diagnosis of AIP at the time of open lung biopsy.

Differential Diagnosis. In most cases, the histologic pattern of DAD is readily apparent. The presence of hyaline membranes is a very helpful clue to the diagnosis of DAD since they are not seen in either UIP or organizing pneumonia (see Table 3-7). They are seen in most cases of AIP, but since these patients are often biopsied during the organizing phase, they may be inconspicuous or absent (264). Cases lacking hyaline membranes are most likely to be confused with organizing pneumonia or UIP.

After recognizing the pattern of DAD, pathologists must thoroughly search for histologic clues to an etiology. The presence of granulomas, viral inclusions, foci of necrosis, or neutrophilic abscesses suggests infection. Special stains for microorganisms should be routinely performed to exclude an infection.

The diffuse nature of DAD distinguishes it from the patchy lesions of UIP and COP (see Table 3-7). In addition, the fibrosis of UIP is temporally heterogeneous, with patchy scarring and scattered fibroblastic foci, in contrast to the temporally uniform fibroblastic connective tissue seen in the proliferative phase of DAD. The histologic pattern of DAD shows more fibroblastic connective tissue within the alveolar septal interstitium, while in organizing pneumonia, it is predominantly within airspaces and rarely in alveolar septal interstitium. The type 2 pneumocyte proliferation is also much more prominent than in the organizing pneumonia pattern.

The cellular and/or fibrosing pattern of NSIP may be confused with the organizing or fibrosing patterns of DAD. Several patients with NSIP in a study by Katzenstein et al. (266), had a previous clinical history of ARDS.

Treatment and Prognosis. Patients who survive the initial illness generally have a favorable outcome (285). Olson et al. (285) reported that 5 of 6 survivors in their series had normal or improving lung spirometry 12 to 24 months following AIP. AIP can be recurrent and can progress to chronic interstitial lung disease (292,304). Persistent physiologic abnormalities, both on spirometry and comprehensive lung function testing, were found in 5 of the 6 survivors in a recent study (304).

There is no effective treatment for patients with AIP. Corticosteroids are commonly used as first-line therapy, but mortality remains high. Recent studies indicate a potential benefit for corticosteroids in the fibroproliferative phase of ARDS (277). Olson (285) found that corticosteroids had little impact on patient survival. Virtually all patients require mechanical ventilation. Overall survival rates range from 25 to 65 percent. Vourlekis and coworkers (304) reported that the serum creatinine level and hematocrit correlated with in-hospital survival. Both have been shown to predict mortality in intensive care patients, and renal dysfunction predicts mortality in ARDS patients. Therefore, both serve as markers of disease severity, but neither variable likely is related to disease pathogenesis (304).

RESPIRATORY BRONCHIOLITIS–INTERSTITIAL LUNG DISEASE

Definition. Respiratory bronchiolitis–interstitial lung disease (RB-ILD) is a mild form of interstitial lung disease characterized histologically by chronic bronchiolitis in which pigmented macrophages accumulate within respiratory bronchioles and adjacent alveolar spaces.

The histologic lesion of respiratory bronchiolitis (RB) is commonly encountered as an incidental finding in lung specimens removed from cigarette smokers. This lesion may be the sole abnormality in patients presenting with interstitial lung disease (ILD). In this setting, the appropriate clinical term is RB-ILD (323).

Numerous papers have described the histologic changes in the bronchioles of cigarette smokers. Many of these papers have used the descriptive term "small airways disease." Niewoehner (319), Cosio (310), Hogg (313), Thurlbeck (322), and Eidelman (311) have described histologic changes in the airways of smokers and attempted to correlate them with clinical and morphologic abnormalities. In 1985, Myers et al. (318) reported on six cigarette-smoking patients with RB who presented with ILD. Subsequent studies have shown that some cases previously diagnosed as DIP actually represent RB-ILD (324).

The strong relationship between smoking and both RB-ILD and DIP has led these diseases to be regarded as a spectrum of smoking-induced DPLD. DIP is considered to be a more extensive form of pigmented alveolar macrophage accumulation while in RB-ILD the macrophages are peribronchiolar (312,315,318, 323). However, due to the differences in the clinical presentation, imaging findings, and prognosis between the two patterns, the ATS/ERS Panel for Classification of Idiopathic Interstitial Pneumonias addressed them separately.

Clinical Features. The incidence and prevalence of RB-ILD are unknown. The cause and pathogenesis are also unknown, however, virtually all patients with RB-ILD are current or past heavy cigarette smokers (316,317). The rare nonsmoker may have a history of other inhalational exposures such as occupational exposure to fumes of solder flux (317). The mean age at onset for RB-ILD is 36 years (range, 22 to 53 years), and there is no sex predilection (318,324). Presenting symptoms include cough and dyspnea. Fine, bibasilar, end-inspiratory crepitations are common findings on chest examination. The rales are said to be coarser than those heard in other interstitial lung diseases (such as IPF); they occur throughout inspiration and sometimes continue into expiration. Clubbing is rare (317, 321). Routine laboratory studies are nonspecific and generally not helpful. Pulmonary function tests may be normal, or show only an increase in residual volume. When abnormal, a mixed obstructive-restrictive pattern with a slightly reduced diffusing capacity is common. Few studies of gas exchange have been reported. Mild hypoxemia may be present at rest or with exercise.

The diagnosis of RB-ILD requires the proper clinical setting (specifically, a patient with a history of cigarette smoking within the last 6 months), appropriate clinical and radiologic manifestations, and a lung biopsy that identifies RB-ILD and rules out more serious causes of DPLD, especially idiopathic pulmonary fibrosis (312,317).

Radiologic Findings. The radiographic abnormalities usually consist of poorly defined hazy areas of increased density (ground-glass opacities) and bronchial wall thickening (fig. 3-48) (312). Less common findings include a fine reticular or reticulonodular pattern and small peripheral ring shadows (314,324). The chest radiograph is normal in 20 to 30 percent of patients (314,324). The main findings on HRCT are bilateral areas of ground-glass attenuation and centrilobular nodular opacities (fig. 3-48) (312,320). These abnormalities may be diffuse or have an upper or lower lung zone predominance. The findings often resemble those of DIP and hypersensitivity pneumonitis. Reticular opacities may be present and, occasionally, are the predominant finding (312,314).

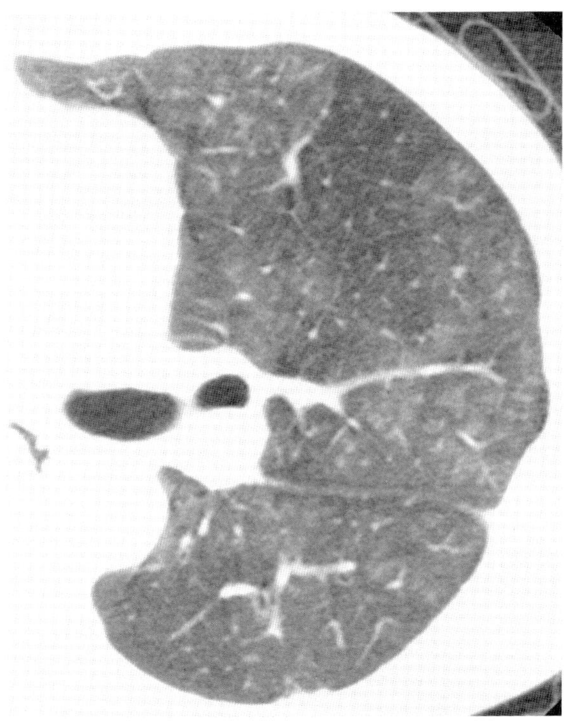

Figure 3-48

RESPIRATORY BRONCHIOLITIS–ASSOCIATED INTERSTITIAL LUNG DISEASE

HRCT of the left lung demonstrates patchy areas of ground-glass attenuation and a few poorly defined nodular opacities.

Histologic Findings. The histologic lesion of RB consists of numerous finely pigmented macrophages within the lumen of the respiratory bronchiole and the surrounding alveolar spaces (318,324). The wall of the bronchioles may show mild chronic inflammation and fibrosis

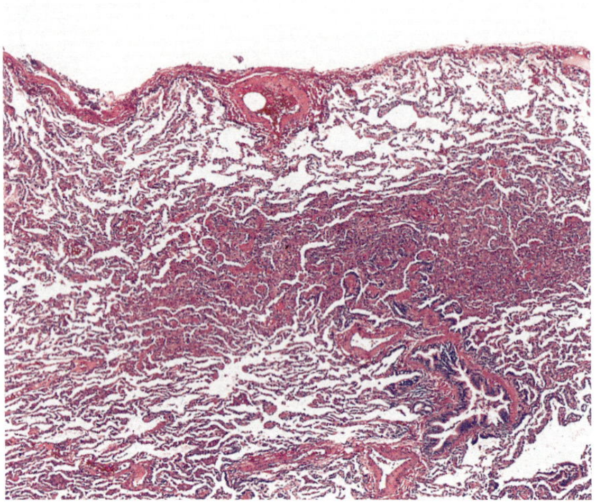

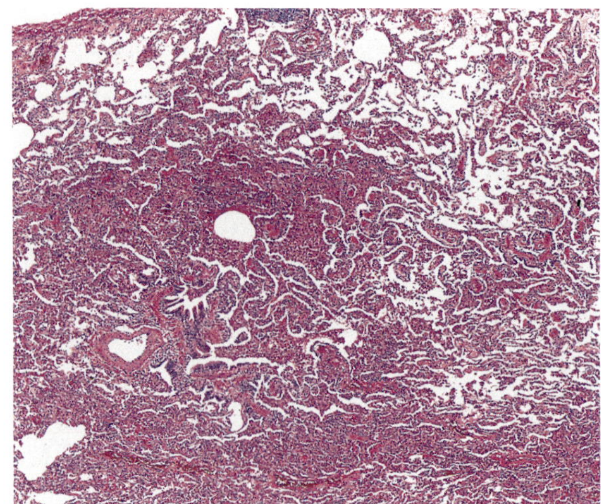

Figure 3-49

RESPIRATORY BRONCHIOLITIS

Low magnification shows a nodular area of macrophage accumulation (left). There is marked peribronchiolar alveolar macrophage accumulation (right). This patient presented with interstitial lung disease and had no other finding on lung biopsy.

(figs. 3-49, 3-50). The macrophages typically have a fine brown cytoplasmic pigment with some black particles. The bronchiolar epithelial cells may show goblet cell metaplasia. Cuboidal cell hyperplasia may be seen along alveolar ducts and alveoli adjacent to the bronchioles. In some cases, the bronchiolar wall shows remodeling, with interstitial fibrosis extending along the surrounding alveolar walls. The epithelium lining these airspaces ranges from cuboidal to bronchiolar-type, pseudostratified and ciliated respiratory epithelium. The alveolar parenchyma between the bronchioles is relatively normal, without interstitial fibrosis or extensive alveolar macrophage accumulation. The histologic features of RB are identical in the setting of ILD or in other pathologic settings such as pulmonary Langerhans' cell histiocytosis or lung cancer.

Differential Diagnosis. The primary differential diagnoses for RB are DIP, asbestosis, and Langerhans' cell histiocytosis. Peribronchiolar lesions similar to those of RB are seen in DIP, however, the intervening alveolar spaces are also diffusely filled with alveolar macrophages. There may be a continuum in the extent of airspace macrophage accumulation, so in some cases the distinction between RB and DIP may be difficult (324). Bronchiolar fibrosis and asbestos bodies in the lung biopsy specimen characterize early asbestosis. A careful search for asbestos bodies on H&E- and iron-stained sections as well as correlation with the history for any evidence of occupational exposure should help in excluding asbestosis. Since virtually all patients with Langerhans' cell histiocytosis are cigarette smokers, the lesion of RB will be present in their lung biopsies. Occasionally, an open lung biopsy has only a focal lesion of Langerhans' cell histiocytosis. Therefore, lung biopsies from patients with RB should be carefully examined for focal, peribronchiolar, stellate scars or cellular infiltrates of Langerhans' cells that may suggest Langerhans' cell histiocytosis. The chest radiograph and HRCT may highlight the distinctive findings in Langerhans' cell histiocytosis. The DIP-like reaction described by Bedrossian et al. (309) probably represents RB in many cases.

Treatment and Prognosis. The clinical course and prognosis of most patients with RB-ILD is favorable.

Smoking plays a role in the pathogenesis, therefore, cessation of smoking is probably important in the resolution of these lesions (321). Respiratory symptoms may improve if the patients stop smoking (321). A favorable response to corticosteroids, with documented improvement in lung function and chest radiographs,

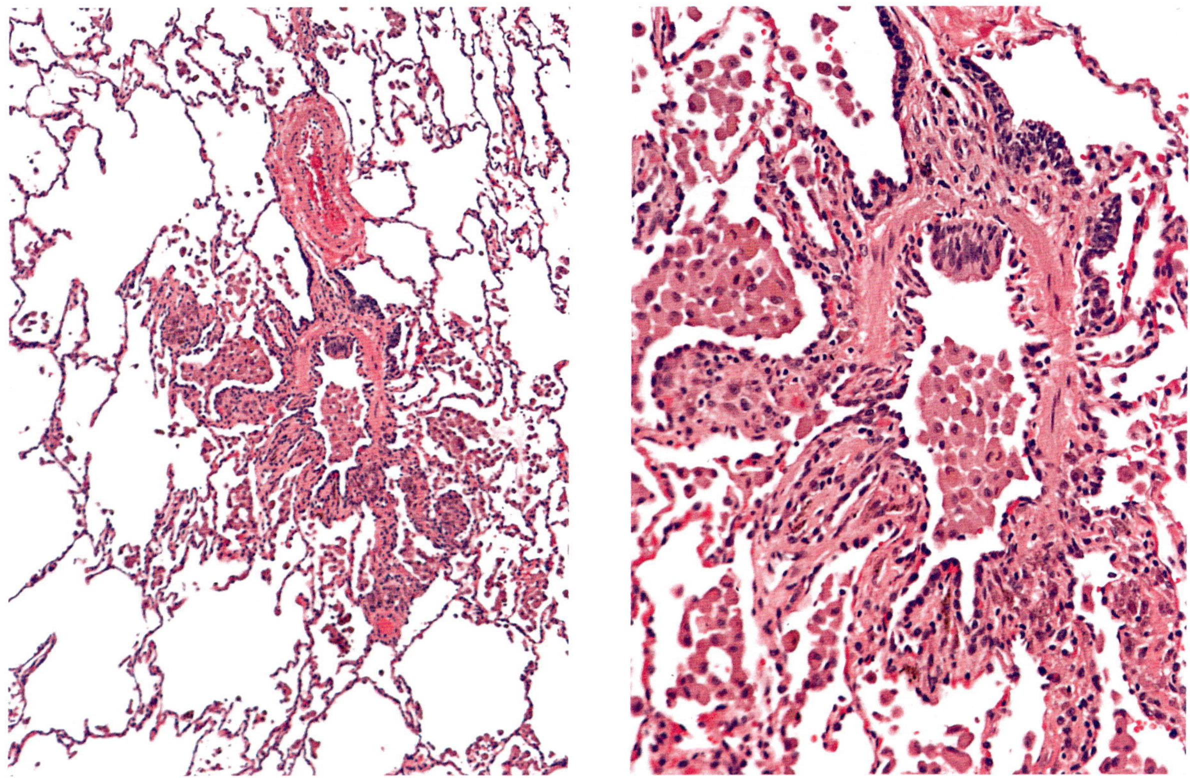

Figure 3-50

RESPIRATORY BRONCHIOLITIS

Left: There is marked alveolar macrophage accumulation concentrated in and around this bronchiole.

Right: The wall of the bronchiole shows mild fibrous thickening and chronic inflammation. The macrophages are faintly pigmented.

has been noted in a small number of patients (317,318,321,324). However, some patients deteriorate despite therapy (317).

The prognosis for RB-ILD patients is excellent. Given this very favorable prognosis, it is important to distinguish this syndrome from other interstitial pneumonias, for which the prognosis is much worse (321).

DESQUAMATIVE INTERSTITIAL PNEUMONIA

Definition. Desquamative interstitial pneumonia (DIP) is a clinical and pathologic entity found almost exclusively in current or former cigarette smokers. It is characterized by mononuclear cell infiltration of the airspaces without prominent fibrosis or honeycombing.

DIP is used to describe a clinicopathologic entity and a histologic pattern (359). Liebow (346) first described DIP in 1965 and thought that most of the desquamated cells were epithelial cells rather than macrophages. It was subsequently shown that most of the intra-alveolar cells are alveolar macrophages (329,346, 362). DIP and UIP were thought to be part of the spectrum of idiopathic pulmonary fibrosis (IPF). It was commonly regarded that DIP was the early, cellular phase and UIP the later, fibrotic phase of the same disease (332,342). Early studies showed a significantly better prognosis for patients with the DIP pattern compared to those with the UIP pattern (330). They are now accepted as separate clinicopathologic entities, with the radiologic and histologic pattern of UIP being required for the diagnosis of IPF (359). DIP also shares many histologic features with RB-ILD (325,352,353,365). The shared morphologic features and the strong epidemiologic link to cigarette smoking in both RB-ILD and DIP

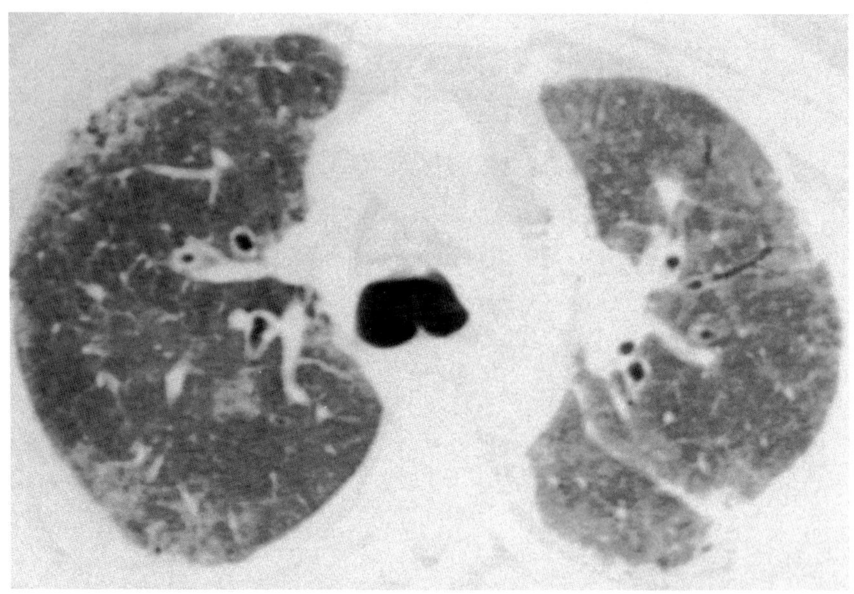

Figure 3-51

DESQUAMATIVE INTERSTITIAL PNEUMONIA

HRCT in a 53-year-old man demonstrates extensive bilateral areas of ground-glass attenuation. Localized irregular linear opacities are present in the subpleural regions, consistent with mild fibrosis. The diagnosis of DIP was proven by open lung biopsy.

suggest that they both may represent points along a spectrum of smoking-related interstitial lung disease (341). The ATS/ERS Panel for Classification of Idiopathic Interstitial Pneumonia recommends using the same term, DIP, for both the pathologic pattern and the clinical diagnosis (359). However, there was considerable debate about replacing the term DIP with a more technically correct term such as alveolar macrophage pneumonia (359).

Clinical Features. The incidence and prevalence of DIP are not known. In the past decade the histologic criteria for DIP have been narrowed after the description of the histologic pattern of RB-ILD and refinement of criteria for UIP (360). Consequently, the clinicopathologic entity of DIP is rare (359). DIP was found in only 8 percent of cases of idiopathic interstitial pneumonia in a recent review from the Mayo Clinic (328), and was seen in less than 3 percent of the patients in a specialized ILD program in Denver (343). The etiology of DIP is unknown, however, the strong epidemiologic link to cigarette smoking suggests its role in causation.

Most patients with DIP present in the fourth to fifth decade of life (mean, 42 years; range, 27 to 79 years) (330,341,359,360). DIP is more common in men, with a male to female ratio of 2 to 1. Rare cases of DIP are reported in children (327,347,355,356,361). These cases probably represent a different disorder than adult DIP and may actually be another entity, such as surfactant deficiency or alveolar proteinosis, which can show prominent alveolar macrophage accumulation (327,333,340,354,356).

Most patients present with a subacute (weeks to months) illness characterized by dyspnea or cough. Physical examination shows crackles on auscultation of the chest that are not as prominent as in other idiopathic interstitial pneumonias. Clubbing can be found. Laboratory investigations are usually unremarkable. Lung function tests show a restrictive pattern with reduced DLCO and hypoxemia on arterial blood gas analysis. BAL shows a marked increase in total cells recovered with a predominance of macrophages.

Radiologic Findings. The predominant finding on the chest radiograph and HRCT is the presence of bilateral symmetric areas of ground-glass opacification involving mainly the lower lung zones (fig. 3-51) (338,346,349). Mild, localized areas of fibrosis cause a reticular pattern that can be seen on the radiograph and CT in approximately 50 percent of patients (fig. 3-51) (330,338). The fibrosis is usually limited to the subpleural lung regions of the lower lung zones. The areas of ground-glass attenuation seen on HRCT have a predominantly peripheral distribution in 60 percent of patients, a patchy distribution in 25 percent, and are diffuse in 15 percent (338). With treatment, in the

Table 3-20

HISTOLOGIC FEATURES OF DESQUAMATIVE INTERSTITIAL PNEUMONIA PATTERN

Major Features
- Uniform involvement of lung parenchyma
- Prominent accumulation of alveolar macrophages
- Mild to moderate fibrotic thickening of alveolar septa
- Mild interstitial chronic inflammation

Minor Features
- Cuboidal hyperplasia of type 2 pneumocytes
- Lymphoid aggregates
- Vascular medial and intimal thickening
- Bronchiolar fibrosis and mild inflammation
- Pleural fibrosis and/or pleuritis
- Blue bodies
- Rare eosinophils
- Dilated pleural lymphatics

Pertinent Negative Findings
- Lack of lung architecture remodeling
- Dense extensive fibrosis: inconspicuous or absent
- Smooth muscle proliferation: inconspicuous or absent
- Honeycomb fibrosis: absent
- Fibroblast foci and organizing pneumonia: inconspicuous or absent
- Eosinophils: inconspicuous, absent, or only focal

majority of cases, the areas of ground-glass attenuation improve or resolve (338). In approximately 20 percent of cases, the areas of ground-glass attenuation progress to a reticular pattern, reflecting the presence of fibrosis (337,338).

Pathologic Findings. The histologic hallmark of the DIP pattern is diffuse, marked, intra-alveolar macrophage accumulation (Table 3-20; figs. 3-52–3-54). The macrophage accumulation may be accentuated around respiratory bronchioles, however, it extends diffusely throughout the lung parenchyma. There is little fibrosis with only mild or moderate thickening of the alveolar walls. Unlike the UIP pattern, there is no scarring fibrosis causing remodeling of the lung architecture. The fibrous connective tissue that is present is all about the same age. Therefore, fibroblastic foci are absent or inconspicuous.

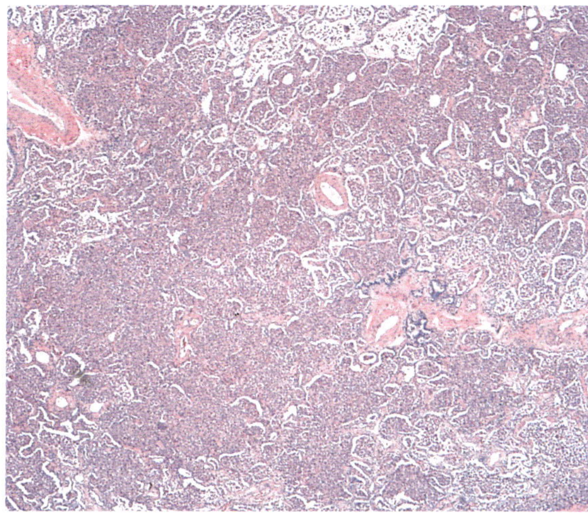

Figure 3-52

DESQUAMATIVE INTERSTITIAL PNEUMONIA PATTERN

The lung is diffusely involved by prominent accumulation of alveolar macrophages. There is minimal interstitial fibrosis and the architecture of the lung is well preserved.

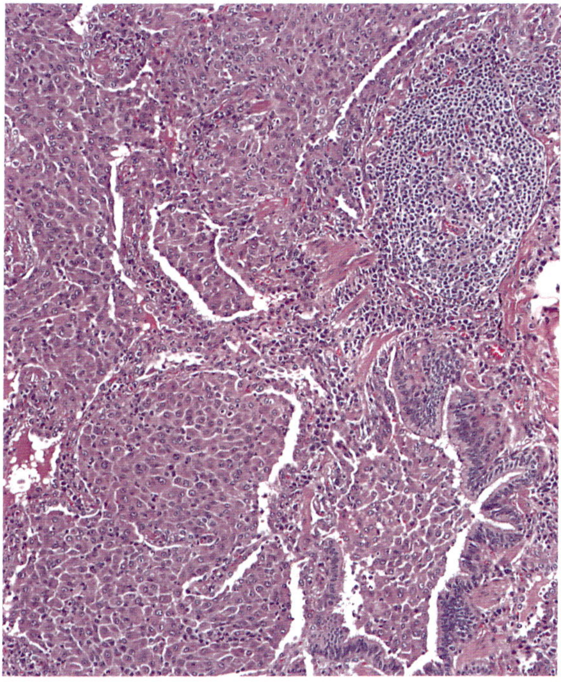

Figure 3-53

DESQUAMATIVE INTERSTITIAL PNEUMONIA PATTERN

In addition to the numerous alveolar macrophages, there is mild thickening of the alveolar septa by fibrosis and a mild chronic inflammatory infiltrate. A hyperplastic lymphoid follicle is present.

Table 3-21

DIFFERENTIAL DIAGNOSIS OF DESQUAMATIVE INTERSTITIAL PNEUMONIA PATTERN

Histologic Patterns
- Usual interstitial pneumonia
- Respiratory bronchiolitis (RB) or RB-interstitial lung disease (RB-ILD)
- Nonspecific interstitial pneumonia, cellular or fibrosing patterns
- Eosinophilic pneumonia
- Chronic hemorrhage, hemosiderosis
- Histiocyte-rich infections
- Giant cell interstitial pneumonia
- Veno-occlusive disease
- Focal nonspecific "DIP-like" reaction
- Carcinoma with intra-alveolar spread

Etiologic Possibilities
- Cigarette smoking
- Pneumoconioses—especially asbestosis
- Idiopathic

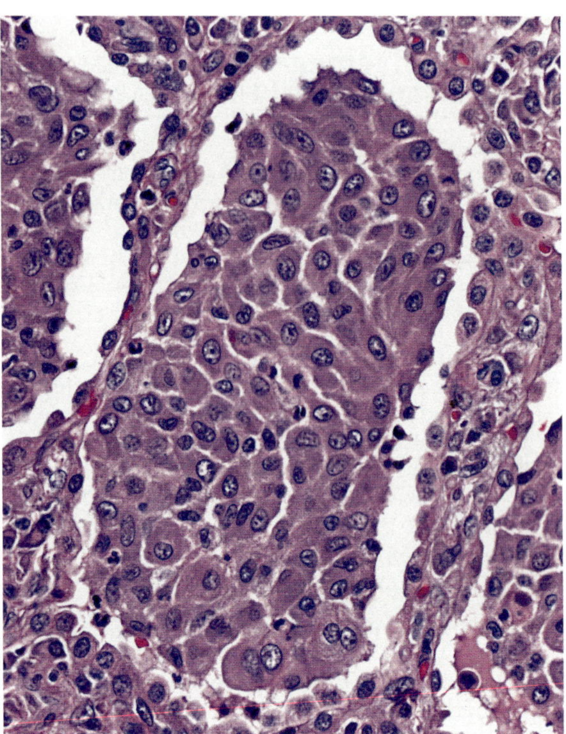

Figure 3-54

DESQUAMATIVE INTERSTITIAL PNEUMONIA PATTERN

The alveolar space is filled with macrophages and there is cuboidal hyperplasia of type 2 pneumocytes lining the fibrotically thickened alveolar wall.

Interstitial inflammation is usually only mild and consists of lymphocytes and a few plasma cells. Occasional eosinophils and mast cells are seen. Neutrophils are absent or rare. Scattered lymphoid aggregates may be seen. The epithelial cells lining the alveolar walls may show cuboidal hyperplasia and may have nuclear cytoplasmic inclusions.

In smokers, the cytoplasm of the alveolar macrophages has a golden brown pigment flecked with tiny black particles (fig. 3-55, left). A few multinucleated macrophages may be seen, however, the nuclei are small and round. Occasional mitotic figures are seen in the macrophages. A finely granular hemosiderin pigment may be detected if examined with a Prussian blue stain for iron (fig. 3-55, right). In some cases, intra-alveolar laminated basophilic concretions ("blue bodies") may be present (see fig. 2-10) (345). These are nonspecific inclusions consisting mostly of calcium carbonate with lesser amounts of mucopolysaccharide matrix and iron, and may be seen in any disorder associated with alveolar macrophage accumulation (345).

Differential Diagnosis. The differential diagnostic considerations for the DIP pattern include the patterns of UIP and RB, as well as DIP-like reactions, histiocyte-rich infections, chronic eosinophilic pneumonia with few eosinophils, cellular and fibrosing NSIP, giant cell interstitial pneumonia (hard metal pneumoconiosis), and carcinoma with alveolar spread (Table 3-21). The major clinical, HRCT, and pathologic differences between IPF (UIP) and DIP are summarized in Table 3-22. In contrast to the UIP pattern, the DIP pattern should not show patchy scarring and remodeling of lung architecture (honeycombing).

The alveolar macrophage accumulation in RB is primarily peribronchiolar while in DIP it is diffuse. It is likely that several of the cases reported by Liebow et al. (346) were actually RB-ILD since less than 50 percent of the lung was consolidated in 4 of the 18 cases. Yousem and Colby (366) retrospectively reviewed lung biopsies from patients included in the series of DIP reported by Carrington et al. in 1978 (330), and reclassified eight of these cases as RB-ILD.

The term DIP-like reaction was proposed by Bedrossian et al. (326) to describe the alveolar macrophage accumulation that can occur as a

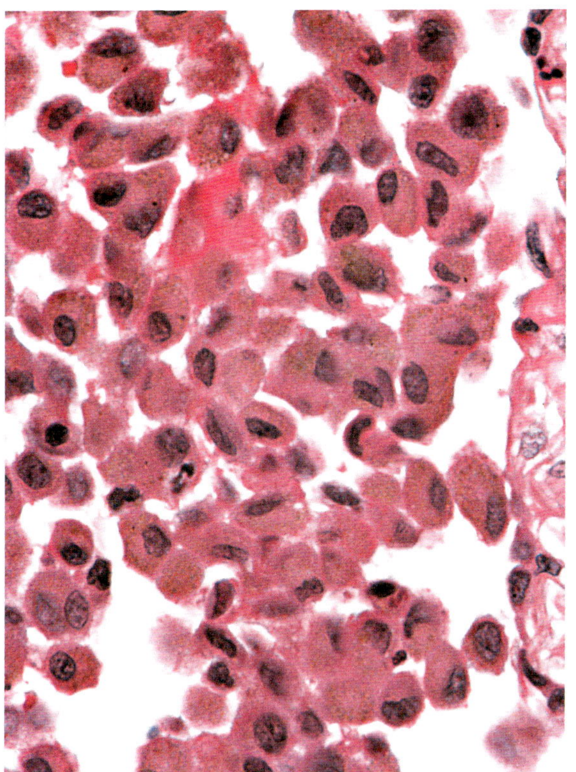

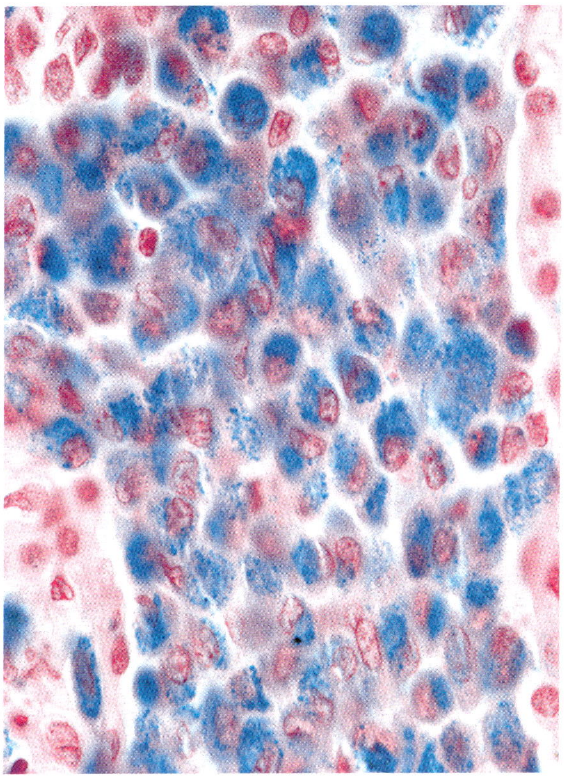

Figure 3-55

DESQUAMATIVE INTERSTITIAL PNEUMONIA PATTERN

Left: The alveolar macrophages contain finely granular brown pigment.

Right: This brown pigment is positive with the Prussian blue iron stain, however, the granules are fine in contrast to the coarse brown hemosiderin granules associated with pulmonary hemorrhage.

nonspecific reaction adjacent to a variety of pathologic lesions, the most well known of which is Langerhans' cell histiocytosis (331, 339,357). However, it is now recognized that most of these cases of DIP-like reaction actually represent RB-ILD (331,357). Focal DIP-like reactions can be seen around mass lesions such as tumors, scars, or infarcts.

"DIP" has been described in a wide variety of conditions that may represent DIP-like reactions. These include asbestosis (334), HIV infection, and certain drug reactions. Lung biopsies with a DIP-like reaction should be carefully examined for asbestos bodies and other dust deposits.

DIP may also come into the differential diagnosis of histiocyte-rich infections such as with *Mycobacterium avium-intracellulare, Cryptococcus,* and *Rhodococcus equi* (see chapter 12), especially in HIV-infected patients.

Chronic eosinophilic pneumonia may resemble DIP, especially in patients who have received steroids prior to the lung biopsy, since eosinophils may rapidly disappear after steroid therapy. In such cases the only way to know the patient had eosinophilic pneumonia is to correlate the clinical presentation with peripheral eosinophilia. The presence of residual focal eosinophilia in a lung biopsy may be a histologic clue.

Occasionally, based on a lung biopsy stained for iron from a patient with DIP, a diagnosis of idiopathic pulmonary hemosiderosis will be made (335). However, the iron granules are finely granular (fig. 3-55, right) in contrast to the coarse granules seen in hemosiderosis due to chronic hemorrhage (discussed later) (358).

Both the cellular and fibrosing patterns of NSIP may be confused with the DIP pattern. In NSIP, the dominant histologic finding is not diffuse alveolar macrophage accumulation: the

Table 3-22

DIFFERENTIAL DIAGNOSIS OF DESQUAMATIVE INTERSTITIAL PNEUMONIA AND USUAL INTERSTITIAL PNEUMONIA[a]

Features	DIP[b]	UIP/IPF
Clinical		
Mean age (years)	42	51
Cigarette smoking	90%	71%
Response to steroids	60%	10%
Survival		
5 year	90–100%	50%
10 year	70–100%	20%
HRCT		
Main findings	Ground-glass attenuation, irregular lines (mild)	Irregular lines, honeycombing
Predominant distribution	Middle and lower lung zones, subpleural in 60% of cases	Middle and lower lung zones, subpleural in 90% of cases
Pathology		
Distribution	Diffuse	Patchy, subpleural, paraseptal
Patchy scarring	No	Yes
Fibroblastic foci	No	Yes
Temporal appearance	Uniform	Heterogeneous
Alveolar macrophages	Diffuse, prominent	Focal

[a]Modified from references 330, 331, 339, 350, and 360.
[b]DIP = desquamative interstitial pneumonia; IPF/UIP = interstitial pulmonary fibrosis/usual interstitial pneumonia.

cellular pattern shows more interstitial inflammation and the fibrosing pattern shows interstitial fibrosis. Giant cell interstitial pneumonia also may have a prominent DIP-like pattern, however, the presence of prominent multinucleated alveolar macrophages and/or epithelial cells as well as the detection of hard metal in the lung biopsy specimen help establish the diagnosis of a hard metal pneumoconiosis (see chapter 16). Giant cell interstitial pneumonia also typically shows a centrilobular pattern of scarring. A few multinucleated alveolar macrophages may be seen in DIP, but they are usually inconspicuous.

Rarely, lung carcinomas have an intra-alveolar growth pattern that mimics DIP (351). The greater degree of nuclear atypia and clustering of the epithelial tumor cells should distinguish them from the intra-alveolar macrophages of DIP. If there is doubt, immunohistochemistry for keratin may highlight the epithelial nature of the intra-alveolar tumor cells (351).

Treatment and Prognosis. Cessation of smoking is the primary treatment for patients with DIP, often leading to spontaneous regression of the disease (344,348). In those with moderate to severe symptoms and gas exchange abnormalities, corticosteroid therapy may be indicated (363). A greater percentage of patients with DIP respond to steroid therapy than do patients with UIP. There may be recurrences, especially if the patient starts smoking cigarettes or is exposed to passive smoke.

The prognosis of patients with DIP is much better than for those with other idiopathic interstitial pneumonias, especially UIP. In the classic study by Carrington et al. (330) the 5- and 10-year survival rates were 95.2 percent and 69.6 percent for patients with DIP in contrast to 65.4 percent and 28.5 percent for those with UIP. However, in this study honeycombing was present in 12.5 percent of cases. In the more recent studies by Travis et al. (360) and Nicholson et al. (198) where cases with honeycombing were excluded, the 5-year survival rate was 100 percent. Nevertheless, DIP is known to progress and a small number of patients do poorly (337). Fulminant DIP leading to death is rare (336). Lung transplantation has been performed successfully in patients with

Table 3-23

HYPERSENSITIVITY PNEUMONITIS: INCITING ANTIGENS AND EXPOSURES

Disease	Antigen	Source
Farmer's lung	*Thermophilic actinomyces*	Moldy hay, grain, silage
Bird fancier's lung	Parakeet, chicken, pigeon proteins	Avian droppings or feathers
Humidifier or air conditioner lung	*Thermophilic actinomyces*	Contaminated water in humidifier or air conditioning units
Bagassosis	*Thermoactinomyces sacchari*	Moldy sugar cane
Maple bark stripper's disease	*Cryptostroma corticale*	Moldy maple bark
Malt worker's lung	*Aspergillus clavatus*	Moldy barley
Humidifier lung	*Bacillus cereus*	Water
Summer type hypersensitivity pneumonitis (Japan)	*Trichosporon cutaneum* or *Cryptococcus albidus*	Home environment

endstage disease from DIP, however, disease recurrence in the transplanted lung has been reported (364).

HYPERSENSITIVITY PNEUMONITIS

Definition. Hypersensitivity pneumonitis (HP), also known as *extrinsic allergic alveolitis,* is a diffuse interstitial granulomatous lung disease that represents an immunologic reaction to inhaled organic antigens or, rarely, to simple chemicals.

Hypersensitivity or allergic processes involving the lung include HP, allergic bronchopulmonary aspergillosis (see chapter 9), and drug reactions (see chapter 7). HP is a complex syndrome of varying intensity, clinical presentation, and natural history rather than a single, uniform disease (368,388,411,415,418). A classic example of HP is "farmer's lung," which occurs in farmers exposed to *Saccharopolyspora rectivirgula,* a bacterium found in "moldy" hay. Other well-known HP syndromes include "bagassosis" which occurs in sugar cane workers exposed to *Thermoactinomyces sacchari* in moldy sugar cane and "maple bark stripper's disease," which occurs in workers exposed to the fungus *Cryptostroma corticale* from moldy maple bark. "Bird fanciers' lung" occurs in bird keepers chronically exposed to the proteins from bird feathers, serum, and excrement. HP can be caused by fungi growing in stagnant water in air conditioners, swimming pools, hot tubs, and central heating units (see Table 3-23 for other causes) (399). The number of known causes of HP continues to grow. For example, *Mycobacterium avium* has recently been implicated as a cause of HP in patients using hot tubs with water contaminated with the organism (379).

Clinical Features. The prevalence and incidence of HP are unknown and vary from country to country and within certain regions of a country. The prevalence rates vary due to the local climate, season, geographic conditions, local customs, and the presence of industrial manufacturing plants (370). Farmer's lung is most common in cold, wet climates and varies with local farming practices (370). It is one of the most common forms of HP, affecting 0.4 to 7.0 percent of the farming population (388). The reported prevalence of HP among bird fanciers is even more variable: estimates range from 20 to 20,000 affected individuals per 100,000 persons at risk (388). The prevalence of HP is likely to be higher among bird fanciers than among farmers because contact with the inciting avian antigens is less limited by season or geographic location (388).

Only a minority of individuals exposed to potential antigens that cause HP actually develop clinical disease and only after the weeks to months of exposure required to induce sensitization. A history of allergic disease is uncommon and not a predisposing factor for the development of HP. Many persons with mild or subclinical HP escape detection or are misdiagnosed as suffering from viral illnesses or asthma, either of which may have nonspecific clinical findings which mimic HP (388). High attack rates of HP have been documented during sporadic outbreaks, for example, 52 percent of exposed office workers developed humidifier lung (381) and 37 percent of lifeguards exposed to a public swimming pool developed HP (414). Cigarette smoking is less prevalent in patients with HP. HP can manifest in acute, subacute, and chronic forms (369,411,418).

HP represents a combination of immune complex–mediated (type III) and T cell–mediated, delayed (type IV) hypersensitivity reactions, although the precise contribution of each is still debated (369,420). In most cases, precipitating immunoglobulin (Ig) G antibodies against the offending agent are demonstrated in the serum. It is important to note, however, that the large majority of persons with serum precipitins to inhaled antigens do not develop HP on exposure, a fact that suggests a genetic component in host susceptibility.

Acute HP. An acute reaction usually follows heavy exposure in a previously sensitized individual. Clinically, it is characterized by the abrupt onset (4 to 6 hours following the exposure) of fever, chills, malaise, cough, chest tightness, and dyspnea without wheezing. Anorexia, nausea, and vomiting may occur. These symptoms subside over hours or days. Diffuse fine rales are heard throughout the chest. Laboratory tests are of limited use (369,386). The erythrocyte sedimentation rate and quantitative immunoglobulins are elevated in many patients. A positive rheumatoid factor, elevated C-reactive protein, and elevated circulating immune complexes also may be found. The serum lactic dehydrogenase (LDH) level may be high in the acute phase of the disease and may decline as the illness resolves. Lung function testing shows a restrictive ventilatory defect and mild hypoxemia during these symptomatic episodes.

Subacute HP. This pattern of HP usually develops insidiously and manifests clinically with cough and breathlessness over days or weeks. Often the course is progressive or there is an acute component that leads to urgent hospitalization. Diffuse crackles are heard throughout the chest. Lung function testing shows a restrictive ventilatory defect and mild hypoxemia.

Chronic HP. An insidious or chronic form results from continued, usually low-level, antigen exposure. A patient with chronic HP may not remember or experience any acute episodes (407). Disabling and frequently irreversible respiratory findings, such as pulmonary fibrosis, are characteristic. Pulmonary function studies show a restrictive pattern, characterized by decreased compliance, reduced diffusion capacity, and hypoxemia (369,411,418). In the chronic stage of HP, airway obstruction may become troublesome (405). In many cases the inciting antigen may be very difficult to detect or never identified (369,411,418). Diagnosis at this stage usually requires lung biopsy. Early diagnosis is critical since irreversible or progressive disease can occur (405).

Confirming the diagnosis of HP can be difficult (Tables 3-24, 3-25) (375,387). Several different diagnostic criteria have been proposed and all have significant problems that limit their usefulness (375,387,413,422). It is common that a lung biopsy is obtained in a patient with DPLD without HP being considered in the differential diagnosis. In these instances, the pathologist plays an important role in suggesting the diagnosis. Skin tests and serum precipitins to a general panel of possible antigens are not helpful in confirming the diagnosis of HP at any stage.

BAL analysis can support the diagnosis of HP (416). A marked lymphocytosis (often exceeding 50 percent of the cells recovered) is a nonspecific but helpful finding since this level of lymphocytosis is uncommon in diseases often considered in the differential diagnosis. The CD4+/CD8+ ratio is usually decreased (less than 1.0). The alveolitis of HP appears to be characterized by cells with the CD3+/CD8+/CD56+/CD57+/CD10- phenotype (369,416). BAL neutrophils are elevated after recent exposure or in advanced cases (389,404), and BAL eosinophilia may be seen in advanced cases, usually associated with the increased neutrophils (389). The finding of substantial numbers of mast cells (more than 1 percent), especially if associated with a marked lymphocytosis, is specific for HP. The presence of mast cells helps monitor ongoing exposure to the responsible antigen. Mast cells are usually increased following acute exposure and decline toward normal 1 to 3 months after removal of exposure (419). BAL

Table 3-24

DIAGNOSTIC CRITERIA FOR HYPERSENSITIVITY PNEUMONITIS[a]

Criteria	Specific Features
1. Known exposure to offending antigen(s)	A. History of appropriate exposure B. Aerobiologic or microbiologic investigations of the environment ment which confirm the presence of an inciting antigen C. The presence of specific IgG antibodies in serum against the identified antigen (serum precipitins)[b]
2. Compatible clinical, radiologic, or physiologic findings	A. Respiratory (± constitutional) symptoms and signs, especially suggestive if they appear or worsen several hours after antigen exposure. B. Compatible chest radiograph or HRCT findings C. Altered lung function or gas exchange either at rest or with exercise testing
3. BAL with lymphocytosis	A. Usually with low CD4 to CD8 ratio B. Positive specific immune response to the antigen by lymphocyte transformation testing[c]
4. Positive inhalation challenge test	A. Reexposure to the environment B. Inhalation challenge to the suspected antigen
5. Histopathology showing compatible changes	A. Poorly formed, noncaseating granulomas B. Mononuclear cell infiltrates

[a]Adapted from reference 387.
[b]A positive precipitin test, even in the presence of a clear history of exposure to the identified antigen, is merely suggestive of, rather than diagnostic of, a potential etiology.
[c]This test is not available in most centers.

Table 3-25

DIAGNOSIS OF HYPERSENSITIVITY PNEUMONITIS[a]

Diagnosis	Criteria Present from Table 3-24	Comments
Definite HP	1, 2, 3	Histopathologic confirmation of the diagnosis is not needed in the majority of such cases
	1, 2, 4A	BAL or histopathologic confirmation of the diagnosis is not needed in the majority of these cases but may be important to allow decision making regarding management
	1, 2A, 3, 5	These patients are usually identified as part of a case cluster; the index cases usually have more severe disease
	2, 3, 5	Diagnosis is first suspected after BAL or transbronchial lung biopsy
Probable HP	1, 2A, 3	
Subclinical HP	1, 3A	
Sensitization	1	

[a]Adapted from reference 387.

fluid also contains increased levels of IgG, IgA, and IgM in some patients (410). The presence of plasma cells, a higher IgG to albumin ratio, and an increased hyaluronic acid or procollagen-III N-terminal peptide level in BAL fluid may be signs of active alveolitis in HP (377,393).

Inhalation challenge by reexposure of the patient to the environment can demonstrate a relationship between symptoms and a particular antigen and thus support the diagnosis of HP (380,383,387,412). Inhalation challenge to a preparation of a suspected antigen in a hospital setting may be helpful but is not generally performed because it may induce progressive disease, and because there are no standardized antigen preparations available (403,407).

Tissue obtained by transbronchial lung biopsy may yield abnormalities suggestive of HP. The findings are often subtle and must be interpreted with knowledge of the clinical and other laboratory findings. Multiple biopsies (5 to 7 samples of tissue) must be obtained to increase the likelihood of a diagnosis. Step sectioning of the tissue specimens is frequently necessary to identify the essential histopathologic features. It is important for clinicians to carefully review the occupational and environmental history of any patient found to have usually small, poorly formed and noncaseating granulomas or ill-defined epithelioid macrophage aggregates, with or without multinucleated giant cells, on lung biopsy. Diagnosis of the chronic form of HP usually requires surgical lung biopsy.

There are several important clinical syndromes that occur as a result of inhalation of organic agents but are not true forms of HP: inhalation fever, organic dust toxic syndrome, chronic bronchitis, asthma, and chronic airflow limitation have been found in patients with exposure to agricultural products, wood dust, and to a lesser extent, other exposures (386). Inhalation fevers ("Monday morning miseries," "humidifier lung") are characterized by fevers, chills, malaise, headaches, and myalgias without prominent pulmonary findings. Mild dyspnea, cough, and chest tightness may occur. The onset usually occurs 4 to 12 hours after exposure, and attack rates can be very high. There are no long-term sequelae. Organic dust toxic syndrome (ODTS or pulmonary mycotoxicosis) results from the deleterious actions of mycotoxins (394,397,398). The toxins enter the body after exposure to bioaerosols contaminated with toxin-producing fungi. The syndrome has been associated with exposure to grains, moldy hay, and textile materials contaminated with *Fusarium,* an aflatoxin-producing fungus (397). Fever, chills, dyspnea, and myalgias occur 4 to 6 hours after exposure (often a first exposure) to contaminated dust. Leukocytosis, diffuse opacities on chest radiography, restrictive ventilatory defects, and reduced DLCO are common laboratory abnormalities. Obliterative bronchiolitis without granulomas is usually present on lung biopsy; DIP and DAD may also be seen (394). These cases are thought not to represent true cases of HP because no prior sensitization is required and there is a lack of serologic response to common fungal antigens. Chronic obstructive lung disease is the most common respiratory syndrome among agricultural workers and the most common cause of severe lung disease (376,423).

Radiologic Findings. Heavy exposure to an inciting antigen can result in an acute presentation with bilateral airspace consolidation resembling pulmonary edema. A fleeting, micronodular, interstitial pattern in the lower and mid-lower zones may be identified on chest roentgenogram. The chest radiograph is frequently normal in population outbreaks of acute HP (e.g., in 10 of 11 patients in one study of biopsy proven HP [396]). The findings characteristic of the subacute stage consist of poorly defined nodular or ground-glass opacities (374, 401). In the chronic stage, there are progressive fibrotic changes with fewer reticular or nodular densities and loss of lung volume. The opacities may be patchy and random in distribution, but most commonly involve the middle or lower lung zones (fig. 3-56) (367,395).

In the acute or subacute stages of HP the characteristic HRCT findings consist of poorly defined centrilobular nodular opacities, which reflect the presence of bronchiolitis, and areas of ground-glass attenuation, which reflect the presence of alveolitis (fig. 3-57) (382,408). These abnormalities are usually diffuse. In chronic HP, with the development of fibrosis, a reticular pattern is seen, which tends to involve mainly the middle and lower lung zones (367,395). The reticular pattern often has a patchy distribution or central predominance; however, occasionally, it is predominantly peripheral, similar to UIP. Identification of areas of decreased attenuation and mosaic perfusion are important ancillary CT findings in HP, and obstructive functional abnormalities indicate that these are caused by bronchiolitis (382).

Pathologic Findings. HP has a broad spectrum of histologic manifestations (371–374,402, 417). Since most patients who have lung biopsies are in the chronic phase, little is known about the histologic findings of acute HP. Acute HP is characterized by a neutrophilic infiltrate in

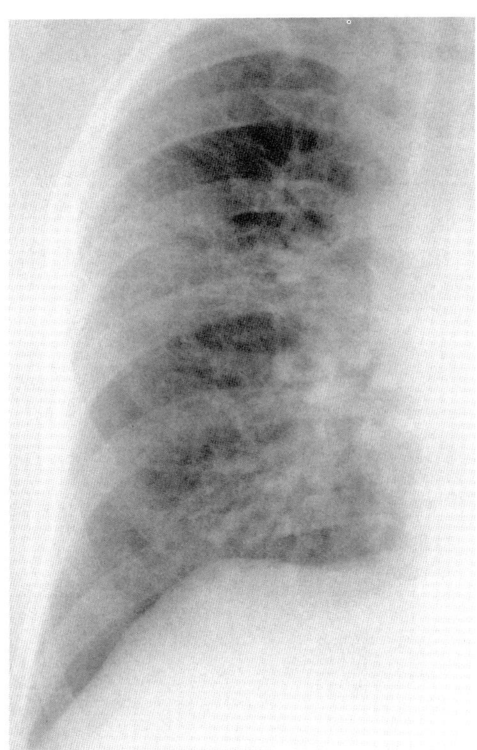

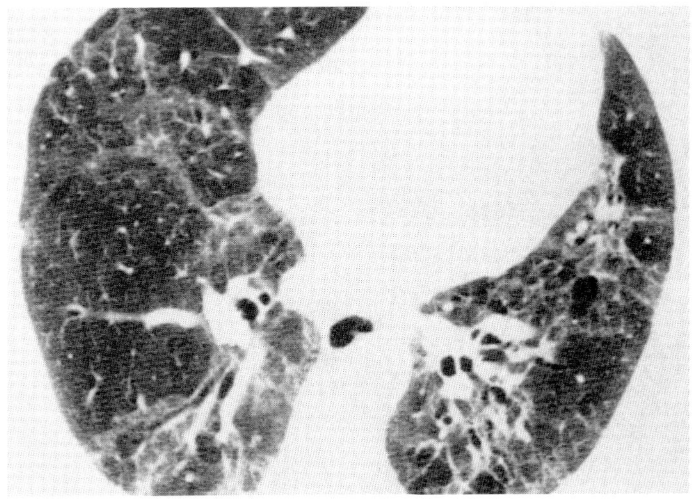

Figure 3-56

CHRONIC HYPERSENSITIVITY PNEUMONITIS

Left: The view of the right lung from a chest radiograph shows a reticular pattern involving mainly the middle and lower lung zones.

Above: HRCT demonstrates patchy areas of ground-glass attenuation and a few irregular linear opacities. The findings are characteristic of subacute changes (ground-glass attenuation) superimposed on a background of fibrosis.

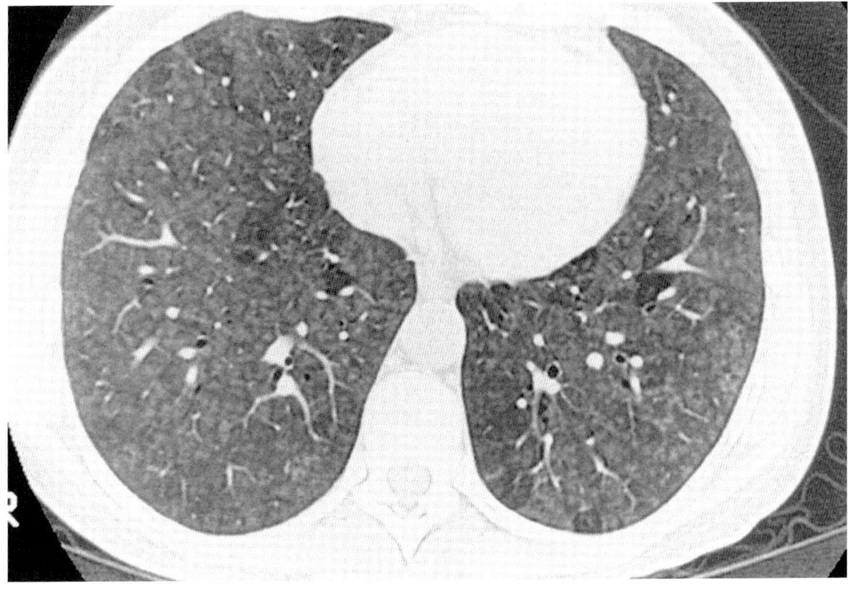

Figure 3-57

SUBACUTE HYPERSENSITIVITY PNEUMONITIS

HRCT demonstrates poorly defined, centrilobular nodular opacities and patchy areas of ground-glass attenuation. The findings are characteristic of the subacute stage of hypersensitivity pneumonitis.

the alveoli and respiratory bronchioles (acute bronchiolitis); sometimes a pattern of DAD is reported (417). A temporally uniform, nonspecific, chronic interstitial pneumonia is commonly seen in these cases (370). Subacute HP shows lymphocytic interstitial pneumonitis, granulomas, organizing pneumonia, and fibrosis (370).

Chronic HP can have a distinctive histologic appearance (372) when all three of the characteristic features are present: 1) bronchiolocentric cellular interstitial pneumonia, 2) noncaseating granulomas, and 3) intraluminal budding fibrosis or organizing pneumonia (figs. 3-58–3-62) (372,385). However, subtle cases may

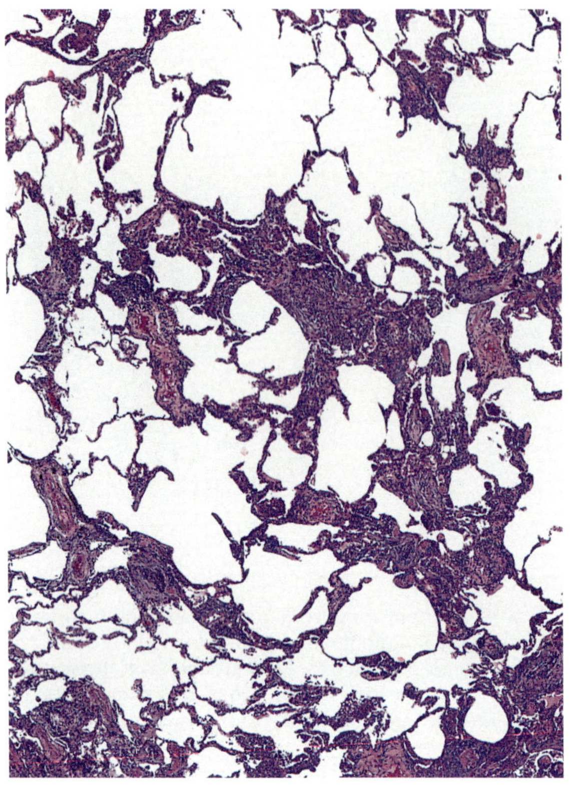

Figure 3-58

HYPERSENSITIVITY PNEUMONITIS

The biopsy shows a moderate, diffuse, peribronchiolar chronic inflammatory infiltrate.

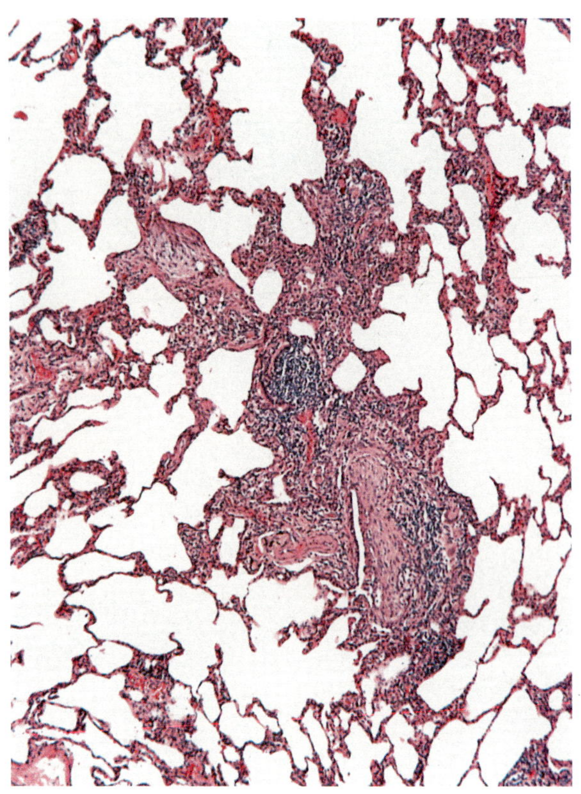

Figure 3-59

HYPERSENSITIVITY PNEUMONITIS IN MAPLE BARK STRIPPER'S DISEASE

This case shows a peribronchiolar chronic inflammatory infiltrate and intraluminal budding fibrosis involving a bronchiole as well as several surrounding airspaces.

require careful clinical correlation and the diagnosis may remain tentative. Open lung biopsy is usually required to detect the histologic features of HP since they are difficult to recognize on transbronchial biopsy (392). When this pattern is encountered a descriptive diagnosis such as *bronchocentric cellular interstitial pneumonia with poorly formed granulomas or organizing pneumonia* is appropriate depending on which features are present. The final diagnosis of HP is not based on pathology alone, but includes clinical information to document an exposure history. Nevertheless, it is likely that in some cases the antigen exposure remains undetected.

The most consistent histologic feature of HP is a cellular chronic bronchiolitis with peribronchiolar interstitial inflammation (fig. 3-58) (405). At low magnification, scattered nodules of inflammation appear centered on bronchioles (figs. 3-58, 3-59). The inflammatory infiltrate consists mostly of lymphocytes, with some plasma cells and histiocytes (fig. 3-60). Eosinophils are scant or absent (372). The inflammation may be extensive, making the bronchiolar distribution difficult to appreciate. The granulomas, found in about two thirds of cases, tend to be poorly formed (figs. 3-60–3-62) (385,409). They consist of loose clusters of epithelioid cells and in about half of the cases giant cells are absent. Intraluminal budding fibrosis consists of polypoid plugs of loose, organizing connective tissue that protrudes into the lumens of alveolar ducts and bronchioles (figs. 3-59, 3-61); it is seen in approximately two thirds of cases (385). As HP progresses it may result in a nonspecific fibrotic histologic picture resembling UIP or endstage fibrosis. In such cases, clues to the diagnosis come from examination of less fibrotic

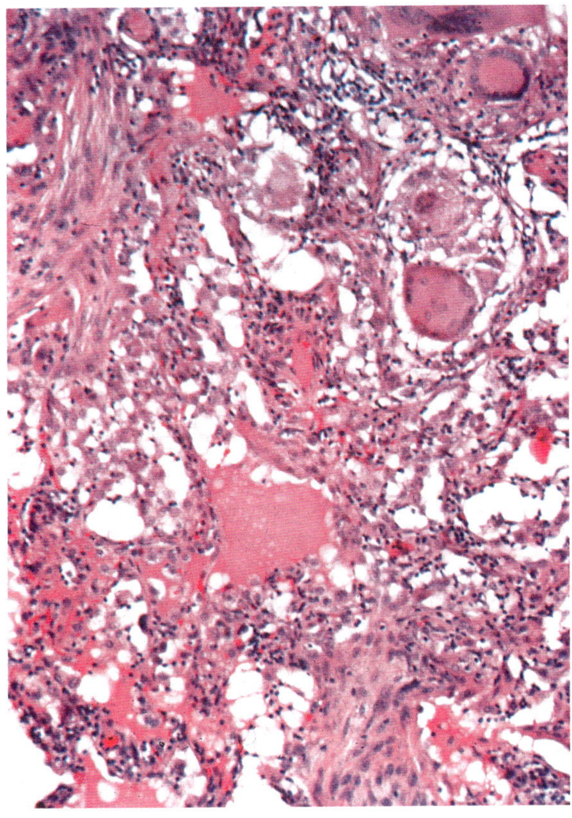

Figure 3-60

HYPERSENSITIVITY PNEUMONITIS IN FARMER'S LUNG

Poorly formed granulomas and intraluminal budding fibrosis are present.

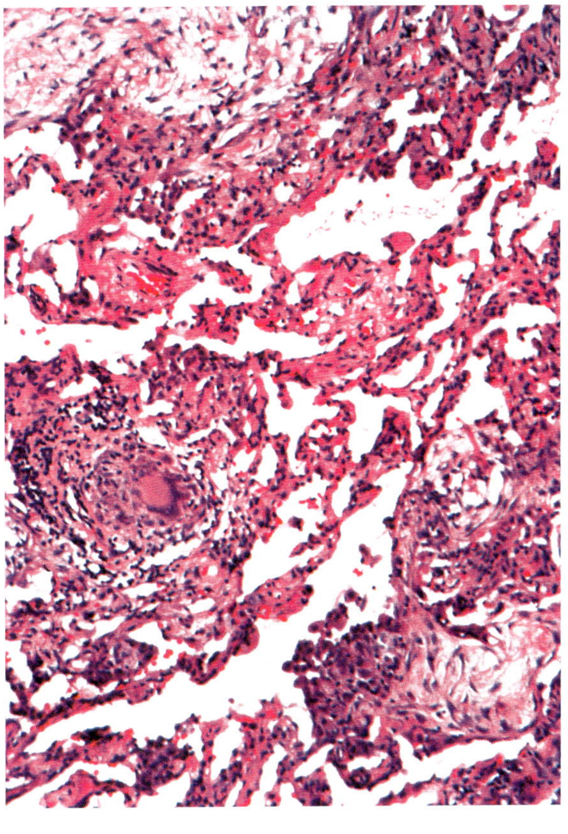

Figure 3-61

HYPERSENSITIVITY PNEUMONITIS

There is prominent intraluminal budding fibrosis as well as a poorly formed granuloma.

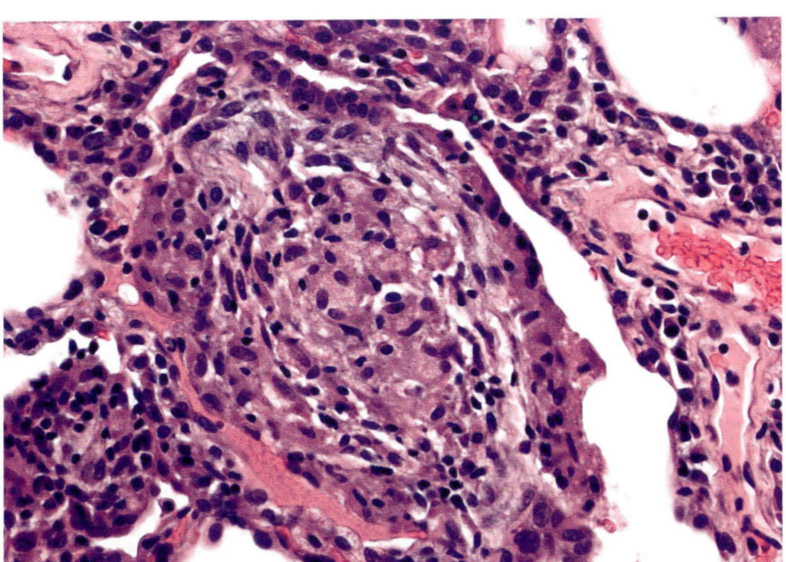

Figure 3-62

HYPERSENSITIVITY PNEUMONITIS

This poorly formed granuloma consists of a loose cluster of epithelioid and giant cells.

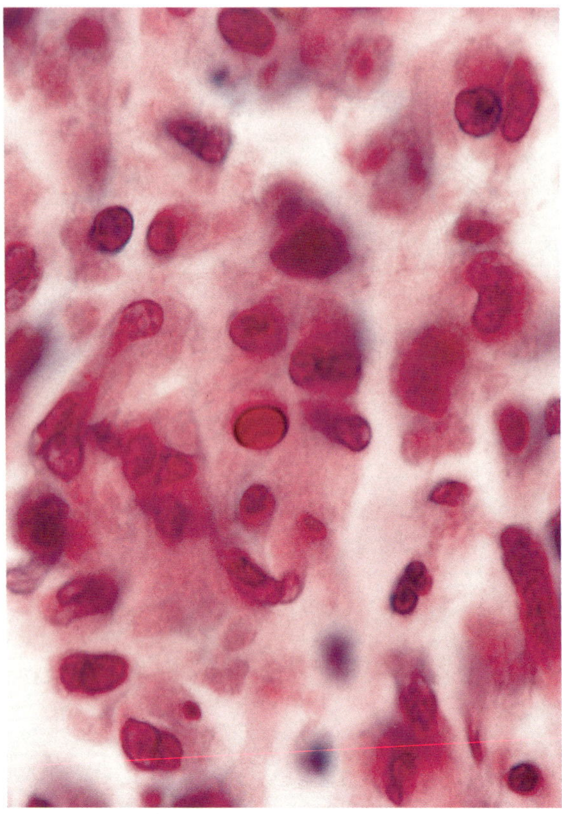

Figure 3-63

HYPERSENSITIVITY PNEUMONITIS: MAPLE BARK STRIPPER'S DISEASE

The brown fungal organism in this biopsy is *Crytostroma corticale.*

areas where characteristic lesions of cellular bronchiolitis, granulomas, or intraluminal fibrosis are more likely to be found.

Occasional lymphoid aggregates may be seen, but they are usually not prominent. Foamy macrophages are common within the peribronchiolar airspaces; they are prominent in approximately 5 percent of cases (409). Crystalline inclusions or cholesterol clefts may be seen within giant cells. Pleural fibrosis may also be seen. In patients with maple bark stripper's disease, *Cryptostroma corticale* may be seen in the lung biopsy (fig. 3-63) (378).

Differential Diagnosis. HP must be separated histologically from LIP, sarcoidosis, infection, NSIP, and UIP. An interstitial lymphoid infiltrate is much more prominent in LIP than HP, and extensively involves alveolar septa. Granulomas and intraluminal budding fibrosis are more common in HP than LIP (Table 3-26). In most cases the separation of sarcoidosis and HP is straightforward, but in rare cases it may be difficult. The granulomas of HP are usually poorly formed and randomly distributed in the alveolar interstitium while the granulomas of sarcoidosis tend to be tightly packed and distributed along bronchovascular bundles and the pleura. It is unusual to see substantial chronic inflammation in sarcoidosis, and intraluminal fibrosis is absent (Table 3-26). Since infection could potentially produce the histologic picture of HP, special stains should be performed to rule out the presence of acid-fast bacilli, fungi, and *Pneumocystis carinii.*

The NSIP pattern can considerably overlap with the HP pattern. The presence of granulomas and an exposure history in the latter help distinguish the two. In some series of patients with NSIP, cases of clinically documented HP have been included (384). The fibrotic phase of HP could potentially be confused with UIP. The typical UIP pattern of temporal heterogeneity with dense fibrosis and scattered fibroblastic foci may even be encountered in HP. The presence of granulomas and/or intraluminal fibrosis is helpful in such cases.

The same constellation of histologic features seen in HP, including peribronchiolar inflammation, scattered poorly formed granulomas, and intraluminal fibrosis, may be seen in collagen vascular disease, drug reactions, and infection. While lung biopsy findings are suggestive, the ultimate diagnosis of HP requires correlation with clinical findings to identify the offending antigen. Clinical information is required to exclude a collagen vascular disease and drug reaction.

Treatment and Prognosis. The majority of patients with HP experience near total recovery of lung function, which in some cases may take several years after the inciting exposure ceases (424). Bird fanciers have a worse prognosis than farmers with HP. The poorer outcome of the former patients may be due to a higher degree of exposure to the HP antigens and the persistence of avian antigens in the home environment despite attempts at decontamination (406,424). Once dense fibrosis has developed with honeycomb changes, the disease may be irreversible.

Table 3-26

DIFFERENTIAL DIAGNOSIS OF HYPERSENSITIVITY PNEUMONITIS

Histologic Feature	Hypersensitivity Pneumonitis	Sarcoidosis	Lymphocytic Interstitial Pneumonia
Granulomas			
Frequency	2/3 of open biopsies	100% of cases	5-10% of cases; well formed or poorly formed
Morphology	Poorly formed	Well formed	Random
Distribution	Mostly random, some peribronchiolar	Lymphangitic, peribronchiolar, perivascular	
Intraluminal fibrosis	2/3 of open biopsies	Very rare	Unusual
Lymphocyte infiltrates	Mild-moderate, peribronchiolar	Absent or minimal	Extensive, diffuse
Dense fibrosis	In advanced cases	In advanced cases	Unusual
BAL lymphocytosis	CD8>CD4	CD4>CD8	Usually B cells

The primary treatment for patients with HP is removal of the antigen exposure, which usually results in complete resolution of the acute stage of the disease (369,411,418,421). Corticosteroids are given for some patients with acute, subacute, and chronic HP. They appear to accelerate initial recovery from farmer's lung and bird fancier's lung, particularly in severely ill patients (400). The long-term outcome for patients with farmer's lung appears unchanged by corticosteroid treatment (390,391,400).

SARCOIDOSIS

Definition. Sarcoidosis is a multiorgan disease of unknown etiology which frequently affects the lung but also commonly involves the lymph nodes, liver, spleen, skin, heart, eye, and other organs. The diagnosis is established when clinical and radiologic findings are supported by histologic evidence of noncaseating granulomatous inflammation. Granulomas of known cause and local sarcoid reactions must be excluded.

Sarcoidosis was first described in 1877 (510). It primarily affects the lung and lymphatic system. A diagnosis of sarcoidosis usually requires the histopathologic demonstration of typical lesions in more than one organ system and exclusion of other disorders known to cause granulomatous disease (510). Importantly, sarcoid-like reactions can be seen in association with a wide variety of conditions (Table 3-27).

Much remains unknown regarding the epidemiology and genetic factors that contribute to the development and expression of the disease, or the appropriate management of its many manifestations. However, considerable progress has been made in understanding the protean clinical and unique immunologic and pathologic features of the disorder (510).

Clinical Features. Sarcoidosis occurs worldwide, affecting persons of all ages, races, and both sexes. It occurs most commonly in young adults between the ages of 20 and 40 years. Most populations show a slight female predominance (447,511). Sarcoidosis has a particular proclivity for blacks in the United States, the Irish, and Scandinavians, although the incidence and prevalence rates vary according to the country and state (510). For unknown reasons, most patients present in the winter and early spring (510). Estimates of prevalence range from less than 1 to 40 cases per 100,000 population (510). The age-adjusted annual incidence rate in the United States is 10.9 per 100,000 for whites and 35.5 per 100,000 for blacks (510). Based on cumulative incidence estimates, the lifetime risk of acquiring sarcoidosis in the United States is 2.4 percent for blacks and 0.85 percent for whites (510).

The precise etiology and pathogenesis of sarcoidosis are not known. However, most evidence suggests that an exaggerated cellular immune response to an unidentified antigen (self or foreign) is responsible. Reports of community outbreaks, a work-related risk of sarcoidosis for nurses, and an epidemiologic study

Table 3-27

CONDITIONS ASSOCIATED WITH SARCOID-LIKE DISORDERS

Malignancies (436)
- Lymphomas
  - Hodgkin's disease (485,513)
  - Non-Hodgkin's lymphoma (507)
- Lung carcinoma (462,506)
- Carcinoid tumors (473, 489)
- Testicular germ cell tumors (452,468,470)
- Granular cell tumor (476)

Collagen Vascular Disease
- Systemic lupus erythematosus (429,456)
- Sjögren's syndrome (488)
- Primary biliary cirrhosis (465,471,478)
- Familial granulomatous arthritis (486)

HIV Infection (440,449,477)

Vasculitis Syndromes
- Wegener's granulomatosis (428)
- Disseminated visceral giant cell arteritis (475,480)
- Systemic necrotizing vasculitis (469,508)
- Takayasu's arteritis (505)

Transplantation
- Recurrence in lung transplant allograft (460)

involving case contacts on the Isle of Man strongly suggest that the disease is spread by person-to-person transmission or shared exposure to an environmental agent (510). A number of studies have used microbiologic and molecular techniques to identify various organisms, including mycobacteria, *Chlamydia, Borrelia burgdorferi, Propionibacterium acnes,* mycoplasma and viruses, in tissues from patients with sarcoidosis (435,445,451,481,494,499, 515). Unfortunately, the data are often conflicting, with some studies showing positive and others negative results. A multicenter study designed to determine the etiology of sarcoidosis is in progress in the United States. The study organization (A Case Control Etiologic Study of Sarcoidosis [ACCESS]) includes 10 clinical centers, a clinical coordinating center, specialized core laboratories, a central specimen repository, and a project office at the National Heart, Lung, and Blood Institute. In addition to etiology, ACCESS will examine the socioeconomic status and clinical course of patients with sarcoidosis (426,457).

There appears to be a genetic predisposition to develop sarcoidosis with increasing recognition of familial clustering of cases (427, 510). It is also likely that genetic factors define the pattern of disease presentation and progression as well as its overall prognosis (457,479,483, 498,510).

Several immunologic features are observed in patients with sarcoidosis including depression of cutaneous delayed-type hypersensitivity, a heightened helper T-cell type 1 (Th1) immune response at sites of disease, elevated circulating immune complexes, and signs of B-cell hyperactivity (427,510). The granulomatous reaction is characterized by a marked cellular immune response on the part of helper/inducer T lymphocytes (455). These cells accumulate in the affected organs, where they secrete lymphokines and recruit macrophages, which participate in the formation of noncaseating granulomas. The organs that contain sarcoid granulomas exhibit a helper/inducer to suppressor/cytotoxic T-cell ratio of 10 to 1, compared with a ratio of 2 to 1 in uninvolved tissues (455).

These T lymphocytes spontaneously release interferon gamma and interleukin 2 (IL-2) and other cytokines. In addition, sarcoid alveolar macrophages behave as secretory cells that release a great variety of cytokines, including tumor necrosis factor-alpha, IL-12, IL-15, and growth factors. Nonspecific polyclonal activation of B cells by helper T cells leads to hyperglobulinemia, which is characteristic of active sarcoidosis. It is also possible that genetic alterations in the immune system play a role in determining the type of T-cell response in the different tissues.

Patients with sarcoidosis present with a wide variety of signs and symptoms. The lung is affected in 90 to 95 percent of patients. The most common presentation is as an incidental finding on a routine chest radiograph in an asymptomatic patient. When symptomatic, the patient most commonly presents with dyspnea with or without exertion, nonproductive cough, or nonspecific chest pain.

There are two major presentations of sarcoidosis in symptomatic patients. Patients with acute sarcoidosis usually present with an abrupt onset of the pulmonary symptoms often associated with fatigue, anorexia, weight loss, and fever (446). The constellation of erythema nodosum, bilateral hilar lymphadenopathy on chest radiograph, and polyarthralgias, known as

Lofgren's syndrome, occurs in 20 to 50 percent of these patients. There is a high frequency of spontaneous remission within 2 years and an excellent response to steroids. Chronic sarcoidosis has an insidious onset, and patients are more likely to have persistent or progressive disease. More than half of the patients in the United States present with chronic respiratory symptoms and few constitutional symptoms (510). Physical exam may show a variety of findings depending on the organ involvement. On chest examination, crackles are present in a minority of patients (less than 20 percent) and clubbing is rare. Sarcoidosis affects the skin (erythema nodosum and lupus pernio) more commonly in women. Black patients tend to have more severe uveitis, skin disease, and lacrimal gland involvement. Hemoptysis is rare and when present suggests the presence of a mycetoma (447,511). Spontaneous resolution is common, but progressive and disabling organ failure occurs in up to 10 percent of patients.

No laboratory test is specific for the diagnosis of sarcoidosis. Peripheral blood eosinophilia occurs commonly (500). The serum level of angiotensin converting enzyme is elevated in two thirds of patients with active sarcoidosis, and the 24-hour urine calcium excretion is frequently increased (447,496,511).

Pulmonary function tests are helpful in establishing the extent of lung function impairment. Restrictive physiology (manifested by reduced lung volumes) and impaired diffusing capacity are common abnormalities. Occasionally, pulmonary function may be normal despite radiographic abnormalities, or mild airflow obstruction may be present. Airway hyperreactivity occurs in up to 20 percent of patients.

The diagnosis of sarcoidosis requires confirmation of the presence of noncaseating granulomas by biopsy of the most accessible organ with the least invasive method. At one time, histologic examination of the Kveim-Siltzbach skin test following the intradermal injection of Kveim antigen (an extract of spleen from a patient with sarcoidosis) was employed in suggesting the diagnosis of sarcoidosis. However, this test is no longer available. Transbronchial lung biopsy, a procedure in which granulomas are demonstrated in lung tissue obtained through a fiberoptic bronchoscope, is the most frequent method used today (447,511). BAL specimens obtained during the same procedure often demonstrate an increase in the proportion of T lymphocytes, which show a predominance of CD4+ cells with a helper/inducer function (447,511). A high CD4/CD8 ratio (greater than 3.5) in BAL lymphocyte counts is of positive predictive value (approximately 75 percent) and high negative predictive value (85 percent) even if the transbronchial biopsy is not diagnostic. Occasionally, the diagnosis is based on the finding of multiple noncaseating granulomas in a biopsy of a skin lesion or a mediastinal lymph node obtained by mediastinoscopy. An increased uptake of gallium 67, a material phagocytosed by activated macrophages, can demonstrate areas of sarcoid involvement. The laboratory data, taken together with the clinical and radiologic findings, allow the diagnosis of sarcoidosis to be established with a high degree of probability.

Radiologic Findings. The characteristic radiologic manifestation of sarcoidosis is symmetric bilateral hilar and mediastinal lymph node enlargement, with or without associated interstitial abnormalities (fig. 3-64). In one survey of 3,676 patients from nine countries, 51 percent had hilar and mediastinal lymphadenopathy without parenchymal abnormalities (also known as stage 1 sarcoidosis), 29 percent had associated parenchymal abnormalities (stage 2), 12 percent had parenchymal findings without radiographic evidence of lymphadenopathy (stage 3), and 8 percent had a normal radiograph (458). The parenchymal abnormalities are usually bilateral and symmetric; although they may be diffuse, they tend to involve mainly the middle and upper lung zones (fig. 3-65) (450,484). The pattern of abnormality is most commonly nodular or reticulonodular. Development of fibrosis results in coarse linear opacities or a reticular pattern.

On HRCT, small nodules are seen at presentation in 90 to 100 percent of patients with parenchymal abnormalities (450,491). The nodules usually are well circumscribed, have irregular margins, and measure 2 to 5 mm in diameter (fig. 3-66). These nodules represent a conglomeration of sarcoid granulomas. The nodules have a characteristic perilymphatic distribution. They are most numerous along the bronchi and pulmonary vessels but can also be

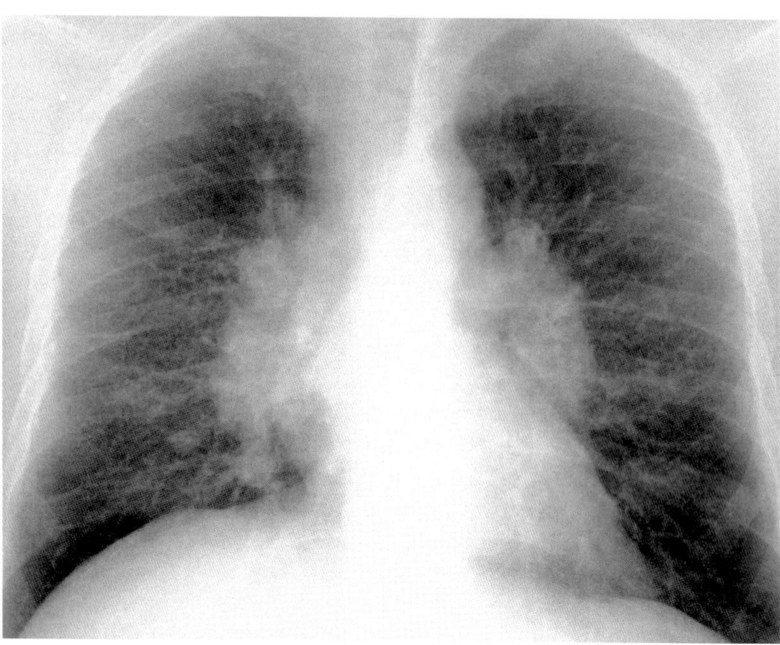

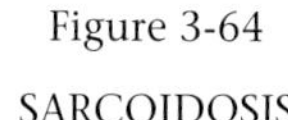

Figure 3-64

SARCOIDOSIS

Chest radiograph in a 43-year-old man with sarcoidosis demonstrates marked, symmetric, bilateral hilar and mediastinal lymphadenopathy. A mild reticulonodular interstitial infiltrate is present in the perihilar regions.

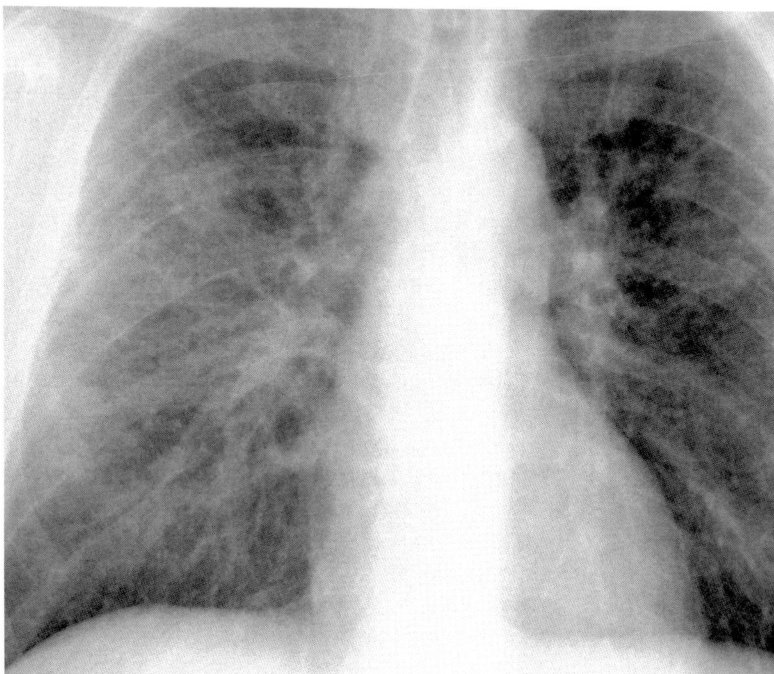

Figure 3-65

SARCOIDOSIS

Chest radiograph demonstrates a bilateral reticulonodular pattern and small, poorly defined areas of consolidation. The abnormalities are most severe in the middle and upper lung zones with relative sparing of the lung bases. There is only mild lymphadenopathy.

seen along the interlobar fissures, subpleural regions, and interlobular septa (450). Less common findings include areas of ground-glass attenuation, consolidation, interlobular septal thickening, and irregular linear opacities (437).

Gross Findings. The gross appearance of pulmonary sarcoidosis depends on the stage of disease. In early stages, the lungs appear grossly normal or small nodules may be seen along the pleura, interlobular septa, and bronchovascular bundles (figs. 3-67, 3-68). In later stages, the lungs show interstitial fibrosis and cavitary lesions (fig. 3-69). In less than 5 percent of cases, sarcoidosis may manifest as solitary or multiple nodules (fig. 3-70) (425,444,493). Such cases are sometimes called *nodular sarcoidosis*.

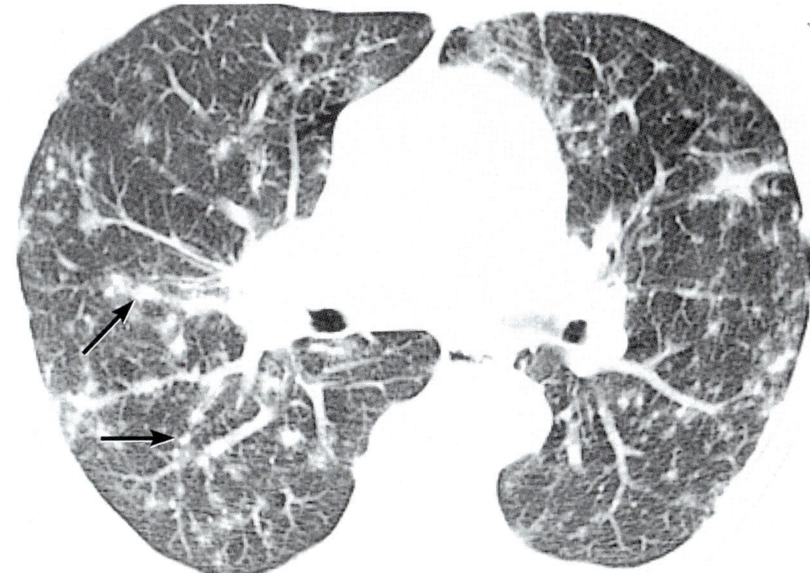

Figure 3-66

SARCOIDOSIS

HRCT demonstrates small nodules, which have irregular margins and are located mainly along the pulmonary vessels (arrows) and bronchi.

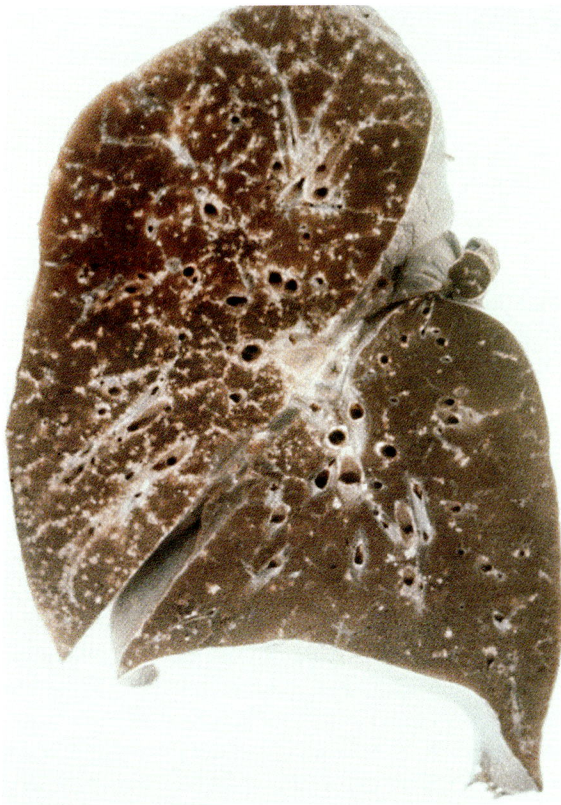

Figure 3-67

SARCOIDOSIS: GROSS SPECIMEN

The lung shows multiple white nodules or granulomas distributed along bronchovascular bundles. The upper lobe is more affected than the lower lobe.

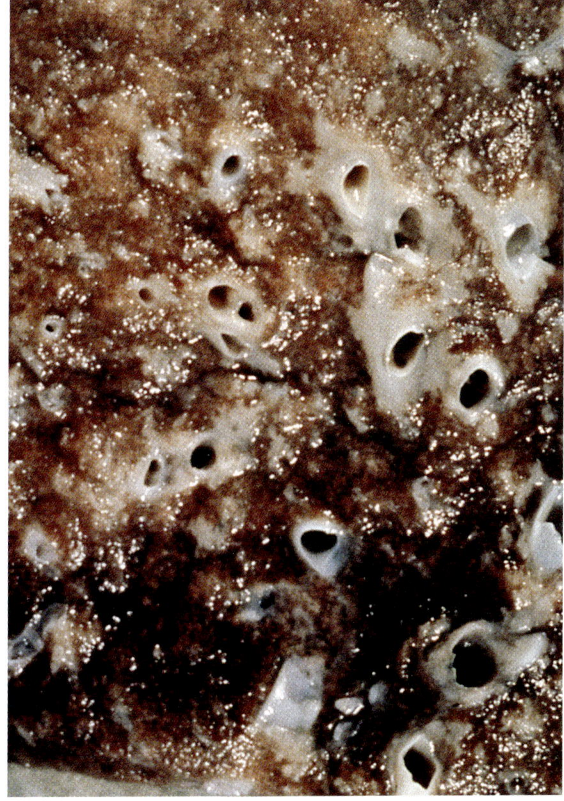

Figure 3-68

SARCOIDOSIS: GROSS SPECIMEN

There are innumerable, millimeter-sized, yellow-white nodules distributed along bronchovascular bundles.

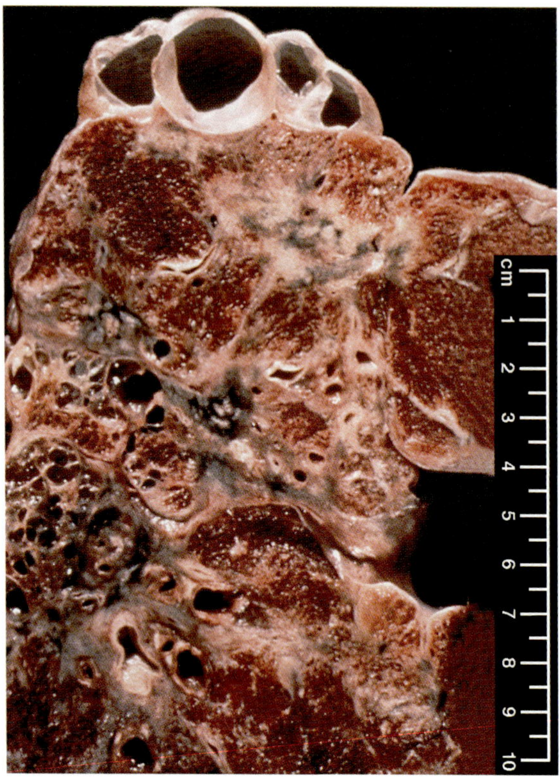

Figure 3-69

SARCOIDOSIS: GROSS SPECIMEN

The lung shows multiple small white nodules which become confluent around some bronchovascular bundles. In addition, there is marked fibrosis and honeycomb change with subpleural cystic change, especially in the apex of this upper lobe.

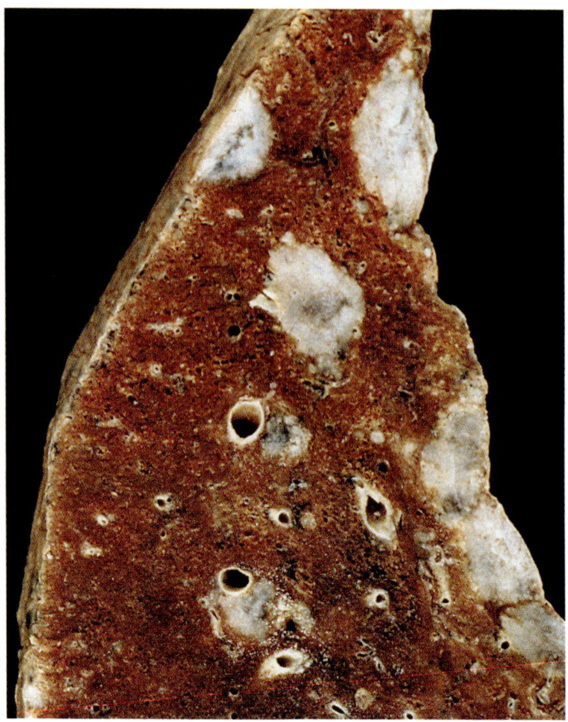

Figure 3-70

NODULAR SARCOIDOSIS: GROSS SPECIMEN

This case primarily shows large nodules with a few scattered, smaller, millimeter-sized nodules.

Histologic Findings. Histologically, multiple noncaseating granulomas are distributed in the interstitium along the pleura and interlobular septa, and around the bronchovascular bundles (Table 3-28, figs. 3-71–3-73) (504). In nodular sarcoidosis, the primary finding is confluent nodular granulomas with relative sparing of the intervening lung (fig. 3-74). The granulomas are often situated in the bronchial or bronchiolar submucosa, accounting for the high diagnostic yield (over 90 percent) on bronchoscopic biopsy (figs. 3-75, 3-76) (454, 487). In small biopsies, one may see only a single giant cell or small granuloma. These may be difficult to identify due to crush artifact and the small tissue sampling. If the clinical diagnosis of sarcoidosis is suspected and granulomas are not initially identified in a bronchoscopic biopsy, deeper sections of the tissue should be evaluated.

Rarely, the granulomas infiltrate the airways so prominently that they cause airway obstruction (*endobronchial sarcoidosis*) (fig. 3-77), or the fibrosis associated with the sarcoid granulomas causes marked bronchial narrowing (fig. 3-78) (504). Interstitial chronic inflammation is usually inconspicuous, although in some cases of early sarcoidosis, a mild to moderate interstitial pneumonitis consisting of lymphocytes may precede the development of granulomas (502). However, if prominent interstitial chronic inflammation is seen, it should raise concern for hypersensitivity pneumonitis, collagen vascular disease, drug-induced pneumonitis, or infection.

The granulomas of sarcoidosis consist of clusters of epithelioid histiocytes and/or multinucleated giant cells (504). The granulomas are well formed in that the epithelioid and giant cells are typically tightly clustered (figs. 3-75,

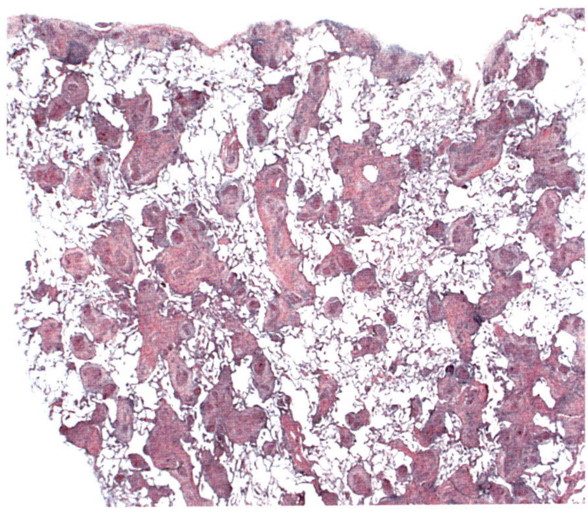

Figure 3-71

SARCOIDOSIS: PLEURAL AND BRONCHOVASCULAR DISTRIBUTION

This low-power view shows extensive infiltration by noncaseating granulomas distributed along the pleura, interlobular septa, and bronchovascular bundles.

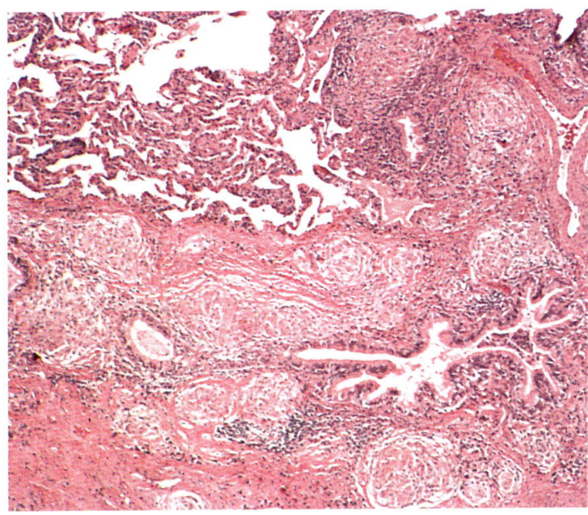

Figure 3-72

SARCOIDOSIS: BRONCHOVASCULAR DISTRIBUTION

The bronchovascular distribution is highlighted by the multiple noncaseating granulomas situated around this terminal bronchiole and its adjacent arteriole.

3-76). As the disease progresses, these granulomas may be replaced by hyalinized fibrosis (fig. 3-78) that may show a concentric lamellar appearance, often beginning at the periphery of the granuloma (fig. 3-73) (504).

Necrosis is usually absent, but small foci of necrosis may be seen in up to one third of open lung biopsies from patients with sarcoidosis (fig. 3-79). Their presence should heighten concern to exclude an infectious etiology (438,504).

Vasculitis can be encountered in up to two thirds of open lung biopsy specimens (438,439, 503,504), and approximately half of transbronchial biopsy specimens (512). The vasculitis may vary, ranging from a granulomatous reaction with epithelioid histiocytes and/or giant cells (fig. 3-80) to a chronic inflammatory infiltrate consisting of lymphocytes and plasma cells. The vasculitis is usually seen in areas of granulomatous inflammation. Pulmonary hypertension with cor pulmonale has been attributed to granulomatous vasculitis (472,509). Pulmonary hypertension has also been attributed to compression of large pulmonary arteries by granulomatous lymph node enlargement (442, 482). Rare reports have documented pulmonary hypertension and veno-occlusive disease due to a sarcoidal granulomatous venulitis (441,453).

Table 3-28

HISTOLOGIC FEATURES OF SARCOIDOSIS

Major Features
- Noncaseating granulomas
  - Characteristics: well formed or tightly packed, may become hyalinized
  - Distribution: along lymphatic routes—bronchovascular bundles, pleura, and septa
- Nodular presentation in less than 5 percent of cases

Minor Features
- Vasculitis in up to 2/3 of open lung biopsies
- Punctate necrosis in up to 1/3 of open lung biopsies
- Inclusions
  - Schaumann bodies
  - Asteroid bodies
  - Birefringent calcium carbonate or calcium oxalate crystals
  - Microcalcifications
  - Hamazaki-Wesenberg bodies

Pertinent Negatives
- Lack of organisms on cultures or special stains
- Lack of exposure to mineral dust such as beryllium, talc, or aluminum
- Paucity of interstitial chronic inflammation

Complications
- Interstitial fibrosis with honeycombing in advanced stages
- Cavitation/cystic changes
  - Aspergillomas

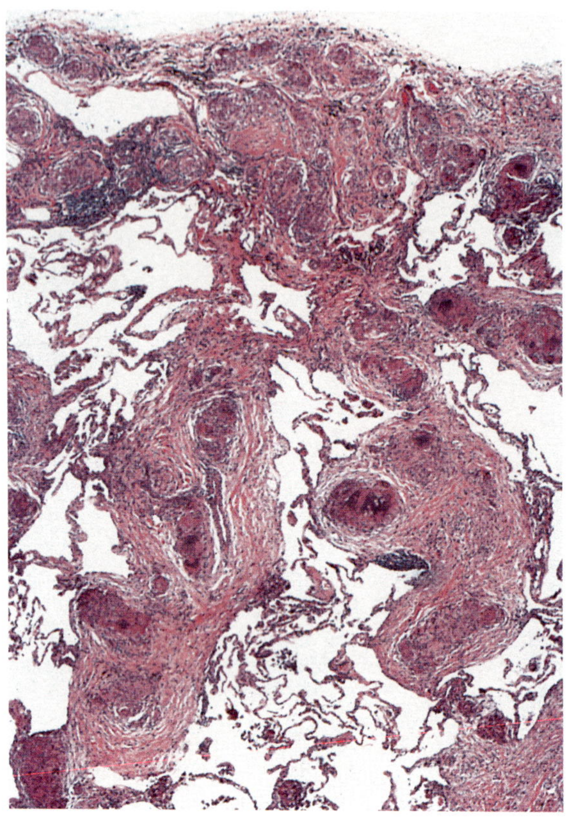

Figure 3-73

SARCOIDOSIS: CONCENTRIC FIBROSIS

In addition to infiltrating the pleura and the interlobular septa, these noncaseating granulomas are surrounded by concentric fibrosis.

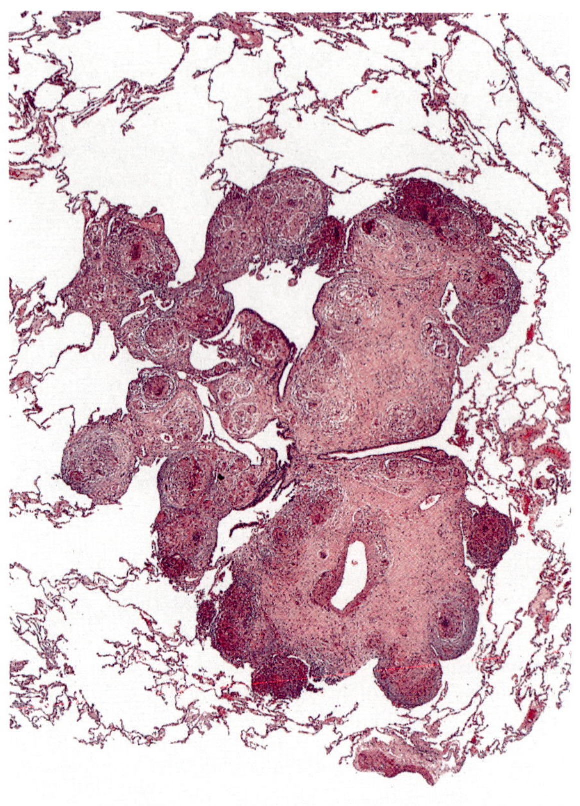

Figure 3-74

NODULAR SARCOIDOSIS

This case was characterized by multiple large nodules of confluent noncaseating granulomas, with a few granulomas in the intervening bronchovascular bundles.

A variety of inclusions may be seen in sarcoidosis. Asteroid bodies, consisting of star-shaped crystals, are seen in granulomas in 2 to 9 percent of patients (fig. 3-81) (504). By electron microscopy these structures consist of an amorphous matrix embedded with microfilaments, microtubules, mature centrioles, and paracentrioles (501). Azar et al. (430) suggested by ultrastructural study that asteroid bodies are crossing bundles of extracellular collagen fibrils. Schaumann bodies, or conchoidal bodies, consisting of small calcifications with a lamellar morphology, are seen in up to 70 percent of cases (fig. 3-82) (454). These are composed of calcium salts and iron within a mucopolysaccharide matrix (443,501). Hamazaki-Wesenberg bodies are oval or spindle shaped, and seen in up to 16 percent of lung biopsies or 11 to 68 percent of involved lymph nodes from patients with sarcoidosis (fig. 3-83) (454,504). They are yellow-brown, with the properties of lipofuscin. They stain with the Gomori methenamine silver (GMS) stain and are acid fast with the Ziehl-Neelsen stain (454,504). They may be mistaken for fungi since they appear to have a yeast-like budding morphology. Small calcifications that are easily mistaken for fungi or *Pneumocystis carinii* can be seen in necrotic or hyalinized areas of old sarcoid granulomas (fig. 3-84). However, they are basophilic and appear calcified. The irregular size and lack of budding are features against fungal yeast. These microcalcifications stain with GMS, but they are also positive with the von Kossa stain for calcium. Birefringent calcium oxalate and calcium carbonate crystals may be seen in two thirds of lung

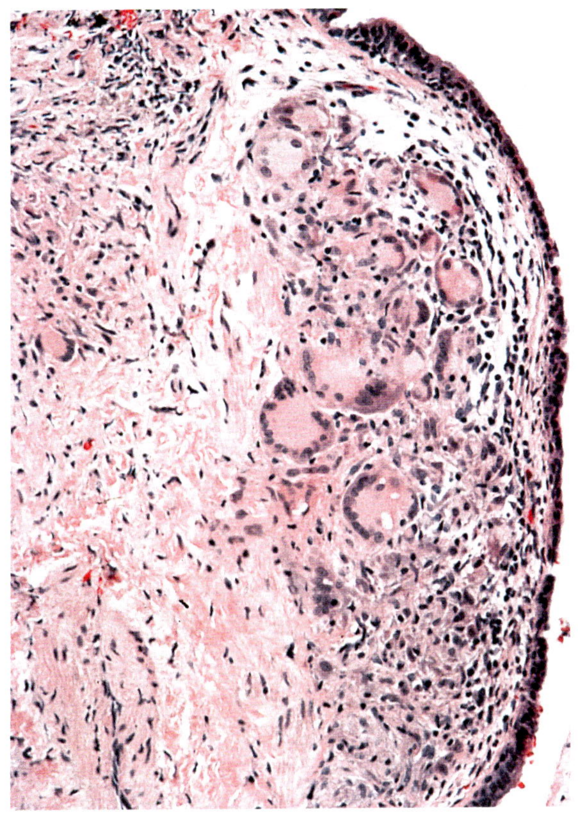

Figure 3-75

SARCOIDOSIS: SUBMUCOSAL GRANULOMA

The submucosa of this bronchiole shows a noncaseating granuloma consisting of a nodular cluster of epithelioid cells and giant cells.

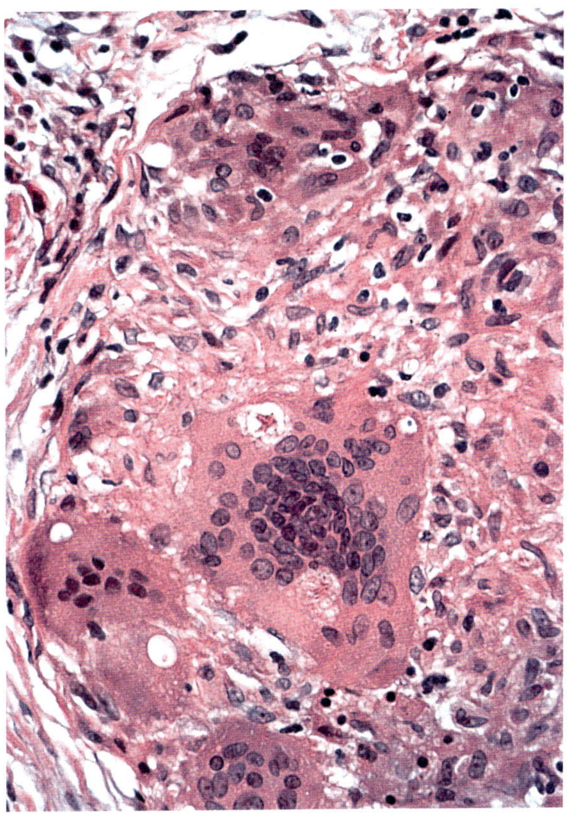

Figure 3-76

SARCOIDOSIS: NONCASEATING GRANULOMA

High-power view of noncaseating granuloma consisting of a cluster of epithelioid cells and giant cells. Two asteroid bodies can be seen in one of the giant cells.

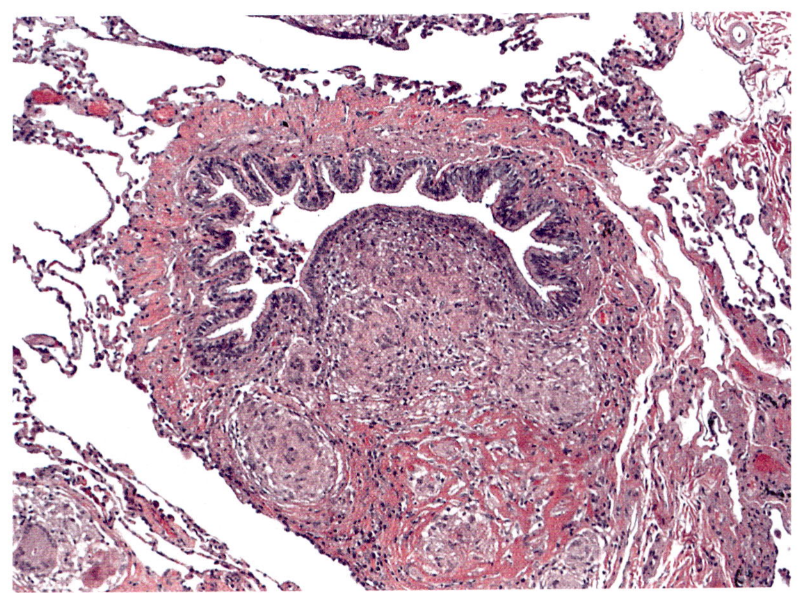

Figure 3-77

SARCOIDOSIS: AIRWAY OBSTRUCTION

This bronchiole shows a noncaseating granuloma protruding into and causing marked narrowing of the airway lumen.

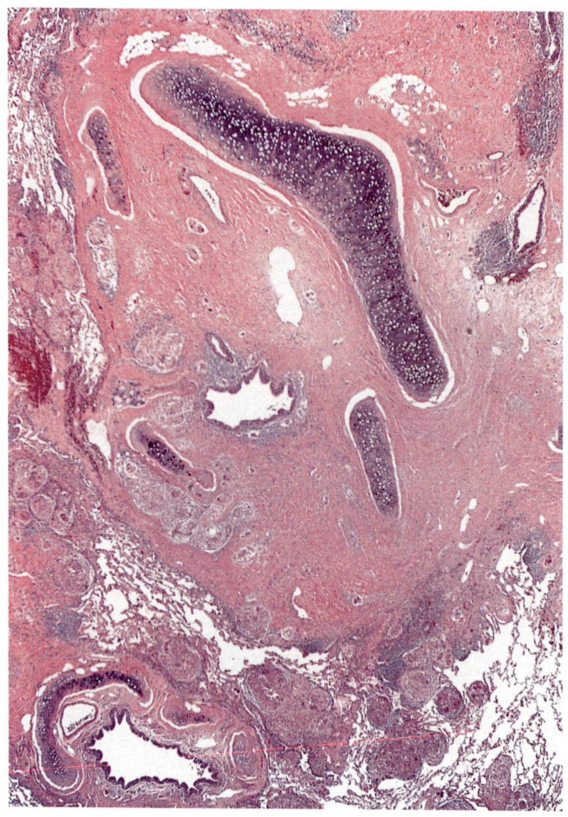

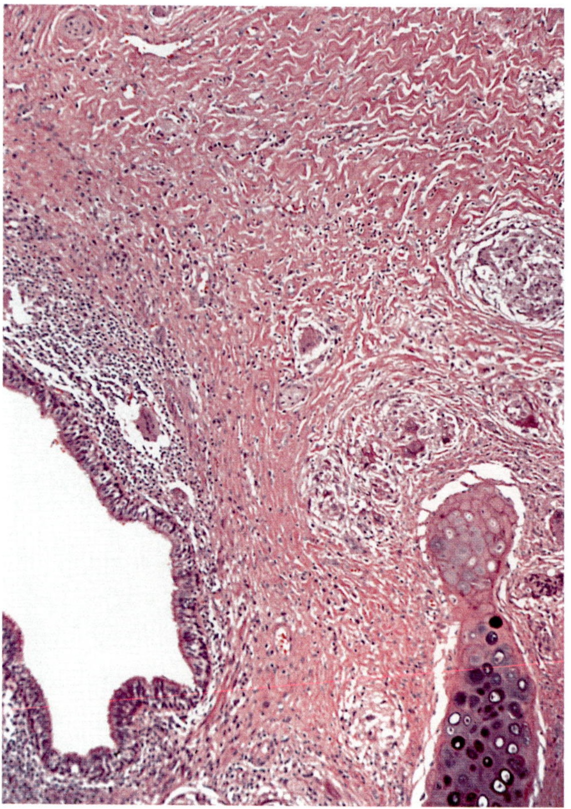

Figure 3-78

SARCOIDOSIS: FIBROSIS

Left: This bronchus is markedly narrowed by extensive fibrosis.

Right: The lumen of this bronchus is markedly narrowed by the submucosal fibrosis that accompanies the granulomatous inflammation. A few residual noncaseating granulomas are present among the extensive areas of dense fibrosis.

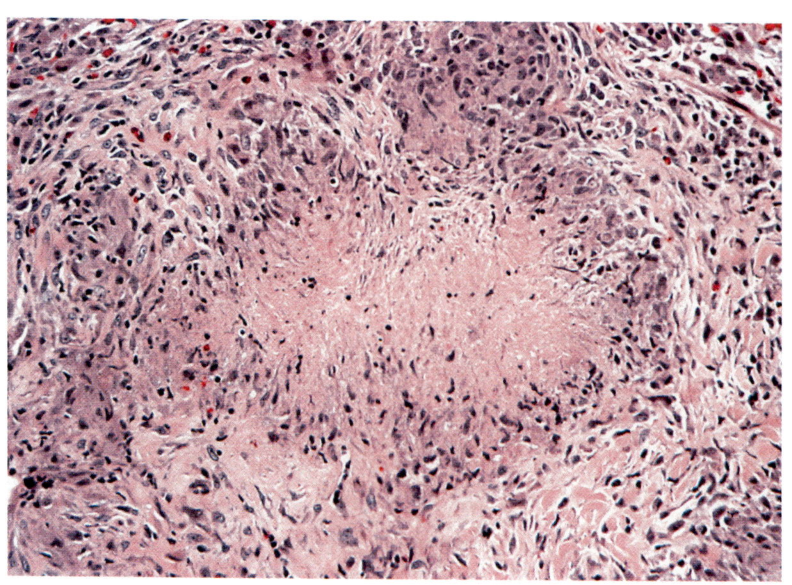

Figure 3-79

SARCOIDOSIS: FOCAL NECROSIS

This granuloma shows punctate necrosis.

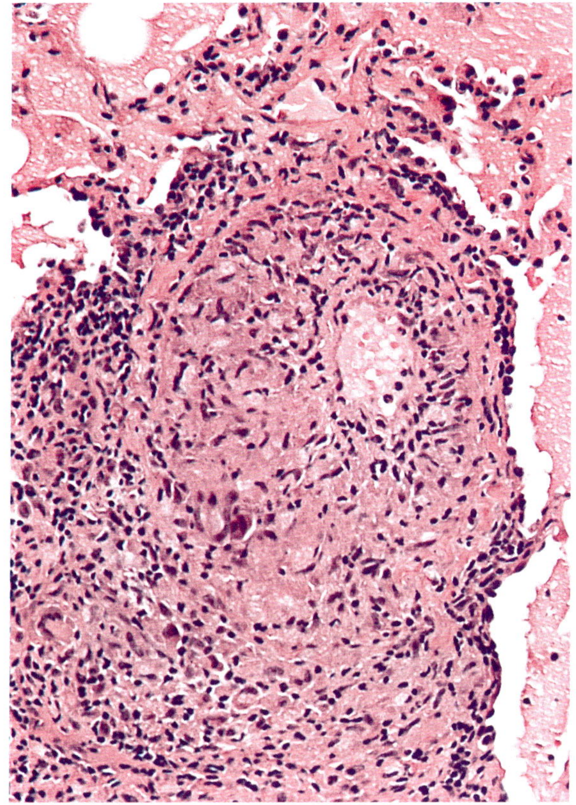

Figure 3-80

SARCOIDOSIS: VASCULITIS

This arteriole is infiltrated by granulomatous inflammation consisting of epithelioid cells and a few giant cells.

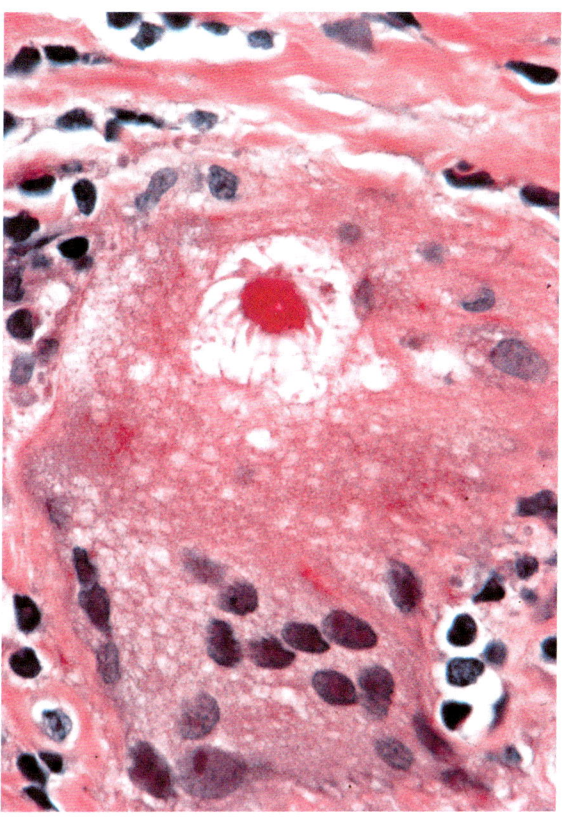

Figure 3-81

SARCOIDOSIS: ASTEROID BODY

This star-shaped, densely eosinophilic structure represents an asteroid body.

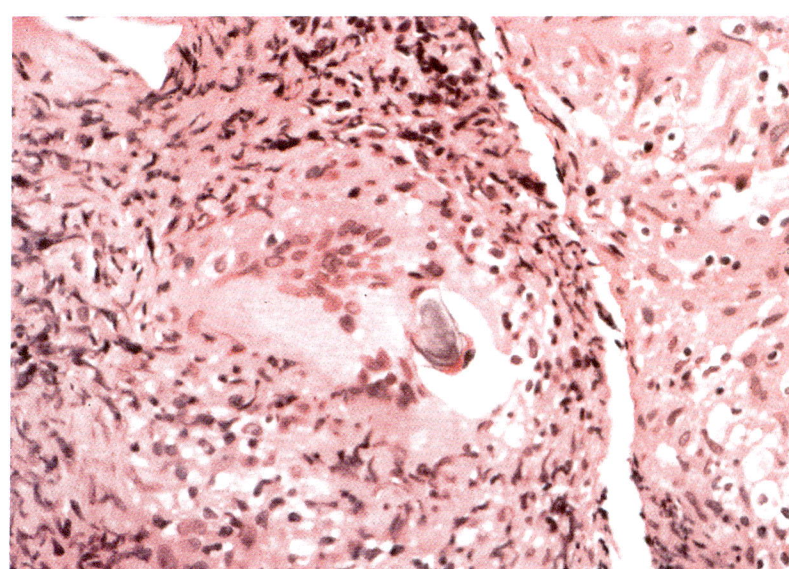

Figure 3-82

SARCOIDOSIS: SCHAUMANN BODY

The concentric laminated calcification within this granuloma is a Schaumann body.

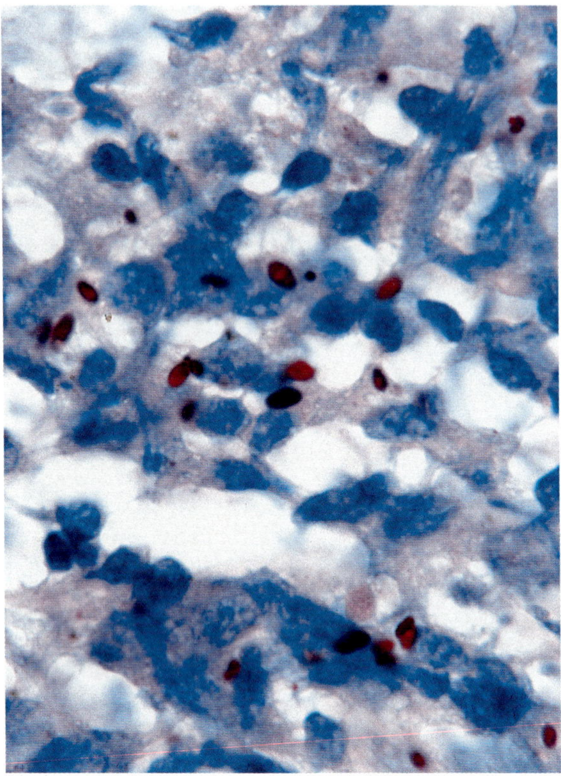

Figure 3-83

SARCOIDOSIS: HAMAZAKI-WESENBERG BODIES

These round to oval bodies were found in a lymph node from a patient with pulmonary sarcoidosis. They are acid fast with the Ziehl-Neelsen stain.

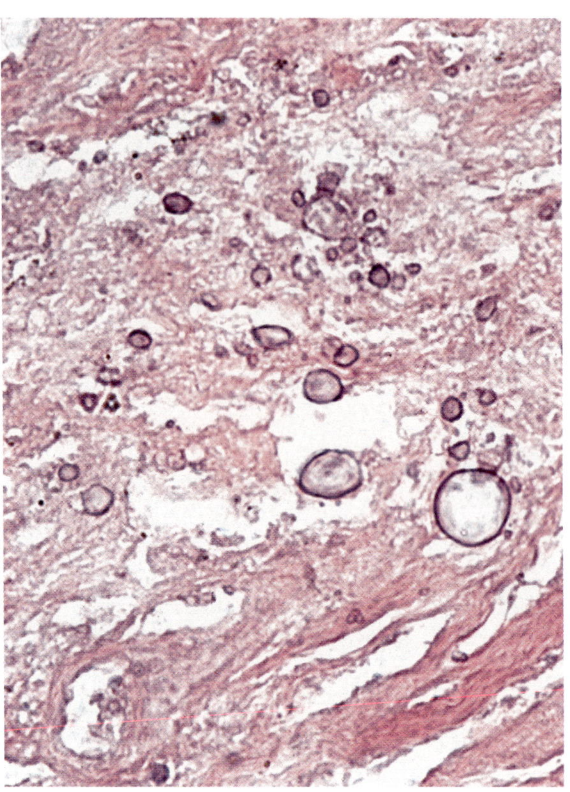

Figure 3-84

SARCOIDOSIS: CALCIFICATIONS

These rounded basophilic calcifications may occur in hyalinized fibrotic granulomas and can be mistaken for fungal organisms.

biopsies from patients with sarcoidosis, and rarely, these are so prominent that they can be mistaken for a pneumoconiosis (fig. 3-85) (514).

The cellular granulomatous phase of sarcoidosis can progress to a fibrotic phase (fig. 3-86). In most cases of pulmonary sarcoidosis, interstitial fibrosis is not a prominent feature. However, progressive pulmonary fibrosis with endstage honeycomb lung develops in a small percentage of cases. In such cases one may need to search carefully to identify the granulomas. In a small percentage of patients who develop severe honeycomb fibrosis, cavitary lesions become complicated by *Aspergillus* infection, usually in the form of a fungus ball (fig. 3-87) (448). This can result in hemorrhage that may cause hemoptysis, which can be life threatening.

Diagnosis. The final diagnosis of sarcoidosis is usually made by the clinician rather than the pathologist, after excluding other etiologies and putting the total picture together including the clinical presentation, and radiologic and pathologic features. For a pathologic diagnosis, the term "non-necrotizing (or noncaseating) granulomatous inflammation, etiology undetermined" is most appropriate, with a comment about the differential diagnosis including infection and berylliosis. In addition, some comment should be made that no organisms were seen on special stains for acid-fast bacteria and fungi and that this could be "consistent with sarcoidosis in the appropriate clinical setting."

Cultures may be useful in excluding infection if an open lung biopsy is performed on a patient suspected of having sarcoidosis. However, bronchoscopic biopsy tissue is difficult to culture and it should be processed entirely for histologic examination to search for granulomas, unless there is a high index of suspicion for infection.

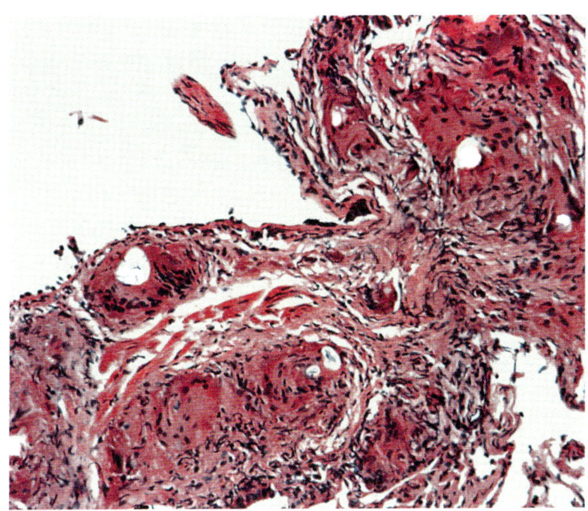

Figure 3-85

SARCOIDOSIS: BIREFRINGENT ENDOGENOUS CALCIFICATIONS

The calcifications within the granulomas of sarcoidosis were initially mistaken for pneumoconiosis.

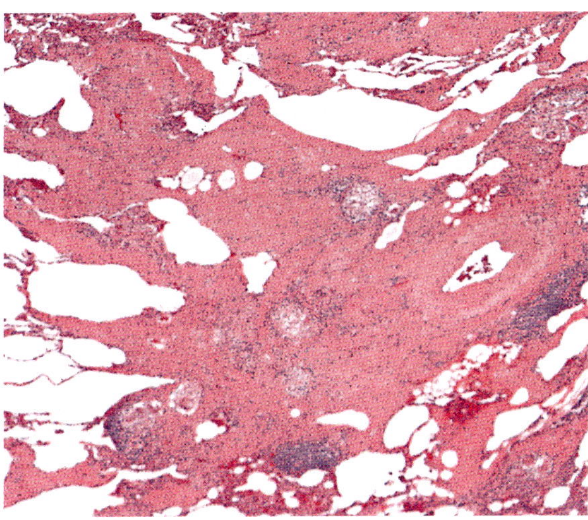

Figure 3-86

SARCOIDOSIS: INTERSTITIAL FIBROSIS

The interstitium is thickened with hyalinized fibrous tissue in addition to a few noncaseating granulomas.

Differential Diagnosis. The differential diagnosis of sarcoidosis includes infection, hypersensitivity pneumonitis, necrotizing sarcoidosis, and reactions to inhaled substances such as beryllium, talc, and aluminum. It is essential that special stains be performed to exclude a fungal or mycobacterial infection, since sarcoid-like granulomas can be seen in these infections. If punctate foci of necrosis are seen, particular attention should be given to special stains to exclude infection. *Mycobacterium avium-intracellulare* infection should be considered if the granulomas are distributed around airways, but do not appear to have a lymphangitic pattern (see chapter 12). Berylliosis can show an identical histologic pattern to sarcoidosis, however, this diagnosis is excluded based on a careful exposure history and in some cases the beryllium lymphocyte stimulation test (see chapter 7). Rarely, exposure to aluminum is associated with a sarcoid-like reaction. The differential diagnosis with hypersensitivity pneumonitis is discussed in detail earlier in this chapter. In necrotizing sarcoidosis the noncaseating granulomas form large nodules associated with large areas of necrosis and vascular inflammation (see chapter 4). This differs from nodular sarcoidosis in which necrosis is minimal or absent.

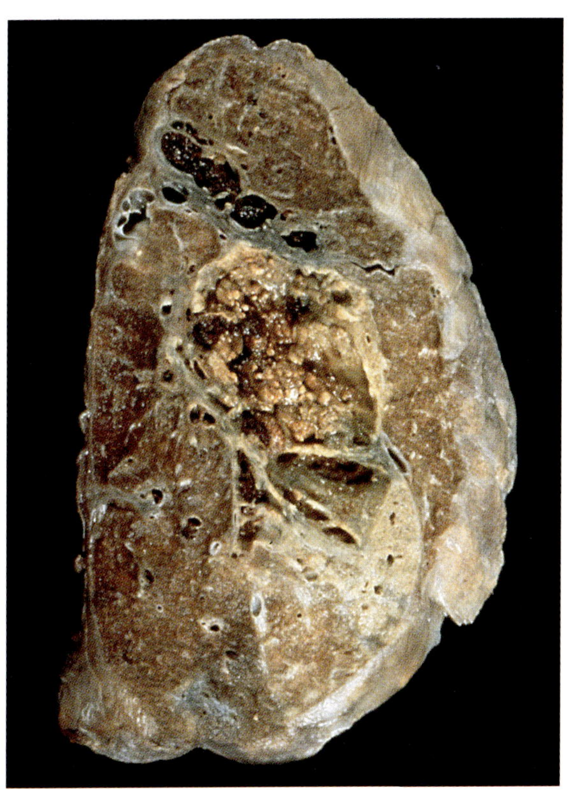

Figure 3-87

SARCOIDOSIS: ASPERGILLOMA

An *Aspergillus* fungus ball complicates this case of cavitary and fibrotic sarcoidosis.

Treatment and Prognosis. Mortality secondary to sarcoidosis occurs in 1 to 5 percent of patients, usually secondary to lung, central nervous system, or cardiac involvement. Deciding when to treat sarcoidosis can be difficult because almost 50 percent of cases spontaneously remit, especially in patients with Lofgren's syndrome.

Corticosteroids are effective in the treatment of patients with sarcoidosis, especially those with stages 2 and 3 disease (moderate to severe or progressive symptoms, or chest radiographic changes and other systemic complications) (459,466,497). The usual dosage of prednisone is 0.5 to 1.0 mg/kg/day or every other day for 6 weeks followed by a slow dosage taper over 3 to 6 months. Many patients require maintenance therapy with 5 to 10 mg/day of prednisone; often higher-dose therapy may be required if the disease activity flares. Oral steroids improve the symptoms and radiologic features over 6 to 24 months (497). There is limited evidence of an improvement in lung function. There are no data beyond 2 years to indicate whether oral steroids have any modifying effect on long-term disease progression (497). Short-term (less than 6 months) use of inhaled steroids may improve symptoms, perhaps in patients who mainly have cough (497). There is growing concern that corticosteroid therapy may be associated with more episodes of chronic disease or relapses. In general, patients with severe symptoms, persistent pulmonary opacities, hypoxemia, and severe lung function impairment should be treated with corticosteroids.

Extrapulmonary manifestations that require therapy include ocular disease, hypercalcemia, cardiac dysrhythmia, neurologic involvement, arthritis, and disfiguring skin lesions. Aspergilloma is a complication that can result in life-threatening pulmonary hemorrhage.

Several alternative approaches have been proposed, such as the use of immunosuppressive, cytotoxic, and antimalarial drugs (467). Specific agents include methotrexate, azathioprine, cyclophosphamide, colchicine, chlorambucil, cyclosporine, chloroquine, hydroxychloroquine, nonsteroidal anti-inflammatory drugs, and pentoxifylline (431–433,474,490). In addition, radiation has been used for neurosarcoidosis.

Organ transplantation has been performed successfully for endstage hepatic, renal, cardiac, or respiratory failure complicating sarcoidosis (461,492,495). There are several concerns about the usefulness of lung transplantation in this setting: 1) the disease can recur in the transplanted lung; 2) patients with sarcoidosis have a high rate of invasive fungal infection after lung transplantation despite prophylaxis with itraconazole, inhaled amphotericin B, or both before the transplant; 3) optimal transplantation procedure (single or bilateral) is unclear; and most concerning, 4) the recent data suggest an increased rate of obliterative bronchiolitis (a form of chronic allograft rejection which contributes substantially to post-transplantation morbidity and mortality) in patients with sarcoidosis (434,460,463,464,492,495).

LANGERHANS' CELL HISTIOCYTOSIS AND OTHER HISTIOCYTIC DISORDERS

Langerhans' Cell Histiocytosis

Definition. Pulmonary Langerhans' cell histiocytosis (PLCH) is a chronic, progressive disorder characterized by a proliferation of Langerhans' cell infiltrates which form multiple, bilateral, interstitial peribronchiolar nodules that frequently cavitate. Langerhans' cells are differentiated cells of monocyte-macrophage lineage that function as antigen-presenting cells. PLCH is strongly associated with cigarette smoking. Although PLCH may be limited to the lung, it can be multifocal and involve other organs, especially bone and lymph nodes. Synonyms include *histiocytosis X, eosinophilic granuloma,* and *Langerhans' cell granulomatosis.*

PLCH is a form of interstitial lung disease that affects the lung either in isolation or in addition to other organ systems (536,561,581). The concept of histiocytosis X was proposed by Lichtenstein in 1953 (560) to embrace three major localized and generalized patterns of histiocytosis including eosinophilic granuloma, Hand-Schüller-Christian disease, and Letterer-Siwe disease. Letterer-Siwe disease is a potentially fatal systemic disease in children under 3 years of age. It is characterized by involvement of the skin, lymph nodes, bone, liver, and spleen. Pneumothorax is a common pulmonary complication. Hand-Schüller-Christian disease is a multifocal disease of early childhood that commonly affects the lungs and bones. A classic triad of bone defects, exophthalmos, and diabetes insipidus can be seen. This multisystem disease is treated with systemic chemotherapy. However, this concept of histiocytosis X is no longer used due to the imprecise definitions of these terms, the recognition that the proliferating cells are Langerhans' cells, and the growing recognition that there are profound differences in organ involvement, clinical course, and therapeutic response (543,561). The World Health Organization Committee on Histiocytic/Reticulum Cell Proliferations recently proposed that Langerhans' cell histiocytosis (LCH) replace the many previous terms for this disorder (543).

Clinical Features. The true incidence and prevalence of PLCH are unknown, although it is thought to be a rare disorder. It is seen in less than 5 percent of lung biopsies from patients with DPLD (548) and in less than 2 percent of the patients presenting to the Denver Specialized Center of Research program in Interstitial Lung Disease (a total of approximately 3,000 patients over 14 years) (535). PLCH primarily afflicts young adults between the ages of 20 and 40 years (546). It is more common in men, although as more women take up the smoking habit the prevalence in women has risen. Virtually all cases of PLCH in adults occur in cigarette smokers (546). The disease has rarely been reported in blacks. PLCH also can occur in children, either as an isolated pulmonary disease (516,531) or in the setting of a multisystem disorder (529,545,576).

The pathogenesis of PLCH is unknown. There are no clear genetic, occupational, or geographic risk factors. Several nonspecific findings consistent with generalized activation of immune effectors have been found including nonspecific increase in IgG in BAL fluid (570), immune complexes in the circulation and bound to tissue (555), and abnormalities in T-cell function (573,577). The pulmonary lesions demonstrate abundant expression of transforming growth factor-beta-1 (TGF-beta-1) and granulocyte-macrophage–colony-stimulating factor (GM-CSF) (519,581). Tumor necrosis factor-alpha (TNF-alpha) and granulocyte GM-CSF may have a critical role in the pathogenesis of the disease, since they make possible in vitro generation of Langerhans' cells from CD34+ hematopoietic stem cells and are key mediators of lung injury in animal models of lung fibrosis (519,581). A role for activation of latent TGF-beta-1 and, in turn, the enhanced production of interleukin resulting in impaired remodeling of bone in patients with LCH, has been reported (528).

The near universal association with cigarette smoking in adults strongly implies some causative role. One hypothesis contends that increased bombesin-like peptide production plays a central role (517). Bombesin is a neuropeptide produced by neuroendocrine cells, which are increased in the lungs of smokers. Bombesin-like peptides are chemotactic for monocytes, are mitogenic for epithelial cells and fibroblasts, and stimulate cytokine secretion (517). Tobacco glycoprotein, a constituent of tobacco, and other regulatory glycopeptides (e.g., GM-CSF) may also contribute to disease pathogenesis (588,590). There appears to be no association of smoking with extrapulmonary LCH.

The clinical presentation is variable, from an asymptomatic state (up to 25 percent) to a rapidly progressive condition. Extrapulmonary involvement, such as bone lesions, occurs in 10 to 15 percent of patients (546). The most common clinical manifestations at presentation are dyspnea (40 to 87 percent); nonproductive cough (56 to 70 percent); chest pain, which is frequently pleuritic (10 to 21 percent); fatigue (approximately 30 percent); weight loss (20 to 30 percent); and fever (15 percent) (534). Pneumothorax occurs in about 25 percent of patients and is occasionally the first manifestation of the illness. Hemoptysis and diabetes insipidus are rare manifestations (about 5 percent of cases each) (546). The physical examination is usually normal. Even crackles are uncommon on chest examination (about 20 percent of patients) (546,563).

Routine laboratory studies are not helpful and the peripheral eosinophil count is normal. Physiologically, the most prominent and frequent pulmonary function abnormality reported is a markedly reduced DLCO (present in 60 to 90 percent of cases). The total lung capacity and expiratory flow rates are both well preserved in PLCH, although a subgroup of patients shows predominantly restrictive disease, with reduced total lung volume and increased

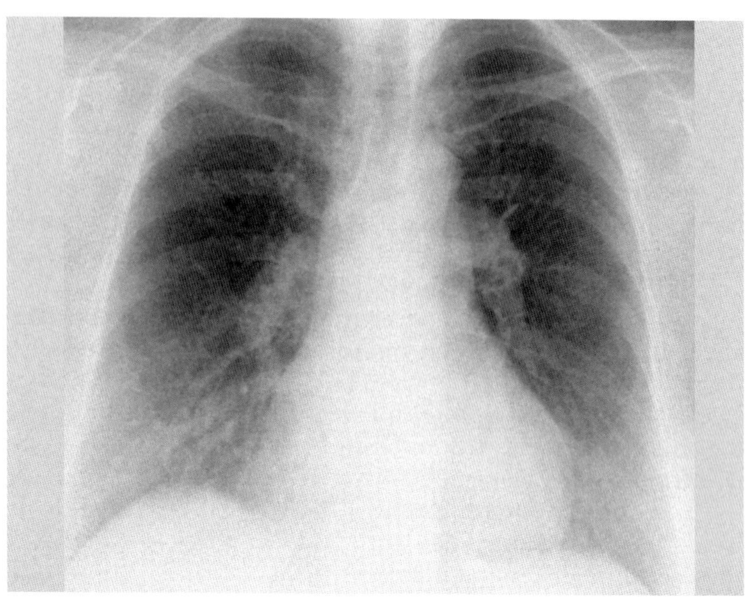

Figure 3-88

PULMONARY LANGERHANS' CELL HISTIOCYTOSIS

Chest radiograph of a 49-year-old woman demonstrates a diffuse reticulonodular pattern with relative sparing of the lung bases. Central pulmonary arteries are enlarged due to pulmonary arterial hypertension.

elastic recoil. Airflow limitation and hyperinflation occur in a minority of patients, and can sometimes be associated with reactive airways and significant improvement after bronchodilator administration (534).

Arterial blood gases measured at rest may be normal despite extensive radiographic abnormalities, and are insensitive indicators of disease (534). Pulmonary hypertension and manifestations of cor pulmonale are seen in advanced stages. Pulmonary arteriopathy and veno-occlusive disease can occur relatively independently of parenchymal and airway disease, and may impair diffusing capacity and exercise capacity to a degree disproportionate to radiographic findings (534,542,552).

The diagnosis of PLCH is often strongly suspected by the clinical and radiographic findings (see below). In most situations, HRCT is the most useful radiologic test in the evaluation of patients with suspected PLCH (581). Fiberoptic bronchoscopy with BAL and transbronchial lung biopsy are often the first procedures of choice to obtain lung cells and tissue. An increased number of Langerhans' cells in BAL has been suggested as a diagnostic feature (521,524,585). However, slightly increased Langerhans' cells in BAL fluid can occur in patients with other interstitial lung disorders (521,524,585) and in smokers without interstitial lung diseases (530,575).

Radiologic Findings. The radiologic manifestations typically consist of a symmetric, bilateral nodular or reticulonodular pattern that is diffuse throughout the upper and mid-lung zones but spares the costophrenic angles (fig. 3-88) (546,559). HRCT demonstrates small nodules and cystic airspaces (fig. 3-89) (526,527, 565,574). The nodules often have a centrilobular (peribronchiolar) distribution and usually measure 1 to 10 mm in diameter. The cysts can range from a few millimeters to 3 cm in diameter and often have bizarre shapes. The parenchymal abnormalities typically have a patchy or diffuse distribution throughout the upper and mid-lung zones but tend to spare the lung bases.

In the majority of patients, the characteristic pattern and distribution of PLCH allow distinction from other infiltrative diseases and confident diagnosis based on HRCT findings (549,553,567). The main considerations in the differential diagnosis are sarcoidosis, silicosis, hypersensitivity pneumonitis, and lymphangioleiomyomatosis (558,581).

Gross Findings. PLCH typically shows multiple, bilateral nodules with varying degrees of cavitation (fig. 3-90). Rarely, a single nodule predominates. It may manifest as an endobronchial mass (562). The upper lobes tend to be more affected, and the lung bases may be spared. The nodules are irregular in shape with a stellate border (fig. 3-91). Pigmentation may be seen

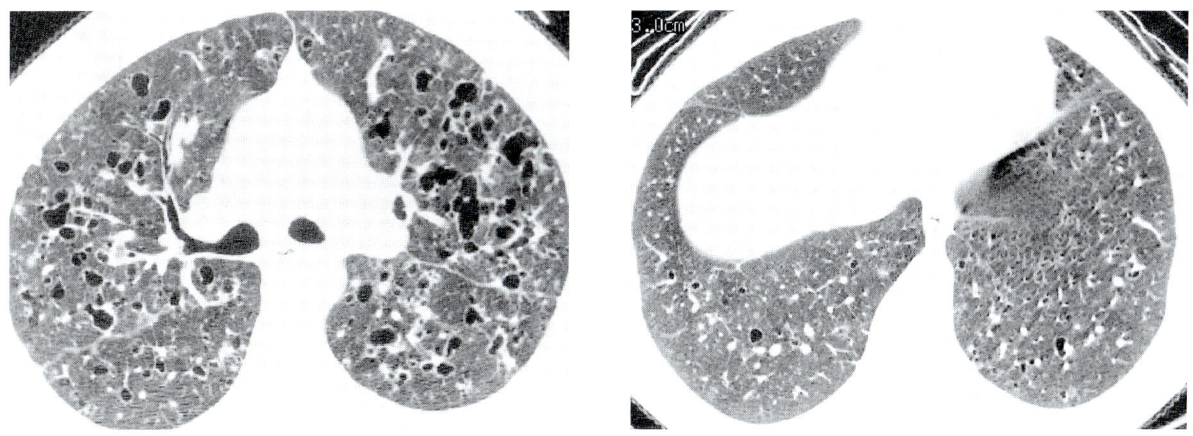

Figure 3-89

PULMONARY LANGERHANS' CELL HISTIOCYTOSIS

Left: HRCT at the level of the right upper lobe bronchus in a 30-year-old man demonstrates numerous irregular cystic spaces and a few small nodules.

Right: HRCT through the lung bases shows only a few cysts.

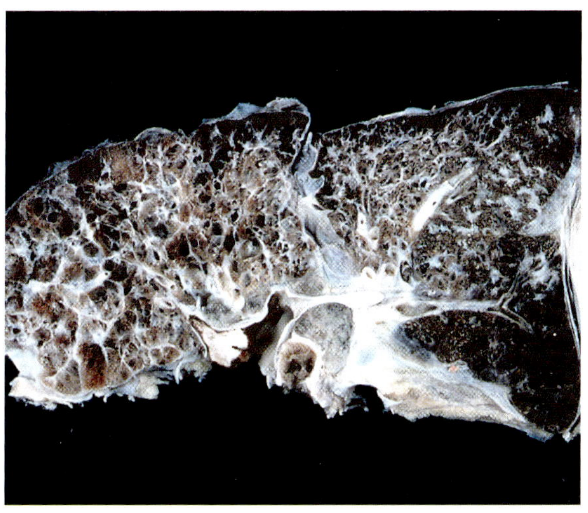

Figure 3-90

PULMONARY LANGERHANS' CELL HISTIOCYTOSIS

The lung shows diffuse nodular and cavitary lesions, especially in the upper lobe.

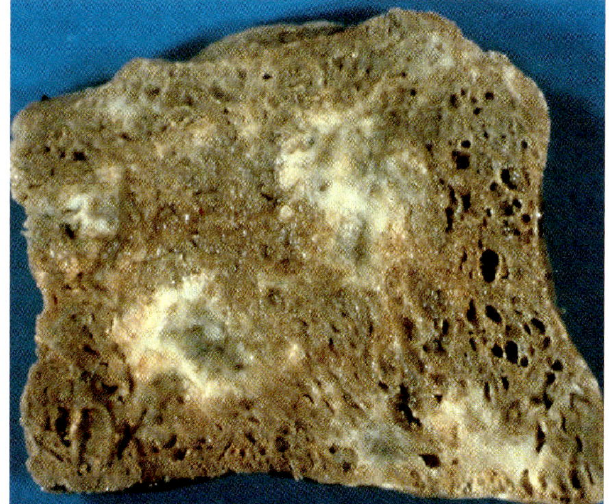

Figure 3-91

PULMONARY LANGERHANS' CELL HISTIOCYTOSIS

This open lung biopsy shows several irregularly shaped, tan-gray nodules with relatively uninvolved intervening lung.

centrally within the nodules. The fibrosing phase may show dense fibrosis and cavitary changes that give a honeycomb appearance.

Histologic Findings. PLCH has a distinctive low-power appearance consisting of multiple nodular infiltrates with a stellate border extending into the surrounding interstitium (figs. 3-92–3-95) (532,580). The lesions are centered on bronchioles, although this may be difficult to appreciate on a given histologic section. Central cavitation is common (figs. 3-93, 3-95). PLCH infiltrates may also be seen along the pleura and interlobular septa. The cellular infiltrates extend into the adjacent alveolar septal interstitium in a stellate pattern (fig. 3-95). The Langerhans' cells appear uniform with moderate eosinophilic cytoplasm and prominently grooved nuclear membranes (fig. 3-96). Organizing pneumonia may

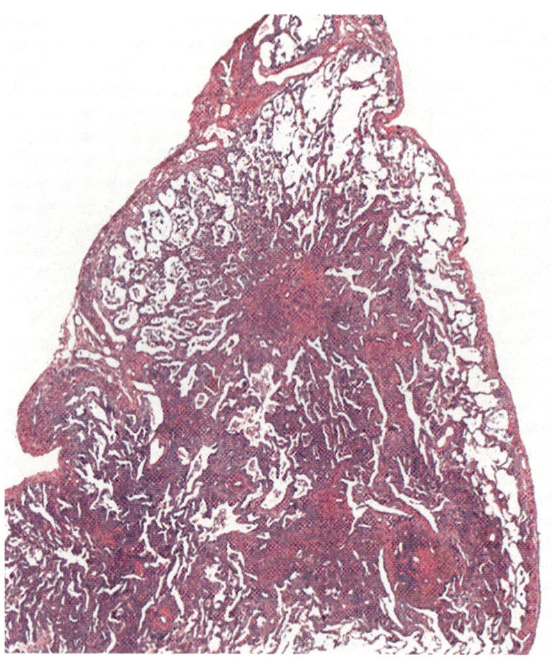

Figure 3-92

PULMONARY LANGERHANS' CELL HISTIOCYTOSIS

Low-power microscopy shows multiple stellate-shaped, nodular interstitial infiltrates.

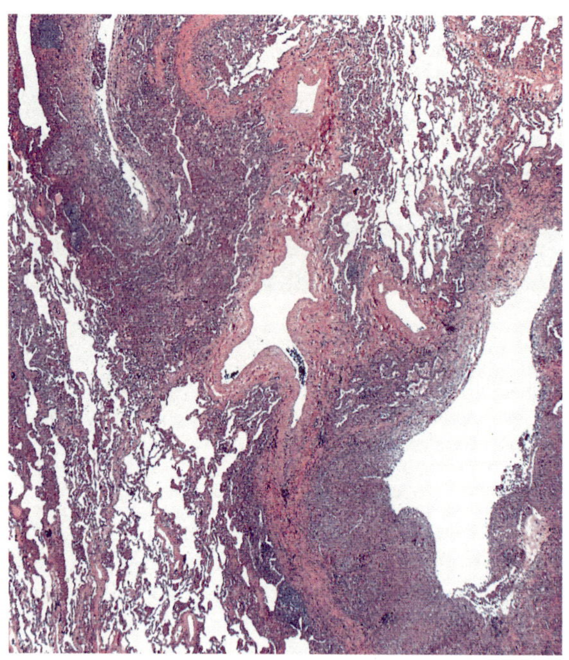

Figure 3-93

PULMONARY LANGERHANS' CELL HISTIOCYTOSIS

Multiple nodular infiltrates show prominent cavitation.

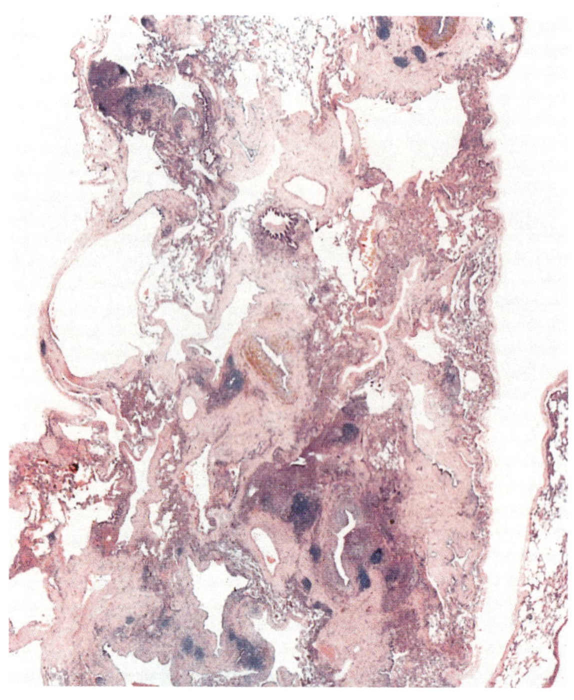

Figure 3-94

PULMONARY LANGERHANS' CELL HISTIOCYTOSIS

Interstitial fibrosis is present in addition to several nodular infiltrates.

be seen at the edge of the nodular infiltrates (fig. 3-97). In most cases the nodular infiltrates are readily apparent, but in some cases they may be difficult to find. The diagnosis can be established based on a bronchoscopic biopsy if diagnostic lesions are sampled, but this occurs in less than 50 percent of cases (532,580). Surgical lung biopsy has the highest diagnostic yield (581).

PLCH lesions progress from a cellular process to fibrotic scars, which may be nondiagnostic (fig. 3-98). Often, a spectrum of cellular, intermediate, and fibrotic lesions is seen in the same biopsy specimen. The cellular lesions consist of varying numbers of Langerhans' cells mixed with macrophages, lymphocytes, and eosinophils (fig. 3-96). The number of eosinophils is highly variable and they may be difficult to find in some cases. The fibrotic scars often maintain the stellate shape of the cellular lesions. This may provide a clue to the diagnosis in cases where only fibrotic lesions are sampled in an open biopsy. Severe cases may progress to honeycomb fibrosis, but this is uncommon.

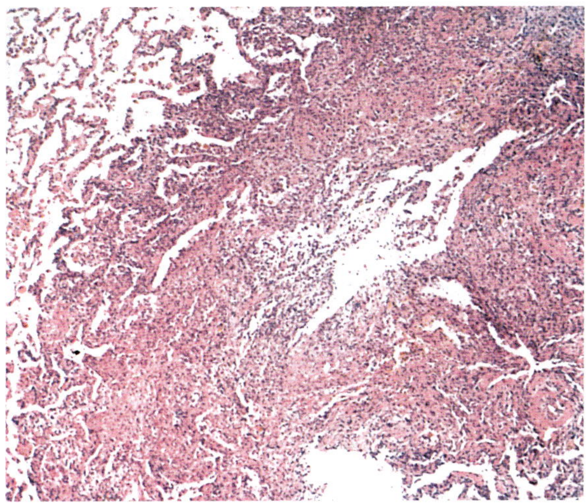

Figure 3-95

PULMONARY LANGERHANS' CELL HISTIOCYTOSIS

This stellate and cavitated nodular infiltrate extends at the periphery into the alveolar septal interstitium. There is central cavitation.

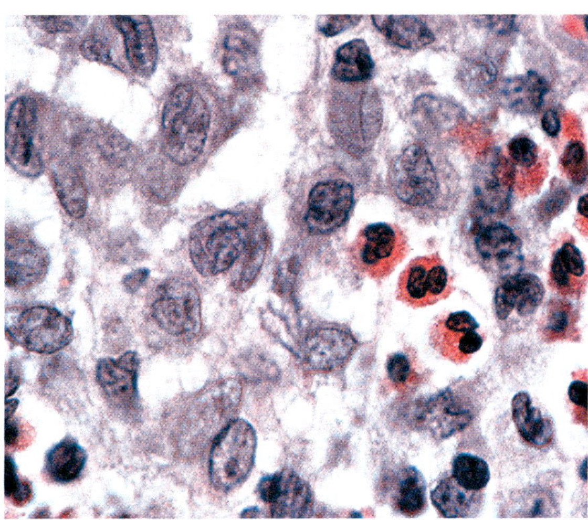

Figure 3-96

PULMONARY LANGERHANS' CELL HISTIOCYTOSIS

The cellular infiltrate consists of a sheet of Langerhans' cells which have a uniform appearance consisting of moderate eosinophilic cytoplasm and prominent nuclear grooves. A few eosinophils are also present.

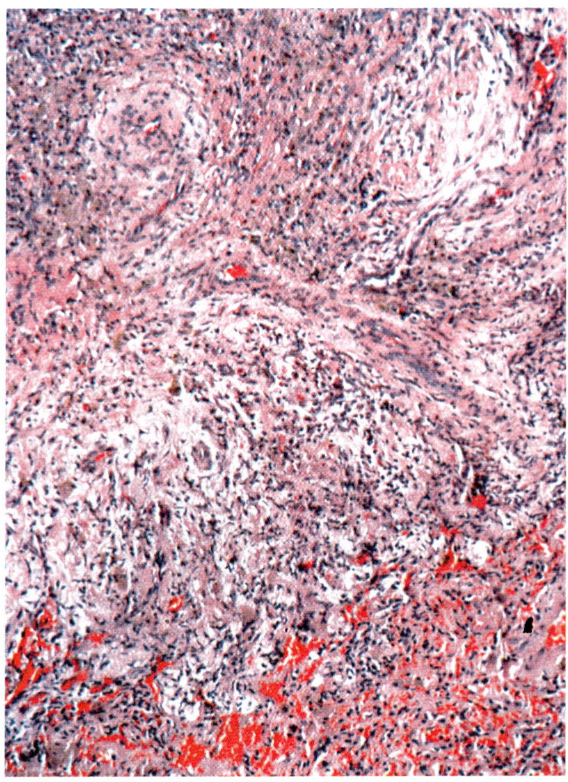

Figure 3-97

PULMONARY LANGERHANS' CELL HISTIOCYTOSIS

Organizing pneumonia is present at the edge of this Langerhans' cell infiltrate.

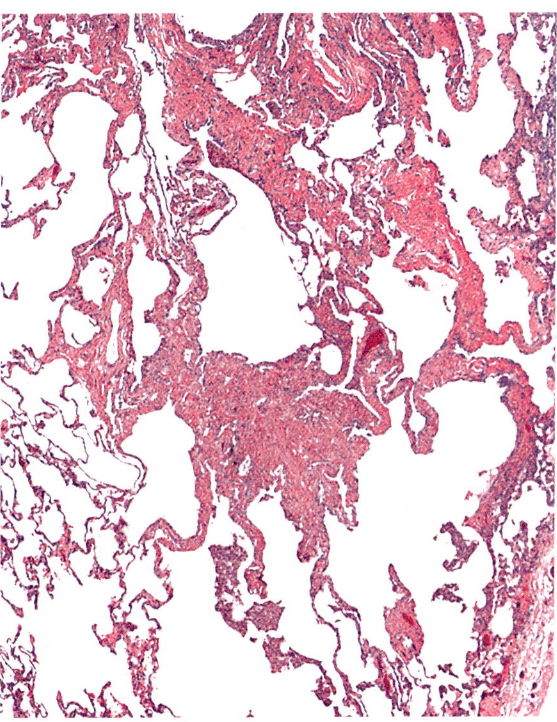

Figure 3-98

PULMONARY LANGERHANS' CELL HISTIOCYTOSIS

This scar is an old fibrotic lesion of PLCH in which Langerhans' cells are no longer present. In this case the scar retains the stellate shape typically seen in active cellular lesions.

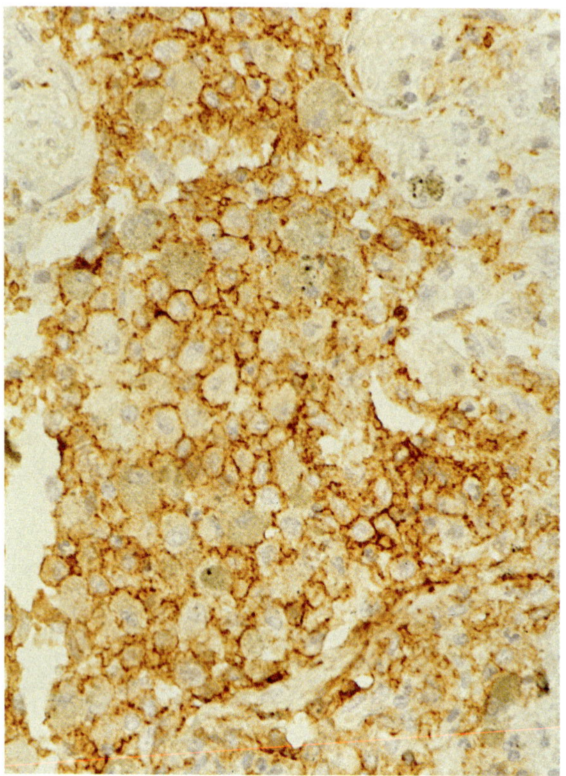

Figure 3-99

PULMONARY LANGERHANS' CELL HISTIOCYTOSIS

Immunohistochemistry for CD1a (O10) antibody in a formalin-fixed, paraffin-embedded section shows positive staining of the Langerhans' cells with a membranous pattern.

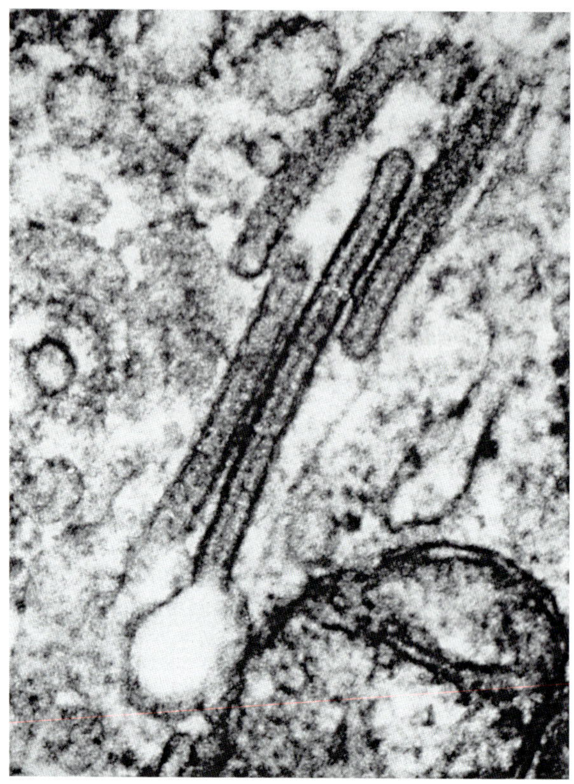

Figure 3-100

PULMONARY LANGERHANS' CELL HISTIOCYTOSIS

Electron microscopy shows the pentilaminar configuration of the Birbeck granule with a bulbous end.

The Langerhans' cells stain with S-100 protein and 010 (CD1a) in formalin-fixed paraffin-embedded tissue sections (fig. 3-99). By electron microscopy, the Langerhans' cells show distinctive structures called Birbeck granules (fig. 3-100). Other characteristic properties of the Langerhans' cells include the presence of C3, IgG-Fc receptors, and Ia antigen (HLA-DR) (522,551,556,580,586).

The clonality that has been demonstrated in LCH raises the possibility of a neoplastic disorder (533,583,589). However, it is also possible that LCH represents a proliferation of activated Langerhans' cells in response to certain immunologic stimuli (525,536,561). Increased proliferation of Langerhans' cells in LCH has been identified by proliferating cell nuclear antigen (PCNA) and Ki-67 antibodies, as well as increased apoptosis in spontaneously regressing LCH lesions (525,536).

The lung surrounding PLCH lesions typically shows the respiratory bronchiolitis associated with cigarette smoking. Vascular changes consisting of medial thickening and intimal proliferation are often present and may account for the clinical finding of pulmonary hypertension in some patients (542,552,580). The pleura may also show lesions of reactive eosinophilic pleuritis if the patient has had pneumothoraces (580).

The histology of PLCH in children (fig. 3-101) is virtually identical to that in adults, although in the setting of diffuse multisystem infiltrates the pulmonary lesions may appear more cellular, with a denser infiltration of Langerhans' cells compared to adults. However, respiratory bronchiolitis and smoker's macrophages are not seen.

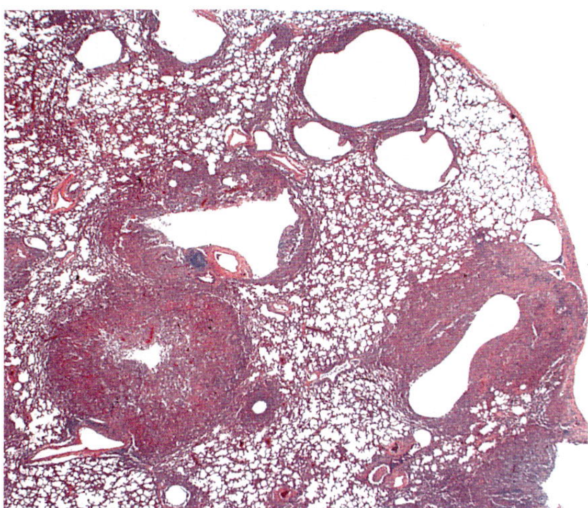

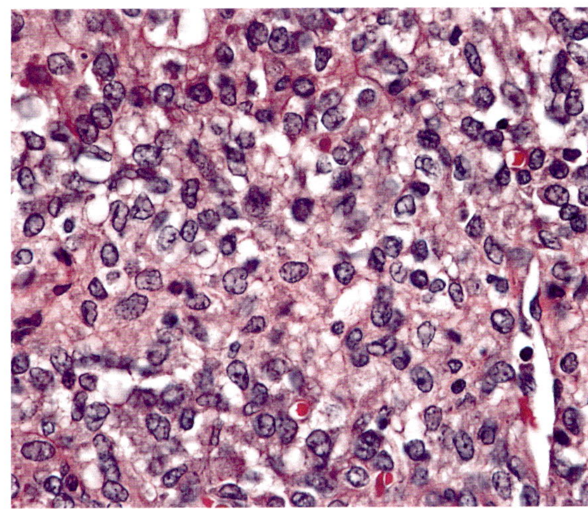

Figure 3-101

PULMONARY LANGERHANS' CELL HISTIOCYTOSIS IN CHILD WITH DISSEMINATED DISEASE

Left: The morphology of the lung infiltration is very similar to that seen in adults, with multiple nodular and cavitated lesions.

Right: The Langerhans' cells have moderate eosinophilic cytoplasm and prominent nuclear grooves.

Differential Diagnosis. The differential diagnosis includes RB, chronic eosinophilic pneumonia, UIP, and reactive eosinophilic pleuritis. Lesions of RB consist of faintly brown pigmented alveolar macrophages surrounding and within respiratory bronchioles. However, pure RB lacks the cellular and nodular interstitial lesions of PLCH. Eosinophilic pneumonia consists of an intra-alveolar accumulation of eosinophils and contrasts with PLCH in which the cellular infiltrates are interstitial. Fibrotic cases of PLCH may be confused with UIP, but the fibrotic scars often retain a stellate shape, show a bronchiolocentric distribution, and typically do not show a UIP-like pattern of temporal heterogeneity. Correlation with the chest radiographs and HRCT should also be very helpful. Reactive eosinophilic pleuritis is a nonspecific pleural reaction seen in association with pneumothorax of any cause (see chapter 18). It differs from PLCH in that it is restricted to the pleura and consists of proliferating mesothelial cells admixed with chronic inflammation and prominent eosinophils (520).

Treatment and Prognosis. The natural history of PLCH is quite variable, with some patients experiencing spontaneous remission of symptoms and others progressing to endstage fibrotic lung disease (535). Most demonstrate gradual progression with continued cigarette smoking, while the disease may regress with the cessation of smoking (564). Relapse of active disease is often associated with relapse in cigarette smoking (578). Patients with radiographic sparing of the lung base adjacent to costophrenic angle are more likely to remain stable or improve than those with lung involvement near the costophrenic angle (559). Delobbe and coworkers (537) found that age older than 26 years, FEV1/FVC ratio lower than 0.66, and RV/TLC ratio higher than 0.33 were associated with poorer prognosis.

Corticosteroids and cytotoxic agents are of limited value in the treatment of this disorder. The most impressive positive response to corticosteroid therapy occurs when nodular opacities are prominent. Chemotherapeutic agents such as vinblastine, methotrexate, cyclophosphamide, etoposide, and cladribine have been used in patients with progressive disease who are unresponsive to corticosteroids or in those with multiorgan involvement (554, 581). Radiotherapy for symptomatic bone lesions can be palliative, but it is not useful for treating the pulmonary manifestations.

Several cancers, including hematologic and solid-organ cancers, have been reported in association with PLCH (554,572,579). The explanation for this association is not clear and may be multifactorial (581). Lung transplantation should be considered in patients with advanced, progressive disease unless contraindications are present (539,587). The condition may recur in the transplanted lung, but it is unclear if this affects overall post-transplant survival (541,547,550). Ten percent of patients die of respiratory failure (554).

Erdheim-Chester Disease

Definition. Erdheim-Chester disease is a rare, histiocytic infiltrative disorder that frequently affects the long bones, but may also involve other viscera including lung.

Clinical Features. Erdheim-Chester disease is extremely rare, with fewer than 100 reported cases (538,571,582,584). The mean age is 53 years (range, 7 to 84 years) and there is a slight male predominance (582). The diaphyses of the long bones typically show symmetrical osteosclerosis. Dyspnea is the most common pulmonary symptom. Other potential manifestations include fever, weight loss, diabetes insipidus, lower limb bone pain, exophthalmos, and periorbital xanthomas.

Radiologic Findings. The characteristic radiographic findings are reticular interstitial opacities and thickening of the fissures and interlobular septa (571,582,584). CT also shows interlobular septal thickening, areas of ground-glass attenuation, and centrilobular nodular opacities. Bullous or cystic lesions, pleural thickening, pleural effusions, and pericardial thickening or effusions may be present (571,582,584). Sclerosis of thoracic vertebrae may be seen on chest CT scans.

Pathologic Findings. The lung shows diffuse infiltration by foamy histiocytes along lymphatic routes including the pleura, septa, and perivascular and peribronchiolar interstitium (fig. 3-102) (571,584). Varying degrees of fibrosis accompany the histiocytic infiltrates. The histiocytes have round to oval nuclei and moderate to abundant cytoplasm; they may be multinucleated. The cytoplasm is usually eosinophilic and foamy. A few lymphocytes, plasma cells, and eosinophils may be present (571,584).

The histiocytes are negative with the PAS stain but positive when stained immunohistochemically for CD68 and factor XIIIa. S-100 protein may be positive, but CD1a, CD45RB, CD21, and keratin are negative. Electron microscopy shows histiocytic cells with phagolysosomes containing lipid, but no Birbeck granules (571,584).

Differential Diagnosis. The main differential diagnosis includes Langerhans' cell histiocytosis and sinus histiocytosis with massive lymphadenopathy. The nuclei of the histiocytes lack the prominent grooves typical of Langerhans' cells and the cells do not stain for CD1a, although they may be variably positive for S-100 protein. Birbeck granules are also absent. Erdheim-Chester disease differs from sinus histiocytosis with massive lymphadenopathy (see below), a condition in which lymphocyte emperipolesis and S-100 protein–positive staining are consistent features. The histiocytes of Erdheim-Chester disease also stain for factor XIIIa, a feature that distinguishes it from the other two diseases (571).

Treatment and Prognosis. In the review by Veyssier-Belot et al. (582), 22 of 59 patients died after a mean follow-up of 1.3 years. A high percentage of patients with extensive pulmonary involvement die from their respiratory complications (571,582). Various forms of treatment have been attempted including corticosteroids, chemotherapy, radiotherapy, surgery, and immunotherapy, but is not clear that any of these are very effective (582).

Sinus Histiocytosis with Massive Lymphadenopathy

Definition. Sinus histiocytosis and massive lymphadenopathy (SHML), also known as *Rosai-Dorfman disease*, is a rare histiocytic proliferative disorder of unknown origin characterized by frequent involvement of lymph nodes (mostly cervical) and less frequent extranodal involvement of sites such as the skin, nasal cavity, soft tissue, eyelid/orbit, bone, and salivary gland. Lower respiratory tract involvement is uncommon.

Rosai and Dorfman described SHML in 1969 and 1972 (568,569). Over the subsequent two decades they established a registry and collected data on a group of 423 patients. This was reviewed in detail in 1990 by Foucar et al. (544). At that time, only nine cases of pulmonary involvement were recorded (2 percent of all cases).

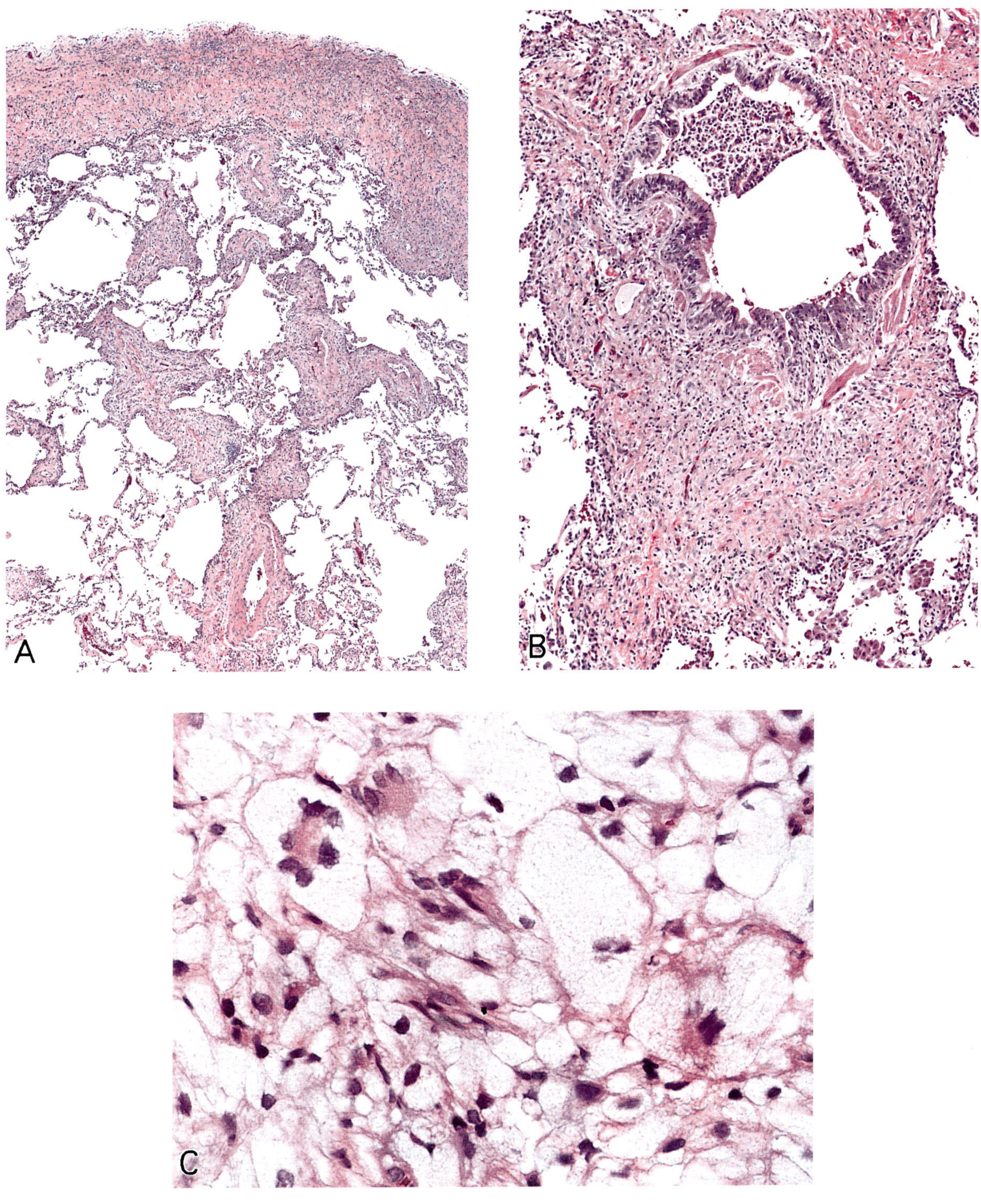

Figure 3-102

ERDHEIM-CHESTER DISEASE

A: There is an extensive infiltrate along the pleura, septa, and bronchovascular interstitium.

B: The interstitium surrounding this bronchiole is markedly infiltrated by histiocytes.

C: The infiltrate consists of histiocytes with abundant foamy cytoplasm. Most of the cells have single small nuclei but several multinucleated histiocytes are also present.

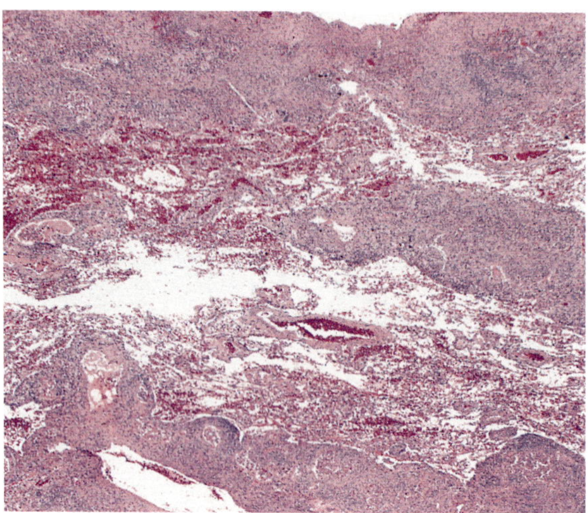

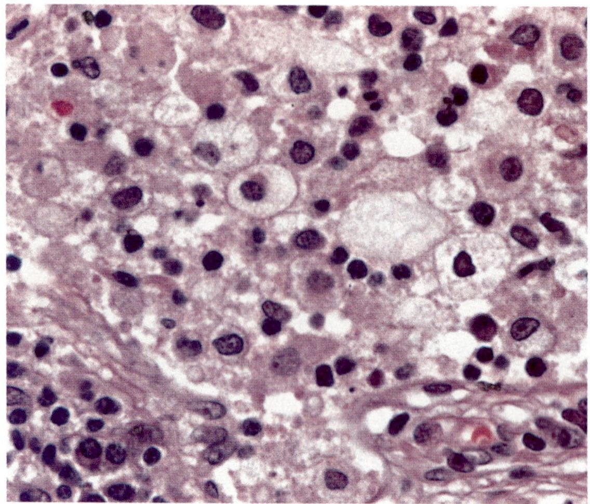

Figure 3-103

SINUS HISTIOCYTOSIS WITH MASSIVE LYMPHADENOPATHY

Left: There is extensive histiocytic infiltration of the pleura and underlying interstitium surrounding bronchovascular bundles.

Right: The histiocytes have abundant eosinophilic cytoplasm, which contains several lymphocytes.

Clinical Features. The mean age of onset is 21 years (range, congenital to 76 years) (544). The race distribution is 44 percent black, 44 percent white, 5 percent oriental, and 7 percent other. There is a male predominance (58 to 42 percent) (544). All of the nine patients with lower respiratory tract involvement summarized by Foucar et al. (544) had evidence of nodal disease.

Pathologic Findings. There is little published data regarding the pathology of SHML with lower respiratory tract involvement. However, based on the review by Foucar et al. (544), infiltration of large airways is the most common pattern of involvement and diffuse lung parenchymal lesions occur less often. There may be mass-like submucosal infiltration of the trachea and main bronchi or polypoid lesions causing varying degrees of airway obstruction. These airway lesions may be solitary or multicentric and have an erythematous granular appearance. Lung parenchymal involvement may consist of diffuse infiltration with involvement of the pleura, septa, and interstitium around bronchovascular bundles (fig. 3-103). Lung parenchymal involvement may resemble a diffuse pneumonia or may consist of fibrous-appearing nodules ranging up to 8 cm in diameter (544).

The pathologic features of lymph node involvement by SHML are much better described. Sinuses are infiltrated by distinctive histiocytes that have abundant, pink to clear cytoplasm; emperipolesis or lymphophagocytosis is seen in well-preserved lymphocytes (fig. 3-103) (544, 568,569). In addition, the cytoplasm may contain a few plasma cells, neutrophils, or red blood cells. The nuclei are round to oval. Most often there is a single small nucleolus, but there may be multiple nucleoli or a single prominent nucleolus. Microabscesses may be present. The lymph node capsule may be fibrotically thickened and the fibrosis may extend into the perinodal soft tissues.

In addition, the histiocytes stain strongly for S-100 protein as well as histiocytic markers such as KP-1 (CD68), but they are negative for CD1a (523,540). The plasma cells are polyclonal (540).

Differential Diagnosis. SHML must be separated from Erdheim-Chester disease and Langerhans' cell histiocytosis (see above), diffuse panbronchiolitis (see chapter 8), Whipple's disease (see chapter 12), malakoplakia (see chapter 12), and inflammatory lesions such as inflammatory pseudotumor with fibroxanthomatous features (see chapter 17). The distinctive features

Table 3-29

PULMONARY LESIONS RELATED TO LYMPHANGIOLEIOMYOMATOSIS: ASSOCIATION WITH TUBEROUS SCLEROSIS

Lesion	Occurs in TSC Patients?	Reported in Non-TSC Patients?
Lymphangioleiomyomatosis	Yes (613,647,672)	Yes (613,647,672)
Micronodular pneumocyte hyperplasia	Yes (623,629,654)	Yes (654)
Regional proliferation of HMB45 clear cells	Not yet	Yes (635)
Clear cell micronodules	Yes (610)	Yes (see fig. 3-120)
Clear cell (sugar) tumor	Yes (610,623,636)	Yes (626)
Angiomyolipoma	Yes (678)	Yes (631,636)
Localized angiomyolipoma-like infiltrative lesion	Yes (see figs. 3-118, 3-119)	Not yet

TSC = Tuberous sclerosis.

of the histiocytes in SHML, the lymphophagocytosis, and the S-100 protein-positive staining are lacking in each of these conditions.

Treatment and Prognosis. Many approaches have been used to treat patients with SHML, although a uniformly effective therapy remains to be established. Localized airway lesions may be amenable to surgical resection (544). Radiation therapy has been attempted for localized lesions (557). Medical therapy including interferon-alpha or a combination of steroids, vinca alkaloids, or alkylating agents may be helpful (518,557,566).

Tracheostomy followed by surgery or local radiation has been successful in several patients with obstructing lesions of the upper trachea (544). One patient with diffuse lung parenchymal involvement treated with tracheostomy followed by prednisone and chlorambucil had a good response (544).

LYMPHANGIOLEIOMYOMATOSIS

Definition. Lymphangioleiomyomatosis (LAM) is a rare disorder that affects women primarily of reproductive age. It is characterized by an abnormal proliferation of smooth muscle cells (LAM cells) in the lungs as well as in the lymphatics and lymph nodes of the thorax and retroperitoneum.

Pulmonary LAM has very distinctive clinical, radiologic, and pathologic features. In recent years with the development of a LAM Foundation and a National Heart Lung and Blood Institute, National Institutes of Health (NIH)-sponsored LAM registry, there has been renewed interest in studying the clinical, radiologic, pathologic, genetic, and molecular features of this interesting disorder (593,606,609,641,647–650, 674). In addition, in recent years a growing number of pulmonary lesions have been recognized to occur in association with LAM or tuberous sclerosis, including micronodular pneumocyte hyperplasia, angiomyolipoma, clear cell tumor, and regional proliferation of HMB45-positive clear cells (Table 3-29).

Clinical Features. LAM is a rare lung disease that afflicts young women of childbearing age (617,639,667,672). A single case of LAM was reported in a male with tuberous sclerosis (592).

The incidence and prevalence of pulmonary LAM are unknown, but this disorder probably represents less than 1 percent of the cases of DPLD. Caucasians are afflicted much more commonly than other racial groups, especially Asians and individuals of African descent. The LAM Foundation estimates that there may be up to 1,000 women with the disease in the United States.

The pathogenesis of LAM is unknown (617, 622,671). Recent studies suggest a role for the loss of tumor suppression functions of certain cellular enzymes, or abnormalities in proteins involved in the synthesis of catecholamines (638,664). Increased expression of matrix metalloproteinase 2 (MMP-2) by the LAM cells suggests an important role in the cystic destruction of the lung parenchyma (634). LAM occurs in women with tuberous sclerosis (TSC) but most LAM patients do not have this disease (see below). TSC also affects the skin and central nervous system and demonstrates a clear Mendelian inheritance. It is possible that patients with LAM are mosaic, with *TSC2* mutations in the lung (and sometimes the kidney) but not elsewhere, or that environmental factors play a critical role in the development of clinically apparent LAM (616,617). It is likely that estrogen plays a central role in disease progression, since the disease does not manifest prior to menarche and only rarely after menopause. LAM is also known to accelerate during pregnancy and to abate after oophorectomy. Furthermore, estrogen and progesterone receptors have been demonstrated in a subpopulation of LAM cells (597, 649,657). The institution of hormonal therapy may downregulate these receptors (649).

Clinically, radiologically, and physiologically, LAM has more in common with pulmonary emphysema than with classic interstitial lung diseases, such as IPF or sarcoidosis. In fact, it is often misdiagnosed as asthma or chronic obstructive pulmonary disease (COPD) because of significant airflow limitation. Pulmonary LAM is seen almost exclusively in premenopausal women (639,667). More than 70 percent of patients are between the ages of 20 and 40 years at the onset of symptoms or at the time of diagnosis; only 6 percent of patients are more than 50 years of age at presentation, and are often taking estrogen replacement therapy (595,642,663).

Nearly all patients complain of dyspnea at the time of diagnosis; other common complaints include cough and chest pain. The physical examination can be normal or demonstrate end-expiratory rales, hyperinflation, decreased or absent breath sounds, ascites, and intra-abdominal or adnexal masses (639,667). Clubbing is uncommon.

A variety of intrathoracic and extrathoracic complications have been associated with pulmonary LAM: spontaneous pneumothorax (often recurrent, can be bilateral, and may necessitate pleurodesis); hemoptysis (may be life-threatening); chylothorax (due to obstruction of the thoracic duct or rupture of the lymphatics in the pleura or mediastinum by proliferating smooth muscle cells); chyloperitoneum (chylous ascites occurs in approximately 10 percent of patients); chyluria (due to abnormal connections between dilated retroperitoneal lymphatics and the renal collecting system); and chylopericardium (620). Renal angiomyolipomas occur in as many as 60 percent of patients and are a characteristic finding in those with tuberous sclerosis (598,609). They may grow to enormous size prior to clinical detection, but only uncommonly affect renal function.

Pulmonary function testing usually reveals an "obstructive" or "mixed" pattern (598, 605,609,617,642,667,670). The lungs are often hyperinflated, with an increased TLC and increased thoracic gas volume. Gas trapping, as evident by an increase in RV and RV/TLC ratio, is commonly present. Airflow limitation and reductions in diffusing capacity occur in the majority of patients. Studies of pulmonary mechanics show that mean elastic recoil is reduced and upstream resistance is increased (615,617), both of which contribute to the observed airflow limitation. Gas exchange is often abnormal, with a markedly reduced DLCO and an increase in the alveolar-arterial oxygen difference (615,617). Diminished exercise performance is found in most patients. The primary determinants of the exercise limitation are related to airflow limitation, mechanical factors (e.g., decreased breathing reserve, increased work of breathing), and pulmonary vascular dysfunction/destruction (615,617).

The diagnosis of LAM should be strongly suspected in any young woman who presents with emphysema, recurrent pneumothorax, or a chylous pleural effusion. HRCT often confirms the diagnosis, and tissue confirmation may not always be necessary.

Radiologic Findings. The radiographic manifestations include a diffuse, bilateral, reticular pattern; cystic airspaces; hyperinflation; pneumothorax; and pleural effusion (fig. 3-104). A reticular pattern is seen in approximately 80 percent of patients, pneumothorax in 30 to 40 percent, and unilateral or bilateral pleural effusion in 10 to 20 percent (642,644, 655,670). Hyperinflation with an associated increase in the retrosternal airspace and flattening of the diaphragm is a relatively late manifestation. In up to 20 percent of patients, the radiograph is normal (642,655,670).

The characteristic finding on HRCT consists of numerous thin-walled cysts, usually

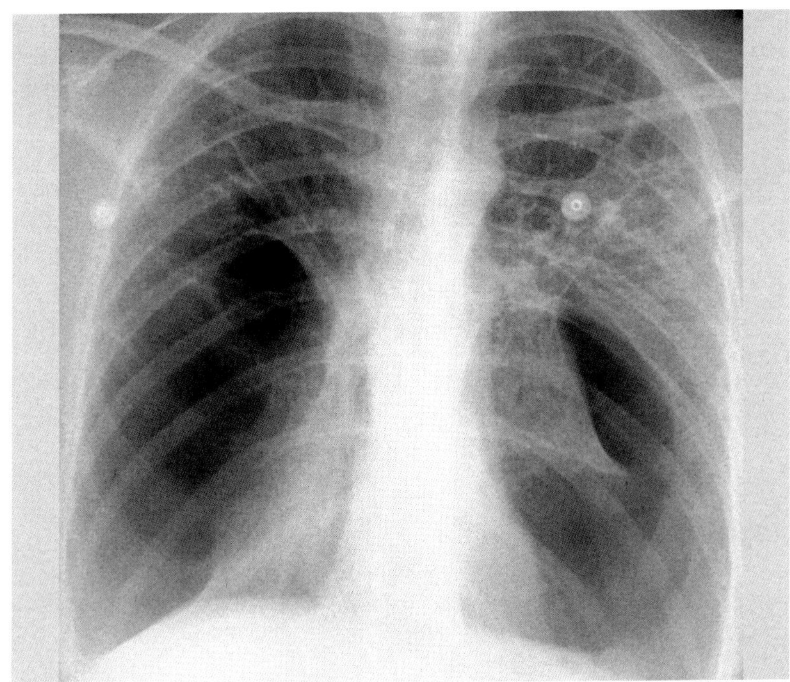

Figure 3-104

LYMPHANGIOLEIOMYOMATOSIS

The chest radiograph demonstrates a reticular pattern, large cystic spaces, and loculated bilateral pneumothoraces.

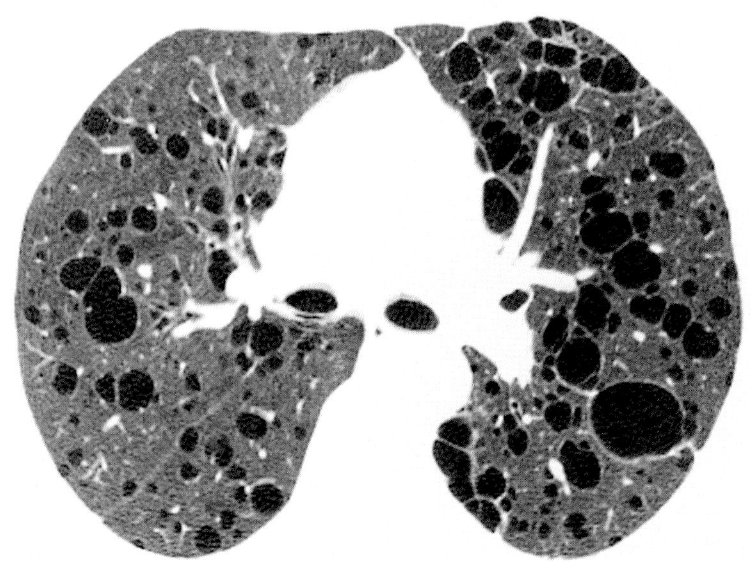

Figure 3-105

LYMPHANGIOLEIOMYOMATOSIS

HRCT demonstrates cystic airspaces randomly distributed in both lungs. The cysts have thin walls. The parenchyma between the cysts appears normal.

measuring 0.2 to 2.0 cm in diameter and distributed diffusely throughout the lungs (fig. 3-105) (641,645,655,670). This abnormality can be detected on HRCT even in patients with normal chest radiographs (655). The typical appearance on HRCT allows ready distinction from other interstitial diseases in the vast majority of cases (601).

Gross Findings. The gross pathology in the lungs is distinctive, with diffuse, bilateral cystic changes throughout (fig. 3-106). The lungs are enlarged, as in severe emphysema. Most cysts are 0.5 to 2.0 cm in size, but in some cases are over 10 cm (605,613).

Histologic Findings. The two key histologic features of pulmonary LAM are the cystic

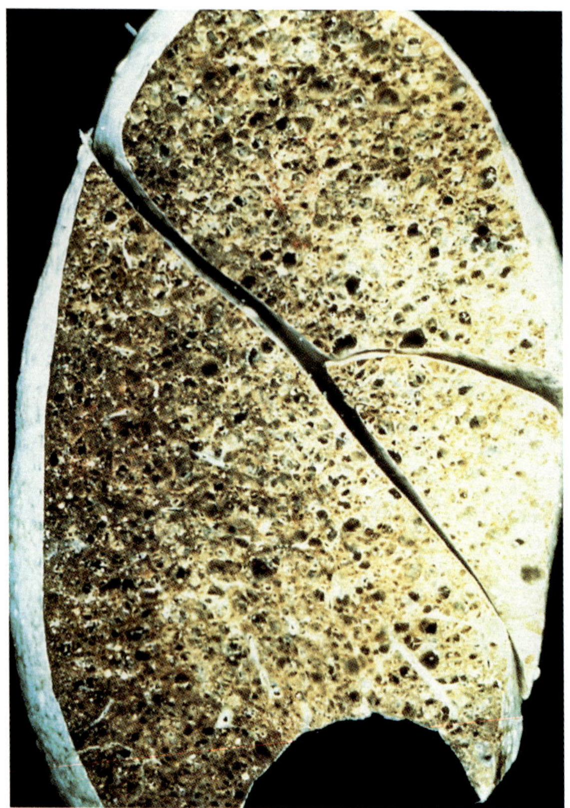

Figure 3-106

LYMPHANGIOLEIOMYOMATOSIS

The lung shows diffuse cystic changes throughout the parenchyma.

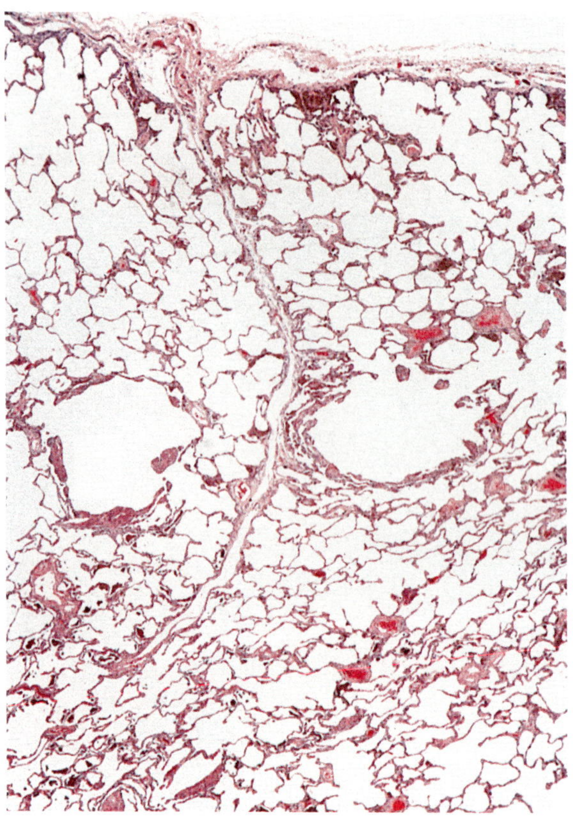

Figure 3-107

LYMPHANGIOLEIOMYOMATOSIS: LAM HISTOLOGY SCORE (LHS)-1

The lung shows several cystic spaces with few LAM cells around the periphery of the spaces. The cystic spaces are empty, without cellular or fluid contents. The intervening lung parenchyma appears normal. The LAM lesion (cysts and muscle) affects less than 25 percent of the lung parenchyma.

changes and LAM cell infiltrates (figs. 3-107–3-109) (605,613,647,672). In the early stages of the disease, the cysts and LAM cells may be inconspicuous. At this stage, the LAM cell infiltrates can be easily overlooked and the biopsy may be misinterpreted as showing either emphysema or normal lung. The LAM cells are typically found as small clusters or nests at the edges of the cysts and along pulmonary lymphatics (figs. 3-107–3-111). In advanced cases, the LAM cells can become so prominent that it is difficult to identify normal lung architecture. LAM cells infiltrate the walls of vessels and distal airways, leading to vascular destruction and microscopic foci of hemosiderosis (fig. 3-112). Bronchiolar obliteration is occasionally seen (613).

Matsui et al. (647) recently defined the LAM Histology Score (LHS) as a way to make a semiquantitative assessment of the severity of the lung involvement. The LHS is based on the involvement, in surgical lung biopsies, of the two major morphologic features of the disease: the cystic lesions and the infiltration by LAM cells. The total percentage of lung tissue involved by these two histologic components determines the extent of the LAM lesion. These amounts are estimated semiquantitatively, using low-power magnification. The LHS is graded as follows: LHS-1, less than 25 percent (fig. 3-107); LHS-2, 25 to 50 percent (fig. 3-108); and LHS-3, more than 50 percent involvement (fig. 3-109).

The proliferating LAM cells are round, oval, or spindle shaped (fig. 3-111). They grow in a haphazard arrangement, unlike the orderly,

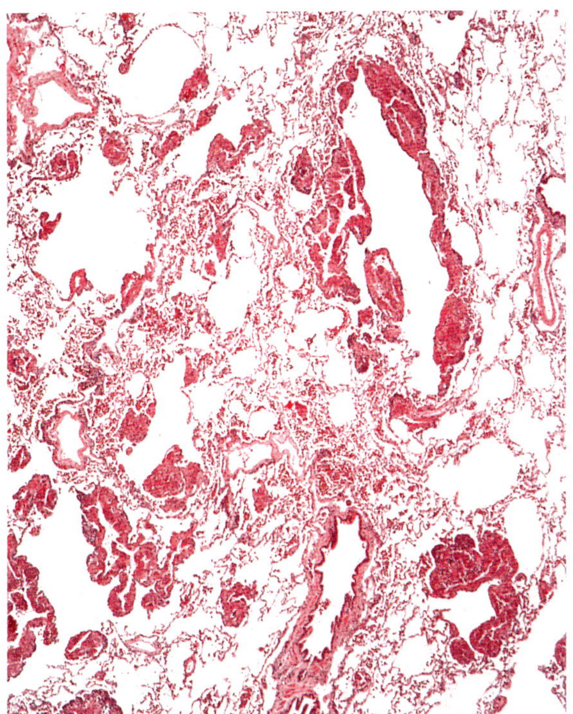

Figure 3-108

LYMPHANGIOLEIOMYOMATOSIS: LHS-2

The lung shows multiple cystic spaces with moderate amounts of LAM cells around the periphery of the spaces. Some of these cells protrude into the cyst lumen in a polypoid fashion. The LAM lesion (cysts and muscle) affects between 25 and 50 percent of the lung parenchyma.

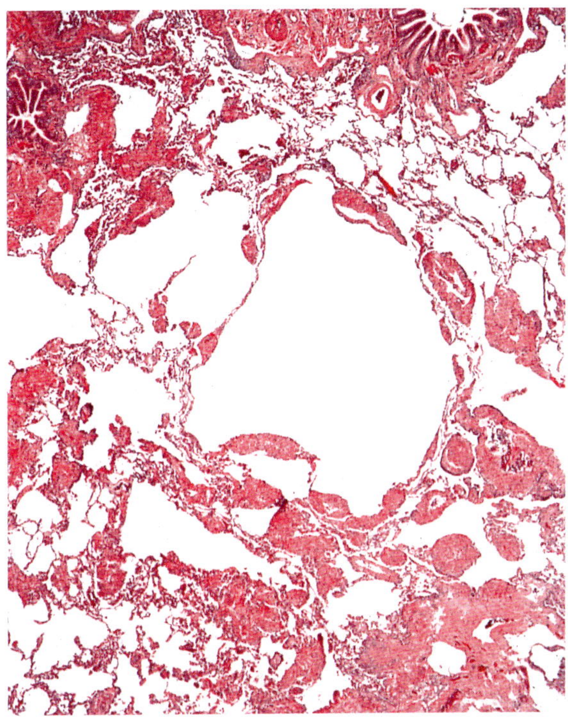

Figure 3-109

LYMPHANGIOLEIOMYOMATOSIS: LHS-3

The lung shows a few cystic spaces with substantial amounts of proliferating LAM cells around the periphery of the spaces and in the intervening interstitium. The cystic spaces are empty, without cellular or fluid contents. The LAM lesion (cysts and muscle) affects more than 50 percent of the lung parenchyma.

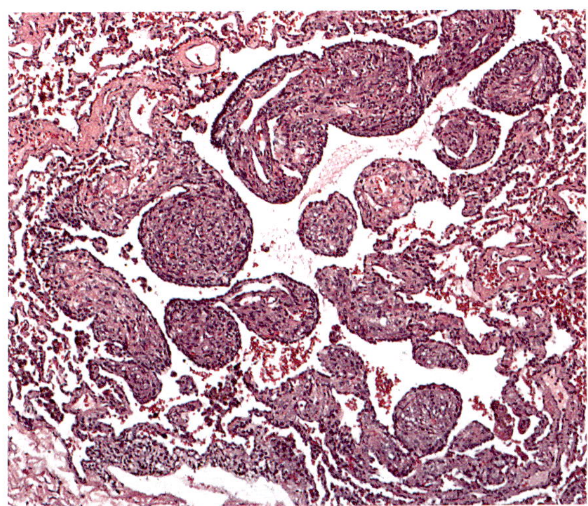

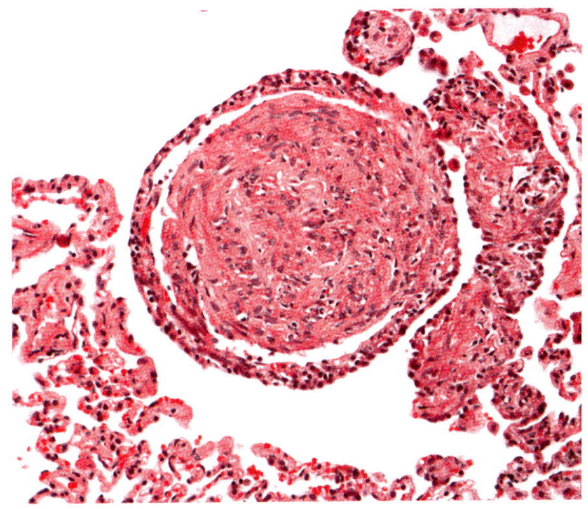

Figure 3-110

LYMPHANGIOLEIOMYOMATOSIS

Left: Several large bundles of LAM cells are more conspicuous than the cystic change in this field.
Right: This rounded bundle of LAM cells has a cleft-like lymphatic space at the periphery.

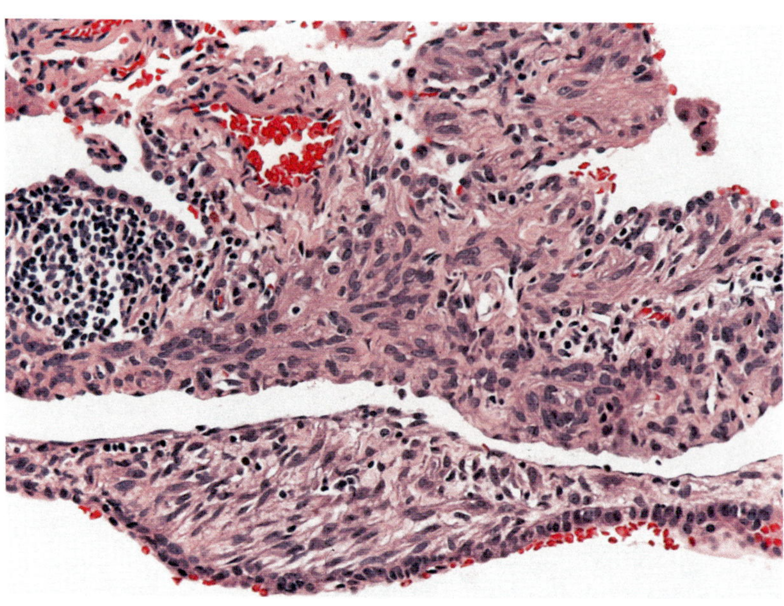

Figure 3-111

LYMPHANGIOLEIOMYOMATOSIS

This LAM cell infiltrate shows a mixture of spindle-shaped and rounded cells resembling smooth muscle.

concentric or parallel pattern of the smooth muscle cells that are normally present in the airways and blood vessels (596,605,613,630). The LAM cells have a moderate amount of eosinophilic cytoplasm and their nuclei have fine or vesicular chromatin. They are morphologically heterogeneous, with a spectrum ranging from small and round to spindle-shaped, oval, and large epithelioid cells (fig. 3-111) (603,605, 613). Rare mitotic figures and cytologically atypical cells may be seen. The diagnosis of LAM can be established based on bronchoscopic biopsy if LAM cells are obtained in the specimen (602,630). The histologic features of LAM in males are indistinguishable from those in females (fig. 3-113).

LAM cells also may infiltrate the thoracic duct and lymph nodes of the thorax or retroperitoneum (605,613,627). In such cases, the cellular proliferation tends to form masses of LAM cells (fig. 3-114). In these masses, the cells are often round to oval rather than spindle shaped, and often grow in papillary clusters (fig. 3-114) (599). In the setting of pneumothorax, reactive eosinophilic pleuritis may be seen in the pleura (see chapter 18) (591,651,653).

Immunohistochemical and Electron Microscopic Findings. LAM cells are immunohistochemically similar to normal smooth muscle cells in that they stain for alpha-smooth muscle actin, desmin, and vimentin. However, they also show reactivity for HMB45 antibody (fig. 3-115). This reactivity is absent in other smooth muscle lesions of the lung (602,608,630). The HMB45 staining is typically localized to cytoplasmic granules and not all cells stain. Estrogen and progesterone receptors are demonstrated in some cases by immunohistochemistry (597,612).

Electron microscopic studies have shown that the immunoreactivity for HMB45 in melanocytes is localized in stages 1 and 2 melanosomes (premelanosomes) and in the nonmelanized portion of stage 3 melanosomes (661). As described by Fukuda et al. (625), LAM cells share many ultrastructural features with normal smooth muscle cells (596,602). Electron microscopic reports have documented the occurrence of inclusions structurally similar to stages 1 and 2 melanosomes in LAM cells (602) and these inclusions were shown by ultrastructure to be immunoreactive with HMB45 conjugated with gold particles.

Lung Pathology in Tuberous Sclerosis. While patients with TSC are not exempt from other types of lung disease, LAM is regarded as the primary form of pulmonary involvement in women with TSC (607,633,644,646). Costello et al. (614) recently showed that 26 percent of women with TSC have LAM as detected by HRCT. Pulmonary abnormalities have previously been reported in men with TSC (618,632), but only recently has the first well-documented

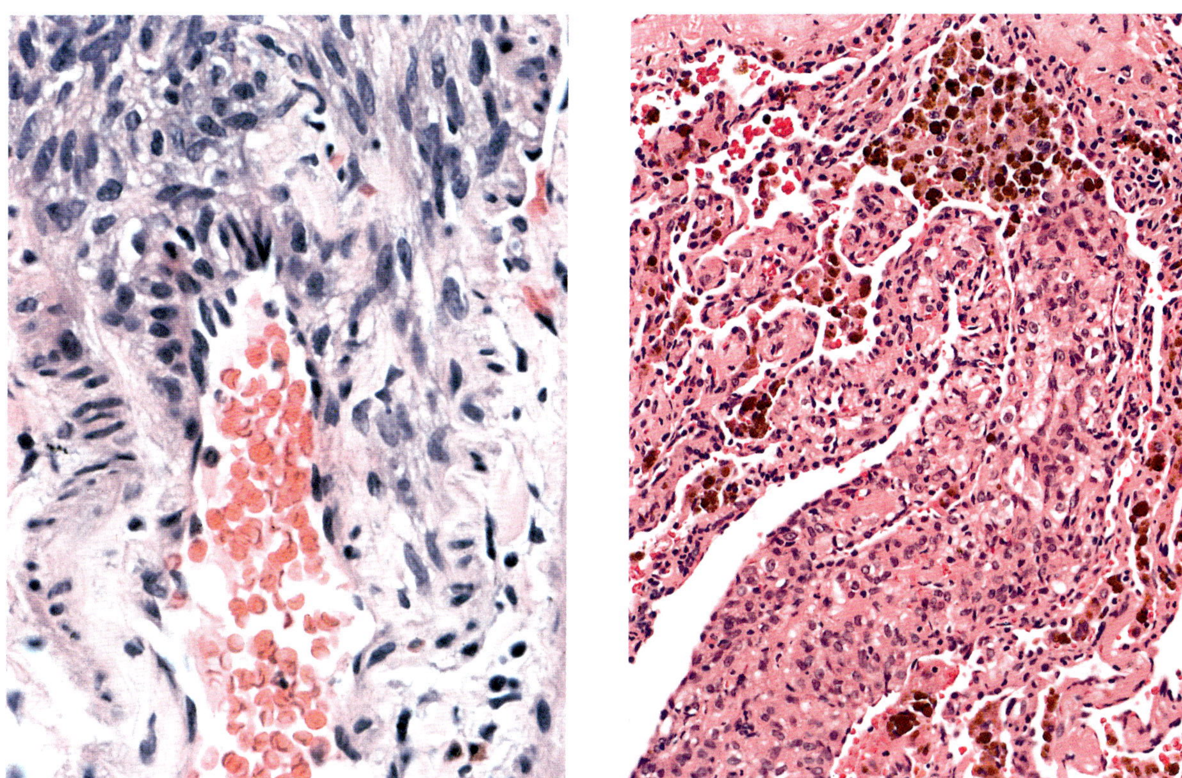

Figure 3-112

LYMPHANGIOLEIOMYOMATOSIS: VASCULAR INFILTRATION

Left: LAM cells are infiltrating the wall of this blood vessel.
Right: Hemosiderin-laden macrophages are present within alveolar spaces adjacent to a LAM lesion.

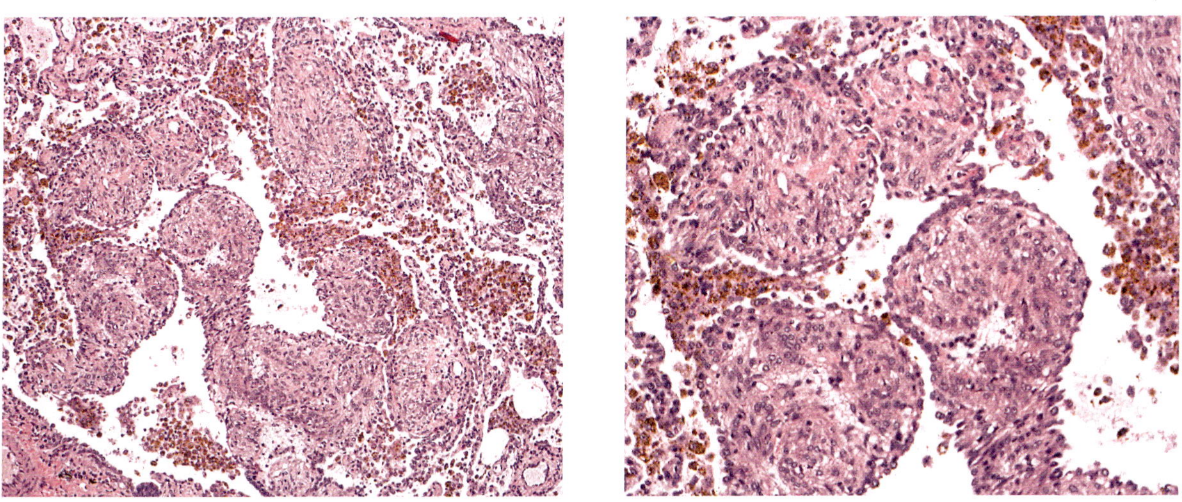

Figure 3-113

LYMPHANGIOLEIOMYOMATOSIS IN A MALE

Left: The lung shows cyst formation associated with polypoid nodules of LAM cells.
Right: The nodules of LAM cells protrude into the cyst lumen and consist of round to oval cells.

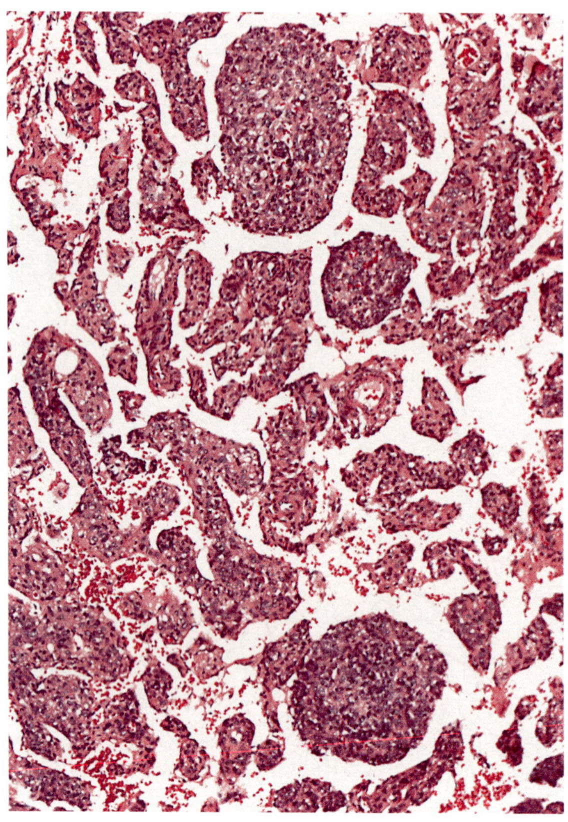

Figure 3-114

LYMPHANGIOLEIOMYOMATOSIS: LYMPH NODE INVOLVEMENT

The LAM cells diffusely infiltrate the lymph node in a mass-like fashion. The infiltrate shows a papillary morphology with cleft-like lymphatic spaces between the cords of LAM cells.

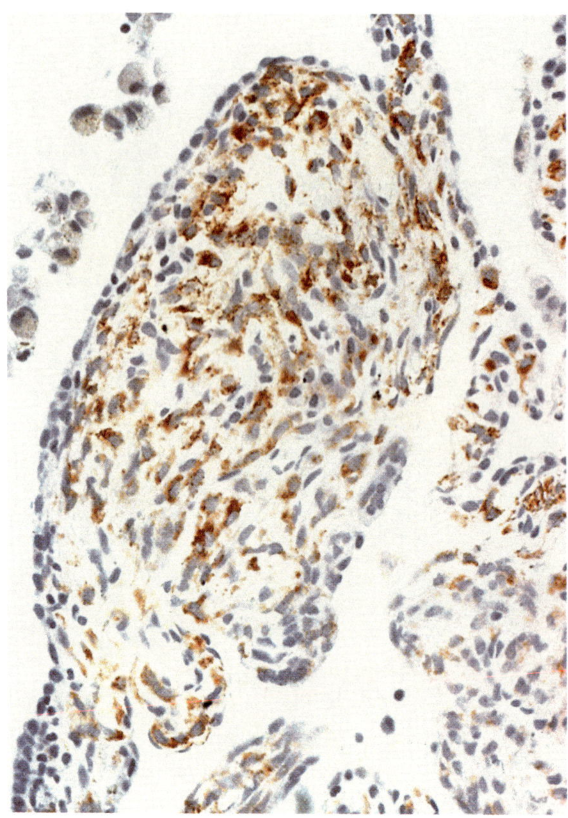

Figure 3-115

LYMPHANGIOLEIOMYOMATOSIS: HMB45 STAINING

The LAM cells are positive with HMB45.

case of LAM in a male TSC patient been reported (592). We have also recently seen two more cases (see fig. 3-113).

The only distinguishing feature seen in lung biopsies from TSC patients is the lesion of multifocal micronodular pneumocyte hyperplasia (MMNPH) (629,654). This lesion is so distinctive that it is virtually pathognomonic for TSC when identified in patients with LAM (629). The lesion can occur in males or females with TSC in the absence of LAM as well. At low-power magnification, the lesions appear as multiple, ill-defined, nodular areas of interstitial thickening measuring several millimeters in size (fig. 3-116, left). The alveolar walls are slightly thickened by fibrous connective tissue and lined by hyperplastic cuboidal type 2 pneumocytes (fig. 3-116, right) (629). Flieder et al. (623) recently described a patient with TSC who had pulmonary LAM, micronodular pneumocyte hyperplasia, and a clear cell tumor (so-called sugar tumor). Wu et al. (678) reported on a pulmonary angiomyolipoma associated with micronodular pneumocyte hyperplasia in a patient with TSC.

We recently encountered a peculiar pulmonary lesion localized to the right upper lobe in a 3-year-old female with TSC. In this case the lung showed diffuse multicentric infiltration by a process that shared some features with angiomyolipoma (AML) and LAM, but more closely resembled a diffuse infiltrative AML-like process (fig. 3-117). Abnormal smooth muscle cells resembling those seen in LAM and AML infiltrated blood vessel walls and the perivascular interstitium. These were accompanied by varying amounts of adipose and vascular tissue.

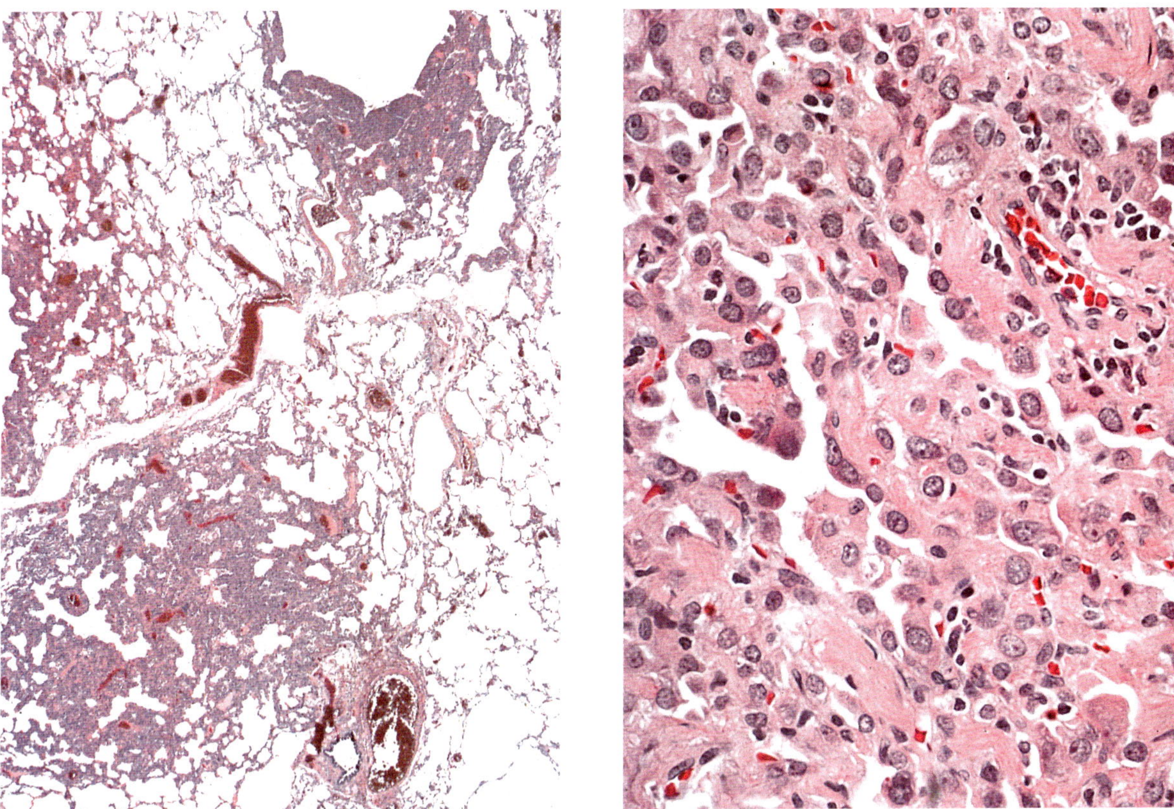

Figure 3-116

LYMPHANGIOLEIOMYOMATOSIS: MICRONODULAR PNEUMOCYTE HYPERPLASIA

Left: Adjacent to the LAM lesion (top) is a discrete but poorly circumscribed proliferation of type 2 pneumocytes forming the lesion of micronodular pneumocyte hyperplasia.

Right: This lesion consists of cuboidal, hobnail-shaped type 2 pneumocytes proliferating along the surface of the alveolar wall.

The abnormal smooth muscle cells were HMB45 positive. This lesion lacked the characteristic combination of cystic changes and abnormal smooth muscle cell infiltrates of LAM.

Recurrent intrapleural cysts have also been reported in patients with TSC (604).

Localized Regional Proliferation of HMB45 Cells with Cystic Changes. Hironaka and Fukayama (635) recently reported on a patient without TSC who had a localized pulmonary lesion consisting of a nodular proliferation of clear HMB45-positive cells associated with cystic parenchymal destruction (figs. 3-118, 3-119). We have recently seen a similar case that appears to represent part of the expanding spectrum of proliferations of HMB45-positive epithelioid cells in the lung. Hironaka and Fukayama proposed that this lesion reflects a proliferation of hybrid clear cell tumor and LAM cells. Chuah et al. (610) described a TSC patient with pulmonary LAM, micronodular pneumocyte hyperplasia, and clear cell micronodules scattered throughout the lung parenchyma. We have also observed micronodules of clear cells (Table 3-29) within the lung of a patient with pulmonary LAM without TSC (fig. 3-120). Such a lesion could be confused with localized emphysema with bullous changes, clear cell carcinoma (primary or metastatic), and granulomatous inflammation.

Differential Diagnosis. Pulmonary LAM must be distinguished from other disorders characterized by an abnormal proliferation of smooth muscle cells in the lung. These include the hyperplasia of interstitial smooth muscle cells that occurs in honeycomb fibrosis of various

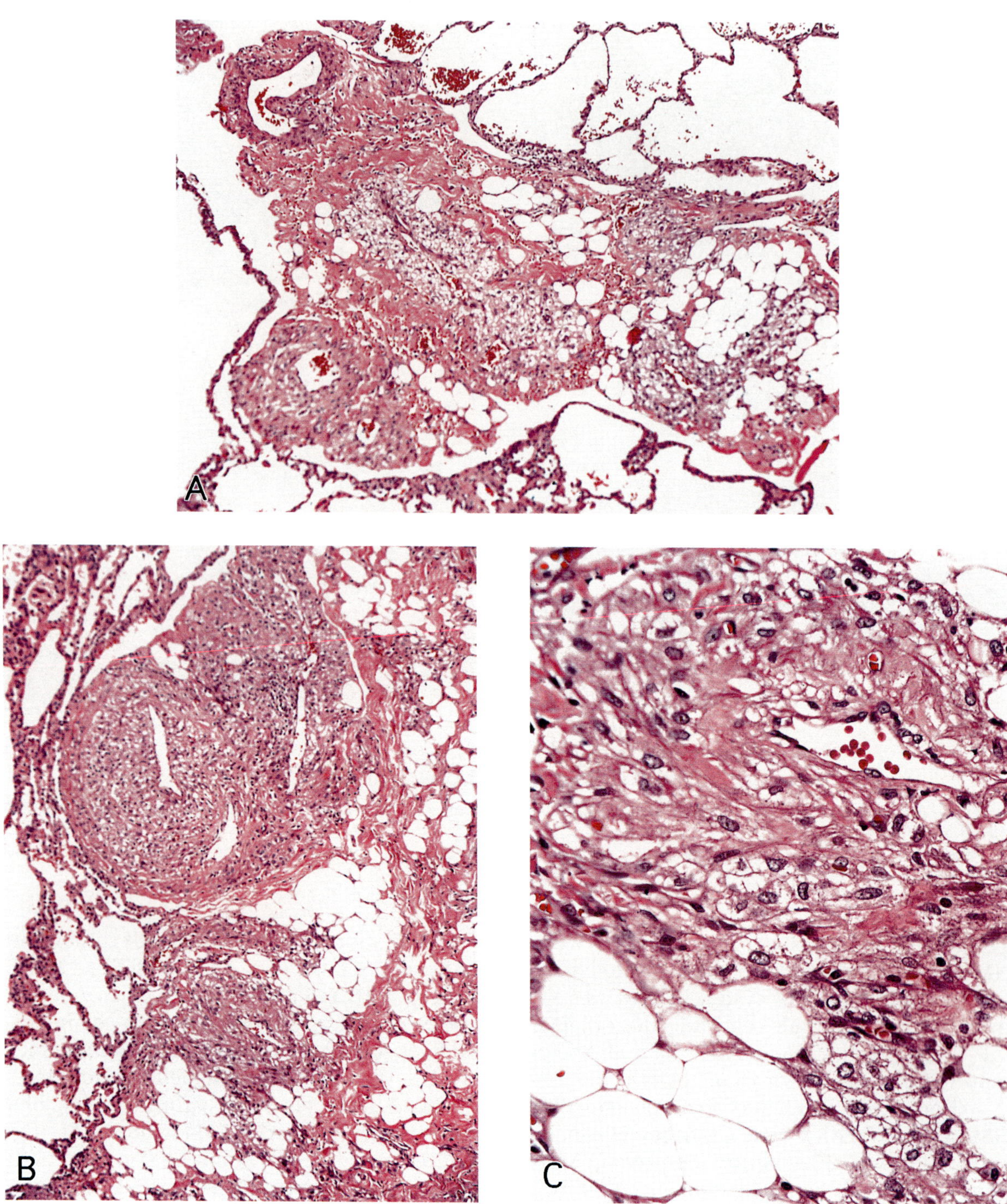

Figure 3-117

TUBEROUS SCLEROSIS

Localized right upper lobe angiomyolipoma-like infiltrative lesion.

A: The perivascular interstitium is infiltrated by an angiomyolipoma-like process consisting of fat, abnormal smooth muscle cells, and blood vessels.

B: The abnormal smooth muscle cells permeate the blood vessel walls and infiltrate the fat.

C: The smooth muscle cells are oval to spindled in shape, with small regular nuclei and moderate to abundant eosinophilic cytoplasm.

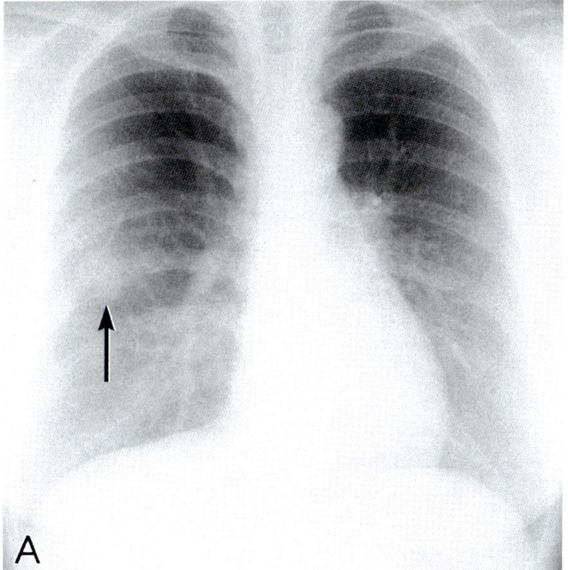

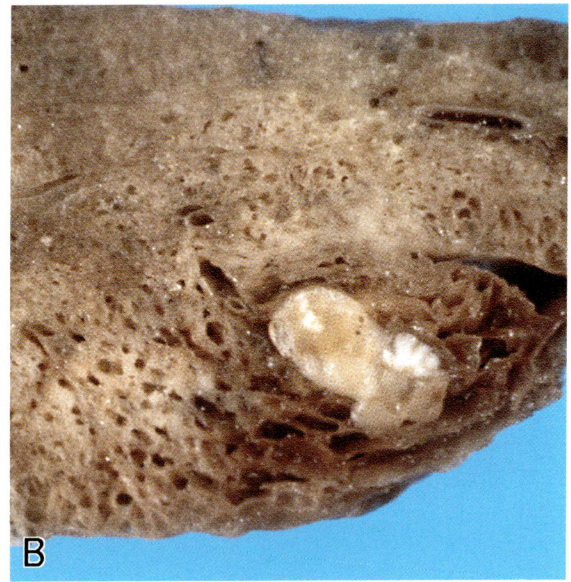

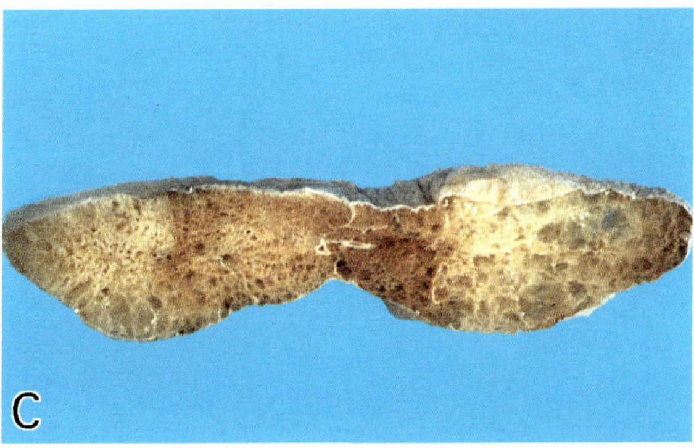
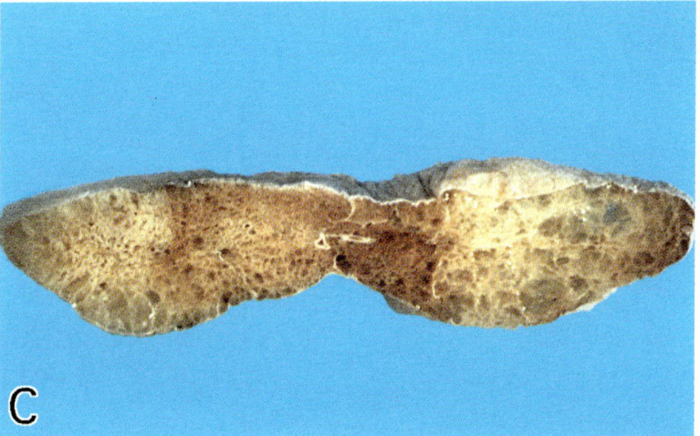

Figure 3-118

REGIONAL PROLIFERATION OF HMB45-POSITIVE CLEAR CELLS

A: Chest radiograph of a 27-year-old woman shows a nodular (arrow) lesion in the right mid-lung.

B: Cut surface of resected right upper lobe shows a circumscribed nodule within cystic lesions.

C: Cut surface of resected right middle lobe shows multiple cystic lesions with septa of variable thickness. (Figures 1A, 2A, and 3A from Hironaka M, Fukayama M. Regional proliferation of HMB-45-positive clear cells of the lung with lymphangioleiomyomatosislike distribution, replacing the lobes with multiple cysts and a nodule. Am J Surg Pathol 1999;23:1288–93.)

causes (particularly in IPF) (660), pulmonary hypertension (640), and emphysema, as well as smooth muscle cell neoplasms, such as benign metastasizing leiomyoma (BML) (658,665,669, 673), leiomyosarcoma (594,628,652,665,677), and various cystic sarcomas.

BML has been confused with LAM; however, there is little similarity between these conditions, except that both are multicentric and contain smooth muscle cells (658,665,669,673). BML usually occurs in women with a prior history of uterine leiomyoma and typically causes multiple, bilateral, discrete nodules, in contrast to the diffuse parenchymal cystic changes and ill-defined smooth muscle infiltrates of LAM (594,624,658,659,665,666,676). The history of uterine leiomyoma is often so remote that it may be impossible to retrieve the original histologic slides. Distinction of BML from metastatic low-grade leiomyosarcoma or endometrial stromal sarcoma is occasionally difficult if the histologic specimens show atypical features, such as mitotic figures or cytologic atypia. BML and metastatic leiomyosarcoma can have cystic changes (662) and patients can present with pneumothorax (652). Estrogen and progesterone receptors may be positive in BML, and therefore, such markers cannot be relied upon for a distinction from LAM (637). Rarely, the differential diagnosis between LAM, BML, or metastatic leiomyosarcoma may be difficult in a small bronchoscopic biopsy containing a few strands of smooth muscle. Immunohistochemical staining for HMB45, correlation with the clinical history, and the HRCT findings are helpful in making this distinction.

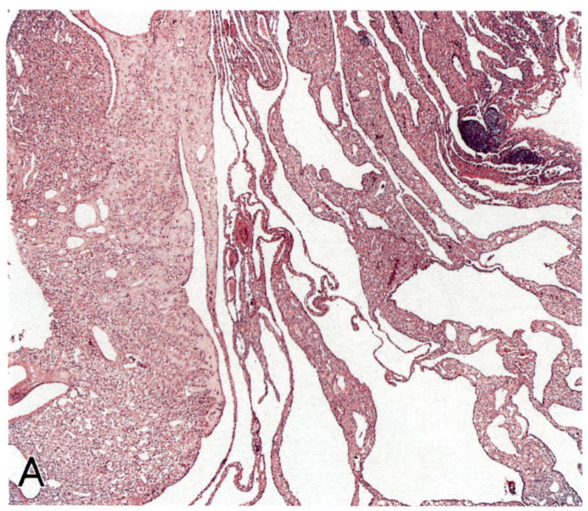

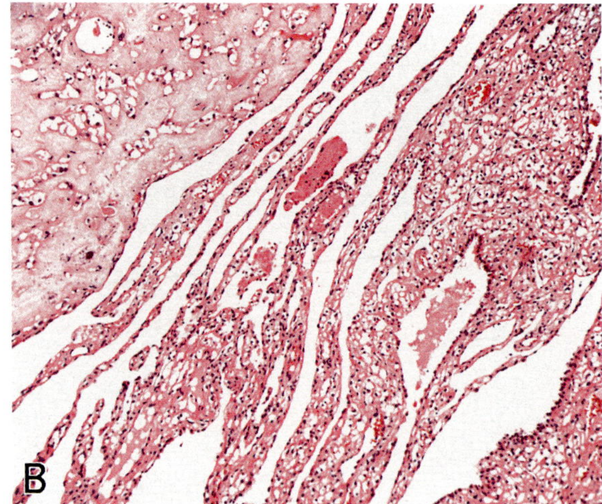

Figure 3-119

REGIONAL PROLIFERATION OF HMB45-POSITIVE CLEAR CELLS

A: The large nodule (left) of clear cells resembles a clear cell tumor, however, the clear cells infiltrate into the interstitium of the adjacent lung in a diffuse manner associated with cystic destruction of the parenchyma.

B: The clear cells infiltrate the interstitium of the alveolar walls in a diffuse pattern.

C: Less involved lung parenchyma shows cystic changes, with focal nodular infiltrates of clear cells more closely resembling lymphangioleiomyomatosis.

D: The clear cells have abundant clear cytoplasm and small regular nucleoli.

E: These clear cells stain for HMB45. (Courtesy of Mitsugu Hironaka and Masashi Fukayama, Jicha Medical School, Tochigi, Japan.)

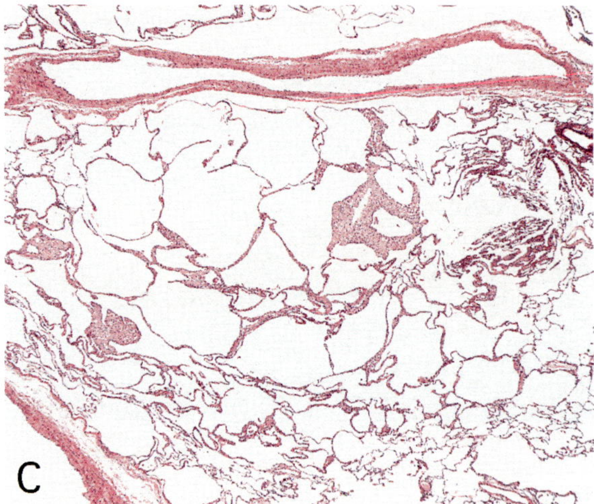

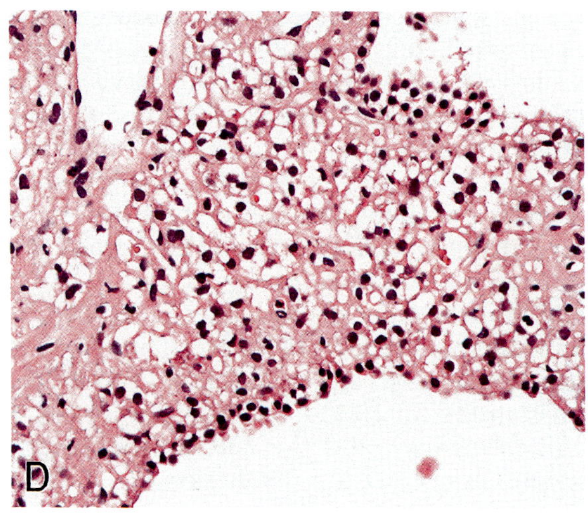

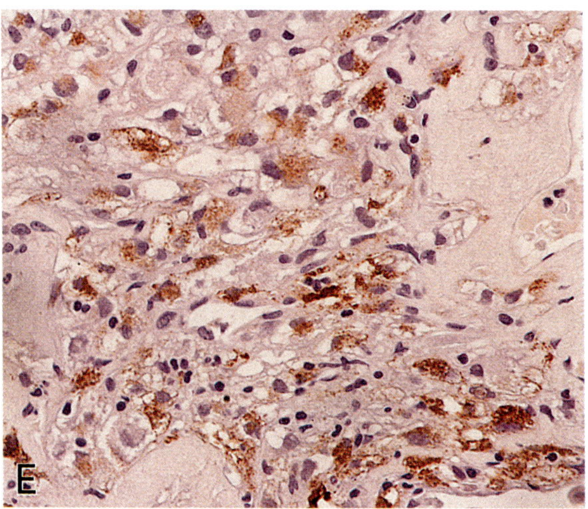

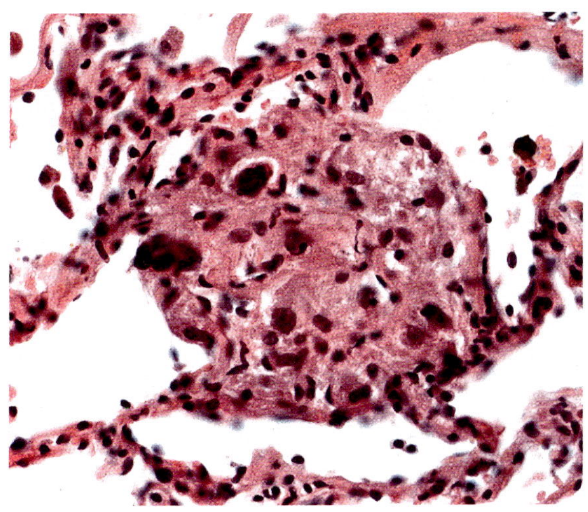

Figure 3-120

CLEAR CELL MICRONODULE IN PATIENT WITH LAM

These micronodular clusters of clear cells were scattered in the pulmonary interstitium adjacent to lesions of LAM. The cells have clear to eosinophilic cytoplasm. The nuclei range from small to large, with hyperchromatic chromatin.

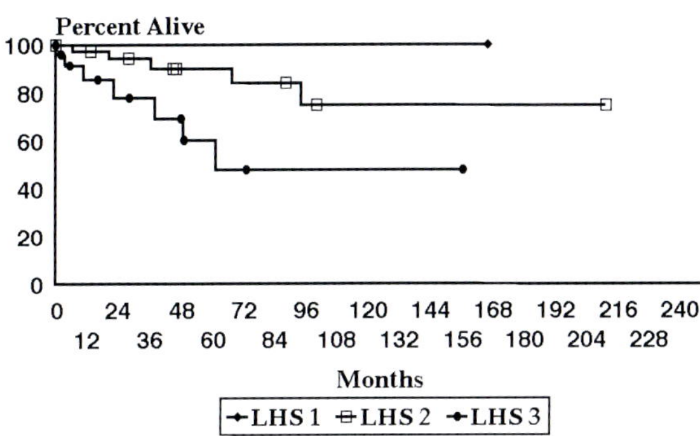

Figure 3-121

LYMPHANGIOLEIOMYOMATOSIS: SURVIVAL BY LHS SCORE

Kaplan-Meier survival curves of 105 patients with pulmonary LAM according to the LHS score. Patients with LHS-1 have an excellent survival with no deaths or need for transplantation. Patients with LHS-3 have the worst survival and those with LHS-2 have an intermediate survival (p=0.002). (Figure 3 from Matsui K, Beasley MB, Nelso WK, et al. Prognostic significance of pulmonary lymphangioleiomyomatosis histologic score. Am J Surg Pathol 2001;25:482.)

Muscular hyperplasia and cystic changes may occur in advanced interstitial fibrosis, but they are found in the presence of extensive and dense collagen deposits and remodeling of the lung architecture. Interstitial fibrosis is absent or inconspicuous in LAM. In emphysema, there is cystic destruction of the lung; however, LAM cell infiltrates are absent. Subtle infiltrates of LAM cells are sometimes overlooked histologically, and for this reason the diagnosis of LAM should be kept in mind when interpreting lung biopsy specimens from women of reproductive age (particularly if they have a history of pneumothorax).

LAM should not be confused with other entities bearing similar names, such as lymphangiomatosis, lymphangioma, and lymphangiectasis (see chapter 11) (621). Lymphangiomatosis is characterized by proliferation of endothelial-lined spaces along lymphatic routes, including those in the pleura, interlobular septa, and bronchovascular bundles (671). It often occurs in infants or young children of either sex. True lymphangiomas of the lung are extremely rare and are manifested by solitary coin lesions rather than by diffuse cystic lung disease (611). Lymphangiectasis simply represents dilatation of lymphatics and is seen most often in children, especially after mechanical ventilation (621).

Treatment and Prognosis. The prognosis for women with pulmonary LAM is variable. Progression is common, with a median survival period of 8 to 10 years from diagnosis (615,617, 642,647,670). Rarely, sudden rapid deterioration complicates the course of the disease, especially during pregnancy or with the use of supplemental estrogen (615,617,642,670). Uncommonly, long-term survival of 20 years from diagnosis has been reported. In several more recent large case series (642,670), there was an apparent improvement in survival compared to earlier series (613). An elevated TLC and a reduced FEV1/FVC ratio are associated with poor survival of 2 to 5 years after initial examination (642). Kitaichi (642) showed that patients with a predominantly cystic type of LAM had a worse prognosis than those with a predominantly muscular type. Matusi et al. (647) recently showed that the 5- and 10-year survival rates for 101 LAM patients were 100 percent and 100 percent for those with LHS-1, 89.9 percent and 74.6 percent for those with LHS-2, and 59.1 percent and 47.3 percent for those with LHS-3, respectively (fig. 3-121). They also found that increasing degrees of hemosiderin deposition were associated with higher LHS scores (p=0.029) and a worse prognosis (p=0.0012).

Hormonal manipulation has been the primary treatment for patients with pulmonary LAM. Such treatment is based on the recognition that female hormones play a possible etiologic role in the pathogenesis of the disease. Oophorectomy, progesterone (10 mg/day), and, more recently, tamoxifen (20 mg/day) and luteinizing hormone-releasing hormone (LHRH) analogs, have been employed (615,617). However, only oophorectomy and treatment with progestational agents appear to provide reliable improvement or stabilization of the disease in a subset of patients (619). It should be noted that response to hormonal manipulation is not universal: only 15 percent of patients in one study responded (674). Chylothorax can be difficult to treat and is typically associated with nutritional wasting and some degree of immune compromise (675). Oophorectomy and treatment with progestins are advocated by some (617). Chemical oophorectomy with LHRH analogs may replace surgical oophorectomy as the primary treatment of this disorder, although data are currently lacking. Alpha-interferon has also been tried for treatment of pulmonary LAM (643). There is no role for either corticosteroids or cytotoxic agents.

Lung transplantation offers the only hope for cure in patients with pulmonary LAM. One retrospective international survey evaluated 34 patients who underwent lung transplantation: 27 received single lung transplants; 6, bilateral lung transplants; and 1, a heart-lung transplant (600). Patient survival was 69 percent at 1 year and 58 percent at 2 years. The main causes of death were acute lung injury (early) and infection and bronchiolitis obliterans (late). Despite the overall benefit, there was a relatively high frequency of disease-related complications, including recurrent LAM in the allograft (656). The multicenter LAM registry is sponsored by the National Heart, Lung, and Blood Institute and seeks to enroll patients with LAM, follow their clinical course, and collect and store biologic specimens for further study (668). Additional registries are being developed in France and the United Kingdom (638).

EOSINOPHILIC PNEUMONIA

The eosinophilic pneumonias are a group of diseases of known and unknown etiology characterized histologically by the accumulation of numerous eosinophils in alveolar spaces and/or the interstitium, and commonly, peripheral blood eosinophilia. They are also known as *pulmonary infiltrates with eosinophilia (PIE) syndrome.*

Eosinophilic pneumonias can be classified by a histologic, clinical, or combined etiologic and clinical approach. Pathologists primarily use the histologic approach by examining lung biopsies for the major and minor histologic features of eosinophilic pneumonia (Table 3-30). Clinicians often base their assessment on the spectrum of clinical syndromes classified according to the severity, duration, and outcome of the illness: chronic eosinophilic pneumonia, acute eosinophilic pneumonia, and simple eosinophilic pneumonia (Table 3-31). Eosinophilic lung diseases can be classified according to a combined etiologic and clinical approach which includes a variety of idiopathic conditions in which no etiology can be determined as well as conditions in which specific causes or associated conditions are identified (Table 3-32). Known causes of eosinophilic pneumonia include infections (see chapter 12), drug-induced pneumonitis (see chapter 7), and systemic diseases (see chapter 6).

Eosinophilic lung diseases can be diagnosed by documenting chest radiographic abnormalities and identifying eosinophilia in peripheral blood, lung biopsy, or BAL fluid (fig. 3-122) (679,680,686,698,702,704,706). The pulmonary opacities on chest radiograph associated with blood eosinophilia are sometimes called the PIE syndrome. In such cases, lung biopsies are often not obtained and a presumptive diagnosis of eosinophilic pneumonia is made.

Several general points are useful to note about the eosinophils and the eosinophilic syndromes (679,696,704). First, blood eosinophilia is defined as a white blood count (WBC) above 11,000/μL, with an absolute eosinophil count exceeding 450/μL. Blood eosinophil numbers do not necessarily indicate the extent of eosinophilic involvement in affected tissues because the eosinophils are primarily tissue dwelling and are several hundred-fold more abundant in tissues than blood (679,704). Eosinophils are most numerous in tissues with a mucosal epithelial interface with the environment, such as the respiratory, gastrointestinal, and lower genitourinary tracts (679,704).

Table 3-30

HISTOLOGIC APPROACH TO EOSINOPHILIC PNEUMONIA

Histologic Lesions of Eosinophilic Pneumonia
- Major Lesions
  - Intra-alveolar accumulation of eosinophils
  - Interstitial accumulation of eosinophils
- Minor Lesions
  - Organizing pneumonia
  - Alveolar macrophage accumulation (may be the only finding after steroid administration)
  - Alveolar fibrin accumulation
  - Zones of necrotic eosinophils
  - Granulomatous inflammation
  - Mild vascular inflammation (secondary vasculitis)

Histologic Lesions of Associated Conditions
- Vasculitis (Churg-Strauss syndrome, drug toxicity)
- Necrotizing ("allergic") granulomas associated with necrotic eosinophils
- Asthmatic bronchitis/bronchiolitis (asthma, chronic eosinophilic pneumonia, allergic bronchopulmonary fungal disease)
- Fungi within mucus plugs of bronchi/bronchioles (allergic bronchopulmonary fungal disease)
- Infectious agents (fungi or parasites)

Table 3-31

ETIOLOGIC AND CLINICAL CLASSIFICATION OF EOSINOPHILIC PNEUMONIA

Idiopathic (unknown cause)
- Chronic eosinophilic pneumonia
- Acute eosinophilic pneumonia
- Simple eosinophilic pneumonia (Löffler's syndrome)
- Incidental eosinophilic pneumonia

Secondary Eosinophilic Pneumonia
- Infection
  - Parasitic
    - Tropical eosinophilic pneumonia
      - *Ascaris lumbricoides, Toxocara canis, filaria*
    - *Dirofilaria*
  - Fungal
    - *Aspergillus*
- Drug induced
  - Antibiotics
  - Cytotoxic drugs
  - Anti-inflammatory agents
  - L-tryptophan
- Immunologic or systemic diseases
  - Allergic bronchopulmonary fungal disease
  - Asthma
  - Collagen vascular disease
  - Churg-Strauss syndrome
  - HIV infection
  - Malignancy
  - Hypereosinophilic syndrome

Second, the roles of eosinophils in these disorders remain unclear and appear to differ among the various disorders. In parasitic infections they play a crucial role in eradicating the infectious pathogen; in allergic bronchopulmonary fungal disease they accumulate in the lung as a result of immune hypersensitivity and are prominent mediators of tissue injury (679,696,704).

Third, eosinophilia in the BAL fluid (more than 5 percent of the differential count), although not diagnostic, can be an extremely valuable method for suggesting the possibility of an eosinophilic syndrome (fig. 3-122) (679,696,697, 704). Eosinophils are not found in the lungs of normal individuals, so their presence in tissue or BAL identifies a pathologic process. Pulmonary eosinophilia may be seen in the absence of peripheral blood eosinophilia. The most common conditions associated with BAL eosinophilia are interstitial lung diseases (e.g., idiopathic pulmonary fibrosis, sarcoidosis, systemic lupus erythematosus, and hypersensitivity pneumonitis [40 percent]), acquired immunodeficiency syndrome (AIDS)-related pneumonia (17 percent), idiopathic eosinophilic pneumonia (15 percent), and drug-induced lung disease (12 percent) (680). Extremely high numbers of eosinophils may be seen in BAL fluid in parasitic infections, drug reactions, allergic bronchopulmonary aspergillosis, acute and chronic eosinophilic pneumonias, hypereosinophilic syndrome, and Churg-Strauss syndrome.

Fourth, the reaction pattern found histopathologically mirrors the cause of the syndrome. For example, in allergic bronchopulmonary fungal disease (ABPFD), the etiologic agent enters the lung via the airways. Consequently, the major pathologic changes are bronchocentric (689,731). ABPFD is frequently associated with eosinophilic pneumonia (see chapters 9 and 12). Conversely, the drug reactions or helminth infections reach the lung via the bloodstream and consequently, the lesions are usually diffuse and angiocentric (centered around blood vessels).

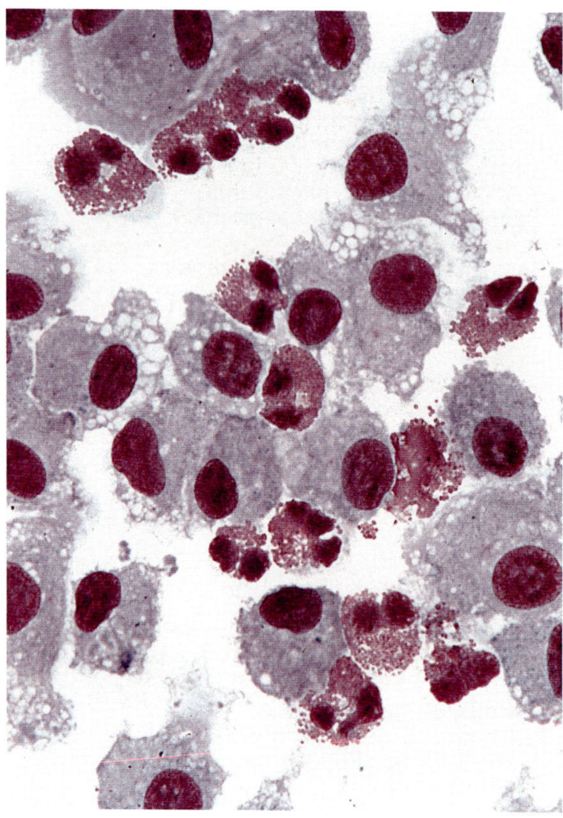

Figure 3-122

TROPICAL EOSINOPHILIC PNEUMONIA

Bronchoalveolar lavage from this patient with tropical eosinophilic pneumonia shows numerous eosinophils within alveolar spaces.

Fifth, the relationship between the blood eosinophilia and total IgE level varies considerably among the many syndromes. The IgE level is almost invariably increased in ABPFD and helminth infections (679,704).

Sixth, asthma is not present in all causes of eosinophilic pneumonia. It is usually absent in drug-induced disease, helminth infections, eosinophilia-myalgia syndrome, acute eosinophilic pneumonia, and the hypereosinophilic syndrome (679,704).

Seventh, the presence of eosinophilia suggests a type I hypersensitivity reaction. However, other features commonly present in this syndrome suggest a type III (e.g., vasculitis) or possibly type IV reaction.

Eighth, the presence of peripheral blood eosinophilia and pulmonary opacities on the chest radiograph are not invariably due to eosinophilic pneumonia. Primary and secondary carcinoma of the lung and malignant lymphomas may have this combination of findings (679,704).

Finally, the eosinophils are exquisitely sensitive to corticosteroids. Consequently, they may dramatically disappear from the bloodstream within a few hours after administration of corticosteroids. The rapid disappearance from the blood may obscure the diagnosis in patients who receive this drug before the diagnostic work-up is instituted.

IDIOPATHIC EOSINOPHILIC PNEUMONIAS

Simple Eosinophilic Pneumonia

Simple eosinophilic pneumonia (*Löffler's syndrome*) is characterized by absent or mild respiratory symptoms; fleeting, migratory pulmonary opacities; and peripheral blood eosinophilia (Table 3-32) (679,686). Immune sensitivity to *Ascaris lumbricoides* has been recognized as the cause of many of the earlier reported cases. Several other parasitic infections and exposures to many drugs and other agents are recognized to cause a similar syndrome (see below). An identifiable etiologic agent is not found in up to one third of patients (696,704). This disorder usually resolves within 1 month.

Histologically, the lung shows eosinophilic pneumonia characterized by numerous eosinophils within alveolar spaces and/or the interstitium. However, lung biopsies are rarely obtained and the diagnosis is usually established clinically, with documentation of the eosinophilia in the peripheral blood and identification of the pulmonary consolidations by chest radiographs.

Chronic Eosinophilic Pneumonia

Chronic eosinophilic pneumonia is the type of eosinophilic pneumonia that most often requires a lung biopsy to confirm the diagnosis (figs. 3-123, 3-124).

Clinical Features. Patients present with fever, night sweats, weight loss, cough productive with eosinophils, and dyspnea (Table 3-32) (690,711). Asthma is present in many of the patients, and circulating eosinophilia may be conspicuous. The etiology of chronic eosinophilic pneumonia is unknown, but an allergic

Table 3-32

COMPARATIVE FEATURES OF THE IDIOPATHIC PULMONARY EOSINOPHILIC SYNDROMES

Feature	Simple Eosinophilic Pneumonia	Chronic Eosinophilic Pneumonia	Acute Eosinophilic Pneumonia
Onset	Acute	Insidious (average duration of symptoms 7.7 months) More common in women	Acute (< 5 days duration) Hypoxemic respiratory failure
Symptoms and signs	Asymptomatic Nonproductive cough, low-grade fever, dyspnea	Cough, low-grade fever, dyspnea, weight loss (10–50 lbs.), drenching night sweats	Fever, dyspnea, cough, myalgias, pleuritic chest pain
Asthma	Absent	30 to 60% (often less than 5-year duration)	Absent
Peripheral blood eosinophilia	Extreme, transient	High (up to 90% of total WBC count)	Normal or high
Elevated serum IgE	+ / -	Moderately elevated about 30% of patients	Moderately elevated in some patients
Chest radiographs	Transient, migratory opacities often peripheral or pleural based	Bilateral airspace consolidation confined to lung periphery	Diffuse alveolar or mixed alveolar-reticular opacities Bilateral pleural effusions
Pulmonary function	Mild to moderate restrictive defects Reduced diffusing capacity Hypoxemia	Mild to moderate restrictive defects Reduced diffusing capacity Hypoxemia	Mild to moderate restrictive defects Reduced diffusing capacity Hypoxemia, may be severe
BAL eosinophilia	Prominent (usually > 20%)	Prominent (usually > 20%)	Prominent (usually > 25 to 50%)
Lung biopsy	Rarely performed Tissue eosinophilia	Tissue eosinophilia Fibrin may be present but not diffuse alveolar damage pattern	Tissue eosinophilia Diffuse alveolar damage
Treatment	Transient, self-limited 1 to 2 weeks)	Prompt and complete response to corticosteroids	Prompt and complete response to corticosteroids within 1 to 2 weeks
	Mebendazole, if *Ascaris* found	Relapse after discontinuation of corticosteroids	Does not relapse after discontinuation of corticosteroids

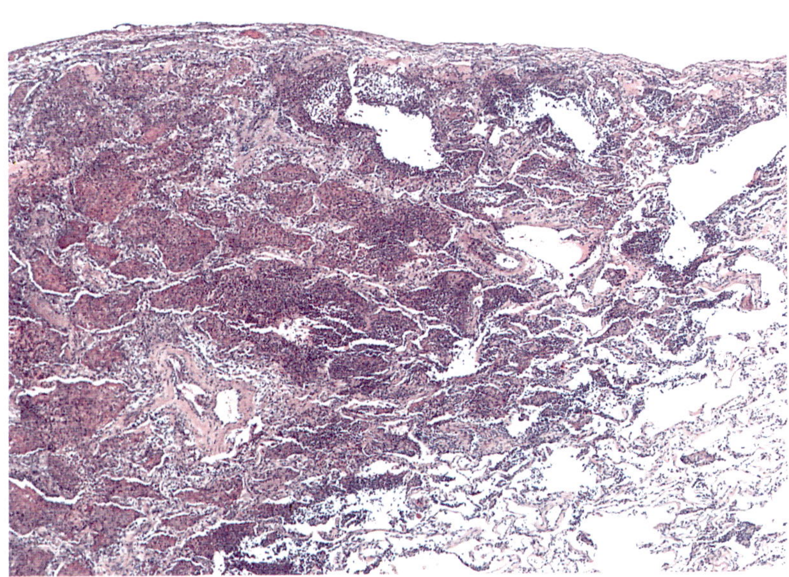

Figure 3-123

CHRONIC EOSINOPHILIC PNEUMONIA

The subpleural parenchyma shows marked intra-alveolar filling by eosinophils. The infiltrate is patchy, with areas of relatively normal lung (bottom right).

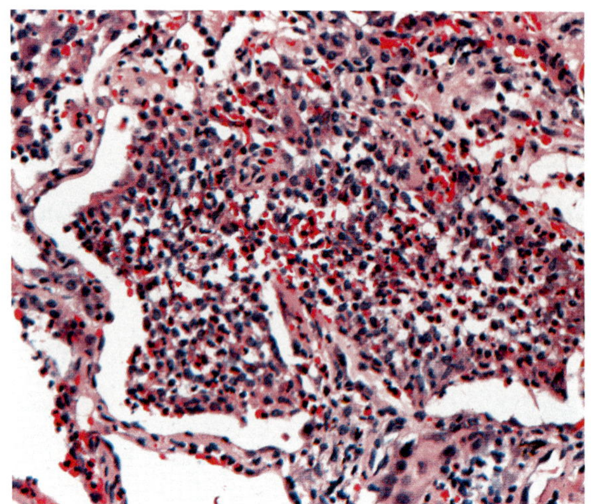
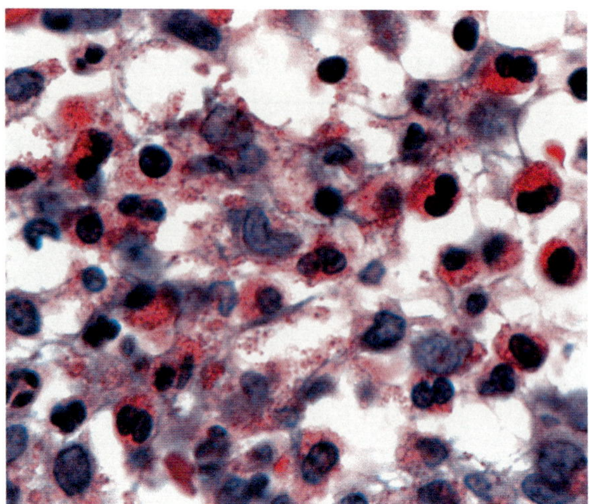

Figure 3-124

CHRONIC EOSINOPHILIC PNEUMONIA

Left: Numerous eosinophils fill the alveolar spaces. There is mild thickening of the alveolar septal interstitium. Right: The alveolar cellular infiltrate is composed of a mixture of eosinophils and macrophages.

diathesis is noted in some patients. Peripheral blood eosinophilia, very high sedimentation rate, iron deficiency anemia, and thrombocytosis are frequent laboratory abnormalities. BAL eosinophilia (more than 40 percent) suggests the diagnosis (679,696,697,704). The eosinophils in BAL fluid show signs of activation with the release of eosinophil proteins (710). Serial BAL specimens may be helpful in following the course of the disease (697). The response to corticosteroids is dramatic and helps confirm the diagnosis (690,711).

Radiologic Findings. The characteristic radiographic pattern consists of bilateral airspace consolidation confined to the lung periphery, a finding often referred to as the reversed pulmonary edema pattern (fig. 3-125) (690,711). This peripheral distribution is evident on the chest radiograph in approximately 60 percent of patients but can be identified on CT in virtually all cases (699,717). The airspace consolidation usually involves mainly the middle and upper lung zones.

Histologic Findings. Histologic examination shows intra-alveolar eosinophils, macrophages, and an amorphous proteinaceous exudate (Table 3-30; figs. 3-123, 3-124) (690,711). Alveolar fibrin may accompany the eosinophils (fig. 3-126). Charcot-Leyden crystals may be present. Eosinophils infiltrate the interstitium in about two thirds of cases, and organizing pneumonia is present in 25 percent (fig. 3-127). Hyperplasia of type 2 pneumocytes may be prominent. In 15 percent of cases, eosinophilic abscesses with foci of necrosis are seen (fig. 3-128) (690,711). The necrotic zones may be surrounded by palisaded macrophages. If the patient has received steroids prior to the biopsy, the eosinophils may be inconspicuous or absent, requiring correlation with the clinical history and laboratory findings of peripheral blood eosinophilia to support the diagnosis. In such cases the alveolar spaces may be filled with macrophages (fig. 3-129). Sarcoid-like granulomas may be seen in approximately 10 percent of cases. There may be a mild chronic or eosinophilic vasculitis (fig. 3-130) (690,711).

Acute Eosinophilic Pneumonia

Clinical Features. The patients present with an acute respiratory illness of usually less than 7 days' duration (Table 3-32) (681,684,726, 730). Manifestations include fever, hypoxemia, and a diffuse interstitial and alveolar infiltrate on the chest radiograph. The peripheral blood usually shows a leukocytosis, but eosinophilia is typically absent. The BAL fluid consistently demonstrates increased eosinophils. Since the

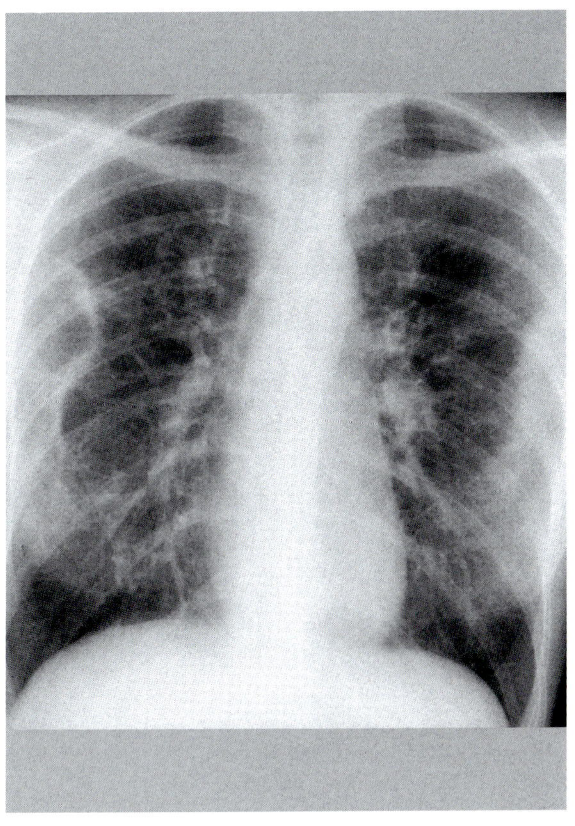

Figure 3-125

CHRONIC EOSINOPHILIC PNEUMONIA

The chest radiograph demonstrates bilateral areas of consolidation involving mainly the subpleural lung regions ("reverse pulmonary edema" pattern).

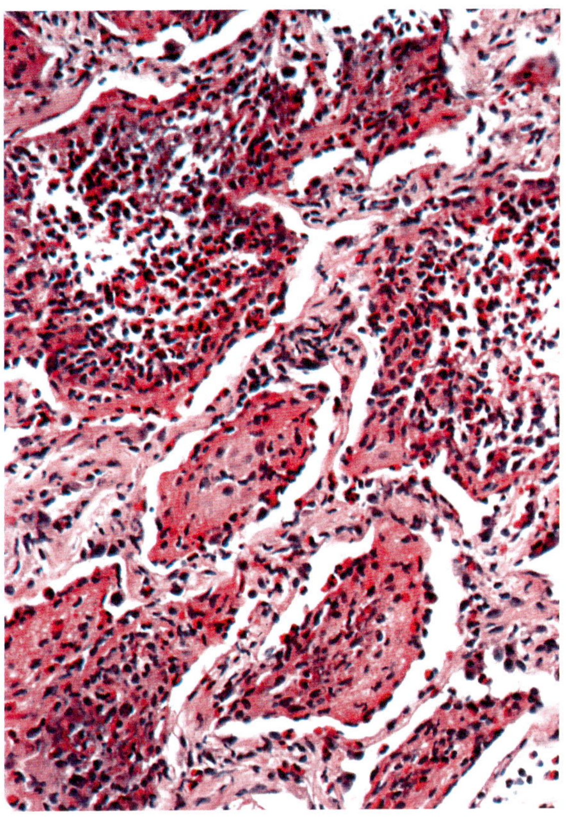

Figure 3-126

CHRONIC EOSINOPHILIC PNEUMONIA

The alveolar spaces are filled with a fibrinous exudate as well as numerous eosinophils.

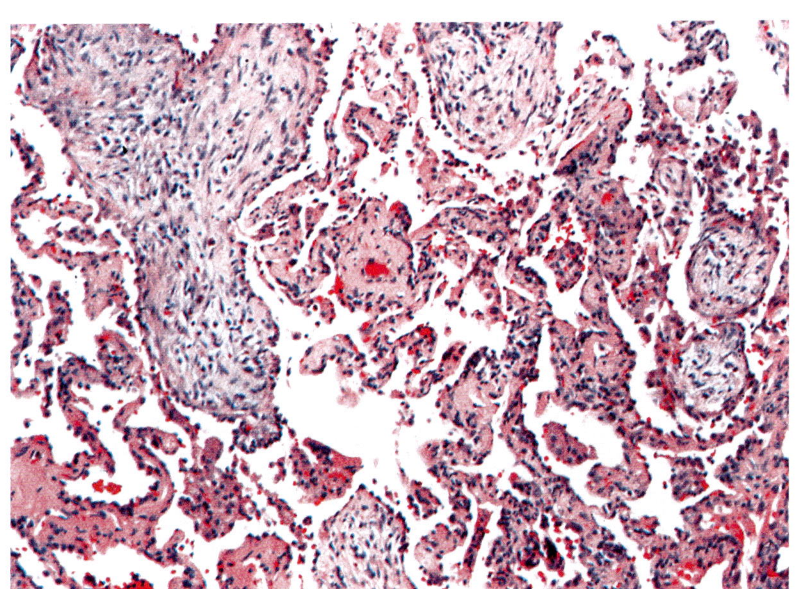

Figure 3-127

CHRONIC EOSINOPHILIC PNEUMONIA

Foci of organizing pneumonia are present.

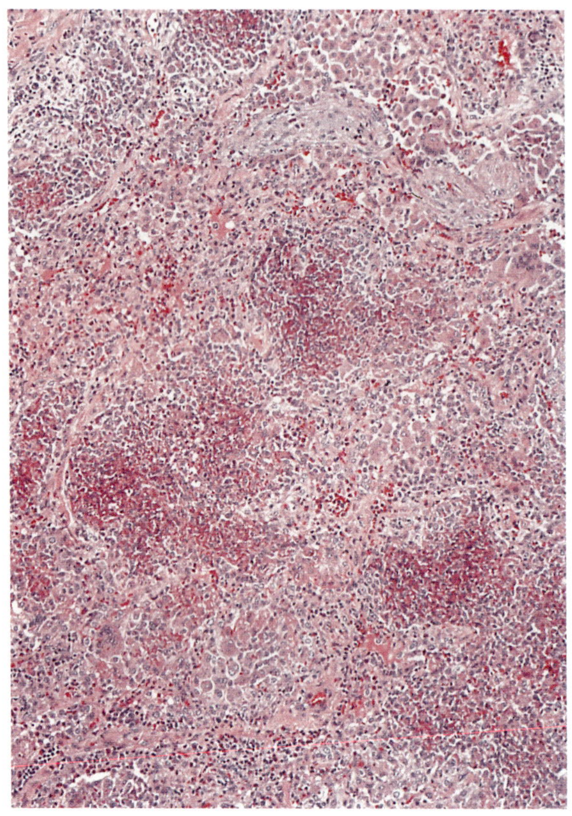

Figure 3-128

CHRONIC EOSINOPHILIC PNEUMONIA

Necrotic abscesses of eosinophils are surrounded by giant cells.

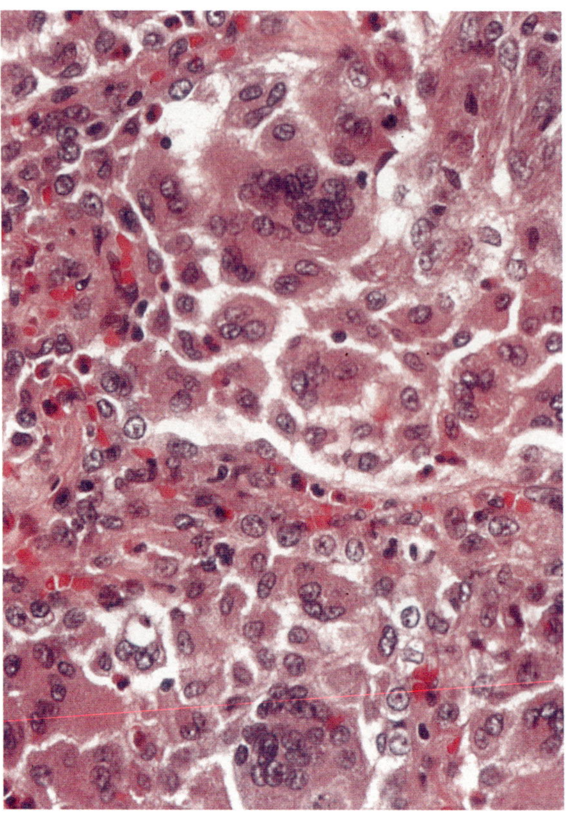

Figure 3-129

CHRONIC EOSINOPHILIC PNEUMONIA

The alveolar spaces are filled with mostly macrophages, some of which are multinucleated. There are few eosinophils in this case since the patient had received steroids prior to the biopsy.

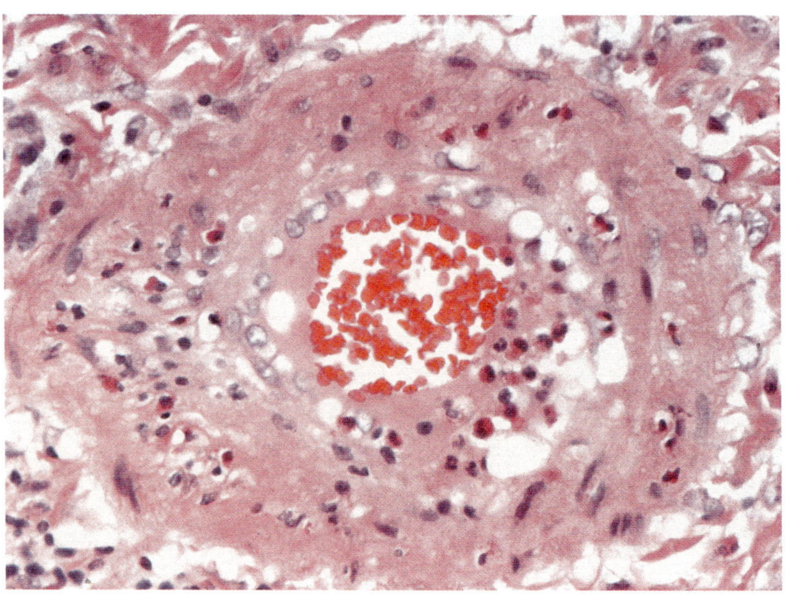

Figure 3-130

CHRONIC EOSINOPHILIC PNEUMONIA

Focal mild secondary vasculitis is present.

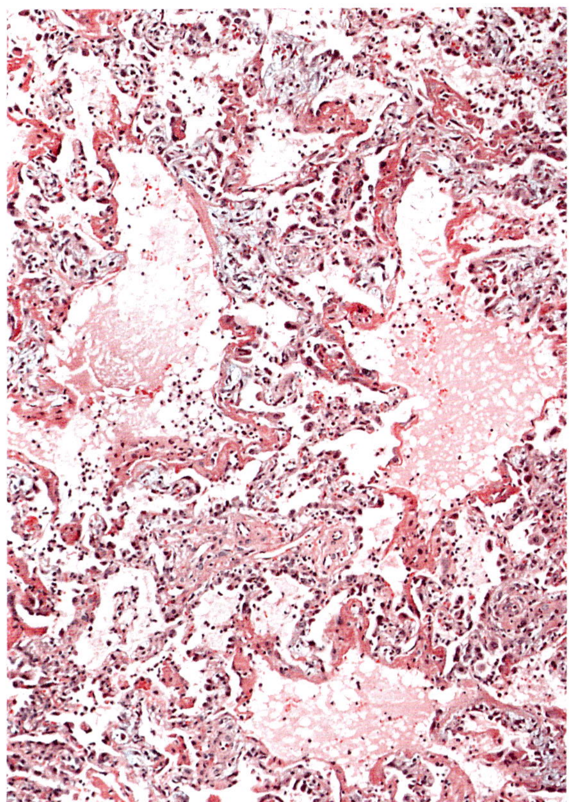

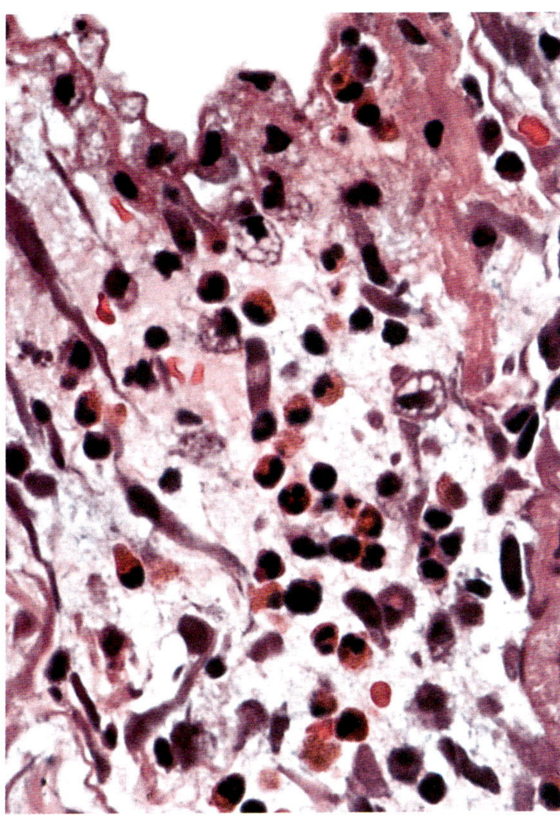

Figure 3-131

ACUTE EOSINOPHILIC PNEUMONIA

Left: The lung shows diffuse alveolar damage with hyaline membranes, mild interstitial thickening, and alveolar edema. Right: Numerous eosinophils are present in the thickened interstitium. Fibrin deposits (top) are also present.

diagnosis is usually established clinically, lung biopsies are seldom obtained. Patients respond dramatically to corticosteroids and in contrast to chronic eosinophilic pneumonia, this condition does not recur. The etiology of idiopathic acute eosinophilic pneumonia is not known, but it is thought to be a type of hypersensitivity reaction (709). A link to cigarette smoke has been proposed (720).

Radiologic Findings. The radiographic findings resemble those of interstitial and airspace pulmonary edema (679,693,714). The earliest radiographic abnormality consists of a reticular pattern, frequently with thickening of interlobular septa (Kerley B lines). This progresses over a few hours or days to bilateral interstitial and airspace opacities involving mainly the lower lung zones (679,693,714). Similar findings are seen on HRCT. Pleural effusion is present at some point during the clinical course in most patients (693,714).

Histologic Findings. Histologically, the lung shows eosinophilic pneumonia accompanied by features of DAD (fig. 3-131) (730). The eosinophilic pneumonia may be obscured by the hyaline membranes and/or organizing fibrosis of DAD.

SECONDARY EOSINOPHILIC PNEUMONIAS

Eosinophilic pneumonia may be associated with a variety of known clinical disorders including parasitic or fungal infection, drug toxicity, and systemic diseases such as Churg-Strauss syndrome (694). These secondary forms can manifest as simple (682,683,685,715), acute (703,713,716), chronic (705,708), or incidental eosinophilic pneumonia.

Infectious Eosinophilic Pneumonia

Parasitic infections can be associated with both *simple eosinophilic pneumonia* and *tropical eosinophilic pneumonia*. Patients with tropical eosinophilic pneumonia have a more severe and prolonged illness (679,704). In the tropics, the most common organism to cause simple eosinophilic pneumonia, or Löffler's syndrome, is *Ascaris lumbricoides*. The larvae pass through the lung tissue and cause disease. Simple eosinophilic pneumonia can also occur with *Ancylostoma duodenale, Clonorchis sinensis, Entamoeba histolytica, Necator americanus,* and *Strongyloides stercoralis*. Tropical eosinophilic pneumonia is most commonly a response to infestation with the filarial nematodes *Wuchereria bancrofti* and *Brugia malayi,* although other parasites such as *A. duodenale, S. stercoralis,* and *Toxocara canis* also produce this syndrome (679,704).

In tropical eosinophilic pneumonia, migration of parasites through the lung is accompanied by an acute, self-limited respiratory illness characterized clinically by marked blood eosinophilia, fever, cough, and transient pulmonary infiltrates (see fig. 3-122) (700,721,723,732). Adenopathy is common. Microfilariae are not found in the blood, but patients have high titers of antifilarial antibodies. IgE levels are also markedly elevated. Lung biopsies show eosinophilic pneumonia. Microfilariae are rarely seen in lung tissue, but are readily found in enlarged lymph nodes. A favorable response to treatment with diethylcarbamazine is seen in most patients.

Drug-Induced Eosinophilic Pneumonia

Many different drugs may cause eosinophilic pneumonia including antibiotics, cytotoxic drugs, anti-inflammatory agents, antihypertensive agents, and L-tryptophan (680,719, 733). A careful drug history should be obtained in any patient with eosinophilic pneumonia.

Immunologic or Systemic Diseases

Eosinophilic pneumonia can occur in the setting of allergic bronchopulmonary fungal disease (ABPFD) (692), asthma (718), collagen vascular disease (724,725), Churg-Strauss syndrome, immunodeficiency (HIV infection [680, 716] and ataxia telangiectasia [736]), malignancy (680,685,688,708,729,735), and idiopathic hypereosinophilic syndrome (695,727). ABPFD, Churg-Strauss syndrome, and collagen vascular disease are described in chapters 6, 9, and 11, respectively.

Idiopathic hypereosinophilic syndrome is a disorder in which mature eosinophils infiltrate multiple organs. Diagnostic criteria include peripheral eosinophilia, disease of longer than 6 months' duration, multiorgan dysfunction, and exclusion of known causes of eosinophilia (695, 701,734). The heart and nervous system are frequently affected. Pulmonary involvement occurs in 30 to 40 percent of patients, usually in the form of cough, pleural effusions, or pulmonary infiltrates (695,728,734). Less often, patients present with features of chronic eosinophilic pneumonia or DAD (734). Histologically, the lung can show interstitial and alveolar infiltration by eosinophils, pulmonary edema, infarcts, and pulmonary arterial infiltration by eosinophils (707). There is very little documentation of the lung pathology of hypereosinophilic syndrome.

Differential Diagnosis of Eosinophilic Pneumonia

The differential diagnosis of eosinophilic pneumonia can be approached from a histologic and an etiologic view. Histologically, eosinophilic pneumonia must be distinguished from other patterns of interstitial lung disease including organizing pneumonia (722), acute fibrinous and organizing pneumonia (687), DIP, pulmonary Langerhans' cell histiocytosis (PLCH), and hypersensitivity pneumonitis. In addition, lung biopsies should be evaluated for histologic clues to other conditions such as Churg-Strauss syndrome, ABPFD, collagen vascular disease, and infection (see Table 3-30). In virtually all cases of eosinophilic pneumonia there is extensive alveolar infiltration by eosinophils. However, there are rare cases where the eosinophils seem restricted to the interstitium (691).

The peribronchiolar stellate scarring and infiltrates of Langerhans' cells characteristic of PLCH are lacking in eosinophilic pneumonia. In DIP, the alveoli are filled with macrophages and only a few eosinophils are seen. The intermixture of eosinophils with macrophages and eosinophilic abscesses is absent in PLCH and DIP. However, if the patient with eosinophilic pneumonia received steroids prior to lung biopsy there may be a marked reduction in eosinophil number, leaving behind alveolar macrophages and resulting in a DIP-like picture (see fig. 3-129). ABPFD may show a focal eosinophilic pneumonia pattern, but the dominant histologic feature is usually necrotizing and/or granulomatous bronchiolitis associated with mucus plugs, which sometimes contain identifiable fungal organisms.

Treatment and Prognosis

Most cases of simple eosinophilic pneumonia are fleeting and may resolve without therapy. Chronic eosinophilic pneumonia responds dramatically to steroids; however, two thirds of patients develop recurrence after tapering of steroids and 20 percent of patients may relapse during tapering of steroids (679, 696,712). If there is an associated underlying clinical disorder, such as infection or drug toxicity, the primary approach to therapy may require antimicrobial agents or discontinuation of the medication. Although acute eosinophilic pneumonia has a fulminant clinical presentation requiring aggressive medical management, most patients recover (679,696).

PULMONARY ALVEOLAR PROTEINOSIS

Definition. Pulmonary alveolar proteinosis (PAP) is a rare condition that is characterized by intra-alveolar accumulation of granular eosinophilic material rich in lipids. Synonyms are *pulmonary alveolar phospholipoproteinosis* and *alveolar lipoproteinosis.*

PAP can occur in a variety of clinical settings including infection, malignancy, immune deficiency, environmental dust exposure, and lysinuric protein intolerance (Table 3-33) (768, 770,783,785).

Clinical Features. The incidence and prevalence of PAP are not known. PAP is a disease of adults; the typical age of presentation is 30 to 50 years (754,770,800). A few cases have been reported in infants and children (737,763, 767,790,799,804); these cases may be due to surfactant deficiency (745,748,749). There is a male to female ratio of 2 to 1. The disease may be more common in whites (754). Many of the patients are current or former cigarette smokers (754). The etiology of PAP remains unknown; however, patients have a high frequency of occupational exposure to dust environments.

Table 3-33

PULMONARY ALVEOLAR PROTEINOSIS: ASSOCIATED CONDITIONS

Infection
Bacteria
Nocardia (784)
Fungi
Viruses (786)
Mycobacteria (802)
Pneumocystis carinii (796)
Neoplasms
Leukemia (746,756)
Lymphoma (742)
Inorganic Dust Exposure
Silicosis (740)
Aluminum (778)
Immunodeficiency
HIV infection (788)
Lung transplantation (803)
IgA deficiency (801)
Other Conditions
Surfactant deficiency (781)
Fanconi's anemia (751,793)
Lysinuric protein intolerance (776)
Idiopathic (785)

PAP has two forms: an idiopathic form and a "secondary" form associated with another condition (800). Historically, there has been some attempt to divide PAP into primary and secondary types based on the presence of surfactant apoprotein and intensity of PAS staining (792). However, this is not a reliable way to distinguish idiopathic cases from those with known associations (747).

It is thought that overproduction of surfactant by type 2 pneumocytes or its impaired clearance by alveolar macrophages contributes to this condition (753,780,782). Most data suggest that the macrophage defect in PAP is secondary (738,758). The alveolar macrophage and type 2 cell clearance mechanisms are overwhelmed by the accumulation of the surfactant-rich material. This leads to impaired phagocytosis and phagolysosome fusion (755). The macrophages themselves may further contribute to the amorphous material upon dying (785). Other causes of impaired macrophage function, such as follows immunosuppression drug therapy or hematologic malignancies, may explain the occasional finding of PAP associated with these disorders (785). Mutant mice lacking the gene for granulocyte-macrophage–colony-stimulating factor (GM-CSF) have a similar accumulation of surfactant and surfactant apoprotein in the alveolar spaces (750). Moreover, reconstitution of the respiratory epithelium of GM-CSF knockout mice with the GM-CSF gene completely corrects the alveolar proteinosis (762,787). Also, PAP has been observed spontaneously occurring in the lungs of mice with severe combined immunodeficiency (764). These studies suggest that a defect in macrophage function, more specifically an impaired ability to process surfactant, may play a role in the pathogenesis of PAP. Recently, it was shown that neutralizing antibodies of immunoglobulin (Ig) G isotype against GM-CSF are present in PAP and likely cause dysfunction of alveolar macrophages, resulting in reduced surfactant clearance (771). The antibody was found to be present in all specimens of BAL fluid obtained from 11 patients but not in 2 patients with secondary PAP, 53 normal subjects, and 14 patients with other lung diseases (771).

The onset of PAP is usually insidious. Approximately one third of patients are asymptomatic at presentation despite extensive radiographic abnormalities. A nonproductive cough is common, but occasionally, expectoration of "chunky" gelatinous material may occur. Other major clinical manifestations are progressive breathlessness with exertion, fatigue, weight loss, hemoptysis, chest pain, and low-grade fever. Physical examination is often normal. Occasionally, clubbing and cyanosis are present (754). Although crackles may be heard on chest examination, the lungs may be clear to auscultation presumably because gas movement is absent in the completely-filled distal airspaces.

Polycythemia, hypergammaglobulinemia, and increased lactate dehydrogenase (LDH) levels are common (774). Markedly elevated serum levels of lung surfactant proteins A and D (SP-A and SP-D) have been found in patients with PAP (759,760,772). This is a nonspecific response since elevated levels are seen in other lung processes, however, measurement of serum SP-A and SP-D may help narrow the diagnosis. A restrictive ventilatory defect is most commonly found on lung function testing. An isolated decrease in DLCO may be present. When present, the decreased DLCO is out of proportion to the degree of reduced lung volume. Varying degrees of hypoxemia and compensated respiratory alkalosis are common and frequently worsen with exercise. An elevated shunt fraction is usually present.

The diagnosis frequently requires tissue examination. Tissue is most often obtained by open or thoracoscopic lung biopsy. Tissue obtained by transbronchial biopsy or material from BAL fluid may obviate the need for surgical lung biopsy (741,754,777,789,800). Examination of sputum may suggest the diagnosis of PAP in the correct clinical context by the identification of PAS-positive macrophages or by finding a significant increase in SP-A (although this latter test is not widely available) (775,798). Findings in the BAL fluid that are characteristic for PAP are: an opaque or milky appearance due to the abundant lipoproteinaceous material (that may settle upon standing), alveolar macrophages that are engorged with the PAS-positive material, large acellular eosinophilic bodies in a background of eosinophilic granules, PAS staining of proteinaceous material, a decrease in the number of alveolar macrophages, and a slight increase in T lymphocytes (with a tendency toward a high CD4/CD8 ratio) (779). Elevated levels of several tumor markers (carcinoembryonic antigen [CEA], carbohydrate antigens sialyl Lewis$_a$ [CA 19-9] and sialyl SSEA-1 [SLX]) have been found in BAL fluid (and serum) from some patients with PAP (752,757). It is possible that these tumor markers may reflect disease activity (752,797). It has been shown that serum or BAL KL-6, a mucin-like glycoprotein, is useful for the diagnosis of PAP and the estimation of its activity (794).

Radiologic Findings. The radiographic manifestations usually consist of bilateral and symmetric areas of airspace consolidation that tend to have a vaguely nodular appearance (fig. 3-132, top) (785,800). In patients with less severe disease, the radiographic findings may consist of hazy areas of ground-glass opacity rather than consolidation (773). The abnormalities tend to involve mainly the perihilar regions and lower lobes (785,800).

The characteristic findings on HRCT are bilateral ground-glass opacities often associated with interlobular septal thickening, a combination

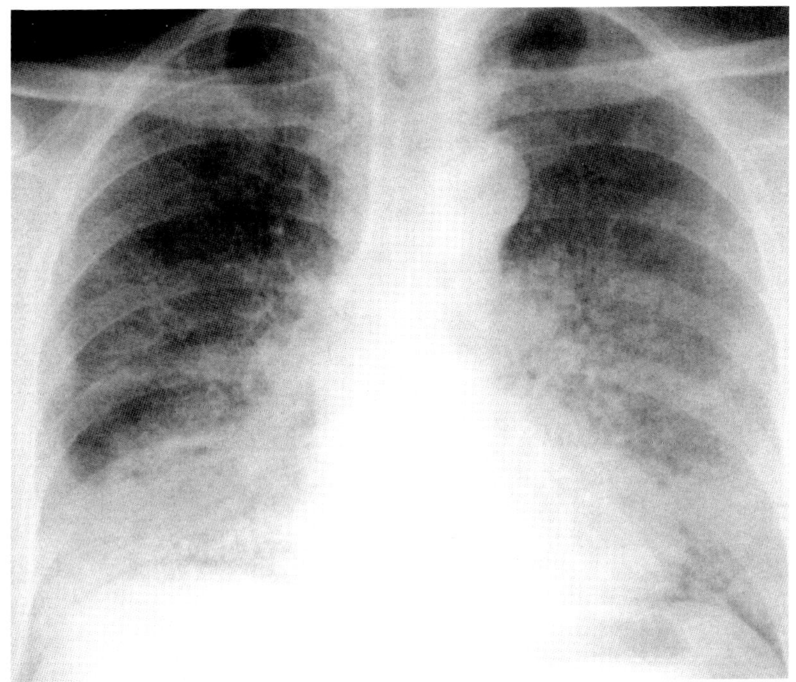

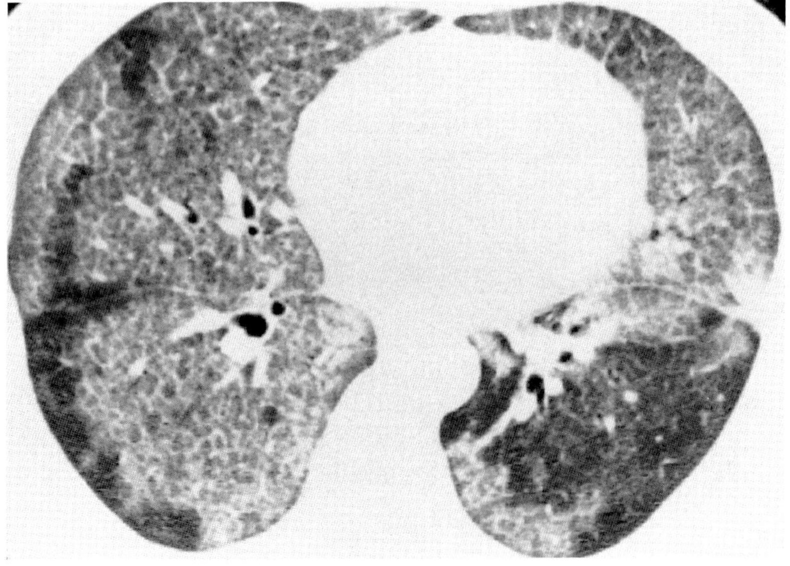

Figure 3-132

ALVEOLAR PROTEINOSIS

Top: Chest radiograph shows bilateral areas of consolidation involving mainly the lower lobes. The consolidation has a vaguely nodular appearance.

Bottom: HRCT demonstrates bilateral ground-glass opacities. Linear opacities are seen within the areas of ground-glass attenuation. Note the sharp demarcation between normal and abnormal parenchyma, giving a geographic appearance, a finding characteristic of alveolar proteinosis. (Courtesy of Dr. Jim Barrie, University of Alberta Medical Centre, Canada.)

that has been described as having the appearance of "crazy paving" (fig. 3-132, bottom) (785,800). Although this pattern, in the appropriate clinical setting, is suggestive of the diagnosis, it may also be seen in a variety of other conditions such as pneumonia, pulmonary hemorrhage, and hydrostatic and increased permeability pulmonary edema (765,773).

Gross Findings. On gross examination, the lungs in PAP are very heavy and viscid, and yellow fluid leaks from the cut surface (fig. 3-133). Scattered, firm, yellowish white nodules vary in size from a few millimeters to 2 cm in diameter.

Histologic Findings. The histologic hallmark consists of an intra-alveolar accumulation of eosinophilic proteinaceous granular material (figs. 3-134–3-138). PAP usually affects the lung diffusely, but in some cases the lesion may be patchy, resulting in areas of normal lung (fig. 3-134). If the biopsy specimen does not sample the affected areas, the lesion may be absent or so subtle that it can be overlooked even in surgical

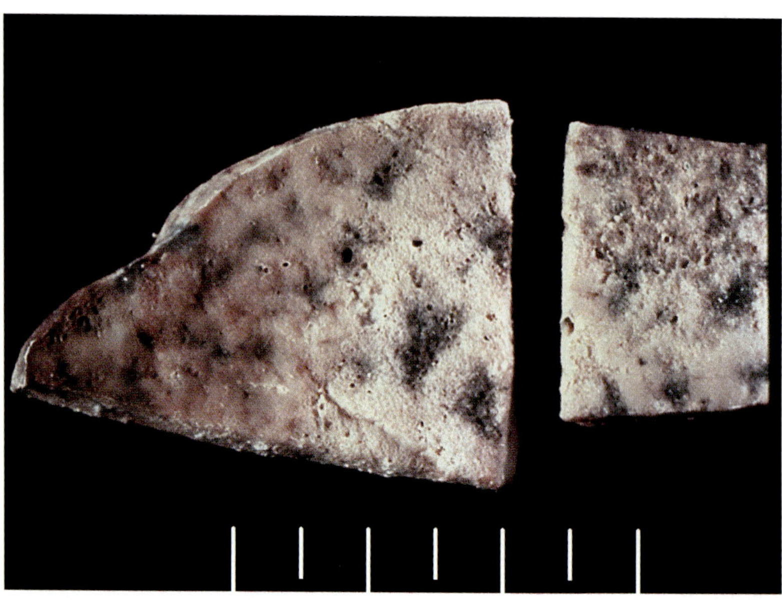

Figure 3-133

ALVEOLAR PROTEINOSIS:
GROSS SPECIMEN

The lung shows yellow-tan discoloration of the parenchyma. The architecture of the lung appears preserved and the process appears to fill the alveolar spaces. The abnormality primarily affects the right portion of the piece of tissue on the left and almost the entire piece of tissue on the right.

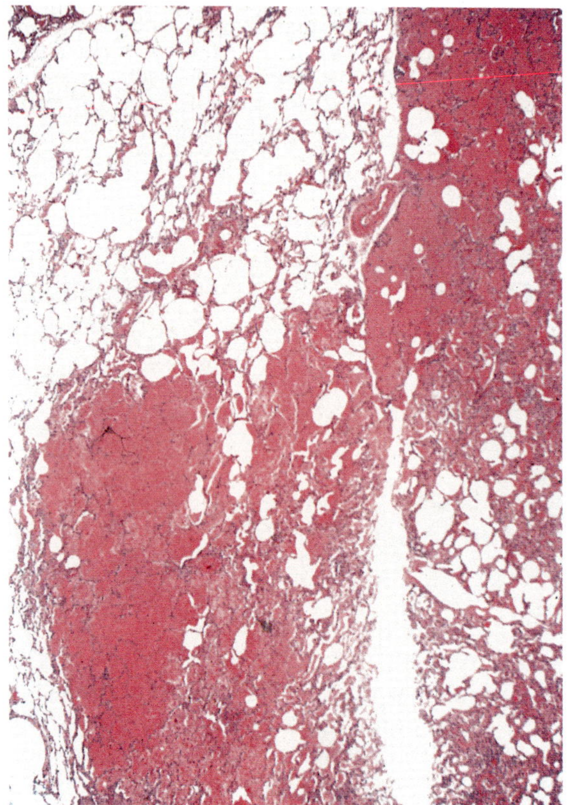

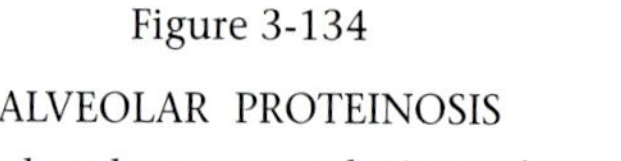

Figure 3-134

ALVEOLAR PROTEINOSIS

The intra-alveolar accumulation of eosinophilic proteinaceous material is extensive but patchy, with areas of normal lung.

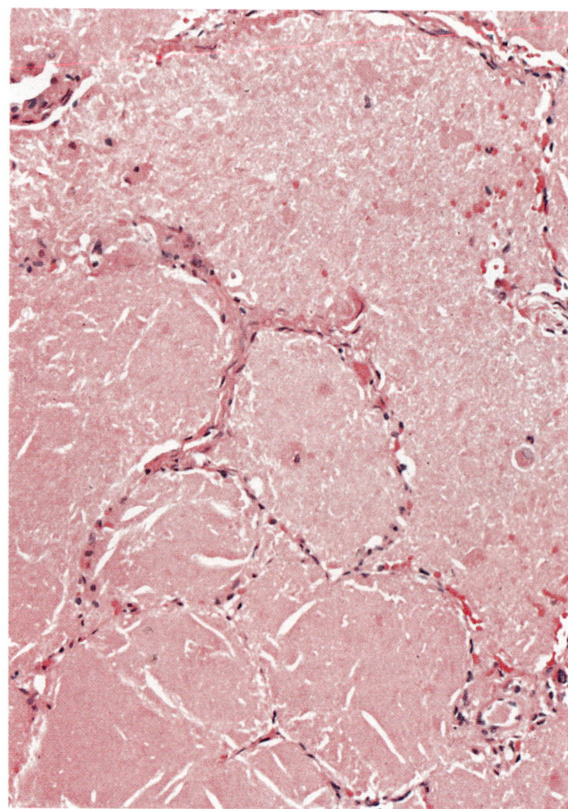

Figure 3-135

ALVEOLAR PROTEINOSIS

The alveolar spaces are filled with eosinophilic proteinaceous material. The interstitium is mildly thickened but does not show fibrosis or inflammation.

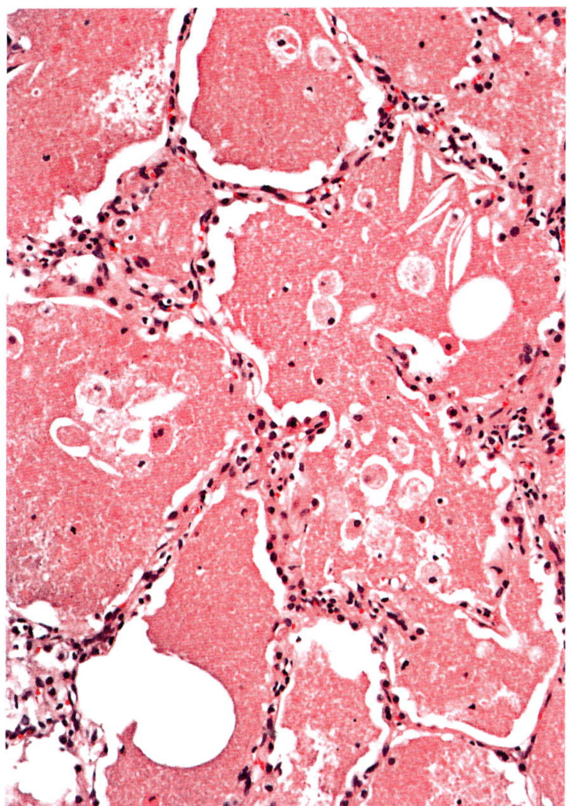

Figure 3-136

ALVEOLAR PROTEINOSIS

The alveolar proteinaceous material has several holes or rounded spaces, which are empty and sharply defined. A few macrophages and cholesterol clefts are present.

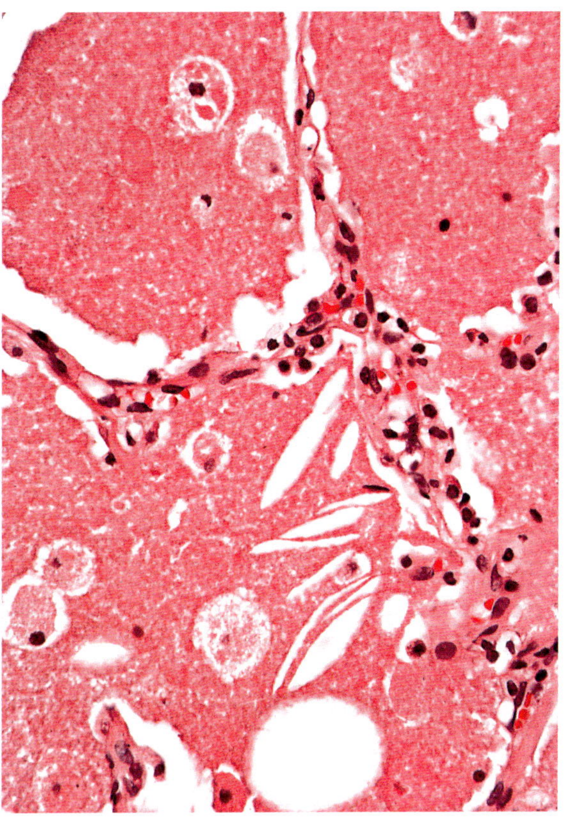

Figure 3-137

ALVEOLAR PROTEINOSIS

Cholesterol clefts and foamy macrophages are present within the proteinaceous material.

lung biopsies. On microscopic examination, the eosinophilic granular material may involve not only the alveolar spaces but also the bronchioles and alveolar ducts. Sharply rounded empty spaces, cholesterol clefts, and small, dense, globular clumps of eosinophilic material are distinctive for PAP (fig. 3-138). The proteinaceous material may stain with the PAS stain (fig. 3-139).

Typically, there is little inflammation or interstitial fibrosis. Within the eosinophilic material may be found cellular debris, foamy macrophages (fig. 3-137), ghosts of degenerated cells, and detached type 2 pneumocytes. Interstitial fibrosis or inflammation should raise the possibility of associated infection, however, it can occur in patients with recurrent or longstanding PAP (fig. 3-140) (743). The intra-alveolar material typically stains with an antibody to surfactant apoprotein (792), and electron microscopy reveals concentrically laminated myelin figures and lamellar bodies identical to the cytoplasmic inclusions of type 2 pneumocytes (fig. 3-141) (761,795). If there is an associated exposure to dust such as silicosis (silicolipoproteinosis), polarization microscopy may reveal birefringent needle-like particles (see chapter 16).

Infection with *Nocardia* is known to be associated with PAP, as are other mycobacterial, fungal, and viral agents (Table 3-33). Most of these infections are thought to be secondary. In some cases, it is speculated that PAP is a secondary reaction to the infection.

Differential Diagnosis. PAP must be separated from pulmonary edema, *Pneumocystis carinii* pneumonia, and alveolar mucinosis. Pulmonary edema lacks the coarse granules, cholesterol clefts, and foamy macrophages of PAP. *Pneumocystis* pneumonia shows an intra-alveolar eosinophilic

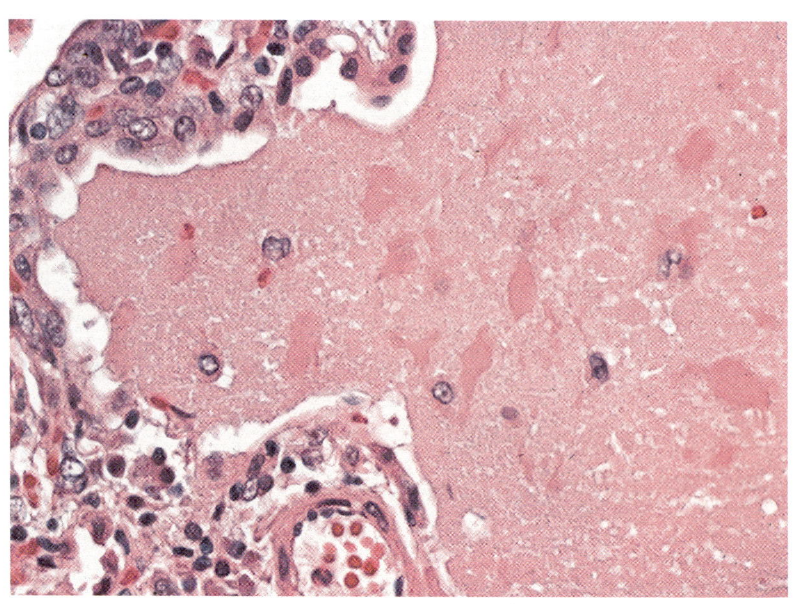

Figure 3-138

ALVEOLAR PROTEINOSIS

Dense clumps of eosinophilic material are present within the proteinaceous exudate.

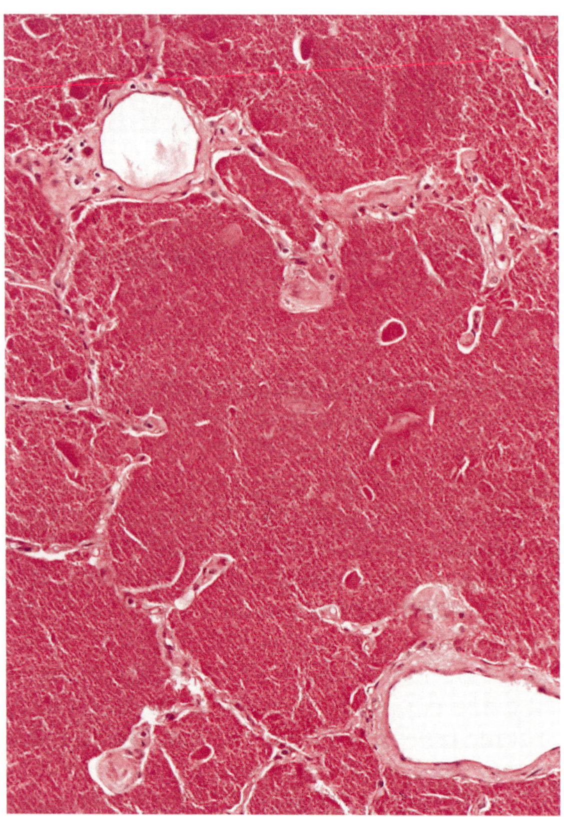

Figure 3-139

ALVEOLAR PROTEINOSIS

The proteinaceous material stains with the PAS stain.

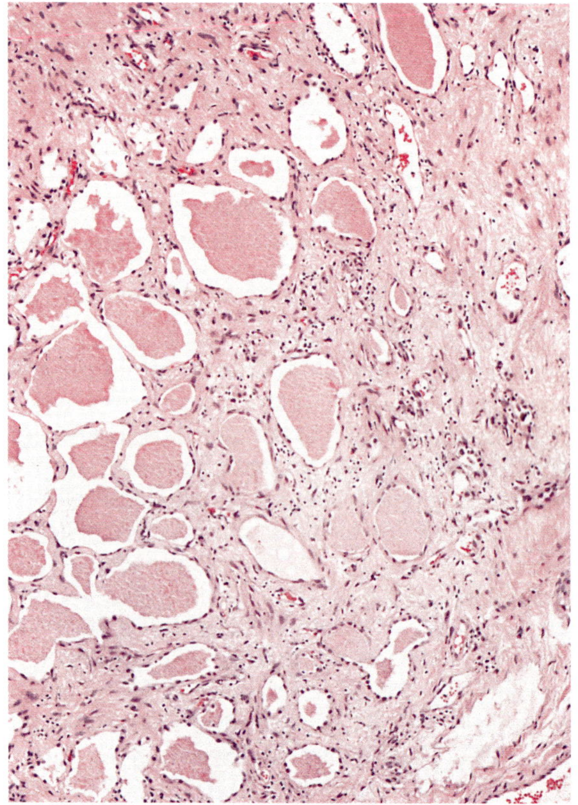

Figure 3-140

ALVEOLAR PROTEINOSIS

Interstitial fibrosis has developed in this patient with longstanding PAP.

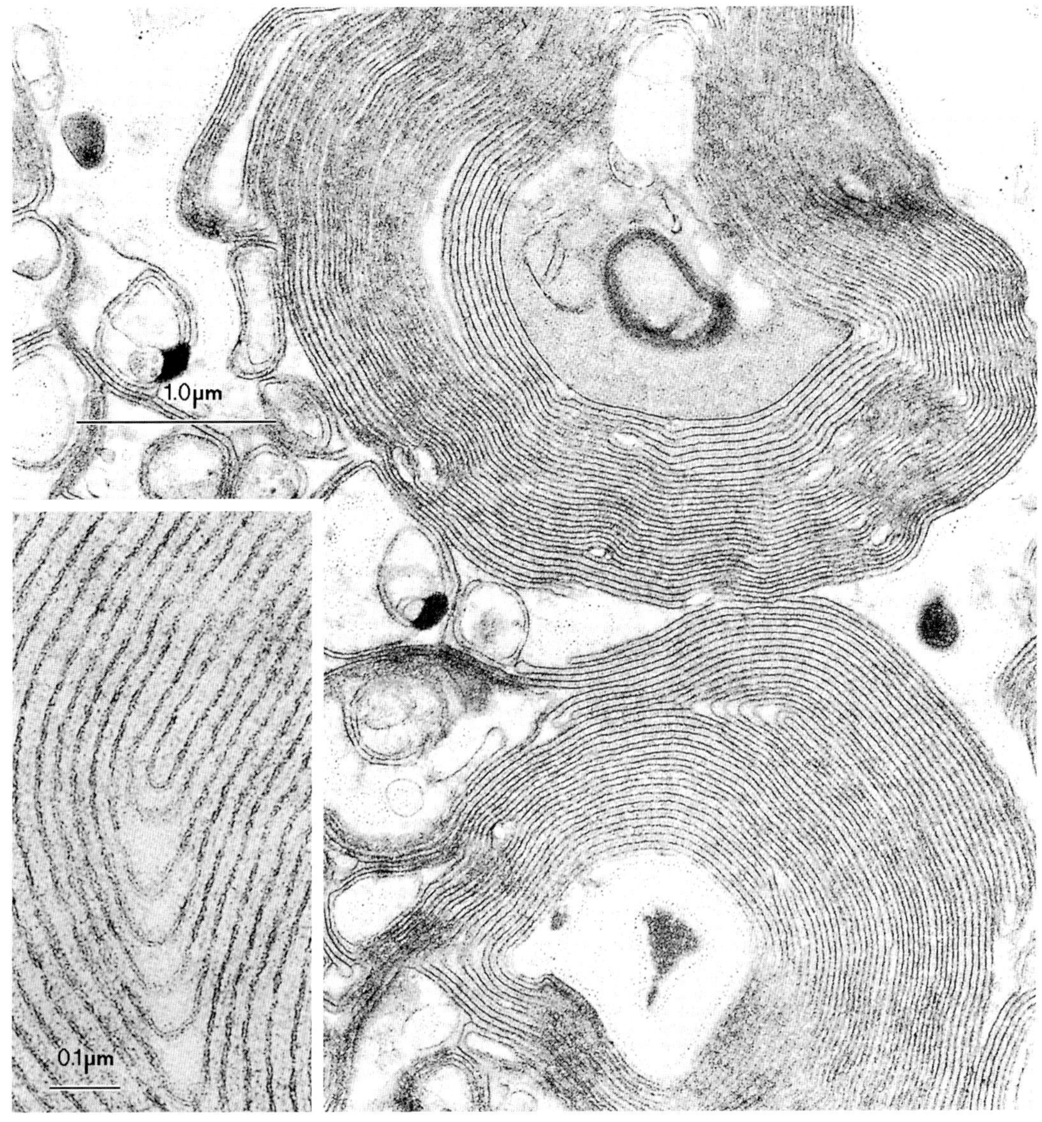

Figure 3-141

ELECTRON MICROSCOPY OF BRONCHOALVEOLAR LAVAGE FLUID FROM PATIENT WITH ALVEOLAR PROTEINOSIS

Multilamellated structures consist of trilaminar membranes separated by amorphous material. Electron dense bodies and membranous vesicles are often found at the center of the multilamellated structures. (Figure 1 from Hook GE, Gilmore LB, Talley FA. Multilamellated structures from the lungs of patients with pulmonary alveolar proteinosis. Lab Invest 1984;50:711-25.)

exudate with "bubbles" that correspond to the cysts or organisms. Intra-alveolar accumulation of mucin may occur in association with mucinous adenocarcinomas or in an obstructive setting such as bronchiectasis or honeycomb fibrosis. Histopathologic findings consistent with PAP can occur in a variety of clinical settings: acute silicosis (silicoproteinosis), aluminum dust exposure, titanium exposure, infections with *Pneumocystis carinii,* and in patients with various hematologic malignancies and immunosuppression (740,746,766,769) (Table 3-33). However, the vast majority of patients with PAP appear not have these underlying disorders or exposures (785). Proteinaceous debris can occasionally be seen in association with interstitial pneumonias, especially in children. Therefore, the presence of such debris, especially in the setting of significant interstitial inflammation or fibrosis, does not always indicate a diagnosis of PAP.

Treatment and Prognosis. Some patients have little or no physiologic impairment despite extensive radiographic abnormalities and do not require immediate treatment. Also, spontaneous remissions have been reported (754). Due to impaired macrophage phagocytic function, there is an increased risk of superinfection in PAP patients by opportunistic organisms such as *Nocardia,* mycobacteria, and various endemic or opportunistic fungi (739,785,802).

Treatment should be instituted with the development of symptoms that are troublesome for the patient, especially severe dyspnea and hypoxemia at rest or on exercise. The most widely accepted and effective form of treatment is therapeutic whole lung lavage via a double-lumen endotracheal tube (744). Complications of whole lung lavage include malpositioning of the endotracheal tube, saline spillover into the unlavaged ventilated lung, and hydropneumothorax. After whole lung lavage, patients often feel dramatically better with improvement in exertional dyspnea. The clinical course is variable, with 30 to 40 percent of patients requiring only one lavage. Some patients, however, require repeat lung lavages at intervals of 6 to 12 months. There is no role for corticosteroids or other immunosuppressives; in fact, there is concern that corticosteroids may increase mortality. A potential role for the administration of GM-CSF in the treatment of PAP patients awaits further study (791).

Table 3-34

VASCULITIC DISORDERS ASSOCIATED WITH DIFFUSE PULMONARY HEMORRHAGE[a]

Wegener's granulomatosis (847)
Churg-Strauss angiitis and granulomatosis (816)
Microscopic polyangiitis (822,826)
Collagen vascular diseases (847)
Systemic lupus erythematosus (838)
Rheumatoid arthritis (847)
Juvenile rheumatoid arthritis (847)
Henoch-Schönlein purpura (835)
Mixed cryoglobulinemia (833)
Behçet's syndrome (840)
Small vessel vasculitis associated with bone marrow transplantation (842)
Systemic sarcoid-like granulomatous vasculitis (844)
Systemic necrotizing vasculitis (hepatitis B infection) (824)
Antiphospholipid antibody syndrome (818)
Antibasement membrane antibody disease (847)
Idiopathic pulmonary hemorrhage (847)
IgA nephropathy (847)
Idiopathic glomerulonephritis (with and without immune complexes) (847)
Circulating IgM antineutrophil antibody (P-ANCA pattern) associated with glomerulonephritis (825)

[a]Although several of these conditions are not considered to be primary vasculitides, histologic evidence of capillaritis in lung biopsy specimens and/or elevated

DIFFUSE ALVEOLAR HEMORRHAGE

Definition. Diffuse alveolar hemorrhage (DAH) is characterized by extensive intra-alveolar hemorrhage that may be acute and/or chronic. Most of these syndromes are associated with a variety of systemic disorders, however, diffuse pulmonary hemorrhage also occurs as an idiopathic condition.

DAH is associated with a wide variety of clinical syndromes (810,841,847). The most common are vasculitic disorders, especially Wegener's granulomatosis (WG), and microscopic polyangiitis (MPA) (847) (Table 3-34) (see chapter 4). Most patients with DAH come to medical attention because of hemoptysis or unexplained dyspnea in the presence of an abnormal chest radiograph. Importantly, hemoptysis may not always be a clinical manifestation even in the presence of severe alveolar hemorrhage.

Clinical Features. The clinical presentation is most often characterized by the abrupt onset of dyspnea. Cough, hemoptysis, and fever are commonly present. For most causes, the duration of illness is less than 7 days. Respiratory distress may progress to respiratory failure requiring respiratory support. Hemoptysis is absent at the time of presentation in one third

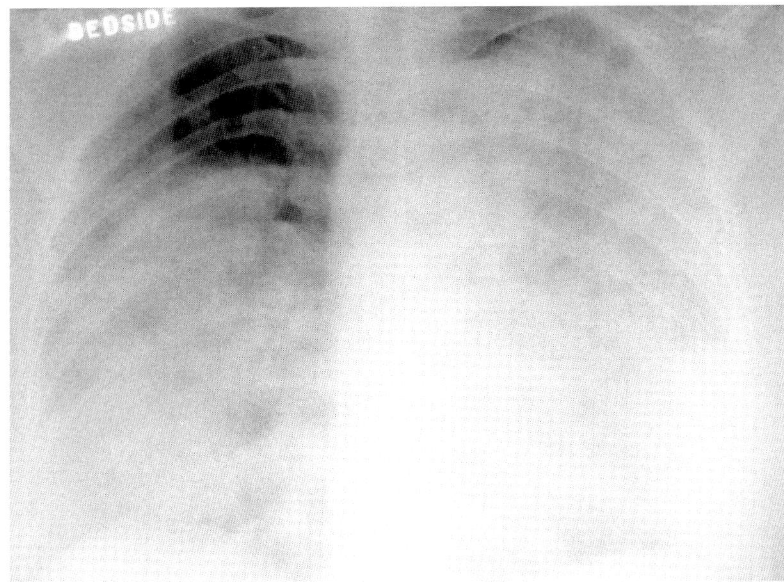

Figure 3-142

GOODPASTURE'S SYNDROME

Chest radiograph demonstrates extensive bilateral areas of consolidation due to diffuse pulmonary hemorrhage.

of the patients, suggesting a community-acquired pneumonia; patients with a more subacute or chronic clinical course may not have hemoptysis. However, the combination of new or progressive alveolar opacities (either localized or diffuse), anemia, and a sequential BAL that is hemorrhagic, point to the diagnosis. Occasionally, a surgical lung biopsy is required to confirm the diagnosis.

The chest examination is nonspecific (crackles, signs of consolidation), but physical evidence of other organ involvement provides important clues to the underlying diagnosis: uveitis, a dermatologic leukocytoclastic vasculitis, myositis, and arthralgias or arthritis point to systemic diseases such as vasculitis or collagen vascular disease.

An elevated erythrocyte sedimentation rate, an elevated white blood cell count, and a falling hematocrit are to be expected. In syndromes where renal involvement is common (systemic lupus erythematosus, Goodpasture's syndrome, and pauci-immune glomerulonephritis) there may be impaired renal function, and urinalysis may reveal red blood cells, protein, and red blood cell casts. Other laboratory evaluations in selected patients include measurement of the serum anticytoplasmic neurophil antibody to myeloperoxidase (ANCA), an echocardiogram to exclude mitral stenosis, and drug screening in suspected crack cocaine abuse.

Hypoxemia is almost always present and is often severe enough to require ventilatory support. A sensitive indicator of DAH is an elevation in the DLCO. This results from the increased availability of hemoglobin within the alveolar compartment. An unexpected increase in the diffusing capacity in the face of severe abnormalities in gas exchange and diffuse lung opacities is also useful for suspecting DAH in new cases. Sequential measurements may detect exacerbations in established cases.

Transbronchial biopsy and BAL evaluations are of limited use in confirming a specific diagnosis, except infection. In any cause of DAH, sequential collection of BAL fluid during bronchoscopy may show a progressive bloody return. As noted above, this is particularly helpful when diagnosing a patient with diffuse pulmonary opacities without hemoptysis.

Radiologic Findings. The radiographic manifestations consist of patchy or diffuse bilateral areas of airspace consolidation (fig. 3-142) (812,837). The areas of consolidation are often widespread but tend to involve mainly the perihilar regions and lower lung zones. Similar findings are seen on HRCT (815,837).

Gross Findings. The pleural and cut surfaces of the lungs appear deep red or purple and spongy when acute hemorrhage is present (fig. 3-143). In chronic hemorrhage, the lung parenchyma appears brown, and it may be firm (fig.

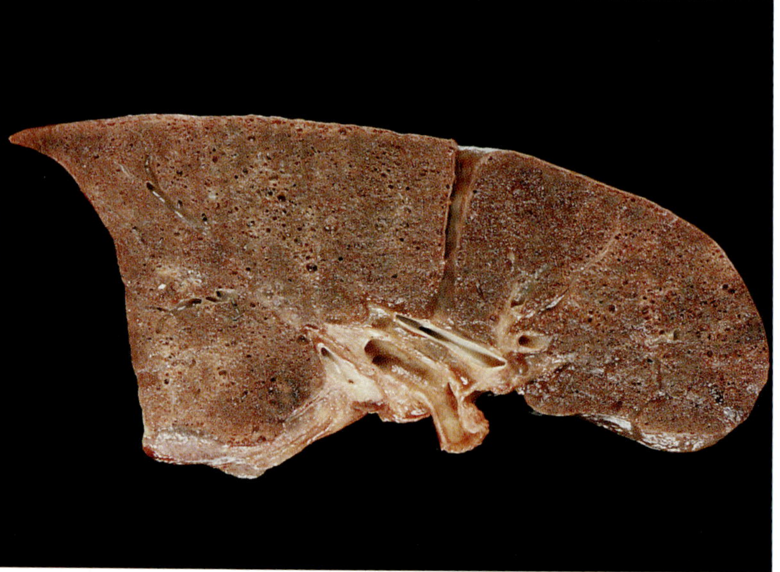

Figure 3-143

IDIOPATHIC PULMONARY HEMORRHAGE: GROSS SPECIMEN

The cut surface of the lung is diffusely dark brown. (Courtesy of Dr. Victor Roggli, Duke University, Durham, NC.)

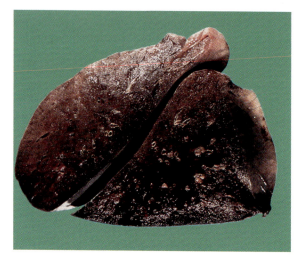

Figure 3-144

GOODPASTURE'S SYNDROME: GROSS SPECIMEN

The cut surface of the lung is dark red to purple. (Courtesy of Dr. Victor Roggli, Duke University, Durham, NC.)

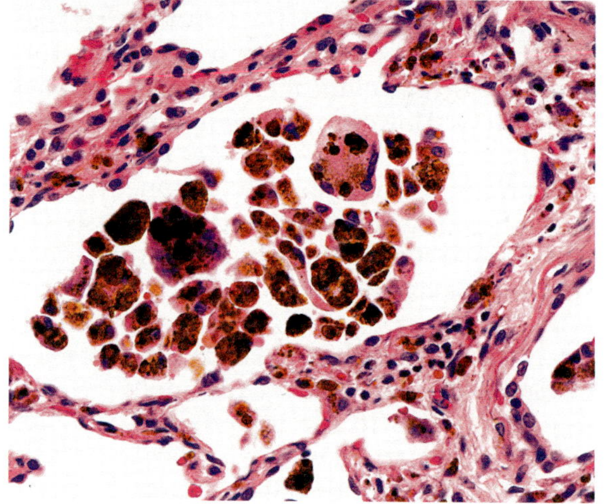

Figure 3-145

IDIOPATHIC PULMONARY HEMORRHAGE

Coarse granules of brown hemosiderin fill these alveolar spaces. Many of the granules are contained within the cytoplasm of macrophages.

3-144). With longstanding chronic hemorrhage, fibrosis may develop. Surgically resected or autopsy specimens may show blood within the airway lumens in the presence of acute hemorrhage. In most cases, open lung biopsies are necessary for diagnosis.

Histologic Findings. Histologically, DAH shows an accumulation of intra-alveolar red blood cells and hemosiderin-laden macrophages. Histologic clues that the hemorrhage is genuine and not a surgical artifact (see fig. 2-5) include the presence of coarse granular hemosiderin deposits (fig. 3-145) and erythrophagocytosis (847). In the absence of these histologic features, there should be some clinical evidence of hemorrhage such as hemoptysis or anemia (847).

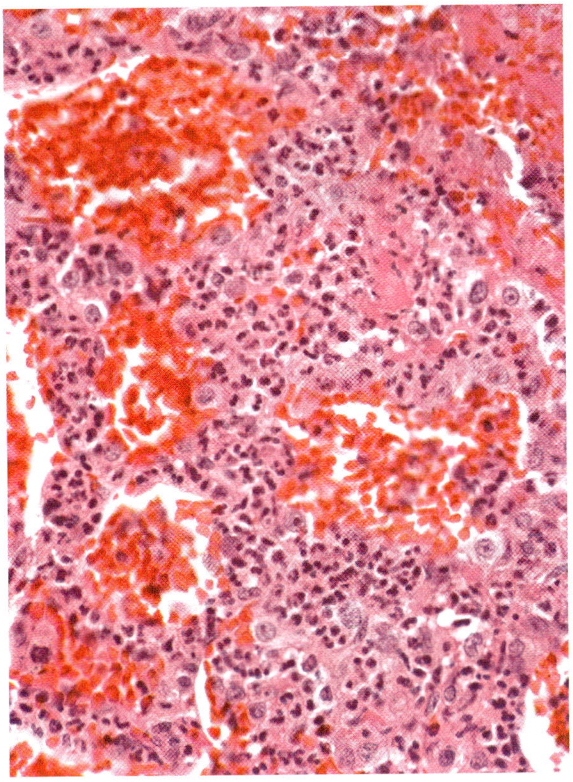

Figure 3-146

HEMORRHAGE AND CAPILLARITIS IN WEGENER'S GRANULOMATOSIS

The alveolar walls are diffusely infiltrated by neutrophils.

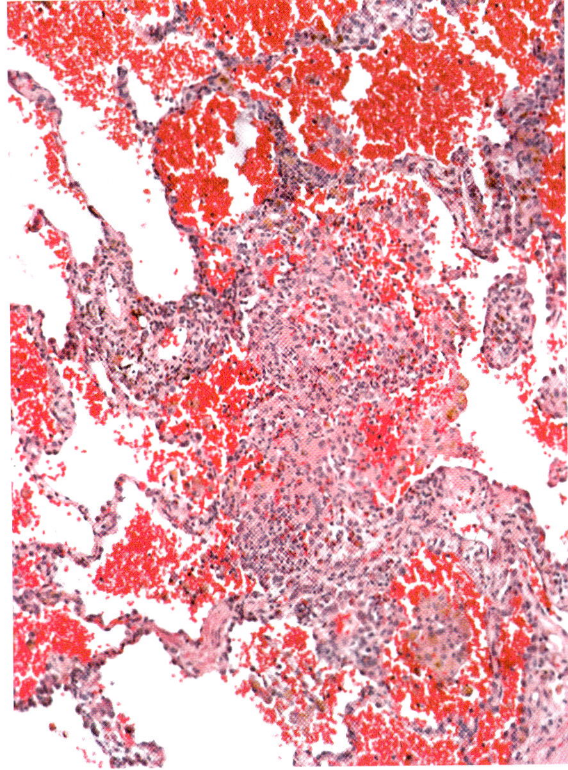

Figure 3-147

HEMORRHAGE AND CAPILLARITIS IN WEGENER'S GRANULOMATOSIS

The alveolar hemorrhage and capillaritis appear as a nodular lesion.

A variety of other lesions may cause chronic hemorrhage including lymphangioleiomyomatosis, DIP, and RB (all described earlier in this chapter), pulmonary veno-occlusive disease (see chapter 15), and asbestos and welder's pneumoconioses (see chapter 16). In lymphangioleiomyomatosis the abnormal smooth muscle cell infiltrates that are usually associated with cystic parenchymal changes are seen. In pulmonary veno-occlusive disease, sclerosis of veins should be identified. In DIP and RB, the intra-alveolar iron pigment is finely granular and differs from the coarse hemosiderin granules seen in chronic hemorrhage. A Prussian blue stain for iron may help highlight the hemosiderin but usually is not needed to recognize the coarse hemosiderin granules of chronic hemorrhage.

Neutrophilic capillaritis (figs. 3-146, 3-147), consisting of neutrophilic infiltration of alveolar septal walls, can be found in lung biopsies from patients with any of the diffuse pulmonary hemorrhage syndromes (847). In cases of Wegener's granulomatosis (WG) and systemic lupus erythematosus the capillaritis may be severe (847). Capillaritis is often patchy and found within nodular areas of hemorrhage (fig. 3-147). Alveolar capillaries may show endothelial swelling, thrombosis, and fibrinoid necrosis. Nuclear dust or karyorrhectic debris, eosinophils, and histiocytes may accompany the neutrophils (834).

Dumbbell-shaped fibrin clots may project from the capillary wall into the alveolar space (834). In most cases, the neutrophils are concentrated primarily around the alveolar wall (fig. 3-

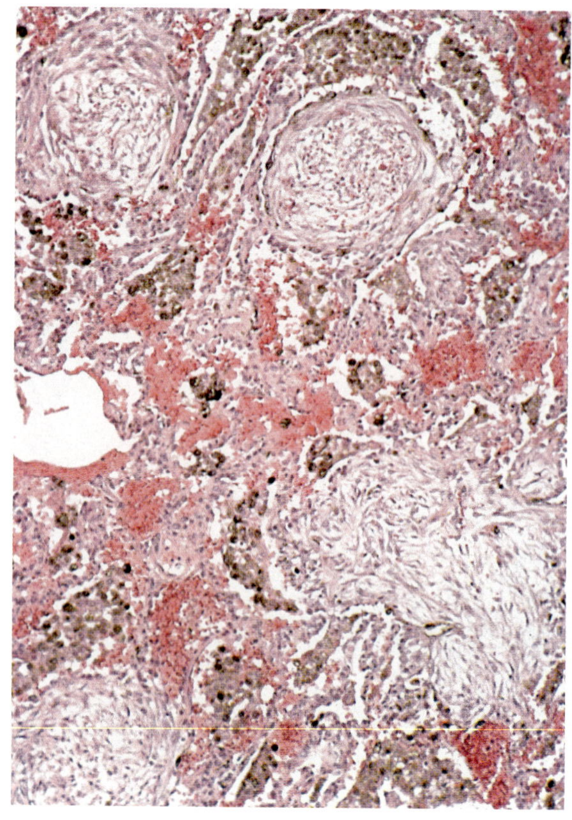

Figure 3-148

IDIOPATHIC PULMONARY HEMORRHAGE: ORGANIZING PNEUMONIA

In addition to chronic hemorrhage with hemosiderin deposits, there is prominent organizing pneumonia.

146). However, the capillaritis may be so severe that the neutrophils spill over into the surrounding alveoli making it difficult to distinguish from a hemorrhagic infectious pneumonia. In such cases the biopsy should be scrutinized for other distinctive areas of capillaritis or histologic lesions of WG.

Hemorrhage is often associated with an organizing pneumonia consisting of intra-alveolar plugs of loose, organizing fibroblastic connective tissue reminiscent of the BOOP pattern (figs. 3-148, 3-149) (822). However, this represents a nonspecific reaction of the lung, a healing phase of alveolar hemorrhage, or capillaritis. Hemosiderin, and in cases of WG, giant cells may be seen within these plugs of fibroblastic connective tissue (fig. 3-149) (847).

Vascular encrustation by hemosiderin may be seen in association with chronic hemorrhage due to any cause (see fig. 2-9). The term *endogenous pneumoconiosis* has been used for this lesion. It can cause degeneration of the vascular walls with fragmentation of the elastic laminae and may elicit a granulomatous reaction (848). The giant cells of this reaction should not be mistaken for the granulomatous inflammatory lesion of WG.

Specific classification of diffuse pulmonary hemorrhage syndromes requires correlation with the clinical history and laboratory results as well as the lung biopsy findings (847). WG is the only syndrome that has distinctive

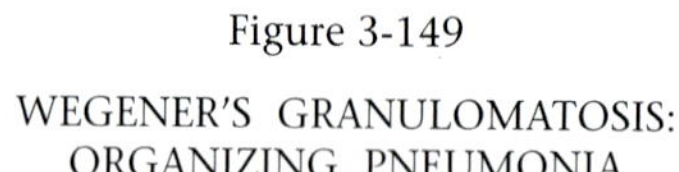

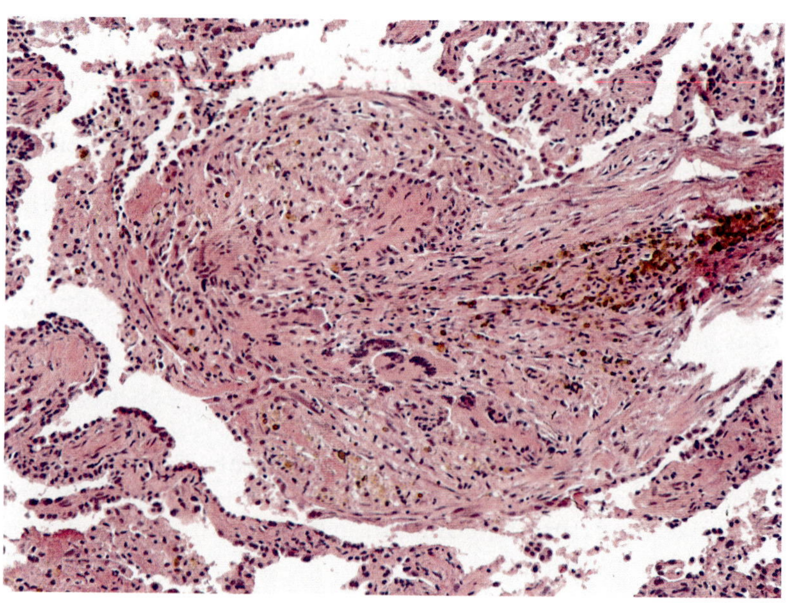

Figure 3-149

WEGENER'S GRANULOMATOSIS: ORGANIZING PNEUMONIA

This focus of organizing pneumonia contains several multinucleated giant cells. In addition, hemosiderin deposits are incorporated within the organizing connective tissue.

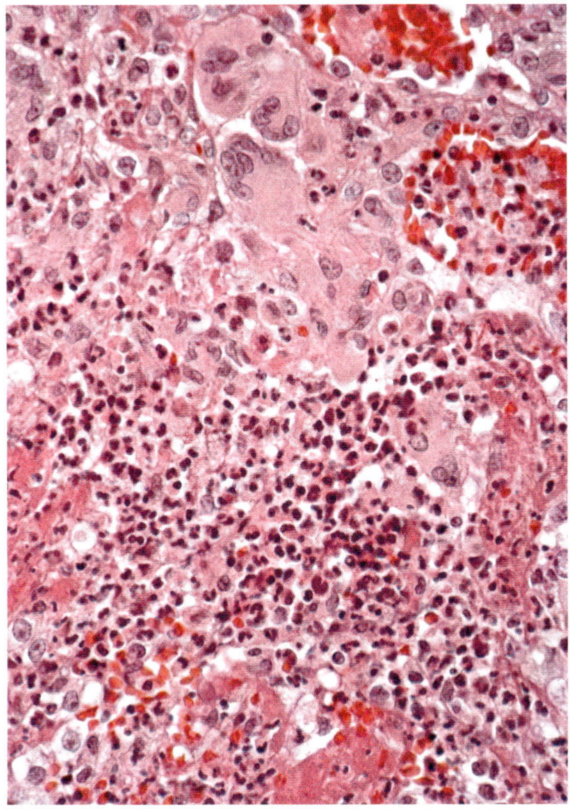

Figure 3-150

WEGENER'S GRANULOMATOSIS: FOCAL GRANULOMATOUS INFLAMMATION

This lung biopsy showed extensive alveolar hemorrhage and after careful search this focus of a neutrophilic microabscess and a cluster of multinucleated giant cells provided clues to the diagnosis of Wegener's granulomatosis.

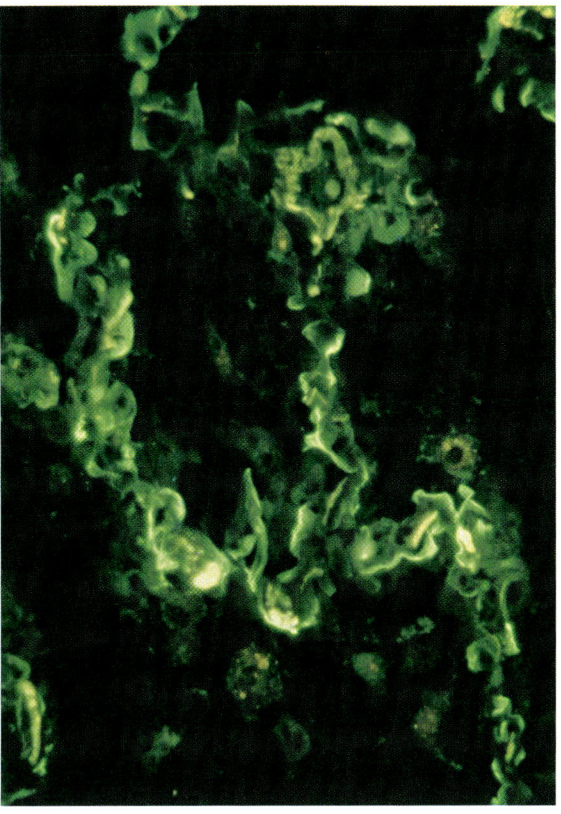

Figure 3-151

IMMUNOFLUORESCENCE OF FROZEN SECTION OF LUNG BIOPSY IN GOODPASTURE'S SYNDROME

Direct immunofluorescence shows linear IgG staining of alveolar septa. (Courtesy of Dr. Victor Roggli, Duke University, Durham, NC.)

findings in lung biopsies: foci of necrosis (fig. 3-150), granulomatous inflammation (fig. 3-150), and vasculitis involving arterioles or venules. These lesions may be focal and require a careful search that includes evaluation of serial sections. Demonstration of antibasement membrane antibody (ABMA) in the serum or in kidney or lung biopsies is required for the diagnosis of Goodpasture's syndrome (fig. 3-151) (807,829). ANCA tests are valuable in the diagnosis of vasculitis syndromes (see chapter 4). Biopsies of the kidney, nasal sinus, or skin may be helpful in making the diagnosis of WG, Goodpasture's syndrome, or collagen vascular diseases such as systemic lupus erythematosus (811). Kidney biopsies may be studied with immunofluorescence and electron microscopy for the separation of ABMA-mediated diffuse pulmonary hemorrhage, IgA nephropathy, and systemic lupus erythematosus. These studies are more difficult to perform on lung biopsy specimens. Nevertheless, in lung biopsies showing DAH it is useful to set aside a small piece of snap-frozen unfixed lung tissue and a small piece of glutaraldehyde-fixed lung tissue for electron microscopy.

Sometimes, the DAH syndromes are difficult to diagnose. For example, some patients do not show all of the clinical or pathologic features of WG, and the best one can do is make a diagnosis of "probable WG." Some cases may completely defy classification, and for such cases the term "unclassified pulmonary renal syndrome" is appropriate. A classification proposed

Table 3-35

CLASSIFICATION OF DIFFUSE PULMONARY HEMORRHAGE SYNDROMES[a]

Immunologic Mechanism	Immuno-fluorescence Pattern	Common Terminology
Antibasement membrane antibody	Linear	Goodpasture's syndrome
Immune complexes	Granular	Systemic lupus erythematosus, mixed cryoglobulinemia, Henoch-Schönlein purpura, IgA disease, pulmonary-renal syndrome, idiopathic necrotizing glomerulonephritis with immune complexes
Antineutrophil cytoplasmic antibody	Negative or pauci-immune	Wegener's granulomatosis, microscopic polyangiitis, Churg-Strauss syndrome, idiopathic necrotizing glomerulonephritis without immune complexes
None detected	Negative or pauci-immune	Idiopathic pulmonary hemorrhage

[a]Modified from reference 811.

by Bosch et al. (811) suggested the following categories of pulmonary hemorrhage: ANCA-associated disorders are pauci-immune, antibody-mediated hemorrhage syndromes of ABMA diseases show linear immunofluorescence patterns, and immune-complex associated diseases show a granular pattern of immunofluorescence (Table 3-35).

Jennings et al. (827) recently described eight patients with DAH and underlying pauci-immune pulmonary capillaritis. These patients lacked extrapulmonary vasculitic manifestations, and other diffuse pulmonary hemorrhage syndromes were excluded by a thorough evaluation including negative test results for ANCA and ABMA. These cases appear to represent a form of capillaritis and hemorrhage limited to the lungs. The study was remarkable for the clinical recovery of seven of the eight patients.

Differential Diagnosis. The differential diagnosis of DAH can be classified immunologically by the immunofluorescence or electron microscopic findings (Table 3-35) or histologically by the findings on lung biopsy. Evaluation of either lung or renal tissue by immunofluorescence techniques will indicate an absence of immune complexes (pauci-immune) in some processes, such as WG, microscopic polyangiitis pauci-immune glomerulonephritis, and isolated pulmonary capillaritis. In others, either a granular pattern is found in collagen vascular diseases, particularly systemic lupus erythematosus (fig. 3-152) or Henoch-Schönlein purpura, or a characteristic linear deposition is found in Goodpasture's syndrome (fig. 3-151) (810,841,847).

Commonly, the patient with DAH has a known predisposing condition such as vasculitis or connective tissue disease (810,841,847). Even so, a careful history and serologic studies are important to rule out other causes, especially exposure to drugs such as penicillamine, crack cocaine (fig. 3-153), nitrofurantoin, and amiodarone (806,809), or environmental exposures (paraquat, pesticides, leather conditioners, trimellitic anhydride or isocyanates, toxic fungi such as *Stachybotrys atra*) (819,820,823, 828). Bone marrow and heart lung transplantation may be associated with DAH (805). Localized lesions such as neoplasms (808,813,843, 845), infarcts, or bronchiectasis may also cause extensive hemorrhage. The presence of vascular malformations in the bronchus, known as Dieulafoy's disease, is also a potential cause of DAH (846,849). Iatrogenic causes such as pulmonary artery perforation secondary to insertion of a Swan Ganz catheter must be considered (821). In general, when the above evaluation process fails to identify a cause of the DAH, four possibilities remain: Goodpasture's syndrome confined to the lung; isolated pulmonary capillaritis with P-ANCA; isolated pulmonary capillaritis without autoantibodies; and idiopathic pulmonary hemorrhage (810,841,847).

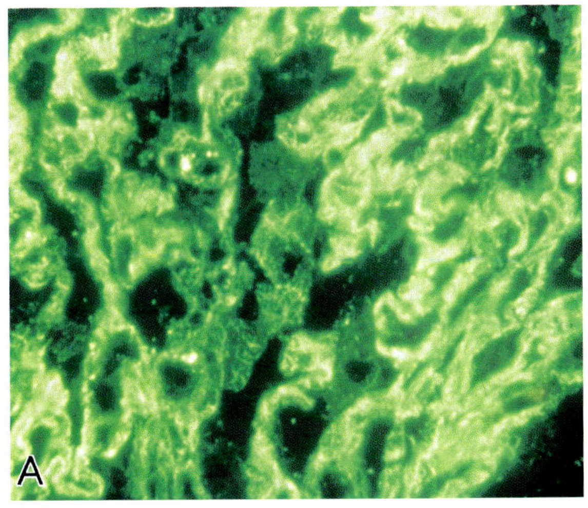

Figure 3-152

IMMUNOFLUORESCENCE OF FROZEN SECTION OF LUNG BIOPSY IN SYSTEMIC LUPUS ERYTHEMATOSUS

A: Direct immunofluorescence with anti-IgG shows bright granular staining of the alveolar septa.

B: Frozen section of the same lung stained with fluorescein-labeled C3 shows granular deposits in the alveolar septa but at a lower density and intensity than IgG.

C: This blood vessel shows bright granular intimal staining with anti-C1q. (Courtesy of Dr. Wilbur Franklin, University of Colorado, Denver, CO.)

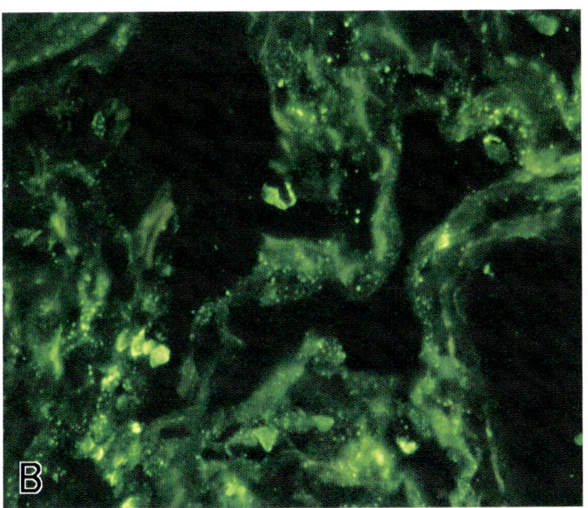

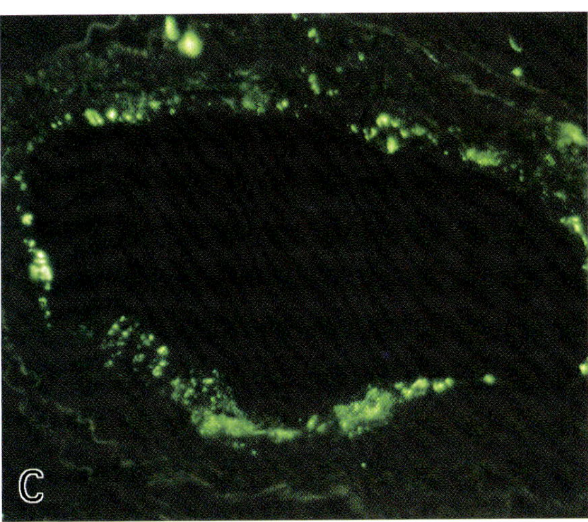

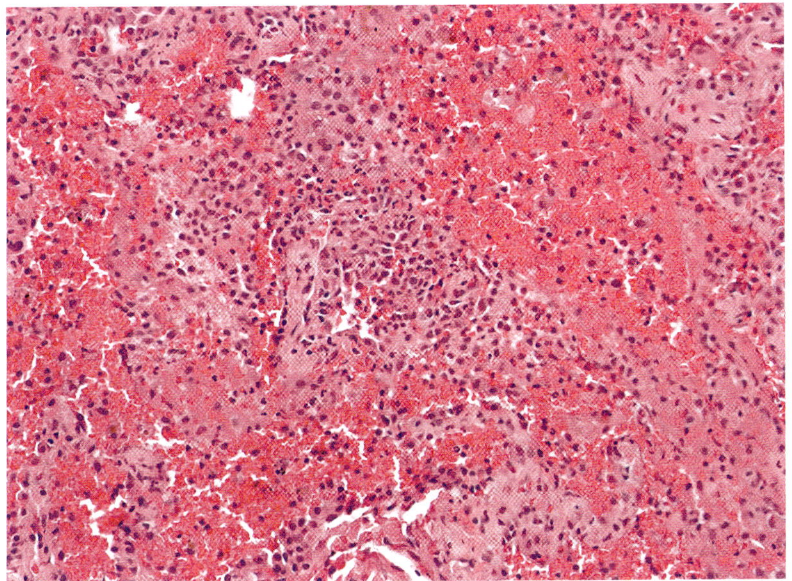

Figure 3-153

DIFFUSE PULMONARY HEMORRHAGE ASSOCIATED WITH SMOKING CRACK COCAINE

There is extensive intra-alveolar hemorrhage. A history of cocaine exposure was apparent only after questioning the patient following lung biopsy.

Treatment and Prognosis. Generally, the prognosis and treatment depend on the underlying associated disease. A fulminant clinical course is often encountered. Such patients require aggressive management. The mainstay of therapy for patients with DAH is a corticosteroid preparation. Most experts recommend intravenous methylprednisolone (500 to 2,000 mg in divided doses daily) for up to 5 days, followed by gradual tapering and then maintenance on an oral preparation. Therapy must be instituted promptly, particularly if renal insufficiency is present, since permanent kidney damage appears more likely than lung disease. The decision to start additional immunosuppressive therapy (cyclophosphamide or azathioprine) depends on the severity of illness and the underlying cause. Plasmapheresis has been recommended but has no proven efficacy in vasculitis or collagen vascular disease associated DAH or renal disease. The role of intravenous immunoglobulin therapy for this group of disorders is unknown. The development of interstitial fibrosis has been well documented, particularly in patients with underlying idiopathic pulmonary hemorrhage and WG. Recently, severe progressive obstructive lung disease, most compatible with the development of emphysema, has been seen in some patients with and without recurrent DAH secondary to microscopic polyangiitis, the small vessel variant of polyarteritis nodosa (810,841,847).

Antibasement Membrane Antibody Disease (Goodpasture's Syndrome)

Definition. Goodpasture's syndrome is an antibasement membrane antibody disease (ABMABD) that affects the lung and kidney. Lung involvement consists of DAH while the kidney typically shows a rapidly progressive glomerulonephritis (807,829).

Both kidney and lung involvement are seen in 60 to 80 percent of patients (807). ABMABD may affect the kidney alone in 20 to 40 percent of cases; the lungs are the only site involved in less than 10 percent (807).

Clinical Features. Most patients are young men; the male to female ratio ranges from 2:1 to 9:1. ABMABD can occur in children or adults, but the mean age is 35 years (807). There is a bimodal distribution: most patients are young Caucasian men presenting with lung and renal disease (807); however, ABMABD also presents in elderly women who have mostly renal disease. Hemoptysis is the primary presenting pulmonary manifestation (807). Iron deficiency anemia may be seen in patients with persistent pulmonary hemorrhage. The diagnosis is made on the basis of a kidney or pulmonary biopsy or serologic demonstration of circulating ABMAs. Approximately one third of patients have positive serum ANCAs with either the C- or the P- pattern (807).

Other presenting signs and symptoms include cough, dyspnea, hematuria, fever, and a recent viral illness (841). Hemoptysis occurs in 80 to 90 percent of patients and can range from mild to life-threatening. The most common physical finding is pallor due to anemia. Chest examination may show crackles or rhonchi in 30 to 50 percent of patients (841).

Azotemia is often present and urinalysis reveals hematuria, proteinuria, and granular casts (841). More than 90 percent of patients with ABMABD have antiglomerular basement membrane (GBM) antibodies, the initial level of which often correlates with the severity of the renal morphologic changes. Circulating anti-GBM antibodies may disappear in successfully treated patients. The chest radiograph typically shows bilateral, symmetric, alveolar-filling opacities in the middle and lower lung zones. Acute alveolar hemorrhage is associated with hypoxemia, respiratory alkalosis, and an increased DLCO. The opacities usually resolve over 2 to 3 weeks once the hemorrhage stops.

Radiologic Findings. The radiographic abnormalities are similar to those of other DAH syndromes: bilateral areas of consolidation which may be patchy in distribution or diffuse (see fig. 3-142) (815,837).

Pathologic Findings. Lung biopsies show extensive intra-alveolar hemorrhage with accumulation of red blood cells and/or hemosiderin-laden macrophages (fig. 3-154). Neutrophilic capillaritis may also be seen, although it is usually not extensive (832,847). The alveolar septa can be mildly thickened by interstitial fibrosis and hyperplasia of type 2 pneumocytes (fig. 3-155). Inconspicuous venular inflammation may be present, but florid vasculitis is absent. Alveolar damage in the form of hyaline membranes, type 2 pneumocyte hyperplasia, and in-

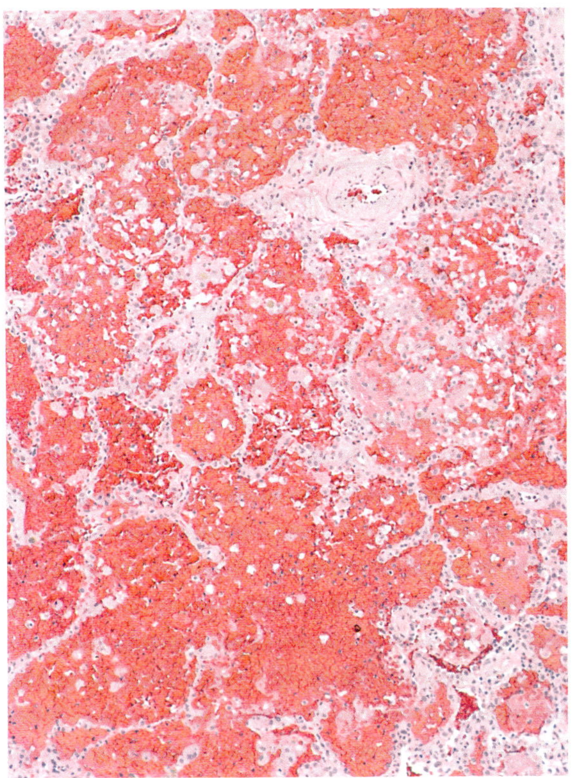

Figure 3-154

GOODPASTURE'S SYNDROME

There is extensive acute hemorrhage with focal interstitial thickening.

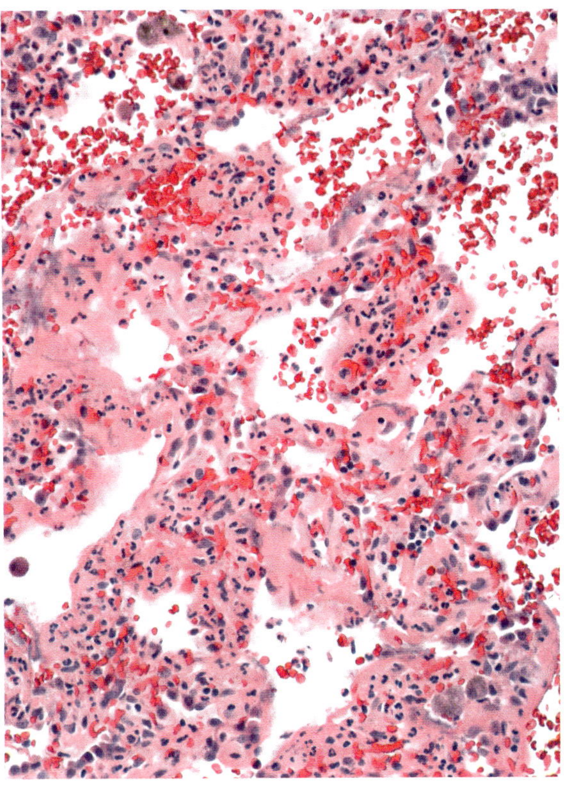

Figure 3-155

GOODPASTURE'S SYNDROME

In addition to acute hemorrhage, there is interstitial thickening and pneumocyte hyperplasia.

terstitial thickening by loose connective tissue is present focally in most cases and on rare occasion may be the dominant lesion with only focal hemorrhage (832). Linear deposition of IgG and complement can be demonstrated in the basement membranes of the alveoli or glomeruli by immunofluorescence.

Pathogenesis. Recent data have shown that the antibodies of ABMABD are directed against the noncollagenous domain of the alpha 3 chain of type IV collagen (829,831). Although it is not known what initiates ABMABD, associations with influenza A and exposure to volatile hydrocarbons, chlorine gas, and hard metal dust have been reported. Genetic factors may also play a role since ABMABD is reported in siblings, cousins, and identical twins. Almost 90 percent of patients have HLA-DR2 (807).

Treatment and Prognosis. Therapy for patients with ABMABD consists of a combination of plasmapheresis to remove the circulating antibodies and immunosuppressive medication including corticosteroids and cytotoxic drugs. Patients who develop endstage renal disease may need renal transplantation (807).

Idiopathic Pulmonary Hemorrhage

Definition. Idiopathic pulmonary hemorrhage (IPH), also known as *idiopathic pulmonary hemosiderosis,* lacks renal involvement, immune complexes, ANCAs, and ABMAs (817,836).

Clinical Features. IPH primarily affects children, however, 20 percent of patients are adults who are usually less than 30 years of age (817, 830,836). There is a 2 to 1 male predominance in adults, but an equal sex distribution in children. The patients present with cough (with or without hemoptysis), dyspnea, substernal chest pain, and fatigue due to iron-deficiency anemia. Episodes of pulmonary hemorrhage are recurrent

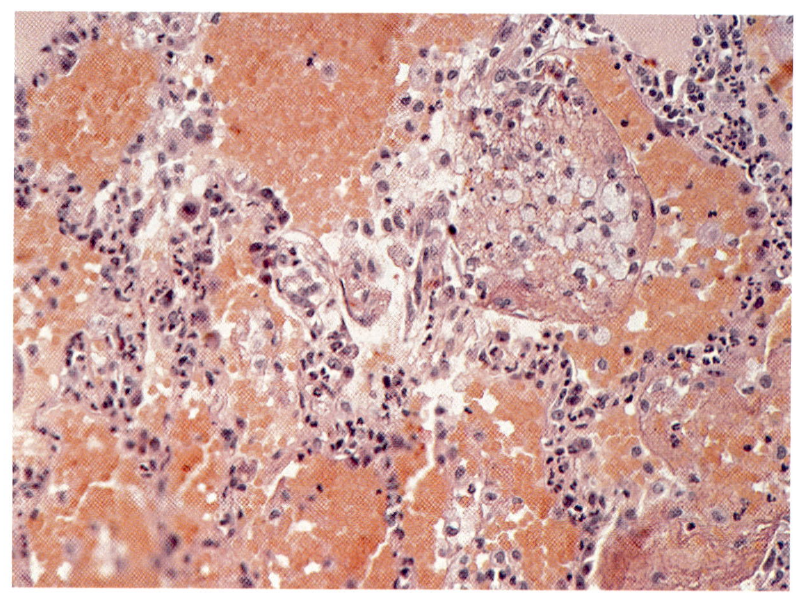

Figure 3-156

IDIOPATHIC PULMONARY HEMORRHAGE

There is acute and chronic hemorrhage with intra-alveolar accumulation of both red blood cells and hemosiderin-laden macrophages. In addition there is mild neutrophilic capillaritis.

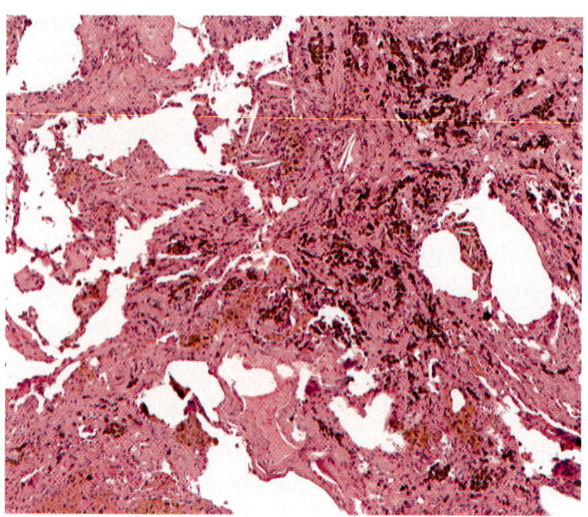

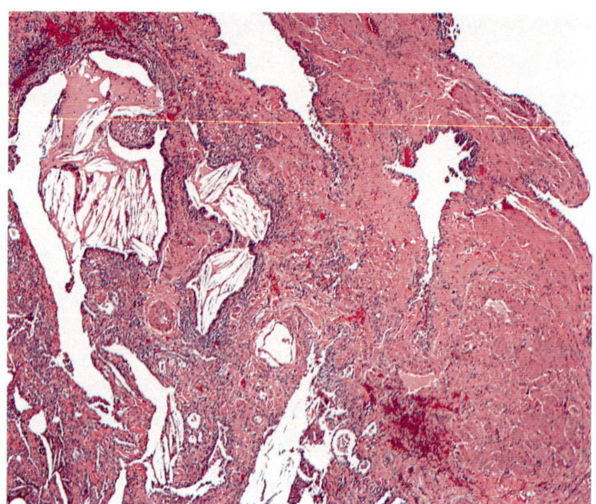

Figure 3-157

IDIOPATHIC PULMONARY HEMORRHAGE WITH FIBROSIS

Left: There are extensive interstitial deposits of hemosiderin granules associated with fibrosis. Right: Elsewhere in this same lung biopsy there is severe fibrosis with honeycomb change.

and intermittent (817,836). Rarely, IPH is associated with celiac disease (830,839).

Radiologic Findings. The radiographic abnormalities are similar to those of other DAH syndromes: bilateral areas of consolidation which may be patchy in distribution or diffuse (815,837).

Histologic Findings. Microscopically, IPH shows diffuse intra-alveolar red blood cell and/or hemosiderin-laden macrophage accumulation (see figs. 3-145, 3-156). Patients with chronic long-term pulmonary hemorrhage may develop interstitial fibrosis (fig. 3-157) (814). Neutrophilic capillaritis is also seen (fig. 3-156), but is uncommon and tends not to be severe (847).

Treatment and Prognosis. The response to corticosteroids is variable. The mean survival period is 3 to 5 years (841). One fourth of patients die rapidly of massive hemorrhage. Another fourth have persistent, active disease with repeated episodes of hemoptysis resulting in interstitial fibrosis and cor pulmonale. Another fourth have inactive disease, but persistent dyspnea and anemia. The remaining patients recover completely without recurrence (841). Hypersensitivity to cow's milk in infants and children generally younger than 2 years of age can result in diffuse pulmonary hemorrhage similar to IPH (841). This condition improves after removal of milk from the diet.

ASPIRATION

Definition. Aspiration results from the inhalation of particulate matter, fluids, or secretions from the stomach, esophagus, oral and nasal cavities, or the oropharynx into the lungs. Aspiration pneumonia is the pathologic consequence of the abnormal entry of this material into the lower airways.

Aspiration is a common event in children and adults. However, the volume is usually small and the normal body defenses (glottic closure, cough reflex, and other clearing mechanisms) are adequate to clear the inoculum without any clinical sequelae. Pathologic consequences leading to aspiration pneumonia occur when there has been a failure of these usual defenses and when the aspirated inoculum produces a direct toxic effect (chemical pneumonitis), stimulates an inflammatory process from a large enough bacterial inoculum (bacterial infection), or obstructs the airway due to the large volume of material or particulate matter that was aspirated (airway obstruction) (854,855,857,900).

Aspiration into the lower respiratory tract can cause a wide variety of effects ranging from airway obstruction to bronchiolitis obliterans, acute pneumonia, organizing pneumonia, abscess formation, and interstitial fibrosis (868, 882). Most community-acquired pneumonias arise following the subtle "aspiration" of highly virulent microorganisms (such as *Streptococcus pneumoniae, Haemophilus influenzae,* Gram-negative bacilli, and *Staphylococcus aureus*) from the oral cavity or nasopharynx into the lower respiratory tract. Therefore, by convention, the term aspiration pneumonia is reserved for pneumonitis that results from less virulent bacteria, primarily anaerobes, which are common constituents of the normal flora, in a susceptible host prone to aspiration, usually in the presence of altered clearance defenses (854).

Aspiration in adults occurs mostly in patients with the following abnormalities: impaired consciousness, usually due to anesthesia, alcohol, or drugs; dysphagia from neurologic disorders; upper gastrointestinal tract abnormalities including esophageal disease, surgery involving the upper airways or esophagus, and gastric reflux; mechanical disruption of the glottic closure or cardiac sphincter due to tracheostomy, endotracheal intubation, bronchoscopy, upper endoscopy, and nasogastric feeding; and miscellaneous conditions such as protracted vomiting, large volume tube feedings, feeding gastrostomy, and the recumbent position (854,862,863,865).

Clinical Features. The clinical manifestations of aspiration depend on the type of aspiration (868). The four major aspiration syndromes are bacterial infection, chemical pneumonitis, airway obstruction, and lipoid pneumonia.

Bacterial Infection. If aspiration results in patients with acute pneumonia or abscess, the usual pathogens are the anaerobic bacteria that colonize the oropharynx (see chapter 12). The onset and progression may be insidious, with symptoms such as fever, cough, shortness of breath, and purulent sputum, which evolve over a period of several days or weeks instead of hours. Many patients have accompanying weight loss and anemia (854). Rigors and shaking chills are commonly absent. Lung abscess, necrotizing pneumonia, or empyema secondary to a bronchopleural fistula are later stages of untreated aspiration pneumonia (854). The presence of putrid discharge in sputum or pleural fluid is regarded as diagnostic of anaerobic infection.

Chemical Pneumonitis. When the aspirated material is directly toxic to the lung it can lead to an acute illness in which the patient presents with acute shortness of breath, tachypnea, and tachycardia. The classic description is that following the aspiration of a large volume of acidic (pH less than 2.5) gastric secretions (*Mendelson's syndrome*) (885). Common associated signs and symptoms include: cyanosis, bronchospasm, fever, and pink and frothy sputum. Hypoxemia is common, with normal or low partial pressure of carbon dioxide (PCO_2) and respiratory alkalosis. Factors that contribute to hypoxemia include pulmonary edema, reduced surfactant activity, reflex airway closure, alveolar hemorrhage, and hyaline membrane formation. Pulmonary function tests may show decreased compliance, abnormal ventilation-perfusion, and reduced diffusing capacity (854).

Airway Obstruction. Inhalation of foreign objects occurs mostly in children and consists of items such as peanuts, other vegetable particles, inorganic materials, beads, teeth, or pieces of toys (890). Large objects may be lodge in the larynx or trachea and lead to sudden respiratory distress, cyanosis, and aphonia; this can quickly cause death if the obstruction is not immediately reversed ("cafe coronary syndrome"). Since the right mainstem bronchus has a straighter branch off the trachea than the left, large aspirated objects tend to lodge on the right side and smaller objects are found most often in the right basilar bronchi (862,868,890). Smaller particles and liquids may reach the smaller airways or alveolar spaces. In such cases, the materials elicit a histologic reaction such as bronchopneumonia or DAD. These patients often present with an irritating cough, unilateral wheezing, or recurrent pneumonia distal to the obstruction, usually in the same segment (854).

Lipoid Pneumonia and Chronic Fibrosis. Gastroesophageal reflux with aspiration is frequently considered in the differential diagnosis of recurrent pneumonia or atypical, diffuse interstitial opacities (851,861,862). Exogenous lipoid pneumonia is an uncommon finding secondary to the aspiration or inhalation of fat-like material of animal, vegetable, or mineral origin (850,856, 869,870,872,873,897,899). Mineral oil is the most common irritant because it can inhibit the cough reflex and ciliary motility, thus facilitating "silent" inhalation (872). In a recent retrospective study in France (872), fever (39 percent), weight loss (34 percent), cough (64 percent), dyspnea (50 percent), and crepitations (45 percent) were the most frequent symptoms and signs identified in patients with lipoid pneumonia. In many patients (41 percent), the finding was incidental. Lung function is normal or may show a restrictive pattern. The DCLO is frequently reduced (872).

When chronic aspiration is suspected, BAL should be performed in the area of greatest radiographic abnormality (usually the dependent lung zones) (875). The cellularity of the BAL fluid is often quite high and the differential reveals nonspecific increases in lymphocytes, eosinophils, and macrophages. BAL cellular analysis in 39 patients with exogenous lipoid pneumonia showed: 23 percent had an isolated lymphocytic alveolitis; 14 percent had isolated neutrophilic lavage; and 31 percent had a mixed alveolitis (lymphocytic and neutrophilic) (872). However, the most important diagnostic finding is the presence of large numbers of lipid-laden macrophages, which is suggestive of chronic aspiration or lipoid pneumonia (861). Marked vacuolization of the alveolar macrophages is appreciated on routine modified Wright's staining; fat staining with oil red O or Sudan black demonstrates the lipid nature of the vacuoles (861). Multinucleated giant cells may be recovered in the BAL specimen and frequently contain lipid droplets within their cytoplasm (876,888,893).

Radiologic Findings. The radiologic manifestations are influenced by the type and severity of aspiration (880). Aspiration of sterile gastric secretions at a low pH results in patchy areas of airspace consolidation involving mainly the dependent regions (fig. 3-158). Because the aspiration usually occurs with the subject supine, the consolidation tends to involve mainly the posterior segments of the upper lobes or the superior segments of the lower lobes (886). Aspiration of large amounts of gastric secretions results in extensive bilateral consolidation similar to that seen in ARDS. A similar appearance is seen in aspiration of large amounts of water (near-drowning). If aspiration results in acute bronchopneumonia or abscess formation, the radiologic manifestations may reflect features characteristic of these disorders as reviewed in chapter 12.

Aspiration of lipid (lipoid pneumonia) can result in a variety of patterns, depending on the amount of aspirated substance (867,877–879). Acute aspiration of large amounts of oil, as seen with aspiration of shark liver oil, can result in extensive ground-glass opacities or areas of consolidation. These areas may have CT attenuation values lower than those of soft tissue but greater than fat (877,879). Repeated aspiration of small amounts of lipid, as typically seen with chronic aspiration of mineral oil, can result in focal or multifocal consolidation or a mass-like lesion that often contains localized areas of fat attenuation evident on HRCT (fig. 3-159) (877, 879). Patients with lipoid

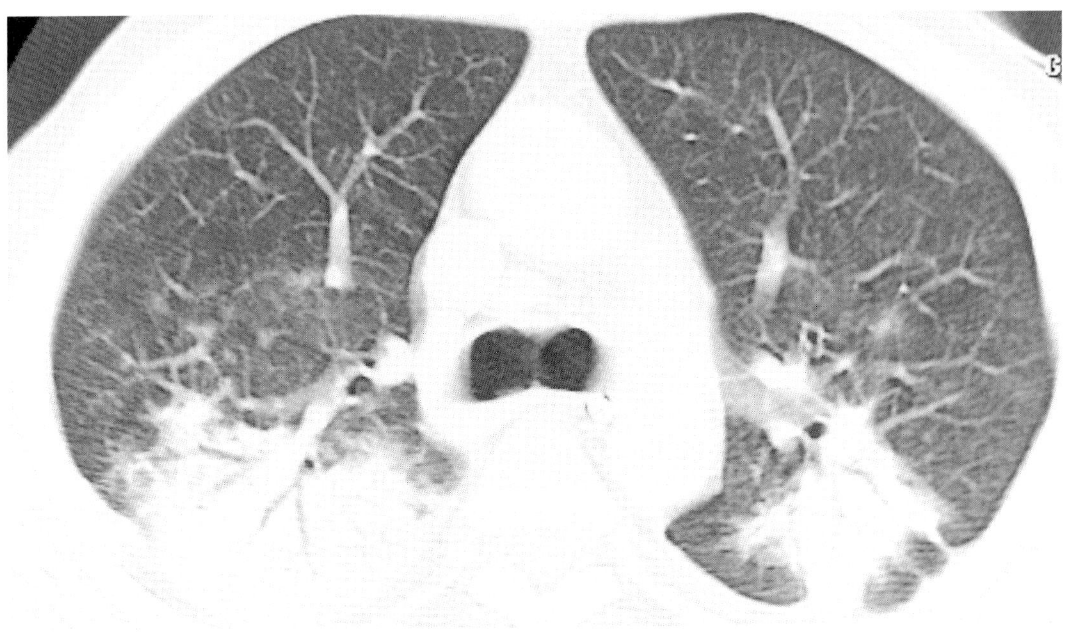

Figure 13-158

ASPIRATION OF GASTRIC SECRETIONS

Chest CT demonstrates bilateral areas of consolidation involving the dependent regions of the upper lobes. The patient had repeated episodes of aspiration following cervical spinal cord injury.

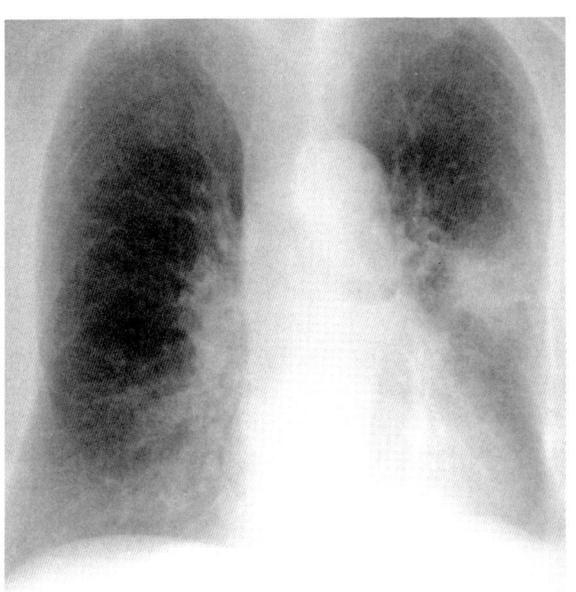

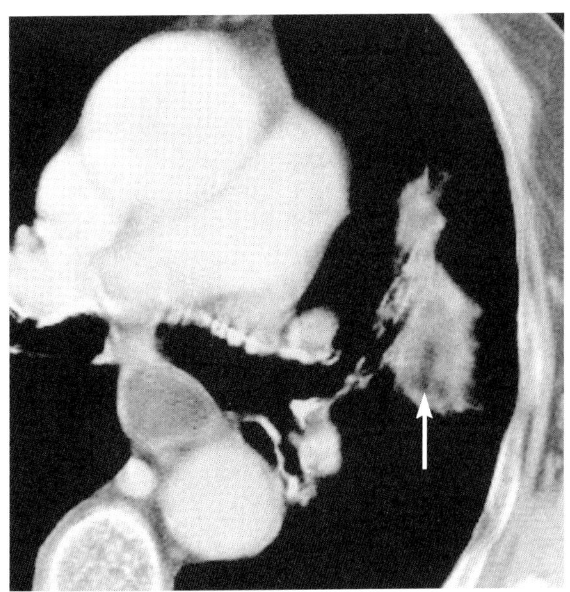

Figure 3-159

LIPOID PNEUMONIA

Left: Chest radiograph shows focal consolidation in the left upper lobe and lingula, and areas of scarring in the left lower lobe.

Right: Chest CT demonstrates focal fat attenuation (arrow) in the consolidation, consistent with lipoid pneumonia. The diagnosis was confirmed by fine-needle aspiration biopsy. The patient was an 81-year-old woman who developed lipoid pneumonia due to long-term intake and repeated aspiration of mineral oil.

pneumonia due to mineral oil aspiration may present with a lung mass that resembles lung cancer (874,880,891). This is frequently associated with aspiration of mineral oil–based laxatives in the elderly. The pattern of crazy paving, consisting of ground-glass consolidation with septal lines, may also be seen (867,877,878).

The aspiration of vegetable materials, including peanuts, is problematic because these substances are not visualized on chest radiography. The chest radiograph may show atelectasis or obstructive emphysema, with a cardiac shift and elevated diaphragm (best seen with an expiratory radiograph). Aspiration of leguminous vegetables can cause a granulomatous pneumonitis known as "lentil aspiration pneumonia" that manifests on radiologic studies with small, poorly defined nodular opacities or some nodules that are large and simulate metastases (883).

Pathologic Findings. *Bacterial Infection.* The pathologic features are described in chapter 12.

Chemical Pneumonitis. Acute aspiration of gastric acid (Mendelson's syndrome) results in pulmonary edema, hemorrhage, and diffuse alveolar damage (857,862,900). Patients with chronic aspiration of gastric secretions who recover from an acute aspiration episode may develop nonspecific pulmonary fibrosis (884).

Hydrocarbons such as kerosene or turpentine may cause congestion, hemorrhage, DAD, or bronchopneumonia.

Airway Obstruction. Foreign objects may be identified within large airways, but in most cases these are removed bronchoscopically. If the obstruction has been prolonged there may be a postobstructive pneumonia distal to the foreign object. If smaller materials have been aspirated, the gross specimen may show a pattern of bronchopneumonia or abscess formation. Only small aspirated particles that reach the bronchioles or alveoli are seen by histologic exam.

Certain aspirated substances such as vegetables (fig. 3-160), lentils (fig. 3-161), or meat (fig. 3-162) have a distinctive appearance (860,862). In the acute phase, the inflammatory reaction may consist of many neutrophils and an acute bronchopneumonia. In the chronic phase, the reaction may consist of lymphocytes, histiocytes, and a foreign body reaction (862). An organizing pneumonia pattern may be seen with chronic aspiration. This may mimic the histologic pattern associated with COP or BOOP (fig. 3-163). Polarization microscopy may be helpful in identifying aspirated foreign particles (fig. 3-163, right) (862).

Lipoid Pneumonia. Lipoid pneumonia due to aspiration of exogenous mineral oil may grossly cause an irregular, firm, yellow consolidation (fig. 3-164) (862). Histologically, the lung shows multiple cystic spaces surrounded by varying amounts of histiocytic infiltration or fibrosis (fig. 3-165). The empty cystic spaces represent lipid vacuoles that washed out during processing. The histiocytes may be finely vacuolated or may form multinucleated giant cells. Histologic examination can also show a granulomatous form of inflammatory reaction suggesting a foreign body reaction (862,870,872).

Unusual aspirated substances include kayexalate or sodium polystyrene sulfonate (fig. 3-166), barium (fig. 3-167), and charcoal (fig. 3-168). In kayexalate aspiration, there is little tissue reaction to the foreign material, which appears as basophilic, irregular, sharply angulated particles of varying size (fig. 3-166) (866, 887). The particles have parallel laminations, which probably represent artifact due to sectioning. In barium aspiration, multiple, irregular, polarizable crystals are found within the interstitium and alveolar spaces (fig. 3-167) (871,881,889,892). In chronic cases, the inflammatory reaction may consist only of histiocytes and a minimal lymphocytic infiltrate. In charcoal aspiration, multiple, large, black, irregular-sized particles are found within bronchioles and the adjacent alveolar spaces (864). There is an associated inflammatory reaction, which in chronic cases consists mostly of a histiocytic infiltrate with foreign body giant cells ingesting the charcoal particles (fig. 3-168).

Differential Diagnosis. Some types of aspiration reaction can be confused with other lesions. Exogenous lipoid pneumonia must be separated from endogenous lipoid pneumonia and pseudolipoid pneumonia. Endogenous lipoid pneumonia consists of an intra-alveolar accumulation of foamy macrophages and is sometimes associated with cholesterol clefts. This is typically seen in the setting of proximal or distal airway obstruction and does not show the rounded empty tissue spaces, association with fibrosis, and foreign body giant cell reaction typical of exogenous lipoid pneumonia.

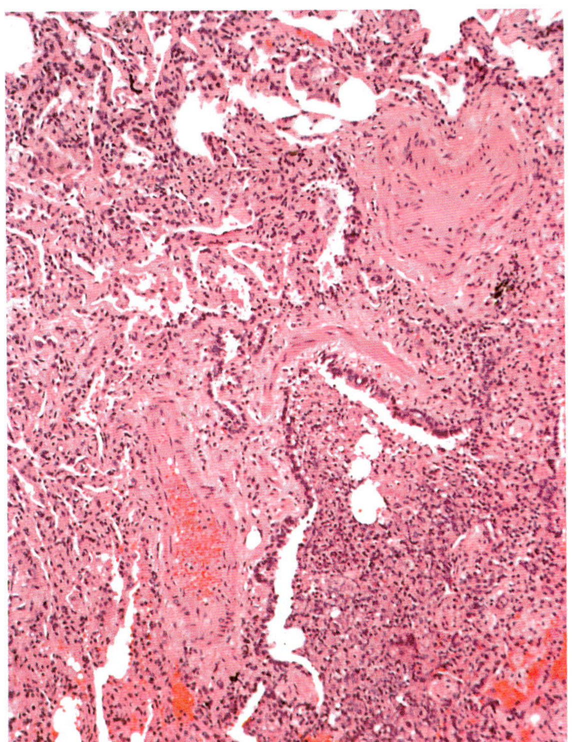

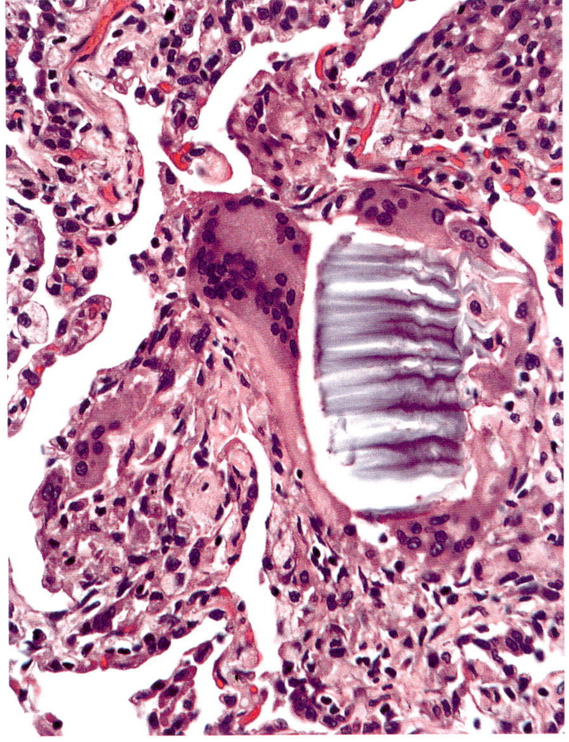

Figure 3-160

ACUTE ASPIRATION PNEUMONIA WITH VEGETABLE FIBERS

Left: Marked acute inflammation involves this bronchiole and the surrounding alveolar spaces. Right: Higher power magnification shows a vegetable fiber surrounded by a giant cell reaction.

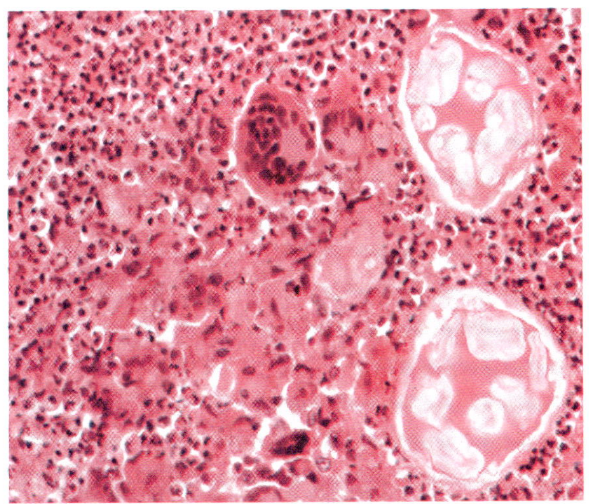

Figure 3-161

PNEUMONIA DUE TO ASPIRATION OF LENTILS

The rounded vegetable particles resemble lentils. They are surrounded by a marked acute inflammatory and giant cell reaction.

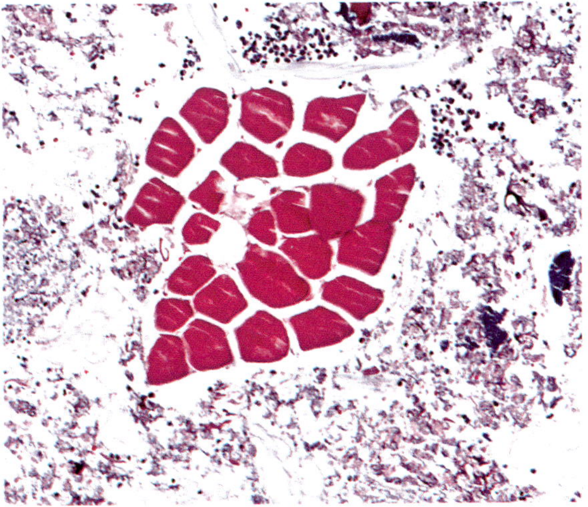

Figure 3-162

ASPIRATED MEAT WITH SKELETAL MUSCLE FIBERS

Within this bronchiole is a fragment of meat with skeletal muscle fibers. The surrounding acute inflammation was associated with *Klebsiella* pneumonia.

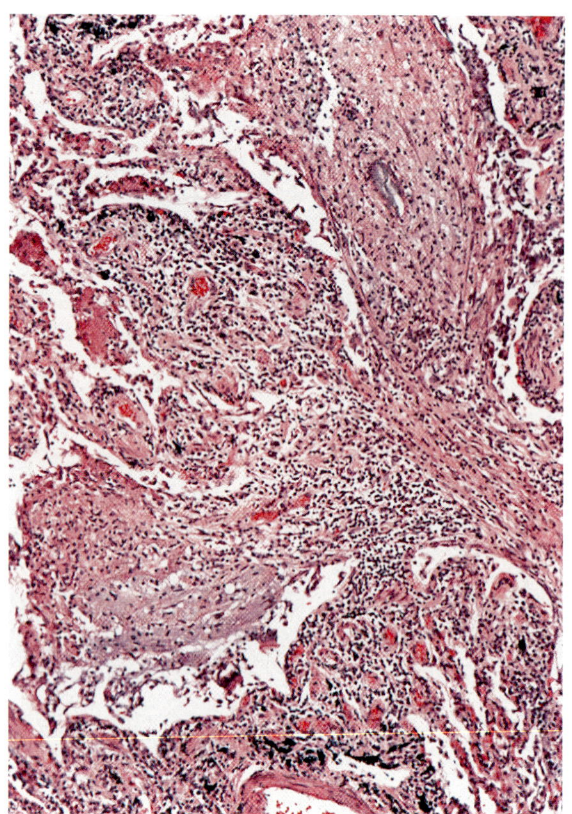

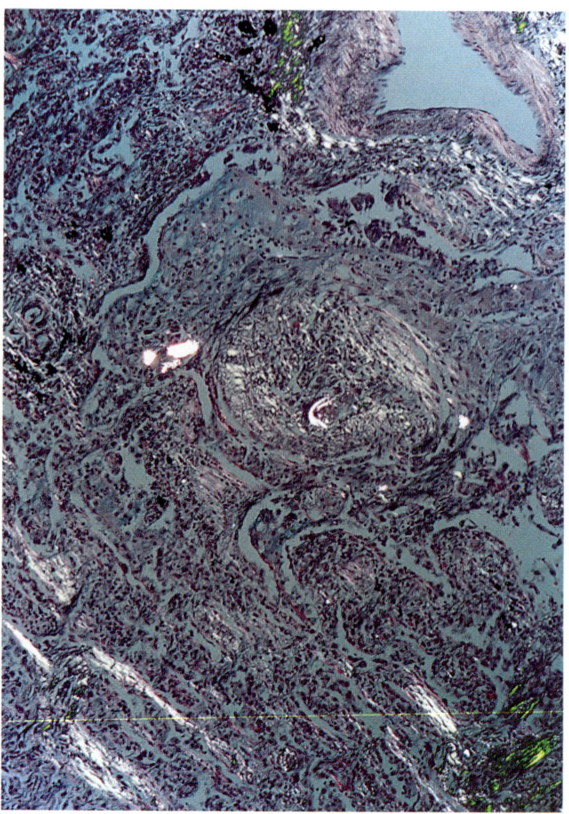

Figure 3-163

ORGANIZING PNEUMONIA WITH ASPIRATED FOREIGN MATERIAL

Left: This organizing pneumonia pattern was originally called bronchiolitis obliterans organizing pneumonia. Several crystalline particles are present within the organizing connective tissue.

Right: Polarizing microscopy highlights the multiple birefringent particles within airspaces, consistent with aspiration.

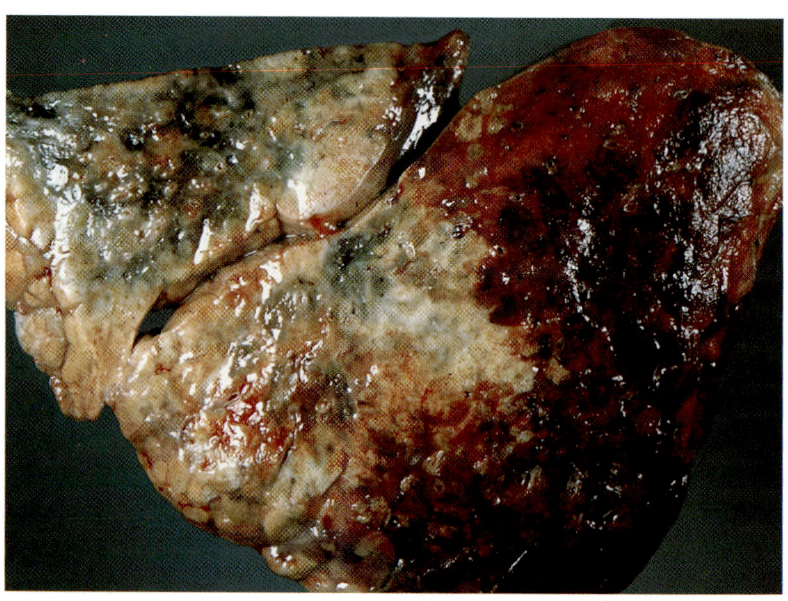

Figure 3-164

LIPOID PNEUMONIA: GROSS SPECIMEN

The lung parenchyma shows an extensive area of yellow, firm consolidation with irregular borders.

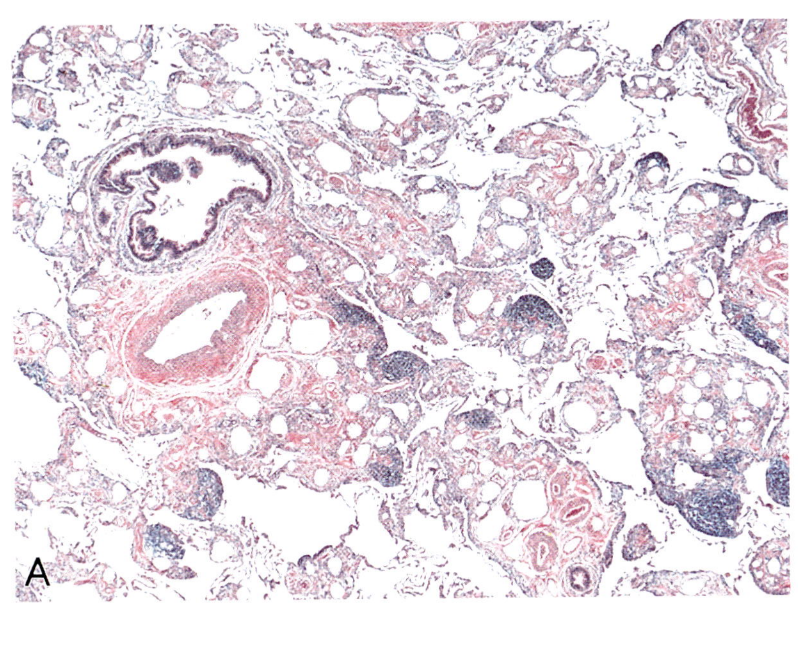

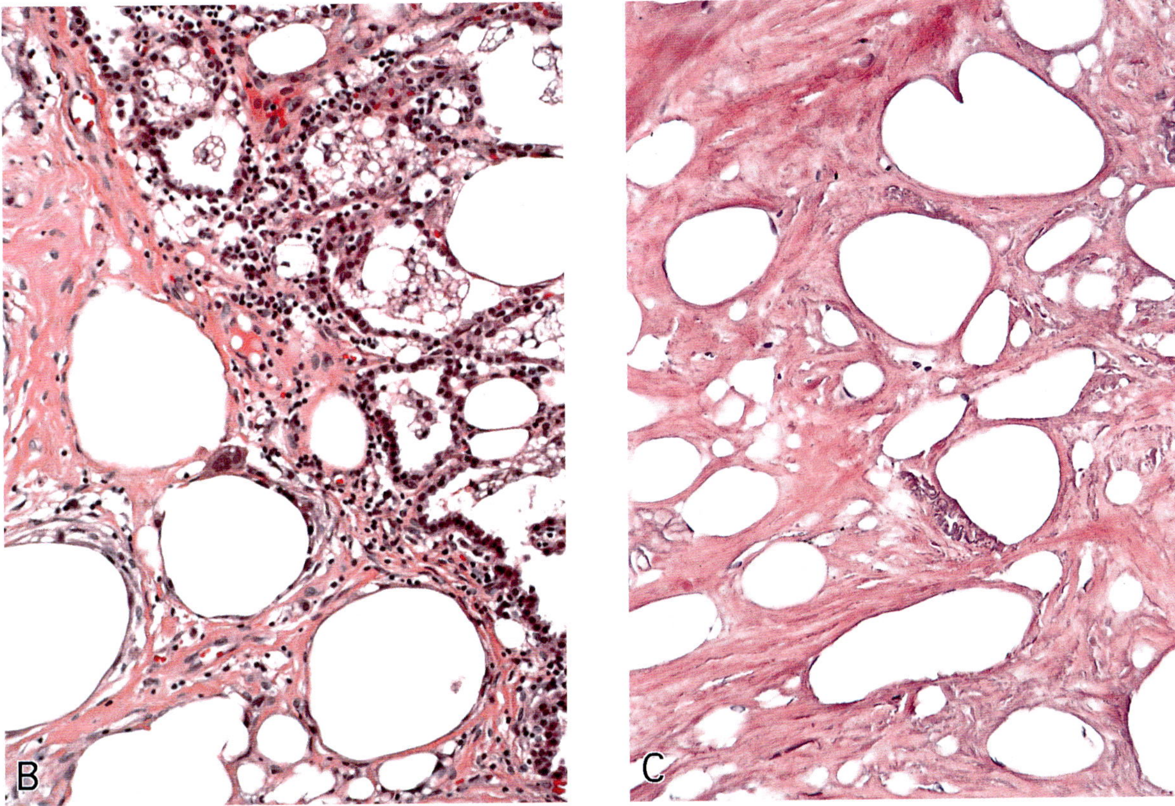

Figure 3-165

LIPOID PNEUMONIA: HISTOLOGY

A: The lung is diffusely altered by numerous round to oval vacuolar spaces.

B: These spaces are surrounded by fibrosis and histiocytes, some of which are finely vacuolated.

C: This area shows only interstitial fibrosis surrounding the vacuolar spaces.

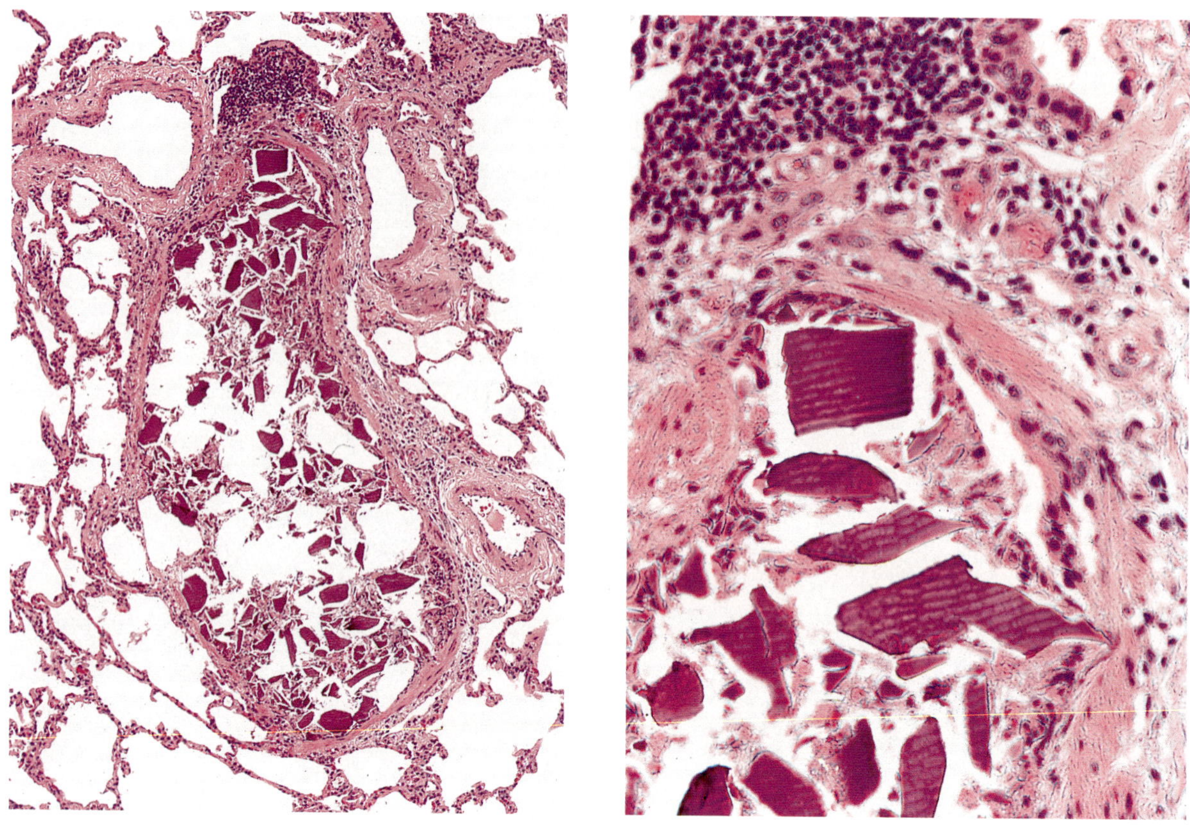

Figure 3-166

KAYEXALATE ASPIRATION

Left: Within the bronchiole are numerous basophilic, irregular, sharply angulated particles of varying size. Right: The particles have parallel laminations, which probably represent artifact due to sectioning.

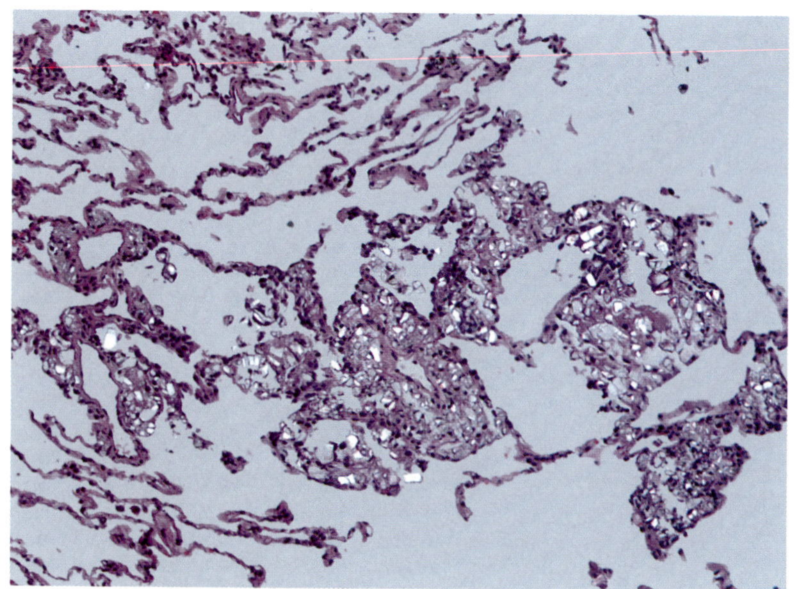

Figure 3-167

BARIUM ASPIRATION

Numerous polarizable, crystalline particles are present within the interstitium. There is little inflammatory reaction.

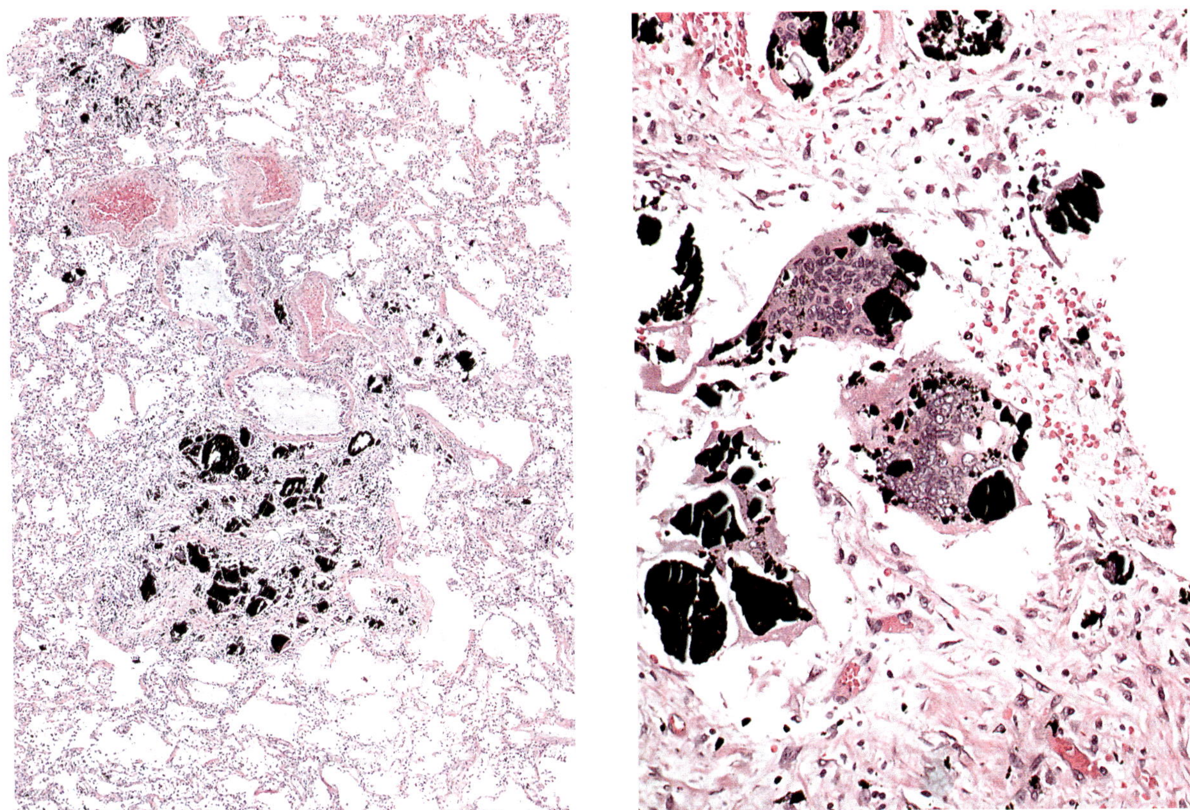

Figure 3-168

CHARCOAL ASPIRATION

Left: Within the bronchiole and surrounding spaces are multiple black particles.
Right: The black particles are associated with foreign body giant cells.

Pseudolipoid pneumonia is an air-bubble artifact associated with the collapse of airspaces (see fig. 2-2). Another potential problem is the endogenous calcium oxalate crystals seen in granulomas of sarcoid (see fig. 3-84) since these can be mistaken for aspirated foreign material.

Treatment and Prognosis. Mortality is high in patients with acute aspiration of gastric acid (30 to 50 percent). There can be rapid improvement, with clearing of the chest radiograph in some patients (up to 62 percent of cases); others develop acute lung injury and progress to ARDS (approximately 12 percent). In about a quarter of patients there is initial rapid clinical improvement, followed by the appearance of new or expanding opacities on chest radiograph which probably represent secondary bacterial infection (854,857). In patients with chemical pneumonitis, the most appropriate therapy is supportive care, usually with intubation and mechanical ventilation. Tracheal suction should be performed to remove aspirated particulate material if the event is witnessed. Corticosteroids are not helpful and antibiotics should only be given if a secondary infection is suspected or develops. Long-term follow-up of patients who survive severe aspiration pneumonia shows either complete recovery or radiographic evidence of pulmonary fibrosis (854,894,896).

Patients with bacterial infection should be treated with antibiotics directed at the pathogen shown to be the cause of the pneumonia. This may be difficult to determine. Clindamycin is now the preferred drug for anaerobic pulmonary infections (852,853). Alternative regimens include amoxicillin-clavulanate and penicillin combined with metronidazole (never use this drug alone in this setting) (852–854). In patients with airway obstruction, the primary therapeutic modality is extraction of the foreign object, usually with fiberoptic or rigid bronchoscopy (901,902).

The most important treatment of lipoid pneumonia is removal of the offending agent and correction of any underlying defect that may favor aspiration (859,895,899). Oral steroids have resulted in improvement of chest radiographic abnormalities in these patients (859). Diffuse lipoid pneumonia has been successfully managed with prednisone and whole lung lavage (858,898).

ALVEOLAR MICROLITHIASIS

Definition. Alveolar microlithiasis is a very rare idiopathic disorder characterized by intra-alveolar accumulation of calcium phosphate which forms laminated concretions.

Pulmonary alveolar microlithiasis is a rare disease of unknown pathogenesis (912,913,921, 931). Friedrich first described it in 1856 (909, 934). It is characterized by the development of heavily calcified laminar microspheres within the alveolar spaces. These lesions slowly progress, growing to diameters of 0.01 to 3.0 mm, and can fill up large portions of the airspaces. Secondary alveolar wall fibrosis develops and eventually the lungs become rock hard (912,913,921,931).

Clinical Features. Pulmonary alveolar microlithiasis has no particular geographic distribution although many cases have been reported from Turkey (915,918,922,923,934). It has been speculated that the disease may be due to a genetically determined metabolic disorder or acquired defects in calcium and phosphorous metabolism (926). A familial association is seen in about 50 percent of patients, often in siblings, with the remaining cases being sporadic (917,926,930). An autosomal recessive pattern of inheritance has been proposed (914,923).

Alveolar microlithiasis typically manifests in the third to fifth decade, although it can occur in children (912). There is no sex predilection although more women are seen among the familial cases. Most patients are asymptomatic at presentation and the diagnosis is discovered incidentally on a chest radiograph. Dyspnea, cough, and chest pain are the most common symptoms (910,933). Expectorated microliths have been infrequently reported (926). In patients with advanced disease, crackles may be heard on chest examination, and clubbing and signs of cor pulmonale may develop (926).

Serum calcium and phosphate levels are normal. Erythrocytosis may develop in patients with hypoxemia, usually in the late stages of the disease. Lung function is normal in most cases at the time of first recognition (926). In advanced disease, a restrictive ventilatory defect with reduced diffusing capacity may be found.

The diagnosis is established by demonstrating a typical chest radiographic appearance and microliths in sputum (905) or BAL fluid (925). The diagnosis can also be established by transbronchial biopsy or open lung biopsy, or a positive technetium bone scintigraphy scan with heavy uptake of technetium in the lungs (904, 905,933). Hypertrophic pulmonary osteoarthropathy has been reported (908). A variety of associated conditions have been reported including nephrolithiasis (924), renal transplantation (928), lymphocytic interstitial pneumonia (925,927), achalasia (925,929), and hypertrophic pulmonary osteoarthropathy (908).

Because of the miliary pattern often seen on chest radiography, the initial differential diagnosis is frequently with disseminated tuberculosis, fungal infection, sarcoidosis, pneumoconioses, hemosiderosis, amyloidosis, or with other forms of pulmonary calcification and ossification. The latter include metastatic calcification associated with hyperparathyroidism, chronic renal failure, vitamin D intoxication, malignancy (e.g., multiple myeloma); dystrophic calcification associated with healed varicella pneumonia; intra-alveolar ossification found with chronic left heart failure or mitral stenosis; interstitial ossification associated with chronic pneumonia or fibrosis (926).

Radiologic Findings. The characteristic radiographic manifestation consists of sharply defined nodules measuring less than 1 mm in diameter and diffusely distributed throughout both lungs (fig. 3-169) (926). Kerley B lines may occasionally be present (920). The "sandstorm" appearance on the radiograph is virtually diagnostic. The opacities are alveolar in character, often with air bronchograms and radiographic obliteration of the heart borders, pulmonary vessels, and diaphragmatic surfaces (903). Pulmonary hypertension may be seen in late stages of the disease.

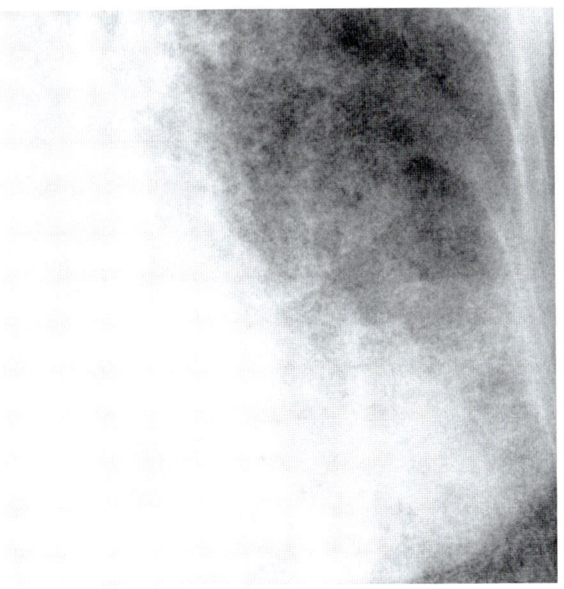

Figure 3-169

ALVEOLAR MICROLITHIASIS

View of the left lower lung from a PA chest radiograph demonstrates numerous sharply defined small nodules. Confluence of the nodules is present in the most dependent lung. (Courtesy of Dr. Jim Barrie, University of Alberta Medical Centre, Canada.)

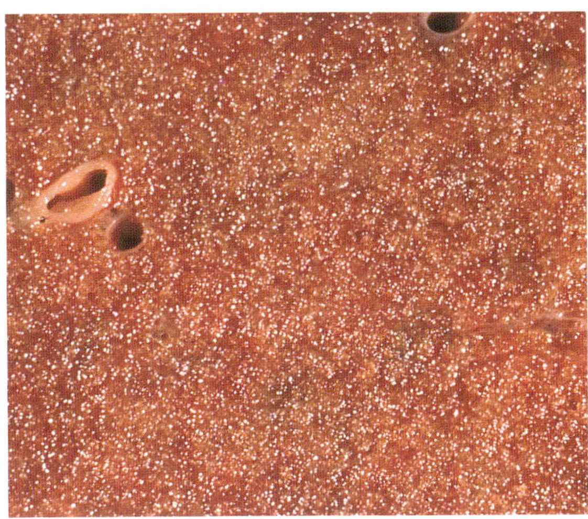

Figure 3-170

ALVEOLAR MICROLITHIASIS

The gross cut surface of the lung shows diffuse granularity due to the numerous microliths.

On HRCT, the tiny calcific nodules tend to be distributed mainly along the cardiac borders and dependent portions of the lower lung zones (906,912,916). HRCT shows that the so-called black pleural line seen on chest radiographs is caused by thin-walled subpleural cysts, ranging from 5 to 10 mm in diameter (916).

Gross Findings. The lungs appear gritty and hard due to the extensive calcospherites within the alveolar spaces (fig. 3-170). This can make the lungs difficult to cut, requiring decalcification procedures. Varying degrees of interstitial fibrosis may be seen (919).

Histologic Findings. The alveoli are filled with calcospherites within alveolar spaces (fig. 3-171). They typically measure 250 to 750 μm in diameter. The concretions have a lamellar appearance and a concentric onion-skin morphology.

The alveolar walls are often histologically normal. In some patients, interstitial fibrosis develops and may appear extensive (919). The diagnosis is established by transbronchial biopsy if the diagnostic lesions of alveolar microliths are seen (904,905,935).

Mineral Analysis. Chemical and X-ray diffraction analyses have shown the intra-alveolar material to represent calcium and phosphorous salts (921). A 2 to 1 calcium to phosphate composition was shown in microliths retrieved by BAL in one case (925).

Differential Diagnosis. The primary differential diagnosis is with corpora amylacea and pulmonary ossification. Corpora amylacea are intra-alveolar lamellar bodies commonly seen in the lungs of older individuals (see fig. 2-6). They are not calcified or ossified although they are birefringent with polarized light. They consist of carbohydrates. Pulmonary ossification consists of spicules of mature bone typically situated within the interstitium. The bone shows osteocytes within lacunar spaces, a feature not seen in alveolar microlithiasis.

Treatment and Prognosis. The clinical course is usually stable although some patients show gradual deterioration. Rapid clinical progression is uncommon. Therapeutic BAL (914,923, 925) and oral administration of disodium etidronate have been used without proven benefit (911,918). Nasal continuous positive airway pressure (nCPAP) and oxygen administration improve the severe pulmonary hypertension and hypoxemia seen in advanced disease by reducing the intrapulmonary shunt. Lung transplantation has been successful in some cases (907,932).

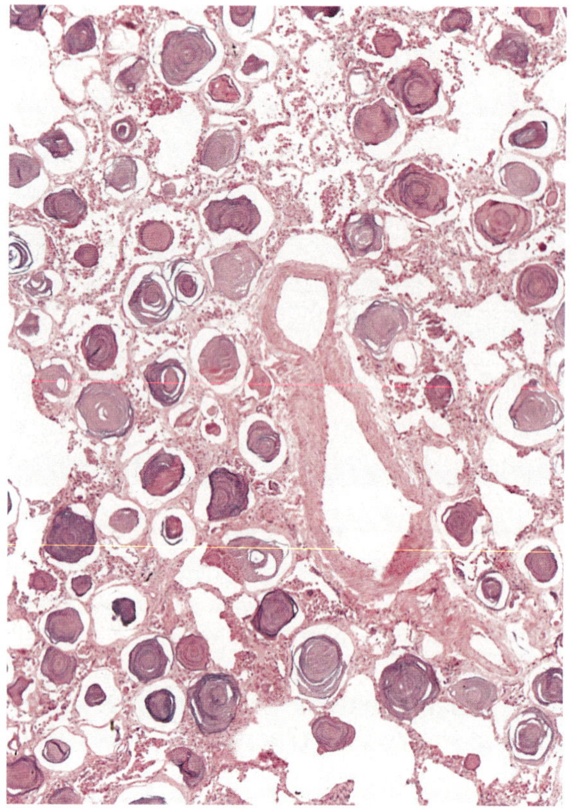

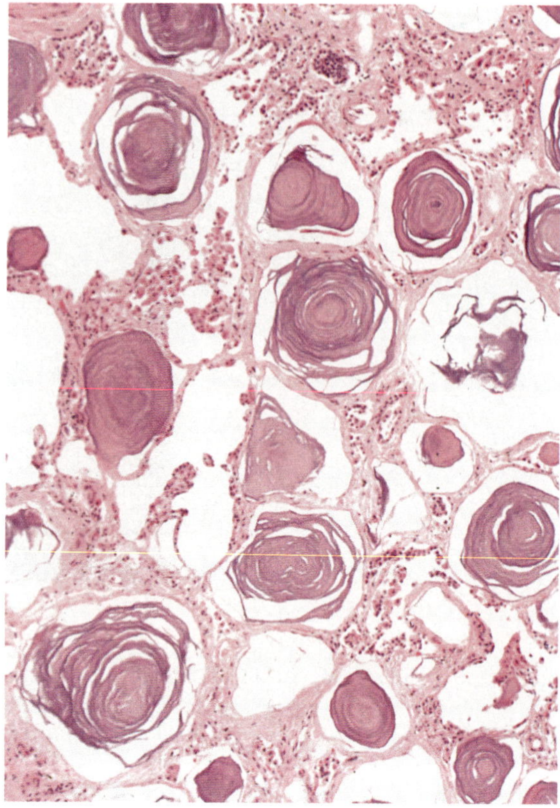

Figure 3-171

ALVEOLAR MICROLITHIASIS

Left: The calcified microliths fill the alveolar spaces.
Right: The microliths are concentrically laminated.

REFERENCES

DPLD: Introduction and Classification

1. American Thoracic Society. Idiopathic pulmonary fibrosis: diagnosis and treatment. Am J Respir Crit Care Med 2000;161:646–64.
2. Anttila S, Sutinen S, Paananen M, et al. Hard metal lung disease: a clinical, histological, ultrastructural and X-ray microanalytical study. Eur J Respir Dis 1986;69:83–94.
3. Arima K, Ando M, Ito K, et al. Effect of cigarette smoking on prevalence of summer-type hypersensitivity pneumonitis caused by Trichosporon cutaneum. Arch Environ Health 1992;47:274–8.
4. Bateman ED, Turner-Warwick M, Haslam PL, Adelmann-Grill BC. Cryptogenic fibrosing alveolitis: prediction of fibrogenic activity from immunohistochemical studies of collagen types in lung biopsy specimens. Thorax 1983;38:93–101.
5. Baumgartner KB, Samet JM, Stidley CA, Colby TV, Waldron JA. Cigarette smoking: a risk factor for idiopathic pulmonary fibrosis. Am J Respir Crit Care Med 1997;155:242–8.
6. Bjoraker JA, Ryu JH, Edwin MK, et al. Prognostic significance of histopathologic subsets in idiopathic pulmonary fibrosis. Am J Respir Crit Care Med 1998;157:199–203.
7. Cantin A, Crystal RG. Interstitial pathology: an overview of the chronic interstitial lung disorders. Int Arch Allergy Appl Immunol 1985;76 [Suppl 1]:83–91.
8. Carrington CB, Gaensler EA. Clinical-pathologic approach to diffuse infiltrative lung disease. In: Thurlbeck WM, Abell MR, eds. The lung: structure, function and disease. Baltimore: Williams and Wilkins; 1978:58–87.

9. Carrington CB, Gaensler EA, Coutu RE, FitzGerald MX, Gupta RG. Natural history and treated course of usual and desquamative interstitial pneumonia. N Engl J Med 1978;298:801–9.
10. Chechani V, Landreneau RJ, Shaikh SS. Open lung biopsy for diffuse infiltrative lung disease. Ann Thorac Surg 1992;54:296–300.
11. Colby TV, Carrington CB. Interstital lung disease. In: Thurlbeck WM, Churg AM, eds. Pathology of the lung, 2nd ed. New York: Thieme Medical Publishers; 1995:589–737.
12. Colby TV, Carrington CB. Lymphoreticular tumors and infiltrates of the lung. Pathol Annu 1983;18[Pt 1]:27–70.
13. Colby TV, Swensen SJ. Anatomic distribution and histopathologic patterns in interstitial lung disease. In: Schwarz MI, King TE Jr, eds. Interstitial lung disease, 3rd ed. Hamilton: BC Decker; 1998:31–50.
14. Coultas DB, Zumwalt RE, Black WC, Sobonya RE. The epidemiology of interstitial lung diseases. Am J Respir Crit Care Med 1994;150:967–72.
15. Crystal RG, Bitterman PB, Rennard SI, Hance AJ, Keogh BA. Interstitial lung diseases of unknown cause. Disorders characterized by chronic inflammation of the lower respiratory tract (first of two parts). N Engl J Med 1984;310:154–66.
16. Crystal RG, Bitterman PB, Rennard SI, Hance AJ, Keogh BA. Interstitial lung diseases of unknown cause. Disorders characterized by chronic inflammation of the lower respiratory tract (second of two parts). N Engl J Med 1984;310:235–44.
17. Crystal RG, Fulmer JD, Roberts WC, Moss ML, Line BR, Reynolds HY. Idiopathic pulmonary fibrosis. Clinical, histologic, radiographic, physiologic, scintigraphic, cytologic, and biochemical aspects. Ann Intern Med 1976; 85:769–88.
18. Davison AG, Heard BE, McAllister WA, Turner-Warwick ME. Cryptogenic organizing pneumonitis. Q J Med 1983;207:382–94.
19. The diagnosis, assessment and treatment of diffuse parenchymal lung disease in adults. Thorax 1999;54:S1–14.
20. Epler GR, Colby TV, McLoud TC, Carrington CB, Gaensler EA. Bronchiolitis obliterans organizing pneumonia. N Engl J Med 1985;312: 152–8.
21. Erbes R, Schaberg T, Loddenkemper R. Lung function tests in patients with idiopathic pulmonary fibrosis. Are they helpful for predicting outcome? Chest 1997;111:51–7.
22. Flaherty KR, Martinez FJ. The role of pulmonary function testing in pulmonary fibrosis. Curr Opin Pulm Med 2000;6:404–10.
23. Flaherty KR, Travis WD, Colby TV, et al. Histological variability in patients with suspected idiopathic pulmonary fibrosis. Am J Respir Crit Care Med 2001:164:1722–7.
24. Hance AJ, Basset F, Saumon G, et al. Smoking and interstitial lung disease. The effect of cigarette smoking on the incidence of pulmonary histiocytosis X and sarcoidosis. Ann N Y Acad Sci 1986;465:643–56.
25. Hartman TE, Primack SL, Kang EY, et al. Disease progression in usual interstitial pneumonia compared with desquamative interstitial pneumonia. Assessment with serial CT. Chest 1996;110:378–82.
26. Haviv YS, Breuer R, Sviri S, Libson E, Safadi R. CT-guided biopsy of peripheral lung lesions associated with BOOP. Eur J Med Res 1997;2:44–6.
27. Hunninghake GW, Costabel U, Ando M, et al. ATS/ERS/WASOG statement on sarcoidosis. American Thoracic Society/European Respiratory Society/World Association of Sarcoidosis and other Granulomatous Disorders. Sarcoidosis Vasc Diffuse Lung Dis 1999;16:149–73.
28. Johkoh T, Müller NL, Cartier Y, et al. Idiopathic interstitial pneumonias: diagnostic accuracy of thin-section CT in 129 patients. Radiology 1999;211:555–60.
29. Johnston ID, Gomm SA, Kalra S, Woodcock AA, Evans CC, Hind CR. The management of cryptogenic fibrosing alveolitis in three regions of the United Kingdom. Eur Respir J 1993;6:891–3.
30. Johnston ID, Prescott RJ, Chalmers JC, Rudd RM. British Thoracic Society study of cryptogenic fibrosing alveolitis: current presentation and initial management. Fibrosing Alveolitis Subcommittee of the Research Committee of the British Thoracic Society. Thorax 1997;52:38–44.
31. Katzenstein AL. Idiopathic interstitial pneumonia: classification and diagnosis. In: Churg A, Katzenstein AL, eds. The lung. Current concepts. Baltimore: Williams & Wilkins; 1993:1–31.
32. Katzenstein AL, Askin FB. Katzenstein and Askin's surgical pathology of non-neoplastic lung disease, 3rd ed. Philadelphia: WB Saunders; 1997.
33. Katzenstein AL, Askin FB. Surgical pathology of non-neoplastic lung disease. Major Probl Pathol 1982;13:1–430.
34. Katzenstein AL, Askin FB. Surgical pathology of non-neoplastic lung disease, 2nd ed. Philadelphia: WB Saunders; 1990.
35. Katzenstein AL, Fiorelli RF. Nonspecific interstitial pneumonia/fibrosis. Histologic features and clinical significance. Am J Surg Pathol 1994;18:136–47.
36. Katzenstein AL, Myers JL. Idiopathic pulmonary fibrosis: clinical relevance of pathologic classification. Am J Respir Crit Care Med 1998; 157:1301–15.

37. Katzenstein AL, Myers JL, Mazur MT. Acute interstitial pneumonia. A clinicopathologic, ultrastructural, and cell kinetic study. Am J Surg Pathol 1986;10:256–67.
38. Kawakami Y, Munakata M. Interstitial pneumonia—with special reference to idiopathic interstitial pneumonia (IIP). Kokyu To Junkan 1983; 31:867–74.
39. Kilburn KH, Lilis R, Anderson HA, Miller A, Warshaw RH. Interaction of asbestos, age, and cigarette smoking in producing radiographic evidence of diffuse pulmonary fibrosis. Am J Med 1986;80:377–81.
40. King TE Jr. Approaches to the patient with interstitial lung diseases. In: Rose BD, ed.Uptodate in medicine. Wellesley: BDR-Uptodate; 2001.
41. King TE Jr. Connective tissue disease. In: Schwarz MI, King TE Jr, eds. Interstitial lung disease, 3rd ed. Hamilton: BC Decker; 1998:451–506.
42. King TE Jr. Idiopathic pulmonary fibrosis. In: Schwarz MI, King TE Jr, eds. Interstitial lung disease, 3rd ed. Hamilton: BC Decker; 1998:597–644.
43. King TE Jr. The role of lung biopsy in the diagnosis of interstitial lung disease. In: Rose BD, ed. UpToDate in medicine. Wellesley: BDR-UpToDate; 2001.
44. Kitaichi M. Pathologic features and the classification of interstitial pneumonia of unknown etiology. Bull Chest Dis Res Inst Kyoto Univ 1990;23:1–18.
45. Kitaichi M, Nishimura K, Itoh H, Izumi T. Pulmonary lymphangioleiomyomatosis: a report of 46 patients including a clinicopathologic study of prognostic factors. Am J Respir Crit Care Med 1995;151:527–33.
46. Lacronique J, Roth C, Battesti JP, Basset F, Chretien J. Chest radiological features of pulmonary histiocytosis X: a report based on 50 adult cases. Thorax 1982;37:104–9.
47. Liebow AA. Definition and classification of interstitial pneumonias in human pathology. Prog Resp Res 1975;8:1–33.
48. Liebow AA, Carrington CB. The interstitial pneumonias. In: Simon M, Potchen EJ, LeMay M, eds. Frontiers of pulmonary radiology. New York: Grune and Stratton; 1969:102–41.
49. Müller NL, Colby TV. Idiopathic interstitial pneumonias: high-resolution CT and histologic findings. Radiographics 1997;17:1016–22.
50. Müller NL, Guerry-Force ML, Staples CA, et al. Differential diagnosis of bronchiolitis obliterans with organizing pneumonia and usual interstitial pneumonia: clinical, functional, and radiologic findings. Radiology 1987;162:151–6.
51. Nagai S, Kitaichi M, Itoh H, Nishimura K, Izumi T, Colby TV. Idiopathic nonspecific interstitial pneumonia/fibrosis: comparison with idiopathic pulmonary fibrosis and BOOP. Eur Respir J 1998;12:1010–9.
52. Nicholson AG, Colby TV, Dubois RM, Hansell DM, Wells AU. The prognostic significance of the histologic pattern of interstitial pneumonia in patients presenting with the clinical entity of cryptogenic fibrosing alveolitis. Am J Respir Crit Care Med 2000;162:2213–7.
53. Nicholson AG, Wotherspoon AC, Diss TC, et al. Pulmonary B-cell non-Hodgkin's lymphomas. The value of immunohistochemistry and gene analysis in diagnosis. Histopathology 1995;26:395–403.
54. Nishimura K, Izumi T, Kitaichi M, Nagai S, Itoh H. The diagnostic accuracy of high-resolution computed tomography in diffuse infiltrative lung diseases. Chest 1993;104:1149–55.
55. Nishimura K, Kitaichi M, Izumi T, Nagai S, Kanaoka M, Itoh H. Usual interstitial pneumonia: histologic correlation with high-resolution CT. Radiology 1992;182:337–42.
56. Raghu G, Mageto YN. Genetic predisposition of interstitial lung disease. In: Schwarz MI, King TE Jr, eds. Interstitial lung disease, 3rd ed. Hamilton: BC Decker; 1998:119–32.
57. Raghu G, Mageto YN, Lockhart D, Schmidt RA, Wood DE, Godwin JD. The accuracy of the clinical diagnosis of new-onset idiopathic pulmonary fibrosis and other interstitial lung diseases: a prospective study. Chest 1999;116:1168–74.
58. Schwarz MI. Approach to the understanding, diagnosis, and management of interstitial lung disease. In: Schwarz MI, King TE Jr, eds. Interstitial lung disease, 3rd ed. Ontario: BC Decker; 1998:1–30.
59. Selman M, King TE, Pardo A. Idiopathic pulmonary fibrosis: prevailing and evolving hypotheses about its pathogenesis and implications for therapy. Ann Int Med 2001;134:136–51.
60. Travis WD, Colby TV, Corrin B, Shimosato Y, Brambilla E, in collaboration with Sobin LH and pathologists from 14 countries. Histological typing of lung and pleural tumors, 3rd ed. Berlin: Springer-Verlag; 1999.
61. Travis WD, King TE, Bateman ED, et al. ATS/ERS International Multidisciplinary Consensus Classification of Idiopathic Interstitial Pneumonia. Am J Respir Crit Care Med 2002;165:277–304.
62. Travis WD, Matsui K, Moss JE, Ferrans VJ. Idiopathic nonspecific interstitial pneumonia: prognostic significance of cellular and fibrosing patterns. Survival comparison with usual interstitial pneumonia and desquamative interstitial pneumonia. Am J Surg Pathol 2000;24:19–33.
63. Turner-Warwick M. Interstitial lung disease. New York: Thieme-Stratton; 1984.

64. Turner-Warwick M, Burrows B, Johnson A. Cryptogenic fibrosing alveolitis: clinical features and their influence on survival. Thorax 1980;35:171–80.
65. Weiss W. Smoking and pulmonary fibrosis. J Occup Med 1988;30:33–9.
66. World Health Organization. Histological typing of lung tumours. Geneva: World Health Organization; 1967.
67. World Health Organization. Histological typing of lung tumors, 2nd ed. Geneva: World Health Organization; 1981.
68. Yamanaka A, Saiki S, Hebisawa A, et al. Idiopathic interstitial pneumonia (including lymphatic interstitial pneumonia). Nippon Rinsho 1983;41:532–43.
69. Zitnik RJ, Matthay RA. Drug-induced lung disease. In: Schwarz MI, King TE Jr, eds. Interstitial lung disease, 3rd ed. Hamilton: BC Decker; 1998:423–50.

Usual Interstitial Pneumonia

70. Agostini C, Siviero M, Semenzato G. Immune effector cells in idiopathic pulmonary fibrosis. Curr Opin Pulm Med 1997;3:348–55.
71. Akira M, Hamada H, Sakatani M, Kobayashi C, Nishioka M, Yamamoto S. CT findings during phase of accelerated deterioration in patients with idiopathic pulmonary fibrosis. AJR Am J Roentgenol 1997;168:79–83.
72. Akira M, Sakatani M, Ueda E. Idiopathic pulmonary fibrosis: progression of honeycombing at thin-section CT. Radiology 1993;189:687–91.
73. American Thoracic Society. Idiopathic pulmonary fibrosis: diagnosis and treatment. Am J Respir Crit Care Med 2000;161:646–64.
74. Barrios R, Pardo A, Ramos C, Montano M, Ramirez R, Selman M. Upregulation of acidic fibroblast growth factor during development of experimental lung fibrosis. Am J Physiol 1997;273:L451–8
75. Basset F, Ferrans VJ, Soler P, Takemura T, Fukuda Y, Crystal RG. Intraluminal fibrosis in interstitial lung disorders. Am J Pathol 1986;122:443–61.
76. Bateman ED, Turner-Warwick M, Haslam PL, Adelmann-Grill BC. Cryptogenic fibrosing alveolitis: prediction of fibrogenic activity from immunohistochemical studies of collagen types in lung biopsy specimens. Thorax 1983;38:93–101.
77. Baughman RP. Bronchoalveolar lavage. St. Louis: Mosby Year Book; 1992.
78. Baumgartner KB, Samet JM, Coultas DB, et al. Occupational and environmental risk factors for idiopathic pulmonary fibrosis: a multicenter case-control study. Collaborating Centers. Am J Epidemiol 2000;152:307–15.
79. Baumgartner KB, Samet JM, Stidley CA, Colby TV, Waldron JA. Cigarette smoking: a risk factor for idiopathic pulmonary fibrosis. Am J Respir Crit Care Med 1997;155:242–8.
80. Bensadoun ES, Burke AK, Hogg JC, Roberts CR. Proteoglycan deposition in pulmonary fibrosis. Am J Respir Crit Care Med 1996;154:1819–28.
81. Bensard DD, McIntyre RC Jr, Waring BJ, Simon JS. Comparison of video thoracoscopic lung biopsy to open lung biopsy in the diagnosis of interstitial lung disease. Chest 1993;103:765–70.
82. Betsholtz C, Raines EW. Platelet-derived growth factor: a key regulator of connective tissue cells in embryogenesis and pathogenesis. Kidney Int 1997;51:1361–9.
83. Bjoraker JA, Ryu JH, Edwin MK, et al. Prognostic significance of histopathologic subsets in idiopathic pulmonary fibrosis. Am J Respir Crit Care Med 1998;157:199–203.
84. Burkhardt A. Alveolitis and collapse in the pathogenesis of pulmonary fibrosis. Am Rev Respir Dis 1989;140:513–24.
85. Burkhardt A, Cottier H. Cellular events in alveolitis and the evolution of pulmonary fibrosis. Virchows Arch [Cell Pathol] 1989;58:1–13.
86. Carrington CB, Gaensler EA, Coutu RE, FitzGerald MX, Gupta RG. Natural history and treated course of usual and desquamative interstitial pneumonia. N Engl J Med 1978;298:801–9.
87. Cherniack RM, Colby TV, Flint A, et al. Quantitative assessment of lung pathology in idiopathic pulmonary fibrosis. The BAL Cooperative Group Steering Committee. Am Rev Respir Dis 1991;144:892–900.
88. Colby TV, Carrington CB. Interstital lung disease. In: Thurlbeck WM, Churg AM, eds. Pathology of the lung, 2nd ed. New York: Thieme Medical Publishers; 1995:589–737.
89. Coultas DB, Zumwalt RE, Black WC, Sobonya RE. The epidemiology of interstitial lung diseases. Am J Respir Crit Care Med 1994;150:967–72.
90. Davies D, Macfarlane A, Darke CS, Dodge OG. Muscular hyperplasia ("cirrhosis") of the lung and bronchial dilatations as features of chronic diffuse fibrosing alveolitis. Thorax 1966;21:272–89.
91. Douglas WW, Ryu JH, Bjoraker JA, et al. Colchicine versus prednisone as treatment of usual interstitial pneumonia. Mayo Clin Proc 1997;72:201–9.
92. Egan JJ, Stewart JP, Hasleton PS, Arrand JR, Carroll KB, Woodcock AA. Epstein-Barr virus replication within pulmonary epithelial cells in cryptogenic fibrosing alveolitis. Thorax 1995;50:1234–9.

93. Egan JJ, Woodcock AA, Stewart JP. Viruses and idiopathic pulmonary fibrosis. Eur Respir J 1997;10:1433–7.
94. Erbes R, Schaberg T, Loddenkemper R. Lung function tests in patients with idiopathic pulmonary fibrosis. Are they helpful for predicting outcome? Chest 1997;111:51–7.
95. Flaherty KR, Travis WD, Colby TV, et al. Histological variability in patients with suspected idiopathic pulmonary fibrosis. Am J Respir Crit Care Med 2001:164:1722–7.
96. Fulmer JD, Roberts WC, von Gal ER, Crystal RG. Morphologic-physiologic correlates of the severity of fibrosis and degree of cellularity in idiopathic pulmonary fibrosis. J Clin Invest 1979;63:665–76.
97. Fulmer JD, Sposovska MS, von Gal ER, Crystal RG, Mittal KK. Distribution of HLA antigens in idiopathic pulmonary fibrosis. Am Rev Respir Dis 1978;118:141–7.
98. Gay SE, Kazerooni EA, Toews GB, et al. Idiopathic pulmonary fibrosis: predicting response to therapy and survival. Am J Respir Crit Care Med 1998;157:1063–72.
99. Grenier P, Chevret S, Beigelman C, Brauner MW, Chastang C, Valeyre D. Chronic diffuse infiltrative lung disease: determination of the diagnostic value of clinical data, chest radiography, and CT and Bayesian analysis. Radiology 1994;191:383–90.
100. Grossman RF, Frost A, Zamel N, et al. Results of single-lung transplantation for bilateral pulmonary fibrosis. The Toronto Lung Transplant Group. N Engl J Med 1990;322:727–33.
101. Hanley ME, King TE Jr, Schwarz MI, Watters LC, Shen AS, Cherniack RM. The impact of smoking on mechanical properties of the lungs in idiopathic pulmonary fibrosis and sarcoidosis. Am Rev Respir Dis 1991;144:1102–6.
102. Hartman TE, Primack SL, Kang EY, et al. Disease progression in usual interstitial pneumonia compared with desquamative interstitial pneumonia. Assessment with serial CT. Chest 1996;110:378–82.
103. Hayashi T, Stetler-Stevenson WG, Fleming MV, et al. Immunohistochemical study of metalloproteinases and their tissue inhibitors in the lungs of patients with diffuse alveolar damage and idiopathic pulmonary fibrosis. Am J Pathol 1996;149:1241–56.
104. Hogg JC, Hegele RG. Adenovirus and Epstein-Barr virus in lung disease. Semin Respir Infect 1995;10:244–53.
105. Homma S, Nagaoka I, Abe H, et al. Localization of platelet-derived growth factor and insulin-like growth factor I in the fibrotic lung. Am J Respir Crit Care Med 1995;152:2084–9.
106. Hubbard R, Lewis S, Richards K, Johnston I, Britton J. Occupational exposure to metal or wood dust and aetiology of cryptogenic fibrosing alveolitis. Lancet 1996;347:284–9.
107. Iwai K, Mori T, Yamada N, Yamaguchi M, Hosoda Y. Idiopathic pulmonary fibrosis. Epidemiologic approaches to occupational exposure. Am J Respir Crit Care Med 1994;150:670–5.
108. Johkoh T, Müller NL, Cartier Y, et al. Idiopathic interstitial pneumonias: diagnostic accuracy of thin-section CT in 129 patients. Radiology 1999;211:555–60.
109. Johnston ID, Prescott RJ, Chalmers JC, Rudd RM. British Thoracic Society study of cryptogenic fibrosing alveolitis: current presentation and initial management. Fibrosing Alveolitis Subcommittee of the Research Committee of the British Thoracic Society. Thorax 1997;52:38–44.
110. Kaarteenaho-Wiik R, Tani T, Sormunen R, Soini Y, Virtanen I, Paakko P. Tenascin immunoreactivity as a prognostic marker in usual interstitial pneumonia. Am J Respir Crit Care Med 1996;154:511–8.
111. Kanematsu T, Kitaichi M, Nishimura K, Nagai S, Izumi T. Clubbing of the fingers and smooth-muscle proliferation in fibrotic changes in the lung in patients with idiopathic pulmonary fibrosis. Chest 1994;105:339–42.
112. Katzenstein AL, Askin FB. Katzenstein and Askin's surgical pathology of non-neoplastic lung disease, 3rd ed. Philadelphia: WB Saunders; 1997.
113. Katzenstein AL, Myers JL. Idiopathic pulmonary fibrosis: clinical relevance of pathologic classification. Am J Respir Crit Care Med 1998;157:1301–15.
114. Khalil N, O'Connor RN, Flanders KC, Unruh H. TGF-beta 1, but not TGF-beta 2 or TGF-beta 3, is differentially present in epithelial cells of advanced pulmonary fibrosis: an immunohistochemical study. Am J Respir Cell Mol Biol 1996;14:131–8.
115. King TE Jr. Idiopathic pulmonary fibrosis. In: Schwarz MI, King TE Jr, eds. Interstitial lung disease, 2nd ed. St. Louis: Mosby Year Book; 1993:367–403.
116. King TE Jr. Idiopathic pulmonary fibrosis. In: Schwarz MI, King TE Jr, eds. Interstitial lung disease, 3rd ed. Hamilton: BC Decker; 1998:597–644.
117. King TE Jr. Role of bronchoalveolar lavage in the diagnosis of interstitial lung disease. In: Rose BD, ed. UpToDate in medicine. Wellesley: UpToDate; 2001.
118. King TK, Costabel U, Cordier JF, et al. Idiopathic pulmonary fibrosis: guidelines for diagnosis and treatment. Am J Respir Crit Care Med 2000;161:646–64.

119. Kitaichi M. Pathologic features and the classification of interstitial pneumonia of unknown etiology. Bull Chest Dis Res Inst Kyoto Univ 1990;23:1–18.
120. Kondoh Y, Taniguchi H, Kawabata Y, Yokoi T, Suzuki K, Takagi K. Acute exacerbation in idiopathic pulmonary fibrosis. Analysis of clinical and pathologic findings in three cases. Chest 1993;103:1808–12.
121. Kuhn C. The pathogenesis of pulmonary fibrosis. Monogr Pathol 1993:78–92.
122. Kuhn C, Boldt J, King TE Jr, Crouch E, Vartio T, McDonald JA. An immunohistochemical study of architectural remodeling and connective tissue synthesis in pulmonary fibrosis. Am Rev Respir Dis 1989;140:1693–703.
123. Kuhn C, McDonald JA. The roles of the myofibroblast in idiopathic pulmonary fibrosis. Ultrastructural and immunohistochemical features of sites of active extracellular matrix synthesis. Am J Pathol 1991;138:1257–65.
124. Kuwano K, Nomoto Y, Kunitake R, et al. Detection of adenovirus E1A DNA in pulmonary fibrosis using nested polymerase chain reaction. Eur Respir J 1997;10:1445–9.
125. Lee HJ, Im JG, Ahn JM, Yeon KM. Lung cancer in patients with idiopathic pulmonary fibrosis: CT findings. J Comput Assist Tomogr 1996;20:979–82.
126. Lee JS, Im JG, Ahn JM, Kim YM, Han MC. Fibrosing alveolitis: prognostic implication of ground-glass attenuation at high-resolution CT. Radiology 1992;184:451–4.
127. Leung AN, Miller RR, Müller NL. Parenchymal opacification in chronic infiltrative lung diseases: CT-pathologic correlation. Radiology 1993;188:209–14.
128. Liebow AA. Definition and classification of interstitial pneumonias in human pathology. Prog Resp Res 1975;8:1–33.
129. Liebow AA, Carrington CB. The interstitial pneumonias. In: Simon M, Potchen EJ, LeMay M, eds. Frontiers of pulmonary radiology. New York: Grune and Stratton; 1969:102–41.
130. Line BR, Fulmer JD, Reynolds HY, et al. Gallium-67 citrate scanning in the staging of idiopathic pulmonary fibrosis: correlation and physiologic and morphologic features and bronchoalveolar lavage. Am Rev Respir Dis 1978;118:355–65.
131. Mageto YN, Raghu G. Genetic predisposition of idiopathic pulmonary fibrosis. Curr Opin Pulm Med 1997;3:336–40.
132. Mapel DW, Samet JM, Coultas DB. Corticosteroids and the treatment of idiopathic pulmonary fibrosis. Past, present, and future. Chest 1996;110:1058–67.
133. Marshall RP, McAnulty RJ, Laurent GJ. The pathogenesis of pulmonary fibrosis: is there a fibrosis gene? Int J Biochem Cell Biol 1997; 29:107–20.
134. Mason RJ, Schwarz MI, Hunninghake GW, Musson RA. NHLBI Workshop Summary. Pharmacological therapy for idiopathic pulmonary fibrosis. Past, present, and future. Am J Respir Crit Care Med 1999;160:1771–7.
135. Massaro D, Katz S. Fibrosing alveolitis: its occurrence, roentgenographic, and pathologic features in von Recklinghausen's neurofibromatosis. Am Rev Respir Dis 1966;93:934–42.
136. Mathieson JR, Mayo JR, Staples CA, Müller NL. Chronic diffuse infiltrative lung disease: comparison of diagnostic accuracy of CT and chest radiography. Radiology 1989;171:111–6.
137. McAdams HP, Rosado-de-Christenson ML, Wehunt WD, Fishback NF. The alphabet soup revisited: the chronic interstitial pneumonias in the 1990s. Radiographics 1996;16:1009–33.
138. McAnulty RJ, Laurent GJ. Pathogenesis of lung fibrosis and potential new therapeutic strategies. Exp Nephrol 1995;3:96–107.
139. McLoud TC, Carrington CB, Gaensler EA. Diffuse infiltrative lung disease: a new scheme for description. Radiology 1983;149:353–63.
140. Meliconi R, Andreone P, Fasano L, et al. Incidence of hepatitis C virus infection in Italian patients with idiopathic pulmonary fibrosis. Thorax 1996;51:315–7.
141. Meyers BF, Lynch JP, Trulock EP, Guthrie T, Cooper JD, Patterson GA. Single versus bilateral lung transplantation for idiopathic pulmonary fibrosis: a ten-year institutional experience. J Thorac Cardiovasc Surg 2000;120:99–107.
142. Miller JD, Urschel JD, Cox G, et al. A randomized, controlled trial comparing thoracoscopy and limited thoracotomy for lung biopsy in interstitial lung disease. Ann Thorac Surg 2000;70:1647–50.
143. Müller NL, Colby TV. Idiopathic interstitial pneumonias: high-resolution CT and histologic findings. Radiographics 1997;17:1016–22.
144. Müller NL, Guerry-Force ML, Staples CA, et al. Differential diagnosis of bronchiolitis obliterans with organizing pneumonia and usual interstitial pneumonia: clinical, functional, and radiologic findings. Radiology 1987;162:151–6.
145. Müller NL, Miller RR, Webb WR, Evans KG, Ostrow DN. Fibrosing alveolitis: CT-pathologic correlation. Radiology 1986;160:585–8.
146. Müller NL, Staples CA, Miller RR, Vedal S, Thurlbeck WM, Ostrow DN. Disease activity in idiopathic pulmonary fibrosis: CT and pathologic correlation. Radiology 1987;165:731–4.

147. Myers JL, Katzenstein AL. Epithelial necrosis and alveolar collapse in the pathogenesis of usual interstitial pneumonia. Chest 1988;94: 1309–11.
148. Nagai A, Chiyotani A, Nakadate T, Konno K. Lung cancer in patients with idiopathic pulmonary fibrosis. Tohoku J Exp Med 1992;167:231–7.
149. Nicod LP. Pirfenidone in idiopathic pulmonary fibrosis. Lancet 1999;354:268–9.
150. Nishimura K, Kitaichi M, Izumi T, Nagai S, Kanaoka M, Itoh H. Usual interstitial pneumonia: histologic correlation with high-resolution CT. Radiology 1992;182:337–42.
151. Orens JB, Kazerooni EA, Martinez FJ, et al. The sensitivity of high-resolution CT in detecting idiopathic pulmonary fibrosis proved by open lung biopsy. A prospective study. Chest 1995; 108:109–15.
152. Panos RJ, Mortenson RL, Niccoli SA, King TE Jr. Clinical deterioration in patients with idiopathic pulmonary fibrosis: causes and assessment. Am J Med 1990;88:396–404.
153. Raghu G. Interstitial lung disease: a diagnostic approach. Are CT scan and lung biopsy indicated in every patient? Am J Respir Crit Care Med 1995;151:909–14.
154. Raghu G, Johnson WC, Lockhart D, Mageto Y. Treatment of idiopathic pulmonary fibrosis with a new antifibrotic agent, pirfenidone: results of a prospective, open-label phase II study. Am J Respir Crit Care Med 1999;159:1061–9.
155. Raghu G, Mageto YN. Genetic predisposition of interstitial lung disease. In: Schwarz MI, King TE Jr, eds. Interstitial lung disease, 3rd ed. Hamilton: BC Decker; 1998:119–32.
156. Raghu G, Mageto YN, Lockhart D, Schmidt RA, Wood DE, Godwin JD. The accuracy of the clinical diagnosis of new-onset idiopathic pulmonary fibrosis and other interstitial lung diseases: a prospective study. Chest 1999;116:1168–74.
157. Reynolds SP, Davies BH, Gibbs AR. Diffuse pulmonary fibrosis and the Hermansky-Pudlak syndrome: clinical course and postmortem findings. Thorax 1994;49:617–8.
158. Saleh D, Furukawa K, Tsao MS, et al. Elevated expression of endothelin-1 and endothelin-converting enzyme-1 in idiopathic pulmonary fibrosis: possible involvement of proinflammatory cytokines. Am J Respir Cell Mol Biol 1997;16:187–93.
159. Scadding JG, Hinson KF. Diffuse fibrosing alveolitis (diffuse interstitial fibrosis of the lungs). Thorax 1967;22:291–304.
160. Schwartz DA, Merchant RK, Helmers RA, Gilbert SR, Dayton CS, Hunninghake GW. The influence of cigarette smoking on lung function in patients with idiopathic pulmonary fibrosis. Am Rev Respir Dis 1991;144:504–6.
161. Scott J, Johnston I, Britton J. What causes cryptogenic fibrosing alveolitis? A case-control study of environmental exposure to dust. Br Med J 1990;301:1015–7.
162. Selman M, King TE Jr, Pardo A. Idiopathic pulmonary fibrosis: prevailing and evolving hypotheses about its pathogenesis and implications for therapy. Ann Intern Med 2001;134:136-51.
163. Staples CA, Müller NL, Vedal S, Abboud R, Ostrow D, Miller RR. Usual interstitial pneumonia: correlation of CT with clinical, functional, and radiologic findings. Radiology 1987;162: 377–81.
164. Terriff BA, Kwan SY, Chan-Yeung MM, Müller NL. Fibrosing alveolitis: chest radiography and CT as predictors of clinical and functional impairment at follow-up in 26 patients. Radiology 1992;184:445–9.
165. Travis WD, King TE, Bateman ED, et al. ATS/ ERS international multidisciplinary consensus classification of idiopathic interstitial pneumonia. Am J Respir Crit Care Med 2002:165;277–304.
166. Travis WD, Matsui K, Moss J, Ferrans VJ. Idiopathic nonspecific interstitial pneumonia: prognostic significance of cellular and fibrosing patterns. Survival comparison with usual interstitial pneumonia and desquamative interstitial pneumonia. Am J Surg Pathol 2000;24:19–33.
167. Vergnon JM, Vincent M, de The G, Mornex JF, Weynants P, Brune J. Cryptogenic fibrosing alveolitis and Epstein-Barr virus: an association? Lancet 1984;2:768–71.
168. Warnock ML, Press M, Churg A. Further observations on cytoplasmic hyaline in the lung. Hum Pathol 1980;11:59–65.
169. Watters LC, King TE, Schwarz MI, Waldron JA, Stanford RE, Cherniack RM. A clinical, radiographic, and physiologic scoring system for the longitudinal assessment of patients with idiopathic pulmonary fibrosis. Am Rev Respir Dis 1986;133:97–103.
170. Wells AU, Cullinan P, Hansell DM, et al. Fibrosing alveolitis associated with systemic sclerosis has a better prognosis than lone cryptogenic fibrosing alveolitis. Am J Respir Crit Care Med 1994;149:1583–90.
171. Wells AU, Hansell DM, Rubens MB, Cailes JB, Black CM, du Bois RM. Functional impairment in lone cryptogenic fibrosing alveolitis and fibrosing alveolitis associated with systemic sclerosis: a comparison. Am J Respir Crit Care Med 1997;155:1657–64.

172. Wells AU, Hansell DM, Rubens MB, Cullinan P, Black CM, du Bois RM. The predictive value of appearances on thin-section computed tomography in fibrosing alveolitis. Am Rev Respir Dis 1993;148:1076–82.
173. Wells AU, Hansell DM, Rubens MB, et al. Fibrosing alveolitis in systemic sclerosis. Bronchoalveolar lavage findings in relation to computed tomographic appearance. Am J Respir Crit Care Med 1994;150:462–8.
174. Wells AU, King AD, Rubens MB, Cramer D, du Bois RM, Hansell DM. Lone cryptogenic fibrosing alveolitis: a functional-morphologic correlation based on extent of disease on thin-section computed tomography. Am J Respir Crit Care Med 1997;155:1367–75.
175. Wright PH, Heard BE, Steel SJ, Turner-Warwick M. Cryptogenic fibrosing alveolitis: assessment by graded trephine lung biopsy histology compared with clinical, radiographic, and physiological features. Br J Dis Chest 1981;75:61–70.
176. Yoshimura K, Nakatani T, Nakamori Y, et al. Acute exacerbation in idiopathic interstitial pneumonia. Nippon Kyobu Shikkan Gakkai Zasshi 1984;22:1012–20.
177. Ziesche R, Hofbauer E, Wittmann K, Petkov V, Block LH. A preliminary study of long-term treatment with interferon gamma-1b and low-dose prednisolone in patients with idiopathic pulmonary fibrosis. N Engl J Med 1999;341:1264–9.

Nonspecific Interstitial Pneumonia

178. Bjoraker JA, Ryu JH, Edwin MK, et al. Prognostic significance of histopathologic subsets in idiopathic pulmonary fibrosis. Am J Respir Crit Care Med 1998;157:199–203.
179. Carrington CB, Gaensler EA, Coutu RE, FitzGerald MX, Gupta RG. Natural history and treated course of usual and desquamative interstitial pneumonia. N Engl J Med 1978;298:801–9.
180. Coleman A, Colby TV. Histologic diagnosis of extrinsic allergic alveolitis. Am J Surg Pathol 1988;12:514–8.
181. Cottin V, Donsbeck AV, Revel D, Loire R, Cordier JF. Nonspecific interstitial pneumonia. Individualization of a clinicopathologic entity in a series of 12 patients. Am J Respir Crit Care Med 1998;158:1286–93.
182. Daniil ZD, Gilchrist FC, Nicholson AG, et al. A histologic pattern of nonspecific interstitial pneumonia is associated with a better prognosis than usual interstitial pneumonia in patients with cryptogenic fibrosing alveolitis. Am J Respir Crit Care Med 1999;160:899–905.
183. Dreisin RB, Schwarz MI, Theofilopoulos AN, Stanford RE. Circulating immune complexes in the idiopathic interstitial pneumonias. N Engl J Med 1978;298:353–7.
184. Flaherty KR, Travis WD, Colby TV, et al. Histological variability in patients with suspected idiopathic pulmonary fibrosis. Am J Respir Crit Care Med 2001;164:1722–7.
185. Fujita J, Yamadori I, Suemitsu I, et al. Clinical features of non-specific interstitial pneumonia. Respir Med 1999;93:113–8.
186. Fujita J, Yoshinouchi T, Ohtsuki Y, et al. Nonspecific interstitial pneumonia as pulmonary involvement of systemic sclerosis. Ann Rheum Dis 2001;60:281–3.
187. Griffiths MH, Miller RF, Semple SJ. Interstitial pneumonitis in patients infected with the human immunodeficiency virus. Thorax 1995; 50:1141–6.
188. Hartman TE, Swensen SJ, Hansell DM, et al. Nonspecific interstitial pneumonia: variable appearance at high-resolution chest CT. Radiology 2000;217:701–5.
189. Katzenstein AL, Askin FB. Katzenstein and Askin's surgical pathology of non-neoplastic lung disease, 3rd ed. Philadelphia: WB Saunders; 1997.
190. Katzenstein AL, Fiorelli RF. Nonspecific interstitial pneumonia/fibrosis. Histologic features and clinical significance. Am J Surg Pathol 1994;18:136–47.
191. Katzenstein AL, Myers JL. Idiopathic pulmonary fibrosis: clinical relevance of pathologic classification. Am J Respir Crit Care Med 1998; 157:1301–15.
192. Kawanami O, Basset F, Barrios R, Lacronique JG, Ferrans VJ, Crystal RG. Hypersensitivity pneumonitis in man. Light- and electron-microscopic studies of 18 lung biopsies. Am J Pathol 1983;110:275–89.
193. Kim EY, Lee KS, Chung MP, Kwon OJ, Kim TS, Hwang JH. Nonspecific interstitial pneumonia with fibrosis: serial high-resolution CT findings with functional correlation. AJR Am J Roentgenol 1999;173:949–53.
194. Kim TS, Lee KS, Chung MP, et al. Nonspecific interstitial pneumonia with fibrosis: high-resolution CT and pathologic findings. AJR Am J Roentgenol 1998;171:1645–50.
195. Kitaichi M. Pathologic features and the classification of interstitial pneumonia of unknown etiology. Bull Chest Dis Res Inst Kyoto Univ 1990;23:1–18.
196. Müller NL, Colby TV. Idiopathic interstitial pneumonias: high-resolution CT and histologic findings. Radiographics 1997;17:1016–22.

197. Nagai S, Kitaichi M, Itoh H, Nishimura K, Izumi T, Colby TV. Idiopathic nonspecific interstitial pneumonia/fibrosis: comparison with idiopathic pulmonary fibrosis and BOOP. Eur Respir J 1998;12:1010–9.
198. Nicholson AG, Colby TV, Dubois RM, Hansell DM, Wells AU. The prognostic significance of the histologic pattern of interstitial pneumonia in patients presenting with the clinical entity of cryptogenic fibrosing alveolitis. Am J Respir Crit Care Med 2000;162:2213–7.
199. Ognibene FP, Masur H, Rogers P, et al. Nonspecific interstitial pneumonitis without evidence of Pneumocystis carinii in asymptomatic patients infected with human immunodeficiency virus (HIV). Ann Intern Med 1988;109:874–9.
200. Park CS, Chung SW, Ki SY, et al. Increased levels of interleukin-6 are associated with lymphocytosis in bronchoalveolar lavage fluids of idiopathic nonspecific interstitial pneumonia. Am J Respir Crit Care Med 2000;162:1162–8.
201. Park JS, Lee KS, Kim JS, et al. Nonspecific interstitial pneumonia with fibrosis: radiographic and CT findings in seven patients. Radiology 1995;195:645–8.
202. Sattler F, Nichols L, Hirano L, et al. Nonspecific interstitial pneumonitis mimicking Pneumocystis carinii pneumonia. Am J Respir Crit Care Med 1997;156:912–7.
203. Schwarz MI, Dreisin RB, Pratt DS, Stanford RE. Immunofluorescent patterns in the idiopathic interstitial pneumonias. J Lab Clin Med 1978; 91:929–38.
204. Travis WD, King TE, Bateman ED, et al. ATS/ERS International Multidisciplinary Consensus Classification of Idiopathic Interstitial Pneumonia. Am J Respir Crit Care Med 2002;165:277–304.
205. Travis WD, Matsui K, Moss J, Ferrans VJ. Idiopathic nonspecific interstitial pneumonia: prognostic significance of cellular and fibrosing patterns. Survival comparison with usual interstitial pneumonia and desquamative interstitial pneumonia. Am J Surg Pathol 2000;24:19–33.
206. Wright PH, Heard BE, Steel SJ, Turner-Warwick M. Cryptogenic fibrosing alveolitis: assessment by graded trephine lung biopsy histology compared with clinical, radiographic, and physiological features. Br J Dis Chest 1981;75:61–70.

Organizing Pneumonia

207. Alasaly K, Müller N, Ostrow DN, Champion P, FitzGerald JM. Cryptogenic organizing pneumonia. A report of 25 cases and a review of the literature. Medicine (Baltimore) 1995;74:201–11.
208. Bartter T, Irwin RS, Nash G, Balikian JP, Hollingsworth HH. Idiopathic bronchiolitis obliterans organizing pneumonia with peripheral infiltrates on chest roentgenogram. Arch Intern Med 1989;149:273–9.
209. Beasley MB, Franks TJ, Galvin JR, Travis WD. Acute fibrinous and organizing pneumonia. Arch Pathol Lab Med 2002:126(in press).
210. Chandler PW, Shin MS, Friedman SE, Myers JL, Katzenstein AL. Radiographic manifestations of bronchiolitis obliterans with organizing pneumonia vs usual interstitial pneumonia. AJR Am J Roentgenol 1986;147:899–906.
211. Colby TV. Pathologic aspects of bronchiolitis obliterans organizing pneumonia. Chest 1992; 102:38S–43S.
212. Cordier JF. Cryptogenic organizing pneumonia. Clin Chest Med 1993;14:677–92.
213. Cordier JF, Loire R, Brune J. Idiopathic bronchiolitis obliterans organizing pneumonia. Definition of characteristic clinical profiles in a series of 16 patients. Chest 1989;96:999–1004.
214. Costabel U, Teschler H, Guzman J. Bronchiolitis obliterans organizing pneumonia (BOOP): the cytological and immunocytological profile of bronchoalveolar lavage. Eur Respir J 1992;5:791–7.
215. Davison AG, Heard BE, McAllister WA, Turner-Warwick ME. Cryptogenic organizing pneumonitis. Q J Med 1983;207:382–94.
216. Domingo JA, Pérez-Calvo JI, Carretero JA, Ferrando J, Cay A, Civeira F. Bronchiolitis obliterans organizing pneumonia. An unusual cause of solitary pulmonary nodule. Chest 1993;103:1621–3.
217. Epler GR. Bronchiolitis obliterans organizing pneumonia: definition and clinical features. Chest 1992;102:2S–6S.
218. Epler GR, Colby TV, McLoud TC, Carrington CB, Gaensler EA. Bronchiolitis obliterans organizing pneumonia. N Engl J Med 1985; 312:152–8.
219. Gosink BB, Friedman PJ, Liebow AA. Bronchiolitis obliterans. Roentgenologic-pathologic correlation. Am J Roentgenol Radium Ther Nucl Med 1973;117:816–32.
220. Grinblat J, Mechlis S, Lewitus Z. Organizing pneumonia-like process: an unusual observation in steroid responsive cases with features of chronic interstitial pneumonia. Chest 1981;80:259–63.
221. Izumi T. The global view of idiopathic bronchiolitis obliterans organizing pneumonia. In: Epler GR, ed. Diseases of the bronchioles. New York: Raven Press; 1994:307–12.
222. Katzenstein AL, Myers JL, Prophet WD, Corley LS, Shin MS. Bronchiolitis obliterans and usual interstitial pneumonia. A comparative clinicopathologic study. Am J Surg Pathol 1986;10:373–81.

223. King TE Jr, Mortenson RL. Cryptogenic organizing pneumonitis. The North American experience. Chest 1992;102:8S–13S.
224. Kitaichi M. Differential diagnosis of bronchiolitis obliterans organizing pneumonia. Chest 1992;102:44S–9S.
225. Lee KS, Kullnig P, Hartman TE, Müller NL. Cryptogenic organizing pneumonia: CT findings in 43 patients. AJR Am J Roentgenol 1994;162:543–6.
226. Liebow AA, Carrington CB. The interstitial pneumonias. In: Simon M, Potchen EJ, LeMay M, eds. Frontiers of pulmonary radiology. New York: Grune and Stratton; 1969:102–41.
227. Lohr RH, Boland BJ, Douglas WW, et al. Organizing pneumonia. Features and prognosis of cryptogenic, secondary, and focal variants. Arch Intern Med 1997;157:1323–9.
228. Müller NL, Guerry-Force ML, Staples CA, et al. Differential diagnosis of bronchiolitis obliterans with organizing pneumonia and usual interstitial pneumonia: clinical, functional, and radiologic findings. Radiology 1987;162:151–6.
229. Müller NL, Staples CA, Miller RR. Bronchiolitis obliterans organizing pneumonia: CT features in 14 patients. AJR Am J Roentgenol 1990;154:983–7.
230. Pesci A, Majori M, Piccoli ML, et al. Mast cells in bronchiolitis obliterans organizing pneumonia. Mast cell hyperplasia and evidence for extracellular release of tryptase. Chest 1996;110:383–91.
231. Poletti V, Castrilli G, Romagna M, et al. Bronchoalveolar lavage, histological and immunohistochemical features in cryptogenic organizing pneumonia. Monaldi Arch Chest Dis 1996;51:289–95.
232. Travis WD, Colby TV, Corrin B, Shimosato Y, Brambilla E, in collaboration with Sobin LH and pathologists from 14 countries. Histological typing of lung and pleural tumors, 3rd ed. Berlin: Springer; 1999.
233. Travis WD, King TE, Bateman ED, et al. ATS/ERS International Multidisciplinary Consensus Classification of Idiopathic Interstitial Pneumonia. Am J Respir Crit Care Med 2002;165:277–304.
234. Travis WD, Matsui K, Moss J, Ferrans VJ. Idiopathic nonspecific interstitial pneumonia: prognostic significance of cellular and fibrosing patterns. Survival comparison with usual interstitial pneumonia and desquamative interstitial pneumonia. Am J Surg Pathol 2000;24: 19–33.
235. Yamamoto M, Ina Y, Kitaichi M. Bronchiolitis obliterans organizing pneumonia (BOOP): profile in Japan. In: Harasawa M, Fukuchi Y, Morinari H, eds. Interstitial pneumonia of unknown etiology. Tokyo: University of Tokyo Press; 1989:61–70.

Diffuse Alveolar Damage

236. Abel SJ, Finney SJ, Brett SJ, Keogh BF, Morgan CJ, Evans TW. Reduced mortality in association with the acute respiratory distress syndrome (ARDS). Thorax 1998;53:292–4.
237. Akikusa B, Kondo Y, Irabu N, Yamamoto S, Saiki S. Six cases of microscopic polyarteritis exhibiting acute interstitial pneumonia. Pathol Int 1995;45:580–8.
238. Ash N, Cohen Y, Liokumovich P, Wollner A. Acute interstitial pneumonia: a case of Hamman-Rich syndrome. Isr J Med Sci 1995; 31:367–70.
239. Askin FB. Back to the future: the Hamman-Rich syndrome and acute interstitial pneumonia [Editorial]. Mayo Clin Proc 1990;65:1624–6.
240. Bachofen M, Weibel ER. Structural alterations of lung parenchyma in the adult respiratory distress syndrome. Clin Chest Med 1982;3:35–56.
241. Basset F, Ferrans VJ, Soler P, Takemura T, Fukuda Y, Crystal RG. Intraluminal fibrosis in interstitial lung disorders. Am J Pathol 1986; 122:443–61.
242. Beasley MB, Franks TJ, Galvin JR, Travis WD. Acute fibrinous and organizing pneumonia. Arch Pathol Lab Med 2002:126(in press).
243. Bitterman PB. Pathogenesis of fibrosis in acute lung injury. Am J Med 1992;92(Suppl 6A):39S–43S.
244. Brower RG, Shanholtz CB, Fessler HE, et al. Prospective, randomized, controlled clinical trial comparing traditional versus reduced tidal volume ventilation in acute respiratory distress syndrome patients. Crit Care Med 1999;27:1492–8.
245. Burkhardt A. Alveolitis and collapse in the pathogenesis of pulmonary fibrosis. Am Rev Respir Dis 1989;140:513–24.
246. Carmichael LC, Dorinsky PM, Higgins SB, et al. Diagnosis and therapy of acute respiratory distress syndrome in adults: an international survey. J Crit Care 1996;11:9–18.
247. Churg A, Golden J, Fligiel S, Hogg JC. Bronchopulmonary dysplasia in the adult. Am Rev Respir Dis 1983;127:117–20.
248. Doyle RL, Szaflarski N, Modin GW, Wiener-Kronish JP, Matthay MA. Identification of patients with acute lung injury. Predictors of mortality. Am J Respir Crit Care Med 1995; 152:1818–24.
249. Fukuda Y, Ishizaki M, Masuda Y, Kimura G, Kawanami O, Masugi Y. The role of intraalveolar fibrosis in the process of pulmonary structural remodeling in patients with diffuse alveolar damage. Am J Pathol 1987;126:171–82.

250. Gattinoni L, Bombino M, Pelosi P, et al. Lung structure and function in different stages of severe adult respiratory distress syndrome. JAMA 1994;271:1772–9.
251. Gattinoni L, Pelosi P, Pesenti A, et al. CT scan in ARDS: clinical and physiopathological insights. Acta Anaesthesiol Scand 1991;95(Suppl):87–94.
252. Gattinoni L, Pelosi P, Vitale G, Pesenti A, D'Andrea L, Mascheroni D. Body position changes redistribute lung computed-tomographic density in patients with acute respiratory failure. Anesthesiology 1991;74:15–23.
253. Greene R. Adult respiratory distress syndrome: acute alveolar damage. Radiology 1987;163:57–66.
254. Guinee D Jr, Brambilla E, Fleming M, et al. The potential role of BAX and BCL-2 expression in diffuse alveolar damage. Am J Pathol 1997;151: 999–1007.
255. Guinee D Jr, Fleming M, Hayashi T, et al. Association of p53 and WAF1 expression with apoptosis in diffuse alveolar damage. Am J Pathol 1996;149:531–8.
256. Hamman L, Rich AR. Acute diffuse interstitial fibrosis of the lungs. Bull Johns Hopkins Hosp 1944;74:177.
257. Hansen-Flaschen JH, Siegel MD. The acute respiratory distress syndrome: definition, diagnosis and etiology. In: Rose BD, ed. Uptodate in medicine. Wellesley: Uptodate; 2001.
258. Hasleton PS, Roberts TE. Adult respiratory distress syndrome–an update. Histopathology 1999;34:285–94.
259. Hayashi T, Stetler-Stevenson WG, Fleming MV, et al. Immunohistochemical study of metalloproteinases and their tissue inhibitors in the lungs of patients with diffuse alveolar damage and idiopathic pulmonary fibrosis. Am J Pathol 1996;149:1241–56.
260. Hudson LD, Steinberg KP. Epidemiology of acute lung injury and ARDS. Chest 1999;116: 74S–82S.
261. Ichikado K, Johkoh T, Ikezoe J, et al. Acute interstitial pneumonia: high-resolution CT findings correlated with pathology. AJR Am J Roentgenol 1997;168:333–8.
262. Johkoh T, Müller NL, Taniguchi H, et al. Acute interstitial pneumonia: thin-section CT findings in 36 patients. Radiology 1999;211:859–63.
263. Katzenstein AL. Idiopathic interstitial pneumonia: classification and diagnosis. In: Churg A, Katzenstein AL, eds. The lung. Current concepts. Baltimore: Williams & Wilkins; 1993:1–31.
264. Katzenstein AL, Askin FB. Katzenstein and Askin's surgical pathology of non-neoplastic lung disease, 3rd ed. Philadelphia: WB Saunders; 1997.
265. Katzenstein AL, Bloor CM, Leibow AA. Diffuse alveolar damage—the role of oxygen, shock, and related factors. A review. Am J Pathol 1976; 85:209–28.
266. Katzenstein AL, Fiorelli RF. Nonspecific interstitial pneumonia/fibrosis. Histologic features and clinical significance. Am J Surg Pathol 1994;18:136–47.
267. Katzenstein AL, Myers JL, Mazur MT. Acute interstitial pneumonia. A clinicopathologic, ultrastructural, and cell kinetic study. Am J Surg Pathol 1986;10:256–67.
268. Kuhn C. The pathogenesis of pulmonary fibrosis. Monogr Pathol 1993;78–92.
269. Lamy M, Fallat RJ, Koeniger E, et al. Pathologic features and mechanisms of hypoxemia in adult respiratory distress syndrome. Am Rev Respir Dis 1976;114:267–84.
270. Lesur O, Berthiaume Y, Blaise G, et al. Acute respiratory distress syndrome: 30 years later. Can Respir J 1999;6:71–86.
270a. Liebow AA, Carrington CB. The interstitial pneumonias. In: Simon M, Potchen EJ, LeMay M, eds. Frontiers of pulmonary radiology. New York: Grune and Stratton; 1969:102–41.
271. Luhr OR, Antonsen K, Karlsson M, et al. Incidence and mortality after acute respiratory failure and acute respiratory distress syndrome in Sweden, Denmark, and Iceland. The ARF Study Group. Am J Respir Crit Care Med 1999;159: 1849–61.
272. Martinez M, Diaz E, Joseph D, et al. Improvement in oxygenation by prone position and nitric oxide in patients with acute respiratory distress syndrome. Intensive Care Med 1999; 25:29–36.
273. Maunder RJ, Shuman WP, McHugh JW, Marglin SI, Butler J. Preservation of normal lung regions in the adult respiratory distress syndrome. Analysis by computed tomography. JAMA 1986;255:2463–5.
274. McAdams HP, Rosado-de-Christenson ML, Wehunt WD, Fishback NF. The alphabet soup revisited: the chronic interstitial pneumonias in the 1990s. Radiographics 1996;16:1009–33.
275. Meduri GU. Late adult respiratory distress syndrome. New Horiz 1993;1:563–77.
276. Meduri GU, Eltorky M, Winer-Muram HT. The fibroproliferative phase of late adult respiratory distress syndrome. Semin Respir Infect 1995;10:154–75.
277. Meduri GU, Headley AS, Golden E, et al. Effect of prolonged methylprednisolone therapy in unresolving acute respiratory distress syndrome: a randomized controlled trial. JAMA 1998;280:159–65.
278. Milberg JA, Davis DR, Steinberg KP, Hudson LD. Improved survival of patients with acute respiratory distress syndrome (ARDS): 1983-1993. JAMA 1995;273:306–9.

279. Milne EN, Pistolesi M, Miniati M, Giuntini C. The radiologic distinction of cardiogenic and noncardiogenic edema. AJR Am J Roentgenol 1985;144:879–94.
280. Mols G, Brandes I, Kessler V, et al. Volume-dependent compliance in ARDS: proposal of a new diagnostic concept. Intensive Care Med 1999;25:1084–91.
281. Morgan PW, Goodman LR. Pulmonary edema and adult respiratory distress syndrome. Radiol Clin North Am 1991;29:943–63.
282. Moss M, Goodman PL, Heinig M, Barkin S, Ackerson L, Parsons PE. Establishing the relative accuracy of three new definitions of the adult respiratory distress syndrome. Crit Care Med 1995;23:1629–37.
283. Nash G, Blennerhassett JB, Pontoppidan H. Pulmonary lesions associated with oxygen therapy and artifical ventilation. N Engl J Med 1967;276:368–74.
284. Nash G, Foley FD, Langlinais PC. Pulmonary interstitial edema and hyaline membranes in adult burn patients. Electron microscopic observations. Hum Pathol 1974;5:149–60.
285. Olson J, Colby TV, Elliott CG. Hamman-Rich syndrome revisited. Mayo Clin Proc 1990;65:1538–48.
286. Ostendorf P, Birzle H, Vogel W, Mittermayer C. Pulmonary radiographic abnormalities in shock. Roentgen-clinical-pathological correlation. Radiology 1975;115:257–63.
287. Pittet JF, Mackersie RC, Martin TR, Matthay MA. Biological markers of acute lung injury: prognostic and pathogenetic significance. Am J Respir Crit Care Med 1997;155:1187–205.
288. Pratt PC. Pathology of adult respiratory distress syndrome. Monogr Pathol 1978;19:43–57.
289. Pratt PC. Pathology of adult respiratory distress syndrome: implications regarding therapy. Semin Respir Med. 1982;4:79–85.
290. Pratt PC, Vollmer RT, Shelburne JD, Crapo JD. Pulmonary morphology in a multihospital collaborative extracorporeal membrane oxygenation project. I. Light microscopy. Am J Pathol 1979;95:191–214.
291. Primack SL, Hartman TE, Ikezoe J, Akira M, Sakatani M, Müller NL. Acute interstitial pneumonia: radiographic and CT findings in nine patients. Radiology 1993;188:817–20.
292. Robinson DS, Geddes DM, Hansell DM, et al. Partial resolution of acute interstitial pneumonia in native lung after single lung transplantation. Thorax 1996;51:1158–9.
293. Roupie E, Lepage E, Wysocki M, et al. Prevalence, etiologies and outcome of the acute respiratory distress syndrome among hypoxemic ventilated patients. SRLF Collaborative Group on Mechanical Ventilation. Société de Reanimation de Langue Française. Intensive Care Med 1999;25:920–9.
294. Rubenfeld GD, Caldwell E, Granton J, Hudson LD, Matthay MA. Interobserver variability in applying a radiographic definition for ARDS. Chest 1999;116:1347–53.
295. Suchyta MR, Elliott CG, Colby T, Rasmusson BY, Morris AH, Jensen RL. Open lung biopsy does not correlate with pulmonary function after the adult respiratory distress syndrome. Chest 1991;99:1232–7.
296. Tagliabue M, Casella TC, Zincone GE, Fumagalli R, Salvini E. CT and chest radiography in the evaluation of adult respiratory distress syndrome. Acta Radiol 1994;35:230–4.
297. Teplitz C. The core pathobiology and integrated medical science of adult acute respiratory insufficiency. Surg Clin North Am 1976;56:1091–133.
298. Teplitz C. The ultrastructural basis for pulmonary pathophysiology following trauma. Pathogenesis of pulmonary edema. J Trauma 1968;8:700–14.
299. Thomsen GE, Morris AH. Incidence of the adult respiratory distress syndrome in the state of Utah. Am J Respir Crit Care Med 1995;152:965–71.
300. Tomashefski JF Jr. Pulmonary pathology of the adult respiratory distress syndrome. Clin Chest Med 1990;11:593–619.
301. Tomashefski JF Jr, Davies P, Boggis C, Greene R, Zapol WM, Reid LM. The pulmonary vascular lesions of the adult respiratory distress syndrome. Am J Pathol 1983;112:112–26.
302. Travis WD, King TE, Bateman ED, et al. ATS/ERS International Multidisciplinary Consensus Classification of Idiopathic Interstitial Pneumonia. Am J Respir Crit Care Med 2002;165:277–304.
303. Ventilation with lower tidal volumes as compared with traditional tidal volumes for acute lung injury and the acute respiratory distress syndrome. The Acute Respiratory Distress Syndrome Network. N Engl J Med 2000;342:1301–8.
304. Vourlekis JS, Brown KK, Cool CD, et al. Acute interstitial pneumonia: case series and review of the literature. Medicine (Baltimore) 2000;79: 369–78.
305. Vracko R. Significance of basal lamina for regeneration of injured lung. Virchows Arch [A] 1972;355:264–74.
306. Ware LB, Matthay MA. The acute respiratory distress syndrome. N Engl J Med 2000;342:1334–49.
307. Yazdy AM, Tomashefski JF Jr, Yagan R, Kleinerman J. Regional alveolar damage (RAD). A localized counterpart of diffuse alveolar damage. Am J Clin Pathol 1989;92:10–5.
308. Zapol WM, Trelstad RL, Coffey JW, Tsai I, Salvador RA. Pulmonary fibrosis in severe acute respiratory failure. Am Rev Respir Dis 1979; 119:547–54.

Respiratory Bronchiolitis

309. Bedrossian CW, Kuhn C III, Luna MA, Conklin RH, Byrd RB, Kaplan PD. Desquamative interstitial pneumonia-like reaction accompanying pulmonary lesions. Chest 1977;72:166–9.
310. Cosio MG, Hale KA, Niewoehner DE. Morphologic and morphometric effects of prolonged cigarette smoking on the small airways. Am Rev Respir Dis 1980;122:265–21.
311. Eidelman D, Saetta MP, Ghezzo H, et al. Cellularity of the alveolar walls in smokers and its relation to alveolar destruction. Functional implications. Am Rev Respir Dis 1990;141:1547–52.
312. Heyneman LE, Ward S, Lynch DA, Remy-Jardin M, Johkoh T, Müller NL. Respiratory bronchiolitis, respiratory bronchiolitis-associated interstitial lung disease, and desquamative interstitial pneumonia: different entities or part of the spectrum of the same disease process? AJR Am J Roentgenol 1999;173:1617–22.
313. Hogg JC, Macklem PT, Thurlbeck WM. The resistance of small airways in normal and diseased human lungs. Aspen Emphysema Conf 1967;10:433–41.
314. Holt RM, Schmidt RA, Godwin JD, Raghu G. High resolution CT in respiratory bronchiolitis-associated interstitial lung disease. J Comput Assist Tomogr 1993;17:46–50.
315. Katzenstein AL, Myers JL. Idiopathic pulmonary fibrosis: clinical relevance of pathologic classification. Am J Respir Crit Care Med 1998;157:1301–15.
316. King TE Jr, Mortenson RL. Syndromes that mimic idiopathic pulmonary fibrosis. Immunology Allergy Clinics of North America. 1992;12:461–89.
317. Moon J, du Bois RM, Colby TV, Hansell DM, Nicholson AG. Clinical significance of respiratory bronchiolitis on open lung biopsy and its relationship to smoking related interstitial lung disease. Thorax 1999;54:1009–14.
318. Myers JL, Veal CF, Jr., Shin MS, Katzenstein AL. Respiratory bronchiolitis causing interstitial lung disease. A clinicopathologic study of six cases. Am Rev Respir Dis 1987;135:880–4.
319. Niewoehner DE, Kleinerman J, Rice DB. Pathologic changes in the peripheral airways of young cigarette smokers. N Engl J Med 1974;291:755–8.
320. Park J, Brown K, Tuder R, Hale V, King TE, Lynch D. Respiratory bronchiolitis associated interstitial lung disease: radiologic features with clinical and pathologic correlation. Radiology 2002;26:13–20.
321. Sadikot RT, Johnson J, Loyd JE, Christman JW. Respiratory bronchiolitis associated with severe dyspnea, exertional hypoxemia, and clubbing. Chest 2000;117:282–5.
322. Thurlbeck WM. Small airways disease. Hum Pathol 1973;4:150–2.
323. Travis WD, King TE Jr, Bateman ED, et al. ATS/ERS International Multidisciplinary Consensus Classification of Idiopathic Interstitial Pneumonia. Am J Respir Crit Care Med 2002;165:277–304.
324. Yousem SA, Colby TV, Gaensler EA. Respiratory bronchiolitis-associated interstitial lung disease and its relationship to desquamative interstitial pneumonia. Mayo Clin Proc 1989;64:1373–80.

Desquamative Interstitial Pneumonia

325. Adesina AM, Vallyathan V, McQuillen EN, Weaver SO, Craighead JE. Bronchiolar inflammation and fibrosis associated with smoking. A morphologic cross-sectional population analysis. Am Rev Respir Dis 1991;143:144–9.
326. Bedrossian CW, Kuhn C, Luna MA, Conklin RH, Byrd RB, Kaplan PD. Desquamative interstitial pneumonia-like reaction accompanying pulmonary lesions. Chest 1977;72:166–9.
327. Bhagwat AG, Wentworth P, Conen PE. Observations on the relationship of desquamative interstitial pneumonia and pulmonary alveolar proteinosis in childhood: a pathologic and experimental study. Chest 1970;58:326–32.
328. Bjoraker JA, Ryu JH, Edwin MK, et al. Prognostic significance of histopathologic subsets in idiopathic pulmonary fibrosis. Am J Respir Crit Care Med 1998;157:199–203.
329. Brewer DB, Heath D, Asquith P. Electron microscopy of desquamative interstitial pneumonia. J Pathol 1969;97:317–23.
330. Carrington CB, Gaensler EA, Coutu RE, Fitzgerald MX, Gupta RG. Natural history and treated course of usual and desquamative interstitial pneumonia. N Engl J Med 1978; 298:801–9.
331. Colby TV, Carrington CB. Interstital lung disease. In: Thurlbeck WM, Churg AM, eds. Pathology of the lung, 2nd ed. New York: Thieme Medical Publishers; 1995:589–737.
332. Crystal RG, Bitterman PB, Rennard SI, Hance AJ, Keogh BA. Interstitial lung diseases of unknown cause. Disorders characterized by chronic inflammation of the lower respiratory tract. N Engl J Med 1984;310:154–66.
333. Cutz E, Wert SE, Nogee LM, Moore AM. Deficiency of lamellar bodies in alveolar type II cells associated with fatal respiratory disease in a full-term infant. Am J Respir Crit Care Med 2000;161:608–14.
334. Freed JA, Miller A, Gordon RE, Fischbein A, Kleinerman J, Langer AM. Desquamative interstitial pneumonia associated with chrysotile asbestos fibres. Br J Ind Med 1991;48:332–7.

335. Gaensler EA, Goff AM, Prowse CM. Desquamative interstitial pneumonia. N Engl J Med 1966;274:113–28.
336. Gould TH, Buist MD, Meredith D, Thomas PD. Fulminant desquamative interstitial pneumonitis. Anaesth Intensive Care 1998;26:677–9.
337. Hartman TE, Primack SL, Kang EY, et al. Disease progression in usual interstitial pneumonia compared with desquamative interstitial pneumonia. Assessment with serial CT. Chest 1996;110:378–82.
338. Hartman TE, Primack SL, Swensen SJ, Hansell D, McGuinness G, Müller NL. Desquamative interstitial pneumonia: thin-section CT findings in 22 patients. Radiology 1993;187:787–90.
339. Katzenstein AL, Askin FB. Katzenstein and Askin's surgical pathology of non-neoplastic lung disease, 3rd ed. Philadelphia: WB Saunders; 1997.
340. Katzenstein AL, Gordon LP, Oliphant M, Swender PT. Chronic pneumonitis of infancy. A unique form of interstitial lung disease occurring in early childhood. Am J Surg Pathol 1995;19:439–47.
341. Katzenstein AL, Myers JL. Idiopathic pulmonary fibrosis: clinical relevance of pathologic classification. Am J Respir Crit Care Med 1998;157:1301–15.
342. King TE Jr. Idiopathic pulmonary fibrosis. In: Schwarz MI, King TE Jr, eds. Interstitial lung disease, 2nd ed. St. Louis: Mosby Year Book; 1993:367–403.
343. King TE Jr, Schwarz MI. Chronic diffuse parenchymal lung diseases. In: Davis G, ed. Medical management of pulmonary diseases. New York: Marcel Decker; 1999:487–529.
344. Kitaichi M. Desquamative interstitial pneumonia: an idiopathic interstitial pneumonia with a possibility of spontaneous regression [Editorial]. Intern Med 1997;36:672–3.
345. Koss MN, Johnson FB, Hochholzer L. Pulmonary blue bodies. Hum Pathol 1981;12:258–66.
346. Liebow AA, Steer A, Billingsley JG. Desquamative interstitial pneumonia. Am J Med 1965;39:369–404.
347. Lynch DA, Hay T, Newell JD Jr, Divgi VD, Fan LL. Pediatric diffuse lung disease: diagnosis and classification using high- resolution CT. AJR Am J Roentgenol 1999;173:713–8.
348. Matsuo K, Tada S, Kataoka M, et al. Spontaneous remission of desquamative interstitial pneumonia. Intern Med 1997;36:728–31.
349. McAdams HP, Rosado-de-Christenson ML, Wehunt WD, Fishback NF. The alphabet soup revisited: the chronic interstitial pneumonias in the 1990s. Radiographics 1996;16:1009–33.
350. Müller NL, Colby TV. Idiopathic interstitial pneumonias: high-resolution CT and histologic findings. Radiographics 1997;17:1016–22.
351. Mutton AE, Hasleton PS, Curry A, et al. Differentiation of desquamative interstitial pneumonia (DIP) from pulmonary adenocarcinoma by immunocytochemistry. Histopathology 1998; 33:129–35.
352. Myers JL, Veal CF Jr, Shin MS, Katzenstein AL. Respiratory bronchiolitis causing interstitial lung disease. A clinicopathologic study of six cases. Am Rev Respir Dis 1987;135:880–4.
353. Niewoehner DE, Kleinerman J, Rice DB. Pathologic changes in the peripheral airways of young cigarette smokers. N Engl J Med 1974;291:755–8.
354. Nogee LM, de Mello DE, Dehner LP, Colten HR. Brief report: deficiency of pulmonary surfactant protein B in congenital alveolar proteinosis. N Engl J Med 1993;328:406–10.
355. Paul K, Klettke U, Moldenhauer J, et al. Increasing dose of methylprednisolone pulse therapy treats desquamative interstitial pneumonia in a child. Eur Respir J 1999;14:1429–32.
356. Stillwell PC, Norris DG, O'Connell EJ, Rosenow EC III, Weiland LH, Harrison EG Jr. Desquamative interstitial pneumonitis in children. Chest 1980;77:165–71.
357. Travis WD, Borok Z, Roum JH, et al. Pulmonary Langerhans cell granulomatosis (histiocytosis X). A clinicopathologic study of 48 cases. Am J Surg Pathol 1993;17:971–86.
358. Travis WD, Colby TV, Lombard C, Carpenter HA. A clinicopathologic study of 34 cases of diffuse pulmonary hemorrhage with lung biopsy confirmation. Am J Surg Pathol 1990;14:1112–25.
359. Travis WD, King TE, Bateman ED, et al. ATS/ERS International Multidisciplinary Consensus Classification of Idiopathic Interstitial Pneumonia. Am J Respir Crit Care Med 2002;165:277–304.
360. Travis WD, Matsui K, Moss JE, Ferrans VJ. Idiopathic nonspecific interstitial pneumonia: prognostic significance of cellular and fibrosing patterns. Survival comparison with usual interstitial pneumonia and desquamative interstitial pneumonia. Am J Surg Pathol 2000;24:19–33.
361. Tsukahara M, Yoshii H, Imamura T, Kamei T, Koga M, Furukawa S. Desquamative interstitial pneumonia in sibs. Am J Med Genet 1995; 59:431–4.
362. Tubbs RR, Benjamin SP, Osborne DG, Barenberg S. Surface and transmission ultrastructural characteristics of desquamative interstitial pneumonitis. Hum Pathol 1978;9:693–703.

363. Vedal S, Welsh EV, Miller RR, Müller NL. Desquamative interstitial pneumonia. Computed tomographic findings before and after treatment with corticosteroids. Chest 1988;93:215–7.
364. Verleden GM, Sels F, Van Raemdonck D, Verbeken EK, Lerut T, Demedts M. Possible recurrence of desquamative interstitial pneumonitis in a single lung transplant recipient. Eur Respir J 1998;11:971–4.
365. Wright JL, Lawson LM, Pare PD, Wiggs BJ, Kennedy S, Hogg JC. Morphology of peripheral airways in current smokers and ex-smokers. Am Rev Respir Dis 1983;127:474–7.
366. Yousem SA, Colby TV, Gaensler EA. Respiratory bronchiolitis-associated interstitial lung disease and its relationship to desquamative interstitial pneumonia. Mayo Clin Proc 1989;64:1373–80.

Hypersensitivity Pneumonitis

367. Adler BD, Padley SP, Müller NL, Remy-Jardin M, Remy J. Chronic hypersensitivity pneumonitis: high-resolution CT and radiographic features in 16 patients. Radiology 1992;185:91–5.
368. Ando M, Suga M. Hypersensitivity pneumonitis. Curr Opin Pulm Med 1997;3:391–5.
369. Ando M, Suga M, Kohrogi H. A new look at hypersensitivity pneumonitis. Curr Opin Pulm Med 1999;5:299–304.
370. Bertorelli G, Bocchino V, Olivieri D. Hypersensitivity pneumonitis. Eur Respir Mon 2000;14:120–36.
371. Bessis L, Callard P, Gotheil C, Biaggi A, Grenier P. High-resolution CT of parenchymal lung disease: precise correlation with histologic findings. Radiographics 1992;12:45–58.
372. Colby TV, Coleman A. The histologic diagnosis of extrinsic allergic alveolitis and its differential diagnosis. Prog Surg Pathol 1989;10:11–25.
373. Coleman A, Colby TV. Histologic diagnosis of extrinsic allergic alveolitis. Am J Surg Pathol 1988;12:514–8.
374. Cook PG, Wells IP, McGavin CR. The distribution of pulmonary shadowing in farmer's lung. Clin Radiol 1988;39:21–7.
375. Cormier Y, Lacasse Y. Keys to the diagnosis of hypersensitivity pneumonitis: the role of serum precipitins, lung biopsy, and high-resolution computed tomography. Clin Pulm Med 1996;3:72–7.
376. Dalphin JC, Debieuvre D, Pernet D, et al. Prevalence and risk factors for chronic bronchitis and farmer's lung in French dairy farmers. Br J Ind Med 1993;50:941–4.
377. Drent M, Wagenaar S, Velzen-Blad H, Mulder PG, Hoogsteden HC, van den Bosch JM. Relationship between plasma cell levels and profile of bronchoalveolar lavage fluid in patients with subacute extrinsic allergic alveolitis. Thorax 1993;48:835–9.
378. Emanuel DA, Wenzel FJ, Lawton BR. Pneumonitis due to Cryptostroma corticale (Maple-bark disease). N Engl J Med 1966;274:1413–8.
379. Embil J, Warren P, Yakrus M, et al. Pulmonary illness associated with exposure to Mycobacterium-avium complex in hot tub water. Hypersensitivity pneumonitis or infection? Chest 1997;111:813–6.
380. Fink JN. The use of bronchoprovocation in the diagnosis of hypersensitivity pneumonitis. J Allergy Clin Immunol 1979;64:590–1.
381. Ganier M, Lieberman P, Fink J, Lockwood DG. Humidifier lung. An outbreak in office workers. Chest 1980;77:183–7.
382. Hansell DM, Wells AU, Padley SP, Müller NL. Hypersensitivity pneumonitis: correlation of individual CT patterns with functional abnormalities. Radiology 1996;199:123–8.
383. Hendrick DJ. Bronchopulmonary disease in the workplace. Challenge testing with occupational agents. Ann Allergy 1983;51:179–84.
384. Katzenstein AL, Fiorelli RF. Nonspecific interstitial pneumonia/fibrosis. Histologic features and clinical significance. Am J Surg Pathol 1994;18:136–47.
385. Kawanami O, Basset F, Barrios R, Lacronique JG, Ferrans VJ, Crystal RG. Hypersensitivity pneumonitis in man. Light- and electron-microscopic studies of 18 lung biopsies. Am J Pathol 1983;110:275–89.
386. King TE Jr. Classification and clinical manifestations of hypersensitivity pneumonitis (extrinsic allergic alveolitis). In: Rose BD, ed. Uptodate in medicine. Wellesley: Uptodate; 2001.
387. King TE Jr. Diagnosis of hypersensitivity pneumonitis (extrinsic allergic alveolitis). In: Rose BD, ed. Uptodate. Wellesley: Uptodate; 2001.
388. King TE Jr. Epidemiology and causes of hypersensitivity pneumonitis (extrinsic allergic alveolitis). In: Rose BD, ed. Uptodate in medicine. Wellesley: Uptodate; 2001.
389. Klech HH, Pohl WW. Use of bronchoalveolar lavage in interstitial lung disease. In: Bone RC, ed. Pulmonary and critical care medicine. St.Louis: Mosby; 1993:1–23.
390. Kokkarinen JI, Tukiainen HO, Terho EO. Effect of corticosteroid treatment on the recovery of pulmonary function in farmer's lung. Am Rev Respir Dis 1992;145:3–5.
391. Kokkarinen JI, Tukiainen HO, Terho EO. Recovery of pulmonary function in farmer's lung. A five-year follow-up study. Am Rev Respir Dis 1993;147:793–6.

392. Lacasse Y, Fraser RS, Fournier M, Cormier Y. Diagnostic accuracy of transbronchial biopsy in acute farmer's lung disease. Chest 1997;112:1459–65.
393. Larsson K, Eklund A, Malmberg P, Bjermer L, Lundgren R, Belin L. Hyaluronic acid (hyaluronan) in BAL fluid distinguishes farmers with allergic alveolitis from farmers with asymptomatic alveolitis. Chest 1992;101:109–14.
394. Lougheed MD, Roos JO, Waddell WR, Munt PW. Desquamative interstitial pneumonitis and diffuse alveolar damage in textile workers. Potential role of mycotoxins. Chest 1995;108:1196–200.
395. Lynch DA, Newell JD, Logan PM, King TE Jr, Müller NL. Can CT distinguish hypersensitivity pneumonitis from idiopathic pulmonary fibrosis? AJR Am J Roentgenol 1995;165:807–11.
396. Lynch DA, Rose CS, Way D, King TE Jr. Hypersensitivity pneumonitis: sensitivity of high-resolution CT in a population-based study. AJR Am J Roentgenol 1992;159:469–72.
397. Malmberg P. Health effects of organic dust exposure in dairy farmers. Am J Ind Med 1990;17:7–15.
398. Malmberg P, Rask-Andersen A, Hoglund S, Kolmodin-Hedman B, Read GJ. Incidence of organic dust toxic syndrome and allergic alveolitis in Swedish farmers. Int Arch Allergy Appl Immunol 1988;87:47–54.
399. Miyagawa T, Hamagami S, Tanigawa N. Cryptococcus albidus-induced summer-type hypersensitivity pneumonitis. Am J Respir Crit Care Med 2000;161:961–6.
400. Monkare S. Influence of corticosteroid treatment on the course of farmer's lung. Eur J Respir Dis 1983;64:283–93.
401. Monkare S, Ikonen M, Haahtela T. Radiologic findings in farmer's lung. Prognosis and correlation to lung function. Chest 1985;87:460–6.
402. Murayama J, Yoshizawa Y, Ohtsuka M, Hasegawa S. Lung fibrosis in hypersensitivity pneumonitis. Association with CD4+ but not CD8+ cell dominant alveolitis and insidious onset. Chest 1993;104:38–43.
403. Ohtani Y, Kojima K, Sumi Y, et al. Inhalation provocation tests in chronic bird fancier's lung. Chest 2000;118:1382–9.
404. Pardo A, Barrios R, Gaxiola M, et al. Increase of lung neutrophils in hypersensitivity pneumonitis is associated with lung fibrosis. Am J Respir Crit Care Med 2000;161:1698–704.
405. Perez-Padilla R, Gaxiola M, Salas J, Mejia M, Ramos C, Selman M. Bronchiolitis in chronic pigeon breeder's disease. Morphologic evidence of a spectrum of small airway lesions in hypersensitivity pneumonitis induced by avian antigens. Chest 1996;110:371–7.
406. Perez-Padilla R, Salas J, Chapela R, et al. Mortality in Mexican patients with chronic pigeon breeder's lung compared with those with usual interstitial pneumonia. Am Rev Respir Dis 1993;148:49–53.
407. Ramirez-Venegas A, Sansores RH, Perez-Padilla R, Carrillo G, Selman M. Utility of a provocation test for diagnosis of chronic pigeon breeder's disease. Am J Respir Crit Care Med 1998;158:862–9.
408. Remy-Jardin M, Remy J, Wallaert B, Müller NL. Subacute and chronic bird breeder hypersensitivity pneumonitis: sequential evaluation with CT and correlation with lung function tests and bronchoalveolar lavage. Radiology 1993;189:111–8.
409. Reyes CN, Wenzel FJ, Lawton BR, Emanuel DA. The pulmonary pathology of farmer's lung disease. Chest 1982;81:142–6.
410. Reynolds HY. Hypersensitivity pneumonitis. Clin Chest Med 1982;3:503–19.
411. Reynolds HY. Hypersensitivity pneumonitis: correlation of cellular and immunologic changes with clinical phases of disease. Lung 1988;166:189–208.
412. Reynolds SP, Jones KP, Edwards JH, Davies BH. Inhalation challenge in pigeon breeder's disease: BAL fluid changes after 6 hours. Eur Respir J 1993;6:467–76.
413. Richerson HB, Bernstein IL, Fink JN, et al. Guidelines for the clinical evaluation of hypersensitivity pneumonitis. Report of the Subcommittee on Hypersensitivity Pneumonitis. J Allergy Clin Immunol 1989;84:839–44.
414. Rose CS, Martyny JW, Newman LS, et al. "Lifeguard lung": endemic granulomatous pneumonitis in an indoor swimming pool. Am J Public Health 1998;88:1795–800.
415. Rose CS, Newman LS. Hypersensitivity pneumonitis and chronic beryllium disease. In: Schwarz MI, King TE Jr., eds. Interstitial lung disease, 2nd ed. St. Louis: Mosby Year Book; 1993:231–54.
416. Satake N, Nagai S, Kawatani A, et al. Density of phenotypic markers on BAL T-lymphocytes in hypersensitivity pneumonitis, pulmonary sarcoidosis and bronchiolitis obliterans with organizing pneumonia. Eur Respir J 1993;6:477–82.
417. Seal RM, Hapke EJ, Thomas GO, Meek JC, Hayes M. The pathology of the acute and chronic stages of farmer's lung. Thorax 1968;23:469–89.
418. Selman M. Hypersensitivity pneumonitis. In: Schwarz MI, King TE Jr, eds. Interstitial lung disease, 3rd ed. Hamilton: BC Decker; 1998:393–422.
419. Semenzato G, Bjermer L, Costabel U, Haslam PL, Olivieri D, Trentin L. Clinical role of bronchoalveolar lavage in extrinsic allergic alveolitis. Eur Respir Review 1992;2:69–74.

420. Semenzato G, Zambello R, Trentin L, Agostini C. Cellular immunity in sarcoidosis and hypersensitivity pneumonitis. Recent advances. Chest 1993;103:139S–43S.
421. Sharma OP, Fujimura N. Hypersensitivity pneumonitis: a noninfectious granulomatosis. Semin Respir Infect 1995;10:96–106.
422. Terho EO. Diagnostic criteria for farmer's lung. Am J Ind Med 1986;10:329.
423. Terho EO. Work-related respiratory disorders among Finnish farmers. Am J Ind Med 1990;18:269–72.
424. Weill D, Rose C, King TE Jr. Treatment and prognosis of hypersensitivity pneumonitis (extrinsic allergic alveolitis). In: Rose BD, ed. Uptodate in medicine. Wellesley: Uptodate; 2001.

Sarcoidosis

425. Abramowicz MJ, Ninane V, Depierreux M, de Francquen P, Yernault JC. Tumour-like presentation of pulmonary sarcoidosis. Eur Respir J 1992;5:1286–7.
426. ACCESS Research Group. Design of a case control etiologic study of sarcoidosis (ACCESS). J Clin Epidemiol 1999;52:1173–86.
427. Agostini C, Adami F, Semenzato G. New pathogenetic insights into the sarcoid granuloma. Curr Opin Rheumatol 2000;12:71–6.
428. Ahuja TS, Mattana J, Valderrama E, Sankaran R, Singhal PC, Wagner JD. Wegener's granulomatosis followed by development of sarcoidosis. Am J Kidney Dis 1996;28:893–8.
429. Askari A, Thompson P, Barnes C. Sarcoidosis: atypical presentation associated with features of systemic lupus erythematosus. J Rheumatol 1988;15:1578–9.
430. Azar HA, Lunardelli C. Collagen nature of asteroid bodies of giant cells in sarcoidosis. Am J Pathol 1969;57:81–92.
431. Baltzan M, Mehta S, Kirkham TH, Cosio MG. Randomized trial of prolonged chloroquine therapy in advanced pulmonary sarcoidosis. Am J Respir Crit Care Med 1999;160:192–7.
432. Baughman RP, Lower EE. A clinical approach to the use of methotrexate for sarcoidosis. Thorax 1999;54:742–6.
433. Baughman RP, Winget DB, Lower EE. Methotrexate is steroid sparing in acute sarcoidosis: results of a double blind, randomized trial. Sarcoidosis Vasc Diffuse Lung Dis 2000;17:60–6.
434. Bjortuft O, Foerster A, Boe J, Geiran O. Single lung transplantation as treatment for end-stage pulmonary sarcoidosis: recurrence of sarcoidosis in two different lung allografts in one patient. J Heart Lung Transplant 1994;13:24–9.
435. Blasi F, Rizzato G, Gambacorta M, et al. Failure to detect the presence of Chlamydia pneumoniae in sarcoid pathology specimens. Eur Respir J 1997;10:2609–11.
436. Bogaerts Y, Van der Straeten M, Tasson J, Pauwels R. Sarcoidosis or malignancy: a diagnostic dilemma. Eur J Respir Dis 1983;64:541–50.
437. Brauner MW, Grenier P, Mompoint D, Lenoir S, de Cremoux H. Pulmonary sarcoidosis: evaluation with high-resolution CT. Radiology 1989;172:467–71.
438. Carrington CB, Gaensler EA, Mikus JP, Schachter AW, Burke GW, Goff AM. Structure and function in sarcoidosis. Ann N Y Acad Sci 1976;278:265–83.
439. Churg A. Vasculitis in sarcoidosis. In: Churg A, Churg J, eds. Systemic vasculitides. New York: Igaku-Shoin; 1991:299–304.
440. Coots LE, Lazarus AA. Bronchoalveolar lavage in sarcoidosis and HIV infection [Letter]. Chest 1990;98:517–8.
441. Crissman JD, Koss M, Carson RP. Pulmonary veno-occlusive disease secondary to granulomatous venulitis. Am J Surg Pathol 1980;4:93–9.
442. Damuth TE, Bower JS, Cho K, Dantzker DR. Major pulmonary artery stenosis causing pulmonary hypertension in sarcoidosis. Chest 1980;78:888–91.
443. De Vuyst P, Dumortier P, Schandene L, Estenne M, Verhest A, Yernault JC. Sarcoidlike lung granulomatosis induced by aluminum dusts. Am Rev Respir Dis 1987;135:493–7.
444. Dhakhwa B, Harman E, Safirstein BH. Sarcoidosis presenting as multiple pulmonary nodules. JAMA 1976;236:2529–30.
445. Di Alberti L, Piattelli A, Artese L, et al. Human herpesvirus 8 variants in sarcoid tissues. Lancet 1997;350:1655–61.
446. Drent M, Wirnsberger RM, de Vries J, Dieijen-Visser MP, Wouters EF, Schols AM. Association of fatigue with an acute phase response in sarcoidosis. Eur Respir J 1999;13:718–22.
447. Fanburg BL, Villa O. Sarcoidosis. In: Murray JF, Nadel JA, eds. Textbook of respiratory medicine, 3rd ed. Philadelphia: WB Saunders; 2000:1717–32.
448. Fujimura M, Ishiura Y, Kasahara K, et al. Necrotizing bronchial aspergillosis as a cause of hemoptysis in sarcoidosis. Am J Med Sci 1998;315:56–8.
449. Gowda KS, Mayers I, Shafran SD. Concomitant sarcoidosis and HIV infection. Can Med Assoc J 1990;142:136–7.
450. Grenier P, Valeyre D, Cluzel P, Brauner MW, Lenoir S, Chastang C. Chronic diffuse interstitial lung disease: diagnostic value of chest radiography and high-resolution CT. Radiology 1991;179:123–32.

451. Grosser M, Luther T, Muller J, et al. Detection of M. tuberculosis DNA in sarcoidosis: correlation with T-cell response. Lab Invest 1999;79:775–84.
452. Heffner JE, Milam MG. Sarcoid-like hilar and mediastinal lymphadenopathy in a patient with metastatic testicular cancer. Cancer 1987;60:1545–7.
453. Hoffstein V, Ranganathan N, Mullen JB. Sarcoidosis simulating pulmonary veno-occlusive disease. Am Rev Respir Dis 1986;134:809–11.
454. Hsu RM, Connors AF Jr, Tomashefski JF Jr. Histologic, microbiologic, and clinical correlates of the diagnosis of sarcoidosis by transbronchial biopsy. Arch Pathol Lab Med 1996;120:364–8.
455. Hunninghake GW, Crystal RG. Pulmonary sarcoidosis: a disorder mediated by excess helper T- lymphocyte activity at sites of disease activity. N Engl J Med 1981;305:429–34.
456. Hunter T, Arnott JE, McCarthy DS. Features of systemic lupus erythematosus and sarcoidosis occurring together. Arthritis Rheum 1980;23:364–6.
457. Ishige I, Usui Y, Takemura T, Eishi Y. Quantitative PCR of mycobacterial and propionibacterial DNA in lymph nodes of Japanese patients with sarcoidosis. Lancet 1999;354:120–3.
458. James DG, Neville E, Siltzbach LE. A worldwide review of sarcoidosis. Ann N Y Acad Sci 1976;278:321–34.
459. Johns CJ, Michele TM. The clinical management of sarcoidosis. A 50-year experience at the Johns Hopkins Hospital. Medicine (Baltimore) 1999;78:65–111.
460. Johnson BA, Duncan SR, Ohori NP, et al. Recurrence of sarcoidosis in pulmonary allograft recipients. Am Rev Respir Dis 1993;148:1373-7.
461. Judson MA. Lung transplantation for pulmonary sarcoidosis. Eur Respir J 1998;11:738–44.
462. Kamiyoshihara M, Hirai T, Kawashima O, Ishikawa S, Morishita Y. Sarcoid reactions in primary pulmonary carcinoma: report of seven cases. Oncol Rep 1998;5:177–80.
463. Kazerooni EA, Cascade PN. Recurrent miliary sarcoidosis after lung transplantation. Radiology 1995;194:913.
464. Kazerooni EA, Jackson C, Cascade PN. Sarcoidosis: recurrence of primary disease in transplanted lungs. Radiology 1994;192:461–4.
465. Keeffe EB. Sarcoidosis and primary biliary cirrhosis. Literature review and illustrative case. Am J Med 1987;83:977–80.
466. King TE Jr. Treatment of pulmonary sarcoidosis with corticosteroids. In: Rose BD, ed. Uptodate in medicine. Wellesley: Uptodate; 2001.
467. King TE Jr. Treatment of pulmonary sarcoidosis with alternatives to corticosteroids. In: Rose BD, ed. Uptodate in medicine. Wellesley: Uptodate; 2001.
468. Kok TC, Haasjes JG, Splinter TA, ten Kate FJ. Sarcoid-like lymphadenopathy mimicking metastatic testicular cancer. Cancer 1991;68:1845–7.
469. Kwong T, Valderrama E, Paley C, Ilowite N. Systemic necrotizing vasculitis associated with childhood sarcoidosis. Semin Arthritis Rheum 1994;23:388–95.
470. Leatham EW, Eeles R, Sheppard M, et al. The association of germ cell tumours of the testis with sarcoid-like processes. Clin Oncol (R Coll Radiol) 1992;4:89–95.
471. Leff JA, Ready JB, Repetto C, Goff JS, Schwarz MI. Coexistence of primary biliary cirrhosis and sarcoidosis. West J Med 1990;153:439–41.
472. Levine BW, Saldana M, Hutter AM. Pulmonary hypertension in sarcoidosis. A case report of a rare but potentially treatable cause. Am Rev Respir Dis 1971;103:413–7.
473. Levy NT, Rubin J, DeRemee RA, Aughenbaugh GL, Unni KK, Kahn MJ. Carcinoid tumors and sarcoidosis–does a link exist? Mayo Clin Proc 1997;72:112–6.
474. Lewis SJ, Ainslie GM, Bateman ED. Efficacy of azathioprine as second-line treatment in pulmonary sarcoidosis. Sarcoidosis Vasc Diffuse Lung Dis 1999;16:87–92.
475. Lie JT. Combined sarcoidosis and disseminated visceral giant cell angiitis: a third opinion. Arch Pathol Lab Med 1991;115:210–1.
476. Liebman J, Linthicum CM. Granular cell myoblastoma (schwannoma) of the carina in a patient with sarcoidosis. South Med J 1976;69:1613–5.
477. Lowery WS, Whitlock WL, Dietrich RA, Fine JM. Sarcoidosis complicated by HIV infection: three case reports and a review of the literature. Am Rev Respir Dis 1990;142:887–9.
478. Maddrey WC. Sarcoidosis and primary biliary cirrhosis. Associated disorders? [Editorial]. N Engl J Med 1983;308:588–90.
479. Maliarik MJ, Chen KM, Sheffer RG, et al. The natural resistance-associated macrophage protein gene in African Americans with sarcoidosis. Am J Respir Cell Mol Biol 2000;22:672–5.
480. Marcussen N, Lund C. Combined sarcoidosis and disseminated visceral giant cell vasculitis. Pathol Res Pract 1989;184:325–30.
481. Martens H, Zollner B, Zissel G, Burdon D, Schlaak M, Muller-Quernheim J. Anti-Borrelia burgdorferi immunoglobulin seroprevalence in pulmonary sarcoidosis: a negative report. Eur Respir J 1997;10:1356–8.

482. Martin JME, Dowling GP. Sudden death associated with compression of pulmonary arteries in sarcoidosis. Can Med Assoc J 1985;133:423–4.
483. Martinetti M, Tinelli C, Kolek V, et al. "The sarcoidosis map": a joint survey of clinical and immunogenetic findings in two European countries. Am J Respir Crit Care Med 1995;152:557–64.
484. Mathieson JR, Mayo JR, Staples CA, Müller NL. Chronic diffuse infiltrative lung disease: comparison of diagnostic accuracy of CT and chest radiography. Radiology 1989;171:111–6.
485. Merchant TE, Filippa DA, Yahalom J. Sarcoidosis following chemotherapy for Hodgkin's disease. Leuk Lymphoma 1994;13:339–47.
486. Miller JJ III. Early onset "sarcoidosis" and "familial granulomatous arthritis (arteritis)": the same disease. J Pediatr 1986;109:387–8.
487. Mitchell DM, Mitchell DN, Collins JV, Emerson CJ. Transbronchial lung biopsy through fibreoptic bronchoscope in diagnosis of sarcoidosis. Br Med J 1980;280:679–81.
488. Miyata M, Takase Y, Kobayashi H, et al. Primary Sjögren's syndrome complicated by sarcoidosis. Intern Med 1998;37:174–8.
489. Miyazaki Y, Miyake S, Taki R, Ohkouchi Y, Matsubara O, Yoshizawa Y. Sarcoid reactions scattered in the tumor-bearing lung parenchyma and regional lymph nodes associated with pulmonary carcinoid. Intern Med 1998;37:304–6.
490. Muller-Quernheim J, Kienast K, Held M, Pfeifer S, Costabel U. Treatment of chronic sarcoidosis with an azathioprine/prednisolone regimen. Eur Respir J 1999;14:1117–22.
491. Müller NL, Kullnig P, Miller RR. The CT findings of pulmonary sarcoidosis: analysis of 25 patients. AJR Am J Roentgenol 1989;152:1179–82.
492. Nunley DR, Hattler B, Keenan RJ, et al. Lung transplantation for end-stage pulmonary sarcoidosis. Sarcoidosis Vasc Diffuse Lung Dis 1999;16:93–100.
493. Onal E, Lopata M, Lourenco RV. Nodular pulmonary sarcoidosis. Cinical, roentgenographic and physiologic course in five patients. Chest 1977;72:296–300.
494. Ozcelik U, Ozkara HA, Gocmen A, et al. Detection of Mycobacterium tuberculosis DNA in tissue samples of children with sarcoidosis [Letter]. Pediatr Pulmonol 1997;24:122-4.
495. Padilla ML, Schilero GJ, Teirstein AS. Sarcoidosis and transplantation. Sarcoidosis Vasc Diffuse Lung Dis 1997;14:16–22.
496. Papadopoulos KI, Melander O, Orho-Melander M, Groop LC, Carlsson M, Hallengren B. Angiotensin converting enzyme (ACE) gene polymorphism in sarcoidosis in relation to associated autoimmune diseases. J Intern Med 2000;247:71–7.
497. Paramothayan NS, Jones PW. Corticosteroids for pulmonary sarcoidosis. Cochrane Database Syst Rev 2000;4:CD001114.
498. Petrek M, Drabek J, Kolek V, et al. CC chemokine receptor gene polymorphisms in Czech patients with pulmonary sarcoidosis. Am J Respir Crit Care Med 2000;162:1000–3.
499. Popper HH, Klemen H, Hoefler G, Winter E. Presence of mycobacterial DNA in sarcoidosis. Hum Pathol 1997;28:796–800.
500. Renston JP, Goldman ES, Hsu RM, Tomashefski JF. Peripheral blood eosinophilia in association with sarcoidosis. Mayo Clin Proc 2000;75:586–90.
501. Rosen Y. Sarcoidosis. In: Dail DH, Hammar SP, eds. Pulmonary pathology, 2nd ed. New York: Springer-Verlag; 1994:615–45.
502. Rosen Y, Athanassiades TJ, Moon S, Lyons HA. Nongranulomatous interstitial pneumonitis in sarcoidosis. Relationship to development of epithelioid granulomas. Chest 1978;74:122–5.
503. Rosen Y, Moon S, Huang C, Gourin A, Lyons HA. Granulomatous pulmonary angiitis in sarcoidosis. Arch Pathol Lab Med 1977;101:170–4.
504. Rosen Y, Vuletin JC, Pertschuk LP, Silverstein E. Sarcoidosis from the pathologist's vantage point. Pathol Annu 1979;14[Part I]:405–39.
505. Schapiro JM, Shpitzer S, Pinkhas J, Sidi Y, Arber N. Sarcoidosis as the initial manifestation of Takayasu's arteritis. J Med 1994;25:121–8.
506. Segawa Y, Takigawa N, Okahara M, et al. Primary lung cancer associated with diffuse granulomatous lesions in the pulmonary parenchyma. Intern Med 1996;35:728–31.
507. Sharma OP, Meyer PR, Akil B, Nademanee A, Owens CM. Sarcoidosis and lymphoma: an unusual association. Sarcoidosis 1987;4:58–63.
508. Shintaku M, Mase K, Ohtsuki H, Yasumizu R, Yasunaga K, Ikehara S. Generalized sarcoidlike granulomas with systemic angiitis, crescentic glomerulonephritis, and pulmonary hemorrhage. Report of an autopsy case. Arch Pathol Lab Med 1989;113:1295–8.
509. Smith LJ, Lawrence JB, Katzenstein AA. Vascular sarcoidosis: a rare cause of pulmonary hypertension. Am J Med Sci 1983;285:38–44.
510. Statement on sarcoidosis. Joint Statement of the American Thoracic Society (ATS), the European Respiratory Society (ERS) and the World Association of Sarcoidosis and Other Granulomatous Disorders (WASOG) adopted by the ATS Board of Directors and by the ERS Executive Committee, February 1999. Am J Respir Crit Care Med 1999;160:736–55.
511. Stirling RG, Cullinan P, Dubois RM. Sarcoidosis. In: Schwarz MI, King TE Jr, eds. Interstitial lung disease, 3rd ed. Hamilton: BC Decker; 1998:279–324.

512. Takemura T, Matsui Y, Oritsu M, Akiyama O, et al. Pulmonary vascular involvement in sarcoidosis: granulomatous angiitis and microangiopathy in transbronchial lung biopsies. Virchows Arch [A] 1991;418:361–8.
513. van den Berg, Fickers M, Theunissen P, van Noord JA. Pulmonary sarcoid-like granulomata in a patient treated for extrapulmonary Hodgkin's disease. Respiration 1997;64:114–7.
514. Visscher D, Churg A, Katzenstein AL. Significance of crystalline inclusions in lung granulomas. Mod Pathol 1988;1:415–9.
515. Vokurka M, Lecossier D, du Bois RM, et al. Absence of DNA from mycobacteria of the M. tuberculosis complex in sarcoidosis. Am J Respir Crit Care Med 1997;156:1000–3.

Histiocytic Disorders

516. Aggarwal S, Arora NK, Koyyana R, Mukhopadhyay S, Kumar A. Interstitial lung disease in a young child. Chest 1989;96:389–90.
517. Aguayo SM, King TE Jr, Waldron JA Jr, Sherritt KM, Kane MA, Miller YE. Increased pulmonary neuroendocrine cells with bombesin-like immunoreactivity in adult patients with eosinophilic granuloma. J Clin Invest 1990;86:838–44.
518. Antonius JI, Farid SM, Baez-Giangreco A. Steroid-responsive Rosai-Dorfman disease. Pediatr Hematol Oncol 1996;13:563–70.
519. Asakura S, Colby TV, Limper AH. Tissue localization of transforming growth factor-beta1 in pulmonary eosinophilic granuloma. Am J Respir Crit Care Med 1996;154:1525–30.
520. Askin FB, McCann BG, Kuhn C. Reactive eosinophilic pleuritis: a lesion to be distinguished from pulmonary eosinophilic granuloma. Arch Pathol Lab Med 1977;101:187–91.
521. Auerswald U, Barth J, Magnussen H. Value of CD-1-positive cells in bronchoalveolar lavage fluid for the diagnosis of pulmonary histiocytosis X. Lung 1991;169:305–9.
522. Barbey S, Jaubert F, Nogues C, Nezelof C, Gane P. Histiocytes X and X body reactivity with concanavalin A, peanut agglutinin and BSPT. Pathol Res Pract 1987;182:805–9.
523. Bonetti F, Chilosi M, Menestrina F, et al. Immunohistological analysis of Rosai-Dorfman histiocytosis. A disease of S-100 + CD1-histiocytes. Virchows Arch [A] 1987;411:129–35.
524. Bonnet D, Kermarec J, Marotel C, et al. Data of bronchoalveolar lavage and pulmonary histiocytosis X. Rev Pneumol Clin 1987;43:121–30.
525. Brabencova E, Tazi A, Lorenzato M, et al. Langerhans cells in Langerhans cell granulomatosis are not actively proliferating cells. Am J Pathol 1998;152:1143–9.
526. Brauner MW, Grenier P, Mouelhi MM, Mompoint D, Lenoir S. Pulmonary histiocytosis X: evaluation with high-resolution CT. Radiology 1989;172:255–8.
527. Brauner MW, Grenier P, Tijani K, Battesti JP, Valeyre D. Pulmonary Langerhans cell histiocytosis: evolution of lesions on CT scans. Radiology 1997;204:497–502.
528. Brown RE. Angiotensin-converting enzyme, transforming growth factor beta(1), and interleukin 11 in the osteolytic lesions of Langerhans cell histiocytosis. Arch Pathol Lab Med 2000;124:1287–90.
529. Carlson RA, Hattery RR, O'Connell EJ, Fontana RS. Pulmonary involvement by histiocytosis X in the pediatric age group. Mayo Clin Proc 1976;51:542–7.
530. Casolaro MA, Bernaudin JF, Saltini C, Ferrans VJ, Crystal RG. Accumulation of Langerhans' cells on the epithelial surface of the lower respiratory tract in normal subjects in association with cigarette smoking. Am Rev Respir Dis 1988;137:406–11.
531. Chatkin JM, Bastos JC, Stein RT, Gaiger AM. Sole pulmonary involvement by Langerhans' cell histiocytosis in a child. Eur Respir J 1993;6:1226–8.
532. Colby TV, Lombard C. Histiocytosis X in the lung. Hum Pathol 1983;14:847–56.
533. Cotter FE, Pritchard J. Clonality in Langerhans' cell histiocytosis [Editorial]. Br Med J 1995;310:74–5.
534. Crausman RS, Jennings CA, Tuder RM, Ackerson LM, Irvin CG, King TE Jr. Pulmonary histiocytosis X: pulmonary function and exercise pathophysiology. Am J Respir Crit Care Med 1996;153:426–35.
535. Crausman RS, King TE Jr. Primary pulmonary histiocytosis X in the adult: clinical features, diagnosis and treatment. In: Rose BD, ed. Uptodate in medicine. Wellesley: Uptodate; 2001.
536. de Graaf JH, Egeler RM. New insights into the pathogenesis of Langerhans cell histiocytosis. Curr Opin Pediatr 1997;9:46–50.
537. Delobbe A, Durieu J, Duhamel A, Wallaert B. Determinants of survival in pulmonary Langerhans' cell granulomatosis (histiocytosis X). Groupe d'Etude en Pathologie Interstitielle de la Société de Pathologie Thoracique du Nord. Eur Respir J 1996;9:2002–6.
538. Egan AJ, Boardman LA, Tazelaar HD, et al. Erdheim-Chester disease: clinical, radiologic, and histopathologic findings in five patients with interstitial lung disease. Am J Surg Pathol 1999;23:17–26.

539. Egan TM, Detterbeck FC, Keagy BA, Turpin S, Mill MR, Wilcox BR. Single lung transplantation for eosinophilic granulomatosis. South Med J 1992;85:551–3.
540. Eisen RN, Buckley PJ, Rosai J. Immunophenotypic characterization of sinus histiocytosis with massive lymphadenopathy (Rosai-Dorfman disease). Semin Diagn Pathol 1990;7:74–82.
541. Etienne B, Bertocchi M, Gamondes JP, et al. Relapsing pulmonary Langerhans cell histiocytosis after lung transplantation. Am J Respir Crit Care Med 1998;157:288–91.
542. Fartoukh M, Humbert M, Capron F, et al. Severe pulmonary hypertension in histiocytosis X. Am J Respir Crit Care Med 2000;161:216–23.
543. Favara BE, Feller AC, Pauli M, et al. Contemporary classification of histiocytic disorders. The WHO Committee On Histiocytic/Reticulum Cell Proliferations. Reclassification Working Group of the Histiocyte Society. Med Pediatr Oncol 1997;29:157–66.
544. Foucar E, Rosai J, Dorfman R. Sinus histiocytosis with massive lymphadenopathy (Rosai-Dorfman disease): review of the entity. Semin Diagn Pathol 1990;7:19–73.
545. The French Langerhans' Cell Histiocytosis Study Group. A multicentre retrospective survey of Langerhans' cell histiocytosis: 348 cases observed between 1983 and 1993. Arch Dis Child 1996;75:17–24.
546. Friedman PJ, Liebow AA, Sokoloff J. Eosinophilic granuloma of lung. Clinical aspects of primary histiocytosis in the adult. Medicine (Baltimore) 1981;60:385–96.
547. Gabbay E, Dark JH, Ashcroft T, et al. Recurrence of Langerhans' cell granulomatosis following lung transplantation. Thorax 1998;53:326–7.
548. Gaensler EA, Carrington CB. Open biopsy for chronic diffuse infiltrative lung disease: clinical, roentgenographic, and physiological correlations in 502 patients. Ann Thorac Surg 1980;30:411–26.
549. Grenier P, Valeyre D, Cluzel P, Brauner MW, Lenoir S, Chastang C. Chronic diffuse interstitial lung disease: diagnostic value of chest radiography and high-resolution CT. Radiology 1991;179:123–32.
550. Habib SB, Congleton J, Carr D, et al. Recurrence of recipient Langerhans' cell histiocytosis following bilateral lung transplantation. Thorax 1998;53:323–5.
551. Hage C, Willman CL, Favara BE, Isaacson PG. Langerhans' cell histiocytosis (histiocytosis X): immunophenotype and growth fraction. Hum Pathol 1993;24:840–5.
552. Harari S, Brenot F, Barberis M, Simmoneau G. Advanced pulmonary histiocytosis X is associated with severe pulmonary hypertension [Letter]. Chest 1997;111:1142–4.
553. Hartman TE, Tazelaar HD, Swensen SJ, Müller NL. Cigarette smoking: CT and pathologic findings of associated pulmonary diseases. Radiographics 1997;17:377–90.
554. Howarth DM, Gilchrist GS, Mullan BP, Wiseman GA, Edmonson JH, Schomberg PJ. Langerhans cell histiocytosis: diagnosis, natural history, management, and outcome. Cancer 1999;85:2278–90.
555. King TE Jr, Schwarz MI, Dreisin RE, Pratt DS, Theofilopoulos AN. Circulating immune complexes in pulmonary eosinophilic granuloma. Ann Intern Med 1979;91:397–9.
556. Klareskog L, Tjernlund U, Forsum U, Peterson PA. Epidermal Langerhans cells express Ia antigens. Nature 1977;268:248–50.
557. Komp DM. The treatment of sinus histiocytosis with massive lymphadenopathy (Rosai-Dorfman disease). Semin Diagn Pathol 1990;7:83–6.
558. Kulwiec EL, Lynch DA, Aguayo SM, Schwarz MI, King TE Jr. Imaging of pulmonary histiocytosis X. Radiographics 1992;12:515–26.
559. Lacronique J, Roth C, Battesti JP, Basset F, Chretien J. Chest radiological features of pulmonary histiocytosis X: a report based on 50 adult cases. Thorax 1982;37:104–9.
560. Lichtenstein L. Histiocytosis X. Arch Pathol 1953;56:84–102.
561. Lieberman PH, Jones CR, Steinman RM, et al. Langerhans cell (eosinophilic) granulomatosis. A clinicopathologic study encompassing 50 years. Am J Surg Pathol 1996;20:519–52.
562. Loukides S, Karameris A, Lachanis S, Panagou P, Kalogeropoulos N. Eosinophilic granuloma of the lung presenting as an endobronchial mass. Monaldi Arch Chest Dis 2000;55:208–9.
563. Marcy TW, Reynolds HY. Pulmonary histiocytosis X. Lung 1985;163:129–50.
564. Mogulkoc N, Veral A, Bishop PW, Bayindir U, Pickering CA, Egan JJ. Pulmonary Langerhans' cell histiocytosis: radiologic resolution following smoking cessation. Chest 1999;115:1452–5.
565. Moore AD, Godwin JD, Müller NL, et al. Pulmonary histiocytosis X: comparison of radiographic and CT findings. Radiology 1989;172:249–54.
566. Palomera L, Domingo JM, Olave T, Romero S, Gutierrez M. Sinus histiocytosis with massive lymphadenopathy: complete response to low-dose interferon-alpha. J Clin Oncol 1997;15:2176.
567. Primack SL, Hartman TE, Hansell DM, Müller NL. End-stage lung disease: CT findings in 61 patients. Radiology 1993;189:681–6.

568. Rosai J, Dorfman RF. Sinus histiocytosis with massive lymphadenopathy. A newly recognized benign clinicopathological entity. Arch Pathol 1969;87:63–70.
569. Rosai J, Dorfman RF. Sinus histiocytosis with massive lymphadenopathy: a pseudolymphomatous benign disorder. Analysis of 34 cases. Cancer 1972;30:1174–88.
570. Rowden G. The Langerhans cell. Crit Rev Immunol 1981;3:95–180.
571. Rush WL, Andriko JA, Galateau-Salle F, et al. Pulmonary pathology of Erdheim-Chester disease. Mod Pathol 2000;13:747–54.
572. Sadoun D, Vaylet F, Valeyre D, et al. Bronchogenic carcinoma in patients with pulmonary histiocytosis X. Chest 1992;101:1610–3.
573. Shijubo N, Shigehara K, Tsutahara S, Abe S. Increased level of circulating gamma/delta T cells in a patient with eosinophilic granuloma. Chest 1994;105:967–8.
574. Soler P, Bergeron A, Kambouchner M, et al. Is high-resolution computed tomography a reliable tool to predict the histopathological activity of pulmonary Langerhans cell histiocytosis? Am J Respir Crit Care Med 2000;162:264–70.
575. Soler P, Moreau A, Basset F, Hance AJ. Cigarette smoking-induced changes in the number and differentiated state of pulmonary dendritic cells/Langerhans cells. Am Rev Respir Dis 1989;139:1112–7.
576. Stiakaki E, Giannakopoulou C, Kouvidi E, et al. Congenital systemic Langerhans cell histiocytosis (report of two cases). Haematologia (Budap) 1997;28:215–22.
577. Tazi A, Bonay M, Grandsaigne M, Battesti JP, Hance AJ, Soler P. Surface phenotype of Langerhans cells and lymphocytes in granulomatous lesions from patients with pulmonary histiocytosis X. Am Rev Respir Dis 1993;147:1531–6.
578. Tazi A, Montcelly L, Bergeron A, Valeyre D, Battesti JP, Hance AJ. Relapsing nodular lesions in the course of adult pulmonary Langerhans cell histiocytosis. Am J Respir Crit Care Med 1998;157:2007–10.
579. Tomashefski JF, Khiyami A, Kleinerman J. Neoplasms associated with pulmonary eosinophilic granuloma. Arch Pathol Lab Med 1991;115:499–506.
580. Travis WD, Borok Z, Roum JH, et al. Pulmonary Langerhans cell granulomatosis (histiocytosis X). A clinicopathologic study of 48 cases. Am J Surg Pathol 1993;17:971–86.
581. Vassallo R, Ryu JH, Colby TV, Hartman T, Limper AH. Pulmonary Langerhans'-cell histiocytosis. N Engl J Med 2000;342:1969–78.
582. Veyssier-Belot C, Cacoub P, Caparros-Lefebvre D, et al. Erdheim-Chester disease. Clinical and radiologic characteristics of 59 cases. Medicine (Baltimore) 1996;75:157–69.
583. Willman CL, Busque L, Griffith BB, et al. Langerhans'-cell histiocytosis (histiocytosis X)–a clonal proliferative disease. N Engl J Med 1994;331:154–60.
584. Wittenberg KH, Swensen SJ, Myers JL. Pulmonary involvement with Erdheim-Chester disease: radiographic and CT findings. AJR Am J Roentgenol 2000;174:1327–31.
585. Xaubet A, Agusti C, Picado C, et al. Bronchoalveolar lavage analysis with anti-T6 monoclonal antibody in the evaluation of diffuse lung diseases. Respiration 1989;56:161–6.
586. Ye F, Huang SW, Dong HJ. Histiocytosis X. S-100 protein, peanut agglutinin, and transmission electron microscopy study. Am J Clin Pathol 1990;94:627–31.
587. Yeatman M, McNeil K, Smith JA, et al. Lung transplantation in patients with systemic diseases: an eleven-year experience at Papworth hospital. J Heart Lung Transplant 1996;15:144–9.
588. Youkeles LH, Grizzanti JN, Liao Z, Chang CJ, Rosenstreich DL. Decreased tobacco-glycoprotein-induced lymphocyte proliferation in vitro in pulmonary eosinophilic granuloma. Am J Respir Crit Care Med 1995;151:145–50.
589. Yu RC, Chu C, Buluwela L, Chu AC. Clonal proliferation of Langerhans cells in Langerhans cell histiocytosis. Lancet 1994;343:767–8.
590. Zeid NA, Muller HK. Tobacco smoke induced lung granulomas and tumors: association with pulmonary Langerhans cells. Pathology 1995;27:247–54.

Lymphangioleiomyomatosis

591. Askin FB, McCann BG, Kuhn C. Reactive eosinophilic pleuritis: a lesion to be distinguished from pulmonary eosinophilic granuloma. Arch Pathol Lab Med 1977;101:187–91.
592. Aubry MC, Myers JL, Ryu JH, et al. Pulmonary lymphangioleiomyomatosis in a man. Am J Respir Crit Care Med 2000;162:749–52.
593. Avila NA, Kelly JA, Chu SC, Dwyer AJ, Moss J. Lymphangioleiomyomatosis: abdominopelvic CT and US findings. Radiology 2000;216:147–53.
594. Bachman D, Wolff M. Pulmonary metastases from benign-appearing smooth muscle tumors of the uterus. Am J Roentgenol 1976;127:441–6.
595. Baldi S, Papotti M, Valente ML, Rapellino M, Scappaticci E, Corrin B. Pulmonary lymphangioleiomyomatosis in postmenopausal women: report of two cases and review of the literature. Eur Respir J 1994;7:1013–6.
596. Basset F, Soler P, Marsac J, Corrin B. Pulmonary lymphangiomyomatosis: three new cases studied with electron microscopy. Cancer 1976;38:2357–66.

597. Berger U, Khaghani A, Pomerance A, Yacoub MH, Coombes RC. Pulmonary lymphangioleiomyomatosis and steroid receptors. An immunocytochemical study. Am J Clin Pathol 1990;93:609–14.
598. Bernstein SM, Newell JD, Adamczyk D, Mortenson RL, King TE Jr, Lynch DA. How common are renal angiomyolipomas in patients with pulmonary lymphangiomyomatosis? Am J Respir Crit Care Med 1995;152:2138–43.
599. Bhattacharyya AK, Balogh K. Retroperitoneal lymphangioleiomyomatosis. A 36-year benign course in a postmenopausal woman. Cancer 1985;56:1144–6.
600. Boehler A, Speich R, Russi EW, Weder W. Lung transplantation for lymphangioleiomyomatosis. N Engl J Med 1996;335:1275–80.
601. Bonelli FS, Hartman TE, Swensen SJ, Sherrick A. Accuracy of high-resolution CT in diagnosing lung diseases. AJR Am J Roentgenol 1998;170:1507–12.
602. Bonetti F, Chiodera PL, Pea M, et al. Transbronchial biopsy in lymphangiomyomatosis of the lung. HMB45 for diagnosis. Am J Surg Pathol 1993;17:1092–102.
603. Bonetti F, Pea M, Martignoni G, Zamboni G, Iuzzolino P. Cellular heterogeneity in lymphangiomyomatosis of the lung [Letter]. Hum Pathol 1991;22:727–8.
604. Bowen J, Beasley SW. Rare pulmonary manifestations of tuberous sclerosis in children. Pediatr Pulmonol 1997;23:114–6.
605. Carrington CB, Cugell DW, Gaensler EA, et al. Lymphangioleiomyomatosis. Physiologic-pathologic-radiologic correlations. Am Rev Respir Dis 1977;116:977–95.
606. Carsillo T, Astrinidis A, Henske EP. Mutations in the tuberous sclerosis complex gene TSC2 are a cause of sporadic pulmonary lymphangioleiomyomatosis. Proc Natl Acad Sci U S A 2000;97:6085–90.
607. Castro M, Shepherd CW, Gomez MR, Lie JT, Ryu JH. Pulmonary tuberous sclerosis. Chest 1995;107:189–95.
608. Chiodera F, Pea M, Martignoni G, et al. Transbronchial biopsies in lymphangioleiomyomatosis of the lung: MOAB HMB-45 is helpful for the diagnosis [Abstract]. Mod Pathol 1993; 6:129A.
609. Chu SC, Horiba K, Usuki J, et al. Comprehensive evaluation of 35 patients with lymphangioleiomyomatosis. Chest 1999;115:1041–52.
610. Chuah KL, Tan PH. Multifocal micronodular pneumocyte hyperplasia, lymphangiomyomatosis and clear cell micronodules of the lung in a Chinese female patient with tuberous sclerosis. Pathology 1998;30:242–6.
611. Colby TV, Koss MN, Travis WD. Tumors of the lower respiratory tract. Atlas of tumor pathology, 3rd Series, Fascicle 13. Washington, D.C.: Armed Forces Institute of Pathology; 1995.
612. Colley MH, Geppert E, Franklin WA. Immunohistochemical detection of steroid receptors in a case of pulmonary lymphangioleiomyomatosis. Am J Surg Pathol 1989;13:803–7.
613. Corrin B, Liebow AA, Friedman PJ. Pulmonary lymphangiomyomatosis. A review. Am J Pathol 1975;79:348–82.
614. Costello LC, Hartman TE, Ryu JH. High frequency of pulmonary lymphangioleiomyomatosis in women with tuberous sclerosis complex. Mayo Clin Proc 2000;75:591–4.
615. Crausman RS, Jennings CA, Mortenson RL, Ackerson LM, Irvin CG, King TE Jr. Lymphangioleiomyomatosis: the pathophysiology of diminished exercise capacity. Am J Respir Crit Care Med 1996;153:1368–76.
616. Crausman RS, King TE Jr. Pulmonary involvement in tuberous sclerosis. In: Rose BD, ed. Uptodate in medicine. Wellesley: Uptodate; 2001.
617. Crausman RS, King TE Jr. Pulmonary lymphangioleiomyomatosis. In: Rose BD, ed. Uptodate in medicine. Wellesley: Uptodate; 2001.
618. Dwyer JM, Hickie JB, Garvan J. Pulmonary tuberous sclerosis. Report of three patients and a review of the literature. Q J Med 1971; 40:115–25.
619. Eliasson AH, Phillips YY, Tenholder MF. Treatment of lymphangioleiomyomatosis. A meta-analysis. Chest 1989;96:1352–5.
620. Fahy J, Toner M, O'Sullivan J, FitzGerald MX. Haemopericardium and cardiac tamponade complicating pulmonary lymphangioleiomyomatosis. Thorax 1991;46:222.
621. Faul JL, Berry GJ, Colby TV, et al. Thoracic lymphangiomas, lymphangiectasis, lymphangiomatosis, and lymphatic dysplasia syndrome. Am J Respir Crit Care Med 2000;161:1037–46.
622. Ferrans VJ, Yu ZX, Nelson WK, et al. Lymphangioleiomyomatosis (LAM): a review of clinical and morphological features. J Nippon Med Sch 2000;67:311–29.
623. Flieder DB, Travis WD. Clear cell "sugar" tumor of the lung: association with lymphangioleiomyomatosis and multifocal micronodular pneumocyte hyperplasia in a patient with tuberous sclerosis. Am J Surg Pathol 1997;21:1242–7.
624. Ford JM, Pang J, Coutts J, Evans BD. Metastasizing leiomyoma of the uterus. Aust N Z J Obstet Gynaecol 1988;28:154–5.
625. Fukuda Y, Kawamoto M, Yamamoto A, Ishizaki M, Basset F, Masugi Y. Role of elastic fiber degradation in emphysema-like lesions of pulmonary lymphangiomyomatosis. Hum Pathol 1990;21:1252–61.

626. Gaffey MJ, Mills SE, Ritter JH. Clear cell tumors of the lower respiratory tract. Semin Diagn Pathol 1997;14:222–32.
627. Gawad KA, Knoefel WT, Izbicki JR, Schroder S, Broelsch CE. Generalised lymphangioleiomyomatosis presenting as a retroperitoneal tumour. Eur J Surg 1996;162:583–5.
628. Gerst PH, Levy J, Swaminathan K, Kshettry V, Albu E. Metastatic leiomyosarcoma of the uterus: unusual presentation of a case with late endobronchial and small bowel metastases. Gynecol Oncol 1993;49:271–5.
629. Guinee D, Singh R, Azumi N, et al. Multifocal micronodular pneumocyte hyperplasia: a distinctive pulmonary manifestation of tuberous sclerosis. Mod Pathol 1995;8:902–6.
630. Guinee DG Jr, Feuerstein I, Koss MN, Travis WD. Pulmonary lymphangioleiomyomatosis. Diagnosis based on results of transbronchial biopsy and immunohistochemical studies and correlation with high-resolution computed tomography findings. Arch Pathol Lab Med 1994;118:846–9.
631. Guinee DG Jr, Thornberry DS, Azumi N, Przygodzki RM, Koss MN, Travis WD. Unique pulmonary presentation of an angiomyolipoma. Analysis of clinical, radiographic, and histopathologic features. Am J Surg Pathol 1995;19:476–80.
632. Harris JO, Waltuck BL, Swenson EW. The pathophysiology of the lungs in tuberous sclerosis. A case report and literature review. Am Rev Respir Dis 1969;100:379–87.
633. Hauck RW, König G, Permanetter W, Weiss M, Wöckel W, Fruhmann G. Tuberous sclerosis with pulmonary involvement. Respiration 1990;57:289–92.
634. Hayashi T, Fleming MV, Stetler-Stevenson WG, et al. Immunohistochemical study of matrix metalloproteinases (MMPs) and their tissue inhibitors (TIMPs) in pulmonary lymphangioleiomyomatosis (LAM). Hum Pathol 1997;28:1071–8.
635. Hironaka M, Fukayama M. Regional proliferation of HMB-45-positive clear cells of the lung with lymphangioleiomyomatosislike distribution, replacing the lobes with multiple cysts and a nodule. Am J Surg Pathol 1999;23:1288–93.
636. Ito M, Sugamura Y, Ikari H, Sekine I. Angiomyolipoma of the lung. Arch Pathol Lab Med 1998;122:1023–5.
637. Jautzke G, Muller-Ruchholtz E, Thalmann U. Immunohistological detection of estrogen and progesterone receptors in multiple and well differentiated leiomyomatous lung tumors in women with uterine leiomyomas (so-called benign metastasizing leiomyomas). A report on 5 cases. Pathol Res Pract 1996;192:215–23.
638. Johnson S. Rare diseases. 1. Lymphangioleiomyomatosis: clinical features, management and basic mechanisms. Thorax 1999;54:254–64.
639. Kalassian KG, Doyle R, Kao P, Ruoss S, Raffin TA. Lymphangioleiomyomatosis: new insights. Am J Respir Crit Care Med 1997;155:1183–6.
640. Kay JM, Kahana LM, Rihal C. Diffuse smooth muscle proliferation of the lungs with severe pulmonary hypertension. Hum Pathol 1996;27:969–74.
641. Kirchner J, Stein A, Viel K, et al. Pulmonary lymphangioleiomyomatosis: high-resolution CT findings. Eur Radiol 1999;9:49–54.
642. Kitaichi M, Nishimura K, Itoh H, Izumi T. Pulmonary lymphangioleiomyomatosis: a report of 46 patients including a clinicopathologic study of prognostic factors. Am J Respir Crit Care Med 1995;151:527–33.
643. Klein M, Krieger O, Ruckser R, et al. Treatment of lymphangioleiomyomatosis by ovariectomy, interferon alpha 2b and tamoxifen—a case report. Arch Gynecol Obstet 1992;252:99–102.
644. Lenoir S, Grenier P, Brauner MW, et al. Pulmonary lymphangiomyomatosis and tuberous sclerosis: comparison of radiographic and thin-section CT findings. Radiology 1990;175:329–34.
645. Liberman BA, Chamberlain DW, Goldstein RS. Tuberous sclerosis with pulmonary involvement. Can Med Assoc J 1984;130:287–9.
646. Lie JT, Miller RD, Williams DE. Cystic disease of the lungs in tuberous sclerosis: clinicopathologic correlation, including body plethysmographic lung function tests. Mayo Clin Proc 1980;55:547–53.
647. Matsui K, Beasley MB, Nelson WK, et al. Prognostic significance of pulmonary lymphangioleiomyomatosis histologic score. Am J Surg Pathol 2001;25:479–84.
648. Matsui K, Takeda K, Yu ZX, Travis WD, Moss J, Ferrans VJ. Role for activation of matrix metalloproteinases in the pathogenesis of pulmonary lymphangioleiomyomatosis. Arch Pathol Lab Med 2000;124:267–75.
649. Matsui K, Takeda K, Yu ZX, et al. Downregulation of estrogen and progesterone receptors in the abnormal smooth muscle cells in pulmonary lymphangioleiomyomatosis following therapy. An immunohistochemical study. Am J Respir Crit Care Med 2000;161:1002–9.
650. Matsumoto Y, Horiba K, Usuki J, Chu SC, Ferrans VJ, Moss J. Markers of cell proliferation and expression of melanosomal antigen in lymphangioleiomyomatosis. Am J Respir Cell Mol Biol 1999;21:327–36.
651. McDonnell TJ, Crouch EC, Gonzalez JG. Reactive eosinophilic pleuritis. A sequela of pneumothorax in pulmonary eosinophilic granuloma. Am J Clin Pathol 1989;91:107–11.

652. Mehzad M. Leiomyosarcoma of the uterus presenting with pneumothorax. Br J Dis Chest 1977;71:132–4.
653. Michal M, Havlicek F. Immunohistochemical phenotypes of histioeosinophilic granulomas of thymus and reactive eosinophilic pleuritis. Acta Histochem 1993;94:97–101.
654. Muir TE, Leslie KO, Popper H, et al. Micronodular pneumocyte hyperplasia. Am J Surg Pathol 1998;22:465–72.
655. Müller NL, Chiles C, Kullnig P. Pulmonary lymphangiomyomatosis: correlation of CT with radiographic and functional findings. Radiology 1990;175:335–9.
656. Nine JS, Yousem SA, Paradis IL, Keenan R, Griffith BP. Lymphangioleiomyomatosis: recurrence after lung transplantation. J Heart Lung Transplant 1994;13:714–9.
657. Ohori NP, Yousem SA, Sonmez-Alpan E, Colby TV. Estrogen and progesterone receptors in lymphangioleiomyomatosis, epithelioid hemangioendothelioma, and sclerosing hemangioma of the lung. Am J Clin Pathol 1991;96:529–35.
658. Parenti DJ, Morley TF, Giudice JC. Benign metastasizing leiomyoma. A case report and review of the literature. Respiration 1992;59:347–50.
659. Pocock E, Craig JR, Bullock WK. Metastatic uterine leiomyomata. A case report. Cancer 1976;38:2096–100.
660. Scadding JG, Hinson KF. Diffuse fibrosing alveolitis (diffuse interstitial fibrosis of the lungs). Correlation of histology at biopsy with prognosis. Thorax 1967;22:291–304.
661. Schaumburg-Lever G, Metzler G, Kaiserling E. Ultrastructural localization of HMB-45 binding sites. J Cutan Pathol 1991;18:432–5.
662. Shin MS, Fulmer JD, Ho KJ. Unusual computed tomographic manifestations of benign metastasizing leiomyomas as cavitary nodular lesions or interstitial lung disease. Clin Imaging 1996;20:45–9.
663. Sinclair W, Wright JL, Churg A. Lymphangioleiomyomatosis presenting in a postmenopausal woman. Thorax 1985;40:475–6.
664. Smolarek TA, Wessner LL, McCormack FX, Mylet JC, Menon AG, Henske EP. Evidence that lymphangiomyomatosis is caused by TSC2 mutations: chromosome 16p13 loss of heterozygosity in angiomyolipomas and lymph nodes from women with lymphangiomyomatosis. Am J Hum Genet 1998;62:810–5.
665. Sprio RH, McPeak CJ. On the so-called metastasizing leiomyoma. Cancer 1966;19:544–8.
666. Stephenson CA, Henley FT, Goldstein AR. Benign metastasizing leiomyoma. Ala J Med Sci 1984;21:78–81.
667. Sullivan EJ. Lymphangioleiomyomatosis: a review. Chest 1998;114:1689–703.
668. Sullivan EJ, Beck GJ, Peavy HH, Fanburg BL. Lymphangioleiomyomatosis Registry [Letter]. Chest 1999;115:301.
669. Takemura G, Takatsu Y, Kaitani K, et al. Metastasizing uterine leiomyoma. A case with cardiac and pulmonary metastasis. Pathol Res Pract 1996;192:622–9.
670. Taylor JR, Ryu J, Colby TV, Raffin TA. Lymphangioleiomyomatosis. Clinical course in 32 patients. N Engl J Med 1990;323:1254–60.
671. Tazelaar HD, Kerr D, Yousem SA, Saldana MJ, Langston C, Colby TV. Diffuse pulmonary lymphangiomatosis. Hum Pathol 1993;24:1313–22.
672. Travis WD, Usuki J, Horiba K, Ferrans VJ. Histopathologic studies on lymphangioleiomyomatosis. In: Moss J, ed. LAM and other diseases characterized by smooth muscle proliferation. New York: Marcel Dekker; 1999:171–217.
673. Uchida T, Tokumaru T, Kojima H, Nakagawaji K, Imaizumi M, Abe T. A case of multiple leiomyomatous lesions of the lung: an analysis of flow cytometry and hormone receptors. Surg Today 1992;22:265–8.
674. Urban T, Lazor R, Lacronique J, et al. Pulmonary lymphangioleiomyomatosis. A study of 69 patients. Groupe d'Etudes et de Recherche sur les Maladies "Orphelines" Pulmonaires (GERM"O"P). Medicine (Baltimore) 1999;78:321–37.
675. Valentine VG, Raffin TA. The management of chylothorax. Chest 1992;102:586-91.
676. Winkler TR, Burr LH, Robinson CL. Benign metastasizing leiomyoma. Ann Thorac Surg 1987;43:100–1.
677. Wolff M, Silva F, Kaye G. Pulmonary metastases (with admixed epithelial elements) from smooth muscle neoplasms. Report of nine cases, including three males. Am J Surg Pathol 1979;3:325–42.
678. Wu K, Tazelaar HD. Pulmonary angiomyolipoma and multifocal micronodular pneumocyte hyperplasia associated with tuberous sclerosis. Hum Pathol 1999;30:1266–8.

Eosinophilic Diseases

679. Allen JN, Davis WB. Eosinophilic lung diseases. Am J Respir Crit Care Med 1994;150:1423–38.
680. Allen JN, Davis WB, Pacht ER. Diagnostic significance of increased bronchoalveolar lavage fluid eosinophils. Am Rev Respir Dis 1990; 142:642–7.
681. Allen JN, Pacht ER, Gadek JE, Davis WB. Acute eosinophilic pneumonia as a reversible cause of noninfectious respiratory failure. N Engl J Med 1989;321:569–74.
682. Ambrus JL, Klein E. Löffler syndrome and ancylostomiasis brasiliensis. N Y State J Med 1988; 88:498–9.

683. Amsterdam JD. Loeffler's syndrome: an uncommon adverse reaction to imipramine. Int Clin Psychopharmacol 1986;1:260–2.
684. Badesch DB, King TE Jr, Schwarz MI. Acute eosinophilic pneumonia: a hypersensitivity phenomenon? Am Rev Respir Dis 1989;139:249–52.
685. Bailey CC, Campbell RH. Lymphosarcoma presenting as Löffler's syndrome. Br Med J 1973;1:460–1.
686. Bain GA, Flower CD. Pulmonary eosinophilia. Eur J Radiol 1996;23:3–8.
687. Beasley MB, Franks TJ, Galvin JR, Travis WD. Acute fibrinous and organizing pneumonia. Arch Pathol Lab Med 2002:126(in press).
688. Boone AW. Pulmonary infiltrations with eosinophilia as a manifestation of carcinoma. Dis Chest 1969;55:341–4.
689. Bosken CH, Myers JL, Greenberger PA, Katzenstein AL. Pathologic features of allergic bronchopulmonary aspergillosis. Am J Surg Pathol 1988;12:216–22.
690. Carrington CB, Addington WW, Goff AM, et al. Chronic eosinophilic pneumonia. N Engl J Med 1969;280:787–98.
691. Case records of the Massachusetts General Hospital. Weekly clinicopathological exercises. Case 1-1993. A seven-year-old girl with recurrent bouts of sore throat, cough, dyspnea, and fever. N Engl J Med 1993;328:48–55.
692. Chapman BJ, Capewell S, Gibson R, Greening AP, Crompton GK. Pulmonary eosinophilia with and without allergic bronchopulmonary aspergillosis. Thorax 1989;44:919–24.
693. Cheon JE, Lee KS, Jung GS, Chung MH, Cho YD. Acute eosinophilic pneumonia: radiographic and CT findings in six patients. AJR Am J Roentgenol 1996;167:1195–9.
694. Chumbley LC, Harrison EG Jr, DeRemee RA. Allergic granulomatosis and angiitis (Churg-Strauss syndrome). Report and analysis of 30 cases. Mayo Clin Proc 1977;52:477–84.
695. Chusid MJ, Dale DC, West BC, Wolff SM. The hypereosinophilic syndrome: analysis of fourteen cases with review of the literature. Medicine (Baltimore) 1975;54:1–27.
696. Cordier JF. Eosinophilic pneumonias. In: Schwarz MI, King TE Jr, eds. Interstitial lung disease, 3rd ed. Hamilton: BC Decker; 1998:559–96.
697. Danel C, Israel-Biet D, Costabel U, Rossi GA, Wallaert B. The clinical role of BAL in eosinophilic lung diseases. Eur Respir J 1990;3:950, 961–969.
698. Dejaegher P, Demedts M. Bronchoalveolar lavage in eosinophilic pneumonia before and during corticosteroid therapy. Am Rev Respir Dis 1984;129:631–2.
699. Ebara H, Ikezoe J, Johkoh T, et al. Chronic eosinophilic pneumonia: evolution of chest radiograms and CT features. J Comput Assist Tomogr 1994;18:737–44.
700. Enzenauer RJ, Underwood GH Jr, Ribbing J. Tropical pulmonary eosinophilia. South Med J 1990;83:69–72.
701. Fauci AS, Harley JB, Roberts WC, Ferrans VJ, Gralnick HR, Bjornson BH. NIH conference. The idiopathic hypereosinophilic syndrome. Clinical, pathophysiologic, and therapeutic considerations. Ann Intern Med 1982;97:78–92.
702. Fujimura M, Yasui M, Shinagawa S, Nomura M, Matsuda T. Bronchoalveolar lavage cell findings in three types of eosinophilic pneumonia: acute, chronic and drug-induced eosinophilic pneumonia. Respir Med 1998;92:743–9.
703. Godeau B, Brochard L, Theodorou I, et al. A case of acute eosinophilic pneumonia with hypersensitivity to "red spider" allergens. J Allergy Clin Immunol 1995;95:1056–8.
704. Goetzl EJ, Luce JM. Eosinophilic lung diseases. In: Murray JF, Nadel JA, Mason RJ, Boushey HA, eds. Textbook of respiratory medicine, 3rd ed. Philadelphia: WB Saunders; 2000:1757–73.
705. Golstein MA, Steinfeld S. Chronic eosinophilic pneumonia followed by Churg-Strauss syndrome. Rev Rhum Engl Ed 1996;63:624–8.
706. Hardy WR, Anderson RE. The hypereosinophilic syndromes. Ann Intern Med 1968;68:1220–9.
707. Hill R, Wang NS, Berry G. Hypereosinophilic syndrome with pulmonary vascular involvement. Angiology 1984;35:238–44.
708. Hirshberg B, Kramer MR, Lotem M, et al. Chronic eosinophilic pneumonia associated with cutaneous T-cell lymphoma. Am J Hematol 1999;60:143–7.
709. Iwami T, Umemoto S, Ikeda K, Yamada H, Matsuzaki M. A case of acute eosinophilic pneumonia. Evidence for hypersensitivity-like pulmonary reaction. Chest 1996;110:1618–21.
710. Janin A, Torpier G, Courtin P, et al. Segregation of eosinophil proteins in alveolar macrophage compartments in chronic eosinophilic pneumonia. Thorax 1993;48:57–62.
711. Jederlinic PJ, Sicilian L, Gaensler EA. Chronic eosinophilic pneumonia. A report of 19 cases and a review of the literature. Medicine (Baltimore) 1988;67:154–62.
712. Johkoh T, Müller NL, Akira M, et al. Eosinophilic lung diseases: diagnostic accuracy of thin-section CT in 111 patients. Radiology 2000;216:773–80.
713. Kelly KJ, Ruffing R. Acute eosinophilic pneumonia following intentional inhalation of Scotchguard. Ann Allergy 1993;71:358–61.

714. King MA, Pope-Harman AL, Allen JN, Christoforidis GA, Christoforidis AJ. Acute eosinophilic pneumonia: radiologic and clinical features. Radiology 1997;203:715–9.
715. Kinsella DL Jr, Simpson HN. Löffler's pneumonia terminating in fatal periarteritis nodosa. JAMA 1967;202:867–9.
716. Mayo J, Collazos J, Martinez E, Diaz F. Acute eosinophilic pneumonia in a patient infected with the human immunodeficiency virus. Tuber Lung Dis 1995;76:77–9.
717. Mayo JR, Müller NL, Road J, Sisler J, Lillington G. Chronic eosinophilic pneumonia: CT findings in six cases. AJR Am J Roentgenol 1989; 153:727–30.
718. Middleton WG, Paterson IC, Grant IW, Douglas AC. Asthmatic pulmonary eosinophilia: a review of 65 cases. Br J Dis Chest 1977;71:115–22.
719. Myers JL. Diagnosis of drug reactions in the lung. Monogr Pathol 1993:32–53.
720. Nakajima M, Manabe T, Niki Y, Matsushima T. Cigarette smoke-induced acute eosinophilic pneumonia [Letter]. Radiology 1998;207:829–31.
721. Nutman TB, Vijayan VK, Pinkston P, et al. Tropical pulmonary eosinophilia: analysis of antifilarial antibody localized to the lung. J Infect Dis 1989;160:1042–50.
722. Olopade CO, Crotty TB, Douglas WW, Colby TV, Sur S. Chronic eosinophilic pneumonia and idiopathic bronchiolitis obliterans organizing pneumonia: comparison of eosinophil number and degranulation by immunofluorescence staining for eosinophil-derived major basic protein. Mayo Clin Proc 1995;70:137–42.
723. Ong RK, Doyle RL. Tropical pulmonary eosinophilia. Chest 1998;113:1673–9.
724. Papiris SA, Maniati MA, Kalousis JV, Constantopoulos SH. Chronic eosinophilic pneumonia in rheumatoid arthritis. Monaldi Arch Chest Dis 1995;50:360–2.
725. Payne CR, Connellan SJ. Chronic eosinophilic pneumonia complicating long-standing rheumatoid arthritis. Postgrad Med J 1980;56:519–20.
726. Pope-Harman AL, Davis WB, Allen ED, Christoforidis AJ, Allen JN. Acute eosinophilic pneumonia. A summary of 15 cases and review of the literature. Medicine (Baltimore) 1996;75:334–42.
727. Spry CJ. The hypereosinophilic syndrome: clinical features, laboratory findings and treatment. Allergy 1982;37:539–51.
728. Spry CJ, Davies J, Tai PC, Olsen EG, Oakley CM, Goodwin JF. Clinical features of fifteen patients with the hypereosinophilic syndrome. Q J Med 1983;52:1–22.
729. Tan AM, Downie PJ, Ekert H. Hypereosinophilia syndrome with pneumonia in acute lymphoblastic leukaemia. Aust Paediatr J 1987;23:359–61.
730. Tazelaar HD, Linz LJ, Colby TV, Myers JL, Limper AH. Acute eosinophilic pneumonia: histopathologic findings in nine patients. Am J Respir Crit Care Med 1997;155:296–302.
731. Travis WD, Kwon-Chung KJ, Kleiner DE, et al. Unusual aspects of allergic bronchopulmonary fungal disease: report of two cases due to Curvularia organisms associated with allergic fungal sinusitis. Hum Pathol 1991;22:1240–8.
732. Udwadia FE. Tropical eosinophilia: a review. Respir Med 1993;87:17-21.
733. White JP, Ward MJ. Drug-induced adverse pulmonary reactions. Adverse Drug React Acute Poisoning Rev 1985;4:183–211.
734. Winn RE, Kollef MH, Meyer JI. Pulmonary involvement in the hypereosinophilic syndrome. Chest 1994;105:656–60.
735. Wright P, Kelly P, Yazbeck J, Clancy L, Healy T. An association between sputum eosinophilia and carcinoma of the lung: a study of 549 patients. Ir J Med Sci 1994;163:492–3.
736. Zagami AS, Colebatch HJ, Wakefield D. Chronic eosinophilic pneumonia in a patient with ataxia telangiectasia. Aust N Z J Med 1987;17:592–5.

Pulmonary Alveolar Proteinosis

737. Albafouille V, Sayegh N, De Coudenhove S, et al. CT scan patterns of pulmonary alveolar proteinosis in children. Pediatr Radiol 1999; 29:147–52.
738. Alberti A, Luisetti M, Braschi A, et al. Bronchoalveolar lavage fluid composition in alveolar proteinosis. Early changes after therapeutic lavage. Am J Respir Crit Care Med 1996;154:817–20.
739. Bedrossian CW, Luna MA, Conklin RH, Miller WC. Alveolar proteinosis as a consequence of immunosuppression. A hypothesis based on clinical and pathologic observations. Hum Pathol 1980;11:527–35.
740. Buechner HA, Ansari A. Acute silicoproteinosis. A new pathologic variant of acute silicosis in sandblasters, characterized by histologic features resembling alveolar proteinosis. Dis Chest 1969;55:274–8.
741. Burkhalter A, Silverman JF, Hopkins MB, Geisinger KR. Bronchoalveolar lavage cytology in pulmonary alveolar proteinosis. Am J Clin Pathol 1996;106:504–10.
742. Carnovale R, Zornoza J, Goldman AM, Luna M. Pulmonary alveolar proteinosis: its association with hematologic malignancy and lymphoma. Radiology 1977;122:303–6.
743. Clague HW, Wallace AC, Morgan WK. Pulmonary interstitial fibrosis associated with alveolar proteinosis. Thorax 1983;38:865–6.

744. Claypool WD, Rogers RM, Matuschak GM. Update on the clinical diagnosis, management, and pathogenesis of pulmonary alveolar proteinosis (phospholipidosis). Chest 1984;85:550–8.
745. Coleman M, Dehner LP, Sibley RK, Burke BA, L'Heureux PR, Thompson TR. Pulmonary alveolar proteinosis: an uncommon cause of chronic neonatal respiratory distress. Am Rev Respir Dis 1980;121:583–6.
746. Cordonnier C, Fleury-Feith J, Escudier E, Atassi K, Bernaudin JF. Secondary alveolar proteinosis is a reversible cause of respiratory failure in leukemic patients. Am J Respir Crit Care Med 1994;149:788–94.
747. Dail DH. Metabolic and other diseases. In: Dail DH, Hammar SP, eds. Pulmonary pathology, 2nd ed. New York: Springer Verlag; 1994:707–77.
748. de la Fuente AA, Voorhout WF, deMello DE. Congenital alveolar proteinosis in the Netherlands: a report of five cases with immunohistochemical and genetic studies on surfactant apoproteins. Pediatr Pathol Lab Med 1997;17:221–31.
749. deMello DE, Nogee LM, Heyman S, et al. Molecular and phenotypic variability in the congenital alveolar proteinosis syndrome associated with inherited surfactant protein B deficiency. J Pediatr 1994;125:43–50.
750. Dranoff G, Mulligan RC. Activities of granulocyte-macrophage colony-stimulating factor revealed by gene transfer and gene knockout studies. Stem Cells 1994;12[Suppl 1]:173–82.
751. Eldar M, Shoenfeld Y, Zaizov R, et al. Pulmonary alveolar proteinosis associated with Fanconi's anemia. Respiration 1979;38:177–9.
752. Fujishima T, Honda Y, Shijubo N, Takahashi H, Abe S. Increased carcinoembryonic antigen concentrations in sera and bronchoalveolar lavage fluids of patients with pulmonary alveolar proteinosis. Respiration 1995;62:317–21.
753. Golde DW, Territo M, Finley TN, Cline MJ. Defective lung macrophages in pulmonary alveolar proteinosis. Ann Intern Med 1976;85:304–9.
754. Goldstein LS, Kavuru MS, Curtis-McCarthy P, Christie HA, Farver C, Stoller JK. Pulmonary alveolar proteinosis: clinical features and outcomes. Chest 1998;114:1357–62.
755. Gonzalez-Rothi RJ, Harris JO. Pulmonary alveolar proteinosis. Further evaluation of abnormal alveolar macrophages. Chest 1986;90:656–61.
756. Green D, Dighe P, Ali NO, Katele GV. Pulmonary alveolar proteinosis complicating chronic myelogenous leukemia. Cancer 1980;46:1763–6.
757. Hirakata Y, Kobayashi J, Sugama Y, Kitamura S. Elevation of tumour markers in serum and bronchoalveolar lavage fluid in pulmonary alveolar proteinosis. Eur Respir J 1995;8:689–96.
758. Hoffman RM, Dauber JH, Rogers RM. Improvement in alveolar macrophage migration after therapeutic whole lung lavage in pulmonary alveolar proteinosis. Am Rev Respir Dis 1989;139:1030–2.
759. Honda Y, Kuroki Y, Shijubo N, et al. Aberrant appearance of lung surfactant protein A in sera of patients with idiopathic pulmonary fibrosis and its clinical significance. Respiration 1995;62:64–9.
760. Honda Y, Takahashi H, Shijubo N, Kuroki Y, Akino T. Surfactant protein-A concentration in bronchoalveolar lavage fluids of patients with pulmonary alveolar proteinosis. Chest 1993;103:496–9.
761. Hook GE, Gilmore LB, Talley FA. Multilamellated structures from the lungs of patients with pulmonary alveolar proteinosis. Lab Invest 1984;50:711–25.
762. Huffman JA, Hull WM, Dranoff G, Mulligan RC, Whitsett JA. Pulmonary epithelial cell expression of GM-CSF corrects the alveolar proteinosis in GM-CSF-deficient mice. J Clin Invest 1996;97:649–55.
763. Ito T, Sato M, Okubo T, Ono I, Akabane J. Infantile pulmonary alveolar proteinosis with interstitial pneumonia: bilateral simultaneous lung lavage utilizing extracorporeal membrane oxygenation and steroid therapy. Tohoku J Exp Med 1999;187:279–83.
764. Jennings VM, Dillehay DL, Webb SK, Brown LA. Pulmonary alveolar proteinosis in SCID mice. Am J Respir Cell Mol Biol 1995;13:297–306.
765. Johkoh T, Itoh H, Müller NL, et al. Crazy-paving appearance at thin-section CT: spectrum of disease and pathologic findings. Radiology 1999;211:155–60.
766. Kadota J, Nakamura Y, Iwashita T, et al. Pulmonary alveolar proteinosis with lung squamous cell carcinoma. Respir Med 1999;93:138–40.
767. Kajiume T, Yoshimi S, Nagita A, et al. A case of myelodysplastic syndrome complicated by pulmonary alveolar proteinosis with a high serum KL-6 level. Pediatr Hematol Oncol 1999; 16:367–71.
768. Kariman K, Kylstra JA, Spock A. Pulmonary alveolar proteinosis: prospective clinical experience in 23 patients for 15 years. Lung 1984;162:223–31.
769. Keller CA, Frost A, Cagle PT, Abraham JL. Pulmonary alveolar proteinosis in a painter with elevated pulmonary concentrations of titanium. Chest 1995;108:277–80.
770. Kim G, Lee SJ, Lee HP, et al. The clinical characteristics of pulmonary alveolar proteinosis: experience at Seoul National University Hospital, and review of the literature. J Korean Med Sci 1999;14:159–64.

771. Kitamura T, Tanaka N, Watanabe J, et al. Idiopathic pulmonary alveolar proteinosis as an autoimmune disease with neutralizing antibody against granulocyte/macrophage colony–stimulating factor. J Exp Med 1999;190:875–80.
772. Kuroki Y, Tsutahara S, Shijubo N, et al. Elevated levels of lung surfactant protein A in sera from patients with idiopathic pulmonary fibrosis and pulmonary alveolar proteinosis. Am Rev Respir Dis 1993;147:723–9.
773. Lee KN, Levin DL, Webb WR, Chen D, Storto ML, Golden JA. Pulmonary alveolar proteinosis: high-resolution CT, chest radiographic, and functional correlations. Chest 1997;111:989–95.
774. Martin RJ, Rogers RM, Myers NM. Pulmonary alveolar proteinosis: shunt fraction and lactic acid dehydrogenase concentration as aids to diagnosis. Am Rev Respir Dis 1978;117:1059–62.
775. Masuda T, Shimura S, Sasaki H, Takishima T. Surfactant apoprotein-A concentration in sputum for diagnosis of pulmonary alveolar proteinosis. Lancet 1991;337:580–2.
776. McManus DT, Moore R, Hill CM, Rodgers C, Carson DJ, Love AH. Necropsy findings in lysinuric protein intolerance. J Clin Pathol 1996;49:345–7.
777. Mikami T, Yamamoto Y, Yokoyama M, Okayasu I. Pulmonary alveolar proteinosis: diagnosis using routinely processed smears of bronchoalveolar lavage fluid. J Clin Pathol 1997;50:981–4.
778. Miller RR, Churg AM, Hutcheon M, Lom S. Pulmonary alveolar proteinosis and aluminum dust exposure. Am Rev Respir Dis 1984;130:312–5.
779. Milleron BJ, Costabel U, Teschler H, et al. Bronchoalveolar lavage cell data in alveolar proteinosis. Am Rev Respir Dis 1991;144:1330–2.
780. Muller-Quernheim J, Schopf RE, Benes P, Schulz V, Ferlinz R. A macrophage-suppressing 40-kD protein in a case of pulmonary alveolar proteinosis. Klin Wochenschr 1987;65:893–7.
781. Nogee LM, de Mello DE, Dehner LP, Colten HR. Brief report: deficiency of pulmonary surfactant protein B in congenital alveolar proteinosis. N Engl J Med 1993;328:406–10.
782. Nugent KM, Pesanti EL. Macrophage function in pulmonary alveolar proteinosis. Am Rev Respir Dis 1983;127:780–1.
783. Parto K, Kallajoki M, Aho H, Simell O. Pulmonary alveolar proteinosis and glomerulonephritis in lysinuric protein intolerance: case reports and autopsy findings of four pediatric patients. Hum Pathol 1994;25:400–7.
784. Pascual J, Gomez Aguinaga MA, Vidal R, et al. Alveolar proteinosis and nocardiosis: a patient treated by bronchopulmonary lavage. Postgrad Med J 1989;65:674–7.
785. Prakash UB, Barham SS, Carpenter HA, Dines DE, Marsh HM. Pulmonary alveolar phospholipoproteinosis: experience with 34 cases and a review. Mayo Clin Proc 1987;62:499–518.
786. Ranchod M, Bissell M. Pulmonary alveolar proteinosis and cytomegalovirus infection. Arch Pathol Lab Med 1979;103:139–42.
787. Reed JA, Ikegami M, Cianciolo ER, et al. Aerosolized GM-CSF ameliorates pulmonary alveolar proteinosis in GM-CSF-deficient mice. Am J Physiol 1999;276:L556–63.
788. Ruben FL, Talamo TS. Secondary pulmonary alveolar proteinosis occurring in two patients with acquired immune deficiency syndrome. Am J Med 1986;80:1187–90.
789. Rubinstein I, Mullen JB, Hoffstein V. Morphologic diagnosis of idiopathic pulmonary alveolar lipoproteinosis—revisited. Arch Intern Med 1988;148:813–6.
790. Sakai Y, Abo W, Yoshimura H, et al. Pulmonary alveolar proteinosis in infants. Eur J Pediatr 1999;158:424–6.
791. Seymour JF, Begley CG, Dirksen U, et al. Attenuated hematopoietic response to granulocyte-macrophage colony-stimulating factor in patients with acquired pulmonary alveolar proteinosis. Blood 1998;92:2657–67.
792. Singh G, Katyal SL, Bedrossian CW, Rogers RM. Pulmonary alveolar proteinosis. Staining for surfactant apoprotein in alveolar proteinosis and in conditions simulating it. Chest 1983;83:82–6.
793. Steens RD, Summers QA, Tarala RA. Pulmonary alveolar proteinosis in association with Fanconi's anemia and psoriasis. A possible common pathogenetic mechanism. Chest 1992;102:637–8.
794. Takahashi T, Munakata M, Suzuki I, Kawakami Y. Serum and bronchoalveolar fluid KL-6 levels in patients with pulmonary alveolar proteinosis. Am J Respir Crit Care Med 1998;158:1294–8.
795. Takemura T, Fukuda Y, Harrison M, Ferrans VJ. Ultrastructural, histochemical, and freeze-fracture evaluation of multilamellated structures in human pulmonary alveolar proteinosis. Am J Anat 1987;179:258–68.
796. Tran Van Nhieu J, Vojtek AM, Bernaudin JF, Escudier E, Fleury-Feith J. Pulmonary alveolar proteinosis associated with Pneumocystis carinii. Ultrastructural identification in bronchoalveolar lavage in AIDS and immunocompromised non-AIDS patients. Chest 1990;98:801–5.
797. Usui Y, Takayama S, Nakayama M, Miura H, Kimula Y. Interstitial lattice shadow and mediastinal lymphadenopathy with an elevation of carcinoembryonic antigen in severe pulmonary alveolar proteinosis. Intern Med 1992;31:422–5.

798. Villanueva AG, Mark EJ. Case records of the Massachusetts General Hospital. Weekly clinicopathological exercises. Case 24-1996. A 54-year-old woman with infiltrative lung disease and mild dyspnea. N Engl J Med 1996;335:417–24.
799. Wallot M, Wagenvoort C, deMello D, Muller KM, Floros J, Roll C. Congenital alveolar proteinosis caused by a novel mutation of the surfactant protein B gene and misalignment of lung vessels in consanguineous kindred infants. Eur J Pediatr 1999;158:513–8.
800. Wang BM, Stern EJ, Schmidt RA, Pierson DJ. Diagnosing pulmonary alveolar proteinosis. A review and an update. Chest 1997;111:460–6.
801. Webster JR Jr, Battifora H, Furey C, Harrison RA, Shapiro B. Pulmonary alveolar proteinosis in two siblings with decreased immunoglobulin A. Am J Med 1980;69:786–9.
802. Witty LA, Tapson VF, Piantadosi CA. Isolation of mycobacteria in patients with pulmonary alveolar proteinosis. Medicine (Baltimore) 1994;73:103–9.
803. Yousem SA. Alveolar lipoproteinosis in lung allograft recipients. Hum Pathol 1997;28:1383–6.
804. Zontsich T, Helbich TH, Wojnarovsky C, Eichler I, Herold CJ. Pulmonary alveolar proteinosis in a child: HRCT findings before and after bronchoalveolar lavage. Eur Radiol 1998;8:1680–2.

Diffuse Pulmonary Hemorrhage Disorders

805. Agusti C, Ramirez J, Picado C, et al. Diffuse alveolar hemorrhage in allogeneic bone marrow transplantation. A postmortem study. Am J Respir Crit Care Med 1995;151:1006–10.
806. Bailey ME, Fraire AE, Greenberg SD, Barnard J, Cagle PT. Pulmonary histopathology in cocaine abusers. Hum Pathol 1994;25:203–7.
807. Ball JA, Young KR Jr. Pulmonary manifestations of Goodpasture's syndrome. Antiglomerular basement membrane disease and related disorders. Clin Chest Med 1998;19:777–91.
808. Benditt JO, Farber HW, Wright J, Karnad AB. Pulmonary hemorrhage with diffuse alveolar infiltrates in men with high-volume choriocarcinoma. Ann Intern Med 1988;109:674–5.
809. Boggess KA, Benedetti TJ, Raghu G. Nitrofurantoin-induced pulmonary toxicity during pregnancy: a report of a case and review of the literature. Obstet Gynecol Surv 1996;51:367–70.
810. Bosch X, Font J. The pulmonary-renal syndrome: a poorly understood clinicopathologic condition. Lupus 1999;8:258–62.
811. Bosch X, Lopez-Soto A, Mirapeix E, Font J, Ingelmo M, Urbano-Marquez A. Antineutrophil cytoplasmic autoantibody-associated alveolar capillaritis in patients presenting with pulmonary hemorrhage. Arch Pathol Lab Med 1994;118:517–22.
812. Bowley NB, Steiner RE, Chin WS. The chest X-ray in antiglomerular basement membrane antibody disease (Goodpasture's syndrome). Clin Radiol 1979;30:419–29.
813. Briens E, Caulet-Maugendre S, Desrues B, et al. Alveolar haemorrhage revealing epithelioid haemangioendothelioma. Respir Med 1997;91:111–4.
814. Buschman DL, Ballard R. Progressive massive fibrosis associated with idiopathic pulmonary hemosiderosis. Chest 1993;104:293–5.
815. Cheah FK, Sheppard MN, Hansell DM. Computed tomography of diffuse pulmonary haemorrhage with pathological correlation. Clin Radiol 1993;48:89–93.
816. Clutterbuck EJ, Pusey CD. Severe alveolar hemorrhage in Churg-Strauss syndrome. Eur J Respir Dis 1987;71:158–63.
817. Cohen S. Idiopathic pulmonary hemosiderosis. Am J Med Sci 1999;317:67–74.
818. Crausman RS, Achenbach GA, Pluss WT, O'Brien RF, Jennings CA. Pulmonary capillaritis and alveolar hemorrhage associated with the antiphospholipid antibody syndrome. J Rheumatol 1995;22:554–6.
819. Etzel RA, Montana E, Sorenson WG, et al. Acute pulmonary hemorrhage in infants associated with exposure to Stachybotrys atra and other fungi. Arch Pediatr Adolesc Med 1998;152:757–62.
820. Fernandez P, Bermejo AM, Lopez-Rivadulla M, Cruz A, Rodriguez E, Otero A. A fatal case of parenteral paraquat poisoning. Forensic Sci Int 1991;49:215–24.
821. Fraser RS. Catheter-induced pulmonary artery perforation: pathologic and pathogenic features. Hum Pathol 1987;18:1246–51.
822. Gaudin PB, Askin FB, Falk RJ, Jennette JC. The pathologic spectrum of pulmonary lesions in patients with anti-neutrophil cytoplasmic autoantibodies specific for anti-proteinase 3 and anti-myeloperoxidase. Am J Clin Pathol 1995;104:7–16.
823. Hubbs AF, Castranova V, Ma JY, et al. Acute lung injury induced by a commercial leather conditioner. Toxicol Appl Pharmacol 1997;143:37–46.
824. Imoto EM, Lombard CM, Sachs DP. Pulmonary capillaritis and hemorrhage. A clue to the diagnosis of systemic necrotizing vasculitis. Chest 1989;96:927–8.
825. Jayne DR, Jones SJ, Lockwood CM. Severe pulmonary hemorrhage and systemic vasculitis in association with isolated circulating IgM antineutrophil antibody [Abstract]. Kidney Int 1988;33:328.

826. Jennette JC, Falk RJ. Small-vessel vasculitis. N Engl J Med 1997;337:1512–23.
827. Jennings CA, King TE Jr, Tuder R, Cherniack RM, Schwarz MI. Diffuse alveolar hemorrhage with underlying isolated, pauciimmune pulmonary capillaritis. Am J Respir Crit Care Med 1997;155:1101–9.
828. Kayser K, Plodziszewska M, Waitr E, Slodkowska J, Altiner M, Gabius HJ. Diffuse pulmonary hemosiderosis after exposure to pesticides. A case report. Respiration 1998;65:214–8.
829. Kelly PT, Haponik EF. Goodpasture syndrome: molecular and clinical advances. Medicine (Baltimore) 1994;73:171–85.
830. Le Clainche L, Le Bourgeois M, Fauroux B, et al. Long-term outcome of idiopathic pulmonary hemosiderosis in children. Medicine (Baltimore) 2000;79:318–26.
831. Leinonen A, Netzer KO, Boutaud A, Gunwar S, Hudson BG. Goodpasture antigen: expression of the full-length alpha3(IV) chain of collagen IV and localization of epitopes exclusively to the noncollagenous domain. Kidney Int 1999;55:926–35.
832. Lombard CM, Colby TV, Elliott CG. Surgical pathology of the lung in antibasement membrane antibody-associated Goodpasture's syndrome. Hum Pathol 1989;20:445–51.
833. Madrenas J, Vallés M, Ruiz Marcellan MC, Fort J, Garcia Bragado F, Pelegri A. Pulmonary hemorrhage and glomerulonephritis associated with essential mixed cryoglobulinemia. Med Clin (Barc) 1989;93:262–4.
834. Mark EJ, Ramirez JF. Pulmonary capillaritis and hemorrhage in patients with systemic vasculitis. Arch Pathol Lab Med 1985;109:413–8.
835. Markus HS, Clark JV. Pulmonary haemorrhage in Henoch-Schönlein purpura. Thorax 1989;44:525–6.
836. Milman N, Pedersen FM. Idiopathic pulmonary haemosiderosis. Epidemiology, pathogenic aspects and diagnosis. Respir Med 1998;92:902–7.
837. Müller NL, Miller RR. Diffuse pulmonary hemorrhage. Radiol Clin North Am 1991;29:965–71.
838. Myers JL, Katzenstein AA. Microangiitis in lupus-induced pulmonary hemorrhage. Am J Clin Pathol 1986;85:552–6.
839. Pacheco A, Casanova C, Fogue L, Sueiro A. Long-term clinical follow-up of adult idiopathic pulmonary hemosiderosis and celiac disease. Chest 1991;99:1525–6.
840. Salamon F, Weinberger A, Nili M, et al. Massive hemoptysis complicating Behcet's syndrome: the importance of early pulmonary angiography and operation. Ann Thorac Surg 1988;45:566–7.
841. Schwarz MI. Diffuse alveolar hemorrhage. In: Schwarz MI, King TE, eds. Interstitial lung disease, 3rd ed. Hamilton: BC Decker; 1998:535–58.
842. Seiden MV, O'Donnell WJ, Weinblatt M, Licht J. Vasculitis with recurrent pulmonary hemorrhage in a long-term survivor after autologous bone marrow transplantation. Bone Marrow Transplant 1990;6:345–7.
843. Sheppard MN, Hansell DM, du Bois RM, Nicholson AG. Primary epithelioid angiosarcoma of the lung presenting as pulmonary hemorrhage. Hum Pathol 1997;28:383–5.
844. Shintaku M, Mase K, Ohtsuki H, Yasumizu R, Yasunaga K, Ikehara S. Generalized sarcoidlike granulomas with systemic angiitis, crescentic glomerulonephritis, and pulmonary hemorrhage. Report of an autopsy case. Arch Pathol Lab Med 1989;113:1295–8.
845. Smith LJ, Katzenstein AL. Pathogenesis of massive pulmonary hemorrhage in acute leukemia. Arch Intern Med 1982;142:2149–52.
846. Sweerts M, Nicholson AG, Goldstraw P, Corrin B. Dieulafoy's disease of the bronchus. Thorax 1995;50:697–8.
847. Travis WD, Colby TV, Lombard C, Carpenter HA. A clinicopathologic study of 34 cases of diffuse pulmonary hemorrhage with lung biopsy confirmation. Am J Surg Pathol 1990;14:1112–25.
848. Travis WD, Hoffman GS, Leavitt RY, Pass HI, Fauci AS. Surgical pathology of the lung in Wegener's granulomatosis. Review of 87 open lung biopsies from 67 patients. Am J Surg Pathol 1991;15:315–33.
849. van der Werf TS, Timmer A, Zijlstra JG. Fatal haemorrhage from Dieulafoy's disease of the bronchus. Thorax 1999;54:184–5.

Aspiration

850. Asnis DS, Saltzman HP, Melchert A. Shark oil pneumonia. An overlooked entity. Chest 1993;103:976–7.
851. Bandla HP, Davis SH, Hopkins NE. Lipoid pneumonia: a silent complication of mineral oil aspiration. Pediatrics 1999;103:E19.
852. Bartlett JG. Anaerobic bacterial infections of the lung and pleural space. Clin Infect Dis 1993;16 [Suppl 4]:S248–55.
853. Bartlett JG. Antibiotics in lung abscess. Semin Respir Infect 1991;6:103-11.
854. Bartlett JG. Aspiration pneumonia. In: Rose BD, ed. Uptodate in medicine. Wellesley: Uptodate; 2001.
855. Bartlett JG, Gorbach SL. The triple threat of aspiration pneumonia. Chest 1975;68:560–6.
856. Brown AC, Slocum PC, Putthoff SL, Wallace WE, Foresman BH. Exogenous lipoid pneumonia due to nasal application of petroleum jelly. Chest 1994;105:968–9.

857. Bynum LJ, Pierce AK. Pulmonary aspiration of gastric contents. Am Rev Respir Dis 1976;114: 1129–36.
858. Chang HY, Chen CW, Chen CY, et al. Successful treatment of diffuse lipoid pneumonitis with whole lung lavage. Thorax 1993;48:947–8.
859. Chin NK, Hui KP, Sinniah R, Chan TB. Idiopathic lipoid pneumonia in an adult treated with prednisolone. Chest 1994;105:956–7.
860. Colby TV, Lombard C, Yousem SA, Kitaichi M. Atlas of pulmonary surgical pathology. Philadelphia: WB Saunders; 1991.
861. Corwin RW, Irwin RS. The lipid-laden alveolar macrophage as a marker of aspiration in parenchymal lung disease. Am Rev Respir Dis 1985;132:576–81.
862. Dail DH. Bronchial and transbronchial diseases. In: Dail DH, Hammar SP, eds. Pulmonary pathology, 2nd ed. New York: Springer-Verlag; 1994:79–119.
863. Daniels SK, Ballo LA, Mahoney MC, Foundas AL. Clinical predictors of dysphagia and aspiration risk: outcome measures in acute stroke patients. Arch Phys Med Rehabil 2000;81:1030–3.
864. Elliott CG, Colby TV, Kelly TM, Hicks HG. Charcoal lung. Bronchiolitis obliterans after aspiration of activated charcoal. Chest 1989;96:672–4.
865. Engelhardt T, Webster NR. Pulmonary aspiration of gastric contents in anaesthesia. Br J Anaesth 1999;83:453–60.
866. Fenton JJ, Johnson FB, Przygodzki RM, Kalasinsky VF, Al-Dayel F, Travis WD. Sodium polystyrene sulfonate (kayexalate) aspiration: histologic appearance and infrared microspectrophotometric analysis of two cases. Arch Pathol Lab Med 1996;120:967–9.
867. Franquet T, Gimenez A, Bordes R, Rodriguez-Arias JM, Castella J. The crazy-paving pattern in exogenous lipoid pneumonia: CT-pathologic correlation. AJR Am J Roentgenol 1998;170:315–7.
868. Franquet T, Gimenez A, Roson N, Torrubia S, Sabate JM, Perez C. Aspiration diseases: findings, pitfalls, and differential diagnosis. Radiographics 2000;20:673–85.
869. Gattuso P, Reddy VB, Castelli MJ. Exogenous lipoid pneumonitis due to Vicks Vaporub inhalation diagnosed by fine needle aspiration cytology [Letter]. Cytopathology 1991;2:315–6.
870. Glynn KP, Gale NA. Exogenous lipoid pneumonia due to inhalation of spray lubricant (WD-40 lung). Chest 1990;97:1265–6.
871. Gombar KK, Singh B, Chhabra B. Fatal pulmonary aspiration of barium during oesophagography. Trop Doct 1995;25:184–5.
872. Gondouin A, Manzoni P, Ranfaing E, et al. Exogenous lipid pneumonia: a retrospective multicentre study of 44 cases in France. Eur Respir J 1996;9:1463–9.
873. Guntupalli KK, Francis PB. Unilateral lung infiltrate. Lipoid pneumonia. Eur Respir J 1991;4:125–7.
874. Kennedy JD, Costello P, Balikian JP, Herman PG. Exogenous lipoid pneumonia. AJR Am J Roentgenol 1981;136:1145–9.
875. King TE Jr. Role of bronchoalveolar lavage in the diagnosis of interstitial lung disease. In: Rose BD, ed. Uptodate in medicine. Wellesley: Uptodate; 2001.
876. Lauque D, Dongay G, Levade T, Caratero C, Carles P. Bronchoalveolar lavage in liquid paraffin pneumonitis. Chest 1990;98:1149–55.
877. Laurent F, Philippe JC, Vergier B, et al. Exogenous lipoid pneumonia: HRCT, MR, and pathologic findings. Eur Radiol 1999;9:1190–6.
878. Lee JS, Im JG, Song KS, Seo JB, Lim TH. Exogenous lipoid pneumonia: high-resolution CT findings. Eur Radiol 1999;9:287–91.
879. Lee KS, Müller NL, Hale V, Newell JD Jr, Lynch DA, Im JG. Lipoid pneumonia: CT findings. J Comput Assist Tomogr 1995;19:48–51.
880. Lipinski JK, Weisbrod GL, Sanders DE. Exogenous lipoid pneumonitis: pulmonary patterns. AJR Am J Roentgenol 1981;136:931–4.
881. Lopez-Castilla JD, Cano M, Munoz M, et al. Massive bronchoalveolar aspiration of barium sulfate during a radiologic study of the upper digestive tract [Letter]. Pediatr Pulmonol 1997;24:126–7.
882. Marom EM, McAdams HP, Erasmus JJ, Goodman PC. The many faces of pulmonary aspiration. AJR Am J Roentgenol 1999;172:121–8.
883. Marom EM, McAdams HP, Sporn TA, Goodman PC. Lentil aspiration pneumonia: radiographic and CT findings. J Comput Assist Tomogr 1998;22:598–600.
884. Mays EE, Dubois JJ, Hamilton GB. Pulmonary fibrosis associated with tracheobronchial aspiration. A study of the frequency of hiatal hernia and gastroesophageal reflux in interstitial pulmonary fibrosis of obscure etiology. Chest 1976;69:512–5.
885. Mendelson CL. The aspiration of stomach contents into the lungs during obstetrical anesthesia. Am J Obstet Gynecol 1946;52:191–205.
886. Müller NL. Aspiration pneumonia. In: Siegel BA, ed. Chest disease: test syllabus (Fifth series). Reston: American College of Radiology; 1996:378–96.
887. Oi RH. The microscopic appearance of a sodium-potassium exchange resin in histologic sections. Am J Clin Pathol 1978;69:359–61.

888. Pujol JL, Barneon G, Bousquet J, Michel FB, Godard P. Interstitial pulmonary disease induced by occupational exposure to paraffin. Chest 1990;97:234–6.
889. Reich SB. Production of pulmonary edema by aspiration of water-soluble nonabsorbable contrast media. Radiology 1969;92:367–70.
890. Ross AH, McCormack RJ. Foreign body inhalation. J R Coll Surg Edinb 1980;25:104–9.
891. Schwindt WD, Barbee RA, Jones RJ. Lipoid pneumonia. Its protean nature and clinical resemblance to carcinoma of the lung. Arch Surg 1967;95:652–7.
892. Shahar J, Mailman D, Meitzen G. Crystals in pulmonary cytologic preparations in association with aspiration of barium. A case report. Acta Cytol 1994;38:415–6.
893. Silverman JF, Turner RC, West RL, Dillard TA. Bronchoalveolar lavage in the diagnosis of lipoid pneumonia. Diagn Cytopathol 1989;5:3–8.
894. Sladen A, Zanca P, Hadnott WH. Aspiration pneumonitis—the sequelae. Chest 1971;59:448–50.
895. Spickard A III, Hirschmann JV. Exogenous lipoid pneumonia. Arch Intern Med 1994; 154:686–92.
896. Steiner J, Bachofen M, Bachofen H. Recovery from aspiration pneumonitis. Pneumonologie 1974;151:127–34.
897. Varkey B. Lipoid pneumonia due to intranasal application of petroleum jelly. An old problem revisited [Letter]. Chest 1994;106:1311–2.
898. Wong CA, Wilsher ML. Treatment of exogenous lipoid pneumonia by whole lung lavage. Aust N Z J Med 1994;24:734–5.
899. Wright BA, Jeffrey PH. Lipoid pneumonia. Semin Respir Infect 1990;5:314–21.
900. Wynne JW, Modell JH. Respiratory aspiration of stomach contents. Ann Intern Med 1977; 87:466–74.
901. Zavala DC. The threat of aspiration pneumonia in the aged. Geriatrics 1977;32:46–51.
902. Zavala DC, Rhodes ML. Foreign body removal: a new role for the fiberoptic bronchoscope. Ann Otol Rhinol Laryngol 1975;84:650–6.

Alveolar Microlithiasis

903. Balikian JP, Fuleihan FJ, Nucho CN. Pulmonary alveolar microlithiasis. Report of five cases with special reference to roentgen manifestations. Am J Roentgenol Radium Ther Nucl Med 1968;103:509–18.
904. Cale WF, Petsonk EL, Boyd CB. Transbronchial biopsy of pulmonary alveolar microlithiasis. Arch Intern Med 1983;143:358–9.
905. Chatterji R, Gaude GS, Patil PV. Pulmonary alveolar microlithiasis: diagnosed by sputum examination and transbronchial biopsy. Indian J Chest Dis Allied Sci 1997;39:263–7.
906. Cluzel P, Grenier P, Bernadac P, Laurent F, Picard JD. Pulmonary alveolar microlithiasis: CT findings. J Comput Assist Tomogr 1991;15:938–42.
907. Edelman JD, Bavaria J, Kaiser LR, Litzky LA, Palevsky HI, Kotloff RM. Bilateral sequential lung transplantation for pulmonary alveolar microlithiasis. Chest 1997;112:1140–4.
908. Emri S, Coplu L, Selcuk ZT, Sahin AA, Baris YI. Hypertrophic pulmonary osteoarthropathy in a patient with pulmonary alveolar microlithiasis. Thorax 1991;46:145–6.
909. Friedrich N. Corpora amylacea in den Lungen. Arch Pathol Anat 1856;9:613–8.
910. Fuleihan FJ, Abboud RT, Balikian JP, Nucho CK. Pulmonary alveolar microlithiasis: lung function in five cases. Thorax 1969;24:84–90.
911. Gocmen A, Toppare MF, Kiper N, Buyukpamukcu N. Treatment of pulmonary alveolar microlithiasis with a diphosphonate—preliminary results of a case. Respiration 1992;59:250–2.
912. Helbich TH, Wojnarovsky C, Wunderbaldinger P, Heinz-Peer G, Eichler I, Herold CJ. Pulmonary alveolar microlithiasis in children: radiographic and high-resolution CT findings. AJR Am J Roentgenol 1997;168:63–5.
913. Hoshino H, Koba H, Inomata S, et al. Pulmonary alveolar microlithiasis: high-resolution CT and MR findings. J Comput Assist Tomogr 1998;22:245–8.
914. Kanra G, Tanyol E, Gocmen A, et al. Pulmonary alveolar microlithiasis (a case report). Turk J Pediatr 1988;30:61–7.
915. Kiatboonsri S, Charoenpan P, Vathesatogkit P, Boonpucknavig V. Pulmonary alveolar microlithiasis: report of five cases and literature review. J Med Assoc Thai 1985;68:672–7.
916. Korn MA, Schurawitzki H, Klepetko W, Burghuber OC. Pulmonary alveolar microlithiasis: findings on high-resolution CT. AJR Am J Roentgenol 1992;158:981–2.
917. Mariotta S, Guidi L, Mattia P, et al. Pulmonary microlithiasis. Report of two cases. Respiration 1997;64:165–9.
918. Mariotta S, Guidi L, Papale M, Ricci A, Bisetti A. Pulmonary alveolar microlithiasis: review of Italian reports. Eur J Epidemiol 1997;13:587–90.
919. Melamed JW, Sostman HD, Ravin CE. Interstitial thickening in pulmonary alveolar microlithiasis: an underappreciated finding. J Thorac Imaging 1994;9:126–8.
920. Miro JM, Moreno A, Coca A, Segura F, Soriano E. Pulmonary alveolar microlithiasis with an unusual radiological pattern. Br J Dis Chest 1982;76:91–6.

921. Moran CA, Hochholzer L, Hasleton PS, Johnson FB, Koss MN. Pulmonary alveolar microlithiasis. A clinicopathologic and chemical analysis of seven cases. Arch Pathol Lab Med 1997;121:607–11.
922. Nouh MS. Pulmonary alveolar microlithiasis: a report on four cases. East Afr Med J 1991; 68:39-42.
923. O'Neill RP, Cohn JE, Pellegrino ED. Pulmonary alveolar microlithiasis—a family study. Ann Intern Med 1967;67:957–67.
924. Pant K, Shah A, Mathur RK, Chhabra SK, Jain SK. Pulmonary alveolar microlithiasis with pleural calcification and nephrolithiasis. Chest 1990;98:245–6.
925. Pracyk JB, Simonson SG, Young SL, Ghio AJ, Roggli VL, Piantadosi CA. Composition of lung lavage in pulmonary alveolar microlithiasis. Respiration 1996;63:254–60.
926. Prakash UB, Barham SS, Rosenow EC III, Brown ML, Payne WS. Pulmonary alveolar microlithiasis: a review including ultrastructural and pulmonary function studies. Mayo Clin Proc 1983;58:290–300.
927. Ratjen FA, Schoenfeld B, Wiesemann HG. Pulmonary alveolar microlithiasis and lymphocytic interstitial pneumonitis in a ten year old girl. Eur Respir J 1992;5:1283–5.
928. Richardson J, Slovis B, Miller G, Dummer S. Development of pulmonary alveolar microlithiasis in a renal transplant recipient. Transplantation 1995;59:1056–7.
929. Ritchie DA, O'Connor SA, McGivern D. An unusual presentation of pulmonary alveolar microlithiasis and diaphyseal aclasia. Br J Radiol 1992;65:178–81.
930. Sears MR, Chang AR, Taylor AJ. Pulmonary alveolar microlithiasis. Thorax 1971;26:704–11.
931. Singh NK, Gupta A. Pulmonary alveolar microlithiasis. J Assoc Physicians India 1995;43:647–8.
932. Stamatis G, Zerkowski HR, Doetsch N, Greschuchna D, Konietzko N, Reidemeister JC. Sequential bilateral lung transplantation for pulmonary alveolar microlithiasis. Ann Thorac Surg 1993;56:972–5.
933. Turktas H, Ozturk C, Guven M, Ugur P, Erzen C. Pulmonary alveolar microlithiasis with the absence of technetium-99m MDP uptake of lungs. Clin Nucl Med 1988;13:883–5.
934. Ucan ES, Keyf AI, Aydilek R, et al. Pulmonary alveolar microlithiasis: review of Turkish reports. Thorax 1993;48:171–3.
935. Wallis C, Whitehead B, Malone M, Dinwiddie R. Pulmonary alveolar microlithiasis in childhood: diagnosis by transbronchial biopsy. Pediatr Pulmonol 1996;21:62–4.

4
PULMONARY VASCULITIS

Vasculitis is defined as inflammation of the blood vessel walls (80). Pulmonary vasculitis embraces a small group of idiopathic vasculitis syndromes that commonly affect the lung, a much larger number of vasculitic disorders that uncommonly affect the lung, and miscellaneous secondary conditions that cause pulmonary vascular inflammation (Table 4-1) (169).

The idiopathic vasculitis syndromes that commonly affect the lung are Wegener's granulomatosis, Churg-Strauss syndrome, and microscopic polyangiitis (Table 4-1). Bronchocentric granulomatosis (BCG) and lymphomatoid granulomatosis have traditionally been grouped as pulmonary "angiitis and granulomatosis," however, neither of these entities is currently thought to be a vasculitic condition. BCG is a morphologic pattern of airway inflammation that occurs in a variety of conditions, especially infection (see chapter 8). Lymphomatoid granulomatosis is now known to represent a lymphoproliferative disorder with prominent vascular involvement (70,127).

In addition to the major idiopathic vasculitic lung disorders, there are a number that uncommonly affect the lung (Table 4-1). Necrotizing sarcoid granulomatosis was formerly regarded as one of the major vasculitis syndromes, but it is so rare that it is now grouped under syndromes that uncommonly affect the lung. We maintain it in the vasculitis chapter because it is often confused with the other vasculitides. Pulmonary vasculitis also occurs in a variety of miscellaneous systemic disorders, in diffuse pulmonary hemorrhagic syndromes, and in a variety of secondary or localized forms (Table 4-1). The term benign lymphocytic angiitis and granulomatosis is not used since this may include low-grade examples of lymphomatoid granulomatosis.

The diagnosis of these vasculitis syndromes is difficult for the surgical pathologist for several reasons. First, they are clinicopathologic entities so the ultimate diagnosis does not rest on pathology alone, but is based on careful correlation between clinical, radiologic, and pathologic features. Second, these are rare dis-

Table 4-1

PULMONARY VASCULITIS SYNDROMES[a]

Idiopathic vasculitis syndromes which commonly affect the lung
Wegener's granulomatosis
Churg-Strauss angiitis and granulomatosis
Microscopic polyangiitis
Idiopathic vasculitis syndromes which uncommonly affect the lung
Necrotizing sarcoid granulomatosis
Polyarteritis nodosa
Small vessel vasculitis
Takayasu's arteritis
Henoch-Shönlein purpura
Behçet's syndrome
Cryoglobulinemic vasculitis
Hypocomplementemic vasculitis
Idiopathic granulomatous arteritis
Giant cell arteritis
Disseminated visceral giant cell angiitis
Miscellaneous systemic disorders
Classic sarcoidosis
Collagen vascular disease
Inflammatory bowel disease
Malignancy
Diffuse pulmonary hemorrhage syndromes
Secondary or localized vasculitis
Pulmonary infection
Bronchocentric granulomatosis
Pulmonary hypertension
Interstitial lung diseases
Chronic eosinophilic pneumonia
Langerhans' cell histiocytosis
Inflammatory pseudotumors
Sequestration
Embolic material (intravenous drug abuse)
Drugs or toxic substances
Transplantation
Radiation
Vascular involvement in lymphoproliferative disorders
Angiocentric immunoproliferative lesion (lymphomatoid granulomatosis)
Non-Hodgkin's lymphoma
Intravascular malignant lymphoma

[a]Modified from reference 169.

orders, so few pathologists have much experience with them. Third, the pathologic features of these rare conditions overlap with common inflammatory lesions such as necrotizing infectious granulomas due to tuberculosis or fungi such as *Histoplasma capsulatum*. Finally, in many cases, the full-blown histopathologic picture is not present, requiring the recognition of subtle clues to suspect the diagnosis.

WEGENER'S GRANULOMATOSIS

Definition. Wegener's granulomatosis (WG) is a systemic granulomatous inflammatory process. The accompanying vasculitis predominantly affects the upper and lower respiratory tract and kidney.

Clinical Features. In 1936, Friedrich Wegener described the disease that bears his name as a systemic disorder characterized by aseptic necrotizing granulomatous inflammation and vasculitis which affects the upper and lower respiratory tracts and the kidneys (180). WG is a rare disorder, occurring in 0.3 persons per million in the United States (35) and 8.5 per million in the United Kingdom (15). While some studies have suggested an increased occurrence in winter months (15), others have disputed this (35). An association between WG and infection has been postulated but remains to be confirmed (61).

WG typically occurs in adults with a mean age of 50 years, however, it can occur in adolescents and, rarely, in children (73,134,176). It most commonly affects the head and neck region, followed by the lung, kidney, and eye (Table 4-2) (73,97). The most common presenting symptoms are persistent rhinorrhea, purulent/bloody nasal discharge, oral or nasal ulcers, polyarthralgias, myalgias, and sinus pain. Less commonly, patients present with hoarseness, stridor, earache, hearing loss, otorrhea, cough, dyspnea, hemoptysis (due to an alveolar capillaritis, necrotic lesions, or endobronchial disease), and pleuritic pain. Pulmonary symptoms in the absence of upper respiratory tract manifestations are unusual. Destructive inflammation of the nose may result in a saddle nose deformity. In addition, patients may have systemic signs and symptoms such as arthralgias, fever, cutaneous lesions, weight loss, and peripheral neuropathy (Table 4-2) (31). Uncommon sites of involvement include the salivary gland, pancreas, breast, mediastinum, gastrointestinal tract, prostate and urethra, vagina and cervix, heart, spleen, and peripheral or central nervous system (63,164).

Table 4-2

CLINICAL MANIFESTATIONS OF WEGENER'S GRANULOMATOSIS[a]

Manifestation	At Presentation (%)	During Course of Disease (%)
Head and Neck Manifestations	73	92
Sinusitis	51	85
Nasal disease	36	68
Otitis media	25	44
Hearing loss	14	42
Subglottic stenosis	8	16
Ear pain	1	14
Oral lesions	3	10
Pulmonary Manifestations	45	85
Infiltrates	23	66
Nodule	22	59
Cough	19	46
Hemoptysis	12	30
Pleuritis	10	28
Renal Manifestations	18	77
Eye Manifestations	15	52
Conjunctivitis	5	18
Dacryocystitis	1	18
Scleritis	6	16
Proptosis	2	15
Eye pain	3	11
Visual loss	0	8
Retinal lesions	0	4
Corneal ulcers	0	1
Iritis	0	2
Systemic Manifestations		
Joints	32	67
Fever	23	50
Skin	13	46
Weight loss	15	35
Peripheral nervous system	1	15
Central nervous system	1	8
Pericarditis	2	6

[a]Data from reference 73.

Physiologic studies show both restrictive and obstructive patterns. The most frequent abnormality is airflow obstruction, often associated with a reduced diffusing capacity for carbon monoxide (DLCO). Airflow obstruction

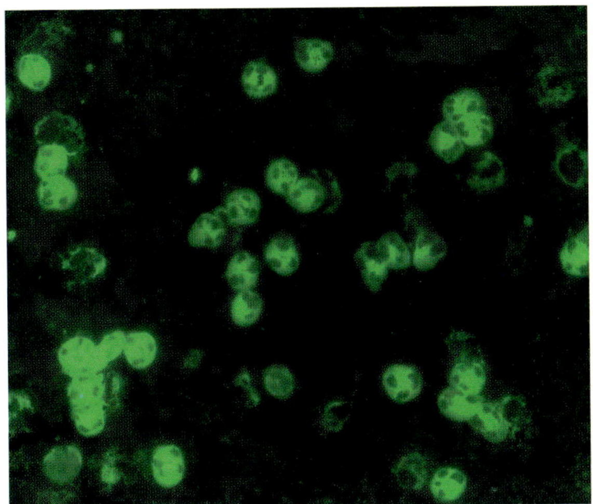
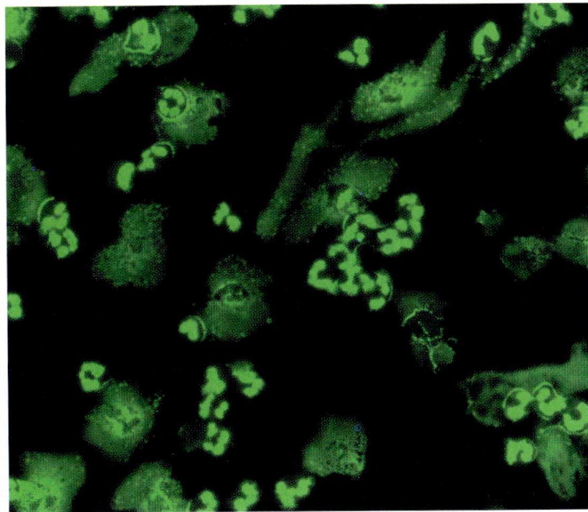

Figure 4-1

ANTINEUTROPHIL CYTOPLASMIC ANTIBODY (ANCA) IMMUNOFLUORESCENCE

Left: Cytoplasmic ANCA shows staining of the neutrophil cytoplasm.

Right: Perinuclear ANCA shows staining in the perinuclear region of the neutrophil cytoplasm. (Courtesy of Dr. Neil Smith, Massachusetts General Hospital, Boston, MA.)

may be a harbinger of tracheal obstruction or lobar collapse.

Antineutrophil Cytoplasmic Antibodies. Routine laboratory results are generally nonspecific in WG and include leukocytosis, thrombocytosis (greater than 400,000/mm^3), marked elevation of the erythrocyte sedimentation rate, and normochromic, normocytic anemia. In the past decade, the diagnosis of WG has been dramatically aided by the discovery and use of the serum antineutrophil cytoplasmic antibody (ANCA) test (65,66,82,142,153). Two major immunofluorescence patterns occur: the cytoplasmic or classic (C-ANCA) or the perinuclear (P-ANCA) pattern (fig. 4-1) (37); the C-ANCA pattern is the more common. C-ANCA typically has specificity for proteinase 3 and is found in 84 to 99 percent of patients with active generalized WG, 50 to 71 percent of patients in partial remission, and 30 to 40 percent of patients in complete remission (129). Although the P-ANCA pattern is seen in WG, but it is more characteristic of idiopathic necrotizing and crescentic glomerulonephritis, microscopic polyangiitis, polyarteritis nodosa, and Churg-Strauss syndrome (79). Most P-ANCAs have a specificity for myeloperoxidase. Recent studies by Gal et al. (56) and Gaudin et al. (59) have shown no significant difference in the lung biopsy findings from patients with C-ANCAs versus P-ANCAs. It is unclear whether an increased level of C-ANCA in the bronchoalveolar lavage (BAL) fluid is a more specific predictor of the diagnosis or the level of disease activity. Importantly, the presence of C-ANCA alone is not sufficiently specific to make or exclude a diagnosis of WG.

Radiologic Findings. The typical radiographic manifestation of WG is that of multifocal pulmonary opacities (figs. 4-2, 4-3). Classically, there are well-marginated nodules or masses of varying sizes, ranging from 0.5 to 10.0 cm, which occur most frequently in the lower lobes (33,46,54). Spiculated or ill-defined nodules may also be observed (156). Cavitation occurs in 25 to 50 percent of cases. Cavity walls are typically thick and irregular, but lesions may evolve into thin-walled cavities or disappear completely with therapy (44,54). Pulmonary lesions may be transient in location and change in appearance with time. Multifocal, ill-defined parenchymal consolidation, with or without cavitation, and diffuse reticular and nodular interstitial opacities have also been reported (1,54). Patients with WG may present initially with diffuse airspace disease representing pulmonary hemorrhage (fig. 4-4). Children typically

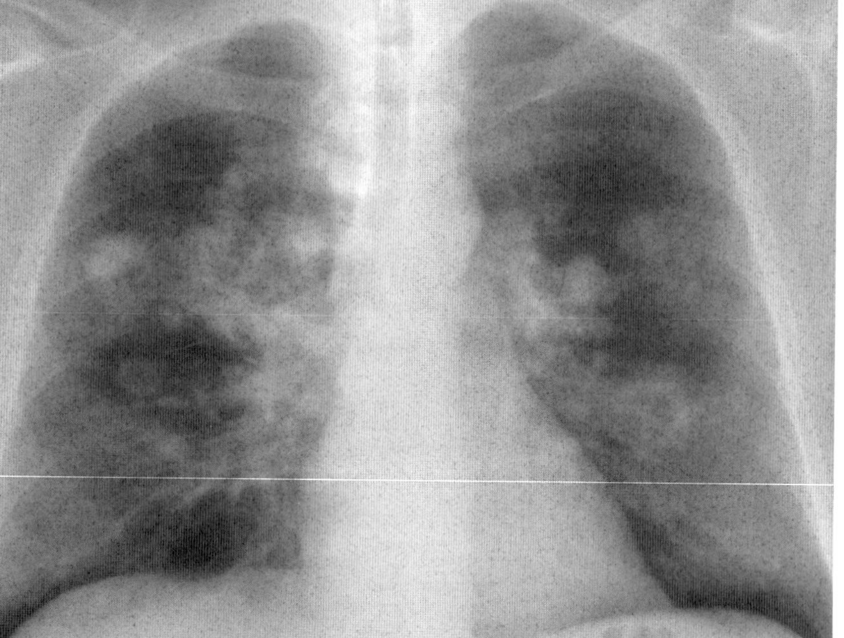

Figure 4-2

WEGENER'S GRANULOMATOSIS

Posteroanterior (PA) chest radiograph in a patient with Wegener's granulomatosis demonstrates multifocal pulmonary nodular opacities, some of which exhibit cavitation.

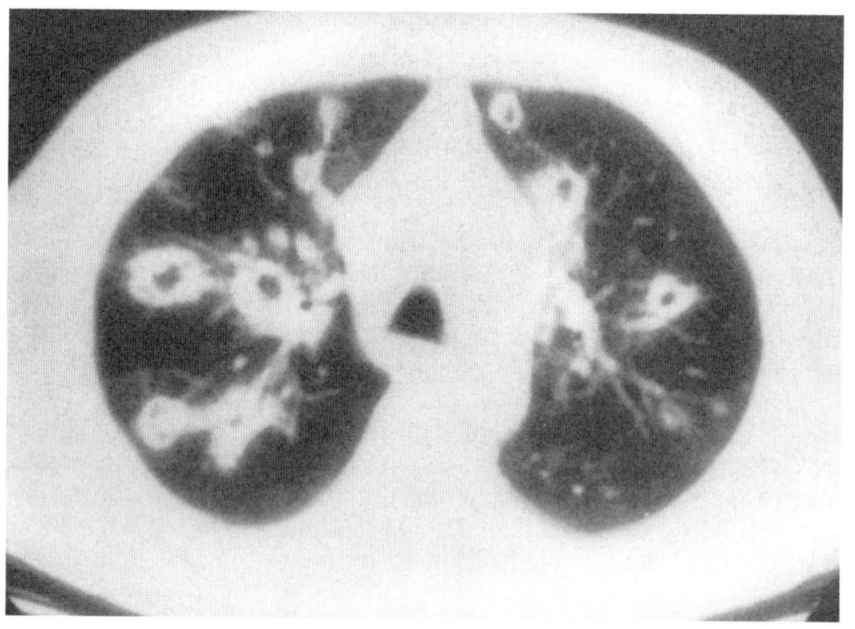

Figure 4-3

WEGENER'S GRANULOMATOSIS

Chest CT (lung window) shows profuse, multifocal cavitary pulmonary nodules and masses. The borders of the lesions vary from irregular to well-marginated. The cavities have thick irregular walls.

present with diffuse interstitial and alveolar opacities frequently secondary to pulmonary hemorrhage. Pulmonary nodules are less frequent in pediatric patients (176). Pleural effusion is seen in 20 to 50 percent of cases, and focal pleural thickening has also been observed. Hilar and/or mediastinal lymphadenopathies are unusual manifestations. Rarely, a solitary pulmonary nodule or consolidation is seen (86).

Computed tomography (CT) affords optimal visualization of the number, morphologic characteristics, and location of the pulmonary abnormalities. Nodules and masses may have well-marginated or spiculated borders. Cavita-

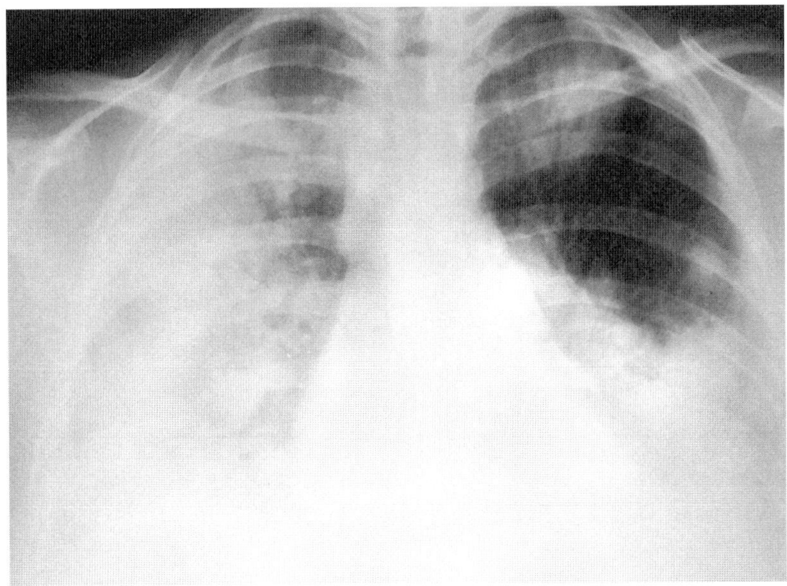

Figure 4-4

WEGENER'S GRANULOMATOSIS WITH DIFFUSE PULMONARY HEMORRHAGE

PA chest radiograph demonstrates bilateral, confluent airspace lung disease and nodular opacities in the left upper lung zone.

tion is identified in 50 percent of cases, and a feeding vascular structure is seen in 88 percent of nodules, consistent with the angiocentric nature of this disorder (92). In addition, in 88 percent of cases, wedge-shaped peripheral opacities have been described which resemble the CT appearance of pulmonary infarction. Air bronchograms, nodules, and the CT halo sign have also been described in WG (92,132). The CT halo sign refers to ground-glass opacity surrounding a pulmonary nodule or mass, and has been correlated with focal hemorrhage around the lesion (132). In children, CT may demonstrate ill-defined centrilobular and perivascular opacities (32). Tracheobronchial involvement by WG manifests as short- or long-segment stenosis of the airways on CT and may be complicated by lobar or complete atelectasis (1,36, 114). Rarely, a solitary nodule or mass with or without cavitation may be seen (86). Lymphadenopathy is a rare manifestation (114).

Gross Findings. The classic pattern of pulmonary involvement by WG is that of multiple bilateral pulmonary nodules with frequent cavitation (fig. 4-5, left) (167). Most open lung biopsies sample only a single nodule, so multiple nodules may be seen grossly only in autopsy or large surgical specimens, such as lobectomies or pneumonectomies. Solid nodular zones of consolidation with foci of punctate or geographic necrosis are often seen (fig. 4-5, right). WG can rarely manifest as a solitary lung lesion, but most solitary necrotizing granulomas are infectious (173) and the classic histologic findings are required in addition to typical clinical findings to support the diagnosis (86). Rarely, the lesions may be centered on bronchi. The cut surface of the lung is dark red and bloody in patients presenting with acute pulmonary hemorrhage.

Histologic Findings. Histologically, the pulmonary lesions of WG typically consist of consolidated nodules of inflammation and necrosis (figs. 4-6–4-8). The major histologic manifestations are often regarded as diagnostic criteria (Table 4-3) and consist of parenchymal necrosis (figs. 4-6–4-8), vasculitis (figs. 4-9–4-11), and granulomatous inflammation (figs. 4-6–4-8, 4-12, 4-13). The surrounding inflammatory infiltrate consists of a mixture of neutrophils, lymphocytes, plasma cells, macrophages, giant cells, and eosinophils. Parenchymal necrosis can take the form of either neutrophilic microabscesses (fig. 4-8) or large zones of geographic necrosis (fig. 4-6). The geographic necrosis is frequently basophilic due to the numerous necrotic neutrophils. Several types of granulomatous inflammation can be seen including giant cells scattered randomly or in loose clusters (fig. 4-12), palisading histiocytes (fig. 4-13) or giant

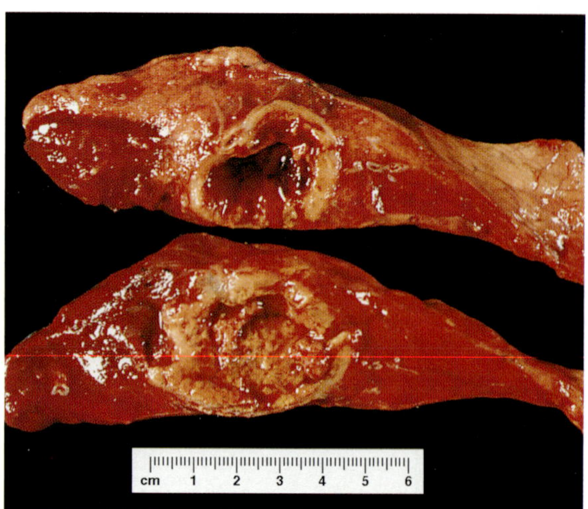
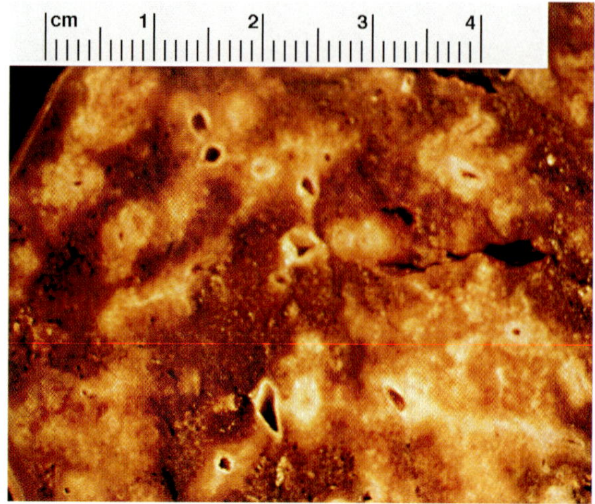

Figure 4-5

WEGENER'S GRANULOMATOSIS: GROSS SPECIMEN

Left: This necrotizing granuloma is cavitated with a necrotic center and an inflammatory border.
Right: There are multiple, scattered, nodular foci of consolidation, with punctate and large zones of necrosis.

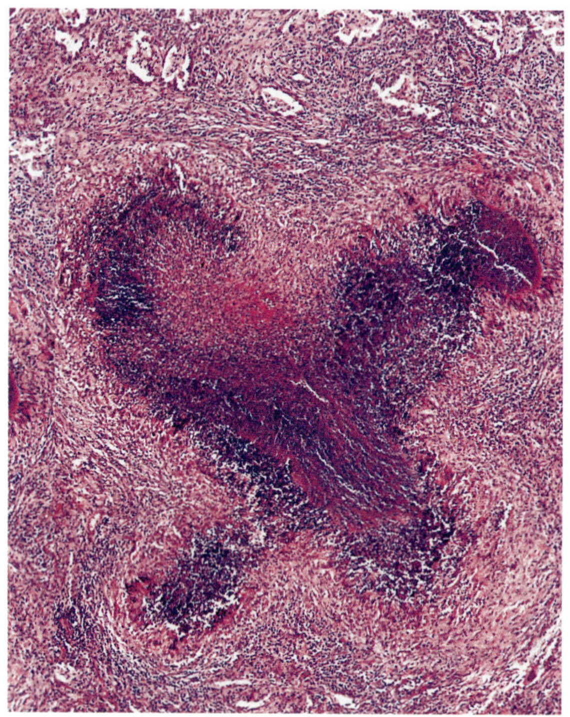

Figure 4-6

WEGENER'S GRANULOMATOSIS: GEOGRAPHIC NECROSIS

Large zones of basophilic necrosis with an irregular, serpiginous border give the appearance of geographic necrosis. The central necrotic zone is surrounded by a dense mixed inflammatory infiltrate.

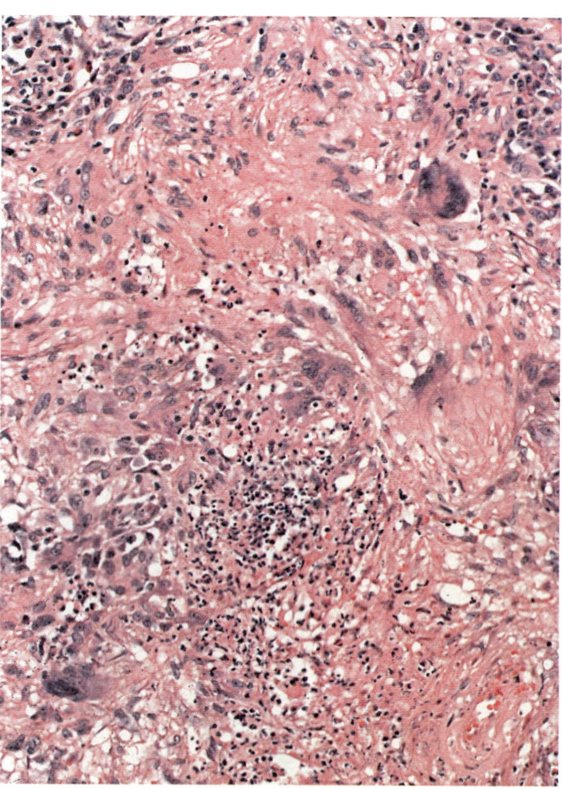

Figure 4-7

WEGENER'S GRANULOMATOSIS: NECROTIZING GRANULOMA

Multinucleated giant cells and a mixture of acute and chronic inflammation surround the central necrosis.

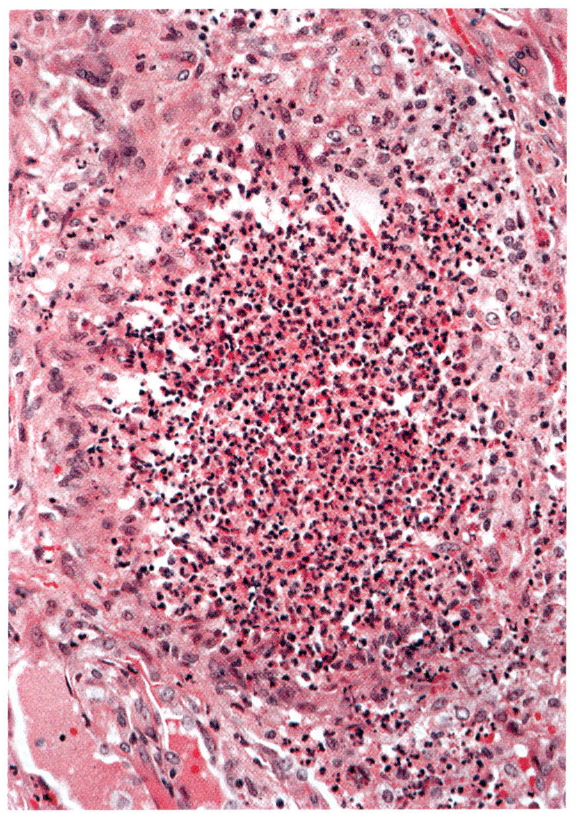

Figure 4-8

WEGENER'S GRANULOMATOSIS: NEUTROPHILIC MICROABSCESS

This collection of neutrophils forms a microabscess that is surrounded by histiocytes and giant cells.

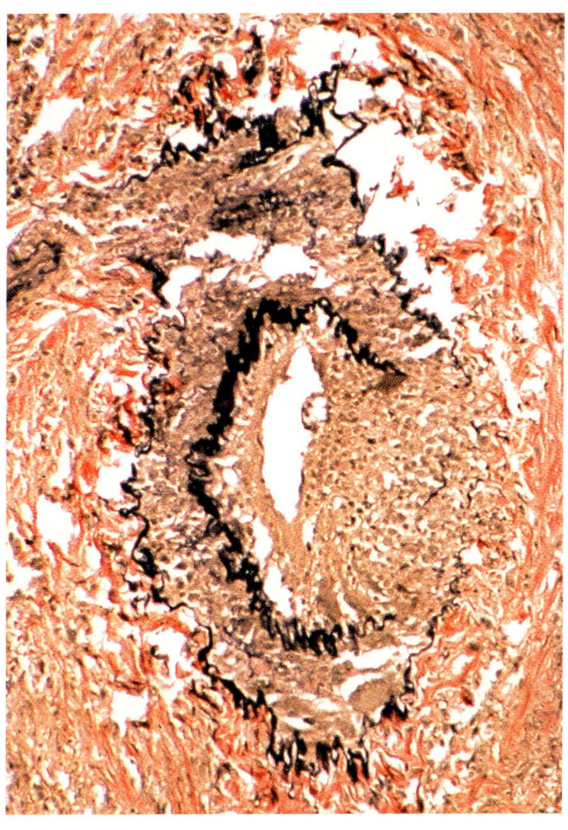

Figure 4-9

WEGENER'S GRANULOMATOSIS: VASCULITIS

This arteriole shows an eccentric, transmural inflammatory infiltrate destroying the vessel wall. The inner elastic lamina is completely destroyed and the outer layer is mostly gone (elastic stain).

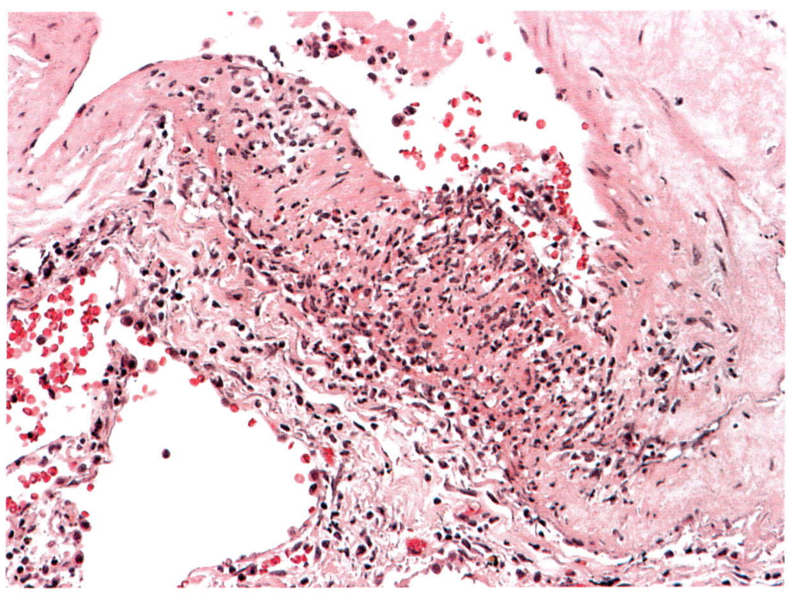

Figure 4-10

WEGENER'S GRANULOMATOSIS: VASCULITIS

This vein shows a focal, eccentric, transmural, chronic inflammatory infiltrate.

Figure 4-11

WEGENER'S GRANULOMATOSIS: VASCULITIS

This arteriole shows marked inflammation in the vessel wall with focal fibrinoid necrosis.

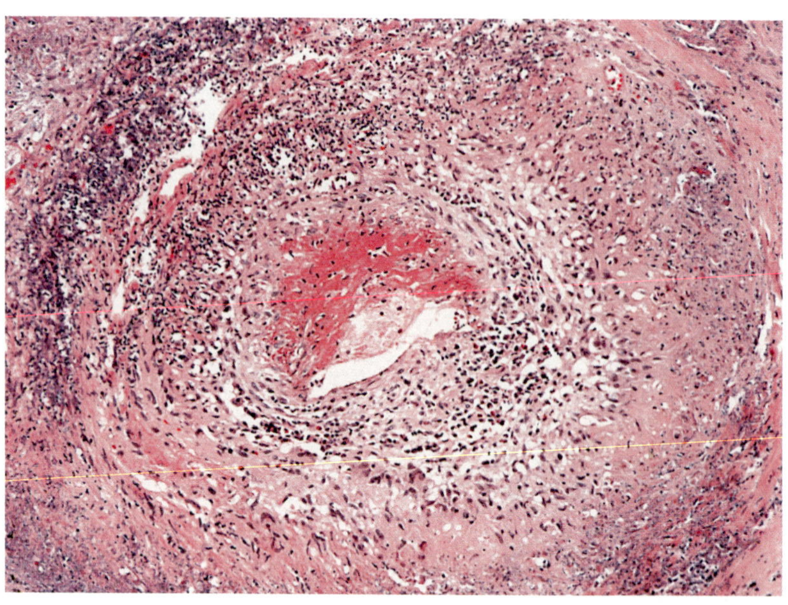

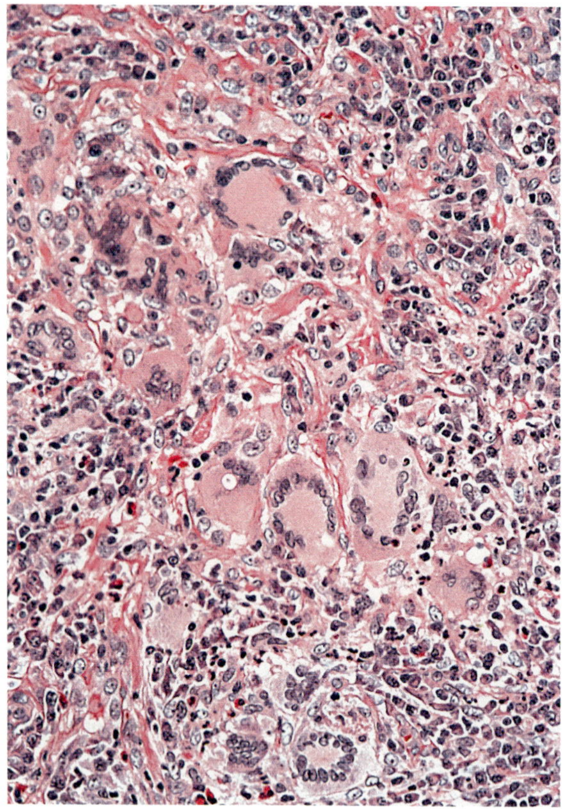

Figure 4-12

WEGENER'S GRANULOMATOSIS: GRANULOMATOUS INFLAMMATION

Loosely clustered giant cells are scattered within a marked inflammatory background.

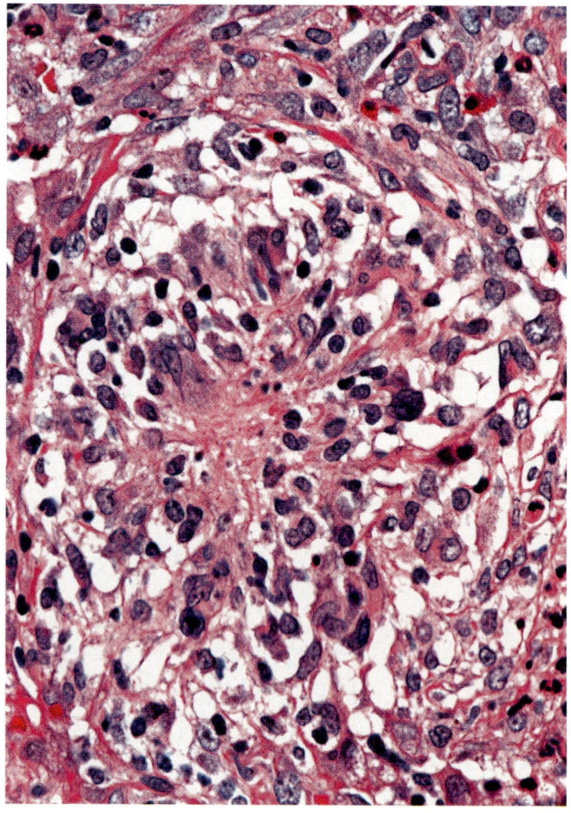

Figure 4-13

WEGENER'S GRANULOMATOSIS: PALISADING MICROGRANULOMA

This granuloma consists of a cartwheel-shaped arrangement of palisading histiocytes surrounding a central eosinophilic focus.

Table 4-3

MAJOR PATHOLOGIC MANIFESTATIONS (DIAGNOSTIC CRITERIA) OF WEGENER'S GRANULOMATOSIS[a]

I. **Vasculitis**
   A. Arteritis, venulitis, capillaritis[b]
   B. Six types: acute, chronic, necrotizing granulomatous, non-necrotizing granulomatous, fibrinoid necrosis, cicatricial changes[c]

II. **Parenchymal Necrosis**
   A. Microabscess
   B. Geographic necrosis

III. **Granulomatous Inflammation (Mixed Inflammatory Infiltrate)**
   A. Microabscess surrounded by granulomatous inflammation
   B. Palisading histiocytes
   C. Scattered giant cells
   D. Poorly formed granulomas
   E. Sarcoid-like granulomas (rare)

[a]Data from references 167 and 169.

[b]Capillaritis was characterized primarily by acute inflammation. Veins and arteries demonstrated all the types of inflammation listed in IB.

[c]Cicatricial vascular changes are nonspecific and should not be used as a diagnostic criterion.

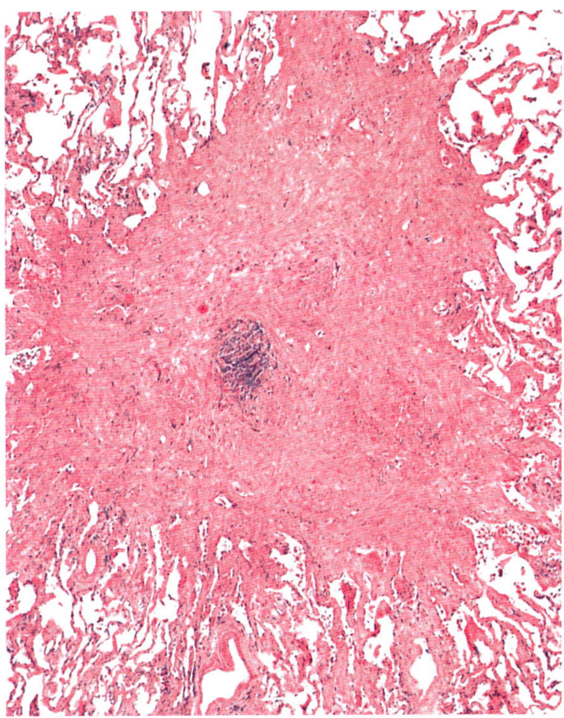

Figure 4-14

WEGENER'S GRANULOMATOSIS: INTERSTITIAL FIBROSIS

This nodular scar consists of dense acellular fibrosis. It was removed from a patient with Wegener's granulomatosis who underwent therapy and had a persistent pulmonary nodule.

cells (fig. 4-7) lining the border of the geographic necrosis or microabscesses, and microgranulomas consisting of small foci of palisading histiocytes arranged in a cartwheel pattern (fig. 4-13). Tightly packed sarcoid-like granulomas are rare and suggest a diagnosis other than WG, such as infection or necrotizing sarcoidosis.

The vasculitis of WG may affect arteries, veins, or capillaries in the form of capillaritis (figs. 4-11, 4-14). The inflammation is often focal and eccentrically involves the vessel wall (figs. 4-9, 4-10). Destruction of the vascular elastic laminae is frequently seen (fig. 4-9). Sometimes the inflammation is limited to the endothelium (endotheliolitis) and subendothelium of the vessel wall. All types of inflammatory cells, including neutrophils, lymphocytes, plasma cells, eosinophils, histiocytes, and giant cells, may inflame vessels. Occasionally, the inflammatory infiltrate consists mostly of mononuclear cells (fig. 4-10). Capillaritis is discussed in more detail in the section on microscopic polyangiitis. Necrotizing granulomas may also involve vessel walls. Cicatricial vascular changes may be seen (fig. 4-14), especially in patients who received prior therapy.

In addition to these major histologic features, there are a variety of minor histologic features including alveolar hemorrhage, interstitial fibrosis (figs. 4-9–4-15), lipoid pneumonia, organizing pneumonia (fig. 4-16), lymphoid hyperplasia, eosinophilia, and xanthomatous lesions (Table 4-4). WG can involve the airways and cause chronic bronchiolitis, acute bronchiolitis/bronchopneumonia, the histologic pattern of bronchiolitis obliterans (with or without organizing pneumonia [BOOP]) (fig. 4-16), bronchocentric granulomatosis (fig. 4-17), follicular bronchiolitis, and bronchial stenosis (Table 4-4) (167,184). Occasionally, one of these minor lesions may be the dominant finding at biopsy (167). Diffuse pulmonary hemorrhage

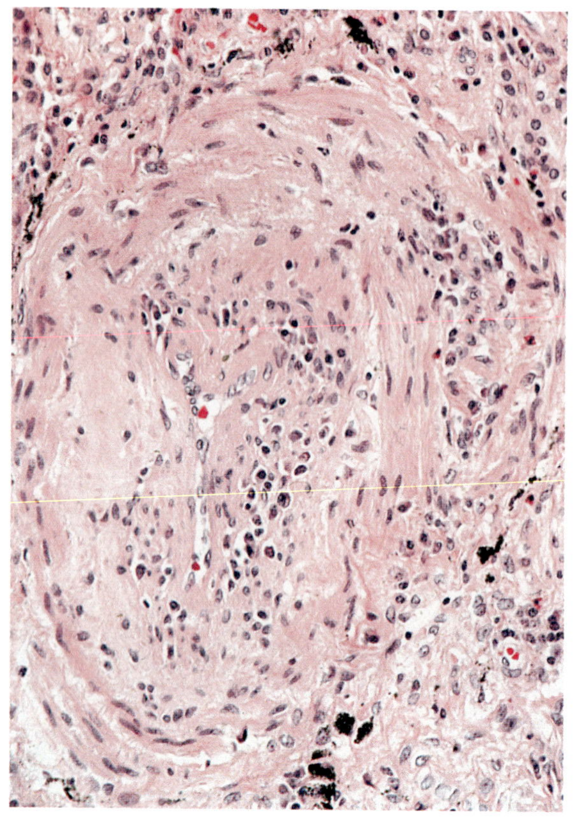

Figure 4-15

WEGENER'S GRANULOMATOSIS: CICATRICIAL VASCULAR CHANGE

This blood vessel shows marked medial thickening due to fibrosis. The lung biopsy is from a patient who had been treated previously.

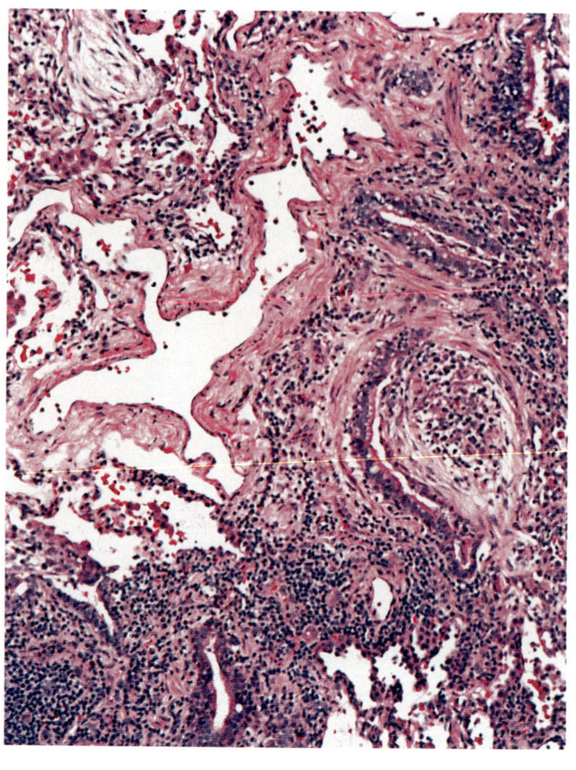

Figure 4-16

WEGENER'S GRANULOMATOSIS: ORGANIZING PNEUMONIA PATTERN WITH FOCAL BRONCHIOLITIS OBLITERANS

Polypoid plugs of loose organizing fibrosis are present within the bronchiole and adjacent airspaces. There is also marked chronic bronchiolar inflammation. This was the predominant finding in this lung biopsy that also showed focal giant cells and vasculitis.

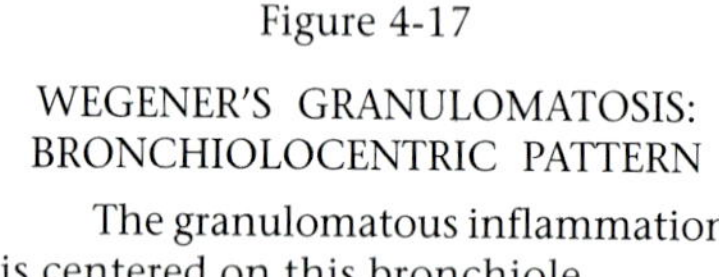

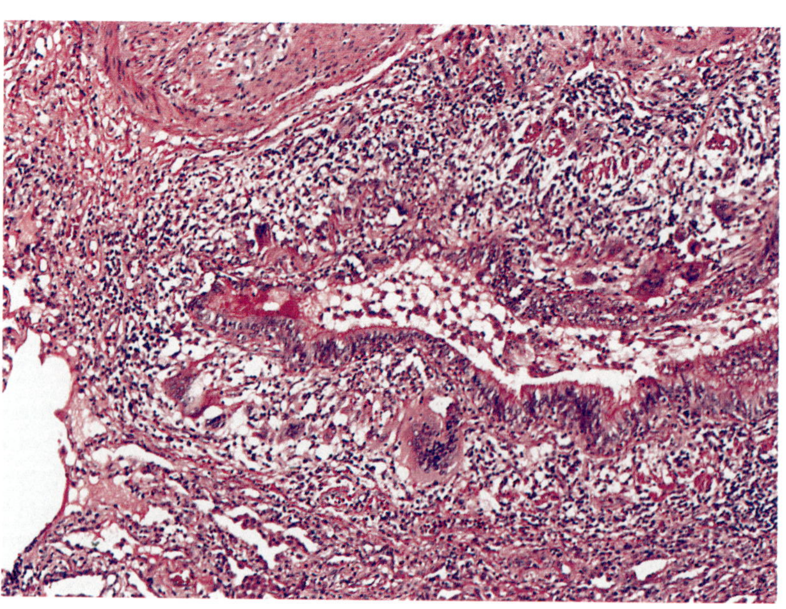

Figure 4-17

WEGENER'S GRANULOMATOSIS: BRONCHIOLOCENTRIC PATTERN

The granulomatous inflammation is centered on this bronchiole.

is a severe life-threatening manifestation of WG (see Diffuse Alveolar Hemorrhage in chapter 3). The pattern of bronchocentric granulomatosis is another rare manifestation encountered in 1 percent of cases (167,184). Organizing pneumonia is seen in 70 percent of lung biopsies from patients with WG (167) and, rarely, may be so prominent that it gives a BOOP-like histologic pattern (167,174).

Classic histologic findings may not be seen if the lung is biopsied very early in the course of disease or following therapy (117,167). Interstitial fibrosis (sometimes with scattered giant cells but without necrosis), bronchial and/or bronchiolar scarring, and cicatricial vascular changes are common in lung biopsies from patients who have received therapy (117,167).

Differential Diagnosis. The differential diagnosis of WG based on lung biopsy evaluation includes lymphomatoid granulomatosis (90,112), Churg-Strauss syndrome (CSS) (19,28, 88,101), sarcoidosis, necrotizing sarcoid granulomatosis (20,22,89), granulomatous infection (173), rheumatoid nodules (20), bronchocentric granulomatosis (20,91,184), and diffuse pulmonary hemorrhage syndromes (118,166). Lymphomatoid granulomatosis is characterized by multiple necrotic pulmonary nodules showing vasocentricity and vasodestruction, and necrotic zones surrounded by a mixed inflammatory infiltrate, and this may resemble WG. However, in lymphomatoid granulomatosis, the lymphoid infiltrate consists of lymphoid cells showing varying degrees of atypia. These are typically B cells (CD20 positive) and often contain the Epstein-Barr virus (70,124). In addition, granulomatous inflammation is comparatively rare in lymphomatoid granulomatosis, and the presence of granulomas is more suggestive of another diagnosis, such as infection or WG.

Prominent tissue eosinophilia occurs in about 5 percent of cases of WG. This finding often raises the possibility of CSS or fungal or parasitic infection (19,23,28,88,100,101). Peripheral eosinophilia is characteristic of CSS and is uncommon in WG (154). Asthma is not a characteristic feature of WG, although it can occur. The distinction between WG and CSS is usually straightforward but some cases may require careful assessment of all of the clinical, pathologic, and laboratory data (Table 4-5). CSS is discussed in detail below.

Table 4-4

MINOR PATHOLOGIC MANIFESTATIONS OF WEGENER'S GRANULOMATOSIS[a,b]

I. Parenchymal
- A. Nodular interstitial fibrosis
- B. Endogenous lipoid pneumonia
- C. Alveolar hemorrhage
- D. Organizing intraluminal fibrosis
- E. Lymphoid aggregates
- F. Tissue eosinophils
- G. Xanthogranulomatous lesions
- H. Alveolar macrophage accumulation

II. Bronchial/Bronchiolar Lesions
- A. Chronic bronchiolitis
- B. Acute bronchiolitis/bronchopneumonia
- C. Bronchiolitis obliterans or a BOOP histologic pattern[c]
- D. Bronchocentric granulomatosis
- E. Follicular bronchiolitis
- F. Bronchial stenosis

[a]Data from references 167 and 169.
[b]May uncommonly represent a dominant pathologic feature.
[c]BOOP = Bronchiolitis obliterans with organizing pneumonia.

One of the most important considerations in the diagnosis of WG is the exclusion of infection. Both tuberculosis and fungal infection can cause a necrotizing granulomatous inflammation and vasculitis resembling that seen in WG. Solitary necrotizing granulomas are associated with vasculitis in 87 percent of cases due to mycobacterial infection and 57 percent of cases due to fungal infection (173). Neutrophilic microabscesses can be seen in certain infections such as blastomycosis or nocardiosis. It is important to evaluate the possibility of infection by performing special stains for acid-fast bacilli and fungi in biopsies with granulomatous inflammation when the diagnosis of WG is being considered. One histologic clue in favor of infection is the presence of sarcoid-like granulomas (167). The presenting manifestation of WG as a solitary lung nodule, as noted above, is extremely rare; this is a setting in which one must be especially cautious to rule out infection (86).

Since WG can have a bronchocentric pattern of lung involvement, bronchocentric

Table 4-5

DISTINGUISHING FEATURES: WEGENER'S GRANULOMATOSIS VERSUS CHURG-STRAUSS SYNDROME

Clinical/Pathologic Feature	Wegener's Granulomatosis	Churg-Strauss Syndrome
Asthma	Rare	Characteristic (diagnostic criterion)
Eosinophilia		
Peripheral	Up to 12%	Characteristic[a]
Tissue	Up to 6%	Characteristic[a]
Sinus disease	Destructive, often causing saddle nose deformity	Less severe, usually allergic rhinitis
Renal disease	More severe	Usually mild
Cardiac disease	Rare	Common
ANCA[b]	Usually C-ANCA	Usually P-ANCA

[a]Eosinophilia may be fleeting and difficult to demonstrate during steroid therapy.
[b]ANCA = Antineutrophil cytoplasmic antibody; C = cytoplasmic; P = perinuclear.

granulomatosis must be considered in the differential diagnosis (167,184). Patients with bronchocentric WG should have other distinguishing features of WG such as renal or sinus involvement and a positive ANCA test.

Diagnosis. The histologic features of WG can be very suggestive of the diagnosis. However, one must rely on careful clinical and pathologic correlation for confirmation. In cases in which the clinical and pathologic features are full-blown, the diagnosis is uncomplicated. However, the diagnosis can be very difficult in cases where only partial clinical and/or pathologic criteria are present. In such cases the ANCA test can be helpful, although one must be careful since ANCAs are not specific for WG (49).

Treatment and Prognosis. Untreated WG is fatal, with up to 90 percent of patients dying within 2 years, usually due to respiratory or renal failure. However, therapy with cyclophosphamide and prednisone is very effective in achieving remissions: 85 to 90 percent of patients respond, with approximately 75 percent experiencing complete remission (45). The median time to remission is 12 months, with occasional patients requiring treatment for more than 2 years before all symptoms have resolved. Relapses are common, with up 50 percent of responders experiencing at least one relapse requiring another course of therapy. Trimethoprim/sulfamethoxazole, pulse cyclophosphamide, and methotrexate are additional ways to treat WG (38,73,98,99). Trimethoprim/sulfamethoxazole may reduce relapses in WG patients in remission (157). Although the clinical manifestations appear similar, the outcome for patients over 60 years of age appears significantly worse than that of younger patients, despite a similar treatment regimen (175). Lung function frequently improves following treatment, although the diffusing capacity may not return to normal.

CHURG-STRAUSS SYNDROME

Definition. Churg-Strauss syndrome (CSS) is a multisystem disorder defined by the presence of asthma, peripheral blood eosinophilia, and systemic vasculitis (19,23,28,100,101,144,154,168,169). Although CSS was initially defined pathologically by Drs. Churg and Strauss based on a series of autopsy cases (28), it is now recognized primarily as a clinical entity and in most cases is diagnosed on the basis of clinical findings (101). More recently, a subcommittee of the American College of Rheumatology proposed two approaches to the diagnosis of CSS (ACR 1990 Criteria): a traditional format classification and a classification tree (109,119). According to the traditional format classification, six criteria are identified: 1) asthma, 2) eosinophils greater than 10 percent of the white blood cell differential count, 3) mononeuropathy (including multiplex) or polyneuropathy, 4) nonfixed radiographic pulmonary infiltrates, 5) paranasal sinus abnormalities, and 6) a biopsy containing a blood vessel with extravascular eosinophils (119). If four of these six criteria are present, the diagnosis can be established with a sensitivity of 85 percent and a specificity of 99.7 percent (119). The major criteria used in the classification tree include: asthma, eosinophilia greater than 10 percent, and a history of allergy (119). According to this method, patients with well-documented systemic vasculitis who do not have a history of asthma can be diagnosed as having CSS if they have peripheral eosinophilia greater than 10 percent and a history of allergy other than drug sensitivity. This seems appropriate, since patients without asthma but with a history of allergic disease can develop CSS (57,113,141). Both classification methods appear to be useful, with greater sensitivity provided by the classification tree and greater specificity by the traditional approach.

Clinical Features. The incidence and epidemiology of CSS remain unclear. Approximately 10 percent of patients with a major form of vasculitis are recognized to have CSS. Among the major vasculitides, the frequency of CSS is second only to that of WG. CSS does not exhibit a gender predominance. The mean age at diagnosis is 50 years, but the systemic vasculitic phase is frequently apparent in patients who are in their late 30s. The exact etiology of CSS is unknown, but the disease is most likely due to an autoimmune process. The upper respiratory tract, lungs, skin, and peripheral nerves are the main sites of involvement (Table 4-6) (19,100,101). Involvement of the heart and kidney can also occur.

CSS progresses through three phases. Initially patients have a prodrome which manifests as allergic rhinitis, asthma, peripheral eosinophilia, and/or eosinophilic infiltrative disease (19, 100,101,154). Recurrent episodes of asthma may occur over a period of years prior to the onset of vasculitis (19,28,101). Tissue infiltration by eosinophils can affect the lungs or gastrointestinal tract. Pulmonary eosinophilia may take the form of Löffler's syndrome with fleeting pulmonary infiltrates or chronic eosinophilic pneumonia.

The prodrome is followed by the vasculitis phase. During this phase patients develop systemic signs and symptoms of vasculitis such as mononeuritis multiplex and cutaneous leukocytoclastic vasculitis. Only during this phase can the diagnosis of CSS be established (100). This is followed by a postvasculitis phase. In this phase patients may experience neuropathy and hypertension, and have continued asthma and allergic rhinitis (100,101). Proteinuria and gastrointestinal involvement are poor prognostic indicators (69).

Table 4-6

CLINICAL MANIFESTATIONS OF CHURG-STRAUSS SYNDROME[a]

Manifestation	Percent of Patients
Pulmonary infiltrates	72
Mononeuritis multiplex	66
Abdominal pain	59
Arthritis/arthralgias	51
Mild/moderate renal disease	49
Purpura	48
Cardiac failure	47
Myalgia	41
Löffler's syndrome	40
Erythema/urticaria	35
Diarrhea	33
Pericarditis	32
Skin nodules	30
Pleural effusion	29
Hypertension	29
Central nervous system abnormalities	27
Gastrointestinal bleeding	18
Renal failure	9

[a]Modified from reference 100.

A major difference from WG is the frequency of cardiac involvement, which occurs in up to 47 percent of CSS patients (100,101). CSS can cause cardiac failure, pericarditis, hypertension, and acute myocardial infarction (19, 28,101). Another major difference from WG is that the renal disease is less frequent and less severe (19,29,100,101). Peripheral neuropathy, often in the form of mononeuritis multiplex, is seen in about two thirds of patients. The most common cutaneous manifestation is leukocytoclastic vasculitis (62). Central nervous system involvement occurs in 25 percent of cases (100,

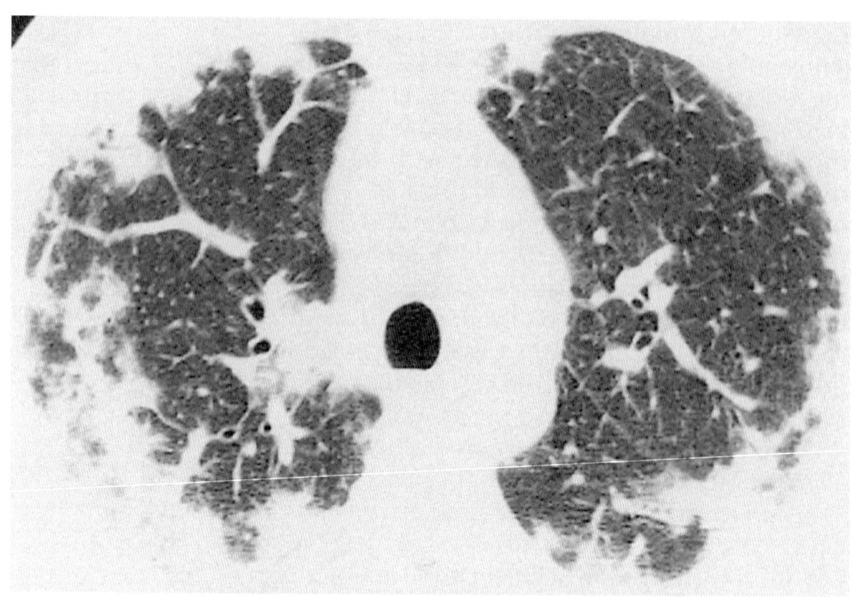

Figure 4-18

CHURG-STRAUSS SYNDROME

Chest CT (lung window) in a patient with a 10-year history of asthma and peripheral eosinophilia demonstrates bilateral multifocal, peripheral, subpleural consolidations. The diagnosis of Churg-Strauss syndrome was confirmed at open lung biopsy.

101,144). Gastrointestinal hemorrhage and perforation are potential complications (53). Patients usually show the P-ANCA pattern, although C-ANCA can also be seen (71). Elevated serum IgE is a characteristic finding (19,88,100,101).

A CSS-like syndrome develops as a rare complication in steroid-dependent asthmatics successfully treated with the leukotriene receptor antagonists (e.g., pranlukast) (27,55,64,75, 179). This complication probably is related to the steroid withdrawal facilitated by the drugs, which unmasks underlying CSS, rather than to the drugs themselves, as similar recognition of CSS has occurred in patients whose withdrawal of oral steroids was facilitated by inhaled steroids (179). An unusual association between a CSS-like vasculitis and the use of free-base cocaine has been noted (131).

There are no laboratory tests that are specific for CSS. Peripheral blood eosinophilia (usually 5,000 to 9,000/μL) is the most characteristic finding. Other, nonspecific laboratory abnormalities include: normochromic, normocytic anemia; markedly elevated erythrocyte sedimentation rate; leukocytosis; elevated IgE level; and hypergammaglobulinemia. BAL shows a high percentage of eosinophils (usually more than 33 percent). An obstructive defect consistent with asthma has been reported on lung function testing.

Radiologic Findings. CSS manifests radiologically as multifocal parenchymal consolidations, which may change in location and appearance over time (fig. 4-18) (21,28,54). The consolidations may exhibit a peripheral distribution and mimic eosinophilic pneumonia. Lung involvement by pulmonary consolidation may be widespread. Diffuse miliary nodules are also reported (21,46). Cavitation is rarely seen, and its presence should suggest superimposed infection (5). Eosinophilic pleural effusions are seen in 29 percent of cases (21,54). Hilar lymphadenopathy is infrequent. The chest radiograph is normal in 25 percent of patients (54).

The high-resolution computed tomography (HRCT) features of CSS consist mostly of parenchymal opacification (consolidation or ground-glass attenuation), followed in frequency by pulmonary nodules, bronchial wall thickening or dilatation, interlobular septal thickening, and normal findings (183). One reported case exhibited "stellate-shaped" peripheral pulmonary arteries and peribronchial and septal interstitial thickening (13). Small patchy opacities were also noted. These HRCT abnormalities correlated with eosinophilic infiltration and foci of eosinophilic pneumonia, respectively.

Pathologic Findings. Lung biopsies from CSS patients may show asthmatic bronchitis, eosinophilic pneumonia (fig. 4-19), extravascular

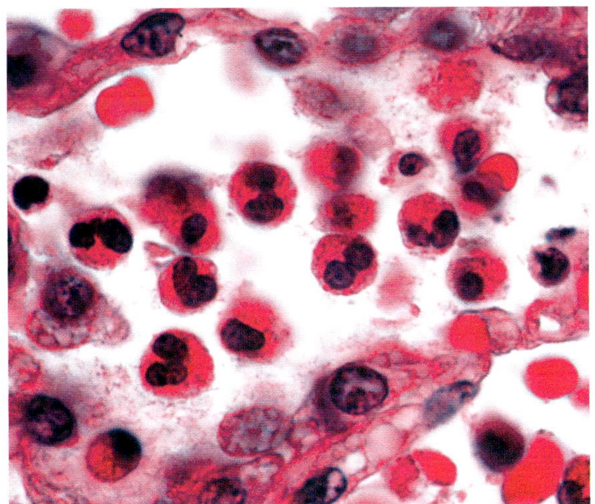

Figure 4-19

CHURG-STRAUSS SYNDROME:
EOSINOPHILIC PNEUMONIA

The alveolar spaces are filled with eosinophils.

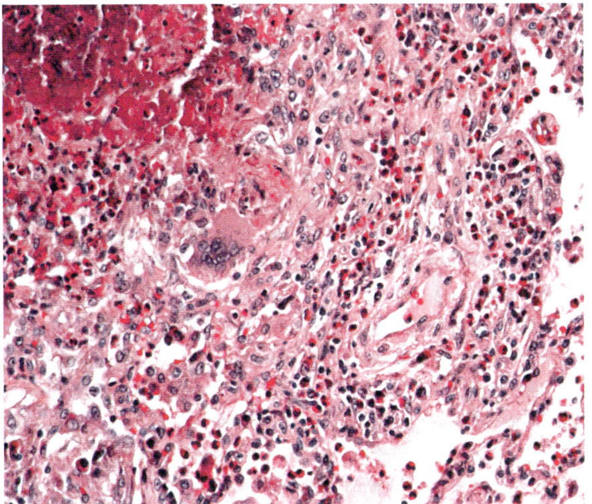

Figure 4-20

CHURG-STRAUSS SYNDROME:
NECROTIZING GRANULOMA

This necrotizing granuloma has a central eosinophilic necrotic zone (upper left) surrounded by marked chronic and eosinophilic inflammation with multinucleated giant cells.

granulomas (fig. 4-20), and vasculitis (fig. 4-21) (28,100). In some cases the inflammatory lesions extend along the pleura and interlobular septa. Extravascular granulomas, sometimes called allergic granulomas, have a border of palisading histiocytes and multinucleated giant cells surrounding a central necrotic zone consisting of necrotic eosinophils (fig. 4-20). Vasculitis can affect arteries, veins, or capillaries (figs. 4-21, 4-22). The vascular inflammatory infiltrates are composed of chronic inflammatory cells, eosinophils, epithelioid cells, multinucleated giant cells, and/or neutrophils. Diffuse pulmonary hemorrhage and capillaritis can be seen (30,94). In patients who are partially treated, the pathologic (and clinical) features may be less than complete (21).

Differential Diagnosis. The differential diagnosis of CSS includes WG (167), eosinophilic pneumonia, allergic bronchopulmonary fungal disease (ABPFD) (170), infection (especially parasitic and fungal) (11), Hodgkin's disease, and drug-induced vasculitis (77). The features distinguishing CSS from WG are summarized in Table 4-5. Eosinophilic pneumonia and ABPFD lack systemic vasculitis. Some patients with eosinophilic pneumonia have a mild nonnecrotizing vasculitis and allergic granulomas. Pathologic features similar to CSS can be mimicked by infection with certain parasites, such as *Strongyloides stercoralis* (159) and *Toxocara canis* (11), so parasitic infection should be carefully excluded. Some fungal infections, especially with *Aspergillus* sp. and *Coccidioides immitis,* may be associated with granulomatous inflammation, prominent eosinophilia, and vasculitis. Rarely, Hodgkin's disease with prominent eosinophils and vascular inflammation may be confused with CSS. Drugs such as carbamazepine can cause a CSS-like syndrome, so attention should be paid to the patient's drug history (77).

Treatment and Prognosis. Most patients with CSS are responsive to corticosteroids. However, in order to avoid irreversible organ injury, some have favored treatment from the outset with immunosuppressive agents such as cyclophosphamide (100). Azathioprine, interferon-alpha, and high-dose intravenous immune globulin have been used with apparent benefit in patients with severe, fulminant disease or in patients unresponsive to corticosteroids. Plasma exchange occasionally has been used but appears to have no added benefit to treatment with corticosteroids, with or without cyclophosphamide (67).

Most patients who die from CSS have cardiac complications such as heart failure or myocardial infarction. Less often, death occurs from

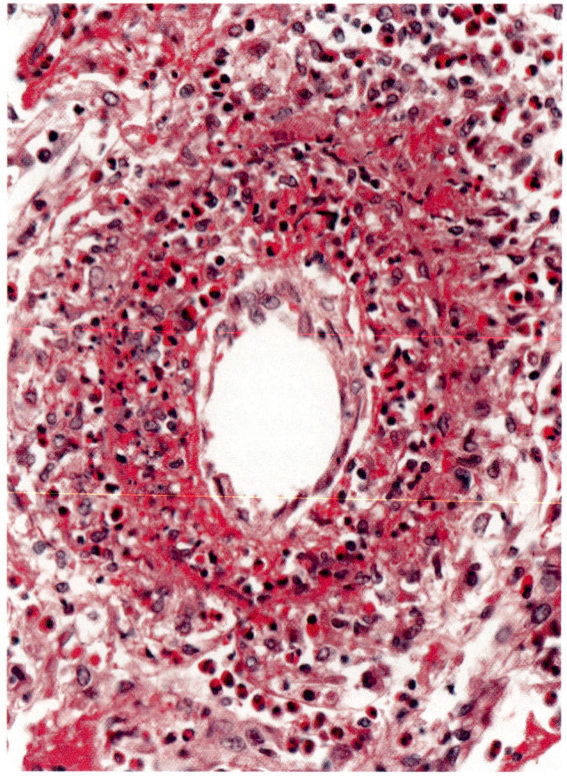

Figure 4-21

CHURG-STRAUSS SYNDROME: EOSINOPHILIC VASCULITIS

The wall of this arteriole shows fibrinoid necrosis as well as an eosinophilic infiltrate.

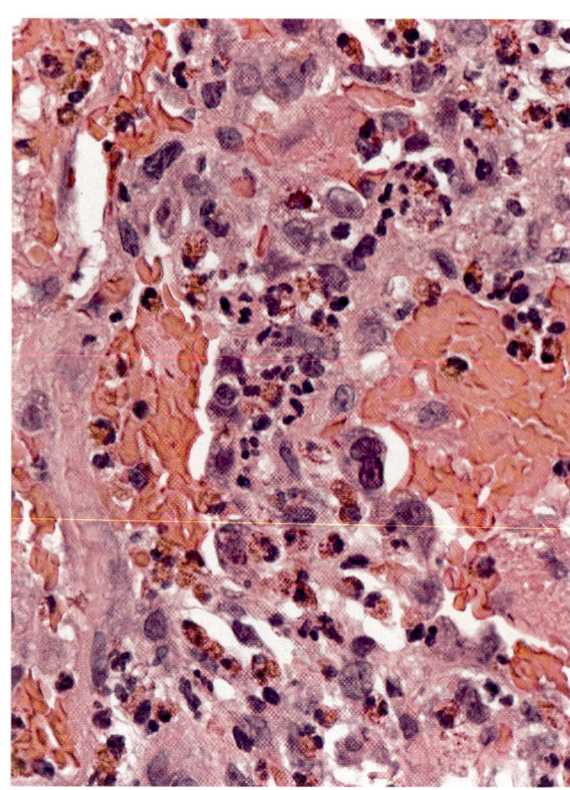

Figure 4-22

CHURG-STRAUSS SYNDROME: CAPILLARITIS

This alveolar wall is infiltrated by eosinophils forming the lesion of eosinophilic capillaritis.

renal failure, cerebral hemorrhage, gastrointestinal perforation or hemorrhage, status asthmaticus, or respiratory failure (2,100).

MICROSCOPIC POLYANGIITIS

Definition. Microscopic polyangiitis is a necrotizing vasculitis with few or no immune deposits that involves small vessels (arterioles, venules, and capillaries). Necrotizing arteritis involving small and medium-sized arteries may be present (80,81).

The concept of microscopic polyangiitis has existed for many years but the definition given above was proposed at a Chapel Hill International Consensus Conference on the Nomenclature of Systemic Vasculitides (80,81). The term microscopic polyangiitis was favored over microscopic polyarteritis since venules are affected as well as arterioles. Although there is better recognition of this entity, a universally accepted definition for microscopic polyangiitis is lacking (96). This is emphasized by the problems related to the variable interpretation of how to distinguish between WG and microscopic polyangiitis. According to the Chapel Hill criteria, granulomatous inflammation is required for the diagnosis of WG, but biopsies from patients with WG do not always demonstrate granulomatous inflammation (40,96,165,167). Furthermore, some studies of microscopic polyangiitis include patients with upper respiratory tract involvement, while such patients are excluded in other studies (68,74,96). Also, patients initially presenting with microscopic polyangiitis may subsequently be found to have WG (9). While these issues remain to be resolved, the concept of microscopic polyangiitis is very useful for classifying patients who present with diffuse pulmonary hemorrhage and capillaritis.

Clinical Features. Microscopic polyangiitis occurs in approximately 1 of 100,000 individuals (68,80,83); the lung is affected in 50 percent of such patients (80). Patients with pulmonary involvement average 56 years of age (+/-17 years), and there is an approximately 1.5 to 1 female predominance (103). Most patients have a rapid onset of symptoms but up to 28 percent may have symptoms for more than 1 year (103). The most common clinical manifestation is glomerulonephritis (97 percent), followed by fever (62 percent), myalgia and arthralgia (52 percent), weight loss (45 percent), ear, nose, and throat symptoms (31 percent), and skin involvement (17 percent) (Table 4-7) (80,103). BAL typically shows acute hemorrhage or hemosiderin-laden macrophages. Over 80 percent of patients have a positive ANCA titer, most often P-ANCA (80). Microscopic polyangiitis is the most common cause of the pulmonary-renal syndrome (80).

Radiologic Findings. Since most patients with pulmonary involvement by microscopic polyangiitis have diffuse pulmonary hemorrhage, the typical radiographic finding is bilateral alveolar opacities without nodules. The lower lungs are most frequently affected (103).

Pathologic Findings. The most common lung biopsy findings in patients with microscopic polyangiitis are pulmonary hemorrhage and neutrophilic capillaritis (fig. 4-23) (59,80). Neutrophilic capillaritis often appears as scattered, patchy foci of inflammation in a background of alveolar hemorrhage. Closer examination reveals thickening of the alveolar walls with many neutrophils infiltrating the septal interstitium and sometimes spilling over into the surrounding alveolar spaces. The neutrophils often show karyorrhexis. In severe cases, the neutrophils may fill the alveoli and resemble acute infectious pneumonia. Identification of the distinctive lesions of capillaritis in the adjacent lung may be helpful in recognizing the vasculitic rather than infectious nature of the process. Alveolar fibrin may accompany the capillaritis, sometimes in a polypoid fashion surrounding the alveolar wall. As the capillaritis heals, polypoid plugs of organizing fibrosis may be seen, sometimes resulting in an organizing pneumonia pattern. There may be hemosiderin deposits with chronic hemorrhage.

Hyaline membranes may show a pattern of diffuse alveolar damage (DAD) (4,59). In some cases it may be difficult to distinguish a pattern of hemorrhagic DAD from a diffuse pulmonary hemorrhagic syndrome with capillaritis. Pulmonary fibrosis (56,59) and progressive obstructive airway disease with emphysematous features (12,143) have been reported in patients with microscopic polyangiitis. The pathology of microscopic polyangiitis in other

Table 4-7

MICROSCOPIC POLYANGIITIS: CLINICAL FEATURES AT PRESENTATION[a]

Manifestation	Number of Patients	Percentage
Pulmonary	29	100
Dyspnea	26	90
Cough	26	90
Hemoptysis	23	79
Chest pain	5	17
Crackles	13	45
Renal	28	97
Fever (>37.5° C)	18	62
Weight loss	13	45
Musculoskeletal	15	52
Arthralgias	13	45
Arthritis	4	14
Myalgia	6	21
Ear, nose, and throat	9	31
Epistaxis	5	17
Sore throat	1	3
Mouth ulcers	2	7
Hearing loss	1	3
Skin	5	17
Purpura	4	14
Nodules	1	3
Erythema elevatum diutinum	1	3
Bullae	1	3
Hypertension	7	25
Ocular	7	25
Episcleritis	5	17
Xerophthalmia	2	7
Peripheral neuropathy	2	7
Gastrointestinal bleeding	1	3

[a]Modified from reference 103.

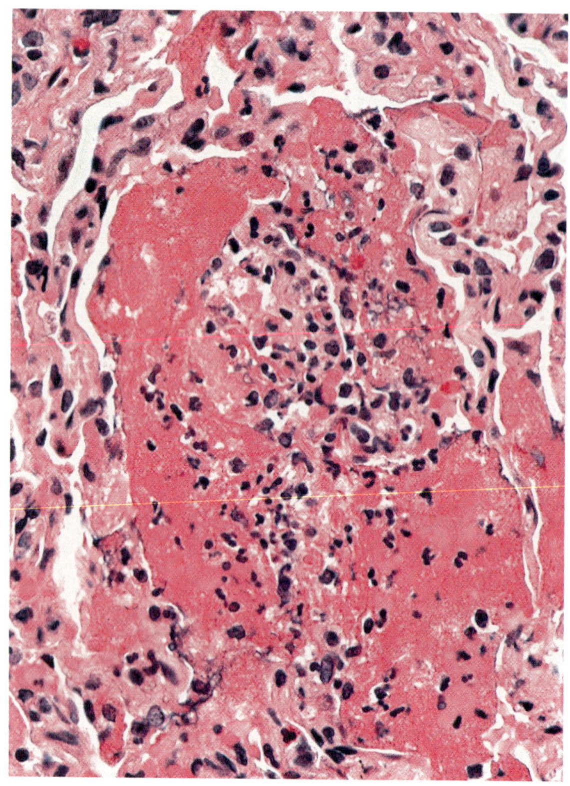

Figure 4-23

MICROSCOPIC POLYANGIITIS

Alveolar red blood cell and fibrin accumulation corresponds to diffuse pulmonary hemorrhage. The alveolar wall is infiltrated by neutrophils that spill over slightly into the adjacent alveolar space.

Table 4-8

DIFFERENTIAL DIAGNOSIS OF MICROSCOPIC POLYANGIITIS

Feature	Microscopic Polyangiitis	Wegener's Granulomatosis	Polyarteritis Nodosa
Size of vessels:			
Medium-sized arteries	Yes or No	Yes or No	Yes (bronchial arteries)
Arterioles, venules, capillaries	Yes	Yes	No
Granulomatous inflammation	No	Yes	No
Lung involvement	Common	Common	Uncommon
ANCA[a]	Mostly P-ANCA	Mostly C-ANCA	Mostly P-ANCA

[a]ANCA = Antineutrophil cytoplasmic antibody.

organs such as kidney and skin has been recently reviewed (83). Kidney biopsies show a necrotizing glomerulonephritis (80,83,103); skin biopsies often show a leukocytoclastic vasculitis (80,83).

Differential Diagnosis. Microscopic polyangiitis is separated from WG by the lack of granulomatous inflammation. It is distinguished from polyarteritis nodosa by the involvement of vessels smaller than the medium-sized arteries involved in microscopic polyangiitis (arterioles, venules, and capillaries) (Table 4-8) (80). Polyarteritis nodosa rarely affects the lung and when it does, it primarily involves bronchial arteries (121,169). As mentioned above, the requirement of granulomatous inflammation for the diagnosis of WG rather than microscopic polyangiitis is a somewhat controversial issue. Granulomatous inflammation may not be identified in patients with WG if a conservative approach is taken to obtaining tissue biopsies, if only small tissue samples are obtained such as bronchoscopic biopsies, or if biopsies are obtained during a phase of disease in which granulomas are not prominent. Therefore, some patients may be classified as having microscopic polyangiitis when in fact they have WG, but granulomas were not obtained in the biopsy specimens.

Microscopic polyangiitis must be separated from other small vessel vasculitides that represent a heterogeneous group of disorders affecting venules, capillaries, and arterioles, several of which are not caused by hypersensitivity reactions to drugs or other agents (Table 4-9) (25,26, 106,160). There are few or no immune deposits in microscopic polyangiitis compared to other types of small vessel vasculitides that have immune complex deposits, such as Henoch-Schönlein purpura, cryoglobulinemic vasculitis, serum sickness, and lupus vasculitis (80,81). Microscopic polyangiitis encompasses the spectrum of vasculitic disorders that have been called systemic necrotizing vasculitis, leukocytoclastic vasculitis, and hypersensitivity vasculitis (14,25,106,160).

Treatment and Prognosis. Similar to WG, the primary approach to therapy for patients with microscopic polyangiitis consists of cyclophosphamide and prednisone (80). Relapses occur in 35 to 40 percent of patients (60,103). Lauque et al. (103) treated their patients with corticosteroids (100 percent), cyclophosphamide (79 percent), plasmapheresis (24 percent), dialysis (28 percent), and mechanical ventilation (10 percent). They found a 5-year survival rate of 68 percent, with causes of death equally divided between vasculitis and the side effects of treatment. Complete recovery occurred in 69 percent of patients, but 24 percent had persistent pulmonary function abnormalities.

NECROTIZING SARCOID GRANULOMATOSIS

Definition. Necrotizing sarcoid granulomatosis (NSG) is a disorder that primarily affects the lung and shows nodular masses of confluent sarcoid-like or epithelioid granulomas with extensive areas of necrosis and vasculitis. There is debate whether NSG should be regarded as a vasculitic syndrome, since it is not a systemic disorder and the lung pathology is primarily that of necrotizing granulomatous inflammation rather than vasculitis.

Clinical Features. The average patient is 50 years of age, but the disease can occur from adolescence throughout adulthood (111,140, 163,168,169). Women are twice as often affected (7,150). Patients present with cough, fever, chest pain, dyspnea, malaise, and weight loss (7,22,158). Up to one quarter of patients are asymptomatic at presentation. NSG primarily affects the lung; extrapulmonary manifestations are uncommon, with rare reports of uveitis and hypothalamic insufficiency (20,41,104, 128). Upper airway disease, glomerulonephritis, and systemic vasculitis are not features of NSG. To date, positive ANCAs have not been reported in these patients.

Radiologic Findings. NSG usually manifests as bilateral, multifocal, parenchymal nodular opacities with well-marginated or ill-defined borders (Table 4-10; figs. 4-24, 4-25). Lesions are typically located in peribronchovascular and subpleural areas and may be more numerous in the lower lung zones (fig. 4-24) (18,22,51,54, 168,169). Solitary lesions and parenchymal consolidations (fig. 4-24) have also been described, but are unusual manifestations.

CT may demonstrate cavitation and/or heterogeneous contrast enhancement of the lesions, which correlates with intralesional necrosis (128). Pleural involvement with thickening or effusion may also be observed (18). Hilar lymphadenopathy is variable and not as frequently seen as in sarcoidosis (89).

Pathologic Findings. NSG is characterized histologically by large nodules of confluent, nonnecrotizing granulomas with large zones of necrosis (fig. 4-26), and vasculitis (fig. 4-27). A sarcoid-like pattern is seen in the granulomas, with tight clusters of giant cells and epithelioid cells (fig. 4-28). There is a sarcoidal pattern of lung involvement with a lymphangitic distribution of

Table 4-9

MICROSCOPIC POLYANGIITIS AND OTHER CONDITIONS ASSOCIATED WITH SMALL VESSEL VASCULITIS[a]

Idiopathic Microscopic Polyangiitis (Small Vessel Vasculitis)[b]
Systemic (80)
Localized pulmonary small vessel vasculitis (84)
Small Vessel Vasculitis Associated with Known Conditions
Hypersensitivity vasculitis (drug-induced) (50)
Penicillin
Sulfonamides
Diuretics
Nonsteroidal anti-inflammatory agents
Anticonvulsants
Infection (106,160)
Hepatitis B
Upper respiratory tract streptococcal infections
Other diseases
Collagen vascular diseases (25,26)
Malignancy (52,87)
Henoch-Schönlein purpura (48,115,181)
Mixed cryoglobulinemia (8,24,122)
Pulmonary interstitial fibrosis in elderly patients (125)
Cystic fibrosis (50)
Bone marrow transplantation (145)

[a]Data from references 14, 25, 26, 80, and 160.
[b]The terms microscopic polyangiitis, microscopic polyarteritis, and hypersensitivity vasculitis have all been used for idiopathic small vessel vasculitis syndromes (14,80).

Table 4-10

CLINICAL AND ROENTGENOGRAPHIC FEATURES OF PATIENTS WITH NECROTIZING SARCOID GRANULOMATOSIS

	Liebow (111)	Saldana (140)	Churg (22)	Koss (89)	Case Reports[b]
No. of cases	11	30	32	13	8
Men:Women	Approximately 1:1	12:18	1:4	3:10	3:5
Bilateral (%)	82	12	72	62	50
Solitary (%)	18[a]	88	22	15	25
Hilar adenopathy (%)	9	7	65	8	25
Cavitation (%)	NA[c]	3	0	23	13
Patients with recurrence (%)	25	11	12	15	13
Died (%)	0	0	4[d]	0	13[e]

[a]Described as "localized, unilateral disease."
[b]Case reports (from references 7,16,51,136,150,155,158).
[c]NA = Data not available.
[d]One patient died of pneumonia several months postresection of a solitary nodule.
[e]One patient died of oat cell carcinoma.

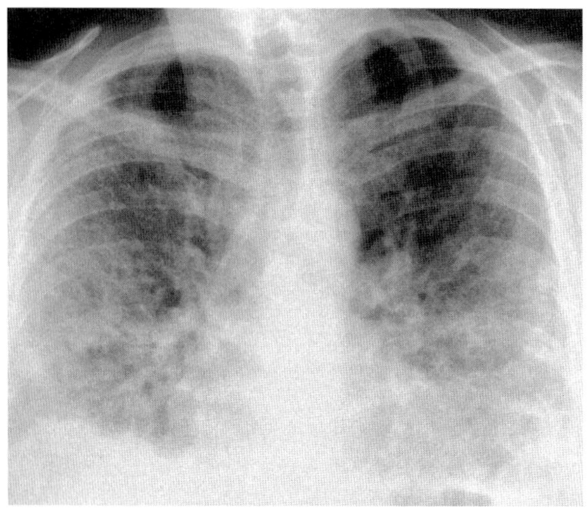
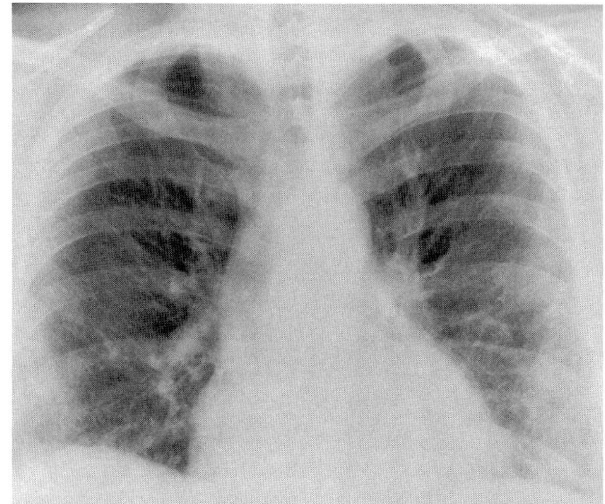

Figure 4-24

NECROTIZING SARCOID GRANULOMATOSIS

Left: PA chest radiograph of a 40-year-old male with fatigue, fever, and dyspnea demonstrates diffuse bilateral airspace consolidation with a predilection for the bases and the mid-lung zones.

Right: PA chest radiograph obtained following biopsy and steroid therapy demonstrates marked improvement with residual parenchymal consolidation in the lung periphery and lower lobes.

the granulomas (22,89,150). In addition to the large zones, there are small foci of necrosis (89).

The vasculitis of NSG can affect both arteries and veins. Three patterns of vasculitis are seen: necrotizing granulomas (fig. 4-28), giant cell vasculitis, and infiltration by chronic inflammatory cells (111). Sometimes the necrotizing granulomas are seen circumferentially along the vascular walls (fig. 4-27).

Differential Diagnosis. The most important differential diagnosis of NSG is granulomatous infection. For this reason the presence of mycobacteria or fungi must be carefully ruled out. Granulomatous infections can cause both vas-

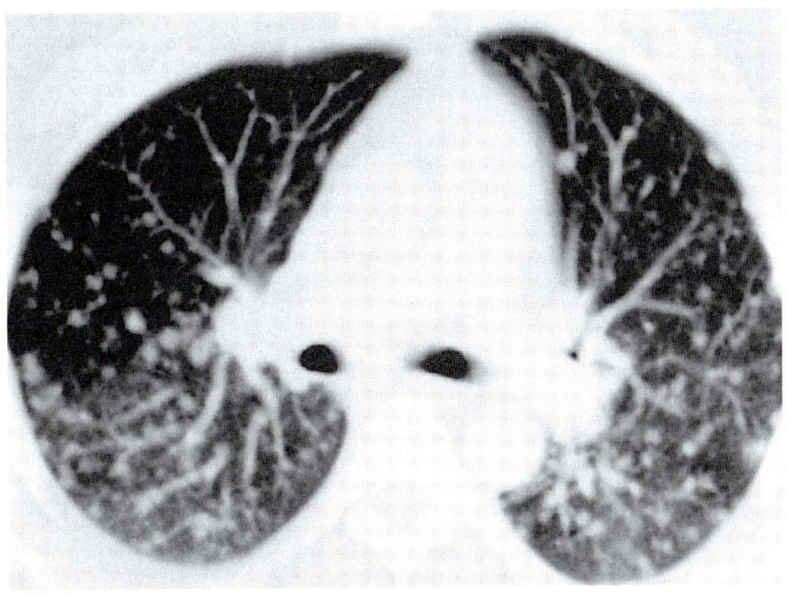

Figure 4-25

NECROTIZING SARCOID GRANULOMATOSIS

Chest CT (lung window) in a 41-year-old male with cough demonstrates bilateral multifocal small nodules.

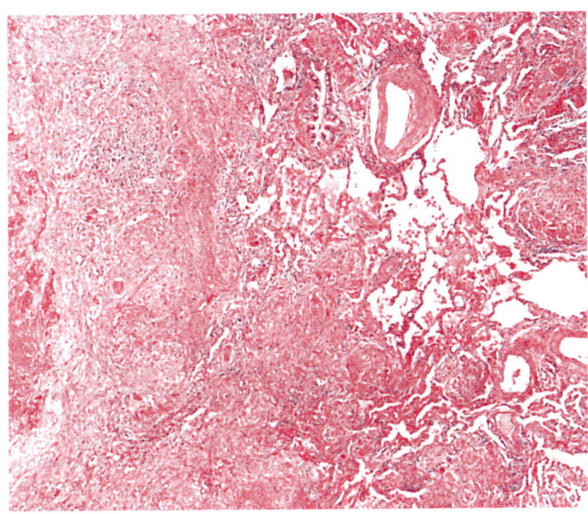

Figure 4-26

NECROTIZING SARCOID GRANULOMATOSIS: NECROTIZING GRANULOMA

A large zone of necrosis is surrounded by an intense inflammatory infiltrate consisting of multiple noncaseating granulomas.

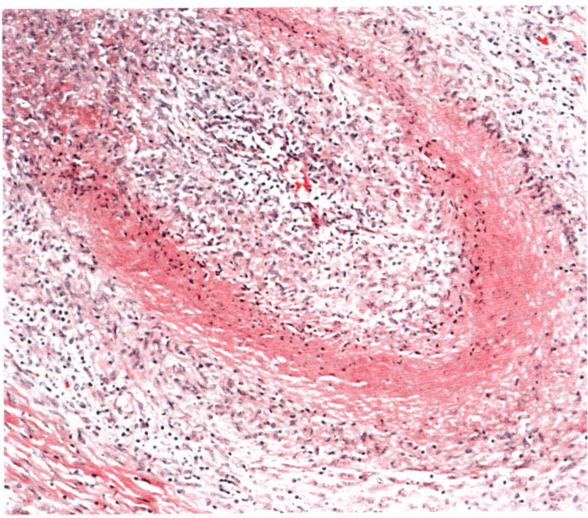

Figure 4-27

NECROTIZING SARCOID GRANULOMATOSIS: VASCULITIS

The wall of this arteriole shows marked inflammation and a necrotic zone that circumferentially involves the vessel wall.

culitis and sarcoid-like granulomas (167,173). The key features distinguishing NSG from WG are summarized in Table 4-11. Some regard NSG as a subset of sarcoidosis known as nodular sarcoidosis. It has also been suggested that some cases of NSG are inactive granulomatous infections (20,89).

Treatment and Prognosis. The clinical outcome for patients with NSG is excellent (136, 150). Localized NSG can be cured by surgical resection. Patients with bilateral opacities or nodules may respond to corticosteroids. A small percentage of patients have persistent opacities (20,22) or a relapse (89,155). Other immunosuppressive therapy should be avoided since the only deaths reported in patients with NSG have been due to opportunistic infections (22).

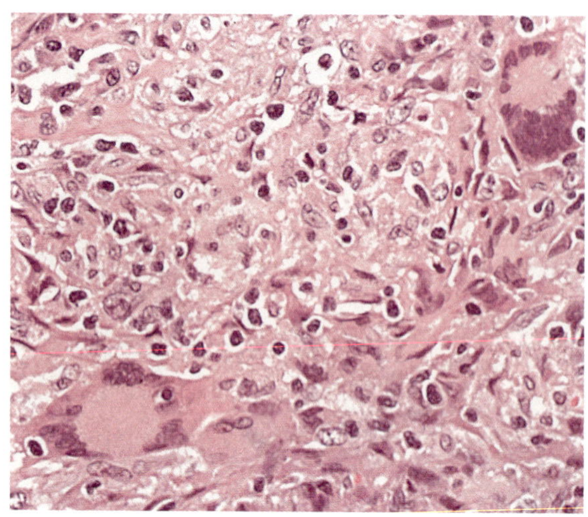

Figure 4-28

NECROTIZING SARCOID GRANULOMATOSIS: GRANULOMAS

The granulomas consist of confluent clusters of epithelioid cells and giant cells.

Table 4-11

DISTINGUISHING FEATURES: WEGENER'S GRANULOMATOSIS VERSUS NECROTIZING SARCOIDOSIS

Clinical/Pathologic Feature	Wegener's Granulomatosis	Necrotizing Sarcoidosis
Lung involvement	66-85%	100%
Extrapulmonary involvement	90-100% ENT[a], kidney, skin, neurologic	10% or less Ocular, neurologic
ANCA[b]	Yes	No
Histology		
Sarcoidal granulomas	Rare	Characteristic
Vasculitis	Characteristic	Characteristic

[a]ENT = Ear, nose, and throat.
[b]ANCA = Antineutrophil cytoplasmic antibody.

OTHER RARE CAUSES OF GRANULOMATOUS ARTERITIS

Giant Cell Arteritis

Giant cell (temporal) arteritis is a vasculitis that includes giant cells and involves the temporal artery. It is associated with upper respiratory tract symptoms in about 10 percent of patients; lower respiratory tract involvement is extremely rare (102). Radiographically, lung nodules (10,135), interstitial opacities (85), and unilateral pleural effusions (102) are seen. Although rare, giant cell arteritis can affect the pulmonary trunk and main pulmonary arteries as well as large and medium-sized intrapulmonary elastic arteries (93).

Histologically, the vasculitis shows medial and adventitial chronic inflammation with giant cells. This causes destruction of the elastic laminae, sometimes with focal fibrinoid medial necrosis (93). Bronchoscopic biopsies may show granulomatous inflammation of pulmonary arteries and fragmented elastic fibers (93,135). Unlike WG, NSG, CSS, and granulomatous infections, there is no parenchymal inflammation (93). The temporal artery involvement and older age of the patients distinguish pulmonary giant cell arteritis from Takayasu's arteritis (93).

The rare disorder called *idiopathic isolated pulmonary giant cell arteritis* (130,177,178) is characterized by a lack of systemic vasculitis and lesions that are limited to the lung. Dyspnea on exertion may be a presenting finding, but patients usually lack hemoptysis, fever, or an elevated erythrocyte sedimentation rate. The lesion is usually an unsuspected finding in a surgical or autopsy specimen (177,178). Histologically, there are organized thrombi with recanalization and narrowing of large pulmonary arteries. The vasculitis is characterized by a destructive inflammatory infiltrate of giant cells, histiocytes, and lymphocytes causing fragmentation of elastic laminae (130,177,178). Peripheral infarcts may also be seen.

Disseminated Visceral Giant Cell Angiitis

Disseminated visceral giant cell angiitis is a form of giant cell arteritis that affects extracranial small arteries and arterioles. This is a very rare condition with only five reported cases, all in males, three of which involved lung (108,123). All of these cases were recognized as incidental autopsy findings (108). Extracranial small arteries and arterioles are affected, and each case involved at least three of the following organs: heart, lung, kidneys, liver, pancreas, and stomach. The vasculitis shows prominent multinucleated giant cells of both the foreign body and Langhans' types, but most of the inflammatory cells consist of histiocytes, lymphocytes, and plasma cells. A relationship has been proposed between sarcoidosis and disseminated visceral giant cell arteritis, but these cases are so rare it is difficult to be certain (107,116,149).

POLYARTERITIS NODOSA

Classic polyarteritis nodosa (PAN) is a vasculitis that involves medium-sized and small arteries. It can involve virtually any organ.

PAN rarely affects the lungs. Most cases previously reported as PAN with lung involvement probably are examples of CSS (39,105, 106,138) or perhaps small vessel vasculitis. PAN differs from CSS in that only arteries are affected, and the hallmark features of tissue eosinophilia and extravascular granulomas are not seen. When PAN affects the lung, the bronchial arteries are primarily involved (121,138). PAN differs from microscopic polyangiitis in that medium-sized arteries are affected while in microscopic polyangiites only arterioles, venules, and capillaries are affected (80,81).

TAKAYASU'S ARTERITIS

Definition. Takayasu's arteritis is a large vessel vasculitis that primarily affects the aorta and its branches. The arteritis consists of lymphocytes, macrophages, and giant cells infiltrating the adventitia, media, and intima.

Clinical Features. Pulmonary arterial involvement occurs in 12 to 86 percent of patients with Takayasu's arteritis (6,72,147,148). Rarely, pulmonary artery involvement may be the presenting manifestation (126). It occurs most commonly in patients less than 40 years of age and in women (6). Systemic manifestations affect the kidney, heart, skin, and gastrointestinal tract (146).

It is difficult to obtain tissue biopsy specimens from large vessels such as the aorta or pulmonary artery so the diagnosis is usually established by angiography. Findings include pulmonary artery stenosis, irregular narrowing, and occlusion (72,110,147). Fistulas between pulmonary arteries and bronchial, coronary, or systemic arteries may occur (76).

Radiologic Findings. Takahashi et al. (161) recently reviewed CT findings of the lungs of patients with Takayasu's arteritis and found frequent areas of low attenuation, subpleural reticulolinear changes, and pleural thickening. The low attenuation areas were thought to represent regional hypoperfusion due to pulmonary arteritis.

Pathologic Findings. Large elastic pulmonary arteries are usually affected with adventitial, medial, and intimal infiltration by lymphocytes, macrophages, and giant cells (fig. 4-29). Thrombi may also be seen. This can progress to diffuse or nodular fibrosis of the artery wall and disintegration or loss of elastic fibers (120,137). The fibrosis can result in stenosis or obliteration of the vascular lumen (fig. 4-29B) and cause aneurysm formation or dilatation of the artery. Matsubara et al. (120) described stenosis-recanalization and so-called blood vessels-in-blood vessels of the pulmonary elastic and muscular arteries (fig. 4-29C).

Treatment. Corticosteroid therapy is often effective, but some patients require cyclophosphamide for management. Surgical correction of stenotic lesions may be successful (78).

BEHÇET'S SYNDROME

Definition. Behçet's syndrome is a systemic vasculitic syndrome characterized by oral and genital ulcers and iridocyclitis.

Clinical Features. The majority of cases of Behçet's syndrome occur in the Mediterranean basin, the Middle East, and Japan, although the distribution is worldwide (43,133). The diagnosis is based primarily on clinical criteria. It requires the presence of recurrent oral aphthosis and at least two of the following five clinical manifestations: recurrent genital aphthosis, uveitis, synovitis, cutaneous vasculitis, and meningoencephalitis, plus the absence of inflammatory bowel or other collagen vascular diseases (17).

The common clinical feature in patients with Behçet's disease is the presence of recurrent, painful, aphthous oral or genital ulcers. Recurrent oral ulceration, more than three times in 1 year, is required to meet the diagnostic criteria for Behçet's disease. These lesions must be distinguished from ulcers related to herpes simplex, inflammatory bowel disease, or other systemic diseases such as systemic lupus erythematosus.

Pulmonary symptoms include dyspnea, cough, chest pain, and hemoptysis (133). Males

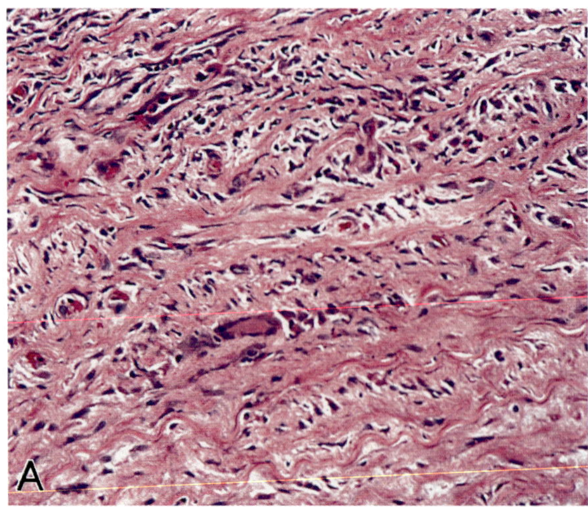

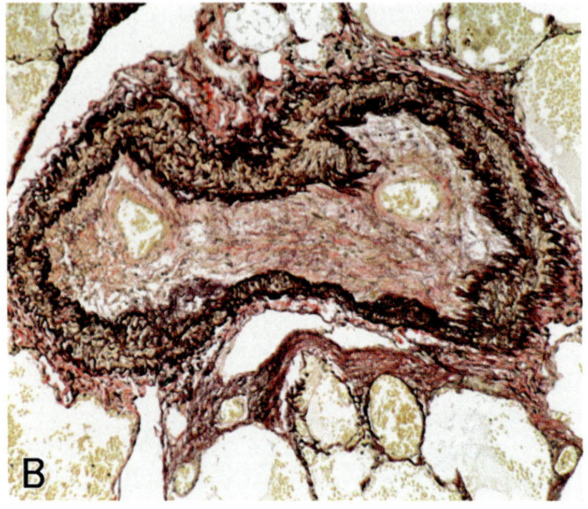

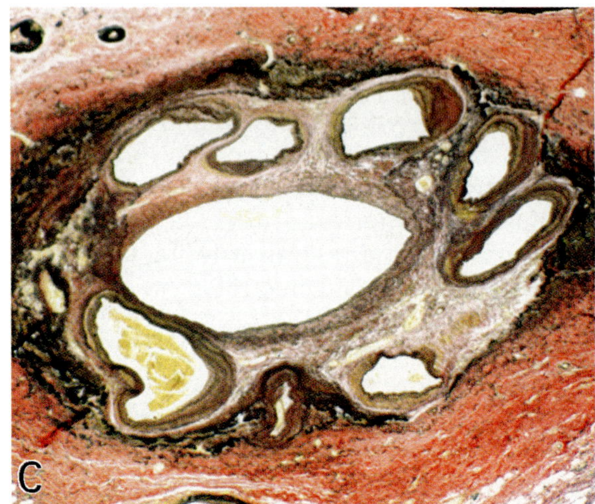

Figure 4-29

TAKAYASU'S ARTERITIS

A: The wall of this pulmonary artery is infiltrated by lymphocytes and giant cells.

B: This elastic stain highlights marked intimal fibrosis with obliteration of the arteriolar lumen.

C: This artery shows "stenosis-recanalization" with blood vessels within blood vessels, highlighted by an elastic stain. (Figures B and C courtesy of Dr. Osamu Matsubara, National Defense Medical College, Japan.)

are more likely to have pulmonary involvement and hemoptysis (42,133). Demonstration of circulating immune complexes in association with active pulmonary disease suggests that immune complexes may be important in the pathogenesis of pulmonary involvement (42,58).

Radiologic Findings. The airspace consolidation seen on chest radiographs and CT images is thought to reflect pulmonary hemorrhage, infarction, and pulmonary artery aneurysms (3,172). CT can be especially helpful in the assessment of thoracic Behçet's syndrome by showing thrombosis of the pulmonary artery or superior vena cava and characteristic aneurysms of the pulmonary arteries (3,172). Angiography may demonstrate pulmonary aneurysms and thromboses (133).

Pathologic Findings. Behçet's syndrome causes a lymphocytic and necrotizing vasculitis involving pulmonary arteries of all sizes, veins, and alveolar septal capillaries (fig. 4-30). In addition, it causes aneurysms of elastic pulmonary arteries, arterial and venous thromboses (fig. 4-31), pulmonary infarcts (fig. 4-32), bronchial erosion by pulmonary artery aneurysms, and arteriobronchial fistulas (95,133,151). Perivascular adventitial fibrosis may be prominent. Collateral vessels lacking elastic lamellae may develop in the periadventitial fibrous tissues around thrombosed arteries and aneurysms (fig. 4-33). Pulmonary hemorrhage (139) and acute interstitial pneumonia (34) may be life-threatening complications.

Treatment and Prognosis. The mucocutaneous manifestations can be treated with oral colchicine, topical anesthetics, topical or intralesional steroids, or systemic steroids. Thalidomide and dapsone have also been shown to

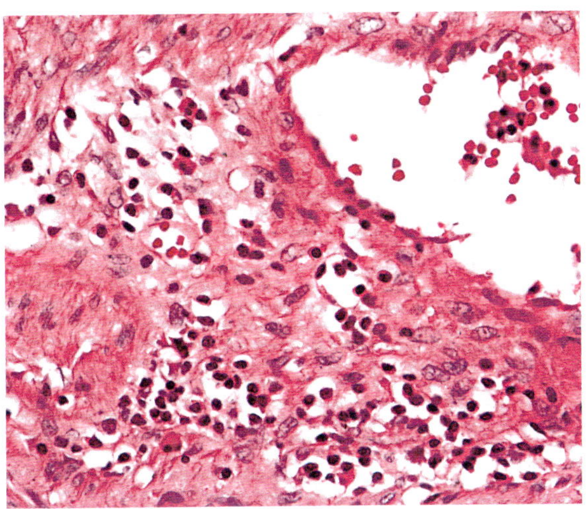

Figure 4-30

BEHÇET'S SYNDROME: VASCULITIS

The wall of this small artery is infiltrated by lymphocytes.

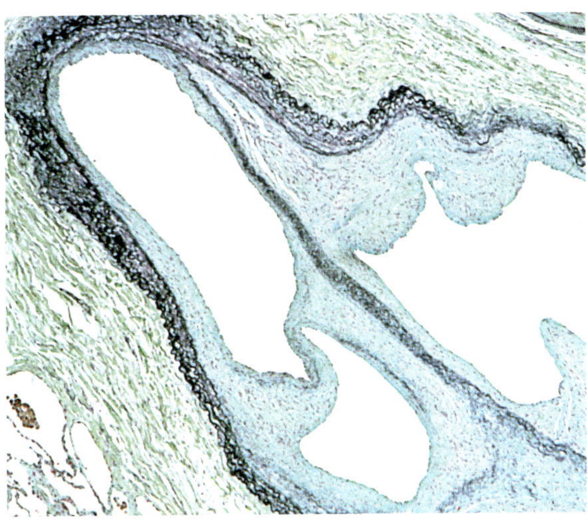

Figure 4-31

BEHÇET'S SYNDROME: ORGANIZING THROMBUS

The web of fibrosis traversing the lumen of this elastic artery is a recanalized thrombus.

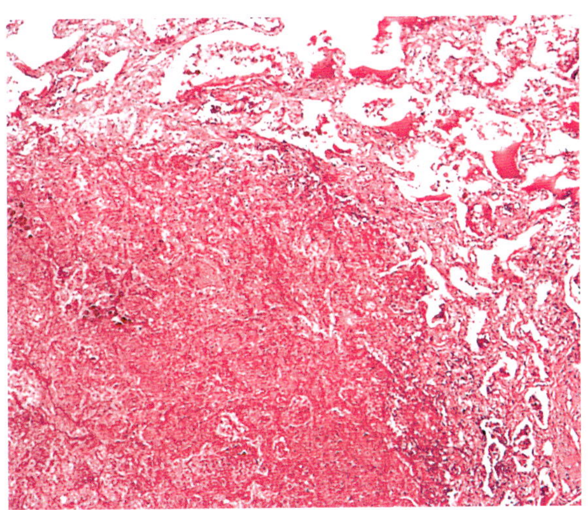

Figure 4-32

BEHÇET'S SYNDROME: INFARCT

The red nodular area represents an acute infarct.

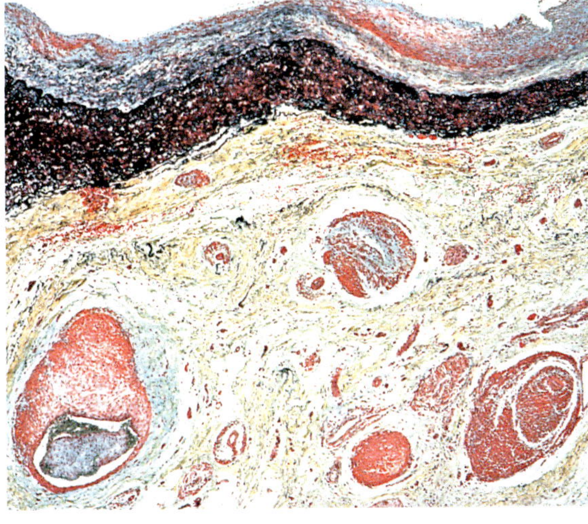

Figure 4-33

BEHÇET'S SYNDROME: COLLATERAL VESSELS

The collateral vessels in the periadventitial tissues surrounding this large elastic artery lack elastic lamellae.

be effective. Significant ocular, neurologic, gastrointestinal, and vascular manifestations typically require treatment with steroids, usually along with another immunosuppressive drug such as azathioprine, cyclophosphamide, cyclosporine, or chlorambucil. Anticoagulation is required for patients who develop thromboses (42). Surgical intervention may be necessary for severe hemoptysis (139). Behçet's disease has an undulating course of exacerbations and remissions, and may become less severe after approximately 20 years.

SECONDARY VASCULITIS

Pulmonary Infection and Septic Emboli

Pulmonary infection can cause a secondary vasculitis. Bacteria like *Pseudomonas aeruginosa* (152) and *Legionella pneumophila* (182) are known for their propensity to invade and cause necrosis of blood vessel walls. Fungal and mycobacterial necrotizing granulomas also cause a secondary vasculitis (173). A necrotizing vasculitis can result from angioinvasive fungal infections due to *Aspergillus* and *Mucor* in immunocompromised patients. This vasculitis may be granulomatous and is frequently associated with pulmonary infarction. Pulmonary vasculitis is also associated with certain parasitic pulmonary infections caused by *Dirofilaria immitis, Schistosoma,* and *Wuchereria*. Vasculitis is a rare complication of *Pneumocystis carinii* pneumonia in human immunodeficiency virus (HIV)-infected patients (171).

Classic Sarcoidosis

Vasculitis is a common incidental histologic finding in surgical lung biopsies from patients with classic sarcoidosis (see chapter 3) (162), however, rarely, systemic vasculitis can also occur. Fernandes et al. (47) recently described six patients with features of both sarcoidosis and vasculitis and reviewed 22 previously reported cases. In total, there were 13 children and 15 adults. Clinical manifestations included fever, peripheral adenopathy, hilar adenopathy, rash, pulmonary parenchymal disease, musculoskeletal symptoms, and scleritis or iridocyclitis.

Medium or large vessel disease is detected by arteriography in half of the patients with sarcoidosis; the other half have findings of small vessel vasculitis (47). Pathologic findings consist of sarcoid-like granulomas, which may show foci of necrosis. These can be found in the skin, lymph nodes, lung, synovium, bone, bone marrow, liver, trachea, or sclera. Patients may respond to treatment with prednisone alone, however, relapses tended to occur if the medication is tapered or withdrawn (47).

REFERENCES

1. Aberle DR, Gamsu G, Lynch D. Thoracic manifestations of Wegener granulomatosis: diagnosis and course. Radiology 1990;174:703–9.
2. Abu-Shakra M, Smythe H, Lewtas J, Badley E, Weber D, Keystone E. Outcome of polyarteritis nodosa and Churg-Strauss syndrome. An analysis of twenty-five patients. Arthritis Rheum 1994;37:1798–803.
3. Ahn JM, Im JG, Ryoo JW, et al. Thoracic manifestations of Behcet syndrome: radiographic and CT findings in nine patients. Radiology 1995;194:199–203.
4. Akikusa B, Kondo Y, Irabu N, Yamamoto S, Saiki S. Six cases of microscopic polyarteritis exhibiting acute interstitial pneumonia. Pathol Int 1995;45:580–8.
5. Amundson DE. Cavitary pulmonary cryptococcosis complicating Churg-Strauss vasculitis. South Med J 1992;85:700–2.
6. Arend WP, Michel BA, Bloch DA, et al. The American College of Rheumatology 1990 criteria for the classification of Takayasu arteritis. Arthritis Rheum 1990;33:1129–34.
7. Beach RC, Corrin B, Scopes JW, Graham E. Necrotizing sarcoid granulomatosis with neurologic lesions in a child. J Pediatr 1980;97:950–3.
8. Bombardieri S, Paoletti P, Ferri C, Di Munno O, Fornai E, Giuntini C. Lung involvement in essential mixed cryoglobulinemia. Am J Med 1979;66:748–56.
9. Bosch X. Microscopic polyangiitis (microscopic polyarteritis) with late emergence of generalised Wegener's granulomatosis. Ann Rheum Dis 1999;58:644–7.
10. Bradley JD, Pinals RS, Blumenfeld HB, Poston WM. Giant cell arteritis with pulmonary nodules. Am J Med 1984;77:135–40.
11. Brill R, Churg J, Beaver PC. Allergic granulomatosis associated with visceral larva migrans. Am J Clin Pathol 1953;23:1208–15.

12. Brugiere O, Raffy O, Sleiman C, et al. Progressive obstructive lung disease associated with microscopic polyangiitis. Am J Respir Crit Care Med 1997;155:739–42.
13. Buschman DL, Waldron JA Jr, King TE Jr. Churg-Strauss pulmonary vasculitis. High-resolution computed tomography scanning and pathologic findings. Am Rev Respir Dis 1990;142:458–61.
14. Calabrese LH, Michel BA, Bloch DA, et al. The American College of Rheumatology 1990 criteria for the classification of hypersensitivity vasculitis. Arthritis Rheum 1990;33:1108–13.
15. Carruthers DM, Watts RA, Symmons DP, Scott DG. Wegener's granulomatosis—increased incidence or increased recognition? Br J Rheumatol 1996;35:142–5.
16. Chabalko JJ. Solitary lung lesion with cavitation due to necrotizing sarcoid granulomatosis. Del Med J 1986;58:15–6.
17. Chajek T, Fainaru M. Behcet's disease. Report of 41 cases and a review of the literature. Medicine (Baltimore) 1975;54:179–96.
18. Chittock DR, Joseph MG, Paterson NA, McFadden RG. Necrotizing sarcoid granulomatosis with pleural involvement. Clinical and radiographic features. Chest 1994;106:672–6.
19. Chumbley LC, Harrison EG Jr, DeRemee RA. Allergic granulomatosis and angiitis (Churg-Strauss syndrome). Report and analysis of 30 cases. Mayo Clin Proc 1977;52:477–84.
20. Churg A. Pulmonary angiitis and granulomatosis revisited. Hum Pathol 1983;14:868–83.
21. Churg A, Brallas M, Cronin SR, Churg J. Formes frustes of Churg-Strauss syndrome. Chest 1995;108:320–3.
22. Churg A, Carrington CB, Gupta R. Necrotizing sarcoid granulomatosis. Chest 1979;76:406–13.
23. Churg J. Allergic granulomatosis and granulomatous-vascular syndromes. Ann Allergy 1963;21:619–28.
24. Churg J. Cryoglobulinemic vasculitis. In: Churg A, Churg J, eds. Systemic vasculitides. New York: Igaku-Shoin; 1991:293–8.
25. Churg J. Nomenclature of vasculitic syndromes: a historical perspective. Am J Kidney Dis 1991;18:148–53.
26. Churg J, Churg A. Idiopathic and secondary vasculitis: a review. Mod Pathol 1989;2:144–60.
27. Churg J, Churg A. Zafirlukast and Churg-Strauss syndrome [Letter]. JAMA 1998;279:1949–50.
28. Churg J, Strauss L. Allergic granulomatosis, allergic angiitis and periarteritis nodosa. Am J Pathol 1951;27:277–94.
29. Clutterbuck EJ, Evans DJ, Pusey CD. Renal involvement in Churg-Strauss syndrome. Nephrol Dial Transplant 1990;5:161–7.
30. Cluttterbuck EJ, Pusey CD. Severe alveolar hemorrhage in Churg-Strauss syndrome. Eur J Respir Dis 1987;71:158–63.
31. Colby TV, Specks U. Wegener's granulomatosis in the 1990s—a pulmonary pathologist's perspective. In: Churg A, Katzenstein AL, eds. The lung. Current concepts. Baltimore: Williams & Wilkins; 1993:195–218.
32. Connolly B, Manson D, Eberhard A, Laxer RM, Smith C. CT appearance of pulmonary vasculitis in children. AJR Am J Roentgenol 1996;167:901–4.
33. Cordier JF, Valeyre D, Guillevin L, Loire R, Brechot JM. Pulmonary Wegener's granulomatosis. A clinical and imaging study of 77 cases. Chest 1990;97:906–12.
34. Corren J. Acute interstitial pneumonia in a patient with Behcet's syndrome and common variable immunodeficiency. Ann Allergy 1990;64: 15–20.
35. Cotch MF, Hoffman GS, Yerg DE, Kaufman GI, Targonski P, Kaslow RA. The epidemiology of Wegener's granulomatosis. Estimates of the five-year period prevalence, annual mortality, and geographic disease distribution from population-based data sources. Arthritis Rheum 1996;39:87–92.
36. Daum TE, Specks U, Colby TV, et al. Tracheobronchial involvement in Wegener's granulomatosis. Am J Respir Crit Care Med 1995;151:522–6.
37. Davenport A, Lock RJ, Wallington TB. Clinical relevance of testing for antineutrophil cytoplasm antibodies (ANCA) with a standard indirect immunofluorescence ANCA test in patients with upper or lower respiratory tract symptoms. Thorax 1994;49:213–7.
38. DeRemee RA, McDonald TJ, Weiland LH. Wegener's granulomatosis: observations on treatment with antimicrobial agents. Mayo Clin Proc 1985;60:27–32.
39. DeRemee RA, Weiland LH, McDonald TJ. Respiratory vasculitis. Mayo Clin Proc 1980;55:492–8.
40. Devaney KO, Travis WD, Hoffman GS, Leavitt RY, Lebovics R, Fauci AS. Interpretation of head and neck biopsies in Wegener's granulomatosis. A pathologic study of 126 biopsies in 70 patients. Am J Surg Pathol 1990;14:555–64.
41. Dykhuizen RS, Smith CC, Kennedy MM, McLay KA, Cockburn JS, Kerr KM. Necrotizing sarcoid granulomatosis with extrapulmonary involvement. Eur Respir J 1997;10:245–7.
42. Efthimiou J, Johnston C, Spiro SG, Turner-Warwick M. Pulmonary disease in Behcet's syndrome. Q J Med 1986;58:259–80.

43. Fairley C, Wilson JW, Barraclough D. Pulmonary involvement in Behcet's syndrome. Chest 1989;96:1428–9.
44. Farrelly CA. Wegener's granulomatosis: a radiological review of the pulmonary manifestations at initial presentation and during relapse. Clin Radiol 1982;33:545–51.
45. Fauci AS, Haynes BF, Katz P, Wolff SM. Wegener's granulomatosis: prospective clinical and therapeutic experience with 85 patients over 21 years. Ann Intern Med 1983;98:76–85.
46. Feigin DS. Vasculitis in the lung. J Thorac Imaging 1988;3:33–48.
47. Fernandes SR, Singsen BH, Hoffman GS. Sarcoidosis and systemic vasculitis. Semin Arthritis Rheum 2000;30:33–46.
48. Fiegler W, Siemoneit KD. Pulmonary manifestations in anaphylactoid purpura (Henoch-Schönlein syndrome). ROFO Fortschr Geb Rontgenstr Nuklearmed 1981;134:269–72.
49. Fienberg R, Mark EJ, Goodman M, McCluskey RT, Niles JL. Correlation of antineutrophil cytoplasmic antibodies with the extrarenal histopathology of Wegener's (pathergic) granulomatosis and related forms of vasculitis. Hum Pathol 1993;24:160–8.
50. Finnegan MJ, Hinchcliffe J, Russell-Jones D, et al. Vasculitis complicating cystic fibrosis. Q J Med 1989;72:609–21.
51. Fisher MR, Christ ML, Bernstein JR. Necrotizing sarcoid-like granulomatosis: radiologic-pathologic correlation. J Can Assoc Radiol 1984;35:313–5.
52. Fortin PR, Esdaile JM. Vasculitis and malignancy. In: Churg A, Churg J, eds. Systemic vasculitides. New York: Igaku-Shoin; 1991:327–41.
53. Fraioli P, Barberis M, Rizzato G. Gastrointestinal presentation of Churg Strauss syndrome. Sarcoidosis 1994;11:42–5.
54. Fraser RS, Pare JA, Fraser RG, Pare PD. Diseases of altered immunologic activity. In: Fraser RS, Pare JA, Fraser RG, Pare PD, eds. Synopsis of diseases of the chest, 2nd ed. Philadelphia: WB Saunders; 1994:392–443.
55. Frosi A, Foresi A, Bozzoni M, Ubbiali A, Vezzoli F. Churg-Strauss syndrome and antiasthma therapy [Letter]. Lancet 1999;353:1102.
56. Gal AA, Salinas FF, Staton GW Jr. The clinical and pathological spectrum of antineutrophil cytoplasmic autoantibody-related pulmonary disease. A comparison between perinuclear and cytoplasmic antineutrophil cytoplasmic autoantibodies. Arch Pathol Lab Med 1994;118:1209–14.
57. Gambari PF, Ostuni PA, Lazzarin P, Fassina A, Todesco S. Eosinophilic granuloma and necrotizing vasculitis (Churg-Strauss syndrome?) involving a parotid gland, lymph nodes, liver and spleen. Scand J Rheumatol 1989;18:171–5.
58. Gamble CN, Wiesner KB, Shapiro RF, Boyer WJ. The immune complex pathogenesis of glomerulonephritis and pulmonary vasculitis in Behcet's disease. Am J Med 1979;66:1031–9.
59. Gaudin PB, Askin FB, Falk RJ, Jennette JC. The pathologic spectrum of pulmonary lesions in patients with anti-neutrophil cytoplasmic autoantibodies specific for anti-proteinase 3 and anti-myeloperoxidase. Am J Clin Pathol 1995;104:7–16.
60. Gayraud M, Guillevin L, le Toumelin P, et al. Long-term follow-up of polyarteritis nodosa, microscopic polyangiitis, and Churg-Strauss syndrome: analysis of four prospective trials including 278 patients. French Vasculitis Study Group. Arthritis Rheum 2001;44:666–75.
61. George J, Levy Y, Kallenberg CG, Shoenfeld Y. Infections and Wegener's granulomatosis—a cause and effect relationship? QJM 1997;90:367–73.
62. Gibson LE. Granulomatous vasculitides and the skin. Dermatol Clin 1990;8:335–45.
63. Goulart RA, Mark EJ, Rosen S. Tumefactions as an extravascular manifestation of Wegener's granulomatosis. Am J Surg Pathol 1995;19:145–53.
64. Green RL, Vayonis AG. Churg-Strauss syndrome after zafirlukast in two patients not receiving systemic steroid treatment [Letter]. Lancet 1999;353:725–6.
65. Gross WL, Csernok E. Immunodiagnostic and pathophysiologic aspects of antineutrophil cytoplasmic antibodies in vasculitis. Curr Opin Rheumatol 1995;7:11–9.
66. Gross WL, Schnabel A, Trabandt A. New perspectives in pulmonary angiitis. From pulmonary angiitis and granulomatosis to ANCA associated vasculitis. Sarcoidosis Vasc Diffuse Lung Dis 2000;17:33–52.
67. Guillevin L, Cohen P, Gayraud M, Lhote F, Jarrousse B, Casassus P. Churg-Strauss syndrome. Clinical study and long-term follow-up of 96 patients. Medicine (Baltimore) 1999;78:26–37.
68. Guillevin L, Durand-Gasselin B, Cevallos R, et al. Microscopic polyangiitis: clinical and laboratory findings in eighty-five patients. Arthritis Rheum 1999;42:421–30.
69. Guillevin L, Lhote F, Gayraud M, et al. Prognostic factors in polyarteritis nodosa and Churg-Strauss syndrome. A prospective study in 342 patients. Medicine (Baltimore) 1996;75:17–28.
70. Guinee D Jr, Jaffe E, Kingma D, et al. Pulmonary lymphomatoid granulomatosis. Evidence for a proliferation of Epstein-Barr virus infected B-lymphocytes with a prominent T-cell component and vasculitis. Am J Surg Pathol 1994;18:753–64.

71. Harrison DJ, Simpson R, Kharbanda R, Abernethy VE, Nimmo G. Antibodies to neutrophil cytoplasmic antigens in Wegener's granulomatosis and other conditions. Thorax 1989;44:373–7.
72. He NS, Liu F, Wu EH, et al. Pulmonary artery involvement in aorto-arteritis. An analysis of DSA. Chin Med J (Engl) 1990;103:666–72.
73. Hoffman GS, Kerr GS, Leavitt RY, et al. Wegener's granulomatosis: an analysis of 158 patients. Ann Intern Med 1992;116:488–98.
74. Hogan SL, Nachman PH, Wilkman AS, Jennette JC, Falk RJ. Prognostic markers in patients with antineutrophil cytoplasmic autoantibody-associated microscopic polyangiitis and glomerulonephritis. J Am Soc Nephrol 1996;7:23–32.
75. Holloway J, Ferriss J, Groff J, Craig TJ, Klinek M, Klinik M. Churg-Strauss syndrome associated with zafirlukast. J Am Osteopath Assoc 1998;98:275–8.
76. Horimoto M, Igarashi K, Aoi K, Okamoto K, Takenaka T. Unilateral diffuse pulmonary artery involvement in Takayasu's arteritis associated with coronary-pulmonary artery fistula and bronchial-pulmonary artery fistula: a case report. Angiology 1991;42:73–80.
77. Imai H, Nakamoto Y, Hirokawa M, Akihama T, Miura AB. Carbamazepine-induced granulomatous necrotizing angiitis with acute renal failure. Nephron 1989;51:405–8.
78. Jakob H, Volb R, Stangl G, Reifart N, Rumpelt HJ, Oelert H. Surgical correction of a severely obstructed pulmonary artery bifurcation in Takayasu's arteritis. Eur J Cardiothorac Surg 1990;4:456–8.
79. Jennette JC, Charles LA, Falk RJ. Antineutrophil cytoplasmic autoantibodies: disease associations, molecular biology, and pathophysiology. Int Rev Exp Pathol 1991;32:193–221.
80. Jennette JC, Falk RJ. Small-vessel vasculitis. N Engl J Med 1997;337:1512–23.
81. Jennette JC, Falk RJ, Andrassy K, et al. Nomenclature of systemic vasculitis. Proposal of an international speakers conference. Arthritis Rheum 1994;37:187–92.
82. Jennette JC, Falk RJ, Wilkman AS. Anti-neutrophil cytoplasmic autoantibodies—a serologic marker for vasculitides. Ann Acad Med Singapore 1995;24:248–53.
83. Jennette JC, Thomas DB, Falk RJ. Microscopic polyangiitis (microscopic polyarteritis). Semin Diagn Pathol 2001;18:3–13.
84. Jennings CA, King TE, Tuder R, Cherniack RM, Schwarz MI. Diffuse alveolar hemorrhage with underlying isolated, pauciimmune pulmonary capillaritis. Am J Respir Crit Care Med 1997;155:1101–9.
85. Karam GH, Fulmer JD. Giant cell arteritis presenting as interstitial lung disease. Chest 1982;82:781–9.
86. Katzenstein AL, Locke WK. Solitary lung lesions in Wegener's granulomatosis. Pathologic findings and clinical significance in 25 cases. Am J Surg Pathol 1995;19:545–52.
87. Komadina KH, Houk RW. Polyarteritis nodosa presenting as recurrent pneumonia following splenectomy for hairy-cell leukemia. Semin Arthritis Rheum 1989;18:252–7.
88. Koss MN, Antonovych T, Hochholzer L. Allergic granulomatosis (Churg-Strauss syndrome). Am J Surg Pathol 1981;5:21–8.
89. Koss MN, Hochholzer L, Feigin DS, Garancis JC, Ward PA. Necrotizing sarcoid-like granulomatosis: clinical, pathologic, and immunopathologic findings. Hum Pathol 1980;11S:510–9.
90. Koss MN, Hochholzer L, Langloss JM, Wehunt WD, Lazarus AA, Nichols PW. Lymphomatoid granulomatosis: a clinicopathologic study of 42 patients. Pathology 1986;18:283–8.
91. Koss MN, Robinson RG, Hochholzer L. Bronchocentric granulomatosis. Hum Pathol 1981;12:632–8.
92. Kuhlman JE, Hruban RH, Fishman EK. Wegener granulomatosis: CT features of parenchymal lung disease. J Comput Assist Tomogr 1991;15:948–52.
93. Ladanyi M, Fraser RS. Pulmonary involvement in giant cell arteritis. Arch Pathol Lab Med 1987;111:1178–80.
94. Lai RS, Lin SL, Lai NS, Lee PC. Churg-Strauss syndrome presenting with pulmonary capillaritis and diffuse alveolar hemorrhage. Scand J Rheumatol 1998;27:230–2.
95. Lakhanpal S, Tani K, Lie JT, Katoh K, Ishigatsubo Y, Ohokubo T. Pathologic features of Behcet's syndrome: a review of Japanese autopsy registry data. Hum Pathol 1985;16:790–5.
96. Langford CA. Treatment of polyarteritis nodosa, microscopic polyangiitis, and Churg-Strauss syndrome: where do we stand? Arthritis Rheum 2001;44:508–12.
97. Langford CA, Hoffman GS. Wegener's granulomatosis. Thorax 1999;54:629–37.
98. Langford CA, Sneller MC. New developments in the treatment of Wegener's granulomatosis, polyarteritis nodosa, microscopic polyangiitis, and Churg-Strauss syndrome. Curr Opin Rheumatol 1997;9:26–30.
99. Langford CA, Sneller MC. Update on the diagnosis and treatment of Wegener's granulomatosis. Adv Intern Med 2001;46:177–206.
100. Lanham JG, Churg J. Churg-Strauss syndrome. In: Churg A, Churg J, eds. Systemic vasculitides. New York: Igaku-Shoin; 1991:101–20.

101. Lanham JG, Elkon KB, Pusey CD, Hughes GR. Systemic vasculitis with asthma and eosinophilia: a clinical approach to the Churg-Strauss syndrome. Medicine (Baltimore) 1984;63:65–81.
102. Larson TS, Hall S, Hepper NG, Hunder GG. Respiratory tract symptoms as a clue to giant cell arteritis. Ann Intern Med 1984;101:594–7.
103. Lauque D, Cadranel J, Lazor R, et al. Microscopic polyangiitis with alveolar hemorrhage. A study of 29 cases and review of the literature. Groupe d'Etudes et de Recherche sur les Maladies "Orphelines" Pulmonaires. Medicine (Baltimore) 2000;79:222–33.
104. Le Gall F, Loeuillet L, Delaval P, Thoreux PH, Desrues B, Ramee MP. Necrotizing sarcoid granulomatosis with and without extrapulmonary involvement. Pathol Res Pract 1996;192:306–13.
105. Leavitt RY, Fauci AS. Pulmonary vasculitis. Am Rev Respir Dis 1986;134:149–66.
106. Leavitt RY, Travis WD, Fauci AS. Vasculitis. In: Shelhamer J, Pizzo PA, Parrillo JE, Masur H, eds. Respiratory disease in the immunosuppressed host. Philadelphia: JB Lippincott; 1991:703–27.
107. Lie JT. Combined sarcoidosis and disseminated visceral giant cell angiitis: a third opinion [Letter]. Arch Pathol Lab Med 1991;115:210–1.
108. Lie JT. Disseminated visceral giant cell arteritis. Histopathologic description and differentiation from other granulomatous vasculitides. Am J Clin Pathol 1978;69:299–305.
109. Lie JT. Illustrated histopathologic classification criteria for selected vasculitis syndromes. American College of Rheumatology Subcommittee on Classification of Vasculitis. Arthritis Rheum 1990;33:1074–87.
110. Lie JT. Takayasu's arteritis. In: Churg A, Churg J, eds. Systemic vasculitides. New York: Igaku-Shoin; 1991:159–79.
111. Liebow AA. The J. Burns Amberson lecture—pulmonary angiitis and granulomatosis. Am Rev Respir Dis 1973;108:1–18.
112. Lipford EH Jr, Margolick JB, Longo DL, Fauci AS, Jaffe ES. Angiocentric immunoproliferative lesions: a clinicopathologic spectrum of post-thymic T-cell proliferations. Blood 1988;72:1674–81.
113. Lipworth BJ, Slater DN, Corrin B, Kesseler ME, Haste AR. Allergic granulomatosis without asthma: a rare 'forme fruste' of the Churg-Strauss syndrome. Respir Med 1989;83:249–50.
114. Maguire R, Fauci AS, Doppman JL, Wolff SM. Unusual radiographic features of Wegener's granulomatosis. AJR Am J Roentgenol 1978;130:233–8.
115. Marandian MH, Ezzati M, Behvad A, Moazzami P, Rakhchan M. Pulmonary involvement in Schönlein-Henoch's purpura. Arch Fr Pediatr 1982;39:255–7.
116. Marcussen N, Lund C. Combined sarcoidosis and disseminated visceral giant cell vasculitis. Path Res Pract 1989;184:325–30.
117. Mark EJ, Flieder DB, Matsubara O. Treated Wegener's granulomatosis: distinctive pathological findings in the lungs of 20 patients and what they tell us about the natural history of the disease. Hum Pathol 1997;28:450–8.
118. Mark EJ, Ramirez JF. Pulmonary capillaritis and hemorrhage in patients with systemic vasculitis. Arch Pathol Lab Med 1985;109:413–8.
119. Masi AT, Hunder GG, Lie JT, et al. The American College of Rheumatology 1990 criteria for the classification of Churg-Strauss syndrome (allergic granulomatosis and angiitis). Arthritis Rheum 1990;33:1094–100.
120. Matsubara O, Yoshimura N, Tamura A, et al. Pathological features of the pulmonary artery in Takayasu arteritis. Heart Vessels Suppl 1992;7:18–25.
121. Matsumoto T, Homma S, Okada M, et al. The lung in polyarteritis nodosa: a pathologic study of 10 cases. Hum Pathol 1993;24:717–24.
122. Monti G, Galli M, Cereda UG, Cannatelli G, Invernizzi F. Mycosis fungoides with mixed cryoglobulinemia and pulmonary vasculitis. A case report. Boll Ist Sieroter Milan 1987;66:324–8.
123. Morita T, Kamimura A, Koizumi F. Disseminated visceral giant cell arteritis. Acta Pathol Jpn 1987;37:863–70.
124. Myers JL, Kurtin PJ, Katzenstein AL, et al. Lymphomatoid granulomatosis. Evidence of immunophenotypic diversity and relationship to Epstein-Barr virus infection. Am J Surg Pathol 1995;19:1300–12.
125. Nada AK, Torres VE, Ryu JH, Lie JT, Holley KE. Pulmonary fibrosis as an unusual clinical manifestation of a pulmonary-renal vasculitis in elderly patients. Mayo Clin Proc 1990;65:847–56.
126. Nakabayashi K, Kurata N, Nangi N, Miyake H, Nagasawa T. Pulmonary artery involvement as first manifestation in three cases of Takayasu arteritis. Int J Cardiol 1997;54[Suppl]:S177–83.
127. Nicholson AG, Wotherspoon AC, Diss TC, et al. Lymphomatoid granulomatosis: evidence that some cases represent Epstein-Barr virus-associated B-cell lymphoma. Histopathology 1996;29:317–24.
128. Niimi H, Hartman TE, Müller NL. Necrotizing sarcoid granulomatosis: computed tomography and pathologic findings. J Comput Assist Tomogr 1995;19:920–3.
129. Nölle B, Specks U, Ludemann J, Rohrbach MS, DeRemee RA, Gross WL. Anticytoplasmic autoantibodies: their immunodiagnostic value in Wegener's granulomatosis. Ann Intern Med 1989;111:28–40.

130. Okubo S, Kuneida T, Ando M, Nakajima N, Yutani C. Idiopathic isolated pulmonary arteritis with chronic cor pulmonale. Chest 1988;94:665–6.
131. Orriols R, Munoz X, Ferrer J, Huget P, Morell F. Cocaine-induced Churg-Strauss vasculitis. Eur Respir J 1996;9:175–7.
132. Primack SL, Hartman TE, Lee KS, Müller NL. Pulmonary nodules and the CT halo sign. Radiology 1994;190:513–5.
133. Raz I, Okon E, Chajek-Shaul T. Pulmonary manifestations in Behcet's syndrome. Chest 1989;95:585–9.
134. Roberti I, Reisman L, Churg J. Vasculitis in childhood. Pediatr Nephrol 1993;7:479–89.
135. Rodat O, Buzelin F, Weber M, et al. Manifestations broncho-pulmonaires de la maladie de Horton: a propos d'une observation. Rev Med Interne 1983;4:225–30.
136. Rolfes DB, Weiss MA, Sanders MA. Necrotizing sarcoid granulomatosis with suppurative features. Am J Clin Pathol 1984;82:602–7.
137. Rose AG, Sinclair-Smith CC. Takayasu's arteritis. A study of 16 autopsy cases. Arch Pathol Lab Med 1980;104:231–7.
138. Rosen S, Falk RJ, Jennette JC. Polyarteritis nodosa, including microscopic form and renal vasculitis. In: Churg A, Churg J, eds. Systemic vasculitides. New York: Igaku-Shoin; 1991:57–77.
139. Salamon F, Weinberger A, Nili M, et al. Massive hemoptysis complicating Behcet's syndrome: the importance of early pulmonary angiography and operation. Ann Thorac Surg 1988;45:566–7.
140. Saldana MJ. Necrotizing sarcoid granulomatosis: clinicopathologic observations in 24 patients [Abstract]. Lab Invest 1978;38:364.
141. Sasaki A, Hasegawa M, Nakazato Y, Ishida Y, Saitoh S. Allergic granulomatosis and angiitis (Churg-Strauss syndrome). Report of an autopsy case in a nonasthmatic patient. Acta Pathol Jpn 1988;38:761–8.
142. Schultz DR, Diego JM. Antineutrophil cytoplasmic antibodies (ANCA) and systemic vasculitis: update of assays, immunopathogenesis, controversies, and report of a novel de novo ANCA-associated vasculitis after kidney transplantation. Semin Arthritis Rheum 2000;29:267–85.
143. Schwarz MI, Mortenson RL, Colby TV, et al. Pulmonary capillaritis. The association with progressive irreversible airflow limitation and hyperinflation. Am Rev Respir Dis 1993;148: 507–11.
144. Sehgal M, Swanson JW, DeRemee RA, Colby TV. Neurologic manifestations of Churg-Strauss syndrome. Mayo Clin Proc 1995;70:337–41.
145. Seiden MV, O'Donnell WJ, Weinblatt M, Licht J. Vasculitis with recurrent pulmonary hemorrhage in a long-term survivor after autologous bone marrow transplantation. Bone Marrow Transplant 1990;6:345–7.
146. Sharma BK, Jain S, Sagar S. Systemic manifestations of Takayasu arteritis: the expanding spectrum. Int J Cardiol 1997;54[Suppl]:S149–54
147. Sharma S, Kamalakar T, Rajani M, Talwar KK, Shrivastava S. The incidence and patterns of pulmonary artery involvement in Takayasu's arteritis. Clin Radiol 1990;42:177–81.
148. Sharma S, Rajani M, Shrivastava S, et al. Non-specific aorto-arteritis (Takayasu's disease) in children. Br J Radiol 1991;64:690–8.
149. Shintaku M, Mase K, Ohtsuki H, Yasumizu R, Yasunaga K, Ikehara S. Generalized sarcoidlike granulomas with systemic angiitis, crescentic glomerulonephritis, and pulmonary hemorrhage. Report of an autopsy case. Arch Pathol Lab Med 1989;113:1295–8.
150. Singh N, Cole S, Krause PJ, Conway M, Garcia L. Necrotizing sarcoid granulomatosis with extrapulmonary involvement. Clinical, pathologic, ultrastructural, and immunologic features. Am Rev Respir Dis 1981;124:189–92.
151. Slavin RE, de Groot WJ. Pathology of the lung in Behcet's disease. Case report and review of the literature. Am J Surg Pathol 1981;5:779–88.
152. Soave R, Murray HW, Litrenta MM. Bacterial invasion of pulmonary vessels. Pseudomonas bacteremia mimicking pulmonary thromboembolism with infarction. Am J Med 1978;65:864–7.
153. Specks U. Pulmonary vasculitis. In: Schwarz MI, King TE Jr, eds. Interstitial lung disease, 3rd ed. Hamilton: BC Decker; 1998:507–34.
154. Specks U, DeRemee RA. Granulomatous vasculitis. Wegener's granulomatosis and Churg-Strauss syndrome. Rheum Dis Clin North Am 1990;16:377–97.
155. Spiteri MA, Gledhill A, Campbell D, Clarke SW. Necrotizing sarcoid granulomatosis. Br J Dis Chest 1987;81:70–5.
156. Staples CA. Pulmonary angiitis and granulomatosis. Radiol Clin North Am 1991;29:973–82.
157. Stegeman CA, Cohen Tervaert JW, de Jong PE, Kallengerg CG. Trimethoprim-sulfamethoxazole (co-trimoxazole) for the prevention of relapses of Wegener's granulomatosis. Dutch Co-Trimoxazole Wegener Study Group. N Engl J Med 1996;335:16–20.
158. Stephen JG, Braimbridge MV, Corrin B, Wilkinson SP, Day D, Whimster WF. Necrotizing 'sarcoidal' angiitis and granulomatosis of the lung. Thorax 1976;31:356–60.
159. Strazzella WD, Safirstein BH. Asthma due to parasitic infestation. N J Med 1989;89:947–9.

160. Swerlick RA, Lawley TJ. Small-vessel vasculitis and cutaneous vasculitis. In: Churg A, Churg J, eds. Systemic vasculitides. New York: Igaku-Shoin; 1991:193–201.
161. Takahashi K, Honda M, Furuse M, Yanagisawa M, Saitoh K. CT findings of pulmonary parenchyma in Takayasu arteritis. J Comput Assist Tomogr 1996;20:742–8.
162. Takemura T, Matsui Y, Saiki S, Mikami R. Pulmonary vascular involvement in sarcoidosis: a report of 40 autopsy cases. Hum Pathol 1992;23:1216–23.
163. Tauber E, Wojnarowski C, Horcher E, Dekan G, Frischer T. Necrotizing sarcoid granulomatosis in a 14-yr-old female. Eur Respir J 1999;13:703–5.
164. Travis WD. Common and uncommon manifestations of Wegener's granulomatosis. Cardiovasc Pathol 1994;3:217–25.
165. Travis WD, Carpenter HA, Lie JT. Diffuse pulmonary hemorrhage. An uncommon manifestation of Wegener's granulomatosis. Am J Surg Pathol 1987;11:702–8.
166. Travis WD, Colby TV, Lombard C, Carpenter HA. A clinicopathologic study of 34 cases of diffuse pulmonary hemorrhage with lung biopsy confirmation. Am J Surg Pathol 1990;14:1112–25.
167. Travis WD, Hoffman GS, Leavitt RY, Pass HI, Fauci AS. Surgical pathology of the lung in Wegener's granulomatosis. Review of 87 open lung biopsies from 67 patients. Am J Surg Pathol 1991;15:315–33.
168. Travis WD, Koss MN. Pulmonary angiitis and granulomatosis: necrotizing sarcoid granulomatosis and Churg-Strauss syndrome. In: Saldana MJ, ed. Pathology of pulmonary disease. Philadelphia: JB Lippincott; 1994:803–9.
169. Travis WD, Koss MN. Vasculitis. In: Dail DH, Hammar SP, eds. Pulmonary pathology, 2nd ed. New York: Springer-Verlag; 1994:1027–95.
170. Travis WD, Kwon-Chung KJ, Kleiner DE, et al. Unusual aspects of allergic bronchopulmonary fungal disease: report of two cases due to Curvularia organisms associated with allergic fungal sinusitis. Hum Pathol 1991;22:1240–8.
171. Travis WD, Pittaluga S, Lipschik GY, et al. Atypical pathologic manifestations of Pneumocystis carinii pneumonia in the acquired immune deficiency syndrome. Review of 123 lung biopsies from 76 patients with emphasis on cysts, vascular invasion, vasculitis, and granulomas. Am J Surg Pathol 1990;14:615–25.
172. Tunaci A, Berkmen YM, Gokmen E. Thoracic involvement in Behcet's disease: pathologic, clinical, and imaging features. AJR Am J Roentgenol 1995;164:51–6.
173. Ulbright TM, Katzenstein AL. Solitary necrotizing granulomas of the lung: differentiating features and etiology. Am J Surg Pathol 1980;4:13–28.
174. Uner AH, Rozum-Slota B, Katzenstein AL. Bronchiolitis obliterans-organizing pneumonia (BOOP)-like variant of Wegener's granulomatosis. A clinicopathologic study of 16 cases. Am J Surg Pathol 1996;20:794–801.
175. Vassallo M, Shepherd RJ, Iqbal P, Feehally I. Age-related variations in presentation and outcome in Wegener's granulomatosis. J R Coll Physicians Lond 1997;31:396–400.
176. Wadsworth DT, Siegel MJ, Day DL. Wegener's granulomatosis in children: chest radiographic manifestations. AJR Am J Roentgenol 1994;163:901–4.
177. Wagenaar SS, van den Bosch JM, Westermann CJ, Bosman HG, Lie JT. Isolated granulomatous giant cell vasculitis of the pulmonary elastic arteries. Arch Pathol Lab Med 1986;110:962–4.
178. Wagenaar SS, Westermann CJ, Corrin B. Giant cell arteritis limited to large elastic pulmonary arteries. Thorax 1981;36:876–7.
179. Wechsler ME, Finn D, Gunawardena D, et al. Churg-Strauss syndrome in patients receiving montelukast as treatment for asthma. Chest 2000;117:708–13.
180. Wegener F. [Generalized septic vascular diseases]. Verh Dtsch Path Ges 1936;29:202–10.
181. White RH. Henoch-Schönlein purpura. In: Churg A, Churg J, eds. Systemic vasculitides. New York: Igaku-Shoin; 1991:203–17.
182. Winn WC, Myerowitz RL. The pathology of the Legionella pneumonias. A review of 74 cases and the literature. Hum Pathol 1981;12:401–22.
183. Worthy SA, Müller NL, Hansell DM, Flower CD. Churg-Strauss syndrome: the spectrum of pulmonary CT findings in 17 patients. AJR Am J Roentgenol 1998;170:297–300.
184. Yousem SA. Bronchocentric injury in Wegener's granulomatosis: a report of five cases. Hum Pathol 1991;22:535–40.

5
REACTIVE LYMPHOID LESIONS

INTRODUCTION

Reactive lymphoid lesions of the lung are a group of lymphoid processes of known and unknown etiology characterized by the accumulation of numerous lymphocytes in the alveolar spaces and/or interstitium. Often, the lymphoid aggregates appear, with or without germinal centers, along lymphatic routes or vessels. These lesions must be distinguished from lymphomas.

Lymphoproliferative disorders involving the lung are rare. When they occur, the patients usually have an underlying systemic disease (Table 5-1). Uncommonly, the lung may be the only organ initially involved. This is the case in reactive lesions such as lymphocytic interstitial pneumonia (LIP), follicular bronchiolitis, and nodular lymphoid hyperplasia.

The clinical diagnosis is often suspected when a systemic disease is present. However, there are no pathognomonic clinical features for these processes; usually the differential diagnosis includes many other possible forms of lung injury. Consequently, tissue examination, usually from an open or thoracoscopic biopsy, is required to make or confirm the diagnosis. Indeed, this situation often requires that a large specimen be examined to identify all the features necessary for diagnosis and to perform requisite special studies (24). Occasionally, analysis of a specimen from a transbronchial biopsy is sufficient to confirm recurrent disease in a patient with a known lymphoproliferative disorder, particularly when supported by immunohistochemical or similar studies on cells retrieved from concomitant bronchoalveolar lavage (BAL) (24). In these cases, small specimens retrieved by transbronchial biopsy, fine needle aspiration, or closed pleural biopsy, may be sufficient (24).

LIP is a benign polyclonal proliferation (usually of mature B cells) that either diffusely involves the lung or is multifocal. Its malignant potential is poorly defined. It appears to be linked to other disorders described in this chapter. In particular, nodular lymphoid hyperplasia is likely a localized form of LIP, given the similar histology and clinical outcome of the two disorders. Further, the separation of LIP and follicular bronchitis/bronchiolitis (pulmonary lymphoid hyperplasia), in which the lymphoid cells are largely confined to peribronchial and lobular septal areas, can be viewed as arbitrary since the disorders can have an overlapping microscopic appearance (87). This chapter describes these disorders, as well as a histogenetically unrelated disease, Castleman's disease; the

Table 5-1

DISEASES ASSOCIATED WITH A LYMPHOCYTIC INTERSTITIAL PNEUMONIA PATTERN IN LUNG[a]

Collagen Vascular Disease
Systemic lupus erythematosus (11,76,125)
Sjögren's syndrome (29,38,106)
Rheumatoid arthritis (121)
Autoimmune Diseases
Primary biliary cirrhosis (63)
Myasthenia gravis (72)
Hashimoto's thyroiditis (58)
Celiac sprue (85)
Autoerythrocyte sensitization (28)
Pernicious anemia (70)
Immunodeficiency
Acquired immunodeficiency syndrome (14,46, 56,81,102,108,114)
Common variable immunodeficiency (62)
Virus-Associated (excluding HIV infection)
Epstein-Barr virus infection (9,64,74)
Human herpesvirus 8 (119)
Chronic active hepatitis (48)
Drug-Induced
Dilantin (19)
Miscellaneous
Crohn's disease (27)
Tuberculosis (77)
Graft versus host disease (93)
Allogeneic bone marrow transplantation (93)
Familial (89)

[a]Excluding animal hosts.

problem posed by intrapulmonary lymph nodes is briefly mentioned. A discussion of pulmonary lymphomas, lymphomatoid granulomatosis (an angioimmunoproliferative lesion) believed by many to be a T-cell–rich B-cell lymphoma, and angioimmunoblastic lymphadenopathy, also believed to be a T-cell lymphoma in most patients with lymphoma (i.e., angioblastic lymphadenopathy [AILD]-like T-cell lymphoma), is beyond the scope of this chapter (24).

LYMPHOCYTIC INTERSTITIAL PNEUMONIA

Definition. Lymphocytic interstitial pneumonia (LIP) is a clinicopathologic term used to describe several disorders that are associated with dysproteinemia, autoimmunity (especially of the connective tissue diseases), or viral infections, such as due to human immunodeficiency virus (HIV) (26,63). However, rarely LIP may be an idiopathic disorder. Histologically, it is characterized by diffuse infiltration of the alveolar septa by a dense lymphocytic infiltrate. Synonyms include *lymphoid interstitial pneumonitis, diffuse hyperplasia of bronchial bronchus-associated lymphoid tissue (BALT), lymphoplasmacytic pneumonia, plasmacytic interstitial pneumonia,* and *plasma cell interstitial pneumonitis.*

LIP is part of a spectrum of pulmonary lymphoid proliferations that includes follicular bronchitis/bronchiolitis, nodular lymphoid hyperplasia, and low-grade malignant lymphoma (60). These lesions may be difficult to differentiate from each other. Indeed, a substantial percentage of the lesions that were initially classified by Liebow (72) as LIP were subsequently recognized to be low-grade B-cell lymphomas, in modern terminology, MALT lymphomas, or extranodal low-grade marginal zone B-cell lymphomas (23,72,87). As a result, LIP was excluded from the classification of idiopathic interstitial pneumonias for several decades. Today, it is clear that the majority of patients with LIP have associated immunologic disorders, dysproteinemias or viral infections, particularly (HIV) infection, so that LIP can therefore be viewed as a morphologic pattern of lung injury that results from multiple etiologies with varying pathogenetic mechanisms (63). In a small subset of cases, however, LIP presents as an idiopathic, inflammatory, non-neoplastic process. LIP, therefore, has been included in the American Thoracic Society/European Respiratory Society (ATS/ERS) international multidisciplinary consensus classification of idiopathic interstitial pneumonias (115).

Clinical Features. The incidence of LIP is unknown, but it appears rare: a Mayo Clinic review found 13 cases during a 10-year experience (110). LIP is most often seen in HIV-positive children (56,81,83,90,103,108). One autopsy series suggested an incidence of 6 percent (81). It was estimated that LIP occurred in 30 to 50 percent of pediatric patients with acquired immunodeficiency syndrome (AIDS), but more recently it is reported to involve only 17 percent (75,107,114). Still, the presence of LIP in a child who is HIV positive and under 13 years of age is now part of the case definition of AIDS, even when no opportunistic infection is present (18,22).

LIP occurs more commonly in children who acquire HIV infection perinatally than in those infected by contaminated blood products (43). Adults who are infected with HIV can develop LIP, but this is rare, occurring in only 1 percent or fewer (57,73,114). Most adults usually have either minimal or mild interstitial lymphoid infiltrates (so-called nonspecific interstitial pneumonitis; see chapter 13) (45,100,108).

Clinically, HIV-infected patients are usually black. They typically have AIDS-related complex (ARC) and polyclonal hypergammaglobulinemia (79,83,100,108). Presenting symptoms include indolent onset of dyspnea, nonproductive cough, and fever. Auscultation of the chest may be normal or it may reveal respiratory crackles. Children may show clubbing, hepatosplenomegaly, salivary gland enlargement, or lymphadenopathy.

LIP can also occur in both children and adults who do not have HIV infection. Affected children usually have congenital immune deficiencies, particularly hypogammaglobulinemia. A familial form of LIP has been reported (89). The adults can have a variety of underlying diseases, but the most common is Sjögren's syndrome. About 0.9 percent of patients with Sjögren's syndrome have LIP and up to 25 percent of adults with LIP have Sjögren's syndrome (38,106). In one study of 20 patients with Sjögren's syndrome, 9 had radiographic evidence of interstitial opacities, and LIP was one of a number of findings, ranging from follicular bronchiolitis to fibrosis with honeycombing (29). A large number of other disorders, primarily autoimmune diseases but also viral infections, have been reported with LIP (Table 5-1). Infrequently, the disease is an isolated idiopathic disorder.

Most adult patients with LIP, whether secondary to a systemic disease or idiopathic, are women in the fourth through seventh decades of life (63,72,87,109,110). The clinical presentation is that commonly found with diffuse interstitial lung diseases, but it may be dominated by the underlying systemic disease. Most patients have cough, dyspnea, or a combination (50 to 80 percent) (122). Weight loss, pleuritic chest pain, arthralgias, and fever can be seen. Other symptoms and signs are related to the associated immunologic diseases such as Sjögren's syndrome or myasthenia gravis (109). Physical examination may show bibasilar crackles. Clubbing is uncommon.

The most remarkable laboratory abnormality is the presence of dysproteinemia, occurring in at least 60 percent of adult patients. Most frequently, there is hypergammaglobulinemia (112); in about 10 percent of cases, there is hypogammaglobulinemia (63,109). If there is a monoclonal gammopathy or hypogammaglobulinemia, the index of suspicion for a lymphoproliferative malignancy should increase. Lung function testing shows features typical of diffuse parenchymal lung disease: reduced lung volumes and lowered diffusing capacity for carbon monoxide (DLCO) (45). Hypoxemia is common. Analysis of BAL shows a striking increase in both the number and percentage of lymphocytes.

Radiologic Findings. Chest radiographic findings are typically nonspecific. They include bilateral reticular and nodular opacities as well as ground-glass opacities and parenchymal consolidation (fig. 5-1) (41,58). These abnormalities usually occur in the lower lung zones. Nodular patterns are also described, particularly in patients with AIDS.

Computed tomography (CT) may demonstrate ground-glass attenuation and poorly defined, 2- to 4-mm centrilobular nodules (fig. 5-2) (16,79). Parenchymal abnormalities can be present in patients with normal chest radiographs (79). Thickening of the bronchovascular interstitium and interlobular septa, cystic spaces, and lymph node enlargement are also described in studies using thin section and high-resolution (HR) CT techniques (54).

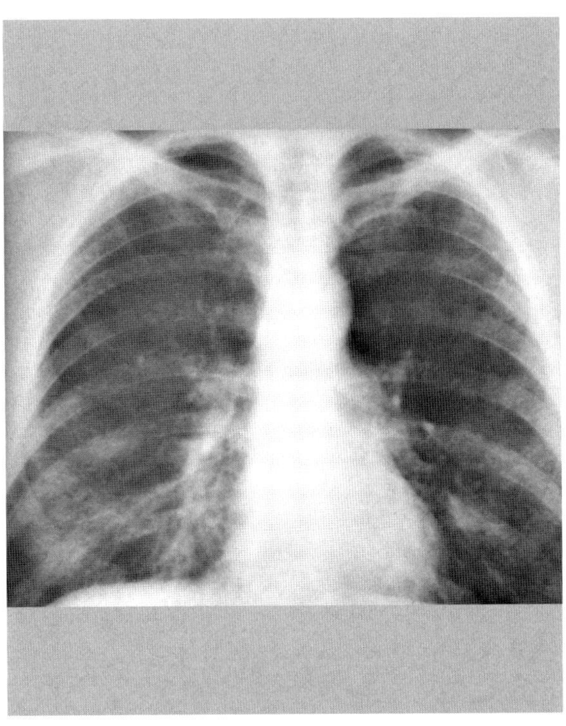

Figure 5-1

LYMPHOCYTIC INTERSTITIAL PNEUMONIA

PA chest radiograph demonstrates diffuse, bilateral, reticular opacities.

Lymphadenopathy may be more common in patients who have concomitant AIDS. In rare cases, fibrosis and honeycomb lung may be demonstrated. Pleural effusion is rare (49). It is unclear whether the radiographic abnormalities in idiopathic LIP differ from those in LIP associated with underlying systemic disease.

Gross Findings. Typically, the lung is pink-tan or tan-gray and is diffusely firm to palpation. In late stages of disease, the lung may contract and the pleural surface may show a cobblestone pattern. There may be subpleural cysts with surrounding gray, firm tissue due to honeycombing fibrosis.

Histologic Findings. LIP is characterized by a prominent interstitial lymphoid infiltrate.

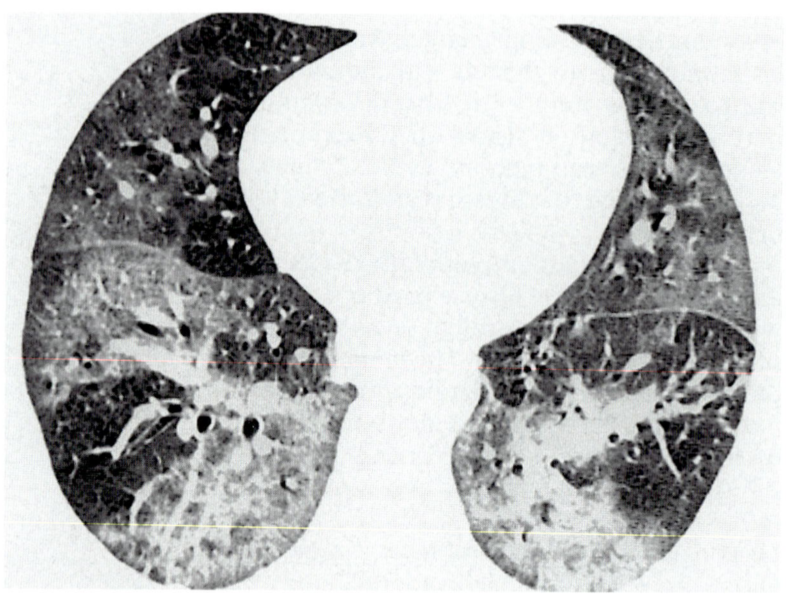

Figure 5-2

LYMPHOCYTIC INTERSTITIAL PNEUMONIA IN A 31-YEAR-OLD WOMAN WITH DYSPNEA

Chest CT (lung window) demonstrates bilateral, patchy, ground-glass opacities that are worse in the lower lobes. (Courtesy of Dr. Mark S. Parker, Richmond, VA.)

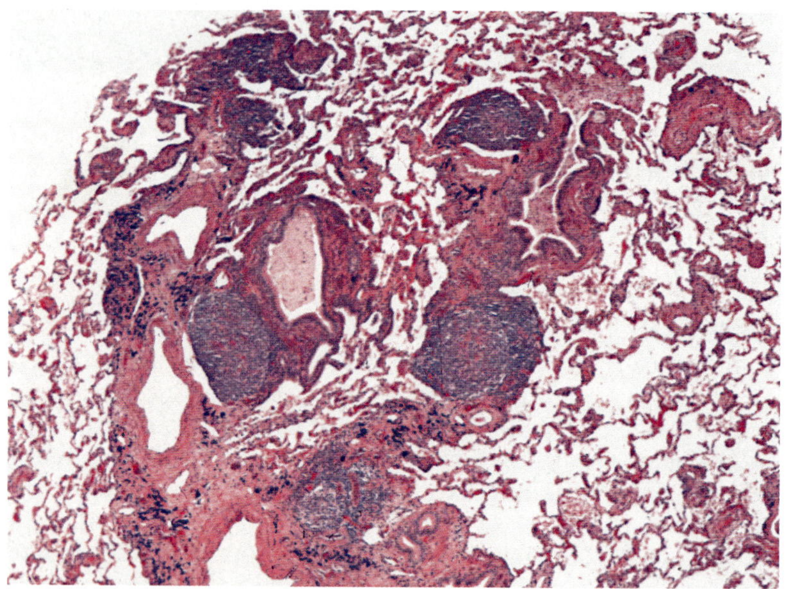

Figure 5-3

FOLLICULAR BRONCHITIS

There are lymphoid nodules, including lymphoid follicles, adjacent to airways.

The infiltrate diffusely spreads into alveolar septa, although occasionally there may be some sparing of the lung (72). When lymphoid nodules are centered about airways, vessels, and interlobular septa (i.e., the pathways of lymphatic vessels in lung), the disease is termed *follicular bronchitis/bronchiolitis* (or *pulmonary lymphoid hyperplasia* in the pediatric AIDS literature) (fig. 5-3) (55). As the disease becomes more florid, the lymphoid infiltrate extends into and extensively involves the pulmonary interstitium; this is the classic form of LIP described by Liebow and Carrington (figs. 5-4–5-6) (72).

The interstitial infiltrate is usually composed of small lymphocytes with variable numbers of plasma cells (fig. 5-6). HIV-infected patients, in particular, usually have moderate to severe infiltrates composed of small and mature lymphocytes, with few plasma cells, and they may have accompanying type 2 pneumocyte hyperplasia. Noncaseating granulomas may be present, but they are usually inconspicuous (114).

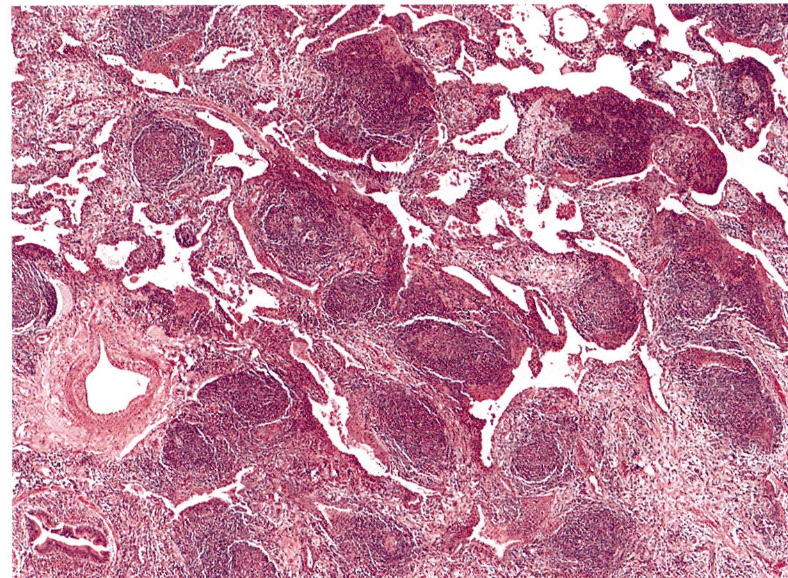

Figure 5-4

LYMPHOCYTIC INTERSTITIAL PNEUMONIA

There is a diffuse lymphoid infiltrate, replete with reactive follicles, that extends through the pulmonary interstitium.

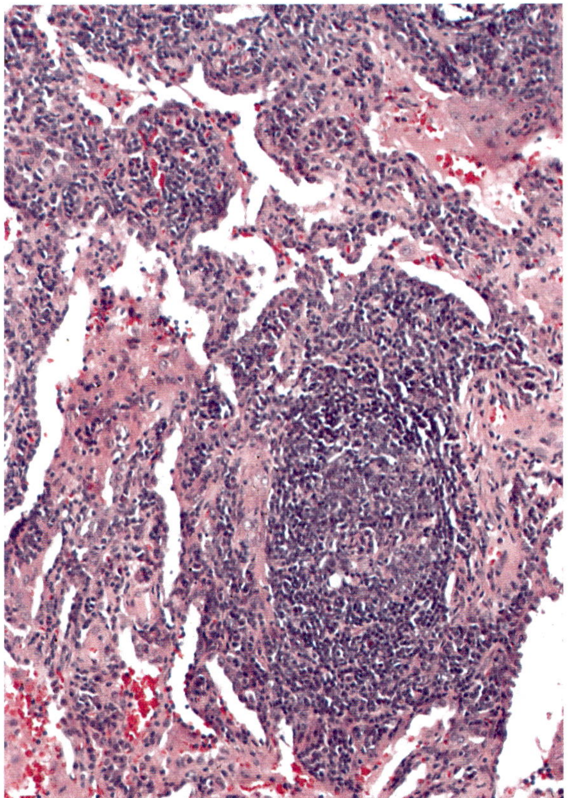

Figure 5-5

LYMPHOCYTIC INTERSTITIAL PNEUMONIA

The lymphoid infiltrate percolates through the alveolar interstitium. A small lymphoid follicle is present.

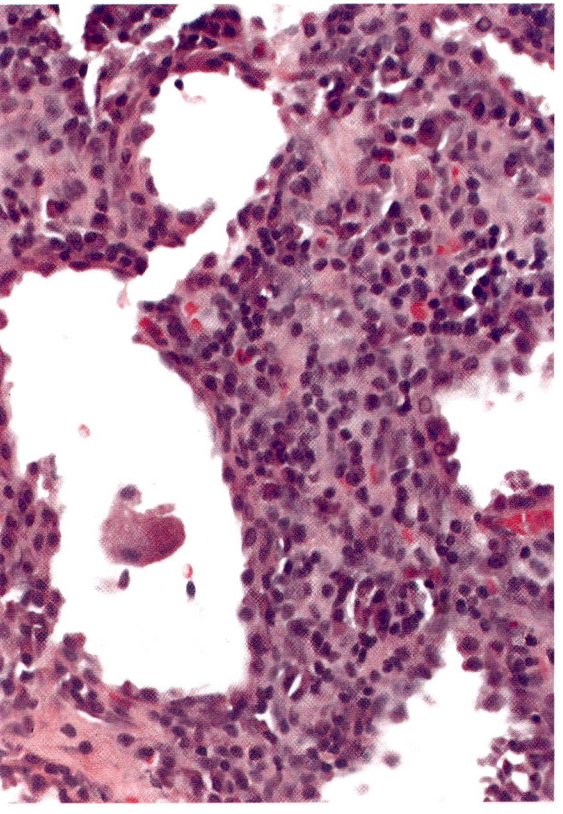

Figure 5-6

LYMPHOCYTIC INTERSTITIAL PNEUMONIA

A mixture of lymphocytes and plasma cells is present within the interstitium.

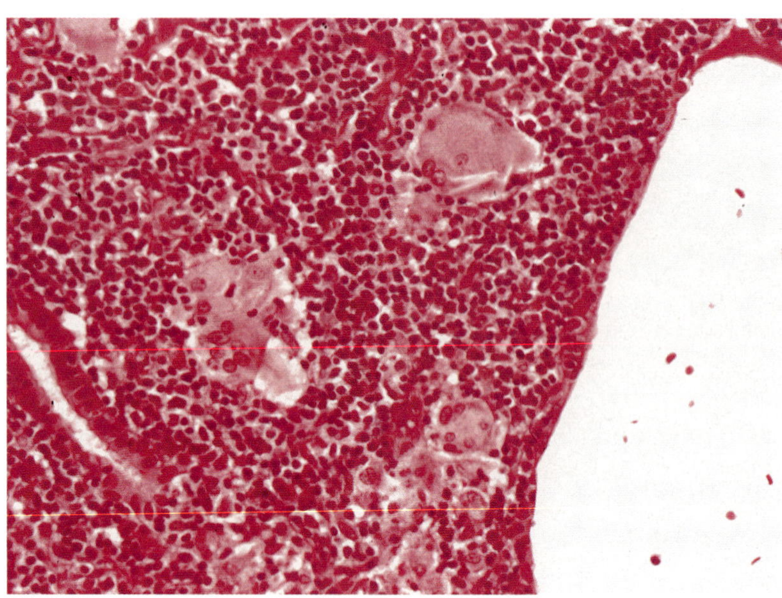

Figure 5-7

LYMPHOCYTIC INTERSTITIAL PNEUMONIA WITH GIANT CELLS

There are a few multinucleated giant cells embedded in the lymphoid infiltrate. Note the cholesterol clefts in the cytoplasm of one of the giant cells.

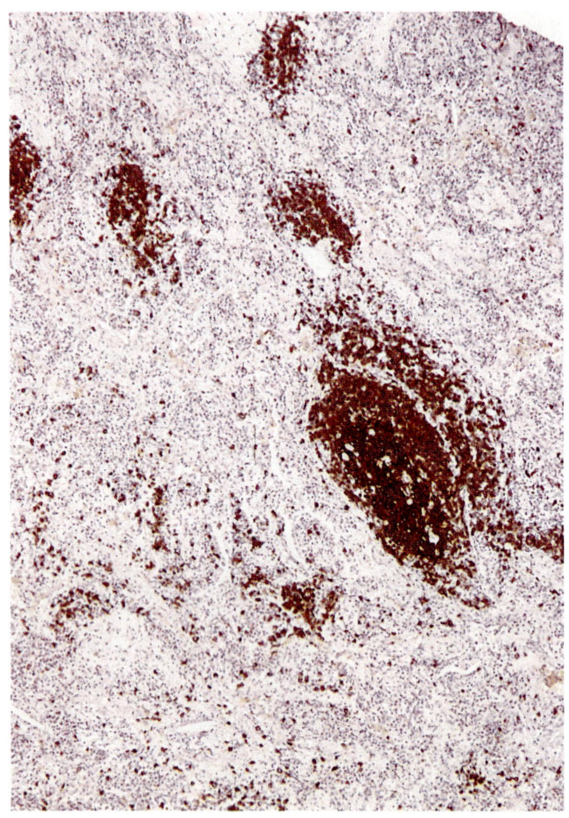

Figure 5-8

LYMPHOCYTIC INTERSTITIAL PNEUMONIA STAINED FOR THE B-CELL MARKER L26

The B cells appear in nodules corresponding to lymphoid follicles.

In non-AIDS patients, there can be more of an admixture of plasma cells within the lymphoid infiltrates. Indeed, occasional cases of LIP in non-AIDS patients are so rich in plasma cells that they have been given names such as lymphoplasmacytic pneumonia (44) or plasma cell interstitial pneumonitis (82,122).

Germinal centers occur in up to half of non-AIDS patients (figs. 5-4, 5-5), but they are usually inconspicuous in patients with AIDS (63,72,110). Scattered, multinucleated giant cells or ill-formed granulomas are also found in the lymphoid infiltrate in up to 50 percent of cases (fig. 5-7) (63). Why giant cells occur is unclear, but they are also seen in malignant lymphomas of the lung (64). Giant cells may be a reaction to lipid released by cellular breakdown, and indeed, they may contain cholesterol clefts (fig. 5-7). In late stages, LIP can produce advanced interstitial fibrosis with honeycombing; small foci of organizing pneumonia also may be seen.

LIP usually shows a mixture of B and T cells. The B cells often appear in nodules corresponding to lymphoid follicles (fig. 5-8), while T cells are present in the pulmonary interstitium (fig. 5-9). The B cells show polyclonal staining for immunoglobulin light chains (7, 63,65). The lymphoid infiltrates of a few cases of LIP associated with hypogammaglobulinemia

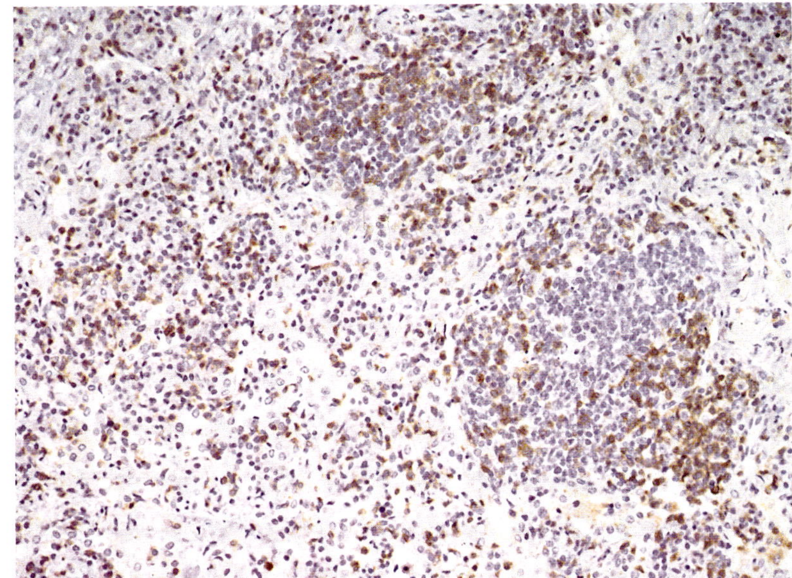

Figure 5-9

LYMPHOCYTIC INTERSTITIAL PNEUMONIA STAINED FOR THE T-CELL MARKER CD3

T cells are present diffusely in the pulmonary parenchyma.

have been studied using frozen tissues: they appear to consist largely of T cells (62), predominantly of T-helper cells (21). The predominant phenotype of the lymphocytes in patients with LIP and AIDS is usually the T cell (36,83).

The definitive diagnosis of LIP requires surgical lung biopsy. Surgical lung biopsies are more likely to yield a diagnosis than transbronchial biopsies due to difficulties in sampling of the latter. However, if there is extensive alveolar septal infiltration, transbronchial biopsy can be diagnostic. In HIV-infected children, there has been a reluctance to perform lung biopsies since the mid-1980s, when the disease was initially recognized to represent a common pulmonary complication of HIV infection, and the diagnosis is often made clinically. The clinical evidence includes the presence of a reticulonodular infiltrate, with or without hilar and mediastinal lymphadenopathy, that does not change after treatment with antibiotics for 2 months (3,43).

Etiology and Pathogenesis. *Autoimmunity.* An autoimmune etiology for LIP is attractive, given its association with many autoimmune processes (especially those with dysproteinemias) (93,97,123). These include systemic lupus erythematosus (11), autoerythrocyte sensitization (28), Hashimoto's thyroiditis (72), pernicious anemia (70), myasthenia gravis (80), chronic active hepatitis (48), primary biliary cirrhosis (63), and Crohn's disease (Table 5-1) (27). Sjögren's syndrome is associated with 25 percent of the reported cases of LIP (29,38,106), often with a marked gammopathy, either monoclonal or polyclonal (see chapter 6). When associated with dysproteinemia or autoimmune processes, LIP may predate the establishment of the protein or other abnormality. Rarely, circulating immune complexes have been reported in patients with LIP.

One recent study favored autoimmunity as the pathogenetic mechanism based on the finding of minor clones of lymphoid cells with a high homology to autoreactive lymphocytes (rheumatoid factor, anti-DNA antibody, and G6-positive lymphocytes) (67). This, in turn, suggests that immature B cells stimulated by autoantigens might play some role in the pathogenesis of true LIP.

Viral Infection. Since disorders in T-cell regulation induced by retroviruses, such as HIV, can produce polyclonal B-cell activation and hyperplasia, the relationship of viral infection to LIP is of great interest. In fact, there appears to be an association between LIP and several different viruses, especially HIV-1, Epstein-Barr virus (EBV), and human herpesvirus 8 (HHV-8).

A potential role for HIV infection is suggested by the markedly increased incidence of LIP in persons infected with the HIV virus, especially children (14,46,56,81,102,108,114).

Table 5-2

DIFFUSE INFILTRATIVE LYMPHOCYTOSIS SYNDROME (DILS) IN INFECTION VERSUS SJÖGREN'S SYNDROME[a]

	Sjögren's Syndrome	DILS
Glandular manifestations	Moderate parotid enlargement	Massive parotid enlargement
Extraglandular manifestations	Infrequent; may have pulmonary, gastrointestinal, renal, and neurologic involvement	Prominent pulmonary, gastrointestinal, neural, or neurologic involvement
Infiltrative lymphocytic phenotype	CD4 predominant	CD8 predominant
Autoantibodies	High frequency; rheumatoid factor, ANA[b], anti-RO/SSA, anti-LA/SSB	Low frequency; rheumatoid factor, ANA, anti-RO/SSA, anti-LA/SSB
HLA association	B8, DR2, DR3, DR4 (rheumatoid arthritis)	DR5, DR6 (blacks), DR6 (whites)

[a]Table 1 from Itescu S. Diffuse infiltrative lymphocytosis syndrome in children and adults infected with HIV-1: a model of rheumatic illness caused by acquired viral infection. Am J Reprod Immunol 1992;28:248.

[b]ANA = antinuclear antibody; HLA = human leukocyte antigen.

While the etiology of LIP in these patients is not completely clarified, reports of improvement with antiviral therapy alone suggest that the virus itself may be driving the proliferation of immune cells (98,105). HIV has been found in BAL fluids and lung tissues of some patients with AIDS (20,100,127). Reverse transcriptase activity and HIV-specific IgG have also been isolated in BAL specimens from several adults (111). HIV has been shown to infect alveolar macrophages, CD4+ lymphocytes, fibroblasts, and dendritic cells, both in vivo and in vitro (78,96). Through the use of in situ hybridization, HIV was shown to be concentrated in the germinal centers of one patient with LIP (114). This correlates with data from lymphoid tissue, which shows that lymphoid germinal centers are reservoirs of HIV (39). In some adults, a transient nonspecific pneumonitis has been reported to be related to an immunologic response to the HIV virus itself (46).

A possibly significant insight into the pathogenesis of LIP in HIV-infected patients has been provided by the recognition that children and adults who are infected with HIV may have infiltration of CD8 lymphocytes in lung tissue, producing an LIP-like appearance (51,52). There may also be CD8 lymphocytosis in BAL fluid, peripheral blood, and salivary gland, producing bilateral parotid enlargement, xerostomia, and xerophthalmia (51,52). This Sjögren syndrome-like disorder has been termed *diffuse infiltrative lymphocytosis syndrome (DILS)* (Table 5-2). Immunologic and genetic factors appear to be important in DILS (51,52).

Black children have the human leukocyte antigen (HLA)-DR5 haplotype or HLA-DR6, while Caucasians have only HLA-DR6 (52). In one case (61), epithelial cells lining the airspaces expressed HLA-DR, while lymphocytes and macrophages in the alveolar spaces strongly expressed transforming growth factor (TGF)-beta. This suggests that abnormal expression of HLA-DR in nonimmune cells and exaggerated production of TGF-beta played important roles in the pathogenesis of LIP in this patient.

A variety of other cytokines are also abnormally expressed in vitro by HIV-infected cells, including interleukin (IL)-1, IL-2, IL-6, IL-8, IL-10, tumor necrosis factor (TNF)-alpha, and granulocyte-monocyte–colony-stimulating factor (GM-CSF) (32,33,69,78). They may be mediators of lung injury, inflammatory cell recruitment, or HIV replication (78). Finally, immune complexes are present in the BAL fluid of HIV-infected children and adults (88).

It is well known that chronic EBV infection can induce a prominent chronic interstitial pneumonitis with abundant lymphocytes. Using Southern blot hybridization EBV DNA was found in lung tissues from 8 of 10 children with LIP and AIDS (4). It has also been found in lung tissue from adults with LIP in greater frequency than in control lung tissues

Table 5-3

DIFFERENTIAL DIAGNOSIS OF NODULAR LYMPHOID HYPERPLASIA (NLH), LYMPHOCYTIC INTERSTITIAL PNEUMONIA (LIP), FOLLICULAR BRONCHIOLITIS (FB), EXTRANODAL MARGINAL ZONE LYMPHOMA (MALTOMA), AND NONSPECIFIC INTERSTITIAL PNEUMONITIS (NSIP)

Feature	NLH	LIP	FB	MALToma	NSIP
Chest Radiograph					
Mass	+[a]	–	–	+	–
Diffuse	–	+	+	+	+
Histologic Findings					
Localized	+	–	–	+	–
Diffuse interstitial	–	+	–	+	+/–
Lymphangitic	+/–	–	–	+	–
Peribronchial only	–	–	+	–	–
Infiltrate	poly	poly	poly	mono or poly	poly
Germinal centers	+	+/–	+/–	+/–	–
Plasma cells	+	+/–	+/–	+/–	+/–
Dutcher bodies	–	–	–	+	–
Monoclonality	–	–	–	+	–
Monocytoid B cells	–	–	–	+	–

[a]+ = present; – = absent; +/– = may be present or absent; poly = polymorphous; mono = monomorphic.

(9,64,74). Interestingly, EBV latent membrane protein-1 appears to be most prevalent in bronchiolar epithelial cells and not in lymphoid cells (64). The mechanism of EBV action to produce LIP is still unclear.

There is also a single case report of a patient who had LIP and simultaneous HHV-8 infection, without demonstrable Kaposi's sarcoma (119). The possibility that HHV-8 might have played a pathogenic role was suggested by the absence of HIV infection, but other potential viral infections were not excluded.

Differential Diagnosis. The differential diagnosis of LIP includes benign lymphoid processes in the lung, low-grade marginal zone B-cell lymphomas presenting as diffuse lung disease, nodular lymphoid hyperplasia, angioimmunoblastic lymphadenopathy, hypersensitivity pneumonitis, and nonspecific interstitial pneumonitis (Table 5-3). In AIDS patients, it is also important to exclude certain infectious pneumonias.

Primary lymphomas of the lung are rare: they comprise approximately 0.3 percent of all primary pulmonary neoplasms. Among primary lymphomas, MALTomas are the most common, comprising 50 to 90 percent of cases (24). These tumors can occasionally assume a widespread interstitial pattern on the chest X ray and histologic sections (figs. 5-10, 5-11). Creating additional confusion, reactive lymphoid follicles or their remnants can be present in MALTomas (fig. 5-12), and the lesions can be surrounded by interstitial reactive lymphoid cells, heightening the resemblance to LIP (35). In fact, it is probable that some cases classified as LIP on purely morphologic grounds are malignant lymphomas (37). We suspect that this may be particularly true in patients with Sjögren's syndrome. Radiologic features suggestive of lymphoma include pleural effusion, consolidation, and large nodular opacities or masses (54).

Microscopically, in low-grade lymphomas there is expansion of the interstitium by neoplastic B lymphocytes, with frequent lymphoepithelial lesions and lymphomatous colonization of germinal centers (94). As the lesions infiltrate surrounding lung, there is destruction of alveolar walls, but bronchioles and foci of alveolar architecture often remain. Malignant lymphoma is strongly favored if the lymphoid infiltrate shows a distinctly lymphangitic pattern, monomorphism, and/or invasion of parietal pleura or regional lymph nodes (fig. 5-11)

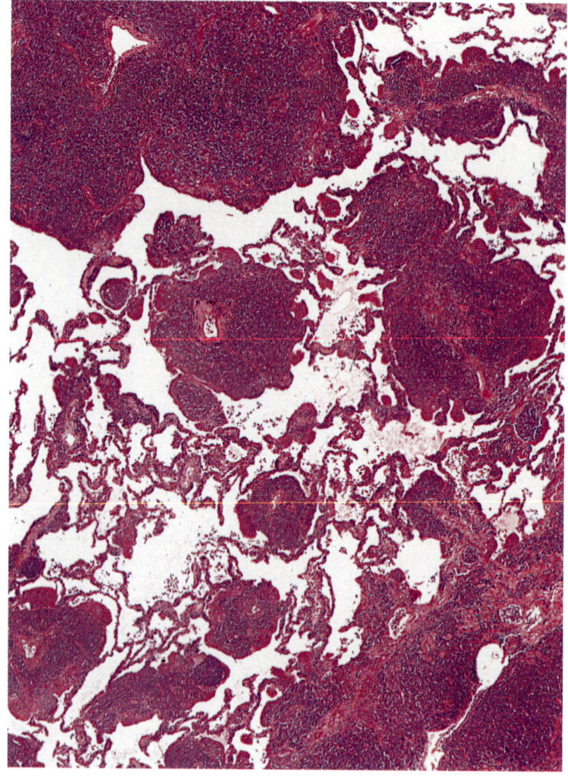

Figure 5-10

LOW-GRADE MARGINAL ZONE B-CELL LYMPHOMA (MALTOMA)

In this low magnification view, the tumor infiltrates extensively through the lung and around vessels and small airways, producing an appearance simulating lymphocytic interstitial pneumonia.

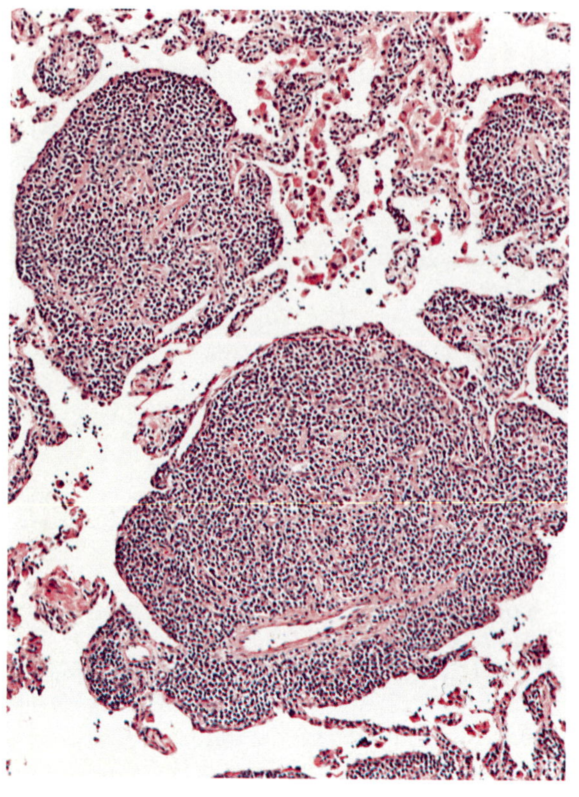

Figure 5-11

LOW-GRADE MARGINAL ZONE B-CELL LYMPHOMA (MALTOMA)

Note the lymphangitic pattern in which the tumor infiltrates around vessels where lymphatics are located. This pattern of growth should suggest the possibility of lymphoma.

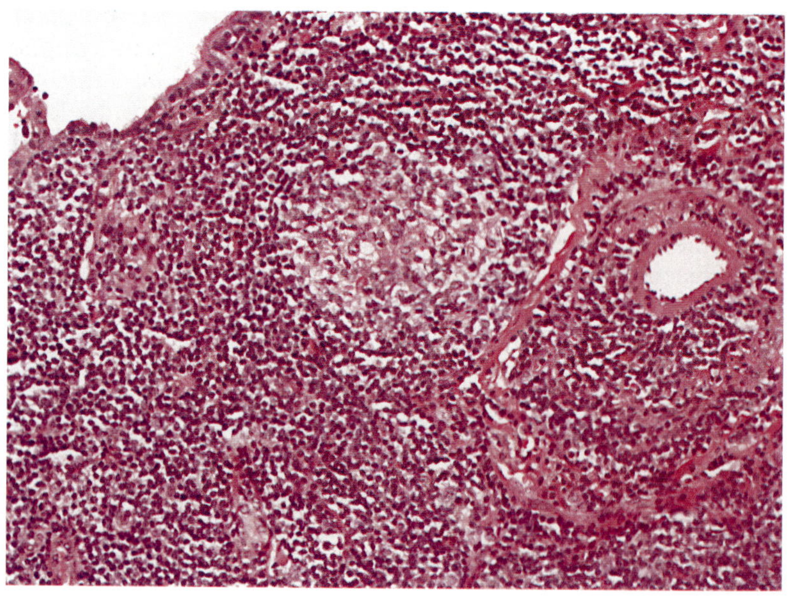

Figure 5-12

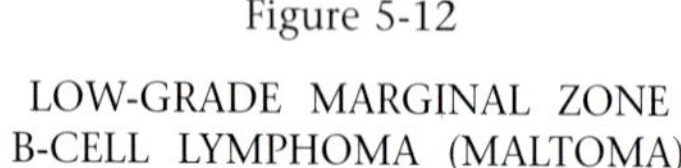

LOW-GRADE MARGINAL ZONE B-CELL LYMPHOMA (MALTOMA)

Note the residual reactive follicle center embedded within the lymphomatous infiltrate. Large reactive follicles are seen occasionally in these lymphomas.

(25). Invasion of bronchial cartilage or visceral pleura by the cellular infiltrate also favors malignant lymphoma, but does not exclude reactive processes. The presence of giant lamellar bodies is a useful indicator of low-grade B-cell lymphoma in the differential diagnosis with reactive pulmonary lymphoid hyperplasia (94). Giant lamellar bodies are rare pulmonary inclusions associated with chronic disease within the lung. They are roughly spherical, eosinophilic, whorled structures occurring singly or in clusters within alveolar ducts and spaces, and stain strongly for surfactant apoprotein (94). Ultrastructurally, they are comprised of concentric laminated layers of extracellular material.

In general, immunohistochemical stains should be done on all cases of LIP to ensure that there is no evidence of a monoclonal lymphoid cell population. In doubtful cases, the polymerase chain reaction (PCR) should be done for immunoglobulin gene rearrangement (35,67). Sometimes, however, these studies produce a result that complicates decision making. For example, a recent evaluation of clonality in five cases morphologically believed to be LIP showed minor monoclonal populations that were interpreted as neoplastic clones hidden in normally reactive lymphocyte clones (67). In these cases, in which the morphology shows an apparently benign lymphoid process and clonality studies show focal clonal cell populations, perhaps the best diagnosis is a descriptive one rather than one of unequivocal lymphoma. If, however, the lymphoid cell population is markedly distorted so that it is uncertain whether it is benign or malignant morphologically, then PCR clonality studies may play an important role in the diagnosis of malignant lymphomas (86).

Nodular lymphoid hyperplasia is microscopically similar to LIP, but it occurs in the lung as one or several localized lesions, rather than as a diffuse bilateral interstitial infiltrate (see section, Nodular Lymphoid Hyperplasia).

Angioimmunoblastic lymphadenopathy (AIBL) can involve the lung in the form of diffuse interstitial infiltrates. Typically, there is little difficulty in distinguishing it from LIP since AIBL has a distinctive set of clinical features, including generalized lymphadenopathy, hepatosplenomegaly, Coombs-positive hemolytic anemia, and skin rash (25).

Hypersensitivity pneumonitis (extrinsic allergic alveolitis) and LIP may be difficult to distinguish from each other (see chapter 3). CT of both conditions may show bilateral ground-glass opacities. Microscopically, hypersensitivity pneumonitis can resemble LIP in showing diffuse interstitial lymphoplasmacytic infiltrates containing ill-formed granulomas, but the lymphoid infiltrate is denser in LIP, and bronchiolitis obliterans, a hallmark of hypersensitivity pneumonitis, is not present.

Prominent peribronchial lymphoid aggregates can be present in interstitial pneumonitides associated with connective tissue diseases, such as systemic lupus erythematosus and rheumatoid arthritis (see chapter 6). The lymphoid infiltrate is typically denser and more diffuse in LIP.

The most recent addition to the histologic differential diagnosis of LIP is nonspecific interstitial pneumonia (NSIP) (see chapter 3). Since this lesion was only described in 1994, prior publications on the topic of LIP probably included cases that would now be called NSIP, cellular pattern (59,117). The cellular pattern of NSIP consists of a mild to moderate interstitial lymphocytic and/or plasma cell infiltrate (117), but it falls short of the extensive alveolar septal infiltration seen in LIP. The lymphoid infiltrate is both less severe and patchier in NSIP than in LIP. Some cases of NSIP with a mixed cellular and fibrosing pattern could be confused with LIP. It is unlikely that the usual interstitial pneumonia pattern would be confused with LIP since the former usually does not show extensive interstitial inflammation (see chapter 3).

Finally, it is important in LIP cases occurring in the setting of HIV infection to exclude pneumonias due to organisms such as *Pneumocystis carinii* or *Mycobacterium avium-intracellulare,* which can be accompanied by prominent interstitial chronic inflammation (84,113, 116,118). In biopsies where the diagnosis of LIP is suspected, one must search carefully for alveolar exudates of *Pneumocystis* pneumonia and examine special stains for *Pneumocystis,* fungi, and acid-fast bacilli.

Treatment and Prognosis. LIP in the non-AIDS patient is usually treated with corticosteroids, but the response is variable. Also, the improvement in symptoms related by some patients after treatment is difficult to assess, since spontaneous remission has been reported (122). Overall, the clinical course is variable (72,110). In our experience, equal numbers of patients die, improve, and remain stable (63). In general, one third to half of non-AIDS adults with LIP die within 5 years (83). Death is most frequently due to infectious complications of treatment with immunosuppressive drugs, but occasionally patients die from respiratory insufficiency or malignant lymphoma.

B-cell lymphomas can develop in patients with LIP, particularly when there is concomitant Sjögren's syndrome. About 5 percent of patients with LIP develop disseminated malignant lymphoma (7,63), in particular B-cell immunoblastic sarcoma (65). Well-differentiated lymphomas associated with prolonged survival can also develop in the setting of LIP (106). As noted above, a minor population of monoclonal lymphoid cells can be present in LIP-like lesions, supporting the idea that evolution of LIP to lymphoma can occur.

Most AIDS patients with LIP have mild disease that may spontaneously resolve, but in those with progressive symptoms corticosteroids are sometimes administered and they may produce significant improvement (83). Some HIV-positive individuals with LIP improve dramatically following highly active antiviral therapy (HAART) alone (98,105). However, rarely, the disease evolves into lymphoma.

Little is known about the clinical behavior of idiopathic LIP. Optimal therapy is administration of corticosteroids, which usually results in improvement or resolution of symptoms (110).

Comparative Lesions in Animals. A member of the lentiretrovirus group, the maedi/visna virus, can induce LIP-like lesions in sheep. Interstitial lymphoid infiltrates can also be induced in cats by feline leukemia virus (15). These animal models suggest that LIP-like reactions may be a common feature of lentivirus infection.

FOLLICULAR BRONCHITIS/BRONCHIOLITIS

Definition. This pattern of lung injury is characterized by the presence of lymphoid nodules, with or without reactive follicles, next to and confined to the walls of the airways and associated peribronchial tissues (126). Synonyms include *follicular hyperplasia of bronchus-associated lymphoid tissue (BALT), hyperplasia of BALT, hyperplasia of mucosa-associated lymphoid tissue (MALT),* and *pulmonary lymphoid hyperplasia (PLH).*

Follicular bronchiolitis (bronchitis) is an inflammatory condition characterized by a proliferation of lymphoid follicles at the bifurcation of the airways and along lymphatic routes (31). This lymphoid tissue has been termed bronchus-associated lymphoid tissue (BALT) or bronchial mucosa-associated tissue (MALT) (12,30,31). Bronchial MALT is a subset of the more general MALT found in the gastrointestinal tract and other sites (12,24). Bronchial MALT is apparent in 10 percent of normal fetuses and infants. It becomes more prominent following an antigenic stimulation such as infection (24). Lymphoid follicles in the alveolar walls and pleura are also part of bronchial MALT, although technically they are not distributed along airways (24). The airway epithelium overlying the lymphoid nodules of bronchial MALT is specialized lymphoepithelium. It is characterized by attenuation and flattening; it often contains infiltrating lymphocytes, especially CD4+ T cells; and it appears to be specialized for antigen transport and presentation (12,24).

Clinical Features. Follicular bronchiolitis can be found in a variety of conditions. These include any of the collagen vascular diseases but particularly rheumatoid arthritis; immunodeficiency syndromes, including AIDS, congenital variable immunodeficiency, IgA deficiency, and Evan's syndrome; nonspecific airway-centered inflammatory conditions such as bronchiectasis, obstructive pneumonias, and chronic infections; and in a heterogeneous group of patients with hypersensitivity-type reactions (12, 30,31,56,65,101,114,126). There is also a report of familial follicular bronchiolitis, termed *familial pulmonary nodular lymphoid hyperplasia* (40).

Follicular bronchiolitis is found most often in adults (126), but it also can be seen in children (87,126). Patients vary in age depending on the underlying condition: the average ages of those with collagen vascular disease, immunodeficiency syndromes, and hypersensitivity syndromes are 44, 16, and 55 years, respectively. Patients have dyspnea, cough, and fever; some may have recurrent pneumonia or weight loss (126). In patients with underlying rheumatoid arthritis, a positive rheumatoid factor is present, often at high levels (1:640 to 1:2,560) (see chapter 6).

Both obstructive and restrictive patterns can be identified by spirometry, but the restrictive pattern is more common; there may be no abnormalities as well. Arterial blood gases show arterial hypoxemia, with a widened $AaPO_2$ gradient, and hypocapnia. Patients with hypersensitivity syndromes can have peripheral blood eosinophilia (126).

Radiologic Findings. The radiographic findings in follicular bronchiolitis are similar to those of LIP. Chest radiographs demonstrate diffuse reticular and nodular opacities. HRCT can show multifocal, bilateral, small (less than 3 mm) nodules or larger (3 to 12 mm) nodules in a centrilobular and peribronchial distribution (41). Centrilobular branching structures, bronchial wall thickening, bronchiectasis, bronchiolectasis, branching opacities and areas of low attenuation have also been described (50,99).

Gross Findings. Grossly, there are numerous minute (1 to 2 mm) nodules located adjacent to airways (50).

Histologic Findings. Microscopically, there are peribronchiolar and/or peribronchial nodular aggregates of lymphoid cells, including lymphocytes and plasma cells, containing reactive germinal centers (figs. 5-3, 5-13) (126). The lymphoid aggregates can be located between bronchioles and pulmonary arterioles, narrowing the small airways by external compression and creating secondary obstructive changes in the form of alveolar foamy macrophages, intrabronchiolar neutrophils, and small foci of organizing pneumonia. Lymphoid follicles may be present along interlobular septa and beneath the pleura—the pathways of the lymphatics.

Immunologic analysis of the lymphoid cells in the hyperplastic BALT in rheumatoid arthritis shows B cells expressing surface IgM in follicular areas and IgA-bearing lymphocytes and numerous T cells, particularly CD4+ cells, expressing alpha/beta, in the parafollicular areas (104).

Differential Diagnosis. It has been suggested that follicular bronchiolitis can be a precursor of lymphocytic interstitial pneumonia and nodular lymphoid hyperplasia (see Table 5-2). The absence of a radiographically explicit nodule or mass helps distinguish follicular bronchitis/bronchiolitis from nodular lymphoid hyperplasia.

The distinction between follicular bronchiolitis, in which the lymphoid cells are largely confined to peribronchial and lobular septal areas, and LIP, in which the lymphoid infiltrate penetrates more diffusely into the alveolar interstitium, is arbitrary, since the appearance of both can overlap.

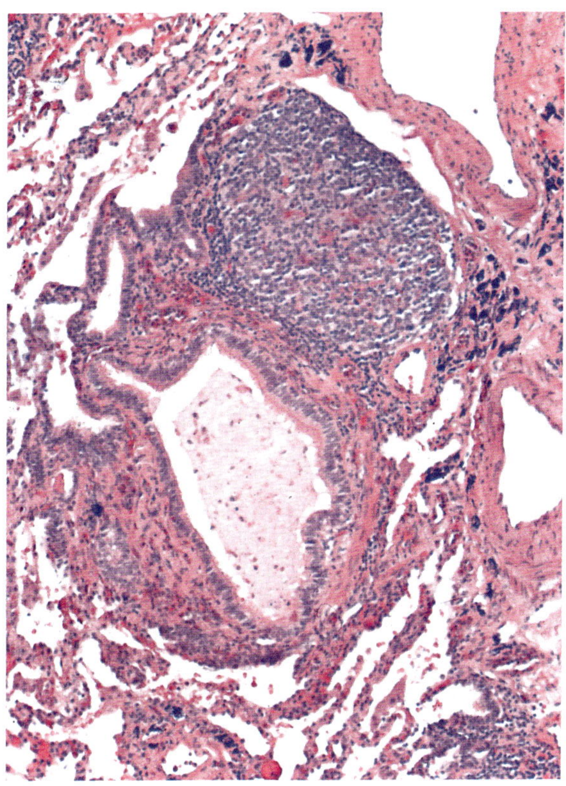

Figure 5-13

FOLLICULAR BRONCHITIS/BRONCHIOLITIS

A reactive lymphoid follicle is present adjacent to a bronchiole.

Treatment and Prognosis. Treatment with corticosteroids has yielded variable results.

NODULAR LYMPHOID HYPERPLASIA OF LUNG

Definition. Nodular lymphoid hyperplasia, also known as *pseudolymphoma,* refers to one or more nodules or localized lung infiltrates consisting of reactive lymphoid cells (65).

The concept of masses composed of reactive lymphoid tissue in lung is controversial because most microscopically low-grade lymphoid proliferations in lung, including those with abundant germinal centers, are now

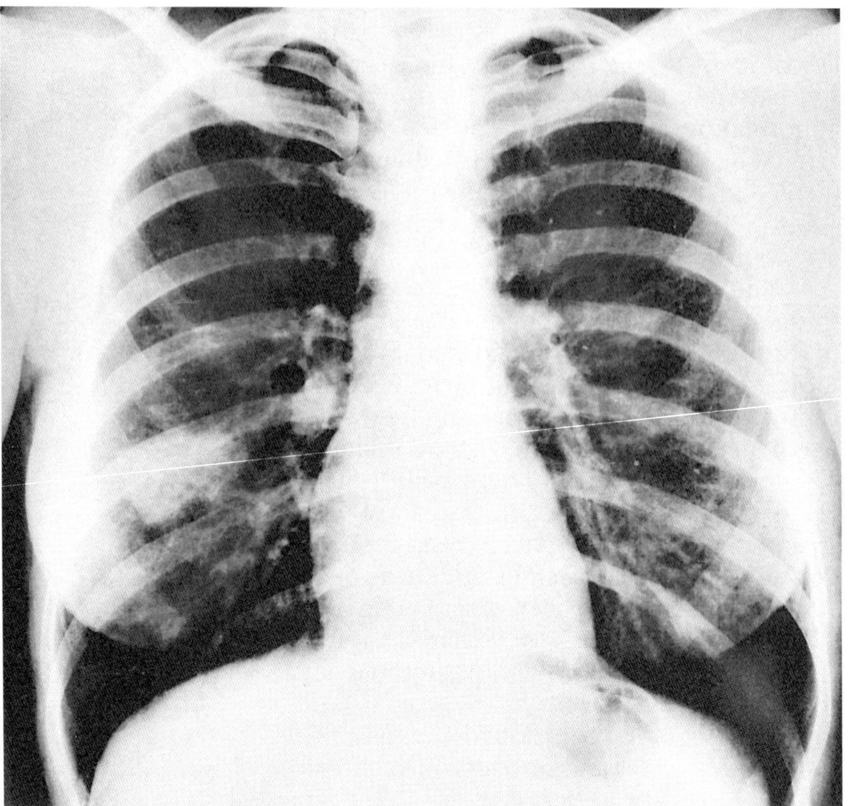

Figure 5-14

NODULAR LYMPHOID HYPERPLASIA

Nodular lymphoid hyperplasia in a 35-year-old woman with right chest discomfort. Posteroanterior chest radiograph demonstrates a mass-like parenchymal consolidation in the right middle lobe with air bronchograms.

known to be extranodal marginal zone B-cell lymphomas (2,63,72). This has lead to suggestions, particularly from Europe, that the term "pseudolymphoma" be disregarded as redundant or inaccurate (2,26,126). However, a recent immunohistochemical and molecular pathologic study has confirmed the existence of pulmonary nodular lymphoid hyperplasia (1).

Clinical Features. Nodular lymphoid hyperplasia is infrequent. In a review of the files of the Department of Pulmonary and Mediastinal Pathology of the Armed Forces Institute of Pathology, only 14 verifiable cases were found (1). Men slightly outnumber women (ratio, 1.3 to 1). The patients range from 19 to 80 years of age (mean, 60 years; median, 65 years). The majority of cases (70 percent) are detected as incidental lesions on radiologic studies obtained for other reasons. Symptoms, when present, include shortness of breath, cough, and pleuritic chest pain. Serologic studies have not been systematically performed.

Radiologic Findings. The most common radiologic pattern is a solitary pulmonary nodule or mass or a focal area of parenchymal consolidation (fig. 5-14). The lesions vary in size from 2 to 5 cm, although masses measuring up to 10 cm have been described. In the vast majority of cases, air bronchograms are present within these lesions. Lymphadenopathy and pleural effusions are rare and their presence should suggest lymphoma. Multifocal lesions have also been described (41).

Gross Findings. The lesions are usually gray, white, or tan nodules or masses with a firm, rubbery or fleshy consistency (1). Most of them are solitary, but occasionally two, three, or even "multiple" lesions occur, the last emphasizing the potential for overlap with lymphocytic interstitial pneumonia. The pulmonary nodules measure from 0.6 to 6.0 cm in greatest dimension; most are 2 to 4 cm (1). There is no predilection for any lobe.

Histologic Findings. The lymphoid lesion is usually subpleural, but it can be peribronchial. Despite the subpleural location of the lesions, the plaque-like invasion of the overlying pleura by the lymphoid infiltrate, seen commonly

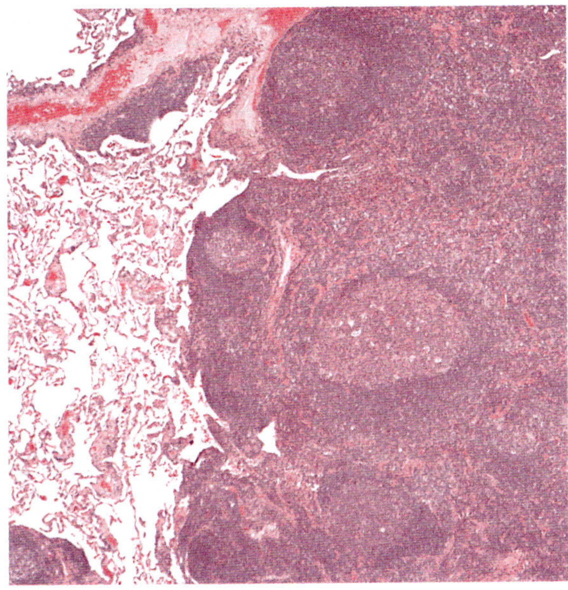

Figure 5-15

MICROSCOPIC VIEW OF THE PERIPHERY OF THE LESION IN NODULAR LYMPHOID HYPERPLASIA

The lesion, which contains numerous reactive follicles, obliterates the underlying lung. It is relatively circumscribed, although there is limited lymphangitic spread into contiguous lung.

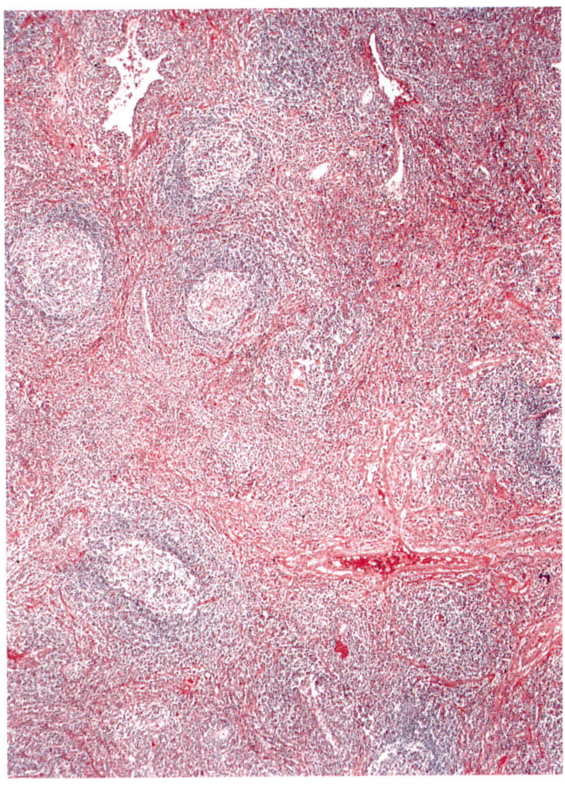

Figure 5-16

MICROSCOPIC VIEW OF THE CENTER LESION IN NODULAR LYMPHOID HYPERPLASIA

Numerous reactive lymphoid follicles are readily evident at this magnification. They are embedded in a collagenous background that for the most part obliterates the alveolar architecture. Only a few residual airways are present.

in low-grade marginal zone B-cell lymphomas, is rarely present.

The lesions are histologically localized (fig. 5-15). The most striking features are the numerous reactive germinal centers with well-preserved mantle zones and the sheets of interfollicular mature plasma cells (figs. 5-15–5-18). There is usually interfollicular fibrosis of varying degree that at least focally obliterates the underlying lung parenchyma (fig. 5-16). The plasma cells may show Russell or Mott bodies, but they do not contain Dutcher bodies (fig. 5-19). Giant cells can be present in the lymphoid infiltrate, but this is a nonspecific feature that is present in low-grade B-cell lymphomas. When the lymphoid lesion is adjacent to an airway, there is no evidence of infiltration of the bronchial cartilage, but limited lymphangitic spread can occur (fig. 5-15). Lymphoepithelial lesions of the type frequently seen in MALTomas are not present. Regional lymph nodes show benign reactive follicular hyperplasia.

Immunohistochemical stains show a reactive pattern of B and T cells. In particular, the germinal centers stain for the B-cell marker CD20, while interfollicular lymphocytes are immunoreactive for CD3, CD43, and CD5 (fig. 5-20) (1). Antibodies to CD45RA stain the mantle zone lymphocytes, but stains for bcl-2 do not decorate the follicles (fig. 5-21). The CD20+ lymphocytes do not coexpress either CD43 or CD5. The immunoglobulin light chain reactivity is polyclonal (fig. 5-22). Molecular genetic analysis shows no rearrangement of the immunoglobulin heavy chain gene (1).

Etiology and Pathogenesis. The etiology of nodular lymphoid hyperplasia is unclear. Unlike LIP, there is no known association with HIV infection, connective tissue diseases, or Sjögren's syndrome. We have found two cases that showed a small microscopic focus of acute

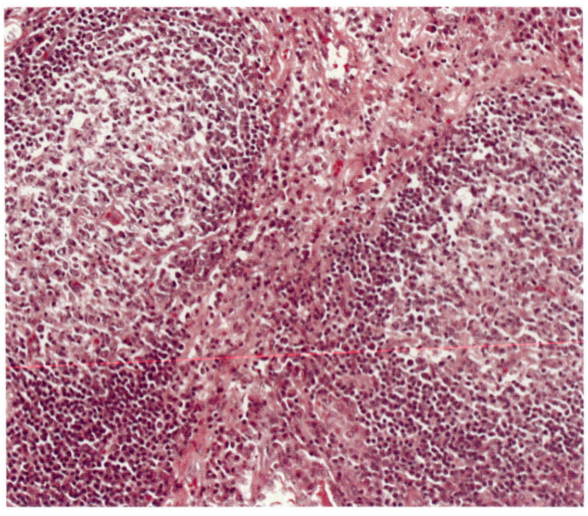

Figure 5-17

NODULAR LYMPHOID HYPERPLASIA

Two large reactive lymphoid follicles, replete with well-preserved mantle zones, are present. A band of fibrosis separates the follicles. (Figures 5-17 to 5-22 courtesy of Dr. Susan Abbondanzo, Washington, DC.)

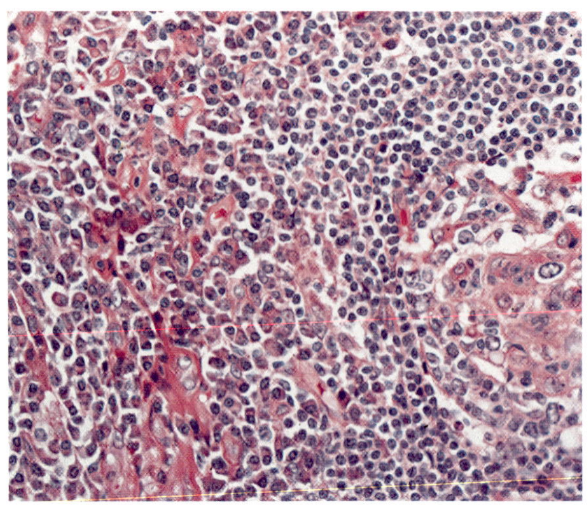

Figure 5-18

NODULAR LYMPHOID HYPERPLASIA

This high magnification view shows the edge of a germinal center and its mantle zone.

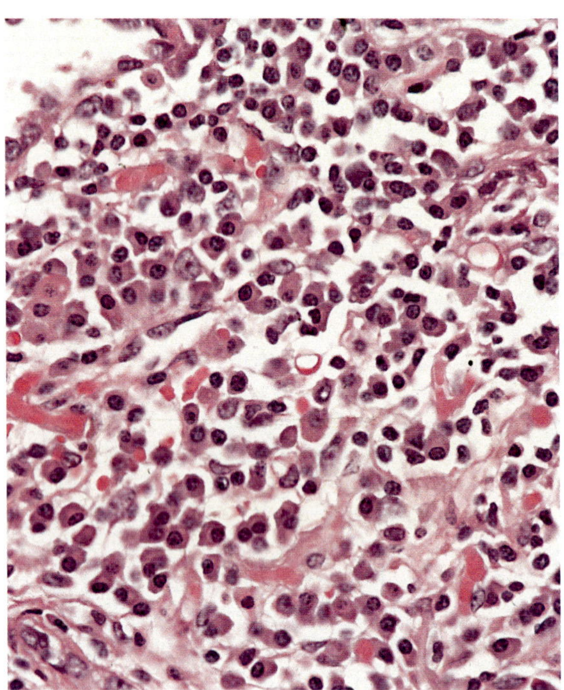

Figure 5-19

INTERFOLLICULAR PLASMA CELLS IN NODULAR LYMPHOID HYPERPLASIA

The plasma cells are cytologically bland. Russell and Mott bodies may be present, but Dutcher bodies are not seen.

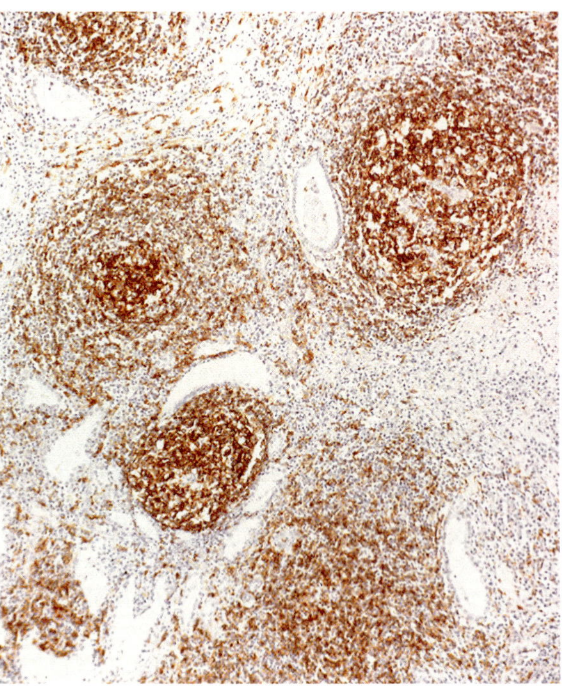

Figure 5-20

NODULAR LYMPHOID HYPERPLASIA: IMMUNOHISTOCHEMICAL STAINING FOR THE B-CELL MARKER CD20

The germinal centers stain intensely. Interfollicular lymphocytes also stained for CD3, CD43, and CD5 (not shown).

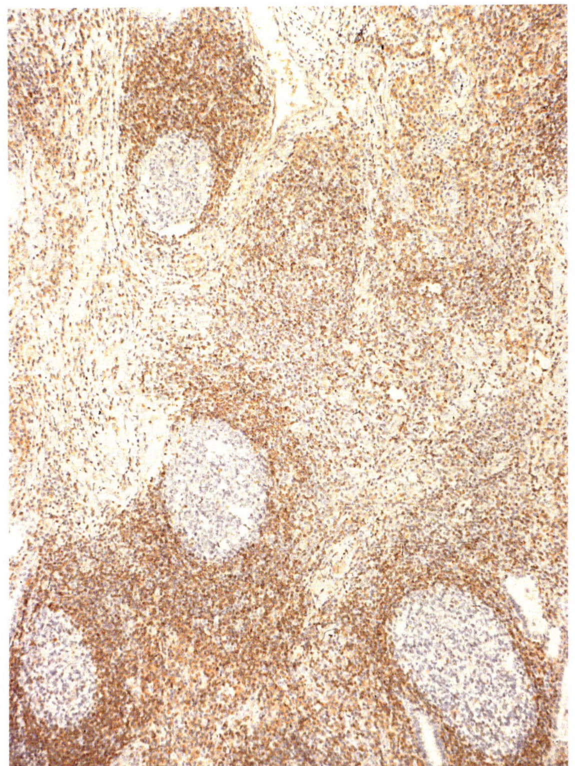

Figure 5-21

NODULAR LYMPHOID HYPERPLASIA: IMMUNOHISTOCHEMICAL STAINING FOR BCL-2

The follicle centers are not stained, a finding in keeping with a reactive follicular hyperplasia.

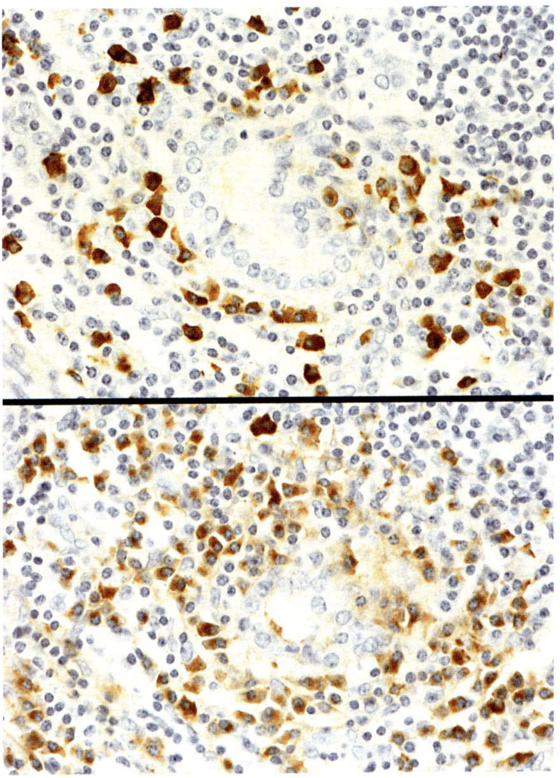

Figure 5-22

NODULAR LYMPHOID HYPERPLASIA: IMMUNOHISTOCHEMICAL STAINING FOR IMMUNOGLOBULIN LIGHT CHAINS

The top panel shows staining for lambda light chains and the bottom panel staining for kappa light chains in the same case. The ratio of staining favors kappa light chain over lambda about 3:1, compatible with a reactive lymphoid process.

inflammation or small foreign body aspiration granulomas, suggesting that inflammatory stimuli may give rise to the prominent follicular lymphoid masses (1).

Differential Diagnosis. The principal differential diagnoses include MALToma, LIP, follicular bronchitis/bronchiolitis, and inflammatory pseudotumor (inflammatory myofibroblastic tumor). Pertinent features of some of the diseases in the differential diagnosis are shown in Table 5-2.

The most important disease in the differential diagnosis is MALToma (63,65,72). This low-grade B-cell lymphoma of lung is far more frequent than nodular lymphoid hyperplasia; hence, any solitary lymphoid mass in the lung is much more likely to be lymphoma than not. The clinical presentation of patients with MALTomas, including the age distribution, symptoms, and chest radiographic appearance, greatly overlaps that of individuals with nodular lymphoid hyperplasia (63,65,72). Typically, these lymphomas are of low histologic grade and often contain reactive germinal centers and admixed plasma cells, which can produce a polymorphous appearance (fig. 5-12) (63,65,71). At times, the follicular proliferation can be exuberant and follicles can show large mantle zones, further mimicking a reactive process. Finally, these follicles are frequently polytypic (72).

Lymphomas differ from nodular lymphoid hyperplasia in showing a sheet-like pattern of growth of small lymphocytes. They are also more invasive of surrounding lung, with penetration of bronchial cartilage plates (occurring in up to 66 percent of cases), plaque-like involvement of pleura over a low-power microscopic field (in over 50 percent of cases), and more extensive lymphangitic spread (figs. 5-10, 5-11) (25,65). Also, lymphoepithelial lesions are frequent and characteristic of MALTomas of lung, but they are not seen in nodular lymphoid hyperplasia (1,23,63,65). Most important, lymphomas usually (about 75 percent of cases) show a monoclonal staining pattern for immunoglobulin light chains in paraffin sections. Still, it has been suggested that lymphomas may arise as a focal process, even in a lesion dominated by a seemingly reactive mass (2,87). In any case, where there is a question, both immunohistochemical and molecular analyses should be used to evaluate for clonality. For cases that are difficult to diagnose because of small tissue size or suboptimal fixation or processing, molecular genetic analysis needs to be done. Even so, there may be lesions in which a definitive diagnosis of benign or reactive cannot be reached with the available pathologic material; the term "atypical lymphoid infiltrate" is appropriate for them (1).

LIP shows a diffuse, prominent interstitial infiltrate of histologically and immunohistochemically reactive plasma cells, lymphocytes, immunoblasts, fibroblasts, and scattered macrophages in lung (fig. 5-4) (64,75). Although germinal centers are less frequent in LIP than in nodular lymphoid hyperplasia, they can occur (figs. 5-4, 5-5). Even when the microscopic appearance is superficially similar to that of nodular lymphoid hyperplasia, the disease is radiographically more diffuse, that is, there are diffuse reticular/nodular or small nodular opacities (figs. 5-1, 5-2). However, there may be reactive lymphoid lesions characterized by several bilateral nodules, making it difficult to decide whether the patient has LIP or multifocal nodular lymphoid hyperplasia. We think that if there is no evidence of interstitial disease radiographically, nodular lymphoid hyperplasia is the better diagnosis in these cases.

Follicular bronchiolitis shows numerous minute (1 to 2 mm) nodules located adjacent to airways (68). Microscopically, the peribronchiolar and/or peribronchial nodular aggregates can contain reactive germinal centers. However, the lesions do not create a radiologically or grossly substantial (larger than 0.5 cm) mass, as in nodular lymphoid hyperplasia (figs. 5-3, 5-13) (126).

Finally, inflammatory pseudotumor/inflammatory myofibroblastic tumor can present as a solitary pulmonary mass radiologically, and it can show an abundant chronic inflammatory infiltrate. However, these inflammatory cells occur in a prominent background of spindled myofibroblastic cells and lymphoid follicles are not a significant component of them.

Treatment and Prognosis. Surgical excision of the nodule(s) appears to be adequate therapy. Despite the concern that these lesions may constitute a precursor lesion of MALToma, in the one small series of cases published to date there was no recurrence of the pulmonary lesion in any patient: all were alive with no evidence of disease or they died of other diseases from 1 to 6 years from presentation (1).

GIANT LYMPH NODE HYPERPLASIA (CASTLEMAN'S DISEASE)

Giant lymph node hyperplasia, or Castleman's disease, is an uncommon lymphoproliferative disorder associated with significant lymphadenopathy that rarely involves the lung. Castleman's disease can be classified as either localized or multicentric in origin (95). There are two histologic subtypes: hyaline vascular and plasma cell. Most cases involving the lung are of the hyaline vascular type. The pulmonary lesion is a solitary, often asymptomatic, hilar mass (5,6,13,17,92).

Patients are 20 to 50 years of age; men and women are equally represented. The plasma cell variant is typically multicentric and associated with systemic features, including fever, splenomegaly, hepatomegaly, and massive lymphadenopathy. Polyclonal hypergammaglobulinemia is found on laboratory testing (53). HIV-seropositive individuals appear at increased risk for the development of multicentric Castleman's disease; in fact, Castleman's disease often arises concurrently with Kaposi's sarcoma (91).

Thin-section chest CT shows poorly defined centrilobular nodules (10, 53). Thin-walled cysts, thickening of the bronchovascular bundles, and interlobular septal thickening are present in most patients. Less common findings include subpleural nodules, ground-glass attenuation, airspace consolidation, and bronchiectasis (53).

Histologically, the hyaline vascular type of Castleman's disease is well circumscribed, typically involves peribronchial or hilar lymph nodes, and often has a thick fibrous capsule (10). The hyaline vascular change of the germinal centers and onion-skin layering of lymphocytes in the mantle zone of the germinal centers are distinctive microscopic features of this variant. The plasma cell variant shows a prominent interfollicular stroma rich in plasma cells and small vessels (fig. 5-23). In cases of multicentric Castleman's disease, the pulmonary parenchyma may show an associated LIP pattern (53). HHV-8 DNA is often detected in the lymph nodes of patients with Castleman's disease (34,47,91). Recently, a 32-year-old woman with multicentric Castleman's disease and lung involvement was reported to have Kaposi sarcoma–associated herpesvirus (KSHV) sequences, demonstrated by both the polymerase chain reaction and in situ hybridization of tissue obtained from her lung (47).

Progression to lymphoma, usually non-Hodgkin's lymphoma, can occur in multicentric Castleman's disease (91). A plasmablastic lymphoma can develop in patients with the plasma cell variant of multicentric Castleman's disease; HHV-8 antigen has been detected in plasmablasts in these patients (91).

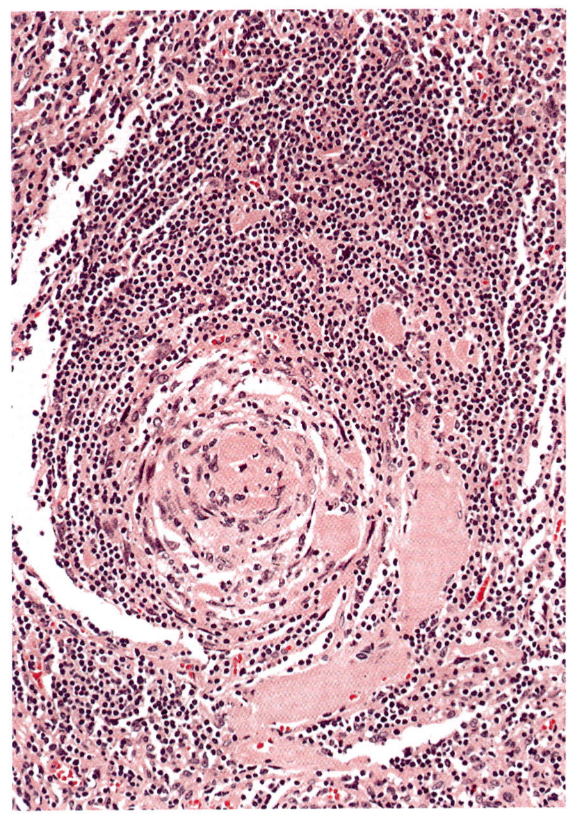

Figure 5-23

CASTLEMAN'S DISEASE

Note the distinctive concentric hyaline sclerosis altering the appearance of the lymphoid follicle.

INTRAPULMONARY LYMPH NODES

Intrapulmonary lymph nodes are most common in the pulmonary hilum, but they can also occur within the lung parenchyma (66, 124). Their clinical significance has until recently been minimal because of their generally small size, but as radiologic imaging has improved they are increasingly likely to be biopsied or resected to exclude primary or metastatic tumor (42,120). The frequency of intrapulmonary nodes visualized by CT scan appears significant, ranging from 18 to 46 percent of those well-circumscribed peripheral nodules that are less than 12 mm in diameter (8,120,124).

Most intrapulmonary lymph nodes occur in the lower lobes and are located close (generally within 20 mm) to the visceral pleura (8,124). They are usually single lesions less than 10 mm in diameter, but over 10 percent of patients have two lesions or more (8). The CT scan findings can sometimes resemble those of lung cancer, including pleural indentation, spicular radiation, and fuzzy margins (120). The usual method of diagnosis is by video-assisted thoracoscopy.

Grossly, the nodes are usually black due to the accumulation of anthracotic pigment. Histologically, intrapulmonary lymph nodes are most often subpleural and show the typical findings of a lymph node, including a capsule, peripheral sinus, cortical zone with lymphoid follicles, and medullary zone (figs. 5-24, 5-25). The nodes most often show accumulation of anthracotic pigment and silica-like particles, as expected in thoracic nodes (fig. 5-25). They can also show the gamut of changes seen in lymph nodes elsewhere, ranging from normal sinusoidal and follicular architecture to Castleman's disease, silicotic nodules, and hyperplastic features.

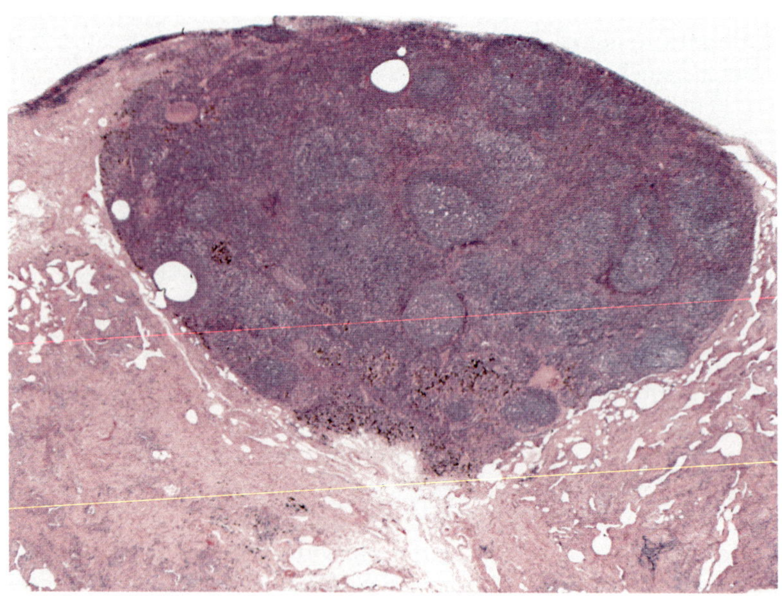

Figure 5-24

INTRAPULMONARY LYMPH NODE

The nodes are most often subpleural and show typical reactive follicles.

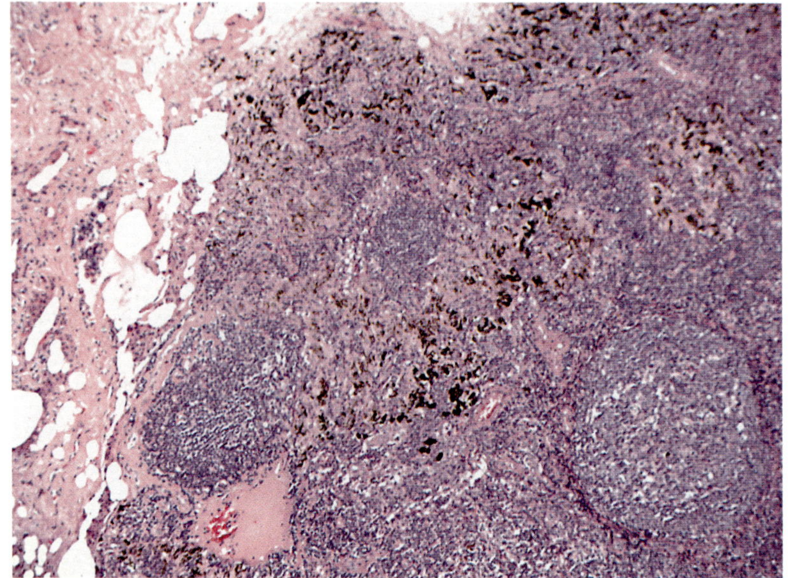

Figure 5-25

INTRAPULMONARY LYMPH NODE

Note the reactive follicles, peripheral sinus, and anthracosis, the latter a common finding in subpleural lymph nodes.

REFERENCES

1. Abbondanzo SL, Rush W, Bijwaard KE, Koss MN. Nodular lymphoid hyperplasia of the lung: a clinicopathologic study of 14 cases. Am J Surg Pathol 2000;24:587–97.
2. Addis B, Hyjek E, Isaacson P. Primary pulmonary lymphoma: a re-appraisal of its histogenesis and its relationship to pseudolymphoma and lymphoid interstitial pneumonia. Histopathology 1988;13:1–17.
3. Amorosa JK, Miller RW, Laraya-Cuasay L, et al. Bronchiectasis in children with lymphocytic interstitial pneumonia and acquired immune deficiency syndrome. Plain film and CT observations. Pediatr Radiol 1992;22:603–6.
4. Andiman W, Martin K, Rubinstein A, et al. Opportunistic lymphoproliferations associated with Epstein-Barr viral DNA in infants and children with AIDS. Lancet 1985;2:1390–3.

5. Atagi S, Sakatani M, Akira M, Yamamoto S, Ueda E. Pulmonary hyalinzing granuloma with Castleman's disease. Intern Med 1994;33:689–91.
6. Awotedu AA, Otulana BA, Ukoli CO. Giant lymph node hyperplasia of the lung (Castleman's disease) associated with recurrent pleural effusion. Thorax 1990;45:775–6.
7. Banerjee D, Ahmad D. Malignant lymphoma complicating lymphocytic interstitial pneumonia: a monoclonal B-cell neoplasm arising in a polyclonal lymphoproliferative disorder. Hum Pathol 1982;13:780–2.
8. Bankoff MS, McEniff NJ, Bhadelia RA, Garcia-Moliner M, Daly BD. Prevalence of pathologically proven intrapulmonary lymph nodes and their appearance on CT. AJR Am J Roentgenol 1996;167:629–30.
9. Barbera J, Hayashi S, Hegele R, Hogg J. Detection of Epstein-Barr virus in lymphocytic interstitial pneumonia by in situ hybridization. Am Rev Respir Dis 1992;145:940–6.
10. Barrie JR, English JC, Müller N. Castleman's disease of the lung: radiographic, high-resolution CT, and pathologic findings. AJR Am J Roentgenol 1996;166:1055–6.
11. Benisch B, Peison B. The association of lymphocytic interstitial pneumonitis and systemic lupus erythematosus. Mt Sinai J Med 1979;46:398–401.
12. Bienenstock J, Johnston N, Perey D. Bronchial lymphoid tissue. I. Morphologic characteristics. Lab Invest 1973;28:686–92.
13. Bragg DG, Chor PJ, Murray KA, Kjeldsberg CR. Lymphoproliferative disorders of the lung: histopathology, clinical manifestations, and imaging features. AJR Am J Roentgenol 1994;163:273–81.
14. Brodie SJ, de la Rosa C, Howe JG, Crouch J, Travis WD, Diem K. Pediatric AIDS-associated lymphocytic interstitial pneumonia and pulmonary arterio-occlusive disease: role of VCAM-1/VLA-4 adhesion pathway and human herpesviruses. Am J Pathol 1999;154:1453–64.
15. Cadore J, Steiner-Laurent S, Greenland T, Mornex J, Loire R. Interstitial lung disease in feline immunodeficiency virus (FIV) infected cats. Res Vet Sci 1997;62:287–8.
16. Carignan S, Staples CA, Müller NL. Intrathoracic lymphoproliferative disorders in the immunocompromised patient: CT findings. Radiology 1995;197:53–8.
17. Castleman B, Iverson L, Menendez V. Localized mediastinal lymph-node hyperplasia resembling thymoma. Cancer 1956;9:822–30.
18. Centers for Disease Control and Prevention. 1993 revised classification system for HIV infection and expanded surveillance case definition for AIDS among adolescents and adults. JAMA 1993;269:729–30.
19. Chamberlain DW, Hyland RH, Ross DJ. Diphenylhydantoin-induced lymphocytic interstitial pneumonia. Chest 1986;90:458–60.
20. Chayt K, Harper M, Marselle L, et al. Detection of HTLV-III RNA in lungs of patients with AIDS and pulmonary involvement. JAMA 1986;256:2356–9.
21. Church J, Nye C, Isaacs H. Lymphocyte subsets in lymphoid interstitial pneumonitis. Arch Pathol Lab Med 1984;108:861–2.
22. Classification system for human immunodeficiency virus (HIV) in children under 13 years of age. MMWR Morb Mortal Wkly Rep 1987;36:225–6.
23. Colby TV, Carrington CB. Lymphoreticular tumors and infiltrates of the lung. Pathol Annu 1983;18[Pt 1]:27–70.
24. Colby TV, Koss MN, Travis WD. Tumors of the lower respiratory tract. Atlas of Tumor Pathology, 3rd Series, Fascicle 13. Washington, D. C.: Armed Forces Institute of Pathology; 1994:419–64.
25. Colby TV, Yousem SA. Pulmonary lymphoid neoplasms. Semin Diagn Pathol 1985;2:183–96.
26. Corrin B. Pathology of the lungs. London: Churchill Livingstone; 2000.
27. Dawson A, Gibbs AR, Anderson G. An unusual perilocular pattern of pulmonary interstitial fibrosis associated with Crohn's disease. Histopathology 1993;23:553–6.
28. DeCoteau W, Tourville D, Ambrus J, Montes M, Adler R, Tomasi TJ. Lymphoid interstitial pneumonitis and autoerythrocyte sensitization syndrome. A case with deposition of immunoglobulins on the alveolar basement membrane. Arch Intern Med 1974;134:519–22.
29. Deheinzelin D, Capelozzi VL, Kairalla RA, Barbas Filho JV, Saldiva PH, de Carvalho CR. Interstitial lung disease in primary Sjögren's syndrome. Clinical-pathological evaluation and response to treatment. Am J Respir Crit Care Med 1996;154:794–9.
30. Delventhal S, Brandis A, Ostertag H, Pabst R. Low incidence of bronchus-associated lymphoid tissue (BALT) in chronically inflamed human lungs. Virchows Arch [Cell Pathol] 1992;62:271–4.
31. Delventhal S, Hensel A, Petzoldt K, Pabst R. Effects of microbial stimulation on the number, size and activity of bronchus-associated lymphoid tissue (BALT) structures in the pig. Int J Exp Pathol 1992;73:351–7.
32. Denis M, Ghadirian E. Alveolar macrophages from subjects infected with HIV-1 express macrophage inflammatory protein-1 alpha (MIP-1 alpha): contribution to the CD8+ alveolitis. Clin Exp Immunol 1994;96:187–92.

33. Denis M, Ghadirian E. Dysregulation of interleukin 8, interleukin 10, and interleukin 12 release by alveolar macrophages from HIV type 1-infected subjects. AIDS Res Hum Retroviruses 1994;10:1619–27.
34. Dupin N, Diss TL, Kellam P, et al. HHV-8 is associated with a plasmablastic variant of Castleman disease that is linked to HHV-8-positive plasmablastic lymphoma. Blood 2000;95:1406–12.
35. Elenitoba-Johnson K, Medeiros LJ, Khorsand J, King TC. Lymphoma of the mucosa-associated lymphoid tissue of the lung. A multifocal case of common clonal origin. Am J Clin Pathol 1995;103:341–5.
36. Fackler J, Nagel J, Adler W, Mildvan PT, Ambinder RF. Epstein-Barr virus infection in a child with acquired immunodeficiency syndrome. Am J Dis Child 1985;139:1000–4.
37. Faguet G, Webb H, Agee J, Ricks W. Immunologically diagnosed malignancy in Sjogren's pseudolymphoma. Am J Med 1978;65:424–9.
38. Fishback N, Koss M. Update on lymphoid interstitial pneumonitis. Curr Opin Pulm Med 1996;2(5):429–33.
39. Fox CH, Tenner-Racz K, Racz P, Firpo A, Pizzo PA, Fauci AS. Lymphoid germinal centers are reservoirs of human immunodeficiency virus type 1 RNA. J Infect Dis 1991;164:1051–7.
40. Franchi LM, Chin TW, Nussbaum E, Riker J, Robert M, Talbert WM. Familial pulmonary nodular lymphoid hyperplasia. J Pediatr 1992; 121:89–92.
41. Fraser RS, Müller NL, Colman N, Pare PD. Lymphoproliferative disorders and leukemia. In: Fraser RF, Müller NL, Colman N, Pare PD, eds. Fraser and Pare's diagnosis of diseases of the chest, 4th ed. Philadelphia: WB Saunders; 1999:1269–330.
42. Fujimoto N, Segewa Y, Takigawa N, et al. Two cases of intrapulmonary lymph node presenting as a peripheral nodular shadow: diagnostic differentiation from lung cancer. Lung Cancer 1998;20:203–9.
43. Grattan-Smith D, Harrison LF, Singleton EB. Radiology of AIDS in the pediatric patient. Curr Probl Diagn Radiol 1992;21:79–109.
44. Greenberg S, Haley M, Jendkins D, Fischer S. Lymphoplasmacytic pneumonia with accompanying dysproteinemia. Arch Pathol 1973;96: 73–80.
45. Grieco M, Chinoy-Acharya P. Lymphocytic interstitial pneumonia associated with the acquired immune deficiency syndrome. Am Rev Respir Dis 1985;131:952–5.
46. Griffiths MH, Miller RF, Semple SJ. Interstitial pneumonitis in patients infected with the human immunodeficiency virus. Thorax 1995;50: 1141–6.
47. Hayashi M, Aoshiba K, Shimada M, Izawa Y, Yasui S, Nagai A. Kaposi's sarcoma-associated herpesvirus infection in the lung in multicentric Castleman's disease. Intern Med 1999;38: 279–82.
48. Helman C, Keeton G, Benatar S. Lymphoid interstitial pneumonia with associated chronic active hepatitis and renal tubular acidosis. Am Rev Respir Dis 1977;115:161–4.
49. Honda O, Johkoh T, Ichikado K, et al. Differential diagnosis of lymphocytic interstitial pneumonia and malignant lymphoma on high-resolution CT. Am J Roentgenol 1999;173:71–4.
50. Howling SJ, Hansell DM, Wells AU, Nicholson AG, Flint JD, Müller NL. Follicular bronchiolitis: thin-section CT and histologic findings. Radiology 1999;212:637–42.
51. Itescu S. Diffuse infiltrative lymphocytosis syndrome in children and adults infected with HIV-1: a model of rheumatic illness caused by acquired viral infection. Am J Reprod Immunol 1992;28:247–50.
52. Itescu S, Brancato L, Buxbaum J, et al. A diffuse infiltrative CD8 lymphocytosis syndrome in human immunodeficiency virus (HIV) infection: a host immune response associated with HLA-DR5. Ann Int Med 1990;112:3–10.
53. Johkoh T, Müller NL, Ichikado K, et al. Intrathoracic multicentric Castleman disease: CT findings in 12 patients. Radiology 1998;209:477–81.
54. Johkoh T, Müller NL, Pickford HA, et al. Lymphocytic interstitial pneumonia: thin-section CT findings in 22 patients. Radiology 1999;212: 567–72.
55. Joshi V, Kauffman S, Oleske J, et al. Polyclonal polymorphic B-cell lymphoproliferative disorder with prominent pulmonary involvement in children with acquired immune deficiency syndrome. Cancer 1987;59:1455–62.
56. Joshi V, Oleske J, Minnefor A, et al. Pathologic pulmonary findings in children with the acquired immunodeficiency syndrome: a study of ten cases. Hum Pathol 1985;16:241–6.
57. Joshi VV, Oleske JM, Saad S, Connor EM, Rapkin RH, Minnefor AB. Pathology of opportunistic infections in children with acquired immune deficiency syndrome. Pediatr Pathol 1986;6:145–50.
58. Julsrud P, Brown L, Li C, et al. Pulmonary processes of mature-appearing lymphocytes: pseudolymphoma, well-differentiated lymphocytic lymphoma and lymphocytic interstitial pneumonitis. Radiology 1978;127:289–96.

59. Katzenstein AL, Fiorelli RF. Nonspecific interstitial pneumonia/fibrosis. Histologic features and clinical significance. Am J Surg Pathol 1994;18:136–47.
60. Kennedy J, Nathwani B, Burke J, Hill LR, Rappoport H. Pulmonary lymphomas and lymphoid lesions. A clinicopathologic and immunologic study of 64 patients. Cancer 1985;56: 539–52.
61. Koga M, Umemoto Y, Nishikawa M, Nakashima K, Ishihara T, Furukawa S. A case of lymphoid interstitial pneumonia in a 3-month-old boy not associated with HIV infection: immunohistochemistry of lung biopsy specimens and serum transforming growth factor-beta 1 assay. Pathol Int 1997;47(10):698–702.
62. Kohler P, Cook R, Brown W, Manguso R. Common variable hypogammaglobulinemia with T-cell nodular lymphoid interstitial pneumonitis and B-cell nodular lymphoid hyperplasia: different lymphocyte populations with a similar response to prednisone therapy. J Allergy Clin Immunol 1982;70:299–305.
63. Koss M, Hochholzer L, Langloss J, Wehunt W, Lazarus A. Lymphoid interstitial pneumonia: clinicopathological and immunopathological findings in 18 cases. Pathology 1987;19:178–85.
64. Koss M, Hochholzer L, Nichols P, Wehunt W, Lazarus A. Primary non-Hodgkin's lymphoma and pseudolymphoma of lung: a study of 161 patients. Hum Pathol 1983;14:1024–38.
65. Kradin R, Mark E. Benign lymphoid disorders of the lung, with a theory regarding their development. Hum Pathol 1983;14:857–967.
66. Kradin RI, Spirn PW, Mark EJ. Intrapulmonary lymph nodes. Clinical, radiologic, and pathologic features. Chest 1985;87:662–7.
67. Kurosu K, Yumoto N, Furukawa M, Kuriyama T, Mikata A. Third complementarity-determining-region sequence analysis of lymphocytic interstitial pneumonia: most cases demonstrate a minor monoclonal population hidden among normal lymphocyte clones. Am J Respir Crit Care Med 1997;155(4):1453–60.
68. L'Hoste R, Filippa D, Lieberman P, Bretsky S. Primary pulmonary lymphomas. A clinicopathologic analysis of 36 cases. Cancer 1984;54:1397–406.
69. Lairmore M, Poulson J, Adducci T, DeMartini JC. Lentivirus-induced lymphoproliferative disease. Comparative pathogenicity of phenotypically distinct ovine lentivirus strain. Am J Pathol 1988;130:80–90.
70. Levinson A, Hopewell P, Stites D, Spitler LE, Fudenberg HH. Co-existent lymphoid interstitial pneumonia, pernicious anemia and aggammaglobulinemia: comment on autoimmune pathogenesis. Arch Intern Med 1976;136:213–6.
71. Li G, Hansmann ML, Zwingers T, Lennert K. Primary lymphoma of the lung: morphological, immunohistochemical and clinical features. Histopathology 1990;16:519–31.
72. Liebow A, Carrington C. Diffuse pulmonary lymphoreticular infiltrations associated with dysproteinemia. Med Clin North Am 1973;57:809–43.
73. Lin RY, Gruber PJ, Saunders R, Perla EN. Lymphocytic interstitial pneumonitis in adult HIV infection. N Y State J Med 1988;88:273–6.
74. Malamou-Mitsi V, Tsai M, Gal A, Koss M, O'Leary T. Lymphoid interstitial pneumonia not associated with HIV infection: role of Epstein-Barr virus. Mod Pathol 1992;5:487–91.
75. Marchevsky A, Padilla M, Kaneko M, Kleinerman J. Localized lymphoid nodules of lung. A reappraisal of the lymphoma versus pseudolymphoma dilemma. Cancer 1983;51:2070–7.
76. Matthay RA, Schwarz MI, Petty TL, et al. Pulmonary manifestations of systemic lupus erythematosus: review of twelve cases of acute lupus pneumonitis. Medicine (Baltimore) 1975;54:397–409.
77. Maurer J, Chei HS. Lymphocytic interstitial pneumonitis manifesting concurrently with active tuberculosis. Arch Intern Med 1984;144: 1855–7.
78. Mayaud CM, Cadranel J. HIV in the lung: guilty or not guilty? [Editorial]. Thorax 1993;48:1191–5.
79. McGuinness G, Scholes JV, Jagirdar JS, et al. Unusual lymphoproliferative disorders in nine adults with HIV or AIDS: CT and pathologic findings. Radiology 1995;197:59–65.
80. Montes M, Tomasi T, Noehren T, Culver G. Lymphoid interstitial pneumonitis with monoclonal gammopathy. Am Rev Respir Dis 1968;98:277–80.
81. Moran CA, Suster S, Pavlova Z, Mullick FG, Koss MN. The spectrum of pathological changes in the lung in children with the acquired immunodeficiency syndrome: an autopsy study of 36 cases. Hum Pathol 1994;25:877–82.
82. Moran T, Totten R. Lymphoid interstitial pneumonia with dysproteinemia. Report of two cases with plasma cell predominance. Am J Clin Pathol 1970;54:747–56.
83. Morris J, Rosen M, Marchevsky A, et al. Lymphocytic interstitial pneumonia in patients as risk for the acquired immune deficiency syndrome. Chest 1987;91:63–7.
84. Murphy PM, Fox C, Travis WD, Koenig S, Fauci AS. Acquired immunodeficiency syndrome may present as severe restrictive lung disease. Am J Med 1989;86:237–40.

85. Neil GA, Lukie BE, Cockroft DW, Murphy F. Lymphocytic interstitial pneumonia and abdominal lymphoma complicating celiac sprue. J Clin Gastroenterol 1986;8:282–5.
86. Nicholson AG, Kim H, Corrin B, et al. The value of classifying interstitial pneumonitis in childhood according to defined histological patterns. Histopathology 1998;33:203–11.
87. Nicholson AG, Wotherspoon A, Diss T, et al. Reactive lymphoid disorders. Histopathology 1995;26:405–12.
88. Nowakowski M, Clarke LM, Amaro R, Pelligrino MG, Sierra MF, Steiner P. Characterization of cells, immunoglobulins, and immune complexes present in the bronchoalveolar lavage of pediatric AIDS patients. Reg Immunol 1992;4:34–40.
89. O'Brodovich H, Moser M, Lu L, et al. Familial lymphoid interstitial pneumonia: a long-term follow-up. Pediatrics 1980;65:523–8.
90. Oleske J, Minnefor A, Cooper R, et al. Immune deficiency syndrome in children. JAMA 1983;249:2345–9.
91. Pauk JS, Corey L. Disease associations, diagnosis, and treatment of human herpesvirus 8. In: Rose BD, ed. Uptodate in medicine. Wellesley: BDR-Uptodate; 2000.
92. Pejaver RK, Watson AH. Castleman's disease. Respir Med 1994;88:309–11.
93. Perreault C, Cousineau S, D'Angelo G, et al. Lymphoid interstitial pneumonia after allogeneic bone marrow transplantation. A possible manifestation of chronic graft-versus-host disease. Cancer 1985;55:1–9.
94. Perry L, Florio R, Dewar A, Nicholson A. Giant lamellar bodies as a feature of pulmonary low-grade MALT lymphomas. Histopathology 2000;36:240–4.
95. Peterson BA, Frizzera G. Multicentric Castleman's disease. Semin Oncol 1993;20:636–47.
96. Plata F, Garcia-Pons F, Ryter A, et al. HIV-1 infection of lung alveolar fibroblasts and macrophages in humans. AIDS Res Hum Retroviruses 1990;6:979–86.
97. Popa V. Lymphocytic interstitial pneumonia of common variable immunodeficiency. Ann Allergy 1988;60:203–6.
98. Principi N, Marchisio P, Massironi E, et al. Effect of zidovudine in HIV-infected children with lymphocytic interstitial pneumonitis [Letter]. AIDS 1991;5:468–9.
99. Reittner P, Fotter R, Lindbichler F, et al. HRCT features in a 5-year-old child with follicular bronchiolitis. Pediatr Radiol 1997;27:877–9.
100. Resnick L, Pitchenik A, Fisher E, Croney R. Detection of HTLV-III/LAV-specific IgG and antigen in bronchoalveolar lavage fluid from two patients with lymphocytic interstitial pneumonitis associated with AIDS-related complex. Am J Med 1987;82:553–6.
101. Roca B, Ferran G, Simon E, Cortes V. Lymphoid hyperplasia of the lung and Evan's syndrome in IgA deficiency [Letter]. Am J Med 1999;106:121–2.
102. Rubinstein A, Morecki R, Silverman B, et al. Pulmonary disease in children with acquired immune deficiency syndrome and AIDS-related complex. J Pediatr 1986;108:498–503.
103. Saldana MJ, Mones J. Pulmonary pathology in AIDS: atypical Pneumocystis carinii infection and lymphoid interstitial pneumonia. Thorax 1994;49:S46–55.
104. Sato A, Hayakawa H, Uchiyama H, Chida K. Cellular distribution of bronchus-associated lymphoid tissue in rheumatoid arthritis. Am J Respir Crit Care Med 1996;154:1903–7.
105. Scarborough M, Lishman S, Shaw P, Fakoya A, Miller RF. Lymphocytic interstitial pneumonitis in an HIV-infected adult: response to antiretroviral therapy. Int J Std Aids 2000;11:119–22.
106. Schwarz M. Lymphoplasmacytic interstitial pneumonias. In: Schwarz M, King TE Jr, eds. Interstitial lung disease, 2nd ed. St. Louis: Mosby Year Book; 1992:405–12.
107. Smith JL, Hodges E, Quin CT, McCarthy KP, Wright DH. Frequent T and B cell oligoclones in histologically and immunophenotypically characterized angioimmunoblastic lymphadenopathy. Am J Pathol 2000;156:661–9.
108. Solal-Celigny P, Couderc L, Herman D, et al. Lymphoid interstitial pneumonitis in acquired immunodeficiency syndrome-related complex. Am Rev Respir Dis 1985;131:956–60.
109. Strimlan CV, Rosenow EC III, Divertie MB, Harrison EG Jr. Pulmonary manifestations of Sjögren's syndrome. Chest 1976;70:354–61.
110. Strimlan CV, Rosenow EC III, Weiland LH, Brown LR. Lymphocytic interstitial pneumonitis. Review of 13 cases. Ann Intern Med 1978;88:616–21.
111. Teirstein A, Rosen MJ. Lymphocytic interstitial pneumonia. Clin Chest Med 1988;9:467–71.
112. Torii K, Ogawa K, Kawabata Y, Yokoi T, Takagi K, Miwa T. Lymphoid interstitial pneumonia as a pulmonary lesion of idiopathic plasmacytic lymphadenopathy with hyperimmunoglobulinemia. Intern Med 1994;33:237–41.
113. Travis WD. Pathologic features. In: Walzer PD, ed. Pneumocystis carinii pneumonia, 2nd ed. New York: Marcel Dekker; 1993:155–80.
114. Travis WD, Fox C, Devaney K, et al. Lymphoid pneumonitis in 50 adult patients infected with the human immunodeficiency virus: lymphocytic interstitial pneumonitis versus nonspecific interstitial pneumonitis. Hum Pathol 1992; 23:529–41.

115. Travis WD, King TE, Bateman ED, et al. ATS/ ERS International Multidisciplinary Consensus Classification of Idiopathic Interstitial Pneumonia. Am J Respir Crit Care Med 2002;165:277–304.
116. Travis WD, Lack EE, Ognibene FP, Suffredini AF, Shelhamer J. Lung biopsy interpretation in the acquired immunodeficiency syndrome: experience of the National Institutes of Health with literature review. Prog AIDS Pathol 1989;1:51–84.
117. Travis WD, Matsui K, Moss JE, Ferrnas VJ. Idiopathic nonspecific interstitial pneumonia: prognostic significance of cellular and fibrosing patterns: survival comparison with usual interstitial pneumonia and desquamative interstitial pneumonia. Am J Surg Pathol 2000;24:19–33.
118. Travis WD, Pittaluga S, Lipschik GY, et al. Atypical pathologic manifestations of Pneumocystis carinii pneumonia in the acquired immune dificiency syndrome. Review of 123 lung biopsies from 76 patients with emphasis on cysts, vascular invasion, vasculitis and granulomas. Am J Surg Pathol 1990;14:615–25.
119. Trovato R, Luppi M, Barozzi P, et al. Cellular localization of human herpesvirus 8 in nonneoplastic lymphadenopathies and chronic interstitial pneumonitis by in situ polymerase chain reaction studies. J Hum Virol 1999;2:38–44.
120. Tsunezuka Y, Sato H, Hiranuma C, et al. Intrapulmonary lymph nodes detected by exploratory video-assisted thoracoscopic surgery: appearance of helical computed tomography. Ann Thorac Cardiovasc Surg 2000;6:369–72.
121. Uziel Y, Hen B, Cordoba M, Wotach B. Lymphocytic interstitial pneumonitis preceding polyarticular juvenile rheumatoid arthritis. Clin Exp Rheumatol 1998;16:617–9.
122. Vath RR, Alexander CB, Fulmer JD. The lymphocytic infiltrative lung diseases. Clin Chest Med 1982;3:619–34.
123. Waters K, Bale P, Isaacs D, Mellis C. Successful chloroquine therapy in a child with lymphoid interstitial pneumonitis. J Pediatr 1991;119:989–91.
124. Yokomise H, Mizuno H, Ike O, Wada H, Hitomi S, Itoh H. Importance of intrapulmonary lymph nodes in the differential diagnosis of small pulmonary nodular shadows. Chest 1998;113:703–6.
125. Yood RA, Steigman DM, Gill LR. Lymphocytic interstitial pneumonitis in a patient with systemic lupus erythematosus. Lupus 1995;4:161–3.
126. Yousem S, Colby T, Carrington C. Follicular bronchitis/bronchiolitis. Hum Pathol 1985;16:700–3.
127. Ziza J, Brun-Vezinet F, Venet A, et al. Lymphadenopathy-associated virus isolated from bronchoalveolar lavage fluid in AIDS-related complex with lymphoid interstitial pneumonitis [Letter]. N Engl J Med 1985;313:183.

6
CONNECTIVE TISSUE AND INFLAMMATORY BOWEL DISEASES

Pleuropulmonary complications are common in patients with systemic disorders, especially connective tissue and inflammatory bowel diseases. All components of the respiratory system can be affected, singly or in combination. In some cases the pleuropulmonary manifestation is the initial finding and the systemic disorder only becomes apparent months to years later. Moreover, the pleuropulmonary manifestations may be the major cause of morbidity and mortality in these patients.

The incidence of pleuropulmonary complications varies for different entities. Almost all patients with scleroderma have some type of lung involvement; in contrast, lung involvement is relatively uncommon in ankylosing spondylitis. Because of improvements in the detection of lung disease (exercise gas exchange, bronchoalveolar lavage, and high-resolution lung scanning), the incidence of pleuropulmonary complications is rising.

There are several general concepts that should guide the evaluation of patients with a systemic disorder and lung involvement. Pulmonary manifestations of connective tissue disorders and inflammatory bowel diseases include many different histologic patterns (Table 6-1) (29,73,90,204,206,218). In most cases, the histologic patterns are the same as those that occur in patients without underlying systemic disorders. Consequently, it is impossible for the pathologist to know about an associated condition based on a review of a lung biopsy and it is essential that there be detailed communication between the clinician and the pathologist regarding the patient's clinical history.

Determination of the precise nature of the lung involvement in most of the connective tissue diseases is often difficult due to the high incidence of lung disease caused by disease-associated complications, for example, esophageal dysfunction predisposing to aspiration and secondary infections, respiratory muscle weakness causing atelectasis, therapeutic complications often leading to opportunistic infections, and associated malignancies. In most cases, the underlying systemic disease is known and the major reason for the lung biopsy is to rule out infection or drug reaction, determine the diagnosis and assess the extent and severity of the pulmonary abnormalities. Transbronchial lung biopsies generally do not provide an adequate sample to definitively confirm a diagnosis or rule out other disorders. Bronchoalveolar lavage (BAL) is a useful tool for evaluating problems frequently encountered in patients with connective tissue disease, such as drug-induced pulmonary dysfunction, infection, pulmonary hemorrhage, alveolar proteinosis, and malignancy. Since drug toxicity and infections may cause the same histologic reaction patterns as the underlying systemic disorder, it is important to carefully correlate the histologic findings with a good clinical history and to routinely examine lung biopsies for organisms using special stains.

Most of the therapeutic reports of the many pleuropulmonary manifestations of the connective tissue diseases have been anecdotal, retrospective, or uncontrolled in which poorly stratified groups are treated for variable lengths of time. Therefore, most treatment is empiric.

HISTOLOGIC SPECTRUM OF THE PLEUROPARENCHYMAL REACTIONS

The pulmonary manifestations of each systemic disorder have their own characteristic histologic patterns, but there is considerable overlap (Table 6-1). Nearly all of the histologic patterns associated with the diffuse parenchymal lung diseases discussed in chapter 3 can be found with connective tissue diseases. In fact, in many cases the lung shows several histologic patterns rather than only one. Most of the literature about interstitial lung disease in systemic disorders was written before current concepts regarding the patterns of usual interstitial pneumonia (UIP) and nonspecific interstitial pneumonia (NSIP) were developed (35, 90,102,133,229). Recent data suggest that the NSIP pattern (previously called cellular interstitial pneumonitis) may be the most common pattern of interstitial lung disease encountered in some of the connective tissue disorders, such as scleroderma, rheumatoid arthritis, polymyositis/

Table 6-1

PATTERNS OF LUNG DISEASE IN CONNECTIVE TISSUE DISORDERS AND INFLAMMATORY BOWEL DISEASE

	RA[a]	SLE	Sclero-derma	PM/DM	SS	MCTD	AS	IBD	PC
Pleural Disease									
Pleuritis +/– effusion	+	+	+	+	+	+	+		
Pleural fibrosis	+	+	+	+	+	+	+		
Sterile or septic empyema	+						+		
Spontaneous pneumothorax				+			+		
Interstitial/Parenchymal Lesions									
Usual interstitial pneumonia (IP)	+	+	+	+	+	+			
Diffuse alveolar damage	+	+	+	+		+			
Nonspecific IP	+	+	+	+	+	+		+	
Organizing pneumonia	+	+	+	+	+	+		+	
Lymphocytic IP/LH	+				+	+			
Granulomatous IP	+	+				+		+	
Apical fibrobullous disease	+		+			+	+		
Aspiration pneumonia			+	+	+	+	+		
Necrobiotic rheumatoid nodule +/– rupture	+					+			
Amyloid deposits	+				+	+	+		
Alveolar Lesions									
Diffuse hemorrhage	+	+	+	+		+			
Eosinophilic pneumonia	+					+		+	
Alveolar proteinosis				+		+			
Vascular Lesions									
Vasculitis	+	+	+	+	+	+		+	
Pulmonary hypertension	+	+	+	+	+	+			
Thromboembolism		+							
Airway Lesions									
Bronchiolitis +/– fibrosis	+	+		+	+	+		+	+
Follicular bronchiolitis	+	+			+	+		+	
Constrictive bronchiolitis	+					+		+	
Bronchiectasis	+					+		+	
Xerotrachea					+				
Bronchocentric granulomatosis	+	+					+	+	
Diffuse panbronchiolitis	+							+	
Indirect Respiratory Effects									
Diaphragmatic or respiratory muscle dysfunction		+		+		+			
Thoracic cage immobility	+						+		
Atelectasis (shrinking)		+		+	+		+		
Neoplasms									
Lung cancer			+			+	+		
Lymphoma		+			+	+			
Kaposi's sarcoma		+							

[a]RA = rheumatoid arthritis, SLE = systemic lupus erythematosus, PM/DM = polymyositis/dermatomyositis, SS = Sjögren's syndrome, MCTD = mixed connective tissue disease, AS = ankylosing spondylitis, IBD = inflammatory bowel disease, PC = polychondritis; LH = lymphoid hyperplasia.

dermatomyositis, and mixed connective tissue disease. This probably accounts for the improved corticosteroid response and better survival of these patients compared to patients with idiopathic pulmonary fibrosis. Also, the organizing pneumonia (OP) pattern is a distinctive histologic lesion that is seen in patients with bronchiolitis obliterans organizing pneumonia (BOOP) associated with connective tissue disease. The OP pattern is particularly problematic because it is often difficult to distinguish clinically from other forms of idiopathic interstitial pneumonia and it has the unique potential to be extremely responsive to treatment. Lymphocytic interstitial pneumonia (LIP) commonly accompanies the primary or secondary form of Sjögren's syndrome. Constrictive or obliterative bronchiolitis, associated with severe and progressive obstructive lung disease, is a complication that is being increasingly recognized in patients with rheumatoid arthritis.

Pulmonary vascular disease is commonly recognized in patients with scleroderma and is seen with increasing frequency in those with systemic lupus erythematosus. Histologically, the vascular lesions may be similar to those found in the syndrome of primary pulmonary hypertension seen in young women without connective tissue disorders (plexogenic arteriopathy; see chapter 15). This form of pulmonary hypertension must be distinguished from the secondary forms induced by hypoxic vasoconstriction secondary to the underlying interstitial lung disease. Patients with systemic lupus erythematosus and the antiphospholipid syndrome may develop recurrent pulmonary emboli, resulting in pulmonary hypertension. Also, a small vessel vasculitis involving the arterioles and small muscular pulmonary arteries may be seen in systemic lupus erythematosus and less often in rheumatoid arthritis, polymyositis/dermatomyositis, and mixed connective tissue disease.

Diffuse alveolar damage (DAD) is the underlying histopathologic lesion in many patients with rapidly progressive lung disease associated with the connective tissue diseases. It can present as a de novo process in acute lupus pneumonitis and polymyositis/dermatomyositis; or it can be secondary to acute lung injury associated with the acute respiratory distress syndrome or drug toxicity.

Diffuse alveolar hemorrhage, sometimes associated with pulmonary capillaritis, can occur in the connective tissue disorders, especially systemic lupus erythematosus. Cases have also been reported in rheumatoid arthritis, Sjögren's syndrome, polymyositis/dermatomyositis, and mixed connective tissue disease.

Since the pathologic features of most lesions that occur in systemic disorders are identical to those seen in patients with no known underlying disease, and are discussed in detail elsewhere in this book, this chapter will emphasize the clinical and radiologic features of the pulmonary manifestations. The clinical and radiographic manifestations of the interstitial lung diseases associated with the connective tissue diseases are virtually identical to those of the idiopathic varieties (see chapter 3). However, with the recent evolution in terminology and criteria for the various patterns of disease, it is helpful to use the term pattern when talking about the lung biopsy histology (i.e., UIP, NSIP, or OP pattern) and to mention the underlying disease (i.e., rheumatoid arthritis) when referring to the clinicopathologic diagnosis (i.e. UIP, NSIP, or OP associated with rheumatoid arthritis). The major systemic disorders discussed include rheumatoid arthritis, systemic lupus erythematosus, scleroderma, polymyositis/dermatomyositis, Sjögren's syndrome, mixed connective tissue disease, ankylosing spondylitis, relapsing polychondritis, and inflammatory bowel disease. Discussion of the features of the less common disorders of Marfan's syndrome and primary biliary cirrhosis can be found elsewhere (29,30,204).

RHEUMATOID ARTHRITIS

Definition. Rheumatoid arthritis is a chronic, nonsuppurative arthritis which often affects the peripheral joints in a symmetric pattern (198). A wide variety of pulmonary manifestations occur in patients with rheumatoid arthritis including pleural, interstitial/parenchymal, alveolar, vascular, and airway lesions (Table 6-1).

Clinical Features. Rheumatoid arthritis is associated with a wide variety of pleural and pulmonary manifestations (Table 6-1). Pleural effusion and pleuritis are the most common. The lung involvement is commonly subclinical; therefore, its identification requires careful surveillance and monitoring of abnormalities to avoid progressive and irreversible injury.

Pleural effusions occur in 3 to 5 percent of rheumatoid arthritis patients, however, pleuritic manifestations can be found in up to 20 percent throughout the course of the disease. Pleuritis is present in up to 40 percent of autopsy cases. Pleural complications occur primarily in men, with a 5 to 1 male to female ratio, and occur most frequently during episodes of active articular disease (90,218). Patients with pleural disease are likely to have severe arthritis, and subcutaneous nodules are seen in approximately 80 percent (90,218). The pleural effusions in patients with rheumatoid arthritis are less often symptomatic, less frequently bilateral, and usually larger than those in patients with systemic lupus erythematosus (90,218).

The best recognized histologic patterns of interstitial lung disease that occur in patients with rheumatoid arthritis are UIP and OP. The NSIP pattern has been reported in a few patients (57,102), however, it is not well described and its frequency is not known. Approximately 1 to 4 percent of rheumatoid arthritis patients develop a UIP pattern of interstitial lung disease (7,56,124,149,210). Such patients have a poor prognosis, with a median survival time of 3.5 years and a 39 percent 5-year survival rate (206). UIP tends to be a relatively early manifestation of rheumatoid arthritis since 70 percent of patients who develop this lesion do so within 4 years of the onset of joint symptoms (218). Cases of BOOP (49,96,148,156,211) are reported and the patients have a good prognosis, similar to patients with cryptogenic organizing pneumonia (idiopathic BOOP). Chronic eosinophilic pneumonia may occur in rheumatoid arthritis patients (34,144,145,177) and it can be difficult to determine whether it is induced by penicillamine or gold therapy, or the underlying rheumatoid arthritis (184).

Pulmonary rheumatoid nodules usually occur in men with advanced seropositive rheumatoid arthritis who frequently have subcutaneous rheumatoid nodules (73,90,218). The nodules rarely present before the arthritis. Pulmonary rheumatoid nodules are usually asymptomatic unless infection, hemorrhage, rupture, or bronchopleural fistulae complicate them. *Caplan's syndrome* occurs when rheumatoid nodules are associated with coal worker's pneumoconiosis or silicosis (11,79,204,218).

Several airway lesions occur in rheumatoid arthritis including constrictive bronchiolitis, follicular bronchiolitis, bronchiectasis, and bronchocentric granulomatosis. Patients with constrictive bronchiolitis (138,174) have a downhill clinical course with severe pulmonary obstruction. Treatment with penicillamine is associated with most but not all cases of constrictive bronchiolitis in patients with rheumatoid arthritis (138). Follicular bronchiolitis or hyperplasia of the bronchial-associated lymphoid tissue (BALT) can be seen in rheumatoid arthritis patients and consists of hyperplastic lymphoid follicles surrounding the bronchioles (see chapter 5) (77,88,229). Bronchiectasis is a potential late complication of rheumatoid arthritis (82, 157,179). Bronchocentric granulomatosis has been reported in a few patients (18,78). The differential diagnosis for this histologic pattern includes mycobacterial and fungal infection.

Pulmonary vascular complications of rheumatoid arthritis are rare and include pulmonary hypertension and vasculitis. Pulmonary hypertension may have features of primary pulmonary hypertension (62,103,139, 226). Pulmonary vasculitis can occur in the context of systemic vasculitis or pulmonary hypertension (10,103).

Diffuse pulmonary hemorrhage in rheumatoid arthritis patients can be associated with penicillamine therapy or it can be a manifestation of the underlying disease (103). These patients may have positive antineutrophil cytoplasmic antibodies (ANCA) (103).

The drugs that are most commonly known to cause pulmonary toxicity in rheumatoid arthritis patients are methotrexate (176), penicillamine (70,186,188), and gold (see chapter 7) (84,144,175,202,223). Patients with pulmonary toxicity to gold usually present within 6 months of initiation of therapy with dyspnea, dry cough, and diffuse bilateral infiltrates (134, 175). Tomioka and King (202) found several features that favor gold-induced pulmonary disease over rheumatoid lung disease: female predominance, presence of fever or rash, absence of subcutaneous nodules or clubbing, low titers of rheumatoid factor at onset of lung disease, lymphocytosis in BAL fluid, and alveolar

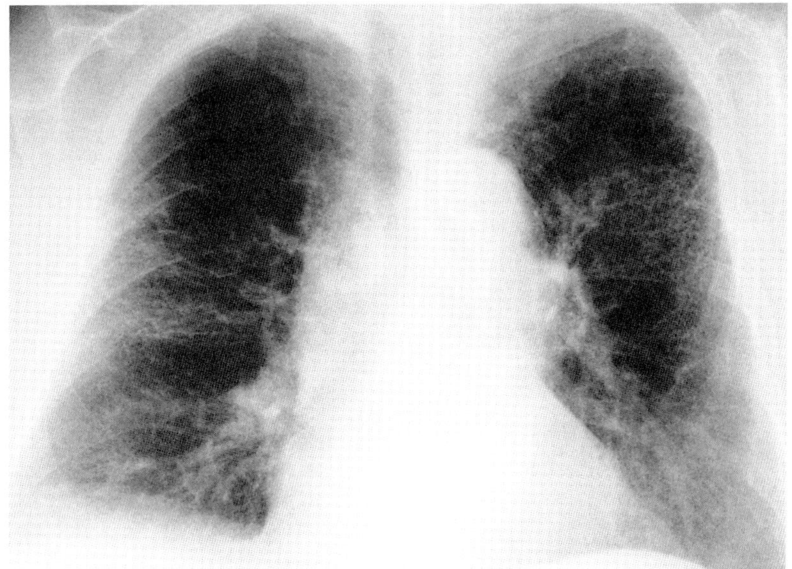

Figure 6-1

INTERSTITIAL FIBROSIS IN RHEUMATOID ARTHRITIS

Posteroanterior chest radiograph demonstrates a reticular pattern throughout both lungs. There is blunting of the right costophrenic sulcus due to chronic pleural thickening. The patient was a 65-year-old man with longstanding rheumatoid arthritis and usual interstitial pneumonia.

opacities distributed along the bronchovascular bundles on chest computed tomography (CT) (202). Constrictive bronchiolitis is a rare complication of penicillamine therapy and is seen in only 1 to 3 percent of patients (187,224). Respiratory symptoms usually occur within 10 months of starting therapy with penicillamine (range, 3 to 10 months) (224). Patients generally present with cough and dyspnea in the presence of a normal chest X ray. On lung function testing there is an obstructive ventilatory defect without bronchodilator response. Other rare complications of penicillamine include a pulmonary-renal syndrome, drug-induced lupus erythematosus, pulmonary hemorrhage, and fibrosis. Methotrexate-associated lung toxicity occurs in 5 to 10 percent of patients (65,169). Patients typically present 3 to 4 months after onset of therapy with a subacute febrile illness associated with peripheral eosinophilia in about 50 percent of cases. Cumulative dose does not appear to be important. Less often, patterns of BOOP, DAD, or pulmonary edema are seen.

Radiologic Findings. The radiologic findings of interstitial fibrosis in patients with rheumatoid arthritis are usually similar to those of idiopathic pulmonary fibrosis (185). Initially, there is a reticular pattern that involves mainly the lower lobes. With disease progression the lung involvement becomes more diffuse and there is progressive volume loss and honeycombing (fig. 6-1) (153). On high-resolution (HR) CT, the abnormalities involve mainly the subpleural lung regions and include intralobular linear opacities, irregular thickening of the interlobular septa, honeycombing, and areas of ground-glass attenuation (fig. 6-2) (153,185).

Pulmonary rheumatoid nodules are uncommon, and only seen on the chest radiograph in 0.2 percent of patients (180). The nodules may be single or multiple, involve mainly the upper or mid-lung zones, and range from 0.5 to 7.0 cm in diameter (180). Fifty percent cavitate.

The chest radiograph of patients with constrictive bronchiolitis may be normal or show hyperinflation (153,180). The HRCT is more sensitive than the radiograph and typically shows focal mosaic areas of decreased attenuation and perfusion (fig. 6-3) (2,153). HRCT performed at end-expiration demonstrates air-trapping (2).

The most common abnormality seen on HRCT in patients with rheumatoid arthritis is bronchiectasis, a finding that has been reported in up to 30 percent of patients (157). The bronchiectasis involves the central and peripheral bronchi, is usually mild, and tends to involve predominantly or exclusively the middle and lower lung zones (157).

Pathologic Findings. Virtually all of the histologic patterns of lung disease that occur in rheumatoid arthritis, except for rheumatoid nodules, are described elsewhere in this book

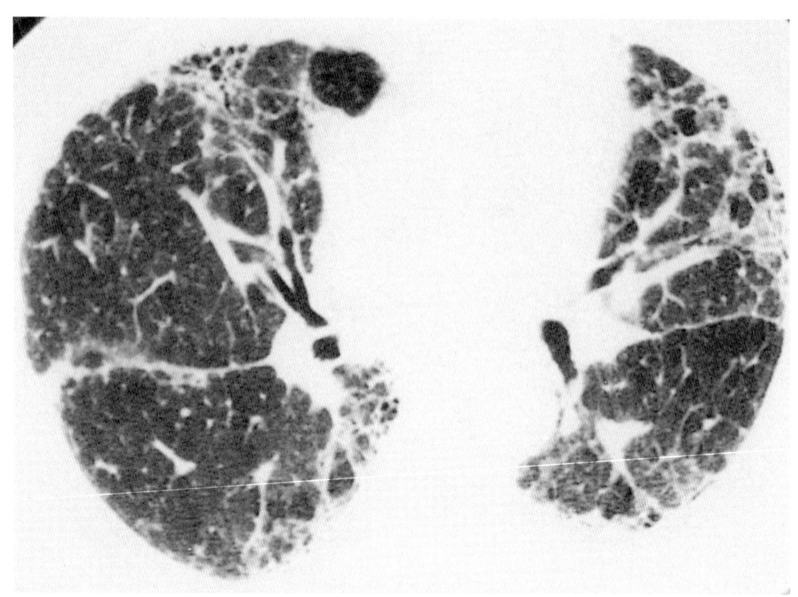

Figure 6-2

INTERSTITIAL FIBROSIS IN RHEUMATOID ARTHRITIS

HRCT demonstrates a reticular pattern and localized ground-glass opacities involving mainly the subpleural lung regions. Note the patchy distribution of the abnormalities with adjacent areas of normal lung. The findings are characteristic of usual interstitial pneumonia.

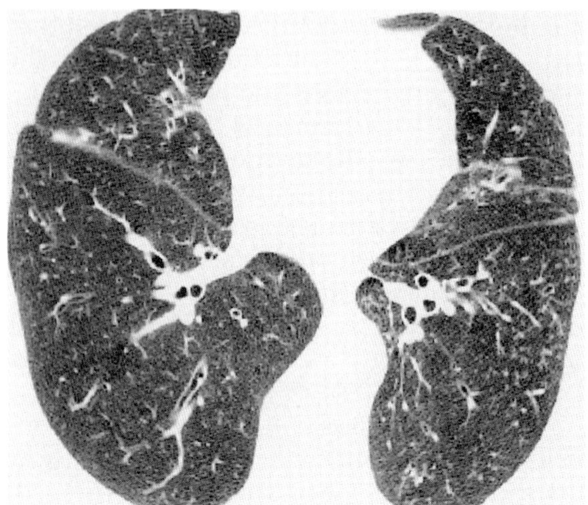

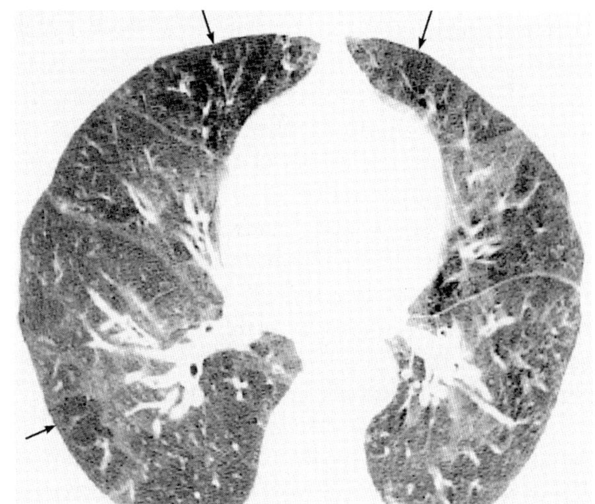

Figure 6-3

CONSTRICTIVE BRONCHIOLITIS IN RHEUMATOID ARTHRITIS

Left: HRCT at end-inspiration shows focal areas of decreased attenuation and perfusion involving mainly the dorsal lung regions. There are a few centrilobular, nodular and branching opacities in the left lower lobe and localized areas of scarring.

Right: Expiratory HRCT demonstrates air-trapping (arrows). The patient was an 84-year-old woman with rheumatoid arthritis and airway obstruction.

(Table 6-1) and they are identical to patterns in patients without rheumatoid arthritis. Some lesions, such as pleuritis (fig. 6-4) and UIP, may have more prominent chronic inflammation or lymphoid aggregates (fig. 6-4) in patients with rheumatoid arthritis, however, this feature is not specific for rheumatoid arthritis.

Pulmonary rheumatoid nodules are frequently situated in a subpleural or paraseptal location (fig. 6-5) (218,229). They consist of necrotizing granulomas with a central eosinophilic or basophilic necrotic center, surrounded by palisading histiocytes (fig. 6-6, left) (218,229). Vasculitis may be identified in the adjacent tissues

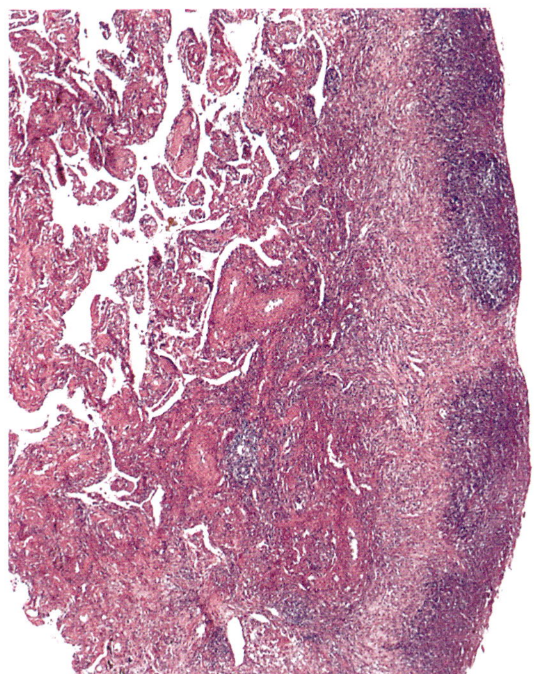

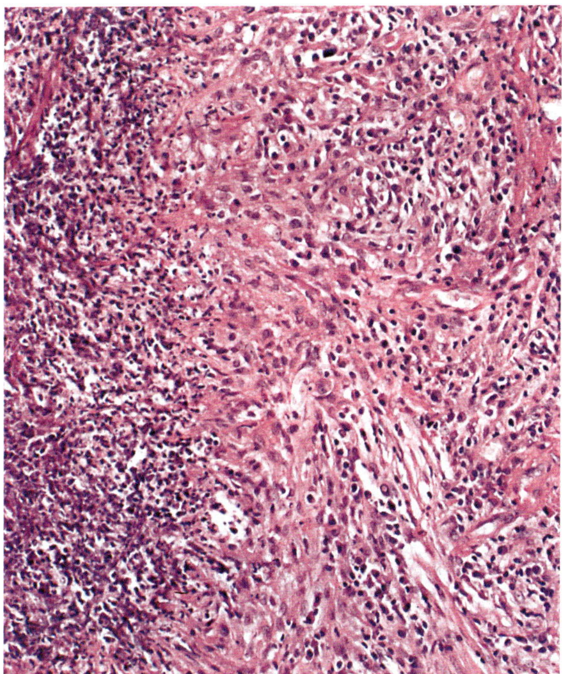

Figure 6-4

CHRONIC PLEURITIS IN RHEUMATOID ARTHRITIS

Left: The pleura is thickened by a marked chronic inflammatory infiltrate.

Right: The infiltrate consists mostly of lymphocytes with scattered plasma cells and there is a proliferation of fibrous connective tissue.

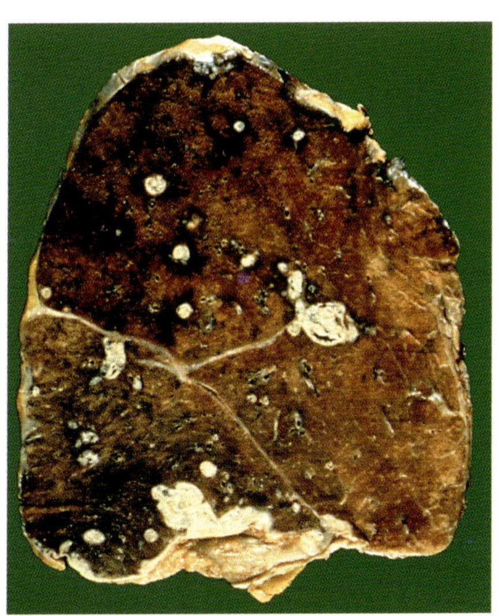

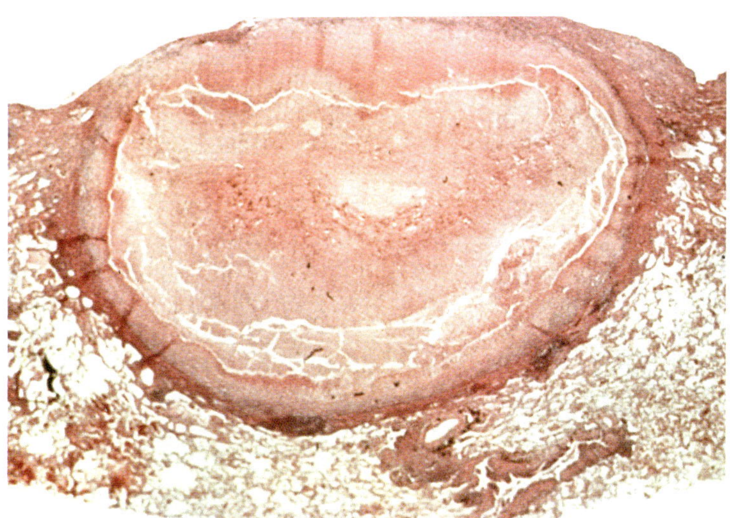

Figure 6-5

RHEUMATOID NODULE

Left: There are multiple, subpleural, yellow nodules measuring up to several centimeters in diameter. (Courtesy of Dr. Andrew Churg, Vancouver, Canada.)

Right: This rhematoid nodule protrudes into the underlying lung parenchyma. It has a necrotic center and a thick fibrous wall.

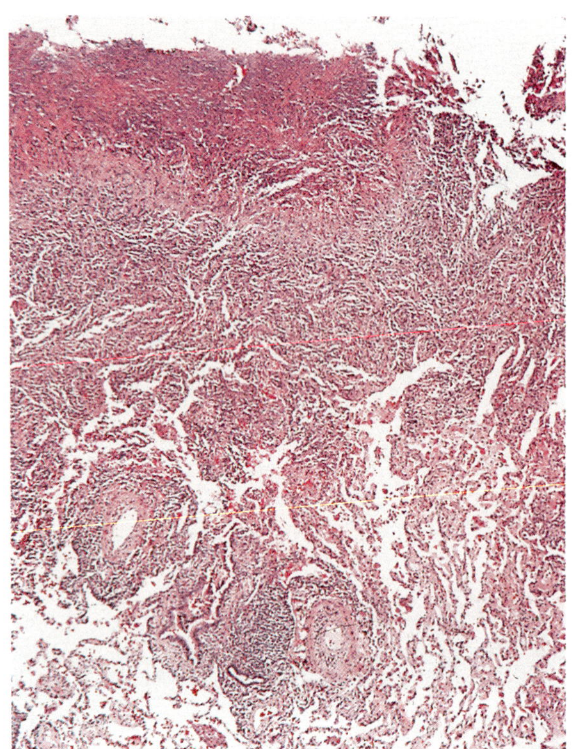

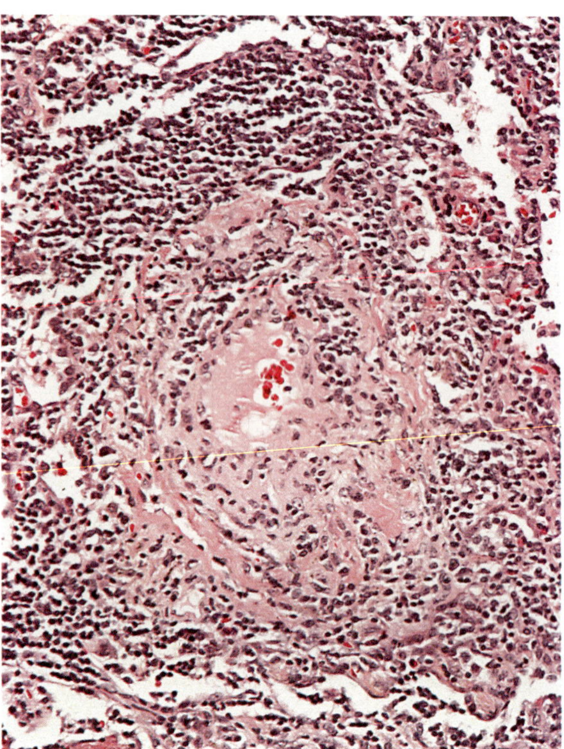

Figure 6-6

RHEUMATOID NODULE: HISTOLOGY

Left: Palisading histiocytes surround the border of the central necrotic cavity.
Right: Vasculitis is present in an adjacent blood vessel.

(fig. 6-6, right). Nodules range from several millimeters to over 7 cm in diameter (90,218). Complications include cavitation, hemorrhage, infection, and rupture forming bronchopleural fistulae. In Caplan's syndrome, anthracotic and silicotic dust deposits may be found within the rheumatoid nodules (see chapter 16). Pulmonary hemorrhage can be either chronic and characterized by prominent hemosiderosis or acute with neutrophilic capillaritis (112,203). The histologic patterns of other lesions in rheumatoid arthritis, such as follicular bronchiolitis, constrictive bronchiolitis (fig. 6-7), OP (fig. 6-8), vasculitis (fig. 6-9), and amyloid deposits (fig. 6-10), are similar to those seen in patients without collagen vascular disease.

It is common for lung biopsies to be performed in rheumatoid arthritis patients in order to determine if the lung disease is due to drug toxicity, underlying disease, or other causes. The principles for diagnosing drug toxicity are summarized in chapter 7. It is important to be familiar with the various patterns of lung injury known to be associated with the medications commonly used for treatment of rheumatoid arthritis. Penicillamine is associated with constrictive bronchiolitis, OP, follicular bronchiolitis, DAD, diffuse pulmonary hemorrhage, peripheral eosinophilia, and drug-induced systemic lupus erythematosus (184,187). Gold toxicity causes constrictive bronchiolitis, BOOP, chronic interstitial pneumonitis (nonspecific), eosinophilic pneumonias, or DAD (138). Lung biopsies from patients with methotrexate toxicity can show interstitial chronic inflammation, granulomas, giant cells, and eosinophilia.

Treatment and Prognosis. Corticosteroids may result in variable subjective and objective improvement in patients with interstitial lung disease associated with rheumatoid arthritis. Patients generally respond to withdrawal of methotrexate or gold, and the prognosis is usually

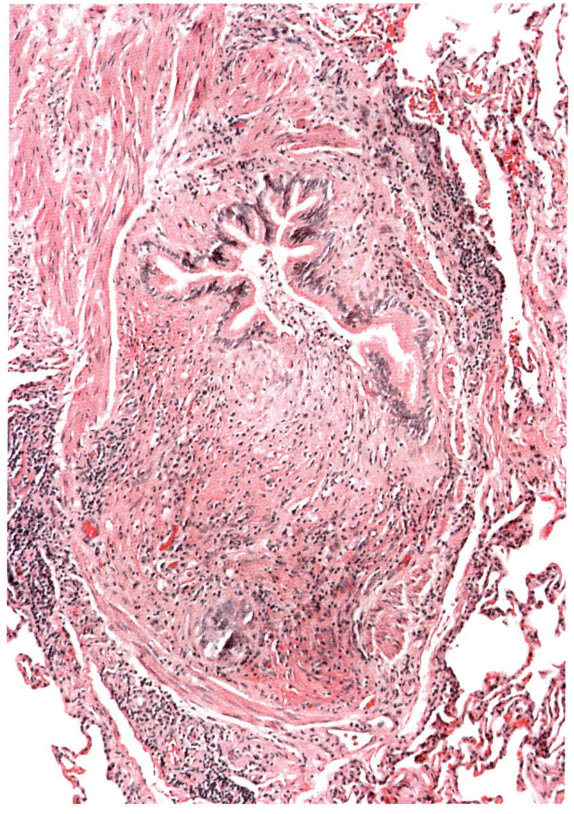

Figure 6-7

CONSTRICTIVE BRONCHIOLITIS IN RHEUMATOID ARTHRITIS

There is marked concentric submucosal fibrosis causing severe narrowing of this bronchiole.

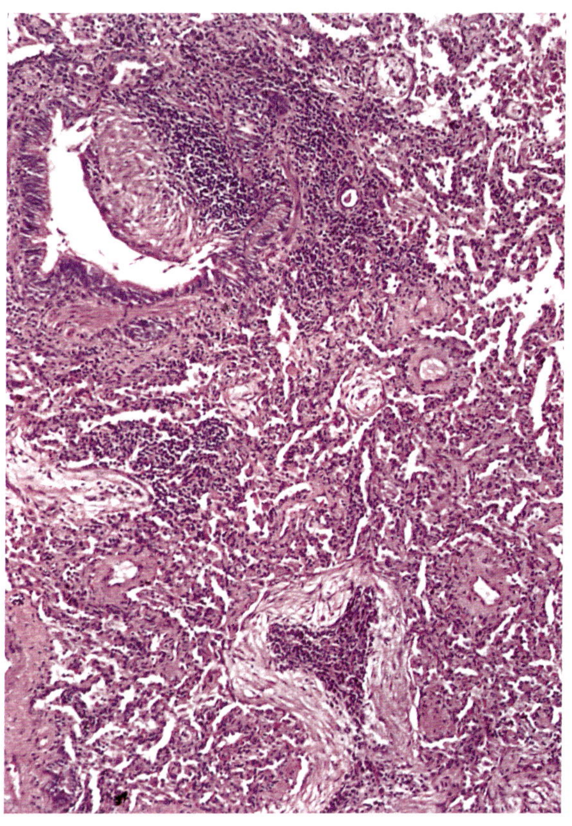

Figure 6-8

ORGANIZING PNEUMONIA IN RHEUMATOID ARTHRITIS

Evenly spaced polypoid plugs of loose organizing connective tissue are present in this bronchiole and in the alveolar ducts and alveoli in the adjacent lung.

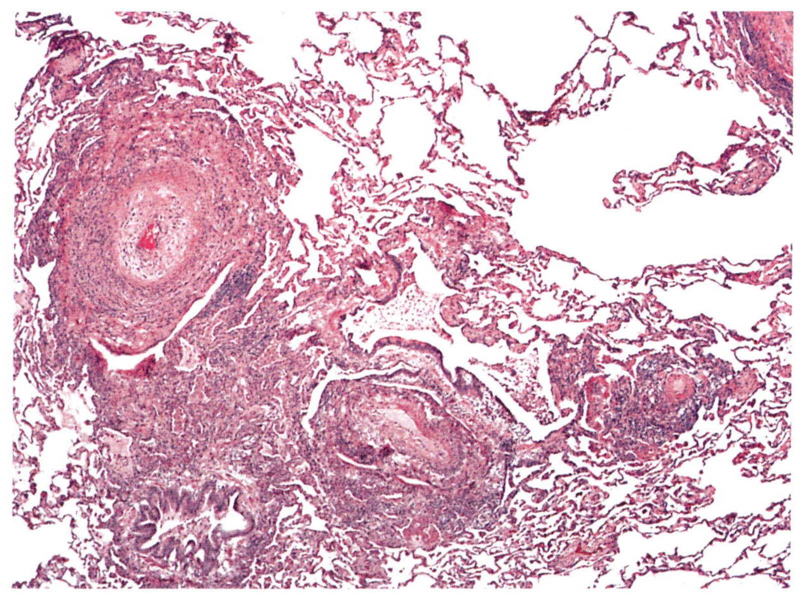

Figure 6-9

VASCULITIS IN RHEUMATOID ARTHRITIS

This patient with rheumatoid arthritis has pulmonary hypertension. Severe medial thickening and fibrinoid necrosis are present in these arterioles.

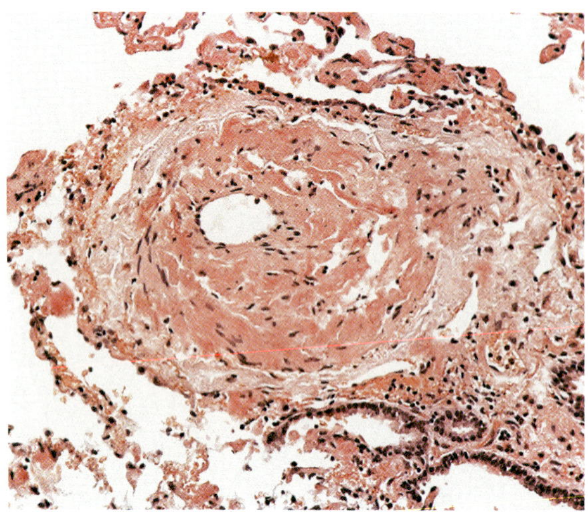

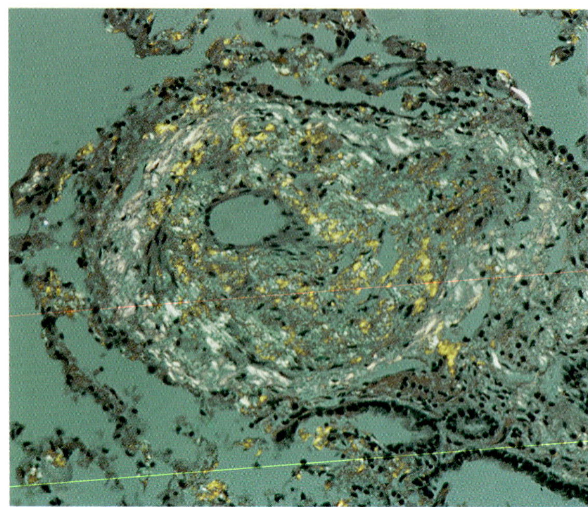

Figure 6-10

VASCULAR AMYLOIDOSIS IN RHEUMATOID ARTHRITIS

Left: The marked thickening of the vascular wall by waxy, eosinophilic, amorphous deposits is seen with the Congo red stain. Right: Polarization microscopy shows the characteristic apple-green birefringence of amyloidosis.

good (although the reaction to methotrexate may be fatal). Uncontrolled studies suggest corticosteroids can hasten recovery to methotrexate toxicity. Rechallenge with methotrexate has been reported without recurrence of lung disease. The prognosis of patients with OP associated with penicillamine treatment is poor, with an estimated mortality of 50 percent. There is little evidence that corticosteroids or any treatment modalities are of benefit for these patients.

SYSTEMIC LUPUS ERYTHEMATOSUS

Definition. Systemic lupus erythematosus (SLE) is a systemic immune disorder characterized by autoantibodies against nuclear antigens and immune-complex deposition. Pulmonary involvement can have many manifestations including pleural, interstitial, alveolar, and airway lesions as well as respiratory muscle weakness and shrinking atelectasis (Table 6-1) (73,76,90,106, 112,126,128,206,218).

Pulmonary involvement occurs in 20 to 90 percent of patients with SLE (73,76,90,106,112, 126,128,206,218) and is associated with a more than two-fold increased mortality risk (133). Infection is the most common pulmonary complication principally because of the common use of immunosuppressive agents in the treatment of the disease. As a result, infection is an important consideration in the differential diagnosis of any SLE patient with acute respiratory failure.

Pleuritis is the most common noninfectious respiratory lesion (Table 6-1). Pleural effusions occur in 5 to 10 percent of SLE patients, but pleural inflammation and/or fibrosis can be found at autopsy in 50 to 83 percent (76,128, 218). Effusions are usually bilateral and small to moderate in size. Pleuritis most often occurs in patients with a preexisting diagnosis, but it can be the initial presenting manifestation of SLE.

Acute lupus pneumonitis is a clinical term that generally corresponds histologically to DAD (122). Patients with SLE develop acute respiratory failure from infection, congestive heart failure, uremia, drug reactions, DAD, acute respiratory distress syndrome (ARDS), and diffuse pulmonary hemorrhage (26). For this reason, lung biopsies are very important for distinguishing infection from underlying disease since the choice between antibiotic versus immunosuppressive therapy is critical (26).

Diffuse alveolar hemorrhage occurs in approximately 2 percent of SLE patients (133). Zamora et al. (231) found pulmonary hemorrhage represented 22 percent of the pulmonary complications of SLE. There is a female predominance: 66 to 79 percent of cases of DAH affect women (231). In up to 20 percent of cases, hemorrhage

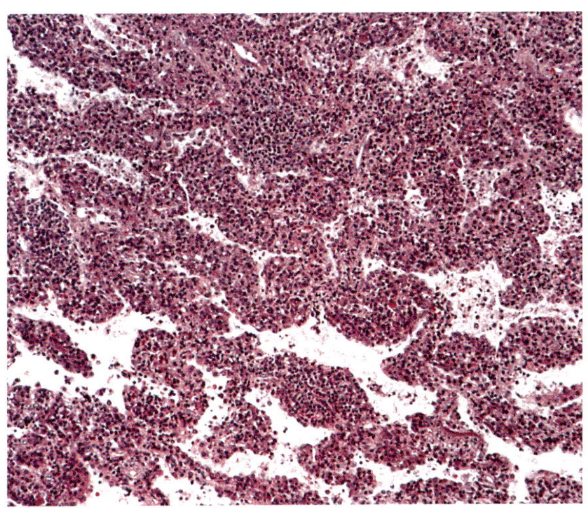

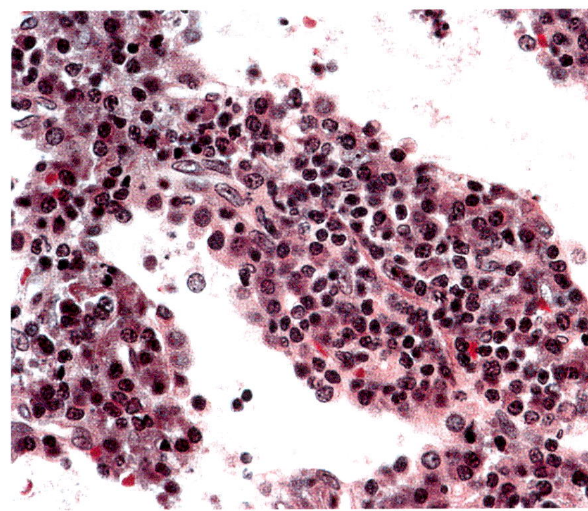

Figure 6-11

LYMPHOCYTIC INTERSTITIAL PNEUMONIA IN SYSTEMIC LUPUS ERYTHEMATOSUS

Left: The alveolar septa are diffusely infiltrated by chronic inflammation.
Right: The inflammation consists of mature lymphocytes and plasma cells.

is the presenting manifestation of SLE (231). The hemorrhage may be acute and life-threatening or chronic (28,44,89,115,135). The hemorrhage caused by SLE must be distinguished from other major causes of hemorrhage including Wegener's granulomatosis, Goodpasture's syndrome, microscopic polyangiitis, and idiopathic pulmonary hemorrhage (203). At initial presentation the clinical picture may resemble idiopathic pulmonary hemosiderosis with subsequent onset of SLE manifestations (45,109). Electron microscopy or immunofluorescence demonstrates immune complexes (28). Renal involvement occurs in 60 to 90 percent of patients. Mortality is 40 to 50 percent and a poor outcome is associated with the need for mechanical ventilation, presence of infection, and lack of therapy with cyclophosphamide (133).

Interstitial lung disease is relatively uncommon in SLE compared to other collagen vascular diseases such as rheumatoid arthritis and scleroderma. A UIP pattern is unusual but cases with a histologic pattern resembling NSIP are reported (102,133). Several cases of BOOP have been described in patients with SLE (60, 117), as well as a variety of lymphoid lesions including LIP (fig. 6-11) (13), nodular lymphoid hyperplasia (230), BALT hyperplasia, and malignant lymphoma (129).

The shrinking lung syndrome is associated with respiratory muscle dysfunction. It is characterized by chest radiographic findings of small lung volumes, elevated hemidiaphragms, and basilar atelectasis (83,164,201,214).

Pulmonary vascular disease, including pulmonary hypertension and vasculitis, can occur in patients with SLE. The vascular pathology of this pulmonary hypertension consists of patterns of plexogenic or thromboembolic arteriopathy and capillary hemangiomatosis (46, 48,101,160,212,225). Necrotizing pulmonary vasculitis is rare and may be associated with pulmonary hypertension and plexogenic arteriopathy (160). Pulmonary hypertension occurs in 0.5 to 14.0 percent of SLE patients (101,113,154, 181,183). It is associated with the presence of rheumatoid factor, lupus anticoagulant, and ribonucleic protein antibody (155,160). Li and Tam (113) found a significant increase in serositis and Raynaud's phenomenon in SLE patients with pulmonary hypertension. Rarely, sarcoidosis and SLE occur together (5,91).

Radiologic Findings. The most common radiologic manifestation of pulmonary SLE is pleural effusion (153,219). The effusion can be unilateral or bilateral and is frequently associated with enlargement of the cardiopericardial silhouette due to pericardial effusion.

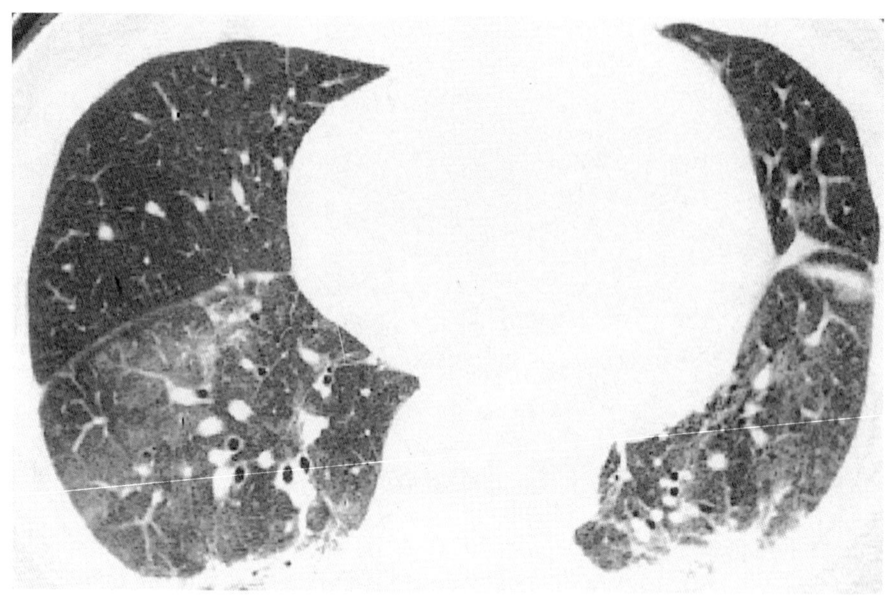

Figure 6-12

ORGANIZING PNEUMONIA PATTERN IN SYSTEMIC LUPUS ERYTHEMATOSUS

HRCT shows ground-glass opacities in the lower lobes and areas of consolidation in the dependent lung regions. The patient was a 46-year-old woman with SLE. The radiologic findings are nonspecific. Surgical lung biopsy demonstrated an organizing pneumonia pattern.

The pulmonary complications in patients with SLE usually result in nonspecific areas of airspace consolidation. The consolidation may be unilateral or bilateral, focal or diffuse, but tends to involve mainly the lower lung zones (153). The most common cause of consolidation is pneumonia (153,219). However, lupus pneumonitis, hemorrhage, ARDS, and, occasionally BOOP can result in similar radiologic findings (fig. 6-12) (60,140,153,219). The chest radiograph, therefore, plays a limited role in diagnosis.

Evidence of interstitial fibrosis is seen on the chest radiograph in approximately 3 percent of patients with SLE (60). However, several studies have demonstrated a considerably higher prevalence of fibrosis with HRCT (6,47,141). In one prospective study of 45 patients with SLE but no prior clinical evidence of lung involvement and normal chest radiographs, 15 (33 percent) had evidence of fibrosis on HRCT (6). The abnormalities involved predominantly or exclusively the lower lobes and consisted of intralobular interstitial thickening and irregular thickening of the interlobular septa. Other HRCT findings include architectural distortion and bronchial dilatation secondary to the fibrosis (traction bronchiectasis), small foci of airspace consolidation, and areas of ground-glass attenuation (6,47).

Histologic Findings. The pulmonary histologic manifestations of SLE are the same patterns seen in patients without SLE, with two minor exceptions: the hematoxylin body, or LE cell, and tuboreticular inclusions. Hematoxylin bodies are so rare they were found in only 1 of 120 autopsies of SLE patients (76). Although not specific for SLE, electron microscopy of lung biopsy specimens from patients with SLE pneumonitis may reveal tubuloreticular inclusions (53,71,116). Even in the presence of these findings, the final diagnosis of SLE is based on a constellation of clinical and laboratory manifestations rather than the presence of LE cells or tubuloreticular inclusions. Therefore, these features are not diagnostically useful. Rare examples of LIP may occur in SLE.

Treatment and Prognosis. Management of infection, the most common case of death, is the important issue in SLE. Corticosteroids may result in a variable degree of subjective and objective improvement in patients with interstitial lung disease. The mortality of patients with acute lupus pneumonitis is 50 percent and survivors have recurrences.

SCLERODERMA

Definition. Scleroderma is a systemic immune disorder characterized by inflammation and fibrosis involving the skin, as well as internal organs such as the vasculature and esophagus. After these sites, the respiratory tract is the next most common organ to be affected

(Table 6-1) (130,158,182). There are diffuse and limited forms of scleroderma in which the lung is affected in 40 and 60 percent of cases, respectively. The limited form is characterized by the CREST syndrome (calcinosis, Raynaud's phenomenon, esophageal dysfunction, sclerodactyly, and telangiectasias). Pulmonary involvement consists most often of interstitial fibrosis, pulmonary arterial hypertension, and aspiration pneumonia, and less often BOOP, amyloid deposits, and diffuse pulmonary hemorrhage. Scleroderma is also known as *progressive systemic sclerosis*.

Clinical Features. Pulmonary complications are the most common cause of death in scleroderma patients but they are rarely the presenting finding. In general, there is a poor correlation between the pulmonary and skin manifestations. Most of the respiratory symptoms occur after the cutaneous involvement, however, the pulmonary symptoms may antedate either Raynaud's phenomenon or cutaneous scleroderma.

Interstitial fibrosis and pulmonary arterial hypertension are the major pulmonary manifestations and are found in 80 percent and 15 to 50 percent of patients, respectively (Table 6-1) (130,132,182,208,227). The UIP and NSIP patterns of diffuse interstitial fibrosis are the most common types of pulmonary involvement in scleroderma patients (68,74,75,107,123,142,182, 217,218). Interstitial fibrosis is found at autopsy in 70 percent of cases (35).

Secondary pulmonary hypertension can occur in the setting of interstitial fibrosis; primary pulmonary arterial hypertension in the absence of interstitial fibrosis occurs almost always in patients with limited scleroderma (130, 227). Pulmonary hypertension can rapidly lead to pulmonary failure, cor pulmonale, and death (132,136,154,218,227,228). A variety of other less common pulmonary lesions occur in scleroderma including BOOP (20), amyloid deposits (12,50, 85), pulmonary hemorrhage (66,104), fibrocystic changes (15,108), sarcoidosis (67), aspiration pneumonia (130,182,218), drug-induced pneumonitis (130,182), pneumoconiosis (130, 182), and spontaneous pneumothorax (182). Whether or not there is an increased risk for lung carcinoma is somewhat controversial (12, 14,80); there appears to be an increased risk in patients with interstitial fibrosis (130,146,163).

Radiologic Findings. Evidence of interstitial fibrosis is present on the chest radiograph in 20 to 65 percent of patients with scleroderma (3,47,141). The fibrosis involves mainly the lower lung zones and is characterized by a fine reticular pattern (3,141). With progression of disease, the reticulation becomes coarser and is associated with honeycombing and volume loss. On HRCT, evidence of interstitial disease is seen in approximately 90 percent of patients, frequently in patients with normal radiographs (170,217). The main finding on HRCT is a fine reticular pattern involving the subpleural regions of the lower lobes (170). Other common findings include ground-glass opacities, honeycombing, and parenchymal micronodules (figs. 6-13, 6-14) (170).

Pleural effusion or thickening is seen less commonly than in other connective tissue disorders (3,153). Diffuse pleural thickening is evident on the chest radiograph in 10 percent of patients (3,123), and on HRCT in 20 percent (217).

Histologic Findings. The most distinctive pulmonary histologic findings in patients with scleroderma are the vascular changes found in pulmonary hypertension in the absence of significant interstitial fibrosis (fig. 6-15). The arterioles in patients with clinical evidence of primary pulmonary hypertension show predominantly concentric laminar fibrosis with relatively few plexiform lesions (33). Yousem et al. (228) proposed a grading scheme for these arteriolar changes: grade 1 consists of medial smooth muscle hypertrophy and concentric intimal thickening; grade 2, concentric intimal fibrosis narrowing the lumen of most arterioles by 50 percent; and grade 3, arteriolar narrowing of least 75 percent. Yousem et al. also found pulmonary vascular changes in 100 percent of autopsies from CREST patients; these were the major pathologic findings in 58 percent of cases. In addition to concentric laminar fibrosis, histologic patterns of veno-occlusive disease and thrombotic arteriopathy are seen (132). Although UIP has been thought to be the most common pattern of interstitial fibrosis in scleroderma, recent studies using current concepts in classification indicate that the NSIP pattern is also common (58,178).

Treatment and Prognosis. There is no good evidence that any drug alters the course of the two main types of lung disease in scleroderma:

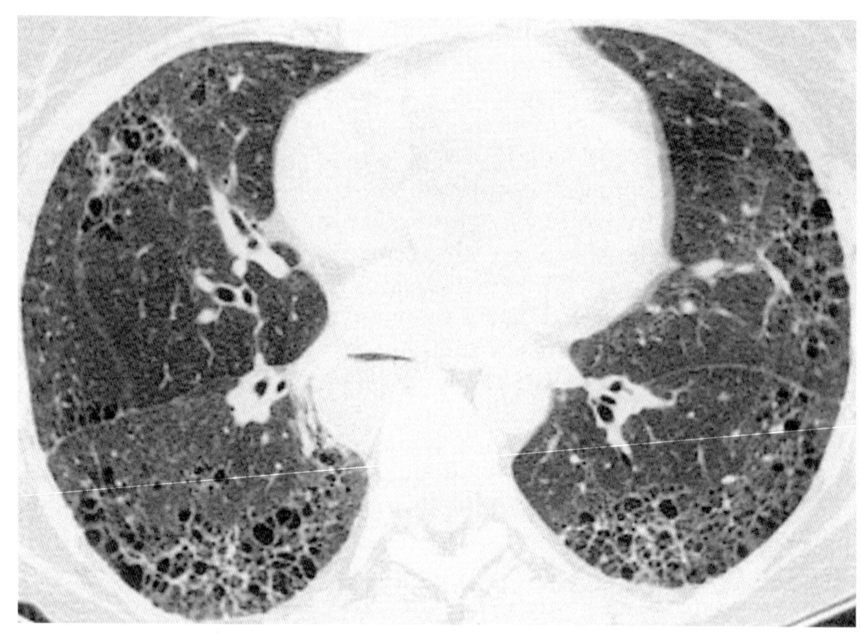

Figure 6-13

ENDSTAGE FIBROSIS IN SCLERODERMA

HRCT demonstrates bilateral subpleural honeycombing. The findings are characteristic of usual interstitial pneumonia. The patient was a 41-year-old woman with scleroderma and endstage interstitial fibrosis.

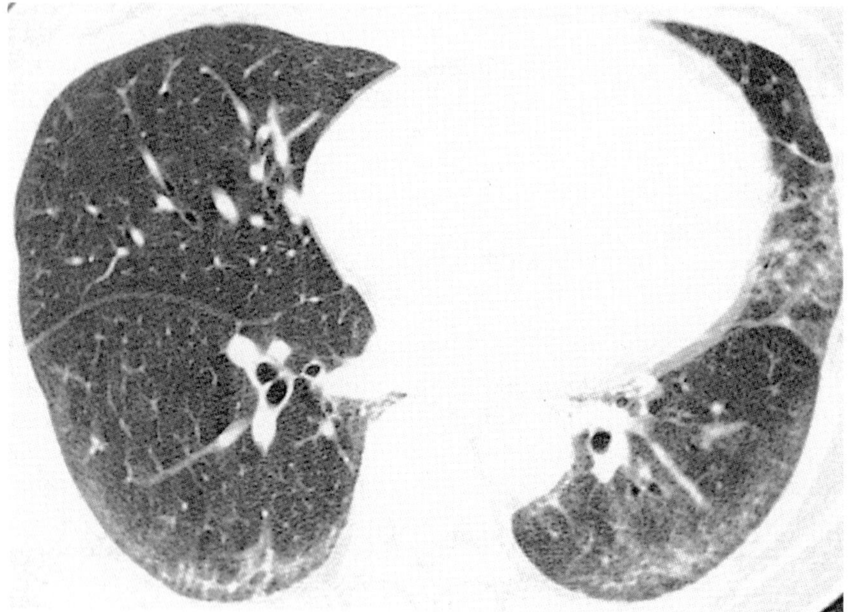

Figure 6-14

NONSPECIFIC INTERSTITIAL PNEUMONIA IN SCLERODERMA

HRCT shows ground-glass opacities and mild reticulation involving the right lower lobe, lingula, and left lower lobe. Surgical lung biopsy demonstrated nonspecific interstitial pneumonia. The patient was a 57-year-old woman with scleroderma.

UIP and pulmonary vascular disease. This apparent failure of therapy may reflect the fact that pulmonary involvement is usually identified at an established or late disease stage. The prognosis of patients with the fibrosing alveolitis associated with scleroderma is better than for those with idiopathic cases. Some of this difference relates to the fact that the fibrosing alveolitis in scleroderma appears to be either a UIP-like pattern or a NSIP pattern. It has been suggested that for fibrosing alveolitis corticosteroids are most effective if given in combination with cyclophosphamide. Penicillamine has been shown to be of some benefit.

POLYMYOSITIS/DERMATOMYOSITIS

Definition. Polymyositis and dermatomyositis (PM/DM) are idiopathic inflammatory myopathies characterized by symmetric proximal muscle weakness, elevated serum muscle

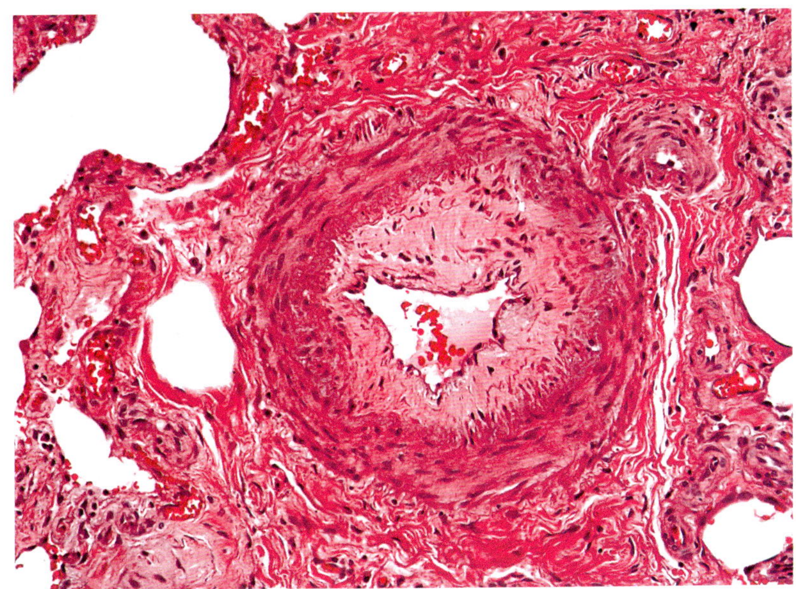

Figure 6-15

PULMONARY HYPERTENSION IN SCLERODERMA

This arteriole shows marked medial thickening and intimal fibrosis.

enzymes, electromyographic changes, and myositis (147,199). Pulmonary involvement consists most often of aspiration pneumonia followed by UIP, NSIP, DAD, and BOOP.

Clinical Features. Clinically significant lung involvement occurs in 5 to 20 percent of PM/DM patients and includes a wide variety of manifestations (Table 6-1) (42,159,172). Lung manifestations precede the muscle or skin manifestations by months to years in up to one third of the patients (42).

The most common pulmonary manifestation is aspiration pneumonia, which occurs in 15 to 20 percent of patients (172). Aspiration pneumonia was found at autopsy in 9 percent of patients by Lakhanpal et al. (110). Weakness of the striated muscle of the upper aerodigestive tract predisposes PM/DM patients to aspiration. Pneumonia is a significant cause of morbidity and mortality in such patients. Lakhanpal found bronchopneumonia caused by a variety of bacterial and fungal organisms in 54 percent of autopsied patients with PM/DM.

Interstitial lung disease occurs in 5 to 30 percent of PM/DM patients and consists of a variety of patterns, including UIP, DAD, BOOP, and NSIP (fig. 6-16) (42,73,118,173,218). The average age of PM/DM patients with interstitial lung disease is 50 years (range, 5 to 77 years) (42,118,173). There is a slight female predominance, with a ratio of 1.6 to 1 (42). Patients present in acute respiratory failure, chronic respiratory failure, or are asymptomatic (55). There is an association between interstitial lung disease and the presence of the serum anti-Jo1 antibody (present in 20 percent of PM/DM patients), which is directed against histidyl-tRNA synthetase (118,173). Interstitial lung disease has been shown to have an adverse effect on the prognosis of PM/DM patients, although this varies depending on the histologic pattern of lung pathology (4,43,166,194,200).

Respiratory insufficiency occurs in 4 to 8 percent of patients due to muscular weakness. When this occurs, the patients usually have severe generalized muscle weakness. Other pulmonary complications of PM/DM include pulmonary arterial hypertension (22), vasculitis (110), alveolar proteinosis (167), and lung cancer (81,215).

PM/DM differs from other connective tissue diseases in that pleuritis and pleural fibrosis occur only in the setting of interstitial lung disease (fig. 6-16) (42).

Radiologic Findings. The radiologic manifestations of aspiration pneumonia consist of unilateral or bilateral segmental areas of airspace consolidation that involve mainly the dependent lung regions (153). Interstitial fibrosis, similar to that of other connective tissue disorders, is characterized radiologically by a reticular pattern involving mainly the lower lung zones

Figure 6-16

DERMATOMYOSITIS, PLEURITIS, AND NONSPECIFIC INTERSTITIAL PNEUMONIA

A: Pleuritis and NSIP. There is a marked, acute fibrinous and chronic fibrous pleuritis associated with a NSIP pattern in the underlying lung.

B: NSIP, cellular pattern and organizing pneumonia. There is a mild to moderate interstitial chronic inflammatory infiltrate and foci of organizing pneumonia.

C: NSIP, cellular and fibrosing pattern. The alveolar walls are thickened by interstitial fibrosis and chronic inflammation.

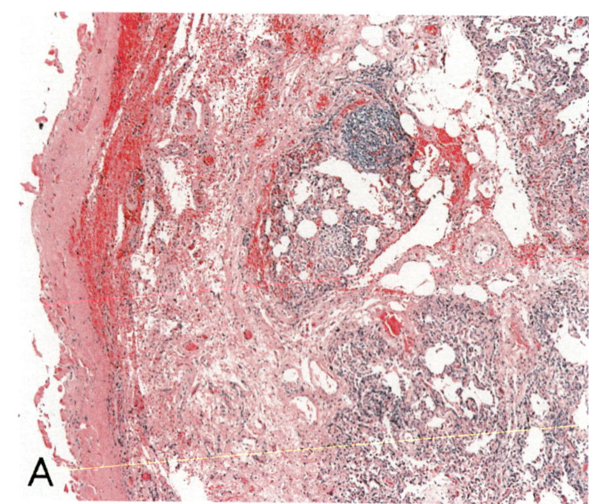

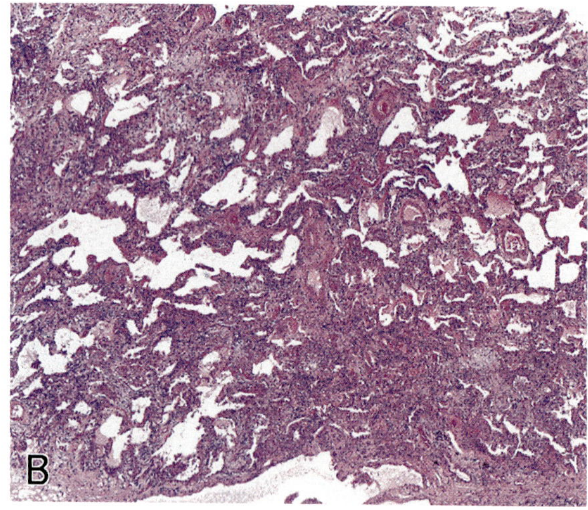

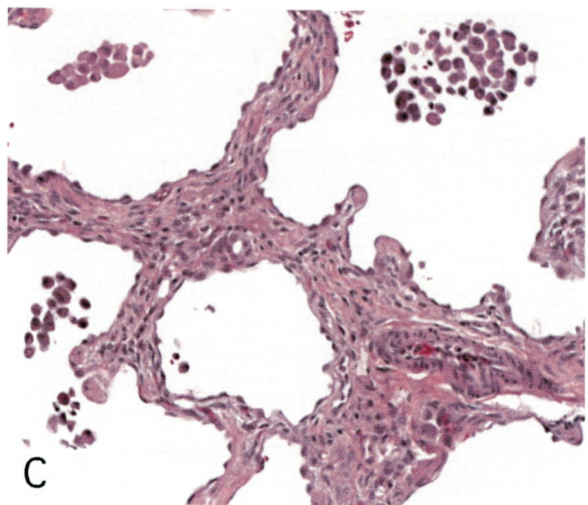

(153,172). With time, there is a progressive increase in the extent of lung involvement, loss of volume, and development of honeycombing and pulmonary arterial hypertension (123,153). BOOP results in patchy bilateral areas of consolidation that, on HRCT, often have a predominantly peribronchial or subpleural distribution (fig. 6-17) (94,131,153).

Pathologic Findings. In the pathologic study of 65 autopsies by Lakhanpal et al. (110), interstitial lung disease was found in 42 percent. The pathologic lesion in these cases was mostly UIP (110). Tazelaar et al. (200) classified a series of lung biopsies from PM/DM patients as showing DAD, BOOP, UIP, or cellular interstitial pneumonia (CIP). The cases of CIP from this study probably would be classified as NSIP by current criteria. NSIP is being recognized as a more common cause of interstitial disease in PM/DM patients than previously thought (fig. 6-16). Pleuritis also may occur (fig. 6-16A).

In patients with respiratory insufficiency due to muscle weakness, biopsies of the intercostal muscles, diaphragm, and accessory muscles of respiration show inflammation and degenerative changes (42).

Treatment and Prognosis. Aspiration pneumonia is the most important cause of mortality in patients with PM/DM. An associated malignancy (lung, ovary, breast, stomach) is present in up to 8 percent of patients. Corticosteroids may result in variable improvement in the interstitial lung disease in these patients.

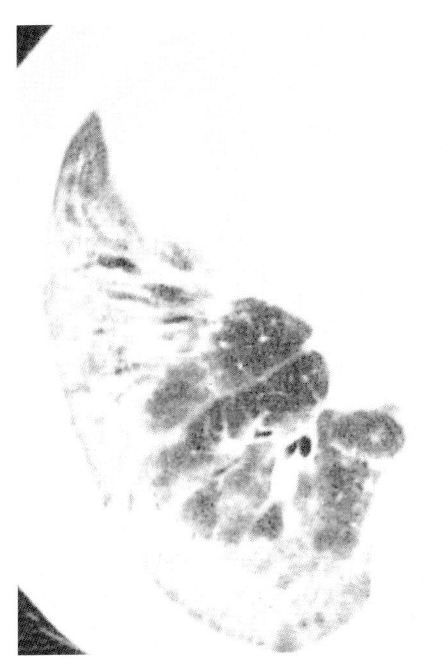
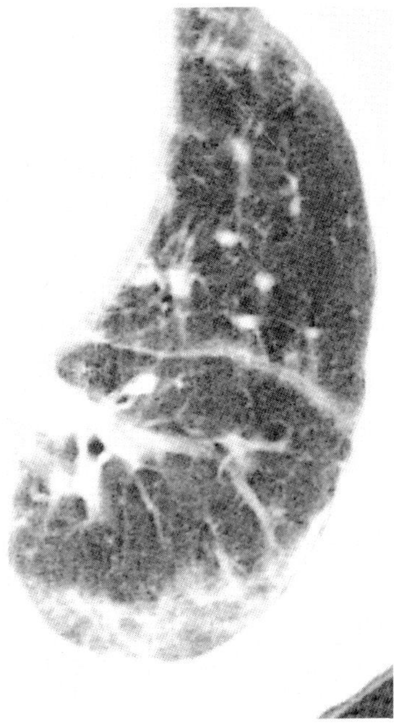

Figure 6-17

POLYMYOSITIS WITH ORGANIZING PNEUMONIA

HRCT shows airspace consolidation involving mainly the subpleural regions of the right middle, right lower, and left lower lobes. Also noted are focal ground-glass opacities. Surgical lung biopsy demonstrated organizing pneumonia. The patient was a 57-year-old man with polymyositis.

SJÖGREN'S SYNDROME

Definition. Sjögren's syndrome (SS) is an autoimmune disorder characterized by the triad of dry eyes (keratoconjunctivitis, sicca or xerophthalmia), dry mouth (xerostomia), and arthritis (24,197). Primary SS occurs in the absence of, while secondary SS occurs in the presence of, another connective tissue disease, usually rheumatoid arthritis.

The most common forms of pulmonary involvement are a variety of airway and lymphoid lesions (Table 6-1).

Clinical Features. The reported frequency of lung involvement in SS is widely variable, ranging from 9 to 90 percent of patients (17, 24,37,61,213). Patients with secondary SS have a higher frequency of lung involvement, which usually reflects the pulmonary manifestations of the associated connective tissue disease (32, 213). Pulmonary involvement is usually a late manifestation and only 5 percent of patients present with it (24).

Airway involvement consists of a variety of lesions including xerotrachea (dessication of the bronchial tree), follicular bronchiolitis (fig. 6-18), bronchiectasis, and obstructive airway disease (24,204). These disorders can contribute to atelectasis, bronchiectasis, and bronchopneumonia (52). A spectrum of lymphoid lesions also occurs in SS, including follicular bronchiolitis or hyperplasia of the BALT (fig. 6-18), mild chronic interstitial pneumonitis (196), LIP (1,190), nodular lymphoid hyperplasia (61,205,218), and malignant lymphoma (61,72,171). Scattered noncaseating granulomas may be present. Nonlymphoid forms of interstitial lung disease are relatively uncommon in patients with SS and include UIP (24,90,190,197,218) and BOOP (121, 209). Other rare lesions include amyloidosis (9, 105,190), multiple bullae (95,105), sarcoidosis (39,196), pulmonary hypertension (24), and vasculitis (21,52).

Radiologic Findings. Interstitial fibrosis is seen radiographically in 10 to 15 percent of patients with SS. It is similar to that seen in other connective tissue disorders (153).

LIP presents on the chest radiograph as a reticulonodular pattern involving mainly the lower lung zones. HRCT frequently demonstrates ground-glass opacities and randomly distributed cystic airspaces (fig. 6-19) (93,98). Occasionally, the cystic lesions may be associated with nodular pulmonary amyloid deposits (41,105).

The most common abnormalities seen on HRCT in patients with SS are bronchiectasis and centrilobular nodular and branching linear opacities suggestive of bronchiolitis (54). Expiratory HRCT may demonstrate areas of air-trapping (125).

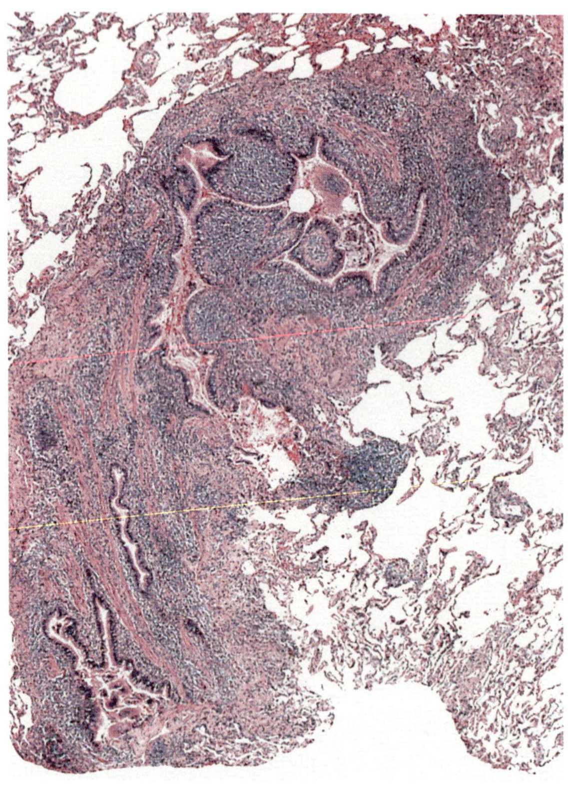

Figure 6-18

SJÖGREN'S SYNDROME: FOLLICULAR BRONCHIOLITIS

There is marked hyperplasia of the lymphoid tissue surrounding this bronchiole.

Histologic Findings. The most distinctive histologic finding in SS is associated with the clinical finding of desiccation of the bronchial tree. The bronchial submucosal glands atrophy and chronic inflammation results in tenacious secretions (8,31,52,137). The frequent pulmonary lymphoid lesions (fig. 6-18) necessitate careful attention to distinguish reactive and neoplastic proliferations. The recently recognized cystic airway lesions associated with LIP are not well known (93,98). Histologically, they consist of dilated bronchioles associated with marked lymphoid interstitial infiltrates.

Treatment and Prognosis. Treatment of the various manifestations of SS is influenced by the treatment required to manage the other associated connective tissue diseases. Corticosteroids and immunosuppressive drugs may result in impressive improvements in patients with LIP and BOOP. Azathioprine has also been used with limited success.

MIXED CONNECTIVE TISSUE DISEASE

Mixed connective tissue disease (MCTD) is characterized by combined features of SLE, scleroderma, and polymyositis, and high titers of a serum antibody to uridine-rich small ribonucleoprotein antigen. The alternative term, *undifferentiated autoimmune rheumatic/connective*

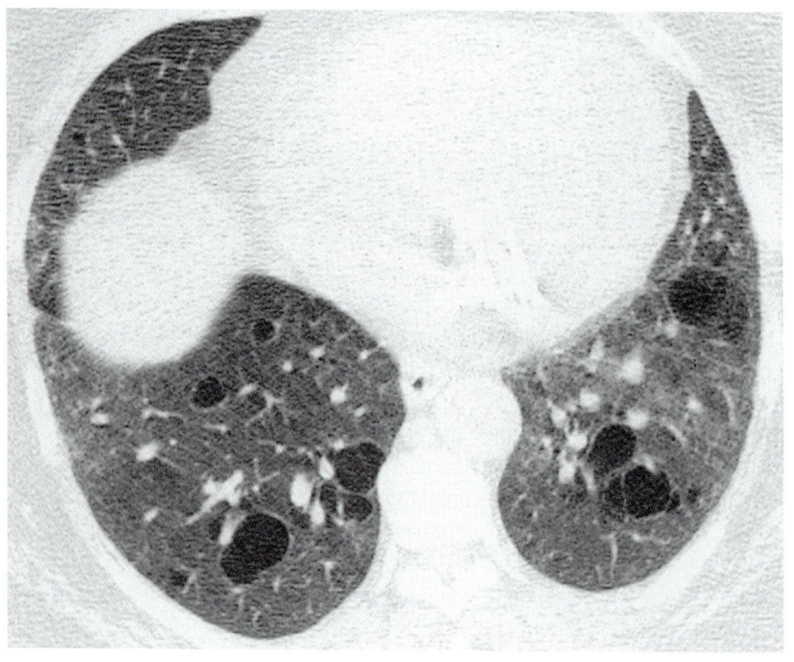

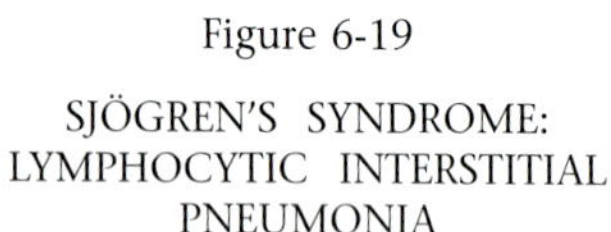

Figure 6-19

SJÖGREN'S SYNDROME: LYMPHOCYTIC INTERSTITIAL PNEUMONIA

HRCT at the level of the right hemidiaphragm shows focal ground-glass opacities and randomly distributed thin-walled cysts. Surgical biopsy demonstrated LIP. The patient was a 50-year-old woman who was a lifelong nonsmoker and who had Sjögren's syndrome.

tissue disorder, has been proposed. Pulmonary involvement consists mostly of pleuritis, UIP, and pulmonary hypertension (Table 6-1).

Pulmonary involvement occurs in 20 to 85 percent of patients with MCTD (151,152,191). The broad spectrum of pulmonary lesions includes all of the lesions encountered in patients with SLE, scleroderma, and PM/DM (Table 6-1).

Pleural effusions occur in up to 50 percent of cases and pleurisy in 35 percent (152). The pleural effusions are usually small and resolve spontaneously (152). The most common type of interstitial lung disease in MCTD is the UIP pattern (152). The fibrosis tends to be worse if there are predominant clinical features of scleroderma.

Pulmonary hypertension occurs mostly in patients with scleroderma-like manifestations (86,99,100,143,161,207). Pulmonary vasculitis is uncommon but can be seen in the setting of pulmonary hypertension (151,220). Alveolar hemorrhage can occur in MCTD patients, especially in those with manifestations of SLE (64,168).

Aspiration pneumonia may occur, particularly in patients with features of scleroderma and PM/DM. Respiratory muscle dysfunction can be associated with respiratory failure, especially in patients with features of PM/DM (119,120).

The pulmonary radiographic and pathologic features of MCTD are identical to those of the particular connective tissue diseases manifested in a given patient, and are therefore nonspecific.

ANKYLOSING SPONDYLITIS

Definition. Ankylosing spondylitis is a chronic inflammatory disease of the axial skeleton manifested by back pain and progressive stiffness of the spine. More than 90 percent of Caucasians with ankylosing spondylitis have human leukocyte antigen (HLA)-B27 positivity. The cause of ankylosing spondylitis remains unknown.

Once considered rare, it is now known that ankylosing spondylitis affects 0.5 to 1.0 percent of the population (197). The onset is insidious and occurs in persons under the age of 40. The male to female ratio is approximately 3 to 1. The disease is rare in nonwhites. Back pain and morning stiffness that improve with exercise are characteristic features useful in differentiating ankylosing spondylitis from mechanical spinal arthritis. The X-ray demonstration of bilateral sacroiliitis is key to the diagnosis. Extra-articular disease is common and includes: fatigue, weight loss, and low-grade fever; uveitis and conjunctivitis; chronic prostatism; and cardiovascular involvement including cardiac conduction defects, aortitis, and aortic insufficiency. Pulmonary involvement consists primarily of apical fibrobullous disease and pneumothorax (Table 6-1).

Clinical Features. The incidence of pleuropulmonary involvement in ankylosing spondylitis is unknown. The most common thoracic complication is fixation of the thoracic cage as a result of costovertebral ankylosis, especially in patients with advanced disease (162, 197). Patients with longstanding, advanced ankylosing spondylitis may present with bilateral apical fibrobullous disease (16,69,92,114). Spontaneous pneumothorax occurs, probably as a result of the rupture of cysts in patients with apical fibrobullous disease. Patients are often asymptomatic but may complain of cough, sputum production, and dyspnea.

Radiologic Findings. The chest roentgenogram reveals diffuse reticulonodular opacities in the upper lung zones. The changes, in general, mimic those found with pulmonary tuberculosis. The opacities progress and eventually cause widespread fibrosis and cyst formation in the upper lobes as a result of the parenchymal destruction. The fibrous portion of the fibrobullous lesions appears as increased interstitial markings. In longstanding disease, there is complete distortion and destruction of the involved lung and retraction of the hilum toward the apex. The process can be complicated by a secondary infection, often by the invasion of *Aspergillus.* Ventilation studies have demonstrated a reduction in ventilation to the lung apices and suggest that this impairment may be a factor in the pathogenesis of apical fibrosis in this disease (189).

Pathologic Findings. Pathologically, the early changes are consistent with a patchy pneumonic process: chronic inflammation and fibrosis that progress in time to extensive fibrosis. Chronic fibrous pleuritis is often associated with pulmonary fibrosis. The fibrosis in the upper lobe can be unilateral or bilateral (19). The etiology of this fibrosis is unknown, although an immune pathogenesis has been postulated (19). Bronchiectasis may also occur.

RELAPSING POLYCHONDRITIS

Definition. Relapsing polychondritis is a chronic, episodic, systemic disorder characterized by recurrent, widespread and potentially destructive inflammatory lesions that involve cartilaginous structures of the external ear, the joints, the nose, and the respiratory tract.

Clinical Features. Approximately 25 percent of patients with relapsing polychondritis have a coexistent connective tissue disease such as adult or juvenile rheumatoid arthritis, SS, SLE, Reiter's disease, psoriatic arthritis, and ankylosing spondylitis. Pulmonary disease occurs in patients who have recurrent involvement of the laryngotracheal bronchial structures, causing obstruction of the upper airways and secondary pneumonia (Table 6-1). Hoarseness and laryngeal tenderness over the thyroid cartilage and anterior trachea are common presenting symptoms. A nonproductive cough, dyspnea, aphonia, inspiratory stridor, or rarely, hemoptysis should also alert the physician to the possibility of this potentially life-threatening complication. Studies of maximal expiratory and inspiratory flow volume curves and airway resistance are often useful in providing information on the site and nature of the obstructive process (111,127).

Radiologic Findings. The chest roentgenogram may reveal atelectasis, pneumonia, or widening of the aortic arch or the ascending or descending aorta. CT is very useful because cartilage and soft tissue components are well visualized and areas of obstruction can be identified (150).

Pathologic Findings. The tracheal and bronchial mucosae may be edematous and their cartilaginous rings exhibit changes varying from mild inflammation to total resorption by granulation tissue (36). The large and medium-sized bronchi show patchy widening or extensive narrowing and collapse. Lesions may be localized or involve the entire upper airway.

Histologically, in the acute phase of relapsing polychondritis, the pericartilaginous tissue is surrounded by lymphocytes, plasma cells, and neutrophils. There is depletion of the matrix proteoglycans, degeneration of the chondrocytes, and destruction of tissue (197). Subsequently, the destroyed cartilage is replaced by granulation and fibrous tissue (197).

Treatment and Prognosis. The management of patients with relapsing polychondritis is directed primarily at maintaining adequate ventilation. Tracheostomy is required if the larynx is significantly involved. Occasionally, surgical treatment of the collapsed airways is successful. Infection, systemic vasculitis, malignancy, and respiratory tract involvement are the most common causes of death (23,111,197). It is not clear whether or not corticosteroid treatment alters the natural course of this disease (23,111,197). Death usually occurs as a result of recurrent attacks that lead to destruction of the cartilage of the tracheal and bronchial rings, causing collapse of these structures with inflammation, edema, and cicatrization. This cartilaginous destruction leads to severe focal or diffuse airway collapse with inadequate ventilation that often is not corrected by tracheostomy and mechanical ventilation. Death then occurs from asphyxiation.

INFLAMMATORY BOWEL DISEASE

Definition. *Crohn's disease* is a disorder of uncertain etiology that is characterized by transmural mucosal inflammation. It may involve the entire gastrointestinal tract from mouth to perianal area. *Ulcerative colitis* is characterized by recurring episodes of inflammation limited to the mucosal layer of the colon. It almost invariably involves the rectum and may extend in a proximal and continuous fashion to involve other portions of the colon.

Pulmonary involvement in inflammatory bowel disease is rare but it can take the form of a variety of airway, interstitial, and pleural lesions in patients with ulcerative colitis and Crohn's disease (25). The lung disease develops after the onset of bowel disease in most patients, but occasionally is the initial manifestation (25). Pulmonary complications of inflammatory bowel disease include airway inflammation at several levels in the tracheobronchial tree (subglottic inflammation and stenosis, chronic bronchitis, bronchiectasis, bronchiolitis), diffuse pulmonary parenchymal disease (BOOP and interstitial lung disease), necrobiotic nodules, and serositis (pleural effusions and pleuropericarditis) (Table 6-1). A pathogenetic relationship between sarcoidosis and Crohn's disease has been suggested since noncaseating granulomas

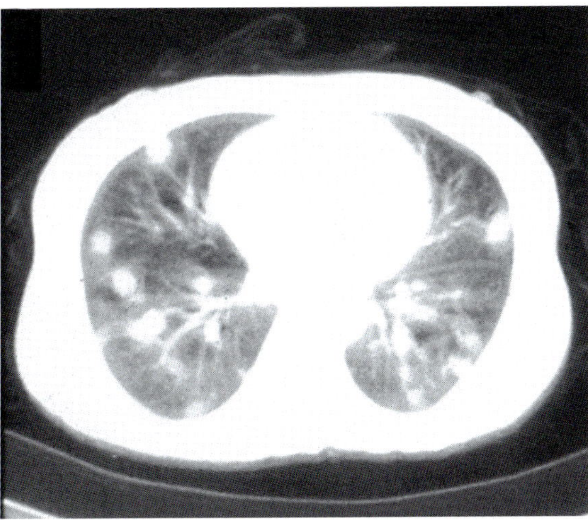

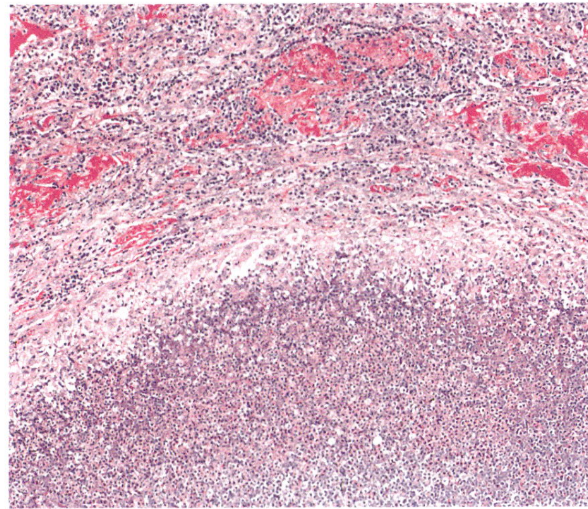

Figure 6-20

CHRONIC ULCERATIVE COLITIS: NODULAR ABSCESSES

Left: This chest CT shows multiple bilateral nodular opacities.

Right: The lung biopsy shows an acute abscess consisting of a nodular accumulation of necrotic neutrophils surrounded by a fibrous wall.

and BAL fluid lymphocytosis (with elevated CD4/CD8 ratios) can be seen in both disorders.

Clinical Features. The airway inflammatory changes are thought to represent the same type of inflammatory changes that occur in the bowel. The primary symptoms are cough and hoarseness, although some patients develop upper airway obstruction with resulting stridor and severe dyspnea. Bronchial involvement may be manifested as unexplained cough with variable amounts of mucopurulent sputum production.

Since these patients require chronic medication it is important to exclude drug-induced lung disease, particularly due to sulfasalazine (27,59,222) or mesalamine (192,195), from pulmonary manifestations related to the underlying disease.

Radiologic Findings. The most common airway abnormalities evident on the chest radiograph are bronchial wall thickening and bronchiectasis (63,221). The most common findings on HRCT are bronchiectasis and centrilobular nodular and branching linear opacities consistent with bronchiolitis (63). Other findings that may be seen on CT include multiple bilateral nodular opacities (fig. 6-20, left), thickening of the wall of the trachea and main bronchi, and tracheal and bronchial stenosis (63).

Pathologic Findings. A spectrum of airway inflammatory and/or fibrotic lesions can occur in inflammatory bowel disease including subglottic stenosis, chronic bronchitis, severe chronic bronchial suppuration, bronchiectasis, chronic bronchiolitis, diffuse panbronchiolitis (40), and constrictive bronchiolitis (25,63,216). Large airway involvement is characterized by inflammation, ulceration, and narrowing of the trachea and/or bronchi. In surgical lung biopsies, this may appear as large nodular abscesses (fig. 6-20, right) or marked bronchiolar inflammation and microabscess formation (fig. 6-21). Several patterns of interstitial lung disease may occur including BOOP (193) and eosinophilic pneumonia (25). Several cases of interstitial lung disease with patterns of interstitial inflammation and/or fibrosis are described in patients with Crohn's disease (38,87). Other pulmonary lesions include necrotic parenchymal nodules with lots of neutrophils (25), vasculitis (51,97), and serositis (25). A vasculitis-like syndrome resembling Wegener's granulomatosis has been described in a patient receiving sulfasalazine for ulcerative colitis (165).

Treatment and Prognosis. If the patient is receiving treatment with sulfasalazine or 5-aminosalicylate (5-ASA), these should be

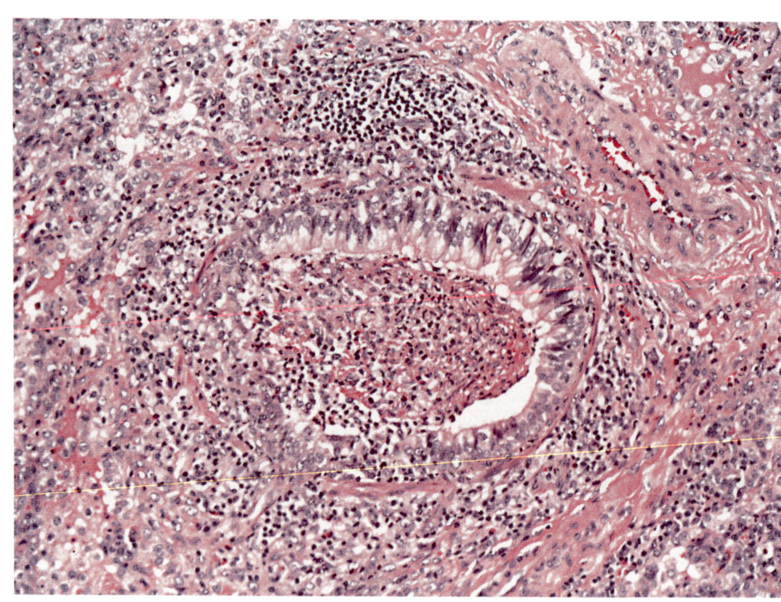

Figure 6-21

CROHN'S DISEASE: BRONCHIOLAR INFLAMMATION AND ABSCESS

There is a neutrophilic exudate in the lumen of this bronchiole and marked chronic inflammation of the airway wall and surrounding lung tissue.

stopped. This is of concern because the inflammatory bowel disease could flare up if the drug is withdrawn. Inhaled or systemic corticosteroids may be effective, depending upon the type of pulmonary complication. Potentially life-threatening airway inflammation, as with subglottic involvement causing upper airway obstruction, may require intravenous steroids. Pleural effusions respond to nonsteroidal anti-inflammatory therapy, but corticosteroids may be necessary in an unresponsive patient.

REFERENCES

1. Anderson LG, Talal N. The spectrum of benign to malignant lymphoproliferation in Sjögren's syndrome. Clin Exp Immunol 1972;10:199–221.
2. Aquino SL, Webb WR, Golden J. Bronchiolitis obliterans associated with rheumatoid arthritis: findings on HRCT and dynamic expiratory CT. J Comput Assist Tomogr 1994;18:555–8.
3. Arroliga AC, Podell DN, Matthay RA. Pulmonary manifestations of scleroderma. J Thorac Imaging 1992;7:30–45.
4. Arsura EL, Greenberg AS. Adverse impact of interstitial pulmonary fibrosis on prognosis in polymyositis and dermatomyositis. Semin Arthritis Rheum 1988;18:29–37.
5. Askari A, Thompson P, Barnes C. Sarcoidosis: atypical presentation associated with features of systemic lupus erythematosus. J Rheumatol 1988;15:1578–9.
6. Bankier AA, Kiener HP, Wiesmayr MN, et al. Discrete lung involvement in systemic lupus erythematosus: CT assessment. Radiology 1995;196:835–40.
7. Banks J, Banks C, Cheong B, et al. An epidemiological and clinical investigation of pulmonary function and respiratory symptoms in patients with rheumatoid arthritis. Q J Med 1992;85:795–806.
8. Bariffi F, Pesci A, Bertorelli G, Manganelli P, Ambanelli U. Pulmonary involvement in Sjögren's syndrome. Respiration 1984;46:82–7.
9. Batra P, Collins JD, Magidson JG. Pulmonary nodular amyloidosis presenting as Sjögren's syndrome. J Natl Med Assoc 1983;75:903–5.
10. Baydur A, Mongan ES, Slager UT. Acute respiratory failure and pulmonary arteritis without parenchymal involvement: demonstration in a patient with rheumatoid arthritis. Chest 1979;75:518–20.
11. Bely M, Apathy A. Changes of the lung in rheumatoid arthritis–rheumatoid pneumonia. A clinicopathological study. Acta Morphol Hung 1991;39:117–56.

12. Benharroch D, Sukenik S, Sacks M. Bronchioloalveolar carcinoma and generalized amyloidosis complicating progressive systemic sclerosis. Hum Pathol 1992;23:839–41.
13. Benisch B, Peison B. The association of lymphocytic interstitial pneumonia and systemic lupus erythematosus. Mt Sinai J Med 1979;46:398–41.
14. Benson CH, Pinkston WC, Woodliff J, Harisdangkul V. Pulmonary malignancy in a 21-year-old male with progressive systemic sclerosis. J Miss State Med Assoc 1983;24:147–9.
15. Bergemann A, Tikly M. Cystic lung disease in systemic sclerosis: a case report with high resolution computed tomography findings. Rev Rhum Engl Ed 1996;63:213–5.
16. Blavia R, Toda MR, Vidal F, Benet A, Razquin S, Richart C. Pulmonary diffuse amyloidosis and ankylosing spondylitis. A rare association. Chest 1992;102:1608–10.
17. Bloch KJ, Buchanan WW, Wohl MJ, Bunim JJ. Sjögren's syndrome. A clinical, pathological, and serological study of sixty-two cases. Medicine 1965;44:187–231.
18. Bonafede RP, Benatar SR. Bronchocentric granulomatosis and rheumatoid arthritis. Br J Dis Chest 1987;81:197–201.
19. Boushea DK, Sundstrom WR. The pleuropulmonary manifestations of ankylosing spondylitis. Semin Arthritis Rheum 1989;18:277–81.
20. Bridges AJ, Hsu KC, Dias-Arias AA, Chechani V. Bronchiolitis obliterans organizing pneumonia and scleroderma. J Rheumatol 1992;19:1136–40.
21. Bucher UG, Reid L. Sjögren's syndrome: report of a fatal case with pulmonary and renal lesions. Br J Dis Chest 1959;53:237–52.
22. Bunch TW, Tancredi RG, Lie JT. Pulmonary hypertension in polymyositis. Chest 1981;79:105–7.
23. Burlew BP, Lippton H, Klinestiver D, Haponik EJ. Relapsing polychondritis: new pulmonary manifestations. J La State Med Soc 1992;144:58–62.
24. Cain HC, Noble PW, Matthay RA. Pulmonary manifestations of Sjögren's syndrome. Clin Chest Med 1998;19:687–99.
25. Camus P, Piard F, Ashcroft T, Gal AA, Colby TV. The lung in inflammatory bowel disease. Medicine (Baltimore) 1993;72:151–83.
26. Carette S, Macher AM, Nussbaum A, Plotz PH. Severe, acute pulmonary disease in patients with systemic lupus erythematosus: ten years of experience at the National Institutes of Health. Semin Arthritis Rheum 1984;14:52–9.
27. Cazzadori A, Braggio P, Bontempini L. Salazopyrin-induced eosinophilic pneumonia. Respiration 1985;47:158–60.
28. Churg A, Franklin W, Chan KL, Kopp E, Carrington CB. Pulmonary hemorrhage and immune-complex deposition in the lung. Complications in a patient with systemic lupus erythematosus. Arch Pathol Lab Med 1980;104:388–91.
29. Colby TV. Pulmonary pathology in patients with systemic autoimmune diseases. Clin Chest Med 1998;19:587–612.
30. Colby TV, Carrington CB. Interstital lung disease. In: Thurlbeck WM, Churg AM, eds. Pathology of the lung, 2nd ed. New York: Thieme Medical Publishers; 1995:589–737.
31. Constantopoulos SH, Drosos AA, Maddison PJ, Moutsopoulos HM. Xerotrachea and interstitial lung disease in primary Sjögren's syndrome. Respiration 1984;46:310–4.
32. Constantopoulos SH, Tsianos EV, Moutsopoulos HM. Pulmonary and gastrointestinal manifestations of Sjögren's syndrome. Rheum Dis Clin North Am 1992;18:617–35.
33. Cool CD, Kennedy D, Voelkel NF, Tuder RM. Pathogenesis and evolution of plexiform lesions in pulmonary hypertension associated with scleroderma and human immunodeficiency virus infection. Hum Pathol 1997;28:434–42.
34. Cooney TP. Interrelationship of chronic eosinophilic pneumonia, bronchiolitis obliterans, and rheumatoid disease: a hypothesis. J Clin Pathol 1981;34:129–37.
35. D'Angelo WA, Fries JF, Masi AT, Shulman LE. Pathologic observations in systemic sclerosis (scleroderma). A study of fifty-eight autopsy cases and fifty-eight matched controls. Am J Med 1969;46:428–40.
36. Dail DH. Metabolic and other diseases. In: Dail DH, Hammar SP, eds. Pulmonary pathology, 2nd ed. New York: Springer Verlag; 1994:707–77.
37. Dalavanga YA, Constantopoulos SH, Galanopoulou V, Zerva L, Moutsopoulos HM. Alveolitis correlates with clinical pulmonary involvement in primary Sjögren's syndrome. Chest 1991;99:1394–7.
38. Dawson A, Gibbs AR, Anderson G. An unusual perilobular pattern of pulmonary interstitial fibrosis associated with Crohn's disease. Histopathology 1993;23:553–6.
39. Deheinzelin D, de Carvalho CR, Tomazini ME, Barbas Filho JV, Saldiva PH. Association of Sjögren's syndrome and sarcoidosis. Report of a case. Sarcoidosis 1988;5:68–70.
40. Desai SJ, Gephardt GN, Stoller JK. Diffuse panbronchiolitis preceding ulcerative colitis. Chest 1989;95:1342–4.
41. Desai SR, Nicholson AG, Stewart S, Twentyman OM, Flower CD, Hansell DM. Benign pulmonary lymphocytic infiltration and amyloidosis: computed tomographic and pathologic features in three cases. J Thorac Imaging 1997;12:215–20.

42. Dickey BF, Myers AR. Pulmonary disease in polymyositis/dermatomyositis. Semin Arthritis Rheum 1984;14:60–76.
43. Duncan PE, Griffin JP, Garcia A, Kaplan SB. Fibrosing alveolitis in polymyositis. A review of histologically confirmed cases. Am J Med 1974;57:621–6.
44. Eagen JW, Memoli VA, Roberts JL, Matthew GR, Schwartz MM, Lewis EJ. Pulmonary hemorrhage in systemic lupus erythematosus. Medicine (Baltimore) 1978;57:545–60.
45. Elliot ML, Kuhn C. Idiopathic hemosiderosis: ultrastructural abnormalities in the capillary walls. Am Rev Respir Dis 1970;102:895–904.
46. Fayemi AO. Pulmonary vascular disease in systemic lupus erythematosus. Am J Clin Pathol 1976;65:284–90.
47. Fenlon HM, Doran M, Sant SM, Breatnach E. High-resolution chest CT in systemic lupus erythematosus. AJR Am J Roentgenol 1996;166:301–7.
48. Fernandez-Alonso J, Zulueta T, Reyes-Ramirez JR, Castillo-Palma MJ, Sanchez-Roman J. Pulmonary capillary hemangiomatosis as cause of pulmonary hypertension in a young woman with systemic lupus erythematosus [Letter]. J Rheumatol 1999;26:231–3.
49. Flowers JR, Clunie G, Burke M, Constant O. Bronchiolitis obliterans organizing pneumonia: the clinical and radiological features of seven cases and a review of the literature. Clin Radiol 1992;45:371–7.
50. Focan C, Swale JL, Borlee-Hermans G, Claessens JJ. Systemic sclerosis, aplastic anemia and amyloidosis associated with lung carcinoma [Letter]. Acta Clin Belg 1985;40:204–5.
51. Forrest JA, Shearman DJ. Pulmonary vasculitis and ulcerative colitis. Digest Dis 1975;20:482–6.
52. Fox RI, Howell FV, Bone RC, Michelson P. Primary Sjögren syndrome: clinical and immunopathologic features. Semin Arthritis Rheum 1984;14:77–105.
53. Fraire AE, Smith MN, Greenberg SD, Weg JG, Sharp JT. Tubular structures in pulmonary endothelial cells in systemic lupus erythematosus. Am J Clin Pathol 1971;56:244–8.
54. Franquet T, Gimenez A, Monill JM, Diaz C, Geli C. Primary Sjögren's syndrome and associated lung disease: CT findings in 50 patients. AJR Am J Roentgenol 1997;169:655–8.
55. Frazier AR, Miller RD. Interstitial pneumonitis in association with polymyositis and dermatomyositis. Chest 1974;65:403–7.
56. Fujii M, Adachi S, Shimizu T, Hirota S, Sako M, Kono M. Interstitial lung disease in rheumatoid arthritis: assessment with high-resolution computed tomography. J Thorac Imaging 1993;8:54–62.
57. Fujita J, Yamadori I, Suemitsu I, et al. Clinical features of non-specific interstitial pneumonia. Respir Med 1999;93:113–8.
58. Fujita J, Yoshinouchi T, Ohtsuki Y, et al. Non-specific interstitial pneumonia as pulmonary involvement of systemic sclerosis. Ann Rheum Dis 2001;60:281–3.
59. Gabazza EC, Taguchi O, Yamakami T, et al. Pulmonary infiltrates and skin pigmentation associated with sulfasalazine. Am J Gastroenterol 1992;87:1654–7.
60. Gammon RB, Bridges TA, al-Nezir H, Alexander CB, Kennedy JI Jr. Bronchiolitis obliterans organizing pneumonia associated with systemic lupus erythematosus. Chest 1992;102:1171–4.
61. Gardiner P, Ward C, Allison A, et al. Pleuropulmonary abnormalities in primary Sjögren's syndrome. J Rheumatol 1993;20:831–7.
62. Gardner DL, Duthie JJ, Macleod J, Allan WS. Pulmonary hypertension in rheumatoid arthritis: report of a case with intimal sclerosis of the pulmonary and digital arteries. Scott Med J 1957;2:183–8.
63. Garg K, Lynch DA, Newell JD. Inflammatory airways disease in ulcerative colitis: CT and high-resolution CT features. J Thorac Imaging 1993;8:159–63.
64. Germain MJ, Davidman M. Pulmonary hemorrhage and acute renal failure in a patient with mixed connective tissue disease. Am J Kidney Dis 1984;3:420–4.
65. Goodman TA, Polisson RP. Methotrexate: adverse reactions and major toxicities. Rheum Dis Clin North Am 1994;20:513–28.
66. Griffin MT, Robb JD, Martin JR. Diffuse alveolar haemorrhage associated with progressive systemic sclerosis. Thorax 1990;45:903–4.
67. Groen H, Postma DS, Kallenberg CG. Interstitial lung disease and myositis in a patient with simultaneously occurring sarcoidosis and scleroderma. Chest 1993;104:1298–300.
68. Guidry GG, Baethge BA, Payne DK, Grafton WD. Pulmonary fibrosis as the initial manifestation of scleroderma. J La State Med Soc 1990;142:33–6.
69. Gupta SM, Johnston WH. Apical pulmonary disease in ankylosing spondylitis. N Z Med J 1978;88:186–8.
70. Haerden J, Coolen L, Dequeker J. The effect of D-penicillamine on lung function parameters (diffusion capacity) in rheumatoid arthritis. Clin Exp Rheumatol 1993;11:509–13.

71. Hammar SP, Winterbauer RH, Bockus D, Remington F, Sale GE, Meyers JD. Endothelial cell damage and tubuloreticular structures in interstitial lung disease associated with collagen vascular disease and viral pneumonia. Am Rev Respir Dis 1983;127:77–84.
72. Hansen LA, Prakash UB, Colby TV. Pulmonary lymphoma in Sjögren's syndrome. Mayo Clin Proc 1989;64:920–31.
73. Harmon KR, Leatherman JW. Respiratory manifestations of connective tissue disease. Semin Respir Infect 1988;3:258–73.
74. Harrison NK, Glanville AR, Strickland B, et al. Pulmonary involvement in systemic sclerosis: the detection of early changes by thin section CT scan, bronchoalveolar lavage and 99mTc-DTPA clearance. Respir Med 1989;83:403–14.
75. Harrison NK, Myers AR, Corrin B, et al. Structural features of interstitial lung disease in systemic sclerosis. Am Rev Respir Dis 1991;144: 706–13.
76. Haupt HM, Moore GW, Hutchins GM. The lung in systemic lupus erythematosus. Analysis of the pathologic changes in 120 patients. Am J Med 1981;71:791–8.
77. Hayakawa H, Sato A, Imokawa S, Toyoshima M, Chida K, Iwata M. Bronchiolar disease in rheumatoid arthritis. Am J Respir Crit Care Med 1996;154:1531–6.
78. Hellems SO, Kanner RE, Renzetti AD Jr. Bronchocentric granulomatosis associated with rheumatoid arthritis. Chest 1983;83:831–2.
79. Helmers R, Galvin J, Hunninghake GW. Pulmonary manifestations associated with rheumatoid arthritis. Chest 1991;100:235–8.
80. Henry DW, Rosenthal A, McCarty DJ. Adenocarcinoma of the lung associated with eosinophilia and hidebound skin. J Rheumatol 1994;21:972–3.
81. Hidano A, Torikai S, Uemura T, Shimizu S. Malignancy and interstitial pneumonitis as fatal complications in dermatomyositis. J Dermatol 1992;19:153–60.
82. Hillarby MC, McMahon MJ, Grennan DM, et al. HLA associations in subjects with rheumatoid arthritis and bronchiectasis but not with other pulmonary complications of rheumatoid disease. Br J Rheumatol 1993;32:794–7.
83. Hoffbrand BI, Vianna J, Khamashta M, Hughes GR, Walters DV. Antiphospholipid antibodies and shrinking lungs in SLE [Letter]. Lupus 1992;1:408.
84. Holness L, Tenenbaum J, Cooter NB, Grossman RF. Fatal bronchiolitis obliterans associated with chrysotherapy. Ann Rheum Dis 1983;42:593–6.
85. Holzmann H, Korting GW. Pericollagenous amyloid deposits in the skin and internal organs in scleroderma. Klin Wochenschr 1969;47:390–1.
86. Hosoda Y, Suzuki Y, Takano M, Tojo T, Homma M. Mixed connective tissue disease with pulmonary hypertension: a clinical and pathological study. J Rheumatol 1987;14:826–30.
87. Hotermans G, Benard A, Guenanen H, Demarcq-Delerue G, Malart T, Wallaert B. Nongranulomatous interstitial lung disease in Crohn's disease. Eur Respir J 1996;9:380–2.
88. Howling SJ, Hansell DM, Wells AU, Nicholson AG, Flint JD, Müller NL. Follicular bronchiolitis: thin-section CT and histologic findings. Radiology 1999;212:637–42.
89. Hsu BY, Edwards DK, Trambert MA. Pulmonary hemorrhage complicating systemic lupus erythematosus: role of MR imaging in diagnosis. AJR Am J Roentgenol 1992;158:519–20.
90. Hunninghake GW, Fauci AS. Pulmonary involvement in the collagen vascular diseases. Am Rev Respir Dis 1979;119:471–503.
91. Hunter T, Arnott JE, McCarthy DS. Features of systemic lupus erythematosus and sarcoidosis occurring together. Arthritis Rheum 1980;23: 364–6.
92. Hurwitz SS, Conlan AA, Krige LP. Fibrocavitating pulmonary lesions in ankylosing spondylitis. S Afr Med J 1982;61:168–70.
93. Ichikawa Y, Kinoshita M, Koga T, Oizumi K, Fujimoto K, Hayabuchi N. Lung cyst formation in lymphocytic interstitial pneumonia: CT features. J Comput Assist Tomogr 1994;18:745–8.
94. Ikezoe J, Johkoh T, Kohno N, Takeuchi N, Ichikado K, Nakamura H. High-resolution CT findings of lung disease in patients with polymyositis and dermatomyositis. J Thorac Imaging 1996;11:250–9.
95. Inase N, Usui Y, Tachi H, et al. Sjögren's syndrome with bronchial gland involvement and multiple bullae. Respiration 1990;57:286–8.
96. Ippolito JA, Palmer L, Spector S, Kane PB, Gorevic PD. Bronchiolitis obliterans organizing pneumonia and rheumatoid arthritis. Semin Arthritis Rheum 1993;23:70–8.
97. Isenberg JI, Goldstein H, Korn AR, Ozeran RS, Rosen V. Pulmonary vasculitis—an uncommon complication of ulcerative colitis. Report of a case. N Engl J Med 1968;279:1376–7.
98. Johkoh T, Müller NL, Pickford HA, et al. Lymphocytic interstitial pneumonia: thin-section CT findings in 22 patients. Radiology 1999;212:567–72.
99. Jolliet P, Thorens JB, Chevrolet JC. Pulmonary vascular reactivity in severe pulmonary hypertension associated with mixed connective tissue disease. Thorax 1995;50:96–7.

100. Jones MB, Osterholm RK, Wilson RB, Martin FH, Commers JR, Bachmayer JD. Fatal pulmonary hypertension and resolving immune-complex glomerulonephritis in mixed connective tissue disease. A case report and review of the literature. Am J Med 1978;65:855–63.
101. Kanemoto N, Sato M, Moriuchi J, Ichikawa Y, Goto Y, Sasadaira H. An autopsied case of systemic lupus erythematosus with pulmonary hypertension—a case report. Angiology 1988;39:187–92.
102. Katzenstein AL, Fiorelli RF. Nonspecific interstitial pneumonia/fibrosis. Histologic features and clinical significance. Am J Surg Pathol 1994;18:136–47.
103. Kay JM, Banik S. Unexplained pulmonary hypertension with pulmonary arteritis in rheumatoid disease. Br J Dis Chest 1977;71:53–9.
104. Kim JH, Follett JV, Rice JR, Hampson NB. Endobronchial telangiectasias and hemoptysis in scleroderma. Am J Med 1988;84:173–4.
105. Kobayashi H, Matsuoka R, Kitamura S, Tsunoda N, Saito K. Sjögren's syndrome with multiple bullae and pulmonary nodular amyloidosis. Chest 1988;94:438–40.
106. Koh WH, Boey ML. Open lung biopsy in systemic lupus erythematosus patients with pulmonary disease. Ann Acad Med Singapore 1993;22:323–5.
107. Konig G, Luderschmidt C, Hammer C, Adelmann-Grill BC, Braun-Falco O, Fruhmann G. Lung involvement in scleroderma. Chest 1984;85:318–24.
108. Kosaka Y, Akizuki M, Yoshida S, Mimori T, Homma M. Large cystic lesions of the upper lobes of the lungs in two patients with CREST syndrome. Arthritis Rheum 1984;27:935–8.
109. Kuhn C. Systemic lupus erythematosus in a patient with ultrastructural lesions of the pulmonary capillaries previously reported in the review as due to idiopathic pulmonary hemosiderosis. Am Rev Respir Dis 1974;106:931–2.
110. Lakhanpal S, Lie JT, Conn DL, Martin WJ. Pulmonary disease in polymyositis/dermatomyositis: a clinicopathological analysis of 65 autopsy cases. Ann Rheum Dis 1987;46:23–9.
111. Lee-Chiong TL Jr. Pulmonary manifestations of ankylosing spondylitis and relapsing polychondritis. Clin Chest Med 1998;19:747–57.
112. Lemley DE, Katz P. Rheumatoid-like arthritis presenting as idiopathic pulmonary hemosiderosis: a report and review of the literature. J Rheumatol 1986;13:954–7.
113. Li EK, Tam LS. Pulmonary hypertension in systemic lupus erythematosus: clinical association and survival in 18 patients. J Rheumatol 1999;26:23–9.
114. Libshitz HI, Atkinson GW. Pulmonary cystic disease in ankylosing spondylitis: two cases with unusual superinfection. J Can Assoc Radiol 1978;29:266–8.
115. Liu MF, Lee JH, Weng TH, Lee YY. Clinical experience of 13 cases with severe pulmonary hemorrhage in systemic lupus erythematosus with active nephritis. Scand J Rheumatol 1998;27:291–5.
116. Lyon MG, Bewtra C, Kenik JG, Hurley JA. Tubuloreticular inclusions in systemic lupus pneumonitis. Report of a case and review of the literature. Arch Pathol Lab Med 1984;108:599–600.
117. Mana F, Mets T, Vincken W, Sennesael J, Vanwaeyenbergh J, Goossens A. The association of bronchiolitis obliterans organizing pneumonia, systemic lupus erythematosus, and Hunner's cystitis. Chest 1993;104:642–4.
118. Marie I, Hatron PY, Hachulla E, Wallaert B, Michon-Pasturel U, Devulder B. Pulmonary involvement in polymyositis and in dermatomyositis. J Rheumatol 1998;25:1336–43.
119. Martens J, Demedts M. Diaphragm dysfunction in mixed connective tissue disease. A case report. Scand J Rheumatol 1982;11:165–7.
120. Martyn JB, Wong MJ, Huang SH. Pulmonary and neuromuscular complications of mixed connective tissue disease: a report and review of the literature. J Rheumatol 1988;15:703–5.
121. Matteson EL, Ike RW. Bronchiolitis obliterans organizing pneumonia and Sjögren's syndrome. J Rheumatol 1990;17:676–9.
122. Matthay RA, Schwarz MI, Petty TL, et al. Pulmonary manifestations of systemic lupus erythematosus: review of twelve cases of acute lupus pneumonitis. Medicine (Baltimore) 1975;54:397–409.
123. McCarthy DS, Baragar FD, Dhingra S, et al. The lungs in systemic sclerosis (scleroderma): a review and new information. Semin Arthritis Rheum 1988;17:271–83.
124. McDonagh J, Greaves M, Wright AR, Heycock C, Owen JP, Kelly C. High resolution computed tomography of the lungs in patients with rheumatoid arthritis and interstitial lung disease. Br J Rheumatol 1994;33:118–22.
125. Meyer CA, Pina JS, Taillon D, Godwin JD. Inspiratory and expiratory high-resolution CT findings in a patient with Sjögren's syndrome and cystic lung disease. AJR Am J Roentgenol 1997;168:101–3.
126. Meyers OL. Pulmonary involvement in systemic lupus erythematosus. Scand J Rheumatol Suppl 1984;54:19–23.
127. Michet CJ Jr, McKenna CH, Luthra HS, O'Fallon WM. Relapsing polychondritis. Survival and predictive role of early disease manifestations. Ann Intern Med 1986;104:74–8.

128. Miller LR, Greenberg SD, McLarty JW. Lupus lung. Chest 1985;88:265–9.
129. Milligan DW, Chang JG. Systemic lupus erythematosus and lymphoma. Acta Haematol 1980;64:109–10.
130. Minai OA, Dweik RA, Arroliga AC. Manifestations of scleroderma pulmonary disease. Clin Chest Med 1998;19:713–31.
131. Mino M, Noma S, Taguchi Y, Tomii K, Kohri Y, Oida K. Pulmonary involvement in polymyositis and dermatomyositis: sequential evaluation with CT. AJR Am J Roentgenol 1997;169:83–7.
132. Morassut PA, Walley VM, Smith CD. Pulmonary veno-occlusive disease and the CREST variant of scleroderma. Can J Cardiol 1992;8:1055–8.
133. Murin S, Wiedemann HP, Matthay RA. Pulmonary manifestations of systemic lupus erythematosus. Clin Chest Med 1998;19:641–65.
134. Myers JL. Diagnosis of drug reactions in the lung. Monogr Pathol 1993;36:32–53.
135. Myers JL, Katzenstein AL. Microangiitis in lupus-induced pulmonary hemorrhage. Am J Clin Pathol 1986;85:552–6.
136. Naeye RL. Pulmonary vascular lesions in systemic scleroderma. Dis Chest 1963;44:374–80.
137. Newball HH, Brahim SA. Chronic obstructive airway disease in patients with Sjögren's syndrome. Am Rev Respir Dis 1977;115:295–304.
138. O'Duffy JD, Luthra HS, Unni KK, Hyatt RE. Bronchiolitis in a rheumatoid arthritis patient receiving auranofin. Arthritis Rheum 1986;29:556–9.
139. Onodera S, Hill JR. Pulmonary hypertension. Report of a case in association with rheumatoid arthritis. Ohio State Med J 1965;61:141–4.
140. Onomura K, Nakata H, Tanaka Y, Tsuda T. Pulmonary hemorrhage in patients with systemic lupus erythematosus. J Thorac Imaging 1991;6:57–61.
141. Ooi GC, Ngan H, Peh WC, Mok MY, Ip M. Systemic lupus erythematosus patients with respiratory symptoms: the value of HRCT. Clin Radiol 1997;52:775–81.
142. Owens GR, Paradis IL, Gryzan S, et al. Role of inflammation in the lung disease of systemic sclerosis: comparison with idiopathic pulmonary fibrosis. J Lab Clin Med 1986;107:253–60.
143. Ozawa T, Ninomiya Y, Honma T, et al. Increased serum angiotensin I-converting enzyme activity in patients with mixed connective tissue disease and pulmonary hypertension. Scand J Rheumatol 1995;24:38–43.
144. Partanen J, van Assendelft AH, Koskimies S, Forsberg S, Hakala M, Ilonen J. Patients with rheumatoid arthritis and gold-induced pneumonitis express two high-risk major histocompatibility complex patterns. Chest 1987;92:277–81.
145. Payne CR, Connellan SJ. Chronic eosinophilic pneumonia complicating long-standing rheumatoid arthritis. Postgrad Med J 1980;56:519–20.
146. Peters-Golden M, Wise RA, Hochberg M, Stevens MB, Wigley FM. Incidence of lung cancer in systemic sclerosis. J Rheumatol 1985;12:1136–9.
147. Plotz PH, Dalakas M, Leff RL, Love LA, Miller FW, Cronin ME. Current concepts in the idiopathic inflammatory myopathies: polymyositis, dermatomyositis, and related disorders. Ann Intern Med 1989;111:143–57.
148. Pommepuy I, Farny M, Billey T, Olivier P, Lassoued S. Bronchiolitis obliterans organizing pneumonia in a patient with rheumatoid arthritis. Rev Rhum Engl Ed 1998;65:65–7.
149. Popp W, Rauscher H, Ritschka L, et al. Prediction of interstitial lung involvement in rheumatoid arthritis. The value of clinical data, chest roentgenogram, lung function, and serologic parameters. Chest 1992;102:391–4.
150. Port JL, Khan A, Barbu RR. Computed tomography of relapsing polychondritis. Comput Med Imaging Graph 1993;17:119–23.
151. Prakash UB. Lungs in mixed connective tissue disease. J Thorac Imaging 1992;7:55–61.
152. Prakash UB. Respiratory complications in mixed connective tissue disease. Clin Chest Med 1998;19:733–46.
153. Primack SL, Müller NL. Radiologic manifestations of the systemic autoimmune diseases. Clin Chest Med 1998;19:573–86.
154. Pronk LC, Swaak AJ. Pulmonary hypertension in connective tissue disease. Report of three cases and review of the literature. Rheumatol Int 1991;11:83–6.
155. Quismorio FP Jr, Sharma O, Koss M, et al. Immunopathologic and clinical studies in pulmonary hypertension associated with systemic lupus erythematosus. Semin Arthritis Rheum 1984;13:349–59.
156. Rees JH, Woodhead MA, Sheppard MN, du Bois RM. Rheumatoid arthritis and cryptogenic organising pneumonitis. Respir Med 1991;85:243–6.
157. Remy-Jardin M, Remy J, Cortet B, Mauri F, Delcambre B. Lung changes in rheumatoid arthritis: CT findings. Radiology 1994;193:375–82.
158. Rocco VK, Hurd ER. Scleroderma and scleroderma-like disorders. Semin Arthritis Rheum 1986;16:22–69.
159. Romans B, Cohen S. A rheumatologist's view of polymyositis/dermatomyositis: extracutaneous and extramuscular involvement and overlap syndromes. Clin Dermatol 1988;6:15–22.
160. Roncoroni AJ, Alvarez C, Molinas F. Plexogenic arteriopathy associated with pulmonary vasculitis in systemic lupus erythematosus. Respiration 1992;59:52–6.

161. Rosenberg AM, Petty RE, Cumming GR, Koehler BE. Pulmonary hypertension in a child with mixed connective tissue disease. J Rheumatol 1979;6:700–4.
162. Rosenow E, Strimlan CV, Muhm JR, Ferguson RH. Pleuropulmonary manifestations of ankylosing spondylitis. Mayo Clin Proc 1977;52:641–9.
163. Roumm AD, Medsger TA Jr. Cancer and systemic sclerosis. An epidemiologic study. Arthritis Rheum 1985;28:1336–40.
164. Rubin LA, Urowitz MB. Shrinking lung syndrome in SLE—a clinical pathologic study. J Rheumatol 1983;10:973–6.
165. Salerno SM, Ormseth EJ, Roth BJ, Meyer CA, Christensen ED, Dillard TA. Sulfasalazine pulmonary toxicity in ulcerative colitis mimicking clinical features of Wegener's granulomatosis. Chest 1996;110:556–9.
166. Salmeron G, Greenberg SD, Lidsky MD. Polymyositis and diffuse interstitial lung disease. A review of the pulmonary histopathologic findings. Arch Intern Med 1981;141:1005–10.
167. Samuels MP, Warner JO. Pulmonary alveolar lipoproteinosis complicating juvenile dermatomyositis. Thorax 1988;43:939–40.
168. Sanchez-Guerrero J, Cesarman G, Alarcon-Segovia D. Massive pulmonary hemorrhage in mixed connective tissue diseases. J Rheumatol 1989;16:1132–4.
169. Schnabel A, Gross WL. Low-dose methotrexate in rheumatic diseases—efficacy, side effects, and risk factors for side effects. Semin Arthritis Rheum 1994;23:310–27.
170. Schurawitzki H, Stiglbauer R, Graninger W, et al. Interstitial lung disease in progressive systemic sclerosis: high-resolution CT versus radiography. Radiology 1990;176:755–9.
171. Schuurman HJ, Gooszen HC, Tan IW, Kluin PM, Wagenaar SS, van Unnik JA. Low-grade lymphoma of immature T-cell phenotype in a case of lymphocytic interstitial pneumonia and Sjögren's syndrome. Histopathology 1987;11:1193–204.
172. Schwarz MI. Pulmonary and cardiac manifestations of polymyositis-dermatomyositis. J Thorac Imaging 1992;7:46–54.
173. Schwarz MI. The lung in polymyositis. Clin Chest Med 1998;19:701–12.
174. Schwarz MI, Lynch DA, Tuder R. Bronchiolitis obliterans: the lone manifestation of rheumatoid arthritis? Eur Respir J 1994;7:817–20.
175. Scott DL, Bradby GV, Aitman TJ, Zaphiropoulos GC, Hawkins CF. Relationship of gold and penicillamine therapy to diffuse interstitial lung disease. Ann Rheum Dis 1981;40:136–41.
176. Searles G, McKendry RJ. Methotrexate pneumonitis in rheumatoid arthritis: potential risk factors. Four case reports and a review of the literature. J Rheumatol 1987;14:1164–71.
177. Seed WA, Fox B. Chronic eosinophilic pneumonia and rheumatoid arthritis—coincidental? [Letter]. J Clin Pathol 1981;34:813.
178. Servi RJ, Albertini RE, Torretti D. Pulmonary hypertension, hypoxemia, and death in a patient with scleroderma. South Med J 1985;78:739–41.
179. Shadick NA, Fanta CH, Weinblatt ME, O'Donnell W, Coblyn JS. Bronchiectasis. A late feature of severe rheumatoid arthritis. Medicine (Baltimore) 1994;73:161–70.
180. Shannon TM, Gale ME. Noncardiac manifestations of rheumatoid arthritis in the thorax. J Thorac Imaging 1992;7:19–29.
181. Shen JY, Chen SL, Wu YX, et al. Pulmonary hypertension in systemic lupus erythematosus. Rheumatol Int 1999;18:147–51.
182. Silver RM, Miller KS. Lung involvement in systemic sclerosis. Rheum Dis Clin North Am 1990;16:199–216.
183. Simonson JS, Schiller NB, Petri M, Hellman DB. Pulmonary hypertension in systemic lupus erythematosus. J Rheumatol 1989;16:918–25.
184. Smith DH, Scott DL, Zaphiropoulos GC. Eosinophilia in D-penicillamine therapy. Ann Rheum Dis 1983;42:408–10.
185. Staples CA, Müller NL, Vedal S, Abboud R, Ostrow D, Miller RR. Usual interstitial pneumonia: correlation of CT with clinical, functional, and radiologic findings. Radiology 1987;162:377–81.
186. Stein HB, Chalmers A, Schroeder ML, Dillon A. Selected adverse reactions of D-penicillamine. Clin Invest Med 1984;7:73–6.
187. Stein HB, Patterson AC, Offer RC, Atkins CJ, Teufel A, Robinson HS. Adverse effects of D-penicillamine in rheumatoid arthritis. Ann Intern Med 1980;92:24–9.
188. Stein HB, Ruedy J, Atkins CJ, Offer RC. Penicillamine and other remittive agents in rheumatoid arthritis: comparisons and interaction. Clin Invest Med 1984;7:59–63.
189. Stewart RM, Ridyard JB, Pearson JD. Regional lung function in ankylosing spondylitis. Thorax 1976;31:433–7.
190. Strimlan CV, Rosenow EC, Divertie MB, Harrison EG Jr. Pulmonary manifestations of Sjögren's syndrome. Chest 1976;70:354–61.
191. Sullivan WD, Hurst DJ, Harmon CE, et al. A prospective evaluation emphasizing pulmonary involvement in patients with mixed connective tissue disease. Medicine (Baltimore) 1984;63:92–107.
192. Sviri S, Gafanovich I, Kramer MR, Tsvang E, Ben-Chetrit E. Mesalamine-induced hypersensitivity pneumonitis. A case report and review of the literature. J Clin Gastroenterol 1997;24:34–6.

193. Swinburn CR, Jackson GJ, Cobden I, Ashcroft T, Morritt GN, Corris PA. Bronchiolitis obliterans organising pneumonia in a patient with ulcerative colitis. Thorax 1988;43:735–6.
194. Takizawa H, Shiga J, Moroi Y, Miyachi S, Nishiwaki M, Miyamoto T. Interstitial lung disease in dermatomyositis: clinicopathological study. J Rheumatol 1987;14:102–7.
195. Tanigawa K, Sugiyama K, Matsuyama H, et al. Mesalazine-induced eosinophilic pneumonia. Respiration 1999;66:69–72.
196. Taniguchi M, Sato A, Honda K, Ohgo S, Yoshimura K. Bronchopulmonary manifestations of Sjögren's syndrome: the findings of the BAL, TBLB, and bronchoscopy. Panminerva Med 1986;28:249–51.
197. Tanoue LT. Pulmonary involvement in collagen vascular disease: a review of the pulmonary manifestations of the Marfan syndrome, ankylosing spondylitis, Sjögren's syndrome, and relapsing polychondritis. J Thorac Imaging 1992;7:62–77.
198. Tanoue LT. Pulmonary manifestations of rheumatoid arthritis. Clin Chest Med 1998;19:667–85.
199. Targoff IN, Arnett FC, Berman L, O'Brien C, Reichlin M. Anti-KJ: a new antibody associated with the syndrome of polymyositis and interstitial lung disease. J Clin Invest 1989;84:162–72.
200. Tazelaar HD, Viggiano RW, Pickersgill J, Colby TV. Interstitial lung disease in polymyositis and dermatomyositis. Clinical features and prognosis as correlated with histologic findings. Am Rev Respir Dis 1990;141:727–33.
201. Thompson PJ, Dhillon DP, Ledingham J, Turner-Warwick M. Shrinking lungs, diaphragmatic dysfunction, and systemic lupus erythematosus. Am Rev Respir Dis 1985;132:926–8.
202. Tomioka R, King TE Jr. Gold-induced pulmonary disease: clinical features, outcome, and differentiation from rheumatoid lung disease. Am J Respir Crit Care Med 1997;155:1011–20.
203. Travis WD, Colby TV, Lombard CM, Carpenter HA. A clinicopathologic study of 34 cases of diffuse pulmonary hemorrhage with lung biopsy confirmation. Am J Surg Pathol 1990;14:1112–25.
204. Travis WD, Koss MN, Ferrans VJ. The lung in connective tissue disorders. In: Hasleton PS, ed. Spencer's pathology of the lung, 5th ed. New York: McGraw-Hill; 1996:803–34.
205. Tsuzaka K, Akama H, Yamada H, Akizuki M, Tojo T, Homma M. Pulmonary pseudolymphoma presented with a mass lesion in a patient with primary Sjögren's syndrome: beneficial effect of intermittent intravenous cyclophosphamide. Scand J Rheumatol 1993;22:90–3.
206. Turner-Warwick M. Connective tissue disorders and the lung. Aust N Z J Med 1986;16:257–62.
207. Ueda N, Mimura K, Maeda H, et al. Mixed connective tissue disease with fatal pulmonary hypertension and a review of literature. Virchows Arch [A] 1984;404:335–40.
208. Ungerer RG, Tashkin DP, Furst D, et al. Prevalence and clinical correlates of pulmonary arterial hypertension in progressive systemic sclerosis. Am J Med 1983;75:65–74.
209. Usui Y, Kimula Y, Miura H, et al. A case of bronchiolitis obliterans organizing pneumonia associated with primary Sjögren's syndrome who died of superimposed diffuse alveolar damage. Respiration 1992;59:122–4.
210. Van Hoeyweghen RJ, De Clerck LS, Van Offel JF, Stevens WJ. Interstitial lung disease and adult-onset Still's disease. Clin Rheumatol 1993;12: 418–21.
211. van Thiel RJ, van der Burg S, Groote AD, Nossent GD, Wills SH. Bronchiolitis obliterans organizing pneumonia and rheumatoid arthritis. Eur Respir J 1991;4:905–11.
212. Wakaki K, Koizumi F, Fukase M. Vascular lesions in systemic lupus erythematosus (SLE) with pulmonary hypertension. Acta Pathol Jpn 1984;34:593–604.
213. Wallaert B, Prin L, Hatron PY, Ramon P, Tonnel AB, Voisin C. Lymphocyte subpopulations in bronchoalveolar lavage in Sjögren's syndrome. Evidence for an expansion of cytotoxic/suppressor subset in patients with alveolar neutrophilia. Chest 1987;92:1025–31.
214. Walz-Leblanc BA, Urowitz MB, Gladman DD, Hanly PJ. The shrinking lungs syndrome in systemic lupus erythematosus—improvement with corticosteroid therapy. J Rheumatol 1992;19:1970–2.
215. Wang YT, Singh D, Poh SC. Diffuse interstitial pulmonary fibrosis, dermatomyositis and lung cancer—a case report. Singapore Med J 1980;21:778–80.
216. Ward H, Fisher KL, Waghray R, Wright JL, Card SE, Cockcroft DW. Constrictive bronchiolitis and ulcerative colitis. Can Respir J 1999;6:197–200.
217. Warrick JH, Bhalla M, Schabel SI, Silver RM. High resolution computed tomography in early scleroderma lung disease. J Rheumatol 1991;18:1520–8.
218. Wiedemann HP, Matthay RA. Pulmonary manifestations of the collagen vascular diseases. Clin Chest Med 1989;10:677–722.
219. Wiedemann HP, Matthay RA. Pulmonary manifestations of systemic lupus erythematosus. J Thorac Imaging 1992;7:1–18.
220. Wiener-Kronish JP, Solinger AM, Warnock ML, Churg A, Ordonez NG, Golden JA. Severe pulmonary involvement in mixed connective tissue disease. Am Rev Respir Dis 1981;124:499–503.

221. Wilcox P, Miller R, Miller G, et al. Airway involvement in ulcerative colitis. Chest 1987;92:18–22.
222. Williams T, Eidus L, Thomas P. Fibrosing alveolitis, bronchiolitis obliterans, and sulfasalazine therapy. Chest 1982;81:766–8.
223. Winterbauer RH, Wilske KR, Wheelis RF. Diffuse pulmonary injury associated with gold treatment. N Engl J Med 1976;294:919–21.
224. Wolfe F, Schurle DR, Lin JJ, et al. Upper and lower airway disease in penicillamine treated patients with rheumatoid arthritis. J Rheumatol 1983;10:406–10.
225. Yokoi T, Tomita Y, Fukaya M, Ichihara S, Kakudo K, Takahashi Y. Pulmonary hypertension associated with systemic lupus erythematosus: predominantly thrombotic arteriopathy accompanied by plexiform lesions. Arch Pathol Lab Med 1998;122:467–70.
226. Young ID, Ford SE, Ford PM. The association of pulmonary hypertension with rheumatoid arthritis. J Rheumatol 1989;16:1266–9.
227. Young RH, Mark EJ. Pulmonary vascular changes in scleroderma. Am J Med 1978;64:998–1004.
228. Yousem SA. The pulmonary pathologic manifestations of the CREST syndrome. Hum Pathol 1990;21:467–74.
229. Yousem SA, Colby TV, Carrington CB. Lung biopsy in rheumatoid arthritis. Am Rev Respir Dis 1985;131:770–7.
230. Yum MN, Ziegler JR, Walker PD, Ridolfo AS, Brashear RE. Pseudolymphoma of the lung in a patient with systemic lupus erythematosus. Am J Med 1979;66:172–6.
231. Zamora MR, Warner ML, Tuder R, Schwarz MI. Diffuse alveolar hemorrhage and systemic lupus erythematosus. Clinical presentation, histology, survival, and outcome. Medicine (Baltimore) 1997;76:192–202.

7
DRUG AND RADIATION REACTIONS

DRUG REACTIONS

Definition and Background

Pulmonary drug reactions are the result of either direct or indirect effects of a drug on the lung. Direct effects can be broadly divided into those that are toxic reactions and those that are idiosyncratic reactions. The histologic manifestations are often not unique to the particular drug and many drugs are associated with more than one clinical or pathologic pattern of disease. For convenience, reactions associated with some illicit drugs are also included in this section.

The criteria for the definitive diagnosis of a drug reaction are quite rigorous: the drug has to have been administered in a temporal fashion consistent with an adverse reaction and other possible causes must have been excluded; the reaction abates when the drug is stopped and recurs with rechallenge; the implicated drug is the only drug being administered; the pattern of disease (clinical, radiologic, and/or pathologic) is characteristic of the drug under question; and, for some drugs, quantitatively abnormal drug levels are present (28). Very few cases fulfill these criteria and most pulmonary drug reactions remain suspected rather than proven. According to Irey (28), one should assign a degree of certainty for a drug in any given case as causative, probable, or possible. In practice, most potential drug reactions fall into the probable or possible categories. A casual review of the literature on pulmonary drug reactions reveals that the criteria for diagnosis are arbitrary and vary considerably from report to report.

Drug reactions in the lung represent a significant clinical problem, the frequency of which is increasing (9,10,11,26,32,36,41,43,52, 67,68), and there are a large number of drugs that have been implicated in causing pulmonary disease. Pharmacologic groups associated with pulmonary toxicity include antimicrobials, anti-inflammatory agents, cancer chemotherapeutic agents, cardiovascular drugs, and illicit drugs. The majority of pulmonary drug reactions are not biopsied, and thus the pathologist's perspective is skewed. The cases that come to biopsy tend to be those that are severe or those in which the clinical diagnosis is in doubt.

Generally, pulmonary drug reactions are the result of either direct or indirect effects of the drug (52). Reactions due to direct effects can be broadly divided into those that are toxic reactions (which to some extent are dose-related, such as reactions to chemotherapeutic agents) and those that are idiosyncratic reactions (which tend not to show a consistent dose-response relationship) (52). Needless to say, this division is artificial and the distinction between toxic reactions and idiosyncratic reactions is not always clear-cut. Amiodarone toxicity is a case in point (12,36,41,45,52). Amiodarone may exert a direct toxic effect on the lung by an acquired phospholipidosis that corresponds to the foamy macrophages so characteristic of this disease. In some cases a lymphocytic alveolitis is also apparent in the bronchoalveolar lavage (BAL) specimen suggesting an immunologic component to the disease. Features reflecting both putative mechanisms may be apparent histologically (fig. 7-1). Similarly, bleomycin has been implicated in both toxic-type and idiosyncratic-type reactions (fig. 7-2) (9,10,36,41,52).

Examples of the indirect effects of drugs in the lung include drug-induced thromboembolic complications, drug-induced central nervous system (CNS) depression and its effect on the lung (for example, aspiration) and, most importantly, drug-induced immunosuppression with secondary opportunistic pulmonary infection (9,33,43,52). For the surgical pathologist, one of the most common differential diagnostic considerations in a suspected drug reaction is opportunistic infection in an immunosuppressed patient.

Very few drugs produce unique (or nearly unique) histologic findings (9,41). This lack of histologic specificity complicates diagnosis. In addition, one drug may be associated with more than one clinical or pathologic pattern of disease (fig. 7-2), and multiple drugs may cause a given clinical or pathologic disease pattern. Nitrofurantoin is a good example of a drug with

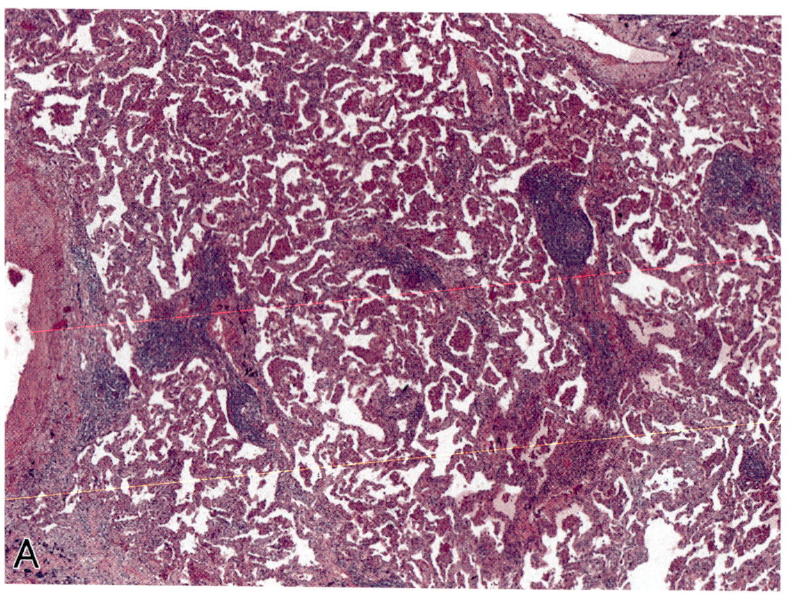

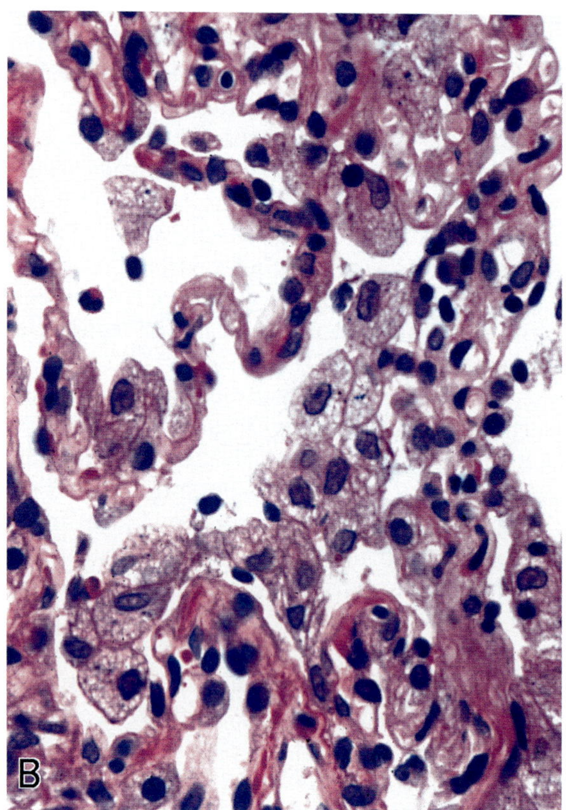

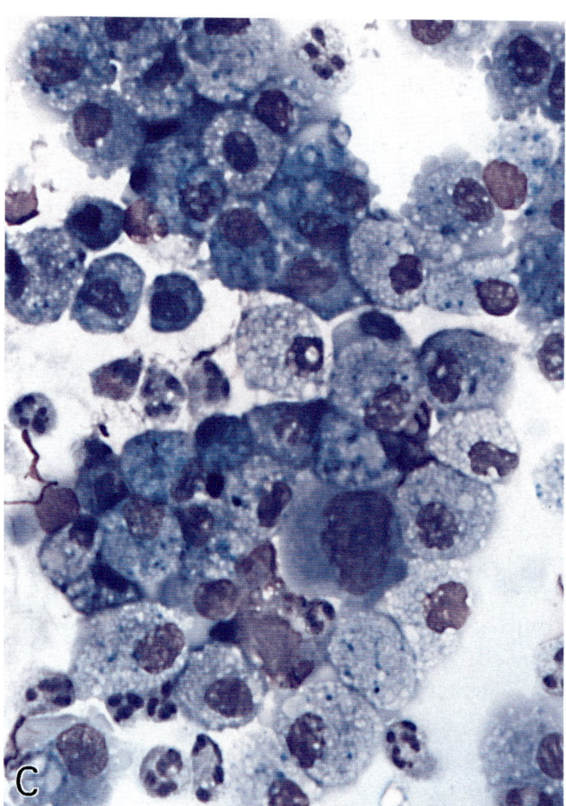

Figure 7-1

AMIODARONE TOXICITY

Amiodarone toxicity shows lymphoid hyperplasia as well as an increase in alveolar macrophages, which impart a desquamative interstitial pneumonia-like appearance at low power (A). The alveolar macrophages show a prominent foamy change in the cytoplasm (the acquired phospholipidosis) which is apparent in both the histologic section (B) and bronchoalveolar lavage material (C).

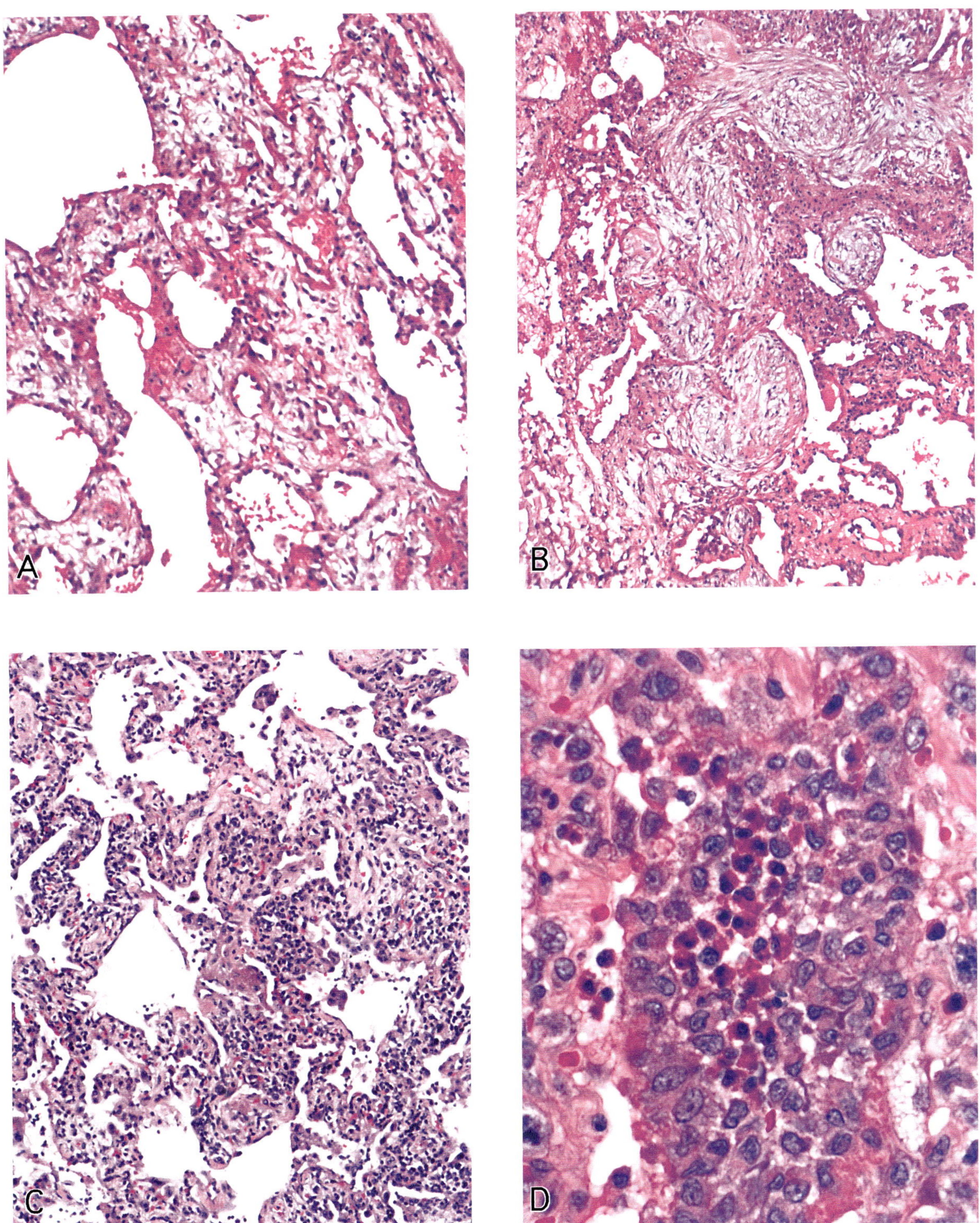

Figure 7-2

BLEOMYCIN PULMONARY TOXICITY: HISTOLOGIC SPECTRUM

Changes associated with bleomycin toxicity include: acute diffuse alveolar damage (A), organizing pneumonia (B), cellular interstitial infiltrates with focal airspace fibrin (C), and eosinophilic pneumonia (D).

multiple pulmonary manifestations: chronic or acute interstitial pneumonitis, pulmonary hemorrhage, bronchoconstriction, anaphylaxis, and pleural effusion (67).

Clinical Syndromes Associated with Pulmonary Drug Reactions

The identification of drug-induced lung disease requires an active consideration of any change in the patient's clinical course as a possible response to medications (67). There are no pathognomonic signs, symptoms, laboratory tests, or pathologic features that identify a drug as the cause of the illness. Further, drug-induced lung disease must be distinguished from more common illnesses or causes of acute exacerbation of an ongoing illness such as asthma, infection, congestive heart failure, pulmonary thromboembolism, or malignancy.

A new and continuously updated web site is available for information on drug-induced pulmonary reactions: http://www.pneumotox.com. This is an effort by the Groupe d'Etudes de la Pathologie Pulmonaire Iatrogène (GEPPI), a study group founded in France in 1995 within the Société de Pneumologie de Langue Française (SPLF) and the Association Française des Centres de Pharmacovigilance (AFCP). The group's stated purpose is to provide information regarding individual cases, collect and update literature on drug-induced lung disease, publish updated lists of offending compounds, and formulate warnings when new side-effects of drugs are reported. This is a useful, readily available resource when drug toxicity is under consideration.

There are a number of recognized cofactors that may enhance the likelihood of a pulmonary drug reaction, particularly reactions associated with chemotherapeutic agents. These include advanced age, prior radiotherapy, and, in the case of bleomycin, elevated inspired oxygen levels; the presence of any or all of these factors increases the likelihood of developing a pulmonary drug reaction (9,67). Surgery may even be a precipitating event (63).

There are also some remarkable peculiarities of pulmonary drug reactions (9). Perhaps analogous to localized fixed drug eruptions in the skin, some pulmonary drug reactions are relatively localized (figs. 7-3, 7-4). Drug reactions in the lung may present as an acute process in a patient who has been on the implicated drug for months or even years. Late complications in the lung due to drug therapy may manifest years after the drug has been stopped; this is best shown in the development of pulmonary fibrosis many years after bischloroethyl nitrosourea (BCNU) therapy for childhood brain tumors (44).

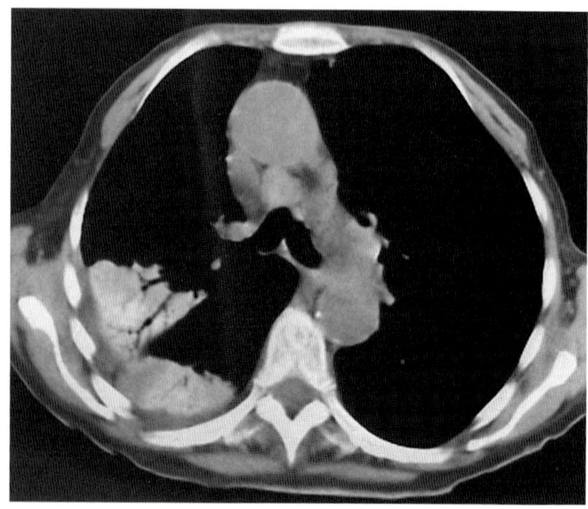

Figure 7-3

AMIODARONE TOXICITY

Amiodarone toxicity associated with a localized infiltrate. Increased attenuation was due to the accumulation of the iodinated compound (amiodarone) in the region of the consolidation.

The spectrum of clinical syndromes associated with pulmonary drug reactions is broad (Table 7-1) and spans most of pulmonary medicine. One useful grouping is by rapidity of onset and rate of progression: acute reactions (onset of clinical manifestations within minutes to hours of taking the drug), for example, anaphylaxis, exacerbation of bronchospasm, alveolar hypoventilation, or pulmonary edema; subacute reactions (days to weeks), characterized by hypersensitivity pneumonitis, drug-induced systemic lupus erythematosus, eosinophilic pneumonitis, alveolar hemorrhage, diffuse alveolar damage, organizing pneumonia with or without obliterans, or pleural processes; and chronic reactions (months to years), seen mainly in patients with interstitial pneumonitis.

The clinical presentation of patients with most drug reactions is nonspecific: cough, dyspnea, fatigue, fever, chest pain, and weight loss

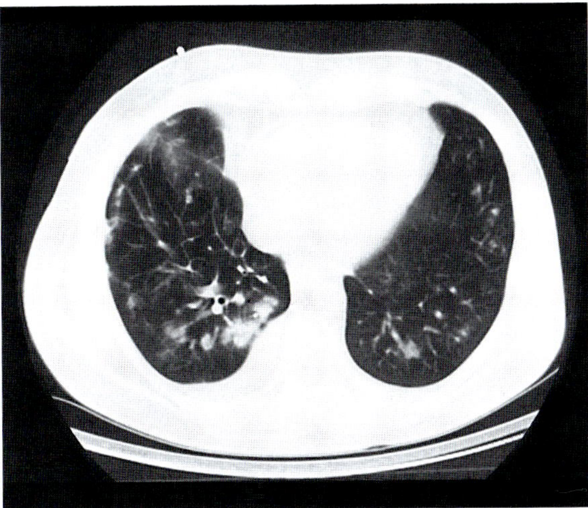

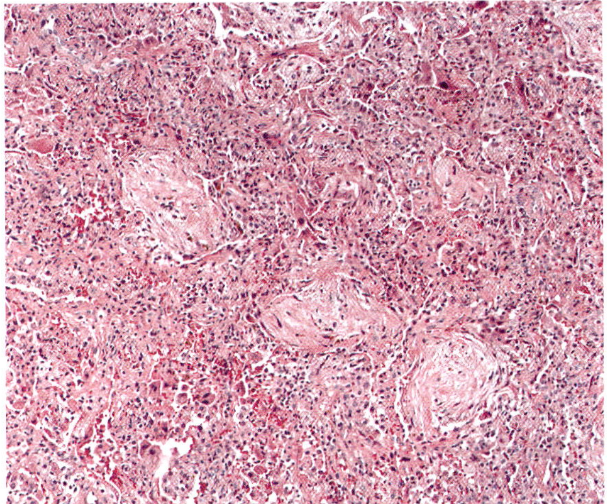

Figure 7-4

BLEOMYCIN TOXICITY

Top: Chest CT demonstrates bilateral nodular opacities, worse in the right lung.

Bottom: Histologically, there is organizing pneumonia.

are the most common manifestations. On physical examination there may be crackles in the chest, rarely rubs or evidence of pleural effusion. Laboratory studies may show eosinophilia. The chest radiograph may show parenchymal opacities and, rarely, pleural effusion. Pulmonary function testing often shows a decrease in the diffusion of carbon monoxide (DLCO), with or without a restrictive pattern (10,32,36,52,67).

A lung biopsy is often required to help establish the diagnosis. An open or thoracoscopic lung biopsy is recommended. BAL may be of value in suggesting drug-induced lung diseases (fig. 7-1C), or more importantly, in ruling out other problems that are more common in this setting, especially infection or malignancy. The BAL findings supporting a drug-related lung reaction include (12,36,45,52): 1) cytotoxic reactions in which the typical finds are atypical cells (cytomegaly, cytoplasmic eosinophilia, bizarre cell shape, nuclear hyperchromasia, prominent

Table 7-1

CLINICAL SYNDROMES AND DISEASES ASSOCIATED WITH PULMONARY DRUG REACTIONS

Airway Dysfunction or Respiratory Insufficiency
Asthma or bronchospasm
Chronic cough
Acute airway obstruction and laryngeal edema (anaphylaxis)
Irreversible airflow obstruction (bronchiolitis obliterans)
Emphysema
Airway burns
Alveolar hypoventilation
Impairment of respiratory muscles
Alveolar Processes
Pulmonary edema (noncardiogenic)
Diffuse alveolar hemorrhage
Diffuse Parenchymal Lung Processes
Acute respiratory distress syndrome
Acute or subacute or chronic interstitial lung disease
Interstitial pneumonitis as part of a hypersensitivity reaction (± eosinophilia)
Systemic lupus erythematosus-like syndromes
Organizing pneumonia
Metastatic calcification involving pulmonary parenchyma
Foreign body granulomatosis
Localized or Nodular Infiltrates
Pulmonary Vascular Disease
Pulmonary hypertension
Pulmonary vasculitis
Pulmonary thromboembolism
Pulmonary veno-occlusive disease
Hemolytic-uremic (thrombotic microangiopathic) syndrome
Pleural Disease
Pleuritis or pleural effusion
Hemothorax
Pneumothorax/pneumomediastinum
Mediastinal Manifestations
Enlarged hilar/mediastinal lymph nodes
Angioimmunoblastic lymphadenopathy-like syndrome
Mediastinal fatty deposits (lipomatosis)
Sclerosing mediastinitis

nucleoli, and multinucleation), increased eosinophils, and extracellular lipoproteinaceous debris; 2) pulmonary hemorrhage with hemosiderin-laden alveolar macrophages; 3) lymphocytic alveolitis in which 40 to 50 percent of retrieved cells are lymphocytes, as well as increased CD8+ cells and a decreased CD4+ to CD8+ ratio suggestive of a hypersensitivity reaction. Gold, methotrexate, and azathioprine have been associated with lymphocytic alveolitis. A predominance of suppressor/cytotoxic T cells with a reduced CD4+/CD8+ ratio is common in methotrexate-induced pneumonitis; 4) neutrophilic alveolitis, consisting of less than 5 percent neutrophils. This may reflect fibrosis; 5) eosinophilic alveolitis, consisting of fewer than 5 percent eosinophils. Several drugs may cause an acute "allergic" or "hypersensitivity" type reaction manifested by the onset of symptoms within days of starting the medication. Fever, chills, dyspnea, pulmonary infiltrates, and peripheral eosinophilia (approximately 40 percent of cases) are seen. BAL and tissue (via transbronchial lung biopsy) eosinophilia may be identified; and 6) lipoid pneumonia due to mineral oil nose-drops or laxatives.

Occasionally, BAL reveals abnormalities associated with a "drug effect" but without the findings of drug toxicity. Gold therapy is a well-established treatment modality in patients with active rheumatoid arthritis. Alveolar macrophages retain gold for prolonged periods but this is not associated with the development of gold-induced pneumonitis or chronic rheumatoid lung disease (20). Amiodarone therapy is associated with the development of lamellar inclusions in alveolar macrophages, indicating a "phospholipidosis"; this finding only indicates that the patient is taking the drug and does not provide any information regarding the possibility of pulmonary toxicity (12,36,45). The cellular profile of the BAL fluid in amiodarone pneumonitis is highly variable: mixed in 33 percent, neutrophilic in 26 percent, lymphocytic in 21 percent, and normal in 20 percent of reported cases (12). In these cases, the BAL pattern was not related to the daily or total dose of amiodarone or to the duration of treatment. No cellular pattern of BAL seems to be predictive of a detrimental outcome or of irreversible fibrosis (12).

Table 7-2

HISTOLOGIC PATTERNS ASSOCIATED WITH PULMONARY DRUG REACTIONS[a]

Pulmonary edema
Acute or chronic alveolar hemorrhage
Alveolar proteinosis-like reaction
Acute, organizing or organized diffuse alveolar damage
Organizing pneumonia
Fibrosing chronic interstitial pneumonitis resembling usual interstitial pneumonia
Diffuse cellular interstitial infiltrates (± foci of organization)
Nonspecific interstitial pneumonia
Lymphocytic interstitial pneumonia
Giant cell interstitial pneumonia
Diffuse lymphoid pneumonia
Granulomatous interstitial pneumonia
Acute or chronic eosinophilic pneumonia
Small vessel angiitis
Metastatic calcification
Foreign body reaction (intravenous drug abuse)
Pulmonary arterial hypertension
Pulmonary veno-occlusive disease
Asthma
Constrictive bronchiolitis (bronchiolitis obliterans with airflow obstruction)
Bronchiectasis
Miliary small nodules
Panacinar emphysema and bullous lung disease
Combinations of these

[a]Modified from references 9, 41, and the text.

Pathologic Patterns Associated with Pulmonary Drug Reactions

As can be seen in Table 7-2, there are many histologic patterns associated with a drug-induced lung injury. While some drugs may produce relatively pure patterns (as described in chapter 2), in many instances drug reactions are somewhat difficult to classify and the patterns may vary from field to field. The reaction may defy classification beyond a histologic descriptive tabulation of the features present. In some instances, there is evidence of acute organizing and chronic disease in the same biopsy and the features do not fit into any well-recognized pattern (figs. 7-5, 7-6).

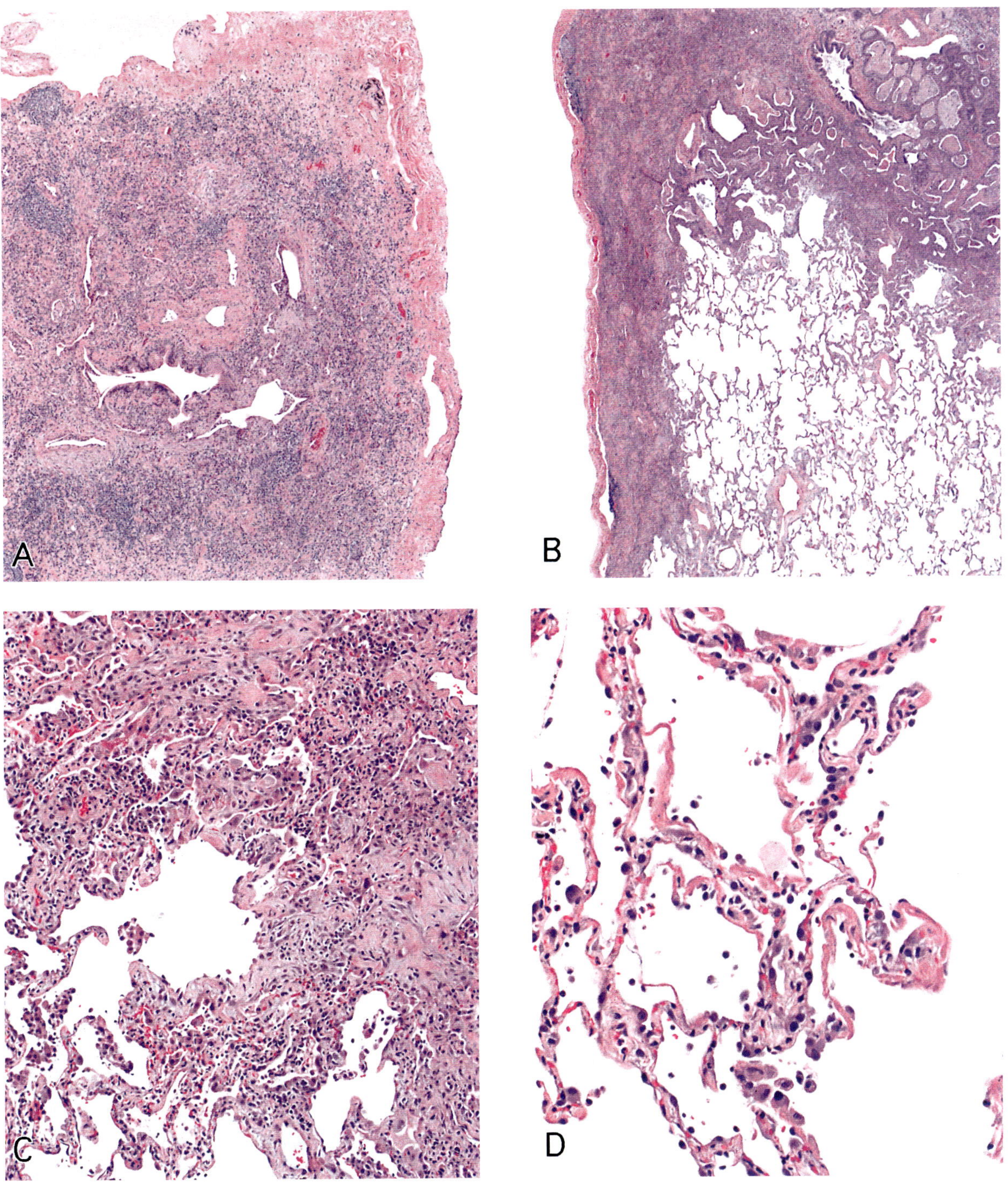

Figure 7-5

NITROFURANTOIN TOXICITY

This patient had been on nitrofurantoin for several years and then developed acute diffuse pulmonary disease. In some regions (A) the lung showed loss of architecture with fibrosis and prominent chronic inflammation. In some regions there was an abrupt transition to architecturally normal lung (B) with some suggestion of subpleural involvement, but without honeycomb change. Much of the involved lung tissue showed fibroblastic proliferation with prominent inflammatory infiltrates (C), whereas some of the intact alveoli showed hyaline membranes (D). This spectrum of chronic, subacute, and acute changes is not uncommon in pulmonary drug reactions.

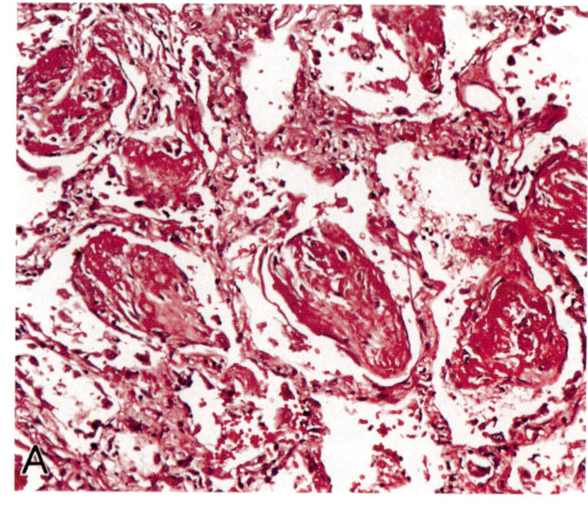

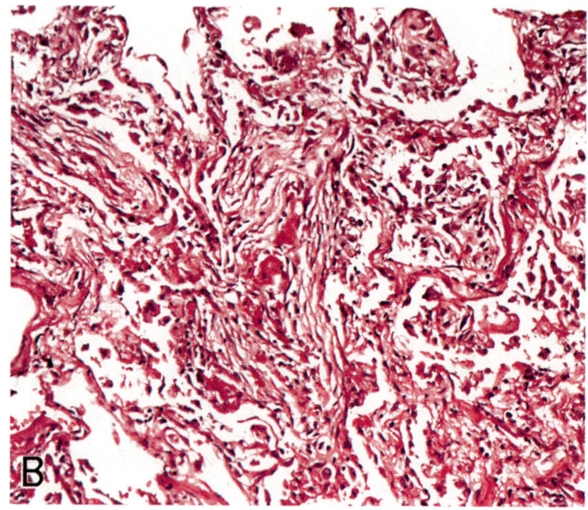

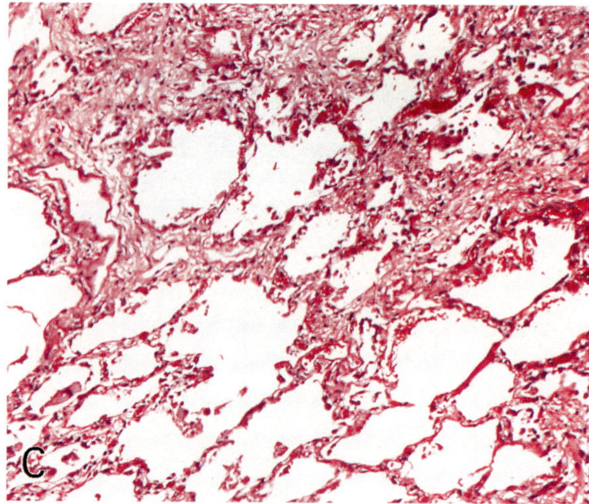

Figure 7-6

BUSULFAN TOXICITY

Busulfan toxicity shows a spectrum of changes from field to field, including acute lung injury with airspace fibrin (A), organizing pneumonia (B), and interstitial fibrosis (C).

Most of the pathologic descriptions of pulmonary drug reactions in the literature predate the current classification of interstitial pneumonias (see chapter 3) so that many cases previously called usual interstitial pneumonia (UIP) might currently be designated nonspecific interstitial pneumonia (NSIP). Similarly, cases that are now be classified as diffuse alveolar damage (DAD) or organizing pneumonia (OP) might have previously been labeled UIP. The most important aspects in considering the reaction of a given drug are whether it has been previously reported to cause lung disease (usually an interstitial pneumonia) and recognizing that subclassification may not necessarily fit with exactly what has been reported previously. In addition, it is common for patients with drug reactions to be taking multiple drugs (e.g., chemotherapeutic agents), and it may be impossible to implicate one specific drug on biopsy.

The following conditions and the drugs associated with them are modified from Myers (41), with additions as noted.

Chronic interstitial pneumonia (resembling UIP, lymphocytic interstitial pneumonia, NSIP, or cellular interstitial infiltrates) (figs. 7-6–7-11): amiodarone, BCNU, busulfan, chlorambucil, cocaine, cyclophosphamide, fluoxetine, gold salts, melphalan, methotrexate, methyl-chloroethyl chlorohexl nitrosourea (CCNU), nilutamide, nitrofurantoin, phenytoin, pindolol, procarbazine, quinidine, sulfasalazine, tocainide, tryptophan, and uracil mustard. Some examples of drug-induced pulmonary fibrosis have developed from lesions that previously showed the pattern of DAD or organizing pneumonia and these patterns

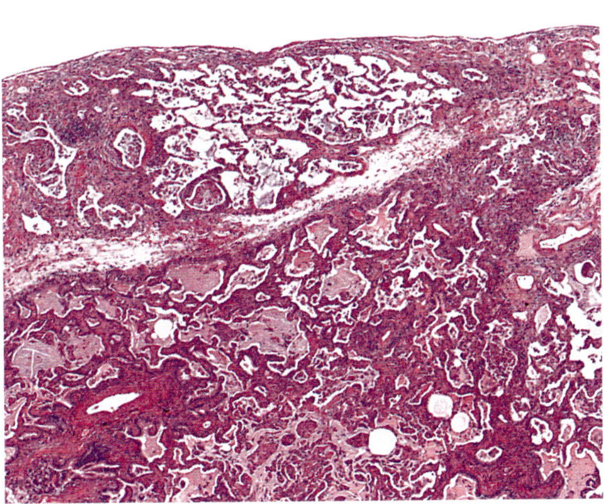

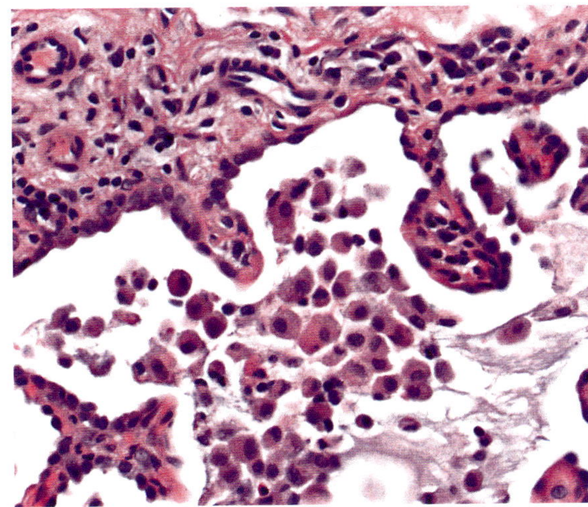

Figure 7-7

AMIODARONE PULMONARY TOXICITY RESEMBLING USUAL INTERSTITIAL PNEUMONIA

Left: This case shows interstitial inflammation and fibrosis with foci of microscopic honeycombing (upper left).
Right: Airspaces contain increased alveolar macrophages with foamy change, characteristic of amiodarone effect.

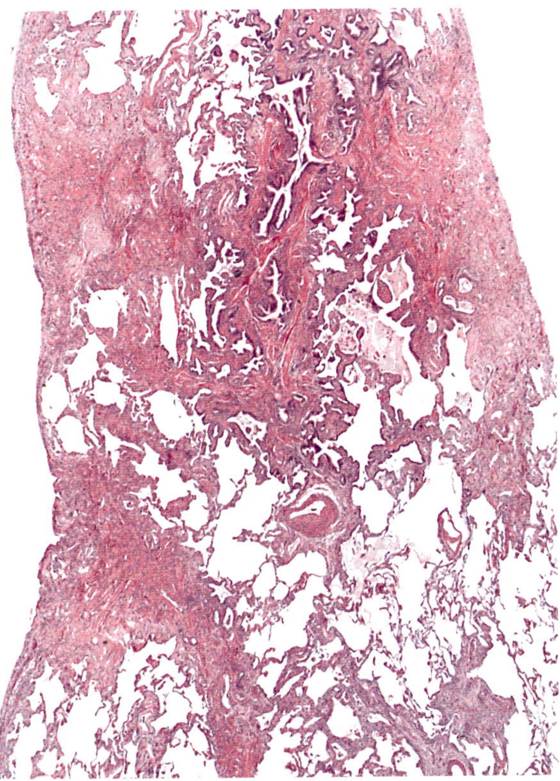

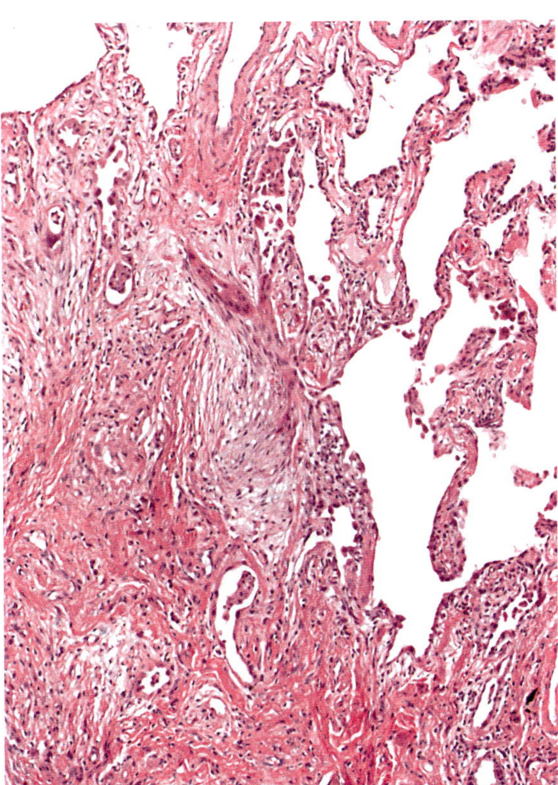

Figure 7-8

CHEMOTHERAPY-RELATED CHRONIC INTERSTITIAL FIBROSIS

Left: There is patchy interstitial fibrosis that is prominent in the subpleural regions.
Right: Fibroblastic foci are present. This patient had been on both BCNU and melphalan therapy and either (or both) could have been responsible for the pulmonary damage.

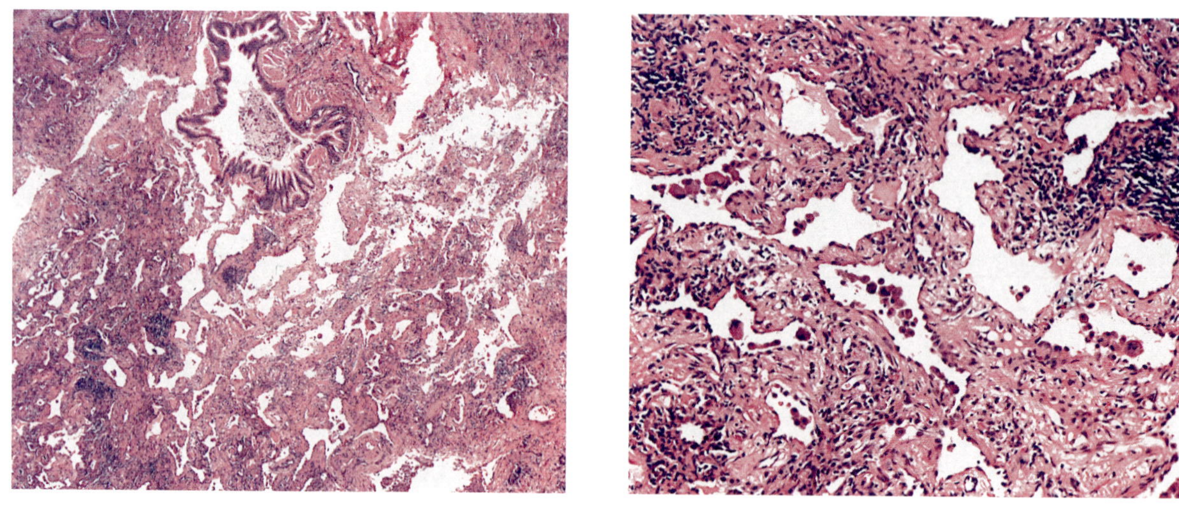

Figure 7-9

METHOTREXATE-RELATED PULMONARY TOXICITY

There is interstitial widening caused by inflammation and fibrosis, without frank honeycomb change. By current criteria, this is nonspecific interstitial pneumonia with fibrosis.

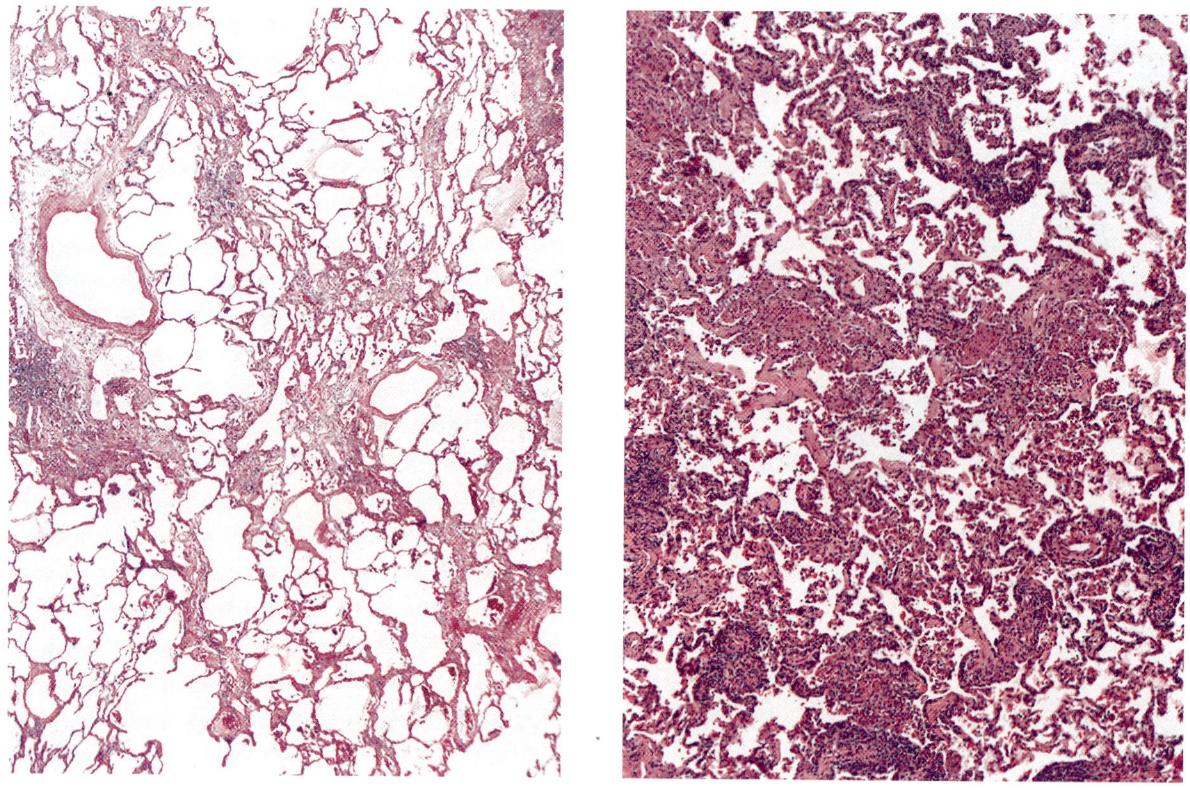

Figure 7-10

METHOTREXATE-RELATED PULMONARY TOXICITY

These two cases illustrate patchy interstitial fibrosis (left) and cellular interstitial inflammation with predilection for perivascular regions (right).

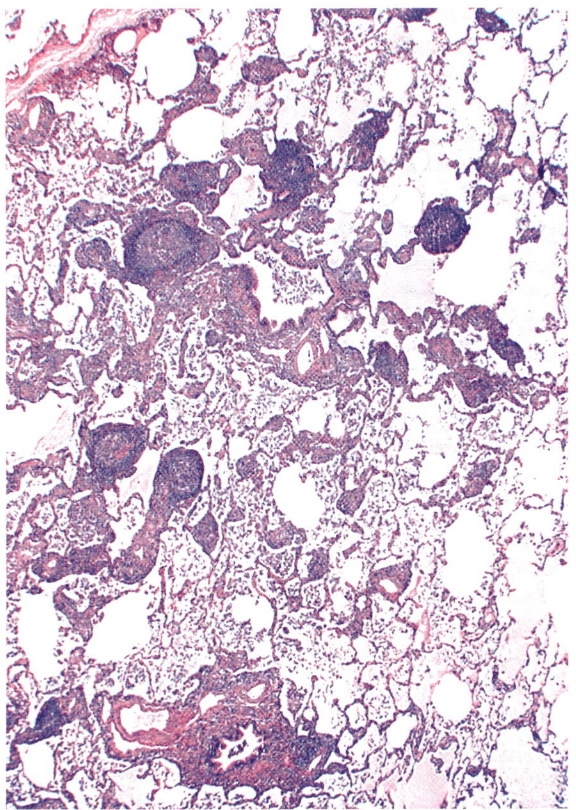

Figure 7-11

SULFASALAZINE PULMONARY TOXICITY

There is prominent lymphoid hyperplasia along lymphatic routes, with mild cellular interstitial inflammation and an increase in alveolar macrophages, resembling diffuse interstitial pneumonia.

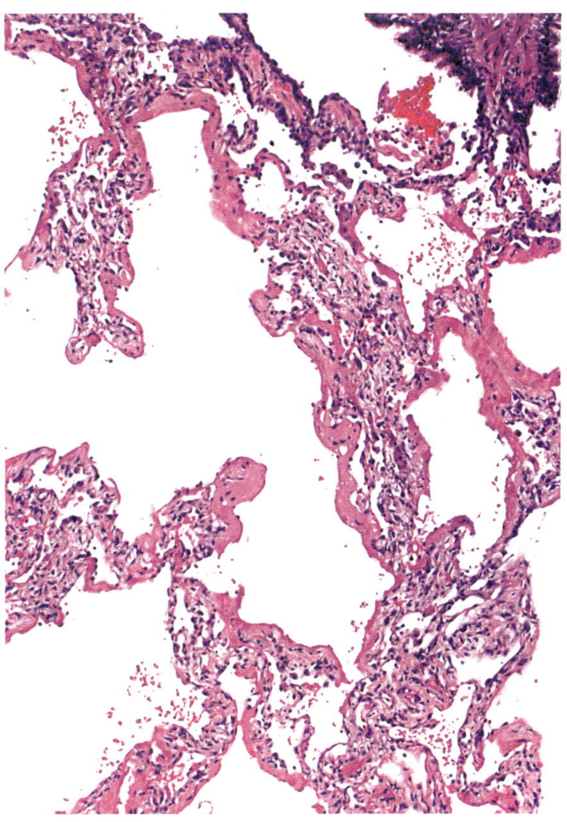

Figure 7-12

METHOTREXATE PULMONARY TOXICITY

Methotrexate pulmonary toxicity manifests here as acute diffuse alveolar damage.

would have been identified had earlier biopsies been performed.

Diffuse alveolar damage (figs. 7-2, 7-12): amiodarone, amitriptyline, azathioprine, BCNU, bleomycin, busulfan, CCNU, cocaine, colchicine, cyclophosphamide, deferoxamine mesylate, gold salts, hexamethonium, melphalan, methotrexate, mitomycin, nitrofurantoin, penicillamine, procarbazine, streptokinase, sulfathiazole, teniposide, tocainide, vinblastine, and zinostatin. The herbicide paraquat ingested accidentally or intentionally (suicide or homicide) is associated with severe hemorrhagic DAD (fig. 7-13).

Organizing pneumonia (bronchiolitis obliterans with organizing pneumonia pattern [figs. 7-14–7-16]): amiodarone, bleomycin, chlorozotocin, cocaine, cromolyn sodium, cyclophosphamide, gold salts, hexamethonium, interferon, mecamylamine, methotrexate, mitomycin, nilutamide, penicillamine, nitrofurantoin, phenytoin, sulfasalazine, and tocainide.

Bronchiolitis obliterans (constrictive bronchiolitis with airflow obstruction [fig. 7-17]): CCNU, gold, and penicillamine. Bronchiolitis obliterans with progressive airway obstruction is a recognized complication in rheumatoid arthritis in the absence of penicillamine or gold therapy. Consequently, it remains unclear whether these drugs are truly an etiologic factor in the development of bronchiolitis obliterans in patients with rheumatoid arthritis (61).

Pulmonary infiltrates with eosinophilia (figs. 7-2, 7-18–7-20): acetaminophen, ampicillin, AVC (vaginal) cream, bleomycin, carbamazepine, chlorpropamide, cocaine, cromolyn sodium,

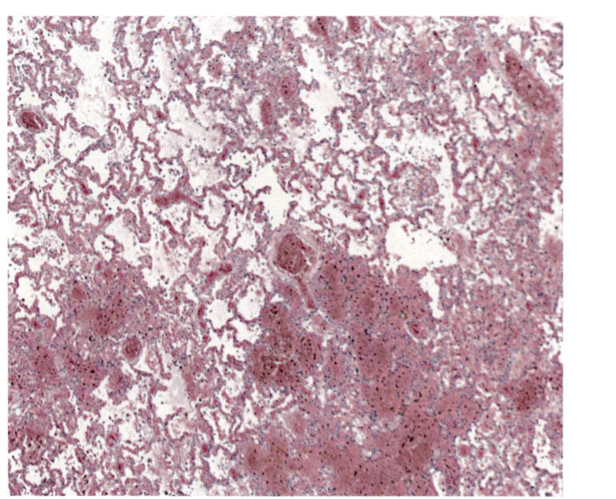

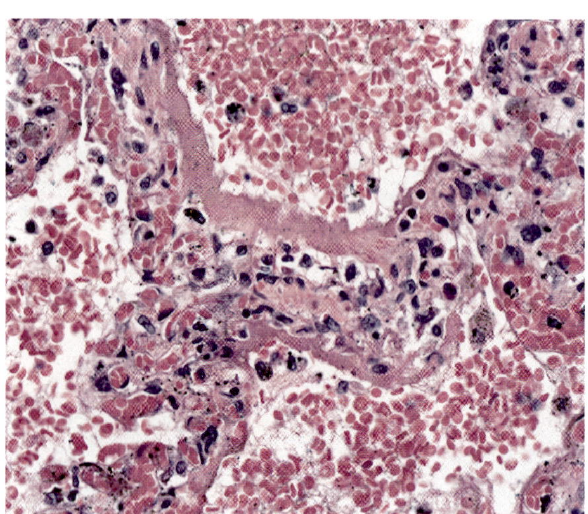

Figure 7-13

PARAQUAT INJURY

Left: Scanning power microscopy shows hemorrhage and edema.
Right: At higher power, hyaline membranes are apparent.

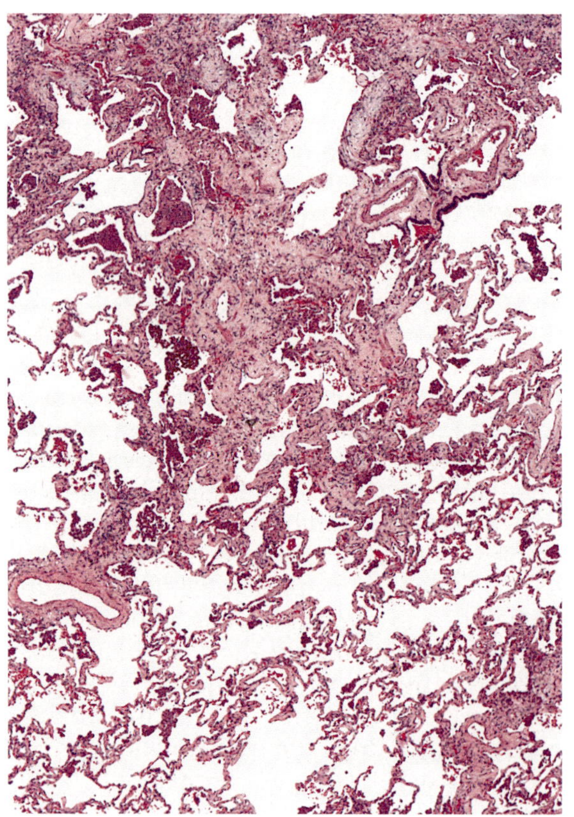

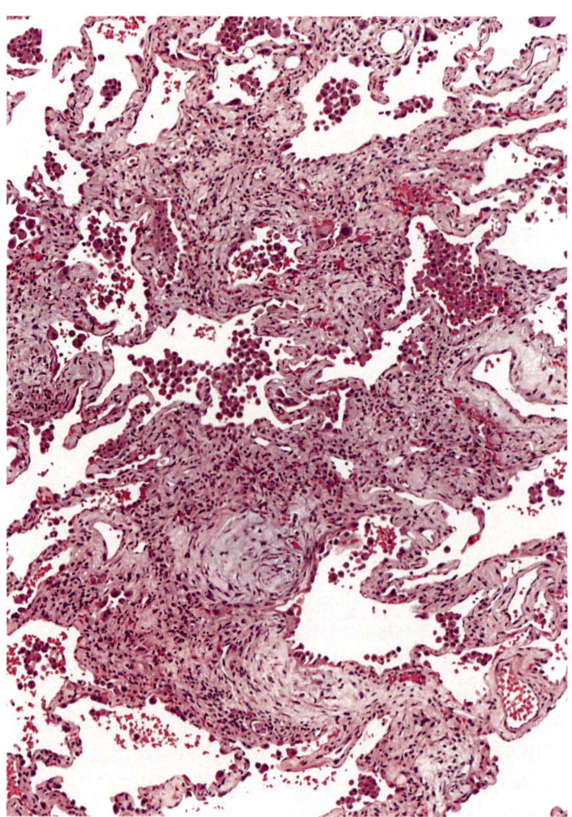

Figure 7-14

AZATHIOPRINE PULMONARY TOXICITY WITH PATCHY ORGANIZING PNEUMONIA

There are patchy areas of organizing intraluminal plugs of loose connective tissue (left and right).

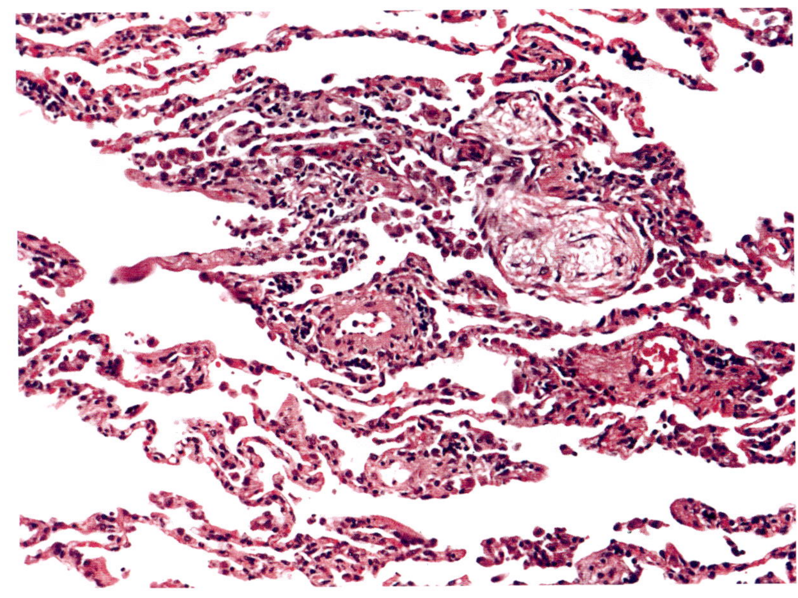

Figure 7-15

METHOTREXATE PULMONARY TOXICITY WITH A FOCUS OF ORGANIZING PNEUMONIA

A mild interstitial chronic inflammatory infiltrate is associated with a polypoid plug of organizing pneumonia.

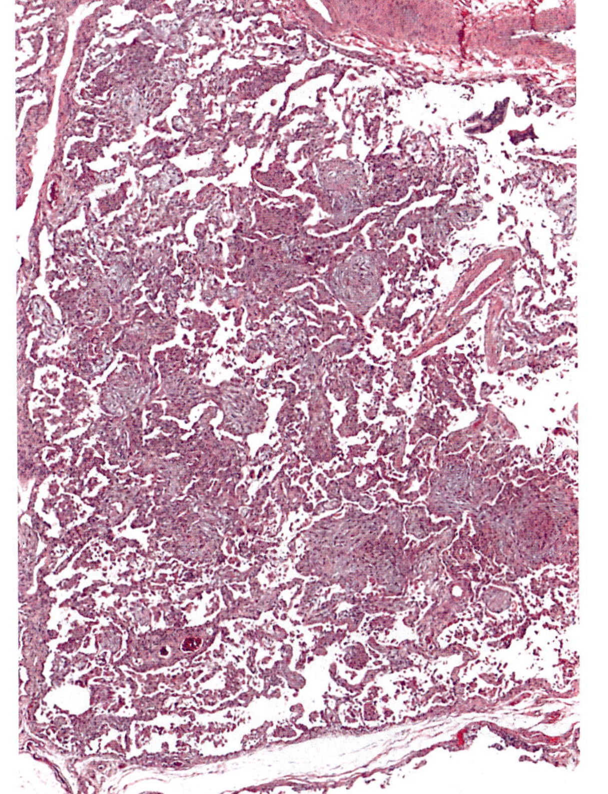

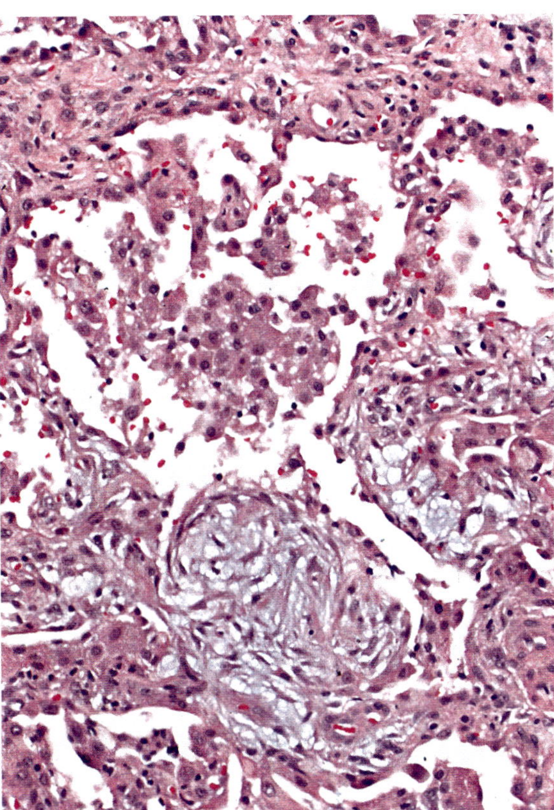

Figure 7-16

AMIODARONE TOXICITY

Amiodarone toxicity with organizing pneumonia (left) and the characteristic foamy alveolar macrophages (right).

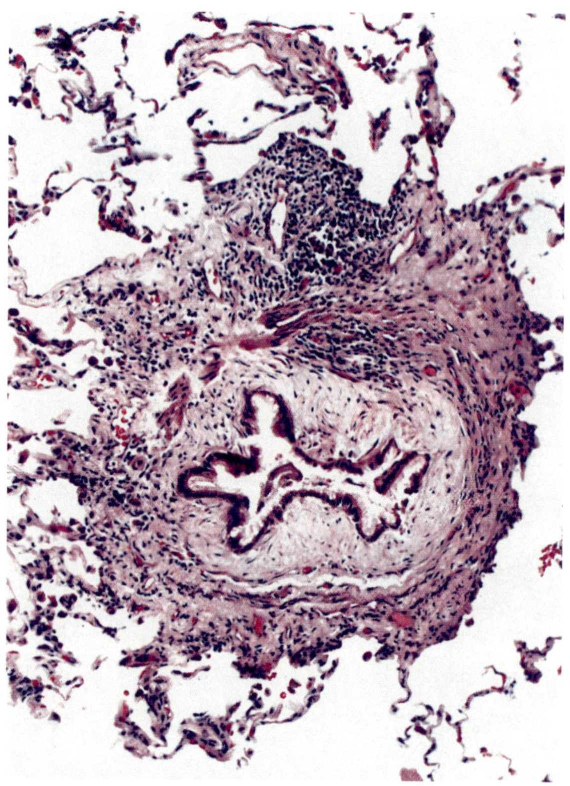

Figure 7-17

PENICILLAMINE-ASSOCIATED CONSTRICTIVE BRONCHIOLITIS

This case was associated with marked clinical evidence of airflow obstruction. There is marked luminal compromise due to submucosal scarring and consequent luminal narrowing.

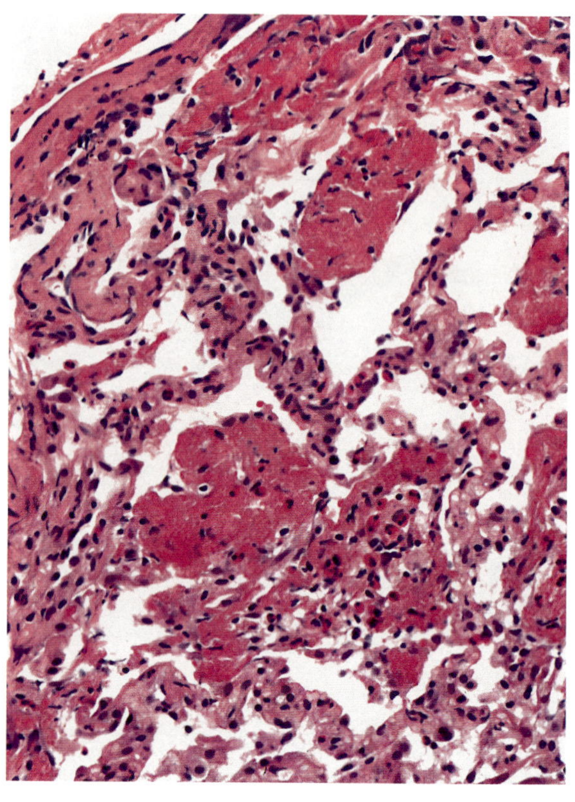

Figure 7-18

SULFASALAZINE-ASSOCIATED PULMONARY TOXICITY

Sulfasalazine-associated pulmonary toxicity manifests here as eosinophilic pneumonia. In this case, in addition to the accumulations of eosinophils (right upper center), there is prominent airspace fibrin, typical of that seen in idiopathic eosinophilic pneumonia.

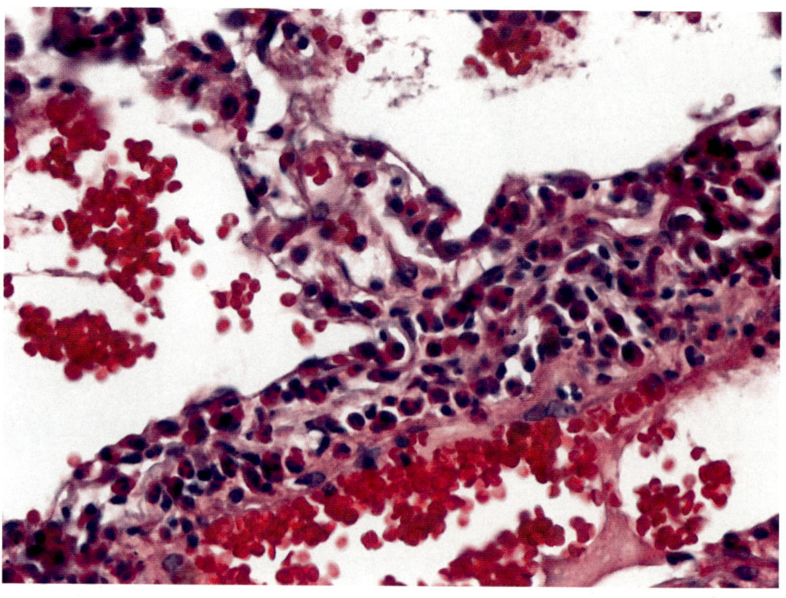

Figure 7-19

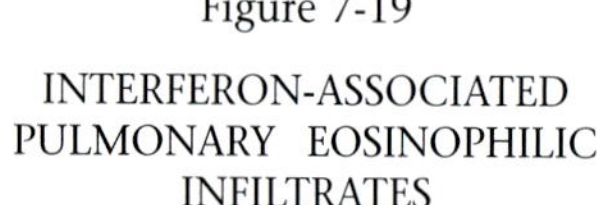

INTERFERON-ASSOCIATED PULMONARY EOSINOPHILIC INFILTRATES

This patient developed pulmonary infiltrates corresponding to courses of interferon therapy. The lung biopsy shows prominent perivascular eosinophils.

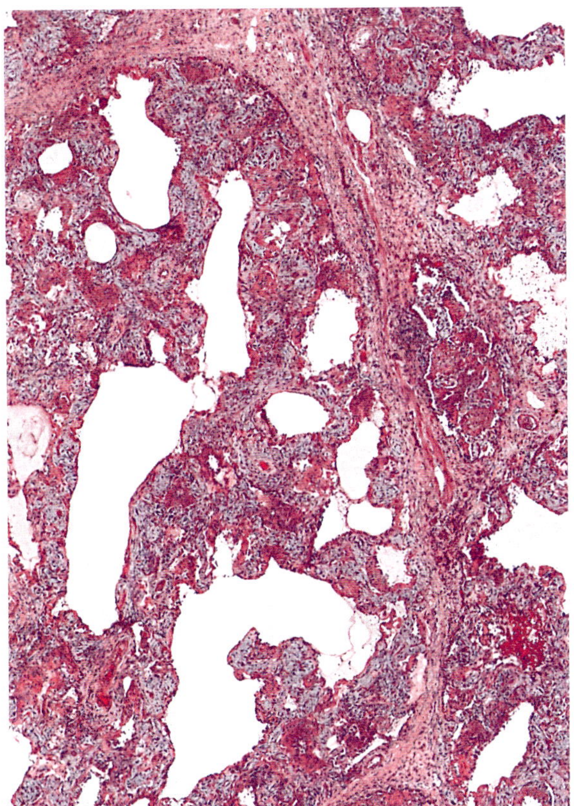

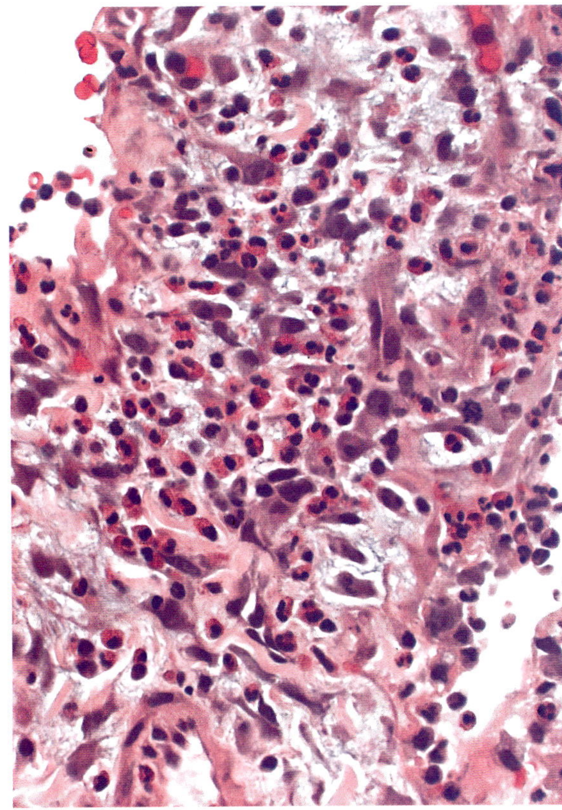

Figure 7-20

COCAINE-ASSOCIATED ACUTE EOSINOPHILIC PNEUMONIA

These two cases illustrate a pattern suggesting acute diffuse lung injury (left) and marked interstitial and airspace eosinophils (right).

imipramine, mephenesin, nabumetone, naproxen, nitrofurantoin, periodic acid–Schiff (PAS) stain, phenylbutazone, procarbazine, prontosil, propranolol, pyrimethamine, sulfasalazine, tetracycline, trazodone, and inhalation abuse of Scotchguard (30).

Pulmonary edema (fig. 7-21): buprenorphine, chlordiazepoxide, cocaine, codeine, cytosine arabinoside, epinephrine, ethchlorvynol, haloperidol, heroin, hydrochlorothiazide, isoxsuprine, lidocaine, magnesium sulfate, methadone, methamphetamine, methotrexate, mitomycin, nalbuphine, naloxone, nifedipine, paraldehyde, penicillin, propoxyphene, propranolol, radiocontrast material, ritodrine, salbutamol, salicylates, sulindac, terbutaline, and tryptophan.

Pulmonary hemorrhage: amphotericin B, anticoagulants, cocaine (1), cyclophosphamide, haloperidol, hydralazine, mitomycin, nitrofurantoin, penicillamine, propylthiouracil, streptokinase, sulfonamides, and urokinase.

Pulmonary hypertension (figs. 7-22, 7-23): aminorex, fenfluramine and phenteramine (fenphen) mitomycin, methamphetamine (also known as "speed" or "crank"), tryptophan, and intravenous drug abuse (43,51,60,66). Drugs with sympathomimetic properties (for example, cocaine or methamphetamine) may cause transient pulmonary vasoconstriction but it is unclear if recurrent episodes can lead to permanent pulmonary hypertension (31).

Pulmonary veno-occlusive disease (fig. 7-24): BCNU, bleomycin, mitomycin, zinostatin.

Granulomatous inflammation (fig. 7-25): acebutolol, Bacillus Calmette Guerin (BCG), cocaine, cromalyn sodium, fluoxetine hydrochloride, methotrexate, nitrofurantoin, procarbazine, pentazocine and tripelennamine ("T's and

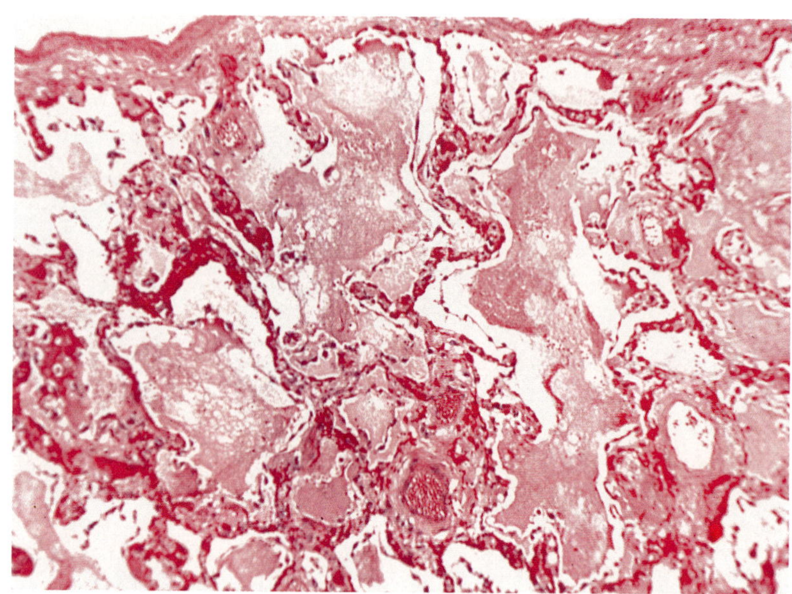

Figure 7-21

CYTOSINE ARABINOSIDE–ASSOCIATED PULMONARY EDEMA

Figure 7-22

L-TRYPTOPHAN–ASSOCIATED PULMONARY HYPERTENSION

A: One case shows mild cellular infiltrates of the intima and media in addition to marked pulmonary vascular mural thickening characteristic of pulmonary hypertension.

B: Eosinophils are relatively prominent.

C: Another case shows only moderate myointimal thickening.

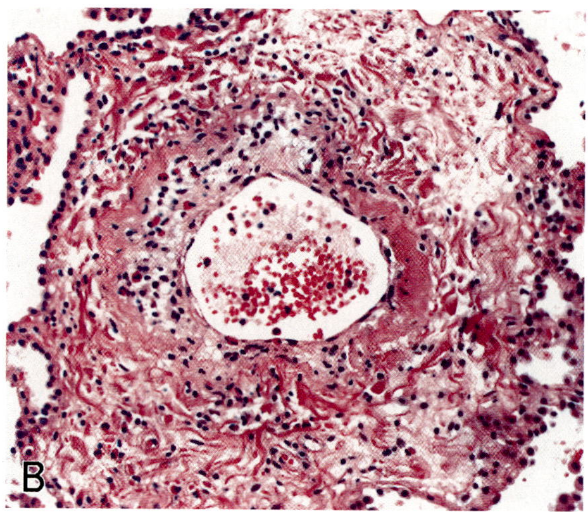

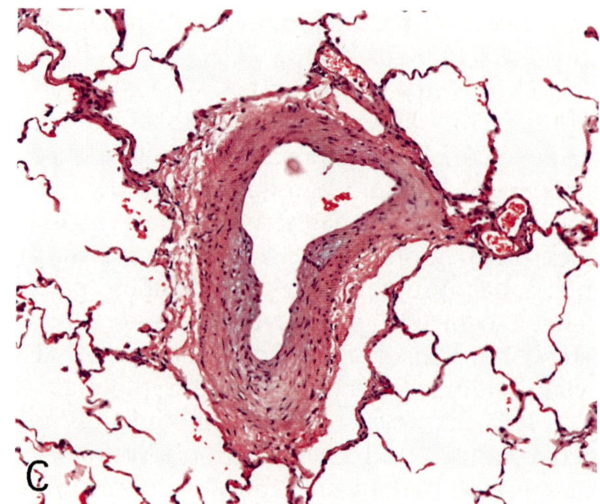

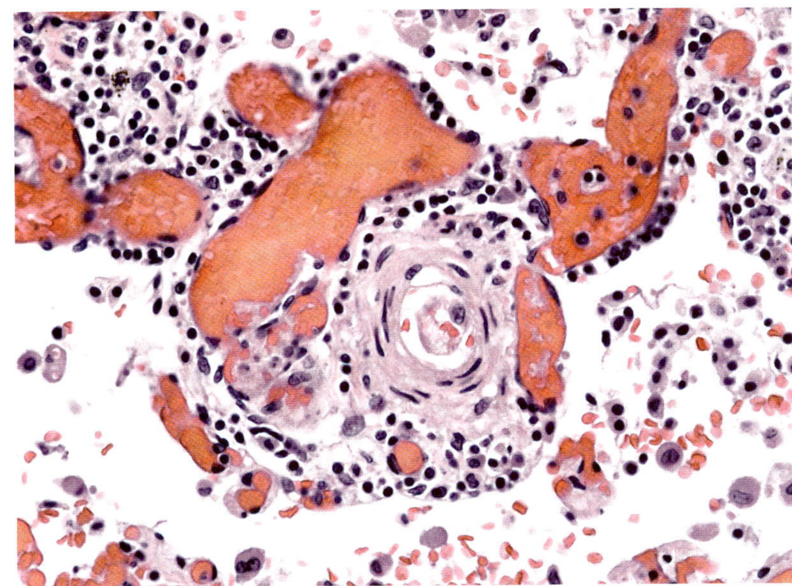

Figure 7-23

PULMONARY HYPERTENSION SECONDARY TO FENFLURAMINE AND PHENTERAMINE (FENPHEN) TOXICITY

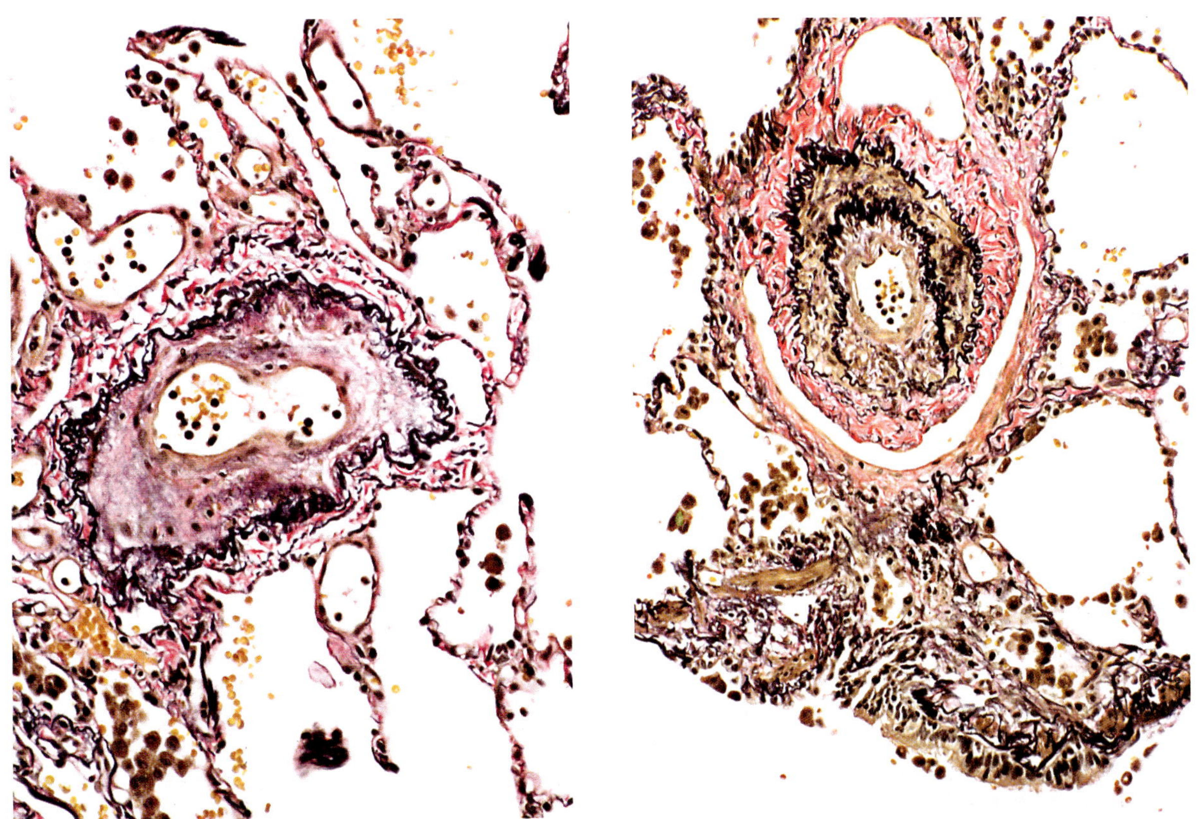

Figure 7-24

MITOMYCIN-ASSOCIATED PULMONARY VENO-OCCLUSIVE DISEASE

In addition to the veno-occlusive lesions (left), there were secondary pulmonary hypertensive changes involving the arterial system (right).

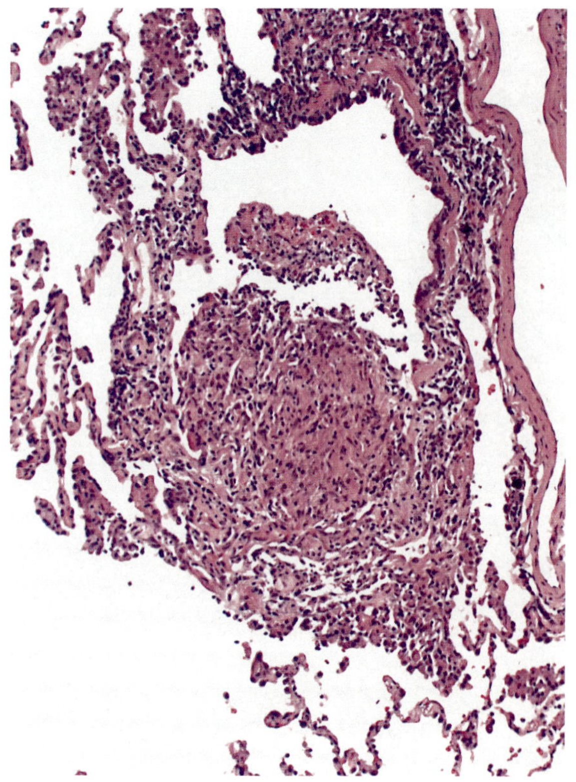

Figure 7-25

METHOTREXATE TOXICITY WITH NON-NECROTIZING GRANULOMAS

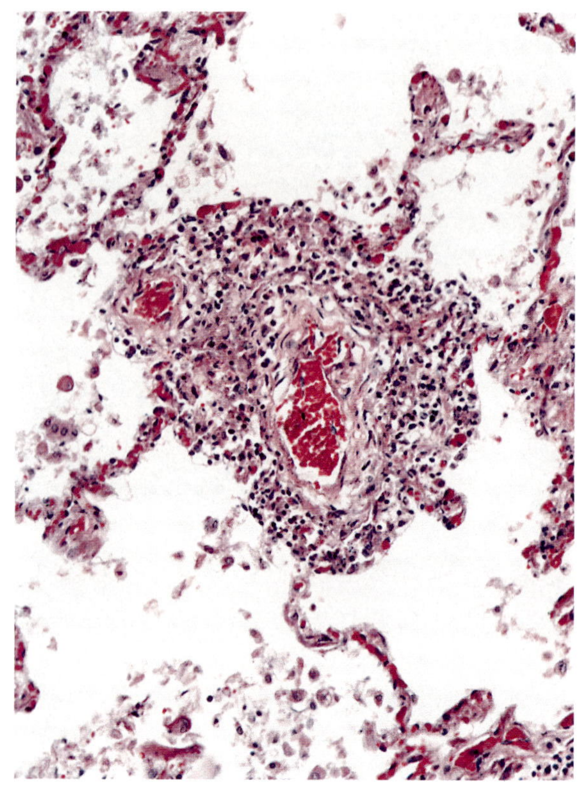

Figure 7-26

SMALL VESSEL (HYPERSENSITIVITY) VASCULITIS

Small vessel (hypersensitivity) vasculitis is associated with a systemic reaction to trimethoprim sulfamethoxazole therapy.

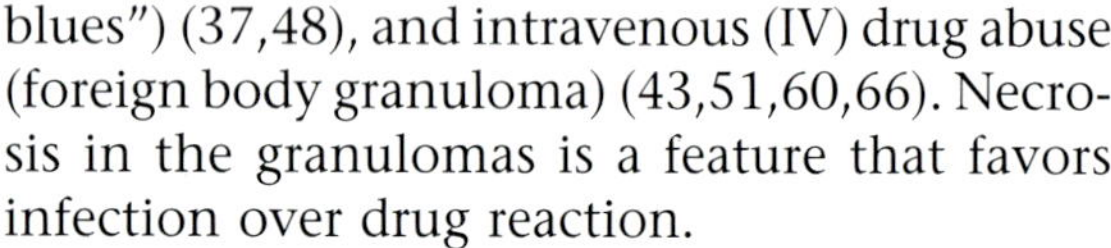

blues") (37,48), and intravenous (IV) drug abuse (foreign body granuloma) (43,51,60,66). Necrosis in the granulomas is a feature that favors infection over drug reaction.

Bullous lung disease and emphysema: IV drug users, particularly when methadone, methylphenidate, or talc-containing drugs have been injected (see chapter 16) (23,46,57–59,65).

Bronchiectasis: extensive and severe bronchiectasis can be found in heroin-addicted individuals with pulmonary symptoms, with or without abnormal chest roentgenograms. It appears to be related to episodes of heroin-induced pulmonary edema, aspiration pneumonia, or infection (2,3,56,64).

Progressive massive fibrosis: IV drug abuse (7).

Pleural disease (38): acyclovir, amiodarone, bleomycin, bromocriptine, clozapine, cyclophosphamide, dantrolene, d-penicillamine, granulocyte-monocyte–colony-stimulating factor (GM-CSF), interleukin-2, isotretinoin, itraconazole, l-tryptophan, methotrexate, methysergide, mesalamine, minoxidil, mitomycin, nitrofurantoin, practolol, propylthiouracil, procarbazine, sclerotherapy agents (absolute alcohol, sodium morrhuate), simvastatin, valproic acid, and talc pleurodesis (49).

Drug-induced lupus pleuritis: procainamide, hydralazine, chlorpromazine, isoniazid, methyldopa, penicillamine, and quinidine.

Vasculitis of the type associated with Wegener's granulomatosis, Churg-Strauss syndrome, or microscopic polyangiitis is generally not associated with drugs. Small vessel injury, which has sometimes been called hypersensitivity vasculitis, can be found in systemic drug reactions, and thus could be seen in many of the patterns above, particularly pulmonary infiltrates with eosinophilia (fig. 7-26). Inflammatory vessel injury may also be a factor in

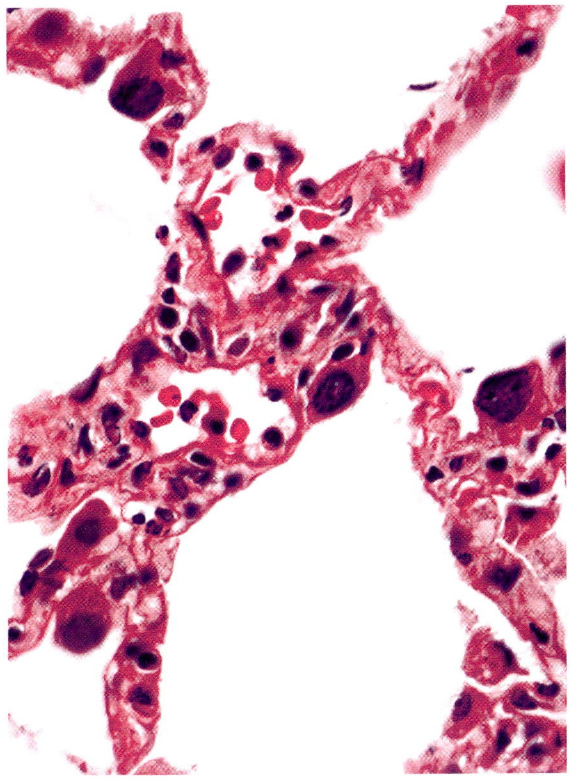

Figure 7-27

CYTOTOXIC EFFECTS

Cytotoxic effects in type 2 cells associated with busulfan therapy.

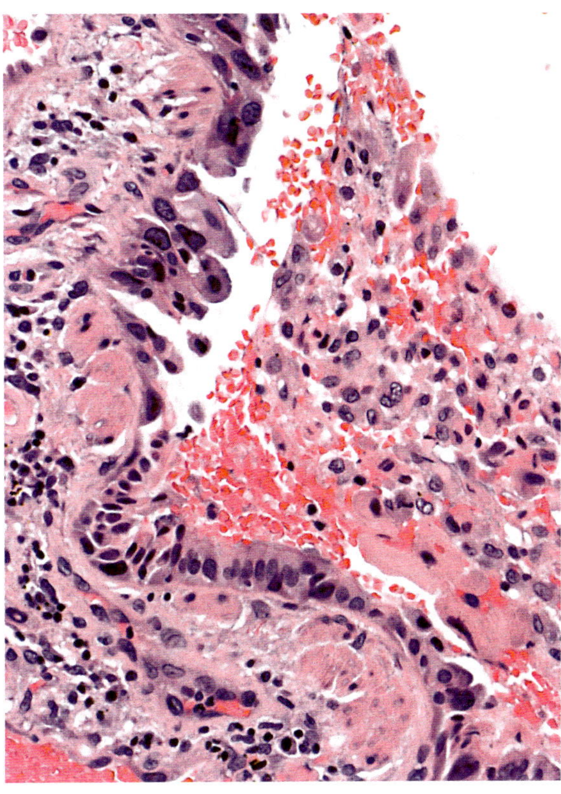

Figure 7-28

CYTOTOXIC EFFECTS

Marked atypia in the bronchiolar epithelium followed induction chemotherapy for bone marrow transplantation.

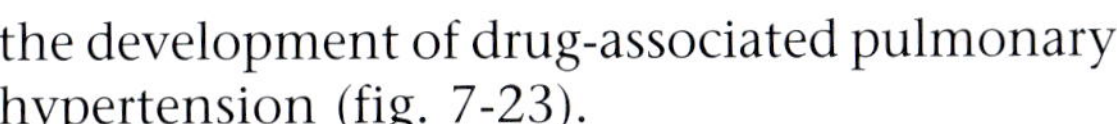

the development of drug-associated pulmonary hypertension (fig. 7-23).

Cytotoxic drugs have been associated with "cytotoxic changes" in pulmonary epithelial cells: nuclear and cytoplasmic enlargement with hyperchromatic, atypical-appearing nuclei and abundant eosinophilic cytoplasm (figs. 7-27, 7-28) (9). The changes are reminiscent of radiation-induced cellular changes. Although nuclear features may be worrisome for malignancy, the clinical history, concomitant increase in cytoplasm, and the overall milieu of an inflammatory and reparative process usually point to cytotoxic effects. Distinction of these changes from viral infections may also be a problem unless one maintains a high threshold for identification of viral inclusions. Immunostaining for specific viruses is also helpful.

The presence at scanning power microscopy of multiple, small inflammatory nodules (miliary nodules), especially in an immunosuppressed patient, should first raise the possibility of infection. Such an appearance is unusual for a drug reaction, but anecdotal experience suggests that the pattern occasionally does occur with drugs. That a drug reaction should be associated with localized or patchy nodular disease makes little sense intuitively, but nonetheless this occurs. As illustrated previously, some drug reactions may even manifest as localized masses or opacities on a chest radiograph, a finding well-described with bleomycin and amiodarone (see figs. 7-3, 7-4).

While the histologic changes for most drug reactions are nonspecific, and the diagnosis rests primarily on clinical and historical features (see below), there are occasional cases in which the histologic findings are sufficiently distinctive as to suggest the possibility of a drug reaction. This is the case with amiodarone which leads to an accumulation of phospholipid in alveolar macrophages and type 2 cells (9,12,36,41, 45). In patients on amiodarone, this change should be considered an amiodarone effect, not necessarily toxicity. Amiodarone toxicity is a diagnosis of exclusion when other possible causes of clinical lung disease have been ruled out.

Diagnosing and Treating Pulmonary Drug Reactions

Most pulmonary drug reactions are diagnosed clinically and only a minority of patients need a biopsy. For the latter cases, the pathologist's job is to provide data for the clinician to work with. As such, the pathologist should attempt to define the pathologic pattern present and determine whether or not it is associated with the drug(s) being implicated. A drug reaction is a diagnosis of exclusion and drug-induced immunosuppression resulting in opportunistic infection is often the most important consideration in the differential diagnosis. Exclusion of infection (with appropriate cultures, special stains, and other studies) is of paramount importance. The pathologist should be aware that cytotoxic changes (which may indeed be due to prior chemotherapy) may be an incidental finding in a patient whose current clinical pulmonary disease is caused by an opportunistic infection or some other process. Opportunistic infections may be associated with relatively low doses of immunosuppressive drugs. A history of any sort of immunosuppression is important in the differential diagnosis and should lead to a routine battery of special stains for organisms, especially *Pneumocystis*.

No specific treatment exists for most drug-induced lung diseases (10,11,32,36,52,67,68). Fortunately, most pulmonary drug reactions abate when the causative drug is stopped. In many instances, concomitant steroid therapy is given and the relative effects of stopping the drugs versus steroid therapy may be difficult to separate.

RADIATION LUNG INJURY

Definition. Radiation induced lung injury—acute, delayed, or chronic—is damage to the lung produced by ionizing therapeutic radiation. The radiation damage is usually confined within the radiation field but may uncommonly result in an immunologic reaction with involvement of lung tissue outside the irradiated field.

Table 7-3

FACTORS IN RADIATION INJURY TO THE LUNG

Volume of radiated lung tissue
Total dose of radiation
Rate of delivery of radiation
History of prior radiation
Previous or concomitant chemotherapy
Steroid withdrawal
Age and preexisting lung disease

The use of radiation to treat malignancies began in the early 1900s and radiation lung injury has been recognized since the 1920s (9). *Radiation pneumonitis* is lung injury caused by therapeutic radiation. A variety of radiotherapeutic modalities may affect the lung but the most common is external beam radiotherapy given for cancers of the breast and intrathoracic organs (6,8,9,13–17,19,21,22,24,25,27,40,53,54,62). The administration of radioisotopes is only rarely associated with lung injury; radiation pneumonitis has been described following administration of iodine 131, and exposure to radioactive dust and paint (9). Thorotrast-induced lung fibrosis has also been described and is of historical interest (15). For the most part, radiation damages that portion of the lung included within the radiation field, although recent clinical and radiologic observations (see below) and immunologic data suggest that the effects of radiation may be more widespread and affect lung tissue outside the irradiated field (27).

The incidence of clinically manifested radiation lung injury varies considerably, usually affecting 5 to 15 percent of patients at risk (6,9, 40). This incidence is directly related to the factors shown in Table 7-3 (9,17,25,53).

The incidence of radiation lung injury increases with the volume of radiated tissue. There is a much greater toxicity associated with larger doses of radiation. Increasing dosage fractionation is associated with a lower incidence of radiation lung injury. The greatest likelihood of radiation lung injury is associated with single large doses. Tissue that has been previously irradiated, including the lung, has an increased likelihood for radiation-induced injury. Just as radiation is a cofactor for lung injury with chemotherapy, a history of prior chemotherapy is associated with a greater likelihood of injury following radiation therapy (6). Some studies have suggested that withdrawal of steroids may "unmask" radiation pneumonitis (5,47). Increasing age and associated preexisting lung disease also increase the likelihood of radiation-induced lung injury (40).

Clinical Features. Three clinical syndromes comprise radiation lung injury (9,13, 17,25,40,53,62):

Acute radiation pneumonitis: patients have insidious development of cough, 2 weeks to 6 months after radiation has been completed (the majority between 2 and 3 months). Hemoptysis may occur. Patients may be febrile with spiking fevers and leukocytosis and, in severe cases, acute respiratory distress syndrome (ARDS) may develop. Acute radiation pneumonitis may mimic infection or recurrent or metastatic neoplasm (8,55).

Radiation fibrosis (chronic radiation pneumonitis): scarring in the radiated fields may follow clinically manifested acute radiation pneumonitis or develop insidiously after the radiation exposure. The fibrosis resembles a fibrosing interstitial pneumonia with signs and symptoms of interstitial lung disease, the severity of which depends on the extent of lung tissue involved and the degree of fibrosis. Radiation fibrosis is generally apparent within a year of completion of radiation therapy (see below).

Migratory pulmonary infiltrates following (relatively localized) radiation: there have been a number of reports of migratory pulmonary infiltrates outside the fields of radiation (13,62). Some have referred to this syndrome as *sporadic radiation pneumonitis* (39). Compared to the above two syndromes, the occurrence of migratory radiation pneumonitis is unpredictable and sporadic, affects only a minority of radiated patients, the dyspnea experienced is out of proportion to the volume of lung tissue that was irradiated, and the symptoms resolve without sequelae in the majority of patients. The clinical findings, radiologic findings, histologic findings, therapy, and response to therapy are all similar to those in cryptogenic organizing pneumonia (13,62).

BAL has been used in an attempt to determine whether serial measurements are useful in the early diagnosis of radiation-induced lung injury. A lymphocytosis is often present in patients following lung irradiation. However, in a recent study of breast cancer patients who received unilateral thoracic radiotherapy, the severity of the BAL lymphocytosis did not differ significantly between patients who did and did not develop subsequent pneumonitis (35). The early lymphocytic alveolitis induced by unilateral thoracic radiotherapy was always bilateral and did not predict the subsequent development of pneumonitis.

Radiologic Findings. The radiologic findings of acute radiation pneumonitis range from subtle hazy areas of increased density (ground-glass opacities) to patchy or homogeneous airspace consolidation (fig. 7-29) (34). These abnormalities usually are first seen approximately 8 weeks after completion of radiotherapy and peak 3 to 4 months after treatment. The radiologic abnormalities usually have sharply defined margins limited to the lung parenchyma within the radiation fields. Acute radiation pneumonitis is seen more commonly and better on high resolution computed tomography (HRCT) than on the chest radiograph (18,27).

Radiation fibrosis first becomes evident radiologically 3 to 4 months after completion of radiotherapy and stabilizes after 9 to 12 months (34). The radiologic manifestations can be subtle, consisting of mild pleural thickening and loss of lung volume, or more obvious and include dense fibrotic strands, traction bronchiectasis, obliteration of normal lung markings, and marked volume loss. Similar to acute radiation pneumonitis, radiation fibrosis has sharply defined boundaries corresponding to the radiation portals (fig. 7-30). The manifestations of radiation fibrosis are better visualized on HRCT than on the chest radiograph (34). In a small number of patients, the manifestations of acute radiation pneumonitis extend outside of the radiation portal (27). The abnormalities consist of ground-glass opacities or areas of consolidation, which are less severe than those seen within the radiation portal.

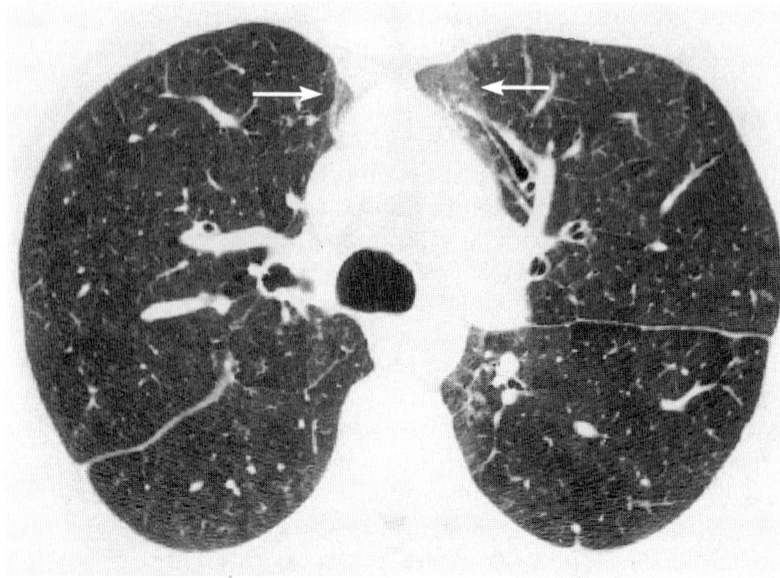

Figure 7-29

ACUTE RADIATION PNEUMONITIS

HRCT demonstrates areas of ground-glass attenuation (arrows) in the paramediastinal regions of both lungs. The patient was a 37-year-old man who had completed a course of radiotherapy for Hodgkin's disease 2 months previously.

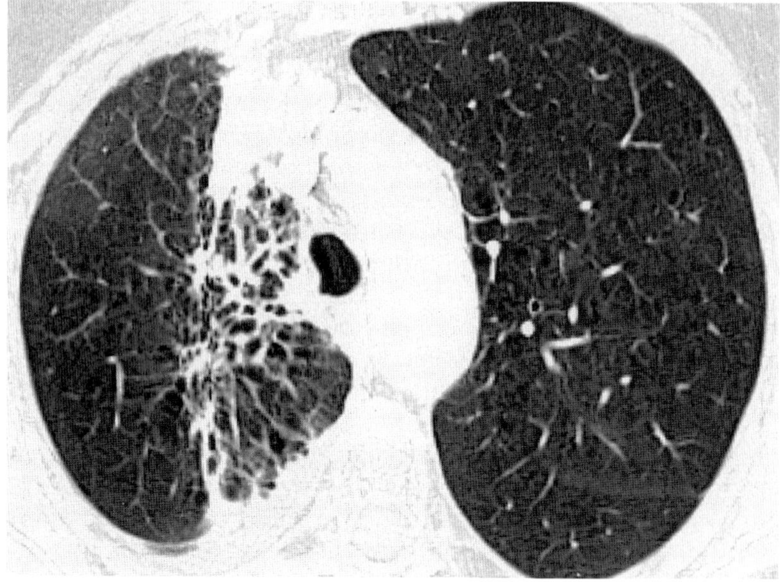

Figure 7-30

RADIATION FIBROSIS

HRCT demonstrates severe fibrosis in the medial region of the right upper lobe, with associated loss of volume. The fibrosis is limited to the lung within the radiation field. The patient had undergone radiotherapy for a right upper lobe bronchogenic carcinoma 7 months previously.

Occasionally, patients may develop migratory pulmonary infiltrates outside of the radiation fields (fig. 7-31). Rarely, limited thoracic radiation may be complicated by ARDS, with rapid development of respiratory failure and diffuse bilateral airspace consolidation (4).

Pathologic Findings. The pathologic findings in acute radiation pneumonitis resemble acute and organizing DAD (figs. 7-32–7-34); in the organizing phase, an organizing pneumonia pattern may be prominent (9,17). Like radiation injury at other sites, large bizarre cells with enlarged hyperchromatic nuclei and abundant, eosinophilic, irregularly shaped cytoplasm may be prominent.

In radiation fibrosis the pathologic findings are those of organized DAD with interstitial fibrosis (figs. 7-35–7-41) (9,17). In addition, the vessels are thickened, and there may be intimal fibrosis and accumulations of foamy macrophages in pulmonary arteries and veins (fig. 7-41). The fibrosis in chronic radiation injury may have an elastic appearance reminiscent of apical caps (figs. 7-37, 7-38). The gross findings

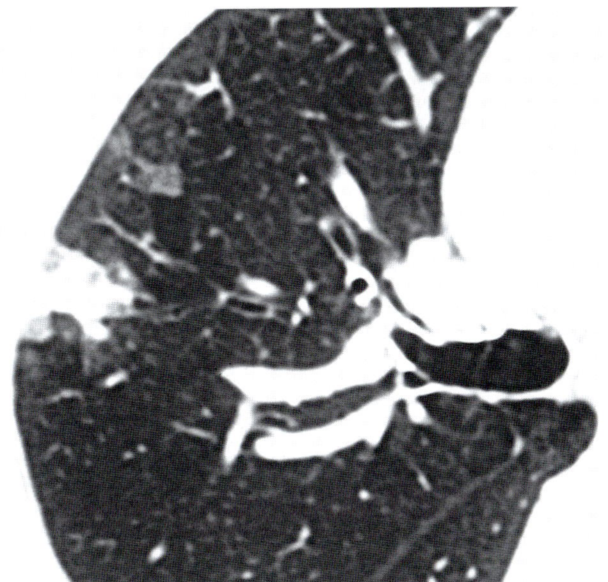

Figure 7-31

MIGRATORY PULMONARY INFILTRATES FOLLOWING RADIATION

HRCT of the right lung shows a focus of consolidation which occurred outside the field of radiation. Clinical presentation and radiologic findings were similar to those of cryptogenic organizing pneumonia.

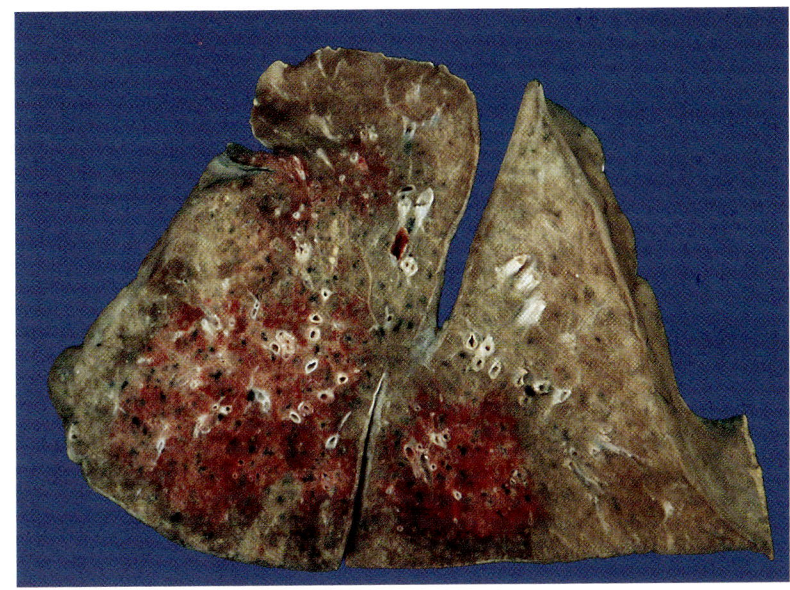

Figure 7-32

ACUTE RADIATION PNEUMONITIS

This gross photograph shows consolidation and hemorrhage in the upper lobe and superior segment of the lower lobe, which corresponded to the regions of recent radiotherapy.

parallel the radiologic features. Associated findings as described for acute radiation pneumonitis may also be present.

Sporadic radiation pneumonitis histologically shows organizing pneumonia (fig. 7-42) (13,62).

Pathogenesis. Radiation directly damages cell membranes, cell proteins, and DNA, resulting in direct tissue damage, tissue injury associated with inflammation, and tissue injury associated with free radical production (9,17,24, 25,39). Acute radiation pneumonitis and radiation fibrosis involving the irradiated fields are the manifestations of these injuries.

Radiation to localized regions of the lung may also be associated with bilateral lymphocytic alveolitis. The activation of T lymphocytes as identified by BAL fluid evaluation and a diffuse increase in uptake in gallium scans suggest more widespread effects in the lungs than expected, given the fields of radiation (29,35,39,40,42,50). These findings have been used to explain, in part, the occurrence of migratory infiltrates following radiation therapy (sporadic radiation pneumonitis).

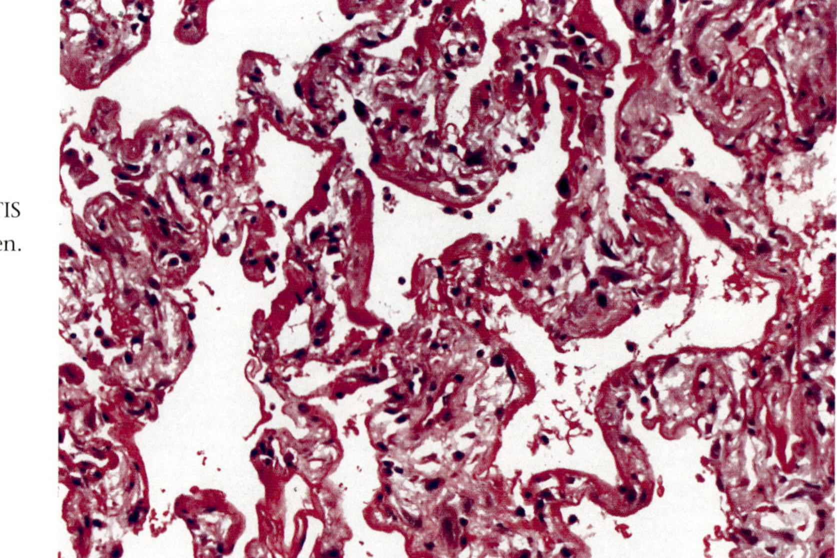

Figure 7-33

ACUTE RADIATION PNEUMONITIS

Acute diffuse alveolar damage is seen.

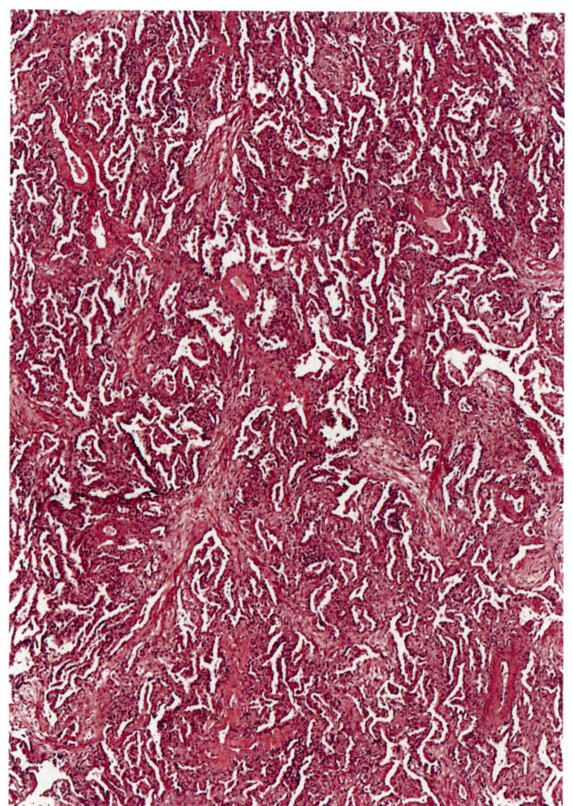

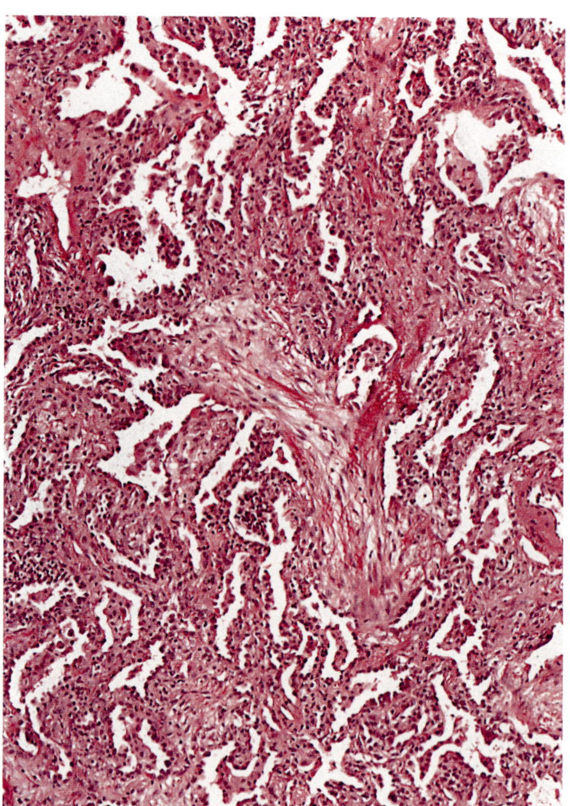

Figure 7-34

ACUTE RADIATION PNEUMONITIS

Acute radiation pneumonitis showing organizing diffuse alveolar damage. While some fields (right) raise the possibility of organizing pneumonia, the diffuse nature of the process (left) is more in keeping with organizing diffuse alveolar damage.

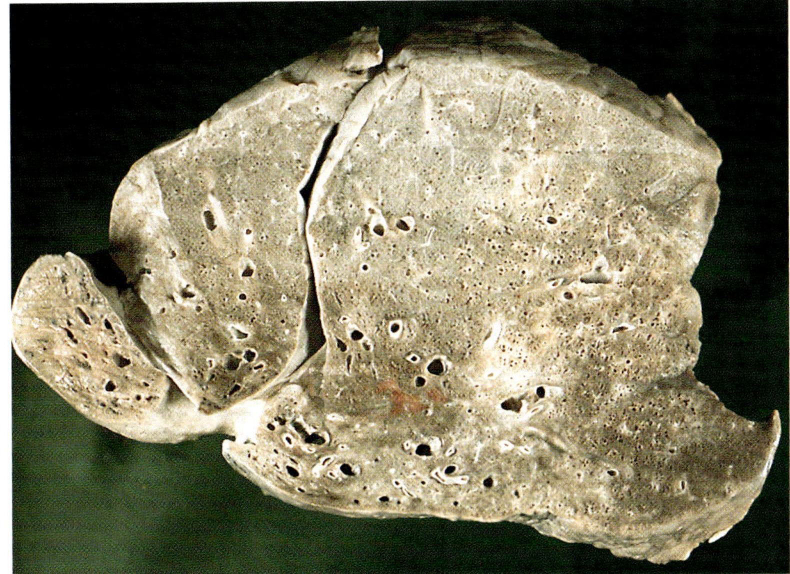

Figure 7-35

RADIATION FIBROSIS

The right upper lobe is markedly atelectatic and fibrotic following radiotherapy for carcinoma of the breast.

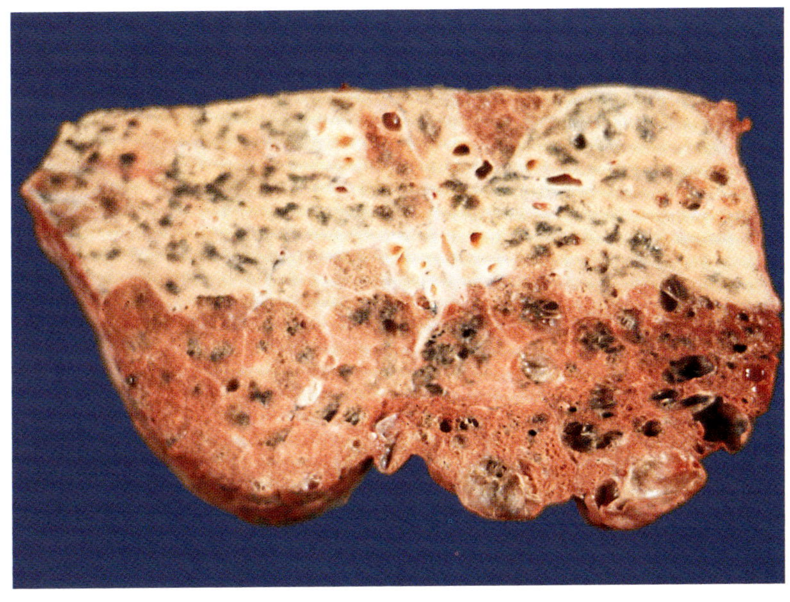

Figure 7-36

RADIATION FIBROSIS

Radiation fibrosis following radiotherapy for primary carcinoma of the lung. The fibrotic irradiated tissue is sharply demarcated from the surrounding lung tissue. No residual carcinoma was identified.

Diagnosis. The diagnosis of acute radiation pneumonitis and radiation fibrosis is often straightforward with knowledge of the history and the radiation ports. The primary concern in the differential diagnosis of acute radiation pneumonitis and migratory infiltrates following radiation is infection. As mentioned, acute radiation pneumonitis may also mimic recurrent or metastatic neoplasm.

Treatment and Prognosis. Most cases of acute radiation pneumonitis are subclinical and relatively mild and do not require therapy (54). In significantly symptomatic patients with acute radiation pneumonitis, corticosteroids are indicated (27). Radiation fibrosis is irreversible. Migratory radiation pneumonitis is treated in the same way as idiopathic bronchiolitis obliterans organizing pneumonia (BOOP) (13,62). Only a small percentage of patients die of radiation lung injury (9).

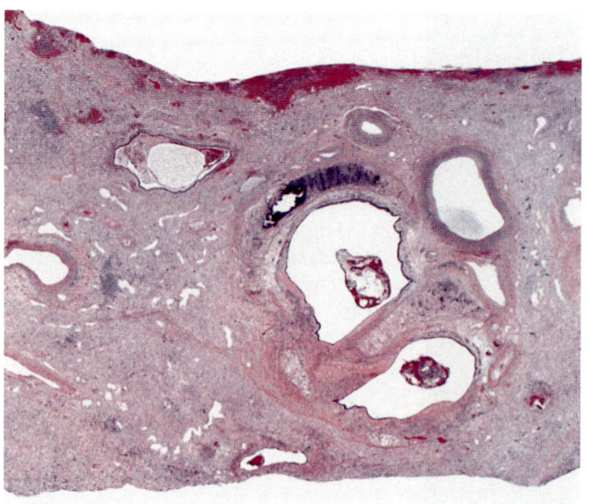

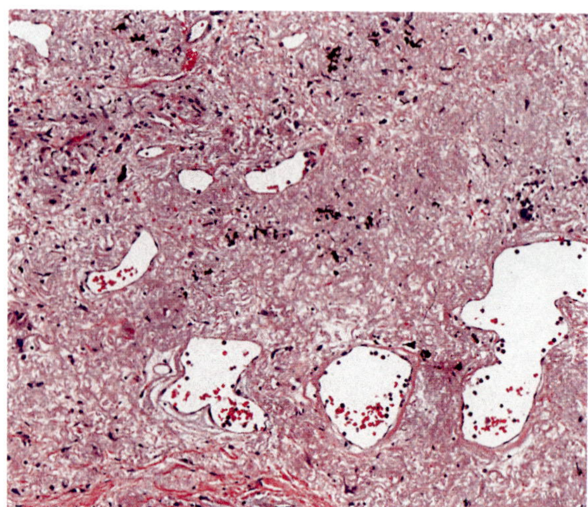

Figure 7-37

RADIATION FIBROSIS

Left: Radiation fibrosis with complete loss of alveolar parenchyma and shrinkage of the lung tissue around a bronchus. Right: The lung tissue is replaced by elastotic tissue containing anthracotic pigment.

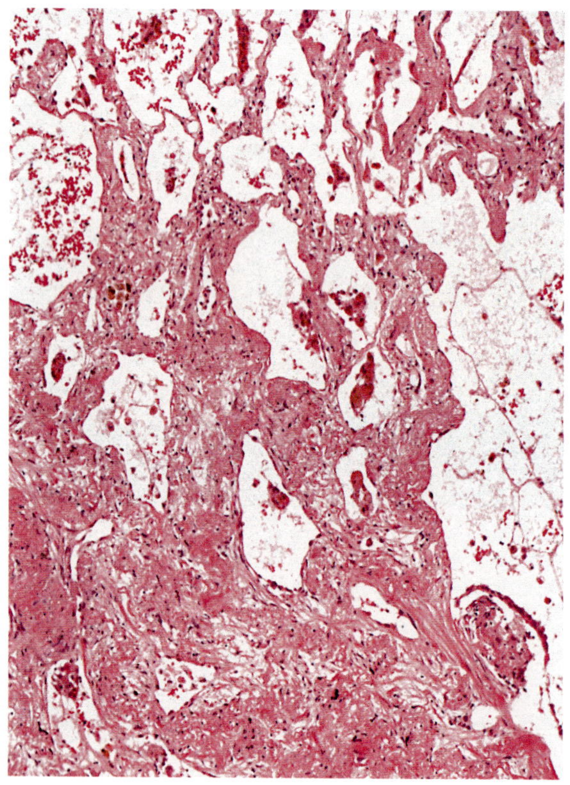

Figure 7-38

RADIATION FIBROSIS

There is patchy fibrosis by acellular elastotic fibrous tissue.

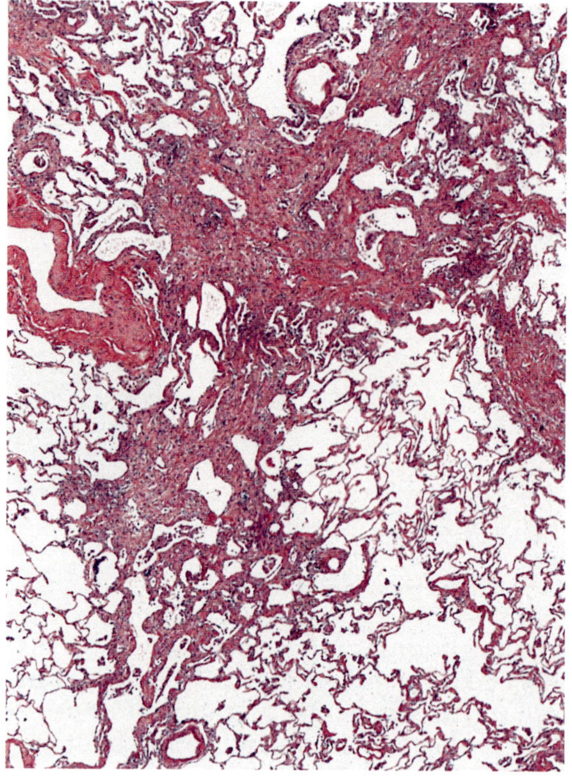

Figure 7-39

RADIATION FIBROSIS

There is patchy interstitial fibrosis resembling that seen in usual interstitial pneumonia.

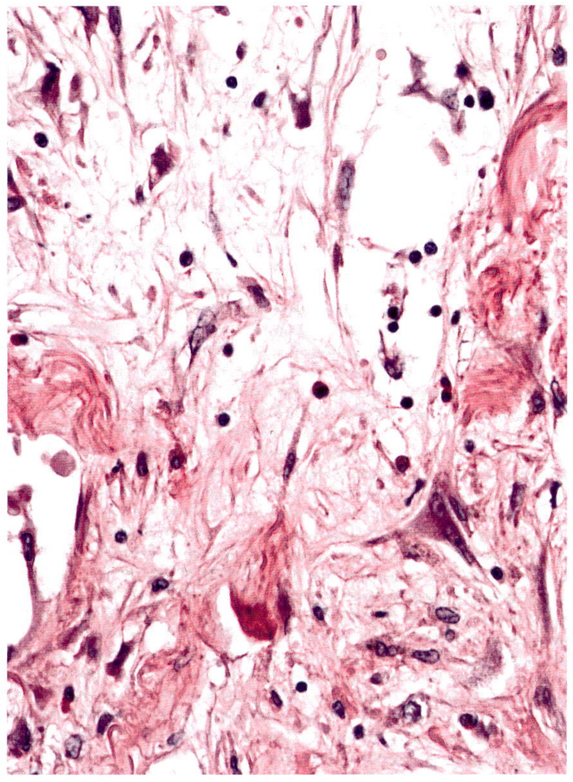

Figure 7-40

RADIATION FIBROSIS

The fibrous tissue demonstrates the bizarre fibroblasts characteristic of chronic radiation effect.

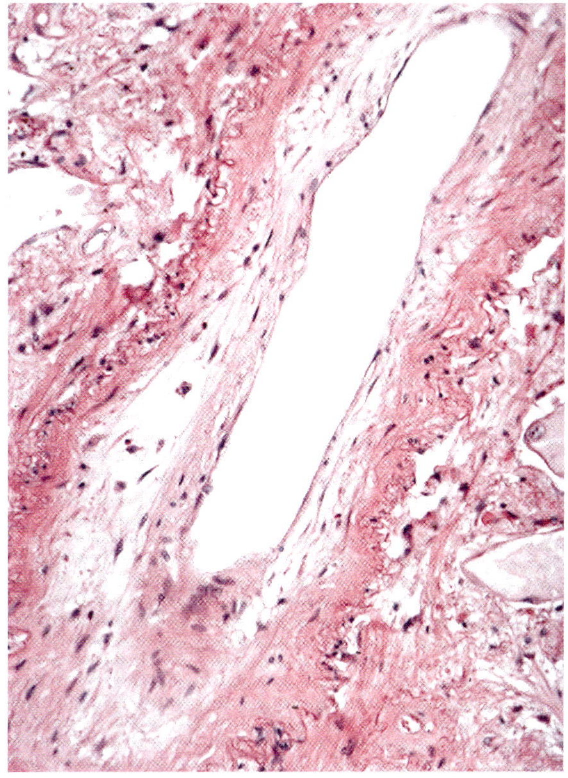

Figure 7-41

RADIATION FIBROSIS

There is myointimal fibrosis in a vein.

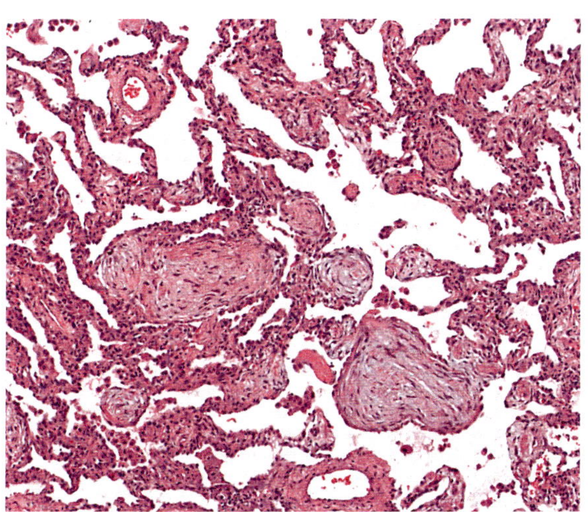

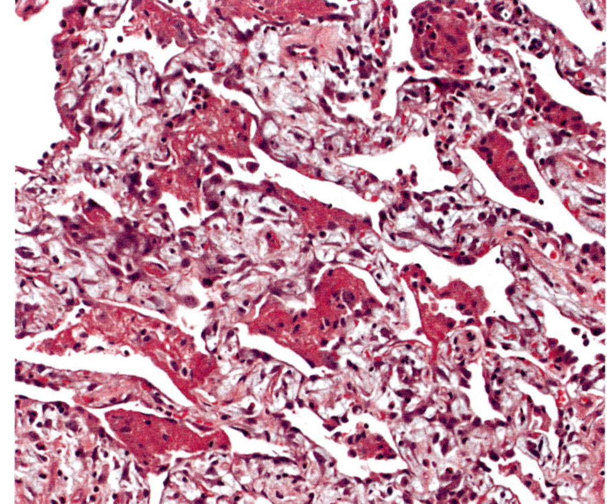

Figure 7-42

RADIATION-ASSOCIATED MIGRATORY PULMONARY INFILTRATES

Left: The infiltrates occurring outside the field of radiation show patchy organizing pneumonia.
Right: In some foci there was acute lung injury with deposition of airspace fibrin and interstitial edema.

REFERENCES

1. Bailey ME, Fraire AE, Greenberg SD, Barnard J, Cagle PT. Pulmonary histopathology in cocaine abusers. Hum Pathol 1994;25:203–7.
2. Banner AS, Muthuswamy P, Shah RS, Rodriguez J, Saksena FS, Addington WW. Bronchiectasis following heroin-induced pulmonary edema. Rapid clearing of pulmonary infiltrates. Chest 1976;69:552–5.
3. Banner AS, Rodriguez J, Sunderrajan EV, Agarwal MK, Addington WW. Bronchiectasis: a cause of pulmonary symptoms in heroin addicts. Respiration 1979;37:232–7.
4. Byhardt RW, Abrams R, Almagro U. The association of adult respiratory distress syndrome (ARDS) with thoracic irradiation (RT). Int J Radiat Oncol Biol Phys 1988;15:1441–6.
5. Castellino RA, Glatstein E, Turbow MM, Rosenberg S, Kaplan HS. Latent radiation injury of lungs or heart activated by steroid withdrawal. Ann Intern Med 1974;80:593–9.
6. Catane R, Schwade JG, Turrisi AT III, Webber BL, Muggia FM. Pulmonary toxicity after radiation and bleomycin: a review. Int J Radiat Oncol Biol Phys 1979;5:1513–8.
7. Churg A, Green FH. Miscellaneous conditions: pulmonary lesions associated with intravenous drug abuse and iatrogenic conditions. In: Churg A, Green FH, eds. Pathology of occupational lung disease, 2nd ed. Baltimore: William & Wilkins; 1998:451–60.
8. Cohen MD, Hornback NB, Mirkin DL, Smith JA, Provisor A, Slabaugh RD. Lung nodules after whole lung radiation. Am J Pediatr Hematol Oncol 1983;5:283–6.
9. Colby TV, Carrington CB. Interstitial lung disease. In: Thurlbeck WM, Churg AC, eds. Pathology of the lung, 2nd ed. New York: Thieme; 1995:589–737.
10. Cooper JA Jr, White DA, Matthay RA. Drug-induced pulmonary disease. Part 1: Cytologic drugs. Am Rev Resp Dis 1986;133:321–40.
11. Cooper JA Jr, White DA, Matthay RA. Drug-induced pulmonary disease. Part 2: Noncytotoxic drugs. Am Rev Resp Dis 1986;133:448–505.
12. Coudert B, Bailly F, Lombard JN, Andre F, Camus P. Amiodarone pneumonitis: bronchoalveolar lavage findings in 15 patients and review of the literature. Chest 1992;102:1005–12.
13. Crestani B, Valeyre D, Roden S, Wallaert B, Dalphin JC. Bronchiolitis obliterans organizing pneumonia syndrome primed by radiation therapy to the breast. The Groupe d'Etudes et de Recherche sur les Maladies Orphelines Pulmonaires. Am J Respir Crit Care Med 1998;158:1929–35.
14. DeGreve J, Warson F, Deleu D, Storme G. Fatal pulmonary toxicity by the association of radiotherapy and medroxyprogesterone acetate. Cancer 1985;56:2434–6.
15. De Vuyst P, Dumortier P, Ketelbant P, Flament-Durand J, Henderson J, Yernault JC. Lung fibrosis induced by Thorotrast. Thorax 1990;45:899–901.
16. Einhorn L, Krause M, Hornback N, Furnas B. Enhanced pulmonary toxicity with bleomycin and radiotherapy in oat cell lung cancer. Cancer 1976;37:2414–6.
17. Fajardo LF. Pathology of radiation injury. Masson monographs in diagnostic pathology, vol. 6. New York: Masson; 1982:34–46.
18. Frija J, Ferme C, Baud L, et al. Radiation-induced lung injuries: a survey by computed tomography and pulmonary function tests in 18 cases of Hodgkin's disease. Europ J Radiol 1988;8:18–23.
19. Fulkerson WJ, McLendon RE, Prosnitz LR. Adult respiratory distress syndrome after limited thoracic radiotherapy. Cancer 1986;57:1941–6.
20. Garcia JG, Munim A, Nugent KM, et al. Alveolar macrophage gold retention in rheumatoid arthritis. J Rheumatol 1987;14:435–8.
21. Gibson PG, Bryant DH, Morgan GW, et al. Radiation-induced lung injury: a hypersensitivity pneumonitis? Ann Intern Med 1988;109:288–91.
22. Goldman AL, Enquist R. Hyperacute radiation pneumonitis. Chest 1975;67:613–5.
23. Goldstein DS, Karpel JP, Appel D, Williams MH. Bullous pulmonary damage in users of intravenous drugs. Chest 1986;89:266–9.
24. Gross NJ. The pathogenesis of radiation-induced lung damage. Lung 1981;159:115–25.
25. Gross NJ. Pulmonary effects on radiation therapy. Ann Intern Med 1977;86:81–92.
26. Heffner JE, Harley RA, Schabel SI. Pulmonary reactions from illicit substance abuse. Clin Chest Med 1990;11:151–62.
27. Ikezoe J, Takashima S, Morimoto S, et al. CT appearance of acute radiation-induced injury in the lung. AJR Am J Roentgenol 1988;150:765–70.
28. Irey NS. Tissue reactions to drugs. Am J Pathol 1976;82:613–47.
29. Kataoka M. Gallium-67 citrate imaging for the assessment of radiation pneumonitis. Ann Nucl Med 1989;3:73–81.
30. Kelly KJ, Ruffing R. Acute eosinophilic pneumonia following intentional inhalation of Scotchguard. Ann Allergy 1993;71:358–61.

31. Kleerup EC, Wong M, Marques-Mgallanes JA, Goldman MD, Tashkin DP. Acute effects of intravenous cocaine on pulmonary artery pressure and cardiac index in habitual crack smokers. Chest 1997;111:30–5.
32. Kreisman H, Wolkove N. Pulmonary toxicity of antineoplastic therapy. Semin Oncol 1992;19:508–20.
33. Lemense GP, Sahn SA. Opportunistic infection during treatment with low dose methotrexate. Am J Respir Crit Care Med 1994;150:258–60.
34. Libshitz HI. Radiation changes in the lung. Semin Roentgenol 1993;28:303–20.
35. Martin C, Romero S, Sanchez-Paya J, Massuti B, Arriero JM, Hernandez L. Bilateral lymphocytic alveolitis: a common reaction after unilateral thoracic irradiation. Eur Respir J 1999;13:727–32.
36. Martin WJ II. Drug-induced lung disease. In: Baughman RP, ed. Bronchoalveolar lavage. St. Louis: Mosby Year Book; 1992:193–211.
37. Monforte JR, Gault R, Smialek J, Goodin T. Toxicological and pathological findings in fatalities involving pentazocine and tripelennamine. J Forensic Sci 1983;28:90–101.
38. Morelock SY, Sahn SA. Drugs and the pleura. Chest 1999;116:212–21.
39. Morgan GW, Breit SN. Radiation and the lung: a reevaluation of the mechanisms mediating pulmonary injury. Int J Radiat Oncol Biol Phys 1995;31:361–9.
40. Movsas B, Raffin TA, Epstein AH, Link CJ Jr. Pulmonary radiation injury. Chest 1997;111: 1061–76.
41. Myers JL, Pathology of drug-induced lung disease. In: Katzenstein AL, ed. Katzenstein and Askin's surgical pathology of non-neoplastic disease, 3rd ed. Philadelphia: WB Saunders; 1997:81–111.
42. Nakayama Y, Makino S, Fududa Y, Min KY, Shimizu A, Ohsawa N. Activation of lavage lymphocytes in lung injuries caused by radiotherapy for lung cancer. Int J Radiat Oncol Biol Phys 1996;34:459–67.
43. O'Donnell AE, Selig J, Aravamuthan M, Richardson MS. Pulmonary complications associated with illicit drug use. An update. Chest 1995;108:460–63.
44. O'Driscoll BR, Hasleton PS, Taylor PM, Poulter LW, Gattameneni HR, Woodcock AA. Active lung fibrosis up to 17 years after chemotherapy with carmustine (BCNU) in childhood N Eng J Med 1990;323:378–382.
45. Ohar JA, Jackson F, Dettenmeier PA, Bedrossian CW, Tricomi SM, Evans RG. Bronchoalveolar lavage cell count and differential are not reliable indicators of amiodarone-induced pneumonitis. Chest 1992;102:999–1004.
46. Pare JP, Cote G, Fraser R. Long-term follow-up of drug abusers with intravenous talcosis. Am Rev Respir Dis 1989;139:233–41.
47. Pezner RD, Bertrand M, Cecchi GR, Paladugu RR, Kendregan BA. Steroid-withdrawal radiation pneumonitis in cancer patients. Chest 1984;85:816–7.
48. Poklis A, Mackell MA. Pentazocine and tripelennamine (T's and Blues) abuse: toxicological findings in 39 cases. J Anal Toxicol 1982;6:109–14.
49. Rehse DH, Aye RW, Florence MG. Respiratory failure following talc pleurodesis. Am J Surg 1999;177:437–40.
50. Roberts CM, Foulcher E, Zaunders JJ, et al. Radiation pneumonitis: a possible lymphocyte-mediated hypersensitivity reaction. Ann Intern Med 1993;118:696–700.
51. Robertson CH Jr, Reynolds RC, Wilson J. Pulmonary hypertension and foreign body granulomas in intravenous drug abusers. Documentation by cardiac catheterization and lung biopsy. Am J Med 1976;61:657–64.
52. Rosenow EC, Myers JL, Swensen SJ, Pisani RJ. Drug-induced pulmonary disease: an update. Chest 1992;102:239–50.
53. Rosiello RA, Merrill WW. Radiation-induced lung injury. Clin Chest Med Arch 1990;11:65–75.
54. Roswit B, White DC. Severe radiation injuries of the lung. Am J Roentgenol 1977;129:127–36.
55. Salinas FV, Winterbauer RH. Radiation pneumonitis: a mimic of infectious pneumonitis. Sem Respir Infect 1995;10:143–53.
56. Schachter EN, Basta W. Bronchiectasis following heroin overdose. A report of two cases. Chest 1973;63:363–6.
57. Schmidt RA, Glenny RW, Godwin JD, Hampson NB, Cantino ME, Reichenbach DD. Panlobular emphysema in young intravenous Ritalin abusers. Am Rev Respir Dis 1991;143:649–56.
58. Sherman CB, Hudson LD, Pierson DJ. Severe precocious emphysema in intravenous methylphenidate (Ritalin) abusers. Chest 1987;92:1085–7.
59. Stern EJ, Frank MS, Schmutz JF, Glenny RW, Schmidt RA, Godwin JD. Panlobular pulmonary emphysema caused by i.v. injection of methylphenidate (Ritalin): findings on chest radiographs and CT scans. AJR Am J Roetgenol 1994;162:555–60.
60. Tomashefski JF Jr, Hirsch CS. The pulmonary vascular lesions of intravenous drug abuse. Hum Pathol 1980;11:133–45.
61. Tomioka R, King TE Jr. Gold-induced pulmonary disease: clinical features, outcome, and differentiation from rheumatoid lung disease. Am J Respir Crit Care Med 1997;155:1011–20.

62. Van Laar JM, Holscher HC, Van Krieken JH, Stolk J. Bronchiolitis obliterans organizing pneumonia after adjuvant radiotherapy for breast carcinoma. Respir Med 1997;91:241–4.
63. Van Mieghem W, Coolen L, Malysse I, Lacquet LM, Deneffe GJ, Demedts MG. Amiodarone and the development of ARDS after lung surgery. Chest 1994;105:1642–45.
64. Warnock ML, Chahremani GG, Rattenborg C, Ginsberg M, Valenzuela J. Pulmonary complication of heroin intoxication. Aspiration pneumonia and diffuse bronchiectasis. JAMA 1972;219:1051–3.
65. Weisbrod GL, Rahman M, Chamberlain D, Herman SJ. Precocious emphysema in intravenous drug abusers. J Thorac Imaging 1993;8:233–40.
66. Yakel DL, Eisenberg MJ. Pulmonary artery hypertension in chronic intravenous cocaine users. Am Heart J 1995;130:398–9.
67. Zitnik RJ, Cooper JA Jr. Drug-induced pulmonary disease. Clin Chest Med 1990;11:139–50.
68. Zitnik RJ, Matthay RA. Drug-induced lung disease. In: Schwarz MI, King TE Jr, eds. Interstitial lung disease, 3rd ed. Hamilton: BC Decker; 1998:423–50.

8
BRONCHIOLAR DISORDERS

INTRODUCTION

Since bronchioles are connected to bronchi at one end and alveoli at the other, bronchiolar pathology frequently accompanies diseases of the large airways as well as diseases of the distal (alveolar) lung parenchyma (4,11,23). Clinicopathologic settings associated with significant pathologic changes in the bronchioles are shown in Table 8-1.

Conditions showing bronchiolar pathology are varied and heterogeneous, and there is overlap with many other areas in lung pathology. A full understanding and characterization of these conditions requires a multidisciplinary (clinical/radiologic/pathologic) approach.

BACKGROUND

The following points set the stage for evaluation of bronchiolar pathology (4,11,23).

"Bronchiolitis" means something different to the clinician, the physiologist, the radiologist, and the pathologist. No one view suffices, and hence our emphasis on a clinical/radiologic/pathologic approach. As an example, the characteristic micronodular pattern seen on high-resolution computed tomography (HRCT) in extrinsic allergic alveolitis is recognized as bronchiolocentric by the radiologist and correlates with bronchiolocentric inflammation histologically, yet the clinician views this condition as an interstitial lung disease (see chapter 3).

Pathologic changes in the bronchioles may be associated with restrictive or obstructive pulmonary functions (or both).

Dramatic clinical (and functional) findings caused by bronchiolar disease may be present with minor radiologic or pathologic changes. Reactive airways disease/asthma is an example. In such a setting, the pathology is not the gold standard.

Pathologic changes in the bronchioles may be primary (i.e., the main pathologic lesion) or secondary. Severe bronchiolitis is often seen distal to bronchiectasis (fig. 8-1) yet it is considered a secondary phenomenon. Conversely, bronchiectasis may develop secondarily in cases of chronic bronchiolitis. This is well described in diffuse panbronchiolitis and transplant-associated bronchiolitis obliterans (fig. 8-2). Late in the course of these diseases it may be difficult to determine (solely on the basis of histology) which was the initial lesion.

Table 8-1

CLINICAL AND PATHOLOGIC SETTINGS ASSOCIATED WITH BRONCHIOLAR PATHOLOGY[a]

Asthma
Infections/postinfections
Allergic reactions (eosinophilic pneumonia, hypersensitivity pneumonitis)
Chronic obstructive pulmonary disease
Respiratory (smoker's) bronchiolitis
Respiratory bronchiolitis–associated interstitial lung disease
Bronchopulmonary dysplasia
Bronchiectasis (regardless of cause)
Collagen vascular diseases
Fume/toxic exposure
Drug reactions
Transplant-associated
Lung transplant rejection
Graft versus host disease following bone marrow transplantation
Conditions associated with cryptogenic organizing pneumonia (Table 8-3)
Aspiration
Diffuse panbronchiolitis
Inflammatory bowel disease
Mineral dust exposure/cobalt lung/nylon flock worker's lung
Vasculitis (esp. Wegener's granulomatosis)
Diffuse idiopathic pulmonary neuroendocrine cell hyperplasia (multiple carcinoid tumorlets)
Idiopathic bronchiolitis (including constrictive bronchiolitis)
Miscellaneous: Stevens-Johnson syndrome, neoplasms, thyroiditis, primary biliary cirrhosis, irradiation, lysinuric protein intolerance, ataxia-telangiectasia

[a]Data from references 11 and 23.

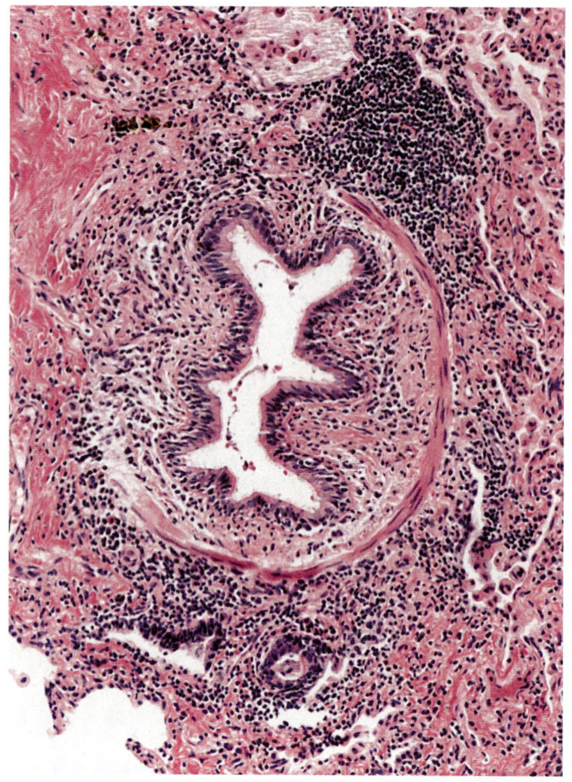

Figure 8-1

CHRONIC BRONCHIOLITIS

Chronic bronchiolitis with transmural inflammation and luminal compromise due to submucosal scarring distal to established bronchiectasis.

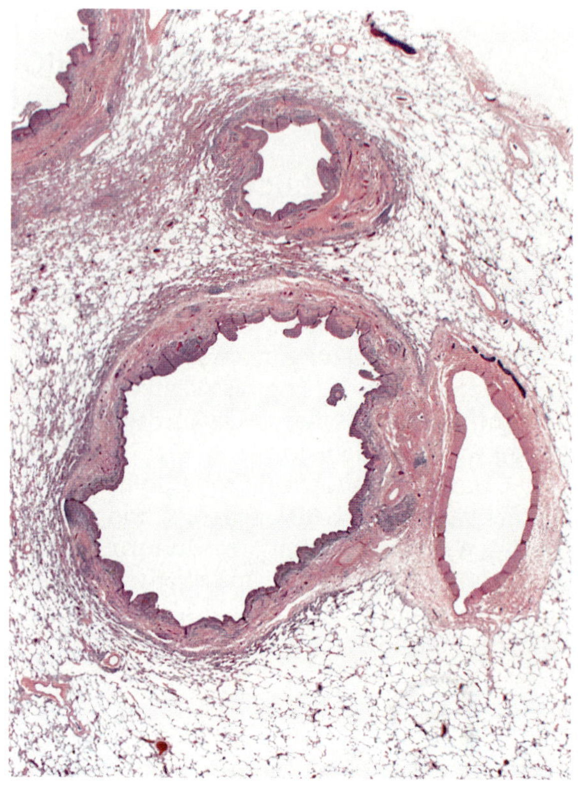

Figure 8-2

SECONDARY BRONCHIECTASIS IN TRANSPLANT-ASSOCIATED BRONCHIOLITIS OBLITERANS SYNDROME

This patient with a lung allograft developed biopsy-proven bronchiolitis obliterans (constrictive bronchiolitis). At autopsy extensive secondary bronchiectasis was seen.

Pathologic changes in the bronchioles may be a component of a constellation of histologic changes. Many interstitial lung diseases, such as extrinsic allergic alveolitis and cryptogenic organizing pneumonia, have bronchiolar changes as an integral part of their histopathology.

Cases of bronchiolitis have a natural history that is reflected in the clinical/radiologic/pathologic features. The findings of bronchiolitis may change over time, as illustrated in cases of infectious bronchiolitis, fume exposure, and transplant-associated bronchiolitis: the early cellular or necrotizing reaction presents an entirely different clinical/radiologic/histologic picture than does the late/chronic lesion which may produce clinical/radiologic/histologic features of bronchiolitis obliterans with airflow obstruction (constrictive bronchiolitis; see below).

The pathologic spectrum of bronchiolar disorders is explained by the complex interplay of various elements. These include inflammatory cells (acute, chronic, granulomatous, and lymphoid hyperplasia in a mural or luminal location); mesenchymal (fibroblastic/fibrotic) reaction (organizing [still capable of resolution] or collagenized [irreversible]) located in intraluminal polyps, as well as submucosal (with luminal narrowing) and peribronchiolar (without luminal narrowing) areas; epithelial changes (necrosis and sloughing, metaplasia, peribronchiolar metaplasia); smooth muscle hypertrophy; basement membrane thickening (e.g., asthma); and secondary changes (e.g., distal acute/organizing pneumonia).

The various combinations and permutations of these features explain the broad clinical and radiologic spectra of bronchiolar disorders.

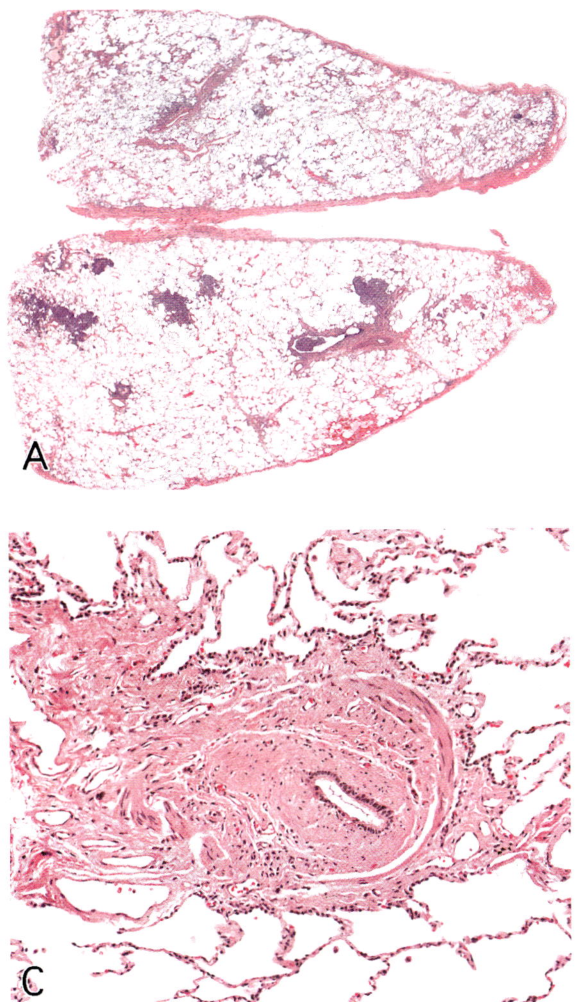

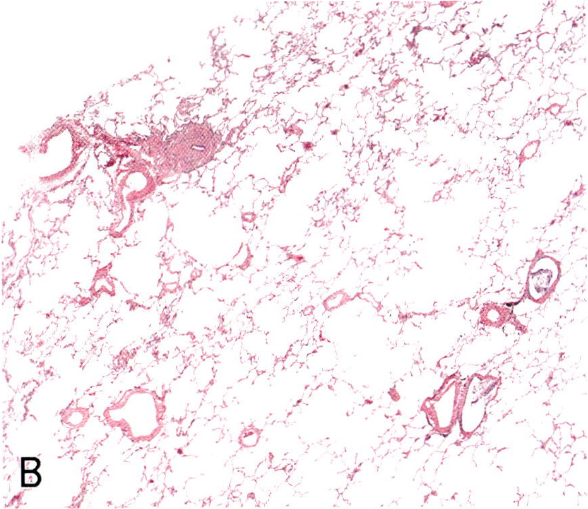

Figure 8-3

CONSTRICTIVE BRONCHIOLITIS

Pathologic changes in the small airways are best appreciated at scanning power microscopy. The changes are obvious when there is prominent inflammation in the bronchioles (A) but may be more difficult to appreciate in cases of constrictive bronchiolitis when more subtle abnormalities are present in the small airways (B). A bronchiole at 4 o'clock shows mucostasis within its lumen and another at 10 o'clock shows almost complete luminal obliteration (C) by submucosal collagen deposition. The lung parenchyma shows mild to moderate histologic emphysema.

PATHOLOGIC PATTERNS OF BRONCHIOLITIS

One must first be able to recognize that the histologic abnormalities are related primarily to the bronchioles. This is accomplished at scanning power microscopy by examining all the tissue and assessing whether the abnormalities identified (inflammation, fibrosis) center on the bronchioles or alveolar duct regions (fig. 8-3). If secondary changes have developed in the more distal lung parenchyma (acute/organizing pneumonia or fibrosis), they tend to be focal (fig. 8-4). An airway-centered distribution may sometimes involve only alveolar ducts, with relatively inconspicuous changes in the bronchioles themselves.

Table 8-2 shows the spectrum of bronchiolar lesions (exclusive of clinical and radiologic

Table 8-2

BRONCHIOLAR HISTOPATHOLOGY GROUPINGS[a]

Asthmatic changes
Chronic bronchitis/emphysema-associated changes
Cellular bronchiolitis
Follicular bronchiolitis; diffuse panbronchiolitis
Respiratory (smoker's) bronchiolitis
Bronchiolitis obliterans with intraluminal polyps (also called bronchiolitis obliterans-see text)
Constrictive bronchiolitis (also called obliterative bronchiolitis and bronchiolitis obliterans–see text)
Mineral dust airways disease
Peribronchiolar fibrosis and bronchiolar metaplasia
Bronchiolocentric nodules

[a]Data from references 3 and 5.

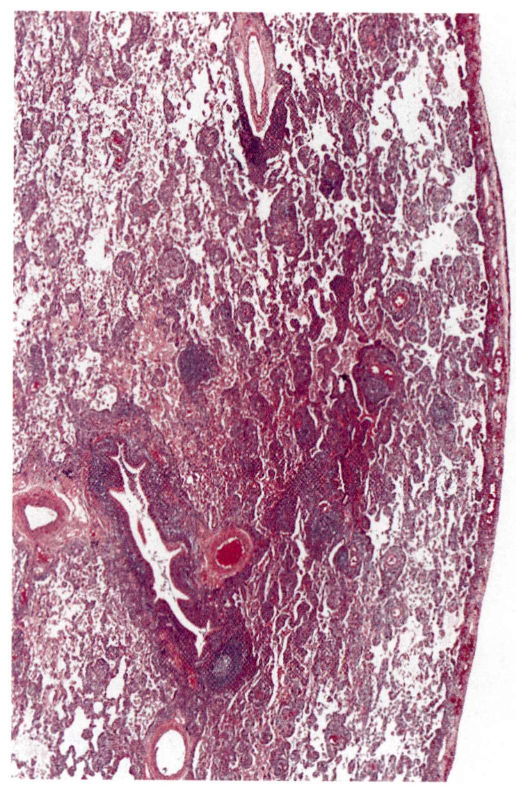

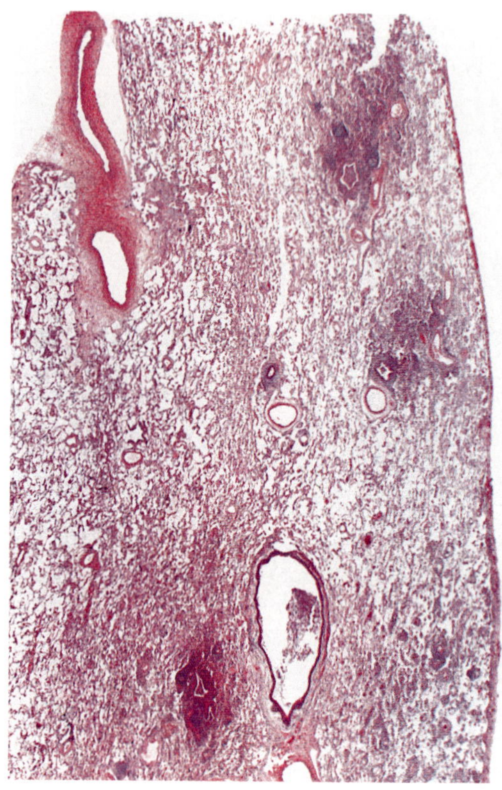

Figure 8-4

SECONDARY ALVEOLAR PARENCHYMAL CHANGES IN CHRONIC BRONCHIOLITIS

Left: This case of inflammatory bowel disease–related chronic bronchiolitis (with associated airflow obstruction) shows some regions where there appears to be an interstitial pneumonia involving the subpleural alveoli in addition to the follicular bronchiolitis noted at 4 o'clock.

Right: The alveolar changes are secondary because multiple other tissue sections in this case showed that the pathologic changes were primarily restricted to bronchioles.

findings) commonly encountered by the surgical pathologist. Table 8-2 is oriented toward histopathology and there are a number of clinical/radiologic/histologic entities that are included in each of the categories. Some are discussed in other sections: asthma and small airway changes in chronic bronchitis/emphysema are discussed in chapter 10; mineral dust airway changes are discussed in chapter 16.

Cellular bronchiolitis (fig. 8-5) is a useful morphologic descriptor for the surgical pathologist even though it is a common pattern seen in many clinicopathologic settings (3–5). The inflammation may be acute or chronic (or both) and there may be associated bronchiolitis obliterans with intraluminal polyps or constrictive bronchiolitis (see below). Two distinctive types of cellular bronchiolitis deserve special attention.

Follicular bronchiolitis has lymphoid follicles with reactive centers along airways (fig. 8-6) (45). Follicular bronchiolitis represents hyperplasia of mucosa-associated lymphoid tissue (MALT) along the airways (bronchus-associated lymphoid tissue [BALT]). Follicular bronchiolitis overlaps with diffuse lymphoid hyperplasia/lymphocytic interstitial pneumonia (see chapters 3 and 5). *Diffuse panbronchiolitis* (DPB), a special subtype of cellular bronchiolitis, is discussed below.

Respiratory bronchiolitis (RB) is a common reaction seen in cigarette smokers and its presence histologically is usually good evidence that the patient is a cigarette smoker (fig. 8-7) (see chapter 3) (32,33,43,46). RB is a mild inflammatory reaction of the respiratory bronchioles and immediately surrounding alveoli consisting of slight fibrosis, smooth muscle hypertrophy, and

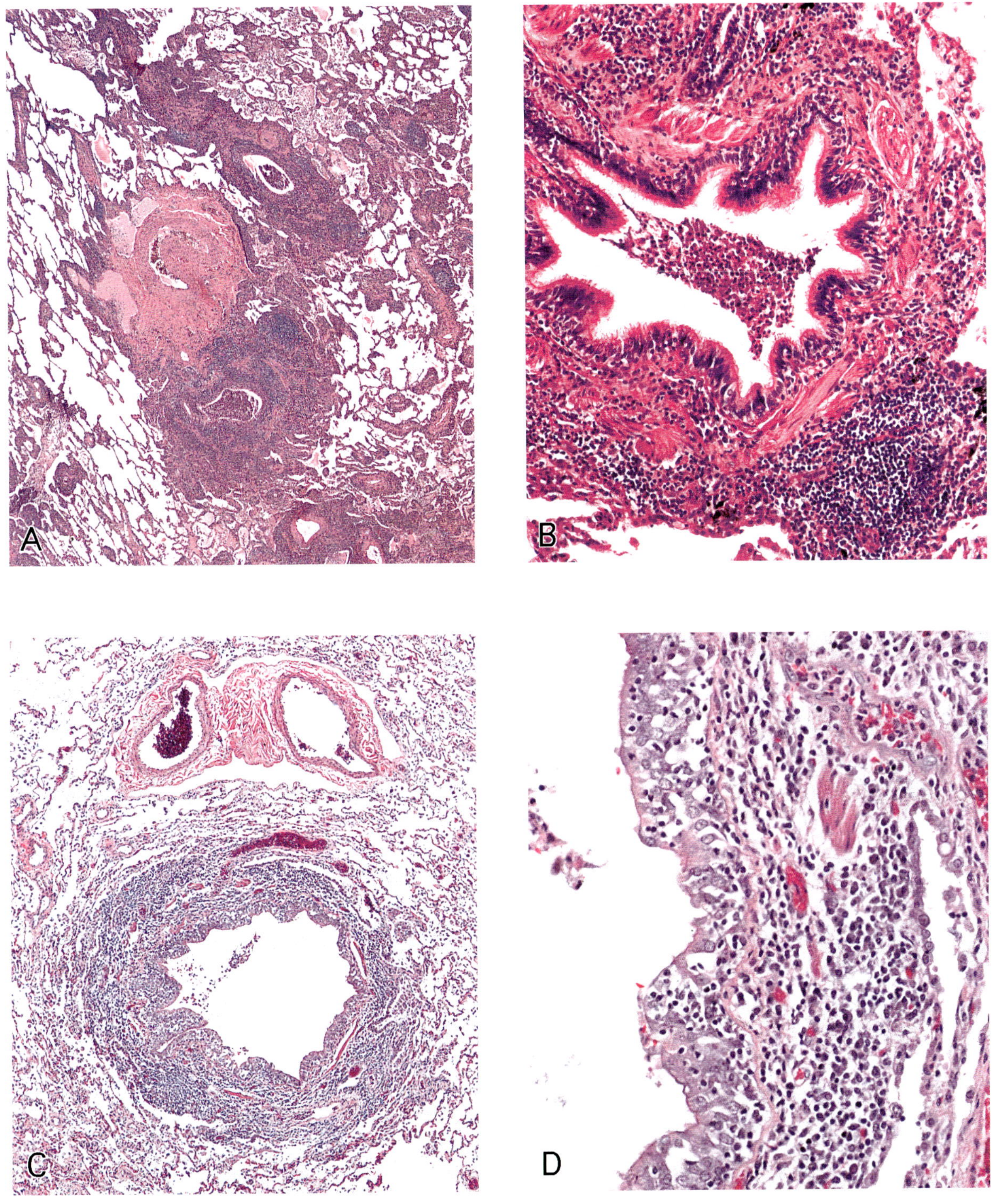

Figure 8-5

CELLULAR BRONCHIOLITIS

A: Acute and chronic cellular bronchiolitis associated with inflammatory bowel disease.

B: Idiopathic acute and chronic cellular bronchiolitis.

C,D: Transplant-associated chronic cellular bronchiolitis as part of post-transplant bronchiolitis obliterans syndrome. Lymphocytic infiltration of the bronchiolar epithelium is shown in D.

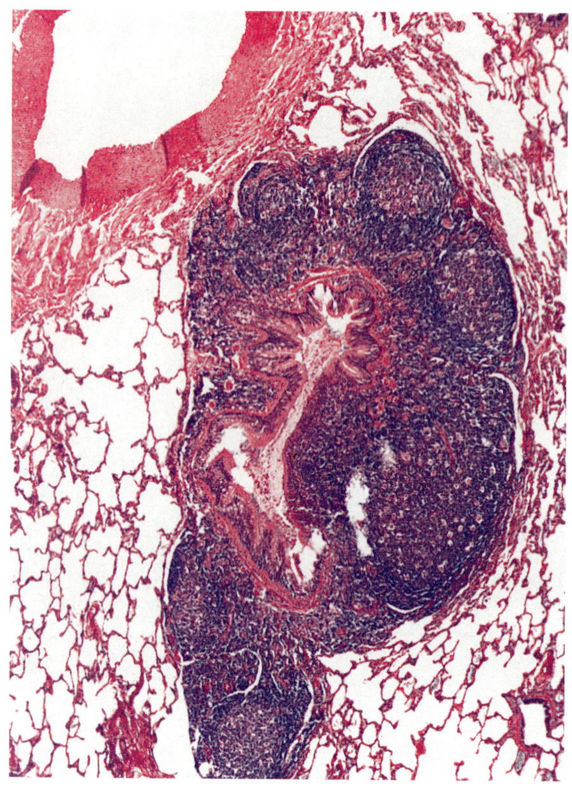

Figure 8-6

FOLLICULAR BRONCHIOLITIS

Lymphoid hyperplasia and reactive germinal centers cuff a bronchiole.

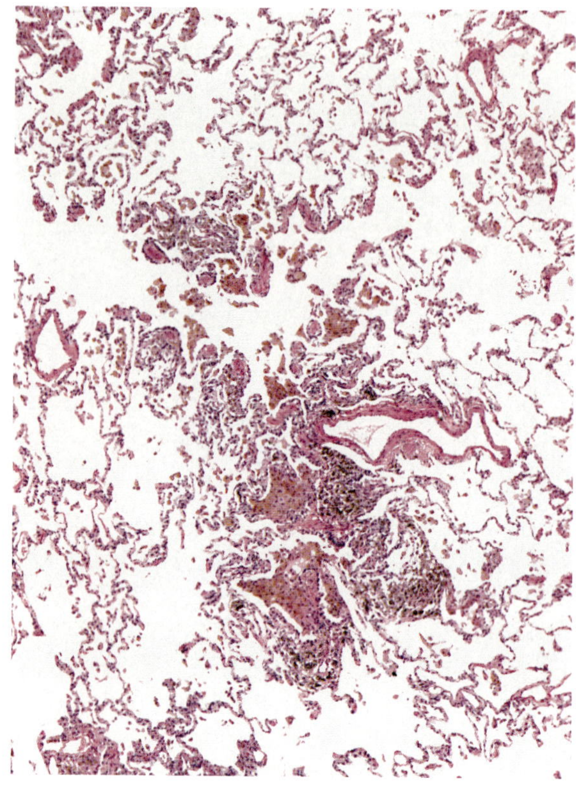

Figure 8-7

RESPIRATORY BRONCHIOLITIS

There is a mild inflammatory infiltrate involving the interstitium of a respiratory bronchiole. Associated accumulations of tan macrophages are seen within the bronchiolar lumen and immediately adjacent to alveoli.

a prominent increase in alveolar macrophages in the respiratory bronchioles and adjacent alveoli. Mucus stasis may be present. The macrophages are lightly pigmented, tan-brown, and usually contain flecks of dark debris; they typically stain with the Prussian blue reaction for iron, resulting in a diffuse fine pattern (in contrast to the coarse granular staining pattern of hemosiderin in alveolar hemorrhage syndromes).

The term *bronchiolitis obliterans* has been used for two histologic lesions: *bronchiolitis obliterans with intraluminal polyps* (fig. 8-8) and the spectrum of changes seen in *constrictive bronchiolitis* (figs. 8-9–8-13) (4,6,43). In this section these two bronchiolar reaction patterns are separated because there is relatively little overlap among the clinical settings in which they are commonly identified. Bronchiolitis obliterans with intraluminal polyps typically includes a reaction in the distal parenchyma called "organizing pneumonia" and the terms *bronchiolitis obliterans organizing pneumonia (BOOP)* or simply *organizing pneumonia* are descriptive of this pattern (6). The AST/ERS classification of idiopathic interstitial pneumonias recommends using the term *organizing pneumonia pattern* for this histologic reaction (39a). Bronchiolitis obliterans with intraluminal polyps is used in this section to emphasize the presence of intraluminal polyps in this type of bronchiolitis obliterans and to contrast it with constrictive bronchiolitis. For practical purposes, bronchiolitis obliterans with intraluminal polyps rarely occurs outside the setting of an organizing pattern, a very common reaction seen in a variety of settings, as shown in Table 8-3. *Cryptogenic organizing pneumonia* (idiopathic BOOP[12]) is discussed in chapter 3.

Constrictive bronchiolitis is a histologic descriptor for the spectrum of morphologic changes typically associated with the clinical syndrome

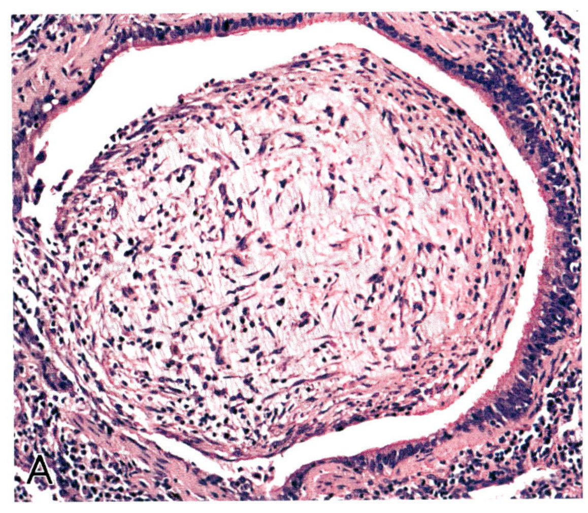

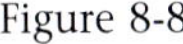

Figure 8-8

BRONCHIOLITIS OBLITERANS WITH INTRALUMINAL POLYPS (ORGANIZING PNEUMONIA PATTERN)

A: The original (classic) description of bronchiolitis obliterans was of intraluminal polypoid fibroblastic tissue, as illustrated here.

B: Bronchiolitis obliterans with intraluminal polyps is commonly associated with organizing pneumonia involving the more distal parenchyma; this is recognized as similar tufts of organizing fibroblastic tissue within alveolar ducts and alveoli.

C: Organizing pneumonia is a histologic term for a relatively common nonspecific reaction in the lung in which there is often bronchiolitis obliterans with intraluminal polyps (10 o'clock) and patchy airspace organization, i.e., organizing pneumonia (right).

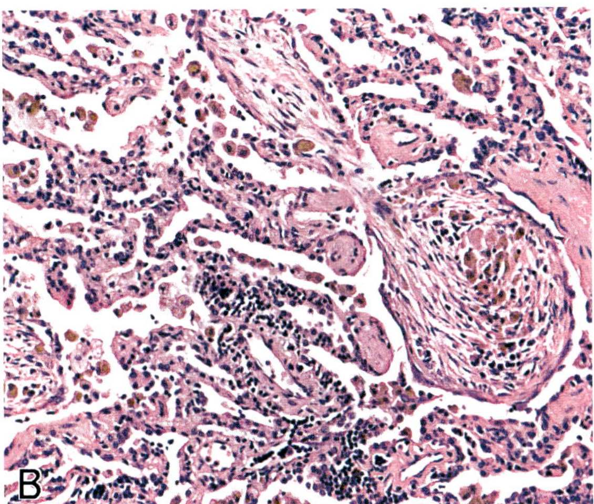

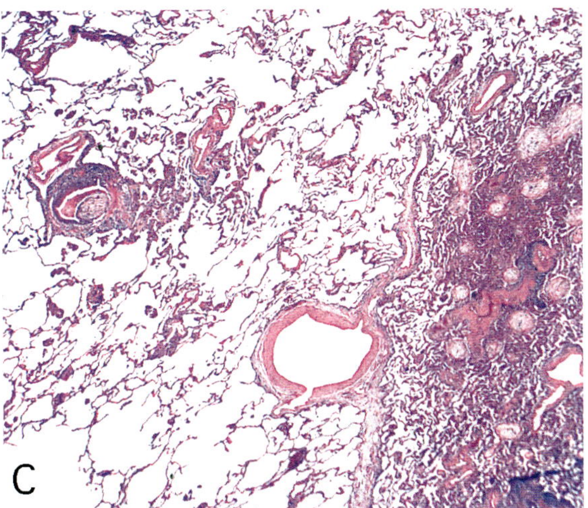

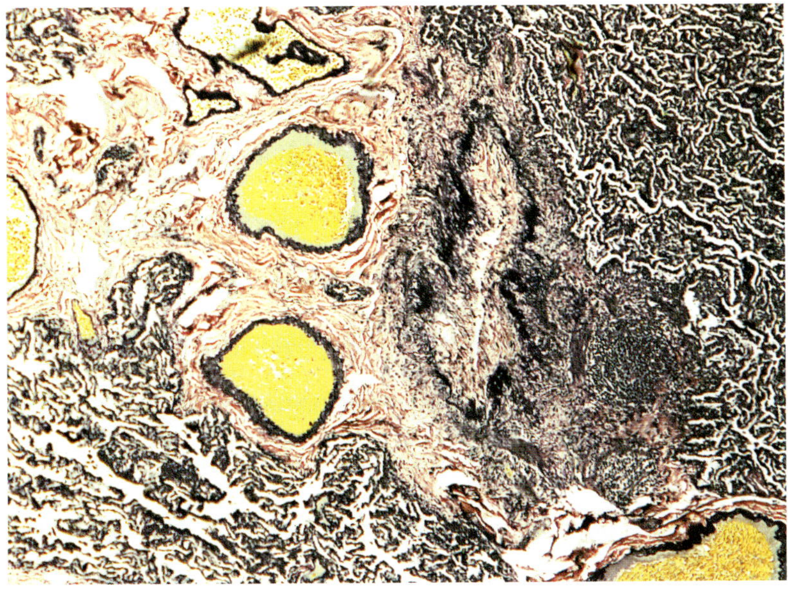

Figure 8-9

POSTINFECTIOUS CONSTRICTIVE BRONCHIOLITIS

The elastic tissue stain highlights the complete bronchiolar obliteration (center) that followed severe adenovirus pneumonia.

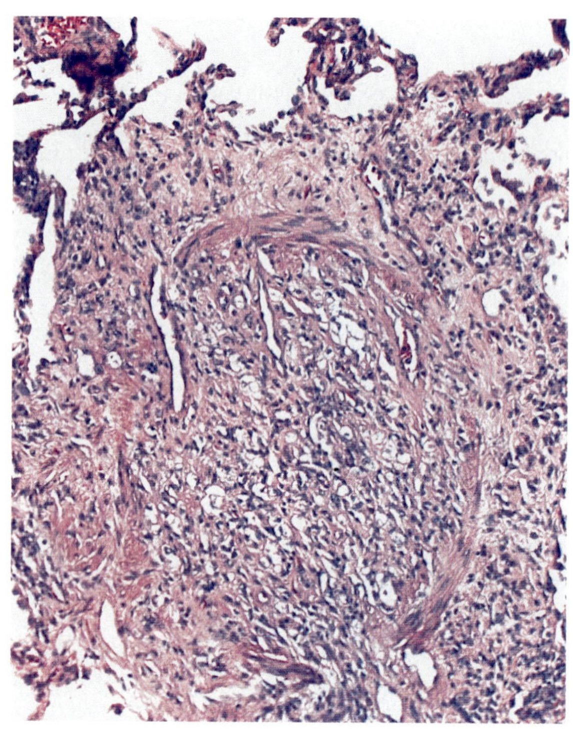

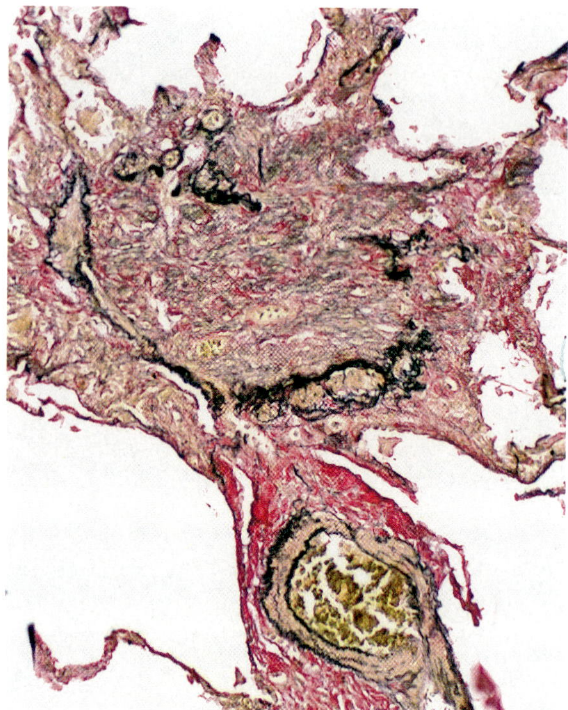

Figure 8-10

TRANSPLANT-ASSOCIATED CONSTRICTIVE BRONCHIOLITIS

Left: This heart-lung allograft shows complete obliteration of a bronchiole by fibrous tissue, with modest associated inflammation.

Right: The preexisting elastica of the bronchiole is highlighted with an elastic tissue stain.

Table 8-3

CONDITIONS ASSOCIATED WITH BRONCHIOLITIS OBLITERANS WITH INTRALUMINAL POLYPS (ORGANIZING PNEUMONIA PATTERN)[a]

Organizing diffuse alveolar damage
Organizing infectious pneumonias
Organization distal to obstruction
Organizing aspiration pneumonia
Organizing reactions, fume or toxic exposures
Connective tissues diseases
Extrinsic allergic alveolitis
Eosinophilic pneumonia
Lung transplantation and graft versus host disease
Secondary reaction distal to chronic bronchiolitis or bronchiectasis
As an idiopathic process, that is either localized (focalorganizing pneumonia) or more widespread (cryptogenic organizing pneumonia–see chapter 3)

[a]Data from references 5 and 23 (see Table 3-16).

of bronchiolitis obliterans (airflow obstruction due to lesions in the small airways) (figs. 8-9–8-13) (4,6,43). *Obliterative bronchiolitis* is a synonym. Changes seen in constrictive bronchiolitis include submucosal scarring, concentric luminal narrowing, adventitial scarring, chronic inflammation (chronic cellular bronchiolitis), decreased bronchiolar lumen size, bronchiolar ectasia with mucus stasis, epithelial metaplasia, smooth muscle hypertrophy, and complete (irreversible) luminal obliteration with replacement of the bronchiole by a relatively acellular scar. The histologic changes of constrictive bronchiolitis may be seen in localized inflammatory processes (e.g., distal to the bronchiectasis). The conditions shown in Table 8-4 are those in which there is widespread narrowing and clinical evidence of airflow obstruction in small airways.

The most distinctive feature of constrictive bronchiolitis is the subtlety of the changes in the face of clinical and radiologic findings

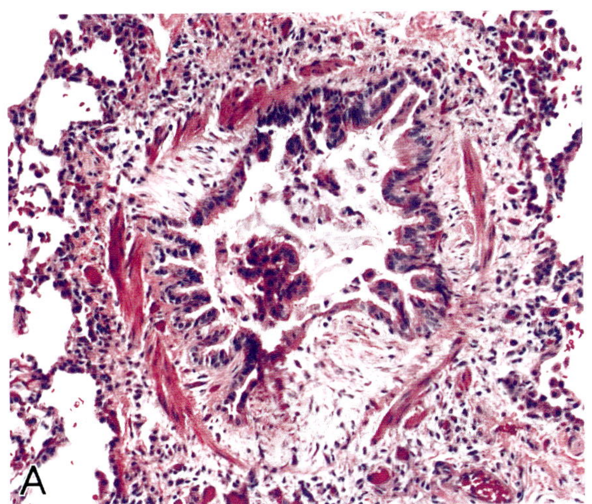

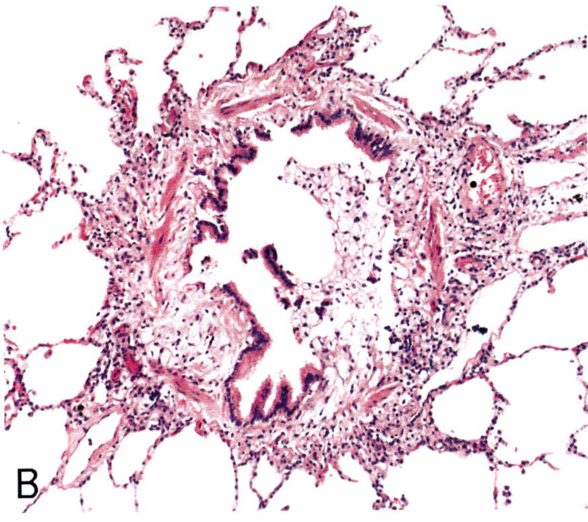

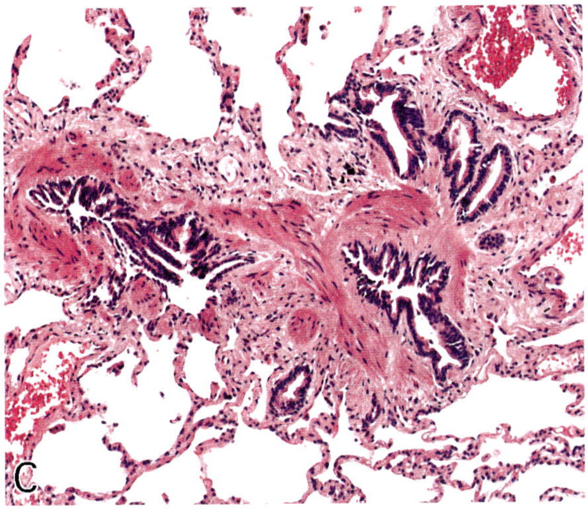

Figure 8-11

CONSTRICTIVE BRONCHIOLITIS

Incomplete luminal compromise is much more commonly seen than complete luminal obliteration, as illustrated in:

A: Bone marrow transplant–associated constrictive bronchiolitis with adventitial and submucosal scarring;

B: *Sauropus androgynus*–associated constrictive bronchiolitis with submucosal scarring, focal mucosal ulceration, and luminal exudate;

C: Idiopathic constrictive bronchiolitis with submucosal scarring, smooth muscle hypertrophy, and irregular and contorted bronchiolar lumens;

D: Inflammatory bowel disease–associated constrictive bronchiolitis with severe airflow obstruction clinically, subtle submucosal scarring, mural chronic inflammation, and luminal stasis of histocytes;

E: Bone marrow transplant–associated constrictive bronchiolitis with only subtle chronic inflammation in the wall. By itself, the bronchiolar lesion shown would be nondiagnostic.

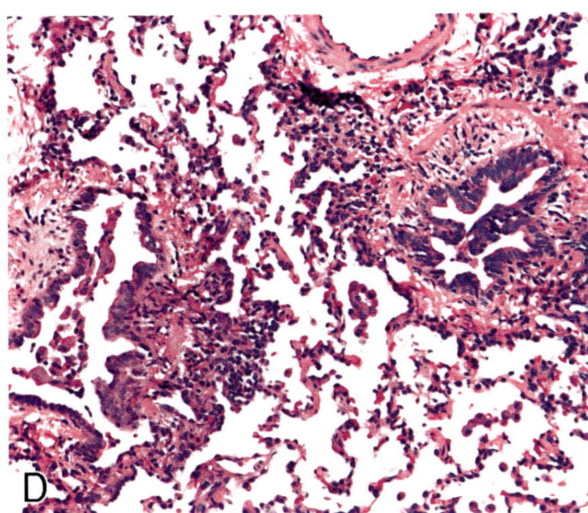

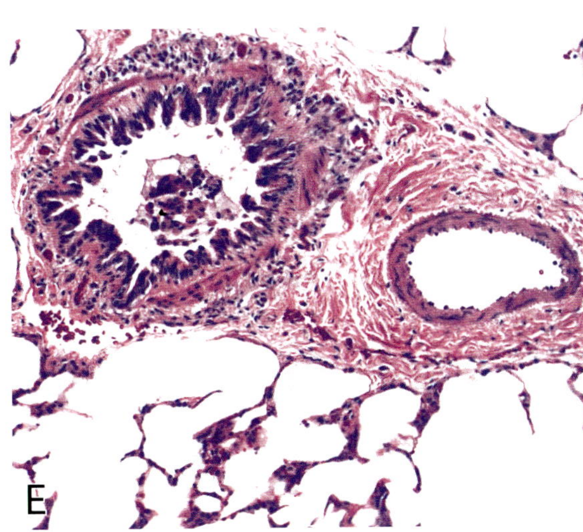

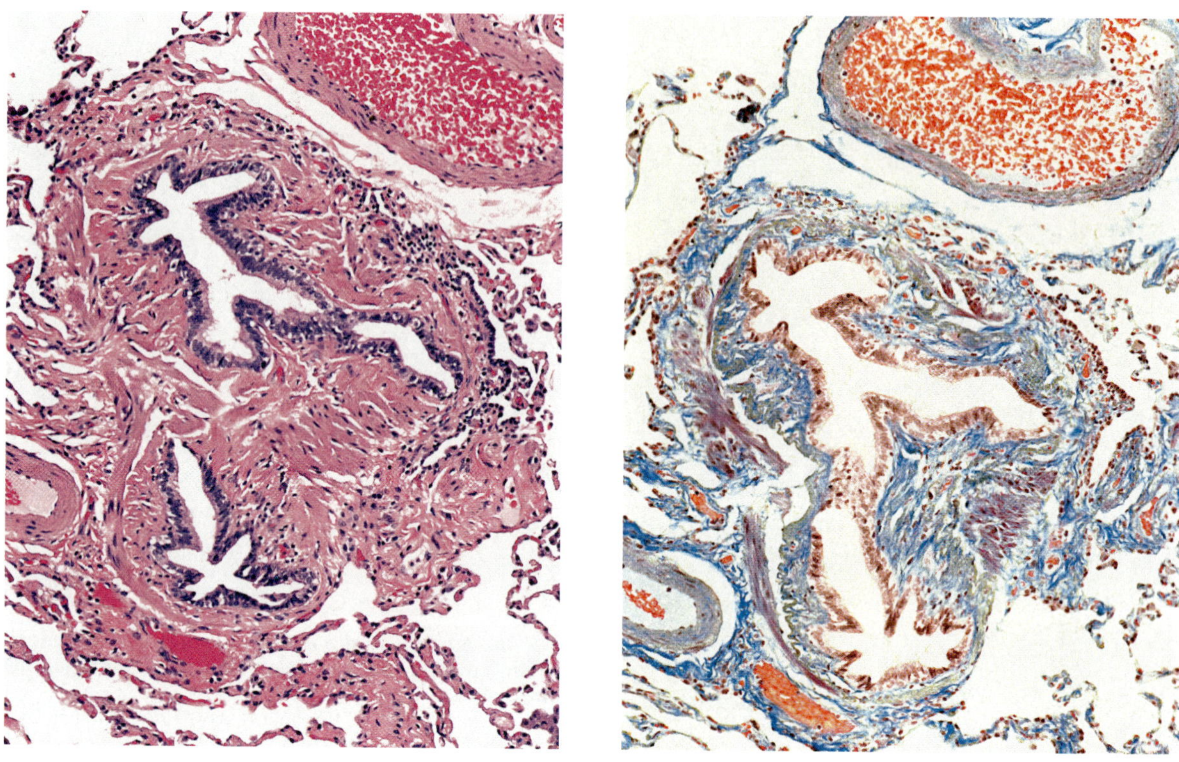

Figure 8-12

CONSTRICTIVE BRONCHIOLITIS

Constrictive bronchiolitis with submucosal scarring (left) highlighted with a trichrome stain (right). The patient had chronic asthma and developed irreversible airflow obstruction.

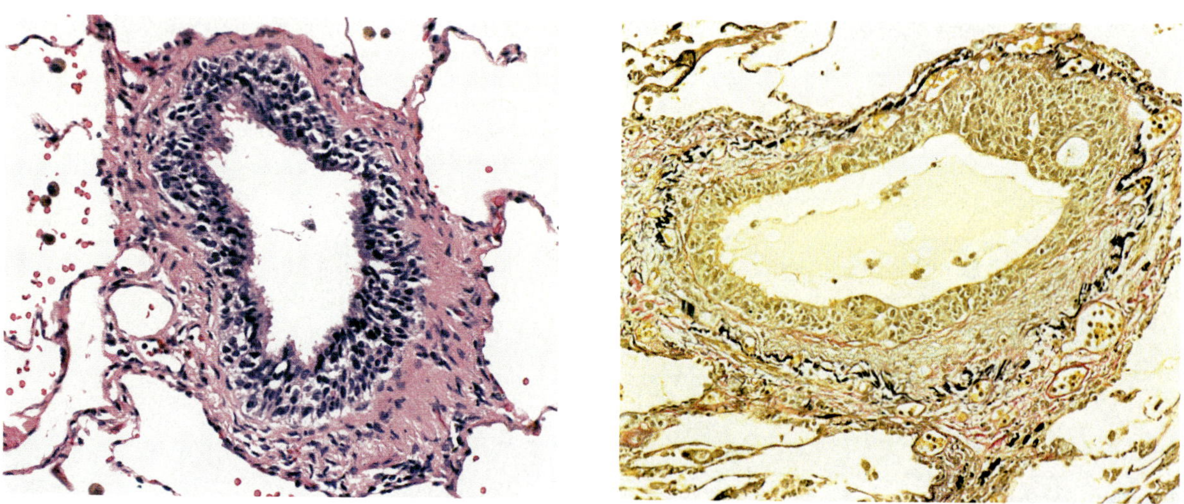

Figure 8-13

CONSTRICTIVE BRONCHIOLITIS SECONDARY TO BRONCHIOLAR NEUROENDOCRINE CELL HYPERPLASIA

Left: There is a proliferation of cells above the basal layer which elevates the bronchiolar mucosa and is associated with subtle mural thickening of the bronchiole.

Right: Elastic tissue stain confirms the presence of a layer of submucosal collagen between the bronchiolar elastica and the overlying neuroendocrine cell proliferation.

that are often quite dramatic. Only a minority of airways in a given biopsy show dramatic or complete bronchiolar luminal narrowing. When constrictive bronchiolitis is found in the setting of neuroendocrine cell hyperplasia and multiple tumorlets (fig. 8-13), the term *diffuse idiopathic neuroendocrine cell hyperplasia* is appropriate (1).

Peribronchiolar metaplasia (bronchiolarization) refers to the growth of bronchiolar epithelium into alveoli surrounding the bronchioles (fig. 8-14) (3–5). It represents a manifestation of bronchiolar injury/scarring and thus may be seen in many settings. Some cases are identified in biopsy material from individuals without any prior history of bronchiolar injury. The exclusive bronchiolocentricity of the injury is usually apparent and should allow distinction of this pattern from chronic fibrosing interstitial pneumonia (which may show this change focally). Biopsies that show these features may

Table 8-4

DIFFUSE LUNG DISEASE WITH CONSTRICTIVE BRONCHIOLITIS[a]

Healed infections (especially adenovirus)
Healed fume or toxin exposures (inhaled or ingested: e.g., *Sauropus androgynus*)
Connective tissue diseases, especially rheumatoid arthritis
Transplant-associated (bone marrow, lung, heart-lung)
Drug reactions (e.g., penicillamine, lomustine)
Inflammatory bowel disease–associated
Diffuse idiopathic pulmonary neuroendocrine cell hyperplasia
Complication of asthma
Extrinsic allergic alveolitis (rare to see histologically)
Idiopathic (idiopathic bronchiolitis obliterans/cryptogenic obliterative bronchiolitis)

[a]Data from references 4, 5, and 23.

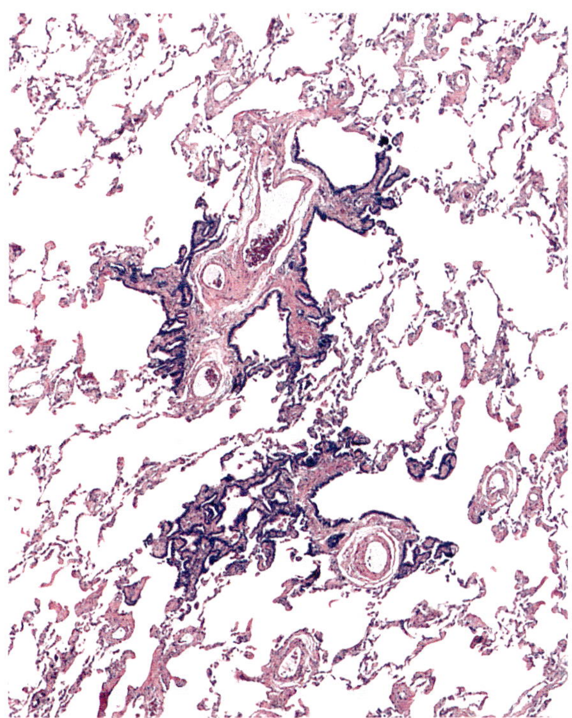

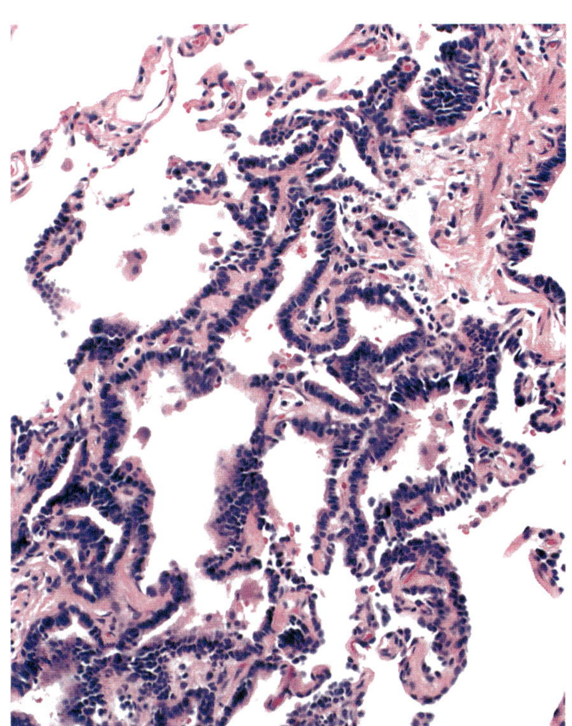

Figure 8-14

PERIBRONCHIOLAR METAPLASIA

Right: Scanning power microscopy illustrates that the pathologic abnormalities show a predilection to involve bronchioles and the immediately adjacent alveolar walls.

Left: The abnormality is seen as extension of metaplastic bronchiolar mucosa over mildly thickened and fibrotic alveolar walls.

come from patients who have clinical evidence of interstitial lung disease and radiologic infiltrates on chest radiographs, despite the histologic finding of bronchiolocentric pathology.

Bronchiolocentric nodules (as identified radiologically, grossly, and at scanning power microscopy) occur in a number of conditions (figs. 8-15–8-17). Nodules composed predominately of inflammatory cells are common in cases of cellular bronchiolitis with relatively localized involvement of the airway. Bronchiolocentric nodules can be divided into differential diagnostic groupings, as shown in Table 8-5. Individual histologic lesions of bronchioles and conditions to consider when they are encountered are shown in Table 8-6.

Table 8-5

BRONCHIOLOCENTRIC NODULES[a]

Primarily Cellular
- Acute, chronic, acute and chronic bronchiolitis (see also Table 8-7)
- Diffuse panbronchiolitis
- Follicular bronchiolitis
- Extrinsic allergic alveolitis
- Respiratory (smoker's) bronchiolitis
- Lymphoreticular neoplasms involving bronchioles

Cellular and Fibrotic
- Pulmonary Langerhans' cell histocytosis (histiocytosis X)
- Giant cell interstitial pneumonia/hard metal pneumoconiosis
- Other pneumoconiosis; dust macules centering on bronchioles/alveolar ducts
- Granulomatous conditions
  - Noninfectious: sarcoidosis, bronchocentric granulomatosis, bronchocentric Wegener's granulomatosis
  - Infectious, especially mycobacterial and fungal

Miscellaneous
- Diffuse idiopathic pulmonary neuroendocrine cell hyperplasia (multiple carcinoid tumorlets)
- Lymphangitic neoplasms involving peribronchiolar lymphatic routes

*Data from reference 5.

CLINICAL MANIFESTATIONS

The manifestations of diffuse lung disease due to bronchiolar pathology vary with the pathologic findings, and multiple clinical syndromes are recognized (23). Some of these are well-defined clinicopathologic entities and are covered in other chapters (asthma, congestive obstructive pulmonary disease [COPD], and emphysema—chapter 10; respiratory bronchiolitis and respiratory bronchiolitis associated interstitial lung disease—chapter 3; mineral dust airway injury—chapter 16). The following are general descriptions; well-characterized clinicopathologic syndromes are discussed later in this chapter.

Cellular bronchiolitis associated with an acute clinical syndrome is typical of infectious causes of bronchiolitis. Patients present with a viral syndrome, coryza, sneezing, cough, dyspnea, tachypnea, tachycardia, chest wall retraction, sibilant and sonorous rales, wheezing, and in severe cases cyanosis (23). Other cases showing cellular bronchiolitis are associated with a more chronic disease (e.g., collagen vascular disease–associated bronchiolitis).

Bronchiolitis obliterans with intraluminal polyps or the organizing pneumonia pattern (as typically seen in cryptogenic organizing pneumonia) is associated with dyspnea and cough of relatively recent onset, with crackles on auscultation (23). Fever is present in some cases. The clinical findings are further described in chapter 3 with cryptogenic organizing pneumonia. Bronchiolitis obliterans with intraluminal polyps is an extremely common finding in localized inflammatory processes of diverse etiology and as one component in a number of interstitial pneumonias (see chapter 3).

Constrictive bronchiolitis is associated with dyspnea, malaise, fatigue, nonproductive cough, and occasional wheezing. An obstructive pulmonary function defect is characteristic. The symptoms may be of relatively recent onset or slowly progressive over months or years (23).

Peribronchiolar metaplasia (peribronchiolar scarring with bronchiolar metaplasia) is primarily associated with radiologically evident infiltrative lung disease. Manifestations include cough, dyspnea, and restrictive pulmonary functions (4). In some cases these findings follow an identifiable clinical syndrome (e.g., infectious bronchiolitis, extrinsic allergic alveolitis).

RADIOLOGIC MANIFESTATIONS

Radiologically, the various forms of bronchiolitis result in one (or more) of three main patterns: centrilobular nodules, mosaic attenuation, and airspace consolidation (30).

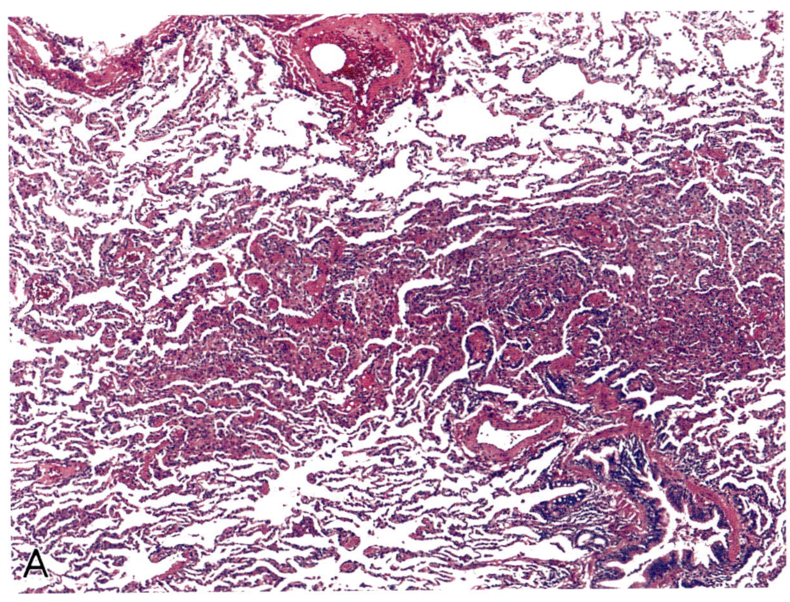

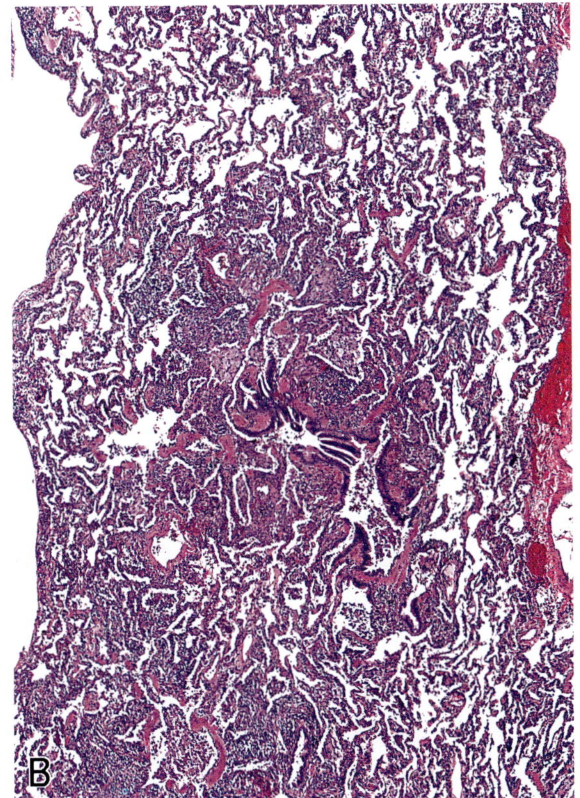

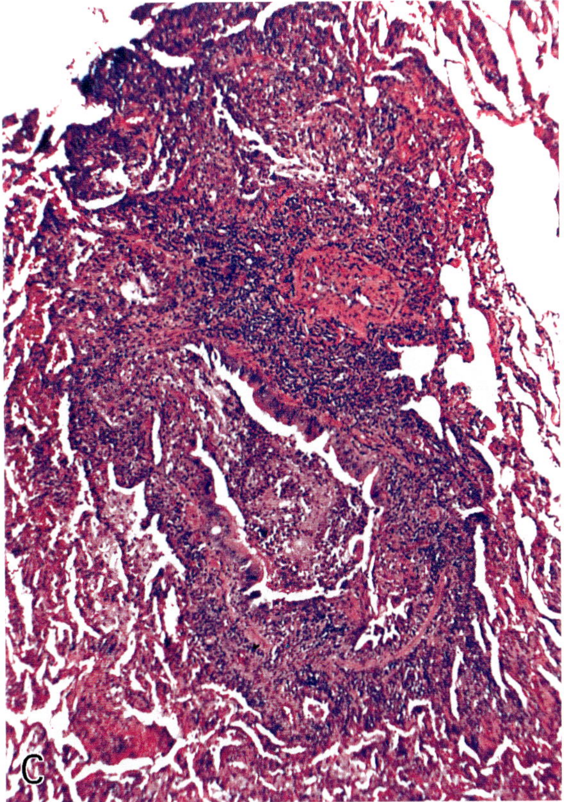

Figure 8-15

CELLULAR BRONCHIOLOCENTRIC NODULES

Cellular bronchiolocentric nodules are subtle and best appreciated at scanning microscopy as illustrated in examples of respiratory bronchiolitis–associated interstitial lung disease (A), extrinsic allergic alveolitis (B), and a T-cell lymphoma with disproportionate bronchovascular bundle involvement (C).

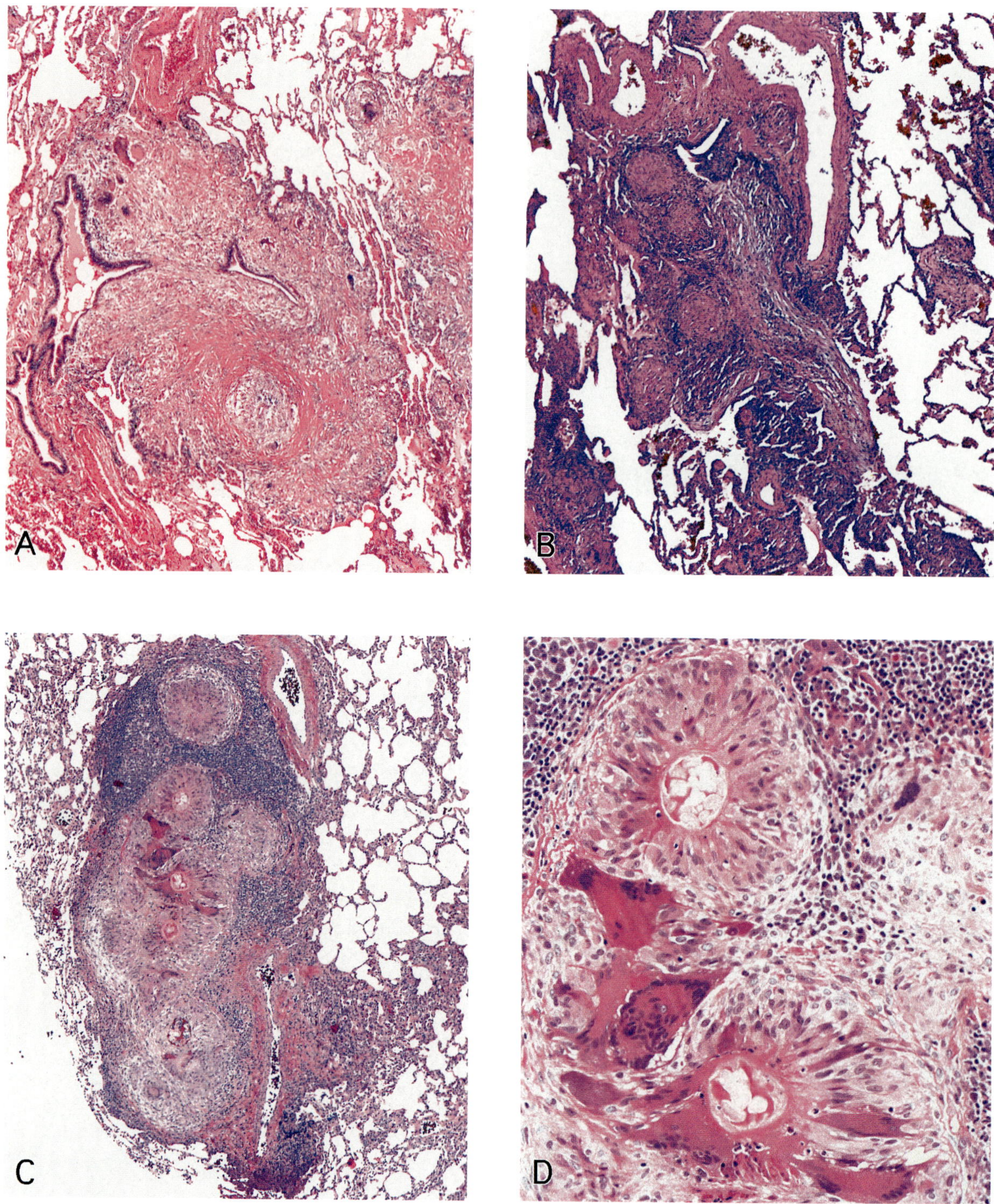

Figure 8-16

BRONCHIOLOCENTRIC NODULES WITH GRANULOMAS

A: Sarcoidosis with prominent associated scarring and some distortion of the bronchiolar lumen.

B: Mycobacterial infection with granulomas associated with relatively prominent chronic inflammation and bronchiolitis obliterans with intraluminal polypoid connective tissue.

C,D: Chronic aspiration in which the granulomas contain foreign material typical of vegetable matter (starch grains).

Table 8-6

INDIVIDUAL HISTOLOGIC LESIONS OF BRONCHIOLES AND CONDITIONS TO BE CONSIDERED WHEN THEY ARE ENCOUNTERED[a]

Acute Bronchiolitis (neutrophils usually luminal; +/- necrosis; +/- epithelial necrosis)
- Infections: bacterial and viral
- Acute fumes/toxic exposure
- Acute aspiration (look for foreign material)
- Wegener's granulomatosis
- Part of a localized reaction—acute bronchopneumonia

Acute and Chronic Bronchiolitis (usually luminal neutrophils with mural chronic inflammation; +/- necrosis or metaplastic epithelial changes; +/- changes of constrictive bronchiolitis and distal organizing pneumonia)
- Infections: bacterial, viral, mycoplasma, fungal
- Distal to bronchiectasis
- Allergic reactions (asthma, extrinsic allergic alveolitis)
- Inflammatory bowel disease–related airway disease
- Diffuse panbronchiolitis
- Collagen vascular diseases
- Aspiration—giant cells and foreign material may be present
- Transplantation-associated (bone marrow/lung)
- Wegener's granulomatosis
- Idiopathic
- Part of a localized inflammatory reaction

Chronic Bronchiolitis (usually mural chronic inflammation; +/- germinal centers; +/- changes of constrictive bronchiolitis)
- Distal to bronchiectasis
- Collagen vascular diseases
- Inflammatory bowel disease–associated airway disease
- Asthma
- Transplantation-associated
- Immunodeficiency states (associated with follicular bronchiolitis)
- Lymphoproliferative diseases
- Respiratory bronchiolitis
- Langerhans' cell histocytosis
- Diffuse panbronchiolitis
- Chronic aspiration-giant cells or foreign material may be apparent
- Idiopathic
- Part of a localized inflammatory reaction

Follicular Bronchiolitis
- Immunodeficiency states
- Congenital
- Acquired (eg., Ig deficiency, HIV infection)
- Collagen vascular diseases
  - Esp. rheumatoid arthritis, Sjögren's syndrome
- Hypersensitivity reactions
- Distal to bronchiectasis (regardless of cause)
- Middle lobe syndrome
- Diffuse panbronchiolitis
- Part of diffuse lymphoid hyperplasia/lymphocytic interstitial pneumonia (chapter 10)
- Accompanying a MALT lymphoma
- Miscellaneous
- Idiopathic

Bronchiolar Necrosis (usually mucosal necrosis; +/- submucosal/mural necrosis)
- Infections: bacterial, viral, mycobacterial, fungal
- Toxic/fume exposure
- Bronchocentric granulomatosis
- Wegener's granulomatosis

Peribronchiolar Metaplasia (bronchiolarization)
- Healed bronchiolitis (regardless of cause)
- Distal to bronchiectasis (regardless of cause)
- Middle lobe syndrome
- Associated with various causes of interstitial fibrosis
- Chronic extrinsic allergic alveolitis
- As a component of constrictive bronchiolitis
- Idiopathic (may be associated with clinical evidence of interstitial lung disease)

Alveolar Duct Fibrosis/Dust Deposition
- Dust macules
- Mineral dust exposure/mineral dust airway disease
- Cigarette smoking/respiratory bronchiolitis
- Healed Langerhans' cell histiocytosis

Luminal Mucus Stasis/Histiocytes in Bronchioles
- Chronic bronchitis/emphysema (often an incidental finding in a smoker)
- Respiratory bronchiolitis
- Asthma (Including status asthmaticus)
- Mucoid impaction/allergic bronchopulmonary aspergillosis (allergic type of mucin may be present)
- Constrictive bronchiolitis
- Distal to bronchiectasis
- As part of a local inflammatory process (e.g., middle lobe syndrome)
- Diffuse panbronchiolitis

Bronchiolar Smooth Muscle Hypertrophy
- Asthma

Component of Constrictive Bronchiolitis
- Component of bronchiolar scarring and peribronchiolar metaplasia
- Associated with chronic interstitial fibrosis/honeycombing

Bronchiolar Fibrosis (submucosal, peribronchiolar; +/- smooth muscle hypertrophy)
- Component of bronchiolar scarring and peribronchiolar metaplasia
- Distal to bronchiectasis
- Associated with chronic interstitial fibrosis/honeycombing
- Part of the localized inflammatory process (e.g., middle lobe syndrome)

(Continued on the next page)

Table 8-6 (Continued)

INDIVIDUAL HISTOLOGIC LESIONS OF BRONCHIOLES AND CONDITIONS TO BE CONSIDERED WHEN THEY ARE ENCOUNTERED[a]

Irregular Bronchiolar Shape/Bronchiolectasis
- Chronic bronchitis/emphysema
- Component of constrictive bronchiolitis
- Distal to bronchiectasis
- Diffuse panbronchiolitis
- Associated with chronic interstitial fibrosis
- Part of a localized inflammatory process (e.g., middle lobe syndrome)

Decreased Bronchiolar Size (in comparison to accompanying artery)
- Constrictive bronchiolitis
- Healed neonatal respiratory distress syndrome/ bronchopulmonary dysplasia

Bronchiolitis Obliterans with Intraluminal Polyps (organizing pneumonia)
- See Table 8-3

Granulomatous Bronchiolitis (with or without necrosis; +/-giant cells)
- Infections: fungal, mycobacteria (including atypical mycobacteria)
- Sarcoidosis
- Extrinsic allergic alveolitis
- Bronchocentric granulomatosis
- Wegener's granulomatosis
- Aspiration—foreign material may be evident
- Giant cell interstitial pneumonia/hard metal pneumoconiosis (giant cells in alveoli)

[a]Data from reference 5.

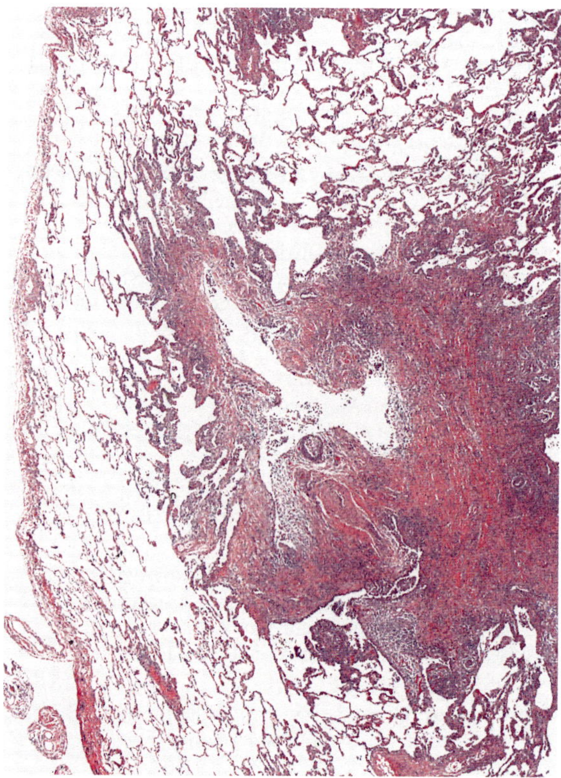

Figure 8-17

BRONCHIOLOCENTRIC NODULE IN LANGERHANS' CELL HISTIOCYTOSIS

This cellular and fibrotic nodule centers on a bronchiole which is ectatic and branches within the center of the lesion.

Centrilobular Nodules. Bronchiolocentric nodules seen histologically (Table 8-5) manifest radiologically as a pattern of centrilobular nodules (15,30). This distribution can be recognized on HRCT by the presence of a cluster of small nodular opacities a few millimeters away from the interlobular septa, pleura, and major vessels (fig. 8-18). Important in the differential diagnosis of the various bronchiolocentric nodular abnormalities is their extent and distribution. For example, the centrilobular nodules in patients who have cellular bronchiolitis due to viral, mycoplasma, or fungal infection usually have a patchy distribution; bronchiolocentric nodules in respiratory bronchiolitis involve predominantly or exclusively the upper lobes while the centrilobular nodules in extrinsic allergic alveolitis tend to involve mainly the mid- and lower lung zones.

Mosaic Attenuation. This pattern is seen in constrictive bronchiolitis and reflects the presence of airway obstruction and the patchy distribution of the abnormalities (30). Bronchiolar obstruction results in reflex vasoconstriction which causes focal areas of decreased attenuation and vascularity on HRCT; blood flow redistribution to relatively normal lung results in focal areas of increased attenuation and vascularity. This combination of findings is known as mosaic attenuation (fig. 8-19) (42). Partial airway obstruction also leads to air-trapping which is best

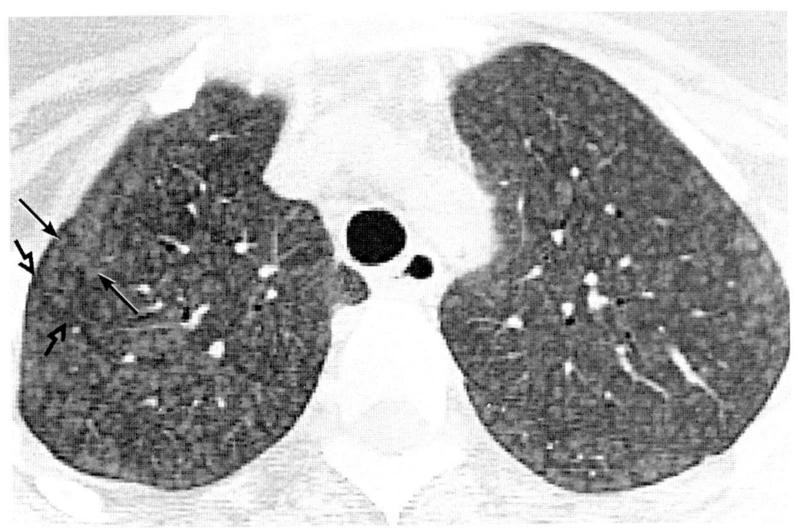

Figure 8-18

CENTRILOBULAR NODULES IN EXTRINSIC ALLERGIC ALVEOLITIS

HRCT demonstrates poorly defined nodules measuring 2 to 4 mm in diameter throughout both lungs. The nodules are distributed in clusters (straight arrows) a few millimeters away from the pleura and major vessels. This distribution is characteristic of centrilobular nodules. Sparing of the parenchyma adjacent to the interlobular septa results in linear bands of normal attenuation (open arrows). The patient was a 44-year-old woman who had subacute extrinsic allergic alveolitis (bird fancier's lung).

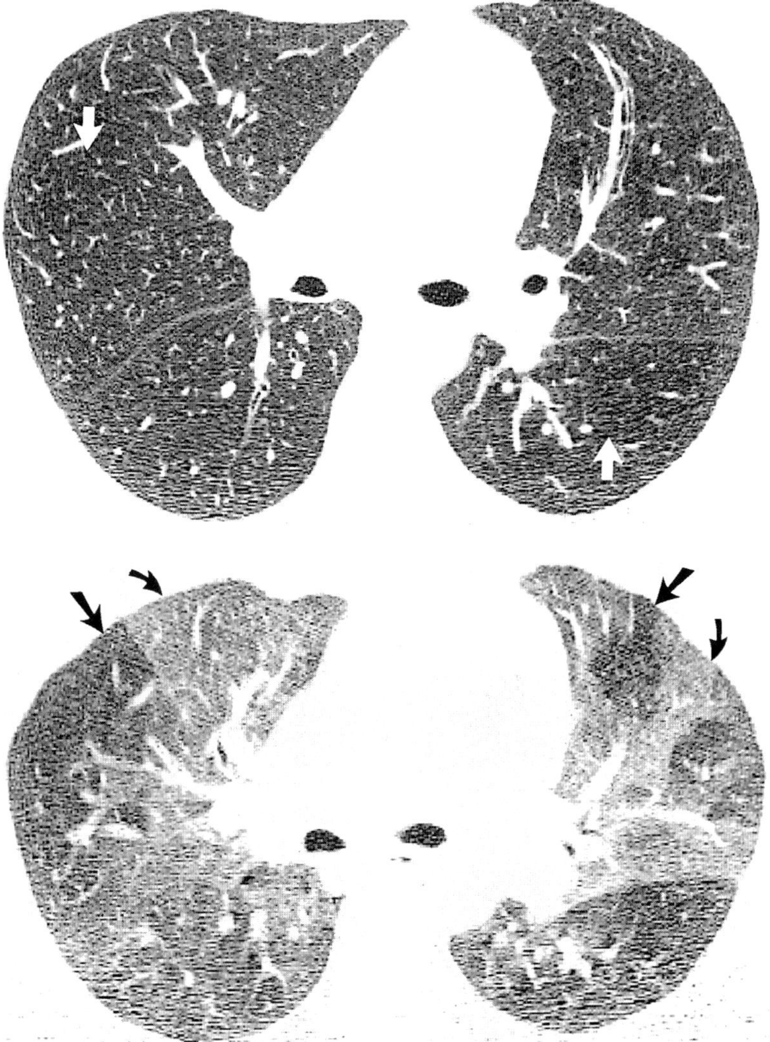

Figure 8-19

MOSAIC ATTENUATION AND AIR-TRAPPING IN CONSTRICTIVE BRONCHIOLITIS

Top: HRCT performed at end-inspiration shows localized areas of decreased attenuation and perfusion (arrows).

Bottom: HRCT performed at the end of maximal expiration accentuates the differences between normal and abnormal lung by demonstrating air-trapping (straight arrows). At the end of expiration the normal lung increases in attenuation (curved arrows) while the areas with air-trapping have decreased attenuation and perfusion (straight arrows). The patient was a 32-year-old woman with constrictive bronchiolitis 5 years following bone marrow transplant.

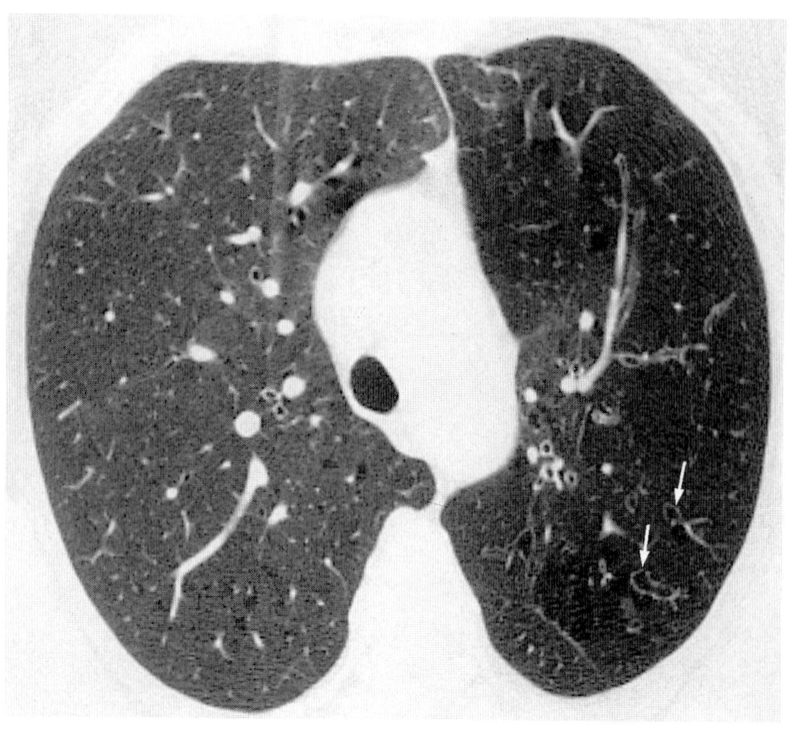

Figure 8-20

SWYER-JAMES (MACLEOD) SYNDROME

HRCT demonstrates decreased volume, attenuation, and vascularity of the left lung. There are localized areas of bronchiectasis (arrows). The findings are characteristic of constrictive bronchiolitis following childhood viral infection. The right lung is normal.

seen on expiratory HRCT scans, even when the radiograph is still normal. In patients who have severe constrictive bronchiolitis, hyperinflation may be evident on the radiograph and HRCT. A variant of postinfection constrictive bronchiolitis is the *Swyer-James (MacLeod) syndrome* which is characterized by the presence of unilateral hyperlucent lung which has decreased volume during inspiration and air-trapping during expiration (fig. 8-20). HRCT of the abnormal lung also demonstrates decreased vascularity and bronchiectasis (29).

Consolidation. Unilateral or bilateral areas of consolidation, usually patchy in distribution, are a characteristic finding of cryptogenic organizing pneumonia. In approximately 60 percent of cases, the consolidation has a predominantly peribronchial or subpleural distribution (fig. 8-21) (27,31). Less common are centrilobular nodules or a reticular pattern.

CLINICOPATHOLOGIC ENTITIES

Asthma

Asthma is primarily a disease of small bronchi, and is discussed in chapter 10. The bronchiolar changes are similar to those in the bronchi and can be grouped as follows (3–5): 1) classic changes (best seen in status asthmaticus) of smooth muscle hypertrophy, submucosal edema, and inflammatory infiltrates composed of eosinophils, submembranous thickening, mucosal sloughing, and luminal mucus stasis; 2) normal or nearly normal histology between attacks and during mild attacks (fig. 8-22); 3) morphologic counterparts of irreversible airflow obstruction that develop in asthmatics such as bronchiectasis and constrictive bronchiolitis (as a complication [fig. 8-12]); and 4) allergic bronchopulmonary fungal disease (usually due to *Aspergillus*) with mucoid impaction (in bronchi) and bronchocentric granulomatosis which may affect bronchioles (see chapter 9).

Infectious Bronchiolitis and Postinfectious Constrictive Bronchiolitis

Definition. This bronchiolar injury is caused by infectious agents, primarily viruses and mycoplasma, and includes acute changes as well as late sequelae.

Clinical Features. Clinically, severe infectious bronchiolitis is rarely seen in individuals older than age 2 years, with the exception of those who are immunosuppressed. Hospitalization or death is a rare complication. The most common pathogens are viral agents, especially respiratory

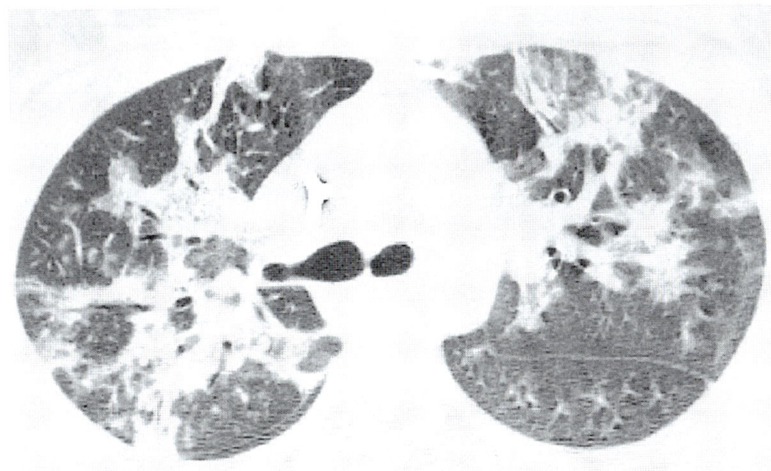

Figure 8-21

BRONCHIOLITIS OBLITERANS ORGANIZING PNEUMONIA (BOOP)

HRCT demonstrates bilateral areas of consolidation in a predominantly peribronchial distribution in a 20-year-old woman. The diagnosis was confirmed by transbronchial biopsy.

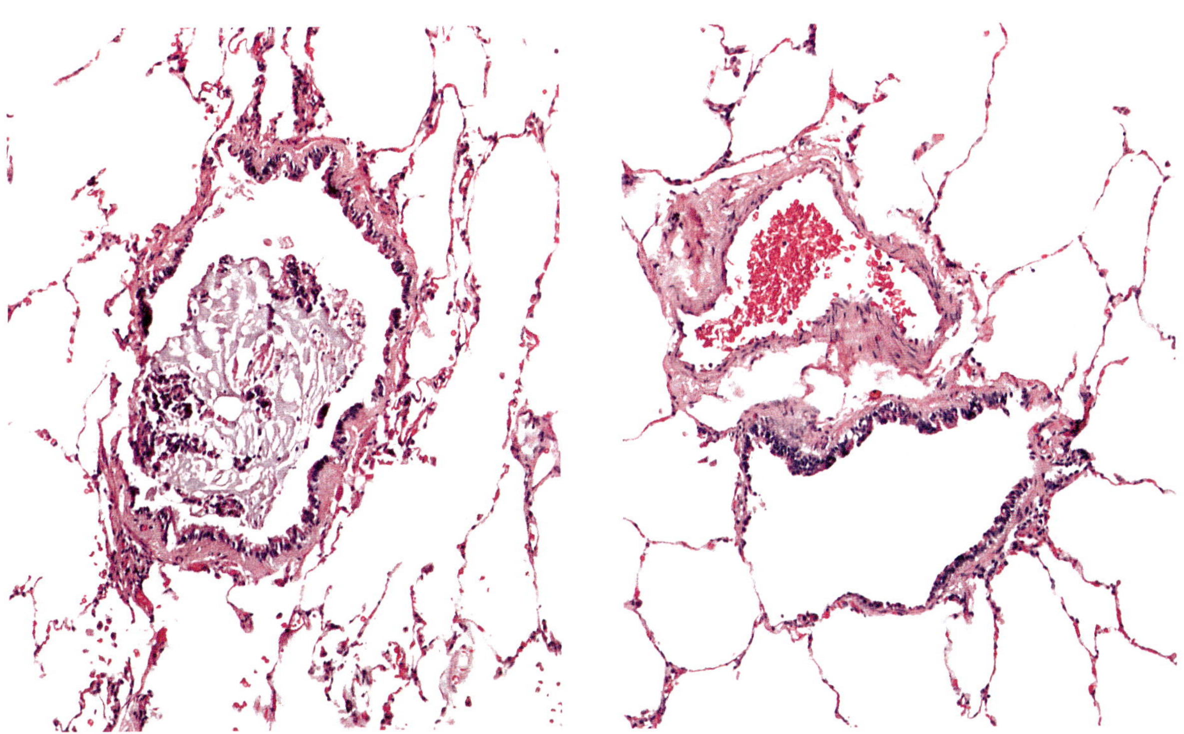

Figure 8-22

ASTHMA

Bronchiolar changes in mild asthma may be subtle (left) with some mucostasis in the lumen, or entirely inapparent (right). Both these airways are from the same patient.

syncytial virus; parainfluenza virus types 1–3; adenovirus types 3, 7, and 21; influenza virus A and B; and measles virus, as well as *Bordetella pertussis* and *Mycoplasma pneumoniae* (16,35, 41). The spectrum of pathology is included in Table 8-6. A relatively small number of agents have been implicated in postinfectious bronchiolitis obliterans with airflow obstruction (postinfectious constrictive bronchiolitis) (Table 8-7). The clinical manifestations of acute infectious bronchiolitis have been summarized under cellular bronchiolitis above. Postinfectious

Table 8-7

AGENTS CAUSING POSTINFECTIOUS CONSTRICTIVE BRONCHIOLITIS[a]

Common	Uncommon
Respiratory syncytial virus	Corona virus
Adenovirus	Rubeola virus
Mycoplasma	Mumps virus
Varicella virus	Varicella-zoster virus
Influenza A and B	Influenza
Parainfluenza II and III	Rhinovirus
Cytomegalovirus	Parvovirus B19
	Eteroviruses

[a]Data from references 7 and 23.

constrictive bronchiolitis is associated with a clinical syndrome of airflow obstruction with air-trapping (i.e., constrictive bronchiolitis). Resting hypoxemia is frequently present.

Only sporadic cases of bronchiolitis obliterans secondary to infection have been reported in the adult population (7,35). Most cases have been associated with *Mycoplasma pneumoniae* and respiratory syncytial virus (especially in the elderly), measles and varicella-zoster viruses, *Bordetella pertussis,* and other bacterial agents. The clinical presentation of postinfectious bronchiolitis obliterans in adults is ill-defined; no systematic study has been reported.

Most patients have a history of an upper respiratory tract illness that precedes the onset of dyspnea with exertion, cough, tachypnea, fever, and wheezing.

Radiologic Findings. The roentgenographic pattern of infectious bronchiolitis is quite variable. The chest X ray may be normal or show hyperinflation with increased bronchial markings. Some patients demonstrate a diffuse nodular or reticular pattern, whereas others show patchy alveolar or ground-glass opacities. The role of HRCT has not been adequately defined, but is important in ruling out other diagnoses, especially bronchiectasis.

The development of a unilateral hyperlucent lung (Swyer-James [MacLeod] syndrome) is a long-term complication of bronchiolitis in children (7,16,23). This syndrome typically follows adenovirus infection (see fig. 8-9). There is an asymptomatic latent period between the acute infection and the development of obstructive lung disease; long-term complications usually manifest as recurrent infections and eventually bronchiectasis (23). Dyspnea on exertion, hemoptysis, and chronic productive cough are seen. Patients may have localized, unilateral, or bilateral involvement. The chest radiograph usually shows a lobar or unilateral hyperlucent lung; normal or reduced volume of the involved lung is noted on full inspiration. Severe airflow obstruction becomes apparent with expiratory views. The involved lung has a diminished pulmonary vascular bed, decreased pulmonary blood flow, and reduced peripheral vascular markings.

HRCT is the procedure of choice for identifying the characteristic changes in Swyer-James syndrome (23). Lung size in this syndrome relates to the age of the patient at the time bronchiolitis occurs: early in life the lung fails to grow normally and is smaller than the opposite lung; later, in childhood, the lung may be of normal size. The Swyer-James syndrome has followed infections by a number of etiologic agents and must be distinguished from congenital absence of the pulmonary artery, pulmonary artery occlusion, partial obstruction of a lobar or main bronchus, and congenital lobar emphysema.

Treatment and Prognosis. Treatment of patients with viral and mycoplasma bronchiolitis is symptomatic, including administration of supplemental oxygen and adequate hydration (23). Few controlled clinical trials have proven the efficacy bronchodilators, antibiotics, antiviral agents, and corticosteroids in management. Recovery is usual and occurs in days or weeks. Lung transplantation has been performed in severe cases.

Fume-Related Bronchiolar Injury

Definition. This bronchiolar injury is associated with the inhalation of toxic fumes or gases, and includes acute changes and chronic sequelae.

Fume inhalation may be identified in the acute, organizing, and chronic phases (9,23). Not all fume exposures progress to a chronic phase which usually shows histologic features of constrictive bronchiolitis. The types of inhalation and fume exposure associated with bronchiolitis

Table 8-8

INHALATION- AND FUME-ASSOCIATED BRONCHIOLAR INJURY[a]

Toxic and irritant gases and fumes: nitrogen dioxide, sulfur dioxide, ammonia, chlorine, phosgene, chloropicrin, trichloroethylene, ozone, cadmium oxide, methyl sulfate, hydrogen sulfide, hydrogen fluoride
Grain dusts
Mineral dusts: talc, stearate of zinc powder, asbestos, iron oxide, aluminum oxide, silica, sheet silicates, coal, activated charcoal
Organic dusts: (e.g., extrinsic allergic alveolitis, nylon flock)
Cigarette smoke
Fire smoke
Free-base cocaine
Incinerator fly ash
Thionyl chloride (in lithium batteries)

[a]Data from references 9 and 23.

are shown in Table 8-8; the severity of the subsequent syndromes varies considerably.

Clinical Features. The classic clinical syndrome of fume exposure follows exposure to nitrogen dioxide in silo filler's disease (23). Three clinical phases may be recognized: an immediate phase right after exposure; an asymptomatic second phase which may last hours, days, or even a few weeks; and then a third phase with the re-emergence of the symptoms. Symptoms in the acute phase depend on the severity of exposure and in very mild cases, patients may be asymptomatic. Typically, there is acute upper airway irritation and visual disturbances; cough, dyspnea, fatigue, cyanosis, hypoxemia, vertigo, somnolence, headache, emotional difficulties, cyanosis, vomiting, hemoptysis, and loss of consciousness may follow. In severe cases pulmonary edema and acute respiratory distress syndrome (ARDS) develop. With very heavy exposures, there may be sudden death from reflex bronchiolar spasm, laryngospasm, and respiratory arrest with associated asphyxiation.

For patients who survive the acute event, recovery is the rule, without long-term sequelae (9,23). In a small proportion of patients (including some who were relatively asymptomatic at the time of initial exposure), a clinical illness may ensue (over a period of a few weeks) with cough, dyspnea, hypoxemia, cyanosis, and rales on auscultation. There is clinical and radiologic evidence of obstructive disease, and the pathologic findings are those of constrictive bronchiolitis (4,9). As the syndrome develops, some of the airways may show bronchiolitis obliterans with intraluminal polyps (associated with a micronodular pattern on chest radiographs), and this is one of the instances in which progression from bronchiolitis obliterans with intraluminal polyps to constrictive bronchiolitis is recognized.

Radiologic Findings. The most common abnormality on the initial chest radiograph following fume exposure is bronchial wall thickening (28). This may be followed by the development of bilateral areas of consolidation due to pulmonary edema or BOOP (14,28). The majority of cases resolve. Rarely, development of constrictive bronchiolitis may result in air-trapping or hyperinflation, evident on the chest radiograph or HRCT.

Pathologic Findings. The pathologic findings in fume exposure parallel the clinical syndromes (9). Early on there is bronchiolar mucosal necrosis and acute inflammation; concomitant pulmonary edema or diffuse alveolar damage may be present. As the process organizes, granulation tissue within the lumens of the bronchioles becomes apparent (fig. 8-23). It is likely that both of these phases heal completely; only a minority of cases progress to a syndrome of airflow obstruction with the histologic features of constrictive bronchiolitis described above (fig. 8-24).

Treatment and Prognosis. The treatment of individuals with significant exposure to toxic gases or fumes should include observation in the hospital for 24 to 48 hours (23). Weekly or biweekly outpatient evaluations should be performed for the next 8 weeks. Corticosteroid therapy is useful in the management of both the acute phase (pulmonary edema) and the late phase (bronchiolitis obliterans). Corticosteroids should be continued until the patient shows full recovery with stable lung function and improved radiographic findings (usually about 8 to 12 weeks of treatment). Relapses have been reported with early cessation of therapy.

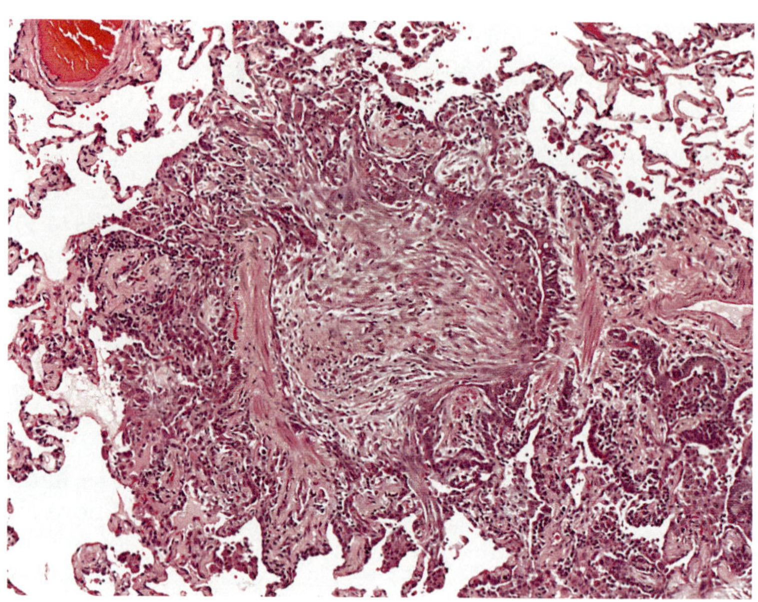

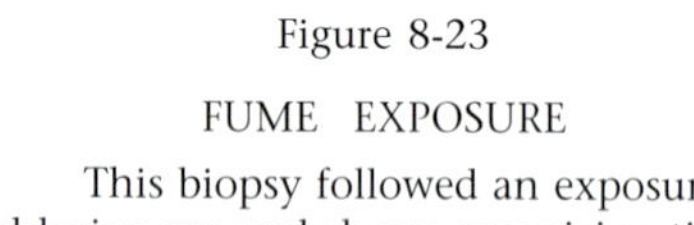

Figure 8-23

FUME EXPOSURE

This biopsy followed an exposure to chlorine gas and shows organizing tissue filling the bronchiolar lumen.

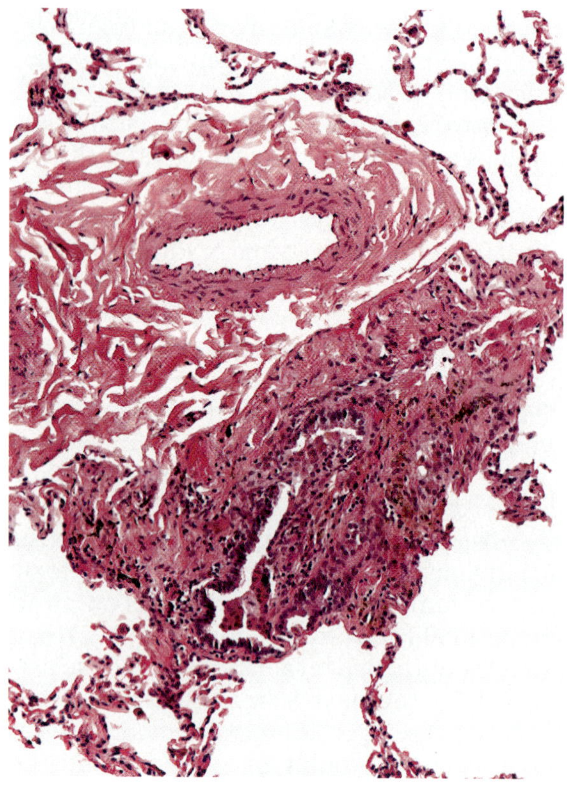

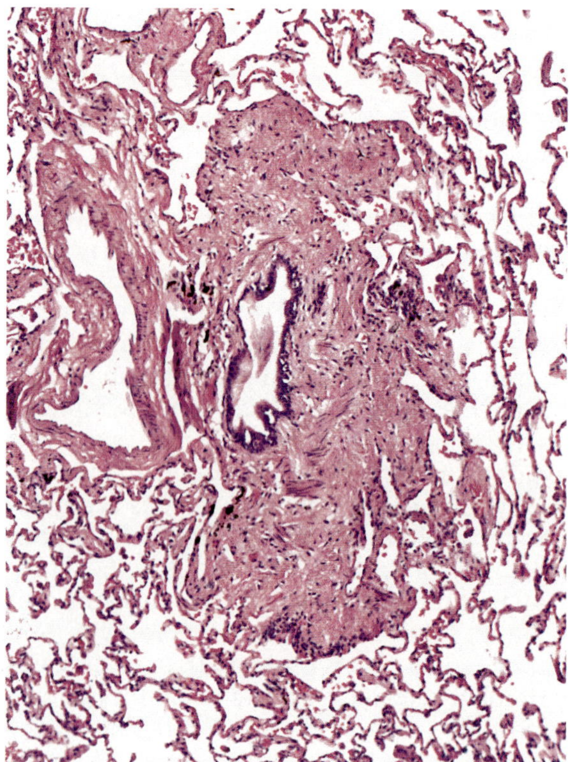

Figure 8-24

POST-FUME EXPOSURE CONSTRICTIVE BRONCHIOLITIS

Both cases are from individuals who developed airflow obstruction following exposure to ammonia gas.

Left: Constrictive bronchiolitis with mild chronic inflammation in the wall, some cellular stasis in the lumen, and some adventitial scarring.

Right: Marked fibrosis which predominantly is adventitial and distorts the bronchiolar smooth muscle.

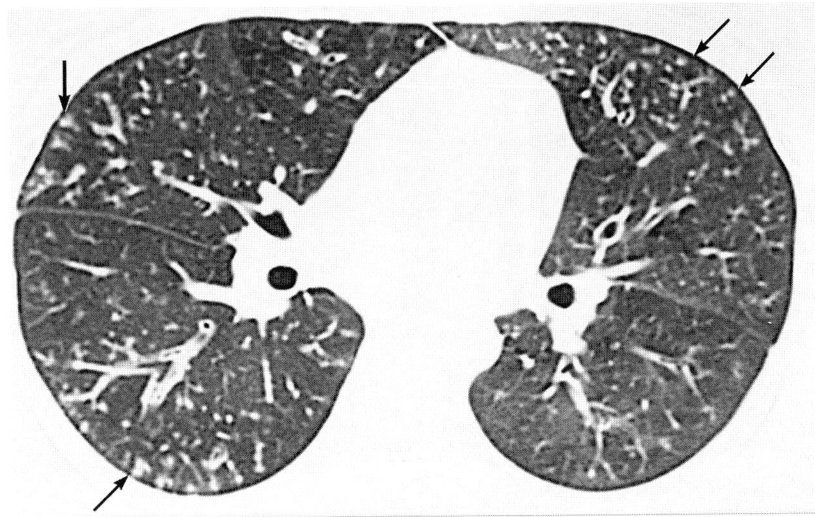

Figure 8-25

PANBRONCHIOLITIS

HRCT in a patient with panbronchiolitis demonstrates centrilobular nodules (arrows), bronchial wall thickening, and mild bronchiectasis.

Bronchodilators are occasionally helpful, but antibiotics should be used only when clinically indicated for secondary infections; they should be directed at specific identified pathogens. In general, the prognosis for survivors of toxic gas or fume inhalation (fewer than one third die acutely) is good. Lasting pulmonary disability is uncommon but may include a wide variety of functional derangements.

Diffuse Panbronchiolitis

Definition. Diffuse panbronchiolitis (DPB) is a distinctive form of chronic bronchiolitis largely restricted to individuals of Japanese heritage. It is often associated with chronic sinusitis. The clinical and radiologic findings are characteristic, as is the histopathology, which shows a prominence of interstitial foam cells.

DPB was first described in 1969 by Yamanaka et al. (44). The large series of Homma et al. (18) in 1983 followed a nationwide survey. Most individuals with DPB are of Japanese heritage (18, 20,44), and the syndrome is rare (but recognized) in non-Asian populations (13,17,19,36,37).

Clinical Features. Males are affected slightly more frequently than females (18,20, 44). The peak incidence occurs between the fourth and seventh decades of life; mean age at presentation is 50 years. Symptoms include chronic productive cough, wheezing, and dyspnea. Copious amounts of purulent sputum are produced late in the course of the disease. Eighty percent of the patients have associated chronic sinusitis. Physical examination reveals coarse crackles in more than 80 percent of the patients. Clubbing is not a typical feature.

The most characteristic laboratory abnormality is persistent, marked elevation of serum cold agglutinins (more than 64 times normal value in some patients); mycoplasma antibody titers are negative (26). Rheumatoid factor may be elevated. Immunoglobulin levels are usually normal. Bronchoalveolar lavage (BAL) studies reveal marked neutrophilia. Pulmonary function tests show obstruction. Arterial blood gases reveal hypoxemia, with or without hypercapnia. The diffusing capacity is usually not severely reduced.

Radiologic Findings. Chest radiography shows bilateral, diffuse nodular shadows in more than 70 percent of patients at first presentation, and in more than 90 percent of patients at a later stage of the disease (26). On HRCT, DPB is characterized by the presence of centrilobular nodules, bronchiolectasis, and bronchiectasis (fig. 8-25) (1a). The abnormalities are usually diffuse throughout both lungs. Other findings include areas of mosaic attenuation, air-trapping, and, in the late stages, hyperinflation.

Diagnosis. The clinical and radiologic criteria for the diagnosis of DPB developed by the Japanese Ministry of the Health and Welfare Diffuse Lung Disease Committee (MHW-DLDC) are shown in Table 8-9 (26). Some patients identified with bronchiectasis may be considered to be in later stages of DPB.

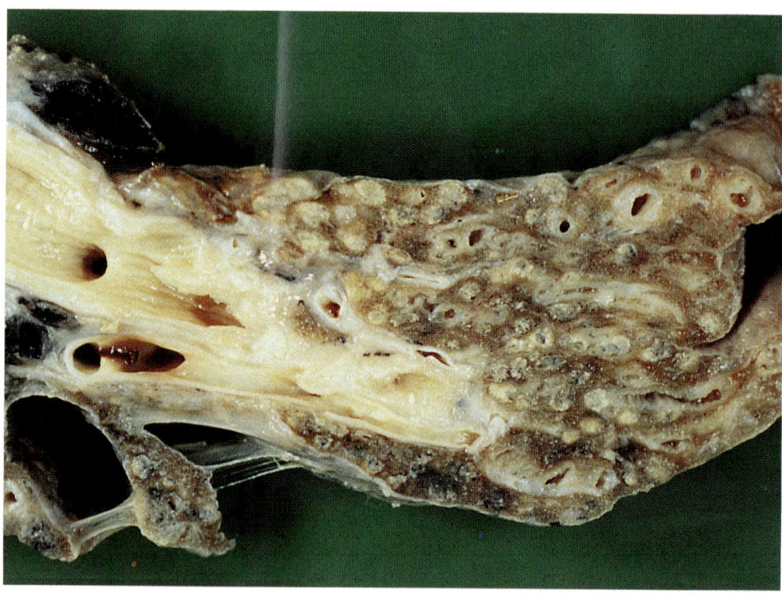

Figure 8-26

DIFFUSE PANBRONCHIOLITIS

Scattered nodules are grossly identified. On close examination these are seen to center on airways.

Table 8-9

CLINICAL AND RADIOLOGIC CRITERIA FOR DIFFUSE PANBRONCHIOLITIS[a]

Symptoms: chronic cough, sputum production, and dyspnea on exertion
Physical signs: coarse crackles, rhonchi
Chest radiographic findings: bilateral fine nodular shadows, mainly in the lower lung fields, often with hyperinflation of the lungs
Pulmonary function tests and blood gas analysis: FEV1 < 70% and PaO_2 < 80 mm Hg[b]
Elevated titers of cold hemagglutinin: X64 and more
Past history or coexistence of chronic parasinusitis
Transbronchial biopsies, if taken, show thickness of the wall of the respiratory bronchiole with infiltration of lymphocytes, plasma cells, and foamy histiocytes expanded into the peribronchiolar area

[a]Data from reference 26.

[b]FEV1 = forced expiratory volume; PaO_2 = arterial oxygen pressure.

Pathologic Findings (18–20,24,36,37,44). Grossly, the lungs of patients with DPB are hyperinflated and often show (secondary) bronchiectasis. Cut sections of the lung parenchyma show yellow nodules, 2 to 3 mm in diameter, centering on bronchioles (fig. 8-26). Bronchopneumonia may be present. Microscopically, the changes are most prominent in the bronchioles, which show marked acute and chronic bronchiolitis (fig. 8-27) and may have associated lymphoid hyperplasia (follicular bronchiolitis). The primary lesion involves the respiratory bronchiole where there is an interstitial infiltrate of lymphocytes, plasma cells, and interstitial foamy macrophages (fig. 8-28) (24). The interstitial foamy macrophages are the most distinctive feature of DPB. Membranous bronchioles also show an acute and chronic bronchiolitis and the alveoli distal to affected bronchioles frequently show foci of secondary acute, organizing, or healed pneumonia.

Bronchiolectasis and bronchiectasis may be present. The pathologic criteria for the diagnosis of DPB are shown in Table 8-10.

Differential Diagnosis. The features of DPB are compared with those of other common chronic airway diseases in Table 8-11. Histologically, interstitial foamy macrophages around respiratory bronchioles is the most distinctive feature. Among non-Japanese, such a finding may be seen in the setting of inflammatory bowel disease–related airway disease.

Pathogenesis. The pathogenesis of DPB is unknown. Most affected individuals are of Japanese ancestry and 63 percent have human leukocyte antigen (HLA)-Bw54 (38). Since HLA-Bw54 or its related haplotype is largely confined to some mongoloid races, e.g., Japanese, Chinese, and Koreans, the genetic and ethnic back-

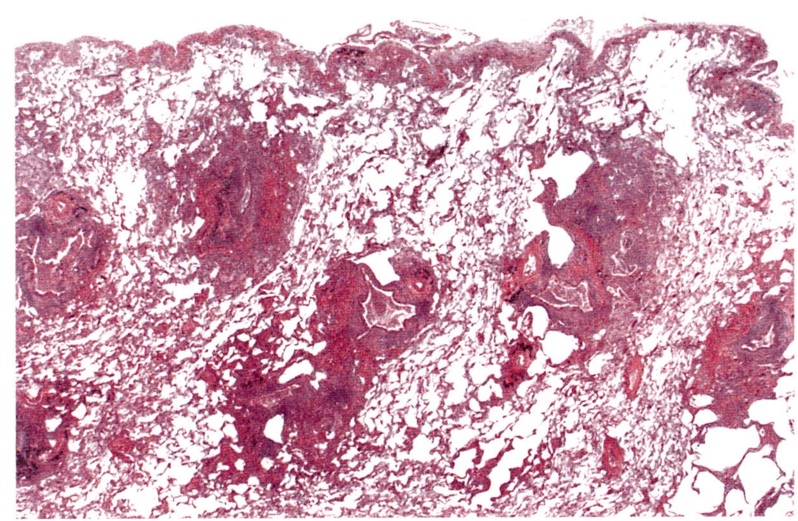

Figure 8-27

DIFFUSE PANBRONCHIOLITIS

Scanning power microscopy confirms the gross impression and the inflammatory process shows an exquisite predilection for bronchioles.

Table 8-10

PATHOLOGIC CRITERIA FOR DIFFUSE PANBRONCHIOLITIS[a]

Lesions are diffusely distributed in both lungs
Lesions are composed of respiratory bronchiolitis and peribronchiolitis
The respiratory bronchioles are narrowed or obstructed as a result of lymphoid follicles and mononuclear cell infiltration and/or intraluminal organization
No pathologic changes are detectable in the alveoli except overinflation in the distal lobular units
Accumulation of foamy macrophages in the interstitial tissue of the respiratory bronchioles, alveolar ducts, septal walls, and alveolar spaces
Chronic inflammatory changes extend to proximal bronchioles and small bronchi
Cell infiltration (acute and chronic bronchiolitis)
Secondary bronchiectasis

[a]Data from references 20 and 24.

ground observed with this unique syndrome may be explained (21,34). HLA-Bw54 may also be a useful marker in the differential diagnosis of DPB since the frequency of this antigen in the general population is low (11.8 percent) (38).

Treatment and Prognosis. The clinical course of patients with DPB is a slow progression, and once the diagnosis is made the 5-year survival rate is in the range of 50 percent (20). Individuals tend to be colonized by a variety of organisms, including *Pseudomonas aeruginosa*. Once *Pseudomonas* infection develops, the mean survival time is less than 3 years (20). Recently, low-dose erythromycin has been shown to considerably improve survival and decrease symptomatology (20,26). Lung transplantation is also an option (2).

Idiopathic Bronchiolitis (Including Cryptogenic Obliterative Bronchiolitis)

Definition. This is a type of bronchiolar injury for which no specific etiology or association can be implicated. The histologic spectrum is comprised of acute or chronic cellular infiltrates to bronchiolar scarring, including constrictive bronchiolitis (4,8,10,22,25,39,40). Cases of idiopathic bronchiolitis have included a variety of different terms: *(idiopathic) bronchiolitis obliterans, cryptogenic obliterative bronchiolitis, bronchiolitis in adults,* and *cryptogenic constrictive bronchiolitis* (4,22,23,25,40).

Idiopathic bronchiolitis is a rare clinicopathologic syndrome seen in adults. It is often confused with asthma, chronic bronchitis, cystic fibrosis, bronchiectasis, or alpha-1-antitrypsin

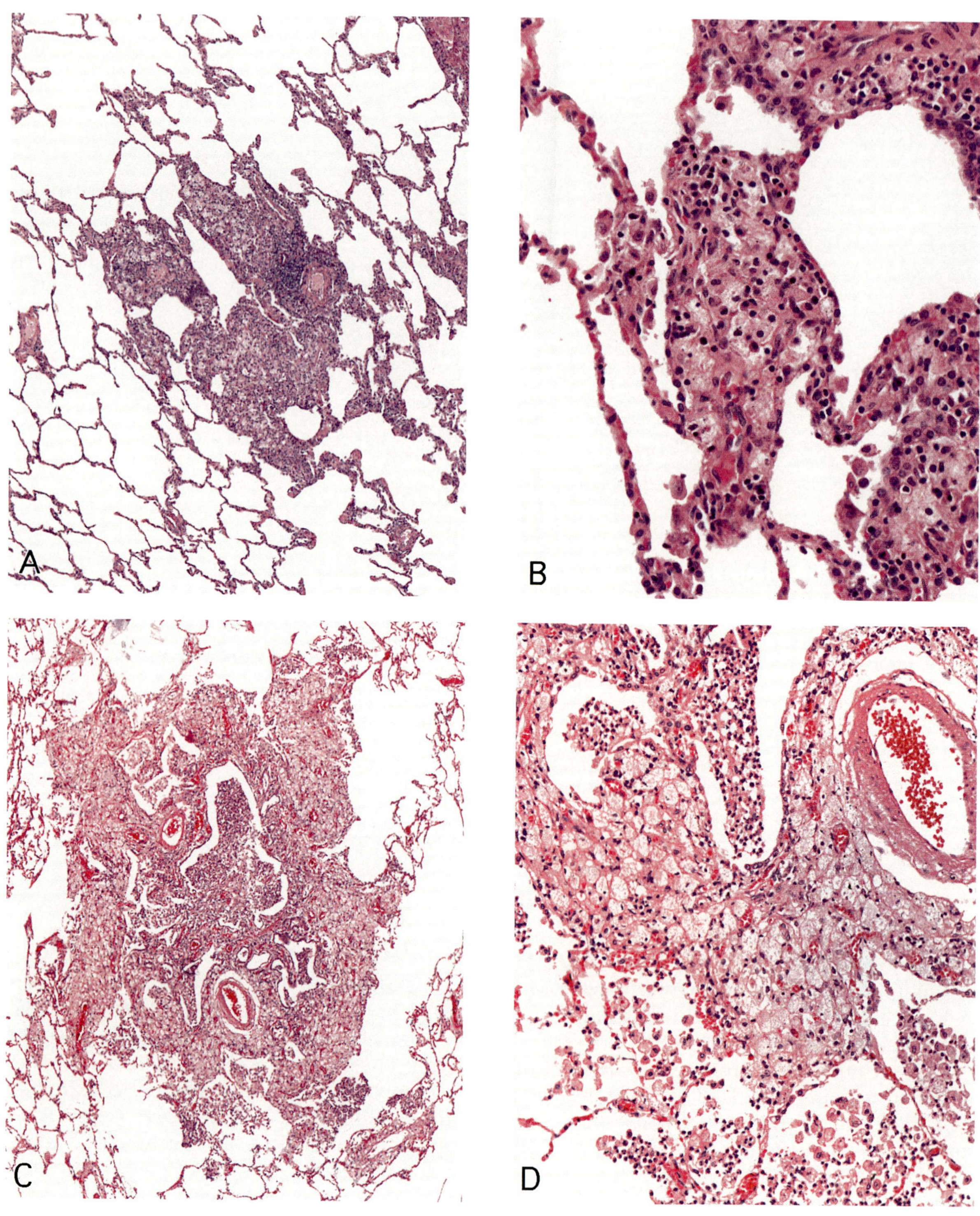

Figure 8-28

DIFFUSE PANBRONCHIOLITIS

The primary lesion is thought to be an inflammatory process of the respiratory bronchiole (A,C) with marked associated interstitial foam cell accumulation (B,D). A and B are from a Caucasian and C and D are from a Japanese individual. Both show acute inflammation in the lumen of the respiratory bronchi with chronic inflammation in the wall, including numerous interstitial foam cells.

Table 8-11

CLINICAL FEATURES OF DIFFUSE PANBRONCHIOLITIS AND OTHER COMMON AIRWAY DISEASES[a]

	Diffuse Panbronchiolitis	Bronchiectasis	Chronic Bronchitis and Emphysema	Idiopathic Constrictive Bronchiolitis	Cystic Fibrosis
Age	>20	All ages	>40	>40	All ages (young)
Sex	M=F[b]	M=F	M>F	M<F	M=F
Symptoms	Cough, sputum, dyspnea	Cough, sputum, hemoptysis	Dyspnea, cough, sputum	Cough, sputum, dyspnea	Cough, sputum, hemoptysis, dyspnea
Respiratory Dysfunction	Mixed (obst>rest) DLCO → RV ↑	Mixed	Obstructive, DLCO? RV ↑	Obstructive	Mixed (obst>rest)
Chest X Ray	Micronodular overinflation (early), ectatic change (late)	Bronchiectasis, tram-tracks	Overinflation or prominent broncho-vascular markings	Overinflation	Diffuse bronchial ectasia
Other	Chronic sinusitis (>90%), cold hemagglutinin ↑, *Pseudomonas* infection	Chronic sinusitis (50%)	Smokers		*Pseudomonas* infection

[a]Data from reference 20.

[b]M = male; F = female; obst = obstructive; rest = restrictive; DLCO = diffusing capacity for carbon monoxide; RV = residual volume.

deficiency. The constellation of findings in reported cases is unique and suggests that idiopathic bronchiolitis in adults represents a distinct, definable clinicopathologic entity but one that remains a diagnostic challenge to clinicians and pathologists.

These cases have generally been defined clinically (yet they show a variety of histologic changes [see below]). They come to attention in a variety of ways, predominantly with airflow obstruction without identifiable causes of the obstruction and without large airway disease (22,23,25,40). The patients tend to be adults (more often females) who have no history of smoking, collagen vascular disease, or other cause of airflow obstruction. Diagnosis may be based on clinical criteria (see below), lavage data, and histologic study.

In studying the pathologic features of idiopathic bronchiolitis, two overlapping histopathologic groups emerge: those that are associated primarily with a cellular reaction involving the bronchioles (cellular bronchiolitis) and those in which the most prominent feature is constrictive bronchiolitis. There is some histologic overlap (for example, constrictive bronchiolitis frequently includes a component of acute or chronic cellular bronchiolitis), as well as clinical and radiologic overlap, and the two broad categories discussed below are intended as conceptual guidelines. The categories of idiopathic cellular bronchiolitis and idiopathic constrictive bronchiolitis are defined on the basis of the histologic findings, although there is a considerable proportion of cases that are diagnosed on the basis of clinical/radiologic functional features (40), and in such cases the histologic findings remain suspected rather than proven.

Idiopathic Cellular Bronchiolitis (see fig. 8-5B). The most prominent histologic finding is inflammatory cell infiltrates involving the airways. The inflammation may be purulent with acute inflammatory cells and debris in the bronchiolar lumen. However, the inflammation in the bronchiolar wall is primarily chronic and there may be follicular hyperplasia (follicular bronchiolitis). Some cases are defined on the basis of clinical data and BAL analysis: patients with obstructive disease of unknown cause with primarily acute inflammatory cells in the BAL material.

Most patients present with symptoms of dyspnea or cough of long duration (mean, 4.7

years) (22). Chronic sputum production, recurrent respiratory infections, or wheezing are uncommon. Lung function tests show an obstructive pattern in most patients, with a few having a mixed obstructive-restrictive pattern (22). A bronchodilator response is uncommon. BAL studies demonstrate a marked increase in neutrophils associated with an increase in the specific neutrophil products, collagenase and myeloperoxidase (22). The majority of patients have a neutrophil level of more than 25 percent (normal for nonsmokers: less than 4 percent); some have levels exceeding 90 percent (22).

Over time, the persistence of idiopathic cellular bronchiolitis can be traced to chronic/recurrent infection, and antibiotic therapy, analogous to that for bronchiectasis and DPB, may be appropriate. Some patients respond to glucocorticoids and/or immunosuppressive therapy (at least for a period of time), presumably because of the lympholytic effect of these forms of therapy (22). Full return of lung function is unusual.

Idiopathic Constrictive Bronchiolitis (see fig. 8-3B,C). The histologic changes are primarily those of constrictive bronchiolitis with relatively little inflammation. Submucosal scarring with luminal narrowing is associated with adventitial scarring, distorted bronchiolar lumens, bronchiolectasis, mucostasis, and foci of complete luminal loss. Most patients are middle-aged women who have a nonproductive cough, shortness of breath, or other nonspecific chest complaints, usually of relatively short duration (6 to 24 months) (23). Most are identified because of an accelerated severe obstructive respiratory disorder. A history of cigarette smoking, chronic sputum production, frequent chest infections, wheezing, known connective tissue disorder, or immunoglobulin deficiency is absent. No association with inhalation injury or viral infection has been identified. Physical findings are often unremarkable, although wheezing or crackles may be heard.

The radiologic manifestations of idiopathic constrictive bronchiolitis consist of hyperinflation and vascular attenuation (39). HRCT shows a mosaic pattern of attenuation with areas of decreased attenuation and vascularity (39). Scans performed at end-expiration demonstrate air-trapping.

The clinical course varies and may be rapid and progressive or slow. Some patients have long periods of stable functional deficits. Anecdotally, steroids may prove helpful.

REFERENCES

1. Aguayo SM, Miller YE, Waldron JA, et al. Brief report: idiopathic diffuse hyperplasia of pulmonary neuroendocrine cells and airways disease. N Engl J Med 1992;327:1285–8.

1a. Akira M, Kitatani F, Lee YS, et al. Diffuse panbronchiolitis: evaluation with high-resolution CT. Radiology 1988;168:433–8.

2. Baz MA, Kussin PS, VanTrigt P, Davis RD, Roggli VL, Tapson VF. Recurrence of diffuse panbronchiolitis after lung transplantation. Am J Resp Crit Care Med 1995;151:895–8.

3. Colby TV. Bronchiolar pathology. In: Epler GR, ed. Diseases of the bronchials. New York: Raven Press; 1994:77–100.

4. Colby TV. Bronchiolitis, pathologic considerations. M J Clin Pathol 1998;109:101–9.

5. Colby TV, Leslie KO. Small airway lesions. In: Cagle PT, ed. Diagnostic pulmonary pathology. New York: Marcel Dekker; 2000:231-49.

6. Colby TV, Myers JL. Clinical and histologic spectrum of bronchiolitis obliterans including bronchiolitis obliterans organizing pneumonia. Semin Respir Med 1992;13:113–9.

7. Coultas DB, Funk LM. Post infectious bronchiolitis obliterans. In: Epler GR, ed. Diseases of the bronchioles. New York: Raven Press; 1994:215–30.

8. Dorinsky PM, Davis WB, Lucas JH, Weiland JE, Gadek JE. Adult bronchiolitis. Evaluation of bronchoalveolar lavage and response to prednisone therapy. Chest 1985;88:58–63.

9. Douglas WW, Colby TV. Fume-related bronchiolitis obliterans. In: Epler GR, ed. Diseases of the bronchioles. New York: Raven Press; 1994: 187–214.
10. Edwards C, Cayton R, Bryan R. Chronic transmural bronchiolitis: non-specific lesion of small airways. J Clin Pathol 1992;45:993–8.
11. Epler GR, ed. Disease of the bronchioles. New York: Raven Press; 1994.
12. Epler GR, Colby TV, McCloud TC, Carrington CB, Gaensler EA. Bronchiolitis obliterans organizing pneumonia N Engl J Med 1985;312:152–8.
13. Fitzgerald JE, King TE Jr, Lynch DA, Tuder RM, Schwarz MI. Diffuse panbronchiolitis in the United States. Am J Respir Crit Care Med 1996;154:497–503.
14. Gosink BB, Friedman PJ, Liebow AA. Bronchiolitis obliterans: roentgenologic-pathologic correlation. AJR Am J Roentgenol 1973;117:816–32.
15. Gruden JF, Webb WR, Warnock M. Centrilobular opacities in the lung on high-resolution CT: diagnostic considerations and pathologic correlation. AJR Am J Roentgenol 1994;162:569–74.
16. Hardy KA. Childhood bronchiolitis obliterans. In: Epler GR, ed. Disease of the bronchioles. New York: Raven Press; 1994:415–26.
17. Homer R, Khoo L, Smith G. Diffuse panbronchiolitis in a Hispanic man with travel history to Japan. Chest 1995;107:1176–8.
18. Homma H, Yamanaka A, Tanimoto S, et al. Diffuse panbronchiolitis: a disease of the transitional zone of the lung. Chest 1983;83:63–9.
19. Iwata M, Colby TV, Kitaichi M. Diffuse panbronchiolitis: diagnosis and distinction from various pulmonary diseases with centrilobular intestinal foam cell accumulations. Hum Pathol 1994;25:357–63.
20. Iwata M, Sato A, Colby TV. Diffuse panbronchiolitis. In: Epler GR, ed. Diseases of the bronchioles. New York: Raven Press; 1994:153–80.
21. Keicho N, Ohashi J, Tamiya G, et al. Fine localization of a major disease-susceptibility locus for diffuse panbronchiolitis. Am J Hum Gen 2000;66:501–7.
22. Kindt GC, Weiland JE, Davis WB, Gadek JE, Dorinsky PM. Bronchiolitis in adults. A reversible cause of airway obstruction associated with airway neutrophils and neutrophil products. Am Rev Respir Dis 1989;140:483–92.
23. King TE Jr. Bronchiolitis. In: Schwartz MI, King TE Jr, eds. Interstitial lung disease, 3rd ed. London: BC Decker; 1998:645–84.
24. Kitaichi M, Nishimura K, Izumi T. Diffuse panbronchiolitis: In: Sharma OP, ed. Lung disease in the tropics. New York: Marcel Dekker; 1991: 479–509.
25. Kraft M, Mortenson RL, Colby TV, Newman L, Waldron JA Jr, King TE Jr. Cryptogenic constrictive bronchiolitis: a clinicopathologic study. Am Rev Respir Dis 1993;148:1093–101.
26. Kudoh S, Azuma A, Yamamoto M. Izumi T, Ando M. Improvement of survival in patients with diffuse panbronchiolitis treated with low-dose erythromycin. Am J Respir Crit Care Med 1998;157:1829–32.
27. Lee KS, Kullnig P, Hartman TE, Müller NL. Cryptogenic organizing pneumonia: CT findings in 43 patients. AJR Am J Roentgenol 1994;162: 543–6.
28. Lee MJ, O'Connell DJ. The plain chest radiograph after acute smoke inhalation. Clin Radiol 1988;39:33–7.
29. Marti-Bonmati L, Perales FR, Catala F, Mata JM, Calonge E. CT findings in Swyer-James syndrome. Radiology 1989;172:477–80.
30. Müller NL, Miller RR. Diseases of the bronchioles: CT and histopathologic findings. Radiology 1995;196:3–12.
31. Müller NL, Staples CA, Miller RR. Bronchiolitis obliterans organizing pneumonia: CT features in 14 patients. AJR Am J Roentgenol 1990;154:983–7.
32. Myers J, Veal C Jr, Shin M, Katzenstein AL. Respiratory bronchiolitis causing interstitial lung disease: a clinicopathologic study of six cases. Am Rev Respir Dis 1987;135:880–4.
33. Niewoehner D, Kleinerman J, Rice D. Pathologic changes in peripheral airways of young cigarette smokers. N Engl J Med 1974;291:755–8.
34. Park MH, Kim YW, Yoon HI, et al. Association of HLA class I antigens with diffuse panbronchilitis in Korean patients. Am J Respir Crit Care Med 1999;159:526–9.
35. Penn CC, Liu C. Bronchiolitis following infection in adults and children. Clin Chest Med 1993;14:645–54.
36. Poletti V, Patelli M, Poletti G, Bertanti T, Spiga L. Diffuse panbronchiolitis observed in an Italian [Letter]. Chest 1990;98(2):515–6.
37. Randhawa P, Hoagland MH, Yousem SA. Diffuse panbronchiolitis in North America. Report of three cases and review of the literature. Am J Surg Pathol 1991;15(1):43–7.
38. Sugiyama Y, Kudoh S, Maeda H, Suzaki H, Takaku F. Analysis of HLA antigens in patients with diffuse panbronchilitis. Am Rev Respir Dis 1990;141:1459–62.
39. Sweatman MC, Millar AB, Strickland B, Turner-Warwick M. Computed tomography in adult obliterative bronchiolitis. Clin Radiol 1990;41:116–9.
39a. Travis WD, King TE, Bateman ED, et al. ATS/ERS international multidisciplinary consensus classification of idiopathic interstitial pneumonia. Am J Respir Crit Care Med 2002;165:277–304.

40. Turton CW, Williams G, Green M. Cryptogenic obliterative bronchiolitis in adults. Thorax 1981;36:805–10.
41. Wohl ME. Bronchiolitis in children. In: Epler GR, ed. Diseases of the bronchioles. New York: Raven Press; 1994:397–407.
42. Worthy SA, Müller NL, Hartman TE, Swensen SJ, Padley SP, Hansell DM. Mosaic attenuation pattern on thin-section CT scans of the lung: differentiation among infiltrative lung, airway, and vascular diseases as a cause. Radiology 1997;205:465–70.
43. Wright JL, Cagle P, Churg A, Colby TV, Myers JL. Diseases of the small airways. Am Rev Respir Dis 1992;146:240–62.
44. Yamanaka A, Saiki S, Tamura S, Saito K. Problems in chronic obstructive bronchial disease, with special reference to diffuse panbronchiolitis. Naika 1969;23:442–51.
45. Yousem SA, Colby TV, Carrington CB. Follicular bronchitis/bronchiolitis. Hum Pathol 1985;16:700–6.
46. Yousem SA, Colby TV, Gaensler EA. Respiratory bronchiolitis-associated interstitial lung disease and its relationship to desquamative interstitial pneumonia. Mayo Clin Proc 1989;64:1373–80.

9
BRONCHIAL DISORDERS

INTRODUCTION

There are many non-neoplastic disorders that affect the bronchi and there is considerable overlap among them (Table 9-1). Many of the conditions in Table 9-1 are discussed elsewhere: asthma and chronic bronchitis in chapter 10, infections in chapter 12, and collagen vascular diseases in chapter 6. Some of these entities are recognized clinically (e.g., asthma and chronic bronchitis), some radiologically (e.g., bronchiectasis), some pathologically (e.g., bronchocentric granulomatosis), and some are defined on the basis of combinations of these features.

The introduction of high-resolution computed tomography (HRCT) scanning has dramatically improved the radiologic evaluation of the bronchi. In fact, bronchiectasis is being redefined radiologically and the traditional pathologic definitions are becoming obsolete as fewer and fewer cases of bronchiectasis come to morphologic assessment (either at resection or at autopsy). Complications of, and adverse reactions to, bronchography and the fact that HRCT scanning can add as much information as bronchography has led to the latter being discontinued in current clinical practice.

The proximal bronchi are accessible to the fiberoptic bronchoscope; cytologic and histologic specimens are readily retrieved and represent the primary source of pathologic material from the large bronchi. The bronchi are not well sampled in peripheral wedge biopsies retrieved by either traditional open lung biopsy or video-assisted thoracic surgical biopsy; bronchi larger than 2 to 3 mm in diameter are rarely sampled.

In routine surgical pathology practice, bronchi are rarely examined beyond evaluation of the bronchial margin in resections for lung neoplasms. More extensive gross and histologic examination is indicated when bronchial pathology is known or suspected. Formalin inflation of resected specimens, specimen radiographs, and specimen bronchography may help define disease states in individual cases and assist in the selection of tissue for histologic evaluation. Dissection of the bronchial tree and serial blocking are also useful.

Table 9-1

NON-NEOPLASTIC DISORDERS OF THE BRONCHI

Asthma
Bronchitis
Infectious
Irritant (e.g., cigarettes, dust, aspiration)
Collagen vascular diseases (especially Sjögren's syndrome)
Miscellaneous (e.g., inflammatory bowel disease-related bronchitis, Wegener's granulomatosis)
Bronchiectasis (see Table 9-3)
Bronchocentric granulomatosis
Mucoid impaction of bronchi
Allergic bronchopulmonary fungal disease
Plastic bronchitis
Tracheobronchomegaly
Congenital bronchial cartilage deficiency
Relapsing polychondritis
Broncholithiasis, bronchostenosis
Miscellaneous (e.g., tracheobronchial amyloid, tracheopathia osteochondroplastica)

Only rarely is there isolated pathology of the bronchi. Evidence of bronchial injury is common in pulmonary disorders that affect the bronchioles as well as those affecting the alveoli. For example, bronchiectasis can be a secondary change in cases of chronic bronchiolitis (e.g., in transplantation-associated bronchiolitis obliterans syndrome or diffuse panbronchiolitis). Scarring of the parenchyma as occurs in pulmonary fibrosis also affects bronchi and results in secondary "traction bronchiectasis." Conversely, diseases that primarily involve the bronchi are often associated with secondary changes in the bronchioles and alveoli.

INFECTIOUS BRONCHITIS

Many infectious agents, especially those that reach the lung by inhalation, cause bronchitis. The changes vary from mild chronic inflammation in the submucosa in normal hosts to fulminant necrotizing bronchitis seen in immunosuppressed individuals. The pathologic changes found in cases of infectious bronchitis are shown in Table 9-2. Pulmonary infections are discussed in chapter 12.

Table 9-2

PATHOLOGIC CHANGES IN INFECTIOUS BRONCHITIS

Lumen
- Mucus, exudate, inflammatory/necrotic debris

Mucosal changes
- Necrosis and sloughing
- Inflammation
- Reparative/metaplastic mucosa

Submucosal (and deeper) changes
- Inflammation
- Necrosis (esp. severe infections in the immunosuppressed)

Inflammatory cell reaction[a]
- Acute (neutrophils)
- Acute and chronic (neutrophils, lymphocytes, plasma cells)
- Chronic (including lymphoid follicles/follicular bronchitis)
- Granulomatous (with or without necrosis)
- Mixtures

Organisms or inclusions (rarely seen except in immunosuppressed individuals); sought at the edge of necrosis and in the luminal exudate

Fibrosis; architectural derangement
- Submucosal fibrosis
- Bronchostenosis/bronchitis obliterans
- Bronchiectasis

[a]Severely immunosuppressed individuals may have little inflammatory reaction and show only hemorrhage, edema, and tissue necrosis.

BRONCHIECTASIS

Background. Other than chronic bronchitis in chronic obstructive pulmonary disease (COPD; chapter 10), the best known benign disease of the bronchi, bronchiectasis, was relatively common and extensively studied in the middle of the 20th century (54,117,134). Antibiotic therapy and prophylaxis for childhood infections have led to a marked decline in the number of cases of bronchiectasis seen clinically. At Massachusetts General Hospital in Boston, the number of patients with bronchiectasis per 10,000 admissions declined from 45 in 1947 to 9 in 1984 (114). Bronchiectasis remains a significant problem in developing countries (53). Some ethnic groups are notable for an increased incidence of bronchiectasis: Native Americans and Eskimos, New Zealand Maori, and Western Samoans (53).

Definition and Classification. Bronchiectasis is defined as permanent abnormal dilatation of the bronchi, usually associated with inflammation (3,26,51,53,54,65,72,114,117,134, 140). Bronchial dilatation in bronchiectasis varies from subtle enlargement that only can be appreciated by comparing the bronchus to its accompanying pulmonary artery (which should be approximately the same size) to massive dilatation with grossly dilated airways extending to a few millimeters from the pleural surface (117,134).

The spectrum of causes of bronchiectasis is broad and includes many entities (Table 9-3); some are associated with localized bronchiectasis (which may be amenable to surgical resection) and some with widespread bronchiectasis. Well-recognized clinicopathologic categories of bronchiectasis (e.g., primary ciliary dyskinesia, cystic fibrosis, and others) are discussed separately. Most historical classification schemes for bronchiectasis were based on observations of radiologic features (primarily bronchography), pathologic findings in resected lobes or lungs obtained at autopsy, or presumed etiology/pathogenesis (Table 9-4).

After a review of the topic, Thurlbeck favored Reid's classification as both simple and applicable (117), but since it is in part based on bronchography, which is now obsolete, the relevance of this classification is being reassessed. The classification is divided into: 1) *saccular (cystic) type* in which the first three or four divisions of segmental bronchi show progressive dilatation toward the periphery of the lung. Typically there is marked luminal narrowing of more distal airways; 2) *varicose type* in which the dilated bronchi show variable combinations of ectasia and constriction with no regular pattern and distal ends are bulbous; and 3) *cylindrical,* in which the ectatic bronchi appear as cylinders and do not taper as do normal bronchi.

There has been a shift in clinical practice from traditional definitions based on bronchography and pathology (gross and/or histologic) to a definition based on HRCT scanning (51,65, 72,140). The HRCT scan has become the gold standard, and the diagnostic procedure of choice for the noninvasive diagnosis of bronchiectasis

Table 9-3

CAUSES AND ASSOCIATIONS OF BRONCHIECTASIS[a]

Conditions Predominantly Affecting the Lung
- Postinfectious bronchial damage (see Table 9-6)
- Abnormal host defense
  - Immune deficiency
    - Primary: selective or panhypogammaglobulinemia, complement deficiency, leukocyte dysfunction
    - Secondary: malignancy, chemotherapy
  - Ciliary dyskinesia: immotile cilia, Kartagener's syndrome, Young's syndrome, secondary ciliary dyskinesia
- Congenital
  - Cystic fibrosis and variants
  - α-1 protease inhibitor deficiency
  - Unilateral hyperlucent lung (Swyer-James syndrome)
  - Tracheobronchomegaly (Mounier-Kuhn syndrome)
  - Congenital cartilage deficiency (Williams-Campbell syndrome)
  - Pulmonary sequestration
  - Miscellaneous anomalies (T:E fistulae, ectopic bronchi, bronchomalacia, bronchial cysts, vascular anomalies)
- Mechanical bronchial obstruction
  - Intrinsic: foreign body, tumor, viscid secretions, COPD, amyloid
  - Extrinsic: adenopathy, tumors
- Asthma
- Middle lobe syndrome
- Postinflammatory pneumonitis (noninfectious)
  - Aspiration
  - Inhalation of toxic gases
- Secondary to bronchiolar disease
  - Post-transplantation (bone marrow or lung)
  - Diffuse panbronchiolitis
- Idiopathic pulmonary fibrosis
- Idiopathic/cause unknown

Systemic Disorders
- Collagen vascular diseases
  - Rheumatoid arthritis
  - Sjögren's syndrome
  - Ankylosing spondylitis
  - Relapsing polychondritis
  - Systemic lupus erythematosus
  - Marfan's syndrome
- Inflammatory bowel disease
- Celiac disease
- Sarcoidosis
- Yellow nail syndrome
- Human immunodeficiency virus (HIV) infection
- Endometriosis
- Amyloidosis

[a]Modified from references 53, 72, 114, and 117.

Table 9-4

HISTORICAL CLASSIFICATION SCHEMES OF BRONCHIECTASIS[a]

Gross/Radiologic
- Cylindrical, saccular
- Saccular, varicose, cylindrical
  - Tubular; early fusiform; late fusiform, commencing saccular; fusosaccular; saccular, congenital

Histologic
- Follicular, saccular, atelectatic

Etiologic/Pathogenic
- Postinfectious, postobstructive (see Table 9-3)

[a]From references 117 and 134.

during life. Although differentiation between the types of bronchiectasis is useful in assessing disease severity, this distinction is less important than establishing the presence and extent of disease. Assessment of the extent of bronchiectasis is of particular importance because surgery is seldom performed in patients with involvement of multiple lobes. Identification of bronchiectasis by HRCT will change the population of patients defined as having bronchiectasis, with a relative increase in mild and subclinical cases.

Clinical Features. Bronchiectasis presents at all ages and affects both sexes (6,26,54,90,91, 108,112). Although most patients have symptoms, some have symptoms only at the time of an exacerbation and some remain asymptomatic and are identified radiologically (90,112). Many patients have an identified pulmonary illness preceding the onset of respiratory symptoms (90). Common symptoms include cough, purulent sputum (worse in mornings), fever, dyspnea, and hemoptysis (which can be massive). Many patients have coexisting sinusitis. Acute exacerbations are characterized by increased breathlessness, cough, and sputum production, often associated with fever and pleuritic chest pain (90).

The clinical features of patients with bronchiectasis, compiled by Nicotra et al. (90), reflect current practice (Table 9-5). They had noted that most of the medical literature was skewed toward rare and genetic diseases, and as shown in Table 9-5, few of these types of cases were encountered in their study. There was a disproportionate number of women (whereas males were more commonly affected in the past), and a relative paucity of nonwhites (in a hospital population that is 30 percent nonwhite).

Laboratory Tests. The initial evaluation of a patient with suspected bronchiectasis includes chest and sinus radiographs, HRCT scan, and lung function testing (3,6,26,51,53,65,72,90,91,108, 112,114,140). Sputum microscopy, culture, and cytology are often useful. A variety of organisms may infect individuals with established bronchiectasis (Tables 9-5, 9-6) and management requires cultures and appropriate sensitivity studies (see below). A number of special studies may be required depending on the clinical setting: skin tests, sweat test (nasal potentials, genotyping), assessment of nasal mucociliary clearance, semen analysis, serum immunoglobulin titers, fiberoptic bronchoscopy, or barium swallow.

Pulmonary function testing is not specific but often shows airflow obstruction, often with air-trapping or hyperreactivity. A recent study has suggested that airflow obstruction in the setting of bronchiectasis is primarily related to intrinsic disease of the small and medium airways (i.e., bronchiolitis), as evidenced by HRCT, and not primarily to bronchiectatic abnormalities in the large airways (101).

Bronchoscopic Findings. Fiberoptic bronchoscopy is not helpful in the identification of bronchiectasis. However, it can be useful in establishing the cause (for example, to obtain tissue to study the ciliary ultrastructure; to identify the presence of an obstructing lesion causing localized bronchiectasis) or for finding the site of hemoptysis.

Clinical Differential Diagnosis. Causes and conditions associated with bronchiectasis are shown in Table 9-5. Infections play a primary or secondary role in most cases. Infections clinically associated with the development of bronchiectasis are shown in Table 9-6. Even though the incidence of bronchiectasis has decreased, the percentage of cases caused by infections has not decreased in the latter half of the 20th century and there remain cases for which no cause is identified (6,90). In Barker and Bardana's review of multiple series of bronchiectasis reported from 1935 to 1981 (6), the percentage of cases of unknown cause was significant in all the series (29 to 78 percent of the cases); in the recent series of Nicotra et al. (90), the figure was 30 percent.

Table 9-5

BRONCHIECTASIS IN CURRENT PRACTICE[a]

Demographics
- Number of patients—123
- Age (57.2 ± 16.7 years)
- Sex (male, 31 percent; female, 70%)
- Race/ethnicity: white—92.7%; black—6.5%; Hispanic—0.8%
  - Smokers present or past—45%; lifetime nonsmokers—55%

Predisposing Factors
- Recognized cause/injury—70%
  - Age at injury or known cause—21.0 ± 23.1 years
  - Age at onset of symptoms—38.6 ± 24.8 years
- No known cause—30%
- Prior pneumonia—35%
- Pertussis—7.3%
- Other childhood disease—3.2%
- Granulomatous disease—9.8%
- Genetic disease—4.1%
- Miscellaneous—10.6%

Clinical Findings
- Stellate sputum—75.6%
- Dyspnea—71.5%
- Recurrent fever—69.9%
- Recurrent pleurisy—46.3%
- Crackles—69.9%
- Wheezes—34.1%
- Squeaks/rhonchi—43.9%
- Clubbing—3.2%

Microbiology
- *Streptococcus pneumoniae*—10.6%
- *Staphylococcus aureus*—7.35%
- Beta-hemolytic strep—7.3%
- *Haemophilus influenzae*—30.1 %
- *Pseudomonas aeruginosa*—30.9 %
- Gram-negative bacilli—13%
- *Moraxella catarrhalis*—2.4%
- Anaerobic organisms—1.6%
- *Nocardia*—3.3%
- Mycobacteria—22.8%
  - *Mycobacterium avium-intracellulare*—17.1%
- *Aspergillus*—4.9%

[a]Modified from reference 90.

Recent work raises the possibility that *Helicobacter pylori* may play a role in the development of bronchiectasis (124). *H. pylori* has been identified in tracheobronchial secretions of subjects with bronchiectasis, although further studies are indicated to evaluate its possible pathogenic role.

Radiologic Findings. The chest radiograph may demonstrate parallel-line opacities (tram tracks) representing thickened bronchial walls, tubular opacities representing mucus-filled bronchi, and cystic spaces which sometimes contain

Table 9-6

INFECTIONS ASSOCIATED WITH THE DEVELOPMENT OF BRONCHIECTATSIS[a]

Bacterial: *Staphylococcus aureus, Haemophilus influenzae, Pertussis, Streptococcus, Mycoplasma pneumoniae,* anaerobes (recurrent aspiration), *Klebsiella, Pseudomonas, Mycobacterium tuberculosis,* and atypical mycobacteria *(Mycobacterium avium* complex*)*

Fungal: *Aspergillus* (including allergic bronchopulmonary aspergillosis), *Histoplasma, Coccidioides, Pneumocystis*

Viral: Measles, pertussis, adenovirus, influenza, herpes, human immunodeficiency virus (HIV)

[a]Modified from references 72 and 114.

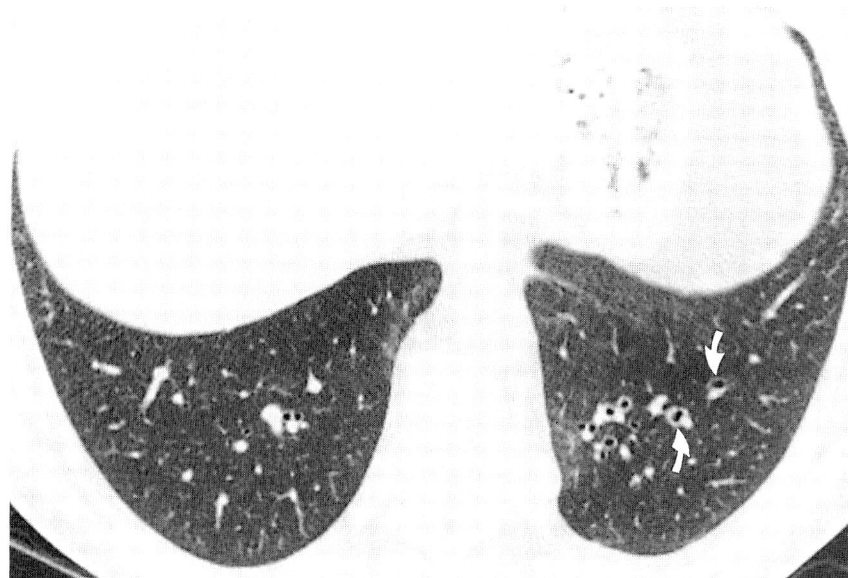

Figure 9-1

CYLINDRICAL BRONCHIECTASIS

HRCT through the lung bases in a 48-year-old man demonstrates cylindrical bronchiectasis involving the posterior and lateral segments of the left lower lobe. The internal diameter of the abnormal left lower lobe bronchi is greater than that of the adjacent pulmonary artery (arrows). The internal diameter of the bronchi in the right lower lobe is less than that of the adjacent pulmonary arteries.

air-fluid levels (114). Less specific findings include indistinctness and crowding of the pulmonary vascular markings caused by the associated loss of volume. Although bronchiectasis can sometimes be recognized on the chest radiograph, in the majority of patients the radiograph is normal or shows nonspecific abnormalities.

The diagnosis of bronchiectasis can be readily made by HRCT (51,65,72,140). The HRCT diagnosis is based on the presence of one or more of the following findings: internal bronchial diameter greater than that of the adjacent pulmonary artery; lack of bronchial tapering considered present when a bronchus maintains the same diameter before and for more than 2 cm after branching; visualization of bronchi within 1 cm of the costal pleura; or visualization of bronchi abutting the mediastinal pleura. The appearance of ectatic bronchi on HRCT depends on the type of bronchiectasis and on the orientation of the bronchi (51,65,72,140). In cylindrical bronchiectasis, bronchi coursing horizontally are visualized as parallel lines (tram tracks) while bronchi coursing vertically are seen as circular lucencies whose internal bronchial diameter is larger than the diameter of the adjacent pulmonary artery, resulting in a "signet-ring" appearance (fig. 9-1). Varicose bronchiectasis is identified by the presence of nonuniform bronchial dilatation (fig. 9-2) while cystic bronchiectasis results in a cluster of thin-walled cystic spaces often containing air-fluid levels (fig. 9-3). Lynch and coworkers (82) showed that patients with cystic bronchiectasis were more likely to have significant airflow obstruction, grow *Pseudomonas* from their sputa, and have purulent sputa than were patients with cylindrical or varicose bronchiectasis.

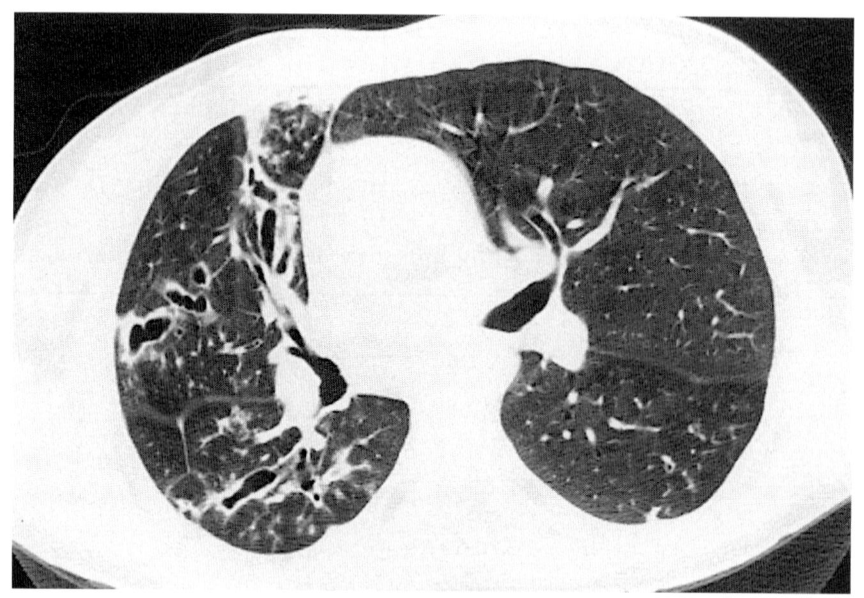

Figure 9-2
VARICOSE BRONCHIECTASIS
HRCT in a 24-year-old woman demonstrates bronchiectasis involving the right middle and lower lobes. The bronchi show nonuniform dilatation, a finding characteristic of varicose bronchiectasis. Note the associated volume loss. Cylindrical bronchiectasis is present in the superior segment of the left lower lobe.

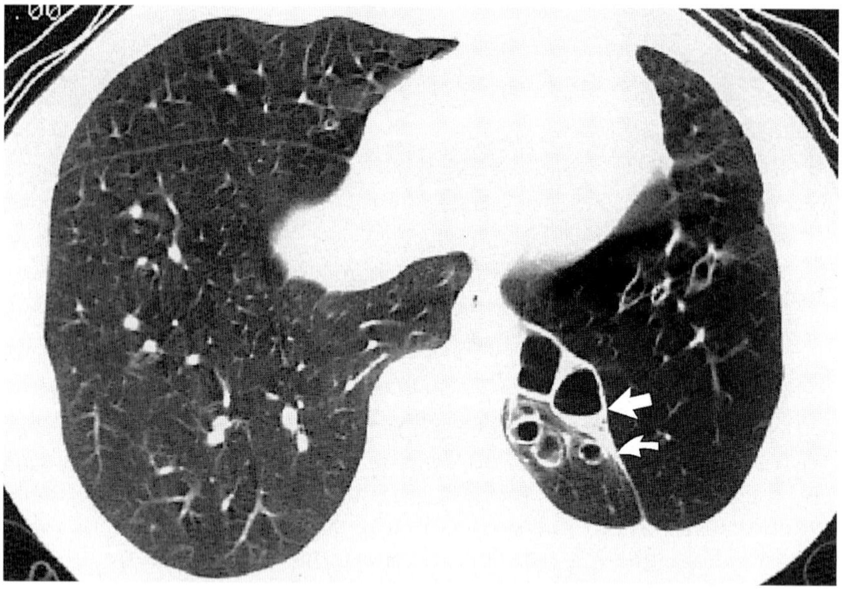

Figure 9-3
CYSTIC BRONCHIECTASIS
HRCT in a 27-year-old man demonstrates cystic left lower lobe bronchiectasis. Some of the cystic areas of bronchiectasis contain air-fluid levels (straight arrow). The bronchiectasis is associated with volume loss of the left lower lobe as noted by the posterior displacement of the left interlobar fissure (curved arrow) and compensatory overinflation of the left upper lobe. Varicose bronchiectasis is present in the left upper lobe.

Several studies have assessed the diagnostic accuracy of HRCT in the diagnosis of bronchiectasis (51,65,72,140). In two large studies that used bronchography as the gold standard, the sensitivity of HRCT in the detection of bronchiectasis was 96 and 98 percent, respectively, and the specificity, 93 and 99 percent, respectively (51,140). In a third study the authors compared the preoperative HRCT findings to the pathologic findings in 47 lobes of 22 patients who had undergone surgical resection of bronchiectasis (65). Using HRCT, abnormalities were detected in all lobes, however, bronchiectasis was only clearly identified in 41 of the 47 lobes (87 percent). The main cause for a false-negative interpretation of HRCT is filling of ectatic bronchi by secretions, mucous plugs, or blood.

In patients who have parenchymal consolidation, normal bronchi may be dilated because of increased elastic recoil. This reversible bronchial dilatation is particularly common in the resolving phase of acute pneumonia. With resolution of the pneumonia the dilatation gradually disappears. Because of this transient

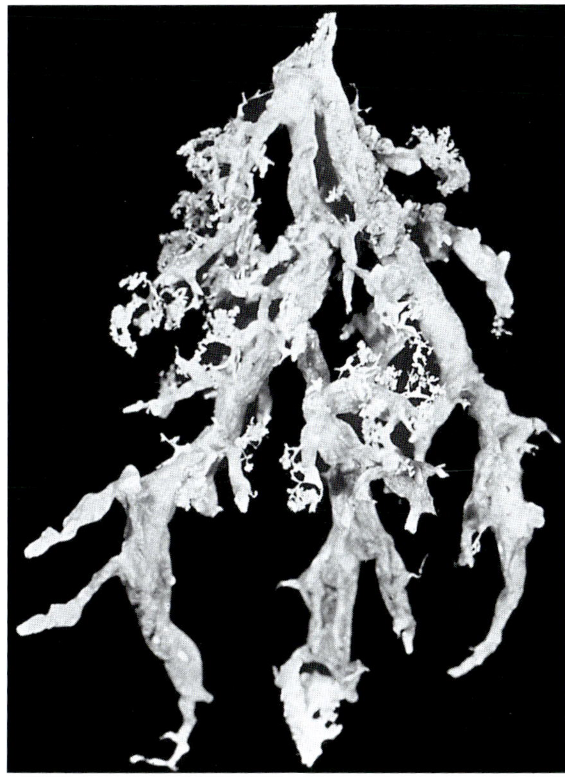

Figure 9-4

BRONCHIAL CAST FROM A CASE OF BRONCHIECTASIS

There is irregularity of the bronchi, zones of dilatation, and abrupt transitions to normal-sized or stenotic airways.

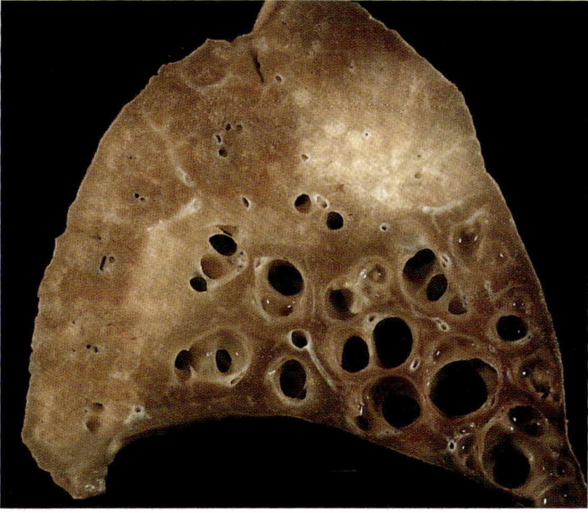

Figure 9-5

SEVERE BRONCHIECTASIS INVOLVING THE LOWER LOBE

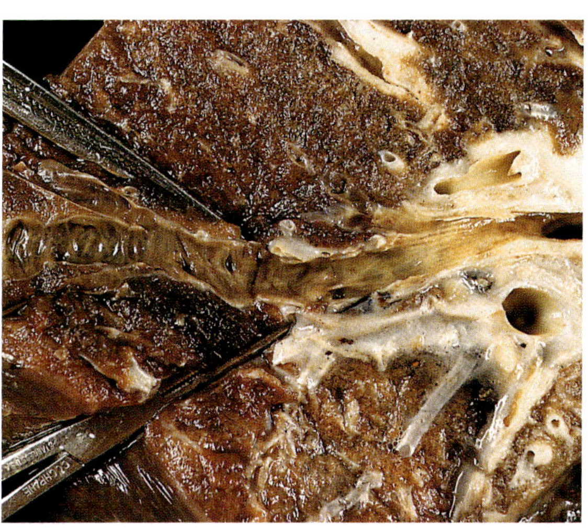

Figure 9-6

BRONCHIECTASIS OF THE LOWER LOBE

Bronchiectasis of the lower lobe shows extension of a dilated airway to within a centimeter of the pleural surface.

bronchial dilatation, an interval of 3 to 6 months should be allowed to elapse after acute pneumonia before making a definitive diagnosis of bronchiectasis based on HRCT results.

Pathologic Findings. The gross descriptions of the forms of bronchiectasis (saccular, varicose, and cylindrical) are included above. The gross findings of bronchiectasis are dramatic (figs. 9-4–9-7) (54,116,117,134). Somewhat less than half the cases are bilateral. The bronchi are dilated, and tenacious mucopurulent secretions may fill the lumens; the lower lobes are more frequently affected, especially the left lower lobe. Transverse ridging by hypertrophied circular smooth muscle bundles and mucosal pits (dilated bronchial gland orifices) may be apparent grossly. Mild bronchiectasis may be difficult to appreciate in collapsed lobes if not specifically sought.

The histologic findings in bronchiectasis vary considerably, with some cases showing minimal changes (tending to correlate with a relative lack of signs and symptoms clinically), and some showing severe acute and chronic inflammatory changes and fibrosis (figs. 9-8–9-13) (54,116,117,134). The lumen may be filled with acute inflammatory and mucopurulent or necrotic debris. The bronchial wall typically shows

Figure 9-7

BRONCHIECTASIS

A: Bronchiectasis distal to an obstructing hilar tumor is shown. The ectatic bronchi are filled with mucus.

B,C: A lobectomy for chronic bronchiectasis following aspiration. The bronchiectatic airways (B, center) were found to contain a seed from Timothy grass. Histologic sections (C) show inflammation and irregularity of the bronchial wall and a small portion of the foreign body (center) surrounded by inflammatory debris.

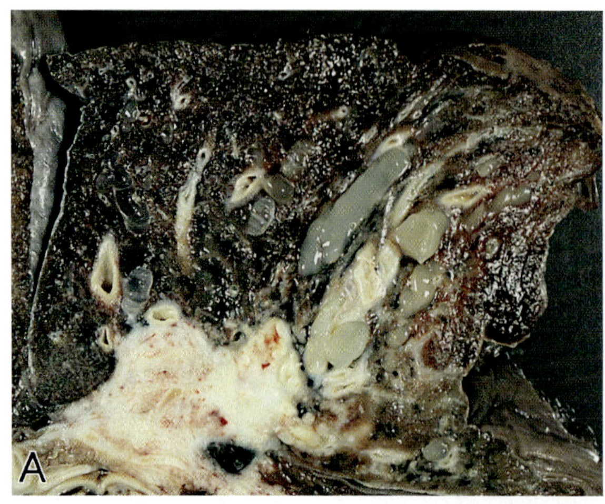

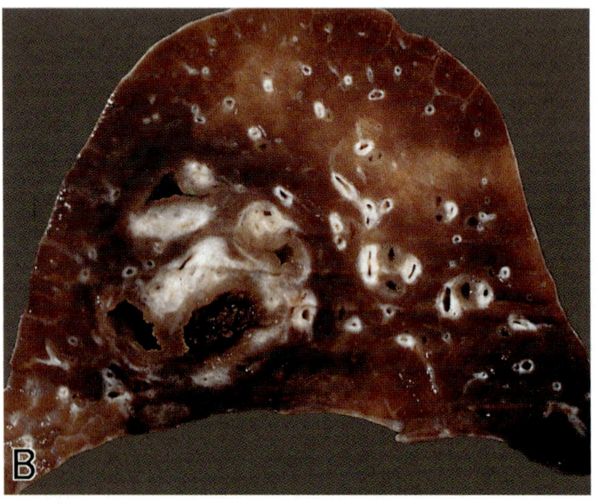

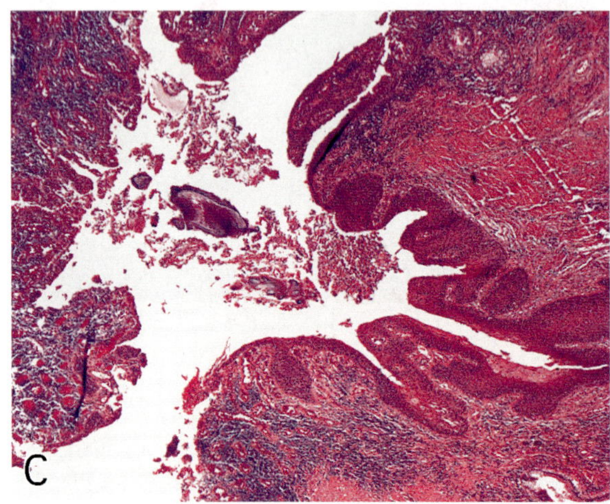

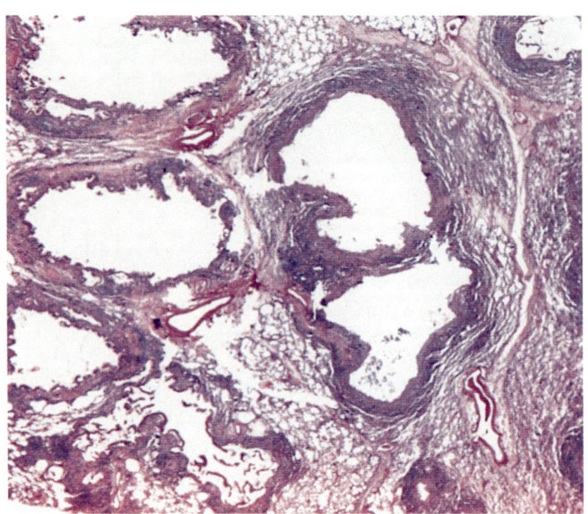

Figure 9-8

BRONCHIECTASIS INVOLVING MULTIPLE AIRWAYS

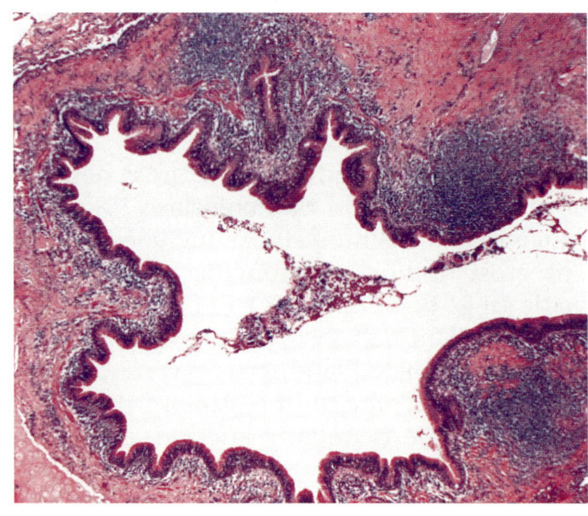

Figure 9-9

BRONCHIECTASIS

There is ectasia of the bronchus, chronic inflammation and fibrosis, and irregular thickening of the wall.

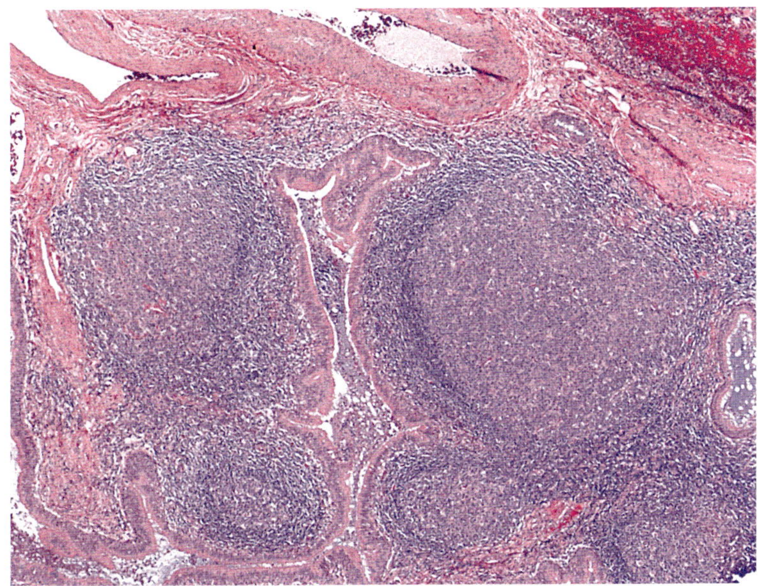

Figure 9-10
BRONCHIECTASIS
Follicular bronchiectasis with marked lymphoid hyperplasia is seen.

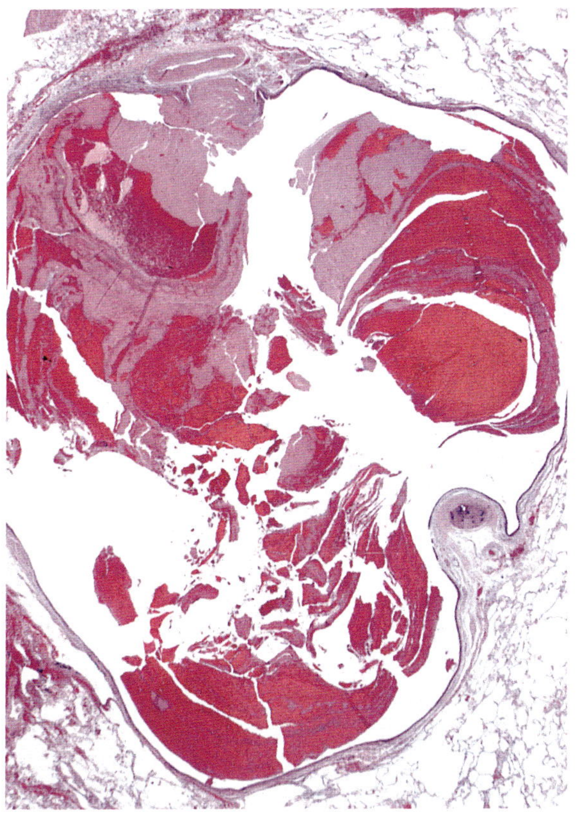

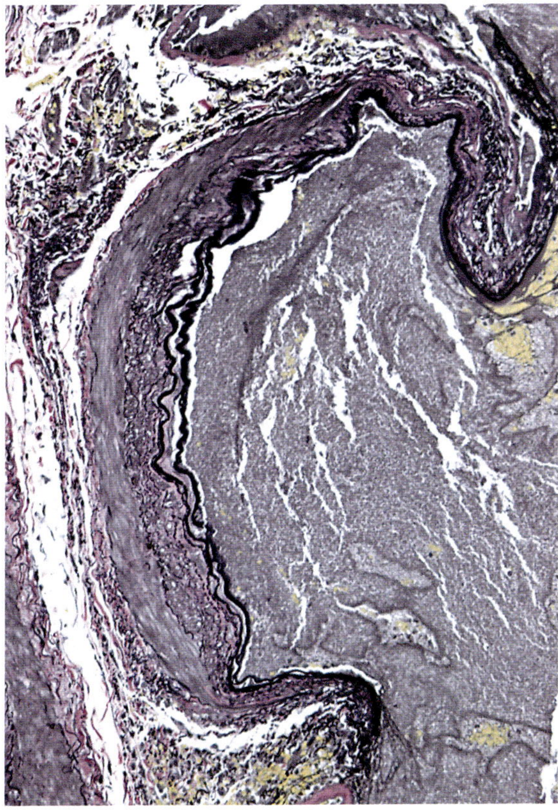

Figure 9-11
BRONCHIECTASIS
Bronchiectasis with massive hemoptysis and blood filling the lumen (left). An eroded artery was found in the wall (top). The arterial nature of the vessel was confirmed with elastic tissue stains (right).

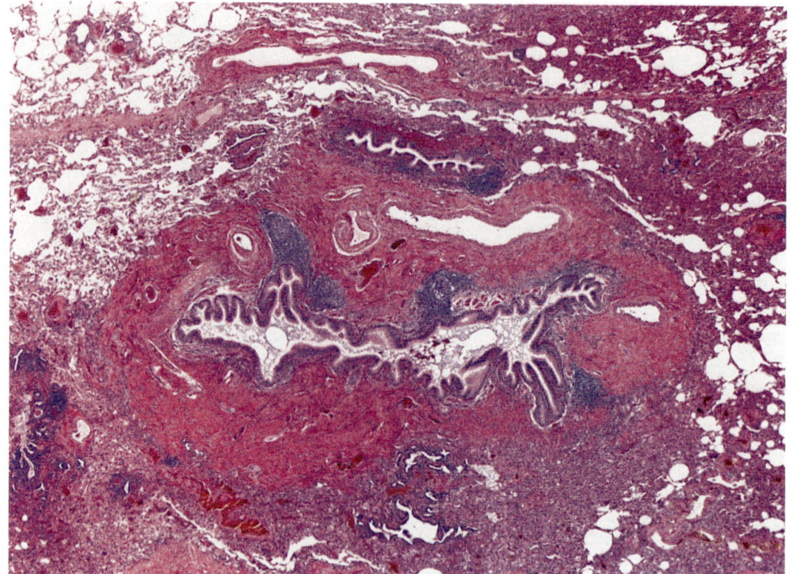

Figure 9-12

CHRONIC BRONCHIECTASIS

There is severe peribronchial and peribronchiolar fibrosis.

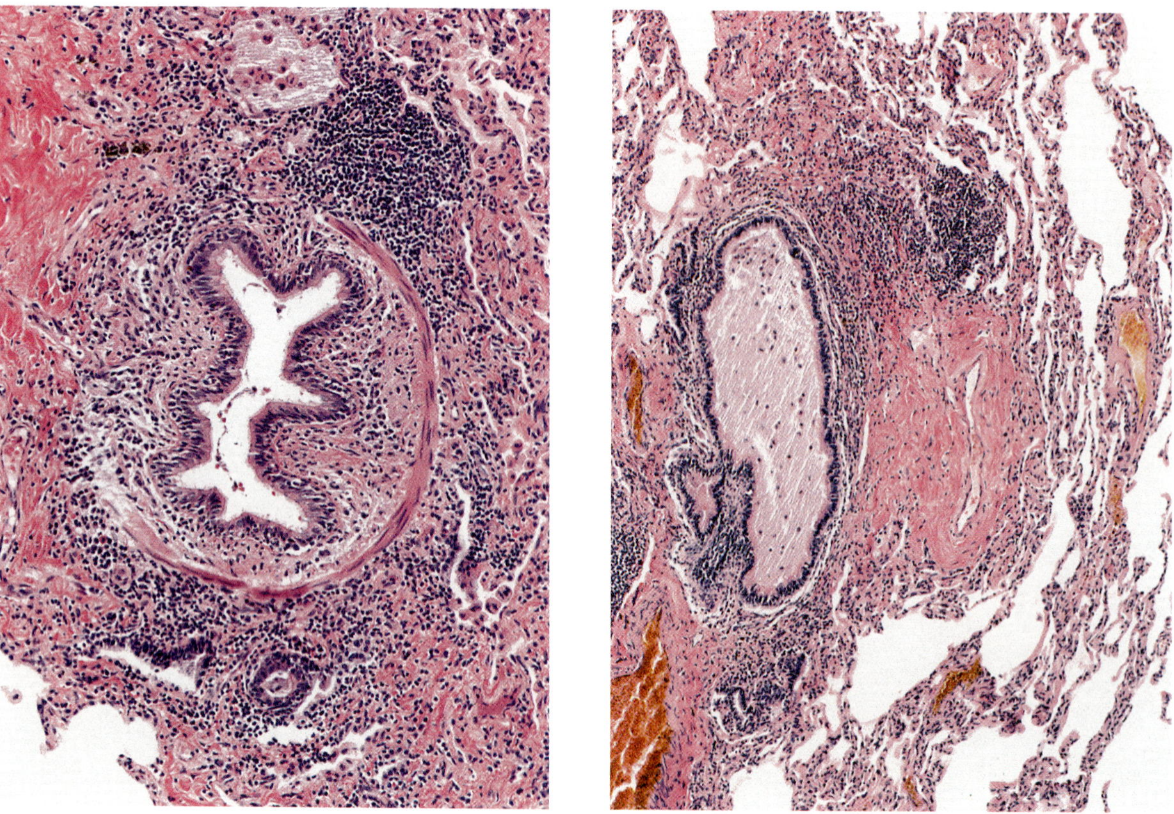

Figure 9-13

BRONCHIOLAR CHANGES IN BRONCHIECTASIS

These bronchioles show chronic constrictive bronchiolitis and mucostasis.

chronic inflammation; the term *follicular bronchiectasis* is appropriate if lymphoid hyperplasia is prominent. The mucosa may be ulcerated or replaced by metaplastic epithelium. In severe cases, there is destruction of all components of the bronchial wall including mucosa, submucosa, muscularis propria, and cartilaginous plates. A similar spectrum of changes may be apparent in the bronchioles distal to the affected bronchi. Some bronchioles may be partially or completely obliterated. Neuroendocrine cell hyperplasia along small bronchi and bronchioles (carcinoid tumorlets) may be found.

Histologic changes in the alveolar parenchyma vary with the activity of the disease and whether secondary pneumonia has supervened. Acute bronchopneumonia, organizing bronchopneumonia, organized pneumonia with septal fibrosis, and obstructive changes in alveoli (with foamy macrophages) may all be seen. Pleural fibrosis and lymphoid hyperplasia may be present. Zones of emphysema/overinflation and zones of atelectasis without associated fibrosis also occur. Fibrotic zones of lung tissue may show all the features of honeycomb change, with metaplastic epithelium and mucous pooling in airspaces.

The pulmonary arteries frequently show endarteritis obliterans in the foci of marked fibrosis. Bronchial arteries and veins are hypertrophied. Massive hemoptysis in bronchiectasis is usually the result of bleeding from eroded bronchial arteries.

Etiology and Pathogenesis. Classically, the proximate cause in most cases of bronchiectasis is necrotizing infection involving the bronchus and/or surrounding lung tissue (114). The infection may be primary (as in severe childhood pneumonia) or secondary to some predisposing factor (many of which are recognized [Table 9-6]). Some of the predisposing factors are decreased mucociliary clearance (such as with cystic fibrosis, primary ciliary dyskinesia) or abnormalities of immune function (such as with immunoglobulin deficiencies or leukocyte abnormalities). Once bronchiectasis develops there is a vicious cycle of recurrent infection and inflammation leading to further anatomic distortion, and in turn further infection and inflammation.

The development of bronchiectasis in patients with collagen vascular diseases (26), following transplantation (115,139), and in other settings suggests infection need not be a proximate cause in all cases. There may be appreciable numbers of cases of bronchiectasis that are unrelated to infection or that follow chronic bronchiolitis (e.g., post lung transplant).

Differential Diagnosis. There are many causes of inflammation in the bronchi and many causes of bronchiectasis. Consequently, the histologic differential diagnosis is impossible without knowledge of the clinical and radiologic findings. In cases showing typical radiologic findings of bronchiectasis, a small bronchial biopsy may show a variety of inflammatory changes (see above) that are all consistent with bronchiectasis.

Parenchymal scarring secondary to bronchiectasis may mimic interstitial fibrosis (e.g., usual interstitial pneumonia). The clinical and radiologic features are helpful in the diagnosis, as is the fact that scarring due to airway disease often appears airway-centered on scanning power microscopy.

In cases in which bronchiectasis is identified, effort should be made to determine if any causes are apparent such as obstructing neoplasm, aspirated foreign body, middle lobe syndrome (see below), or others.

Treatment and Prognosis. Recurrent episodes of acute bronchopneumonia and exacerbations of bronchitis are the most common ongoing problems in most patients (6,90,112, 114). Unfortunately, the infections may be due to antibiotic-resistant organisms. Hemoptysis, mild or life-threatening, is a frequent problem. Chronic respiratory failure associated with cor pulmonale is particularly common when both bronchiectasis and emphysema are present. The prognosis of patients with bronchiectasis is not clearly established. Nicotra and coworkers (90) showed that radiographic progression "was the exception rather than the rule." A European study (71) showed that patients with COPD had a worse prognosis than similar age- and sex-matched patients with bronchiectasis. Bronchiectasis alone was the main cause of death in only 13 percent of bronchiectatic patients followed up to 10 years from diagnosis.

The primary goals in the management of bronchiectasis are to control symptoms, prevent progression, and avoid complications (6,26,90,

112,114). In most cases, management involves treatment of any underlying predisposing factors or conditions (Tables 9-3, 9-6) and control of infection with antibiotic therapy tailored to the individual case. Bronchospasm is a problem in many patients and this can be managed with bronchodilators. A recent double-blind placebo-controlled study showed that the 8-week administration of low-dose erythromycin (500 mg b.i.d.) to patients with steady-state idiopathic bronchiectasis resulted in improved lung function and sputum volume (123).

Surgery is generally reserved for relatively young patients with severe persistent or recurrent symptoms and localized bronchiectasis. Severe hemorrhage from enlarged bronchial arteries may be life-threatening and require urgent or emergent surgical management. In a recent review of 134 patients who underwent pulmonary resection for bronchiectasis during a 17-year period (1), 86 patients (64.2 percent) underwent lobectomy; 21, pneumonectomy; 18, wedge resection or segmentectomy; and 9, a combination of these approaches. The operative mortality rate was 2.2 percent and the morbidity rate was 24.6 percent. Following surgery, 59 percent of the patients were asymptomatic, 29 percent had improved, and 12 percent were unchanged.

Table 9-7

PRESENTING MANIFESTATIONS OF CYSTIC FIBROSIS[a]

Pulmonary
Wheezing
Chronic or productive cough
Recurrent or chronic pneumonia infiltrates
Recurrent bronchiolitis
Atelectasis
Hemoptysis
Infection with *Pseudomonas*
Staphylococcal pneumonia
Other
Family history of cystic fibrosis
Failure to thrive
Salty taste when kissed
Nasal polyps
Unexplained hypochloremic alkalosis
Pansinusitis
Absence of sperm in semen
Pseudotumor cerebri
Gastrointestinal
Meconium ileus, meconium plug syndrome
Steatorrhea, malabsorption
Rectal prolapse
Biliary cirrhosis, portal hypertension, bleeding esophageal varices
Hypoprothrombinemia beyond newborn period
Hypoproteinemia, anasarca
Deficiency of vitamin A, D, E, or K
Recurrent pancreatitis
Acrodermatitis enteropathic-like rash

[a]Data from reference 12.

CYSTIC FIBROSIS

Definition and Background. Cystic fibrosis is a multisystem disease affecting the respiratory and digestive systems, sweat glands, and reproductive tract. Patients have abnormal transport of chloride and sodium across the respiratory epithelium, resulting in thickened, viscous airway secretions. Chronic infection of the respiratory tract with a characteristic array of bacterial flora results in progressive respiratory insufficiency and eventual respiratory failure and death.

Cystic fibrosis is the most common fatal hereditary disease in Caucasians, affecting approximately 1 in 3,000 live births (12,114). The frequency of mutant alleles in the Caucasian population is about 0.02. Among blacks the disease is much less common, seen in 1 in 17,000 births, and among Asians (in Hawaii) it is rare, occurring in 1 in 90,000 live births.

Cystic fibrosis affects exocrine tissue in the lung, pancreas, gastrointestinal tract, liver, salivary glands, and male reproductive system (8, 12,35,38,43,46,58,94,107,110,114,119,120,127). Lung involvement is seen in 100 percent of cases that come to autopsy and it is the cause of death in approximately 95 percent. Bronchiectasis is almost universal among individuals over 6 months of age with cystic fibrosis, and cystic fibrosis is one of the most common causes of bronchiectasis in children.

Clinical Features. Since cystic fibrosis involves several organ systems, many signs and symptoms may be the presenting manifestations of the illness (Table 9-7) (12,114). Many of these manifestations vary with the age at presentation. For example, meconium ileus is present during infancy. Cough is the most common pulmonary symptom; initially it is dry, but later mucopurulent. The physical examination is nonspecific but may show nasal polyps, an increased anterior to posterior chest diameter, and clubbing.

Once the diagnosis is made or suspected, the clinical evaluation of a patient with cystic fibrosis commonly includes: chest radiograph, HRCT scanning, measurements of lung function and gas exchange, sputum cultures (these are often obtained serially), and functional assessment of the liver, pancreas, and reproductive organs (12,114). Pulmonary function studies (at 5 to 6 years of age, and thereafter) show obstruction as the predominant functional manifestation (12).

Gas exchange abnormalities are common (decreased diffusing capacity for carbon monoxide [DLCO] or arterial PaO_2). As gas exchange worsens, hypercapnic respiratory failure and cor pulmonale develop. Many organisms are known to be colonizers or pathogenic in this setting (11,12,114,121). The organisms most commonly cultured from individuals with cystic fibrosis include *Staphylococcus aureus* (although the percentage of positive individuals has decreased in recent years), *Haemophilus influenzae, Pseudomonas aeruginosa* (there is a 60 to 90 percent colonization rate), and *Burkholderia cepacia.* Enterobacteriaceae may also be identified. These organisms produce a host of toxins and chemotactic factors that can contribute to tissue damage. Allergic bronchopulmonary aspergillosis may develop (74).

The diagnostic work-up for patients with cystic fibrosis is usually initiated by finding conditions shown in Table 9-8. The diagnosis is usually confirmed by abnormal chloride secretion: the sweat chloride test is interpreted as diagnostic if greater than or equal to 60 mEq/L; levels between 40 and 60 mEq/L are considered suggestive of cystic fibrosis (12). If a sweat chloride test is normal or inconclusive, chromosome analyses can be performed to confirm a cystic fibrosis genotype in cases that remain clinically suspicious.

Radiologic Findings. The chest radiograph shows thickened bronchial walls, bronchial dilatation, hyperinflation, and, commonly, prominence of the pulmonary hila due to lymph node enlargement or, in the late stages, pulmonary arterial hypertension (12,42, 43,114,138). Bronchiectasis is usually widespread but tends to be most severe in the upper lobes (42,138). When filled with secretions or inspissated mucus, ectatic bronchi are seen as nodular, finger-like or branching, band-like opacities. Recurrent foci of consolidation occur in the majority of patients and segmental or lobar atelectasis in approximately 50 percent.

Table 9-8

PULMONARY COMPLICATIONS OF CYSTIC FIBROSIS[a]

Hyperreactive airways
Atelectasis
Pneumothorax
Hemoptysis
Allergic bronchopulmonary aspergillosis
Acute respiratory failure
Chronic respiratory failure
Cor pulmonale

[a]Data from reference 12.

The abnormalities on chest radiography have been incorporated into semiquantitative scoring schemes. The most commonly used scoring scheme is the Brasfield score which is a 25-point score based on a 0 to 4 grading of air-trapping, linear markings, nodular cystic lesions, large opacities (atelectasis or consolidation), and general severity (an extra point is given for cardiomegaly or evidence of pulmonary hypertension) (18).

HRCT is superior to the radiograph for demonstrating bronchiectasis and is useful for identifying early involvement of the peripheral airways in cystic fibrosis, as manifested by centrilobular nodules and branching linear opacities away from areas affected by bronchiectasis (10,138). These nodules and linear opacities result in a "tree in bud" appearance and reflect the presence of small, branching bronchioles whose walls are thickened by fibrous tissue and inflammatory cells, and whose lumina are filled with secretions. A scoring system for pulmonary abnormalities detected on HRCT has been proposed that involves a 0 to 2 or 0 to 3 score for the presence and extent of bronchiectasis, peribronchial thickening, mucous plugging, atelectasis/consolidation, and cystic or emphysematous changes (10). On HRCT, as on the radiograph, the bronchiectasis in cystic fibrosis typically is diffuse throughout both lungs but is more severe in the upper lobes (fig. 9-14) (24).

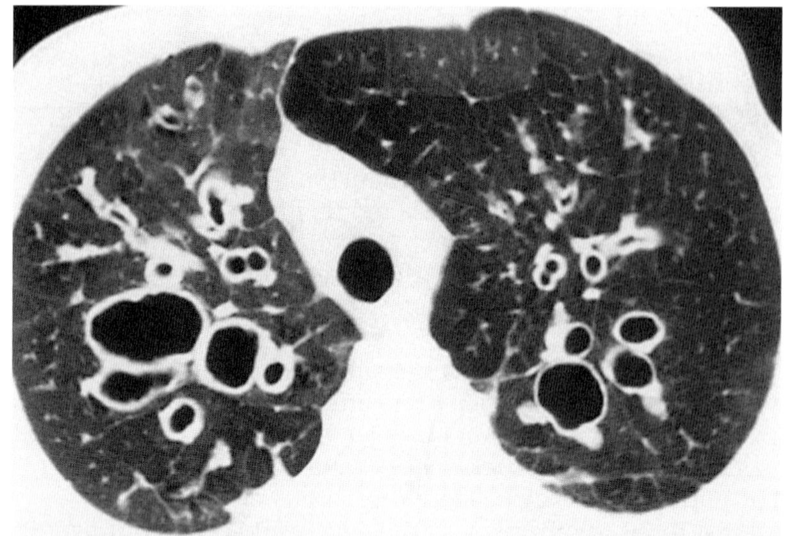

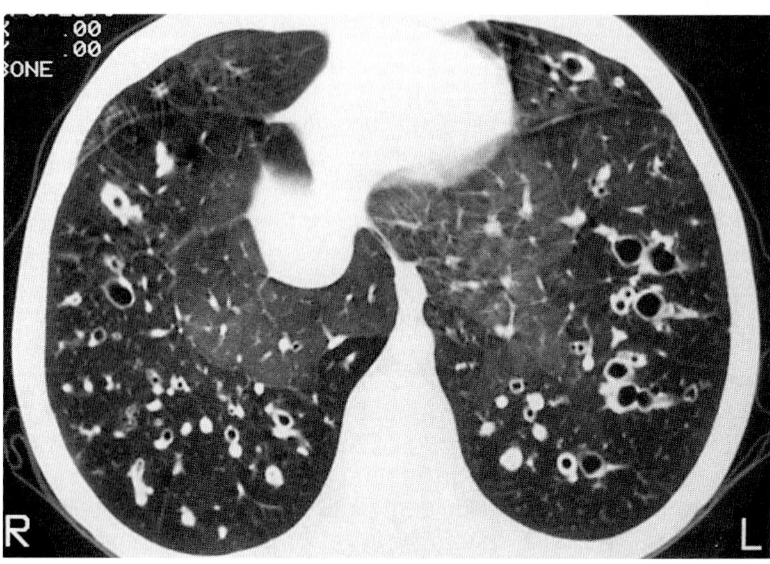

Figure 9-14
CYSTIC FIBROSIS

Top: HRCT in a 15-year-old male with cystic fibrosis demonstrates cystic and varicose bronchiectasis involving both upper lobes.

Bottom: HRCT through the lower lung zones demonstrates extensive but less severe bronchiectasis.

Pathologic Findings. The upper respiratory tract pathology includes nasal polyps and chronic sinusitis, and in specimens from these regions inspissation of secretion product may be identified in minor salivary gland tissue. The pathology in the lung is the major feature of cystic fibrosis and many findings are recognized (Table 9-9); the most distinctive are widespread bronchiectasis involving all lobes (especially upper) and inspissated tenacious mucus secretions (figs. 9-15–9-24).

Genetics and Pathogenesis. The cystic fibrosis gene has been cloned and sequenced (12,107,114). It is on chromosome 7 (7q3); it encodes a 1480 amino acid protein called the cystic fibrosis transmembrane regulator (CFTR), which is expressed in epithelial cells in the lung, gastrointestinal tract, and elsewhere (12,107). Mutations in the CFTR lead to the clinical manifestations of cystic fibrosis. Over eight alleles have been identified (and the number continues to grow) and some produce more severe clinical manifestations than others; the most common mutation in Caucasians (occurring in 70 percent of cases) is a deletion of the phenylalanine residue at amino acid 508 (ΔF-508) (12,46,107).

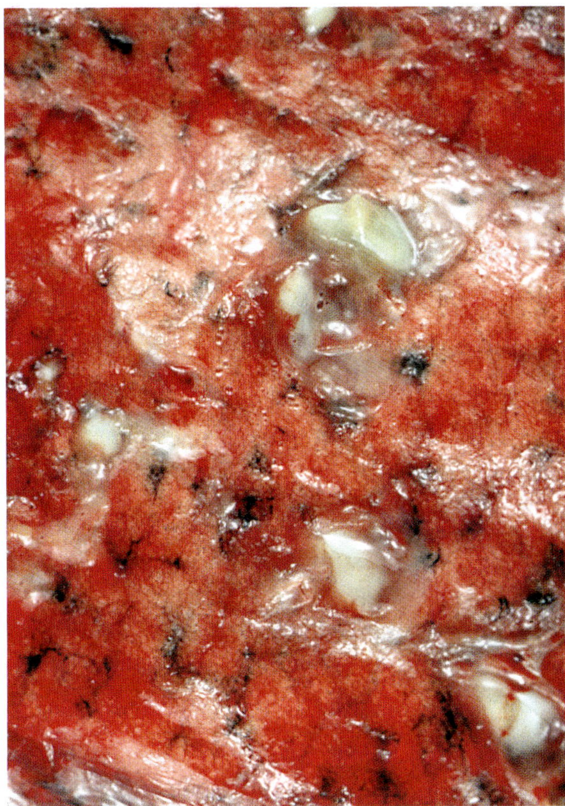

Figure 9-15

CYSTIC FIBROSIS

Cut section of fresh autopsy lung tissue show purulent gray-white mucus in bronchi and bronchioles.

Table 9-9

PULMONARY PATHOLOGY OF CYSTIC FIBROSIS[a]

Gross Pathologic Findings
- Widespread bronchiectasis with purulent tenacious airway mucus
- Pleural adhesions/fibrosis
- Lobar atelectasis
- Lobar overdistention
- Focal/widespread pneumonic consolidation
- Abscess(es)
- Cystic changes
  - Bronchiectatic
  - Interstitial air
  - Emphysematous bullae

Histologic Findings—Large Airways
- Acute and chronic inflammation
- Purulent mucous plugging
- Epithelial sloughing/metaplasia
- Submucosal gland inspissation of secretion/ sclerotic atrophy
- Bronchiectasis
- Bronchostenosis
- Increased Reid index (bronchial gland hypertrophy/hyperplasia)
- Goblet cell hyperplasia
- Bronchial artery hypertrophy

Histologic Findings—Small Airways
- Acute and chronic inflammation
- Epithelial necrosis/metaplasia
- Purulent mucous plugging
- Constrictive bronchiolitis
- Peribronchiolar scarring/metaplasia

Histologic Findings—Alveolar/Parenchymal
- Acute/Organizing/Organized pneumonia
- Abscess(es)
- Atelectasis
- Emphysema/air-trapping
- Septal fibrosis
- Interstitial thickening/fibrosis
- Interstitial inflammatory infiltrate

Histologic Findings—Pleura
- Pleural adhesions
- Fibrous thickening
- Loss of elastica
- Subpleural cysts/blebs (with interstitial air)
- Cuboidal mesothelium

[a]Collated from references 8,12,38,94,110,114,119, 120,127.

Dysfunction of the CFTR leads to an inability on the part of airway epithelial cells to secrete salt (and secondarily water) and excessive reabsorption of salt and water with consequent desiccation of luminal secretions (12). Mucous plugging is a consequence of lack of hydration, with subsequent diminished mucociliary clearance. Mucous plugging and decreased clearance predispose to colonization by bacteria, which sets the stage for recurrent infections and all the complications thereof.

Differential Diagnosis. None of the pathologic changes in the lung (Table 9-9) is specific for cystic fibrosis. Focal biliary cirrhosis and underdevelopment of the male reproductive system are the only morphologic lesions considered specific for cystic fibrosis (127).

Treatment and Prognosis. Survival has dramatically improved for patients with cystic fibrosis (12,114). The clinical severity of the disease varies considerably. Some patients present in the neonatal period and others in late adulthood. The variation in severity is related in part

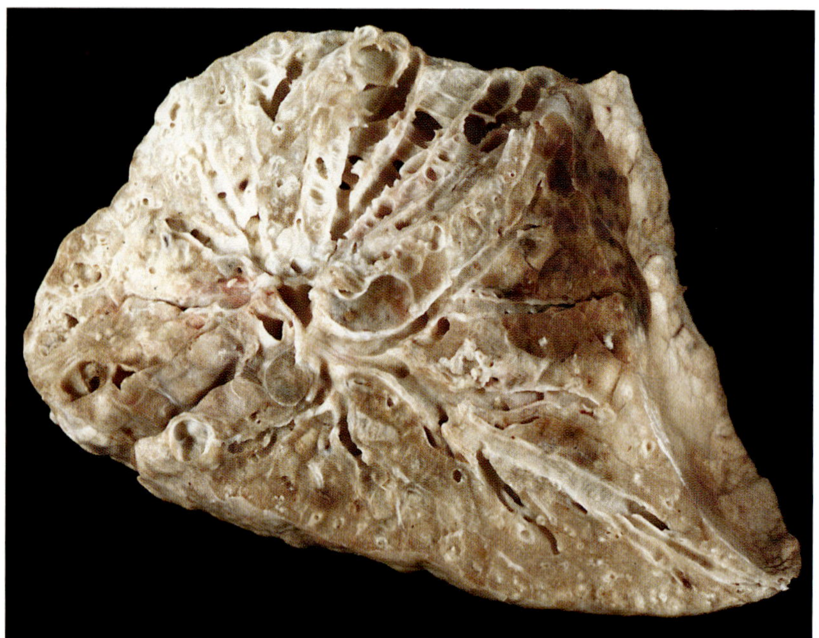

Figure 9-16

CYSTIC FIBROSIS

Cystic fibrosis with extensive bronchiectasis, which is more severe in the upper lobes.

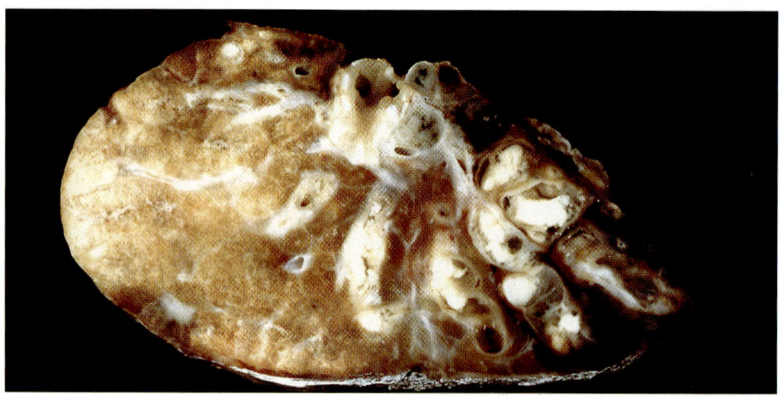

Figure 9-17

CYSTIC FIBROSIS

This lobectomy specimen shows regions of bronchiectasis with gray-white mucous plugs in the bronchi.

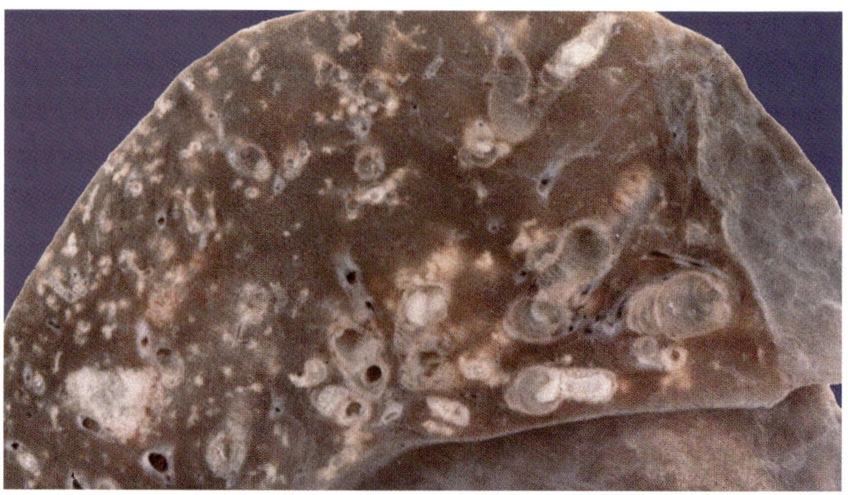

Figure 9-18

CYSTIC FIBROSIS

In addition to the obvious bronchiectasis there are smaller white nodules which represent foci of acute bronchiolitis.

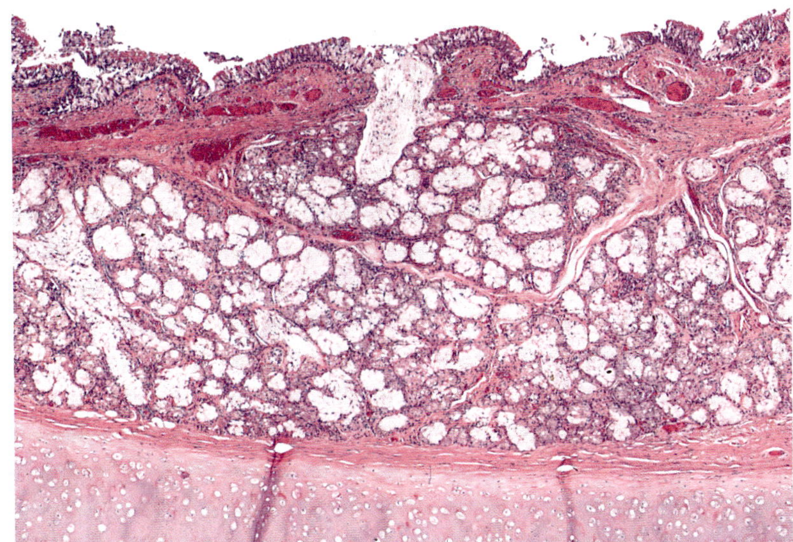

Figure 9-19

CYSTIC FIBROSIS

The large airways show marked submucosal gland hypertrophy; mucous plugging can be seen in one of the ducts (upper center).

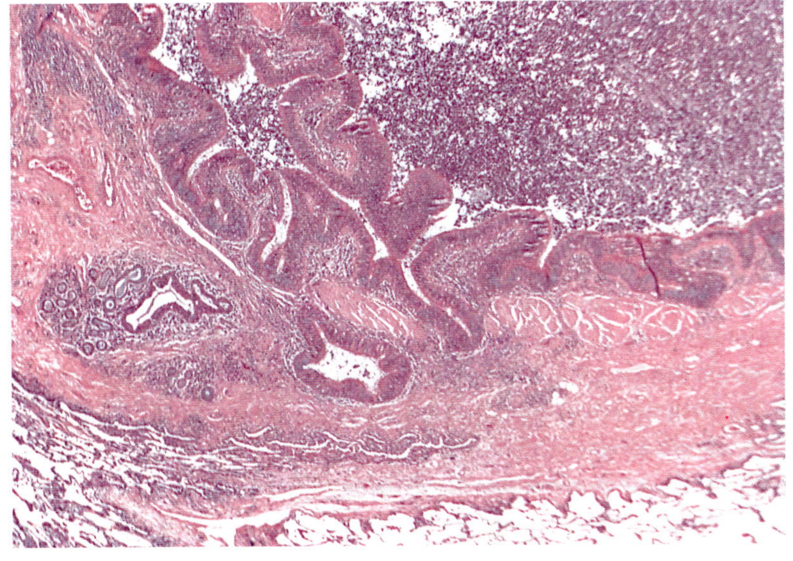

Figure 9-20

CYSTIC FIBROSIS

The bronchial wall is thickened and fibrotic with mucosal thickening and irregularity. Purulent material is seen in the lumen.

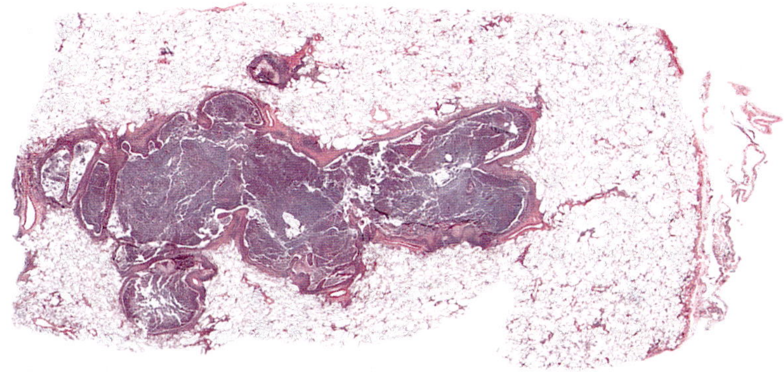

Figure 9-21

CYSTIC FIBROSIS

The small airways show plugging by mucopurulent material.

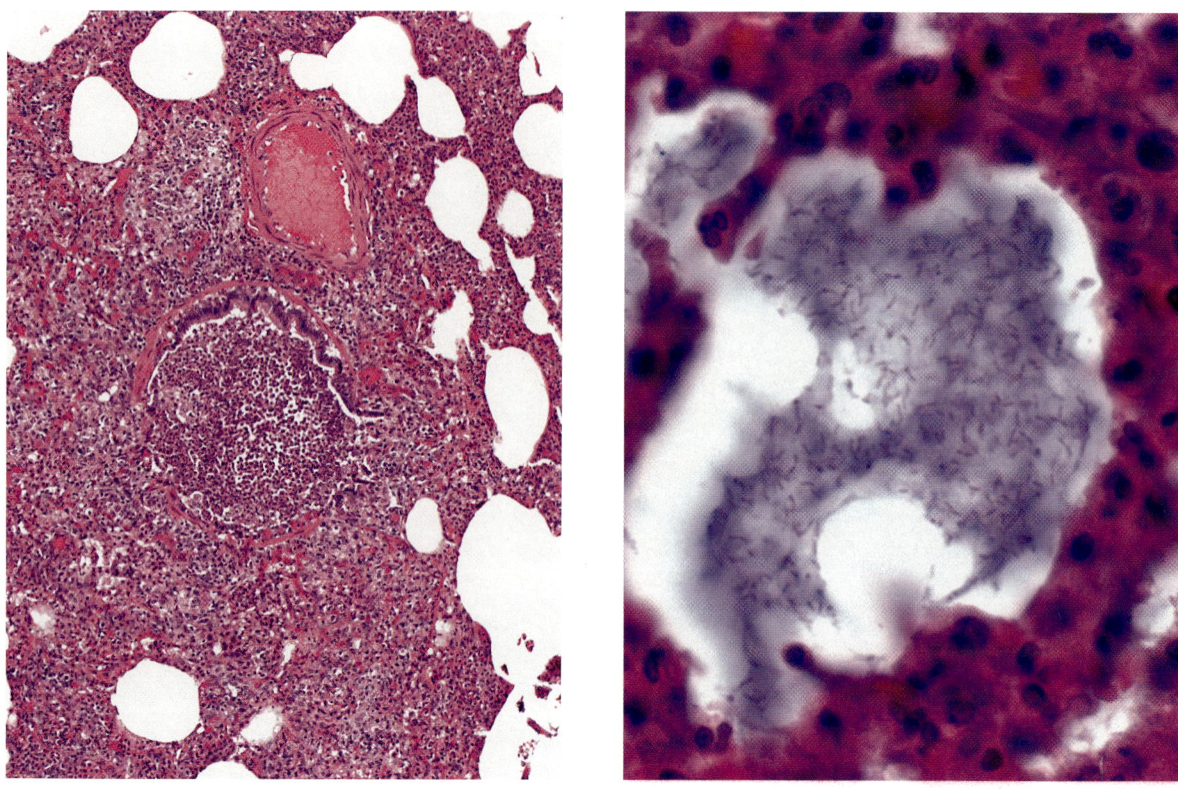

Figure 9-22

CYSTIC FIBROSIS

Left: There is acute and chronic bronchiolitis with purulent material filling the lumen. The bronchiole shows mural chronic inflammation in the wall.

Right: The purulent material in the airways frequently contains readily identifiable colonies of bacteria.

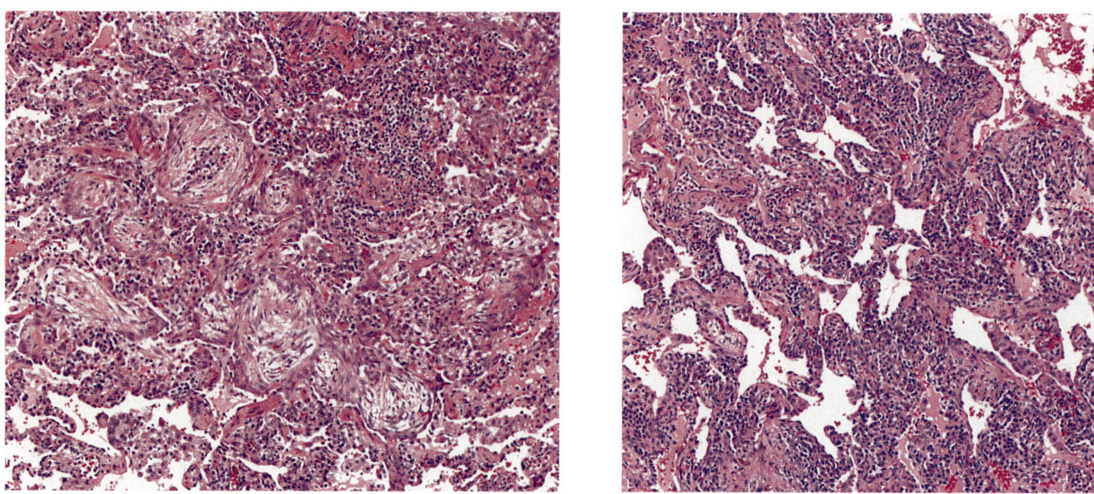

Figure 9-23

CYSTIC FIBROSIS

Interstitial changes identified in cystic fibrosis include foci of organizing pneumonia (left) and interstitial inflammation and fibrosis (right).

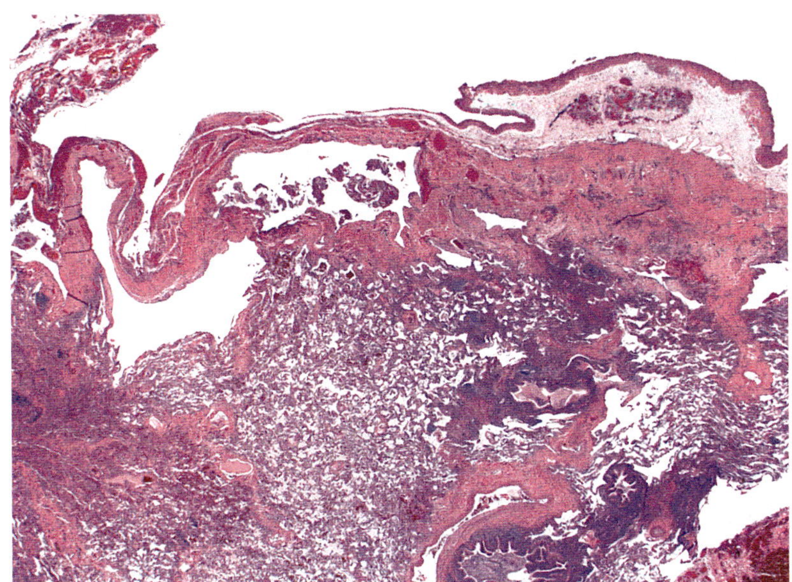

Figure 9-24

PNEUMOTHORAX IN CYSTIC FIBROSIS

Pneumothoraces in this case prompted resection of the subpleural blebs. The underlying lung tissue shows less inflammation than seen at autopsy, although acute and chronic bronchiolitis still is apparent (lower right).

to genetic factors, with some alleles associated with less severe manifestations. Because of the complex nature of this disease and the multiple organ systems that can be affected, it is not possible to describe a "typical" or "classic" clinical course. However, the severity and rate of progression of the lung disease is an important determinant of long-term prognosis. Pulmonary complications are shown in Table 9-8.

Patients with cystic fibrosis present complicated clinical problems and the management of lung disease is only one facet of the clinical approach (12). Management of pulmonary disease includes: 1) maintaining airway clearance; 2) controlling infections; and 3) maintaining adequate nutritional support. The prognosis has improved in recent years, with many individuals surviving into adulthood, occasionally beyond 60 years of age (12,43,58,127).

PRIMARY CILIARY DYSKINESIA

Definition. Primary ciliary dyskinesia represents a group of disorders (13,14,20,21,30,34, 36,57,104,105,113,128) in which there is absent, scattered, or uncoordinated ciliary motility. Synonyms include *immotile cilia syndrome, ciliary dyskinesia syndrome,* and *Kartagener's syndrome*. These disorders are usually associated with: 1) chronic/recurrent upper and lower respiratory infections; 2) absent or deficient tracheobronchial and nasal mucociliary transport; 3) total or near total absence of the dynein arms (or other ultrastructural defects) in cilia of the respiratory tract; and 4) sterility in males due to viable but immotile sperm (fertility in females is also reduced).

The prevalence of this syndrome is approximately 1 in 20,000 (13). Among all patients with bronchiectasis, 1.5 percent have primary ciliary dyskinesia, and among all patients with situs inversus, 15 percent have primary ciliary dyskinesia (114). Primary ciliary dyskinesia affects approximately 10 to 15 percent of children evaluated for chronic suppurative lung disease (20,91).

Kartagener's syndrome is a subset of primary ciliary dyskinesia that includes bronchiectasis, sinusitis, and situs inversus (114). Kartagener's syndrome is found in approximately 50 percent of patients with primary ciliary dyskinesia (114).

Clinical Features. Primary ciliary dyskinesia is a familial condition with an autosomal recessive inheritance pattern and no sex predilection (13,21). Most affected individuals present with chronic sinusitis and respiratory tract infections any time from the newborn period into adulthood. Chronic otitis media is a particularly prominent feature that helps in distinguishing primary ciliary dyskinesia from cystic fibrosis. Pulmonary manifestations include wheezing, productive cough, and recurrent pneumonias. Males may present with infertility.

Table 9-10

CLINICAL SITUATIONS SUSPICIOUS OF PRIMARY CILIARY DYSKINESIA[a]

Neonatal respiratory distress syndrome in term infants with no risk for transient tachypnea of the new born, neonatal pneumonia with no predisposing factors, and any neonate with significant prolonged nasal discharge
Child/adult with bronchiectasis of unknown cause
Child with severe or atypical asthma
Child with severe upper airway disease in whom cystic fibrosis has been excluded
Male infertility with immotile sperm or sperm showing reduced motility and infertile or subfertile females without obvious anatomical or hormonal cause, especially if other features of primary ciliary dyskinesia are known to be present (Note: Fertility does not exclude a diagnosis of primary ciliary dyskinesia in men)
Other clinical features such as dextrocardia, disorders of laterality, deafness, hydrocephalus, biliary atresia, congenital heart disease

[a]Data from reference 21.

Table 9-11

FUNCTIONAL AND ULTRASTRUCTURAL CILIARY ABNORMALITIES IN PATIENTS WITH PRIMARY CILIARY DYSKINESIA AND BRONCHIECTASIS, AND NORMAL CONTROLS[a]

Feature	Normal Controls (n=62)		Bronchiectatic (n=20)		Primary Ciliary Dyskinesia (n=31)	
	Range	(Mean)	Range	(Mean)	Range	(Mean)
Ciliary beat frequency	9.6-15.3Hz	(11.5)	9.6-14.1Hz	(12.0)	0-12.9 Hz	(4.1)
Peripheral microtubular defects	0-9%	(2.2)	0.5-7.3%	(2.0)	0.7-36.5%	(7.2)
Number of inner dynein arms	3.0-7.1	(5.4)	2.7-7.5	(5.0)	0.1-6.5	(2.7)
Number of outer dynein arms	7.4-9.0	(8.5)	6.5-9.0	(8.3)	0.1-8.8	(3.2)
Ciliary disorientation (deviation angles)	8-29°	(14.3°)	10-25°	(15.6°)	14-49°	(29.8°)

[a]Modified from reference 30.

The presence of chronic respiratory tract infections and a right-sided heart is virtually diagnostic of primary ciliary dyskinesia, but situs inversus occurs in only 50 percent of affected individuals. The diagnosis of primary ciliary dyskinesia may be suspected in any individual with chronic, recurring, upper and lower respiratory tract disease (13,20,21,91,114). According to Bush et al. (21), primary ciliary dyskinesia may be suspected in the clinical situations shown in Table 9-10.

Examination of fresh scrapings of nasal mucosa with a light microscope (with the condenser lowered) is a quick screening method to assess ciliary movement and beat frequency. If ciliary beat frequency is less than 10 Hz, ultrastructural examination is indicated (20). Definitive diagnosis is by ultrastructural examination of nasal or bronchial cilia in appropriately fixed (2 percent glutaraldehyde), processed, and transversely sectioned specimens. For a detailed discussion of diagnostic criteria, the reader is referred to the review by Bush et al. (21). It is recommended that specimens be taken no sooner than 2 weeks after an active infection has cleared (13). Recognizing that the abnormalities in primary ciliary dyskinesia can be difficult to separate from the secondary effects of inflammation and infection, the data of de Iongh and Rutland (Table 9-11) are useful (30). Recently, measurement of exhaled nitric oxide, thought to be involved in both the regulation of ciliary motility and host defense, has been recommended as a screening test for this condition (66,98).

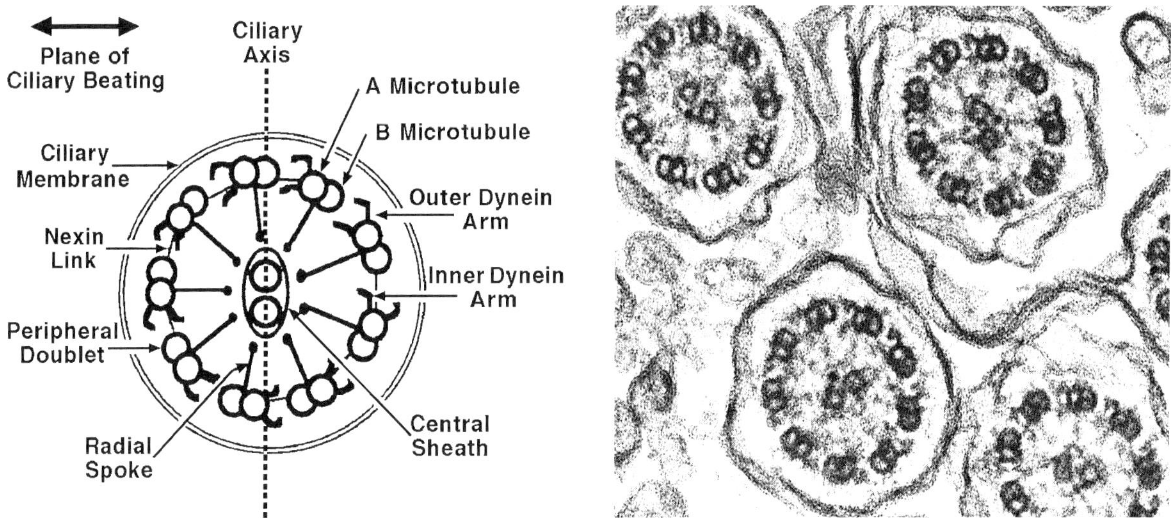

Figure 9-25

NORMAL CILIA

Left: A diagrammatic representation of a normal cilium is depicted. (Figure 1 from Rutland J, de Iongh RU. Random ciliary orientation. N Eng J Med 1990;323:1681.)

Right: The normal structures of a cilium can be discerned from one ultrastructurally normal case (X75,000).

Radiologic Findings. The findings on the chest radiograph and HRCT include bronchial wall thickening, bronchiectasis, hyperinflation, and, commonly, areas of atelectasis or consolidation (13,21,114). Centrilobular small nodules may be seen on HRCT scans and these correspond to bronchiolitis involving membranous bronchioles (57). Approximately 50 percent of patients have situs inversus.

Pathologic Findings. The gross and histologic findings in primary ciliary dyskinesia are nonspecific: bronchitis, bronchiolitis, bronchiectasis, and bronchopneumonia (acute, organizing, or healed). The diagnostic findings of interest are ultrastructural and since the original description of morphologically abnormal cilia in the syndrome, attempts have been made to define the disease ultrastructurally (figs. 9-25–9-27) (13,14,20,21,30,34,36,104, 105,113,114,128,). In general, there is a correlation between ultrastructural abnormalities and ciliary dysfunction (20). The following ultrastructural abnormalities have been noted: absent or shortened dynein arms, absence of radial spokes, microtubular transposition or disarrangement, absence of microtubules, presence of compound cilia, and ciliary disorientation (30,34,36,105,113,128).

Unfortunately, an appreciable percentage of cilia from individuals who do not have primary ciliary dyskinesia are abnormal, particularly during active respiratory tract inflammation (14,23,30,34,41,98). In primary ciliary dyskinesia the defects affect nearly all the cilia (as a congenital defect), whereas only up to 30 percent of cilia are abnormal in infection-related disorders (34). In addition, in primary ciliary dyskinesia nearly all peripheral microtubular doublets are affected in all cilia. In contrast, in acquired conditions only a few of the microtubular doublets are lacking or all the doublets are lacking in but a few cilia (34). Acquired ultrastructural and/or functional abnormalities of cilia may follow viral infection or inhalation of airborne toxins (14). In normal children only 3 to 5 percent of cilia show microtubular disorganization (34).

Ciliary orientation has been assessed by evaluating the cilia originating from a single cell, and has been shown to be abnormal in primary ciliary dyskinesia (30,105). A line is drawn through the centers of two central microtubules for all the cilia in a given cell. The degree of deviation from parallel that these lines make when compared to one another (with the aid of a computer and image analysis on photomicrographs) is the degree of ciliary

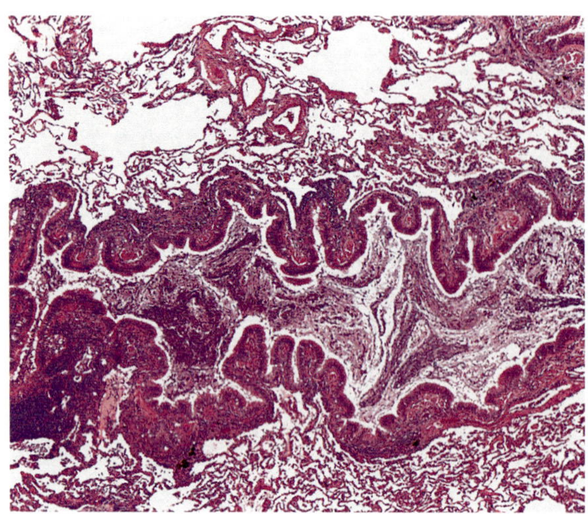

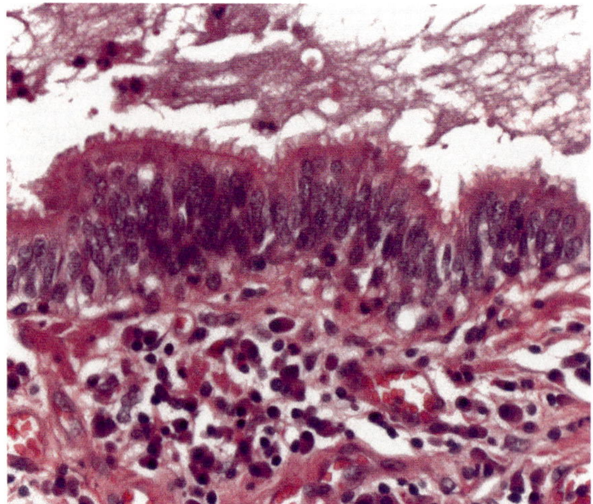

Figure 9-26

PRIMARY CILIARY DYSKINESIA

Histologic sections from an explanted lung from a patient with primary ciliary dyskinesia show nonspecific acute and chronic bronchiolitis (left). Cilia are present and histologically unremarkable (right).

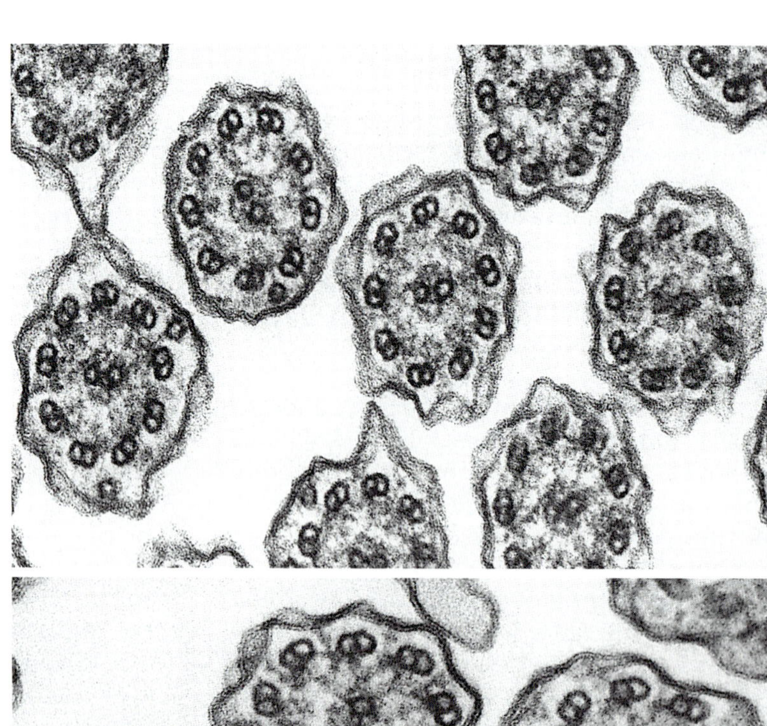

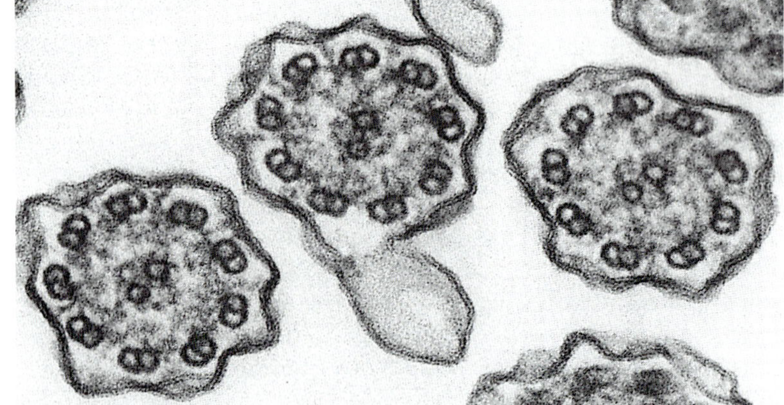

Figure 9-27

PRIMARY CILIARY DYSKINESIA

Ultrastructural features in this case show complete loss of dynein arms, occasional misplaced single tubules near the surface plasma membrane, and some apparent disorganization of radial spokes (top X60,000; bottom X75,000).

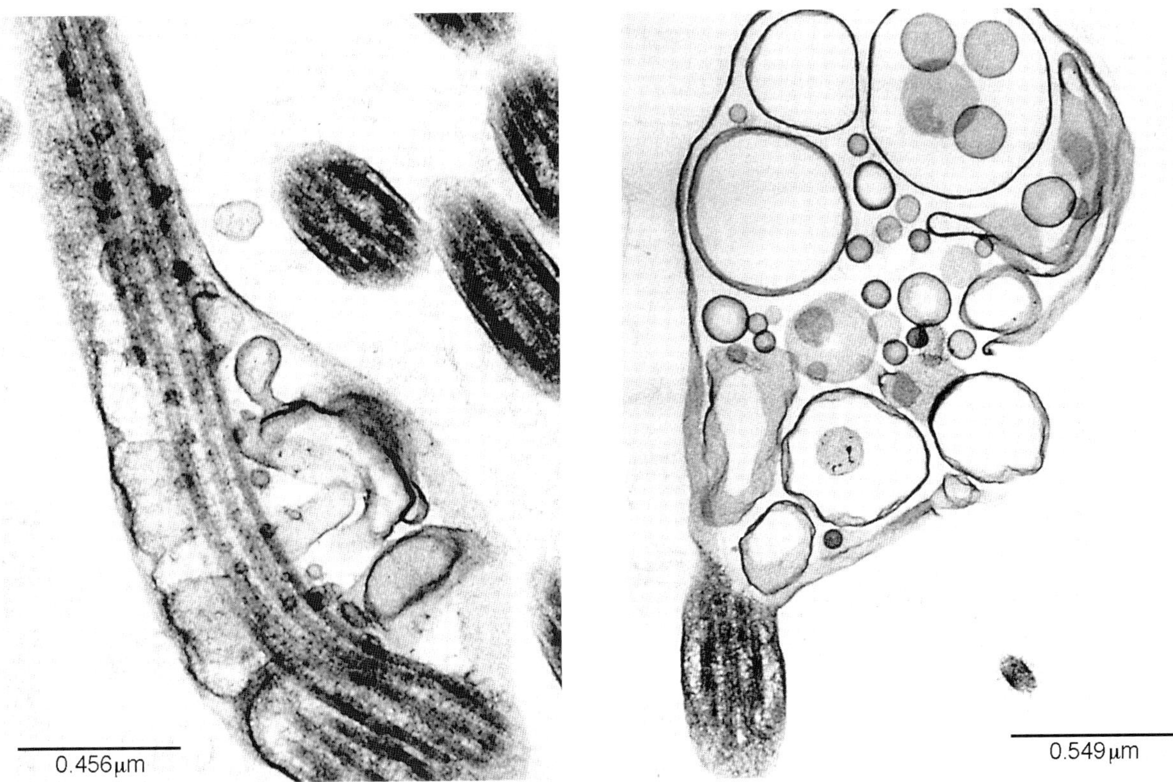

Figure 9-28
BRONCHIECTASIS
Bronchiectasis associated with peculiar cyst-like changes in the cilia. (Figures 3B and 4A from Tsang KW, Tipoe G, Sun J, et al. Severe bronchiectasis in patients with "cystlike" structures within the ciliary shafts. Am J Resp Crit Care Med 2000;161:1300.)

disorientation. Like other ultrastructural abnormalities in primary ciliary dyskinesia (105), ciliary disorientation can also be an acquired abnormality and one that may be reversible with treatment of the inflammatory process (98).

Patients with primary ciliary dyskinesia have been shown to have a significantly lower beat frequency, higher incidence of peripheral and central microtubule defects, and greater ciliary disorientation compared to healthy subjects and those with other respiratory tract diseases, as shown in Table 9-11.

Some other unusual ultrastructural abnormalities in cilia have been reported in bronchiectasis. Kovesi et al. (76) described a patient with bronchiectasis and Down's syndrome in whom there was a partial absence of ciliary walls and peripheral doublets as well as associated abnormal mucociliary transport. Tsang et al. (125) described four young adult patients (ages 18 to 28; 3 female, 1 male) with severe bronchiectasis and a previously undescribed ciliary defect in which there were numerous cyst-like structures within the ciliary shafts (fig. 9-28). The authors interpreted this as a primary defect and postulated that it was the cause of the bronchiectasis in the patients described. Nitric oxide, which can be measured by chemiluminescence, has been found to be reduced in patients with primary ciliary dyskinesia.

Treatment and Prognosis. Treatment of patients with primary ciliary dyskinesia is supportive, with appropriate antibiotic therapy for associated infections (13,114). The prognosis of these patients is much better than for those with cystic fibrosis: individuals may have a normal life span. Approximately 30 percent develop bronchiectasis (13,114).

Table 9-12

CAUSES AND ASSOCIATIONS OF MIDDLE LOBE SYNDROME[a]

Neoplastic Causes
- Benign or malignant
- Primary or metastatic
- They may cause obstruction by:
  - Producing an endobronchial mass or by mural infiltration
  - Extrinsic bronchial compression

Non-Neoplastic Causes and Associations
- Extrinsic bronchial obstruction.
  - Lymphadenopathy/calcification
  - Esophageal traction diverticula
  - Granulomatous infection (tuberculosis), histoplasmosis
  - Occupational dust exposure (e.g., anthraco-silicosis)
  - Reactive lymph node hyperplasia
- Intrinsic bronchial obstruction
  - Foreign body aspiration
  - Edema of bronchial mucosa
  - Submucosal scarring/fibrosis
  - Granulation tissue
  - Mucous plugs/mucoid impaction bronchi (e.g., asthma)
  - Broncholithiasis
  - Endobronchial sarcoidosis
- Nonobstructing conditions (some of which may be secondary)
  - Bronchiectasis
  - Nonspecific chronic inflammation of the bronchus
  - Infarct
  - Bronchial pulmonary cyst

[a]Modified from reference 78.

Table 9-13

CLINICAL FEATURES OF MIDDLE LOBE SYNDROME

Feature		Eskanasay[a] (n = 60)	Kwon et al.[b] (n = 21)
Age:	Mean (Range)	NS[c] (7-59)	47 (5-80)
Sex:	F	37%	71%
	M	63%	29%
Symptoms:			
Cough (+/- productive)		80%	39%
Hemoptysis		32%	29%
Chest pain		47%	20%
Dyspnea		30%	15%
Fever		25%	10%
Other		NS	10%
Asymptomatic		8%	0%
Site:			
Right middle lobe		[d]	53%
Lingula		[d]	19%
Both		[d]	28%

[a]Reference 37.
[b]Reference 78.
[c]NS = not stated.
[d]Only right middle lobes were studied.

MIDDLE LOBE SYNDROME

Definition. Middle lobe syndrome (MLS) is a recurrent or fixed atelectasis or opacification of the right middle lobe or lingula (or both) (9,28,29,37,78,102,106,129). This is a clinical definition that does not necessarily imply recognizable pathology of the large airways, although intrinsic or extrinsic bronchial obstruction is often implicated pathogenetically and bronchiectasis is common. One fourth to half of the cases are caused by malignancies (78,129), and these are excluded from the following discussion.

The term "right middle lobe syndrome" was first used in 1937 to refer to obstructive atelectasis of the right middle lobe by compression from peribronchial lymph nodes (28,78). Tuberculous lymphadenitis was initially implicated. Subsequent studies showed that the lingula could also be affected and that an identifiable obstructive process was not always found (28,78). Causes and associations of MLS from a recent review are shown in Table 9-12. Identifiable causes vary with the series and the population studied. No recognizable pathologic cause for obstruction has been found in an appreciable number of cases (78).

Clinical Features. The signs and symptoms of patients with MLS are primarily those of chronic recurrent atelectasis or inflammation of the right middle lobe or lingula: chronic cough, hemoptysis, chest pain, dyspnea, and fever. Some patients are asymptomatic but have abnormal radiographs. The clinical findings in two large series of patients with MLS are shown in Table 9-13 (37,78). Patients without an identifiable central obstructing lesion tend to be middle-aged or elderly women (78,102). MLS may be a manifestation of severe asthma secondary to mucous plugging of the bronchus (92).

Table 9-14

RADIOLOGIC FINDINGS IN MIDDLE LOBE SYNDROME[a]

Finding	Number Affected (n=9)
Mass-like consolidation	8
Air bronchograms	2
Bronchiectasis	9
Patchy infiltrates	5
Atelectasis	4
Broncholithiasis	1
Bronchostenosis	1
Pleural effusion	1
Volume loss	4
Hilar adenopathy	1

[a]Modified from reference 78.

In the series of Kwon et al. (78), 20 of 21 patients had no identifiable cause for obstruction at the time pathologic evaluation. Thirteen patients had undergone bronchoscopy, and findings included mucosal inflammation, inspissated mucus, and/or narrowing of the bronchi to the middle lobe or lingula; in 2 patients there was severe stenosis with associated broncholithiasis. Thus, an obstructive process was identified more often at bronchoscopy than at gross examination of the resected lobe. In a review by Wagner and Johnson (129), nearly half of the patients with MLS had significant bronchoscopic abnormalities.

Radiologic Findings. The radiographic findings consist of chronic or recurrent atelectasis and consolidation involving the right middle lobe or lingula (Table 9-14; fig. 9-29) (22,78). HRCT frequently shows right middle lobe and lingular bronchiectasis.

Pathologic Findings. The gross and histologic features of MLS (as distinct from those of an obstructing process if one is identified) vary with the activity and chronicity of the inflammatory process at the time of tissue evaluation (figs. 9-29–9-31) (37,78,102,106). The findings of Kwon et al. (78) are shown in Table 9-15.

Table 9-15

PATHOLOGIC FINDINGS IN MIDDLE LOBE SYNDROME[a]

Pathologic Finding	Number Affected (n=21)
Bronchiectasis	10
Bronchiolitis with lymphoid hyperplasia (follicular bronchiolitis)	7
Organizing pneumonia	6
Bronchial lithiasis	1
Atelectasis	5
Granulomatous inflammation	5
Necrotizing granulomas (positive AFB stains in 3; MAI cultured in 2)[b]	3
Non-necrotizing granulomas (*Mycobacterium fortuitum* cultured in 1)	2
Abscesses	4
Hemosiderosis	3
Interstitial fibrosis or honeycomb change	3
Pleural fibrosis	3

[a]Modified from reference 78.
[b]AFB = acid-fast bacilli; MAI = *Mycobacterium avium-intracellulare.*

In individuals with MLS, infection by *Mycobacterium avium-intracellulare* (MAI) or other organisms may be identified and granulomatous inflammation (with or without necrosis) may be apparent histologically (fig. 9-32) (78). This has been termed *Lady Windemere syndrome* (78, 99,129). The traditional view has been that abnormal lung tissue is colonized by these organisms, although recently it has been suggested that the infection may predate, and actually be the cause of, the airway abnormalities (44,103).

Pathogenesis. MLS can result from intrinsic or extrinsic obstruction of the bronchus to the right middle lobe or lingula, causes of which are shown in Table 9-12. MLS can also be found without any identifiable obstruction and many cases in current practice fall into this category (78,102). Poor drainage of the middle lobe bronchus (with secondary transient obstruction and inflammation) and relative anatomic isolation (with decreased collateral ventilation and recurrent atelectasis) have both been pathogenetically implicated in cases of MLS without identifiable obstruction (28,78,102,129). Transient obstruction and/or recurrent atelectasis makes the right middle lobe or lingula prone to recurrent infection, which evolves into a vicious cycle of recurring inflammation and anatomic distortion (28,78,102,129).

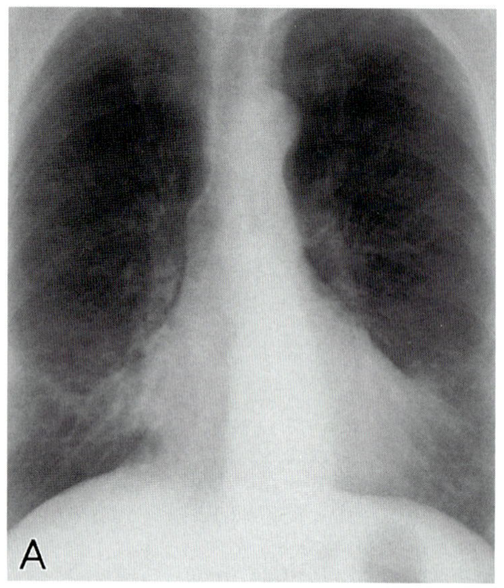

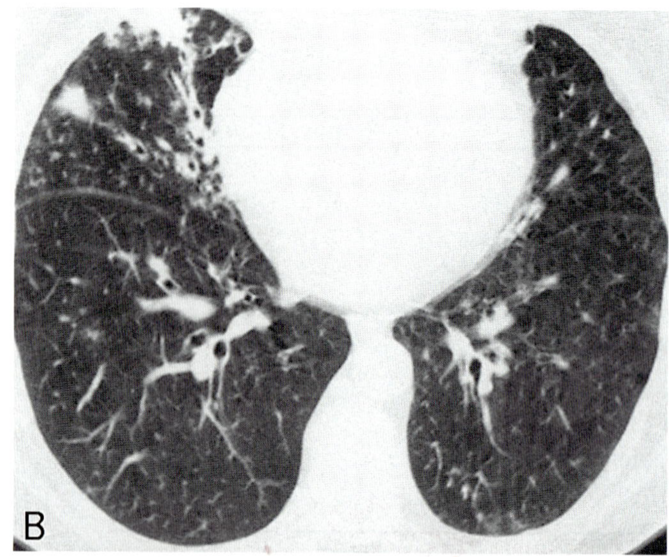

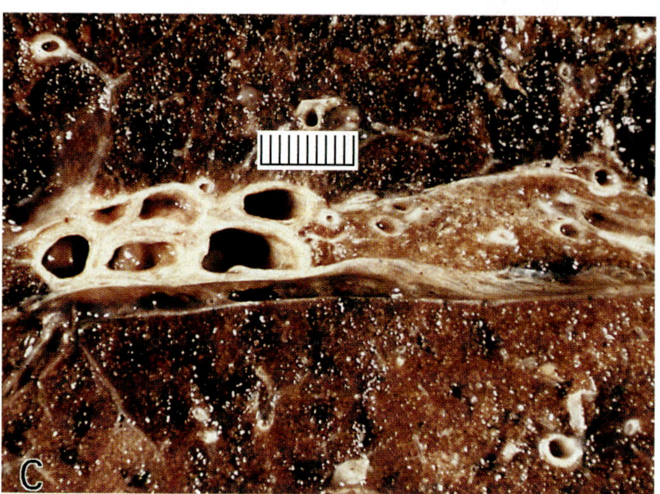

Figure 9-29

MIDDLE LOBE SYNDROME

A: Chest radiograph demonstrates consolidation in the right middle lobe with associated obscuration of the right heart border.

B: HRCT demonstrates bronchiectasis and small foci of consolidation in the right middle lobe.

C: A gross example shows the right middle lobe is severely atelectatic and wedged between the upper and lower lobes. Bronchiectasis is apparent grossly.

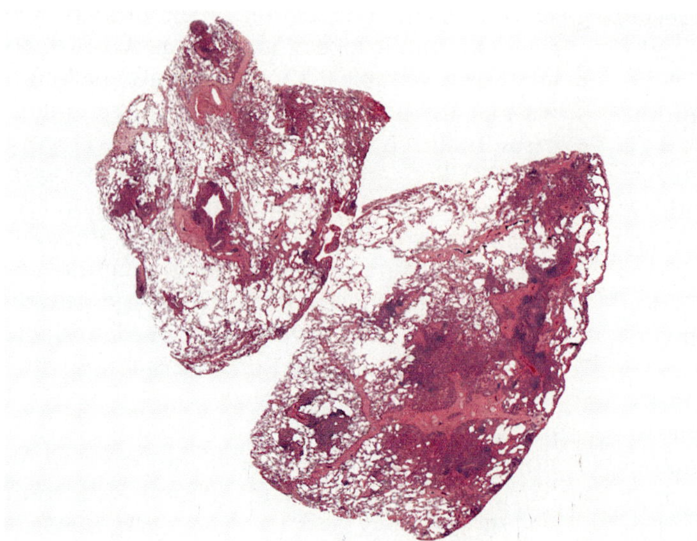

Figure 9-30

MIDDLE LOBE SYNDROME

Scanning power microscopy shows patchy inflammatory changes that include airway-centered inflammation as well as larger zones of inflammation and fibrosis.

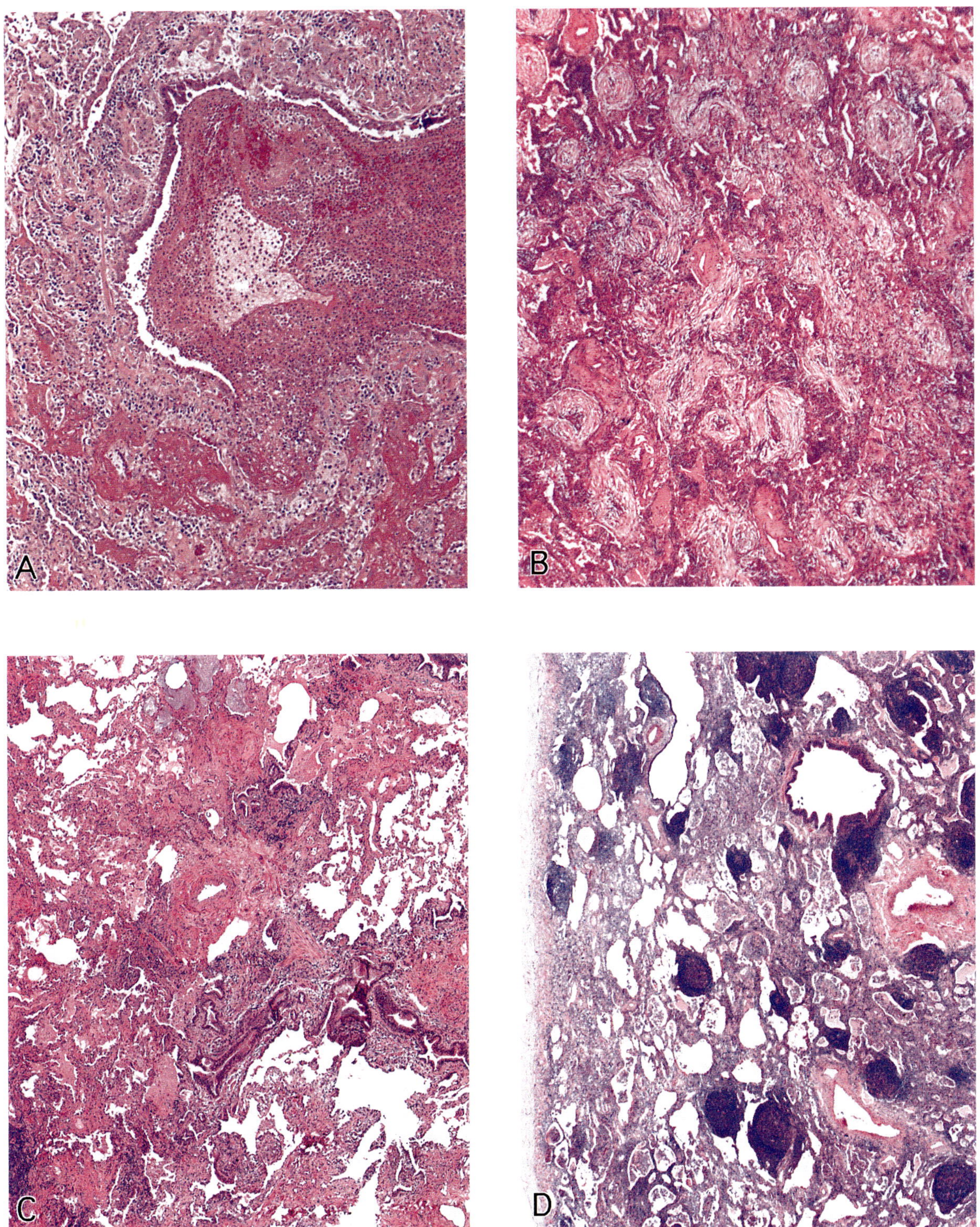

Figure 9-31

MIDDLE LOBE SYNDROME

The spectrum of histologic changes include: acute bronchopneumonia (A), organizing pneumonia (B), chronic interstitial inflammation and fibrosis (C), and lymphoid hyperplasia (D).

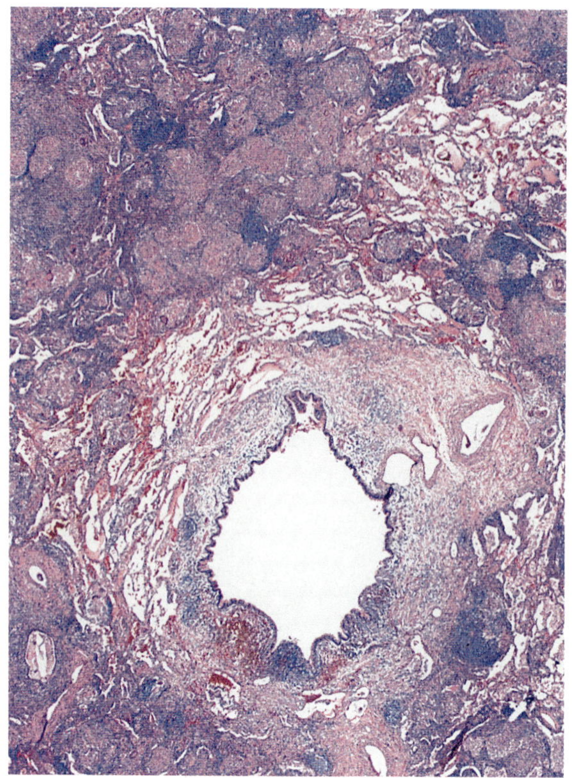
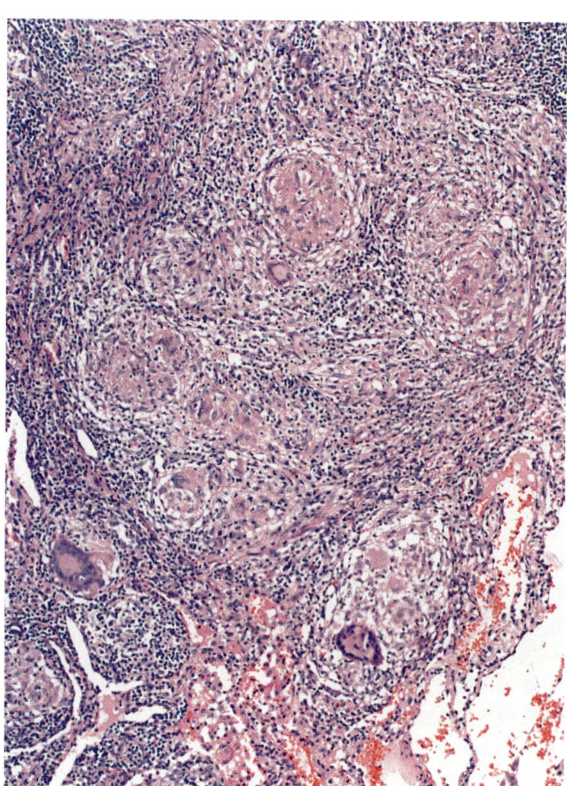

Figure 9-32

MIDDLE LOBE SYNDROME

This is complicated by *Mycobacterium avium-intracellulare* infection which manifests as zones of granulomas. Note the underlying ectatic and inflamed airways.

Diagnosis. The key to making a diagnosis of MLS is the clinical history of disease restricted to the right middle lobe and/or lingula. The histologic findings are nonspecific.

Treatment and Prognosis. Patients with neoplastic causes of MLS should undergo curative surgical resection if feasible (129). Medical management with antibiotics and avoidance of irritating agents (e.g., tobacco) may be associated with clearing of the syndrome. Surgical resection is the treatment of choice for those who fail medical management (129).

BRONCHOCENTRIC GRANULOMATOSIS

Definition. Bronchocentric granulomatosis (BCG) is a bronchocentric and bronchiolocentric necrotizing granulomatous process in which the airway wall is replaced by granulomatous tissue; palisaded histiocytes surround necrotic debris in the airway lumen (68,70,75,87).

BCG can be considered a pathologic reaction pattern with multiple causes that fall into two basic groups: infectious and noninfectious (Table 9-16). The infections that cause BCG are discussed in chapter 12. Noninfectious processes, including primarily allergic bronchopulmonary aspergillosis as well as other rare lesions, are discussed below.

Clinical Features. Most noninfectious cases of BCG are allergic and associated with allergic bronchopulmonary aspergillosis (68,70). About half the patients have a history of chronic asthma. They present with fever, cough, and wheezing. Eosinophilia may be present. Nonasthmatic patients with noninfectious BCG are unusual and are a heterogenous group that may have minimal symptoms or acute fulminant illness (68,70,75). Eosinophilia is generally not present and the radiologic findings resemble those seen in patients with asthma.

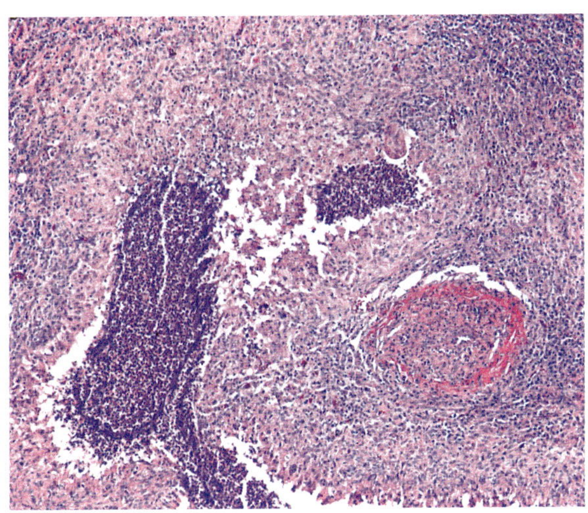
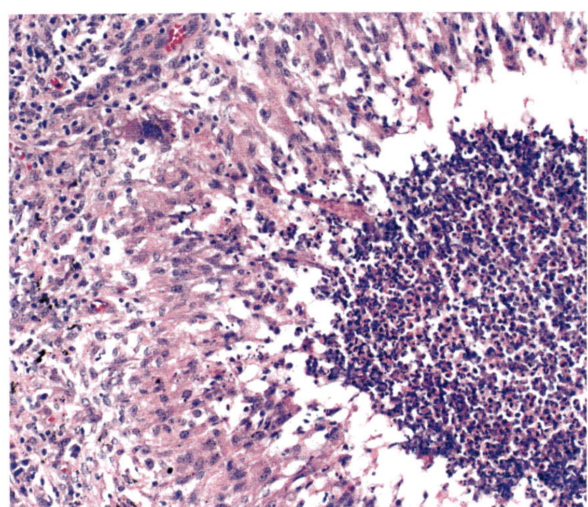

Figure 9-33

BRONCHOCENTRIC GRANULOMATOSIS

Left: Adjacent to a pulmonary artery (lower right) is a zone of bronchiolar destruction with purulent material in the lumen. Right: A palisaded histiocytic reaction replaces the bronchiolar wall.

Mycobacterial cultures should be very carefully followed and bronchocentric Wegener's granulomatosis should be excluded. Many cases of allergic bronchopulmonary aspergillosis are associated with proximal mucoid impaction of the bronchi (see below).

Radiologic Findings. The radiologic findings of BCG associated with mucoid impaction consist of band-like or branching opacities in a precise bronchial distribution. There may be associated airspace consolidation. Manifestations seen mainly in nonasthmatic individuals consist of spiculated nodules or masses measuring 1 to 5 cm in diameter (131). These may occasionally cavitate (131).

Pathologic Findings. BCG is defined histologically by a pattern of necrotizing granulomatous inflammation that destroys the walls of small bronchi and bronchioles (figs. 9-33, 9-34) (68,70,75,87). The airway wall is replaced by a palisading histiocytic reaction with central luminal necrotic debris, including neutrophils and eosinophils. Eosinophils are particularly prominent in cases of allergic bronchopulmonary aspergillosis but they are also a frequent finding in coccidioidomycosis-associated BCG.

BCG can arise from an acute and chronic cellular bronchiolitis in which there is progressive ulceration and loss of the bronchiolar mucosa and wall, with replacement of it by a palisaded histiocytic reaction (fig. 9-34). In BCG associated with mucoid impaction of the bronchi, the proximal airways show impaction with allergic type mucin (see below). The lung parenchyma distal to BCG frequently shows a mixed inflammatory reaction, typical of obstructive pneumonia, as well as scattered granulomas. In allergic cases, eosinophilic pneumonia may be present.

Table 9-16

CAUSES OF BRONCHOCENTRIC GRANULOMATOSIS[a]

Infections
Mycobacterial
Fungal—histoplasmosis, blastomycosis, coccidioidomycosis, mucormycosis, aspergillosis (nonallergic)
Parasitic—echinococcosis
Allergic
Allergic bronchopulmonary fungal disease (especially allergic aspergillosis in association with mucoid impaction of the bronchi)
Noninfectious
Wegener's granulomatosis
Rheumatoid arthritis

[a]Compiled from references 68, 70, 75, 87, and personal experience.

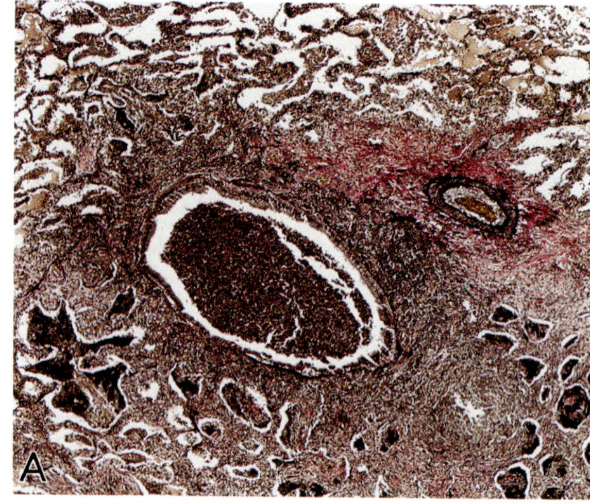

Figure 9-34

BRONCHOCENTRIC GRANULOMATOSIS

The development of bronchocentric granulomatosis can be traced from a chronic bronchiolitis with an intact bronchiolar elastica (A) to partial (B) and then nearly complete (C) destruction of the elastica of the bronchioles and replacement of the bronchiolar wall by a palisaded histiocytic reaction around central necrotic debris.

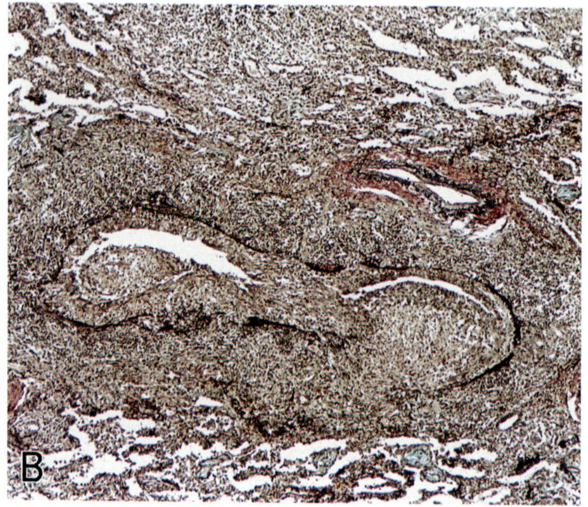

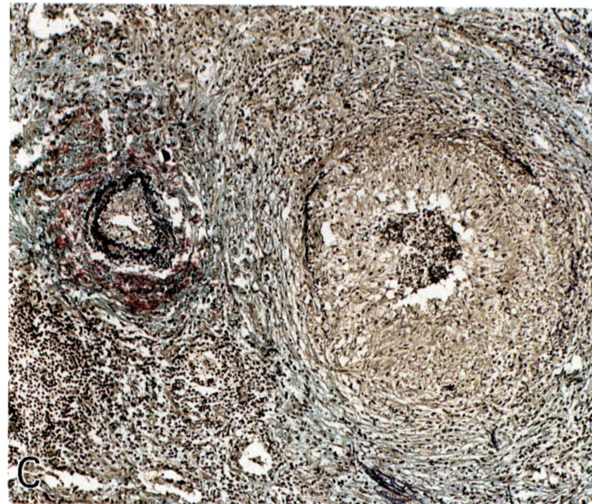

Giant cells may be present. Necrotic eosinophil debris sometimes induces a giant cell reaction resembling a foreign body reaction. While the inflammatory process centers on the airways, there may be some secondary inflammation involving vessel walls. In patients with a history of asthma, asthmatic changes may be noted in airways not involved by the BCG reaction. BCG resembles any infectious granuloma except for its bronchocentric location, which sometimes can only be inferred by identification of the adjacent pulmonary artery. In all cases, a routine battery of special stains for microorganisms is indicated. In some patients with infectious BCG, special stains may be negative and a diagnosis possible only after the results of tissue culture are available. In allergic bronchopulmonary aspergillosis, hyphal fragments may be found in the proximal mucoid impaction and, occasionally, in the BCG reaction itself (68).

Differential Diagnosis. The finding of a BCG pattern should lead to consideration of the lesions shown in Table 9-16. Primary consideration should be given to excluding an infection (fig. 9-35) and Wegener's granulomatosis (fig. 9-36), and determining whether there is evidence of asthma or allergic bronchopulmonary aspergillosis. Features helpful in the last situation include elevated IgE levels and serum precipitins to *Aspergillus*.

The key histologic finding in BCG is destruction of the airway wall and its replacement by a palisaded histiocytic reaction. The presence of chronic bronchitis or chronic bronchiolitis with only scattered necrotizing or non-necrotizing

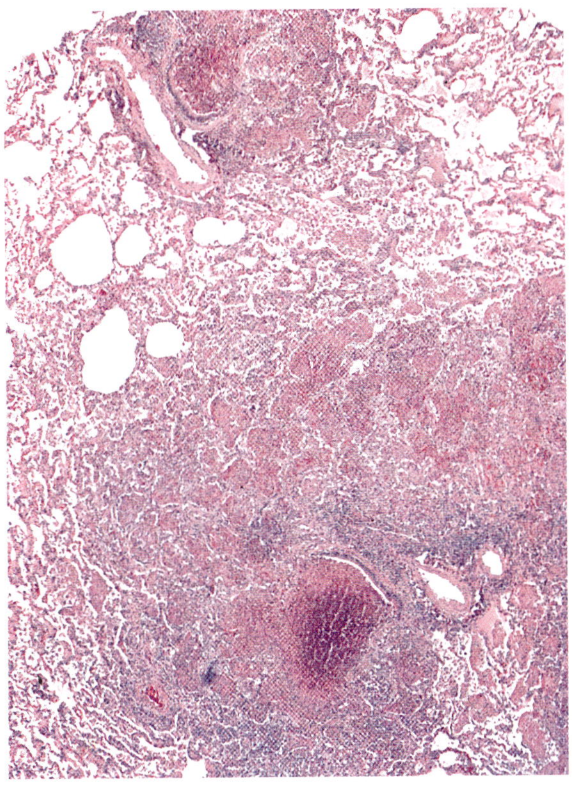

Figure 9-35

COCCIDIOIDOMYCOSIS

Bronchocentric necrotizing lesions of coccidioidomycosis are indistinguishable from noninfectious bronchocentric granulomatosis.

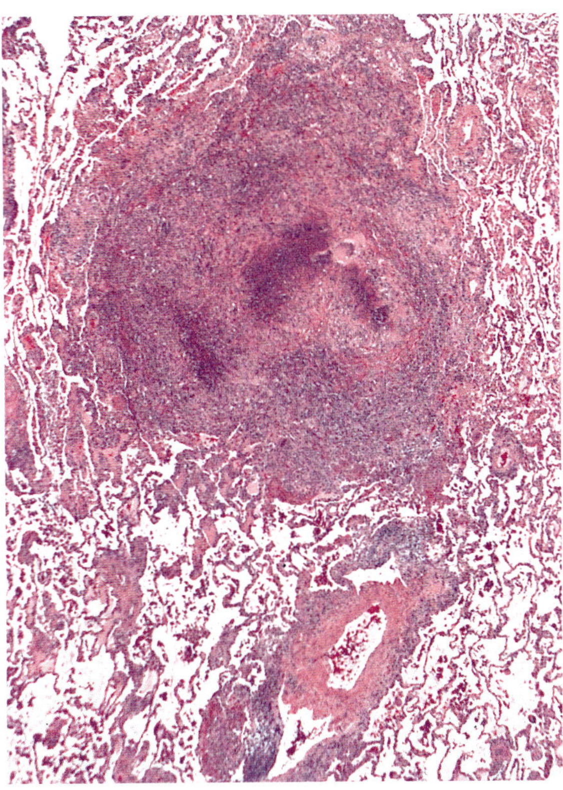

Figure 9-36

BRONCHOCENTRIC WEGENER'S GRANULOMATOSIS

Wegener's granulomatosis with marked bronchiolocentricity. There is destruction of the bronchiole with necrosis surrounded by a palisaded histiocytic rim.

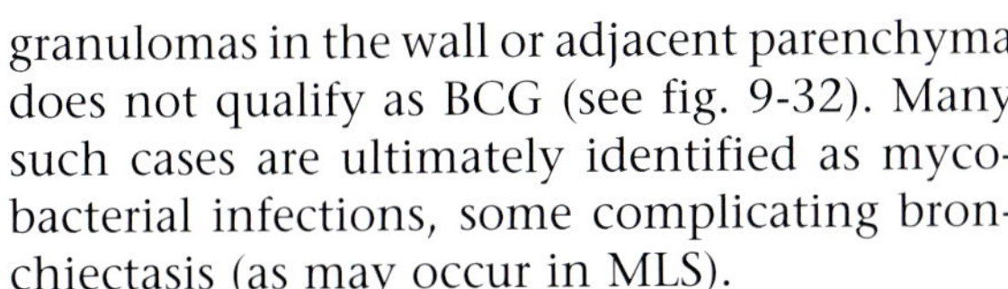

granulomas in the wall or adjacent parenchyma does not qualify as BCG (see fig. 9-32). Many such cases are ultimately identified as mycobacterial infections, some complicating bronchiectasis (as may occur in MLS).

Foreign body aspiration may produce a granulomatous bronchitis or bronchiolitis (fig. 9-37). Foreign debris may be apparent in the lumen and the granulomatous reaction typically manifests as individual or clusters of giant cells associated with foreign material. There is often an acute inflammation that may surround the aspirated material, but complete destruction of the bronchial wall and its replacement by a palisaded histiocytic reaction is unusual.

Wegener's granulomatosis may be bronchocentric or bronchiolocentric (fig. 9-36). In such cases, features of Wegener's granulomatosis are typically present elsewhere: vasculitis, microabscesses, and a necrotizing granulomatous reaction involving consolidated parenchyma.

Sarcoidosis is commonly associated with granulomatous involvement of the airways. Usual features of sarcoidosis include coalescing non-necrotizing granulomas involving the airway wall without associated necrosis and with little associated inflammation. However, in necrotizing sarcoidosis, necrosis is present and may be bronchocentric.

Necrotizing bronchocentric granulomas have also been reported with rheumatoid arthritis (68).

Treatment. Steroids are the treatment of choice for both allergic and nonallergic BCG (68). Lesions associated with extensive parenchymal destruction or that are refractory to treatment (including some that may be associated mucoid impaction) may require resection.

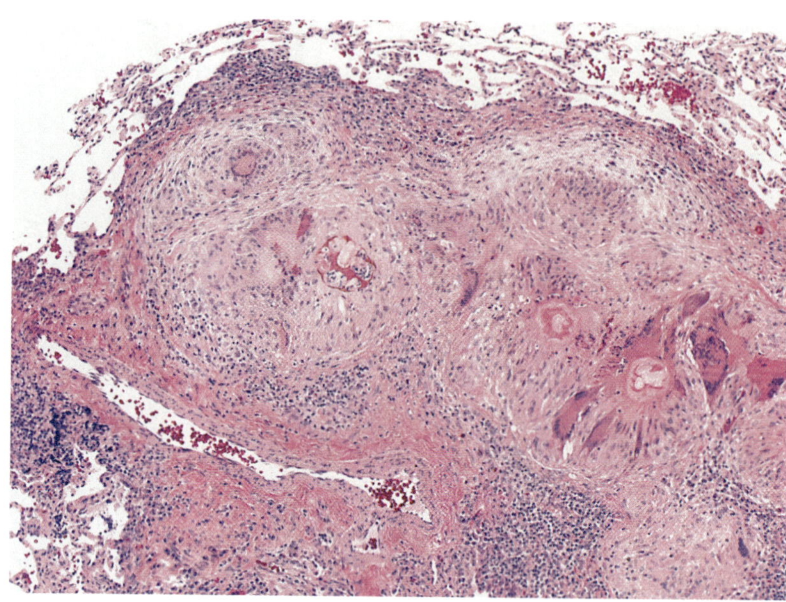

Figure 9-37
CHRONIC ASPIRATION BRONCHIOLITIS

There is a granulomatous reaction around foreign food material in the bronchiolar lumen. The wall is replaced by fibrosis, chronic inflammation, and a granulomatous reaction.

MUCOID IMPACTION OF BRONCHI

Definition. Mucoid impaction of bronchi is used here to refer to a distinctive clinicopathological syndrome consisting of mucous plugs in dilated segmental or subsegmental bronchi and a distinctive mucus appearance, so-called "allergic mucin" (59–61,69,70). Mucoid impaction has been used in the radiologic literature for any process associated with inspissated secretions; the causes are many and heterogeneous (39).

Clinical Features. Most patients with mucoid impaction of bronchi have underlying allergic disease, often asthma and allergic bronchopulmonary aspergillosis with BCG (see above) (59–61,69). In some cases the predisposing condition is chronic bronchitis or cystic fibrosis. Patients may be asymptomatic and found to have a radiologic abnormality, have signs and symptoms associated with obstructive pneumonia distal to the mucoid impaction, or have signs and symptoms related to the underlying condition.

Radiologic Findings. The characteristic radiologic manifestation is the presence of band-like or branching densities in a precise bronchial distribution, usually involving the upper lobes (fig. 9-38). These band-like and branching opacities have been variously described as having a "gloved finger," "inverted Y or V," or "cluster of grapes" appearance. Occasionally, a single focus of mucoid impaction presents as a solitary nodule. Following expectoration of a mucous plug, residual bronchial dilatation may be evident on the chest radiograph or HRCT scan; in the latter, the mucoid impaction and bronchiectasis involve mainly the segmental and subsegmental bronchi of the upper lobes (2,88). Bronchoscopy with bronchial biopsy and washing may detect mucoid impaction and its cause in some patients (5).

Pathologic Findings. Grossly, the affected bronchi are dilated and contain firm, rubbery, and grayish to greenish to brownish mucus (figs. 9-39–9-41) (59–61,69). Similar mucous plugs may be expectorated.

Histologically, the mucus shows a laminated appearance with abundant eosinophilic debris, including Charcot-Leyden crystals (figs. 9-41, 9-42) (5,59,61,69). There are layers of mucus, fibrin, eosinophils, eosinophilic debris, Charcot-Leyden crystals, neutrophils, and necrotic material. Charcot-Leyden crystals are elongated, sometimes hexagonal, bright eosinophilic crystals ranging in size from a few microns to 100 µm. The affected bronchi show underlying changes of asthma as well as mural thinning and fibrosis, muscular and cartilaginous atrophy, and epithelial metaplasia including squamous metaplasia. Submucosal mixed chronic inflammatory infiltrates (including eosinophils) are present. Within the mucin, fungal stains may demonstrate fragments of

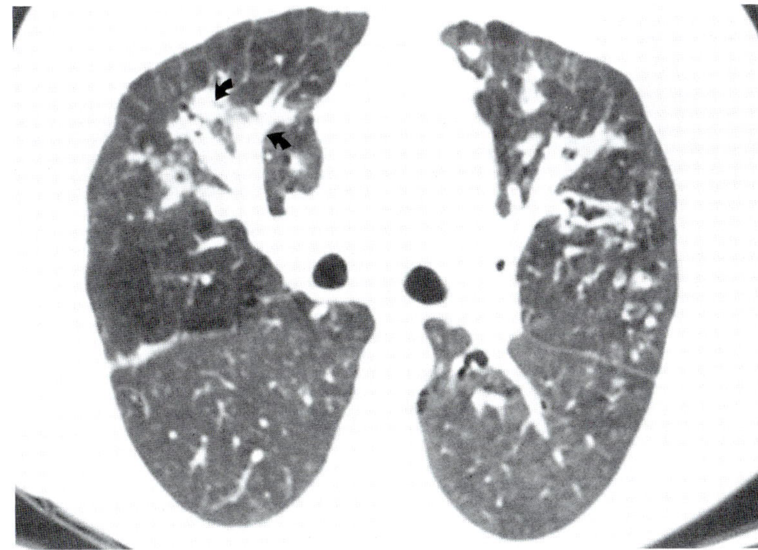

Figure 9-38

MUCOID IMPACTION

HRCT in a 46-year-old woman demonstrates branching finger-like opacities (arrows) involving the anterior segment of the right upper lobe. These were bronchoscopically proven to be due to mucoid impaction. Localized areas of bronchiectasis are present in the left upper lobe.

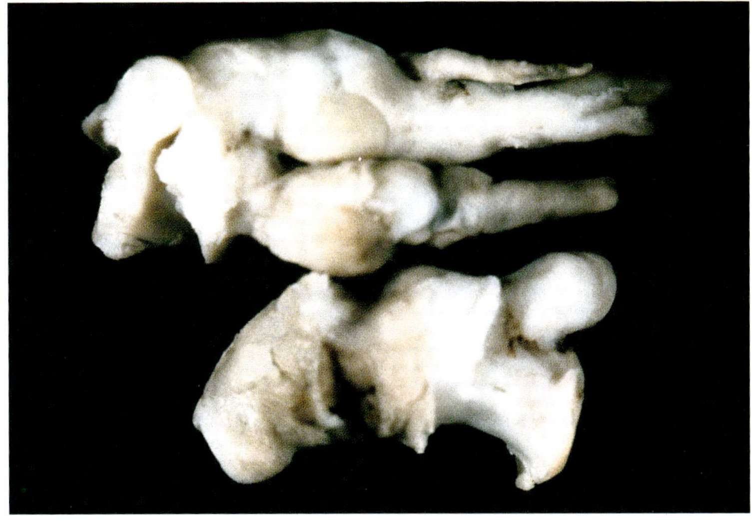

Figure 9-39

MUCOID IMPACTION OF BRONCHI

Mucoid impaction of bronchi with a mucous cast of the bronchiectatic airway from which it originated.

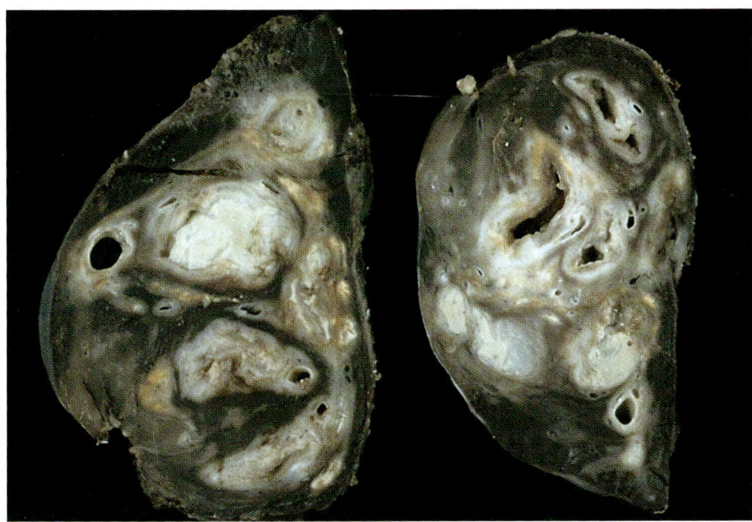

Figure 9-40

MUCOID IMPACTION OF BRONCHI

Mucoid impaction of bronchi with plugs of mucus filling markedly dilated airways.

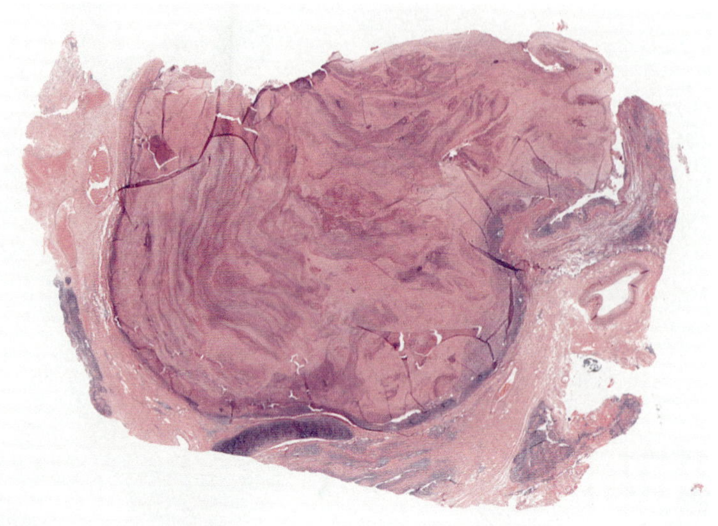

Figure 9-41

MUCOID IMPACTION OF BRONCHI

The layered impacted mucus is apparent histologically.

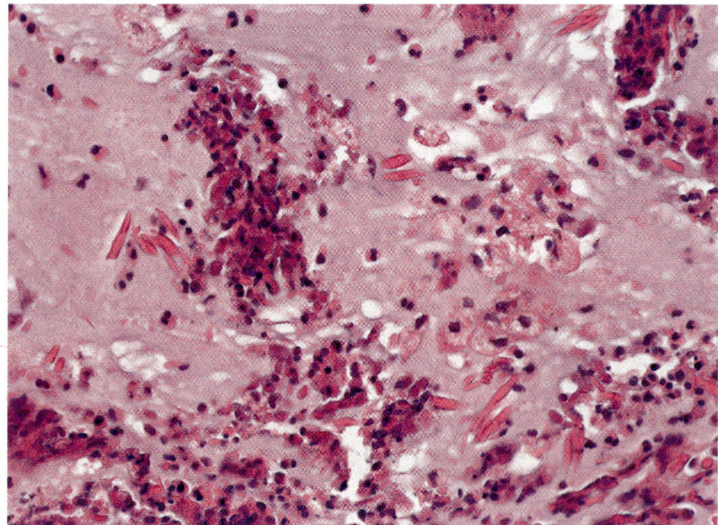

Figure 9-42

MUCOID IMPACTION OF BRONCHI

Allergic mucin is layered and there is cell debris in which brightly eosinophilic Charcot-Leyden crystals were identified.

fungal hyphae in cases of allergic bronchopulmonary fungal disease (fig. 9-43).

Differential Diagnosis. Mucus in airways is extremely common since it may be a feature of cigarette-related COPD and asthma. Mucoid impaction of bronchi must be distinguished from mucous plugs distal to obstruction, mucous plugs in otherwise uncomplicated asthma and COPD, and plastic bronchitis (see below) (69). Mucous plugs may also be seen in cystic fibrosis, a condition that may be complicated by allergic bronchopulmonary fungal disease (74). The feature that sets mucoid impaction of the bronchi apart from these conditions and allows recognition of its allergic nature is its dense laminated character with intervening eosinophils, eosinophilic debris, and Charcot-Leyden crystals. These features are not seen in mucous plugs in COPD, asthma, and distal to an obstruction.

The presence of allergic-type mucin should alert one to the possibility of allergic bronchopulmonary fungal disease, particularly allergic bronchopulmonary aspergillosis (see below). In general, when mucous plugs are submitted to the pathology laboratory, they should be examined for organisms, particularly whether or not fungal hyphae can be identified, and for features of allergic mucin.

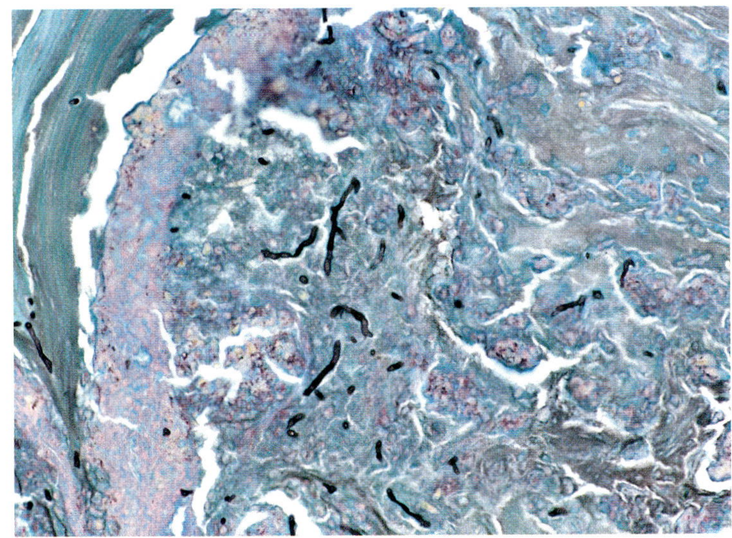

Figure 9-43

MUCOID IMPACTION OF BRONCHI

In allergic bronchopulmonary fungal disease fragments of fungal hyphae are frequently identified in the mucus.

Treatment. Most cases of mucoid impaction of bronchi are associated with allergic bronchopulmonary aspergillosis and treatment for that condition is discussed in the next section.

ALLERGIC BRONCHOPULMONARY FUNGAL DISEASE

Definition. Allergic bronchopulmonary fungal disease (primarily *allergic bronchopulmonary aspergillosis* [ABPA]) is a clinical syndrome typically found in chronic asthmatics who develop hypersensitivity to various fungi, particularly *Aspergillus fumigatus* (17,25,40,49,50,69,70, 100). Other fungi occasionally implicated include *Curvularia lunata, Drechslera hawaiiensis, Helminthosporium, Torulopsis glabrata, Candida albicans, Bipolaris* sp, *Pseudoallescheria boydii,* and *Fusarium vasinfectum* (69).

Clinical Features. Allergic bronchopulmonary aspergillosis may be suspected when an individual with asthma develops eosinophilia, fleeting pulmonary opacities, *A. fumigatus* in the sputum cultures, an immediate cutaneous reaction to *Aspergillus,* elevated serum IgE, precipitating antibodies to *Aspergillus,* elevated antibody levels (particularly IgE and IgG) to *Aspergillus,* and central bronchiectases (17,26,40, 49,50,69,100). Elevated IgE antibodies to *Aspergillus* and central bronchiectasis are almost pathognomonic of allergic bronchopulmonary aspergillosis. Allergic bronchopulmonary aspergillosis may occur in the absence of asthma (48), or manifest as episodic disease with symptom-free intervals between attacks (19). In these patients the diagnosis is best supported by the following criteria: total serum IgE greater than 1,000 ng/mL, an immediate prick test reaction to *Aspergillus,* presence of precipitins against *A. fumigatus,* and presence of bronchiectasis on chest radiograph or HRCT scan.

In patients who clinically appear to have allergic bronchopulmonary fungal disease, but in whom immunoreactivity to *A. fumigatos* is negative or lung biopsy shows an unusual fungal morphology, an unusual fungal species should be suspected.

Radiologic Findings. The radiologic findings in allergic bronchopulmonary fungal disease include all the various combinations of mucoid impaction (fig. 9-44), BCG, and eosinophilic pneumonia. Ward and colleagues (132) showed that the HRCT findings most commonly seen in patients with allergic bronchopulmonary aspergillosis include bronchiectasis (95 percent of the subjects), centrilobular nodules (93 percent), and mucoid impaction (67 percent) (24,132). The bronchiectasis is bilateral and predominantly in the upper lobes.

Pathologic Findings. The pathologic changes include (combinations of) mucoid impaction of bronchi (see above), BCG (see above), eosinophilic pneumonia (chapter 3), and asthma (chapter 10) (figs. 9-45–9-53). The specific features of these patterns are described elsewhere (122a).

Treatment. Allergic pulmonary fungal disease is treated with oral corticosteroids. While

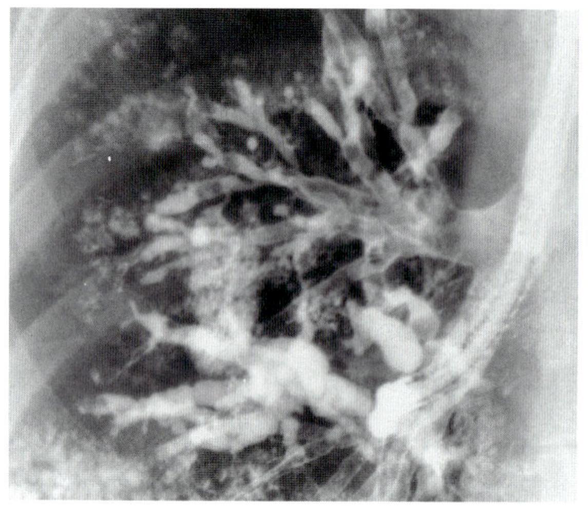

Figure 9-44
ALLERGIC BRONCHOPULMONARY ASPERGILLOSIS
This bronchogram illustrates ectatic bronchi.

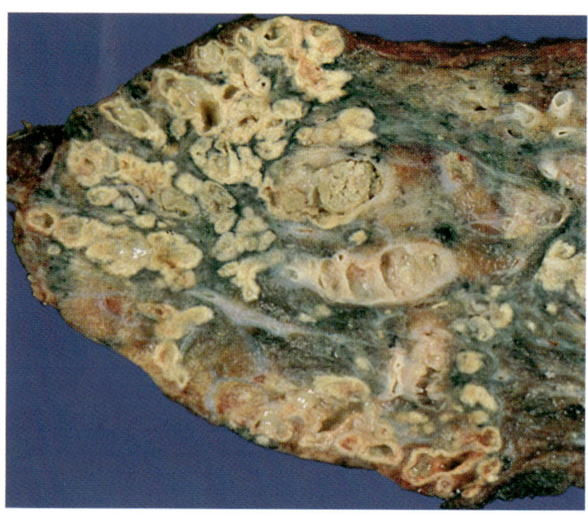

Figure 9-45
ALLERGIC BRONCHOPULMONARY ASPERGILLOSIS
There is marked bronchiectasis and mucoid impaction.

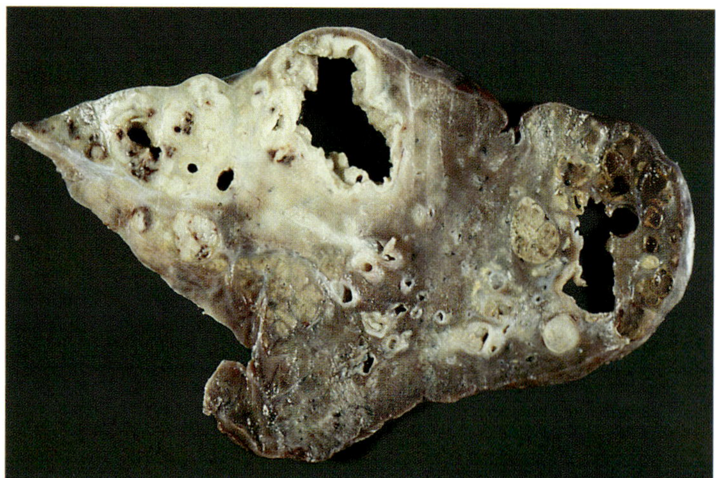

Figure 9-46
ALLERGIC BRONCHOPULMONARY ASPERGILLOSIS

This gross specimen shows bronchiectasia as well as a zone of consolidation and purulent necrosis corresponding to foci of bronchocentric granulomatosis.

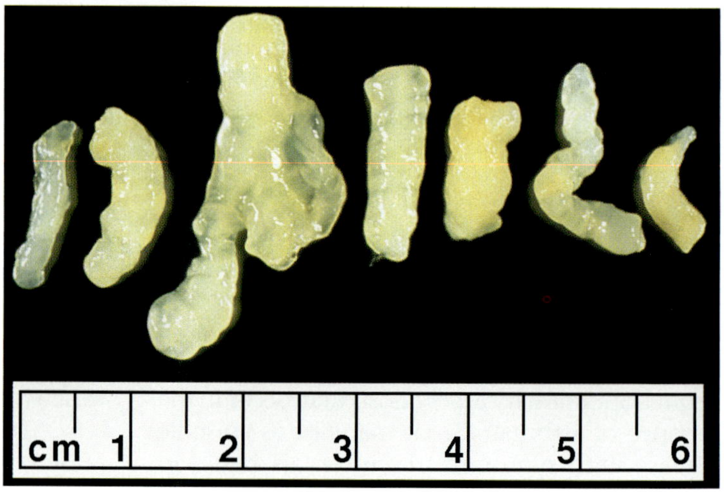

Figure 9-47
ALLERGIC BRONCHOPULMONARY ASPERGILLOSIS

Plugs of allergic mucin retrieved bronchoscopically.

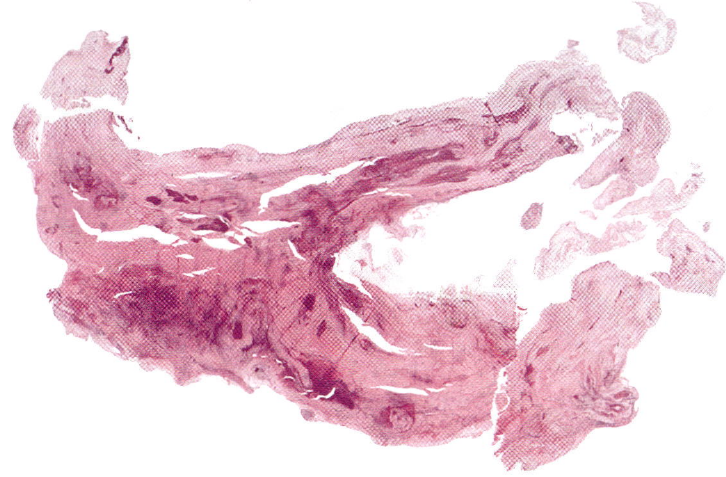

Figure 9-48
ALLERGIC BRONCHOPULMONARY ASPERGILLOSIS
Typical allergic layered mucin and eosinophilic cellular debris.

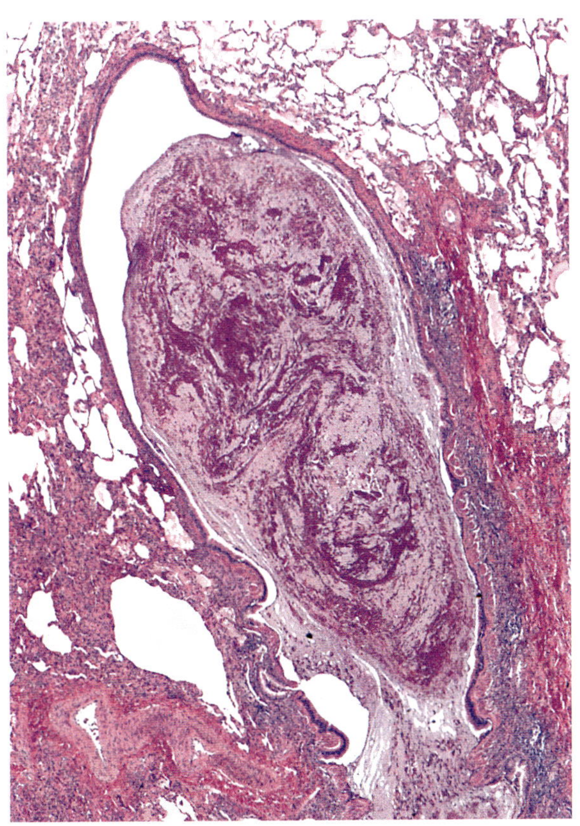

Figure 9-49
ALLERGIC BRONCHOPULMONARY ASPERGILLOSIS
The allergic mucin extends into ectatic bronchioles.

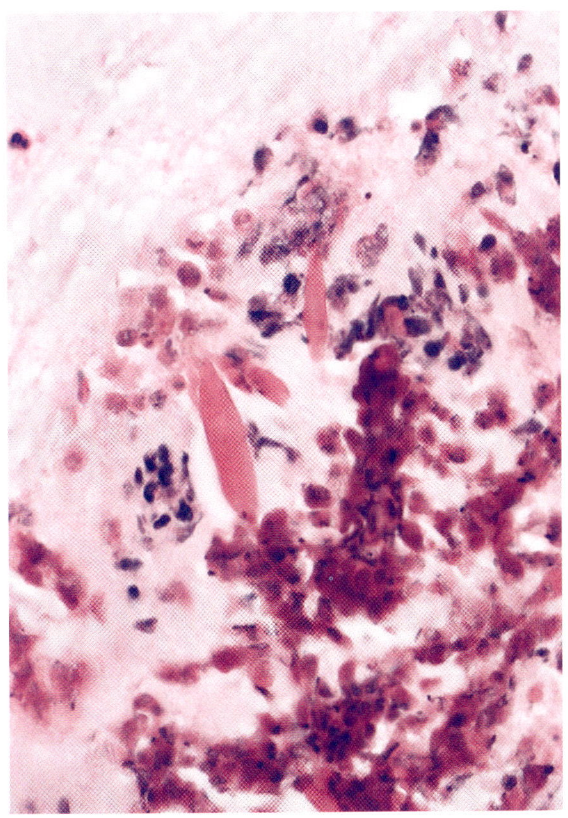

Figure 9-50
ALLERGIC BRONCHOPULMONARY ASPERGILLOSIS
Allergic mucin contains degenerating cellular debris (primarily eosinophils), mucin, and large pink Charcot-Leyden crystals.

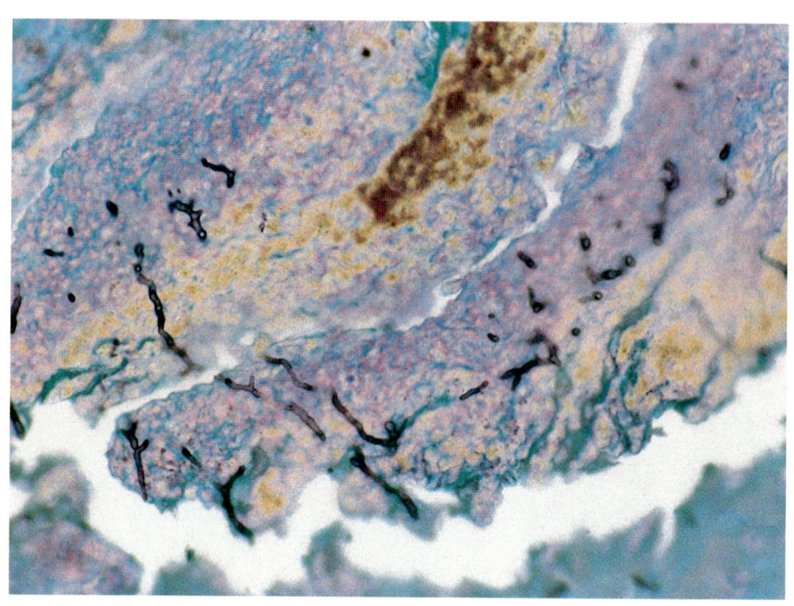

Figure 9-51

ALLERGIC BRONCHOPULMONARY ASPERGILLOSIS

The degenerating hyphae of *Aspergillus* are apparent in the mucin.

A

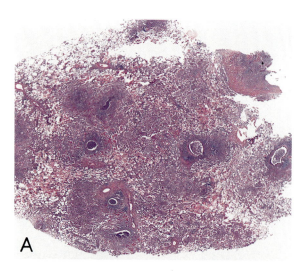

Figure 9-52

ALLERGIC BRONCHOPULMONARY ASPERGILLOSIS: THE SPECTRUM OF HISTOLOGIC CHANGES

Scanning power shows an airway-centered inflammatory process (A) in which some foci of classic bronchocentric granulomatosis are apparent (B,C).

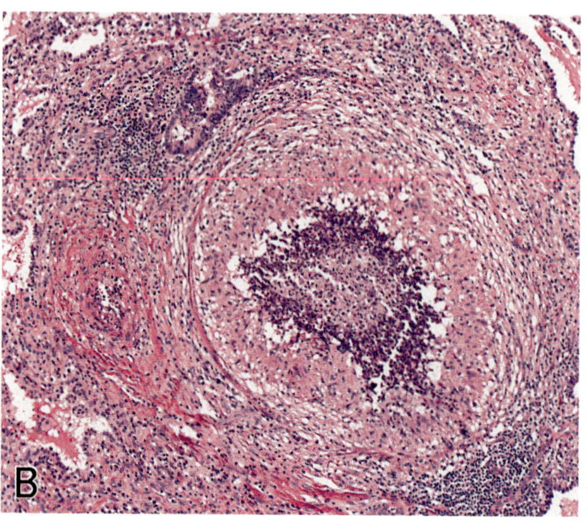

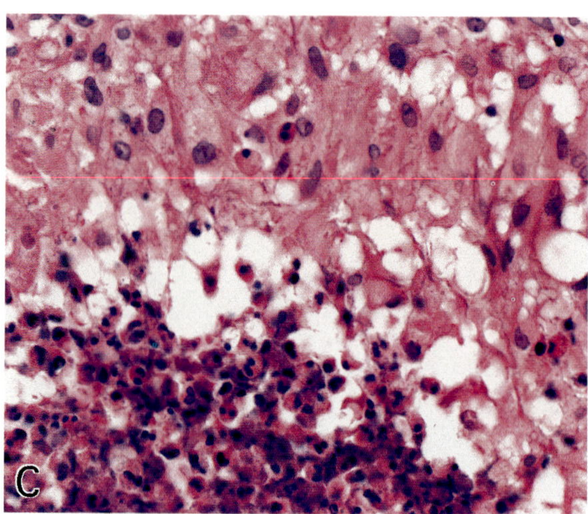

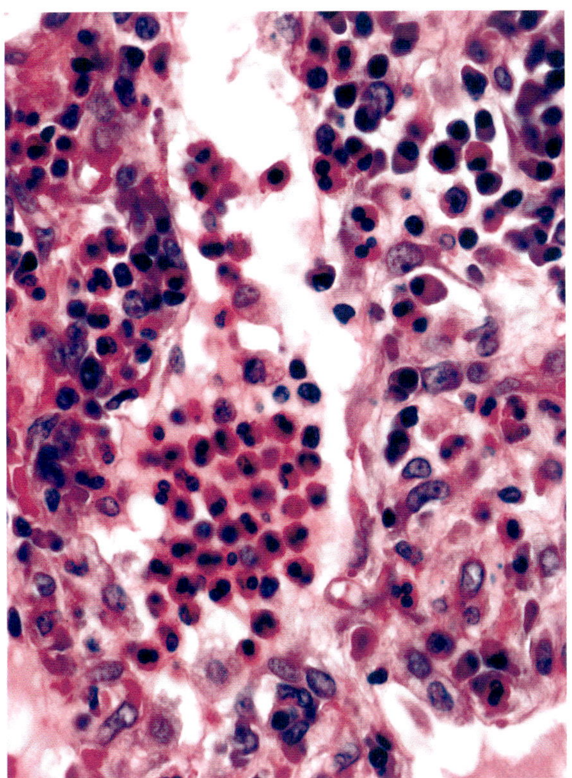

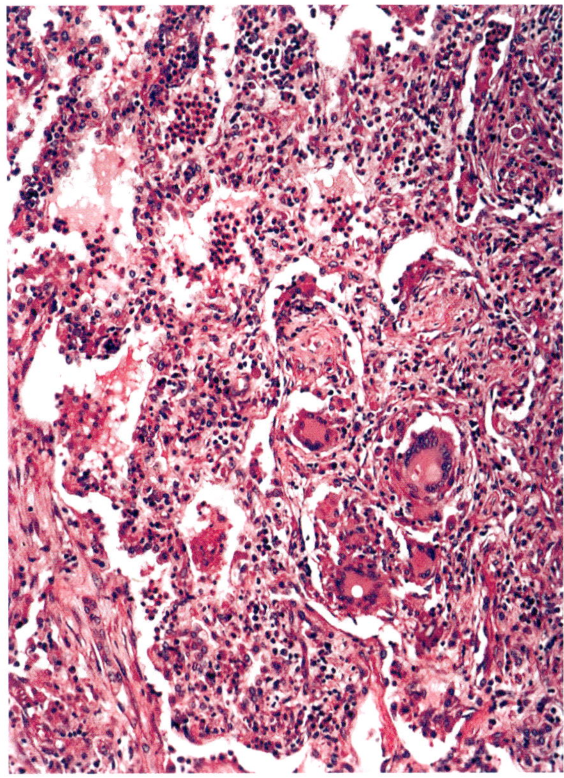

Figure 9-53

ALLERGIC BRONCHOPULMONARY ASPERGILLOSIS: THE SPECTRUM OF HISTOLOGIC CHANGES

Left: A field of eosinophilic pneumonia.

Right: The surrounding lung tissue shows scattered non-necrotizing granulomas.

recurrences are common, early stages of the disease may be reversible (69,100). The chances of cure are decreased in higher stage disease when irreversible damage to the large airways has occurred. Itraconazole may have a role in therapy for patients who have not responded to corticosteroid therapy or who are unable to continue it because of side effects, however, controlled studies are needed (65). Control of the patient's asthma and declines in serum IgE (usually not to normal but to a plateau level that varies from patient to patient) are the best markers to follow in deciding on the dose of prednisone therapy (97).

PLASTIC BRONCHITIS

Definition. Plastic bronchitis is a clinical entity characterized by large bronchial casts of inspissated secretion (16,62,96). Synonyms include *fibrinous bronchitis* and *pseudomembranous bronchitis*.

Clinical Features. Symptoms include dyspnea, wheeze, cough, fever, and hemoptysis (16, 62,96). Some symptoms relate to the underlying bronchopulmonary disease (see below). The large bronchial casts characteristic of plastic bronchitis are usually expectorated, found and removed at bronchoscopy, or identified at the time of surgery or autopsy (24,81,97).

Radiologic Findings. The radiologic findings include segmental, lobar, or occasionally, whole lung consolidation or atelectasis (24,81,97).

Pathologic Findings. The gross features of plastic bronchitis are the most dramatic (and defining of the entity): large branching casts that can be many centimeters in length (fig. 9-54) (16,62,96). Histologically, the casts are composed of fibrin, mucus, and inflammatory cells, primarily lymphocytes and histiocytes (fig. 9-55). Infiltration by eosinophils and features of allergic mucin (see Mucoid Impaction) are lacking (62,96).

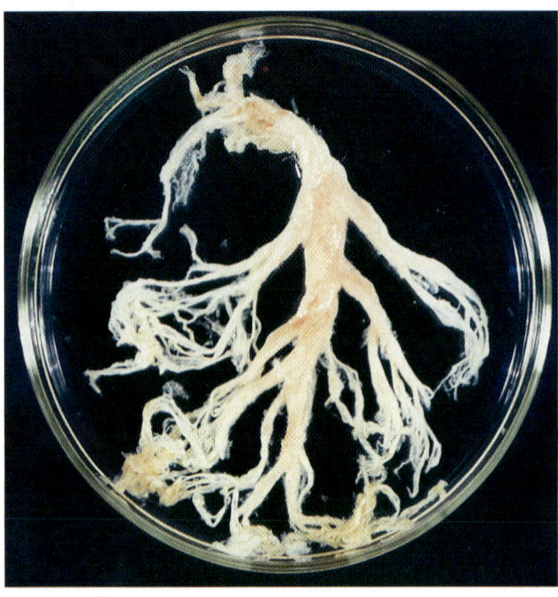

Figure 9-54
BRONCHIAL CAST IN PLASTIC BRONCHITIS

The lung tissue from which the casts are removed may show evidence of obstructive pneumonia and acute and chronic bronchitis or bronchiolitis.

Pathogenesis. Bronchial casts may be found in a variety of bronchopulmonary diseases (39,62,86,96); in some cases there is no apparent underlying disease or association. It is not clear when the designation plastic bronchitis is appropriate in contrast to bronchial casts complicating one of the defined entities shown in Table 9-17. It is reasonable to consider the diagnosis of plastic bronchitis when no obvious underlying cause or association can be identified and to make a designation of secondary bronchial casts when a specific entity can be implicated.

Differential Diagnosis. Plastic bronchitis is defined by the gross appearance and the absence histologically of features of allergic mucin. The main differential diagnosis is mucoid impaction of bronchi, discussed in the previous

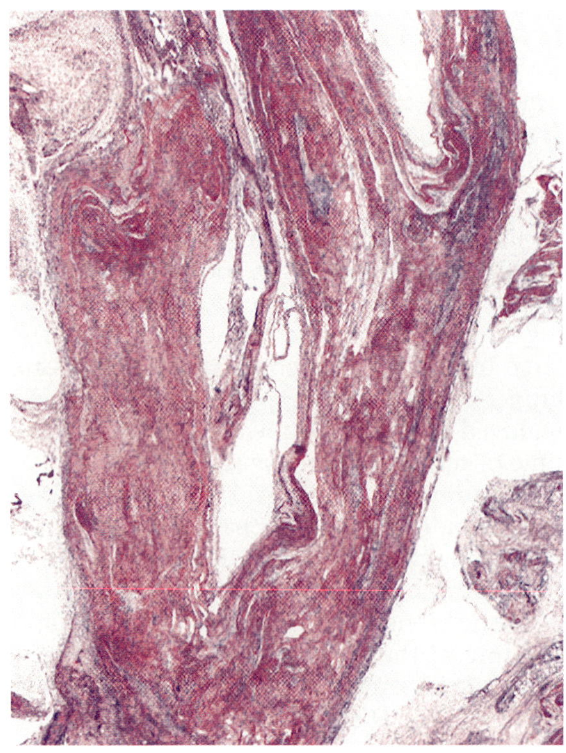

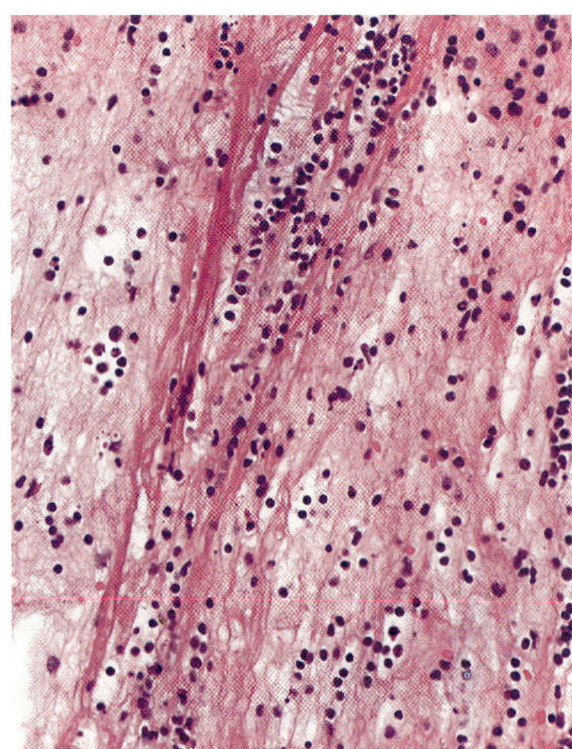

Figure 9-55
PLASTIC BRONCHITIS
The bronchial casts in plastic bronchitis are composed of mucin and scattered inflammatory cells, primarily mononuclear cells. Features of allergic mucin are not apparent.

section. The causes and associations of plastic bronchitis are shown in Table 9-17. Since plastic bronchitis is a clinically defined lesion, a number of clinicopathologic entities are included in this table, and some have questioned the existence of plastic bronchitis as an entity (86).

Treatment and Prognosis. The treatment and prognosis of patients with plastic bronchitis depend on the underlying condition (if any) (16,62,96). For cases without identifiable cause or association treatment is supportive, including bronchodilators, antibiotics, hydration, physical therapy, and postural drainage. The prognosis is favorable. Bronchoscopic or surgical removal of casts may be necessary in some cases. Steroids have been shown to be of some benefit. Spontaneous remission as well as late exacerbations are known to occur.

Table 9-17

CAUSES AND ASSOCIATIONS OF BRONCHIAL CASTS (PLASTIC BRONCHITIS)[a]

Asthma
Mucoid impaction of bronchi (allergic bronchopulmonary fungal disease)
Cystic fibrosis
Bronchiectasis
Infections: *Diphtheria, Hemophilus, Klebsiella,* mycobacteria
Rheumatic fever
Rheumatic heart disease
Constrictive pericarditis
No identified cause or association

[a]Modified from references 16, 62, and 96.

RELAPSING POLYCHONDRITIS

Definition. Relapsing polychondritis (*polychondritis, polychondropathy*) is a rare systemic condition in which the connective tissues, particularly the cartilage of the ears, joints, nose, eyes, respiratory tract, and cardiovascular system, are affected by a progressive inflammatory process (45,73,118,135).

Approximately 25 percent of patients with relapsing polychondritis have a coexistent connective tissue disease such as adult or juvenile rheumatoid arthritis, Sjögren's syndrome, systemic lupus erythematosus, Reiter's disease, psoriatic arthritis, or ankylosing spondylitis (73).

Clinical Features. Caucasians are most commonly affected, with an equal sex predilection and no apparent familial predisposition (45,73,118,135). Onset occurs between the ages of 40 and 60 years. Involvement of extrapulmonary sites, particularly the external ear, is the most common clinical finding. Patients frequently present with sudden onset of pain, tenderness, and a violaceous erythematous swelling of one or both external ears. Two thirds of the patients develop nasal chondritis, which often occurs suddenly and may result in cartilaginous destruction and deformity of the nose. Ocular inflammation (episcleritis, scleritis, conjunctivitis, and iritis) occurs in two thirds of patients. Many patients develop an arthropathy characterized as an episodic, asymmetric, nonerosive, and nondeforming arthritis. Vasculitis with involvement of the medium and large vessels is common and is manifested by aneurysm formation and thrombosis. The vasculitis may be focal or diffuse, indolent or fulminant, and rapidly fatal. Men are more likely to develop cardiovascular complications (present in 25 percent of all patients) consisting of aortic insufficiency secondary to progressive dilatation of the aortic ring in the ascending aorta; mitral and tricuspid insufficiency (occur less frequently); and aneurysms involving the ascending, thoracic, and abdominal aortas (these may rupture and cause sudden death). Pericarditis and myocarditis with conduction disturbances, endocarditis, and myocardial infarction are less common.

Approximately half of the patients have laryngotracheobronchial disease related to cartilaginous inflammation and destruction, with secondary pneumonia (73). Hoarseness and laryngeal tenderness over the thyroid cartilage and anterior trachea are common presenting symptoms. There may be a nonproductive cough, dyspnea, aphonia, inspiratory stridor, or rarely, hemoptysis, which may be life-threatening. Airway stenosis is common and associated with airflow obstruction (118). Assessment of the maximal expiratory and inspiratory flow volume curves and airway resistance may be useful in identifying the site and severity of the obstructive process (52,126). Patients with expiratory obstruction do not have evidence of a loss of elastic force (77).

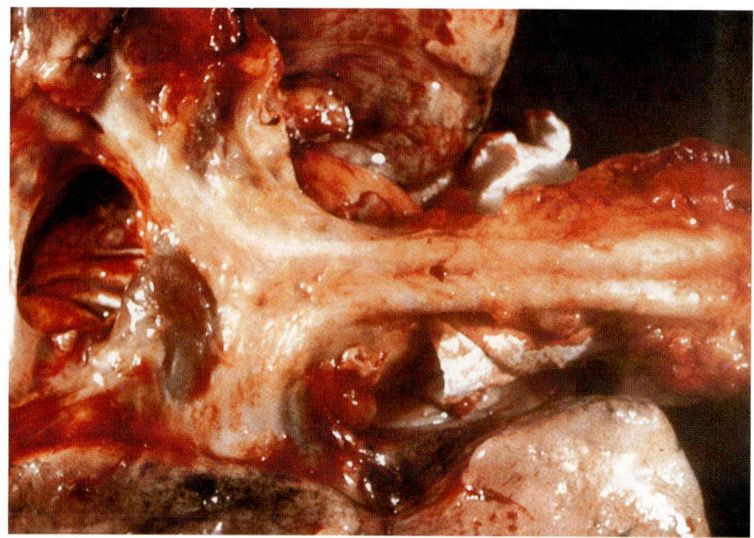

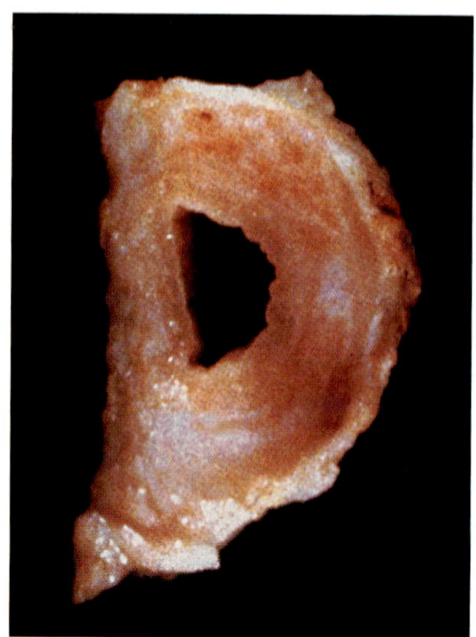

Figure 9-56

RELAPSING POLYCHONDRITIS

Left: The trachea and bronchi appear narrowed, the wall is thickened, and discrete cartilaginous rings are not apparent. Right: Cross section of a bronchus shows luminal narrowing, loss of cartilage, and mural thickening due to inflammatory tissue.

Radiologic Findings. Tracheal tomogram, cinebronchography, and CT scans are useful for identifying an obstruction of the anatomic airways. The characteristic findings on the chest radiograph and CT are circumferential thickening of the wall of the trachea and main bronchi and narrowing of airway lumen. The narrowing may be single or multiple, localized or diffuse (15,79). The chest roentgenogram may also reveal atelectasis, pneumonia, or widening of the aortic arch or of the ascending or descending aorta.

Pathologic Findings. Lung cartilage is rarely studied. Inflammatory destruction, primarily consisting of neutrophils, may be seen; the cartilage is progressively destroyed and replaced by fibrous tissue (figs. 9-56, 9-57) (45). In ear biopsies, there is an infiltration of the perichondrium by lymphocytes and plasma cells, with associated cartilaginous destruction, necrosis, and replacement by granulation tissue (45).

Pathogenesis. The cause of relapsing polychondritis is unknown and both humoral and cell-mediated immunologic reactions are implicated (45,118). Some patients have predisposing conditions such as alcoholism, connective tissue disease, infection, and trauma (including thermal and radiation trauma).

Differential Diagnosis. Cartilaginous destruction in the lung may be a feature of granulomatous infections, Wegener's granulomatosis, and bronchiectasis (45). The features of relapsing polychondritis are not specific. The diagnosis is suggested when there is recurrent inflammatory disease involving two or more cartilaginous sites, with changes consistent with the diagnosis histologically (45). The ear is the preferred site for biopsy and diagnosis.

Treatment and Prognosis. Medical treatment of relapsing polychondritis includes anti-inflammatory agents (nonsteroidal agents, systemic corticosteroids, Dapsone). However, since the disease is rare and prone to spontaneous remissions and relapses (47,55,84,135), the efficacy of therapy is difficult to prove.

Over time the disease may gradually progress and patients with pulmonary involvement have a somewhat worse outlook (118). The major concern is to maintain adequate ventilation. Death usually occurs as a result of recurrent attacks that lead to destruction of the cartilage of the tracheal and bronchial rings, causing collapse of these structures with inflammation, edema, and cicatrization. This cartilaginous destruction may lead to severe focal or diffuse airway collapse and inadequate ventilation.

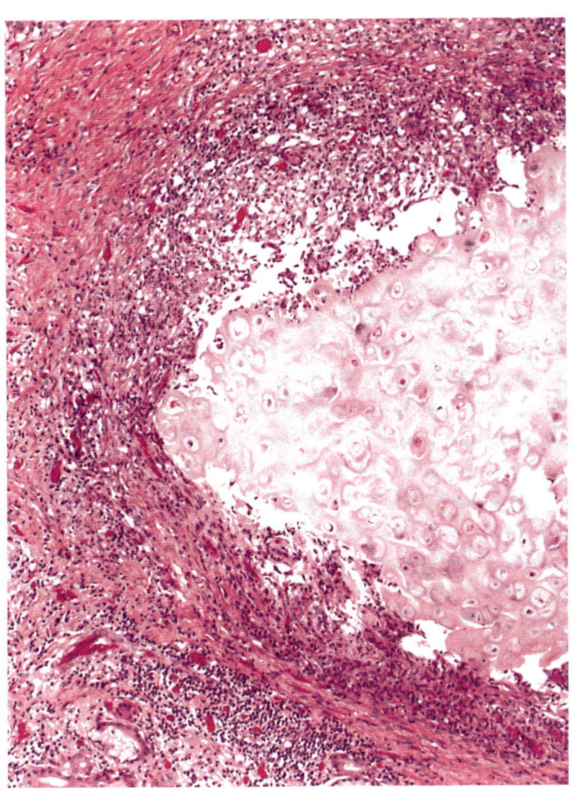

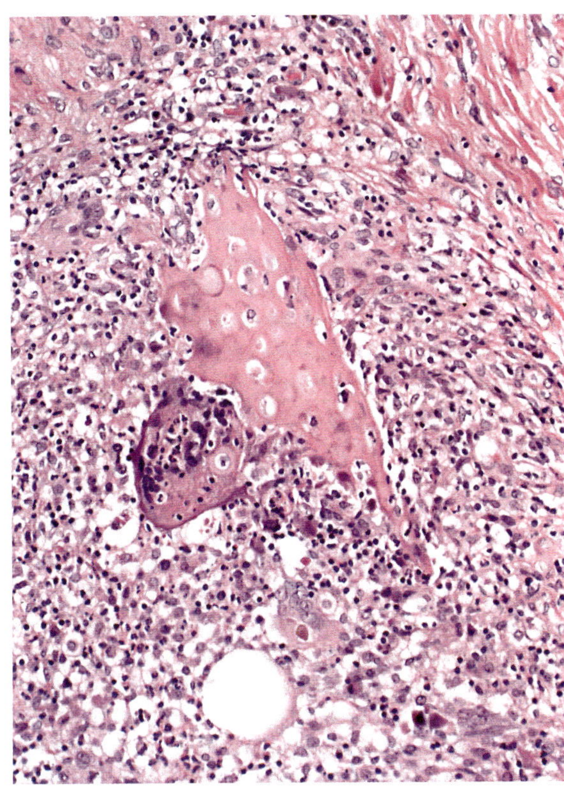

Figure 9-57

RELAPSING POLYCHONDRITIS

Left: Necrotic cartilage is surrounded by an acute and chronic inflammatory reaction.

Right: In other regions there is marked cartilaginous destruction with irregular-shaped remnants of cartilage surrounded by acute and chronic inflammation.

Tracheostomy may be required if the larynx is significantly involved. Surgical treatment of the collapsed airways with stents may be successful. The most common causes of death in relapsing polychondritis are infection, systemic vasculitis, malignancy, and respiratory failure (approximately 10 percent, usually due to asphyxiation) (55,56,84).

TRACHEOBRONCHOMEGALY

Definition. Tracheobronchomegaly (also termed *Mounier-Kuhn syndrome*) is marked symmetrical dilatation of the trachea and major bronchi, usually complicated by repeated bouts of infection (7,63,67,80,111,114).

Clinical Features. Although tracheobronchomegaly is usually identified in adults, symptoms often date from childhood; a few cases in infants have been found (7,63,67,80,111,114). Some cases are familial (autosomal recessive). Tracheobronchomegaly is associated with cutis laxa and Ehlers-Danlos syndrome (111). Patients have recurrent bouts of infection, and a clinical picture resembling and ultimately indistinguishable from bronchiectasis. Airway collapse during expiration is a feature predisposing to infection.

Radiologic Findings. The diagnosis can be readily made on the chest radiograph or CT scan (fig. 9-58). The caliber of the trachea and main bronchi is increased, and the tracheal and bronchial walls have a corrugated appearance caused by protrusion of the redundant mucosal and submucosal tissue between the cartilaginous rings. The diagnosis of tracheomegaly is made when the diameter of the trachea exceeds 3 cm and the diagnosis of bronchomegaly is made when the diameters of the right and left main bronchi exceed 2.4 and 2.3 cm, respectively (109). CT may also demonstrate associated dilation of the intraparenchymal bronchi

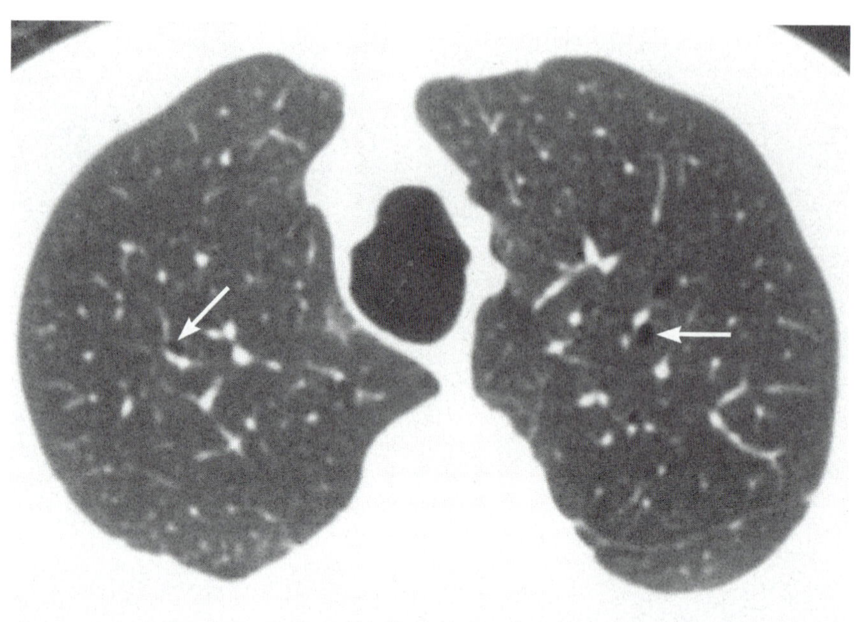

Figure 9-58
TRACHEOBRONCHOMEGALY
Chest CT in a 29-year-old man with tracheobronchomegaly demonstrates marked dilatation of the trachea. Both the coronal and sagittal diameters measured more than 3 cm. Subsegmental bronchi in the upper lobes are dilated (arrows). Note the dilated bronchi have almost imperceptible walls.

(32,33,79). The dilated bronchi, as distinct from bronchiectasis, typically have thin walls. CT allows visualization of tracheal diverticula which manifest as mucosal protrusions between adjacent cartilaginous plates. These mucosal outpouchings produce a corrugated appearance of the airway wall. Thin-walled, air-filled cystic structures of various sizes, representing bronchial diverticula, may be visualized in the central lung parenchyma. Bronchiectasis may also be seen.

Pathologic Findings. Pathologic studies of tracheobronchomegaly are limited and compounded by the effects of secondary infection and bronchiectatic change (111,114). The gross findings may be dramatic (fig. 9-59). Atrophy of bronchial tissue and smooth muscle is thought to characterize the condition and to be the feature that leads to airway enlargement. Diverticula occur between the cartilaginous plates (111). Once secondary features of bronchiectasis have supervened, all the varied histologic patterns described in bronchiectasis may be encountered.

Treatment and Prognosis. Treatment is directed against secondary infections, stasis of secretions, airway obstruction, and complications (e.g., hemoptysis or respiratory failure). A tracheobronchial prosthesis is useful for some patients.

CONGENITAL BRONCHIAL CARTILAGE DEFICIENCY

Definition. Congenital bronchial cartilage deficiency refers to symmetric deficiency of bronchial cartilage in the 3rd through 8th generation bronchi (64,83,85,89,95,111,114,130,136,137). The trachea and proximal bronchi are normal. This is also known as the *Williams-Campbell syndrome.*

Clinical Features. Most patients with congential bronchial cartilage deficiency present in the first year of life with clinical manifestations of bronchiectasis: productive cough, recurrent pneumonia, and clubbing (64,83,85,89,111,114,130,136,137).

Radiologic Findings. The radiologic findings consist of varicose or cystic bronchiectasis typically involving the 3rd through 8th generation bronchi and pulmonary hyperinflation (fig. 9-60). Airway collapse may be demonstrated with expiratory CT scans (83).

Pathologic Findings. There is symmetric absence of cartilaginous rings beyond the first and second bronchial divisions (111,114,136,137). Intact cartilaginous plates may be found at bronchial bifurcations. Grossly, there is dramatic symmetric dilation of the bronchi (fig. 9-60, left). There is a notable absence of destruction of the other wall elements (in contrast to established bronchiectasis) (fig. 9-60, right).

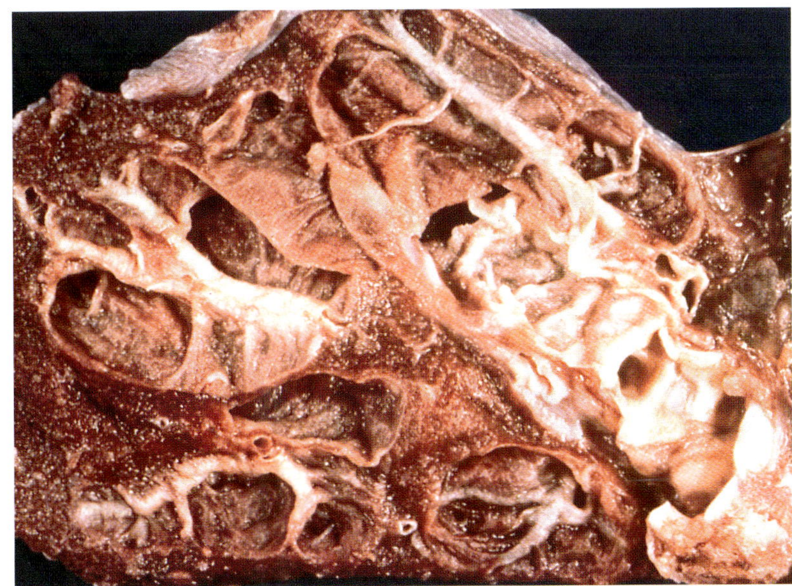

Figure 9-59

TRACHEOBRONCHOMEGALY

This gross photograph dramatically illustrates marked dilatation of the bronchi.

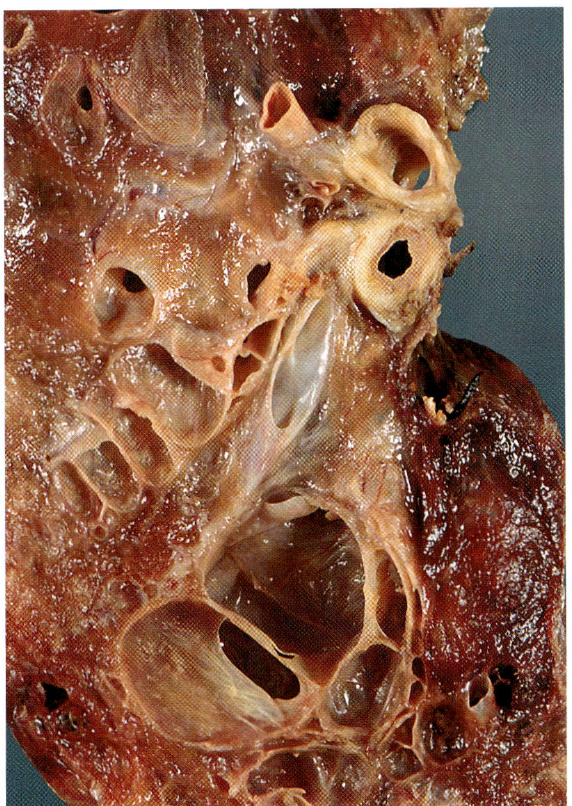

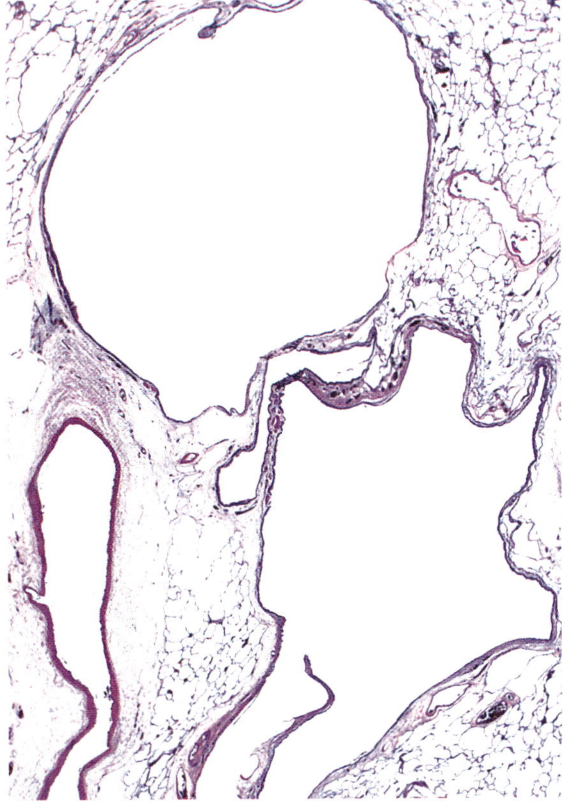

Figure 9-60

CONGENITAL BRONCHIAL CARTILAGE DEFICIENCY

In this example of congenital bronchial cartilage deficiency (Williams-Campbell syndrome) dilated airways are seen. (Courtesy of Dr. Victor Roggli, Durham, NC.)

Once changes of bronchiectasis have supervened, marked inflammatory distortion and destruction are seen.

Differential Diagnosis. The differential diagnosis of congenital bronchial cartilage deficiency primarily includes other causes of bronchiectasis. Symmetric changes extending from the proximal first and second bronchial divisions separate this from cases of acquired bronchiectasis.

Treatment and Prognosis. The management is similar to that described for other causes of bronchiectasis. The prognosis can be serious. A recent report described a lung transplantation in a patient with endstage lung disease (95). Although the patient did not have proximal airway collapse prior to transplantation, his post-transplant course was complicated by the development of bronchomalacia of the right and left mainstem bronchi. This suggests, in contrast to previous reports, that the cartilage deficiency can involve both proximal and distal airways. The authors concluded that bilateral sequential lung transplantation might not be an effective therapeutic option in patients with this syndrome.

BRONCHOLITHIASIS

Definition. Broncholithiasis refers to the erosion into, obstruction of, or significant distortion of, the tracheobronchial tree by calcified lymph nodes (4,27,31,93,122,133). Since calcified lymph nodes are very common in the chest (usually from granulomatous infection), minor degrees of tracheobronchial distortion by calcified lymph nodes are not included in this definition.

Clinical Features. The sex incidence is equal and most patients present in the sixth decade, although there is a wide age range (4). The most distinctive clinical feature of broncholithiasis is expectoration of calcareous material, but this occurs in one third or less of cases (4). Other symptoms include cough (which may be productive), hemoptysis (which is rarely massive), fever, chills, wheezing, and chest pain. Approximately 5 percent of patients are asymptomatic (122). In the series of Arrigoni et al. (4), the average duration of symptoms was 4.5 years.

Findings at bronchoscopy include tracheobronchial distortion in 86 percent of patients, inflammation in 69 percent, visible broncholith in 35 percent, bleeding in 22 percent, purulent secretions in 11 percent, and normal in 4 percent (122). Any of the major airways can be affected by broncholithiasis (4).

Radiologic Findings. The chest radiograph shows hilar calcification. The diagnosis of broncholithiasis can be strongly suspected on the basis of the following CT findings: endobronchial or peribronchial calcified nodes with distal changes due to bronchial obstruction (atelectasis, opacities, bronchiectasis, or air-trapping) and the absence of an associated soft tissue mass (27).

Pathologic Findings. Grossly calcified nodes distort or erode into airways (fig. 9-61) (4). There may be dense associated fibrosis. The bronchial lumen may be eroded or there may be a sinus tract to the calcified lymph node. The calcified material resembles gravel (fig. 9-61). Purulent material, hemorrhage, and surrounding consolidation of the lung parenchyma may all be encountered.

The histologic features are those of an old calcified granuloma involving a lymph node (fig. 9-62), with variable degrees of surrounding fibrosis and chronic inflammation (4). The degree of inflammation varies, but it tends to be acute and marked when there has been erosion into the bronchial lumen (fig. 9-63). Organisms can be sought with special stains in decalcified sections of the lymph nodes. Surrounding lung tissue may show bronchiectasis and/or obstructive pneumonia. One patient in the series of Arrigoni et al. (4) had an associated carcinoma.

Pathogenesis. Dystrophic calcification in an old healed granuloma in a hilar lymph node is thought to erode into adjacent structures as a result of the motion of the heart and lungs (122). The tracheobronchial tree is most commonly affected, but the esophagus and pulmonary vasculature may also be involved. Mycobacterial infection and histoplasmosis are sometimes confirmed by cultures or special stains (4). In most cases, the specific cause is not identified.

Treatment and Prognosis. The aim of treatment of broncholithiasis is to prevent irreversible complications such as bronchiectasis, abscess formation, chronic obstruction, and massive hemoptysis (27). Some patients may expectorate calcified material and have no further symptoms (4). Many patients do well following

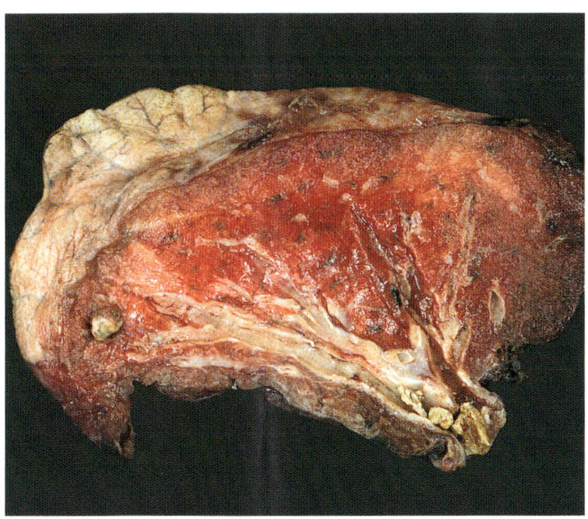

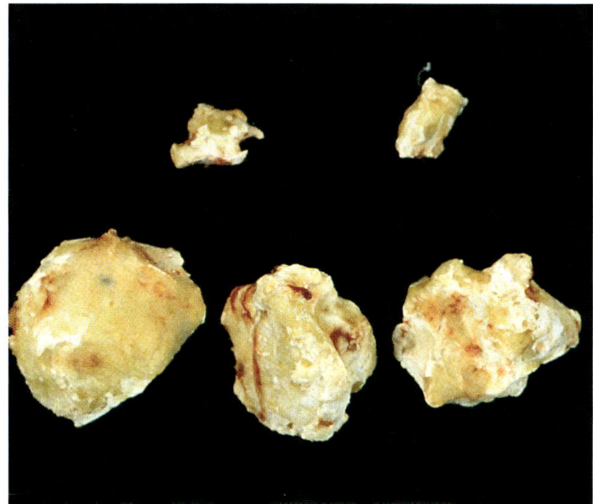

Figure 9-61

BRONCHOLITHIASIS

Left: A resection specimen shows luminal broncholiths near the hilum and one that has been aspirated distally. There is associated bronchiectasis.

Right: Broncholiths from another case.

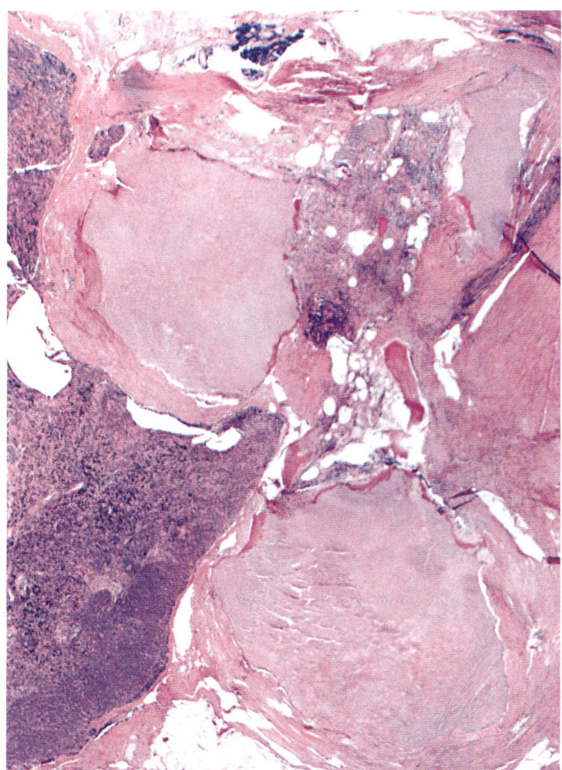

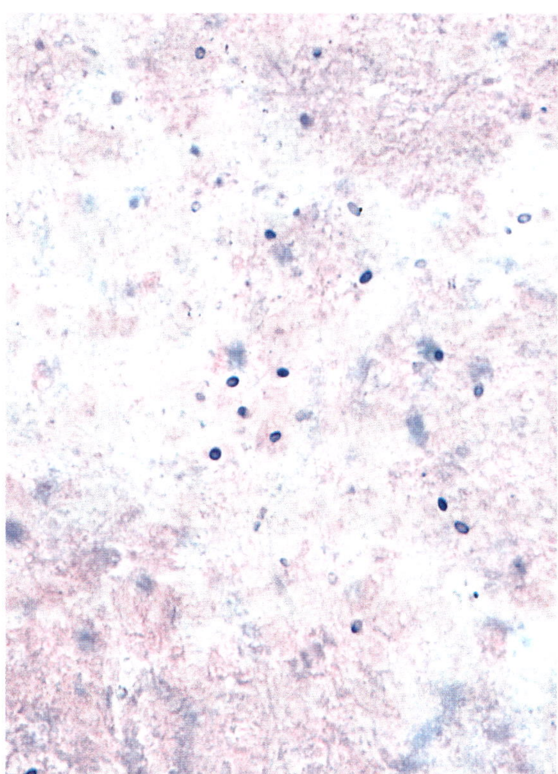

Figure 9-62

BRONCHOLITHIASIS

Left: Calcified peribronchial lymph nodes show typical features of old granulomatous disease.

Right: Broncholiths may be decalcified to reveal organisms, such as the yeast forms of *Histoplasma*.

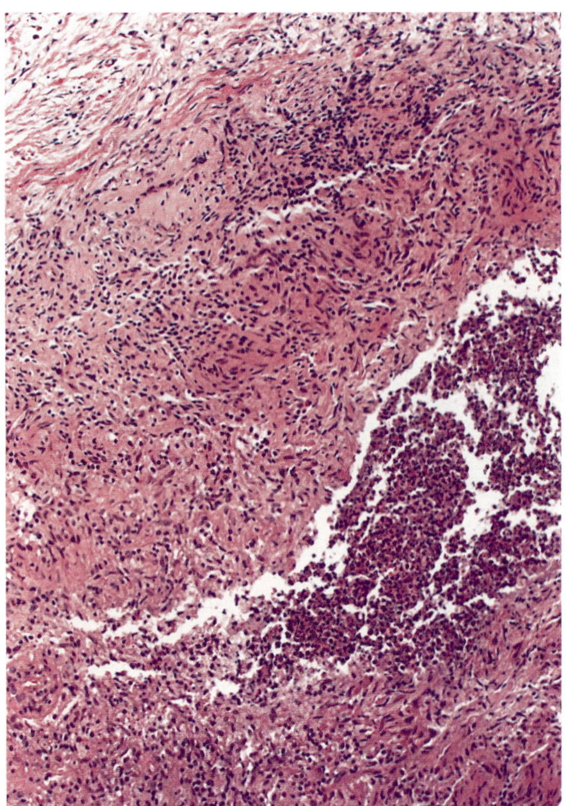

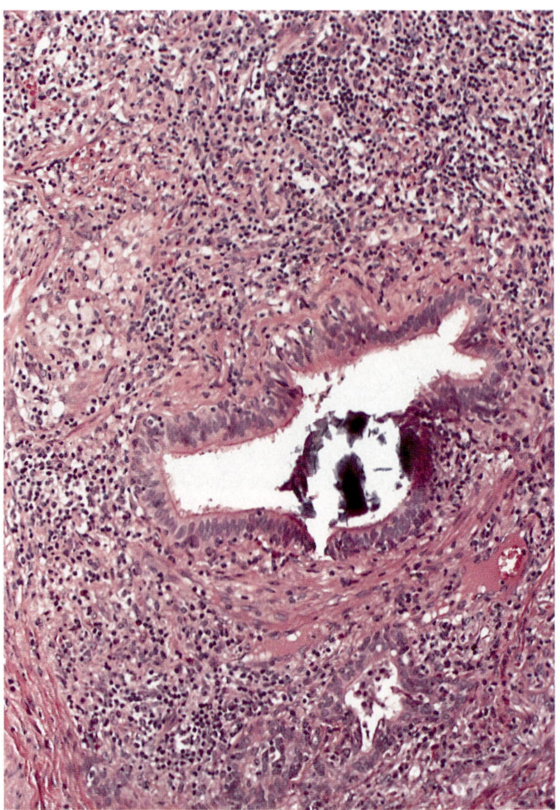

Figure 9-63

BRONCHOLITHIASIS

Left: When the calcified lymph nodes erode the bronchus, acute and chronic inflammatory changes are present in the mucosa. Some granulomatous features may be noted.

Right: In this case there was histologic evidence of aspiration of calcified material into distal airways.

bronchoscopic removal of the stones (4,27,31,93, 122,133). Indications for surgery include intractable cough, recurrent hemoptysis, chronic suppuration fistulae, and stenosis (122). The goal of surgery is removal of all calcified debris and abnormal bronchial and lung tissue. In some cases, bronchotomy and broncholithectomy achieve this. In general, surgery must be individualized depending on the findings. Surgery was performed in approximately one fourth of patients in the large series reported by Arrigoni et al. (4). In most patients the prognosis is favorable; there may be recurrences (4,93,122).

REFERENCES

1. Agasthian T, Deschamps C, Trastek VF, Allen MS, Pairolero PC. Surgical management of bronchiectasis. Ann Thorac Surg 1996;62:976–8; discussion 979–80.
2. Angus RM, Davies ML, Cowman MD, McSharry C, Thomson NC. Computed tomographic scanning of the lung in patients with allergic bronchopulmonary aspergillosis and in asthmatic patients with a positive skin test to Aspergillus fumigatus. Thorax 1994;49:586–9.
3. Annest LS, Kratz JM, Crawford FA. Current results of treatment of bronchiectasis. J Thorac Cardiovasc Surg 1982;83:546–50.
4. Arrigoni MG, Bernatz PE, Donoghue FE. Broncholithiasis. J Thorac Cardiovasc Surg 1971;62:231–7.
5. Aubry MC, Fraser R. The role of bronchial biopsy and washing in the diagnosis of allergic bronchopulmonary aspergillosis. Mod Pathol 1998;11:607–11.
6. Barker AF, Bardana EJ. Bronchiectasis: update of an orphan disease. Am Rev Respir Dis 1988;137:969–78.
7. Bateson EM, Woo-Ming M. Tracheobronchomegaly. Clin Radiol 1973;24:354–8.
8. Bedrossian CW, Greenberg SD, Singer DB, Hansen JJ, Rosenberg HS. The lung in cystic fibrosis. A quantitative study including prevalence of pathologic findings among different age groups. Hum Path 1976;7:195–204.
9. Bertelsen S, Struve-Christensen E, Aasted A, Sparup J. Isolated middle lobe atelectasis: aetiology, pathogenesis, and treatment of the so-called middle lobe syndrome. Thorax 1980;35:449–52.
10. Bhalla M, Turcios N, Aponte V, et al. Cystic fibrosis: scoring system with thin-section CT. Radiology 1991;179:783–8.
11. Bhargava V, Joseph BA, Tomashefski JF, Stern RC, Abramowsky CR. The pathology of fungal infection and colonization in patients with cystic fibrosis. Hum Pathol 1989;20:977–86.
12. Boat TF. Cystic fibrosis. In: Nelson WE, ed. Nelson textbook of pediatrics, 15th ed. Philadelphia: WB Saunders; 1996:1239–51.
13. Boat TF. Primary ciliary dyskinesia. In: Nelson WE, ed. Textbook of pediatrics, 15th ed. Philadelphia: WB Saunders; 1996:1251.
14. Boat TF, Carson JL. Ciliary dysmorphology and dysfunction—primary or acquired? N Engl J Med 1990;323:1700–2.
15. Booth A, Dieppe PA, Goddard PL, et al. The radiological manifestations of relapsing polychondritis. Clin Radiol 1989;40:147–9.
16. Borbely BR, Davies AL, Jones M. Left lung atelectasis in a smoker. Chest 1994;105:1833–5.
17. Bosken CH, Myers JL, Greenberger PA, Katzenstein AL. Pathologic features of allergic bronchopulmonary aspergillosis. Am J Surg Pathol 1988;12:216–22.
18. Brasfield D, Hicks G, Soong S, Peters J, Tiller R. Evaluation of a scoring system of the chest radiograph in cystic fibrosis: a collaborative study. AJR Am J Roentgenol 1980;234:1195–8.
19. Breslin AB, Jenkins CR. Experience with allergic bronchopulmonary aspergillosis: some unusual features. Clinical Allergy 1984;14:21–8.
20. Buchdahl RM, Reiser J, Ingram D, Rutman A, Cole PJ, Warner JO. Ciliary abnormalities in respiratory disease. Arch Dis Child 1998;63:238–43.
21. Bush A, Cole P, Hari M, et al. Primary ciliary dyskinesia: diagnosis and standards of care. Eur Respir J 1998;12:982–8.
22. Byrd R, Payne JL, Roy TM. Lingular and middle lobe infiltrates in an elderly woman. Chest 1995;108:1156–7.
23. Carson JL, Collier AM, Hu SC. Acquired ciliary defects in nasal epithelium of children with acute viral upper respiratory infections. N Engl J Med 1985;212:463–8.
24. Cartier Y, Kavanach PV, Johkoh T, Mason AC, Müller NL. Bronchiectasis: accuracy of high-resolution CT in the differentiation of specific diseases. AJR Am J Roentgenol 1999;173:47–52.
25. Cockrill BA, Hales CA. Allergic bronchopulmonary aspergillosis. Ann Rev Med 1999;50:303–16.
26. Cohen M, Sahn SA. Bronchiectasis in systemic diseases. Chest 1999;116:1063–74.
27. Conces DJ, Tarver RD, Vix VA. Broncholithiasis: CT features in 15 patients. AJR Am J Roentgenol 1991;157:249–53.
28. Culner MM. The right middle lobe syndrome, a non-obstructive complex. Dis Chest 1966;50: 57–66.
29. Dees SC, Spock A. Right middle lobe syndrome in children. JAMA 1966;197:78-84.
30. de Iongh RU, Rutland J. Ciliary defects in health subjects, bronchiectasis, and primary ciliary dyskinesia. Am J Respir Crit Care Med 1995; 151:1559–67.
31. Dixon GF, Donnerberg RL, Schonfeld SA, Whitcomb ME. Advances in the diagnosis and treatment of broncholithiasis. Am Rev Respir Dis 1984;129:1028–30.
32. Doyle AJ. Demonstration on computed tomography of tracheomalacia in tracheobronchomegaly (Mounier-Kuhn syndrome). Brit Radiol 1989;62:176–7.

33. Dunne MG, Reiner B. CT features of tracheobronchomegaly. J Comput Assist Tomogr 1988;12:388–91.
34. Ehouman A, Pinchon MC, Escudier E, Bernaudin JF. Ultrastructural abnormalities of respiratory cilia. Descriptive and quantitative study of respiratory mucosa in a series of 33 patients. Virchows Arch [Cell Pathol] 1985;48:87–95.
35. Elborn JS, Shale DJ. Lung injury in cystic fibrosis. Thorax 1990;45:970–3.
36. Eliasson R, Mossberg B, Camner P, Afzelius BA. The immotile-cilia syndrome. A congenital ciliary abnormality as an etiologic factor in chronic airway infections and male sterility. N Engl J Med 1977;297:1–6.
37. Eskenasy A, Eana-Iorgulescu L. Pathology of the middle lobe syndromes. A histopathological and pathogenetic analysis of sixty surgically-cured cases. Med Interne 1982;20:73–80.
38. Esterly JR, Oppenheimer EH. Observations in cystic fibrosis of the pancreas. 3. Pulmonary lesions. Johns Hopkins Med J 1968;122:94–101.
39. Felson B. Mucoid impaction (inspissated secretions) in segmental bronchial obstruction. Radiology 1979;133:9–16.
40. Fink JN. Allergic bronchopulmonary aspergillosis. Chest 1985;87:81s–4s.
41. Fox B, Bull TB, Makey AR, Rawbone R. The significance of ultrastructural abnormalities of human cilia. J Chest 1981;80S:796S–9S.
42. Friedman PJ. Chest radiographic findings in the adult with cystic fibrosis. Semin Roentgenol 1987;22:114–24.
43. Friedman PJ, Harwood IR, Ellenbogen PH. Pulmonary cystic fibrosis in the adult: early and late radiologic findings with pathologic correlation. AJR Am J Roentgenol 1981;136:1131–44.
44. Fujita J, Ohtsuki Y, Suemitsu I, et al. Pathological and radiological changes in resected lung specimens in Mycobacterium avium intracellulare complex disease. Eur Respir J 1999;13:535–40.
45. Gardner DL. Pathologic basis of the connective tissue diseases. Philadelphia: Lea & Febiger; 1992:711–5.
46. Geddes DM, Alton ER. The CF gene: 10 years on. Thorax 1999;54:1052–3.
47. Gibson GJ, Davis P. Respiratory complications of relapsing polychondritis. Thorax 1974;29:726–31.
48. Glancy JJ, Elder JL, McAleer R. Allergic bronchopulmonary fungal disease without clinical asthma. Thorax 1981;36:345–9.
49. Glimp RA, Bayer AS. Fungal pneumonias. Part 3. Allergic bronchopulmonary aspergillosis. Chest 1981;80:85–94.
50. Greenberger PA, Patterson R. Allergic bronchopulmonary aspergillosis. Model of bronchopulmonary disease with defined serologic, radiologic, pathologic and clinical findings from asthma to fatal destructive lung disease. Chest 1987;91:165s–71s.
51. Grenier P, Maurice F, Musset D, et al. Bronchiectasis: assessment by thin-section CT. Radiology 1986;161:95–9.
52. Grilliat JP, Vautrin DA. Manifestations respiratoires de la polychondrite atrophiante chronique. Presse Med 1969;77:1455–6.
53. Hansell DM. Bronchiectasis. Radiol Clin North Am 1998;36:107–28.
54. Heard BE, Khatchatourov V, Otto H, Putov NV, Sobin L. The morphology of emphysema, chronic bronchitis, and bronchiectasis: definition, nomenclature and classification. J Clin Pathol 1979;32:882–92.
55. Herman JH. Polychondritis. In: Kelley WN, Harris ED, Ruddy S, Sledge CB, eds. Textbook of rheumatology. Philadelphia: WB Saunders; 1985:1458.
56. Higenbottam T, Dixon J. Chondritis associated with fatal intramural bronchial fibrosis. Thorax 1979;34:563–4.
57. Homma S, Kawabata M, Kishi K, et al. Bronchiolitis in Kartagener's syndrome. Eur Respir J 1999;14:1332–9.
58. Hunt B, Geddes DM. Newly diagnosed cystic fibrosis in middle and later life. Thorax 1985;40:23–6.
59. Hutcheson JB, Shaw RR, Paulson DL, Kee JL. Mucoid impaction of the bronchi. Am J Clin Pathol 1960;33:427–32.
60. Irwin RS, Thomas HM. Mucoid impaction of the bronchus. Diagnosis and treatment. Am Rev Respir Dis 1973;108:955–9.
61. Jelihovsky T. The structure of bronchial plugs in mucoid impaction, bronchocentric granulomatosis and asthma. Histopathology 1983;7:153–67.
62. Jett JR, Tazelaar HD, Keim LW, Ingrassia TS. Plastic bronchitis: an old disease revisited. Mayo Clin Proc 1991;66:305–11.
63. Johnston RF, Green RA. Tracheobronchomegaly. Report of 5 cases and demonstration of familial occurrence. Am Rev Respir Dis 1965:91:35–50.
64. Jones VF, Elid NS, Franco SM, Badgett JT, Buchino JJ. Familial congenital bronchiectasis: Williams-Campbell syndrome. Pediatr Pulmonol 1993;16:263–7.
65. Kang EY, Miller RR, Müller NL. Bronchiectasis: comparison of preoperative thin-section CT and pathologic findings in resected specimens. Radiology 1995;195:649–54.

66. Karadag B, James AJ, Gultekin E, Wilson NM, Bush A. Nasal and lower airway level of nitric oxide in children with primary ciliary dyskinesia. Eur Respir J 1999;13:1402–5.
67. Katz I, LeVine M, Herman P. Tracheobronchomegaly. The Mounier-Kuhn syndrome. AJR Am J Roentgenol 1962;88:1084–94.
68. Katzenstein AL. Angiitis and granulomatosis. In: Katzenstein and Askin's surgical pathology of non-neoplastic lung disease, 3rd ed. Philadelphia: WB Saunders; 1997:193–222.
69. Katzenstein AL. Immunologic lung disease. In: Katzenstein and Askin's surgical pathology of non-neoplastic lung disease, 3rd ed. Philadelphia: WB Saunders; 1997:138–67.
70. Katzenstein AL, Liebow AA, Friedman PJ. Bronchocentric granulomatosis, mucoid impaction, and hypersensitivity reactions to fungi. Am Rev Respir Dis 1975;111:497–537.
71. Keistinen T, Saynajakangas O, Tuuponen T, Kivela SL. Bronchiectasis: an orphan disease with a poorly-understood prognosis. Eur Respir J 1997;10:2784–7.
72. Kim JS, Müller NL, Park CS, et al. Cylindrical bronchiectasis: diagnostic findings on thin-section CT. AJR Am J Roentgenol 1997;168:751–4.
73. King TE Jr. Connective tissue disease. In: Schwarz MI, King TE Jr, eds. Interstitial lung diseases. Hamilton: BC Decker, 1998:451–505.
74. Knutsen AP, Slavin RG. Allergic bronchopulmonary aspergillosis in patients with cystic fibrosis. Clin Rev Allergy 1991;9:103–18.
75. Koss M, Robinson R, Hochholzer L. Bronchocentric granulomatosis. Hum Pathol 1981;12:632–8.
76. Kovesi T, Sinclair B, MacCormick J, Matzinger MA, Carpenter B. Primary ciliary dyskinesia associated with a novel microtubule defect in a child with Down's syndrome. Chest 2000; 117:1207–09.
77. Krell WS, Staats BA, Hyatt RE. Pulmonary function in relapsing polychondritis. Am Rev Respir Dis 1986;133:1120–3.
78. Kwon KY, Myers JL, Swensen, SJ, Colby TV. Middle lobe syndrome: a clinicopathological study of 21 patients. Hum Pathol 1995;26:302–7.
79. Kwong JS, Müller NL, Miller RR. Diseases of the trachea and main-stem bronchi: correlation of CT with pathologic findings. Radiographics 1992;12:645–57.
80. Landing BH, Dixson LG. Congenital malformation and genetic disorders of the respiratory tract. Am Rev Respir Dis 1979;120:151–85.
81. Leon EE, Craig TJ. Antifungals in the treatment of allergic bronchopulmonary aspergillosis. Ann Allergy Asthma Immunol 1999;82:511–6.
82. Lynch DA, Newell J, Hale V, et al. Correlation of CT findings with clinical evaluations in 261 patients with symptomatic bronchiectasis. AJR Am J Roentgenol 1999;173:53–8.
83. McAdams P, Erasmus J. Williams-Campbell syndrome. Am J Radiol 1995;165:190–1.
84. Michet CJ, McKenna CH, Luthra HS, O'Fallon WM. Relapsing polychondritis. Survival and predictive role of early disease manifestation. Ann Intern Med 1986;104:74–8.
85. Mitchell RE, Bury RG. Congenital bronchiectasis due to deficiency of bronchial cartilage (Williams-Campbell syndrome). J Pediatr 1975;87:230–4.
86. Morgan AD, Bogomoletz W. Mucoid impaction of the bronchi in relation to asthma and plastic bronchitis. Thorax 1968;23:356–69.
87. Myers JL, Katzenstein AL. Granulomatous infection mimicking bronchocentric granulomatosis. Am J Surg Pathol 1986;10:317–22.
88. Neeld DA, Goodman LR, Gurney JW, Greenberger PA, Fink JN. Computerized tomography in the evaluation of allergic bronchopulmonary aspergillosis. Am Rev Respir Dis 1990;142:1200–5.
89. Newman K, Beam W. Congenital bronchiectasis in an adult. Am J Med 1991;91:198–201.
90. Nicotra NB, Rivera M, Dale AM, Shepherd R, Carter R. Clinical, pathophysiologic, and microbiologic characterization of bronchiectasis in an aging cohort. Chest 1995;108:995–61.
91. Nikolaizik WH, Warner JO. Aetiology of chronic suppurative lung disease. Arch Dis Child 1994;70:141–2.
92. Nuhoglu Y, Bahceciler N, Yuksel M, et al. Thorax high resolution computerized tomography findings in asthmatic children with unusual clinical manifestations. Ann Allergy Asthma Immunol 1999;82:311–4.
93. Olson EJ, Utz JP, Prakash UB. Therapeutic bronchoscopy in broncholithiasis. Am J Respir Crit Care Med 1999;160:766–70.
94. Oppenheimer EH, Esterly JR. Pathology of cystic fibrosis—review of the literature and comparison with 146 autopsied cases. Perspect Pediatr Pathol 1975;2:241–78.
95. Palmer SM, Layish DT, Kussin PS, Oury T, Davis RD, Tapson VF. Lung transplantation for Williams-Campbell syndrome. Chest 1998;113:534–7.
96. Park JY, Elshami AA, Kang DS, Jung TH. Plastic bronchitis. Eur Respir J 1996;9:612–4.
97. Patterson R. Allergic bronchopulmonary aspergillosis and hypersensitivity reactions to fungi. In: Fishman AP, ed. Pulmonary diseases and disorders. Philadelphia: McGraw-Hill; 1998;777–82.

98. Rayner CF, Rutman A, Dewar A, Cole PJ, Wilson R. Ciliary disorientation in patients with chronic upper respiratory tract inflammation. Am J Respir Crit Care Med 1995;151:800–4.
99. Reich JM, Johnson RE. Mycobacterium avium complex. Pulmonary disease presenting as isolated lingular or middle lobe pattern. The Lady Windemere syndrome. Chest 1992;101:1605–9.
100. Ricketti AJ, Greenberger PA, Mintzer RA, Patterson R. Allergic bronchopulmonary aspergillosis. Chest 1984;86:773–8.
101. Roberts HR, Wells AU, Milne DG, et al. Airflow obstruction in bronchiectasis: correlation between computed tomography features and pulmonary function tests. Thorax 2000;55:198–204.
102. Rosenbloom SA, Ravin CE, Putman CE, et al. Peripheral middle lobe syndrome. Radiology 1983;149:17–21.
103. Rossman MD. Colonization with Mycobacterium avium complex—an outdated concept. Eur Respir J 1999;13:479.
104. Rutland J, Cole PJ. Nasal mucociliary clearance and ciliary beat frequency in cystic fibrosis compared with sinusitis and bronchiectasis. Thorax 1981;36:654–8.
105. Rutland J, de Iongh RU. Random ciliary orientation. A cause of respiratory tract disease. N Engl J Med 1990;323:1681–4.
106. Saha SP, May OP, Long GA, McElvein RB. Middle lobe syndrome: diagnosis and management. Ann Thorac Surg 1982;33:28–31.
107. Schwiebert EM, Benos DJ, Fuller CM. Cystic fibrosis: a multiple exocrinopathy caused by dysfunctions in a multifunctional transport protein. Am J Med 1998;104:576–90.
108. Sheikh S, Madiraju K, Steiner P, Rao M. Bronchiectasis in pediatric AIDS. Chest 1997; 112:1202–7.
109. Shin MS, Jackson RM, Ho KJ. Tracheobronchomegaly (Mounier-Kuhn syndrome): CT diagnosis. AJR Am J Roentgenol 1988;150:777–9.
110. Sobonya RE, Taussig LM. Quantitative aspects of lung pathology in cystic fibrosis. Am Rev Respir Dis 1986;134:290–5.
111. Stocker JT. Congenital and developmental diseases. In: Dail DH, Hammar SP, eds. Pulmonary pathology, 2nd ed. New York: Springer-Verlag; 1994:155–90.
112. Stockley RA. Bronchiectasis—new therapeutic approaches based on pathogenesis. Clin Chest Med 1987;8:481–94.
113. Sturgess JM, Chao J, Wong J, Aspin N, Turner JA. Cilia with defective radial spokes: a cause of human respiratory disease. N Engl J Med 1979;300:53–6.
114. Swartz, MN. Bronchiectasis. In: Fishman AP, ed. Fishman's pulmonary disease and disorders, 3rd ed. New York: McGraw Hill; 1998:2045–70.
115. Tazelaar HD, Yousem SA. The pathology of combined heart lung transplantation: an autopsy study. Hum Pathol 1988;19:1403–16.
116. Thurlbeck WM. Chronic airflow obstruction. In: Thurlbeck WM, Churg AM, eds. Pathology of the lung, 2nd ed. New York: Thieme; 1995:739–826.
117. Thurlbeck WM. Chronic airflow obstruction in lung disease. Philadelphia: WB Saunders; 1976.
118. Tillie-Leblond I, Wallaert B, Leblond D, et al. Respiratory involvement in relapsing polychondritis. Clinical, functional, endoscopic, and radiographic evaluations. Medicine 1998;77:168–76.
119. Tomashefski JF Jr, Bruce M, Stern RC, Dearborn DG, Dahms B. Pulmonary air cysts in cystic fibrosis: relation of pathologic features to radiologic findings and history of pneumothorax. Hum Pathol 1985;16:253–61.
120. Tomashefski JF Jr, Konstan MW, Bruce MC, Abramowsky CR. The pathologic characteristics of interstitial pneumonia in cystic fibrosis. A retrospective autopsy study. Am J Clin Pathol 1989;91:522–30.
121. Tomashefski JF, Thomassen MJ, Bruce MC, Goldberg HI, Konstan MW, Stern RC. Pseudomonas cepacia-associated pneumonia in cystic fibrosis. Relation of clinical features to histopathologic patterns of pneumonia. Arch Pathol Lab Med 1988;112:166–72.
122. Trastek VF, Pairolero PC, Ceithaml EL, Piehler JM, Payne WS, Bernatz PE. Surgical management of broncholithiasis. J Thorac Cardiovasc Surg 1985;90:842–8.
122a. Travis WD, Kwon-Chung J, Kleiner DE, et al. Unusual aspects of allergic bronchopulmonary fungal disease: report of two cases due to Curvularia organisms associated with allergic fungal sinusitis. Hum Pathol 1991;22:1240–8.
123. Tsang KW, Ho PI, Chan KN, et al. A pilot study of low-dose erythromycin in bronchiectasis. Eur Respir J 1999;13:361–4.
124. Tsang KW, Lam SK, Lam WK, et al. High seroprevalence of Helicobacter pylori in active bronchiectasis. Am J Respir Crit Care Med 1998;158:1047–51.
125. Tsang KW, Tipoe G, Sun J, et al. Severe bronchiectasis in patients with "cystlike" structures within the ciliary shafts. Am J Respir Crit Care Med 2000;161:1300–5.
126. Vandour X, Payot J, Diebnold J, LeMelletier J. Les manifestations respiratoires de la polychondrite chronique atrophiante. J Fr Med Chir Thorae 1967;21:383.

127. Vawter GF, Shwachman H. Cystic fibrosis in adults. An autopsy study. Path Annu 1979;14: 357–82.
128. Veerman AJ, van Delden L, Feenstra L, Leene W. The immotile cilia syndrome: phase contrast light microscopy, scanning and transmission electron microscopy. Pediatrics 1980; 65:698–702.
129. Wagner RB, Johnston MR. Middle lobe syndrome. Ann Thorac Surg 1983;35:679–86.
130. Wantanabe Y, Nishiyama Y, Kanayama H, Enomoto K, Kato K, Takeichi M. Congenital bronchiectasis due to cartilage deficiency: CT demonstration. J Comp Asst Tomog 1987; 11:701–3.
131. Ward S, Heyneman LE, Flint JD, Leung AN, Kazerooni EA, Müller NL. Bronchocentric granulomatosis: computed tomographic findings in 5 patients. Clin Radiol 2000;55:296–300.
132. Ward S, Heyneman L, Lee MJ, Leung AN, Hansell DM, Müller NL. Accuracy of CT in the diagnosis of allergic bronchopulmonary aspergillosis in asthmatic patients. AJR Am J Roentgenol 1999;173:937–42.
133. Wedel MK, Hanson AS, Heithoff K. Broncholithiasis. Minn Med 1984;67:139–40.
134. Whitwell F. A study of the pathology and pathogenesis of bronchiectasis. Thorax 1952;7:213–39.
135. Wiedemann HP, Matthay RA. Pulmonary manifestations of the collagen vascular diseases. Clin Chest Med 1989;10:677–2.
136. Williams H, Campbell P. Generalized bronchiectasis associated with deficiency of cartilage in the bronchial tree. Arch Dis Child 1960;35:182–91.
137. Williams HE, Landau LI, Phelan PD. Generalized bronchiectasis due to extensive deficiency of bronchial cartilage. Arch Dis Child 1972; 47:423–8.
138. Wood BP. Cystic fibrosis: 1997. Radiology 1997;204:1–10.
139. Worthy SA, Park CS, Kim JS, Müller NL. Bronchiolitis obliterans after heart lung transplantation: high-resolution CT findings in 15 patients. AJR Am J Roentgenol 1997;169:673–7.
140. Young K, Aspestrand F, Kolbenstevdt A. High-resolution CT and bronchography in the assessment of bronchiectasis. Acta Radiologica 1991;32:439–41.

10
OBSTRUCTIVE PULMONARY DISEASES

The major disorders that cause pulmonary airflow obstruction include chronic bronchitis, emphysema, and asthma; a number of other less common disorders are discussed elsewhere in this monograph. In the United States in 1997, obstructive lung disease was the fourth most common cause of death in women and the fifth most common cause in men, accounting for 53,045 and 55,984 deaths, respectively (57).

The two major causes of airflow obstruction are increased airflow resistance and reduced outflow pressure. In chronic bronchitis and asthma, luminal narrowing of the airways produces increased resistance by a variety of mechanisms. In emphysema, loss of elastic recoil results in decreased outflow pressure. In some conditions both mechanisms are at play. The term chronic obstructive pulmonary disease (COPD) is used for patients who have airflow obstruction that is usually the result of both chronic bronchitis and emphysema. The diagnosis of obstructive lung disease is based on clinical, functional, and radiologic features, although it is important to understand the pathologic basis of these disorders. COPD is associated with three main pathologic lesions: emphysema, mucous plugging, and chronic obstructive bronchitis (fig. 10-1). A discussion of the management of COPD is beyond the scope of this chapter; however, consensus guidelines for the management of patients with COPD have been published by the American Thoracic Society (3), the European Respiratory Society (125), and the British Thoracic Society (21), and are widely recognized (44).

CHRONIC BRONCHITIS

Definition. Chronic bronchitis is defined clinically as a productive cough of unknown cause, occurring on most days for 3 or more months for at least 2 successive years in the absence of any known cause of chronic cough. It has proven difficult to define chronic bronchitis pathologically since there is overlap between the histologic findings in airways of asymptomatic smokers and those with chronic bronchitis.

Since there is considerable overlap in the clinical features of chronic bronchitis and emphysema, they are often referred to as COPD. However, patients may have clinical features that are typical of either chronic bronchitis or emphysema (Table 10-1). The primary cause of both is cigarette smoking, although it is not known why some patients develop chronic bronchitis and others emphysema (106).

In addition to the above criteria, the diagnosis of chronic bronchitis requires exclusion of other causes of cough such as tuberculosis, lung carcinoma, bronchiectasis, cystic fibrosis, and congestive heart failure. It is helpful to subdivide chronic bronchitis into three clinical subtypes: 1) chronic simple bronchitis, characterized by a chronic or recurrent increase in the volume of mucoid bronchial secretions associated with

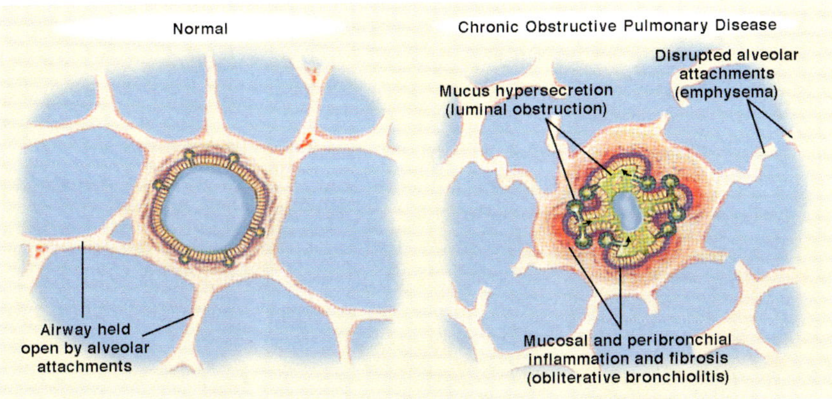

Figure 10-1

MECHANISMS OF AIRFLOW LIMITATION IN COPD

Compared to normal airways (left), in COPD there is airflow limitation in the peripheral airways due to varying degrees of loss of alveolar attachments, inflammatory obstruction of airways, and luminal obstruction due to mucus (right). (Figure 1 from Barnes PJ. Chronic obstructive pulmonary disease. N Engl J Med 2000;343:270.)

Table 10-1

CLINICAL FEATURES OF PREDOMINANT CHRONIC BRONCHITIS AND PREDOMINANT EMPHYSEMA[a]

	Predominant Bronchitis	Predominant Emphysema
General appearance	Mesomorphic, overweight, dusky with suffused conjunctivae, warm extremeties	Thin, often emaciated; pursed-lip breathing; anxious, prominent use of accessory muscles; normal or cool extremities
Age, years	40-55	50-75
Onset	Cough	Dyspnea
Cyanosis	Marked	Slight to none
Sputum	Copious	Scanty
Upper respiratory infections	Common	Occasional
Breath sounds	Moderately diminished	Markedly diminished
Cor pulmonale and right heart failure	Common	Only during bout of respiratory infection, and terminally
Radiograph	Normal diaphragm position; cardiomegaly, lungs normal or with increased bronchovascular markings	Small, pendulous heart; low, flat diaphragm; areas of increased radiolucency
Course	Ambulatory but constantly on verge of right-sided heart failure and coma	Incapacitating breathlessness punctuated by life-threatening bouts of upper respiratory infections; prolonged course, culminating in right heart failure and coma

[a]Modified rom reference 48.

cough; 2) chronic mucopurulent bronchitis, characterized by persistent or intermittent mucopurulent sputum and disease not related to localized destructive pulmonary disease, for example bronchiectasis; and 3) chronic obstructive bronchitis, characterized by cough and sputum sufficient to constitute chronic bronchitis, and associated with persistent widespread narrowing of airways.

Clinical Features. Chronic bronchitis affects an estimated 5.4 percent of the population or 14.2 million people in the United States (44). The prevalence rate is higher in women than men. Although chronic bronchitis most commonly affects those over age 45 years, it can be seen at any age. People who smoke cigarettes are most likely to develop chronic bronchitis. However, those exposed to high concentrations of dust and irritating fumes are also at high risk of developing this disease. Higher rates of chronic bronchitis are found among coal miners, grain handlers, metal molders, welders, asbestos workers, fire fighters, and other workers exposed to dust (caulker/burners, slate workers, textile workers, workers exposed to rice husks or grain) (69,150). The symptoms of chronic bronchitis worsen when atmospheric concentrations of sulfur dioxide and other air pollutants increase.

The patient with predominant bronchitis usually presents with a history of cough and sputum production for many years' duration (Table 10-1) (5,106). In the early stages of the disease, the symptoms are most troubling in the winter months and are attributed to a chronic, persistent "cold" or asthma. As disease severity progresses, the patient comes to medical attention usually because of acute or subacute worsening of dyspnea and productive cough (see below). At this stage, symptoms are present at any time of the year and usually the patient is an active smoker and/or has a viral upper respiratory tract infection. Occasionally, patients present with cyanosis and edema secondary to heart failure (referred to as "blue bloaters"). Such patients may progress to respiratory failure.

Acute bronchitis is commonly encountered in clinical practice (5,106). It should be distinguished from acute exacerbation of COPD. Acute bronchitis is generally caused by a viral infection (e.g., influenza A and B, parainfluenza, coronavirus, rhinovirus, and respiratory syncytial virus) and is characterized by inflammation of the bronchi. It is clinically expressed as cough, usually with sputum production, and evidence of concurrent upper airway infection. The absence of abnormalities on chest radiography distinguishes acute bronchitis from pneumonia.

Acute exacerbation of COPD is characterized by increased frequency and severity of cough, increased volume or change in the character of purulent sputum, increased dyspnea and sometimes wheezing, all in the presence of a normal chest radiograph (5,106). Exacerbations of chronic bronchitis are related to smoking, viral infections, air pollution, allergens, occupational exposure, or asthma. In 50 percent of cases of acute exacerbation of chronic bronchitis, studies have failed to identify a definite pathogen.

Physical examination reveals a patient who is often obese and asymptomatic at rest, although cyanosis may be noted (21,125). The respiratory rate is normal or slightly increased, and unlike patients with emphysema, there is no apparent use of accessory muscles or prolonged expiratory time. Percussion of the chest is normal and auscultation usually shows coarse rhonchi and wheezes. In the late stages of the process, signs of cor pulmonale may be present (sustained heave along the lower left sternal border, an early diastolic gallop, and occasionally, signs of tricuspid regurgitation). Clubbing is unusual.

Erythrocytosis is common. Pulmonary function testing shows a normal total lung capacity (TLC) with moderate elevation of residual volume (RV) (21,125). The vital capacity may be mildly reduced, and maximal expiratory flow rates are low. The elastic recoil properties of the lung are normal or only slightly impaired, and the diffusing capacity for carbon monoxide (DLCO) is either normal or minimally decreased. Arterial blood gases may be severely deranged, with hypoxemia and hypercapnia (the arterial PCO_2 may be 45 to 60 mm Hg). These patients often have sleep apnea with associated severe nocturnal oxygen desaturation; the latter contributes to the development of cor pulmonale and secondary erythrocytosis.

Radiologic Findings. There are no radiographic features that are definitive for chronic bronchitis and in 40 to 50 percent of patients the chest radiograph is normal (126). When present, the radiologic abnormalities are nonspecific and consist of bronchial wall thickening and an increase in lung markings (a finding commonly referred to as "dirty chest") (126,158). Similarly, there are no specific high-resolution computed tomography (HRCT) findings (158). In advanced disease, the main pulmonary arteries may be enlarged and the cardiac silhouette may become more prominent due to enlargement of the right atrium and right ventricle.

Gross Findings. Increased mucus in the airways as a result of mucus hypersecretion is the cardinal feature of chronic bronchitis. The airway lumens contain increased amounts of mucus: approximately 10 times more than normal in central airways and over 20 times more in peripheral airways (2). The bronchial wall is thickened due to the mucosal gland enlargement and sometimes encroaches on the bronchial lumen. The mucosal surface may show loss of normal rugal folds, with edema and focal erosions. Careful examination of the mucosal surface with a hand lens or dissecting microscope reveals pits up to 1 mm in diameter that represent gaping openings of the hyperplastic and hypertrophied tracheal-bronchial glands (155,157). Wang and Ying (155,157) proposed that these pits originate as dilatation of the gland ducts and depression of the epithelium, and ultimately result in herniation of the epithelium through the muscularis. The pits are diverticulum-like outpouchings that are typically present along the inferior border of the major bronchi (140). While the pits are characteristic of chronic bronchitis, they are not specific since they can be seen in bronchiectasis and other disorders (155,157).

Histologic Findings. The primary abnormality of chronic bronchitis is mucus hypersecretion due to an increase in submucosal glands and goblet cell metaplasia/hyperplasia in the surface epithelium. Histologic examination of the lumens of proximal and peripheral airways

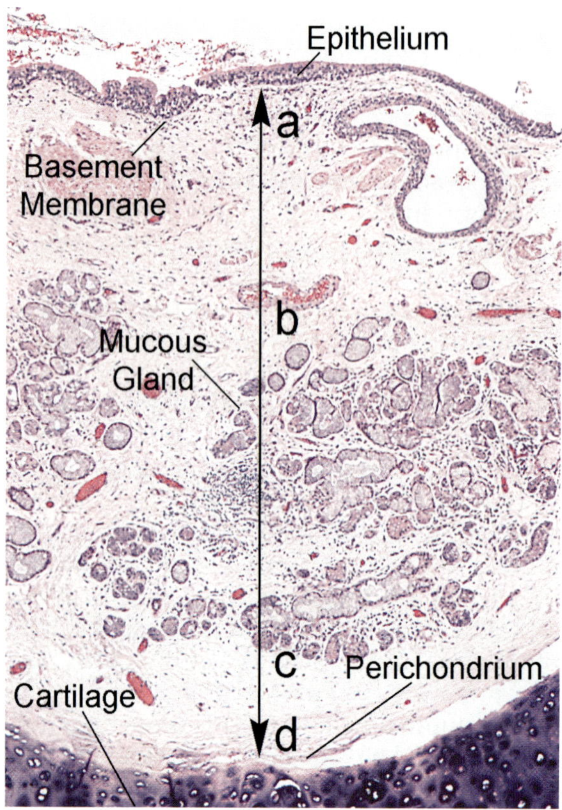

Figure 10-2

CHRONIC BRONCHITIS: REID INDEX

The bronchial submucosa is greatly expanded by hyperplastic submucosal glands, which comprise well over 50 percent of the thickness of the bronchial wall. The Reid index equals the maximum thickness of the bronchial mucous glands internal to the cartilage (b to c) divided by the bronchial wall thickness (a to d).

reveals increased mucus (2,54,71,108,144,147). The tracheobronchial mucous glands in the bronchial submucosa are enlarged (fig. 10-1). There may be enlargement and dilatation of the gland ducts that open on the mucosal surface, accounting for the pits seen grossly. Goblet cell hyperplasia of the surface mucosa is common, but goblet cells are thought to be a relatively minor source of the increased mucus production compared to the bronchial glands.

The most widely accepted method of measuring the mucous gland enlargement is the Reid index (fig. 10-2) (108). This represents the ratio of the thickness of the glands to the thickness of the bronchial wall, from the subepithelial basement membrane to the inner perichondrium. It is important to exclude bronchi showing acute inflammation and hemorrhage and those with submucosa separated from cartilage. Measurements should be taken in areas where the epithelium and cartilage are parallel, and they should be made along the same line for both the gland and wall thickness. A Reid index of 0.4 or less is regarded as normal and more than 0.5 as consistent with chronic bronchitis; however, there is a continuum of mucous gland enlargement that correlates poorly with the presence or absence of chronic bronchitis in the range between 0.36 and 0.55 (140). The Reid index is useful for comparing groups of patients but may not be useful in individual cases.

While chronic inflammation of the mucosa is often present, it is usually mild and does not correlate with mucous gland enlargement (140). Increased numbers of neutrophils and macrophages are present (112,114). The lymphocytes are predominately CD8+ T lymphocytes (99,112,114). Eosinophils are typically inconspicuous but mast cells may be increased in the mucosa and submucosal glands (103, 112). Squamous metaplasia may be present in the bronchial or bronchiolar mucosa. Airway narrowing is common. The bronchial wall smooth muscle is increased (112,140).

Respiratory bronchiolitis is common in cigarette smokers and is probably associated with airflow obstruction. For this reason, it is found in the peripheral airways of patients with chronic bronchitis or emphysema. In patients with mild chronic airflow obstruction who do not have significant chronic bronchitis or emphysema, the histologic abnormality may be respiratory bronchiolitis (98). It is not clear whether the inflammation alone or the associated bronchiolar narrowing and fibrosis cause the obstruction (140). However, studies suggest that cigarette smoke–induced lung inflammation has a pathogenic role in the development of COPD. Neutrophils, eosinophils, alveolar macrophages, and lymphocytes all appear to participate in the inflammatory process. Cosio et al. (25, 26) found that several morphologic features distinguished smokers from nonsmokers: increased goblet cell metaplasia ($p < 0.001$), smooth muscle hypertrophy ($p<0.05$), inflammation in the walls of bronchioles ($p < 0.01$), and respiratory bronchiolitis ($p<0.001$). Wright et al. (165) found that the membranous bronchioles of current smokers and exsmokers displayed increased goblet cell metaplasia when compared with those of nonsmokers (165). In addition, increases were seen in intraluminal and airway wall inflammatory cells, wall fibrosis, and pigment deposition in the respiratory bronchioles of current smokers and exsmokers.

Differential Diagnosis. Since there is considerable overlap in the morphologic findings of the airways in patients with symptomatic chronic bronchitis and asymptomatic smokers, chronic bronchitis is a clinical rather than a pathologic diagnosis. For this reason, the term "chronic bronchitis" is probably best avoided as a pathologic term and more descriptive terminology applied to report chronic inflammation of the airways. The presence of prominent features of asthmatic bronchitis, such as eosinophilia and basement membrane thickening, may raise the consideration of asthma, a relatively common complicating factor in patients with COPD.

Pathogenesis. Although the precise pathogenetic mechanisms are not clearly understood, chronic bronchitis is strongly associated with cigarette smoking. It is found in 5 percent of nonsmokers, 20 percent of light smokers, and 30 percent of smokers of 15 or more cigarettes per day (140). Environmental causes are also important since industrial workers have an increased frequency of chronic bronchitis as well. Chronic irritation/inflammation is thought to play an important role, although it is mild, chronic, and the injury is repetitive. This is consistent with the finding of CD8+ T lymphocytes and macrophages in bronchial biopsies and increased numbers of neutrophils found in these patients (30,99,112). Cytokines and other inflammatory mediators are also involved (fig. 10-3). In addition, proteases are potent stimulants of mucus secretion (fig. 10-4) (5,129,162). Oxidative stress also appears to be important in the pathogenesis of chronic bronchitis (fig. 10-5) (5,24,93,110). Infection, particularly bacterial and possibly viral, was thought to play a major role in the pathogenesis of chronic bronchitis; however, currently, infection is thought to be less important than smoking and infection is mostly regarded as a complication that

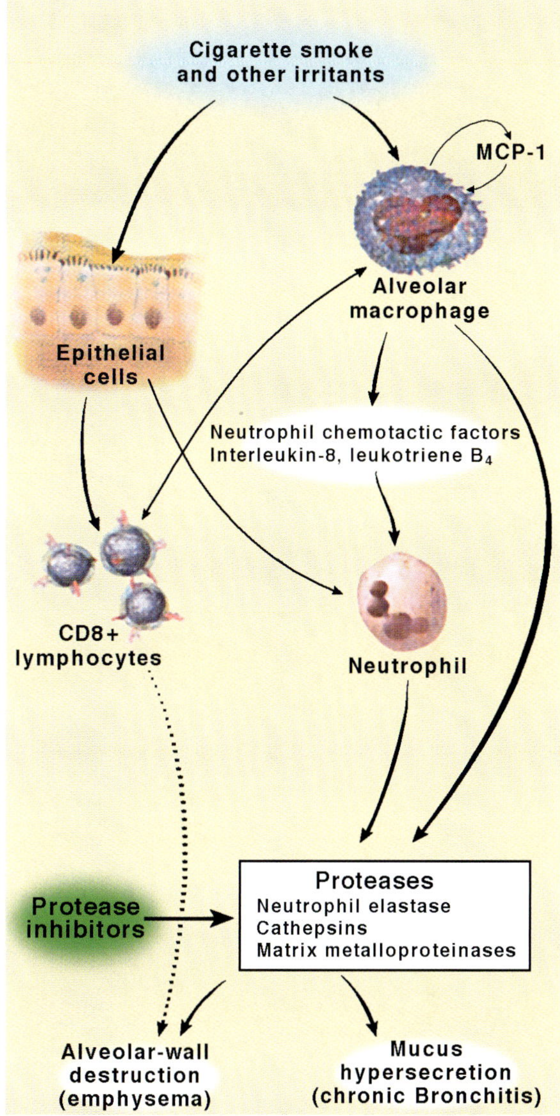

Figure 10-3

INFLAMMATORY MECHANISMS IN CHRONIC OBSTRUCTIVE PULMONARY DISEASE

Cigarette smoke and other irritants activate macrophages and airway epithelial cells in the respiratory tract, which release neutrophil chemotactic factors, including interleukin 8 and leukotriene B4. Neutrophils and macrophages then release proteases that break down connective tissue in the lung parenchyma, resulting in emphysema, and also stimulate mucus hypersecretion. Proteases are normally counteracted by protease inhibitors, including alpha-1-antitrypsin, secretory leukoprotease inhibitor, and tissue inhibitors of matrix metalloproteinases. Cytotoxic T cells (CD8+ lymphocytes) may also be involved in the inflammatory cascade. MCP-1 denotes monocyte chemotactic protein 1, which is released by and affects macrophages. (Figure 3 from Barnes PJ. Chronic obstructive pulmonary disease. N Engl J Med 2000;343:273.)

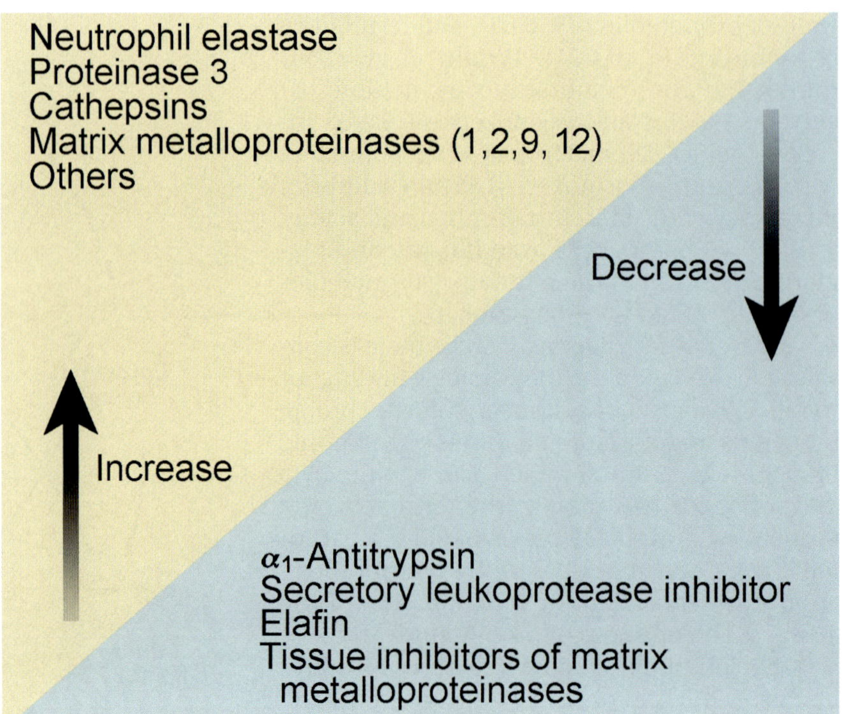

Figure 10-4

PROTEASE-ANTIPROTEASE IMBALANCE IN CHRONIC OBSTRUCTIVE PULMONARY DISEASE

In COPD, the balance appears to be tipped in favor of increased proteolysis, because of either an increase in proteases, including neutrophil elastase, cathepsins, and matrix metalloproteinases, or a deficiency of antiproteases, which may include alpha-1-antitrypsin, elafin, secretory leukoprotease inhibitor, and tissue inhibitors of matrix metallopropteinases. (Figure 4 from Barnes PJ. Chronic obstructive pulmonary disease. N Engl J Med 2000;343:274.)

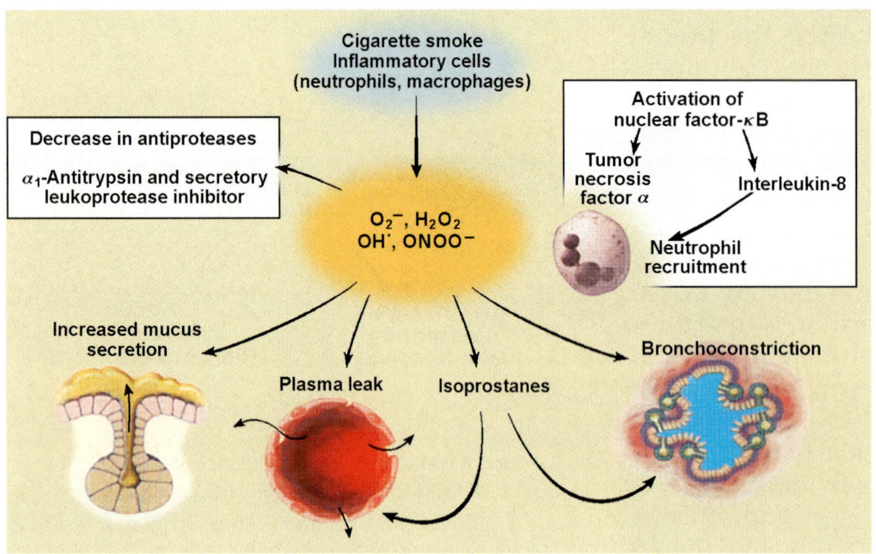

Figure 10-5

OXIDATIVE STRESS IN CHRONIC OBSTRUCTIVE PULMONARY DISEASE

Several damaging effects may result from cigarette smoke or inflammatory cells including decreases in antiproteases; activation of nuclear factor kappa-B, leading to increased secretion of the cytokine interleukin 8 and tumor necrosis factor-alpha; increased production of isoprostanes; and direct effects on airway functions. O_2 = superoxide anion, H_2O_2 = hydrogen peroxide, OH = hydroxyl radical, and ONOO = peroxynitrate. (Figure 5 from Barnes PJ. Chronic obstructive pulmonary disease. N Engl J Med 2000;343:275.)

sometimes causes acute exacerbations (119, 120). Recent studies have suggested that latent adenovirus or rhinovirus may play a role (63,120).

Treatment and Prognosis. There is no cure for chronic bronchitis and an acute exacerbation is the most frequent terminal event. In general, the prognosis of patients with COPD is worst when lung function, as reflected by the forced expiratory volume (FEV1), falls below 50 percent of predicted values. Patients with this degree of impairment have a 5-year survival rate of approximately 50 percent.

Treatment is aimed at relieving symptoms and preventing complications. Smoking cessation is the most important management option. In addition, the patient should be counseled to

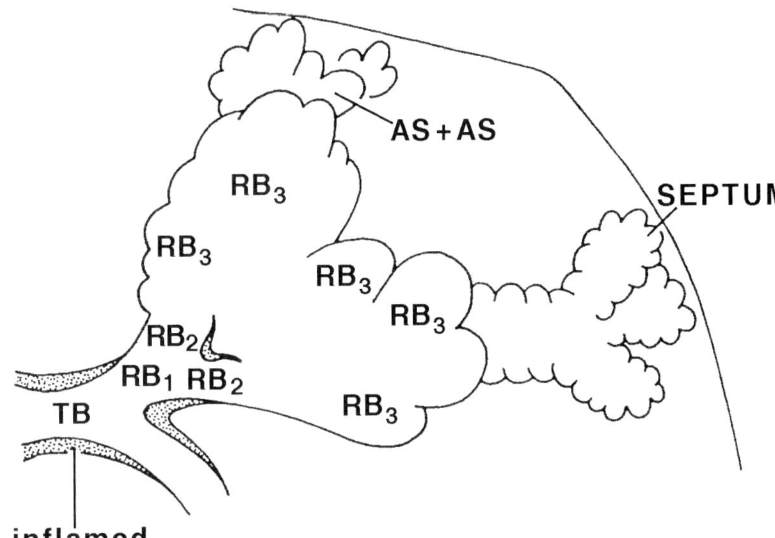

Figure 10-6

PROXIMAL ACINAR (CENTRILOBULAR) EMPHYSEMA

There is dilatation primarily in the respiratory bronchioles. RB = respiratory bronchiole (subscript indicates order), TB = terminal bronchiole. (Figure 9 from Thurlbeck WM. Chronic obstructive lung disease. Pathol Annu 1968;3:378.)

avoid exposure to other irritants. Inhaled long-acting bronchodilators (salmeterol and formoterol) and anticholinergics (ipratropium bromide and tiotropium bromide) are the mainstays of therapy. They relieve airway obstruction but do not alter the progression of COPD. The efficacy of corticosteroids in COPD remains poorly defined. Antibiotics have no role in the management of stable chronic bronchitis but may be prescribed for infections. Respiratory treatments, including nebulizers and postural drainage, facilitate the removal of thick mucus from the airways. Oral mucolytics may cause a small reduction in the number of acute exacerbations and a somewhat greater reduction in the total number of days of disability. Home oxygen therapy, physical exercise programs, and breathing exercises are also helpful.

EMPHYSEMA

The American Thoracic Society defines emphysema as "a condition of the lung characterized by abnormal, permanent enlargement of the airspaces distal to the terminal bronchiole, accompanied by destruction of their walls" (17,18). Fibrosis may be absent or subtle and mild (127,128,140,164).

There are several types of emphysema depending on which part of the pulmonary acinus is primarily affected (8,27,49,145,149,164). In *proximal acinar (centrilobular, centriacinar) emphysema,* only the proximal part of the acinus is involved (fig. 10-6). This pattern is strongly associated with smoking. In *panacinar (panlobular) emphysema,* the entire acinus is affected and this pattern is characteristic of alpha-1-antitrypsin (alpha1AT) deficiency (fig. 10-7). Other forms include *distal acinar (paraseptal) emphysema* which is the least common type (fig. 10-8) and *irregular emphysema,* which is the most common type (fig. 10-9). Blebs represent air-filled spaces within the pleura. A bleb is less than 1 cm in diameter. *Interstitial emphysema* is the accumulation of air within the interstitium and is not emphysema as defined above (see chapter 11). Occasionally in adults, interstitial emphysema is an incidental histologic finding in lung tissue showing some other pathologic process in addition to interstitial pulmonary emphysema. A bulla is defined as an emphysematous space that measures greater than 1 cm in diameter. *Placental transmogrification of the lung* is a very rare and distinctive variant of *giant bullous emphysema* localized to a single lobe (see below). Airspace dilatation associated with aging and compensatory overinflation associated with pneumonectomy should not be confused with emphysema (Table 10-2).

A variety of clinical conditions and toxic exposures are associated with emphysema (Table 10-3).

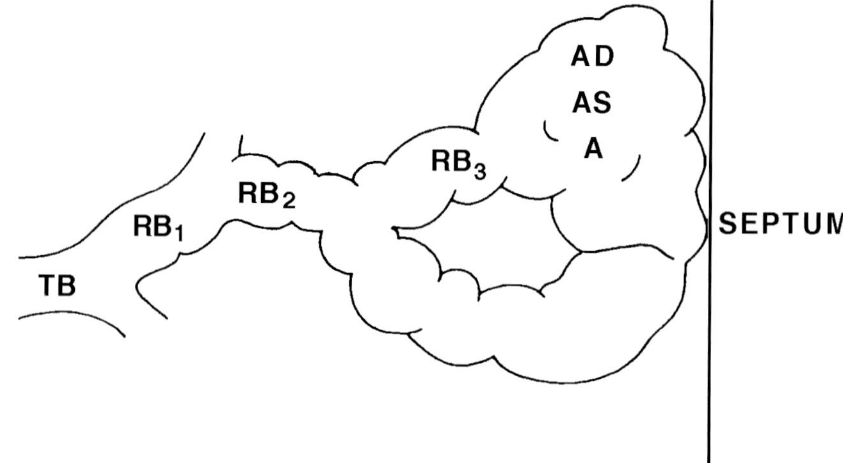

Figure 10-7

PANACINAR (PANLOBULAR) EMPHYSEMA

There is enlargment and destruction of airspaces, with uniform involvement of the acinus. RB = respiratory bronchiole (subscript indicates order), TB = terminal bronchiole, A = alveoli, AD = alveolar duct, AS = alveolar sac. (Figure 12 from Thurlbeck WM. Chronic obstructive lung disease. Pathol Annu 1968;3:381.)

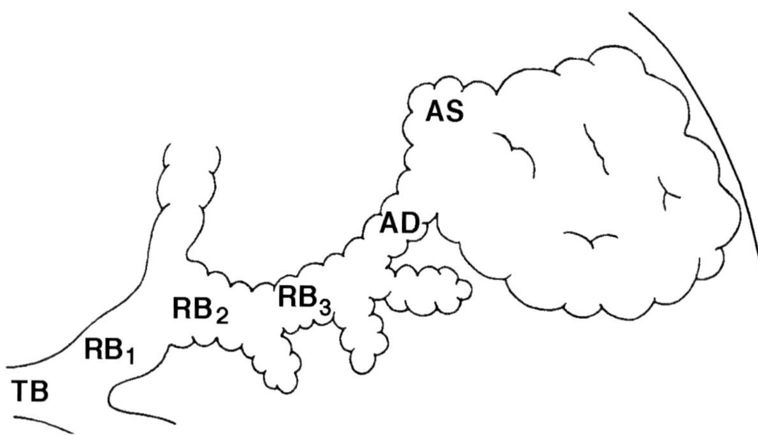

Figure 10-8

DISTAL ACINAR (PARASEPTAL) EMPHYSEMA

There is distension of the peripheral part of the acinus. (Figure 2-4 from Thurlbeck WM. Terminology, definitions and classification. In: Thurlbeck WM, ed. Chronic airflow obstruction in lung disease. Philadelphia: WB Saunders; 1976:16.)

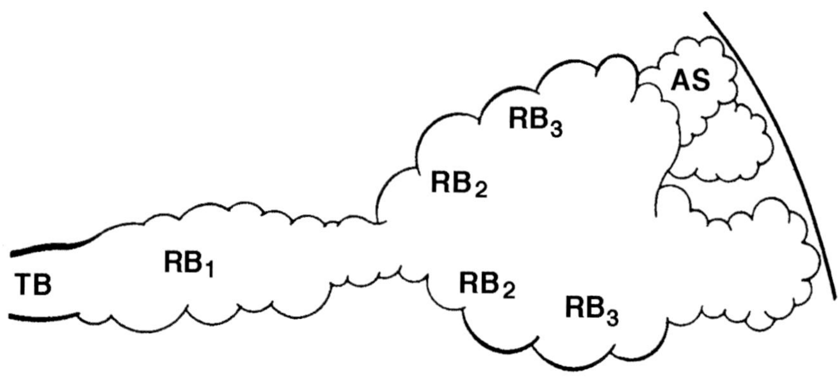

Figure 10-9

IRREGULAR EMPHYSEMA

In irregular emphysema there is variable dilatation of all aspects of the terminal bronchioles, respiratory bronchioles, and alveolar sacs. RB = respiratory bronchiole (subscript indicates order), TB = terminal bronchiole, A = alveoli, AD = alveolar duct, AS = alveolar sac. (Figure 2-5 from Thurlbeck WM. Terminology, definitions and classification. In: Thurlbeck WM, ed. Chronic airflow obstruction in lung disease. Philadelphia: WB Saunders; 1976:17.)

Table 10-2

PATTERNS OF RESPIRATORY AIRSPACE ENLARGEMENT[a]

Simple Airspace Enlargement
Congenital
Down's syndrome
Lobar overinflation
Acquired
Postpneumonectomy (compensatory)
Aging lung
? Starvation lung
Hyperlucent lung ("vanishing lung")
Swyer-James syndrome
Emphysema
Proximal acinar (centrilobular, centriacinar)
Panacinar (panlobular)
Distal acinar (Paraseptal)
Airspace Enlargement with Fibrosis
Irregular emphysema
Fibrotic lung disease
Other Lesions of Airspace Enlargement
Bullae
Bleb
Giant bullous emphysema (placental transmogrification)

[a]Modified from reference 164.

Table 10-3

CONDITIONS AND EXPOSURES ASSOCIATED WITH EMPHYSEMA

Alpha-1-antitrypsin deficiency
Toxic agents/drugs
Cigarette smoking
IV drug abuse—ritalin (118,134)
Cadmium (97)
Connective tissue disorders
Marfan's syndrome (29)
Salla's disease (101)
Congenital cutis laxa (22)

Pathologic Evaluation of the Lung for Emphysema

Optimal pathologic evaluation of the lung for emphysema requires some type of inflation method. The simplest technique involves insertion of a cannula into the bronchus and filling the lung with fixative from a container stored at 30 to 100 cm above the position of inflation. Formalin is a perfectly acceptable fixative although a variety of alternative fixatives include glutaraldehyde, Bouin's (92), and warm agarose (142,164). Several specialized methods can be used to prepare the lungs for evaluation for emphysema including paper-mounted whole-lung sectioning (56,142) and barium sulfate impregnation (60,142). Either a sagittal or transverse approach to sectioning can be used, the latter allowing for correlation with CT scan images (164). Once the specimens have been properly prepared, morphometric methods can be used to evaluate the type, extent, and severity of the emphysema. For routine evaluation, a simple and practical approach involves floating the lungs in a pan filled with enough water to cover a slice of lung tissue (164). Careful gross examination of the lung allows distinction between centriacinar and panacinar emphysema. These methods are reviewed in detail elsewhere (56,60,92,142,146,164).

The Destructive Index (DI) is a method developed for assessing the severity of destruction due to emphysema based on random histologic sections of lung (113). It is comprised of three factors: 1) airspaces with breaks in the alveolar wall; 2) histologic changes: cuboidal change of epithelium lining airspaces; and 3) classic emphysema. The DI has been shown to correlate with the severity of the emphysema and the pulmonary function defects (40,77,90,117,148).

Proximal Acinar Emphysema (Centriacinar or Centrilobular Emphysema)

Definition. Proximal acinar emphysema is defined as distention and destruction mainly limited to the respiratory bronchioles, with relatively less change peripherally in the acinus. Synonyms are *centrilobular* or *centriacinar emphysema.*

Proximal acinar emphysema results from scarring and focal dilation of the bronchioles and adjacent alveoli, which lead to an enlarged airspace or "microbulla" in the center of the secondary lung lobule (140,141). This pattern is frequently associated with long-term cigarette smoking and predominantly involves the upper and posterior portions of the lung (centrilobular emphysema). Another variant, *focal emphysema,* occurs in individuals heavily exposed to dust, especially coal dust. It is uniformly distributed throughout the lung. Inherited forms of proximal acinar emphysema have been reported. A nonsmoking patient with Salla's disease, a rare recessive hereditary disorder of sialic acid metabolism that causes intralysosomal accumulation of free sialic acid in cells of various tissues, developed proximal acinar emphysema (101). Early onset emphysema was also reported in a mother and daughter with autosomal dominant cutis laxa (22).

Clinical Features. Emphysema is less common than chronic bronchitis, and occurs in about 2 million Americans. Patients with proximal acinar emphysema are usually between 50 and 75 years of age. Dyspnea is the presenting manifestation (Table 10-1) (48,106). If cough is present, it is less notable than dyspnea and produces only scant sputum. Mucopurulent exacerbations in association with infections are not frequent. The patients are usually thin (so-called pink puffers), with evidence of weight loss resulting from energy expenditure in excess of caloric intake. Usually, these patients appear in distress, with rapid breaths and frequent use of their accessory muscles of respiration. They have relatively prolonged expiration, breathe with pursed lips, and make a grunting sound with each expiratory maneuver. They often sit leaning forward with extended arms to brace themselves. On chest examination the breath sounds are markedly diminished, with faint, high-pitched rhonchi heard toward the end of expiration (48,106). The percussion note is hyperresonant.

The TLC and RV are invariably increased, the vital capacity is low, and the maximal expiratory flow rates are diminished. The elastic recoil properties of the lung are severely impaired. The diffusing capacity is commonly low. The arterial PaO_2 is often normal or mildly reduced and the PCO_2 is low to normal.

Radiologic Findings. Proximal acinar emphysema involves mainly the upper lobes. The manifestations of emphysema on the chest radiograph relate to hyperinflation and lung destruction (fig. 10-10) (149,158). Hyperinflation results in flattening of the diaphragm and increase in the retrosternal airspace. Lung destruction results in focal lucencies and bullae. Although the majority of patients with moderate and severe emphysema have abnormal radiographs, mild emphysema is usually missed (149,158).

HRCT is superior to the radiograph in the diagnosis of emphysema, in the assessment of the type of emphysema, and in the quantification of the severity of the disease (133,149,158). Proximal acinar emphysema is characterized on HRCT by the presence of focal areas of low attenuation measuring from a few millimeters to approximately 1 cm in diameter (fig. 10-11) (133,149,158). The abnormalities are situated near the center of the secondary lobule. Several studies have shown a good correlation between the pathologic findings and the presence and severity of the HRCT findings (52,67,77, 92,158). It should be noted, however, that very mild focal cases can be missed on HRCT (92, 109), and, therefore, CT cannot be used to rule out the diagnosis.

Gross Findings. The lungs are enlarged and appear overinflated on examination of gross specimens and Gough sections (figs. 10-12–10-14). The emphysematous airspaces are situated midway between the center and periphery of the acini (fig. 10-6). The center of the acinus contains a bronchiole with its paired arteriole (55,60,140). Depending on the severity of the changes, the airspaces at the periphery of the acinus may appear normal or some degree of destruction and enlargement may be seen (fig. 10-14). Pigment deposits are common, although there are fewer than in patients with associated pneumoconiosis (fig. 10-14). Variation of severity between lobules and even within the same lobule is common (figs. 10-13, 10-14). The frequency and severity of proximal acinar emphysema are greatest in the upper lobes (fig. 10-13), and the lesions in the superior segment of the lower lobes are similar to those seen in the upper lobes.

Histologic Findings. The respiratory bronchioles are enlarged and destroyed (fig. 10-15). The enlarged airspaces are seen at the center of the secondary acinus. These emphysematous spaces become confluent (fig. 10-16). The lung tissue distal to the emphysematous areas is often relatively normal, although some generalized airspace enlargement may be present. There tends to be a greater degree of involvement of second and third order rather than first order respiratory bronchioles. Varying degrees of respiratory

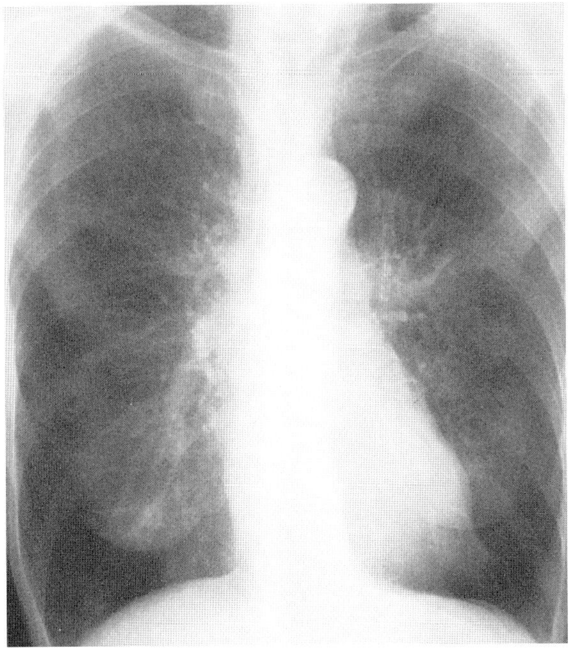

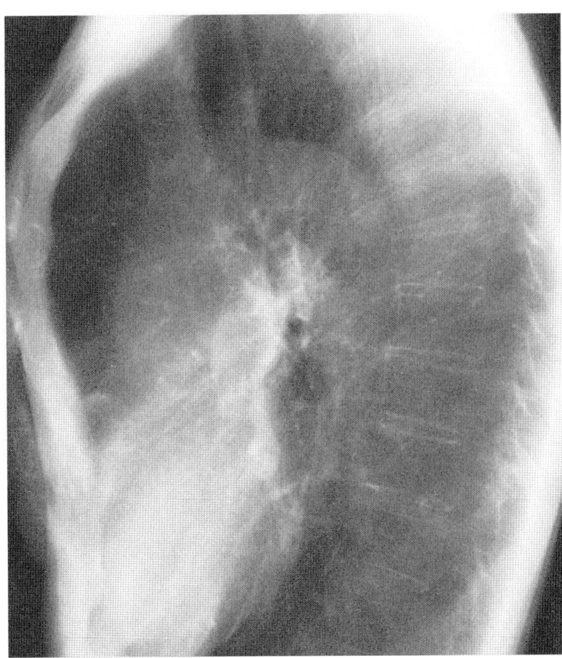

Figure 10-10

PROXIMAL ACINAR (CENTRILOBULAR) EMPHYSEMA

Posteroanterior (left) and lateral (right) chest radiographs demonstrate marked hyperinflation resulting in an increased retrosternal airspace and depression and flattening of the diaphragm. Also note focal lucencies and areas of decreased vascularity due to emphysema. The patient was an 85-year-old woman with severe proximal acinar emphysema.

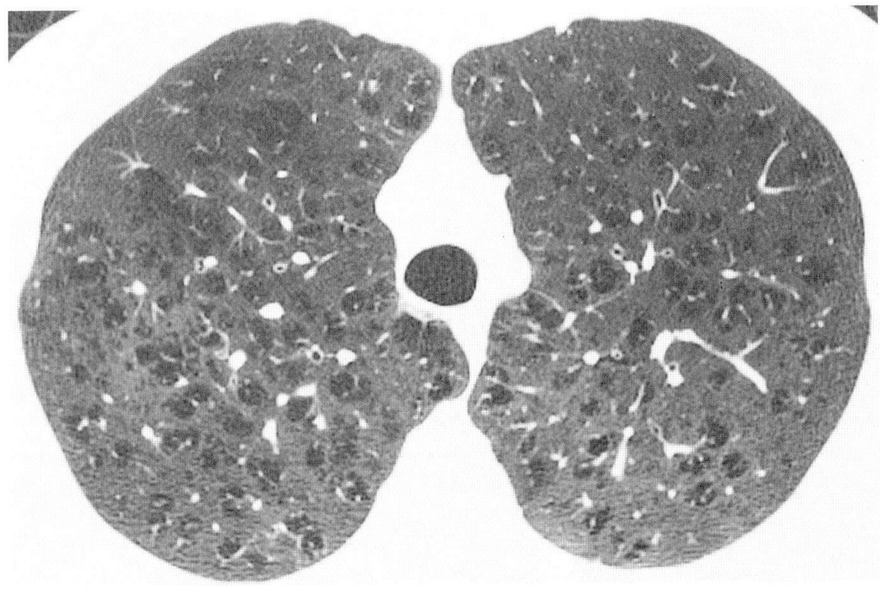

Figure 10-11

PROXIMAL ACINAR (CENTRILOBULAR) EMPHYSEMA

HRCT demonstrates focal areas of decreased attenuation without visible walls. The abnormal areas are sharply circumscribed and measure from a few millimeters to approximately 1 cm in diameter. Note the presence of small centrilobular vessels within the areas of emphysema. The patient was a 49-year-old smoker with proximal acinar emphysema.

bronchiolitis are present (81,86). However, conspicuous central airway inflammation involving bronchial glands is not seen unless there is concomitant chronic bronchitis. The primary lesion consists of destruction of the lung tissue rather than the proximal dilatation that occurs in proximal acinar emphysema due to dust. Some relatively acellular, pink, collagenized fi-

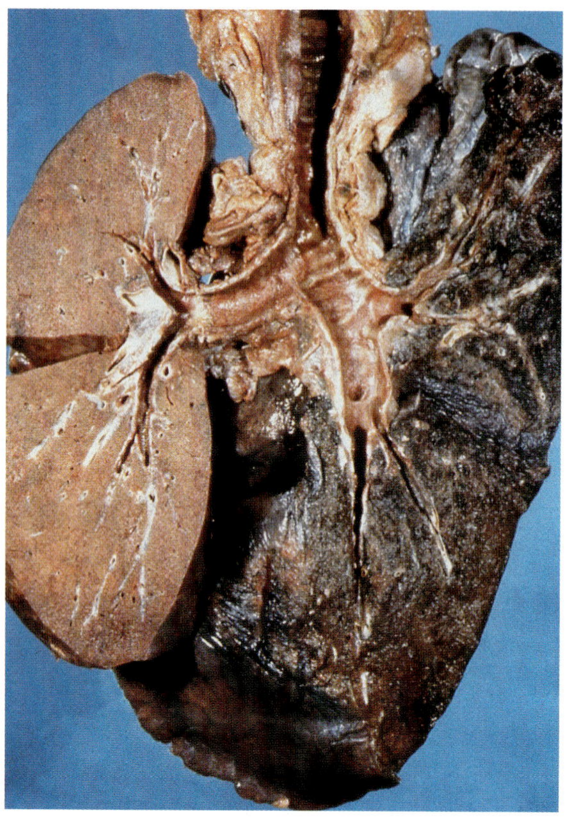

Figure 10-12

EMPHYSEMA POST-TRANSPLANTATION

The native emphysematous lung (right) is much larger and appears overinflated in comparison to the transplanted lung (left). (Courtesy of the Gordon Museum, London, England.)

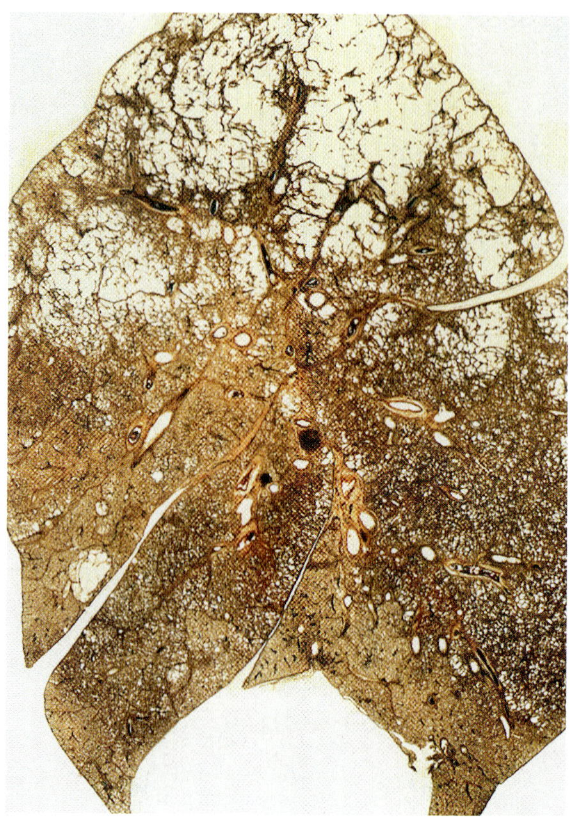

Figure 10-13

PROXIMAL ACINAR EMPHYSEMA

The upper pole of this lung is severely affected by emphysema, which is causing marked dilatation of the centrilobular aspect of the acini. The abnormal emphysematous upper aspect stands in contrast to the relatively preserved lower portion of the lung.

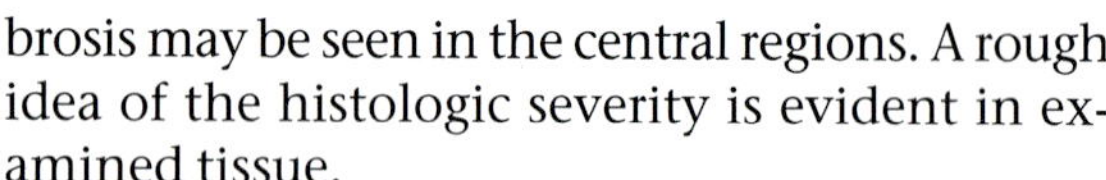

brosis may be seen in the central regions. A rough idea of the histologic severity is evident in examined tissue.

Differential Diagnosis. Lung pathology is not the primary method for diagnosing pulmonary emphysema, although autopsy studies have been very helpful in understanding the morphologic abnormalities. Clinical information, pulmonary function tests, and chest radiographs, especially HRCTs, are the usual methods for diagnosis. The patterns of proximal acinar and panacinar emphysema can be seen with CT but the best way to study the morphology is by evaluating the entire lung following appropriate inflation and fixation either in autopsy material or explanted lungs following transplantation. In routine practice this is rarely necessary. Outside of a research setting or postmortem examination, a pathologist is rarely asked to distinguish these types of emphysema. Gough (56) developed a method for sectioning whole lungs that historically had a major impact on understanding the pathology of emphysema (figs. 10-13, 10-14, 10-17). Honeycomb fibrosis differs from emphysema in that extensive interstitial fibrosis is the primary lesion. In contrast, fibrosis is not a prominent feature of emphysema.

Although small carbon deposits may be seen, significant dust deposits should cause the consideration of pneumoconiosis with focal emphysema, especially coal worker's pneumoconiosis.

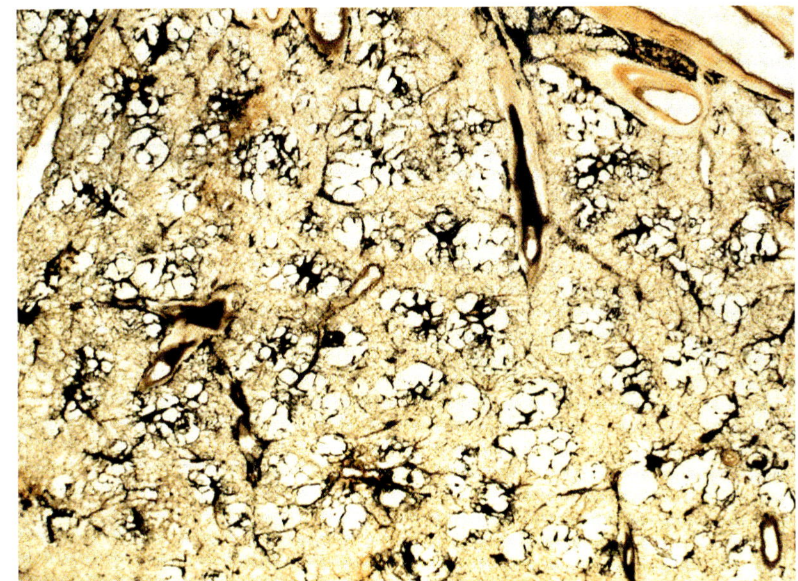

Figure 10-14

PROXIMAL ACINAR EMPHYSEMA

This example of proximal acinar emphysema shows less severe dilation of the centrilobular aspect of the acini. Deposits of anthracotic pigment are present in association with the airways.

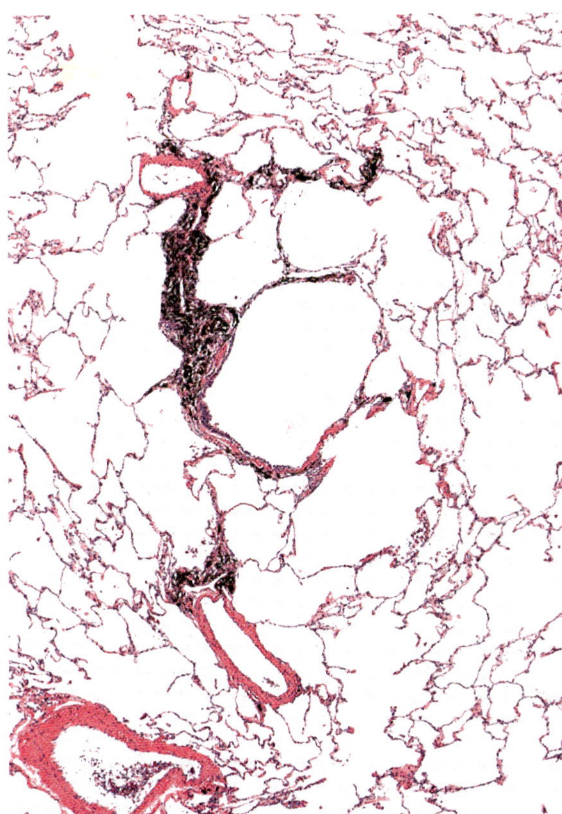

Figure 10-15

PROXIMAL ACINAR EMPHYSEMA

This respiratory bronchiole is dilated and shows an early form of proximal acinar emphysema.

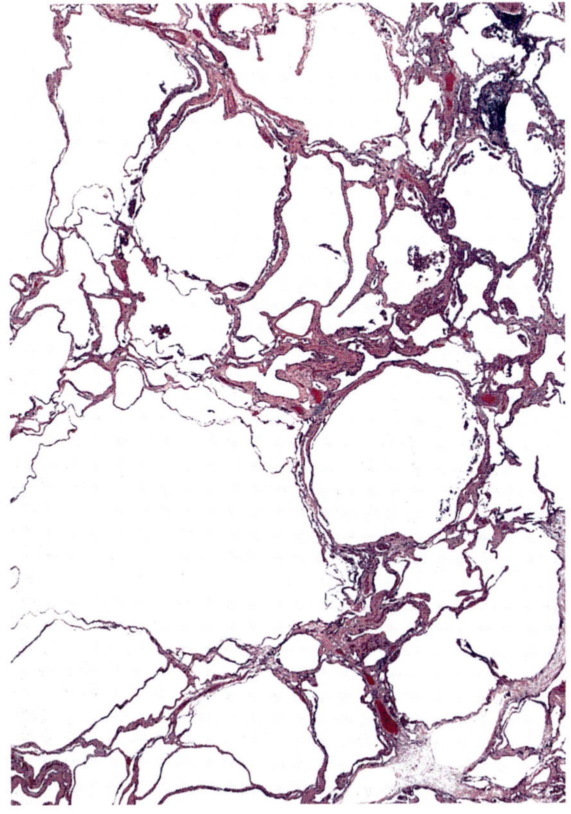

Figure 10-16

PROXIMAL ACINAR EMPHYSEMA

This routine histologic section of proximal acinar emphysema shows severe airspace dilatation.

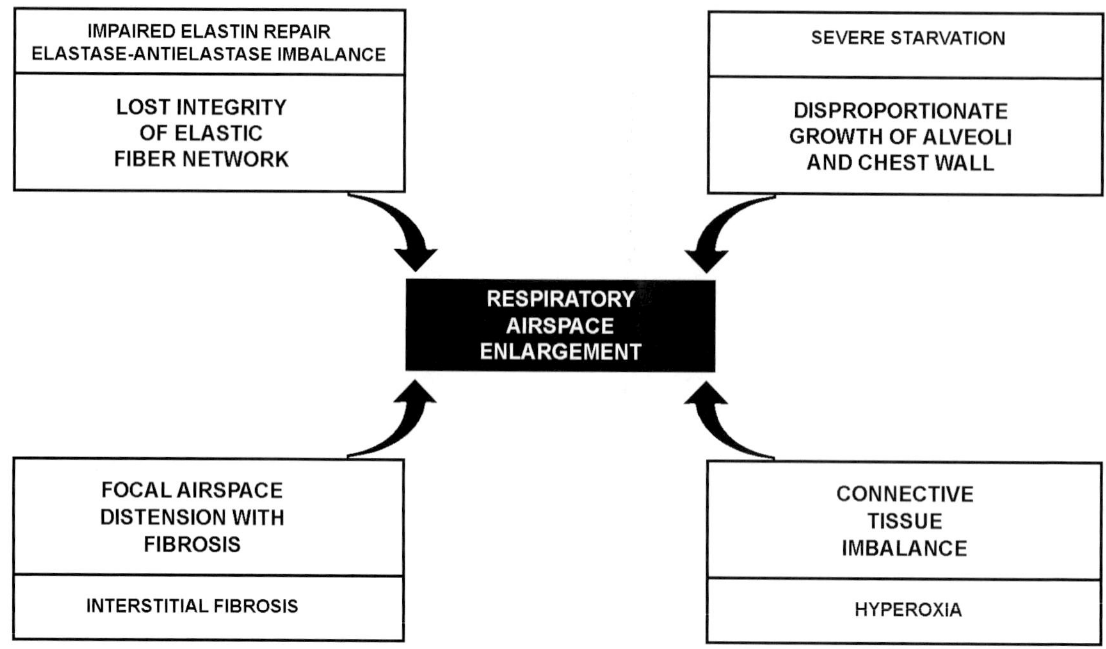

Figure 10-17

RESPIRATORY AIRSPACE ENLARGEMENT

Schema suggesting that respiratory airspace enlargement is a stereotyped response of the lungs to a variety of injuries. Different injuries give rise to airspace enlargement and accompanying loss of alveoli and interstitial fibrosis, by the development of connective tissue imbalance and by altering lung growth. (Figure 10 from Snider GL. Emphysema: the first two centuries–and beyond. A historical overview, with suggestions for future research: part 2. Am Rev Respir Dis 1992;146:1619.)

Pathogenesis. In proximal acinar emphysema there is loss of attachments between alveolar walls and bronchioles, which may result from extension of the inflammation of the peripheral airways (84,140). This lung damage results from a variety of mechanisms (fig. 10-17). When the bronchioles lose their connection with the alveoli and the elastic framework of the lung, they tend to collapse, resulting in airflow obstruction. The loss of alveolar attachments may also be a cause of morphologic changes in the bronchioles, such as increased tortuosity and irregular lumens (84,85,140).

Cigarette smoking plays a major role in the pathogenesis of proximal acinar emphysema (43,123,140). Although the protease-antiprotease hypothesis is a fundamental concept in the development of emphysema (figs. 10-3, 10-4), inflammatory cells and mediators (fig. 10-3) as well as oxidative stress (fig. 10-5) also play important pathogenetic roles (fig. 10-15) (5,59,70,93,110). According to the protease-antiprotease concept, an imbalance of proteases and their inhibitors provides the basis for the lung destruction of emphysema. Ultrastructural studies of the lungs of humans and animals with emphysema following treatment with elastolytic enzymes have demonstrated marked fragmentation of elastic fibers, indicating that the major structural connective tissue component of the lung that is destroyed in emphysema is elastin (46,50,156). Thus, factors that increase the proteinase to antiproteinase ratio favor the development of emphysema (43,122,140).

Serine elastases, primarily from neutrophils and metalloproteinases primarily from macrophages, are thought to be major sources of elastolytic activity (figs. 10-3, 10-4) (47,101,121,123). There are several proteinase and metalloproteinase inhibitors present in the lining fluid of the lung, the most abundant of which is alpha1AT) which inhibits serine elastases. Damage to alpha1AT

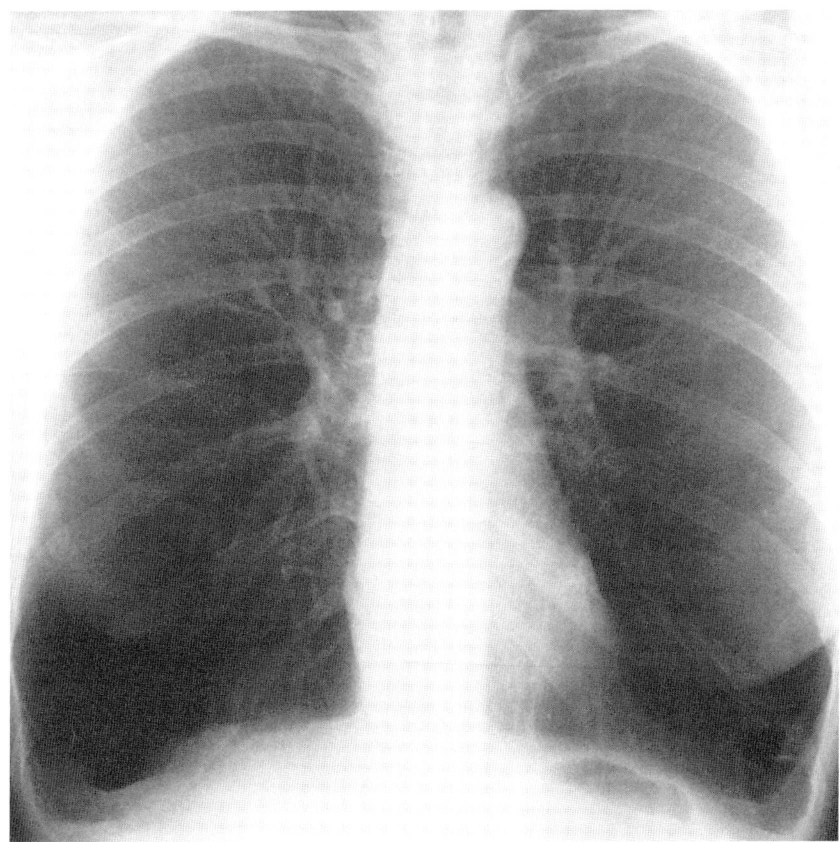

Figure 10-18

PANACINAR EMPHYSEMA

Posteroanterior chest radiograph shows hyperinflation and large areas of increased lucency and decreased vascularity involving mainly the lower lung zones. The increased size and number of vessels in the upper lobes are due to redistribution of blood flow. The patient was a 57-year-old woman with alpha-1-antitrypsin deficiency.

by components of cigarette smoke impairs its ability to inhibit the proteases, resulting in increased elastolytic activity (43,100,123).

It is thought that the emphysema in patients with Salla's disease results from alteration of pulmonary macrophages due to the storage of free sialic acid in the lysosomes (101). In two patients with emphysema associated with cutaneous laxa, it is thought that the combination of cigarette smoking and subnormal alpha1AT levels associated with heterozygosity for the AAT genotype may explain the pulmonary involvement in this usually benign disease limited to the skin (22). Pulmonary emphysema has also been described in Marfan's syndrome (29,35,111) and in association with toxic exposures, such as to cadmium (80,97).

Treatment and Prognosis. The clinical course of proximal acinar emphysema is characterized by progressive, disabling dyspnea for which little can be done. Acute exacerbations are less frequent in the patient with predominant emphysema, however, such relapses frequently lead to severe respiratory failure and death. There has been increasing interest in surgical resection of emphysematous lungs through a median sternotomy (lung volume reduction surgery) and lung transplantation for the management of endstage emphysema. Lung volume reduction surgery appears to offer dramatic improvement in some patients with COPD. However, the long-term benefits and the risk to benefit ratio have not been determined. COPD is now the most common diagnosis for which lung transplantation is carried out.

Panacinar Emphysema

Definition. Panacinar emphysema (*panlobular emphysema*) is characterized by diffuse, bilateral lung involvement in which the alveolar ducts as well as respiratory bronchioles are enlarged, causing uniform destruction of the alveolar tissue.

Panacinar emphysema is less common than proximal acinar emphysema. It is associated with several conditions including familial

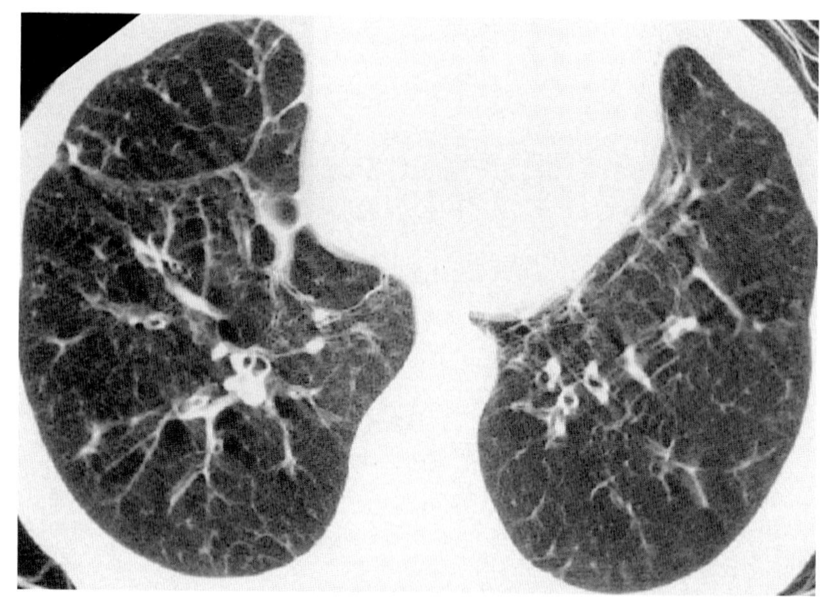

Figure 10-19

PANACINAR EMPHYSEMA

HRCT through the lower lung zones demonstrates a diffuse decrease in attenuation and vascularity. There was blood flow redistribution with increased size and number of vessels in the upper lobes. The patient was a 66-year-old woman with panacinar emphysema.

emphysema associated with alpha1AT deficiency, intravenous drug abuse, and bronchial atresia (140).

Clinical Features. The pulmonary clinical manifestations of panacinar emphysema are similar to those of proximal acinar emphysema. Patients with alpha1AT deficiency may have associated liver disease. Panacinar emphysema occurs at a younger age in alpha1AT patients, especially if the patient smokes cigarettes. Cigarette smoking is the major risk factor for developing emphysema. Patients with severe alpha1AT deficiency who are smokers develop symptoms up to 20 years earlier than their nonsmoking counterparts (136).

Radiologic Findings. Panacinar emphysema is manifested radiologically by hyperinflation and a uniform decrease in vascularity involving predominantly the lower lung lobes (fig. 10-18). Because it involves the entire secondary lobule, panacinar emphysema is characterized on HRCT by the presence of extensive areas of low attenuation and decreased vascularity (fig. 10-19) (133,149,158). The lack of focal abnormalities makes it more difficult to recognize than proximal and distal acinar emphysema (92,132,149). Therefore, mild and even moderately severe panacinar emphysema can be missed on HRCT (92,132).

Gross Findings. Mild panacinar emphysema is best appreciated in lungs that are processed in barium sulfate and immersed in water (140). In early stages, the alveoli are enlarged and flattened, with loss of the normal sharp distinction between alveolar ducts and alveoli (140). The lower lung zones are more severely affected than the upper zones (fig. 10-20) (143). On close examination of the gross specimen, the supporting structures, including airways, vessels, and lobular septa, tend to protrude slightly above the cut surface of the lung because the lung parenchyma falls away from them. As the disease progresses, all airspaces become enlarged and the lung tissue is destroyed. Commonly, strands of tissue, which represent blood vessels, can be seen crossing the emphysematous spaces. There is frequent overlap between the patterns of proximal acinar and panacinar emphysema making it difficult to make a sharp distinction. However, in panacinar emphysema there is no normal lung parenchyma, whereas in proximal acinar emphysema, normal and emphysematous lung can be found side by side.

In intravenous drug abusers the emphysematous changes may be accompanied by interstitial fibrosis, sometimes with the pattern of progressive massive fibrosis.

Histologic Findings. In panacinar emphysema the entire acinus is uniformly enlarged and destroyed (fig. 10-7). The secondary lobules are uniformly affected from the center to the periphery (figs. 10-20, 10-21). In early

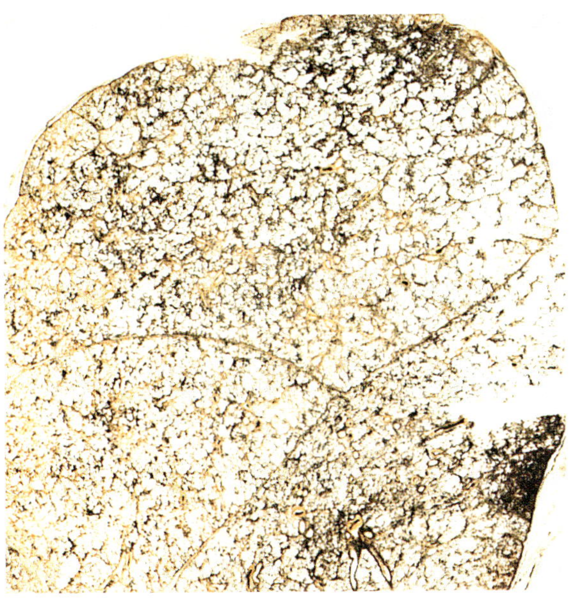

Figure 10-20

PANACINAR EMPHYSEMA

The lung is diffusely and severely affected by panacinar emphysema.

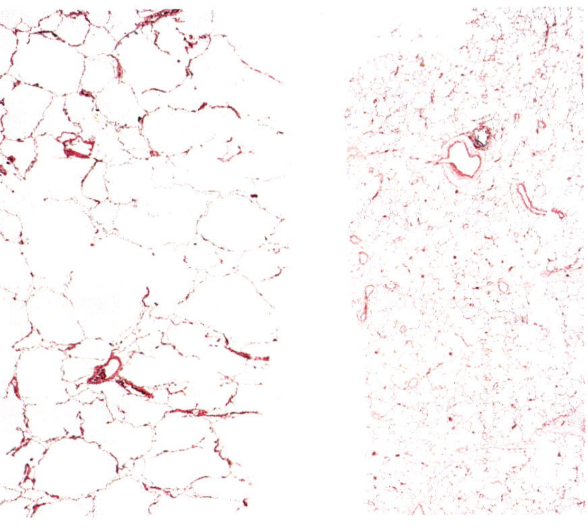

Figure 10-21

PANACINAR EMPHYSEMA

The section on the left is from a patient with panacinar emphysema associated with alpha-1-antitripsin deficiency. It contrasts greatly with the section of normal lung on the right. The emphysematous lung shows diffuse enlargement of the airspaces affecting the entire acinus.

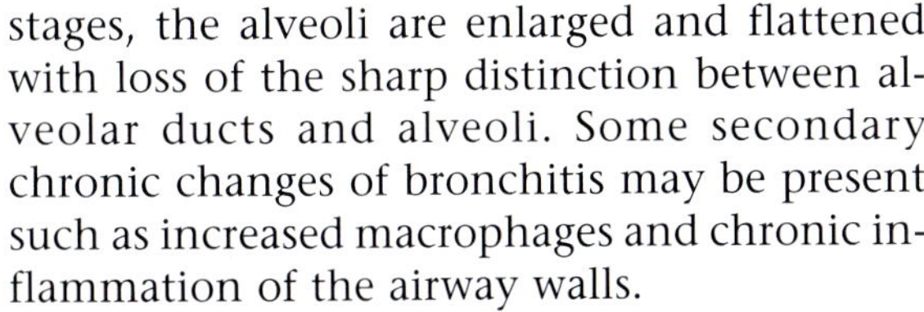

stages, the alveoli are enlarged and flattened with loss of the sharp distinction between alveolar ducts and alveoli. Some secondary chronic changes of bronchitis may be present such as increased macrophages and chronic inflammation of the airway walls.

Panacinar emphysema associated with intravenous drug abuse shows talc granulomas. There may be associated fibrosis that resembles progressive massive fibrosis (fig. 10-22 and chapter 7) (101,118,124,134,159).

Pathogenesis. There are several conditions associated with the pattern of panacinar emphysema, including familial emphysema associated with alpha1AT deficiency and intravenous drug abuse (140). A panacinar pattern of emphysema may also be seen in association with the Swyer-James syndrome or unilateral hyperlucent lung (140).

Differential Diagnosis. The distinction between panacinar and proximal acinar emphysema is based primarily on clinical and radiographic findings or the gross pathology of large specimens if they are available. It is generally not necessary to make this separation on routine surgical specimens. However, pathologists may encounter emphysematous lungs at autopsy or in explanted lungs. If the gross lung specimens are properly prepared it may be possible to make this distinction. In severe proximal acinar emphysema there can be complete destruction of secondary pulmonary lobules. This can lead to confusion with panacinar emphysema, in which the lung destruction is more uniform. In some cases there may be a mixture of patterns, with a pattern of panacinar emphysema in the lower lobes and proximal acinar emphysema in the upper lobes (27,140).

Alpha1AT Deficiency. The most common cause of panacinar emphysema is an autosomal codominant genetic disorder that results in low serum levels of alpha1AT (12,41,42,105, 136). Alpha1AT deficiency occurs when two protease inhibitor (PI) deficiency alleles from the alpha1AT gene locus (designated PI) on chromosomal segment 14q32.1 are inherited (12,41,42, 105,136). Approximately 75 different alleles for alpha1AT variants are recognized but only 10 to 15 are associated with severe alpha1-AT deficiency (136). The most common severe deficient variant is the PI*Z allele. Approximately 95 percent of patients with severe alpha1AT deficiency

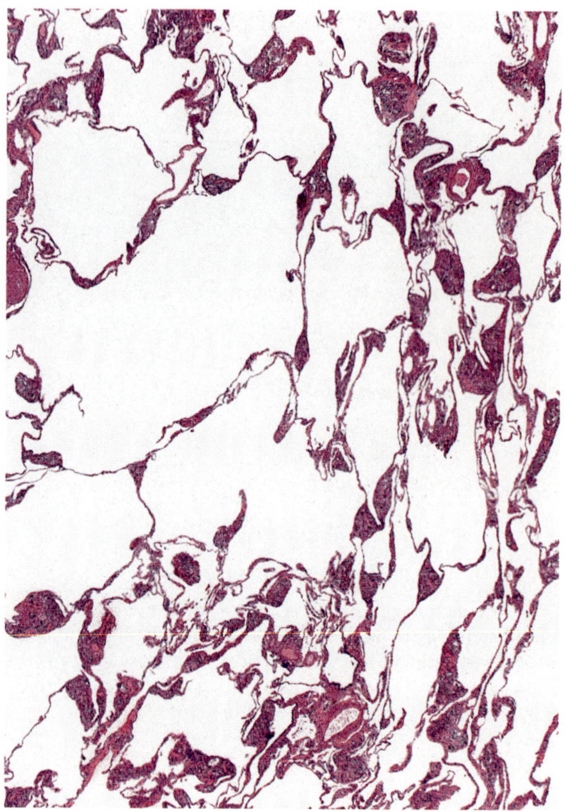

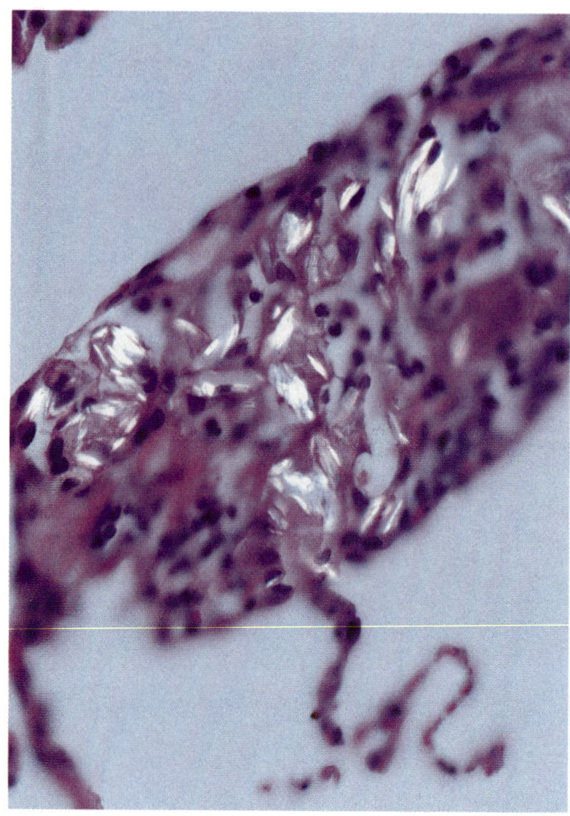

Figure 10-22

PANACINAR EMPHYSEMA ASSOCIATED WITH INTRAVENOUS DRUG ABUSE

Left: The emphysematous lung shows markedly dilated airspaces but there is also mild interstitial thickening due to deposits of talc and slight interstitial fibrosis.

Right: Polarization microscopy highlights the extensive birefringent deposits of talc in the interstitium.

are PI type ZZ (136). Alpha1AT deficiency is present in 2 to 3 percent of patients with COPD and in the United States it occurs in 1 of 3,000 to 1 of 6,000 persons (12,136). COPD with the pattern of panacinar emphysema is the most common manifestation of alpha1AT deficiency and the most frequent cause of disability and death.

Alpha1AT plays a major role in inhibiting serine proteases, especially neutrophil elastase; the latter contributes to elastic fiber degradation in the lung (76,136). After alpha1-AT is cleaved by neutrophil elastase they both combine to form tight complexes that are removed by the liver. The reduced alpha1AT levels allow neutrophil elastase to degrade pulmonary elastic fibers and other structural connective tissues, resulting in emphysema (76,136). Smoking may be an exacerbating factor.

Emphysema in Intravenous Drug Abusers. The cause of emphysema in IV drug abusers is not clear but several mechanisms are possible: 1) ischemic necrosis of alveolar septa due to repeated microembolization of alveolar capillaries by embolic particulate material; 2) widespread septic emboli; 3) a direct elastolytic effect by drugs such as Ritalin; and 4) release of elastases and other proteases by macrophages after phagocytosis of particulate embolic material (102,118). The latter mechanism is favored.

Distal Acinar Emphysema

Definition. Distal acinar emphysema affects the periphery of the acinus, most often in the upper lobes beneath the pleura, lobular septa, or airways and vessels. Alveolar ducts are predominantly enlarged and destroyed.

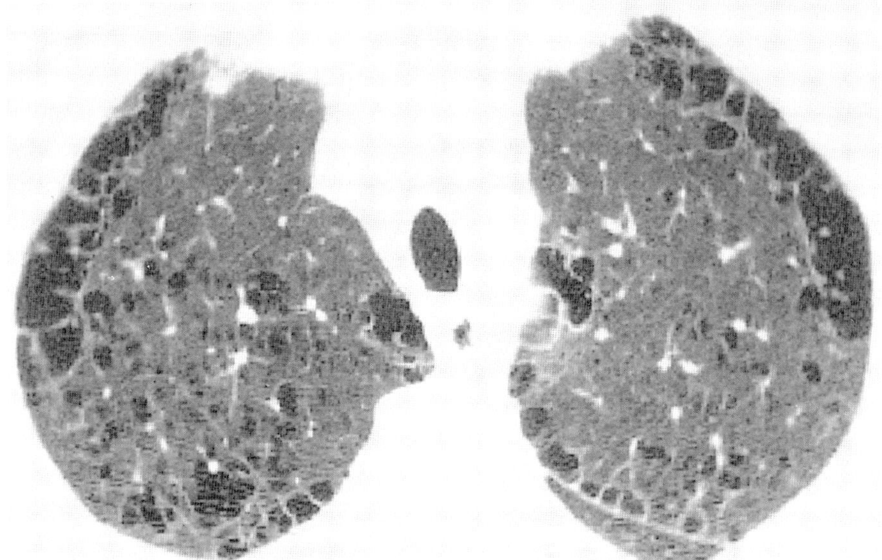

Figure 10-23

DISTAL ACINAR EMPHYSEMA

HRCT demonstrates numerous bullae involving mainly the subpleural lung regions. The patient was a 71-year-old man with mild proximal acinar and extensive distal acinar emphysema.

Synonyms include *paraseptal, subpleural,* or *localized emphysema.*

Clinical Features. Distal acinar emphysema is the type of emphysema that produces apical bullae. It may be a cause of spontaneous pneumothorax in young adults.

Radiologic Findings. On the chest radiograph, distal acinar emphysema is most commonly manifested as bullae near the lung apex. In other areas of the lungs, bullae are difficult to visualize unless they are large and displace the adjacent vessels. On HRCT, distal acinar emphysema is characterized by the presence of areas of low attenuation and bullae in the subpleural lung regions and adjacent to the pulmonary vessels and interlobular septa (fig. 10-23) (133,149). HRCT is superior to the radiograph in the assessment of distal acinar emphysema, frequently demonstrating lesions in patients with normal radiographs (7,75), and identifying the characteristic distribution (92).

Gross Findings. Distal acinar emphysema is typically situated in the subpleural aspect of the upper lobes and is often associated with fibrosis (figs. 10-24, 10-25) (39,140,164). It is usually seen as multiple, subpleural, contiguous emphysematous spaces measuring from less than 1 mm to more than 2 cm in diameter (fig. 10-24). It is often limited in extent although it may be found in association with proximal acinar or panacinar emphysema (fig. 10-25). Bullae are often found if the emphysema is extensive and may appear as thin-walled cystic spaces (fig. 10-26).

Histologic Findings. In distal acinar emphysema the periphery of the acinus is affected beneath the pleura, lobular septa, or airways and vessels (fig. 10-27). Alveolar ducts are predominantly enlarged and destroyed. The walls of the bullae, overlying pleura or emphysematous spaces, may show fibrosis. The adjacent lung is normal unless there is associated proximal acinar or panacinar emphysema.

Pathogenesis. The pathogenesis of distal acinar emphysema is not certain (39). However, there are fewer capillaries in the alveolar walls adjacent to the subpleural connective tissue compared to those surrounded only by airspaces. This could lead to higher compliance in the distal acinar region due to reduced vascularity. In addition, during lung development, elastic fibers are initially found surrounding the bronchioles in the centriacinar region and at birth there are no elastic fibers against the pleura (39). The combination of distribution of vascularity and elastic fibers may contribute to the development of distal acinar emphysema.

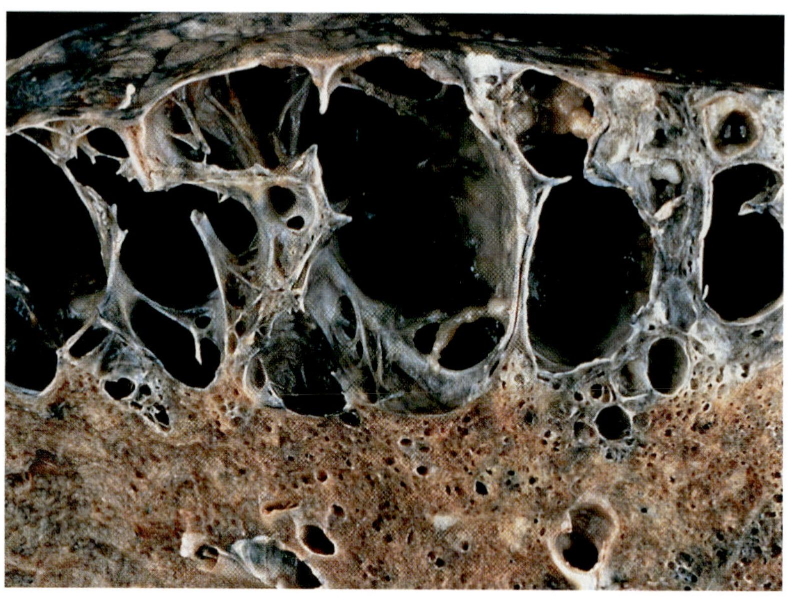

Figure 10-24

DISTAL ACINAR EMPHYSEMA

There is striking subpleural emphysema with marked dilation of the distal acini. The interstitium shows mild fibrosis.

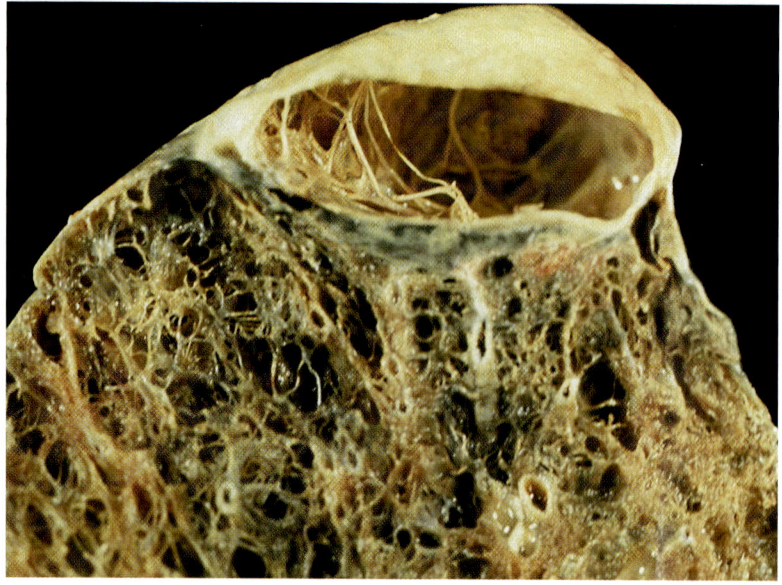

Figure 10-25

DISTAL ACINAR EMPHYSEMA WITH APICAL BULLAE

The apex of this lung shows a large bullous cyst, with fibrous thickening of the pleura and the border with the underlying lung. The underlying lung shows proximal acinar emphysema.

Irregular Emphysema

Definition. Irregular emphysema refers to airspace enlargement and lung destruction associated with a pulmonary scar. The National Heart, Lung and Blood Institute does not regard this as a form of emphysema, but rather as "airspace enlargement with fibrosis" (128). Synonyms are *scar emphysema, paracicatricial emphysema,* and *perifocal emphysema.*

Clinical and Radiologic Findings. Since this type of emphysema is secondary to lung scars, there are no distinctive clinical or radiographic findings.

Gross Findings. At the edge of fibrotic scars the airspaces appear irregularly enlarged.

Histologic Findings. In irregular emphysema (see fig. 10-9) there is airspace enlargement in the lung parenchyma surrounding a scar (fig. 10-28). Morphologically, the acinus shows irregular enlargement and destruction. The scars are often caused by granulomatous inflammation, dust deposits, organizing pneumonia, and pulmonary infarcts.

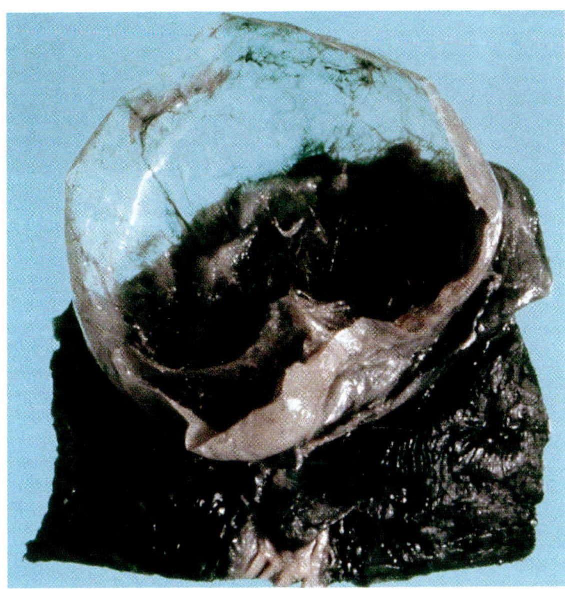

Figure 10-26

DISTAL ACINAR EMPHYSEMA WITH APICAL BULLAE

This apical bulla has a very thin translucent wall. (Courtesy of the Gordon Museum, London, England.)

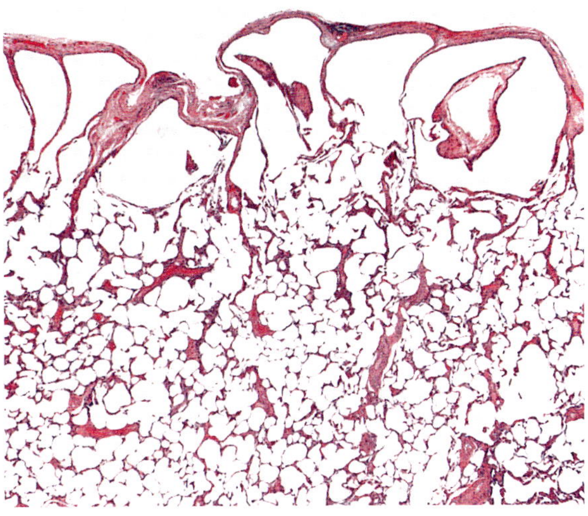

Figure 10-27

DISTAL ACINAR EMPHYSEMA

There is marked dilatation of the subpleural airspaces primarily affecting the distal acini. The emphysema is accompanied by mild interstitial and pleural fibrosis.

Localized Giant Bullous Emphysema

Definition. Giant bullous emphysema is a cystic lesion that typically involves a single lobe in young or middle-aged adults. A rare subset of these patients has unusual histologic findings resembling placental tissues. In such cases, the cystic spaces are unilocular or paucilocular, and microscopically consist of papillae resembling placental villi that contain blood vessels, lymphoid nodules, smooth muscle, and fat. *"Vanishing lung"* is a synonym and cases with placental-like features have been called *placental transmogrification of the lung* and *placentoid bullous lesion of the lung*

Clinical Features. Patients are young to middle-aged adults; there is no sex predilection. Presenting manifestations are dyspnea, chest pain, recurrent spontaneous pneumothorax, or recurrent episodes of pneumonia, or patients may be asymptomatic. Less than 10 cases of this lesion are reported (45,61,89).

Radiologic Findings. The characteristic radiographic and HRCT manifestations consist of large bullae occupying one third or more of the hemithorax (fig. 10-29) (135). The lung

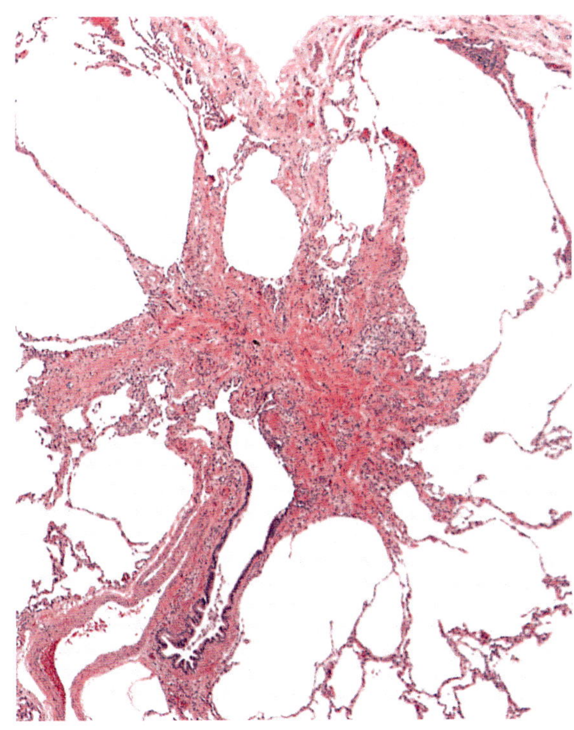

Figure 10-28

IRREGULAR EMPHYSEMA

Irregular emphysema associated with a fibrosing lesion of Langerhans' cell histiocytosis. There is irregular emphysematous dilation of airspaces adjacent to the stellate-shaped scar.

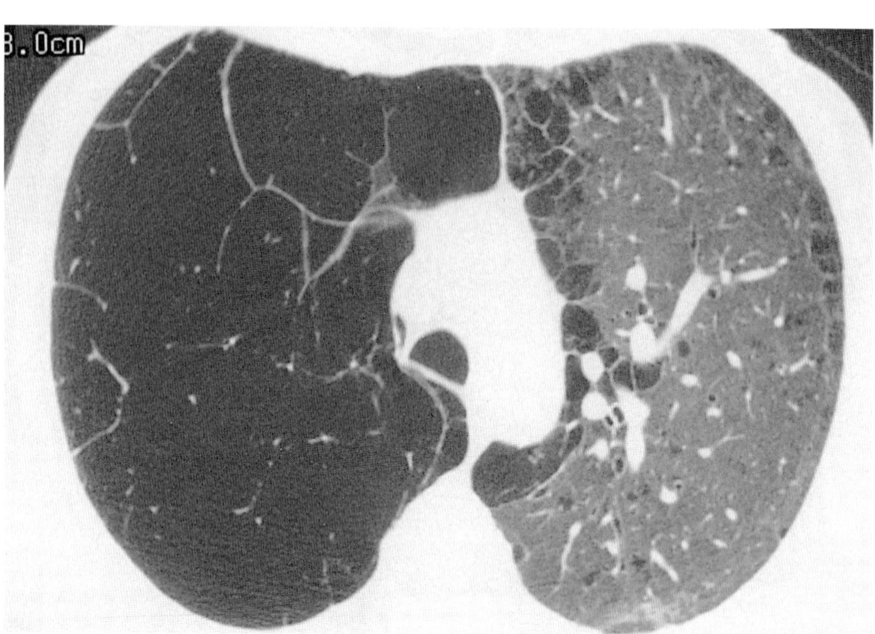

Figure 10-29

GIANT BULLOUS EMPHYSEMA

HRCT shows almost complete destruction of the right upper lobe by severe bullous emphysema. The mediastinum is shifted to the left and there is mild distal acinar emphysema with bullae in the subpleural regions of the left lung. The patient was a 68-year-old man.

adjacent to the bullae can appear compressed due to retraction of the more normal lung by its intact elastica and overexpansion of the emphysematous lung because of increased compliance and decreased elasticity. The bullae may be present for several years and be seen to gradually enlarge before surgical resection. CT allows assessment of the extent of bullous disease, the severity of compression of the adjacent lung, and evidence of emphysema in the remaining lung (51,149,154).

Radiographically, the bullous lesions are unilateral, cystic, and localized to a single lobe of lung. The bullous cystic spaces can be so large that the mediastinum is shifted. They appear to enlarge gradually and may be observed over many years before surgical resection is necessary.

Gross Findings. The cystic lesions most often merge with the adjacent lung parenchyma although they may be sharply demarcated. The lesion may appear spongy or cystic depending on the size of the cystic spaces, which can range from a few millimeters to up to 20 cm. The cystic spaces can be filled with gelatinous material that appears vesicular or grape-like.

Histologic Findings. The histologic features may consist of severe emphysema that is so extensive that it is difficult to classify as proximal, panacinar, or distal acinar in type. In cases with placental features, the cystic spaces are separated by fibrotic septa with papillary structures that resemble placental villi with hydropic degeneration (figs. 10-30, 10-31). The cores of the papillae consist of vascular channels, pale cuboidal to spindled stromal cells, lymphocytes, plasma cells, and bundles of smooth muscle (fig. 10-31); they may be sclerotic and calcified. Lymphoid aggregates and fat may be present.

Differential Diagnosis. Localized giant bullous emphysema needs to be separated from lymphangiomas, hemangiomas, alveolar adenomas, and other cystic lung lesions. However, these lesions do not show placentoid papillary structures nor do they contain fat. Bullous emphysema also lacks these structures. Lymphangiomas and hemangiomas consist primarily of proliferation of vascular spaces rather than emphysematous airspaces. Alveolar adenomas are discrete nodules of several centimeters in size comprised of tissue resembling alveolar spaces. Although there may be cystically dilated airspaces, they do not show features of emphysema.

Treatment and Prognosis. Surgical resection consisting of either lobectomy or pneumonectomy of the affected lobe is curative.

Simple (Nonemphysematous) Airspace Enlargement

There are a variety of types of airspace enlargement that differ from emphysema in that

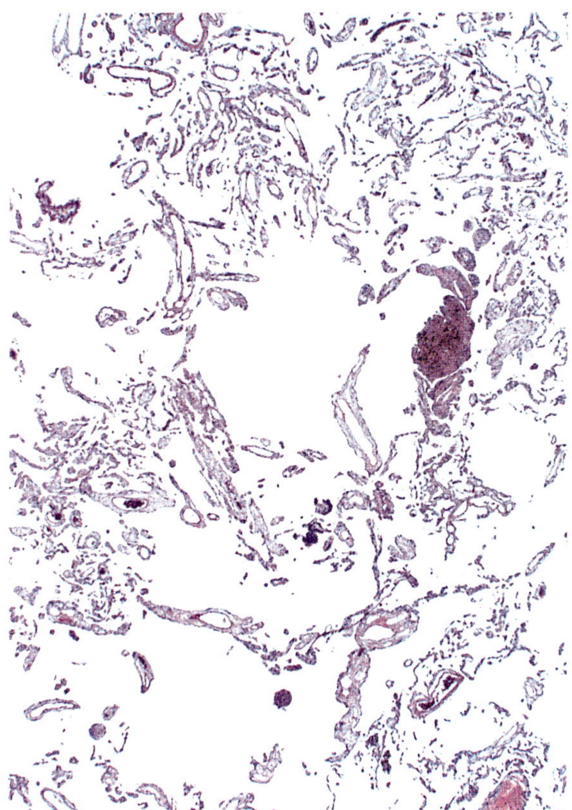

Figure 10-30

LOCALIZED GIANT BULLOUS EMPHYSEMA WITH PLACENTAL HISTOLOGIC FEATURES

The lung shows emphysema with focal thickening of the walls of the cystic spaces.

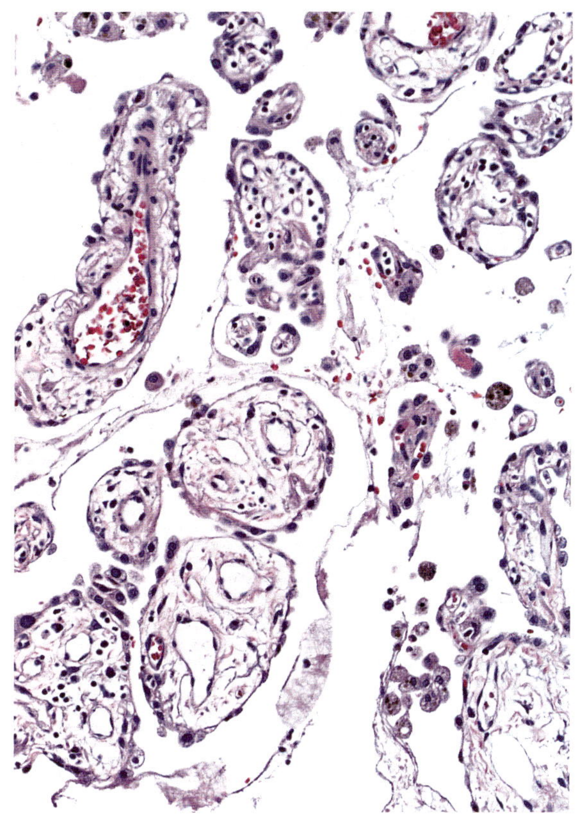

Figure 10-31

LOCALIZED GIANT BULLOUS EMPHYSEMA WITH PLACENTAL HISTOLOGIC FEATURES

Within the cystic spaces are papillae consisting of fibrovascular cores lined by hyperplastic pneumocytes.

they do not involve lung destruction. These include aging, or "senile emphysema" (53,95,151, 152), as well as a few rare disorders such as Down's syndrome (19,20), postpneumonectomy, and severe starvation. In *senile emphysema,* the airspace dilatation is more regular than in emphysematous lungs and there is no destruction of alveolar walls. In addition, there is an increased thickening of alveolar septa, without inflammation or fibrosis (95,152). In children with *Down's syndrome,* the lungs are hypoplastic with a diminished number of alveoli in relation to acini and enlarged alveoli and alveolar ducts (see chapter 11) (19,20). The lungs also have a smaller total number of alveoli and a smaller alveolar surface area (19,20). *Postpneumonectomy,* there can be airspace expansion in the remaining lung. Whether the increase in lung volume is due to multiplication or distension of alveoli is not known (14). Emphysema also occurs in association with *severe starvation,* although most of this data is from experimental rat models (115,116).

ASTHMA

Definition. The National Institutes of Health (NIH) 1997 Guidelines for the Diagnosis and Management of Asthma defined asthma as "a chronic inflammatory disorder of the airways in which many cells and cellular elements play a role, in particular, mast cells, eosinophils, T lymphocytes, neutrophils, and epithelial cells. In susceptible individuals, this inflammation causes recurrent episodes of wheezing, breathlessness, chest tightness, and cough, particularly at night and in the early morning. These episodes are usually associated with widespread but variable airflow obstruction that is often reversible either spontaneously or with treatment. The inflammation also causes an associated increase in the existing bronchial hyperresponsiveness to a variety of stimuli" (96).

Asthma is a major health problem affecting more than 15 million people in the United States (3,14,88). The incidence and prevalence of asthma in children and adults has increased substantially in the last 20 years. Asthma is responsible for 9 million visits to health care providers, over 1.8 million emergency room visits, over 460,000 hospitalizations, and kills over 5,000 Americans each year.

Epidemiologic studies have suggested that the presence of allergy and the degree of atopy (e.g., positive immediate skin test responses) parallel the frequency of asthma in the population (94). In fact, atopy, the genetic predisposition for the development of an IgE-mediated response to common aeroallergens, is the strongest identifiable predisposing factor for developing asthma (94,96). There are strong associations between the development of allergic reactions to certain environmental allergens (house dust mites, cat dander, *Alternaria,* and cockroach antigens) and the development asthma (94). In addition, there is sufficient evidence that environmental tobacco smoke causes exacerbations of asthma in preschool-aged children. Common air pollutants such as ozone, sulfur dioxide, and particulate matter are known to be respiratory irritants and can contribute to an exacerbation of asthma symptoms. Moreover, asthma is the leading work-related lung disease.

Clinical Features. Making the correct diagnosis of asthma is often not easy, but is extremely important. Clinical judgment is required because signs and symptoms vary widely from patient to patient as well as within each patient over time (10,15,96). To establish the diagnosis, the clinician must determine that: episodic symptoms of airflow obstruction are present; airflow obstruction is at least partially reversible; and alternative diagnoses are excluded (96).

Asthma commonly begins in childhood and adolescence. However, it can develop at anytime in life. In adults, asthma occurs in variety of settings. Allergens may play an important role although some adults who develop asthma do not have IgE antibodies to allergens or a family history of asthma. These individuals often have coexisting sinusitis, nasal polyps, and sensitivity to aspirin or related nonsteroidal anti-inflammatory drugs (*nonallergic* or *intrinsic asthma*) (96). Occupational exposure to workplace materials (animal products; biological enzymes; plastic resin; wood dusts, particularly cedar; and metals) can cause airway inflammation, bronchial hyperresponsiveness, and clinical signs of asthma (96,150). Identification of the causative agent and its removal from the workplace can reduce symptoms although some individuals will have persistent asthma even though exposure to the causative agent has stopped (150).

Asthma causes recurrent episodes of wheezing, shortness of breath, chest tightness, and cough that are associated with airflow obstruction in predisposed individuals. These episodes are often associated with increased bronchial hyperreactivity to various stimuli. The airflow obstruction is typically reversible with therapy or spontaneously. In *status asthmaticus,* patients have an acute attack of respiratory failure due to airway inflammation, mucous plugging, and edema (23). Other patients develop *sudden asphyxic asthma* due to a sudden increase in airflow obstruction from bronchospasm rather than airway inflammation, mucous plugging, and edema (23,138). Asthma can be classified according to symptom frequency, severity, and required therapy combined with evaluation of airway function (Table 10-4) (163). It can also be classified according to risk factors or inciting agents (Table 10-5).

Physical examination, especially in children with chronic asthma, often shows hyperexpansion of the thorax, use of accessory chest muscles, appearance of hunched shoulders, and chest deformity. There may be signs of increased nasal secretion, mucosal swelling, and nasal polyps. Breath sounds show wheezing during normal breathing, or a prolonged phase of forced exhalation (typical of airflow obstruction). In mild intermittent asthma or between exacerbations, wheezing may be absent.

Spirometry measurements (forced expiratory volume in 1 second [FEV1], forced vital capacity [FVC], FEV1/FVC) before and after the patient inhales a short-acting bronchodilator

Table 10-4

CLASSIFICATION OF ASTHMA[a]

Persistent Asthma
Obstructed Asthma
Episodic Asthma
Asthma in Remission
Potential Asthma
Trivial Wheeze
Extrinsic (Atopic) Asthma
Occupational Asthma
Intrinsic Asthma

[a]Data from reference 163.

Table 10-5

RISK FACTORS FOR ASTHMA[a]

Allergens and atopy
Animal allergens
House-dust mites
Cockroach allergens
Indoor fungi (molds)
Outdoor allergens
Respiratory infections (particularly viral)
Diet
Genetic factors including race and gender
Passive smoking
Physical exertion
Occupational exposures
Environmental and air pollution
Other factors that can influence asthma severity:
Rhinitis/sinusitis
Gastroesophageal reflux
Sensitivity to aspirin, other nonsteroidal anti-inflammatory drugs, and sulfites
Topical and systemic beta-blockers

[a]Data from references 96 and 163.

are useful to confirm the presence of airflow obstruction and whether it is reversible over the short term (96). Airflow obstruction is indicated by reduced FEV1 and FEV1/FVC values relative to reference or predicted values. Significant reversibility is indicated by an increase of more than 12 percent and 200 mL in FEV1 after inhaling a short-acting bronchodilator. A 2- to 3-week trial of oral corticosteroid therapy may be required to demonstrate reversibility. The spirometry measurements that establish reversibility may not indicate the patient's best lung function (96). Airway hyperresponsiveness can be determined through methacholine, histamine, and/or exercise testing. A positive methacholine challenge demonstrates a fall in FEV1 of 20 percent or greater (PC20) with 8 mg/mL or less of methacholine. The finding of reversible airflow obstruction on spirometry or a positive methacholine challenge is inadequate to diagnose asthma alone as many other diseases are associated with this pattern of abnormality, including COPD, congestive heart failure, bronchiectasis, and seasonal allergic rhinitis. A negative bronchoprovocation test may help to rule out asthma.

If there is any question regarding induction of symptoms due to exposure to indoor allergens, allergy skin testing using the skin-prick method should be undertaken to guide avoidance therapy. Exacerbating factors, such as sinus disease or gastroesophageal reflux, should be sought. A chest X ray may be needed to exclude other diagnoses.

Radiologic Findings. The chest radiograph and HRCT play a limited role in the diagnosis and management of patients with asthma. In the majority of patients the chest radiograph is normal. Abnormalities that may be seen are nonspecific and include bronchial wall thickening, hyperinflation, and prominence of the central pulmonary arteries due to transient pulmonary arterial hypertension (62,158). The main role of chest radiography is in the evaluation of patients with severe acute attacks where it is helpful in ruling out precipitating causes, such as pneumonia, and complications, such as pneumomediastinum, pneumothorax, and atelectasis (104,161).

Pathologic Findings. While much of the classic literature on the pathology of asthma has been derived from autopsies of patients who died from status asthmaticus (36,91), over the past decade there has been an explosion of publications on the use of bronchoscopic biopsies in the assessment of asthma (9,11,16, 32,58,74,79,153,160). This has provided many new insights into the pathology of asthma since patients with mild disease can be studied.

Gross Findings. The gross autopsy findings of patients with status asthmaticus are distinctive: mucous plugs occluding primarily medium-sized and small bronchi, and bronchioles associated with overinflation of the lungs (fig. 10-32) (36–38,91,140). Overinflation can be mistaken for emphysema, but emphysema as defined above, is uncommon. Bronchiectasis is a complication of asthma. The mucus is thick and tenacious. Rarely, it causes occlusion of the airways from the trachea to the respiratory bronchioles. Saccular bronchiectasis and subpleural fibrosis, particularly in the upper lobes, are found in 15 to 20 percent of patients (36, 37,91,140). Coiled mucous plugs from small airways can be expectorated in the form of Curschmann spirals.

Histologic Findings. Mucous plugs fill both bronchi and bronchioles (fig. 10-33). Asthma is usually most severe in small bronchi. Bronchiolar lesions are less prominent, but are nonetheless present. The mucus is infiltrated with many eosinophils, Charcot-Leyden crystals, and whorls of shed epithelium that form Creola bodies (1,37,38,91). Curschmann spirals appear as coiled fragments of inspissated mucus (fig. 10-34). The bronchial epithelium often desquamates, resulting in only a layer of basal cells. Goblet cell metaplasia may be prominent (fig. 10-35) and squamous metaplasia may be seen (1, 37,54,91). The airway wall is thickened due to edema, an increase in smooth muscle, and an increase in the size of the submucosal mucous glands. Thickening of the peripheral airways is due to an increase in submucosal vascular volume as well as increased airway smooth muscle.

By light microscopy basement membranes usually appear thickened, although some studies show thinning or reduplication (fig. 10-35) (37,54,91,140). This is not specific for asthma since basement membrane thickening can be present to a lesser degree in any inflammatory airway condition such as chronic bronchitis or bronchiectasis (37,91,140). The median thickness of the basement membrane in patients who die from asthma is 17.5 µm compared to 7.0 µm in nonasthmatics (32). The degree of basement membrane thickening varies and is not uniform throughout the airways. Although light microscopic studies refer to basement membrane thickening, ultrastructural and immunohistochemical studies have shown that the thickening is actually due to deposition of dense deposits of collagen beneath the true basement membrane that is of normal thickness (32). The subepithelial deposits consist of types III and V collagen with fibronectin (32). In the setting of longstanding asthma, bronchioles may become fibrotic and chronically inflamed (fig. 10-36).

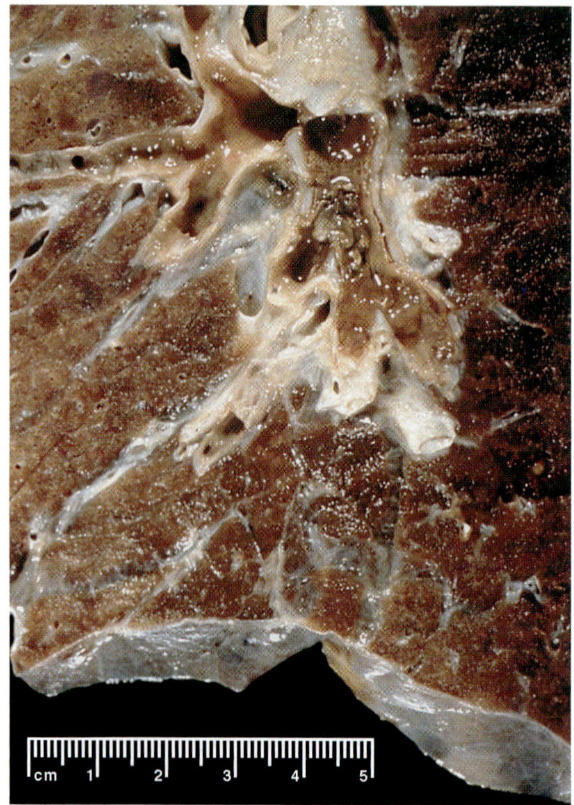

Figure 10-32

ASTHMA: GROSS SPECIMEN

The bronchi are dilated and mucous plugs are present.

The airways are infiltrated by eosinophils, especially in the medium-sized and small bronchi. Bronchial submucosal glands are increased in size. Patients dying of status asthmaticus have a 2- to 3-fold increase in the amount of airway smooth muscle, especially in the medium-sized bronchi (140). Patients with sudden onset fatal asthma may not have mucous plugs in the airways, and it is thought that the obstruction is due to smooth muscle constriction (138). Autopsies from these patients may show more neutrophils and less eosinophils than patients with conventional "slow onset" asthma (138). This suggests that the mechanism may be different and inhalation of *Alternaria* or *Alternaria* contaminated with endotoxin has been suggested as a possible inciting mechanism (138).

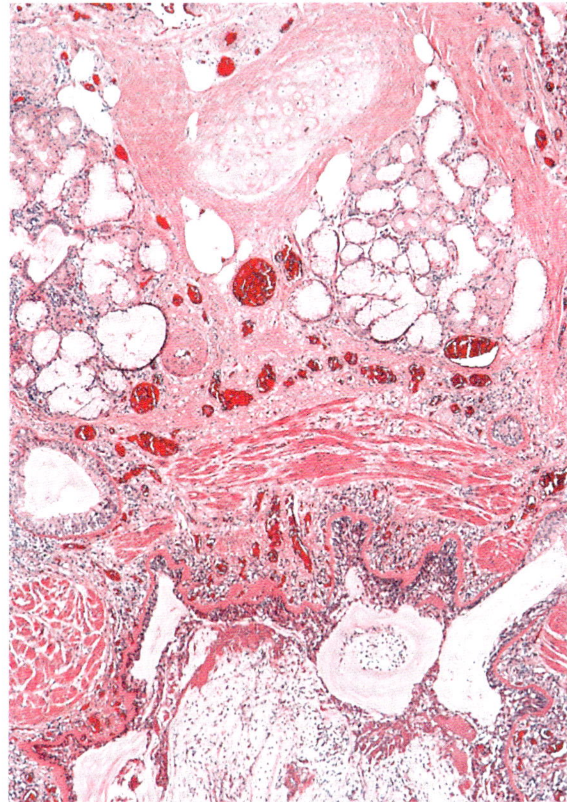

Figure 10-33

ASTHMA: HISTOLOGY

This bronchus is filled with mucus and there is hyperplasia of both submucosal smooth muscle and submucosal glands.

Figure 10-34

ASTHMA: BRONCHIAL HISTOLOGY

There is mucus filling this airway, subepithelial thickening of the basement membrane, and goblet cell hyperplasia.

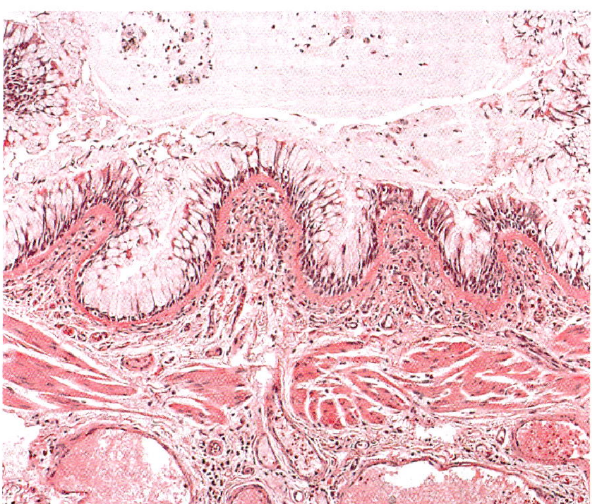

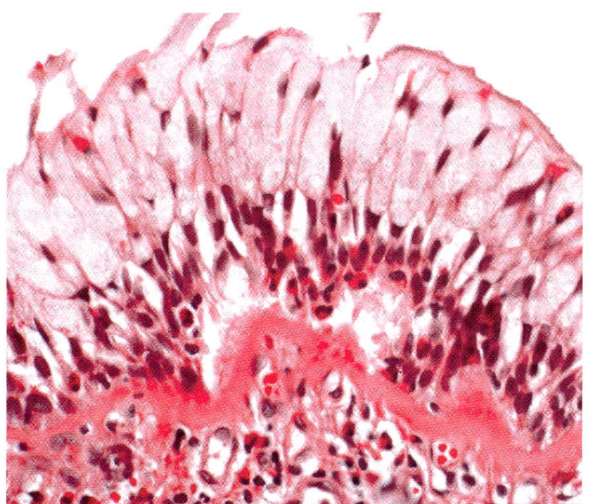

Figure 10-35

ASTHMA: GOBLET CELL HYPERPLASIA

Goblet cell hyperplasia is prominent and the subepithelial basement membrane is thickened.

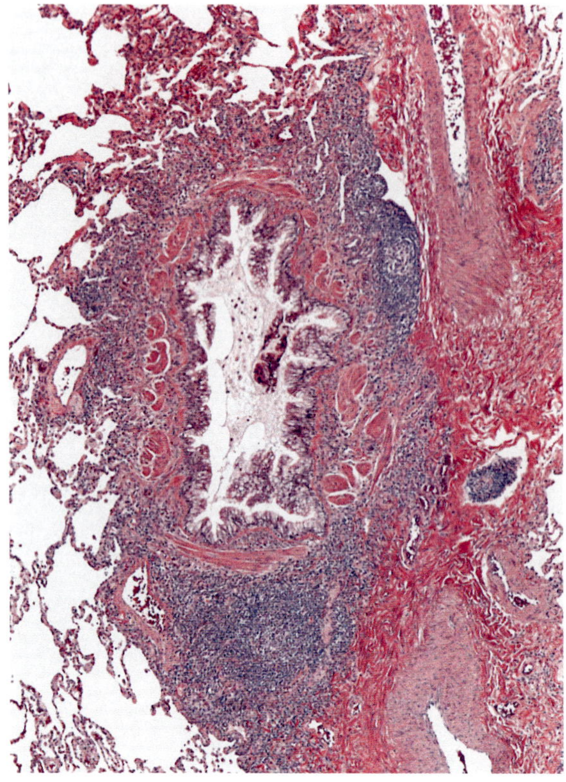

Figure 10-36

ASTHMA: BRONCHIOLAR FIBROSIS

There is fibrosis of the bronchiolar wall with peribronchiolar chronic inflammation and lymphoid aggregates.

Information about the pathology of asthma can be obtained from sputum, bronchoalveolar lavage, and bronchial biopsies (87). Valuable clinical correlations have been made with the histologic findings from bronchial biopsies in a growing number of studies. Many articles have been written about the safety of (34,68) and optimal methods for the bronchoscopic biopsy procedure itself (34,68,139), which is regarded as a safe procedure in these patients (32,131,137). It is beyond the scope of this text to review these studies in detail but one important observation is the finding that prominent histologic changes may be present in patients with mild clinical manifestations of asthma (6,9,28,66). Studies using bronchoscopic biopsies have also correlated various types of medical therapy with the reduction of the inflammatory infiltrate (9,31,33,73,130) and subepithelial fibrosis (9). Most of the above studies refer to status asthmaticus. Between asthmatic attacks the airways may be normal or show only mild histologic changes. Constrictive bronchiolitis and bronchiectasis may be complications. Patients may also develop allergic bronchopulmonary fungal disease or Churg-Strauss syndrome.

Pathogenesis. Asthma, whatever the severity, is a chronic inflammatory disorder of the airways (96). The pathogenesis of asthma involves alterations in airway structure, physiology, neurogenic mechanisms, and immune responses (fig. 10-37). There are two phases of the asthmatic response to inhaled antigen: immediate and late. The immediate allergic response is characterized by mast cell degranulation and causes bronchospasm, edema, and airflow obstruction (fig. 10-38). This may be followed by a late-phase response that involves eosinophil degranulation and an increase in smooth muscle mass accompanied by vasodilatation, vascular congestion (82), and edema; the result is airway wall thickening, inflammation, luminal narrowing, and airway wall remodeling (fig. 10-38) (64, 72,78). Increased mucus production resulting in tenacious plugs that block the airways, contributes to airway obstruction and is a major cause of death in patients with status asthmaticus (64,72,78). Some patients die without mucous plugging. Decreases in the number, length, and motility of cilia in the airway epithelium all contribute to the reduction in the rate of mucus transport and retention (32).

Interactions between CD4+ T cells and B cells are important in IgE synthesis. B cells switch to produce a particular immunoglobulin isotype after two signals: 1) binding of interleukin 4 or interleukin 13 to receptors on B cells and 2) binding of CD40 on B cells to its ligand on T cells (fig. 10-38) (4,13,64,72,78, 107). A complex set of interactions between mast cells, Th2 cells, and eosinophils results in the allergic response. Mast cell and Th2 cell activation in the airways due to inhaled antigen causes the release of mediators such as histamine, leukotrienes, and cytokines including interleukins 4 and 5 (fig. 10-39) (13). Mast cells are activated by an IgE-mediated mechanism. Interleukin 5 causes differentiation of eosinophils, which then migrate from the circulation

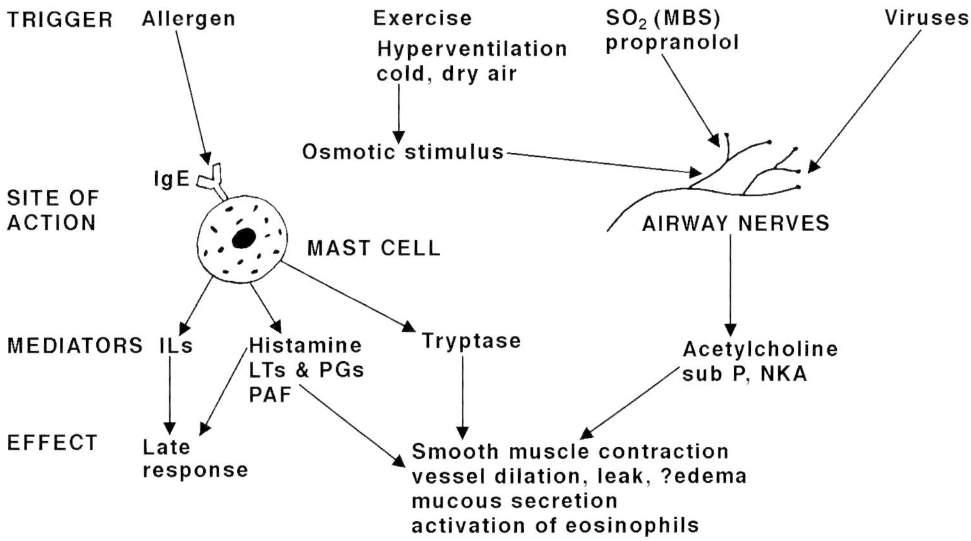

Figure 10-37

ASTHMA: PATHOGENESIS

Postulated mechanisms of provoking stimuli (triggers) of acute airway narrowing are shown in an allergic patient with persistent asthma. IgE = immunoglobulin E, Ils = interleukins, LTs = leukotrienes, NKA = neurokinin A, PAF = platelet-activating factor, PGs = prostaglandins, SO2 (MBS) = sulfur dioxide (metabisulfite), and sub P = substance P. (Figure 40-12 from Woolcock AJ. Asthma. In: Murray JF, Nadel JA, eds. Textbook of respiratory medicine, 2nd ed. Philadelphia: WB Saunders; 1994:1311.)

to the airway after a variety of interactions with integrins and adhesion proteins (vascular cell adhesion molecule 1 and intercellular adhesion molecule 1) (fig. 10-39) (13). Chemokines such as RANES, macrophage inflammatory protein 1-alpha, and eotaxins are important in the migration of eosinophils to the airways (13). Histamine and other mast cell–derived mediators such as prostaglandin D_2, tryptase, and the sulfidopeptide leukotrienes are known to cause smooth muscle contraction resulting in bronchoconstriction (fig. 10-37) (32,65). Neutrophils are also increased in the bronchoalveolar lavage and bronchoscopic biopsy specimens of patients with severe asthma compared to those with mild-moderate asthma and normal controls (160). Epithelial damage and shedding result in increased access of irritant factors to nerve endings, enhanced penetration of allergen particles to mediator-secreting cells in the submucosa, and decreased production of epithelium-derived bronchodilator substances and neural endopeptidases (32).

Treatment and Prognosis. Patients with moderate to severe persistent asthma or a history of severe exacerbations should be given a written action plan based on signs and symptoms and/or peak expiratory flow. Patients should be trained to recognize symptom patterns indicating inadequate asthma control and the need for additional therapy (96). Daily peak flow monitoring is recommended for these patients. Any patient who has persistent asthma requires long-term medications to achieve and maintain control of their disease, in addition to appropriate quick-relief medications to manage asthma exacerbations (96). Use of short-acting beta-2-agonists is the therapy of choice for relief of acute symptoms and prevention of exercise-induced asthma. The most effective medications for long-term control have antiinflammatory effects, for example, inhaled corticosteroids which can improve asthma control, normalize lung function, and possibly prevent irreversible airway injury (96). Long-acting beta-2-agonists are commonly used with antiinflammatory medications for long-term control of symptoms, especially nocturnal symptoms. The cromones (nedocromil sodium or cromolyn sodium, potent mast cell stabilizers in vitro) are

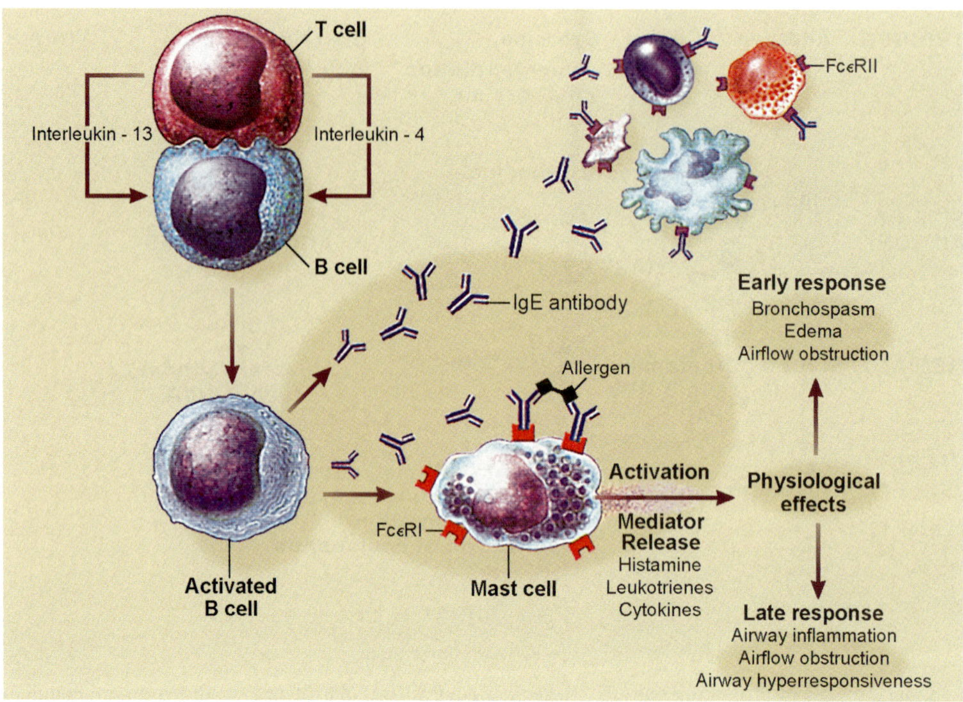

Figure 10-38

INTERACTIONS BETWEEN CD4-POSITIVE T CELLS AND B CELLS THAT ARE IMPORTANT IN IGE SYNTHESIS

The first signal to B cells to switch to the production of the IgE isotype is caused by interleukins 4 and 13. The second signal is provided by accessory pairs of molecules, such as $\alpha_L ß_2$ integrin, intracellular adhesion molecule 1, and CD40 and its ligand. The engagement of allergen by the complex of the T-cell receptor and CD3 on major histocompatibility complex (MHC) class II B cells results in the rapid expression of the CD40 ligand. Once formed, IgE antibody circulates in the blood, eventually binding to both high-affinity IgE receptors (FcεRI, or CD23) and low-affinity IgE receptors (FcεRII, or CD23). After subsequent encounters with antigens, binding of the high-affinity IgE receptors produces the release of preformed and newly generated mediators. Once present in various tissues, mediators may produce various physiologic effects, depending on the target organ. (Figure 2 from Busse WW, Lemanske RF Jr. Asthma. N Engl J Med 2001;344:353.)

moderately efficacious drugs for controlling asthma symptoms. They protect against the physiologic bronchoconstriction following challenges with allergen, ozone, sulfur dioxide, and exercise. Sustained-release theophylline is a mild to moderate bronchodilator used principally as an adjuvant to inhaled corticosteroids for the prevention of nocturnal asthma symptoms. Leukotriene modifiers (for example, zafirlukast, a leukotriene-receptor antagonist, or zileuton, a 5-lipoxygenase inhibitor), may be considered an alternative therapy to low doses of inhaled corticosteroids or cromolyn or nedocromil for patients with mild persistent asthma.

With appropriate management, most patients with asthma have a good prognosis. However, acute attacks represent medical emergencies and may have a fatal outcome. They require aggressive medical therapy, usually with a beta-adrenoceptor agonist (to provide prompt relief of airflow obstruction), systemic corticosteroid (to suppress and reverse airway inflammation), and oxygen (to relieve hypoxemia). Long-term management has the goal of relieving symptoms and preventing long-term risks such as continued symptoms, altered lifestyle, impairment of lung function, drug side effects, and fatal complications. Management includes proper assessment of the type of asthma, pharmacologic therapy, prevention of exacerbations, and patient education (163).

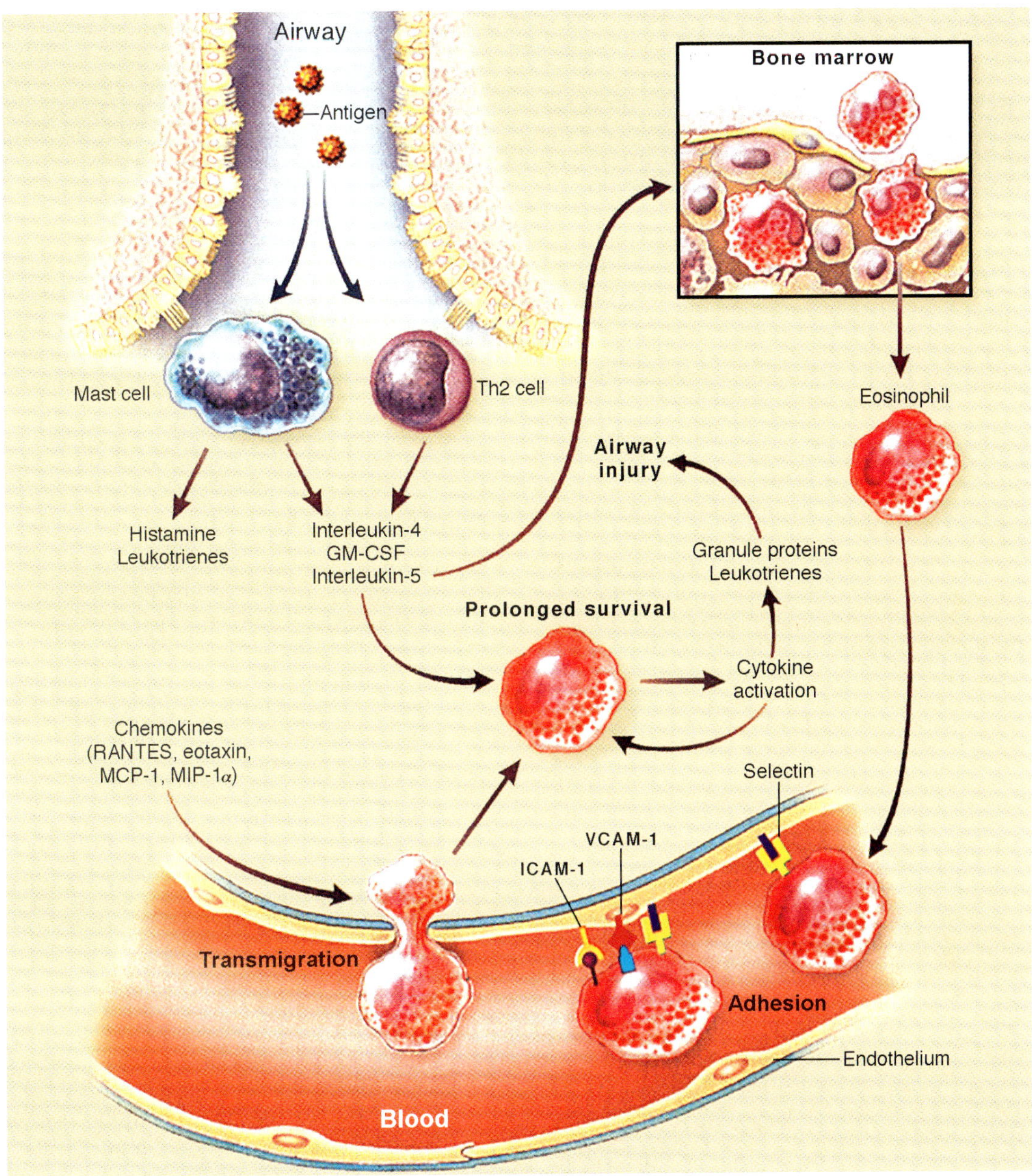

Figure 10-39

THE ROLE OF EOSINOPHILS IN ALLERGIC INFLAMMATION

Inhaled antigen activates mast cells and Th2 cells in the airways. They in turn induce the production of mediators of inflammation (such as histamine and leukotrienes) and cytokines including interleukins 4 and 5. Interleukin 5 travels to the bone marrow and causes terminal differentiation of eosinophils. Circulating eosinophils enter the area of allergic inflammation and begin migrating to the lung by rolling, through interactions with selectins, and eventually adhering to endothelium through the binding of integrins to members of the immunoglobulin superfamily of adhesion proteins: vascular-cell adhesion molecule 1 (VCAM-1) and intercellular adhesion molecule 1 (ICAM-1). As the eosinophils enter the matrix of the airway, through the influence of various chemokines and cytokines, their survival is prolonged by interleukin 5 and granulocyte-macrophage–colony-stimulating factor (GM-CSF). On activation, the eosinophil releases inflammatory mediators such as leukotrienes and granule proteins to injure airway tissues. In addition, eosinophils can generate GM-CSF to prolong and potentiate their survival and contribute to persistent airway inflammation. MCP-1 = monocyte chemotactic protein, MIP-1 = macrophage inflammatory protein. (Figure 3 from Busse WW, Lemanske RF Jr. Asthma. N Engl J Med 2001;344:355.)

REFERENCES

1. Aikawa T, Shimura S, Sasaki H, Ebina M, Takishima T. Marked goblet cell hyperplasia with mucus accumulation in the airways of patients who died of severe acute asthma attack. Chest 1992;101:916–21.
2. Aikawa T, Shimura S, Sasaki H, Takishima T, Yaegashi H, Takahashi T. Morphometric analysis of intraluminal mucus in airways in chronic obstructive pulmonary disease. Am Rev Respir Dis 1989;140:477–82.
3. American Thoracic Society. Standards for the diagnosis and care of patients with chronic obstructive pulmonary disease. Am J Respir Crit Care Med 1995;152:S77–121.
4. Azzawi M, Bradley B, Jeffery PK, et al. Identification of activated T lymphocytes and eosinophils in bronchial biopsies in stable atopic asthma. Am Rev Respir Dis 1990;142:1407–13.
5. Barnes PJ. Chronic obstructive pulmonary disease. N Engl J Med 2000;343:269–80.
6. Beasley R, Roche WR, Roberts JA, Holgate ST. Cellular events in the bronchi in mild asthma and after bronchial provocation. Am Rev Respir Dis 1989;139:806–17.
7. Bense L, Lewander R, Eklund G, Hedenstierna G, Wiman LG. Nonsmoking, non-alpha 1-antitrypsin deficiency-induced emphysema in nonsmokers with healed spontaneous pneumothorax, identified by computed tomography of the lungs. Chest 1993;103:433–8.
8. Bergin C, Müller N, Nichols DM, et al. The diagnosis of emphysema. A computed tomographic-pathologic correlation. Am Rev Respir Dis 1986;133:541–6.
9. Boulet LP, Laviolette M, Turcotte H, et al. Bronchial subepithelial fibrosis correlates with airway responsiveness to methacholine. Chest 1997;112:45–52.
10. Boushey HA, Corry DB, Fahy JV. Asthma. In: Murray JF, Nadel JA, Mason RJ, Boushey HA Jr, eds. Textbook of respiratory medicine, 3rd ed. Philadelphia: WB Saunders; 2000:1247–89.
11. Bousquet J, Chanez P, Lacoste JY, et al. Eosinophilic inflammation in asthma. N Engl J Med 1990;323:1033–9.
12. Browne RJ, Mannino DM, Khoury MJ. Alpha 1-antitrypsin deficiency deaths in the United States from 1979-1991. An analysis using multiple-cause mortality data. Chest 1996;110:78–83.
13. Busse WW, Lemanske RF Jr. Asthma. N Engl J Med 2001;344:350–62.
14. Cagle PT, Thurlbeck WM. Postpneumonectomy compensatory lung growth. Am Rev Respir Dis 1988;138:1314–26.
15. Centers for Disease Control and Prevention. Asthma: United States, 1982-1992. JAMA 1995;273:451–2.
16. Cho SH, Seo JY, Choi DC, et al. Pathological changes according to the severity of asthma. Clin Exp Allergy 1996;26:1210–9.
17. CIBA Foundation Guest Symposium: terminology, definitions and classification of chronic pulmonary emphysema and related conditions. Thorax 1959;14:286–99.
18. Committee on Diagnostic Standards for Nontuberculous Respiratory Diseases. Chronic bronchitis, asthma and pulmonary emphysema. Am Rev Respir Dis 1962;85:762–8.
19. Cooney TP, Thurlbeck WM. Pulmonary hypoplasia in Down's syndrome. N Engl J Med 1982;307:1170–3.
20. Cooney TP, Wentworth PJ, Thurlbeck WM. Diminished radial count is found only postnatally in Down's syndrome. Pediatr Pulmonol 1988;5:204–9.
21. COPD Guidelines Group of the Standards of Care Committee of the BTS. BTS guidelines for the management of chronic obstructive pulmonary disease. Thorax 1997;52 (Suppl 5):S1–28.
22. Corbett E, Glaisyer H, Chan C, Madden B, Khaghani A, Yacoub M. Congenital cutis laxa with a dominant inheritance and early onset emphysema. Thorax 1994;49:836–7.
23. Corbridge TC, Hall JB. The assessment and management of adults with status asthmaticus. Am J Respir Crit Care Med 1995;151:1296–316.
24. Corradi M, Montuschi P, Donnelly LE, Pesci A, Kharitonov SA, Barnes PJ. Increased nitrosothiols in exhaled breath condensate in inflammatory airway diseases. Am J Respir Crit Care Med 2001;163:854–8.
25. Cosio MG, Guerassimov A. Chronic obstructive pulmonary disease. Inflammation of small airways and lung parenchyma. Am J Respir Crit Care Med 1999;160:S21–5
26. Cosio MG, Hale KA, Niewoehner DE. Morphologic and morphometric effects of prolonged cigarette smoking on the small airways. Am Rev Respir Dis 1980;122:265–21.
27. Cosio MG, Majo J. Overview of the pathology of emphysema in humans. Chest Surg Clin N Am 1995;5:603–21.
28. Cutz E, Levison H, Cooper DM. Ultrastructure of airways in children with asthma. Histopathology 1978;2:407–21.
29. Day DL, Burke BA. Pulmonary emphysema in a neonate with Marfan syndrome. Pediatr Radiol 1986;16:518–21.

30. Di Stefano A, Turato G, Maestrelli P, et al. Airflow limitation in chronic bronchitis is associated with T-lymphocyte and macrophage infiltration of the bronchial mucosa. Am J Respir Crit Care Med 1996;153:629–32.
31. Djukanovic R, Homeyard S, Gratziou C, et al. The effect of treatment with oral corticosteroids on asthma symptoms and airway inflammation. Am J Respir Crit Care Med 1997;155:826–32.
32. Djukanovic R, Roche WR, Wilson JW, et al. Mucosal inflammation in asthma. Am Rev Respir Dis 1990;142:434–57.
33. Djukanovic R, Wilson JW, Britten KM, et al. Effect of an inhaled corticosteroid on airway inflammation and symptoms in asthma. Am Rev Respir Dis 1992;145:669–74.
34. Djukanovic R, Wilson JW, Lai CK, Holgate ST, Howarth PH. The safety aspects of fiberoptic bronchoscopy, bronchoalveolar lavage, and endobronchial biopsy in asthma. Am Rev Respir Dis 1991;143:772–7.
35. Dominguez R, Weisgrau RA, Santamaria M. Pulmonary hyperinflation and emphysema in infants with the Marfan syndrome. Pediatr Radiol 1987;17:365–9.
36. Dunnill MS. The pathology of asthma, with special reference to changes in the bronchial mucosa. J Clin Pathol 1960;13:27–33.
37. Dunnill MS. The pathology of asthma. Ciba Foundation Study Group 1971;38:35–46.
38. Dunnill MS, Massarella GR, Anderson JA. A comparison of the quantitative anatomy of the bronchi in normal subjects, in status asthmaticus, in chronic bronchitis, and in emphysema. Thorax 1969;24:176–9.
39. Edge J, Simon G, Reid L. Periacinar (paraseptal) emphysema: its clinical, radiological and physiological features. Brit J Dis Chest 1966;60:10–8.
40. Eidelman DH, Ghezzo H, Kim WD, Cosio MG. The destructive index and early lung destruction in smokers. Am Rev Respir Dis 1991;144:156–9.
41. Eriksson S. Alpha 1-antitrypsin deficiency: lessons learned from the bedside to the gene and back again. Historic perspectives. Chest 1989;95:181–9.
42. Eriksson S. A 30-year perspective on alpha 1-antitrypsin deficiency. Chest 1996;110:237S–42S.
43. Evans MD, Pryor WA. Cigarette smoking, emphysema, and damage to alpha 1-proteinase inhibitor. Am J Physiol 1994;266:L593–611.
44. Ferguson GT. Recommendations for the management of COPD. Chest 2000;117:23S–8S.
45. Fidler ME, Koomen M, Sebek B, Greco MA, Rizk CC, Askin FB. Placental transmogrification of the lung, a histologic variant of giant bullous emphysema. Clinicopathological study of three further cases. Am J Surg Pathol 1995;19:563–70.
46. Finlay GA, O'Donnell MD, O'Connor CM, Hayes JP, FitzGerald MX. Elastin and collagen remodeling in emphysema. A scanning electron microscopy study. Am J Pathol 1996;149:1405–15.
47. Finlay GA, O'Driscoll LR, Russell KJ, et al. Matrix metalloproteinase expression and production by alveolar macrophages in emphysema. Am J Respir Crit Care Med 1997;156:240–7.
48. Fishman AP. The spectrum of chronic obstructive disease of the airways. In: Fishman AP, ed. Pulmonary diseases and disorders, 2nd ed. New York: McGraw-Hill; 1988:1159–71.
49. Foster WL Jr, Gimenez EI, Roubidoux MA, et al. The emphysemas: radiologic-pathologic correlations. Radiographics 1993;13:311–28.
50. Fukuda Y, Masuda Y, Ishizaki M, Masugi Y, Ferrans VJ. Morphogenesis of abnormal elastic fibers in lungs of patients with panacinar and centriacinar emphysema. Hum Pathol 1989;20:652–9.
51. Gaensler EA, Jederlinic PJ, FitzGerald MX. Patient work-up for bullectomy. J Thorac Imaging 1986;1:75–93.
52. Gevenois PA, De Vuyst P, Sy M, et al. Pulmonary emphysema: quantitative CT during expiration. Radiology 1996;199:825–9.
53. Gillooly M, Lamb D. Airspace size in lungs of lifelong non-smokers: effect of age and sex. Thorax 1993;48:39–43.
54. Glynn AA, Michaels L. Bronchial biopsy in chronic bronchitis and asthma. Thorax 1960; 15:142–153.
55. Gough J. Discussion on the diagnosis of pulmonary emphysema: the pathological diagnosis of emphysema. Proc R Soc Med 1952;45:576–7.
56. Gough J. Thin sections of entire organs mounted on paper. Harvey Lect 1958;53:182–5.
57. Greenlee RT, Murray T, Bolden S, Wingo PA. Cancer statistics, 2000. CA Cancer J Clin 2000;50:7–33.
58. Grootendorst DC, Sont JK, Willems LN, et al. Comparison of inflammatory cell counts in asthma: induced sputum vs bronchoalveolar lavage and bronchial biopsies. Clin Exp Allergy 1997;27:769–79.
59. Hanazawa T, Kharitonov SA, Barnes PJ. Increased nitrotyrosine in exhaled breath condensate of patients with asthma. Am J Respir Crit Care Med 2000;162:1273–6.
60. Heard BE. Pathology of pulmonary emphysema: methods of study. Am Rev Respir Dis 1960;82:792–7.
61. Hochholzer L, Moran CA, Koss MN. Pulmonary lipomatosis: a variant of placental transmogrification. Mod Pathol 1997;10:846–9.
62. Hodson ME, Simon G, Batten JC. Radiology of uncomplicated asthma. Thorax 1974;29:296–303.

63. Hogg JC. Childhood viral infection and the pathogenesis of asthma and chronic obstructive lung disease. Am J Respir Crit Care Med 1999;160:S26–8.
64. Hogg JC. The pathology of asthma. APMIS 1997;105:735–45.
65. Holgate ST. Asthma: a dynamic disease of inflammation and repair. Ciba Found Symp 1997;206:5–28.
66. Holgate ST, Roche W, Djukanovic R, Wilson J, Britten K, Howarth P. The need for a pathological classification of asthma. Eur Respir J Suppl 1991;13:113s–22s.
67. Hruban RH, Meziane MA, Zerhouni EA, et al. High resolution computed tomography of inflation-fixed lungs. Pathologic-radiologic correlation of centrilobular emphysema. Am Rev Respir Dis 1987;136:935–40.
68. Humbert M, Robinson DS, Assoufi B, Kay AB, Durham SR. Safety of fibreoptic bronchoscopy in asthmatic and control subjects and effect on asthma control over two weeks. Thorax 1996;51:664–9.
69. Jajosky RA, Harrison R, Reinisch F, et al. Surveillance of work-related asthma in selected U.S. states using surveillance guidelines for state health departments—California, Massachusetts, Michigan, and New Jersey, 1993–1995. Mor Mortal Wkly Rep CDC Surveill Summ 1999;48:1–20.
70. Janoff A. Elastases and emphysema. Current assessment of the protease-antiprotease hypothesis. Am Rev Respir Dis 1985;132:417–33.
71. Jeffery PK. Comparative morphology of the airways in asthma and chronic obstructive pulmonary disease. Am J Respir Crit Care Med 1994;150:S6–13.
72. Jeffery PK. Structural and inflammatory changes in COPD: a comparison with asthma. Thorax 1998;53:129–36.
73. Jeffery PK, Godfrey RW, Adelroth E, Nelson F, Rogers A, Johansson SA. Effects of treatment on airway inflammation and thickening of basement membrane reticular collagen in asthma. A quantitative light and electron microscopic study. Am Rev Respir Dis 1992;145:890–9.
74. Jeffery PK, Wardlaw AJ, Nelson FC, Collins JV, Kay AB. Bronchial biopsies in asthma. An ultrastructural, quantitative study and correlation with hyperreactivity. Am Rev Respir Dis 1989;140:1745–53.
75. Jordan KG, Kwong JS, Flint J, Müller NL. Surgically treated pneumothorax. Radiologic and pathologic findings. Chest 1997;111:280–5.
76. Kalsheker NA. Molecular pathology of alpha 1-antitrypsin deficiency and its significance to clinical medicine. QJM 1994;87:653–8.
77. Kuwano K, Matsuba K, Ikeda T, et al. The diagnosis of mild emphysema. Correlation of computed tomography and pathology scores. Am Rev Respir Dis 1990;141:169–78.
78. Laitinen A, Laitinen LA. Pathology of asthma. Allergy Proc 1994;15:323–8.
79. Laitinen LA, Laitinen A, Altraja A, et al. Bronchial biopsy findings in intermittent or "early" asthma. J Allergy Clin Immunol 1996;98:S3–S6.
80. Lane RE, Campbell AC. Fatal emphysema in two men making copper cadmium alloy. Brit J Industr Med 1954;11:118–22.
81. Leopold JG, Gough J. The centrilobular form of hypertrophic pulmonary emphysema and its relation to chronic bronchitis. Thorax 1957;12:219–35.
82. Li X, Wilson JW. Increased vascularity of the bronchial mucosa in mild asthma. Am J Respir Crit Care Med 1997;156:229–33.
83. Lin YM, Huang WL, Hwang JJ, Ko YL, Lien WP. Swyer-James syndrome associated with Noonan syndrome: report of a case. J Formos Med Assoc 1995;94:742–5.
84. Linhartova A, Anderson AE Jr, Foraker AG. Affixment arrangements of peribronchiolar alveoli in normal and emphysematous lungs. Arch Pathol Lab Med 1982;106:499–502.
85. Linhartova A, Anderson AE Jr, Foraker AG. Further observations on luminal deformity and stenosis of nonrespiratory bronchioles in pulmonary emphysema. Thorax 1977;32:53–9.
86. Linhartova A, Anderson AE Jr, Foraker AG. Site predilection of airway inflammation by emphysema type. Arch Pathol Lab Med 1984;108:662–5.
87. Maestrelli P, Saetta M, Di Stefano A, et al. Comparison of leukocyte counts in sputum, bronchial biopsies, and bronchoalveolar lavage. Am J Respir Crit Care Med 1995;152:1926–31.
88. Mannino DM, Homa DM, Pertowski CA, et al. Surveillance for asthma–United States, 1960-1995. Mor Mortal Wkly Rep CDC Surveill Summ 1998;47:1–27.
89. Mark EJ, Müller KM, McChesney T, Dong-Hwan S, Honig C, Mark MA. Placentoid bullous lesion of the lung. Hum Pathol 1995;26:74–9.
90. Matsuba K, Ikeda T, Nagai A, Thurlbeck WM. The National Institutes of Health intermittent positive-pressure breathing trial: pathology studies. IV. The destructive index. Am Rev Respir Dis 1989;139:1439–45.
91. Messer JW, Peters GA, Bennett WA. Causes of death and pathologic findings in 304 cases of bronchial asthma. Dis Chest 1960;38:616–24.
92. Miller RR, Müller NL, Vedal S, Morrison NJ, Staples CA. Limitations of computed tomography in the assessment of emphysema. Am Rev Respir Dis 1989;139:980–3.

93. Montuschi P, Collins JV, Ciabattoni G, et al. Exhaled 8-isoprostane as an in vivo biomarker of lung oxidative stress in patients with COPD and healthy smokers. Am J Respir Crit Care Med 2000;162:1175–7.
94. Nadel JA, Busse WW. Asthma. Am J Respir Crit Care Med 1998;157:S130–8
95. Nakamura T, Takizawa T, Morone T. Anatomic changes in lung parenchyma due to aging process. Dis Chest 1967;52:518–24.
96. National Heart, Lung and Blood Institute. Expert panel report 2: guidelines for the diagnosis and management of asthma. Bethesda, MD: NIH Publication No. 97-4051; 1997.
97. Nemery B. Metal toxicity and the respiratory tract. Eur Respir J 1990;3:202–19.
98. Niewoehner DE, Kleinerman J, Rice DB. Pathologic changes in the peripheral airways of young cigarette smokers. N Engl J Med 1974;291:755–8.
99. O'Shaughnessy TC, Ansari TW, Barnes NC, Jeffery PK. Inflammation in bronchial biopsies of subjects with chronic bronchitis: inverse relationship of CD8+ T lymphocytes with FEV1. Am J Respir Crit Care Med 1997;155:852–7.
100. Paakko P, Ryhanen L, Rantala H, Autio-Harmainen H. Pulmonary emphysema in a nonsmoking patient with Salla disease. Am Rev Respir Dis 1987;135:979–82.
101. Pardo A, Selman M. Proteinase-antiproteinase imbalance in the pathogenesis of emphysema: the role of metalloproteinases in lung damage. Histol Histopathol 1999;14:227–33.
102. Pare JP, Cote G, Fraser RS. Long-term follow-up of drug abusers with intravenous talcosis. Am Rev Respir Dis 1989;139:233–41.
103. Pesci A, Rossi GA, Bertorelli G, Aufiero A, Zanon P, Olivieri D. Mast cells in the airway lumen and bronchial mucosa of patients with chronic bronchitis. Am J Respir Crit Care Med 1994; 149:1311–6.
104. Pickup CM, Nee PA, Randall PE. Radiographic features in 1016 adults admitted to hospital with acute asthma. J Accid Emerg Med 1994;11:234–7.
105. Pierce JA. Antitrypsin and emphysema. Perspective and prospects. JAMA 1988;259:2890–5.
106. Piquette CA, Rennard SI, Snider GL. Chronic bronchitis and emphysema. In: Murray JF, Nadel JA, Mason RJ, Boushey HA, eds. Textbook of respiratory medicine, 3rd ed. Philadelphia: WB Saunders; 2000:1187–245.
107. Poston RN, Chanez P, Lacoste JY, Litchfield T, Lee TH, Bousquet J. Immunohistochemical characterization of the cellular infiltration in asthmatic bronchi. Am Rev Respir Dis 1992; 145:918–21.
108. Reid L. Measurement of the bronchial mucus gland layer: a diagnostic yardstick in chronic bronchitis. Thorax 1960;15:132–41.
109. Remy-Jardin M, Remy J, Gosselin B, Copin MC, Wurtz A, Duhamel A. Sliding thin slab, minimum intensity projection technique in the diagnosis of emphysema: histopathologic-CT correlation. Radiology 1996;200:665–71.
110. Repine JE, Bast A, Lankhorst I. Oxidative stress in chronic obstructive pulmonary disease. Oxidative Stress Study Group. Am J Respir Crit Care Med 1997;156:341–57.
111. Reye RD, Bale PM. Elastic tissue in pulmonary emphysema in Marfan syndrome. Arch Pathol 1973;96:427–31.
112. Saetta M, Di Stefano A, Turato G, et al. CD8+ T-lymphocytes in peripheral airways of smokers with chronic obstructive pulmonary disease. Am J Respir Crit Care Med 1998;157:822–6.
113. Saetta M, Shiner RJ, Angus GE, et al. Destructive index: a measurement of lung parenchymal destruction in smokers. Am Rev Respir Dis 1985;131:764–9.
114. Saetta M, Turato G, Facchini FM, et al. Inflammatory cells in the bronchial glands of smokers with chronic bronchitis. Am J Respir Crit Care Med 1997;156:1633–9.
115. Sahebjami H, Domino M. Effects of starvation and refeeding on elastase-induced emphysema. J Appl Physiol 1989;66:2611–6.
116. Sahebjami H, Wirman JA. Emphysema-like changes in the lungs of starved rats. Am Rev Respir Dis 1981;124:619–24.
117. Saito K, Cagle P, Berend N, Thurlbeck WM. The "destructive index" in nonemphysematous and emphysematous lungs. Morphologic observations and correlation with function. Am Rev Respir Dis 1989;139:308–12.
118. Schmidt RA, Glenny RW, Godwin JD, Hampson NB, Cantino ME, Reichenbach DD. Panlobular emphysema in young intravenous Ritalin abusers. Am Rev Respir Dis 1991;143:649–56.
119. Seemungal TA, Donaldson GC, Bhowmik A, Jeffries DJ, Wedzicha JA. Time course and recovery of exacerbations in patients with chronic obstructive pulmonary disease. Am J Respir Crit Care Med 2000;161:1608–13.
120. Seemungal TA, Harper-Owen R, Bhowmik A, Jeffries DJ, Wedzicha JA. Detection of rhinovirus in induced sputum at exacerbation of chronic obstructive pulmonary disease. Eur Respir J 2000;16:677–83.
121. Shapiro SD. Elastolytic metalloproteinases produced by human mononuclear phagocytes. Potential roles in destructive lung disease. Am J Respir Crit Care Med 1994;150:S160–4.

122. Shapiro SD. The macrophage in chronic obstructive pulmonary disease. Am J Respir Crit Care Med 1999;160:S29–32.
123. Shapiro SD. The pathogenesis of emphysema: the elastase:antielastase hypothesis 30 years later. Proc Assoc Am Physicians 1995;107:346–52.
124. Sherman CB, Hudson LD, Pierson DJ. Severe precocious emphysema in intravenous methylphenidate (Ritalin) abusers. Chest 1987;92:1085–7.
125. Siafakas NM, Vermeire P, Pride NB, et al. Optimal assessment and management of chronic obstructive pulmonary disease (COPD). The European Respiratory Society Task Force. Eur Respir J 1995;8:1398–420.
126. Simon G. Chronic bronchitis and emphysema: a symposium. III. Radiologic changes in chronic bronchitis. Br J Radiol 1959;32:292–4.
127. Snider GL. Emphysema: the first two centuries–and beyond. A historical overview, with suggestions for future research: part 2. Am Rev Respir Dis 1992;146:1615–22.
128. Snider GL, Kleinerman J, Thurlbeck WM, Bengali ZH. The definition of emphysema. Report of a National Heart, Lung, and Blood Institute, Division of Lung Diseases workshop. Am Rev Respir Dis 1985;132:182–5.
129. Sommerhoff CP, Nadel JA, Basbaum CB, Caughey GH. Neutrophil elastase and cathepsin G stimulate secretion from cultured bovine airway gland serous cells. J Clin Invest 1990;85:682–9.
130. Sont JK, Han J, van Krieken JM, et al. Relationship between the inflammatory infiltrate in bronchial biopsy specimens and clinical severity of asthma in patients treated with inhaled steroids. Thorax 1996;51:496–502.
131. Sont JK, Willems LN, Evertse CE, Hooijer R, Sterk PJ, van Krieken JH. Repeatability of measures of inflammatory cell number in bronchial biopsies in atopic asthma. Eur Respir J 1997;10:2602–8.
132. Spouge D, Mayo JR, Cardoso W, Müller NL. Panacinar emphysema: CT and pathologic findings. J Comput Assist Tomogr 1993;17:710–3.
133. Stern EJ, Frank MS. CT of the lung in patients with pulmonary emphysema: diagnosis, quantification, and correlation with pathologic and physiologic findings. AJR Am J Roentgenol 1994;162:791–8.
134. Stern EJ, Frank MS, Schmutz JF, Glenny RW, Schmidt RA, Godwin JD. Panlobular pulmonary emphysema caused by i.v. injection of methylphenidate (Ritalin): findings on chest radiographs and CT scans. AJR Am J Roentgenol 1994;162:555–60.
135. Stern EJ, Webb WR, Weinacker A, Müller NL. Idiopathic giant bullous emphysema (vanishing lung syndrome): imaging findings in nine patients. AJR Am J Roentgenol 1994;162:279–82.
136. Stoller JK. Clinical features and natural history of severe alpha 1-antitrypsin deficiency. Roger S. Mitchell Lecture. Chest 1997;111:123S–8S.
137. Sullivan P, Stephens D, Ansari T, Costello J, Jeffery P. Variation in the measurements of basement membrane thickness and inflammatory cell number in bronchial biopsies. Eur Respir J 1998;12:811–5.
138. Sur S, Crotty TB, Kephart GM, et al. Sudden-onset fatal asthma. A distinct entity with few eosinophils and relatively more neutrophils in the airway submucosa? Am Rev Respir Dis 1993;148:713–9.
139. ten Hacken NH, Aleva RM, Oosterhoff Y, et al. Submucosa 1.0 x 0.1 mm in size is sufficient to count inflammatory cell numbers in human airway biopsy specimens. Mod Pathol 1998; 11:292–4.
140. Thurlbeck WM. Chronic airflow obstruction. In: Thurlbeck WM, Churg AM, eds. Pathology of the lung, 2nd ed. New York: Thieme Medical Publishers; 1995:739–825.
141. Thurlbeck WM. Chronic obstructive lung disease. Pathol Annu 1968;3:367–98.
142. Thurlbeck WM. Examination of the lung: autopsy. In: Thurlbeck WM, Churg AM, eds. Pathology of the lung, 2nd ed. New York: Thieme Medical Publishers; 1995:129–36.
143. Thurlbeck WM. The incidence of pulmonary emphysema with observations on the relative incidence and spacial distribution of various types of emphysema. Am Rev Respir Dis 1963;87:206–15.
144. Thurlbeck WM. The morphology of chronic bronchitis, asthma, and bronchiectasis. In: Thurlbeck WM, ed. Chronic airflow obstruction in lung disease. Philadelphia: WB Saunders; 1976:31–95.
145. Thurlbeck WM. Morphology of emphysema and emphysema-like conditions. In: Thurlbeck WM, ed. Chronic airflow obstruction in lung disease. Philadelphia: WB Saunders; 1976:96–234.
146. Thurlbeck WM. Quantitative anatomy of the lung. In: Thurlbeck WM, Churg AM, eds. Pathology of the lung, 2nd ed. New York: Thieme Medical Publishers; 1995:89–98.
147. Thurlbeck WM, Angus GE, Pare JA. Mucus gland hypertrophy in chronic bronchitis and its occurrence in smokers. Br J Dis Chest 1963;57:73–8.
148. Thurlbeck WM, Dunnill MS, Hartung W, Heard BE, Heppleston AG, Ryder RC. A comparison of three methods of measuring emphysema. Hum Pathol 1970;1:215–26.

149. Thurlbeck WM, Müller NL. Emphysema: definition, imaging, and quantification. AJR Am J Roentgenol 1994;163:1017–25.
150. Venables KM, Chan-Yeung M. Occupational asthma. Lancet 1997;349:1465–9.
151. Verbeken EK, Cauberghs M, Lauweryns JM, van de Woestijne KP. Anatomy of membranous bronchioles in normal, senile and emphysematous human lungs. J Appl Physiol 1994;77:1875–84.
152. Verbeken EK, Cauberghs M, Mertens I, Clement J, Lauweryns JM, van de Woestijne KP. The senile lung. Comparison with normal and emphysematous lungs. 1. Structural aspects. Chest 1992;101:793–9.
153. Vignola AM, Chanez P, Campbell AM, et al. Airway inflammation in mild intermittent and in persistent asthma. Am J Respir Crit Care Med 1998;157:403–9.
154. Wade JF III, Mortenson R, Irvin CG. Physiologic evaluation of bullous emphysema. Chest 1991;100:1151–4.
155. Wang NS, Ying WL. Morphogenesis of human bronchial diverticulum. A scanning electron microscopic study. Chest 1976;69:201–4.
156. Wang NS, Ying WL. A scanning electron microscopic study of alkali-digested human and rabbit alveoli. Am Rev Respir Dis 1977;115:449–60.
157. Wang NS, Ying WL. The pattern of goblet cell hyperplasia in human airways. Hum Pathol 1977;8:301–11.
158. Webb WR. High-resolution computed tomography of obstructive lung disease. Radiol Clin North Am 1994;32:745–57.
159. Weisbrod GL, Rahman M, Chamberlain D, Herman SJ. Precocious emphysema in intravenous drug abusers. J Thorac Imaging 1993; 8:233–40.
160. Wenzel SE, Szefler SJ, Leung DY, Sloan SI, Rex MD, Martin RJ. Bronchoscopic evaluation of severe asthma. Persistent inflammation associated with high dose glucocorticoids. Am J Respir Crit Care Med 1997;156:737–43.
161. Wilcox P, Miller R, Miller G, et al. Airway involvement in ulcerative colitis. Chest 1987; 92:18–22.
162. Witko-Sarsat V, Halbwachs-Mecarelli L, Schuster A, et al. Proteinase 3, a potent secretagogue in airways, is present in cystic fibrosis sputum. Am J Respir Cell Mol Biol 1999;20:729–36.
163. Woolcock AJ. Asthma. In: Murray JF, Nadel JA, eds. Textbook of respiratory medicine, 2nd ed. Philadelphia: WB Saunders; 1994:1288–330.
164. Wright JL. Emphysema: concepts under change—a pathologist's perspective. Mod Pathol 1995;8:873–80.
165. Wright JL, Lawson LM, Pare PD, Wiggs BJ, Kennedy S, Hogg JC. Morphology of peripheral airways in current smokers and ex-smokers. Am Rev Respir Dis 1983;127:474–7.

11
CONGENITAL ANOMALIES AND PEDIATRIC DISORDERS

INTRODUCTION

Most congenital anomalies manifest within the first year of life. Notable exceptions include bronchogenic cysts and intralobar sequestrations which usually manifest in young adulthood (92,104,106,112,125,154,158). Some congenital anomalies of the lung are incompatible with life and are identified in stillborn infants. Recently, obstetrical ultrasonography has allowed recognition of lesions in utero, and some have been treated by resection and/or shunting prior to birth (36). Congenital anomalies in the lung can be grouped as shown in Table 11-1; the distinct subset that may be associated with cystic lesions in children and neonates is shown in Table 11-2. For some of the lesions discussed in this section, there is controversy regarding whether they should be considered acquired rather than truly congenital; some of these issues are insoluble.

Table 11-1

PULMONARY DEVELOPMENTAL CYSTS, CONGENITAL ANOMALIES, AND RELATED LESIONS[a]

Tracheobronchial
Tracheobronchomegaly
Tracheal atresia, stenosis, and agenesis
Tracheal bronchi and diverticula
Bronchial atresia
Congenital bronchiectasis
Bronchomalacia
Tracheobronchial communication with other foregut derivatives (tracheoesophageal fistulae, bronchobiliary fistulae, etc.)
Bronchial isomerism
Sequestrations (lung tissue without tracheobronchial connection)
Extralobar sequestration
Intralobar sequestration
Bronchopulmonary foregut malformations (tracheobronchial or pulmonary parenchymal, including sequestered tissue with communication with the alimentary tract)
Pulmonary agenesis, aplasia, hypoplasia, hyperplasia, horseshoe lung, acinar dysplasia
Bronchogenic cysts
Infantile lobar emphysema/polyalveolar lobe
Congenital cystic adenomatoid malformation/congenital lung cysts
Vascular anomalies
Vascular sling
Scimitar syndrome (venous drainage from right lung into inferior vena cava)
Arteriovenous fistula(e)
Congenital pulmonary lymphangiectasia, lymphangiomatosis
Persistent pulmonary hypertension
Tissue ectopias
Thyroid, liver, adrenal, pancreatic, glial tissues endometriosis, cardiac muscle, skeletal muscle

[a]Adapted from references 92, 104, 106, 112, 125, 154, and 158.

The term *bronchopulmonary foregut malformation* has been used as an encompassing term for sequestrations associated with bronchopulmonary foregut communications (fig. 11-1) (73,79, 106). According to this concept, pulmonary sequestrations have a common embryologic origin and can be categorized together as bronchopulmonary foregut malformations. This conclusion is based on the observation of hybrid or mixed intralobar and extralobar sequestrations that communicate with portions of the foregut (85).

It is a useful concept for a variety of complex anomalies involving communications between the respiratory and alimentary tracts, but does

Table 11-2

CYSTIC LESIONS IN NEONATES AND CHILDREN[a]

Sequestration/bronchopulmonary foregut malformations
Bronchogenic cyst
Congenital cystic adenomatoid malformation
Interstitial emphysema
Cystic mesenchymal neoplasms (e.g., pleuropulmonary blastomas)
Other cystic lesions
Cystic bronchiectasis
Post-traumatic or postinfarction cysts
Pneumatoceles

[a]Modified from reference 92.

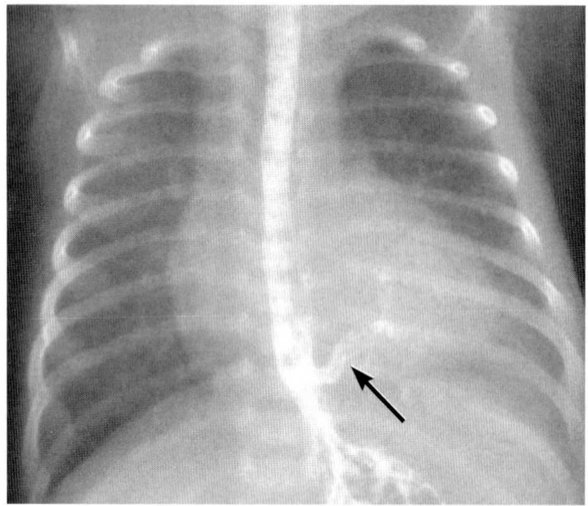

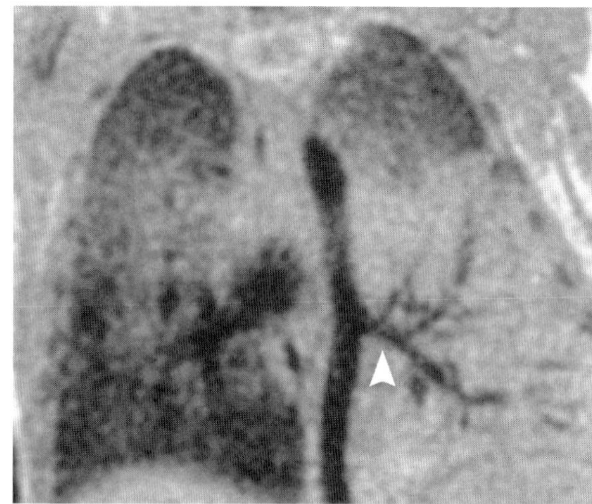

Figure 11-1

BRONCHOPULMONARY FOREGUT MALFORMATION

Bronchopulmonary foregut malformation in a 1-year-old male with respiratory distress since birth aggravated by oral intake.

Left: AP barium esophagram demonstrates a bronchus-like structure (arrow) arising from the distal esophagus, which supplies a consolidated left lower lobe.

Right: Coronal T1-weighted MRI demonstrates an anomalous vessel (arrowhead) that arises from the distal thoracic aorta and supplies the consolidated left lower lobe.

not apply to all sequestrations, particularly the intralobar type (see below). Bronchopulmonary foregut malformations commonly have associated abnormalities of tracheoesophageal septation and components of esophageal atresia and/or tracheoesophageal fistula.

ANOMALIES OF THE TRACHEOBRONCHIAL TREE

Laryngotrachealesophageal Clefts. These vary in length and, because of the communication between the respiratory and the alimentary tracts, are associated with feeding problems and respiratory distress (16,104,154). Nearly half are associated with other congenital anomalies (104,154).

Tracheal Agenesis. Tracheal agenesis is rare and usually is associated with tracheo-esophageal or bronchoesophageal fistulae (66, 101,154). The diagnosis of tracheal agenesis/atresia can be confirmed with computed tomography (CT). Atretic segments are characterized by the absence of the tracheal air column on cross-sectional imaging (101).

Tracheal Stenosis. There are a number of causes of tracheal stenosis, the most common of which is prolonged intubation for mechanical ventilation during the treatment of respiratory distress syndrome (106,154). True congenital tracheal stenosis may be associated with cartilage plate deficiency, complete cartilaginous rings (napkin ring anomaly), or compression by adjacent structures (such as the esophagus or branches of the major vessels) (154). Tracheal stenosis may be segmental, diffuse, or funnel shaped (106).

Tracheobronchomegaly. Also known as *Mounier-Kuhn syndrome,* tracheobronchomegaly usually manifests in adults (although symptoms may begin in childhood) and may be familial (autosomal recessive) (89,91,104,154). Tracheobronchomegaly is discussed in chapter 9.

Congenital Bronchial Cartilage Deficiency. Also known as *Williams-Campbell syndrome,* this manifests as bronchiectasis in the first year of life and is discussed in chapter 9.

Tracheoesophageal Fistulae. These are usually associated with esophageal atresia (104, 106,154). Fistulae may be identified any place along the length of the trachea and esophagus, and a variety of types are described, most commonly esophageal atresia with a fistulous connection between the carina and the distal

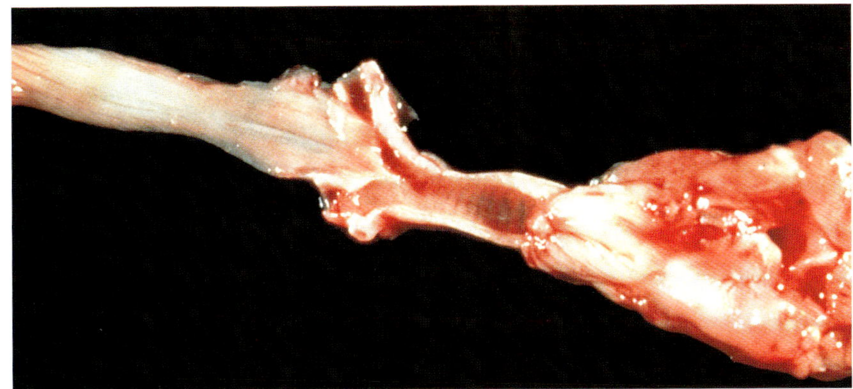

Figure 11-2

TRACHEOESOPHAGEAL FISTULA

Tracheoesophageal fistula demonstrates proximal esophageal atresia (upper center) and origin of the distal esophagus from the carina. (Courtesy of Dr. J.T. Stocker, Bethesda, MD.)

esophagus (fig. 11-2). The diagnosis of esophageal atresia is usually suspected shortly after birth. Radiologic assessment is useful in the identification of a tracheoesophageal fistula (51). The presence of a fistula is inferred from visualization of gas in the gastrointestinal tract. Contrast distention of the atretic proximal esophageal pouch helps exclude additional unsuspected fistulous communications. Diagnosis by prenatal ultrasound is possible based on the presence of polyhydramnios, nonvisualization of the fetal stomach, and direct visualization of a dilated proximal esophageal pouch, which may fill and empty during the study. In some cases, fetal vomiting is witnessed sonographically and indicates a high gastrointestinal obstruction (81). Other associated anomalies are common, including bronchobiliary fistulae (106,154).

Bronchial Anomalies. Bronchial anomalies may be classified according to location (displaced), size, components, or connections, as shown in Table 11-3.

Table 11-3

BRONCHIAL ABNORMALITIES[a]

Abnormality of origin or location
Tracheal bronchus
Pre-eparterial bronchus
Additive bronchus
Isomerism
Bridging bronchus
Abnormal size or components
Bronchial stenosis or atresia
Bronchiectasis
Bronchomalacia
Abnormal connection
Bronchobiliary fistula
Bronchoesophageal fistula
Bronchogenic cysts

[a]Modified from reference 154.

Bronchial Isomerism Syndromes. These syndromes represent peculiar anomalies in which an individual may have bilateral right (3-lobed) lungs or bilateral left (2-lobed) lungs (59,72,103,104,106,122,154). Bronchial isomerism is often associated with splenic abnormalities, including asplenia syndrome, as well as congenital heart disease (106,154). Radiologic assessment of bronchial isomerism is an important step in the evaluation of patients with complex heart disease, as tracheobronchial morphology is a reliable indicator of atrial morphology (59). An eparterial bronchus is one where the first main branch arises superiorly, resides above the morphologic right pulmonary artery, and is associated with an ipsilateral atrial chamber of right-sided morphology. A hyparterial bronchus courses more horizontally below the morphologic left pulmonary artery and is associated with an ipsilateral atrial chamber with left-sided morphology (59). Patients with *asplenia syndrome* typically have bilateral eparterial bronchi and bilateral trilobed lungs (72,59,122). Patients with *polysplenia syndrome* have bilateral hyparterial bronchi and multiple spleens on radiologic imaging (figs. 11-3, 11-4) (59,122). The pattern of bronchial branching can be assessed through a careful review of the chest radiograph, although visualization of the tracheobronchial tree is typically more difficult in infancy.

Bronchial Stenosis. There are a number of etiologies, some congenital and some acquired (104,106,154). Not all affected individuals present as infants. Obstruction may be caused by intrinsic abnormalities, such as fibrosis or meconium

Figure 11-3

POLYSPLENIA

A: A 42-year-old male was evaluated for nodular sclerosing Hodgkin's disease and incidentally found to have polysplenia. AP chest linear tomogram demonstrates an enlarged azygous vein and bilateral hyparterial bronchi consistent with the diagnosis of polysplenia. Note the absence of a right upper lobe bronchus.

B,C: Polysplenia in a 63-year-old female undergoing evaluation for weakness and weight loss. Chest CT (lung window) demonstrates symmetrical (hyparterial) bronchial morphology. The first bronchial branches arise distal to the ipsilateral pulmonary arteries (B). Contrast-enhanced abdominal CT (soft tissue window) demonstrates a right-sided stomach (arrow) and multiple spleens in the right upper quadrant (C).

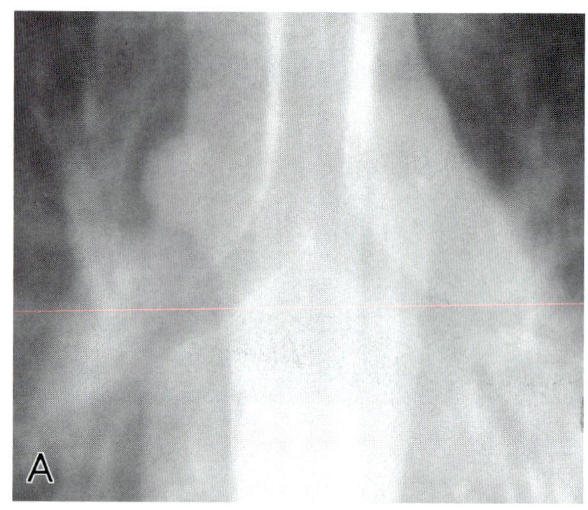

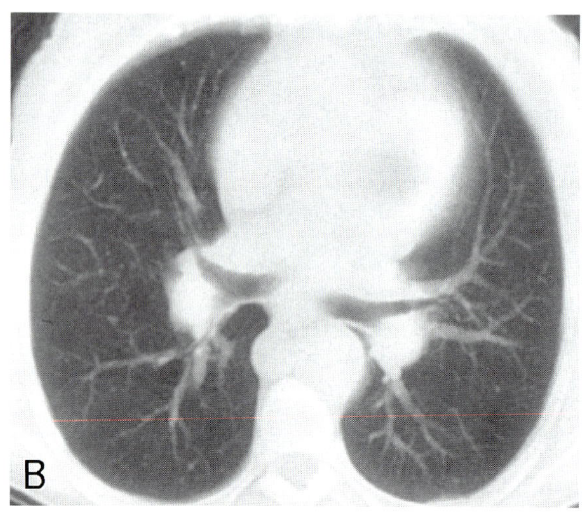

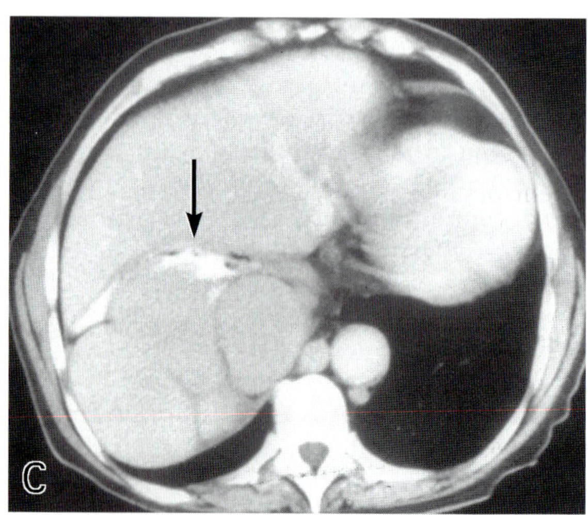

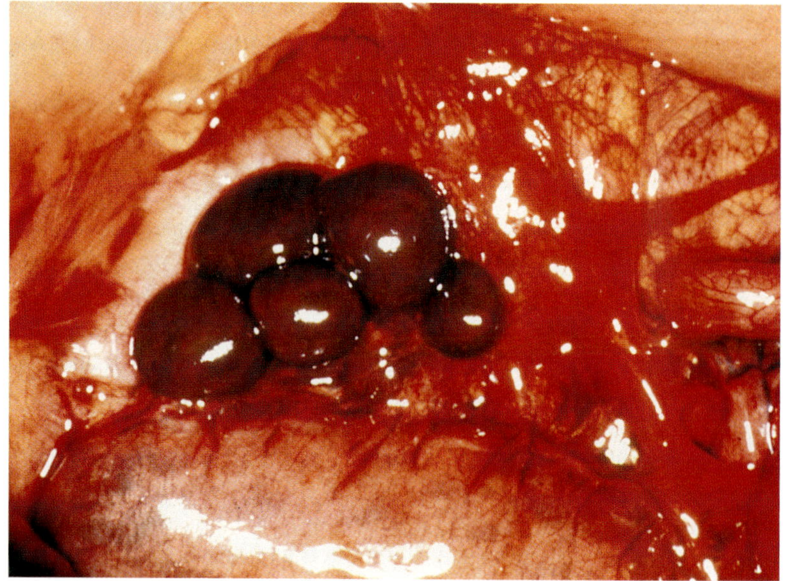

Figure 11-4

POLYSPLENIA

Polysplenia in a newborn female with complex congenital heart disease who died shortly after birth. Postmortem photograph of the abdomen demonstrates multiple spleens.

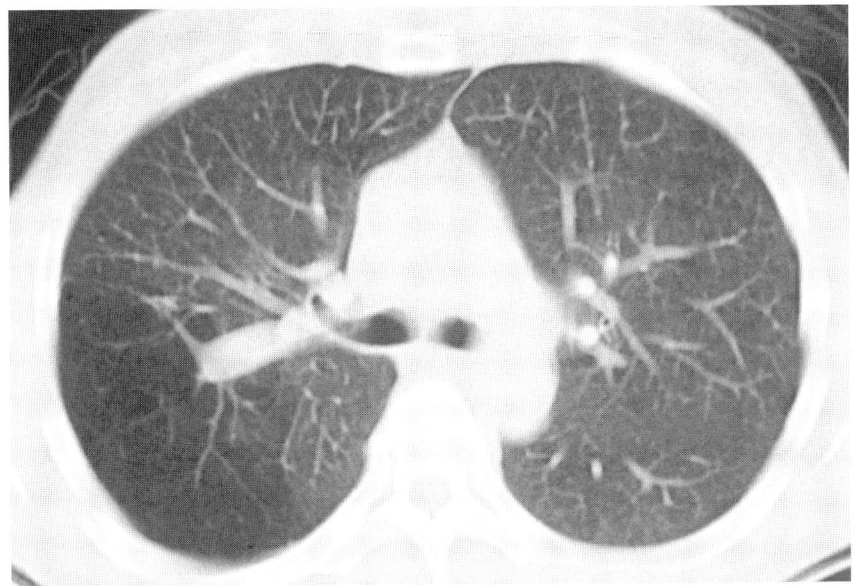

Figure 11-5

BRONCHIAL ATRESIA IN AN ASYMPTOMATIC 40-YEAR-OLD MALE

Chest CT (lung window) demonstrates a tubular opacity in the right upper lobe surrounded by distal hyperlucent lung. (Courtesy of Dr. Gerald F. Abbott, Rhode Island Hospital, Providence, RI.)

aspiration, or extrinsic compression. Involvement of a lobar bronchus may be one of the causes of infantile lobar overinflation (infantile lobar emphysema, see below).

Bronchial Atresia (Regional or Segmental Pulmonary Overinflation). This is a well-characterized clinicopathologic entity that refers to loss of normal bronchial communication due to atresia of a portion of a segmental bronchus (88,104,119). The bronchus distal to the obstruction becomes filled with mucus, and the surrounding lung overinflates. Air-filling and subsequent air-trapping are thought to result from collateral air-drift through the pores of Kohn and canals of Lambert.

Patients with bronchial atresia show a slight male predominance, with an average age at presentation of 17 years (range, birth to 44 years). Sixty percent of patients are asymptomatic; those with symptoms most commonly present with recurrent pneumonia.

A radiologic diagnosis of bronchial atresia is often possible. Chest radiographs typically show segmental hyperinflation in the left upper lobe, most often the apical posterior segment (62). The diagnosis is supported by the identification of a central tubular, ovoid, or branching opacity, which represents a mucous plug that develops distal to the point of atresia (101). CT shows the overinflated hyperlucent lung and delineates the location of the mucous plug or bronchocele, which characteristically has a branching morphology consistent with its endobronchial location (fig. 11-5). The CT attenuation of the mucoid material is low, ranging from –5 to 25 Hounsfield units. High signal intensity on magnetic resonance imaging (MRI) is typical and helps exclude a vascular lesion.

The presence of an air-fluid level within the bronchocele is reported and is associated with infection (97). Bronchography, while rarely performed, may demonstrate lack of filling of the affected bronchus distal to the point of atresia (97).

The pathologic findings depend on whether there has been infection in the tissue distal to the atresia. In the absence of infection, there is a mucus-filled bronchus with surrounding lung tissue that appears grossly normal or overinflated (figs. 11-6, 11-7). If the lesion is infected, acute and chronic inflammation and fibrosis are apparent.

Bronchiectasis. Bronchiectasis in neonates has a variety of etiologies, some acquired, even though the term *congenital bronchiectasis* may be used (154). Affected individuals may have cystic fibrosis, immotile cilia syndrome, or immunoglobulin deficiencies. These entities are discussed in chapter 9.

Bronchomalacia. This anomaly, due to abnormal development of bronchial cartilage with associated bronchiectasis, is rare (154). Bronchomalacia following mechanical ventilation is

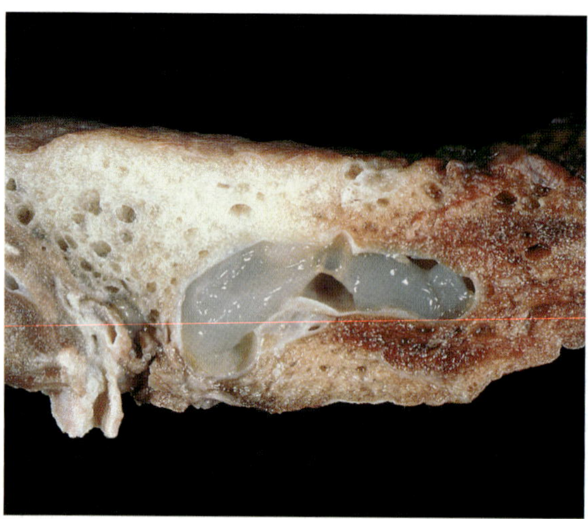

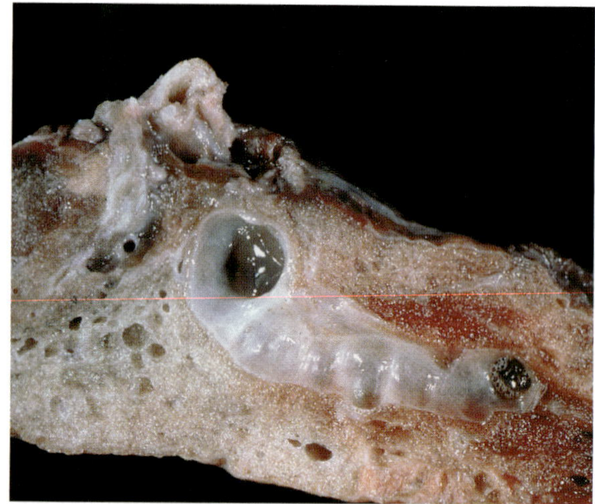

Figure 11-6

BRONCHIAL ATRESIA

Distal to the atresia is bronchial dilatation and a mucous plug. The surrounding airspaces are dilated. (Both figures courtesy Dr. F. G. Askin, Baltimore, MD.)

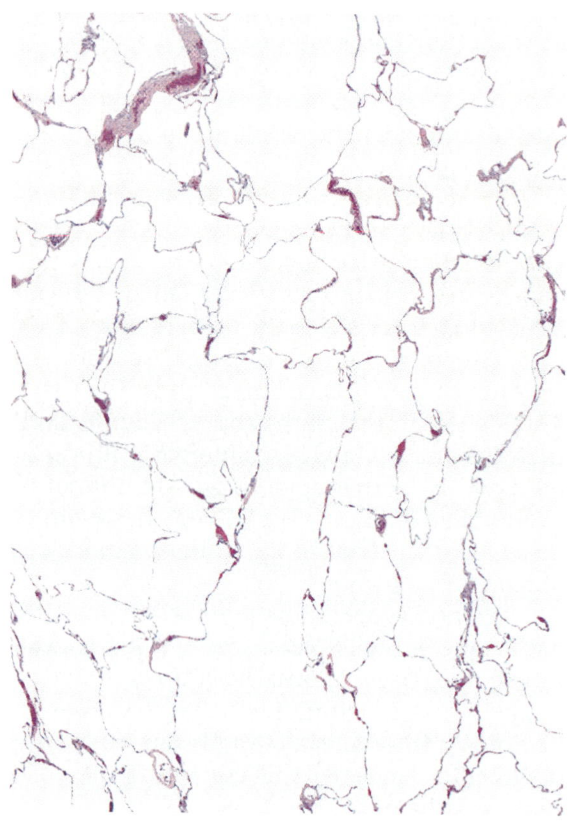

Figure 11-7

BRONCHIAL ATRESIA

The histologic specimen shows alveolar distention.

more common. In patients with developmental abnormalities of the bronchial cartilage, the left mainstem bronchus is more often affected than the right; the cartilaginous plates are grossly small and have an immature appearance histologically. The presence of abnormal cartilaginous plates also predisposes to collapse, secondary infection, and lobar overinflation. Sudden death has been reported (149).

BRONCHOGENIC CYST

Definition. Bronchogenic cysts (also known as *bronchial cysts*) are thought to be supernumerary foregut buds that become separated and disconnected from the tracheobronchial tree and progressively enlarge, forming a cystic mass (4,41, 49,55,92,106,141,142,147,154). Bronchogenic cysts are generally extrapulmonary, and they only rarely occur in the lung. They may connect to the foregut or be identified adjacent to other anomalies, such as extralobar sequestrations.

Clinical Features. Bronchogenic cysts are usually identified in children or young adults, although all age groups are affected. There is no sex predilection. Affected infants present with respiratory distress due to mass effect and compression of the tracheobronchial tree, whereas older patients typically develop symptoms secondary to infection of the cyst. As many as a third of patients are asymptomatic (41).

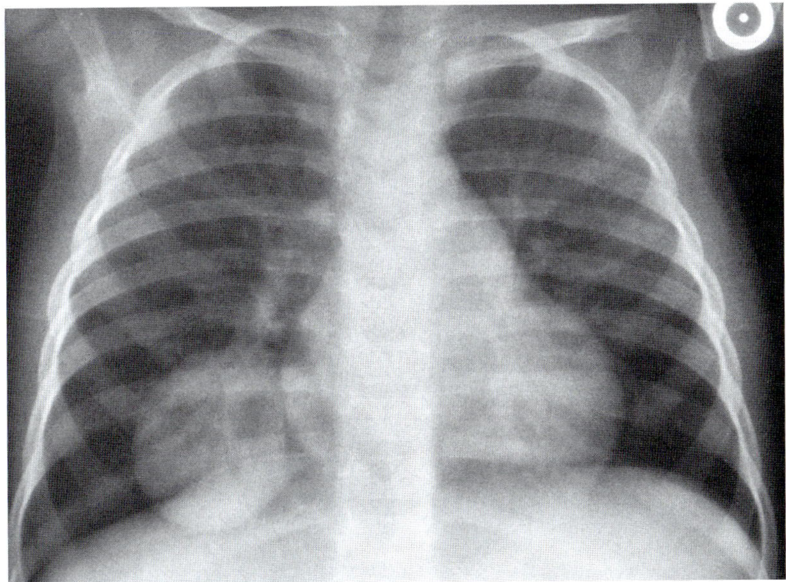

Figure 11-8

BRONCHOGENIC CYST

Bronchogenic cyst in a 1-year-old female who presented with cough and dyspnea. AP chest radiograph demonstrates a well-defined rounded mass, which projects over the medial right hemithorax.

Radiologic Findings. Radiologically, bronchogenic cysts are spherical, well-marginated masses that are typically located in the middle mediastinum in close relationship to the trachea and main-stem bronchi. Unusual locations include the lung, the diaphragm, the neck, and the abdomen (fig. 11-8). On cross-sectional imaging, they are homogeneous, nonenhancing spherical masses, often in close proximity to the carina.

The CT attenuation varies with the composition of the cyst fluid. Approximately half of bronchogenic cysts have water attenuation on CT, but the rest may appear solid or hyperattenuated due to high protein content, hemorrhage, or calcium content. Calcification of the cyst wall on CT and fluid-fluid levels on MRI have been reported; the latter may be due to layering of proteinaceous debris within the cyst (114). Pulmonary bronchogenic cysts manifest as thin-walled, unilocular, spherical masses, which may be fluid-filled, air-filled, or have an air-fluid level (fig. 11-8) (117).

MRI typically demonstrates lesions of relatively high signal intensity on T1-weighted images and very high homogeneous signal intensity on T2-weighted images (126). Rarely, the prenatal diagnosis of bronchogenic cyst is suggested after visualization of a unilocular cystic lesion of the fetal thorax on obstetrical ultrasonography (5).

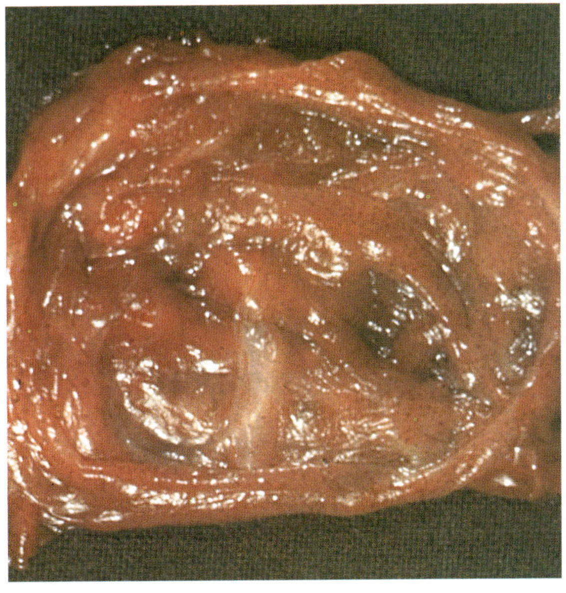

Figure 11-9

BRONCHOGENIC CYST

The cyst has a relatively thin wall and a smooth lining.

Pathologic Findings. Bronchogenic cysts are usually unilocular and filled with mucus (figs. 11-9, 11-10). When infected, they contain grossly purulent material. Histologically, noninfected bronchogenic cysts have a cuboidal to columnar respiratory (ciliated) epithelial lining surrounded by a fibromuscular wall,

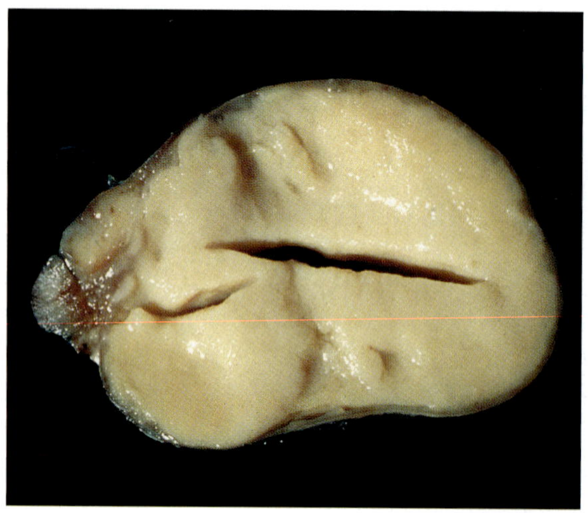

Figure 11-10

BRONCHOGENIC CYST

This bronchogenic cyst is filled with semisolid mucopurulent material. (Courtesy of Dr. J. T. Stocker, Bethesda, MD.)

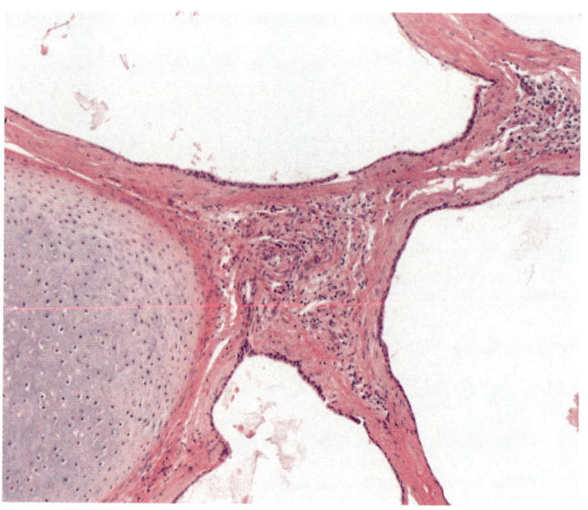

Figure 11-12

BRONCHOGENIC CYST

This multilocular bronchogenic cyst shows cartilage. The lining of the individual cysts is simple columnar epithelium.

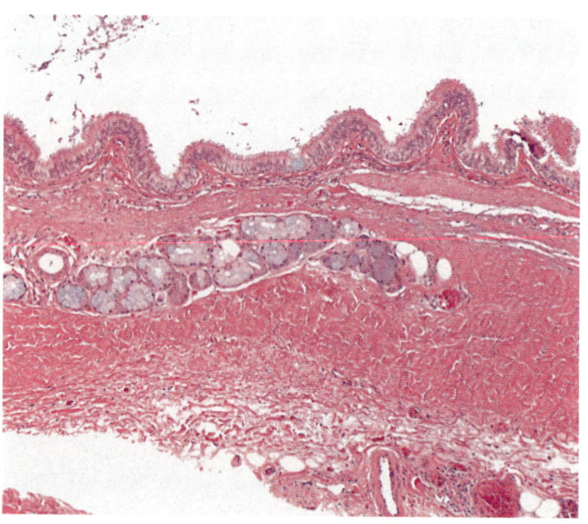

Figure 11-11

BRONCHOGENIC CYST

The epithelial lining is pseudostratified columnar respiratory epithelium. Glands resembling submucosal glands are present.

which may contain islands of cartilage and nests of glands resembling bronchial submucosal glands (figs. 11-11, 11-12). The identification of glands and cartilage may require multiple sections. In the absence of glands and cartilage, it may be impossible to distinguish a bronchogenic cyst from other foregut cysts. If the lesion has been infected, squamous metaplasia, purulent exudate, chronic inflammation, and fibrosis may be present.

Differential Diagnosis. The differential diagnosis of bronchogenic cyst includes abscess, enteric cyst, esophageal cyst, pericardial cyst, and cystic teratoma as well as other lesions listed in Table 11-2. An abscess or other chronic cavity (e.g., an infected sequestration) may be impossible to distinguish from a bronchogenic cyst on morphologic grounds alone, and in such cases the radiologic and surgical findings (including location, morphology, and radiologic appearance, as well as the types of associated bronchial and vascular connections) are extremely helpful in the diagnosis. The presence of cartilage is necessary for a diagnosis of bronchogenic cyst. When cartilage is lacking, the designation of undifferentiated foregut cyst is appropriate. Key features in the differential diagnosis of bronchogenic cysts are shown in Table 11-4.

Treatment. Surgical resection is generally curative (41,112). Percutaneous needle aspiration of the cyst fluid is reported in the literature as a therapeutic option for those patients with bronchogenic cyst who are not good surgical candidates. Transbronchial needle aspiration during bronchoscopy is also reported but has the disadvantage of small needle caliber, which may prove insufficient for draining viscous fluid (2).

PULMONARY SEQUESTRATION

Pulmonary sequestration occurs when lung tissue lacks a connection with the tracheobronchial tree, often with a concomitant anomalous vascular supply from the systemic circulation (92,111,154,156,158,159). Rarely, connections with the alimentary tract occur, and when present, the lesions are termed bronchopulmonary foregut malformations (see fig. 11-1).

Stocker (156) has proposed that sequestrations be defined simply as lung parenchyma not in continuity with the upper respiratory tract (via the normal tracheobronchial tree). This approach allows classification by etiology (congenital, inflammatory, traumatic); site (abdominal, mediastinal, thoracic, intralobar); and vascular connections (pulmonary or systemic arterial, pulmonary or systemic venous). This broad definition may lead to confusion with other entities such as bronchial atresia, but it is simple and easy to apply.

Sequestrations are divided into two types: intralobar and extralobar. These two types have a number of differences as shown in Table 11-5.

Intralobar Sequestrations

Definition. Intralobar sequestrations are found within the normal pleural investment of the lung. They lack a tracheobronchial communication, but may be air-containing and are supplied by anomalous arteries from the systemic circulation. Stocker (156) has postulated that intralobar sequestrations are acquired lesions of inflammatory origin that follow obstruction of

Table 11-4

DIFFERENTIAL DIAGNOSIS OF BRONCHOGENIC CYST[a]

Lesion	Features
Abscess	Intrapulmonary; bronchial communication (often multiple); purulent inflammation
Enteric cyst	Posterior mediastinal location; lined by gastric epithelium; may be associated with vertebral malformations
Esophageal cyst	Squamous lining; double muscle layer characteristic of esophageal wall
Pericardial cyst	Location in right or left cardiophrenic angle; unilocular (resembling a hernia sac) with a mesothelial lining
Cystic teratoma	Anterior mediastinal location; multiloculated; endodermal and ectodermal derivatives in addition to bronchial-type epithelium; cartilage and bronchial-type glands

[a]Modified from reference 92.

Table 11-5

INTRALOBAR VERSUS EXTRALOBAR SEQUESTRATION[a]

Feature	Intralobar Sequestration	Extralobar Sequestration
Age at diagnosis	50 percent over age 20 years (15 percent asymptomatic)	60 percent less than 6 months (10 percent asymptomatic)
Sex (M:F)	1:1	4:1
Side affected	Left, 55 percent	Left, 65 percent
Arterial supply	Systemic	Systemic (rarely pulmonary)
Venous drainage	Pulmonary (rarely systemic)	Systemic or portal (25 percent wholly or in part via pulmonary veins)
Associated anomalies	Uncommon (6-12 percent)	Over 60 percent (e.g., pectus excavatum, diaphragmatic defects)
Pathogenesis	Majority thought to be acquired	Congenital anomaly

[a]Modified from references 9, 154, 156, 158, and 159.

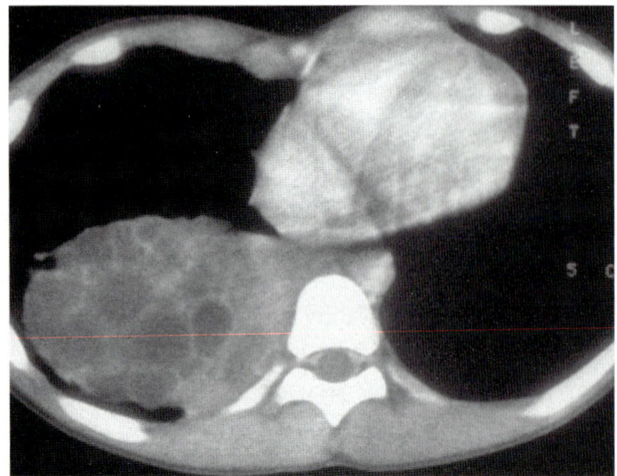

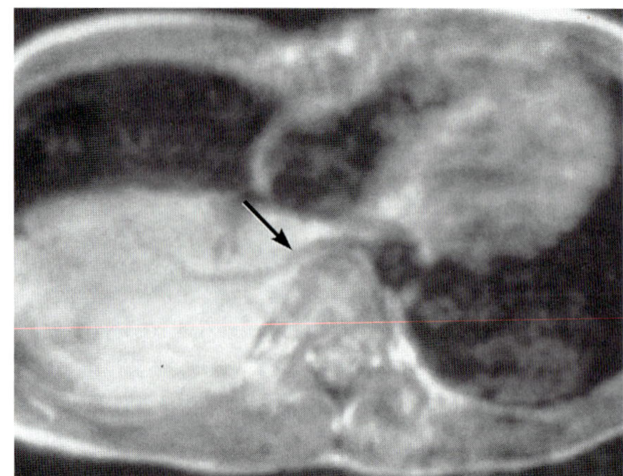

Figure 11-13

INTRALOBAR SEQUESTRATION

Intralobar sequestration in a 13-year-old male with persistent nonproductive cough and fever despite antibiotic therapy.

Left: Contrast-enhanced chest CT (mediastinal window) demonstrates a heterogeneously enhancing, multicystic, right lower lobe mass.

Right: Axial T1-weighted MRI demonstrates an anomalous artery (arrow) that arises from the descending thoracic aorta and supplies the lesion.

the tracheobronchial tree and secondary development of a systemic arterial supply from hypertrophied pulmonary ligament arteries. This theory explains the propensity for intralobar sequestrations to occur in the medial lower lobes.

Clinical Features. There is an equal sex incidence, with most patients presenting after 20 years of age. Symptoms typically include cough, sputum production, and recurrent pneumonia. Fifteen percent of the patients are asymptomatic. Bilateral intralobar sequestrations have been reported, including cases with connections between the two sequestrations (166). An accurate clinical/radiologic diagnosis can often be made on the basis of the history and the cross-sectional imaging or angiographic findings.

Radiologic Findings. Intralobar sequestrations are typically left-sided lesions that affect the lower lobes (usually the posterior basal segments) in up to 98 percent of cases (70). In fact, any persistent consolidation or abnormal opacity in a patient with a history of recurrent pulmonary infection should prompt additional imaging studies for exclusion of intralobar sequestration. Radiographic features of intralobar sequestration include a persistent parenchymal consolidation of irregular borders and a soft tissue mass of smooth or lobulated contour. Lesions may be predominantly cystic and air-filled or may contain fluid or single or multiple air-fluid levels. Another radiographic manifestation is a subtle tubular opacity in the lower lobe, which may represent the anomalous vessel(s) associated with these lesions (70).

CT typically demonstrates a consolidation or mass of homogeneous or heterogeneous attenuation and heterogeneous contrast enhancement. The lesions have an irregular contour against the nonsequestered normal lung. Multiple thin-walled cystic spaces within the lesion, with or without air-fluid levels, are often demonstrated (fig. 11-13). Cross-sectional imaging is particularly helpful in delineating the systemic blood supply to these lesions, which typically originates from the descending thoracic aorta in the region of the pulmonary ligament (fig. 11-13). Tubular opacities with associated emphysematous lung have also been observed. Dynamic thin-section and helical CT have improved preoperative visualization of the anomalous systemic arteries. Angiography of the thoracic aorta can also demonstrate the anomalous pulmonary ligament arteries that supply these lesions. Selective angiography and digital subtraction angiography may demonstrate the pulmonary venous drainage (70).

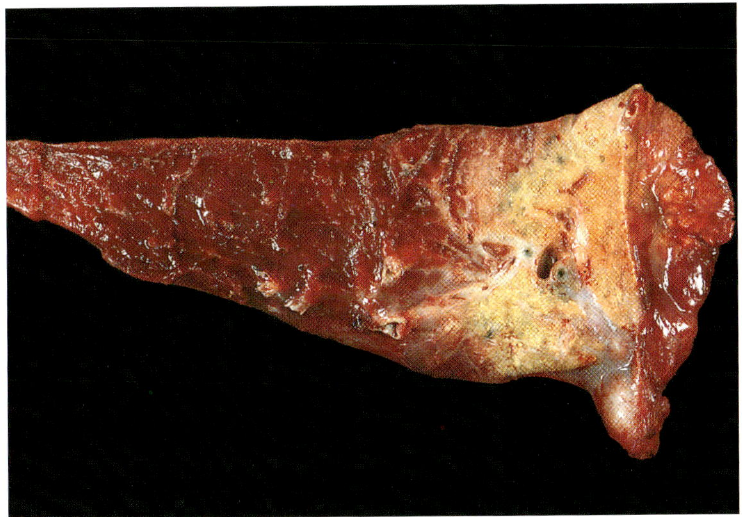
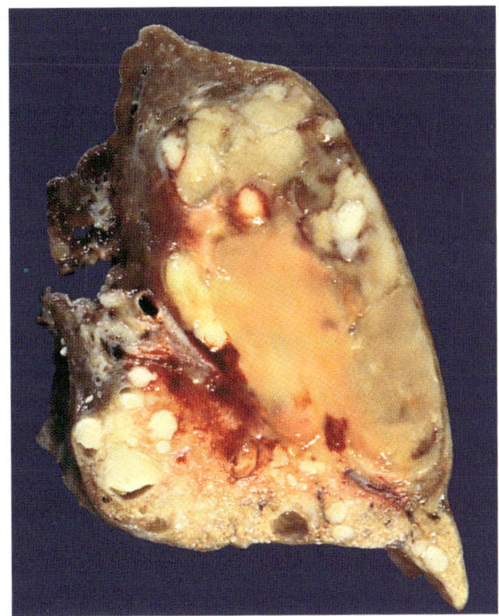

Figure 11-14

INTRALOBAR SEQUESTRATION

There is consolidation of lung tissue with dilated airways (left, right), some containing purulent-appearing mucus (right). Gray-white scarring is also prominent.

Pathologic Findings. Grossly, intralobar sequestrations usually show the effects of chronic inflammation resulting from recurrent or prolonged infection/inflammation (fig. 11-14). The pleura is thickened with associated adhesions, and the parenchyma shows fibrosis with cysts up to 5 cm in diameter. The cysts often contain mucinous or frankly purulent material. Large feeding arteries may be apparent, and these should be sought in gross examination of the specimen. Review of intraoperative or radiologic findings may be necessary to document the anomalous vascular connections.

Histologically, the parenchyma shows the effects of inflammation and fibrosis (fig. 11-15). Remnants of bronchi are dilated and contain mucus or purulent material, and the alveoli are characteristically filled with alveolar macrophages, many of which are foamy. Epithelial metaplasia is common. Interstitial fibrosis may be extensive. Thick-walled vessels, reflecting the systemic vascular supply, can be highlighted with elastic tissue stains. The border between sequestered tissue and adjacent normal lung parenchyma may be abrupt or indistinct. The development of carcinoma in an intralobar sequestration has been described (4).

Differential Diagnosis. The differential diagnosis of intralobar sequestration includes other anomalies and localized inflammatory processes. With full knowledge of the radiologic, intraoperative, and microscopic findings, problems in differential diagnosis can be minimized. Key features are the lack of communication with the tracheobronchial tree and systemic arterial supply. Based solely on the histology, there may be considerable confusion with abscesses, bronchiectasis, and changes distal to bronchial obstruction (such as from neoplasm or aspiration). Marked inflammation and fibrosis secondarily affecting either bronchial atresia or congenital cystic adenomatoid malformation can make these entities difficult to distinguish from sequestration, if examined without correlation with the imaging and gross pathologic findings.

Treatment and Prognosis. The treatment of patients with intralobar sequestration is surgical resection. Following successful resection, the prognosis is excellent, without risk of recurrence. As angiographic examination is performed less frequently, an attempt at preoperative delineation of abnormal feeding vessels with cross-sectional imaging studies may be

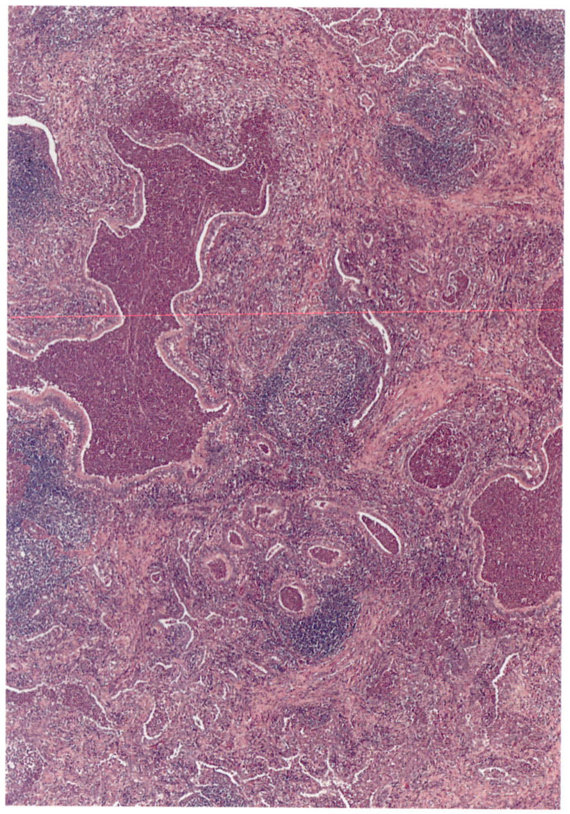

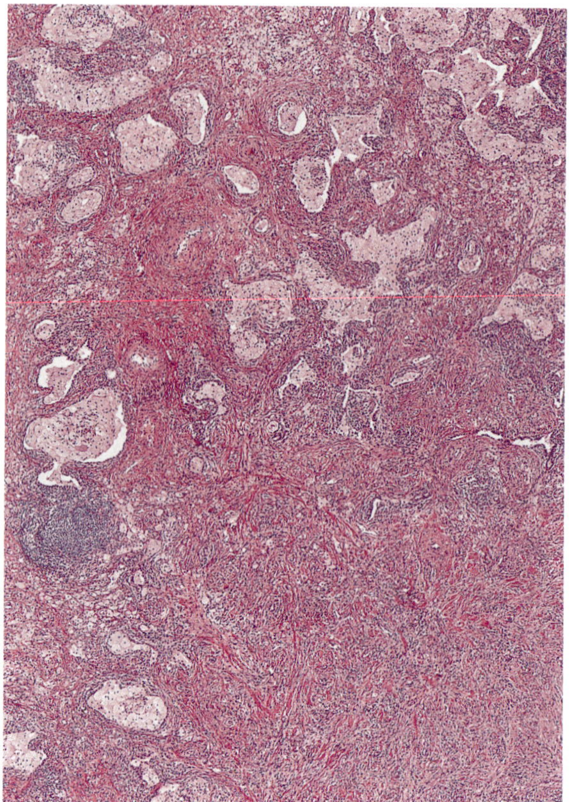

Figure 11-15

INTRALOBAR SEQUESTRATION

Left: Histologically, there is airspace exudate, particularly in airways with associated lymphoid hyperplasia.
Right: Interstitial scarring may be prominent.

helpful for successful identification and ligation of these structures at the time of surgery.

Extralobar Sequestrations

Definition. Extralobar sequestrations *(accessory lung, Rokitansky lobe)* are true congenital anomalies in which accessory (extrapulmonary) lung tissue, usually with its own pleural investment, occurs within the thorax, diaphragm, or abdomen (10,35,92,105,111,123,154,156,158, 159,177). Intradiaphragmatic lesions and peritoneal lesions may not be covered by pleura but by diaphragm or peritoneum, respectively.

Clinical Features. Most cases are identified in male infants under 6 months of age, but some have been described in adults as old as 81 years. Most infants present with dyspnea, cyanosis, and feeding problems. Older individuals may have a history of recurrent pneumonia, especially if there is a communication with the alimentary tract. About 10 percent of patients are asymptomatic.

Radiologic Findings. The typical extralobar sequestration manifests radiographically as a homogeneous, well-marginated, triangular mass in the infant thorax, closely related to the posterior medial diaphragm (fig. 11-16) (143). However, these lesions may occur anywhere in the thorax or below the diaphragm. Air and air-fluid levels are not found unless there is a communication with the gastrointestinal tract, as in the case of bronchopulmonary foregut malformations. Most extralobar sequestrations occur in the left hemithorax. Large masses may manifest as an opaque hemithorax with ipsilateral pleural effusion and mediastinal shift (143).

On cross-sectional imaging with CT, ultrasound, or MRI the lesions are usually homogeneous.

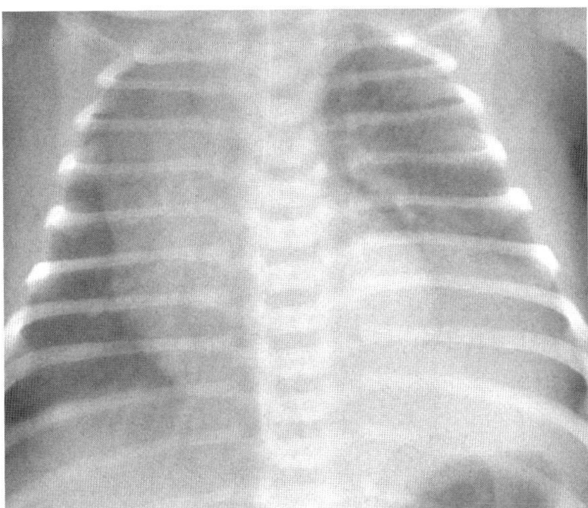

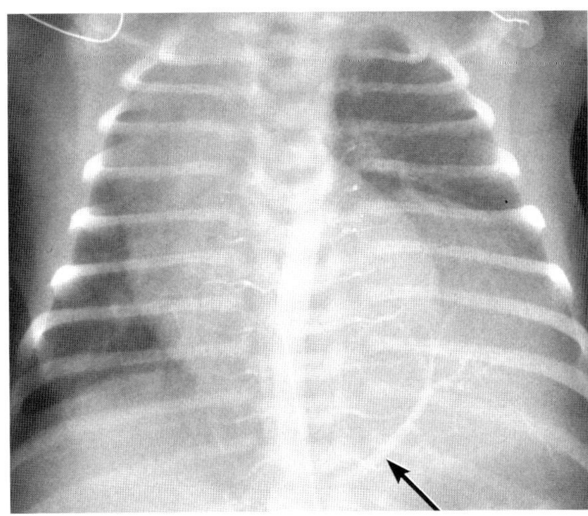

Figure 11-16

EXTRALOBAR SEQUESTRATION

Extralobar sequestration in a newborn male with tachypnea and decreased breath sounds in the left chest.

Left: AP portable chest radiograph demonstrates a large, homogeneous, soft tissue mass of the left lung base, which produces mass effect on the mediastinum.

Right: Thoracic aortogram demonstrates an anomalous artery (arrow), which arises from the distal thoracic aorta and feeds the mass, consistent with the diagnosis of extralobar sequestration.

Ultrasonography typically demonstrates a well-defined echogenic mass and may even show the anomalous vessels that supply it. Antenatal diagnosis with obstetrical ultrasonography is possible and typically demonstrates a homogeneous hyperechoic mass in the fetal thorax, or less commonly, the abdomen. Polyhydramnios may occur from impairment of fetal swallowing. If needle biopsy is undertaken, the identification of normal or near normal lung parenchyma may allow a decision to postpone surgical resection until the infant has grown and is able to withstand surgery (26,143).

Angiography typically demonstrates the anomalous feeding vessels (fig. 11-16). Selective arterial injection and delayed imaging can demonstrate the systemic venous drainage. Digital subtraction angiography is an excellent technique for demonstrating the anomalous vascular supply and venous drainage of these lesions (143).

Pathologic Findings. Extralobar sequestrations are generally single, between 0.5 and 15.0 cm in diameter (usually 3 to 6 cm), and pyramidal or ovoid (figs. 11-15, 11-16). Although they lack a connection with the bronchial tree, remnants of cartilaginous bronchi may be found in approximately half the cases, and the systemic arterial supply should be sought. Those that have been secondarily inflamed or infected are grossly fibrotic, and the pleural covering may be thickened and covered by exudate. The cut surface may reveal normal lung tissue or, when inflamed, cystic change, fibrosis, and purulent secretions.

The microscopic findings vary depending on whether or not secondary infection is present (fig. 11-17). In uninfected cases, dilated airways are lined by bronchiolar-type epithelium, and dilated airspaces are lined by type 1 and type 2 pneumocytes and contain macrophages. Well-formed bronchi may be seen. In premature infants, the tissue is immature-appearing, with interstitial widening. Extramedullary hematopoiesis may be identified, especially in premature infants. The subpleural lymphatics are typically dilated. Thick-walled vessels reflecting systemic vascular supply should be sought. In infected cases, there is nonspecific acute and chronic inflammation, fibrosis, and purulent exudate. Some extralobar sequestrations (up to 25 percent) contain foci that are histologically indistinguishable from (and probably represent)

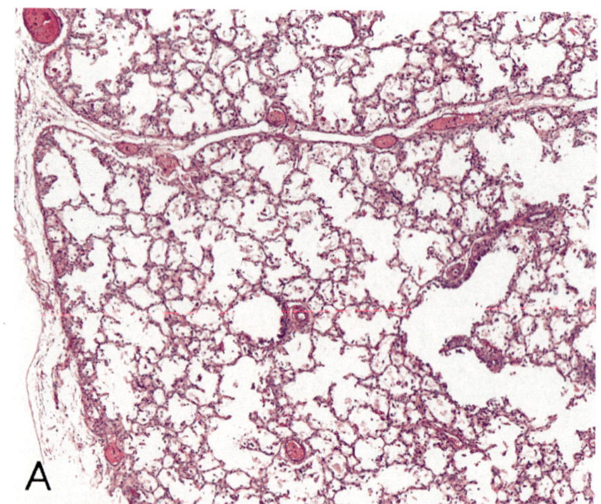

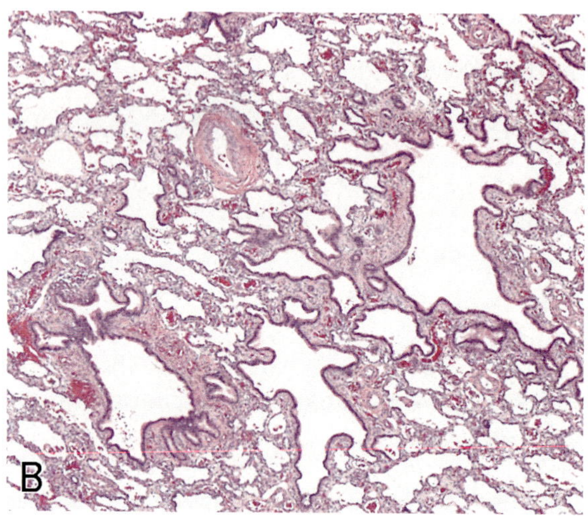

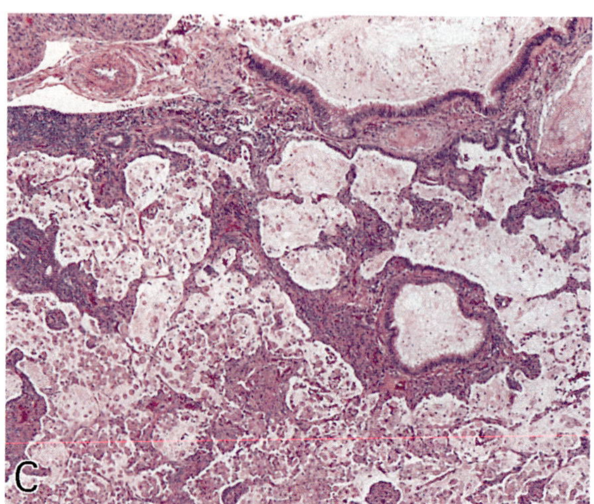

Figure 11-17

EXTRALOBAR SEQUESTRATION

The histologic spectrum varies from nearly normal lung tissue (A), to tissue resembling cystic adenomatoid malformation (B), to inflamed lung tissue with mucin-filled airways in which the underlying architecture is difficult to discern (C).

congenital cystic adenomatoid malformation, type 2 (35,43a,105,123,154,156).

Treatment and Prognosis. The treatment of extralobar sequestration is resection. The outcome is generally excellent unless there are significant associated anomalies, which affect the management and prognosis. Detection by prenatal ultrasound is possible, and spontaneous regression of presumed sequestrations has been shown (19,26,105). In these cases, the differential diagnosis should include neuroblastoma, germ cell tumor, and foregut duplication.

ANOMALIES OF THE LUNG PARENCHYMA

Agenesis. Agenesis of lung tissue is rare (104,106,116,154). It may be unilateral, bilateral, or lobar, and is frequently associated with other anomalies. Complete absence of lung acinar development has been termed *acinar dysplasia* (106), and corresponds to congenital cystic adenomatoid malformation, type 0 (see below), in which there are peculiar bronchial-type structures surrounded by mesenchyme that lacks acinar development (154).

Horseshoe Lung. This refers to a rare anomaly in which the right and left lungs are fused behind the heart by an isthmus of lung parenchyma. The right bronchial tree has a lower lobe branch that crosses the midline into the left lung. Pulmonary angiography is diagnostic, as it demonstrates a right pulmonary artery branch that crosses behind the heart to supply a portion of the left lung (71,92,104,154,174). CT confirms the diagnosis by demonstrating continuity of the right lung and vessels as they cross the midline behind the heart into the left hemithorax.

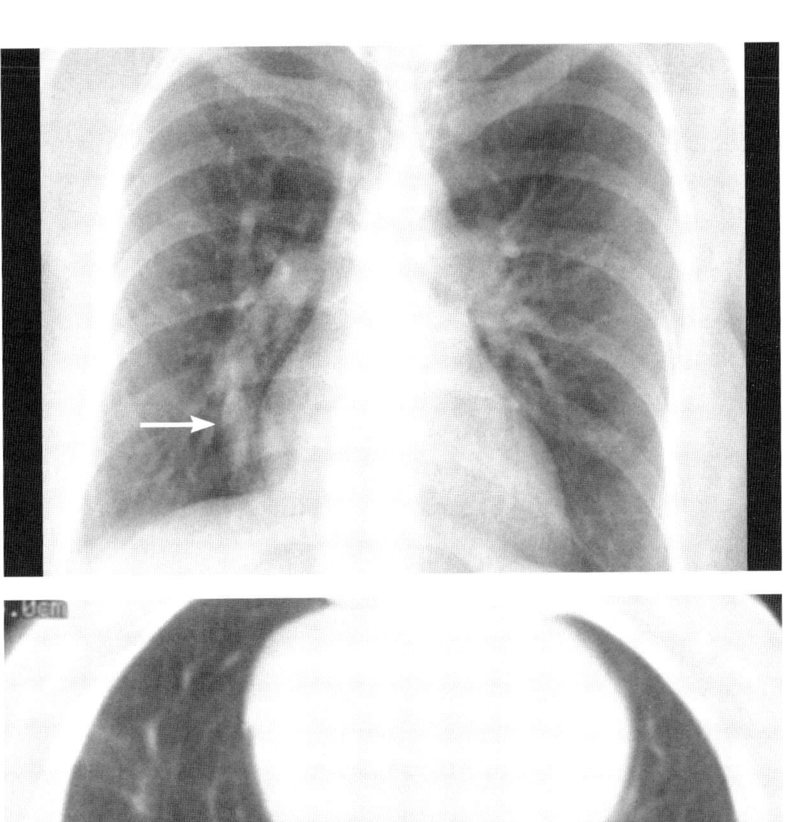

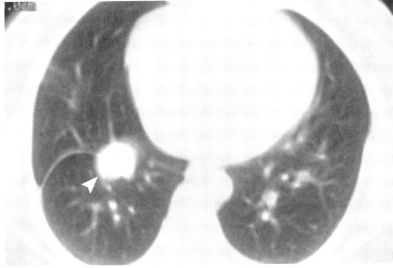

Figure 11-18

SCIMITAR SYNDROME

Scimitar syndrome in a 43-year-old female who was incidentally discovered to have an abnormal chest radiograph.

Top: PA chest radiograph demonstrates accentuation of the central pulmonary vasculature and a small right lung volume. An arcuate vascular structure (arrow) in the right lower lobe courses medially towards the diaphragm.

Bottom: Contrast-enhanced chest CT (lung window) demonstrates the anomalous scimitar vein (arrowhead), which enhanced with contrast and drained into the inferior vena cava.

Horseshoe lung may be found in association with the *scimitar syndrome,* which gets its name from its distinctive radiographic appearance (71,92,154). The scimitar syndrome is characterized by partial anomalous pulmonary venous return and forms part of a series of congenital malformations of the thorax also known as *congenital pulmonary venolobar syndrome* and *hypogenetic lung syndrome.* These anomalies include agenesis, aplasia, or hypoplasia of the lung; partial anomalous pulmonary venous return; absence of the pulmonary artery; sequestration; systemic arterial supply to nonsequestered lung; absence of the inferior vena cava; anomalies of the right hemidiaphragm; abnormalities of lobation, including single lobe or horseshoe lung; and cardiovascular anomalies (27,117,174).

In scimitar syndrome there is anomalous venous drainage from the right lung into the inferior vena cava, or rarely, into the right atrium, the coronary sinus, or the portal or hepatic veins. The anomalous vein manifests radiologically as an arcuate tubular opacity that courses medially toward the inferior vena cava, simulating the shape of a Turkish sword, hence the name (fig. 11-18). Patients with scimitar syndrome may be asymptomatic or have symptoms related to congenital heart disease, pulmonary hypertension, or repeated pulmonary infections.

Table 11-6

METHODS OF DETERMINING PULMONARY HYPOPLASIA[a]

Lung weight
Lung weight/body weight ratio
Radial alveolar count
Alveolar count per unit volume
Lung volume measurement and correlation with crown rump length
Airway branching count using latex injection
DNA content

[a]Modified from reference 154. Details of these methods can be found in references 9, 60, 77, and 170.

Pulmonary Hypoplasia. This has been defined in a variety of ways and is relatively common, seen in approximately 10 percent of neonatal autopsies (fig. 11-19) (92,107,139,154). The methods of determining whether or not pulmonary hypoplasia is present are shown in Table 11-6. The etiology is primarily related to limitations in available space, but many other causes are also recognized (Table 11-7). Two thirds to three quarters of the affected patients have secondary hypoplasia caused by another anomaly that reduces intrathoracic space and prevents normal lung development. Pulmonary hypoplasia is reported in patients with Down's syndrome (44,45,90,175). Studies have shown a decreased total number of alveoli and a smaller than normal alveolar surface area (44,45). These changes appear to result from abnormal postnatal growth and inflation of the lungs, and may produce a distinctive, diffuse, uniform porosity of the cut surfaces of the lungs (45). Grossly and radiographically, these changes may appear as peripheral cystic lung disease. The propensity of such lungs to mechanical trauma has been suggested as an explanation for the occurrence of postoperative respiratory failure in the setting of Down's syndrome (175).

The radiographic recognition of hypoplastic lungs is difficult (102). However, indirect findings include antenatal recognition of pleural effusions or space-occupying pulmonary congenital anomalies. Secondary findings include

Table 11-7

PULMONARY HYPOPLASIA[a]

Etiologic Factors in Pulmonary Hypoplasia
Limitation of available space
Intrathoracic lesions
Thoracic constriction secondary to malformed thorax
Thoracic constriction secondary to disturbance of amniotic and lung fluid volume
Diaphragmatic elevation
Abnormal or absent fetal breathing movements
Environmental agents
Primary mesodermal defect
Unknown

Anomalies Associated with Pulmonary Hypoplasia
Common
Diaphragmatic hernia
Renal agenesis, bilateral
Renal dysgenesis, bilateral
Obstructive uropathy
Polycystic renal disease (Potter, type I)
Large abdominal wall defects
Infrequent
Diaphragmatic hypoplasia or eventration
Hemolytic disease of the newborn
Pleural effusion, as with nonimmune fetal hydrops
Musculoskeletal abnormalities such as thoracic dystrophies
Anencephaly
Scimitar syndrome
Chromosomal anomalies, including trisomy 13, 18, and 21
Rare
Abdominal pregnancy
Ascites secondary to congenital cytomegalovirus infection
Cloacal dysgenesis
Congenital hydropericardium
Down's syndrome
Glutaric acidemia, type II
Laryngotracheoesophageal cleft
Neonatal hypophosphatasia
Pena-Shokeir I syndrome
Phrenic nerve agenesis
Right-sided cardiovascular malformation as with hypoplastic right heart
Thoracic neuroblastoma
Upper cervical spinal cord
Extralobar sequestration

[a]Modified from references 106 and 154.

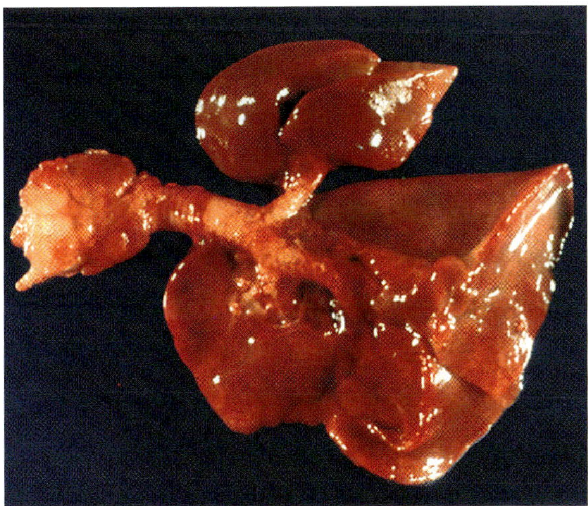

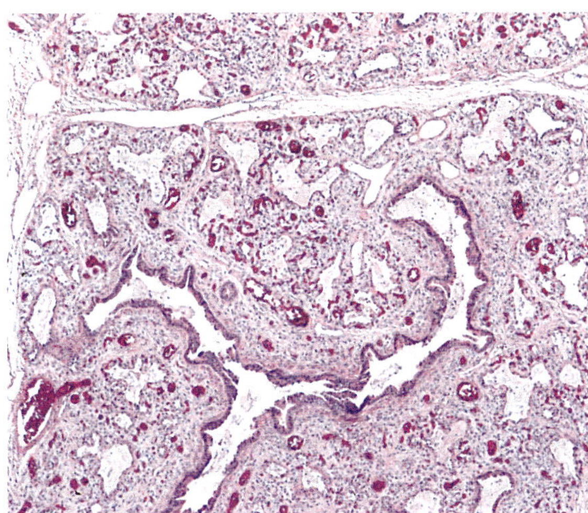

Figure 11-19

PULMONARY HYPOPLASIA

Left: Grossly, the lung is small compared to the opposite lung.

Right: Histologically, another case shows central bronchovascular structures with few surrounding airspaces and marked interstitial widening.

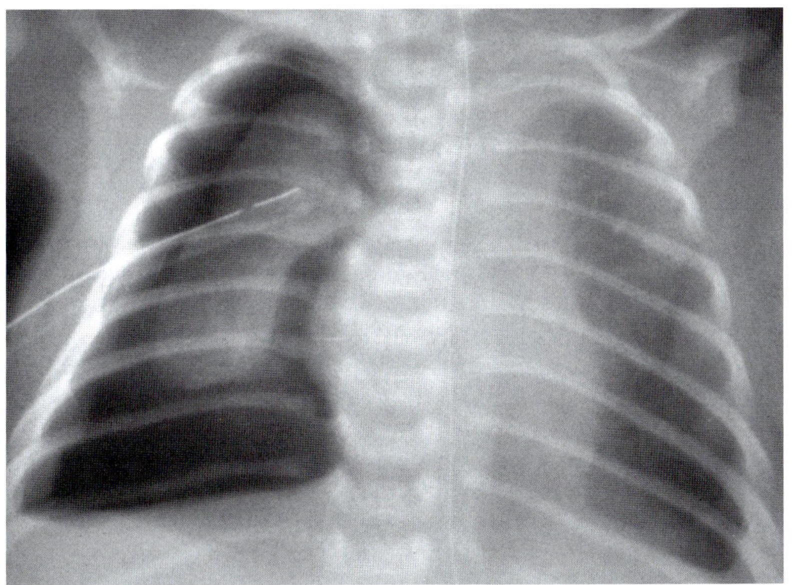

Figure 11-20

PULMONARY HYPOPLASIA

Pulmonary hypoplasia in a 1-month-old female with respiratory distress. AP chest radiograph demonstrates a large right-sided pneumothorax which did not respond to pleural tube drainage.

neonatal pneumothorax or pneumomediastinum that is refractory to therapy (fig. 11-20).

Pulmonary Hyperplasia. In this anomaly, there are more pulmonary acini/alveoli than normal. Lobar involvement has been referred to as *polyalveolar lobe* (154); patients typically present with lobar overinflation (discussed below). Hyperplasia of all lobes may occur as a result of tracheal or laryngeal atresia.

CONGENITAL CYSTIC ADENOMATOID MALFORMATION

Definition. Congenital cystic adenomatoid malformation (CCAM) is a hamartomatous mass of lung tissue that appears disorganized and may have varying degrees of cystic change (14,18,31,36,42,78,104,106,112,120,121,125,138,144,154,158,161). Compared to normal lung, there is an increase in the number of structures

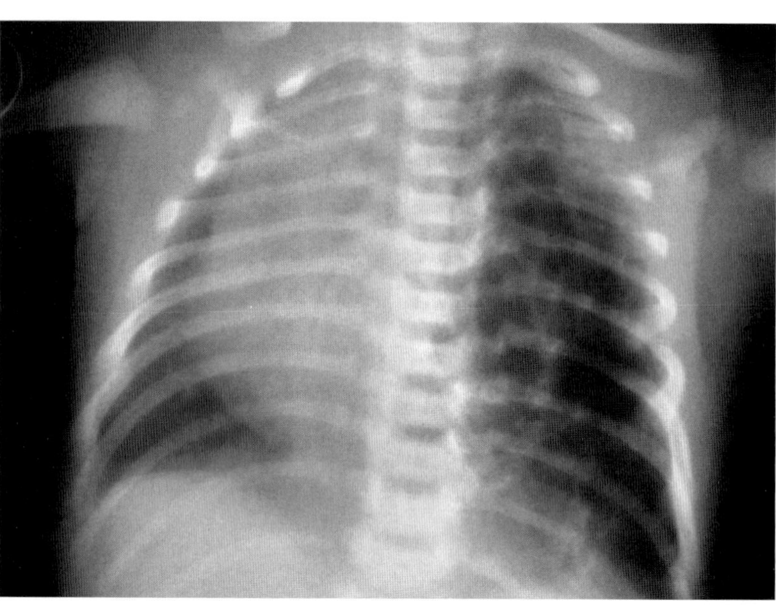

Figure 11-21

CYSTIC ADENOMATOID MALFORMATION

Cystic adenomatoid malformation, type 1, in a newborn female with progressive respiratory distress. PA chest radiograph demonstrates a multicystic air-filled lesion of the left lung, which produces mass effect on the mediastinum.

resembling terminal bronchioles, often with polypoid growths of cuboidal epithelium and increased underlying stromal elastica and smooth muscle. Cystic changes vary with the subtype. There is an absence of inflammation, and cartilage is only rarely present but may dominate some cases (18). The term *congenital pulmonary airway malformation* has been suggested to replace CCAM (156a).

Clinical Features. CCAMs usually occur in stillborn infants or are identified in newborn infants with respiratory distress. Rarely, these lesions manifest in older children and adults (12). There is a slight male predominance, with equal occurrence in the right and left lung. CCAMs are usually unilateral and affect only one lobe. They account for 20 to 40 percent of resected congenital lung lesions. Moerman et al. (121) suggested that segmental bronchial atresia or absence is the primary pathogenetic defect that results in the development of a CCAM distal to the defect.

Radiologic Findings. Chest radiographs typically demonstrate a unilateral, multicystic, air-filled lung lesion (figs. 11-21–11-23) (144). CCAMs may reach large sizes and may produce a mass effect on the adjacent lung and mediastinum, resulting in atelectasis and mediastinal shift, respectively. They may also manifest as areas of hyperlucent lung. In these cases, visualization of thin internal septa provides a clue to the correct preoperative diagnosis (fig. 11-22). Occasionally, retained fetal fluid produces multiple air-fluid levels or a homogeneous mass on chest radiography.

Cross-sectional imaging demonstrates the cystic nature of these lesions, allows visualization of the intervening tissue septa (characteristic of CCAM, type 1), and delineates the extent and distribution of disease (figs. 11-22, 11-23). Large, dominant cysts may also be seen. Type 2 lesions demonstrate the heterogeneity produced by multiple small cysts with intervening normal or atelectatic lung (fig. 11-23). Type 3 lesions are homogeneous masses with an echogenic appearance on ultrasonography (144).

Prenatal diagnosis and follow-up can be performed via obstetrical ultrasonography, which demonstrates a cystic or multicystic mass in the fetal thorax with associated mass effect (fig. 11-24). Fetal hydrops may also be detected and may be associated with anasarca, ascites, pleural effusion, polyhydramnios, and placental edema, particularly with the type 3 lesion. Ultrasonographic evaluation is helpful in the intrauterine surgical management of these lesions (78).

Pathologic Findings. Three types of CCAM (types 1, 2, and 3) have been classically recognized, based on a combination of gross and microscopic features and the presence or absence of associated anomalies (161). Recently, Stocker (154) has expanded the concept of

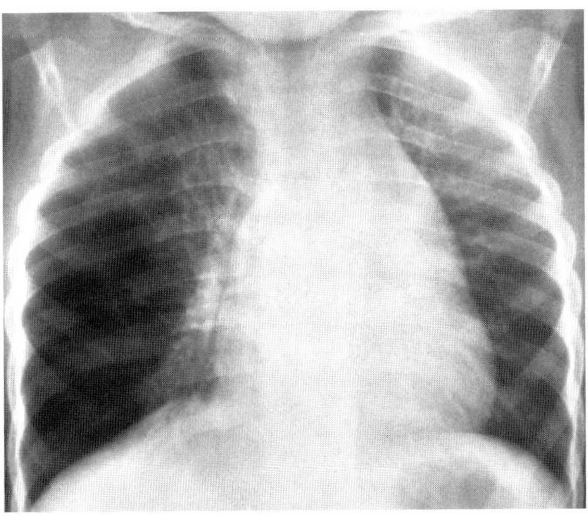

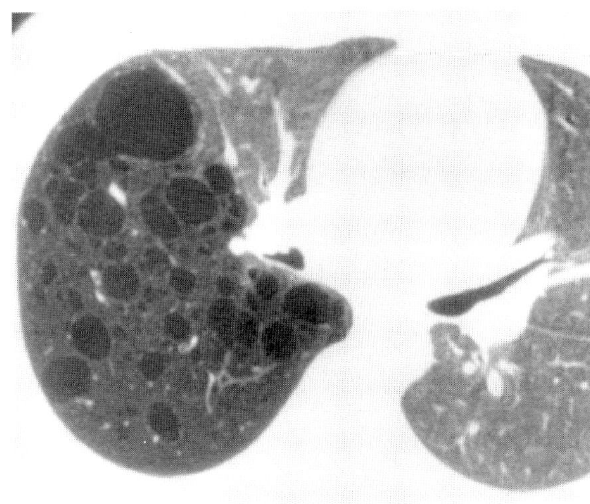

Figure 11-22

CYSTIC ADENOMATOID MALFORMATION

Cystic adenomatoid malformation, type 1, in a 2-year-old male with a history of asthma.

Left: PA chest radiograph demonstrates hyperlucency of the right lower lobe. Unlike the appearance of infantile lobar emphysema, one can perceive rounded lucencies within the area of abnormality. There is mass effect on the rest of the lung.

Right: Chest CT (lung window), obtained at age 13, demonstrates an abnormal right lower lobe with multiple, air-filled, rounded cystic areas of varying sizes.

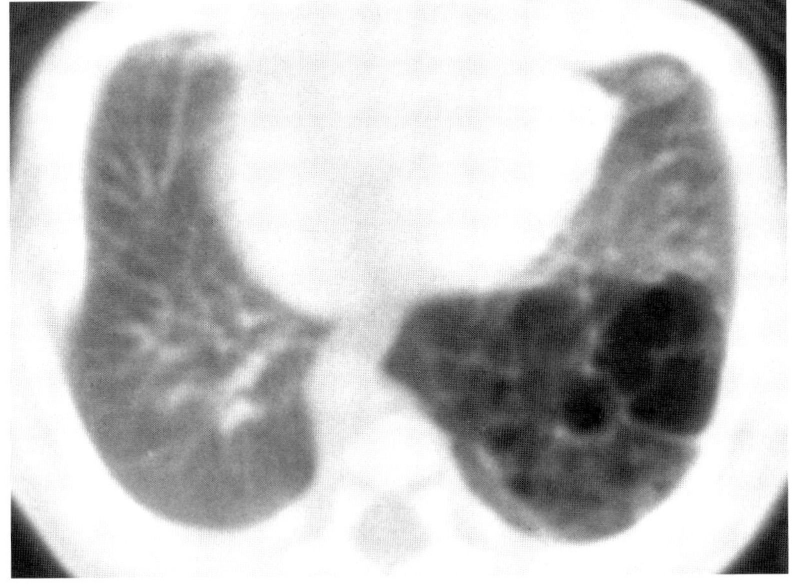

Figure 11-23

CONGENITAL CYSTIC ADENOMATOID MALFORMATION

Congenital cystic adenomatoid malformation, type 2, in a 6-week-old male who was diagnosed by prenatal obstetrical ultrasonography. Chest CT (lung window) demonstrates multiple air-filled cysts that replace the left lower lobe.

CCAM to include five types, adding type 0 and type 4 (Table 11-8) (156a). The hypothesis is that from type 0 to type 4 the abnormalities involve progressively more distal tissue, with type 0 characterized by complete agenesis of acini and type 4 representing cystic change in the peripheral acini; types 1, 2, and 3 are in between. Thus, the presence of cartilage in types 0 and 1 is not surprising, since these anomalies primarily involve proximal airways; whereas the absence of cartilage in types 2 through 4 corresponds to the absence of cartilage in the distal airways and lung parenchyma. While this classification is conceptually useful, it may be difficult to apply in review of individual or small series of cases (36). The gross

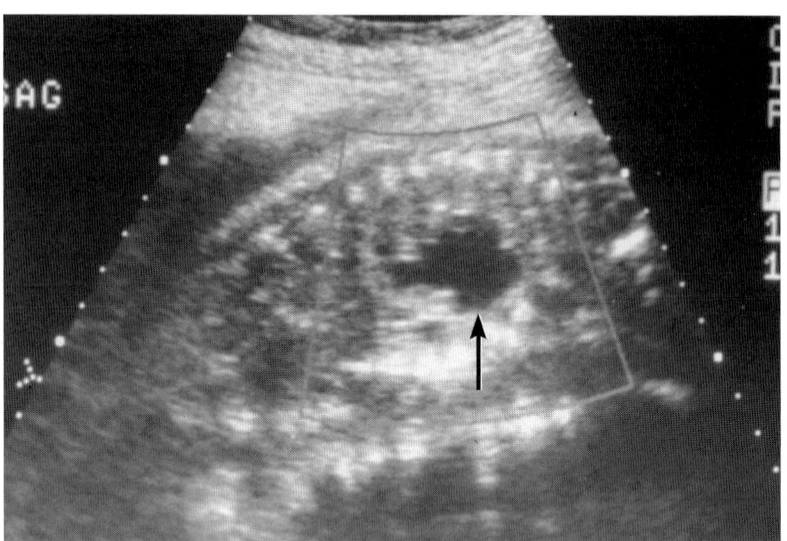

Figure 11-24

CYSTIC ADENOMATOID MALFORMATION

Longitudinal prenatal obstetrical sonogram demonstrates cystic change in the left lung (arrow).

Table 11-8

PATHOLOGIC FEATURES OF CONGENITAL CYSTIC ADENOMATOID MALFORMATION[a]

Features	Type 0	Type 1	Type 2	Type 3	Type 4
Approximate frequency (%)	1–3	>65	20–25	8	2–4
Cyst size (maximum, cm)	0.5	10.0	2.5	1.5	7.0
Epithelial lining (cysts)	Ciliated; pseudostratified; tall columnar with goblet cells	Ciliated; pseudostratified; tall columnar	Ciliated; cuboidal or columnar	Ciliated; cuboidal	Flattened; alveolar lining cells
Muscular wall thickness of cysts (in microns)	100–500	100–300	50–100	0–50	25–100
Mucous cells	Present in all cases	Present (33% of cases)	Absent	Absent	Absent
Cartilage	Present in all cases	Present (5–10% of cases)	Absent	Absent	Rare
Skeletal muscle	Absent	Absent	Present (5% of cases)	Absent	Absent

[a]Modified from reference 154.

findings vary from almost entirely solid to entirely cystic lesions (figs. 11-25–11-27).

CCAM type 0 corresponds to acinar dysplasia or dysgenesis (154,156a). The lung shows only bronchial-like structures, cartilage plates, and loose vascularized mesenchyme. CCAMs types 1,2, and 3 may blend imperceptibly with normal-appearing alveoli, communicate with the bronchial tree, and be aerated. The larger spaces are lined by cuboidal or columnar respiratory epithelium, and the smaller alveolus-like spaces are lined by type 1 or type 2 cells (figs. 11-28–11-32); the latter are common in younger patients with more immature lung tissue. Mucinous cells (fig. 11-32) are seen in all type 0 lesions and in approximately one third of patients with type 1 CCAM as scattered clusters and tufts of well-differentiated goblet cells. The smaller cysts in type 1 lesions and the cysts in type 2 lesions resemble dilated terminal bronchioles. Type 3 lesions are bulky masses which histologically resemble the early canalicular stage of lung development. Type 4 CCAMs are thin-walled cysts in the distal lung tissue

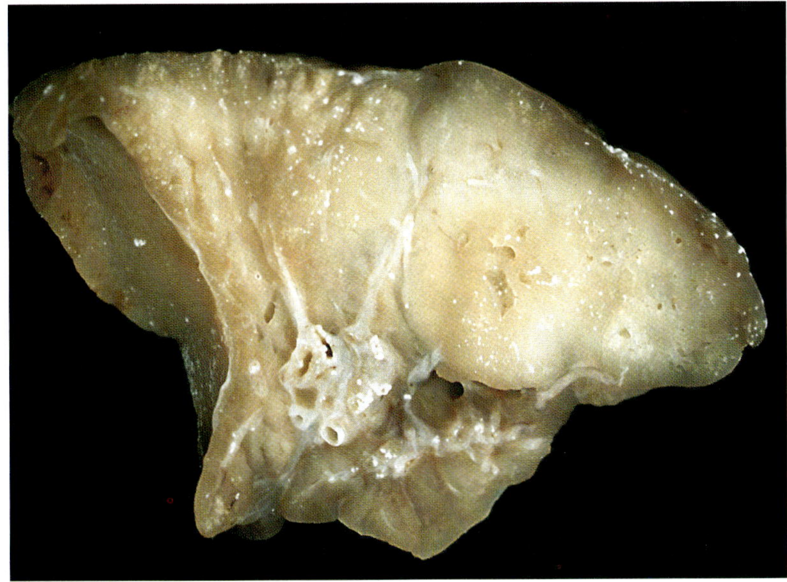

Figure 11-25

CONGENITAL CYSTIC ADENOMATOID MALFORMATION

This lobectomy specimen shows a relatively solid lesion.

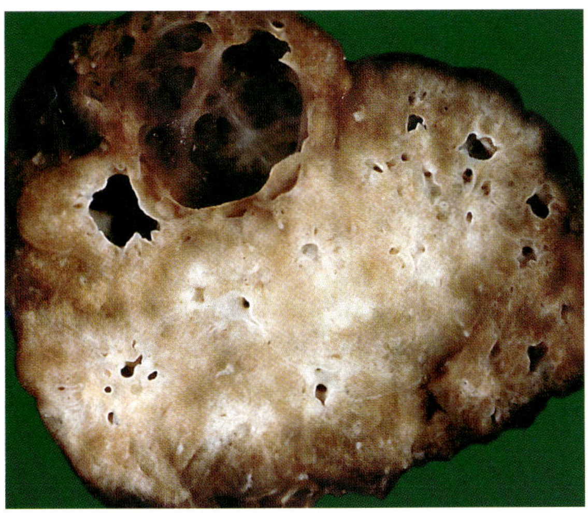

Figure 11-26

CONGENITAL CYSTIC ADENOMATOID MALFORMATION

Congenital cystic adenomatoid malformation with solid areas and cysts of varying size (up to approximately 1.5 cm).

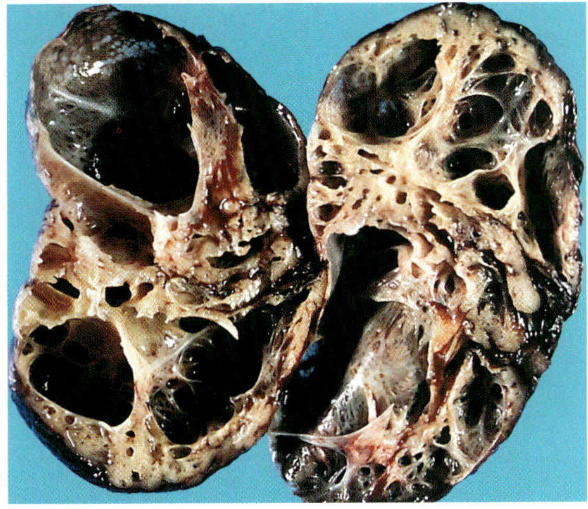

Figure 11-27

CONGENITAL CYSTIC ADENOMATOID MALFORMATION

Congenital cystic adenomatoid malformation with marked cystic change. (Courtesy of Dr. A. Churg, Vancouver, Canada.)

(154,156a). Radiologically, large air-filled cysts that may cause mediastinal shift are seen. Grossly, cystic change is found in the periphery of the lobe and histologically, the abnormal airspaces are lined by type 1 alveolar lining cells and low cuboidal cells. Type 4 lesions lack the primitive interstitial cells seen in pleuropulmonary blastoma.

Treatment and Prognosis. The treatment is resection if other congenital anomalies do not preclude it; CCAMs are thought to predispose to recurring infections if not resected. Examples detected with prenatal ultrasound have successfully undergone resection or drainage while the fetus was still in utero (36). Serial prenatal ultrasonography in other cases has shown apparent

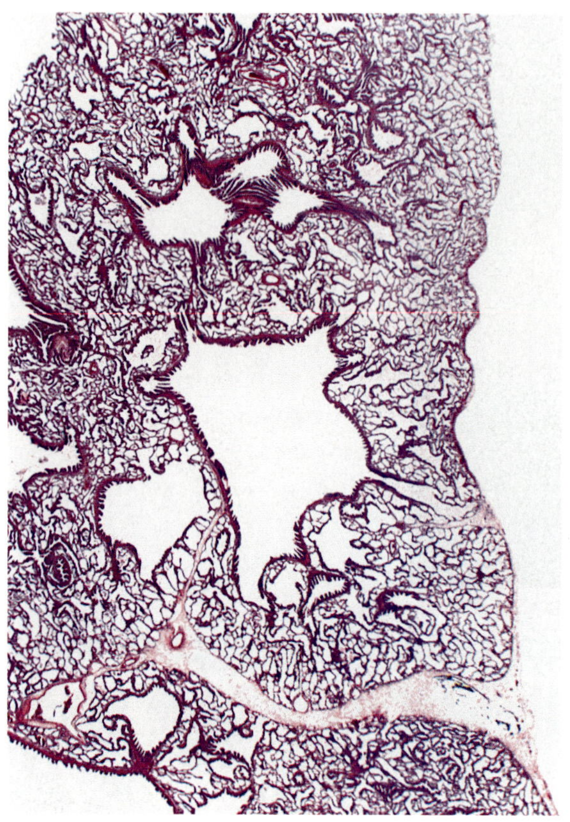

Figure 11-28

CONGENITAL CYSTIC ADENOMATOID MALFORMATION

There is prominent dilatation of bronchiolar-like structures that have papillary change.

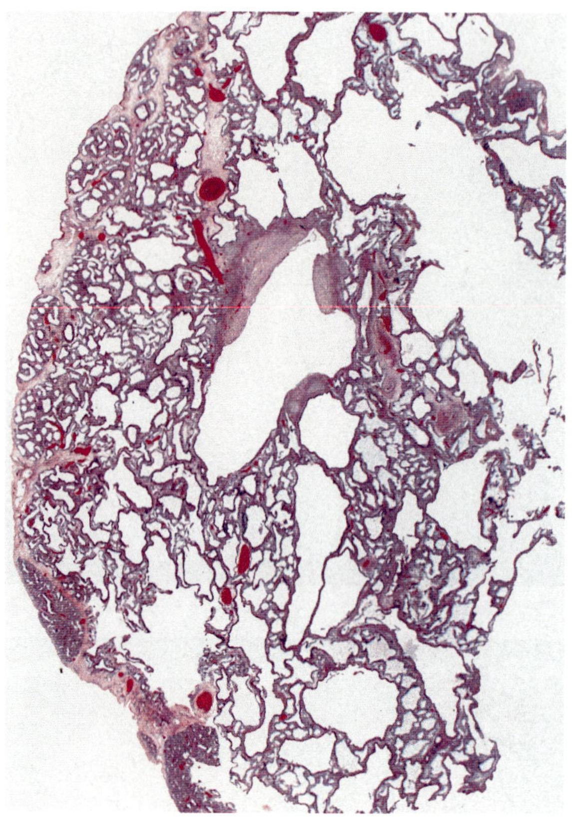

Figure 11-29

CONGENITAL CYSTIC ADENOMATOID MALFORMATION

Congenital cystic adenomatoid malformation with microcysts of varying sizes.

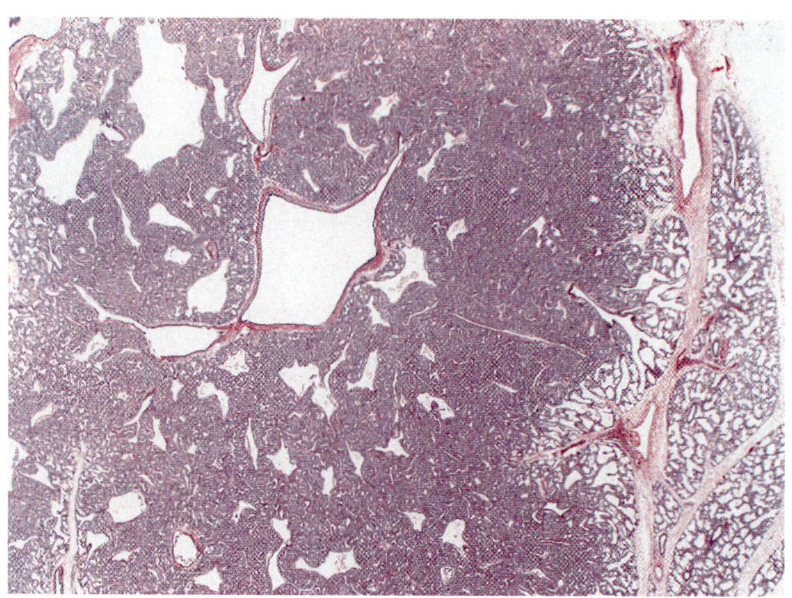

Figure 11-30

CONGENITAL CYSTIC ADENOMATOID MALFORMATION

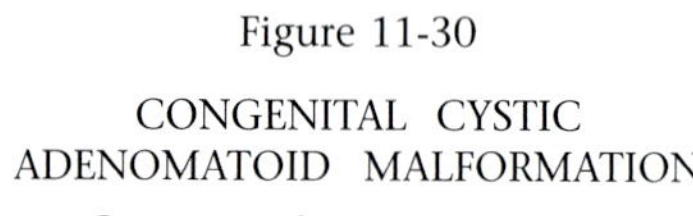

Congenital cystic adenomatoid malformation with variably sized, abnormal, dilated bronchiolar-like structures that merge with adjacent normal lung.

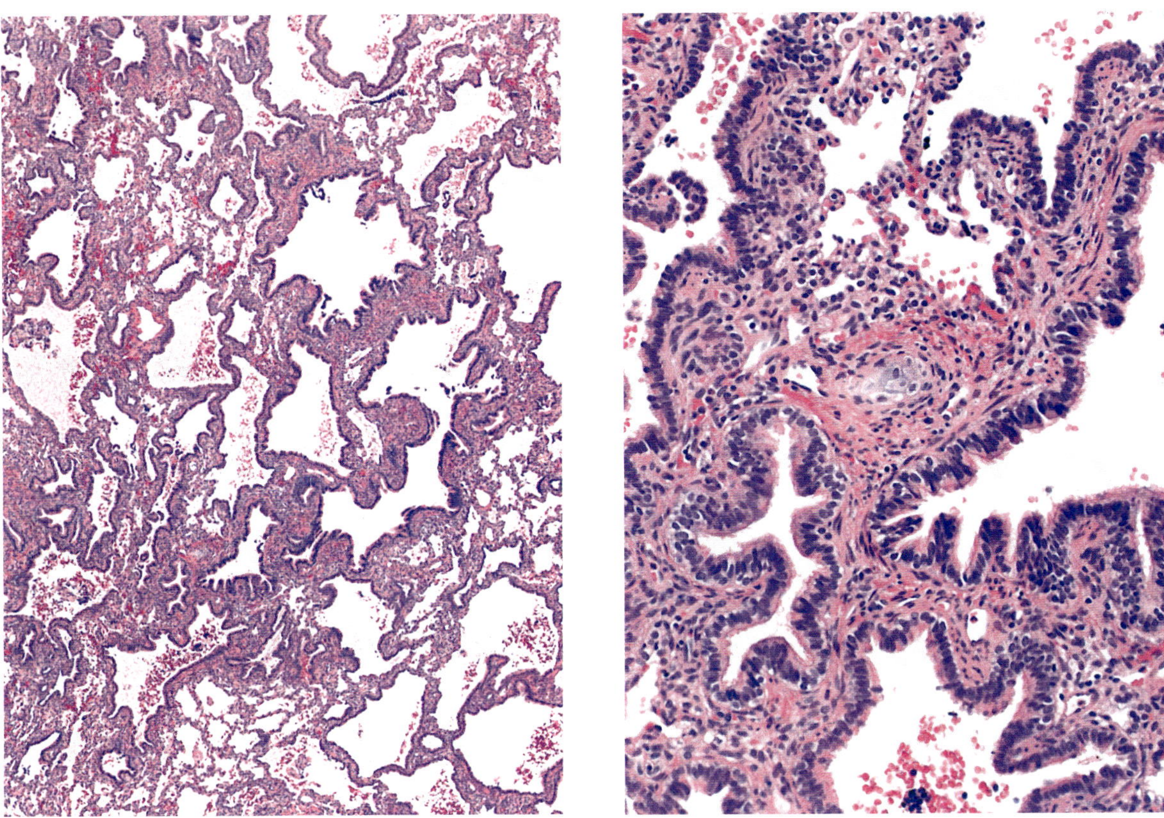

Figure 11-31

CONGENITAL CYSTIC ADENOMATOID MALFORMATION

The bronchiolar-like structures appear remarkably normal, although their shape, dilatation, and crowding together indicate that they are abnormal.

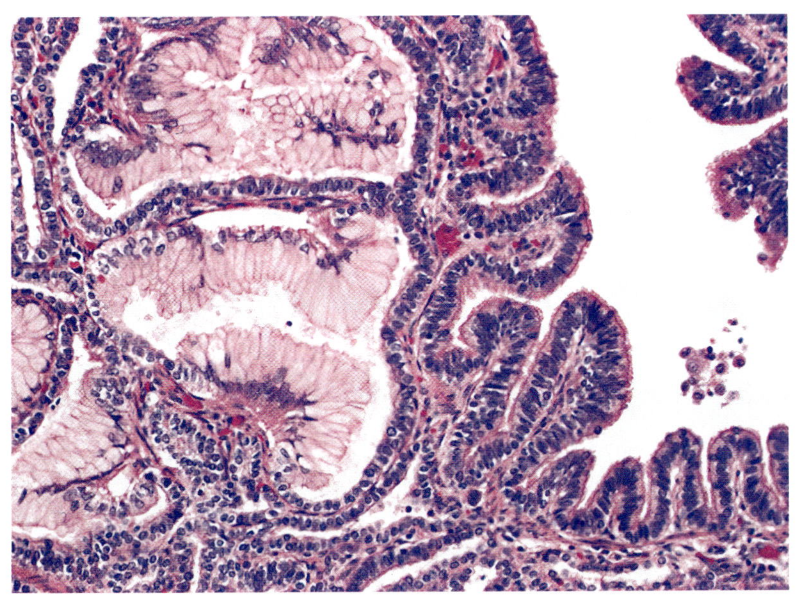

Figure 11-32

CONGENITAL CYSTIC ADENOMATOID MALFORMATION

This case shows well-differentiated mucinous epithelium adjacent to a bronchiolar-like structure (same case as in figure 11-28).

regression of prenatally-detected CCAMs (3,105). The prognosis is favorable with resection. A few patients with (or history of) CCAM have developed carcinomas, particularly mucinous bronchioloalveolar carcinoma (17,151). This has led to the suspicion that the mucinous epithelium in CCAM may be premalignant (151). The number of such cases is small and the association remains to be established.

INFANTILE LOBAR EMPHYSEMA/ POLYALVEOLAR LOBE

Definition and Clinical Features. Infantile lobar emphysema (also known as polyalveolar lobe) results in lobar overinflation with characteristic radiographic and clinical findings (20,50,92,95,109,112,128,154,158). Most patients present in the first 6 months of life with respiratory distress. The condition rarely affects adults (50) and can be thought of as a syndrome that may have a number of causes, primarily, extrinsic or intrinsic obstruction of a bronchus, although in some cases obstruction is not evident (Table 11-9).

Radiologic Findings. Chest radiographs typically demonstrate progressive overinflation and hyperlucency of a lobe, most commonly the left upper lobe, followed by the right middle and right upper lobes (fig. 11-33) (95,109). The overinflated lobe compresses the mediastinal structures, as well as the ipsilateral, and eventually, the contralateral lobes (fig. 11-34). However, infantile lobar emphysema may initially manifest as a homogeneous mass or opacity, which results from retained fetal fluid in the affected lobe. In these cases, clearance of the fluid through the pulmonary lymphatics may result in radiographic progression from parenchymal opacity to increased streaky interstitial opacities in a progressively overinflated lung. Cross-sectional imaging with CT allows visualization of

Table 11-9

CAUSES OF INFANTILE LOBAR EMPHYSEMA[a]

Congenital
Bronchial stenosis
Bronchial atresia
Abnormal origin of bronchus
Tracheal
Eparterial
Obstruction by vascular anomaly
Pulmonary artery sling
Anomalous pulmonary venous return
Obstruction by external mass
Bronchogenic cyst
Pulmonary hyperplasia (polyalveolar lobe)
Acquired
Aspirated meconium
Mucous plug
Granulation tissue
Torsion of bronchus
Bronchial mucosal folds
Respiratory syncytial virus (RSV) infection

[a]Modified from references 128 and 154.

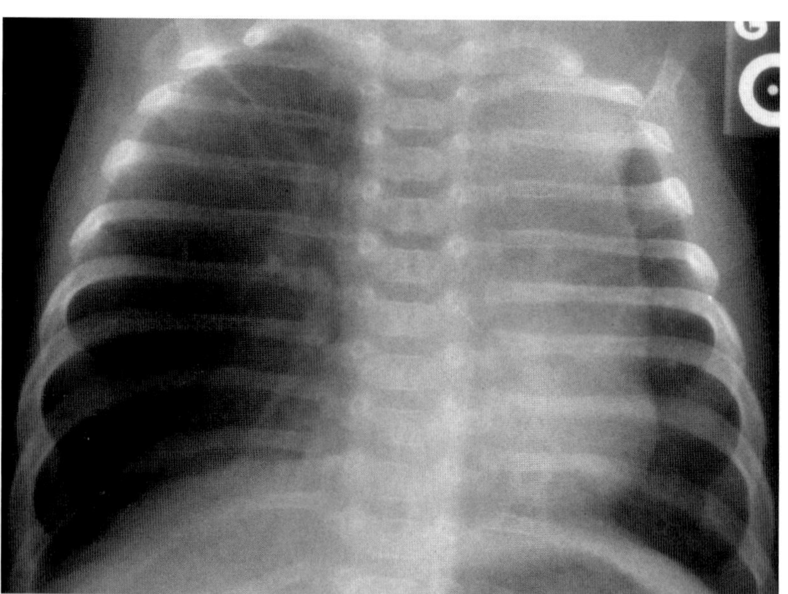

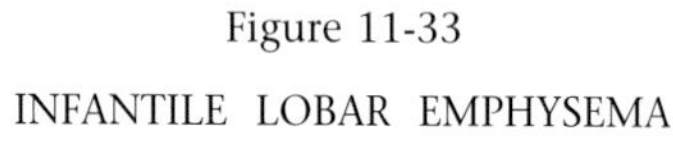

Figure 11-33

INFANTILE LOBAR EMPHYSEMA

Infantile lobar emphysema in a 2-month-old male with recurrent episodes of tachypnea since birth. AP chest radiograph demonstrates overinflation of the right middle lobe with associated atelectasis of the right upper and lower lobes and mass effect on the mediastinum.

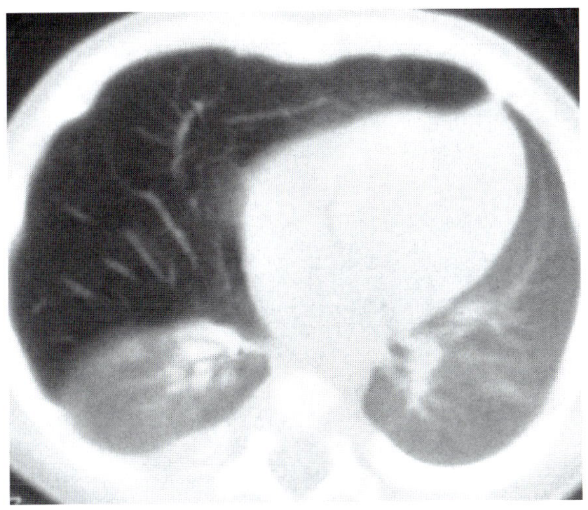

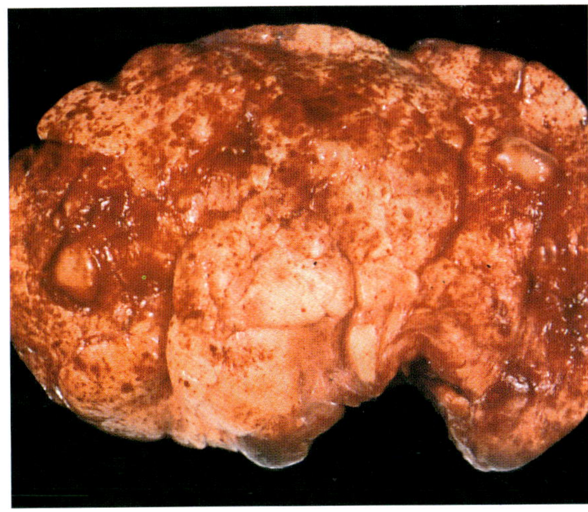

Figure 11-34

INFANTILE LOBAR EMPHYSEMA

Left: Chest CT from the case shown in figure 11-33 demonstrates marked overinflation of the right middle lobe with mass effect on the adjacent lung and mediastinum. The appearance of the right middle lobe lung parenchyma is otherwise normal.

Right: Gross photograph of the resected overinflated right middle lobe demonstrates loss of normal lobar morphology.

the bronchial anatomy and may show the associated lesions, such as anomalous vessels or space-occupying mediastinal masses, responsible for the bronchial obstruction. Ventilation-perfusion pulmonary scintigraphy allows preoperative assessment of lung function. Long-term observation of some patients with infantile lobar emphysema has demonstrated improvement in pulmonary volume and perfusion (95,101).

Pathologic Findings. Grossly and microscopically, the tissue may appear normal for an adult lung. However, for infant lung tissue it is overinflated (figs. 11-34–11-36).

In infantile lobar emphysema, there is an absolute increase in the number of acini/alveoli (fig. 11-37) (92). An alveolar count can be done by radial count or more sophisticated morphometric methods. A radial count is accomplished by making a perpendicular line from the last respiratory bronchiole to the pleura or the closest interlobular septum, and counting the number of alveoli that are transected by that line. Normal fetuses have a radial alveolar count between 2 and 5, normal infants between 5 and 10, and older children between 10 and 12. In infantile lobar emphysema the radial alveolar count is greater, and in one report of a newborn averaged 20 (29).

Treatment and Prognosis. The treatment of infantile lobar emphysema is surgical resection to avoid further respiratory compromise. Some mild cases are managed conservatively, with apparent good results (92).

VASCULAR ANOMALIES

Many of the anomalies already discussed are associated with abnormalities of the pulmonary vascular system. A variety of anomalies originating with the pulmonary arteries are described (106). Pulmonary vascular anomalies are also common with various forms of congenital heart disease.

Vascular Sling Anomaly. Here, the left pulmonary artery arises from the right pulmonary artery, and as it courses between the esophagus and trachea to the left lung, produces a sling around the trachea or main bronchi that may cause obstructive symptoms as a result of compression of these structures (fig. 11-38) (106). Chest radiographs and lateral barium esophagrams demonstrate a soft tissue opacity, which represents the anomalous vessel located between the trachea and the contrast-filled esophagus (68). Cross-sectional imaging with CT or MRI demonstrates the anomalous course of the pulmonary artery and allows assessment of the tracheal lumen to exclude associated congenital

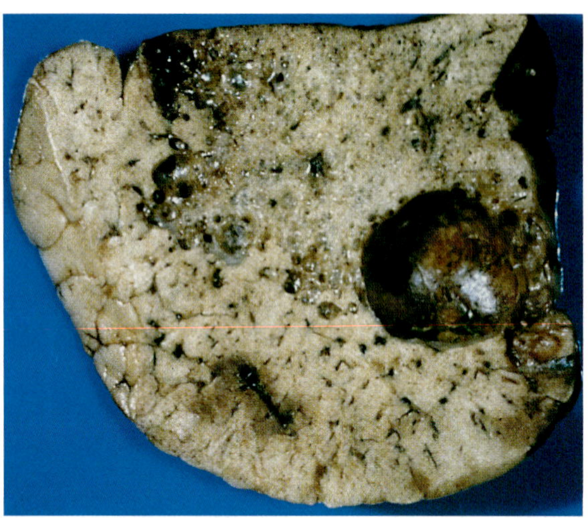

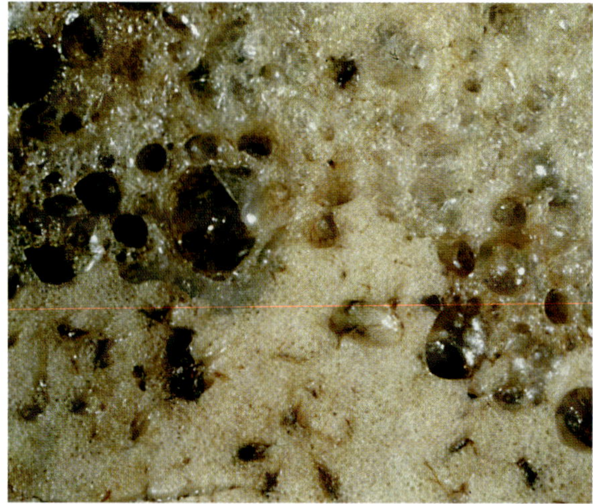

Figure 11-35

INFANTILE LOBAR EMPHYSEMA

Left: This lobectomy specimen measures nearly 8 cm in greatest dimension, which is markedly enlarged for a neonate. Right: Some of the airspaces are markedly dilated.

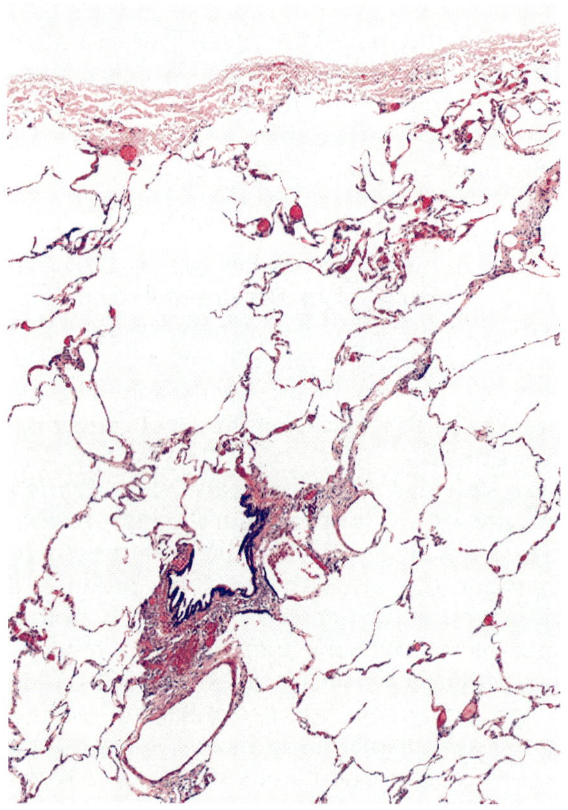

Figure 11-36

INFANTILE LOBAR EMPHYSEMA

There is marked dilatation of the alveoli (far beyond that encountered in normal neonatal lung).

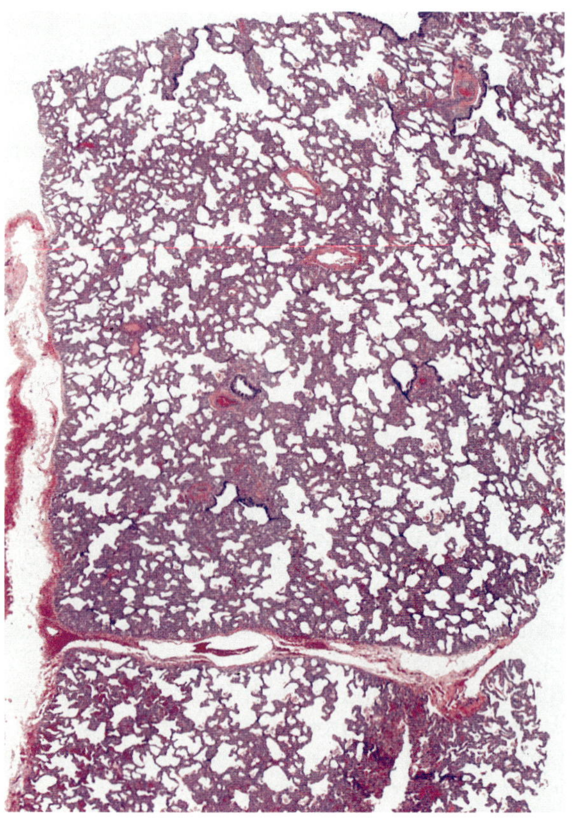

Figure 11-37

INFANTILE LOBAR EMPHYSEMA

This resected lobe is enlarged. The architecture appears nearly normal; however, there is a marked increase in alveoli.

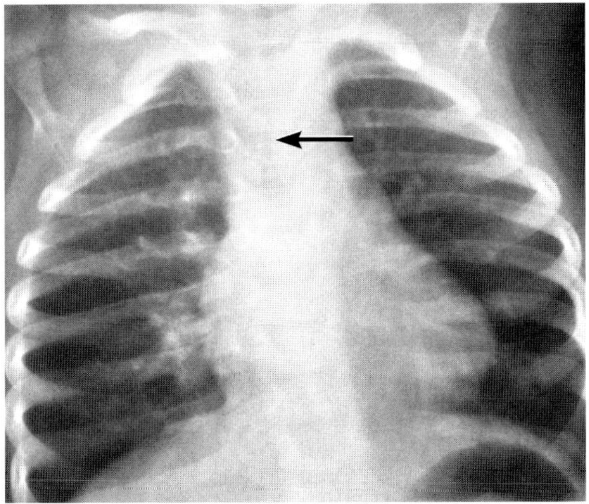

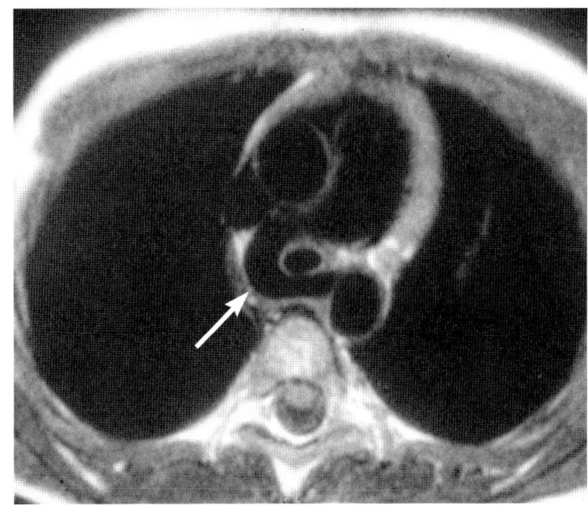

Figure 11-38

PULMONARY ARTERY SLING

Pulmonary artery sling in a 5-year-old male with recurrent respiratory illnesses.

Left: PA chest radiograph demonstrates slightly decreased pulmonary vasculature on the left. Note the poor visualization of the trachea, indicative of tracheal stenosis (arrow).

Right: Axial T1-weighted MRI shows the aberrant left pulmonary artery as it arises from the proximal right pulmonary artery (arrow) and courses behind the trachea to supply the left lung.

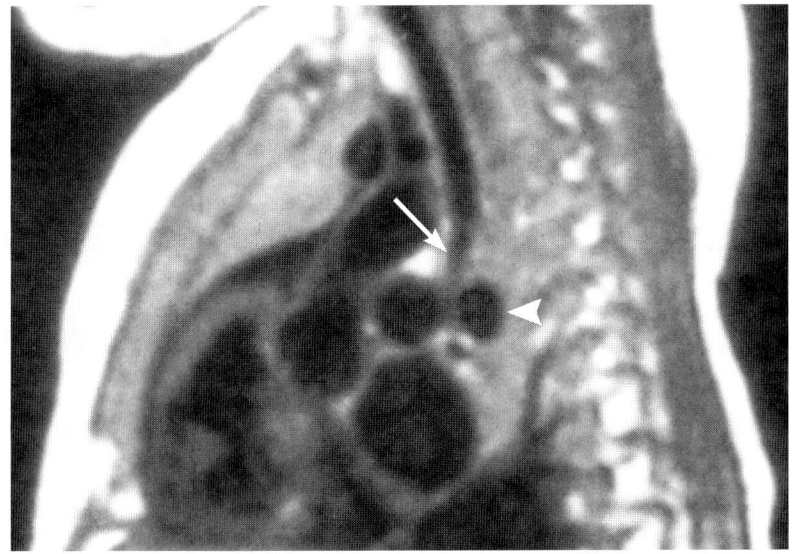

Figure 11-39

PULMONARY ARTERY SLING

Pulmonary artery sling in a 5-month-old male with raspy breathing since birth and recent exacerbation of cough. Sagittal T1-weighted MRI shows the aberrant pulmonary artery (arrowhead) as it courses around and behind the trachea (arrow). Note the resultant tracheal compression.

tracheobronchial stenosis or malacia (fig. 11-39) (68,102).

Arteriovenous Malformations (AVMs). These may be single or multiple, and presentation is generally in older children or adults (106). Cyanosis and heart failure in early childhood are also described. Many affected individuals have Osler-Weber-Rendu syndrome. AVMs are more frequently located in the lower lobe. Chest radiographs usually demonstrate one or more pulmonary nodules or masses (fig. 11-40). Less frequently, there is a parenchymal opacity that mimics a consolidation and represents a tangle of dilated vessels (57,68). Radiologic identification of a feeding artery and a draining vein is virtually pathognomonic for the diagnosis and can be easily confirmed with cross-sectional imaging with CT or MRI (57,68).

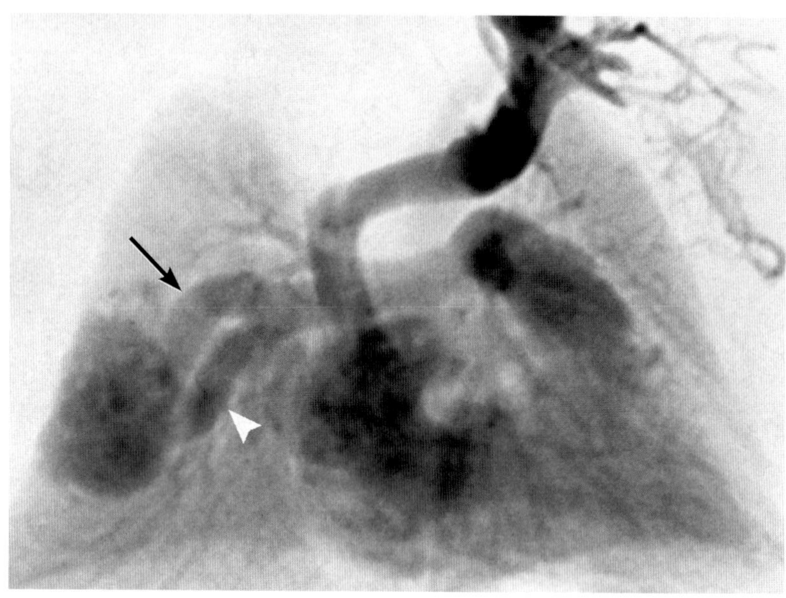

Figure 11-40

PULMONARY ARTERIOVENOUS FISTULA

Pulmonary arteriovenous fistula in a 1-month-old female who developed seizures shortly after birth. Digital subtraction angiography through a left internal jugular venous catheter demonstrates a large arteriovenous malformation, with one large feeding artery (arrow) and a large early draining vein (arrowhead).

Table 11-10

CAUSES OF PERSISTENT PULMONARY HYPERTENSION IN THE NEWBORN[a]

Failure of postnatal decrease in pulmonary vascular resistance; normal prenatal development
Increased blood viscosity
Large ventricular septal defect
Hypoxia
Excessive prenatal muscularization of the distal pulmonary vasculature
Idiopathic
Associated with meconium aspiration
Associated with ductus-dependent systemic blood flow; some congenital cardiac defects
Developmental deficit in cross-sectional area of pulmonary vascular bed
Pulmonary hypoplasia
Congenital diaphragmatic hernia (unilateral hypoplasia)
Misalignment of pulmonary veins with alveolar capillary dysplasia

[a]Modified from reference 106.

Contrast-enhanced chest CT is also diagnostic, as it demonstrates intense (vascular) enhancement of the abnormal vessels. Pulmonary arteriography of both lungs plays a dual role in the evaluation and management of patients with AVMs (fig. 11-40). First, it allows identification of additional and sometimes previously unsuspected lesions in patients with multiple lesions or Osler-Weber-Rendu syndrome. Second, it allows effective conservative therapy with coil embolization. Recurrent AVMs can be repeatedly treated with this method.

Grossly, AVMs show abnormal dilated vessels of varying sizes (figs. 11-41, 11-42). Secondary thrombosis may be present. In some cases the effects of prior embolization therapy may be apparent. Histologically, there is a tangle of abnormal vessels of varying sizes (figs. 11-43, 11-44).

Pulmonary Hypertension. Pulmonary hypertension may be found in patients with Down's syndrome due to hypoplasia and decreased numbers of acinar units. The reduction in the pulmonary capillary bed is a result of lung hypoplasia (40,45).

Persistent Pulmonary Hypertension. Also known as *persistent fetal circulation,* this is a syndrome with a variety of causes, as shown in Table 11-10. Microscopically, persistent pulmonary hypertension of the newborn is associated with muscularization of the small pulmonary arteries, with abnormal extension of vascular smooth muscle into the small intra-acinar arteries (fig. 11-45) (106). There is often an increase in the connective tissue sheaths of these vessels.

One of the more intriguing causes of persistent pulmonary hypertension of the newborn is misalignment of pulmonary veins with alveolar capillary dysplasia (fig. 11-46) (106). This peculiar anomaly is a combined pulmonary vascular and parenchymal abnormality; patients fail to respond to therapeutic measures

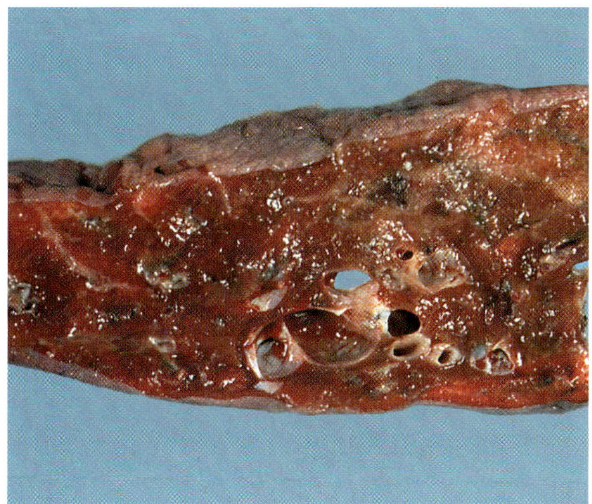

Figure 11-41

ARTERIOVENOUS MALFORMATION

Fresh lobectomy specimen illustrates marked vascular dilatation.

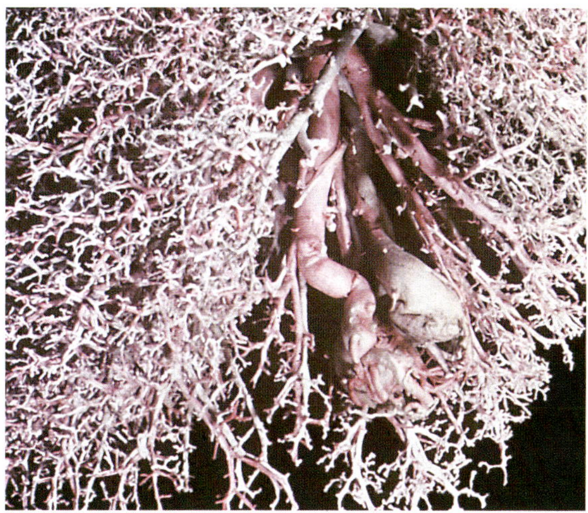

Figure 11-42

ARTERIOVENOUS MALFORMATION

This vascular cast illustrates the markedly enlarged arterial (red) and venous (blue) vessels.

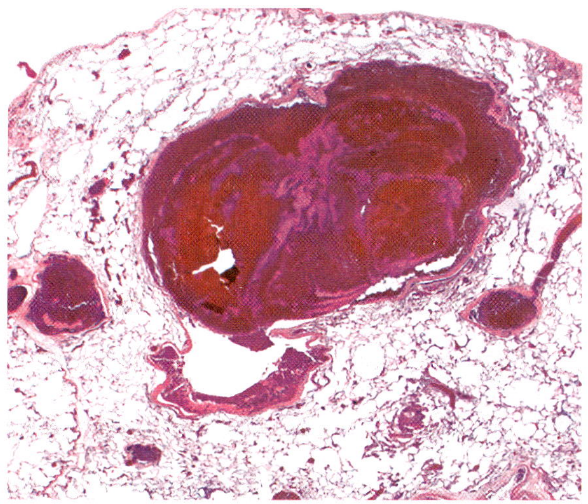

Figure 11-43

ARTERIOVENOUS MALFORMATION

The histologic specimen from figure 11-41 shows a markedly dilated vessel containing a recent blood clot.

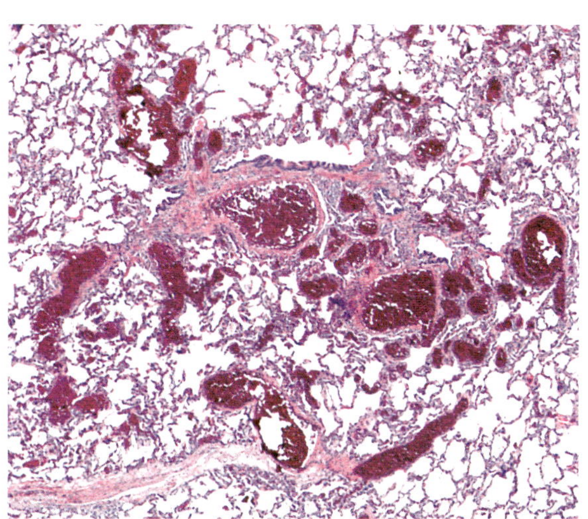

Figure 11-44

ARTERIOVENOUS MALFORMATION

This case of Osler-Weber-Rendu syndrome shows a tangle of abnormal vessels around a bronchovascular bundle.

and usually die a few days or weeks after birth. Histologically, the pulmonary veins run adjacent to pulmonary arteries; there is marked medial hypertrophy and hyperplasia of the pulmonary arterial branches, with extension of arterial smooth muscle into small arterioles; and there is abnormal development of alveolar capillaries and pulmonary acini.

Abnormalities of the Pulmonary Lymphatics. Such anomalies can produce a variety of clinicopathologic syndromes, as shown in Table 11-11. Most of these are rare, although lymphangiectasia and lymphangiomatosis deserve mention.

Diffuse pulmonary lymphangiectasia is a rare condition that is usually fatal (30,80,83,92,104,

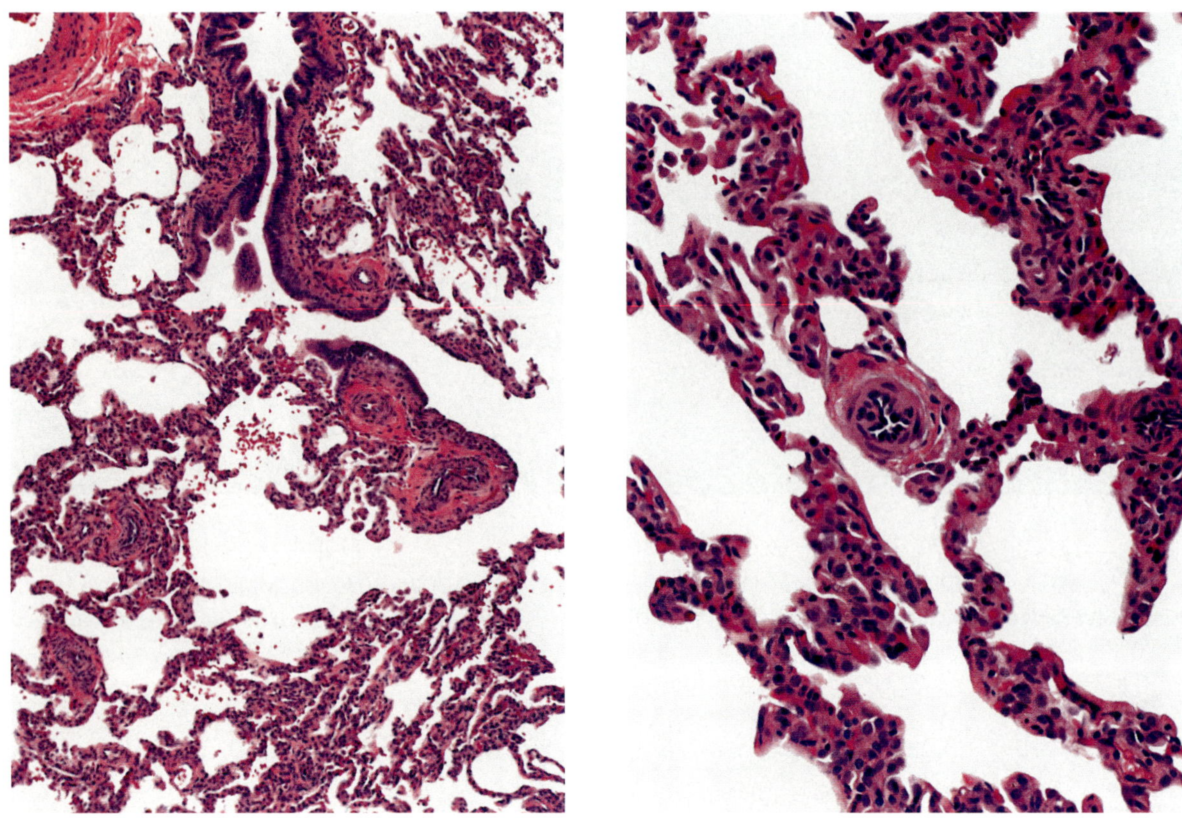

Figure 11-45

PERSISTENT PULMONARY HYPERTENSION

The muscularis of the pulmonary artery is obviously increased (left) and muscularized arterioles are present in the distal alveolar parenchyma (right, center).

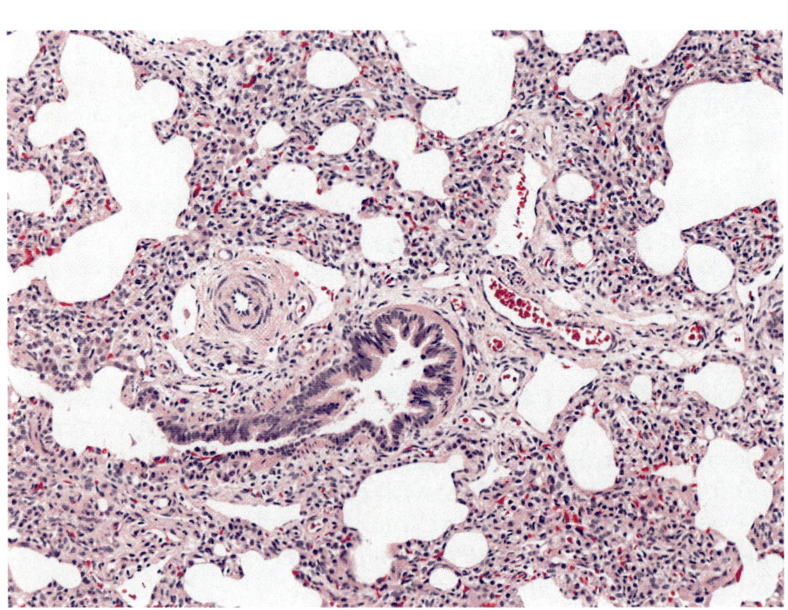

Figure 11-46

PERSISTENT PULMONARY HYPERTENSION

Persistent pulmonary hypertension associated with alveolar capillary dysplasia. A bronchovascular bundle includes a muscularized pulmonary artery (left), a bronchiole (center), and a dilated venous structure (right).

Table 11-11

ABNORMALITIES OF THE PULMONARY LYMPHATIC SYSTEM[a]

Lymphangioma
  Capillary
  Cavernous
  Cystic
	Secondary: due to obstruction or pulmonary venous hypertension

Lymphangiomatosis
  Diffuse pulmonary; may be multifocal in the thorax
  Generalized, with multiorgan involvement including bone
	Lymphatic dysplasia syndrome
	  Primary lymphedema
	  Idiopathic effusions (including pleural)
	  Yellow nail syndrome
	  Congenital chylothorax

Lymphangiectasia
  Primary (congenital)
    Thoracic either limited to the lungs or with lung and mediastinal involvement
    Generalized with intestinal involvement
	Lymphatic injury
	
	Combinations of lymphatic and other tissue
	  Mixed lymphatic and angiomatous lesions
	  Lymphangiomyoma (localized)
	  Lymphangioleiomyomatosis

[a]Modified from references 30, 67, 106, and 165.

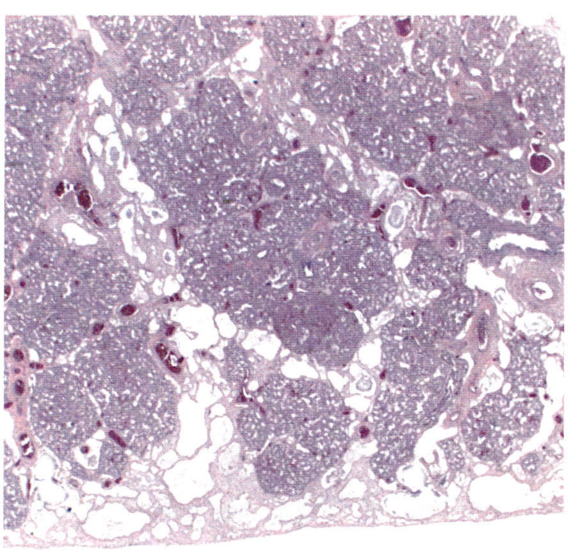

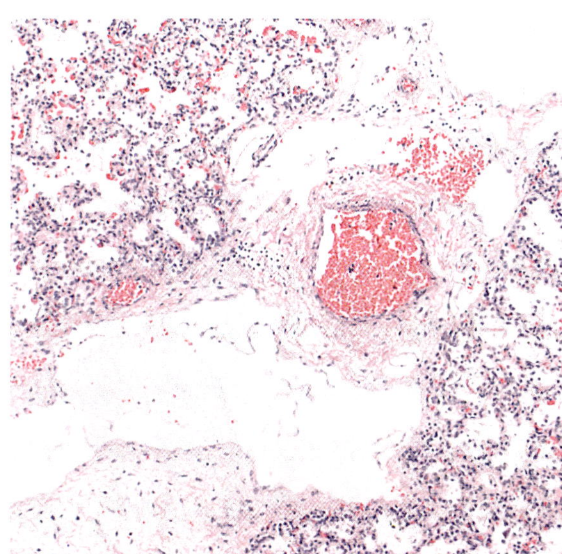

Figure 11-47

DIFFUSE PULMONARY LYMPHANGIECTASIA

There is marked dilatation of the lymphatics in the interlobular septa.

106,112,125,154,158); only occasional patients survive past infancy (80). There is diffuse dilatation of the pulmonary lymphatics (fig. 11-47). This condition is one of dilatation of the normal lymphatics in contrast to lymphangiomatosis in which there is an increased number of anastomosing lymphatic spaces (see below). Diffuse pulmonary lymphangiectasia may be primary, secondary to associated cardiovascular anomalies, or associated with generalized lymphangiectasia. Diffuse pulmonary lymphangiectasia is often confused with interstitial emphysema, since the interstitial air-filled spaces in the latter condition may be misinterpreted as dilated lymphatics. Chest radiographs demonstrate the distended pulmonary lymphatics

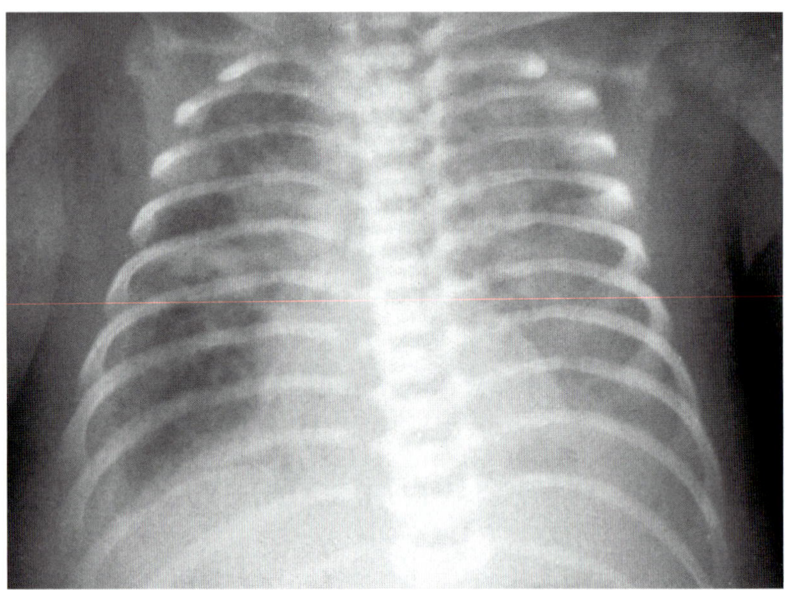

Figure 11-48

GENERALIZED LYMPHANGIECTASIA

Generalized lymphangiectasia in a 1-month-old male with peripheral edema and respiratory distress. AP chest radiograph demonstrates diffusely increased interstitial markings as well as bilateral pleural effusions. (Figures 11-48 and 11-49 are from the same patient.)

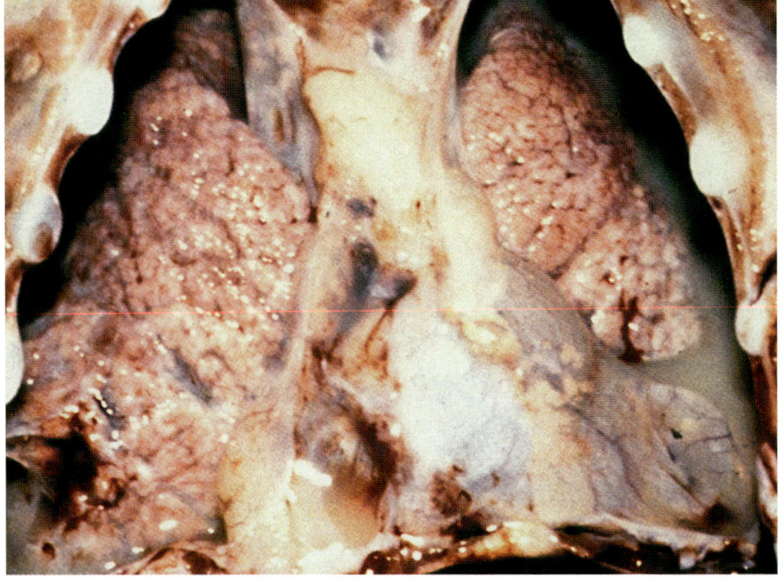

Figure 11-49

GENERALIZED LYMPHANGIECTASIA

Postmortem photograph of the lungs demonstrates bilateral chylous pleural effusions and a cobblestone appearance of the surface of the lung parenchyma.

as diffuse, bilateral, reticular interstitial opacities (fig. 11-48) (102). Kerley-B lines (thickened interlobular septa) and (chylous) pleural effusions may also be seen (fig. 11-49) (102). In cases of generalized lymphangiectasia, associated (chylous) ascites can be demonstrated in cross-sectional imaging of the abdomen. Rarely, lymphangiectasia is a relatively localized process and obstructions at the lobar level should be sought.

Diffuse pulmonary lymphangiomatosis is a rare condition in which the lymphatic routes of the lung (pleura, septa, and bronchovascular bundles) are expanded by an abnormal number of anastomosing lymphatic spaces, sometimes with concomitant fascicles of smooth muscle (67,163,165). Males and females are equally affected, and most patients present in childhood or early adulthood with respiratory distress or dyspnea. Hemoptysis is frequent, probably owing to lymphangiomatous involvement of the airway submucosa, with concomitant friability and bleeding. Chest radiographs demonstrate increased interstitial markings and (chylous) pleural and/or pericardial effusions, sometimes involving the chest wall in the form of multifocal cystic rib lesions (75). Lymphangiomatous involvement of the

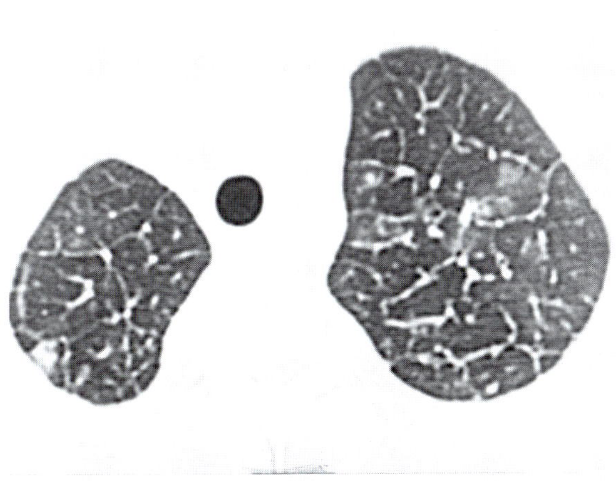

Figure 11-50

DIFFUSE PULMONARY LYMPHANGIOMATOSIS

CT scan highlights the septal and peribronchovascular thickening.

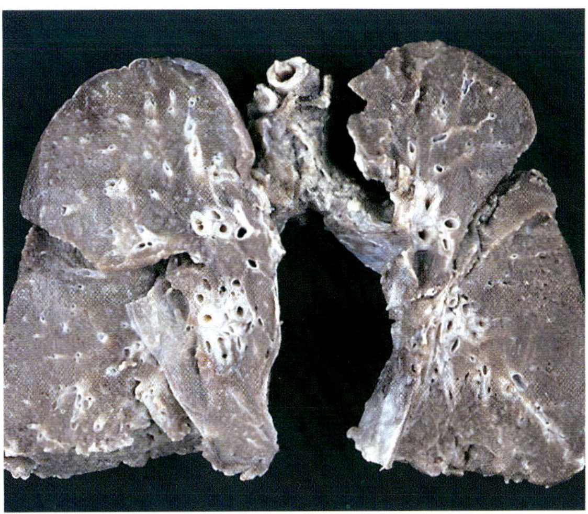

Figure 11-51

DIFFUSE PULMONARY LYMPHANGIOMATOSIS

Autopsy shows increase in lymphatic tissue around the bronchovascular bundles.

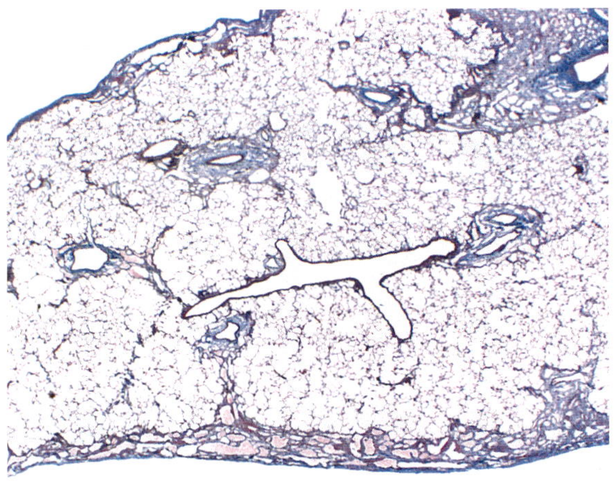

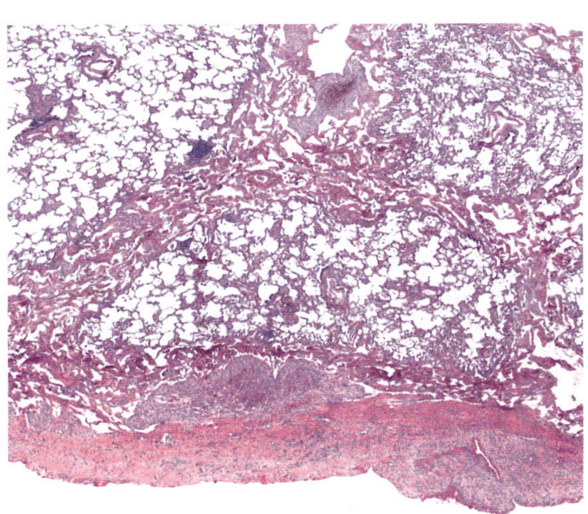

Figure 11-52

DIFFUSE PULMONARY LYMPHANGIOMATOSIS

There is anastomosing lymphatic spaces in the pleura and around bronchovascular bundles (left), associated with prominent septal widening in a second case (right), which also shows a pleural reaction consistent with chronic pleural effusion.

mediastinum or more generalized lymphangiomatosis may be evident with radiologic studies (164) or at the time of surgery. Lymphangiography followed by CT confirms contrast accumulation in affected areas and allows visualization of the extent of involvement. CT scanning also highlights septal and bronchovascular involvement (fig. 11-50).

The condition is progressive, although the rate of progression varies in individual patients. Anecdotal data suggest interferon therapy may be beneficial. Palliative measures to alleviate pleural effusions may be helpful. The gross and histologic findings reflect the proliferation of anastomosing lymphatic structures along lymphatic routes of the lung (figs. 11-51–11-54).

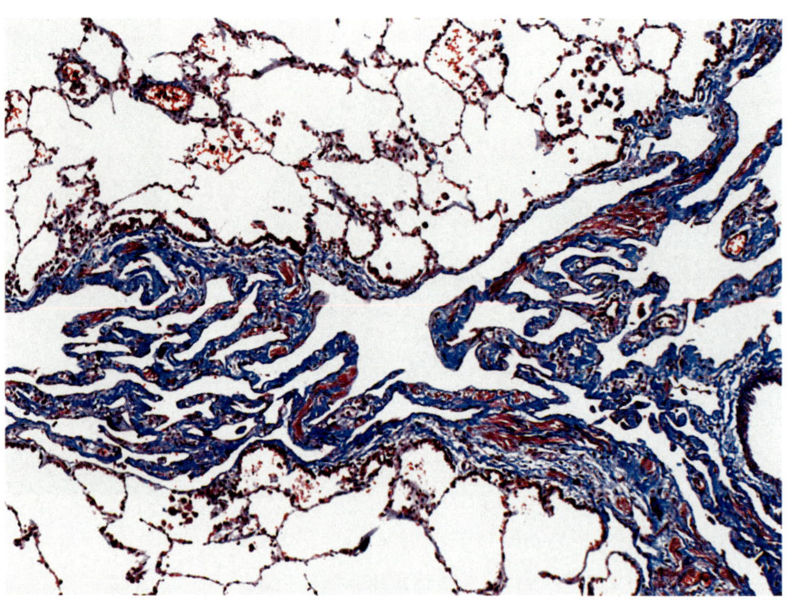

Figure 11-53

DIFFUSE PULMONARY LYMPHANGIOMATOSIS

Trichrome stain highlights the septal widening by anastomosing lymphatic spaces.

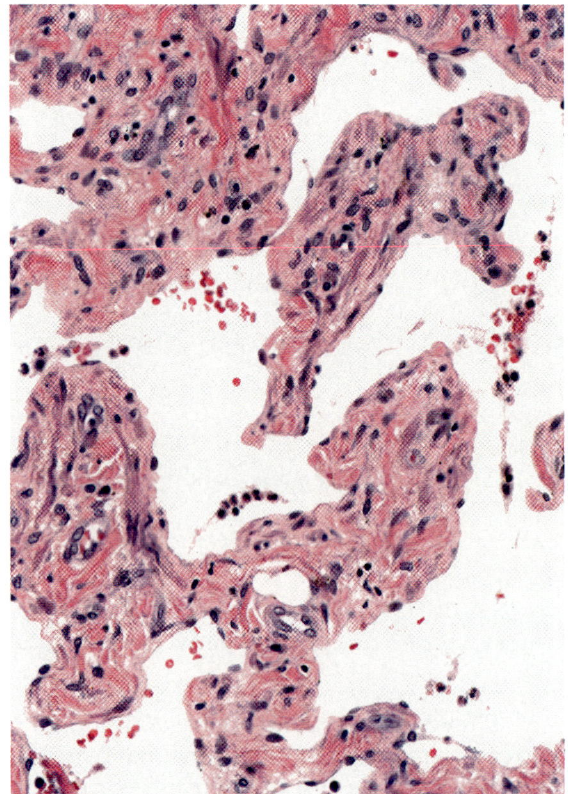

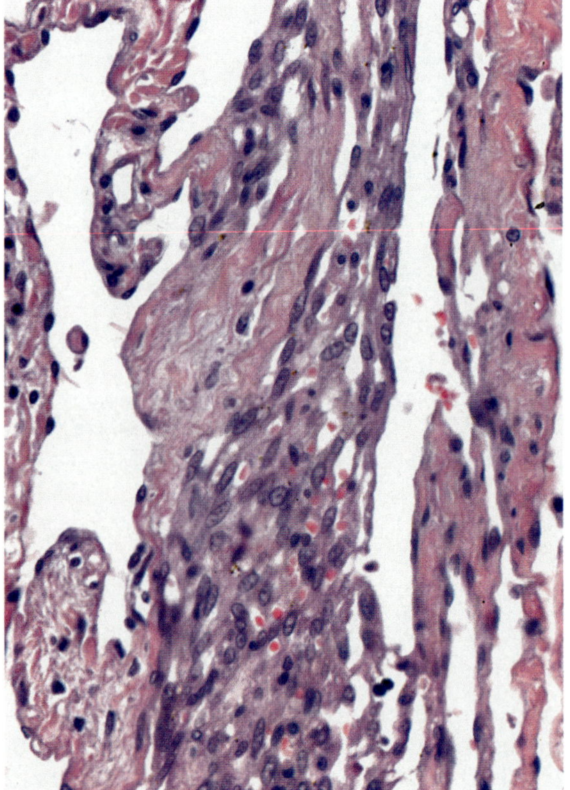

Figure 11-54

DIFFUSE PULMONARY LYMPHANGIOMATOSIS

Left: The lymphatic spaces have a thin endothelial lining and prominent collagenous stroma.
Right: Some cases have fascicles of spindle cells, which stain as smooth muscle cells and are HMB45 negative.

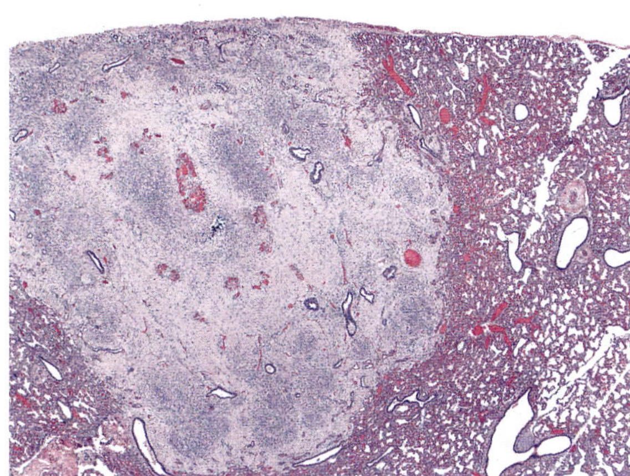

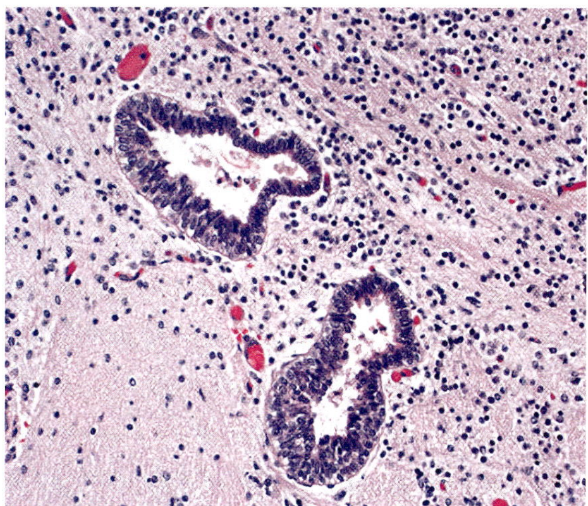

Figure 11-55

GLIAL ECTOPIA IN THE LUNG

There is a nodule of pale glial tissue (left) in which airspaces lined by metaplastic cells are surrounded by typical neuropil (right).

ECTOPIC TISSUES IN THE LUNG

Tissue ectopias in the lung are rare (8,15, 24,28,37,38,40,48,82,94,96,104,118,169). Thyroid tissue has been reported in the trachea (104) and lungs (15). Pancreatic tissue (48,94), neuroglial tissue (fig. 11-55) (28,38,96), liver tissue (118), and adrenocortical tissue (8,24) have been described in the lung, usually in infants. We have seen cardiac muscle in the walls of the pulmonary artery in the hilus of the lung. Skeletal muscle is also seen in the lung, sometimes associated with other anomalies or neoplasms (37, 40,169). Endometriosis occurs in the lung and pleura (82), but whether that should be considered a congenital or acquired tissue ectopia is a matter of controversy. Pleural endometriosis may manifest radiologically as recurrent hemothorax or pneumothorax, usually having a temporal relationship to the menstrual cycle. Endometriosis is not found in all cases of catamenial pneumothorax. The few reports of the radiologic appearance of parenchymal endometriosis describe solitary lung nodules or cysts, which may change in size with the onset of menses (69).

RESPIRATORY DISTRESS SYNDROME OF THE NEWBORN

Definition. The presence of hyaline membranes is the most common histologic finding in premature infants with severe idiopathic respiratory distress syndrome (RDS), for which the term *hyaline membrane disease (HMD)* is classically used (98,106,108,110,135,136,157). Full-term infants may also be affected (63).

Untreated RDS is rarely seen today since most affected infants receive assisted ventilation, oxygen, and surfactant therapy, and either recover or develop bronchopulmonary dysplasia described below. RDS is clinically separated from transient tachypnea of the newborn, the pathology of which is not well described.

Approximately 1 percent of infants born worldwide are affected by RDS (110). RDS and its complications account for about 30 percent of all neonatal deaths; the incidence is inversely proportional to gestational age and birth weight. RDS affects 60 to 80 percent of infants less than 28 weeks of gestational age, 15 to 30 percent of those between 32 to 36 weeks, and 5 percent of infants over 37 weeks. RDS is rare in term and postmature infants (98).

Risk factors for RDS include prematurity, white race, male sex, maternal diabetes, birth by caesarean section, multiple gestation, precipitous delivery, asphyxia, cold stress, and a maternal history of prior affected infants (98,106,110,157).

Clinical Features. In classic RDS, symptoms develop at birth or a few hours thereafter:

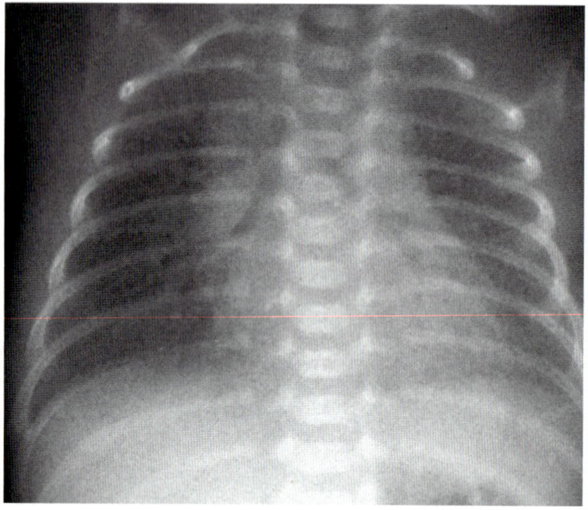

Figure 11-56

RESPIRATORY DISTRESS SYNDROME

AP chest rdiograph in a premature newborn with RDS demonstrates diffuse, bilateral, granular parenchymal opacities. Note the air-filled central bronchi (air bronchograms) made more conspicuous by the parenchymal opacity. The lung volumes are normal. (Courtesy of Lt. Col. Gael J. Lonergan, USAF, MC, Uniformed Services University, Bethesda, MD.)

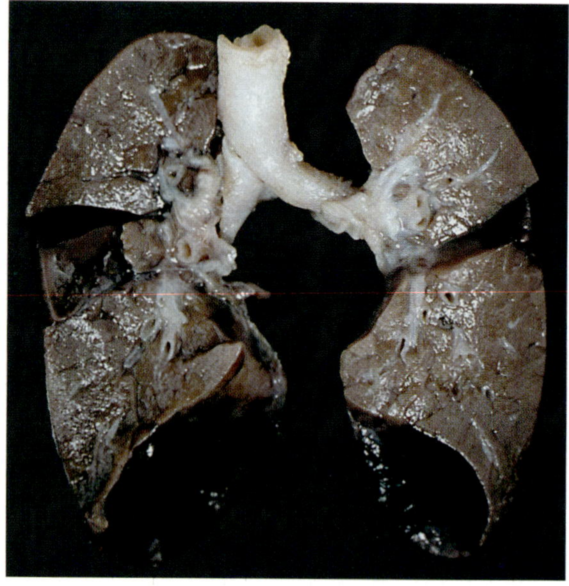

Figure 11-57

RESPIRATORY DISTRESS SYNDROME

The lungs appear firm, rigid, and airless.

tachypnea, flaring of the nostrils, expiratory grunting, intercostal and subcostal retractions, and cyanosis (98,110). These are usually associated with signs of prematurity including low birth weight, reduced muscle tone, thin translucent skin, fine downy hair, smooth soles, small nipples, and immature genitalia. In milder cases, symptoms usually peak at 2 to 3 days of age followed by gradual improvement, and these infants may be on room air by the first week of life (98,110). Infants with more severe involvement may develop bronchopulmonary dysplasia or may die from their disease; death usually occurs between days 2 and 7. The natural history of RDS is rarely observed today because of therapeutic intervention (see Bronchopulmonary Dysplasia).

Radiologic Findings. The typical radiographic finding in infants with RDS is diffuse, bilateral, "granular" opacities throughout the lungs with overimposed "air-filled bronchi" or air bronchograms (fig. 11-56) (102). The granular opacities represent the atelectatic terminal airspaces and retained fetal fluid. The generalized opacity of the lung allows visualization of nonatelectatic areas of air exchange. In addition, the granular appearance may be enhanced by associated early pulmonary interstitial emphysema. Neonatal thoracic ultrasonography in patients with RDS allows demonstration of the collapsed fluid-filled lung, with interspersed bright echoes that represent air-filled airways. The "classic" radiographic appearance of RDS may not be seen in patients who are treated promptly by continuous positive airway pressure (CPAP) or other methods of respiratory assistance. In addition, prophylactic therapy with exogenous surfactant may also alter the radiographic appearance and may produce patchy airspace opacities that result from uneven aeration due to uneven surfactant distribution.

Gross Findings. The lungs are firm, solid, red, and congested, and sink in water (figs. 11-57, 11-58) (108,157). On cut section, they are relatively airless with marked atelectasis, and they have been likened to liver tissue. These gross features are due both to atelectasis and increased lung water that has been documented gravimetrically (54) and ultrastructurally in flash frozen tissue (87).

Histologic Findings. Since most affected infants are premature, the immaturity of the lung tissue is apparent, generally correlating with the gestational age (106,108,157). There is atelectasis of distal airspaces (alveoli) and overdistension of proximal airspaces, primarily respiratory bronchioles that are lined by hyaline membranes (fig. 11-59). Hyaline membranes consist of cellular debris, fibrin, amniotic fluid, and transudate fluid.

Hyaline membranes may make their appearance within 3 to 4 hours after the development of symptoms and are most prominent at approximately 12 hours. The surrounding lung tissue shows congestion, hemorrhage, epithelial desquamation, and lymphatic dilatation. Organization with both airspace and interstitial fibroblastic proliferation may be seen as early as 36 to 38 hours after birth.

Pathogenesis. RDS of the infant is caused by two mechanisms: inadequate amounts of surfactant due to immaturity or insults to the lung that decrease surfactant production, and inadequate resorption of lung liquid at birth (98,

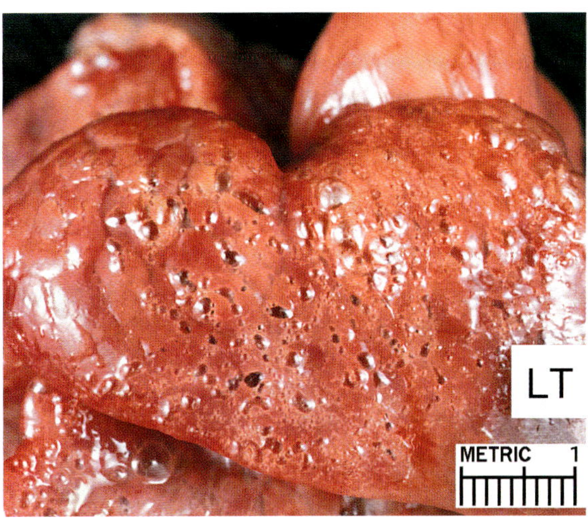

Figure 11-58

RESPIRATORY DISTRESS SYNDROME

Cut section of unfixed lung tissue shows dilated airspaces representing alveolar ducts with surrounding atelectatic and congested lung tissue.

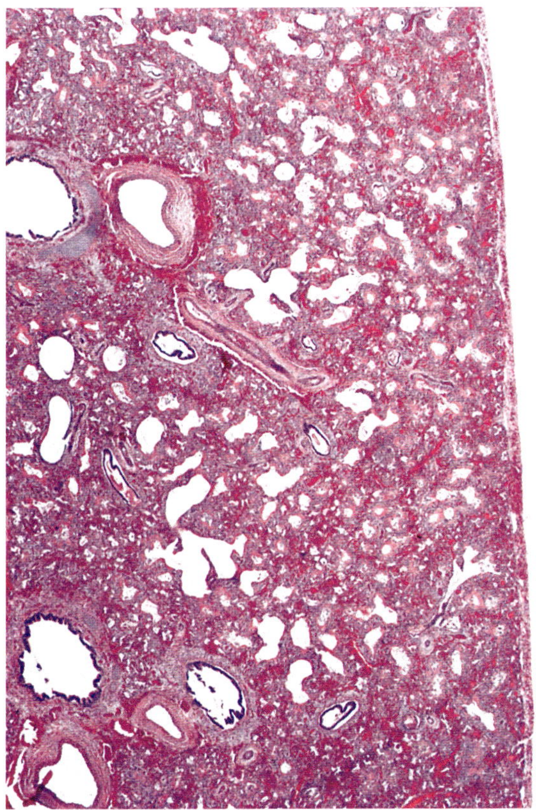

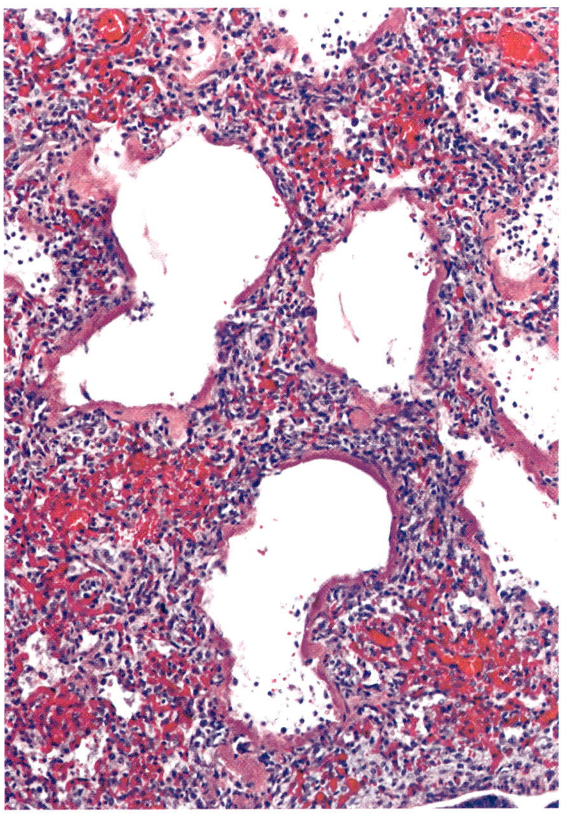

Figure 11-59

RESPIRATORY DISTRESS SYNDROME

The lung tissue is congested and atelectatic with dilated alveolar ducts (left), lined by hyaline membranes (right).

106,110,135,137,157). The consequence of decreased surfactant is inadequate maintenance of surface tension, followed by atelectasis and uneven inflation of the lung tissue, resulting in abnormal ventilation and perfusion. Inadequate resorption of lung water leads to a situation analogous to pulmonary edema in the adult, with consequent respiratory distress (136).

Differential Diagnosis. RDS of the premature infant is similar to diffuse alveolar damage in the adult lung, although superimposed on a lung still undergoing growth and development. It is a reaction pattern with a number of causes. Infections, including those caused by a number of viral and bacterial agents, may produce hyaline membranes, and cultures and special stains may be appropriate. In term and post-term infants with RDS, in addition to infections, aspiration (including meconium aspiration) and associated perinatal complications (such as pre-eclampsia, abruptio placenta, placenta previa, fetomaternal hemorrhage, and abnormalities of the cord) should be carefully sought (63,150).

Prevention, Treatment, and Prognosis. The best prevention of RDS is avoidance of premature labor and delivery. A number of tests of amniotic fluid are available to assess the lung maturity and these have recently been reviewed by Dubin (56). They include the lecithin/sphingomyelin (L/S) ratio, measurement of phosphatidylglycerol levels, and shaking an aliquot of lung fluid and observing the stability of the bubbles (110). An L/S ratio of less than 1 implies a nearly 100 percent risk of RDS, whereas a value greater than 2 is associated with a less than 1 percent risk of RDS. If the phosphatidylglycerol level is more than 1 percent of the total phospholipids, the risk of RDS is less than 1 percent. In the microbubble test, the finding of fewer than five stable bubbles carries a risk of RDS greater than 95 percent.

Antenatal betamethasone therapy is effective in helping to prevent RDS. Additional treatment measures include oxygen therapy, mechanical ventilation, maintenance of thermoneutrality, monitoring of vital signs, fluid and electrolyte management, minimization of stimulation, antibiotic therapy, blood pressure support, correction of metabolic acidosis, continuous positive pressure airway therapy, closure of patent ductus arteriosus (if open), and most importantly, exogenous surfactant therapy (157). Since the advent of exogenous surfactant therapy, the incidence and severity of RDS has been reduced (157). The use of either modified natural surfactant or synthetic surfactant in the treatment of RDS leads to significant improvements in gas exchange and a reduction in air leak complications (100). Some decrease in subsequent bronchopulmonary dysplasia, and improvement in mortality and survival without bronchopulmonary dysplasia have also been noted (100). These findings reflect the use of "rescue therapy" in infants with RDS. Prophylaxis in infants at high risk for RDS (less than 30 weeks' gestation) results in a significant decrease in the incidence of RDS (64 percent versus 36 percent in one study [100]), improvement in ventilatory index and oxygenation, and significantly fewer air leaks (100). There is also improved survival without the development of bronchopulmonary dysplasia (100).

Transient Tachypnea of the Newborn. Also known as *retained fetal lung fluid,* this is a mild self-limited form of respiratory distress seen in newborn infants (11,76,98,106,110). It is seen in normal term or preterm infants following vaginal delivery or caesarean section. Clinical features of transient tachypnea of the newborn resemble those of RDS syndrome but are milder (11,76,98,110). There is early onset of tachypnea after birth. Some affected patients also develop chest retractions, expiratory grunting, and cyanosis. The symptoms tend to be relieved by relatively low dose oxygen therapy and most affected infants recover in 1 to 3 days. The pathologic findings are not well-characterized.

In transient tachypnea of the newborn there tends to be relatively sudden recovery and an absence of the characteristic radiologic findings of RDS (98,110). It is thought to result from persistence of fluid within airspaces, leading to decreased compliance, decreased tidal volume, and increased dead space (110). Immaturity of the lung is probably also a factor (76). Radiographically, there is normal lung volume, small pleural effusions (which may result in thickening of the horizontal fissure), and increased interstitial markings (fig. 11-60) (109). However, these findings may also be seen in neonatal pneumonia and heart failure secondary to

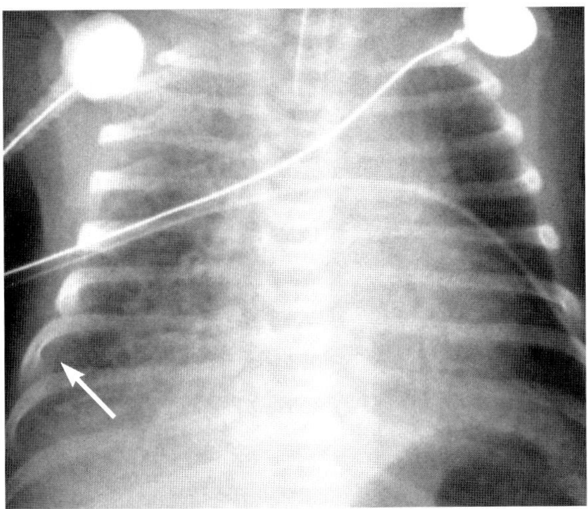

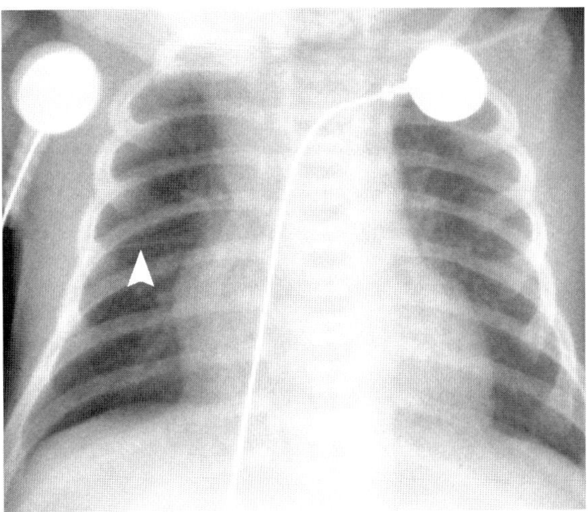

Figure 11-60

TRANSIENT TACHYPNEA OF THE NEWBORN

Left: AP chest radiograph of a term newborn in respiratory distress at 6 hours of age demonstrates coarse reticular opacities throughout the lungs, worse on the right, and a right pleural effusion (arrow). An endotracheal tube is appropriately positioned.

Right: AP chest radiograph of the same infant at 36 hours of age shows marked interval improvement and near resolution of the pleural effusion. The minor fissure (arrowhead) remains visible because of residual pleural fluid. (Courtesy of Lt. Col. Gael J. Lonergan, USAF, MC, Uniformed Services University, Bethesda, MD.)

congenital heart disease. Thus, the diagnosis of transient tachypnea of the newborn is one of exclusion. The rapid resolution of pulmonary abnormalities (within 1 to 2 days) confirms the diagnosis since neonatal pneumonia does not usually resolve this quickly.

BRONCHOPULMONARY DYSPLASIA

Definition. Bronchopulmonary dysplasia (BPD) is a syndrome of injury and repair of the immature lung, and the result of therapeutic interventions, primarily mechanical ventilation and high levels of inspired oxygen, superimposed on the primary disease process, which in most cases is RDS in the premature infant (1,6,7,23,61, 86,98,99,106,110,130,134,145,146,155,157,179). Clinical, radiologic, and pathologic features of BPD are recognizable in infants between 1 and 4 weeks of age, but the diagnosis is often deferred until 28 days of age or 36 weeks postconception and is based on characteristic radiologic abnormalities and persistent oxygen requirements (1).

BPD shows a natural history from acute to chronic pulmonary disease, with characteristic clinical (hypoxemia requiring oxygen therapy in the 28-day-old infant) and radiologic findings. While most cases of BPD follow RDS, some follow other forms of lung injury. BPD has also been described in term infants with RDS and rarely in adults (7). In adults, it is probably best considered as the late stage of diffuse alveolar damage with interstitial fibrosis and honeycomb change. Risk factors for BPD include prematurity, prolonged oxygen therapy, positive pressure ventilation, infection, patent ductus arteriosus, fluid overload, and others (1,7,99,146,179).

Prior to the introduction of surfactant therapy, BPD affected approximately 20 percent of ventilated newborns (146): 15 to 38 percent of infants under 1,500 g were affected, up to 85 percent of those between 500 and 699 g, and only 5 percent of infants over 1,500 g (134,146). The use of surfactant therapy (either modified natural or synthetic surfactant) in infants at high risk for the development of BPD (700 to 2,000 g) decreased the incidence of pneumothorax, bronchopulmonary dysplasia, and mortality.

Clinical Features. The early symptoms of BPD are those of RDS, and patients require oxygen therapy and assisted ventilation (1,7,99, 130,134,145,146,155,179). Over time, some infants improve and are discharged, others worsen and die, and some develop chronic lung disease. Mortality has progressively decreased

Table 11-12

BRONCHOPULMONARY DYSPLASIA: SHORT- AND LONG-TERM COMPLICATIONS AND ASSOCIATIONS[a]

Early:	Pulmonary air leak phenomena
	Patent ductus arteriosus
	Necrotizing enterocolitis
	Gastroesophageal reflux/aspiration
	Complications of hyperalimentation
	Growth failure
	Transient systemic hypertension
	Congestive heart failure
	Asphyxia
Late:	Tracheal stenosis
	Apneic spells
	Sudden infant death
	Respiratory failure during intercurrent viral infection
	Small airways disease
	Bronchial hyperreactivity
	Chronic airflow obstruction as adult
	Poor growth
	Cor pulmonale
	Aspiration
	Social problems

[a]Based on references 1 and 106.

with improvements in management, although in general, the prognosis correlates inversely with birth weight. Survivors are usually discharged between 3 and 6 months of age. Fatalities can occur at any time during the course of the disease, including months or years after discharge.

Established BPD (28 days and thereafter) produces a chronic respiratory disease that may be associated with tachypnea, chest retractions, cough, paroxysmal respirations, wheezing, and rhonchi. Functional deficits at this point include abnormal gas exchange, increased dead space, decreased compliance, maldistribution of ventilation, increased work of breathing, and ventilation-perfusion mismatching. Mild to moderate pulmonary hypertension is usually present.

Early and late complications and associations of BPD are shown in Table 11-12. One of the most significant acute complications is air leak with interstitial emphysema, although the complication rate has dramatically decreased in recent years with improvements in ventilation and ventilator management.

Radiologic Findings. Earlier reviews of the radiographic features of BPD described a progression through different stages (102). Because of changing methods of assisted ventilation, the radiologic features of BPD have changed and include a variety of different findings: diffuse lung haziness, irregular areas of consolidation, interstitial opacities, and "bubble-like" cystic spaces (fig.11-61) (102). The latter may be confused with interstitial emphysema. The appearance of cystic change produces increased lung lucency and may be initially misinterpreted as improvement of RDS. Lobar overinflation, which has been called focal interstitial emphysema, may develop during this process and produce mediastinal shift and mass effect upon the less severely affected lung.

Gross Findings. Early BPD is grossly identical to RDS (6,7,23,61,106,130,155,157,179). Prior to the widespread use of exogenous surfactant, the lungs became firm, congested, heavy, and relatively airless, with uneven airspace distension. As the condition became more chronic, connective tissue increased, architectural destruction took place, and the pleural surface assumed a cobblestone appearance after 1 to 2 weeks (figs. 11-62, 11-63). On cut section, zones of overdistension alternated with zones of fibrosis and contraction (atelectasis). The severity of the changes corresponded to the severity of the clinical disease. Mild cases showed only slight hyperinflation and focal scarring. More recently, patients who have received surfactant therapy and subsequently developed BPD have far less severe and more diffuse alveolar septal fibrosis than patients of the 1970s and 1980s who had not received prior surfactant therapy (86).

Histologic Findings. The histologic findings of nonsurfactant-treated infants of the 1970s and 1980s who developed BPD (6,7,23, 61,106,130,155,157,179) were essentially those of diffuse alveolar damage in the adult, with differences attributed to the occurrence of this reaction in the immature lung: the finding of a necrotizing bronchiolitis, uneven inflation and atelectasis, and frequent interstitial air accumulations (figs. 11-64–11-69) (157). The histologic findings varied with the gestational age/degree of immaturity, the type and duration of ventilation, the duration of oxygen therapy, the degree of associated pulmonary edema, and the presence of any intercurrent disease process (157). While the diagnosis of BPD was usually

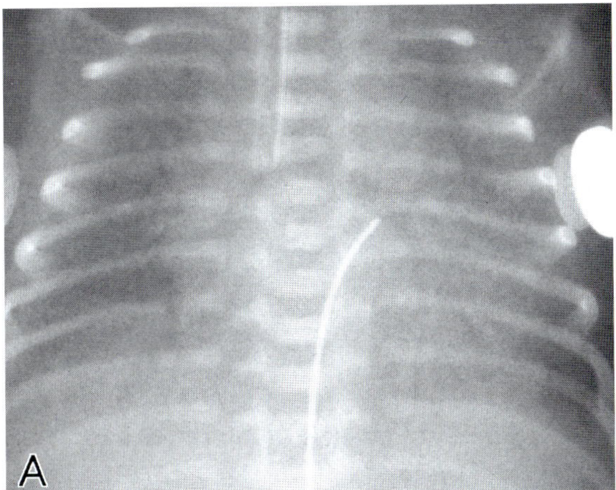

Figure 11-61

BRONCHOPULMONARY DYSPLASIA

A: AP chest radiograph of a preterm newborn with RDS demonstrates diffuse, bilateral, parenchymal granular opacities. There is a right pleural effusion, an unusual finding in RDS.

B: AP chest radiograph of the same infant obtained 2 weeks later demonstrates coarse parenchymal opacities and resolution of the pleural fluid. Mechanical ventilation is likely responsible for the increased lung expansion.

C: AP chest radiograph of the same infant obtained 1 month later demonstrates diffuse, bilateral, coarse reticular opacities and "bubble-like" lung lucencies. Note the large right apical lung cyst (arrow). (Courtesy of Lt. Col. Gael J. Lonergan, USAF, MC, Uniformed Services University, Bethesda, MD.)

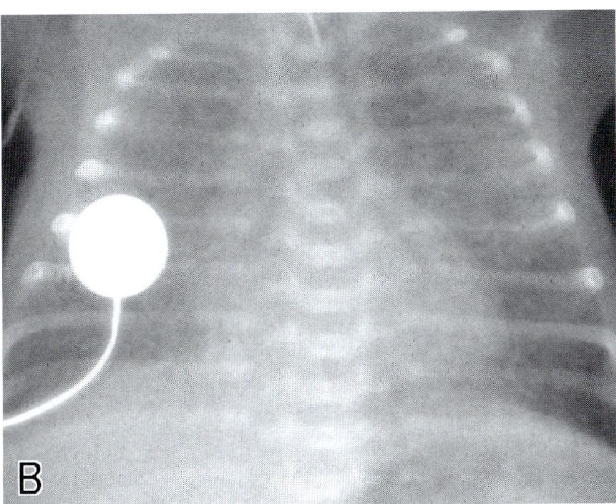

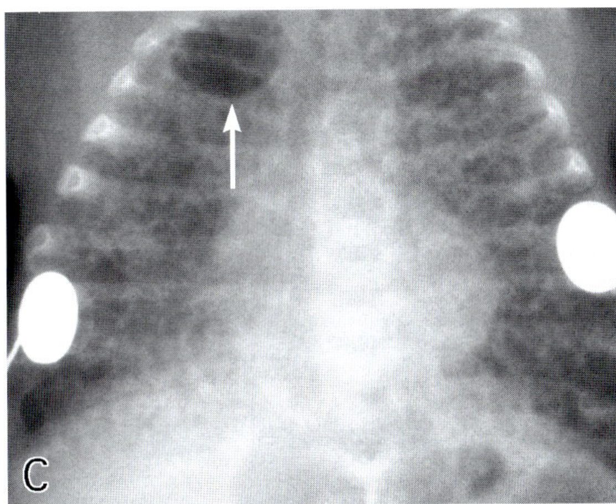

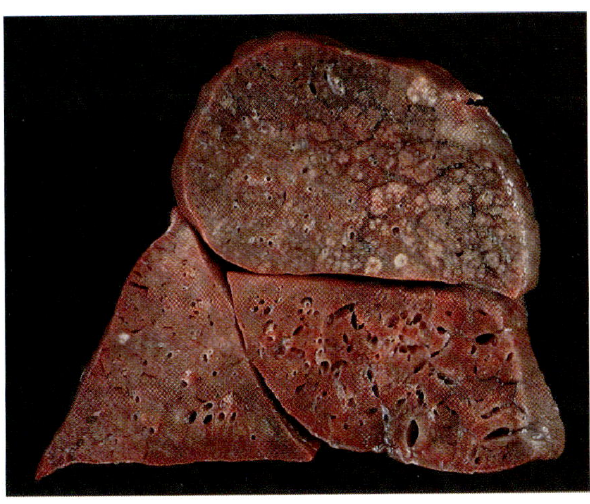

Figure 11-62

BRONCHOPULMONARY DYSPLASIA

The lower lobes are diffusely firm with dilated spaces due to chronic interstitial air. The upper lobe shows some patchy zones of scarring.

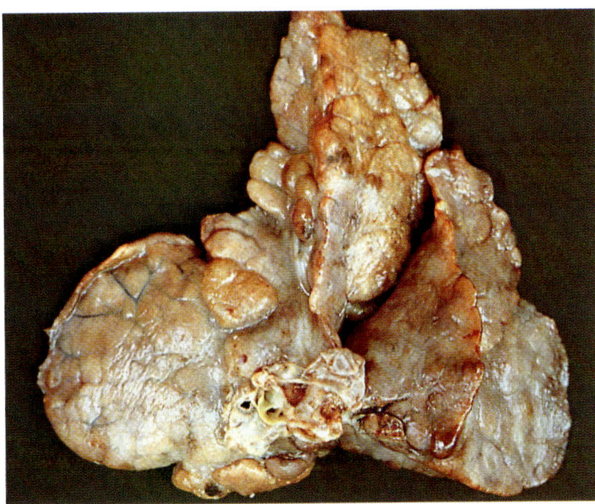

Figure 11-63

BRONCHOPULMONARY DYSPLASIA

The alternating areas of expansion and atelectasis are apparent grossly, imparting a somewhat lobated appearance to the pleural surface.

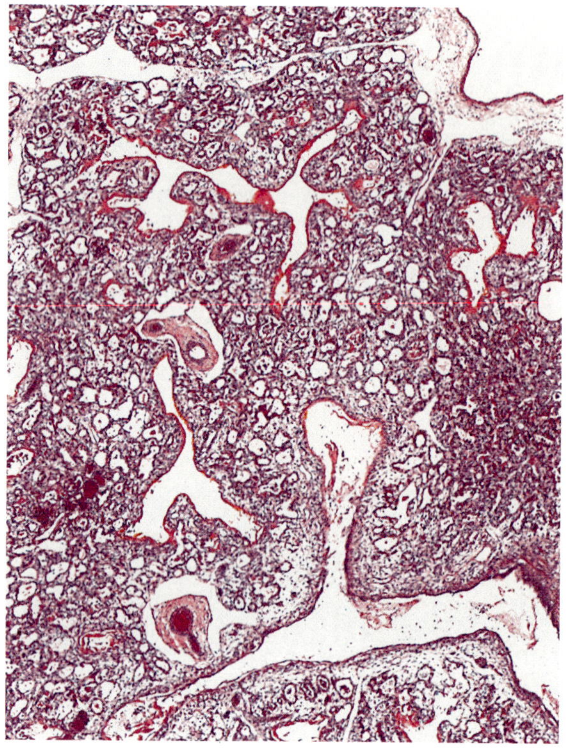

Figure 11-64

BRONCHOPULMONARY DYSPLASIA

In early stages the lung architecture is intact and alveolar ducts are lined by hyaline membranes (left center). The overall appearance is that of immature lung tissue with thickened alveolar septa.

deferred until 28 days of age, histologic changes were apparent much earlier and overlapped with those of acute respiratory distress syndrome (ARDS). Earlier studies had shown a good correlation between pathologic and radiologic staging (58).

Early phases of BPD in nonsurfactant-treated infants were dominated by airspace and interstitial edema, hyaline membranes in alveolar ducts, and necrotizing bronchiolitis (fig. 11-64). Hyaline membranes may be yellow due to bilirubin staining (fig. 11-65) (124). With progression to the reparative phase, metaplastic and even dysplastic-appearing epithelium lined the airways (fig. 11-68), and type 2–like cells repopulated the alveoli. As hyaline membranes and bronchiolitis underwent repair, organization was seen within airways, distal airspaces, and the interstitium (fig. 11-66). Some zones of the lung showed hyperinflation and "cyst" formation with abnormally large airspaces (figs. 11-67, 11-69). In chronic/healed BPD, the cellular fibroblastic tissue was converted into less cellular fibrous tissue (fig. 11-69). Stocker (155, 157) suggested that the lung tissue supplied by bronchioles that had necrotizing bronchiolitis was relatively protected from further injury (e.g., barotrauma) by the occlusive effects of this fibroblastic reaction in the bronchioles.

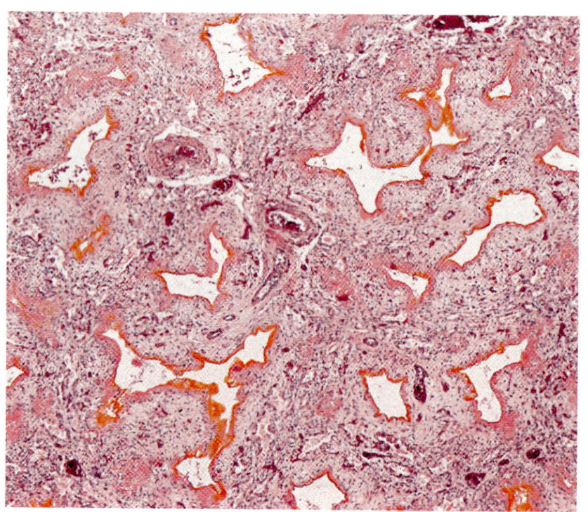

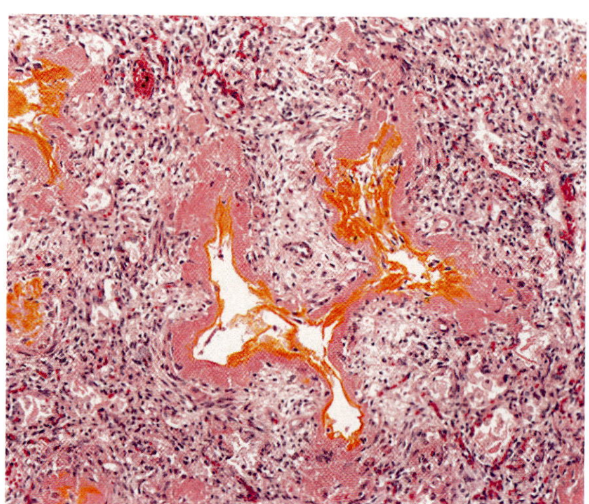

Figure 11-65

BRONCHOPULMONARY DYSPLASIA: ACUTE AND ORGANIZING PHASES

Dilated alveolar ducts are lined by hyaline membranes, which show some yellow staining. The surrounding lung tissue shows fibroblastic proliferation and apparent loss of architecture.

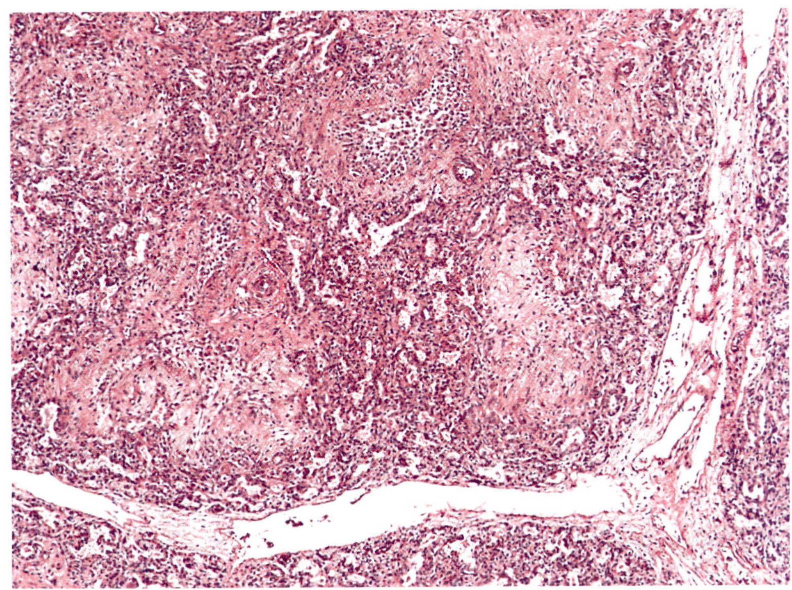

Figure 11-66

BRONCHOPULMONARY DYSPLASIA: ORGANIZING PHASE

The lobular architecture is intact, although there is some fibrosis in the central portions of the lobule corresponding to the alveolar duct regions.

Figure 11-67

BRONCHOPULMONARY DYSPLASIA: CHRONIC PHASE

A: There are zones of irregular alveolar expansion (right) and atelectasis (left).

B: In the atelectatic zones, the paler regions of alveolar duct fibrosis are apparent.

C: In the zones of airspace expansion the architecture appears distorted, with overexpansion of airspaces.

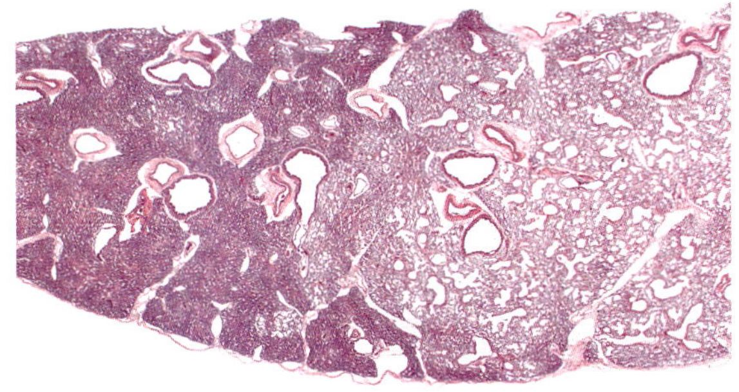

A

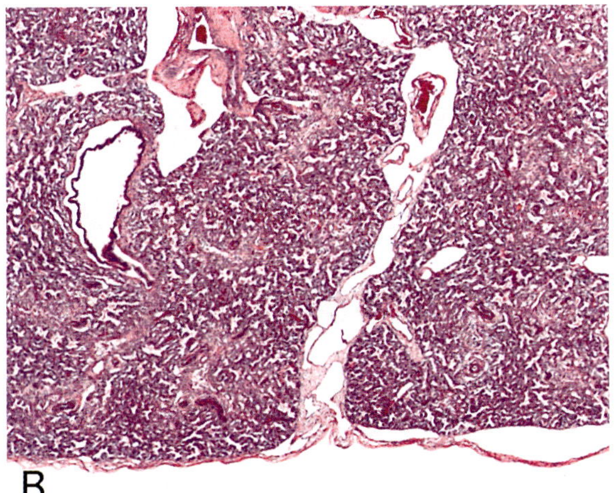

B

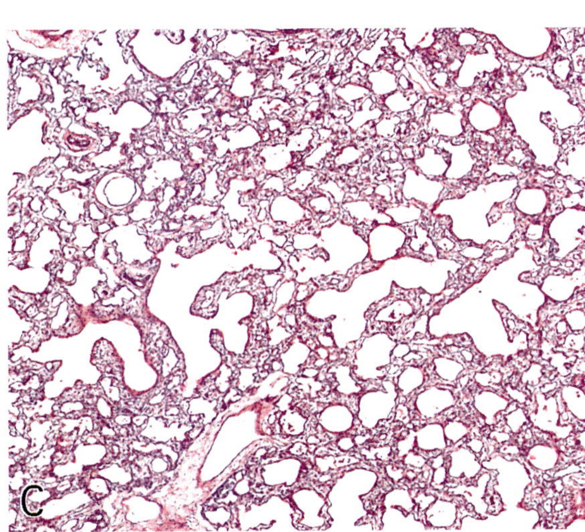

C

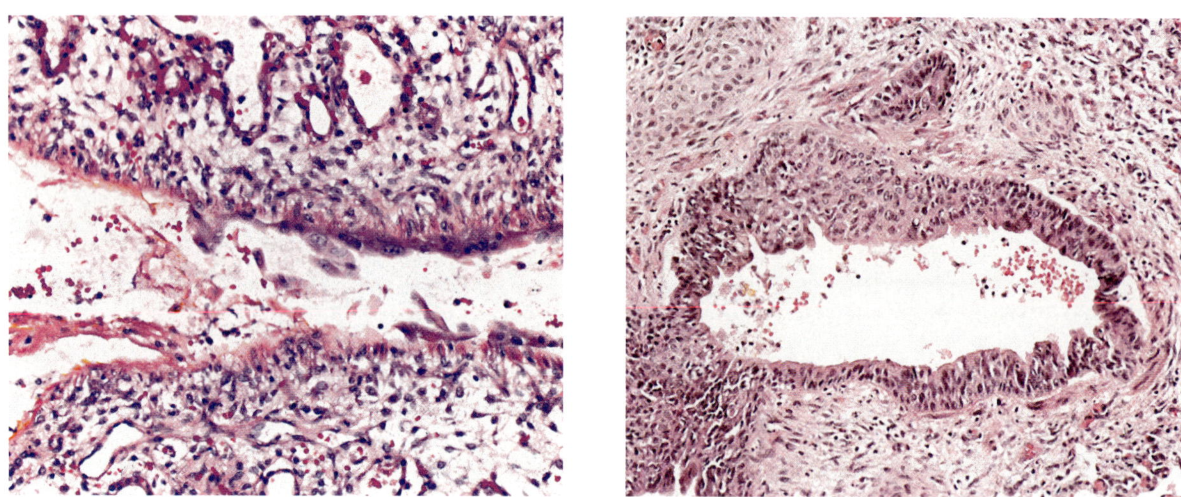

Figure 11-68

AIRWAY CHANGES IN BRONCHOPULMONARY DYPLASIA

Left: Early on there is sloughing of epithelium and hyaline membrane formation.
Right: With time, atypical and somewhat dysplastic-appearing epithelium lines the airways.

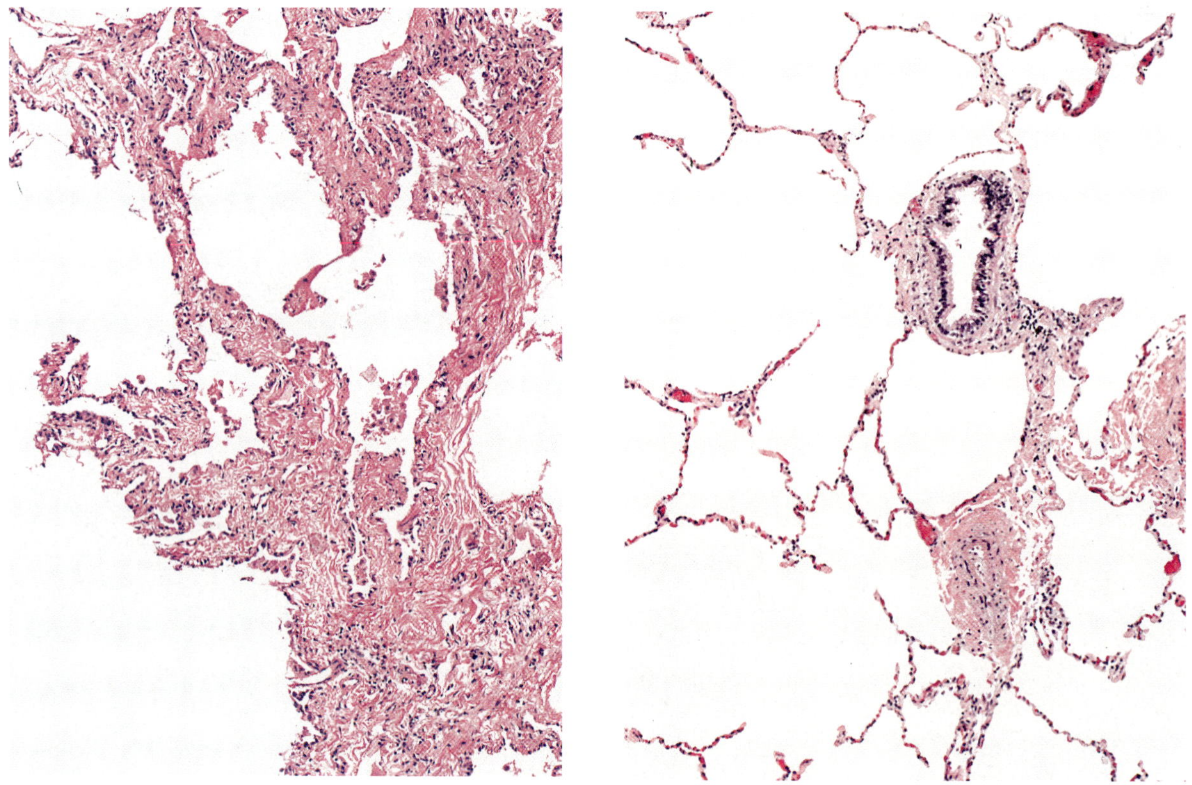

Figure 11-69

BRONCHOPULMONARY DYPLASIA: LATE PHASE

These two cases illustrate lung tissue from patients who had bronchopulmonary dysplasia many years earlier. One case shows marked irregular expansion of airspaces with intervening interstitial fibrosis (left). The other case shows marked alveolar distention and small bronchioles with thickened walls (right).

According to this hypothesis, overinflated lung tissue was supplied by bronchioles that were less severely affected in the acute phase. Following resolution of the bronchiolitis, the supplied parenchyma then became more normally aerated and functional.

Since the advent of surfactant replacement therapy, the necrotizing bronchiolitis and alveolar septal fibrosis of BPD have largely disappeared, and the major change now seen is that of decreased alveolarization in infants following birth (43,61,86,152). Morphometric evidence of decreased alveolarization (for example, by radial alveolar count) can be used to support a diagnosis of BPD and to quantify its severity, particularly in mild cases, which are becoming increasingly frequent with surfactant therapy (86). This is somewhat analogous to the enlarged alveoli associated with hypoplastic lungs in Down's syndrome (44,45,90,175), although the etiology in BPD appears to be an arrest of normal growth (86).

Interstitial accumulations of air (interstitial emphysema) in cases of BPD may be so dramatic that one's first impression is that the tissue has been torn or there is lymphangiectasis. Acute interstitial emphysema is associated with little or no reaction and simply manifests as air dissecting in connective tissue, in septa, and along bronchovascular bundles. With chronicity, a distinctive histiocytic and giant cell reaction develops and the diagnosis is relatively easy.

Pathogenesis. The pathogenesis of BPD is multifactorial, related primarily to immaturity of the lungs with the superimposed effects of hyperoxia (associated with generation of reactive oxygen intermediates), barotrauma, inflammation, and infection (1,7,99,134,146). A number of studies have shown the importance of inflammatory cells and their mediators in the pathogenesis of BPD, especially neutrophils and alveolar macrophages (7,140,178).

Differential Diagnosis. Early stages of BPD cannot be distinguished from (and are indeed synonymous with) RDS. The presence of hyaline membranes and acute lung injury is nonspecific and associated with a number of diseases. Infections should be considered. Late phases of nonsurfactant-treated BPD show features of emphysema, fibrosing interstitial pneumonia, mild pulmonary hypertension, or chronic (constrictive) bronchiolitis. Many years after nonsurfactant-treated BPD only subtle airway or vascular changes may be identified. In small airways, decrease in lumen size, focal ectasia, mucostasis, muscular hypertrophy, and variable degrees of adventitial and submucosal scarring may all be seen; some bronchioles may appear normal in individuals with clinical evidence of small airway disease. Pulmonary arterial changes may manifest only as subtle medial hypertrophy. These changes may all be difficult to interpret without knowledge of the clinical history. Once a history of nonsurfactant-treated BPD is apparent, the diagnosis should be relatively easy in severe cases showing irregular zones of fibrosis and overdistension. In surfactant-treated infants who develop a chronic lung disease, the diagnosis may require correlation of clinical, radiologic, and histologic (and possibly morphometric) findings.

The *Wilson-Mikity syndrome* was described in 1960: premature infants who developed progressive lung disease prior to the introduction of mechanical ventilation and the recognition of BPD (106,171). The radiologic findings in these patients are indistinguishable from those seen in patients with BPD (102). In addition, focal or multifocal areas of overdistention of the lungs may develop. This syndrome is primarily of historical interest only.

Prevention, Treatment, and Prognosis. Prevention of BPD is primarily prevention of RDS, i.e., avoidance of premature delivery. With advances in management, the survival rate for patients with BPD has progressively improved since the disease was originally described in 1967 (1,7,99,134,145,146). While some survivors have no deficits, others have evidence of abnormal lung function and hyperreactive airways (7). In a study of 26 adolescent and young adult long-term survivors, Northway et al. (133) found that individuals with BPD showed significantly more hyperinflation (increased ratio of residual volume to total lung capacity) than did the matched controls (Table 11-13). Six of the patients had severe respiratory dysfunction and/or ongoing symptoms of respiratory disease. The authors concluded that "pulmonary dysfunction is common in adolescents and young adults with a history of bronchopulmonary dysplasia." The results of Blayney et al. (21) are more encouraging: if patients had normal function at age 7, subsequent lung growth was normal, and even patients with mild to moderate lung disease at age 7 tended to have continued lung growth, repair, and functional improvement.

PULMONARY INTERSTITIAL EMPHYSEMA

Definition. Pulmonary interstitial emphysema is an acquired condition in which air gains access to the interstitium and dissects along bronchovascular structures and septa, and into the connective tissue of the visceral pleura (25,32, 92,104,106,112,157,158,160). The presence of interstitial air may lead to pneumothorax, pneumomediastinum, and pneumopericardium; or it may compress the lung tissue and compromise function. Pulmonary interstitial emphysema may be localized or diffuse, acute or chronic (Table 11-14). Most patients have a history of mechanical ventilation (primarily for prematurity).

Table 11-13

LATE PULMONARY SEQUELAE OF BRONCHOPULMONARY DYSPLASIA[a]

Finding	BPD (n=25)	Matched Cohort (n=26)
Normal	24%	69%
Positive methacholine challenge only	8%	31%
Reversible airflow obstruction	44%	0%
Fixed airflow obstruction	24%	0%

[a]Modified from reference 133.

Pulmonary interstitial emphysema affects approximately 20 percent or less of ventilated infants. The incidence increases with decreasing birth weight: slightly over 40 percent of infants less than 1,000 g develop evidence of pulmonary interstitial emphysema (157). Pulmonary interstitial emphysema may complicate RDS even in the absence of assisted ventilation, although the vast majority of affected patients have been on a ventilator.

Clinical Features. Pulmonary interstitial emphysema is usually associated with other conditions, the symptoms of which may dominate the clinical findings (98). It typically occurs in the setting of respiratory distress syndrome or bronchopulmonary dysplasia, and its presence may be associated with decreased compliance, increased hypercarbia, and worsening hypoxia. Localized expansion or air-filled spaces can produce a mass effect, which may be acute or chronic and resemble infantile lobar emphysema with similar symptoms and compromise in lung function.

Radiologic Findings. The early radiographic manifestations of pulmonary interstitial emphysema include distinct rounded and linear, nonbranching lucencies or lucencies with a bizarre, nonbronchial branching pattern (figs. 11-70, 11-71) (102). These are best observed in the medial lung, but when severe, may be diffuse. Once pulmonary interstitial emphysema is suspected radiologically, identification

Table 11-14

FORMS OF INTERSTITIAL PULMONARY EMPHYSEMA[a]

Features	Acute Pulmonary Interstitial Emphysema	Persistent Pulmonary Interstitial Emphysema: Localized	Persistent Pulmonary Interstitial Emphysema: Diffuse
Patient's age (days)	<7	>7	>7
Pneumothorax	++	+	++
Average size of interstitial airspaces (cm)	0.2	1.3	0.7
Shape of interstitial airspaces	Spherical cysts	Irregular cysts	Channels and cysts
Fibrosis of cyst wall	–	++	+
Giant cell reaction along wall	–	++	+

[a]Modified from references 158 and 160.

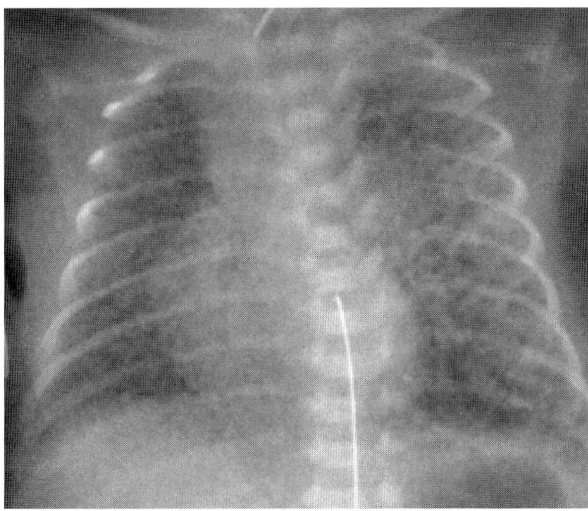

Figure 11-70

PULMONARY INTERSTITIAL EMPHYSEMA

AP chest radiograph of a preterm newborn with RDS who remained on mechanical ventilation. Bilateral linear and rounded lucencies represent early interstitial emphysema.

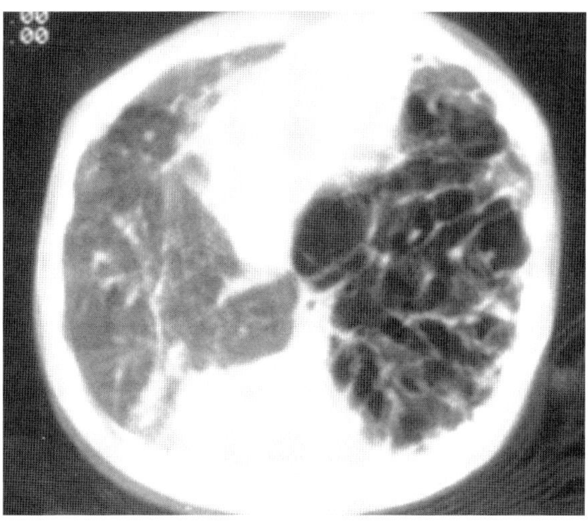

Figure 11-71

UNILATERAL PULMONARY INTERSTITIAL EMPHYSEMA

Chest CT in the same patient demonstrates the large air-filled interstitial spaces in the left lung.

and early treatment of additional complications of air leak, including pneumothorax, pneumomediastinum, pneumopericardium, and pneumoperitoneum, are imperative. Because the lungs have increased stiffness, the classic lung collapse and visualization of a pleural line may not be evident, in spite of the presence of a large pneumothorax. In these cases there may be mass effect on the diaphragm and mediastinum. In cases of pneumomediastinum, elevation of the infant thymus, the so-called spinnaker sail sign, may occur. In cases of pneumopericardium, air surrounding the heart may produce tamponade. Gas embolism is usually a fatal complication characterized by intracardiac, venous, and arterial gas.

Gross Findings. Air bubbles may be noted on the pleural surface of the lungs, particularly where interlobular septa intersect the pleura (figs. 11-72, 11-73) (25,32,92,104,106,157,158,160). Bubbles may also be apparent in the septa and along bronchovascular bundles on cut sections. There may be associated hemorrhage. In the localized form there is gross distortion of the lung parenchyma by air cysts, which may be up to several centimeters in diameter, and the gross appearance may suggest cystic adenomatoid malformation (figs. 11-74, 11-75).

Histologic Findings . The histologic findings of pulmonary interstitial emphysema vary with the age of the lesion (figs. 11-76–11-78) (25,32,92,104,106,157,158,160). In acute cases, there are rents in the interstitium in the septa, pleura, and along bronchovascular bundles, and at first glance these appear as tissue tears or artifacts. With time (usually a week [32,160]) a giant cell and histiocytic reaction may line the abnormal spaces. Later, the air-filled spaces may expand and markedly distort the lung architecture, with markedly atelectatic (yet histologically normal) lung tissue intervening.

Pathogenesis. Pulmonary interstitial emphysema is thought to be due to barotrauma and to arise from a loss of integrity of the epithelium and basement membrane in the distal lung tissue. This allows air to gain access to the interstitium, where it dissects along tissue planes.

Differential Diagnosis. Grossly, localized pulmonary interstitial emphysema may be confused with cystic adenomatoid malformation and infantile lobar emphysema. The distinction between these two entities is histologic. Careful attention needs to be paid as to whether the cystic spaces in a given lesion are lined by epithelium or arise from interstitial tears. The presence of histiocytes and giant cells is a good

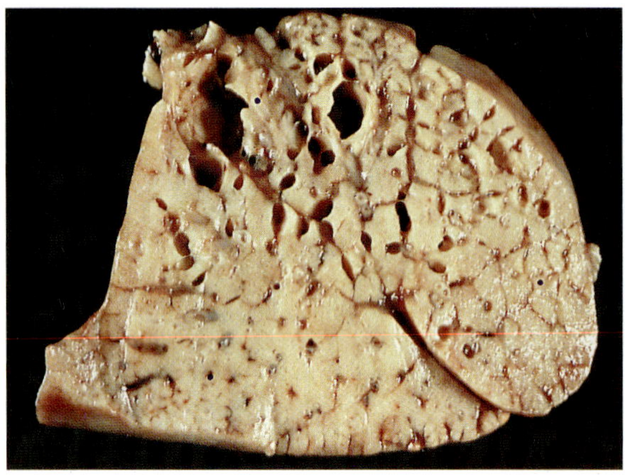

Figure 11-72

PULMONARY INTERSTITIAL EMPHYSEMA

Between the consolidated lung tissue (due to respiratory distress syndrome), there are dilated spaces, some of which are linear and branching, characteristic of pulmonary interstitial emphysema.

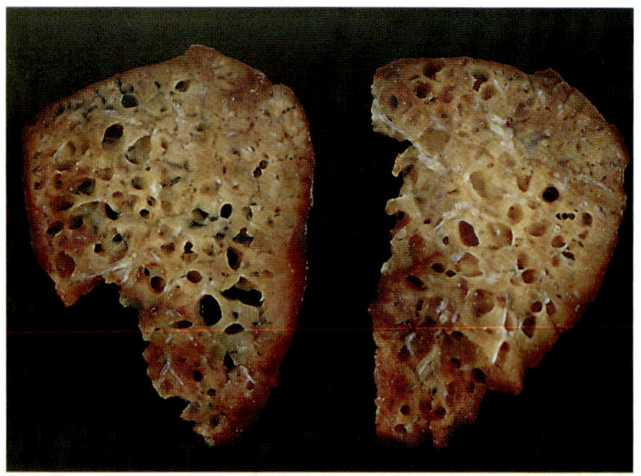

Figure 11-73

LOCALIZED PULMONARY INTERSTITIAL EMPHYSEMA

This lobectomy shows numerous abnormal dilated spaces confirmed histologically as interstitial emphysema.

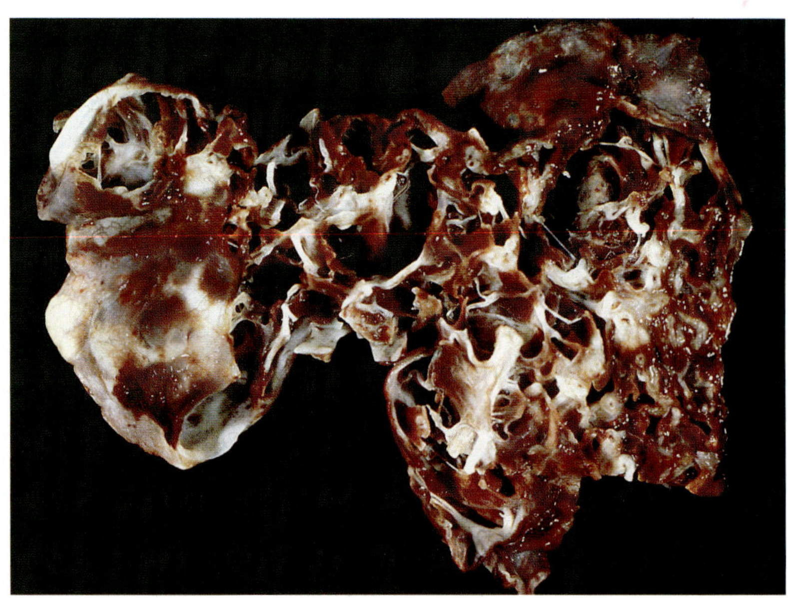

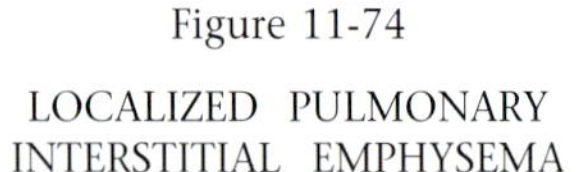

Figure 11-74

LOCALIZED PULMONARY INTERSTITIAL EMPHYSEMA

In this case the lung tissue is markedly distorted and severely compressed, and most of the volume of this lobe was taken up by interstitial air.

clue to interstitial air, although they are not present early on. Diffuse pulmonary lymphangiectasia may resemble pulmonary interstitial emphysema, although the lymphatic nature of the spaces in the former is usually apparent as the lymphatics will be seen both along the interlobular septa and beneath the pleura. In these cases, knowledge of the radiologic findings is helpful. In pulmonary lymphangiectasia there are diffuse interstitial reticular opacities which may be associated with (chylous) pleural effusions. The finding is distinct from that of pulmonary interstitial emphysema where the main abnormality is an interstitial lucency reflecting the abnormal air collections. The differential diagnosis may be aided with immunohistochemistry to clarify the lining cells in the cystic spaces: histiocytic versus endothelial.

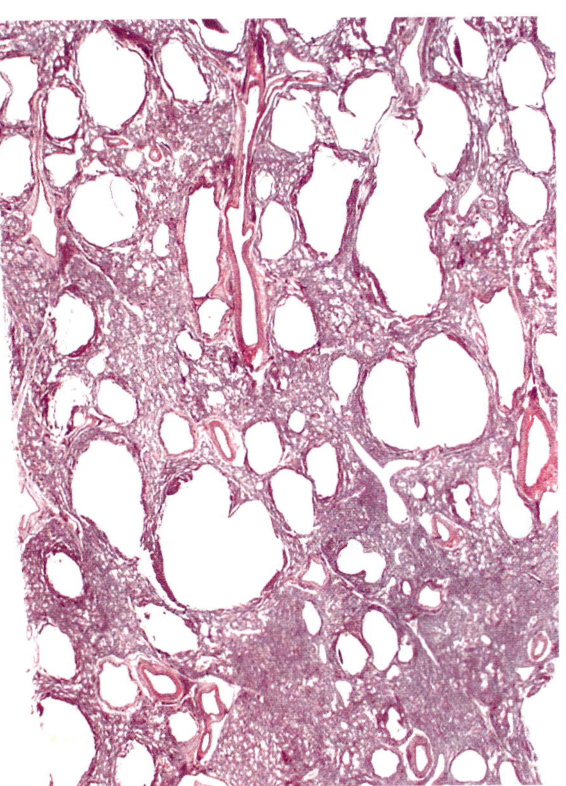

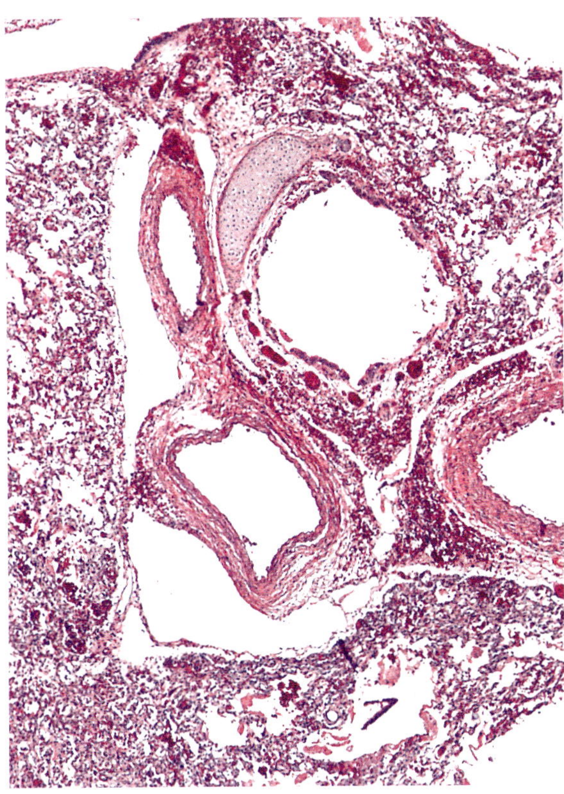

Figure 11-75

PULMONARY INTERSTITIAL EMPHYSEMA

Left: At scanning power microscopy it is difficult to determine the origin of the abnormal spaces in the lung tissue.

Right: Careful evaluation of septa and bronchovascular bundles shows where air has dissected along a bronchovascular bundle separating the lung tissue from the pulmonary artery.

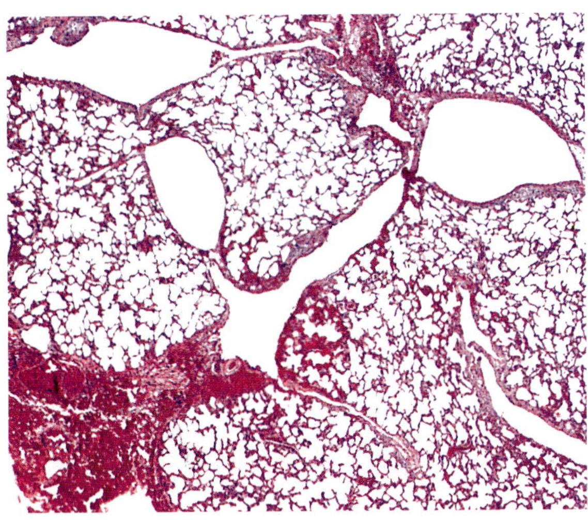

Figure 11-76

PULMONARY INTERSTITIAL EMPHYSEMA WITH PREDILECTION FOR SEPTAL INVOLVEMENT

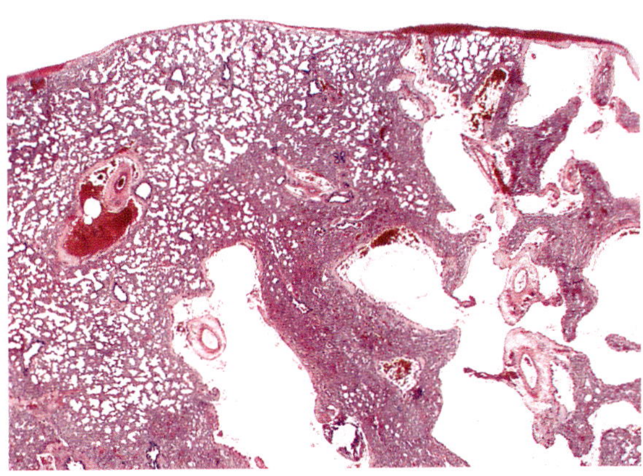

Figure 11-77

CHRONIC PULMONARY INTERSTITIAL EMPHYSEMA

The lung tissue immediately adjacent to the interstitial emphysema shows atelectasis (right) in comparison to the regions of lung tissue that are less affected (left).

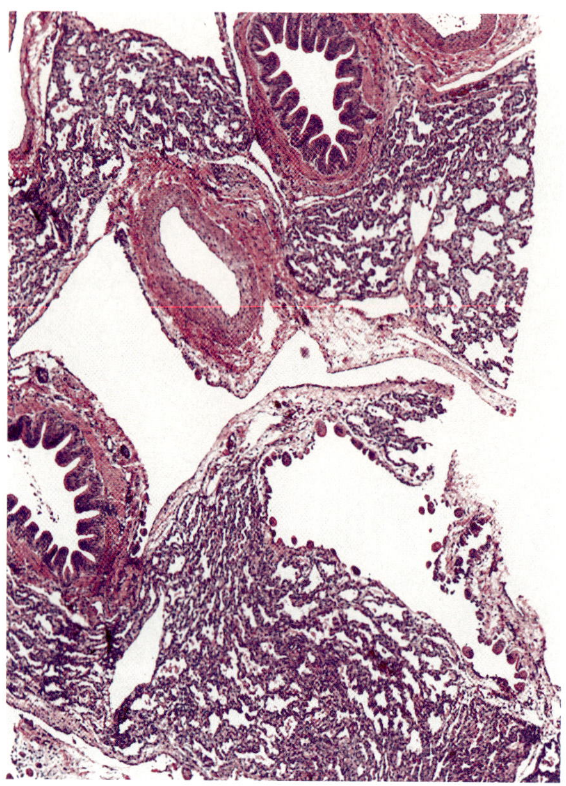

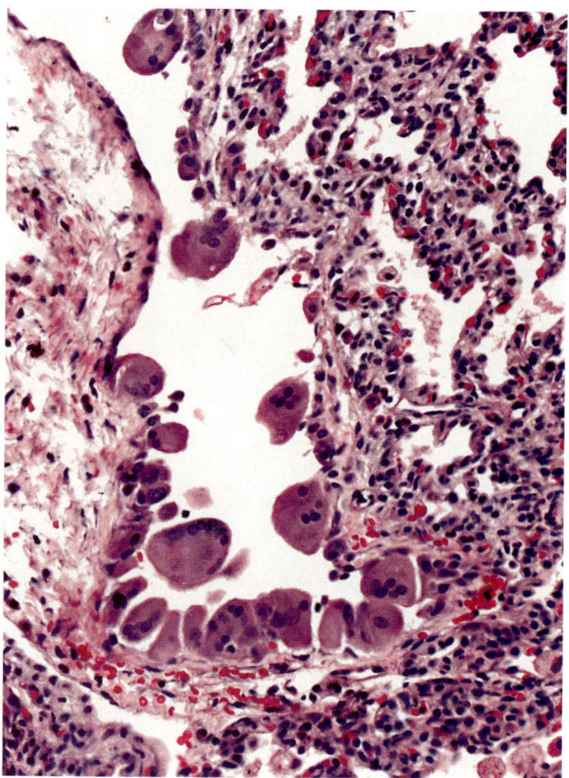

Figure 11-78

CHRONIC PULMONARY INTERSTITIAL EMPHYSEMA

Left: Air dissection has separated a bronchiole from its adjacent pulmonary artery.
Right: The abnormal spaces are lined by giant cells as a chronic reaction to the air.

Prevention and Treatment. Avoidance of barotrauma from increased ventilatory pressure and high-frequency ventilation may help in the prevention of pulmonary interstitial emphysema (63,98).

Interstitial air is slowly resorbed with supportive care. Localized forms that produce mass effect may be treated with selective bronchial intubation of the less affected lung (fig. 11-71) or by placing the affected lung in a dependent position, thus reducing ventilation to this area. However, these abnormalities may recur and may ultimately necessitate surgical resection of the affected area.

MECONIUM ASPIRATION SYNDROME

Definition. The meconium aspiration syndrome (MAS) occurs when there is clinically significant aspiration of meconium into the distal lung parenchyma (13,84,98,106,110,115,127,162, 172,173,176). Approximately 15 percent of births show meconium staining of the amniotic fluid: 2 percent or less before 37 weeks' gestational age and over 40 percent of births after 42 weeks' gestational age. Meconium staining of the amniotic fluid is a marker of fetal distress. Five percent of infants showing meconium staining of the amniotic fluid develop meconium aspiration syndrome: 30 percent require assisted ventilation, and in 5 to 10 percent MAS is fatal.

Clinical Features. Infants affected with MAS tend to be term infants who show meconium staining of the skin and the placental membranes (13,98,106,110). Other signs of postmaturity may be present. The symptoms are similar to those of patients with RDS: tachypnea, retractions, expiratory grunting, and cyanosis, which develop within the first few hours of life. Hyperinflation with an increased anterior-posterior (AP) diameter of the chest, presumably

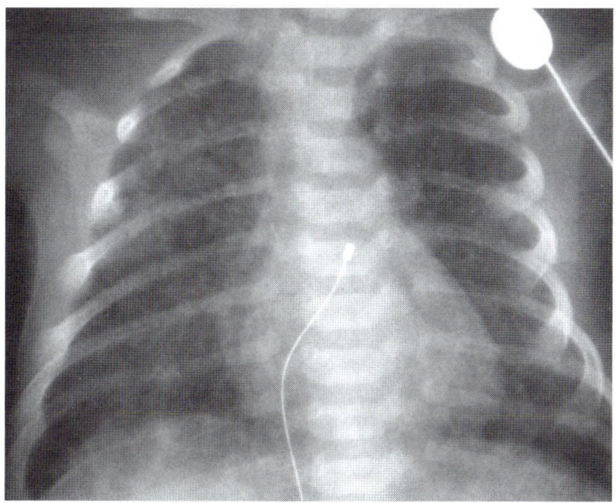

Figure 11-79

MECONIUM ASPIRATION SYNDROME

AP chest radiograph of a post-term meconium-stained infant with respiratory distress demonstrates increased lung volumes with patchy multifocal parenchymal opacities and right upper lobe consolidation. (Courtesy of Lt. Col. Gael J Lonergan, USAF, MC, Uniformed Services University, Bethesda, MD.)

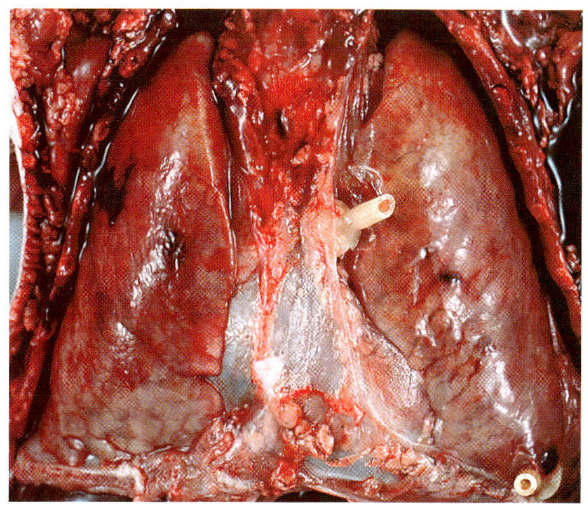

Figure 11-80

MECONIUM ASPIRATION SYNDROME

At autopsy the lungs remain expanded in the chest as a reflection of airflow obstruction.

due to air-trapping, may be found on physical examination. Pneumothorax may be present. Some infants affected with MAS present with unresponsive hypoxemia indicative of persistent pulmonary hypertension. Patients usually improve within 3 days, but in some cases symptoms persist for weeks.

Radiologic Findings. Chest radiographs in patients with MAS may be entirely normal if the meconium only enters the trachea and is successfully suctioned at birth (102). When the meconium is aspirated into the lung(s), there are bilateral and asymmetric patchy opacities and associated overaeration of the lungs (fig. 11-79). These findings may also occur in neonatal pneumonia. While less common, complications of air block, including pneumothorax and pneumomediastinum, may develop and must be monitored with serial radiographs.

Gross Findings. The lungs may be overinflated and have a gray-green appearance, and meconium may be found in the airways (fig. 11-80) (106). Some cases of MAS show gross evidence of interstitial air (84).

Histologic Findings. Meconium is found in the distal airspaces and plugging small airways (figs. 11-81, 11-82) (84,106). Meconium consists of squames, mucus, and amorphous debris. Mucus can be highlighted with mucin stains. The amount of meconium should be appreciable since a small amount of meconium is a common histologic finding in the lungs of infants up to a few weeks old and insufficient for a diagnosis of MAS. A meconium-induced chemical pneumonitis with hyaline membranes may develop a few days after aspiration.

Pathogenesis. Passage of meconium in utero may be physiologic or associated with fetal compromise. Fetal distress, from a variety of causes, may lead to gasping and meconium aspiration (110). If the meconium is finely dispersed in the amniotic fluid, aspiration may be relatively insignificant; but when the meconium is not well dispersed and masses of particulate debris reach the peripheral lung tissue, MAS may develop (110). While meconium aspiration in utero has been reported (115), in the majority of symptomatic cases aspiration occurs in the perinatal and postnatal period as the infant expands its lungs. Once material has been aspirated into the distal lung tissue, obstruction and chemical pneumonitis may develop. Hypoxia and vasoconstriction associated with meconium aspiration is thought to lead to persistent pulmonary hypertension.

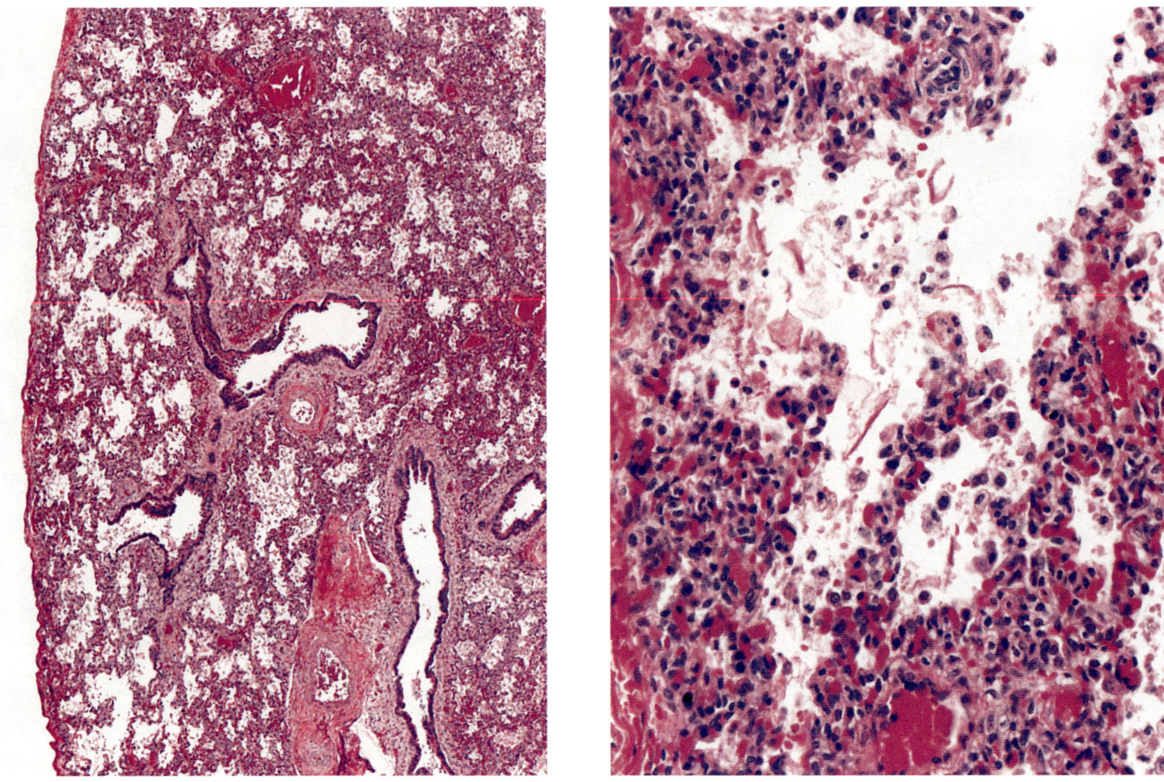

Figure 11-81

MECONIUM ASPIRATION SYNDROME

Left: The underlying lung architecture is intact, although there is increased cellularity in alveolar septa.
Right: In the airspaces, inflammatory cells and keratinous debris can be identified.

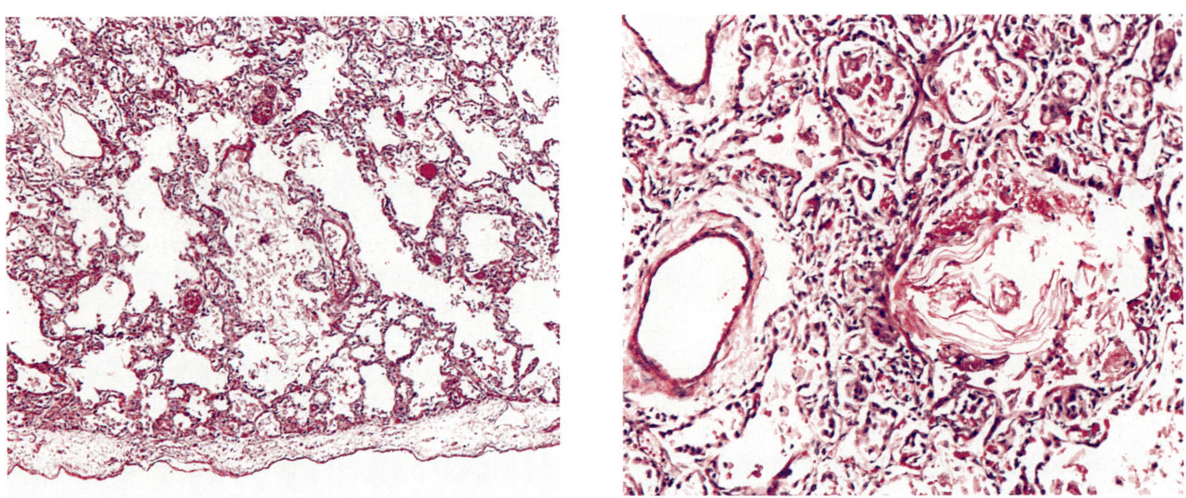

Figure 11-82

MECONIUM ASPIRATION SYNDROME

Left: Meconium aspiration syndrome showing morphologic effects of airflow obstruction with dilated alveolar ducts and alveoli.

Right: Within a small bronchiole is a plug of keratinous debris.

Differential Diagnosis. Clinical evidence of air-trapping and the presence of significant amounts of meconium in the distal airspaces allows separation of this syndrome from RDS and neonatal infectious pneumonia. Radiographically, MAS and neonatal pneumonia may be indistinguishable.

Prevention and Treatment. Suctioning of the trachea and nasopharynx as the head is delivered and after birth has markedly reduced the incidence of MAS, although it is unlikely that the condition can be entirely prevented (172,173,176). Treatment includes suction, oxygen, physical therapy, avoidance of assisted ventilation if possible (because of predisposition to air leaks), surfactant therapy, and, if necessary, extracorporal membrane oxygenation.

Prognosis. Between 90 and 95 percent of patients recover and the majority do not develop long-term problems. A small number of patients have cough, wheezing, and hyperinflation at 5 to 10 years of age. Severely affected infants may also show the effects of central nervous system (CNS) hypoxia during the acute event. Swaminathan et al. (162) studied long-term effects in 11 children. Four of these (36 percent) had long-term sequelae including airway obstruction, hyperinflation, elevated closing volumes, and airway hyperreactivity. The authors noted that these findings are similar, though less severe, than those that follow prematurity and associated BPD.

MASSIVE PULMONARY HEMORRHAGE OF THE NEWBORN

Definition. A rare syndrome of massive pulmonary hemorrhage is seen in newborns (98, 106,168). Affected infants tend to be preterm males that are small for gestational age and have a history of perinatal stress. The pathogenesis is unknown.

Clinical Features. Affected infants may be stillborn or liveborn. Those that are liveborn suddenly collapse with massive pulmonary hemorrhage in the first week of life. Most affected infants die (34,167).

Pathologic Findings. The lungs are diffusely consolidated and hemorrhagic. There is massive airspace and interstitial hemorrhage. There may be associated findings of RDS or BPD.

Differential Diagnosis. The full-blown clinical syndrome of massive pulmonary hemorrhage of the newborn is distinctive and characteristic, allowing differentiation from the minor degrees of alveolar hemorrhage found in RDS and BPD. Aspiration of maternal blood is also included in the differential diagnosis.

PEDIATRIC INTERSTITIAL LUNG DISEASE

Definition. Interstitial lung disease manifesting in the pediatric age group (through 18 years of age).

Background. Pediatric interstitial lung disease can be divided into cases of known versus unknown etiology, as shown in Table 11-15 (22, 47,64,129,131). As in adults, there are many causes of interstitial lung disease, with over 100 described in children. Many of the diseases shown in Table 11-15 never come to biopsy. The cases that do get biopsied represent a subset skewed toward cases in which a clinical or radiologic diagnosis has not been forthcoming. Coren et al. (47) recently described detailed histologic findings in a series of 27 cases of diffuse interstitial lung disease in children (Table 11-16).

Clinical Features. The clinical features of a series of 48 patients with pediatric interstitial lung disease described by Fan et al. (65) are shown in Tables 11-17 and 11-18. There is a considerable difference in age at presentation among pediatric patients and this correlates with the different signs and symptoms encountered.

Radiologic Findings. As in adults, CT scans are more sensitive in identifying and characterizing abnormalities in pediatric diffuse lung disease than are chest radiographs (46, 113). In a study by Lynch et al. (113), five groups of patients were identified on the basis of dominant CT findings: airway disease with geographic hyperlucency, septal disease with septal thickening, infiltrative disease with ground-glass change, airspace disease with consolidation, and nodular/cystic disease; correlation with specific disease entities could be shown. In a separate study by Copley et al. (46), the correct diagnosis was included in the radiologic differential diagnosis in two thirds of 20 cases studied, with CT interpretation being most accurate in cases of alveolar proteinosis, congenital lymphangiectasia, and idiopathic pulmonary hemorrhage. The conditions described below are sufficiently rare that the radiologic findings are not fully characterized.

Table 11-15

PEDIATRIC INTERSTITIAL LUNG DISEASE[a]

Known Cause or Association	
Infectious or postinfectious	Metabolic
Viral	Storage disorders
Mycobacterial fungal	Pulmonary lipidosis
Bacterial	Disorders of ion transport
Parasitic	Congenital surfactant deficiency
Environmental inhalants, toxic	Other
Bronchopulmonary dysplasia (BPD)	Neurocutaneous syndromes with intestinal lung disease
Substances, foreign materials, or antigenic dusts	Interstitial lung disease associated with collagen vascular diseases
Inorganic dusts	Interstitial lung disease associated with pulmonary vasculitides
Organic dusts	
Fumes	Interstitial lung disease associated with inflammatory bowel disease
Gases	
Aspiration syndromes	Interstitial lung disease caused by failure of other organs
Drug-induced disorders	Amyloidosis
Antineoplastic drugs	Graft-versus-host disease/lung transplant rejection
Miscellaneous drugs	Recovering phase of acute respiratory distress syndrome/BPD
Neoplastic diseases	Goodpasture's syndrome
Lymphoproliferative disorders	Hypereosinophilic syndrome
Lymphoid hyperplasia in immunodeficiency states	Pulmonary vascular disease
	Veno-occlusive disease
Unknown Cause	
Idiopathic interstitial pneumonias	Cellular interstitial pneumonitis
Nonspecific interstitial pneumonia	(Usual interstitial pneumonia: see text)
Desquamative interstitial pneumonia	Sarcoidosis
Lymphocytic interstitial pneumonia/diffuse/lymphoid hyperplasia	Idiopathic pulmonary hemorrhage
	Pulmonary alveolar proteinosis
Cryptogenic organizing pneumonia	Pulmonary infiltrates with eosinophilia/eosinophilic pneumonia
Chronic pneumonitis of infancy	Pulmonary alveolar microlithiasis

[a]Modified from references 22, 47, 52, 64, 129, and 131.

Table 11-16

OPEN BIOPSY FINDINGS IN PEDIATRIC DIFFUSE INTERSTITIAL LUNG DISEASE[a]

NSIP[b] – 5 cases	Chronic pneumonitis of infancy – 1 case
Follicular bronchiolitis – 4 cases	DIP – 1 case
LIP – 3 cases	Pulmonary hemosiderosis – 1 case
Lymphangiectasia – 2 cases	Pulmonary veno-occlusive disease – 1 case
Follicular bronchiolitis/pneumocystis – 1 case	Chronic airway inflammation – 1 case
Diffuse pulmonary lymphangiomatosis – 1 case	Normal lung – 1 case
Alveolar proteinosis – 1 case	Nondiagnostic samples – 2 cases
Gaucher's disease – 1 case	

[a]Modified from reference 47.
[b]NSIP = nonspecific interstitial pneumonia; DIP = desquamative interstitial pneumonia; LIP = lymphocytic interstitial pneumonia.

Table 11-17

PEDIATRIC INTERSTITIAL LUNG DISEASE: DEMOGRAPHICS[a]

	Patients No.	Patients %
Gender		
Male	23	48
Female	25	52
Age at onset (yr)		
<1	22	46
1–5	11	23
6–10	9	19
10–18	6	13
Duration of symptoms (yr)		
<1	27	56
1–3	8	17
>3	13	27

[a]Modified from reference 65.

Table 11-18

PEDIATRIC INTERSTITIAL LUNG DISEASE: SIGNS AND SYMPTOMS[a]

	Patients No.	Patients %
Symptoms		
Cough	37	77
Tachypnea	36	75
Dyspnea	34	71
Cyanosis	32	67
Exercise intolerance	31	65
Frequent respiratory infection	21	44
Retractions	20	42
Wheezing	19	40
Hemoptysis	4	8
Signs		
Rales	29	60
Tachypnea	26	54
Retractions	22	46
Weight <5%	17	35
Clubbing	14	29
Wheezing	9	19
Cyanosis	9	19
Height <5%	7	15
Loud P_2	6	13

[a]Modified from reference 65.

Pathologic Findings. Many of the entities shown in Tables 11-15 and 11-16 are covered in other sections. Several, however, deserve specific comment.

Desquamative interstitial pneumonia (DIP) does occur in children (fig. 11-83) (47,129). Children with DIP tend to be steroid responsive and to have a relatively favorable prognosis, compared to those with other interstitial pneumonias (47,129). Foci resembling DIP may occur in congenital surfactant deficiency, including surfactant B deficiency, and the deficiency of lamellar bodies in alveolar type 2 cells (see below). These conditions should be excluded in any neonate in whom a diagnosis of DIP is being considered. Chronic pneumonitis of infancy may show a modest patchy increase in alveolar macrophages (see below), and some cases previously described in the literature as DIP might currently be interpreted as chronic pneumonitis of infancy.

Lymphocytic interstitial pneumonia/diffuse lymphoid hyperplasia has been an acquired immunodeficiency syndrome (AIDS)-defining illness in the pediatric population (see chapters 3 and 13) but it may be associated with other immunodeficiency settings, especially immunoglobulin deficiencies (fig. 11-84) (47,129). Hypersensitivity pneumonitis, infection with *Pneumocystis carinii,* and interstitial lung disease associated with autoimmune disorders (particularly collagen vascular diseases) may all produce the pattern of lymphocytic interstitial pneumonia.

Pulmonary alveolar proteinosis is rare in children. A proteinosis-like pattern may be associated with chronic infections (especially respiratory syncytial virus [RSV]) in the setting of immunodeficiency (especially severe combined immunodeficiency syndrome) and is a finding associated with congenital surfactant protein B deficiency (see chapters 3 and 13).

Congenital surfactant deficiency may be caused by surfactant protein B deficiency or deficiency of lamellar bodies in type 2 cells (39,52, 53,131,132). Patients with these deficiencies present with severe respiratory distress in the neonatal period. Ultrastructurally, type 2 cells in congenital surfactant B deficiency have abnormal lamellar bodies. Immunohistochemistry is negative for mature surfactant protein B, with strong reactivity for surfactant protein A and prosurfactant protein C. In addition to a proteinosis pattern, surfactant protein B deficiency may produce a DIP-like pattern (fig. 11-85). The prognosis is grave and the only available treatment is lung transplantation. The

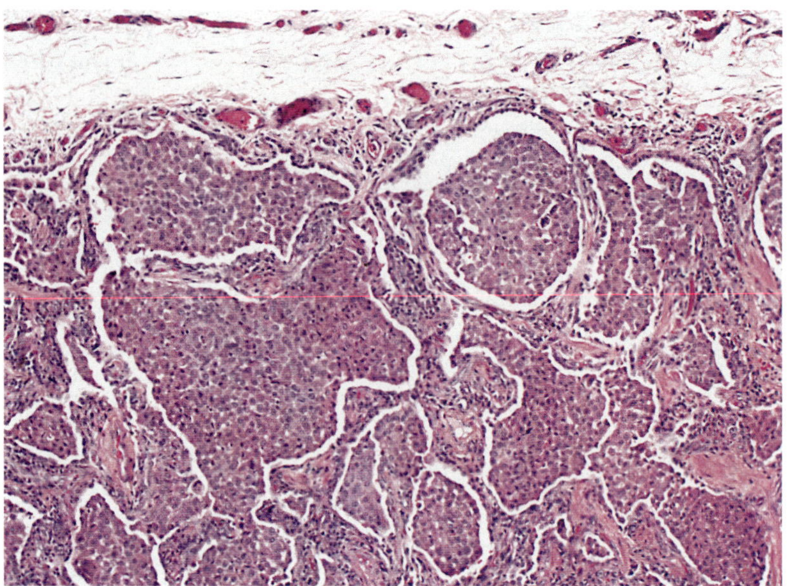

Figure 11-83

DESQUAMATIVE INTERSTITIAL PNEUMONIA

This biopsy is from a nonsmoking teenager with interstitial lung disease. There is uniform filling of alveolar spaces by macrophages and mild alveolar septal widening.

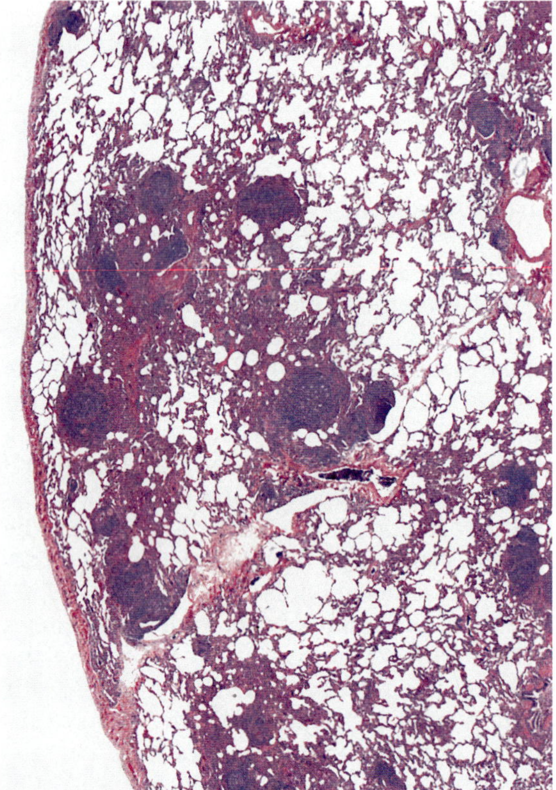

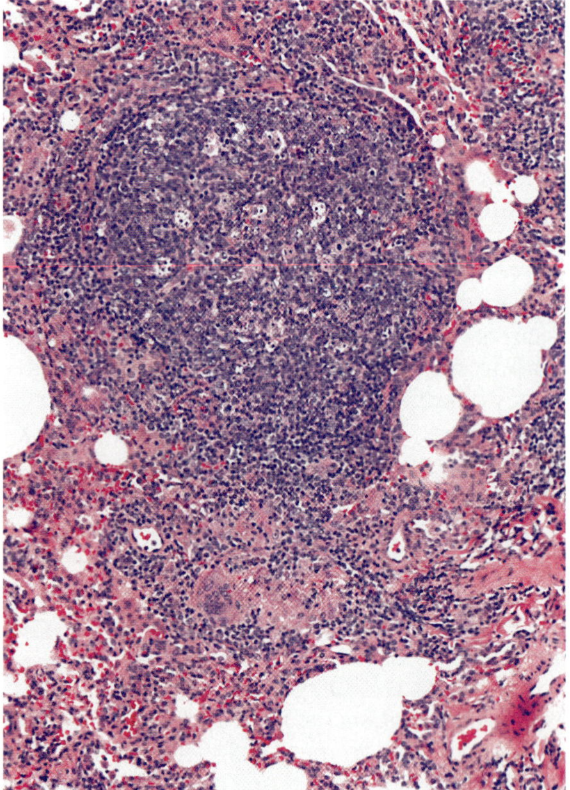

Figure 11-84

DIFFUSE LYMPHOID HYPERPLASIA ASSOCIATED WITH IMMUNOGLOBULIN DEFICIENCY

Left: This 12-year-old with interstitial lung disease was found to have serum deficiencies of both IgG and IgA. Biopsy shows the pattern of diffuse lymphoid hyperplasia.

Right: Detail shows a germinal center and an adjacent giant cell granuloma.

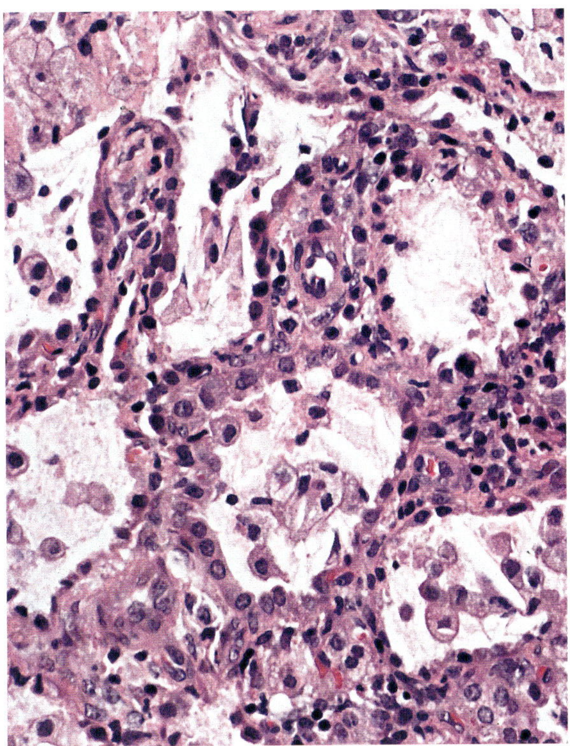

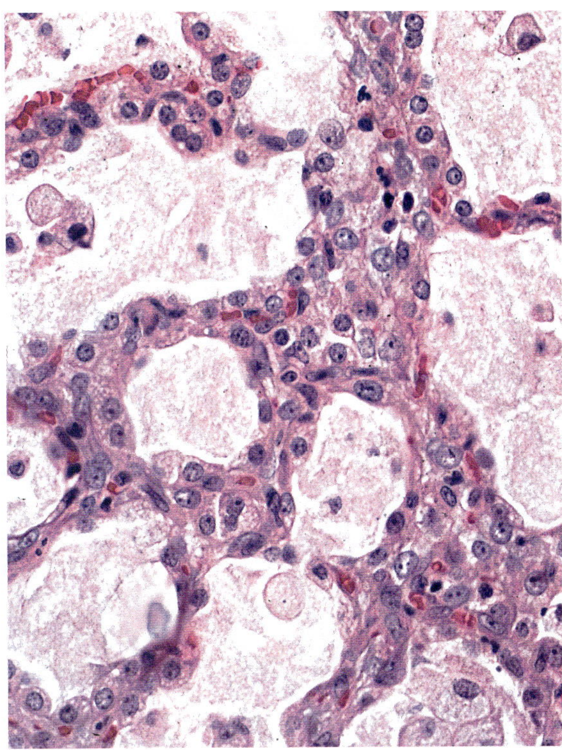

Figure 11-85

CONGENITAL SURFACTANT PROTEIN B DEFICIENCY

Left: Biopsy from a neonate with respiratory distress syndrome shows mild alveolar septal widening and hypercellularity with some increase in alveolar macrophages, some of which are foamy.

Right: In addition, there is material reminiscent of alveolar proteinosis.

diagnosis of surfactant protein B deficiency can be made by bronchoalveolar lavage (BAL), lung biopsy material immunostained for surfactant proteins, or ultrastructural examination. Deficiency of lamellar bodies in alveolar type 2 cells is recognized ultrastructurally and may also show a DIP-like pattern (52).

Vascular disease accounts for a significant proportion of cases of pediatric interstitial lung disease (fig. 11-86) (64). In a review by Sondheimer et al. (153), 8 of 92 children (9 percent) who presented initially as having pediatric interstitial lung disease ultimately were diagnosed as having vascular disease. The diagnoses in this series included total anomalous pulmonary venous return, pulmonary hemangiomatosis, hereditary hemorrhagic telangiectasia, left pulmonary vein stenosis, partial anomalous pulmonary venous return, right pulmonary vein atresia, and pulmonary vein stenosis. In the neonate, alveolar capillary dysplasia with misalignment of pulmonary veins (see above) may manifest as severe respiratory failure.

Cellular interstitial pneumonitis in infants was described in 1992 by Schroeder et al. (33, 148) in five infants who presented in the immediate neonatal period with tachypnea and radiologic findings of interstitial lung disease. The histology showed septal widening by infiltrates of cells resembling histiocytes without significant fibrosis. The authors called attention to distinguishing this condition from usual, desquamative, and lymphocytic interstitial pneumonias. The etiology was not identified. Three of the initial five patients recovered, one had persistent symptoms and radiologic abnormalities, and one died of progressive pulmonary fibrosis. Whether cellular interstitial pneumonitis is an entity or overlaps with other entities described herein is unclear. There are anecdotal reports of chloroquine being associated with improvement in this condition (33).

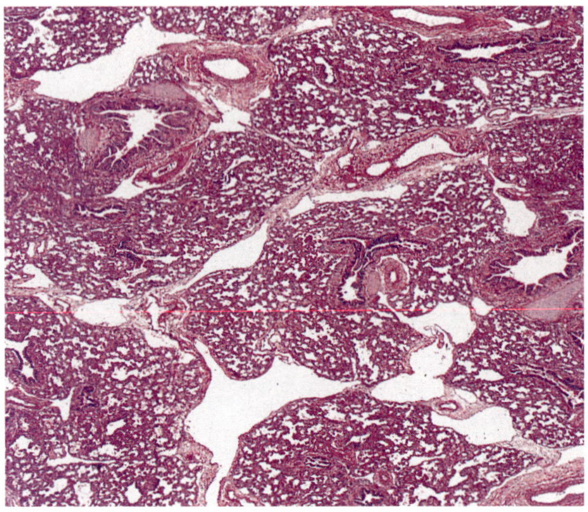

Figure 11-86

LYMPHANGIECTASIA IN CONGENITAL HEART DISEASE

This biopsy is from an infant who presented as having interstitial lung disease but was ultimately shown to have a complex cardiac anomaly with associated lymphangiectasia that resulted in interstitial lung disease.

Chronic pneumonitis of infancy was described by Katzenstein et al. (93) in 1995 in nine infants and young children. Pathologically, these cases were characterized by marked alveolar septal thickening and airspace abnormalities (fig. 11-87). Septa were widened by spindle-shaped cells as well as striking hyperplasia of type 2 pneumocytes. Lymphocytes, plasma cells, and other inflammatory cells were relatively scant and there was no significant scarring. The interstitial cell nuclei and type 2 nuclei imparted the "cellular" appearance to the interstitium. The airspaces showed an increase in alveolar macrophages, at least focally, in all cases and in six they were prominent. Two cases had some hemosiderin in macrophages. Six cases showed patchy airspace material resembling that in pulmonary alveolar proteinosis, particularly in a subpleural distribution, usually focal and affecting only a small percentage of airspaces. Cholesterol clefts were occasionally present. The age at onset was from 2 weeks to 11 months, and the age at biopsy varied from 2 1/2 months to 18 months. Six of the nine patients had follow-up: two died of complications directly (1 patient) or indirectly (1 patient) related to the lung disease, one had a single lung transplantation 15 1/2 months after onset of symptoms, two were stable with persistent symptoms after treatment with steroids and hydroxychloroquine, and one improved on steroids but had relapses when steroids were tapered.

There is probably some overlap between cellular interstitial pneumonitis in infants and chronic pneumonitis of infancy, and it is possible this series could have included cases of congenital surfactant deficiency, either surfactant B deficiency or absence of lamellar bodies in alveolar type 2 cells, since the study predated the description of those entities.

Nonspecific interstitial pneumonia (NSIP) is a recently described pattern that characterizes a portion of cases of interstitial pneumonia, particularly in adults with idiopathic interstitial pneumonia (see chapter 3). NSIP may be seen in children (fig. 11-88), and in the series of Coren et al. (47), 6 of 27 children with diffuse interstitial lung disease who had surgical lung biopsy showed this pattern. One suspects that NSIP would probably be descriptive of cases in older series of pediatric interstitial lung disease that had been given some other label, such as usual interstitial pneumonia.

Extrinsic allergic alveolitis in children is usually due to exposure to avian antigen (bird fancier's lung) (74).

Usual interstitial pneumonia (UIP) rarely, if ever, occurs in children. This diagnosis has been included among reviews of pediatric interstitial lung disease but with the relatively strict definition of UIP currently in use (chapter 3), we have not encountered it in children, and that correlates with the recent experience of others (47,129). Many of the cases previously given a diagnosis of UIP probably would be characterized as cellular interstitial pneumonitis, chronic pneumonitis of infancy, or NSIP.

Interstitial lung disease in general and interstitial pneumonias in particular are much less understood and characterized in children than in adults. Among the interstitial pneumonias there appears to be considerable overlap among the groups described above. Pediatric interstitial lung disease is complicated by the fact that in addition to the idiopathic interstitial pneumonias, there is a subset of patients with

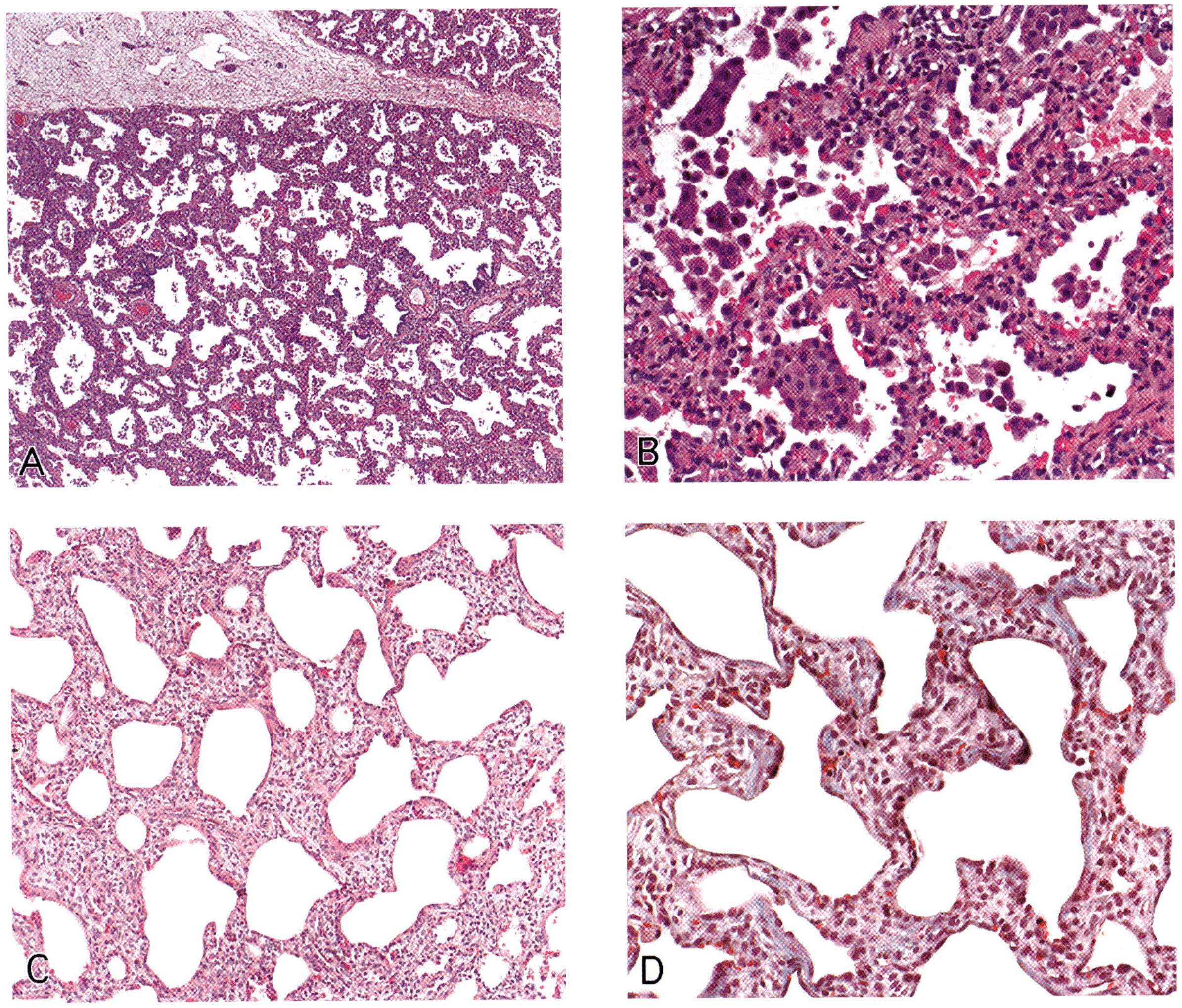

Figure 11-87

CHRONIC PNEUMONITIS OF INFANCY/CELLULAR PNEUMONITIS OF INFANTS

AB: There is hypercellularity of alveolar walls primarily due to type 2 cell and interstitial cell nuclei with relatively little chronic inflammation (A). There is a patchy increase in alveolar macrophages, including some alveoli containing intra-alveolar proteinaceous material reminiscent of proteinosis (B). (This case of chronic pneumonitis of infancy was courtesy of Dr. Anna L. Katzenstein, Syracuse, NY.)

C,D: The alveolar walls are uniformly thickened by chronic inflammatory cells and fibrous tissue. (This case of cellular interstitial pneumonits of infants courtesy of Dr. Eugene Mark, Boston, MA.)

congenital defects (exemplified by surfactant B protein deficiency) who may simulate an idiopathic interstitial pneumonia. From the practical point of view, any neonate with interstitial pneumonia should be rigorously evaluated for the possibility of metabolic defects.

Differential Diagnosis, Treatment, and Prognosis. The differential diagnosis, therapy, and prognosis for patients with pediatric interstitial lung disease vary with the entities, most of which are discussed above or are covered in other sections.

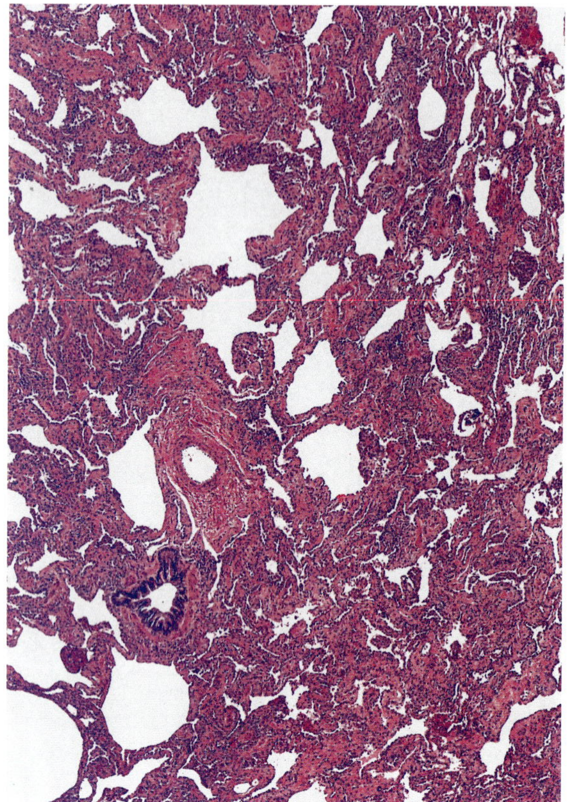

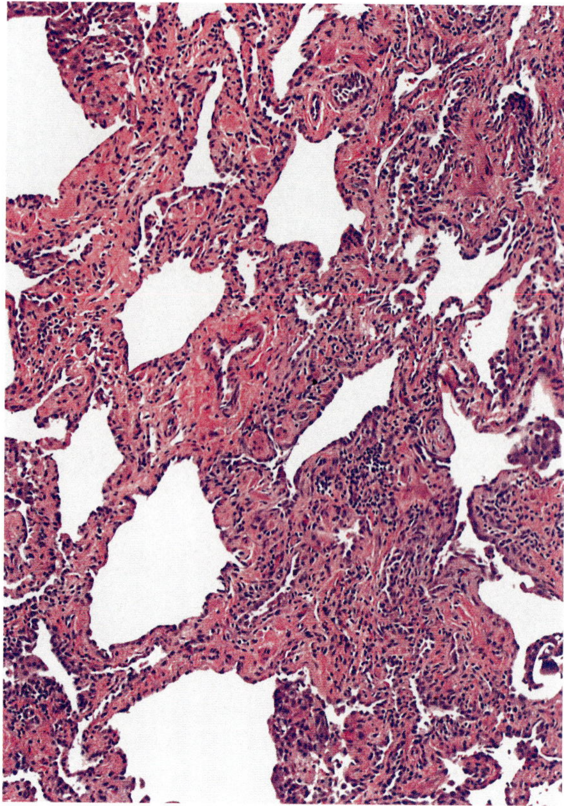

Figure 11-88

NONSPECIFIC INTERSTITIAL PNEUMONIA

Biopsy from this child shows distortion of lung architecture with some simplification of airspaces (left), mild interstitial fibrosis, and an inflammatory infiltrate (right). This patient's brother also had interstitial lung disease, raising the possibility of a familial process.

REFERENCES

1. Abman SH, Groothius JR. Pathophysiology and treatment of bronchopulmonary dysplasia. Current issues. Pediatr Clinics North Am 1994;41:277–315.
2. Adam A, MacSweeney JE, Whyte MK, Smith PL, Ind PW. CT-guided extrapleural drainage of bronchogenic cyst. J Comput Assist Tomogr 1989;13:1065–8.
3. Adzick NS, Harrison MR. Management of the fetus with a cystic adenomatoid malformation. World J Surg 1993;17:342–9.
4. Aktogu S, Yuncu G, Halilcolar H, Ermete S, Buduneli T. Bronchogenic cysts: clinicopathological presentation and treatment. Eur Respir J 1996;9:2017–21.
5. Albright EB, Crane JP, Shackelford GF. Prenatal diagnosis of bronchogenic cyst. J Ultrasound Med 1988;7:91–5.
6. Anderson WR. Bronchopulmonary dysplasia: a correlative study of light, scanning, and transmission electron microscopy. Ultrastruct Pathol 1990;14:221–32.
7. Anderson WR, Engel RR. Cardiopulmonary sequelae of reparative stages of bronchopulmonary dysplasia. Arch Pathol Lab Med 1983;107:603–8.
8. Armin A, Castelli M. Congenital adrenal tissue in the lung with adrenal cytomegaly. Case report and review of the literature. Am J Clin Pathol 1984;82:225–8.
9. Askenazi SS, Perlman M. Pulmonary hypoplasia: lung weight and radial alveolar count as criteria of diagnosis. Arch Dis Child 1979;54:614–8.

10. Aulicino MR, Reis ED, Dolgin SE, Unger PD, Shah KD. Intra-abdominal pulmonary sequestration exhibiting congenital cystic adenomatoid malformation. Report of a case and review of the literature. Arch Pathol Lab Med 1994; 118:1034–7.
11. Avery ME, Gatewood OB, Brumley G. Transient tachypnea of newborn. Possible delayed resorption of fluid at birth. Amer J Dis Child 1966;111:380–5.
12. Avitabile AM, Greco MA, Hulnick DH, Feiner HD. Congenital cystic adenomatoid malformation of the lung in adults. Am J Surg Pathol 1984;8:193–202.
13. Bacsik RD. Meconium aspiration syndrome. Pediatr Clinics North Am 1977;24:463–79.
14. Bale PM. Congenital cystic malformation of the lung. A form of congenital bronchiolar ("adenomatoid") malformation. Am J Clin Pathol 1979;71:411–20.
15. Bando T, Genka K, Ishikawa K, Kuniyoshi M, Kuda T. Ectopic intrapulmonary thyroid. Chest 1993;103:1278–9.
16. Benjamin B, Inglis A. Minor congenital laryngeal clefts: diagnosis and classification. Ann Otol Rhinol Laryngol 1989;98:417–20.
17. Benjamin DR, Cahill JL. Bronchioloalveolar carcinoma of the lung and congenital cystic adenomatoid malformation. Am J Clin Pathol 1991;95:889–92.
18. Benning TL, Godwin JD, Roggli VL, Askin FB. Cartilaginous variant of congenital adenomatoid malformation of the lung. Chest 1987;92:514–6.
19. Benya EC, Bulas DI, Selby DM, Rosenbaum KN. Cystic sonographic appearance of extralobar pulmonary sequestration. Pediatr Radiol 1993;23:605–07.
20. Berlinger NT, Porto DP, Thompson TR. Infantile lobar emphysema. Ann Otol Rhinol Laryngol 1987;96:106–11.
21. Blayney M, Kerem E, Whyte H, O'Brodovich HM. Bronchopulmonary dysplasia: impairment in lung function between 7 and 10 years of age. J Pediatr 1991;1188:201–6.
22. Bokulic RE, Hilman BC. Interstitial lung disease in children. Pediatr Clin North Am 1994;41:543–67.
23. Bonikos DS, Bensch KG, Northway WH, Edwards DK. Bronchopulmonary dysplasia: the pulmonary pathologic sequel of necrotizing bronchiolitis and pulmonary fibrosis. Hum Pathol 1976;7:643–66.
24. Bozic C. Ectopic fetal adrenal cortex in the lung of a newborn. Virchows Arch [A] 1974;363:371–4.
25. Brewer LL, Moskowitz PS, Carrington CB, Bensch KG. Pneumatosis pulmonalis: a complication of the idiopathic respiratory distress syndrome. Am J Pathol 1979;95:171–90.
26. Brink DA, Balsara ZN. Prenatal ultrasound detection of intra-abdominal pulmonary sequestration with postnatal MR correlation. Pediatr Radiol 1991;21:227.
27. Cairns RA, Culham JA, Stringer DA, Murphy JJ. Pediatric case of the day. Hypogenetic lung syndrome (scimitar syndrome) with right-sided congenital diaphragmatic hernia. Radiographics 1995;15:496–9.
28. Campo E, Bombi JA. Central nervous system heterotopia in the lung of a fetus with cranial malformation. Virchows Arch [A] 1981;391:117–22.
29. Case Records of the Massachusetts General Hospital. Weekly clinicopathological exercises. Case 32-1990. A newborn boy with respiratory distress, and opacified left hemithorax and a mediastinal shift. N Engl J Med 1990;323:398–406.
30. Case Records of the Massachusetts General Hospital. Weekly clinicopathological exercises. Case 13-1992. A full-term newborn boy with chronic respiratory distress. N Engl J Med 1992;326:875–84.
31. Case Records of the Massachusetts General Hospital. Weekly clinicopathological exercises. Case 20-1996. A newborn triplet with episodes of respiratory distress and a pulmonary mass. N Engl J Med 1996;334:1726–32.
32. Case Records of the Massachusetts General Hospital. Weekly clinicopathological exercises. Case 30-1997. A preterm newborn female triplet with diffuse cystic changes in the left lung. N Engl J Med 1997;337:916–24.
33. Case Records of the Massachusetts General Hospital. Weekly clinicopathological exercises. Case 40-1999. A four-month-old girl with chronic cyanosis and diffuse pulmonary infiltrates. N Engl J Med. 1999;341:2075–83.
34. Castile RG, Kleinberg F. The pathogenesis and management of massive pulmonary hemorrhage in the neonate. Case report of a normal survivor. Mayo Clin Proc 1976;51:155–8.
35. Cerruti MM, Marmolejos F, Cacciarelli T. Bilateral intralobar pulmonary sequestration with horseshoe lung. Ann Thorac Surg 1993;55:509–10.
36. Cha I, Adzick NS, Harrison MR, Finkbeiner WE. Fetal congenital cystic adenomatoid malformations of the lung: a clinicopathologic study of eleven cases. Am J Surg Pathol 1997;2:537–44.
37. Chen MF, Onerheim R, Wang NS, Huttner I. Rhabdomyomatosis of newborn lung: a case report with immunohistochemical and electron microscopic characterization of striated muscle cells in the lung. Pediatr Pathol 1991;11:123–9.

38. Chen WJ, Kelly MM, Shaw CM, Mottet NK. Pathogenic mechanisms of heterotopic neural tissue associated with anencephaly. Hum Pathol 1982;13:179–82.
39. Chetcuti PA, Ball RJ. Surfactant apoprotein B deficiency. Arch Dis Child Fetal Neonatal Ed 1995;73:F125–7.
40. Chi JG, Shong YK. Diffuse striated muscle heteroplasia of the lung. An autopsy case. Arch Pathol Lab Med 1982;106:641–4.
41. Cioffi U, Bonavina L, De Simone M, et al. Presentation and surgical management of bronchogenic and esophageal duplications cysts in adults. Chest 1998;113:1492–6.
42. Cloutier MM, Schaeffer DA, Hight D. Congenital cystic adenomatoid malformation. Chest 1993;103:761–4.
43. Coalson JJ, Winter V, deLemos RA. Decreased alveolarization in baboon survivors with bronchopulmonary dysplasia. Am J Respir Crit Care Med 1995;152:640–6.
43a. Conran RM, Stocker JT. Extralobar sequestration with frequently associated congenital cystic adenomatoid malformation, type 2: report of 50 cases. Pediatr Dev Pathol 1999;2:454–63.
44. Cooney TP, Thurlbeck WM. Pulmonary hypoplasia in Down's syndrome. N Eng J Med 1982;307:1170–3.
45. Cooney TP, Wentworth PJ, Thurlbeck WM. Diminished radial count is found only postnatally in Down's syndrome. Pediatr Pulmonol 1988;5:204–9.
46. Copley SJ, Coren M, Nicholson AG, Rubens MB, Bush A, Hansell DM. Diagnostic accuracy of thin-section CT and chest radiography of pediatric interstitial lung disease. AJR Am J Roentgenol 2000;174:549–54.
47. Coren ME, Nicholson AG, Goldstraw P, Rosenthal M, Bush A. Open lung biopsy for diffuse interstitial lung disease in children. Eur Respir J 1999;14:817–21.
48. Corrin B, Danel C, Allaway A, Warner J, Lenney W. Intralobar pulmonary sequestration of ectopic pancreatic tissue with gastropancreatic duplication. Thorax 1985;40:637–8.
49. Coselli MP, de Ipolyi P, Bloss RS, Diaz RF, Fitzgerald JB. Bronchogenic cysts above and below the diaphragm: report of eight cases. Ann Thorac Surg 1987;44:491–4.
50. Critchley PS, Forrester-Wood CP, Ridley PD. Adult congenital lobar emphysema in pregnancy. Thorax 1995;50:909–10.
51. Cumming WA. Neonatal radiology. Esophageal atresia and tracheoesophageal fistula. Radiol Clin North Am 1975;13:277–95.
52. Cutz E, Wert SE, Nogee LM, Moore AM. Deficiency of lamellar bodies in alveolar type II cells associated with fatal respiratory disease in a full-term infant. Am J Respir Crit Care Med 2000;161:608–14.
53. deMello DE, Heyman S, Phelps DS, et al. Ultrastructure of lung in surfactant protein B deficiency. Am J Respir Cell Mol Biol 1994;11: 230–9.
54. de Sa DJ. Pulmonary fluid contents in infants with respiratory distress. J Pathol 1969;97:469–78.
55. Doggett RS, Carty SE, Clarke MR. Retroperitoneal bronchogenic cyst masquerading clinically and radiologically as a phaeochromocytoma. Virchows Arch 1997;431:73–6.
56. Dubin SB. Assessment of fetal lung maturity. Practice parameter. Am J Clin Pathol 1998;110:723–32.
57. Dutton JA, Jackson JE, Hughes JM, et al. Pulmonary arteriovenous malformations: results of treatment with coil embolization in 53 patients. AJR Am J Roentgenol 1995;165:1119–25.
58. Edwards DK, Colby TV, Northway WH Jr. Radiographic-pathologic correlation in bronchopulmonary dysplasia. J Pediatr 1979;95:834–6.
59. Elliott LP. Complex heart disease. In: Taveras JM, Ferrucci JT, eds. Radiology: diagnosis, imaging, intervention, vol 2. Philadelphia: Lippincott-Raven; 1996:1–36.
60. Emery JH, Mithal A. The number of alveoli in the terminal respiratory unit of man duirng the late intrauterine life and childhood. Arch Dis Child 1960;35:544–7.
61. Erickson AM, de la Monte SM, Moore GW, Hutchins GM. The progression of morphologic changes in bronchopulmonary dysplasia. Am J Pathol 1987;127:474–84.
62. Evans ED, Kramer SS, Kravitz RM. Pediatric diseases of the lower airways. Semin Roentgenol 1998;33:136–50.
63. Faix FG, Viscardi RM, DiPietro MA, Nicks JJ. Adult respiratory distress syndrome in full-term infants. Pediatrics 1989;83:971–6.
64. Fan LL, Langston C. Chronic interstitial lung disease in children. Pediatr Pulmonol 1993;16:184–96.
65. Fan LL, Mullen AL, Brugman SM, Inscore SC, Parks DP, White CW. Clinical spectrum of chronic interstitial lung disease in children. J Pediatr 1992;121:867–72.
66. Faro RS, Goodwin CD, Organ CH Jr, et al. Tracheal agenesis. Ann Thor Surg 1979;28:295–9.
67. Faul JL, Berry GJ, Colby TV, et al. Thoracic lymphangiomas, lymphangiectasis, lymphangiomatosis, and lymphatic dysplasia syndrome. Am J Respir Crit Care Med 2000;161:1037–46.

68. Fraser RS, Pare JA, Fraser RG, Pare PD. Pulmonary abnormalities of developmental origin. In: Fraser RS, Pare JA, Fraser RG, Pare PD, eds. Synopsis of diseases of the chest, 2nd ed. Philadelphia: WB Saunders; 1994:256–86.
69. Fraser RG, Pare JA, Pare PD, Fraser RS, Genereux GP. Neoplastic disease of the lungs. In: Fraser RG, Pare JA, Pare PD, Fraser RS, Genereux GP, eds. Diagnosis of diseases of the chest, 3rd ed. Philadelphia: WB Saunders; 1989:1327–699.
70. Frazier AA, Rosado de Christenson ML, Stocker JT, Templeton PA. Intralobar sequestration: radiologic-pathologic correlation. Radiographics 1997;17:725–45.
71. Freedom RM, Burrows PE, Moes CA. "Horseshoe" lung: report of five new cases. AJR Am J Roentgenol 1986;146:211–5.
72. Freedom RM, Fellows KE Jr. Radiographic visceral patterns in the asplenia syndrome. Radiology 1973;106:387–91.
73. Gerle RD, Jaretzki A III, Ashley CA, Berne AS. Congenital bronchopulmonary foregut malformation. Pulmonary sequestration communicating with the gastrointestinal tract. N Engl J Med 1968;278:1413–9.
74. Grech V, Vella C, Lenicker H. Pigeon breeder's lung in childhood: varied clinical picture at presentation. Pediatr Pulmonol 2000;30:145–8.
75. Griffin GK, Tatu WF, Fisher LM, Keats TE, Tegtmeyer CJ, Fechner RE. Systemic lymphangiomatosis: a combined diagnostic approach of lymphangiography and computed tomography. J Comput Tomogr 1986;10:335–9.
76. Gross TL, Sokol RJ, Kwong MS, Wilson M, Kuhnert PM. Transient tachypnea of the newborn: the relationship to preterm delivery and significant neonatal morbidity. Am J Obstet Gynecol 1983;146:236–41.
77. Gruenwald P, Minh HN. Evaluation of body and organ weights in perinatal pathology. Am J Clin Pathol 1960;34:247–53.
78. Harrison MR, Adzick NS, Jennings RW, et al. Antenatal intervention for congenital cystic adenomatoid malformation. Lancet 1990;336: 965–7.
79. Heithoff KB, Sane SM, Williams HJ, et al. Bronchopulmonary foregut malformations. A unifying etiological concept. AJR Am J Roentgenol 1976;126:46–55.
80. Hernandez RJ, Stern AM, Rosenthal A. Pulmonary lymphangiectasis in Noonan syndrome. AJR 1980;134:75–80.
81. Hertzberg BS, Bowie JD. Fetal gastrointestinal abnormalities. Radiol Clin North Am 1990;28: 101–14.
82. Hibbard LT, Schumann WR, Goldstein GE. Thoracic endometriosis: a review and report of two cases. Am J Obstet Gynecol 198;140: 227–32.
83. Hilliard RI, McKendry JB, Phillip MJ. Congenital abnormalities of the lymphatic system: a new clinical classification. Pediatrics 1990;86: 988–94.
84. Hoffman RR Jr, Campbell RE, Decker JP. Fetal aspiration syndrome. Clinical, roentgenologic and pathologic features. Am J Roentgenol Radium Ther Nuc Med 1974;122:90–6.
85. Hruban RH, Shumway SJ, Orel SB, Dumler JS, Baker RR, Hutchins GM. Congenital bronchopulmonary foregut malformations. Intralobar and extralobar pulmonary sequestrations communicating with the foregut. Am J Clin Pathol 1989;91:403–9.
86. Husain AN, Siddiqui NH, Stocker JT. Pathology of arrested acinar development in postsurfactant bronchopulmonary dysplasia. Hum Pathol 1998;29:710–7.
87. Jackson JC, Mackenzie AP, Chi EY, Standaert TA, Truog WE, Hodson WA. Mechanisms for reduced total lung capacity at birth during hyaline membrane disease in premature newborn monkeys. Am Rev Resp Dis 1990;142: 413–9.
88. Jederlinic PJ, Sicilian LS, Baigelman W, Gaensler EA. Congenital bronchial atresia. A report of four cases and a review of the literature. Medicine (Baltimore) 1987;66:73–83.
89. Johnston RF, Green RA. Tracheobronchomegaly. Report of five cases and demonstration of familial occurrence. Am Resp Dis 1965; 91:35–50.
90. Joshi VV, Kasznica J, Ali Khan MA, Amato JJ, Levine OR. Cystic lung disease in Down's syndrome. A report of two cases. Pediatric Pathol 1986;5:79–86.
91. Katz I, LeVine M, Herman P. Tracheobronchomegaly. The Mounier-Kuhn syndrome. AJR Am J Roentgenol 1962;88:1084–94.
92. Katzenstein AL. Katzenstein and Askin's surgical pathology of non-neoplastic lung disease, 3rd ed. Philadelphia: WB Saunders; 1997;361–92.
93. Katzenstein AL, Gordon LP, Oliphant M, Swender PT. Chronic pneumonitis of infancy. A unique form of interstitial lung disease occurring in early childhood. Am J Surg Pathol 1995;19:439–47.
94. Kellett HS, Lipphard D, Willis RA. Two unusual examples of heteroplasia in the lung. J Pathol Bacteriol 1962;84:421–5.
95. Kennedy CD, Habibi P, Matthew DJ, Gordon I. Lobar emphysema: long-term imaging follow-up. Radiology 1991;180:189–93.

96. Kershisnik MM, Kaplan C, Craven CM, Carey JC, Townsend JJ, Knisely AS. Intrapulmonary neuroglial heterotopia. Arch Pathol Lab Med 1992;116:1043–6.
97. Kinsella D, Sissons G, Williams MP. The radiological diagnosis of bronchial atresia. Br J Radiol 1992;65:681–5.
98. Kliegman RM. Respiratory tract disorders. In: Nelson WE, ed. Nelson's textbook of pediatrics, 15th ed. Philadelphia: WB Saunders; 1996:476–90.
99. Kraybill EN, Runyan DK, Bose CL, Khan JH. Risk factors for chronic lung disease in infants with birth weights of 751 to 1000 grams. J Pediatr 1989;115:115–20.
100. Kresch MJ, Lin WH, Thrall RS. Surfactant replacement therapy. Thorax 1996;51:1137–54.
101. Kuhn JP, Slovis TL, Silverman FN, Kuhns LR. Diseases of the airways and abnormalities of pulmonary aeration. In: Silverman FN, Kuhn JP, eds. Caffey's pediatric X-ray diagnosis. An integrated imaging approach, 9th ed. St. Louis: Mosby; 1993:465–510.
102. Kuhn JP, Slovis TL, Silverman FN, Kuhns LR. Normal lung and anomalies. In: Silverman FN, Kuhn JP, eds. Caffey's pediatric X-ray diagnosis, 9th ed. St. Louis: Mosby; 1993:443–63.
103. Landing BH. Five syndromes (malformation complexes) of pulmonary symmetry, congenital heart disease, and multiple spleens. Pediatr Pathol 1984;2:125–51.
104. Landing BH, Dixon LG. Congenital malformations and genetic disorders of the respiratory tract (larynx, trachea, bronchi, and lungs). Am Rev Respir Dis 1979;120:151–85.
105. Langer B, Donato L, Riethmuller C, et al. Spontaneous regression of fetal pulmonary sequestration. Ultrasound Obstet Gynecol 1995;6:33–9.
106. Langston C, Askin FB. Pulmonary disorders in the neonate, infant, and child. In: Thurlbeck WM, Churg AM, eds. Pathology of the lung, 2nd ed. New York: Thieme; 1995:151–94.
107. Lauria MR, Gonik B, Romero R. Pulmonary hypoplasia: pathogenesis, diagnosis, and antenatal prediction. Obst Gyn 1995;86:466–75.
108. Lauweryns JM. Hyaline membrane disease in newborn infants. Macroscopic radiographic, light and electron microscopic studies. Hum Pathol 1970;1:175–204.
109. Leonidas JC, Berdon W. The neonatal chest. In: Silverman FN, Kuhn JP, eds. Caffey's pediatric X-ray diagnosis: an integrated imaging approach, 9th ed. St. Louis: Mosby; 1993;1969–2028.
110. Long WA, Corbett A. Respiratory distress syndrome in premature newborn infants. In: Fishman AP, ed. Fishman's pulmonary diseases and disorders, 3rd ed. New York: McGraw-Hill; 1998:2575–87.
111. Louie HW, Martin SM, Mulder DG. Pulmonary sequestration: 17-year experience at UCLA. Am Surg 1993;59:804–5.
112. Luck SR, Reynolds M, Raffensperger JG. Congenital bronchopulmonary malformations. Curr Probl Surg 1986;23:245–314.
113. Lynch DA, Hay T, Newell JD Jr, Divgi VD, Fan LL. Pediatric diffuse lung disease: diagnosis and classification using high-resolution CT. AJR Am J Roentgenol 1999;173:713–18.
114. Lyon RD, McAdams HP. Mediastinal bronchogenic cyst: demonstration of a fluid-fluid level at MR-imaging. Radiology 193;186:427–8.
115. Manning FA, Schreiber J, Turkel SB. Fatal meconium aspiration "in utero": a case report. Am J Obstet Gynecol 1978;132:111–3.
116. Mardini MK, Nyhan WL. Agenesis of the lung: report of four patients with unusual anomalies. Chest 1985;87:522–7.
117. Mata JM, Caceres J, Lucaya J, Garcia-Conesa JA. CT of congenital malformations of the lung. Radiographics 1990;10:651–74.
118. Mendoza A, Voland J, Wolf P, Benirschke K. Supradiaphragmatic liver in the lung. Arch Pathol Lab Med 1986;110:1085–6.
119. Meng RL, Jensik RJ, Faber LP, Matthew GR, Kittle CF. Bronchial atresia. Ann Thor Surg 1978;25:184–92.
120. Miller RK, Sieber WK, Yunis EJ. Congenital adenomatoid malformation of the lung. A report of 17 cases and review of the literature. Pathol Annu 1980;15[Pt 1]:387–402.
121. Moerman P, Fryns JP, Vandenberghe K, Devlieger H, Lauweryns JM. Pathogenesis of congenital cystic adenomatoid malformation of the lung. Histopathology 1992;21:315–21.
122. Moller JH, Nakib A, Anderson RC, Edwards JE. Congenital cardiac disease associated with polysplenia. A developmental complex of bilateral "left-sidedness." Circulation 1967;36:789–99.
123. Morad NA, al-Malki T, e-Tahir M. Intra-abdominal pulmonary sequestration: diagnostic difficulties. Pathology 1997;29:218–20.
124. Morgenstern B, Klionsky B, Doshi N. Yellow hyaline membrane disease. Identification of the pigment and bilirubin binding. Lab Invest 1981;44:514–8.
125. Nakamura Y. Pulmonary disorders in infants. Acta Pathol Jpn 1993;43:347–59.
126. Nakata H. Egashira K, Watanabe H, et al. MRI of bronchogenic cysts. J Comput Assist Tomogr 1993;17:267–370.

127. Nathan L, Leveno KJ, Carmody TJ 3rd, Kelly MA, Sherman ML. Meconium: a 1990's perspective on an old obstetrical hazard. Obstet Gynecol 1994;83:329–32.
128. Newman B, Yunis E. Lobar emphysema associated with respiratory syncytial virus pneumonia. Pediatric Radiol 1995;25:646–8.
129. Nicholson AG, Kim H, Corrin B, et al. The value of classifying interstitial pneumonitis in childhood according to defined histological patterns. Histopathology 1998;33:203–11.
130. Nickerson BG. Bronchopulmonary dysplasia. Chronic pulmonary disease following neonatal respiratory failure. Chest 1985;87:528–35.
131. Nogee L. Surfactant protein B-deficiency. Chest 1997;111[Suppl]:129S–35S.
132. Nogee LM, de Mello DE, Dehner LP, Colten HR. Brief report: deficiency of pulmonary surfactant protein B in congenital alveolar proteinosis. N Engl J Med 1993;328:406–10.
133. Northway WH Jr, Moss RB, Carlisle KB, et al. Late pulmonary sequelae of bronchopulmonary dysplasia. N Engl J Med 1990;323:1793–9.
134. Northway WH Jr, Rosan RC, Porter DY. Pulmonary disease following respiratory therapy of hyaline-membrane disease. Bronchopulmonary dysplasia. N Engl J Med 1967;276:357–68.
135. O'Brodovich HM. Immature epithelial Na+ channel expression is one of the pathogenetic mechanisms leading to human neonatal respiratory distress syndrome. Proc Assoc Am Phys 1996;108:345–55.
136. O'Brodovich HM. Respiratory distress syndrome: the importance of effective transport. J Pediatr 1997;130:342–4.
137. O'Brodovich HM, Mellins RB. Bronchopulmonary dysplasia: unresolved neonatal acute lung injury. Am Rev Respir Dis 1985;132:694–709.
138. Ostor AG, Fortune DW. Congenital cystic adenomatoid malformation of the lung. Am J Clin Pathol 1978;70:595–604.
139. Page DV, Stocker JT. Anomalies associated with pulmonary hypoplasia. Am Rev Respir Dis 1982;125:216–21.
140. Pierce MR, Bancalari E. The role of inflammation in the pathogenesis of bronchopulmonary dysplasia. Ped Pulmonology 1995;19:371–8.
141. Reed JC, Sobonya RE. Morphologic analysis of foregut cysts in the thorax. Am J Roentgen Rad Ther Nucl Med 1976;120:851–60.
142. Rogers LF, Osmer JC. Bronchogenic cyst. A review of 46 cases. Am J Roentgen Rad Ther Nucl Med 1964;91:273–90.
143. Rosado de Christenson ML, Frazier AA, Stocker JT, Templeton PA. Extralobar sequestrations: radiologic-pathologic correlation. Radiographics 1993;13:429–41.
144. Rosado de Christenson ML, Stocker JT. Congenital cystic adenomatoid malformation. Radiographics 1991;11:865–86.
145. Rosan RC. Hyaline membrane disease and a related spectrum of neonatal pneumopathies. Perspect Pediatr Pathol 1975;2:15–60.
146. Rozycki HJ, Kirkpatrick BV. New developments in bronchopulmonary dysplasia. Pediatr Ann 1993;22:532–8.
147. Salyer DC, Salyer WR, Eggleston JC. Benign developmental cysts of the mediastinum. Arch Pathol Lab Med 1977;101:136–9.
148. Schroeder SA, Shannon DC, Mark EJ. Cellular interstitial pneumonitis in infants. A clinicopathologic study. Chest 1992;101:1065–9.
149. Sedivy R. Bankl HC, Stimpfl T, Bankl H, Kurkciyan I. Sudden, unexpected death of a young marathon runner as a result of bronchial malformation. Mod Pathol 1997;10:247–51.
150. Seo IS, Gillim SE, Mirkin LD. Hyaline membranes in post-mature infants. Pediatric Pathol 1990;10:539–48.
151. Sheffield EA, Addis BJ, Corrin B, McCabe MM. Epithelial hyperplasia and malignant change in congenital lung cysts. J Clin Pathol 1987;40:612–4.
152. Sobonya RE, Logvinoff MM, Taussig LM, Theriault A. Morphometric analysis of the lung in prolonged bronchopulmonary dysplasia. Pediatr Res 1982;16:969–72.
153. Sondheimer HM, Lung MC, Brugman SM, Ikle DN, Fan LL, White CW. Pulmonary vascular disorders masquerading as interstitial lung disease. Pediatr Pulmonol 1995;20:284–8.
154. Stocker JT. Congenital and developmental diseases. In: Dail DH, Hammer SP, eds. Pulmonary pathology, 2nd ed. New York: Springer-Verlag; 1994:155–90.
155. Stocker JT. Pathologic features of long-standing "healed" bronchopulmonary dysplasia: a study of 28 3- to 40-month-old infants. Hum Pathol 1986;17:943–61.
156. Stocker JT. Sequestrations of the lung. Semin Diagn Pathol 1986;3:106–21.
156a. Stocker JT. The respiratory tract. In Stocker JT, Dehner LP, eds. Pediatric pathology, 2nd ed. Philadelphia: Lippincott, Williams and Wilkins; 2001:466–73.
157. Stocker JT, Dehner LP. Acquired neonatal and pediatric diseases. In: Dail DH, Hammar SP, eds. Pulmonary pathology, 2nd ed. New York: Springer; 1994:191–254.
158. Stocker JT, Drake RM, Madewell JE. Cystic and congenital lung disease in the newborn. Perspect Pediatr Pathol 1978;4:93–154.

159. Stocker JT, Kagan-Hallet K. Extralobar pulmonary sequestration: analysis of 15 cases. Am J Clin Pathol 1979;72:917–25.
160. Stocker JT, Madewell JE. Persistent interstitial pulmonary emphysema: another complication of the respiratory distress syndrome. Pediatrics 1977;59:847–57.
161. Stocker JT, Madewell JE, Drake RM. Congenital cystic adenomatoid malformation of the lung. Classification and morphologic spectrum. Hum Pathol 1977;8:155–71.
162. Swaminathan S, Quinn J, Stabile MW, Bader D, Platzker AC, Keens TG. Long-term pulmonary sequelae of meconium aspiration syndrome. J Pediatr 1989;114:356–61.
163. Swank DW, Hepper NG, Folkert KE, Colby TV. Intrathoracic lymphangiomatosis mimicking lymphangioleiomyomatosis in a young woman. Mayo Clin Proc 1989;64:1264–8.
164. Swensen SJ, Hartman TE, Mayo JR, Colby TV, Tazelaar HD, Müller NL. Diffuse pulmonary lymphangiomatosis: CT findings. J Comput Assist Tomogr 1995;19:348–52.
165. Tazelaar HD, Kerr D, Yousem SA, Saldana MJ, Langston C, Colby TV. Diffuse pulmonary lymphangiomatosis. Hum Pathol 1993;24: 1313–22.
166. Telander RL, Lennox C, Sieber W. Sequestration of the lung in children. Mayo Clin Proc 1976;51:578–84.
167. Thomas DB. Survival after massive pulmonary hemorrhage in the neonatal period. Acta Paediatr Scand 1975;64:825–9.
168. Trompeter R, Yu VY, Aynsley-Green A, Roberton NR. Massive pulmonary hemorrhage in the newborn infant. Arch Dis Child 1975;50:123–7.
169. Vilanova JR, Burgos-Bretones J, Aguirre JM, Rivera-Pomar JM. Rhabdomyomatous dysplasia of lung and congenital diaphragmatic hernia. J Pediatr Surg 1983;18:201–3.
170. Wigglesworth JS, Desai R. use of DNA estimation for growth assessment in normal and hypoplastic fetal lungs. Arch Dis Child 1981;56: 601–5.
171. Wilson MG, Mikity VG, Shinno NW. A new form of respiratory disease in premature infants. Am J Dis Child 1960;99:489–99.
172. Wiswell TE, Bent RC. Meconium staining and the meconium aspiration syndrome. Unresolved issues. Pediatr Clinics NA 1993;40:955–81.
173. Wiswell TE, Tuggle JM, Turner BS. Meconium aspiration syndrome: have we made a difference? Pediatrics 1990;85:715–21.
174. Woodring JH, Howard TA, Kanga JF. Congenital pulmonary venolobar syndrome revisited. Radiographics 1994;14:349–69.
175. Yamaki S, Horiuchi T, Takahashi T. Pulmonary changes in congenital heart disease with Down's syndrome: their significance as a cause of postoperative respiratory failure. Thorax 1985;40:380–6.
176. Yoder BA. Meconium-stained amniotic fluid and respiratory complications: impact of selective tracheal suction. Obstet Gynecol 1994;83:77–84.
177. Zangwill BC, Stocker JT. Congenital cystic adenomatoid malformation within an extralobar pulmonary sequestration. Pediatric Pathol 1993;13:309–15.
178. Zimmerman JJ. Bronchoalveolar inflammatory pathophysiology of bronchopulmonary dysplasia. Clin Perinatol 1995;22:429–56.
179. Zimmerman JJ, Farrell PM. Advances and issues in bronchopulmonary dysplasia. Curr Probs Pediatr 1994;24:159–70.

12
LUNG INFECTIONS

BACTERIAL PNEUMONIAS

Bacterial pneumonia is an inflammation of the lung that usually affects the distal airspaces such as the respiratory bronchioles, alveolar ducts, and alveoli, but often also affects the larynx, trachea, and bronchi (142). Bacterial pneumonias have been classified in several different ways: according to pathogenesis, epidemiology, anatomic distribution, clinical presentation, and specific bacterial agent (Table 12-1) (142).

Primary and Secondary Pneumonias. Primary bacterial pneumonia can be separated into exogenous or endogenous types. The common organisms that cause these two types are summarized in Table 12-2. *Exogenous pneumonias* are caused by the inhalation of aerosolized organisms such as *Mycobacterium tuberculosis* and *Legionella pneumophila*. *Endogenous pneumonias* are associated with the aspiration of oropharyngeal secretions contaminated with bacteria. Secondary pneumonias are associated with hematogenous dissemination from an infection in another organ such as a subcutaneous abscess leading to staphylococcal pneumonia.

Community-Acquired and Nosocomial Pneumonias. The upper respiratory tract is the source of most community-acquired and nosocomial pneumonias (142). The common bacterial organisms responsible for these two major epidemiologic types are summarized in Table 12-3.

Community-acquired pneumonia in patients that do not require hospitalization is most often caused by *Mycoplasma pneumoniae, Chlamydia pneumoniae,* and viral agents. Organisms associated with more severe illness requiring hospitalization are *Staphylococcus pneumoniae,* followed by *Haemophilus influenzae, Mycobacterium pneumoniae, Legionella* sp, *Staphylococcus aureus,* influenza virus, *C. pneumoniae,* and *Klebsiella pneumoniae.*

Nosocomial pneumonias are most often associated with methicillin-resistant *S. aureus,* enteric Gram-negative bacilli, *Pseudomonas aeruginosa, Acinetobacter baumannii,* and anaerobes (55,103,142). Risk factors for nosocomial pneumonia include old age, immunosuppression, factors predisposing to aspiration (impaired consciousness due to neurologic disorders, anesthesia, prolonged intubation), contaminated respiratory equipment, and colonization after

Table 12-1

BACTERIAL PNEUMONIAS BY ORGANISM

Common Bacterial Pneumonia Organisms
- *Streptococcus pneumoniae* (pneumococcus)
- *Staphylococcus aureus*
- Streptococci other than pneumococcus
- *Haemophilus influenzae*
- *Klebsiella pneumonia*
- *Pseudomonas* sp
- *Legionella* sp
- Anaerobic bacteria
- *Nocardia* sp
- *Actinomyces* sp

Uncommon Bacterial Pneumonia Organisms
- *Burkholderia* (formerly *Pseudomonas*) *pseudomallei* (Melioidosis), *Burkholderia cepacia*
- *Francisella tularensis* (Tularemia)
- *Yersinia pestis* (Plague)
- *Rhodococcus equi* (Malakoplakia)
- *Botryomyces*
- *Bartonella henselae* and *B. quintana* (Bacillary angiomatosis)
- *Tropheryma whippelii* (Whipple's disease)

Table 12-2

BACTERIAL PNEUMONIA ACCORDING TO PATHOGENESIS[a]

Endogenous	Exogenous
Streptococcus pneumoniae	*Mycobacterium tuberculosis*
Haemophilus influenzae	*Mycobacterium* sp
Anaerobic bacteria	*Legionella* sp
Enteric Gram-negative bacilli	*Francisella tularensis*
Pseudomonas sp	*Bacillus anthracis*
Acinetobacter sp	*Yersinia pestis*
Francisella tularensis	
Miscellaneous	

[a]Modified from Table 9-2 from reference 142.

Table 12-3

MOST FREQUENT BACTERIAL CAUSES OF COMMUNITY-ACQUIRED AND NOSOCOMIAL PNEUMONIAS[a]

Location of Acquisition	Causal Organism
Community	*Streptococcus pneumoniae* *Mycoplasma pneumoniae* *Haemophilus influenzae* Anaerobes *Legionella pneumophila* *Chlamydia pneumoniae*
Hospital (nosocomial)	*Staphylococcus aureus* Enteric Gram-negative bacilli *Pseudomonas aeruginosa* Anaerobes

[a]Table 34-1 from Johnson CC, Finegold SM. Pyogenic bacterial pneumonia, lung abscess and empyema. In: Murray JF, Nadel JA, eds. Textbook of respiratory medicine, 2nd ed. Philadelphia: WB Saunders; 1994:1038.

thoracoabdominal surgery (55,103,142). Underlying diseases associated with pneumonia caused by certain bacterial organisms are summarized in Table 12-4. The American Thoracic Society (105), the British Thoracic Society (12), and the Infectious Disease Society of America (6) have published guidelines for the empiric treatment of these patients.

Lobar and Bronchopneumonia or Lobular Pneumonia. Pneumonia can also be categorized according to the morphologic anatomic distribution in the lung. The two major categories are lobar (fig. 12-1) versus bronchopneumonia (fig. 12-2) or lobular pneumonia. *Lobar pneumonia* is a classic manifestation of pneumococcal pneumonia in which an entire lobe is affected by the inflammatory infiltrate, with extension up to the pleura or a major fissure. However, other organisms can also cause this pattern of lung involvement including *K. pneumoniae, L. pneumophila,* and rarely *S. aureus, Neisseria gonorrhoeae,* and *M. pneumoniae.* In patients with lobar pneumonia, the stages of pneumonia progress from edema to red hepatization, gray hepatization, and resolution. The red hepatization phase shows a red, dry, granular cut surface and histologic features of alveolar fibrin, neutrophils, lymphocytes, and pneumocyte hyperplasia. Gray hepatization shows a gray, firm cut surface and histologically, a predominantly neutrophilic infiltrate with lysis of erythrocytes and inflammatory cells. In the resolution phase there is organizing pneumonia, with macrophages and proliferation of loose connective tissue in distal airspaces.

Table 12-4

ORGANISMS PREVALENT IN BACTERIAL PNEUMONIA ACCORDING TO UNDERLYING DISEASE OR SETTING[a]

Alcoholism	*Streptococcus pneumoniae* *Haemophilus influenzae* Anaerobes *Klebsiella pneumoniae*
Risk of aspiration (eg. coma, seizure)	Anaerobes *Staphylococcus aureus* Gram-negative bacilli
Chronic obstructive pulmonary disease	*S. pneumoniae* *Moraxella catarrhalis* *H. influenzae*
Intravenous drug use	*S. aureus*
Neutropenia (granulocytes <1000/µL)	*Pseudomonas aeruginosa* Enteric Gram-negative bacilli *S. aureus*
Cell-mediated immune deficiency	*Legionella* *Nocardia*
Human immunodeficiency (HIV) infection	*S. pneumoniae; H. influenzae;* *S. aureus;* *Rhodococcus equi*
Cystic fibrosis	*P. aeruginosa* *S. aureus* *Burkholderia cepacia*
Pulmonary alveolar proteinosis	*Nocardia*

[a]Modified from Table 34-3 from reference 70.

Lobular pneumonia is also known as *bronchopneumonia* or *focal pneumonia.* It is characterized by centrilobular inflammation that is concentrated around respiratory bronchioles, with spread to the surrounding alveolar ducts and alveolar spaces. When lobular pneumonia becomes confluent, it may be difficult to separate from lobar pneumonia.

Pneumonia may also appear round or circumscribed, and there is a circumscribed nodular

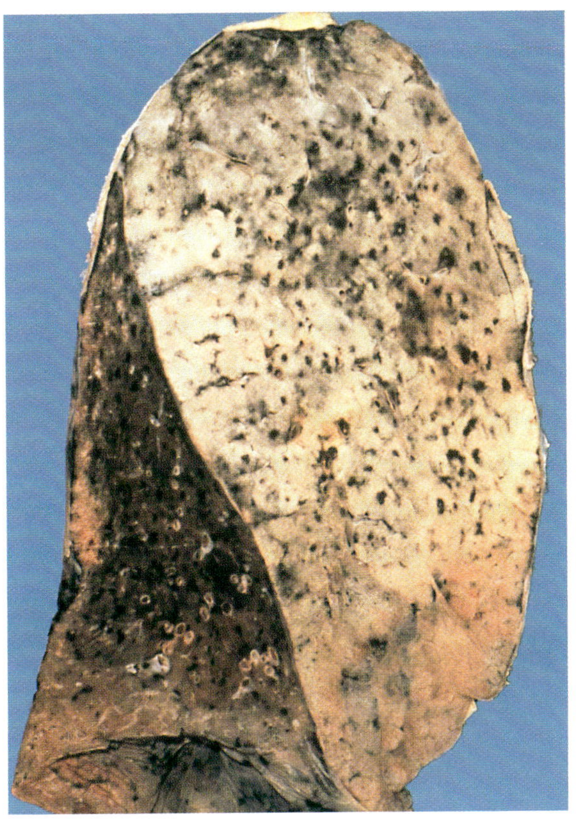

Figure 12-1

LOBAR PNEUMONIA: GROSS SPECIMEN

The lower lobe is diffusely consolidated, with a sharp separation along the interlobar fissure that shows a contrast with the unaffected upper lobe. (Courtesy of the Gordon Museum, London, England.)

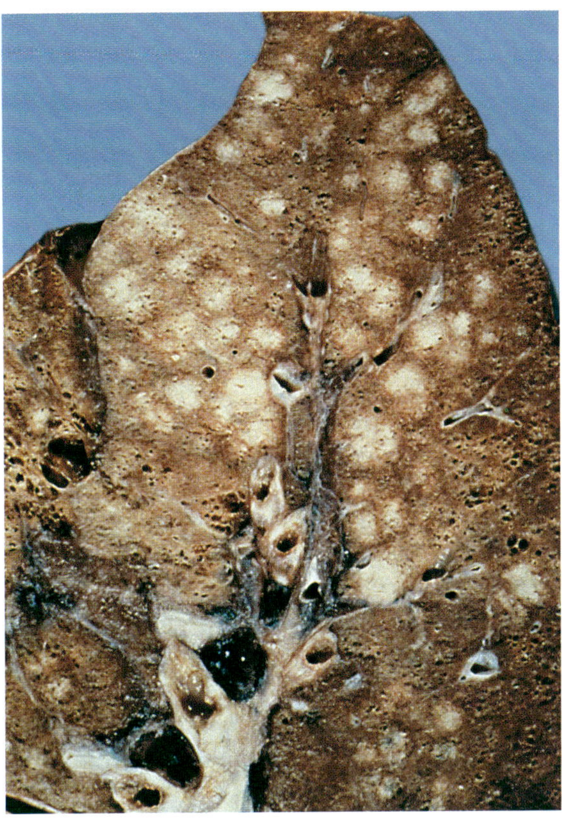

Figure 12-2

LOBULAR BRONCHOPNEUMONIA IN LEGIONNAIRE'S DISEASE

The yellow nodules are centered on the bronchi and the lobular pattern of bronchopneumonia is seen.

area of inflammation and consolidation (fig. 12-3). The radiographic differential diagnosis in these cases is primary neoplasm, metastatic disease, inflammatory pseudotumor, or rounded atelectasis (55,103,142).

Acute and Chronic Pneumonias. Classic examples of acute pneumonia, such as pneumococcal pneumonia, are characterized by prominent neutrophilic infiltrates. Chronic pneumonia, such as caused by fungal or mycobacterial infections, often consists of chronic and/or granulomatous inflammation and/or fibrosis. Bacteria that can cause chronic pneumonias include *Actinomyces* sp, *Nocardia* sp, and *Burkholderia pseudomallei* (55,103,142). The rest of this chapter addresses bacterial pneumonias according to the more commonly recognized or important specific causative organisms.

COMMON BACTERIAL PNEUMONIAS

Streptococcus Pneumoniae

Definition. Pneumococcal pneumonia is an infection of the lung caused by the Gram-positive bacteria *Streptococcus pneumoniae.*

S. pneumoniae is a Gram-positive, catalase-negative coccal bacterium that grows in short chains or pairs (55,142). It has a lancet (pointed) shape and diplococcal morphology. It is the most common cause of community-acquired pneumonia that results in hospital admission and is likely the cause of at least half of all cases of community-acquired pneumonia. It has a capsule that is a virulence factor. Over 80 capsular strains are recognized, although more than 75 percent of human infections are caused by only 12 of them (55,142). The organism is acquired through

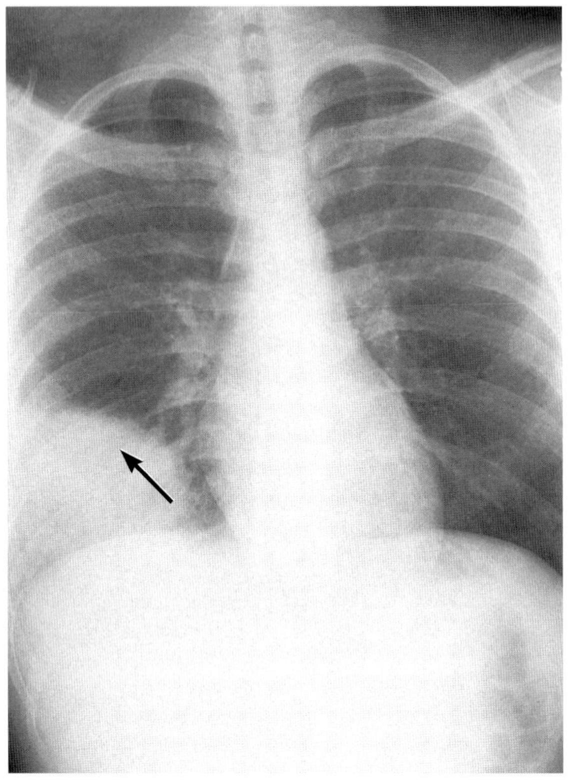

Figure 12-3

STREPTOCOCOCCUS PNEUMONIAE

S. pneumoniae pulmonary infection in a 22-year-old male with cough, fever, and pleuritic chest pain. PA chest radiograph demonstrates a nonsegmental homogeneous consolidation in the right lower lobe. Note the subtle air bronchogram medially (arrow). (Courtesy of Dr. Rosita M. Shah, Philadelphia, PA.)

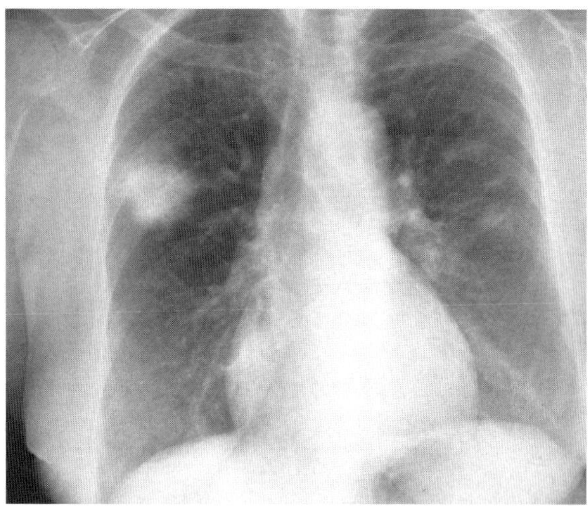

Figure 12-4

STREPTOCOCCUS PNEUMONIAE

Streptococcus pneumoniae causing a round pneumonia in a female with cough and fever. Posteroanterior (PA) chest radiograph demonstrates a mass-like consolidation in the superior segment of the right lower lobe. The lesion exhibits irregular lobular borders and mimics a primary pulmonary neoplasm.

person-to-person transmission by aerosolized droplets, physical contact, or both. Most infections occur in the winter and early spring. It is the most common bacterial pneumonia to follow influenza pneumonia. Pneumococci are colonized in the upper respiratory tract of 5 to 60 percent of the general population (55,142).

Clinical Features. Up to 70 percent of patients have a recent history of an upper respiratory tract infection (55,142). There is a 2 to 1 male to female ratio. Patients have an abrupt onset of rigor followed by fever; productive cough with a rusty mucoid sputum and dyspnea follow. Pleuritic chest pain occurs in up to 75 percent of patients. Extrapulmonary manifestations may include headache and vomiting. Leukocytosis is usually present, with white blood cell (WBC) counts of 15,000 to 25,000 cells/mm^3. Patients with severe infection may have WBC counts of 3,000 or less (55,142).

Radiologic Findings. The classic chest radiographic manifestation of pneumococcal pneumonia is a homogeneous, nonsegmental, parenchymal consolidation involving one lobe (fig. 12-3). The airspace consolidation typically abuts the surrounding visceral pleura. Air bronchograms are commonly seen. Volume loss is minimal in the acute stage of the disease (45,71). Patchy consolidation and interstitial opacities may also be observed. Cavitation is rarely seen (45,71). Round pneumonia (mass-like rounded consolidation) may occur and may mimic a pulmonary neoplasm; clinical evidence of infection is very helpful in these cases (fig. 12-4) (45).

Patients with bacteremia may exhibit a bronchopneumonia pattern of consolidation (60 percent of cases) and pleural effusion (60 percent). Empyema is unusual. The bronchopneumonia pattern of involvement is characterized by peribronchial and peribronchiolar consolidation that affects one lobe or multiple lobes. The resultant opacities measure 4 to 10 mm and are termed "airspace nodules." The

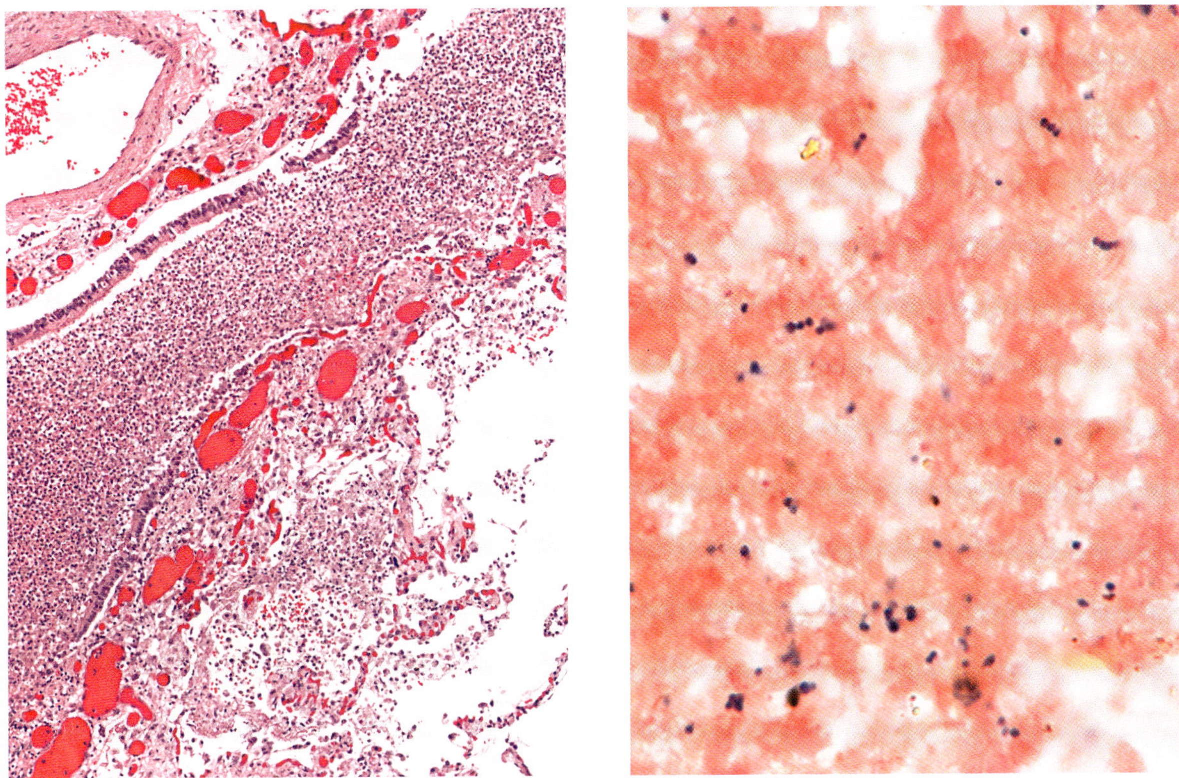

Figure 12-5

STREPTOCOCCUS PNEUMONIAE

Left: There is extensive neutrophilic infiltration involving a bronchiole (top left) and extending into the surrounding alveolar parenchyma.

Right: Numerous Gram-positive streptococci are present.

latter may eventually involve the entire secondary pulmonary lobule (47). Slow clearance of pulmonary consolidation on radiography is seen in both bacteremic and nonbacteremic infections but is more common in the former. This finding does not denote failure to respond to therapy. Typically, radiographic follow-up is done at 6-week intervals (30).

Pathologic Findings. Pneumococcal pneumonia classically causes a lobar consolidation, with pulmonary infiltration by neutrophils and macrophages (figs. 12-1, 12-5, left). This inflammatory infiltrate is surrounded by edema. The bacteria can be found in the inflamed areas in early infection (fig. 12-5, right) (142). Cavitation is uncommon but can occur, especially in patients with bacteremic infection. Necrotizing pneumonia most often occurs with a mixed bacterial infection. Diffuse alveolar damage can be seen in patients with fatal infections. Pneumatoceles are reported to occur in children (142).

Treatment and Prognosis. Penicillin is the treatment of choice for pneumococcal pneumonia. Antibiotic resistance is an increasing problem, with as many as 30 percent of isolates in the United States showing either intermediate or high resistance minimal inhibitory concentration (MIC>2) (6,22,70). Vancomycin is the agent of choice for penicillin-resistant strains. Most patients who receive antibiotics in a timely fashion begin to recover within 24 to 48 hours. Radiographic resolution with appropriate antibiotic therapy is usually rapid, with a significant number of outpatients demonstrating resolution after 2 weeks. Clearance is slower in patients with bacteremia, elderly patients, smokers, patients requiring hospitalization, and those with underlying disease. In such cases, radiographic resolution may take 4 to 8 weeks. Potential complications include metastatic infection and rarely, empyema or pericarditis. Metastatic infection can result in meningitis, endocarditis, arthritis, and cellulitis (70).

Increased mortality is associated with cardiac or chronic pulmonary disease, cirrhosis, malignancy, asplenia, age over 50 years, leukopenia (WBC less than 4,000 cells/mm^3), leukocytosis (WBC more than 20,000 cells/mm^3), multilobar involvement, hypoxemia, bacteremia, and extrapulmonary involvement (70). Patients infected with penicillin-resistant *S. pneumoniae* have a higher mortality rate than those infected with sensitive organisms. The pneumococcal polysaccharide vaccine should be considered for patients at risk for pneumococcal infection: those under the age of 2 years or over the age of 65, patients with certain chronic illnesses, and immunocompromised patients.

Staphylococcus Sp

Definition. Staphylococcal pneumonia is an infection of the lung caused by the Gram-positive bacteria *Staphylococcus* sp, most commonly *Staphylococcus aureus.*

Staphylococcus sp are Gram-positive bacteria that grow in clusters and are catalase positive. The most important species to cause pneumonia is *S. aureus,* although both *S. epidermidis* and *S. saprophyticus* also cause pneumonia. Staphylococci produce a variety of toxins that contribute to tissue injury including alpha-toxin, beta-toxin, gamma-toxin, leukocidin, exfliatins, and enterotoxins (75).

Approximately 20 to 40 percent of older children and adults are nasal carriers of staphylococci (75). Approximately 30 percent of adults are long-term carriers and 50 percent are intermittent carriers (75); however, over 50 percent of health care workers may be carriers (75). Pulmonary infection occurs through hematogenous spread or aspiration of oral secretions.

Clinical Features. Staphylococcal pneumonia is the cause of less than 5 percent of community-acquired pneumonias but it causes approximately 10 percent of nosocomial pneumonias (70). Staphylococcal pneumonia due to aspiration tends to occur in patients with underlying chronic obstructive lung disease, lung carcinoma, or intubation. *Staphylococcus* infection is a known complication of other pulmonary infections such as viral pneumonias, particularly influenza pneumonia in adults, and measles in children and infants (70). Hematogenous spread to the lungs is known to occur in patients with endocarditis, contaminated vascular lines, or intravenous drug abuse (70).

Presenting symptoms include fever, cough, and purulent sputum. Pulmonary symptoms may be minimal despite extensive pulmonary infiltrates (70). Chest pain and hemoptysis occur in patients with pulmonary infarcts. Leukocytosis is common, with WBC counts greater than 15,000 cells/mm^3 with a left shift. If there is underlying endocarditis, patients may also have signs of hematuria, anemia, and renal failure (70).

Radiologic Findings. The typical radiologic manifestation of pulmonary infection with *Staphylococcus* sp is bilateral, multifocal, segmental airspace consolidation affecting the lower lobes, the so-called bronchopneumonia or lobular pattern of infection (fig. 12-6). Volume loss is prominent and air bronchograms are rarely seen. Progression to homogeneous airspace consolidation can occur (fig. 12-6). In some of these cases, there is an increase in the volume of the affected lobe (45,86).

S. aureus has been implicated as an etiologic factor of chronic (slowly resolving) bacterial pneumonia (30). Abscess formation and cavitation may be seen. Cavitary lesions are typically thick-walled with irregular margins (fig. 12-7). Pleural effusions occur in 30 to 50 percent of affected individuals, and in 50 percent there is progression to empyema (30,45,86).

Formation of pneumatoceles is common and particularly affects children. These manifest as multifocal, thin-walled cystic spaces, which may contain air-fluid levels and which typically resolve spontaneously over the course of weeks or months (fig. 12-8) (86,115). However, spontaneous pneumothorax has been described in association with pneumatoceles (86).

High-resolution computed tomography (HRCT) findings include centrilobular nodules and branching linear opacities which typically display a "tree-in-bud" appearance. Secondary pulmonary lobules may become evident as they are outlined by surrounding uninvolved lung. Hematogenous infection of the lung manifests with multifocal nodules or masses, which may exhibit cavitation, or as peripheral and subpleu-

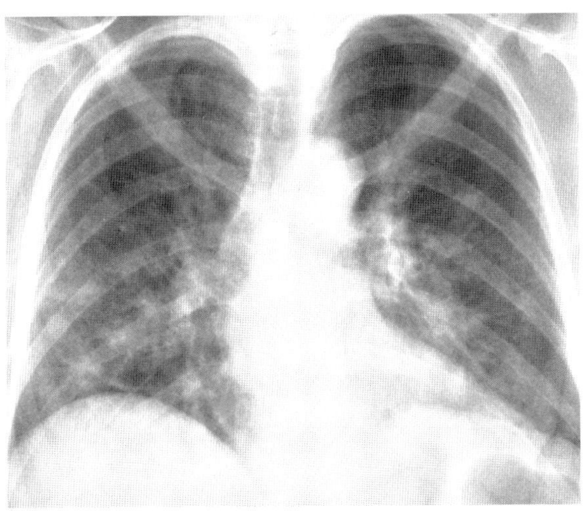

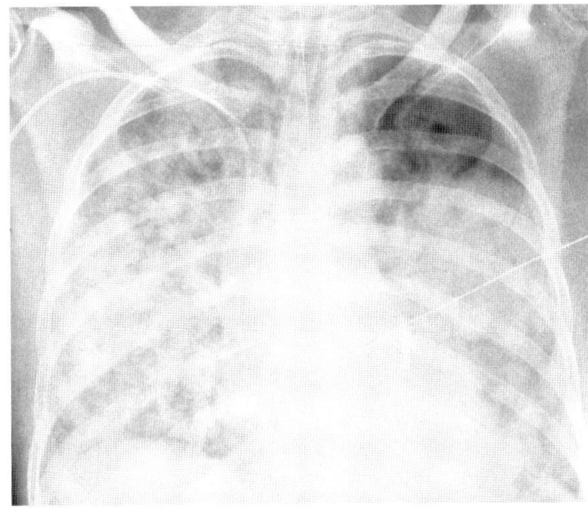

Figure 12-6

STAPHYLOCOCCUS PNEUMONIA

Staphylococcus pneumonia in a 41-year-old female admitted with a flu-like syndrome. The patient had rapid clinical deterioration.

Left: A PA chest radiograph demonstrates multifocal, bilateral, patchy airspace consolidations that predominantly affect the lower lung zones.

Right: AP chest radiograph obtained 3 days later demonstrates confluence of parenchymal consolidation with diffuse bilateral pulmonary involvement. The patient now has endotracheal and nasogastric tubes in place as well as a Swann-Ganz catheter.

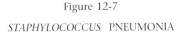

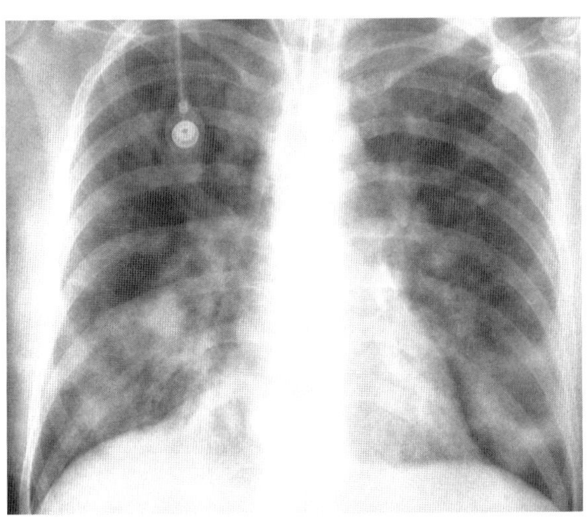

Figure 12-7

STAPHYLOCOCCUS PNEUMONIA

Staphylococcus pneumonia in a 17-year-old diabetic female admitted with a flu-like illness, multiple skin abscesses, and poorly controlled diabetes. PA chest radiograph demonstrates multifocal, bilateral, parenchymal consolidations with early cavitation in the left lower lobe.

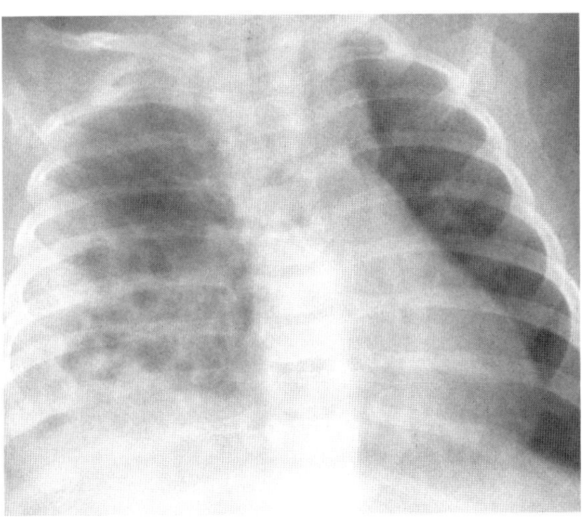

Figure 12-8

STAPHYLOCOCCUS PNEUMONIA

Staphylococcus pneumonia in a 4-month-old female with fever and wheezing. PA chest radiograph demonstrates a large airspace consolidation in the right lung. Note the multifocal lucent areas within the consolidation which represent pneumatoceles.

ral wedge-shaped opacities, which may be associated with a "feeding" artery as visualized on CT (45).

Pathologic Findings. The characteristic histologic lesion of staphylococcal pneumonia is an acute pneumonia with abscess formation

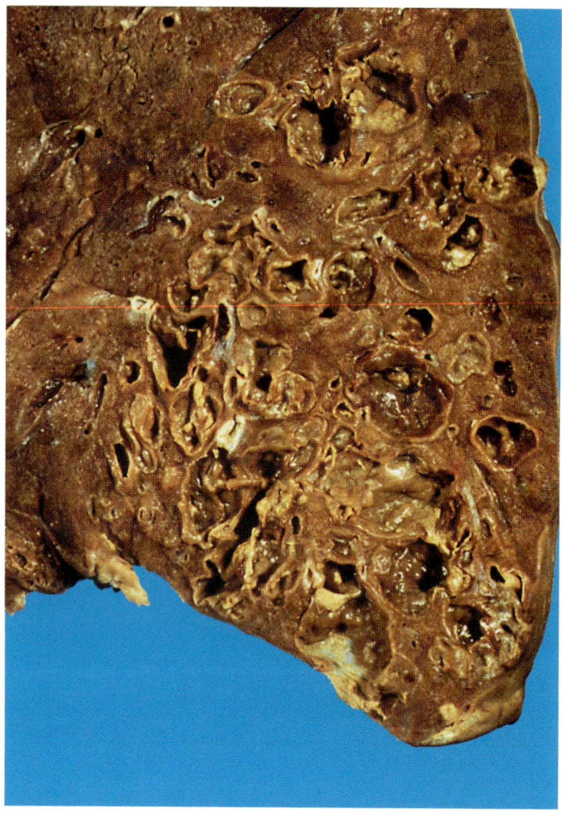

Figure 12-9

STAPHYLOCOCCAL PNEUMONIA: GROSS SPECIMEN

Multiple cavitary abscesses are causing extensive destruction of the lung parenchyma.

(fig. 12-9). Grossly, the lung has yellow to tan nodules that are centered on airways in cases acquired by aspiration or centered on vessels in hematogenous spread to the lungs. The center of the nodule may consist of thick liquid pus. Multiple abscesses are commonly seen and may measure up to many centimeters in diameter (fig. 12-9) (75,142). Histologically, many neutrophils are found within airways and alveolar spaces. The organisms are Gram-positive cocci measuring 0.5 to 1.5 µm in diameter. They grow in grape-like clusters and stain well with the Brown and Brenn and Brown and Hopps stains. The underlying lung becomes necrotic and abscesses begin to form (fig. 12-10). Organizing pneumonia may develop as the process heals. Invasion of the pleura, resulting in pleuritis and empyema, is a common complication (75,142).

In infants, and to a lesser extent adults, abscesses may lead to pneumatoceles, thin-walled cystic spaces lined primarily by respiratory tissue (fig. 12-11) (142). Pneumatoceles may expand rapidly and compress the surrounding lung, or they may rupture into the pleural cavity, thereby causing a pneumothorax (142). It is thought that a pneumatocele develops when an abscess breaks into an airway, thereby allowing its expansion by the pressure of inspired air. The pathologic distinction between a chronic abscess and a pneumatocele may be difficult.

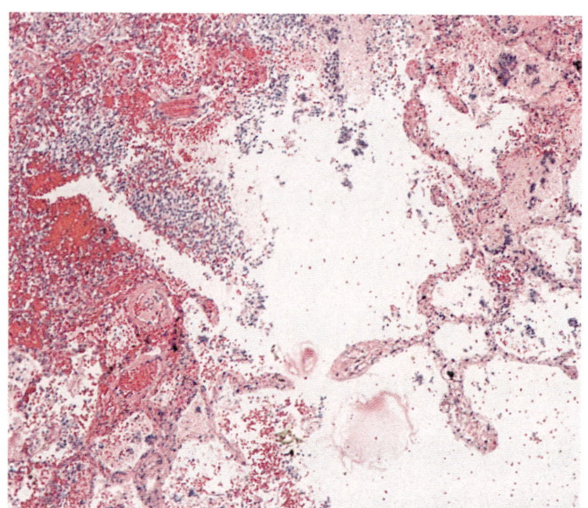

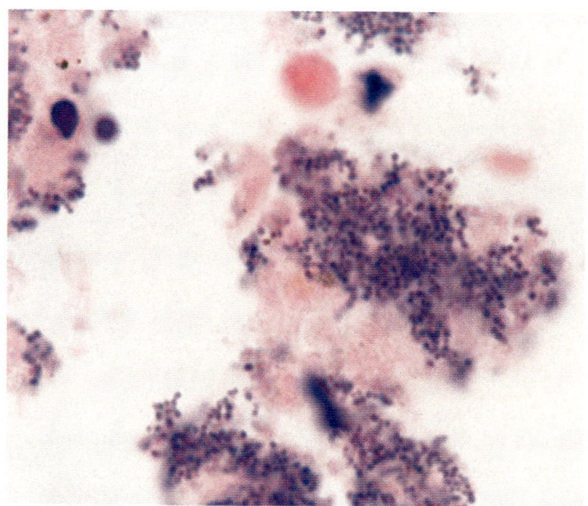

Figure 12-10

STAPHYLOCOCCAL PNEUMONIA: ABSCESS

Left: This staphylococcal pneumonia shows an abscess with cavitary necrosis within acutely inflamed lung parenchyma. Right: Within the abscess cavity are numerous Gram-positive bacteria growing in clusters.

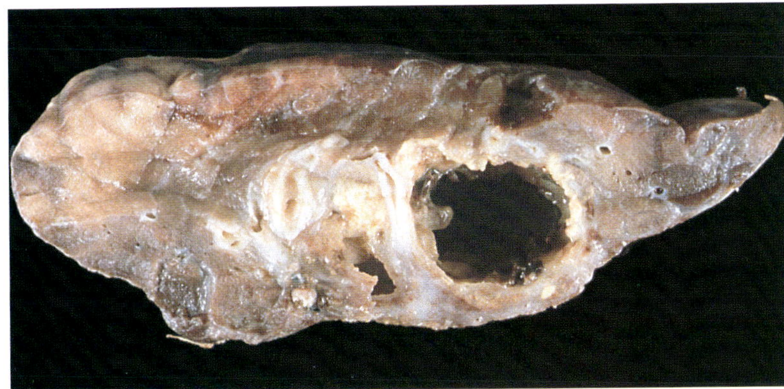

Figure 12-11

PNEUMATOCELE: GROSS SPECIMEN

This thin-walled cavity developed following a severe bacterial pneumonia in a young child. It has a thin fibrous wall and adjacent areas of consolidation. This probably evolved from an abscess.

Treatment and Prognosis. Patients with primary *S. aureus* pneumonia have a mortality rate of 25 to 30 percent, which may increase to over 80 percent if there is associated bacteremia (142). Empyema can be seen in 20 percent of adults and 75 percent of children; abscess formation in 15 to 20 percent. Pneumatoceles are a potential complication in up to 40 percent of children but are rare in adults (142).

Staphylococcal pneumonia requires aggressive antibiotic treatment, particularly in view of the numerous antibiotic-resistant strains of *S. aureus*. The optimal therapy for bacteremia is the intravenous administration of a beta-lactam agent such as nafcillin or oxacillin or a first-generation cephalosporin such as cefazolin. Vancomycin therapy is the preferred alternative in patients with methicillin-resistant strains of *S. aureus*.

Streptococcus Sp (Nonpneumococcal)

Definition. Streptococcal pneumonia is an infection of the lung caused by the Gram-positive, catalase-negative bacteria, *Streptococcus* sp.

Streptococcal pneumonia is an uncommon cause of pneumonia, accounting for less than 1 percent of cases in adults and slightly more in children. Group A beta-hemolytic (*S. pyogenes*), group B (*S. agalactiae*), group D (*Enterococcus*), and alpha-hemolytic nonpneumococcal *(S. viridans)* organisms can all cause pneumonia. *S. pyogenes* colonizes the oropharynx in 20 percent of children and 2 to 3 percent of adults. It is readily transmitted through direct contact. Group A streptococcal pneumonia can be complicated by empyema, pneumothorax, pericarditis, mediastinitis, and bronchopleural fistula.

Group B streptococcus colonizes the lower reproductive tract in 20 to 40 percent of adult women (72a,76). There is evidence that heavy colonization with group B streptococcus leads to premature birth and is a frequent cause of chorioamnionitis, postpartum endometritis, and sepsis in women in the peripartum period. This organism is increasingly recognized as a cause of sepsis, soft tissue infections, and other focal infections in adults, especially those with diabetes mellitus, malignancy, and other immunocompromising conditions.

Clinical Features. Pneumonia due to *S. pyogenes* typically occurs in late winter and spring, and often follows a viral infection, both in children and adults. It is thought to have been a major cause of the bacterial pneumonia complicating the influenza of the 1918-19 pandemic. Group B streptococcal organisms are an important cause of neonatal pneumonia and sepsis. Neonatal pneumonia is associated with infection acquired during labor or delivery (10). Group B streptococci can also cause congenital pneumonia when the amniotic fluid becomes contaminated, either due to premature rupture of membranes or during prolonged labor (70,76).

Radiologic Findings. Pulmonary infection caused by *S. pyogenes* manifests radiologically with homogeneous or patchy, parenchymal airspace consolidation in a segmental distribution. Bilateral lower lobe involvement with volume loss is typical. Lung abscess, cavitation, and empyema may occur (45,76).

Pathologic Findings. *S. pyogenes* can cause a focal lobular pattern or an extensive lobar pattern of pneumonia. The lungs may show a gray-purple cut surface and the exudate in the

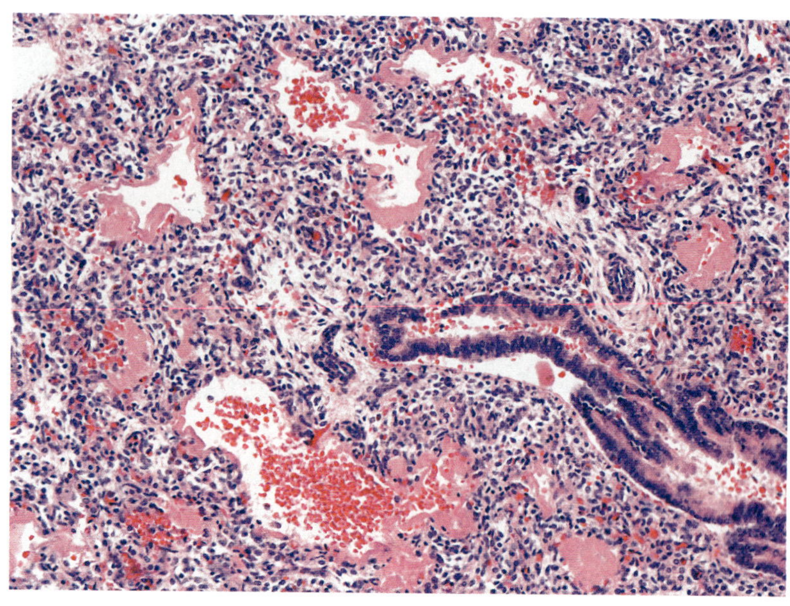

Figure 12-12

GROUP B STREPTOCOCCAL PNEUMONIA

The lung shows diffuse alveolar damage with hyaline membranes accompanied by a neutrophilic infiltrate.

bronchioles may consist of pus. The organisms are Gram-positive with Brown and Brenn and Brown and Hopps stains, measure less than 2 µm in diameter, and grow in chains. The histologic reaction to *S. pyogenes* consists of a marked neutrophilic bronchopneumonia. Extensive suppuration can result in abscess formation, particularly if there is bronchial obstruction (119).

Neonatal pneumonia caused by group B streptococci produces diffuse alveolar damage, which may be associated with a prominent neutrophilic infiltrate (fig. 12-12). Numerous Gram-positive streptococci are characteristically seen in the hyaline membranes (72a). Congenital pneumonia caused by group B streptococci causes a lobar pattern with a marked neutrophilic infiltrate and edema without fibrin (76). Squamous cells and other debris from the amniotic fluid are seen. Interstitial inflammation is present (76).

Treatment and Prognosis. Penicillin is the treatment of choice. Vancomycin is used for those who are allergic to penicillin. There is significant resistance among some group B streptococcal isolates to macrolide agents.

Haemophilus Influenzae

Definition. *Haemophilus* pneumonia is an infection of the lung caused by small Gram-negative bacteria, *Haemophilus influenzae* (Pfeiffer bacillus).

H. influenzae organisms are small, thin, nonmotile, Gram-negative, and pleomorphic, and range from coccobacilli to short filaments (70,89,142). Organisms are acquired through the nasopharynx and transmitted from person-to-person through aerosol inhalation of coccobacilli (70,89,142). The nasopharynx is colonized in up to 90 percent of children at 5 years of age (70). Patients with chronic obstructive pulmonary disease (COPD) are frequently colonized. Most *Haemophilus* organisms that colonize are unencapsulated and nontypeable. Debilitated or immunosuppressed patients who are colonized by an encapsulated strain are at high risk for developing an invasive infection. The encapsulated type B strain is the most common cause of bacteremic pneumonia, but the latter can also be caused by multiple other strains of *H. influenzae* including types c, d, e, and f (142). Most strains that cause pulmonary infection are encapsulated, but nonencapsulated strains also cause pneumonia that tends to be of lesser clinical severity (70,142). In a study of *H. influenzae* pneumonia in adults, Farley et al. (40) found that 50 percent of cases were due to serotype b; 47.5 percent were nontypeable; and 2.5 percent were of serotype f. In addition to pneumonia, *H. influenzae* causes meningitis and bacteremia (70,89,142).

Clinical Features. *H. influenzae* is a major cause of pneumonia in children and adults, although its frequency has been reduced due to the introduction of a vaccine for *H. influenzae* type b (62,85,110). It is one of the major causes of pneumonia resulting in hospital admission. Children are at risk since they do not have immunity to the capsule of the encapsulated strains. *H. influenzae* pneumonia is more likely to occur in adults with COPD, chronic alcoholism, age over 50 years, diabetes mellitus, hypogammaglobulinemia, multiple myeloma, asplenia, sickle cell anemia, and human immunodeficiency virus (HIV) infection (70,142). *H. influenzae* is one of the most common bacterial causes of acute exacerbation of COPD (120).

Patients present with bronchopneumonia, which may be preceded by an upper respiratory tract infection (70,142). Symptoms typically include fever, cough, dyspnea, and purulent sputum. Children may have a subacute clinical presentation with cough and low-grade fever over a period of weeks (70,142). Leukocytosis is absent in up to 25 percent of patients and when present is relatively mild, ranging between 10,000 and 15,000 cells/mm^3. In children, leukopenia is a poor prognostic indicator, often correlating with death (70).

Radiologic Findings. The radiologic manifestations of *H. influenza* pulmonary infection include bronchopneumonia (patchy airspace opacities), lobar consolidation, or combinations of these two patterns. Lobar consolidation is more common in patients with abnormal immunity. Volume expansion is uncommon (28,45,109). Reticular and nodular interstitial opacities may be seen and are associated with consolidation. Pleural effusion occurs in 40 to 50 percent of cases (28,30). Empyema is uncommon. Cavitation is rare and when present usually complicates lobar consolidation (28). Resolution of radiographic abnormalities is usually slow and may be related to the accuracy of the initial diagnosis and the choice and duration of antibiotic therapy (30).

Pathologic Findings. *H. influenzae* causes an acute bronchiolitis and bronchopneumonia (4,142). The bronchi and bronchioles contain a purulent exudate with numerous neutrophils, necrotic cellular debris, and fibrin (142). The small, pleomorphic, Gram-negative coccobacilli are best seen with tissue Gram stains in the airways rather than the alveoli (142). Abscess formation and empyema are uncommon. Rarely, pneumatoceles can be seen (142).

Treatment and Prognosis. A study of *H. influenzae* pneumonia found the overall mortality was 28 percent, and over half of pregnancy-related infections resulted in fetal death (40). In children mortality is only 5 percent. Empyema occurs in 10 percent of children, but is uncommon in adults. The most active drugs for treatment are third-generation cephalosporins and combinations of penicillins with a beta-lactamase inhibitor. Most patients respond to therapy within 24 hours. All children should be immunized to *H. influenza* type b according to current recommendations.

Klebsiella Pneumoniae

Definition. *Klebsiella* pneumonia, also known as *Friedländer's pneumonia,* is caused by the bacteria *Klebsiella pneumoniae.*

K. pneumoniae is a Gram-negative, lactose-fermenting, nonmotile bacillus of the *Enterobacteriaceae* family which has a thick polysaccharide capsule (55). It is normally found in the intestinal flora of humans. It was first described by Friedländer in 1882, hence the term Friedländer's pneumonia (48). Pulmonary infection is usually acquired by aspiration.

Clinical Features. *Klebsiella* is the cause of 1 to 5 percent of community-acquired lobar pneumonia and up to 30 percent of Gram-negative nosocomial pneumonias (55,70). Males are affected in 90 percent of cases and most patients are over 40 years of age (55,70). Predisposing conditions include alcoholism, diabetes mellitus, and COPD (55,70).

Patients present with sudden onset of cough, pleuritic chest pain, dyspnea, fever, and rigors. The cough produces a thick, mucoid, bloody sputum (described as "currant jelly" in quality) (55,70). Patients may be very ill with prostration and hypotension. The WBC count may be high, low, or normal; however, neutropenia is a poor prognostic sign (55,70). *Klebsiella* may also cause bronchitis or bronchopneumonia.

Radiologic Findings. Acute *Klebsiella* pneumonia manifests radiographically with a lobar pattern of consolidation characterized by nonsegmental, homogeneous consolidation with air bronchograms. Characteristically, lobar expansion and bulging fissures accompany

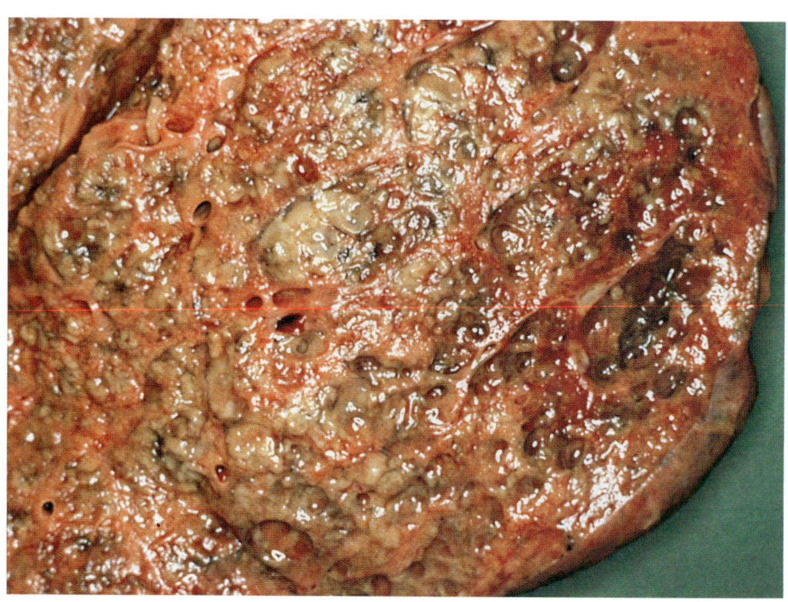

Figure 12-13

KLEBSIELLA PNEUMONIAE: GROSS SPECIMEN

The cut surface of the lung shows extensive consolidation with a mucoid, yellow appearance.

these consolidations due to the large amount of inflammatory exudate produced by this infection (28). Bilateral disease may occur (100). Abscesses form in up to 50 percent of cases. Pulmonary gangrene may occur and is characterized by cavitation, which affects an entire lobe or lung and contains mobile soft tissue (100). Pleural effusion occurs in 70 percent of cases, and empyema is frequent (45,100).

CT is useful in visualization of early cavitation, abscess, and the complication of pulmonary gangrene. Differentiation between abscess formation and pulmonary gangrene is important for management, as surgical intervention may be required in the latter, particularly when the entire lung is affected and a single cavity forms (100). Pleural effusion and lymphadenopathy have also been described (45).

Pathologic Findings. Acute *Klebsiella* pneumonia usually has the pattern of a patchy, lobar or bronchopneumonia (119,142). The lobar pattern results from extensive acute inflammatory infiltration through the entire lobe of lung. In this setting, the affected lobe may be enlarged, causing the fissure to bulge toward the uninvolved lobe (119,142). The cut surface of the lung characteristically has a mucoid appearance due to the thick, gelatinous capsule of the organism (fig. 12-13) (119,142).

Histologically, the bronchioles and alveoli are filled with neutrophils and macrophages. The large, Gram-negative bacilli are seen within the cytoplasm of some of the inflammatory cells. The bacilli can be seen with tissue Gram stains such as the Brown and Hopps and Brown and Brenn, and they may also stain with the periodic acid-Schiff (PAS) stain due to the thick capsule (119). Areas of necrosis may be present and in some cases abscesses develop (fig. 12-14) and are multicentric (119,142). When extensive necrosis occurs, pulmonary gangrene can develop. Acute vasculitis (fig. 12-15) and thrombosis can occur (119,142).

Chronic *Klebsiella* pneumonia may be associated with interstitial fibrosis, organizing pneumonia, bronchiolitis, and necrotizing bronchitis (119,142).

Treatment and Prognosis. The mortality rate for patients with *Klebsiella* pneumonia is high, ranging from 25 to 50 percent (70). Patients in intensive care units have an especially poor prognosis. Antibiotic therapy must be aggressive and include an aminoglycoside combined with either a cephalosporin or broad-spectrum penicillin (70). Complications include abscesses, cavitation, bronchiectasis, empyema, and pleural adhesions (119). It is uncommon to encounter *Klebsiella* pneumonia in neonates and infants, but it is fatal in approximately 50 percent of this population (119).

Pseudomonas Aeruginosa

Definition. *Pseudomonas* pneumonia is an infection of the lung caused by the Gram-negative

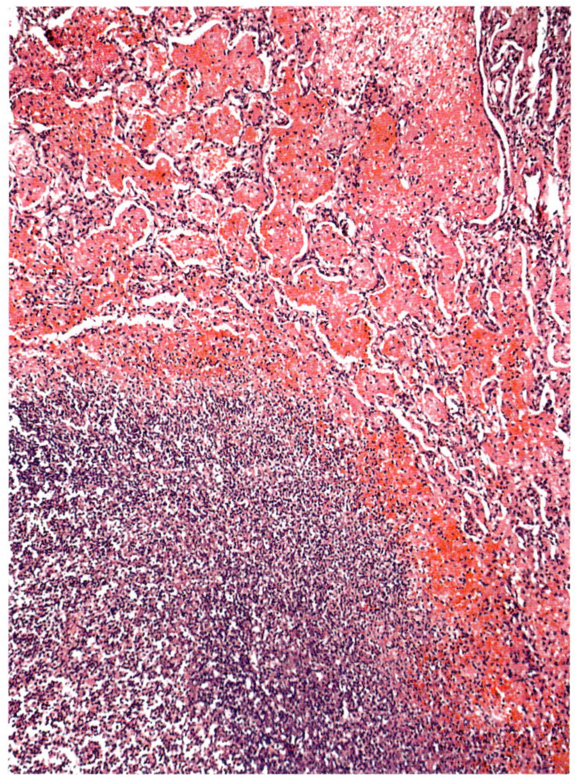

Figure 12-14

KLEBSIELLA PNEUMONIAE: HISTOLOGY

The lung shows an acute rounded abscess (bottom) consisting of extensive necrosis and accumulation of neutrophils.

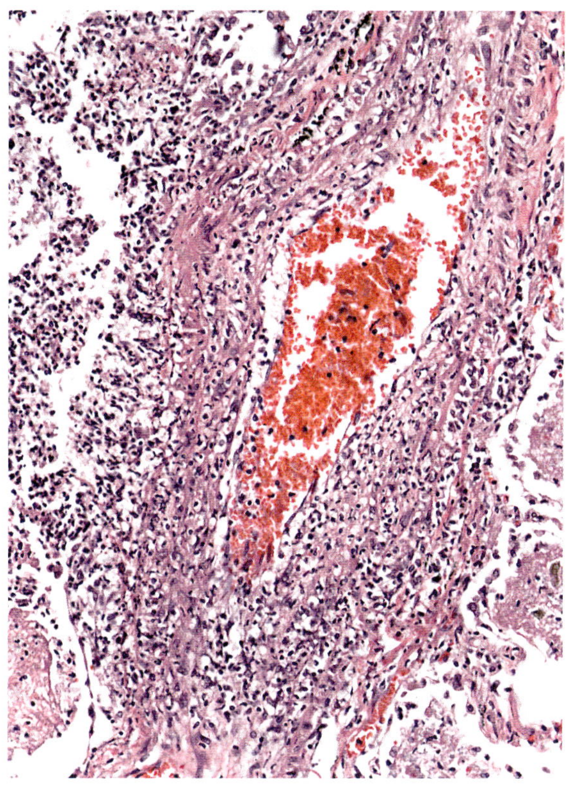

Figure 12-15

KLEBSIELLA PNEUMONIAE: VASCULITIS

This blood vessel shows extensive infiltration by neutrophils.

bacteria *Pseudomonas* sp, most commonly *P. aeruginosa*. Most pulmonary infections are caused by *P. aeruginosa,* but *P. pseudoalcaligenes, P. cepacia,* and *P. maltophilia* also cause pneumonia.

Pseudomonas is a Gram-negative, aerobic (nonfermentative) bacterium found worldwide (95). It has a single polar flagellum that makes it motile and it produces oxidase. It is ubiquitous, with the ability to survive in water, vegetation, and soil. It is also resistant to many disinfectants. All of these features allow the organism to survive in a hospital environment, making it a well-known cause of nosocomial infection. Other modes of infection include exposure to contaminated hot tubs, whirlpools, nails, splinters, and plant material such as salads, vegetables, and flowers (95). *Pseudomonas* colonizes the gastrointestinal tract in 5 percent of adults, but it is found in 50 percent of hospitalized patients with an underlying malignancy (70).

Most pulmonary infections are caused by *P. aeruginosa,* but *P. pseudoalcaligenes* can also cause pneumonia (132). Species formerly known as *P. cepacia* and *P. maltophilia* are now known as *Burkholderia cepacia* (8) and *Stenotrophomonas maltophilia* (54).

Clinical Features. *Pseudomonas* causes two major types of pneumonia: bacteremic and nonbacteremic (70). The bacteremic form occurs mostly in patients with underlying hematologic or lymphoreticular malignancies.

Patients with nonbacteremic *Pseudomonas* pneumonia are usually elderly and debilitated, with underlying chronic pulmonary or cardiovascular disease (70,131). The organism is usually acquired through aspiration of oropharyngeal secretions (70). Patients with COPD who are receiving steroid therapy are well known for getting *Pseudomonas* pneumonia. *Pseudomonas* pneumonia is a major complication of patients

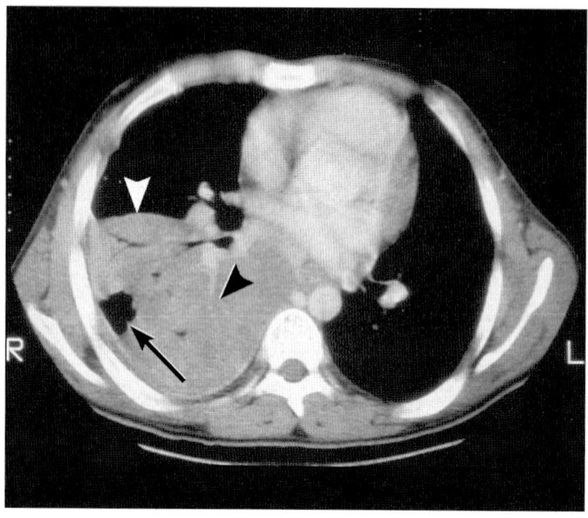

Figure 12-16

PSEUDOMONAS PNEUMONIA

Pseudomonas pneumonia in a 29-year-old male admitted to the hospital after failed therapy for outpatient pneumonia. Contrast-enhanced chest CT (mediastinal window) demonstrates lobar expansion and bulging of the major fissure (white arrowhead). Note the vascular markings within the consolidated lobe (black arrowhead) and the area of cavitation (arrow). (Courtesy of Dr. Rosita M. Shah, Philadelphia, PA.)

with cystic fibrosis and diffuse panbronchiolitis (49). In addition to aspiration, another mechanism of infection is via contaminated respiratory therapy equipment (70,131). Patients with nonbacteremic pneumonia present with systemic toxicity, fever, chills, cough, and abundant purulent sputum (70,131). Initially, leukocytosis may be absent, but it eventually develops in almost all patients. Abscess formation and empyema are common complications (70,131).

Patients with bacteremic *Pseudomonas* pneumonia usually are debilitated or immunocompromised (70). Neutropenia is an important risk factor and is often induced by chemotherapy for malignancy. Patients may also be immunocompromised due to steroid therapy or HIV infection (70). The organism reaches the bloodstream through breaks in the skin, the gastrointestinal tract mucosa, or the respiratory tract. Patients with severe burns are also at risk for developing bacteremic *Pseudomonas* pneumonia. Patients typically present with high fever, dyspnea, systemic toxicity, and confusion. Cough is frequent, but in contrast to the nonbacteremic form, the sputum is usually scant and nonpurulent. Cutaneous lesions of ecthyma gangrenosum may be present. Patients often have worse symptoms than one would suspect based on the chest radiographs. Due to the tendency to invade blood vessels and cause a vasculitis, patients may present with features resembling pulmonary thromboembolism (125,130).

The diagnosis of *Pseudomonas* pneumonia is usually established by culture. In an appropriate clinical setting the presence of numerous, thin, Gram-negative bacilli in sputum or pleural fluid allows a presumptive diagnosis.

Radiologic Findings. The radiologic features of nonbacteremic *Pseudomonas* pulmonary infection are typically those of bronchopneumonia with multifocal, bilateral, segmental, lower lobe pulmonary consolidation (28,45). All lobes may be affected. Nodular and reticular opacities also occur. Abscess formation may complicate this infection (fig. 12-16). Small pleural effusions are common, but empyema is unusual (45). Bacteremic *Pseudomonas* infection may manifest with multifocal pulmonary nodules, which may progress to confluent consolidation (45,56).

P. aeruginosa is the most frequent organism to produce pneumonia in patients undergoing mechanical ventilation. In this patient population, multifocal opacities, emphysema, and cavitation are frequent manifestations of pulmonary infection (141).

Pathologic Findings. The pathology of *Pseudomonas* pneumonia depends on whether the infection is bacteremic or nonbacteremic and on the presence of pathologic features caused by underlying disease. The nonbacteremic form shows a bronchocentric distribution compatible with the acquisition of the organism through the airways (fig. 12-17) (95). The histologic reaction consists of a prominent infiltrate of neutrophils, with frequent abscess formation and necrosis (fig. 12-18, left) (95). The bacteremic form shows a vasocentric distribution with necrosis, hemorrhage, and frequent vasculitis with organisms situated within vessel walls (fig. 12-18, right) (95,125,130). Hemorrhagic infarcts may be seen as well as thromboemboli (125,130). Numerous small, thin, Gram-negative bacilli measuring 1.5–5.0 x 0.5–1.0 µm can be demonstrated in tissue sections using tissue Gram stains such as the Brown and Hopps stain.

Differential Diagnosis. Other causes of fulminant pneumonia similar to that seen with *Pseudomonas* include the community-acquired *Staphylococcus aureus, Streptococcus pyogenes* (group A streptococcus), and *Klebsiella pneumoniae*. In addition, the opportunistic infections that can cause a rapidly progressive pneumonia with frequent cavitation include *Escherichia coli, Proteus* sp, *Enterobacter,* and *Serratia marcescens* (70).

Treatment and Prognosis. The mortality from *Pseudomonas* pneumonia ranges from 36 to 81 percent. Patients with bacteremic pneumonia and those in intensive care units are particularly at risk. An aminoglycoside and antipseudomonal penicillin, cephalosporin, carbapenem, or monobactam antibiotic are helpful but not always effective. Disseminated infection can occur in patients with bacteremic pneumonias.

Legionella Sp

Definition. *Legionella* pneumonia is a pulmonary infection caused by the Gram-negative bacteria *Legionella* sp, most commonly *Legionella pneumophila.*

L. pneumophila was discovered as a result of an outbreak of pneumonia in 1976 at an American Legion convention in Philadelphia. Since that time, more than 50 species of *Legionella* have been recognized (136,142). *Legionella* are aerobic,

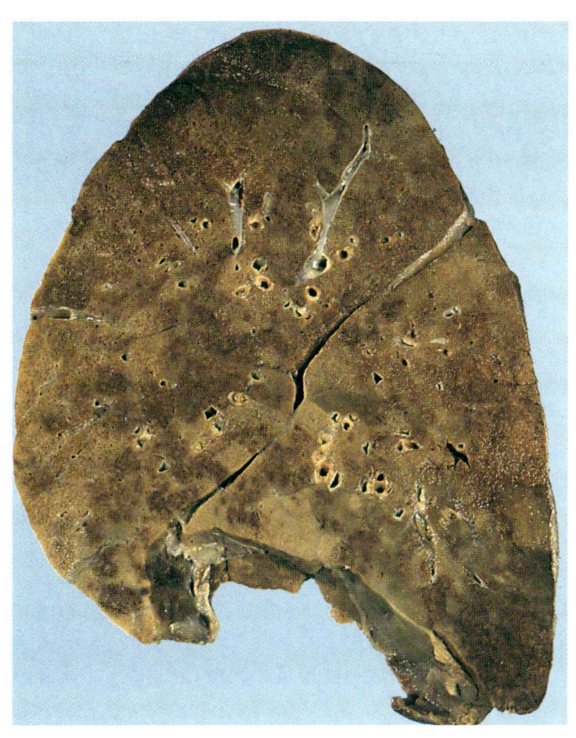

Figure 12-17

PSEUDOMONAS PNEUMONIA: GROSS SPECIMEN

The lung shows extensive bronchopneumonia with large areas of confluent necrosis which appear pale yellow on the cut surface. *Pseudomonas maltophilia* was cultured.

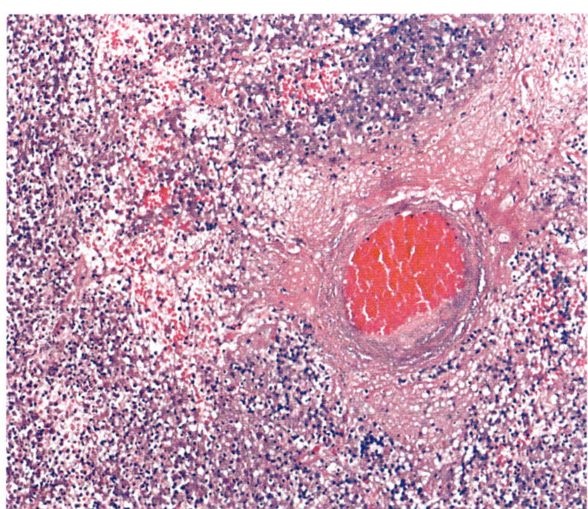

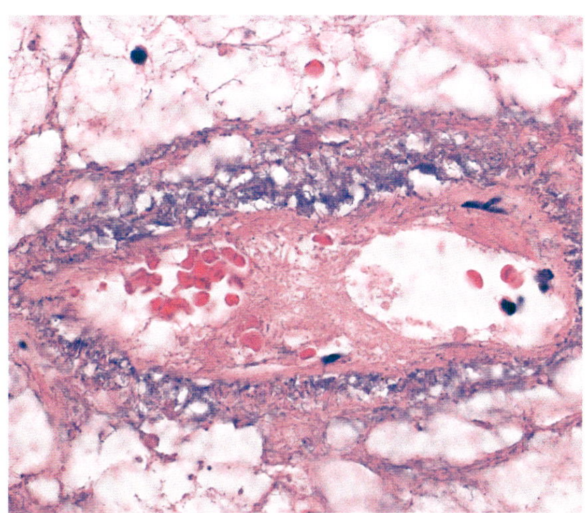

Figure 12-18

PSEUDOMONAS BRONCHOPNEUMONIA: HISTOLOGY

Left: The lung is extensively infiltrated by neutrophils.
Right: The wall of this blood vessel is permeated by numerous bacteria.

Gram-negative bacilli measuring 0.3–1.0 x 2.5 µm. They are most often found as single bacilli, or they may form chains or long filaments (136,142). *Legionella* dwell in an aquatic environment and human infection is acquired through aerosolized droplets from contaminated evaporator pans, cooling towers of air conditioners, humidifiers, respiratory therapy equipment, whirlpool spas, and decorative fountains (136,142). *Legionella* can cause nosocomial outbreaks as well as sporadic pneumonia. However, the organism is not thought to be transmitted from person to person. *Legionella* is thought to cause approximately 1 percent of all pulmonary infections and 15 percent of cases requiring hospitalization.

Pontiac fever is a milder clinical syndrome that may be caused by *L. pneumophila, L. feeleii, L. micdadei,* and *L. anisa* (70,73,142). *L. micdadei* is recognized as the cause of *Pittsburgh pneumonia* (3,29,63,142).

Clinical Features. *Legionella* sp can cause two major types of infections: *Legionella* pneumonia and Pontiac fever. Legionella pneumonia occurs more often in men, with a 2:1 to 3:1 male to female ratio (70,136,142). Most patients are adults, but children and neonates are also affected. In a recent study, *Legionella* pneumonia accounted for 8 percent of community-acquired pneumonia (117). Predisposing factors include age over 50 years, immunosuppressive therapy, malignancy, diabetes mellitus, chronic pulmonary or renal disease, and cigarette smoking.

Patients usually present after a 2- to 10-day incubation period with constitutional symptoms including lethargy, headache, fever, and myalgia (70,136,142). Pulmonary symptoms include nonproductive cough that may evolve to producing watery or purulent sputum. Shortness of breath and pleuritic chest pain develop in 50 and 33 percent of patients, respectively (70,136,142). Up to one third of patients have hemoptysis. Fever is as high as 40.5° C in up to one third of patients. Diarrhea is present in 50 percent of cases and approximately one fourth of patients develop nausea, vomiting, and abdominal pain. Neurologic findings of headache, confusion, delirium, seizures, and hallucinations may develop. Hyponatremia and hypophosphatemia are present in 50 percent of patients (70,136,142). Most patients have a leukocytosis with a left shift in the neutrophils, however, patients who are very sick may have leukopenia and thrombocytopenia.

Pontiac fever is an acute, febrile, self-limited illness, with upper respiratory tract symptoms (70,73,142). Affected patients exhibit a short incubation period and a good prognosis.

Radiologic Findings. Chest radiographs of patients with *Legionella* pneumonia are typically abnormal and demonstrate patchy, peripheral, nonsegmental consolidation. Initial involvement is usually unilateral and limited to one lobe. Progression to extensive lobar involvement, involvement of contiguous and noncontiguous lobes, and bilateral disease occurs commonly (fig. 12-19). Progression is usually rapid and may occur in spite of appropriate antibiotic therapy (26, 78,87). Nodular and mass-like consolidations have also been reported (14,101). Cavitation is unusual in immunocompetent individuals but is common in immunocompromised patients (fig. 12-19) (101). Pleural effusions are reported in half to two thirds of affected patients, are typically small, and may resolve spontaneously (26). Pneumothorax is rare. Lymphadenopathy typically does not occur (87). Radiologic resolution is usually slow and characteristically lags behind clinical improvement.

Pneumonia caused by *L. micdadei* is characterized by segmental to lobar consolidations, although nodular opacities are also reported (102). Progression to multilobar disease is recognized and is particularly severe when there is co-infection with *L. pneumophila* or when infection occurs in an immunocompromised patient (102,114).

Pathologic Findings. Grossly, *Legionella* pneumonia most often causes a focal and lobular pattern of lung involvement (see fig. 12-2) (142,143). Commonly, involvement is multilobar. A pattern of lobar pneumonia is described, but this may represent extensive confluence of a lobular pattern (142,143). Poorly marginated or distinct rounded lesions may be seen. Abscesses occur but they are usually small. Occasionally, however, cavitary lesions may be seen (142,143).

Histologically, in one third of cases the infiltrate is predominantly neutrophilic, in one third the infiltrate is mostly of monocytes or macrophages, and in the remaining third a combination of neutrophils and macrophages are seen (fig. 12-20, left) (142,143). Intra-alveolar fi-

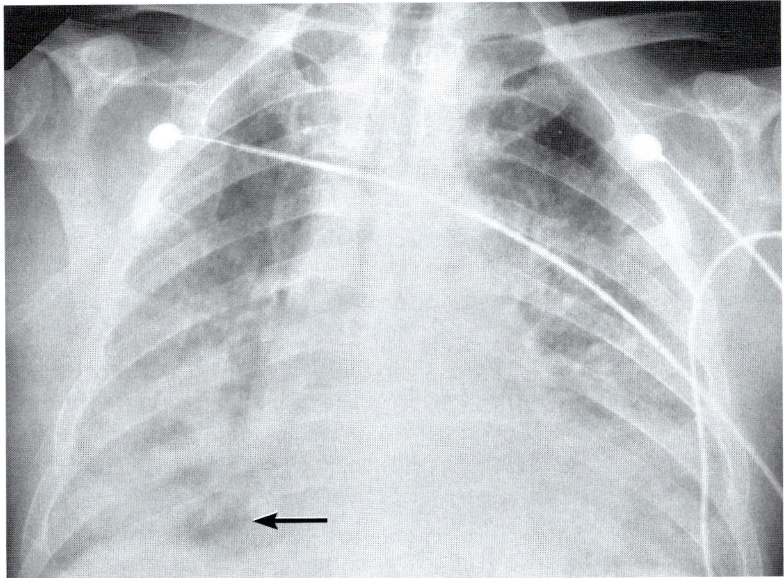

Figure 12-19

LEGIONELLA PNEUMONIA

Legionella pneumonia in a 59-year-old male with a 10-year history of chronic lymphocytic leukemia who developed chest pain, productive cough, headache, and malaise. PA portable chest radiograph obtained 10 days later demonstrates confluent parenchymal consolidations with early cavitation (arrow) in the right lower lobe.

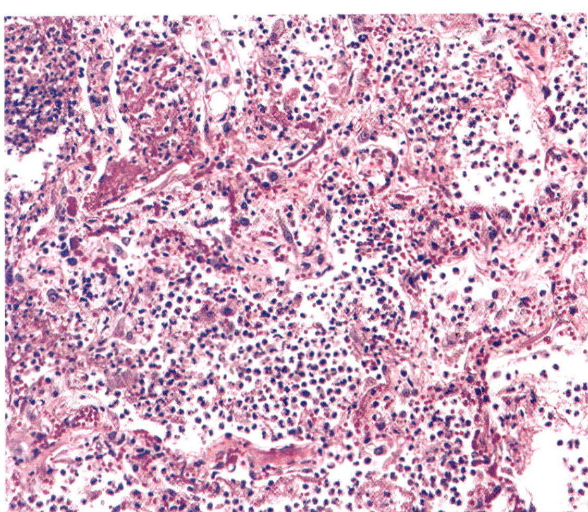

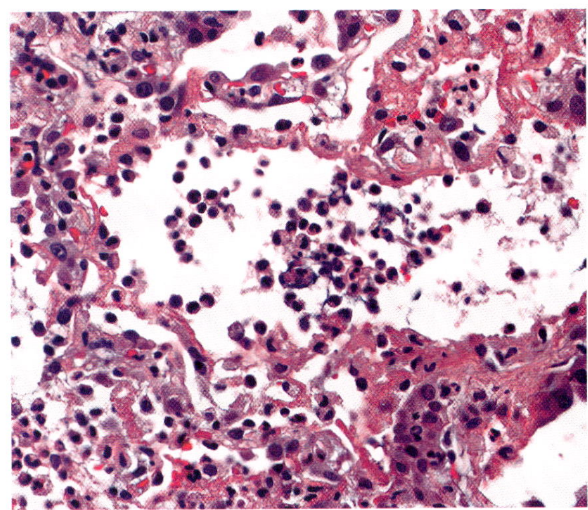

Figure 12-20

LEGIONELLA PNEUMONIA: HISTOLOGY

Left: There is extensive neutrophilic infiltration of the alveolar parenchyma in this bronchopneumonia. Focal intra-alveolar fibrin is present (top left).

Right: Focal hyaline membranes, in addition to marked neutrophil infiltrates, are present.

brin (fig. 12-20, left) and hemorrhage are common. There is prominent nuclear debris due to necrosis of neutrophils, resulting in a "dusty" appearance. The cellular lysis may be so prominent that the alveolar exudate appears acellular and fibrinoserous (138,142). Diffuse alveolar damage may be seen away from the active pneumonia in 20 percent of cases, and rarely, is the only finding on open lung biopsy (fig. 12-20, right) (142). Occasional cases show necrosis that may resemble infarcts. Vasculitis is seen in up to 30 percent of cases. It may be associated with thrombi, but bacteria are usually not seen in the vessel walls (142,143).

Electron microscopy shows the organisms within macrophages and neutrophils, and within vacuoles that are closely apposed to ribosome-like structures (142). It can be difficult

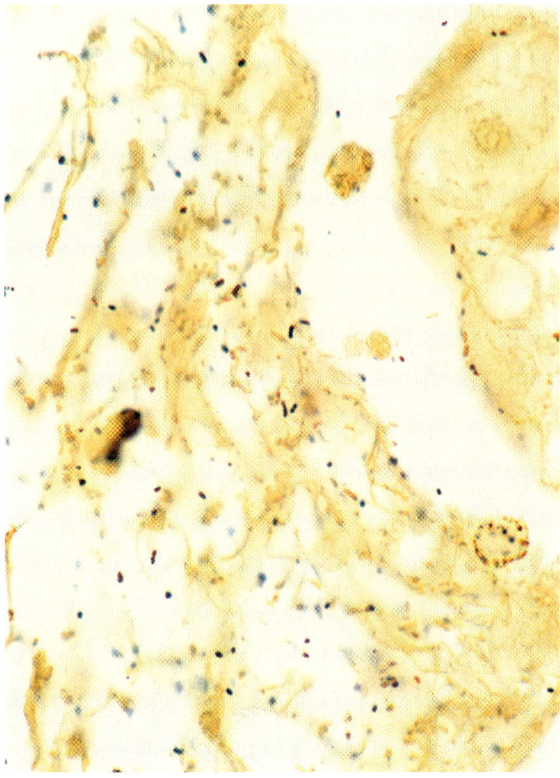

Figure 12-21

LEGIONELLA PNEUMONIA: DIETERLE STAIN

Multiple small bacilli are highlighted with this Dieterle stain.

to see the bacteria with the Brown and Hopps stain but they are usually discernable within macrophages with careful observation. The organisms are seen well with tissue silver stains such as the Steiner, Warthin-Starry, or Dieterle stains (fig. 12-21) (136,142). Immunoperoxidase and immunofluorescence methods are also useful and can be applied to deparaffinized, formalin-fixed tissue samples (136,142).

Interstitial fibrosis may be a long-term complication (20,66). Bullous emphysema followed *Legionella* pneumonia in a 2-year-old child (51).

Treatment and Prognosis. Patients respond rapidly to antibiotic therapy. Erythromycin has been supplanted by newer macrolides such as azithromycin and quinolones which penetrate macrophages (5,34,55,134,136). Patients may have severe extrapulmonary manifestations including gastrointestinal tract, central nervous system, bone marrow, renal, and hepatic abnormalities. Acute renal failure develops in 10 percent of patients. Even in patients who receive antibiotic therapy, however, in previous epidemics there has been a 5 to 25 percent mortality rate and in sporadic cases the mortality rate is 19 percent (55,136,142).

Anaerobic Bacteria

Definition. Lung infection can be caused by anaerobic bacteria: bacteria that grow poorly in the presence of oxygen (room air).

The diagnosis of pulmonary anaerobic bacterial infection requires methods that do not expose the samples to oxygen. This can be achieved with cultures of blood or pleural fluid, or in some cases biopsy specimens specially processed under anaerobic conditions. The most common cause of pulmonary anaerobic bacterial infection is aspiration (55). Consequently, many infections are mixed.

Clinical Features. Many anaerobic organisms are normal commensals of the oral cavity, especially in patients with poor dental hygiene (55). These include certain streptococci, fusobacteria, and *Bacteroides* species. Aspiration of these organisms commonly occurs with swallowing disorders, as seen in stuporous alcoholics, anesthetized patients, and persons subject to seizures. Infections by anaerobic organisms frequently cause pneumonia that is complicated by lung abscess, empyema, or both. Anaerobes are recovered in up to 89 percent of patients with lung abscesses (mixed anaerobic and aerobic infections are common). Anaerobes are also commonly isolated alone or with other aerobic bacteria in most empyemas. The clinical presentation is usually an indolent one characterized by fever, sweats, cough, dyspnea, weight loss, and pleurisy. A foul breath odor is common.

Pathologic Findings. Pulmonary infection with anaerobic organisms leads to necrotizing pneumonias, which are frequently complicated by lung abscesses. Necrotizing pneumonias are characterized by massive neutrophil accumulation causing extensive necrosis and abscess formation. The necrotic tissue may cavitate. The pathology of lung abscess is addressed in more detail below. Many anaerobes have peculiar morphologies.

The most dramatic complication is gangrene of the lung, a result of thrombosis of a branch of the pulmonary artery and consequent infarction. This is regarded as a medical emergency and requires resection of the affected lung.

Treatment and Prognosis. Antimicrobial therapy based on the microbiology, chest physical therapy, and postural drainage are the key approaches to the management of lung abscesses. Untreated, mortality of patients with lung abscess approaches 33 percent; however, up to 90 percent recover with treatment, although a long course of therapy may be required (55). Surgical resection of the necrotic lung may occasionally be necessary if there is a poor response to antibiotics or if airway obstruction limits adequate drainage. Drainage of the infected fluid or pus and antimicrobial treatment are the keys to effective management of empyema.

Nocardia Sp

Definition. Nocardiosis of the lung is caused by infection with the bacteria, *Nocardia* sp.

Nocardia are aerobic, Gram-positive bacilli with a filamentous, beaded morphology (16,43, 55). The organism is found in the soil and is distributed throughout the world. Pulmonary infection is usually acquired through inhalation of saprophytic organisms in the soil or decaying vegetable matter (16,43,55,142). Rarely, the organisms reach the lungs via the bloodstream from other infected sites such as a contaminated catheter (97). There are multiple species of *Nocardia,* but pneumonia is caused most often by *N. asteroides,* which accounts for 80 percent of pulmonary or disseminated infections (18,43, 55). *N. brasiliensis* and *N. otitidiscaviarum* (previously *N. caviae*) are the next most common causes of pneumonia (118,123). Rarely, *N. transvalensis, N. nova,* or *N. farcinica* cause pneumonia (93,97, 99,133). Approximately 500 to 1,000 new cases of nocardiosis are diagnosed each year in the United States (18,43).

Clinical Features. Nocardiosis is more common in adults than children. There is a male predominance, with a 2:1 to 3:1 male to female ratio (18,43,55). Patients usually have a subacute clinical presentation over a period of one to several weeks, although an acute onset may occur in immunocompromised patients. Nocardiosis bears some resemblance to actinomycosis, but it is more likely to occur in immunosuppressed hosts and to disseminate hematogenously. The main risk factor for nocardiosis is immunodeficiency, especially associated with lymphoreticular malignancy, Cushing's disease, acquired immunodeficiency syndrome (AIDS), corticosteroid therapy, and chronic granulomatous disease (18,43,55). Presenting symptoms consist of fatigue, low-grade fever, weight loss, and productive cough. Less often patients have dyspnea, pleuritic chest pain, or hemoptysis (18, 55). Patients often experience exacerbations and remissions over periods of days to weeks and the diagnosis is often delayed. In approximately 50 percent of cases of *Nocardia* pneumonia the infection disseminates to other organs, especially the brain, skin, kidney, and bone (43,55).

Radiologic Findings. Radiographs of patients with pulmonary nocardiosis typically demonstrate nonsegmental and homogeneous parenchymal consolidation, which may involve large areas (41). Parenchymal disease is often peripheral and abuts the adjacent pleura (fig. 12-22). Multifocal peripheral nodules or masses with irregular borders also occur (fig. 12-22) (27, 41,116,144). Cavitation is seen in over one third of patients and may occur within nodular opacities, masses, or areas of consolidation (fig. 12-22). Small nodular and interstitial opacities are less commonly described (41). Cross-sectional imaging with CT demonstrates internal low attenuation, cavitation, and peripheral enhancement of lesions after intravenous contrast administration (28). Pleural effusions are common, and empyema and chest wall involvement have been reported. Immunocompromised patients may demonstrate rapid progression of radiologic abnormalities (fig. 12-23). Chronic disease may extend to adjacent structures to include the chest wall and mediastinum (28). Lymphadenopathy is not common (46).

Pathologic Findings. Grossly, the lungs typically show multiple abscesses, which may be confluent. The abscesses may contain thick green pus (fig. 12-24). Histologically, there is extensive suppuration and necrosis (fig. 12-25). Numerous neutrophils form microabscesses, which may be associated with varying numbers of macrophages (fig. 12-25). In chronic cases, there may be epithelioid cells and multinucleated giant cells. The organisms are seen within the areas of necrosis and suppuration (fig. 12-26). Large abscesses and cavitation may occur. Endobronchial nocardiosis is reported (64).

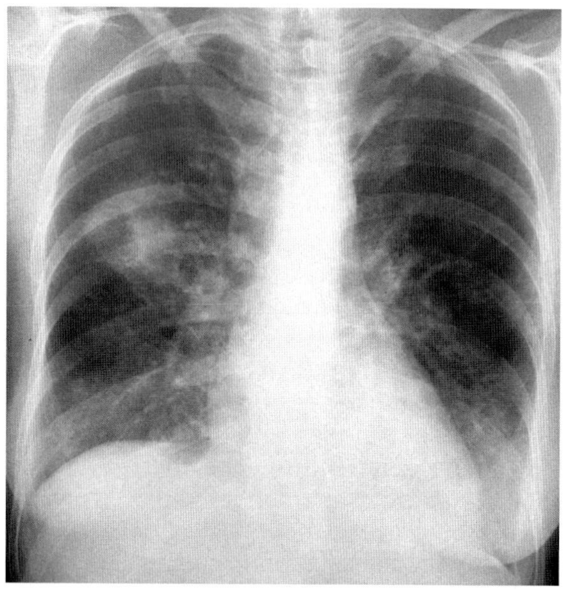

Figure 12-22

PULMONARY NOCARDIOSIS

Nocardiosis in a 53-year-old female with renal insufficiency, rheumatoid arthritis, and anemia who became febrile. PA chest radiograph demonstrates a confluent consolidation in the left lower lobe and a mass-like consolidation in the superior segment of the right lower lobe, with internal cavitation. Small bilateral pleural effusions are also present.

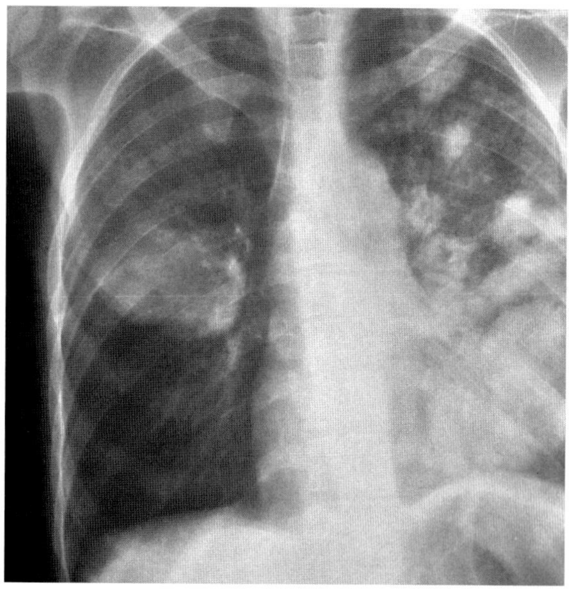

Figure 12-23

PULMONARY NOCARDIOSIS

Nocardiosis in a 27-year-old male with AIDS and a 3-week history of fever, cough, dyspnea, and weight loss. PA chest radiograph obtained 3 months later demonstrates marked progression of pulmonary disease, with confluent pulmonary masses in the left lower lobe and additional nodules and masses throughout the rest of the lungs bilaterally.

Rarely, *Nocardia* sp forms "fungus balls" within preexisting cavities (fig. 12-27) (7,84). A case of superior vena cava syndrome associated with *Nocardia* pneumonia and mediastinitis is reported (112). Alveolar proteinosis may be associated with *Nocardia* pulmonary infection (107).

Nocardia consists of long, thin, beaded, bacterial filaments measuring approximately 1 µm in thickness (figs. 12-26, 12-27, right) (16, 142). They branch at right angles and have so many branches they are said to have a "Chinese character" pattern. The organisms can be demonstrated with the Gomori methenamine silver (GMS), Brown and Brenn, and Brown and Hopps stains (16,142). However, the organisms can be difficult to detect and are easily overlooked unless one specifically searches for the somewhat unusual morphology. It is difficult to see the organisms in sections stained with hematoxylin and eosin (H&E), PAS, and Gridley fungal stains. The organisms are weakly acid-fast, requiring the use of modified acid-fast stains such as Coates-Fite, Kinyoun, or Fite-Faraco which use less decolorization than the routine acid-fast stain for mycobacteria (16,142).

Differential Diagnosis. The definitive diagnosis is established by culture of lung biopsy tissue or bronchoalveolar lavage fluid. Since cultures usually require 1 to 2 weeks to confirm the diagnosis, a more rapid diagnosis may be pursued through other methods such as direct examination of respiratory specimens, including sputum, with the Gram or Coates-Fite stain (106).

The most difficult problem in the diagnosis of *Nocardia* in lung biopsy specimens is simply recognizing that the organisms are present. It is important to suspect *Nocardia,* to perform appropriate stains such as the Brown and Brenn or Coates-Fite stain. The filamentous branching bacteria of *Nocardia* are often overlooked since they may be difficult to see with routine special stains. The major differential diagnosis is with *Actinomyces. Actinomyces* may form sulfur granules in the lung while *Nocardia* does not.

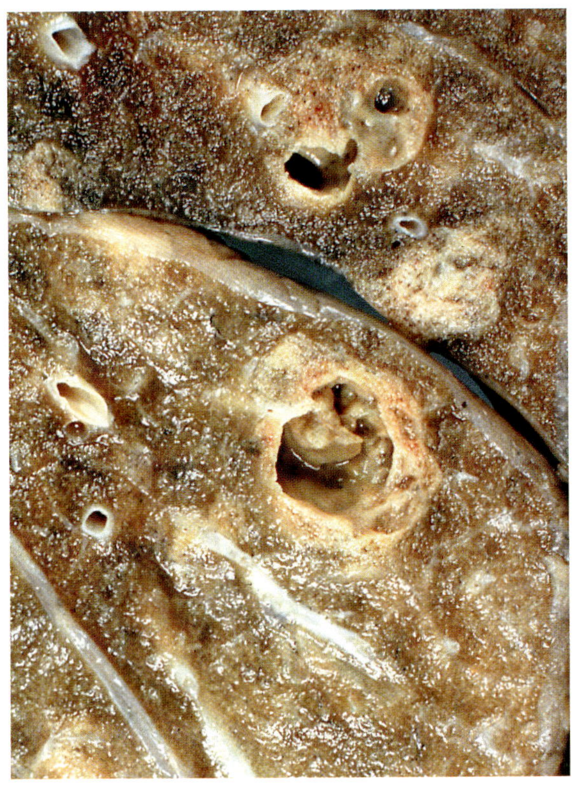

Figure 12-24

NOCARDIA PNEUMONIA: GROSS SPECIMEN

Cavitary abscesses are seen in this *Nocardia* bronchopneumonia.

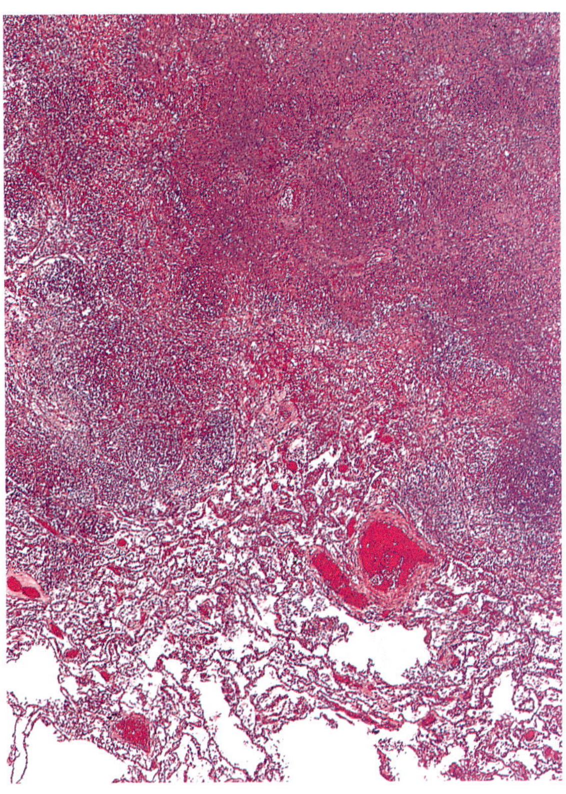

Figure 12-25

NOCARDIA PNEUMONIA: HISTOLOGY

This necrotizing pneumonia is characterized by extensive acute inflammation and a large zone of necrosis.

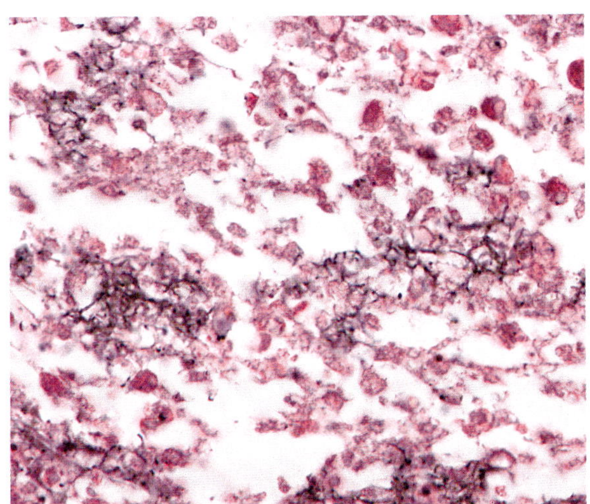

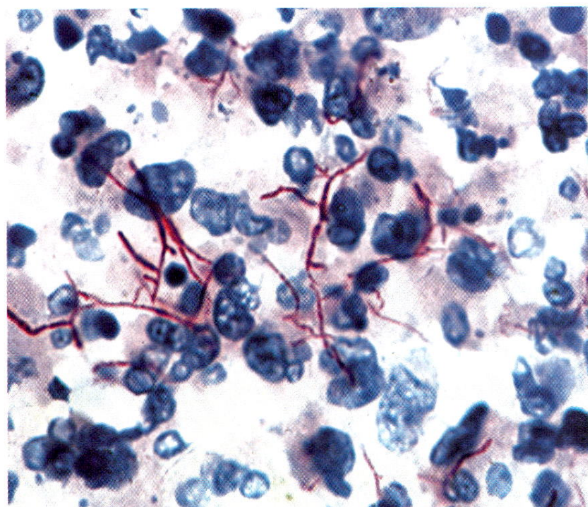

Figure 12-26

NOCARDIA ORGANISMS

Left: The complex branching pattern of the filamentous bacteria is highlighted by the GMS stain.
Right: The acid-fast nature of these long, branching, filamentous bacteria is highlighted by Coates-Fite stain.

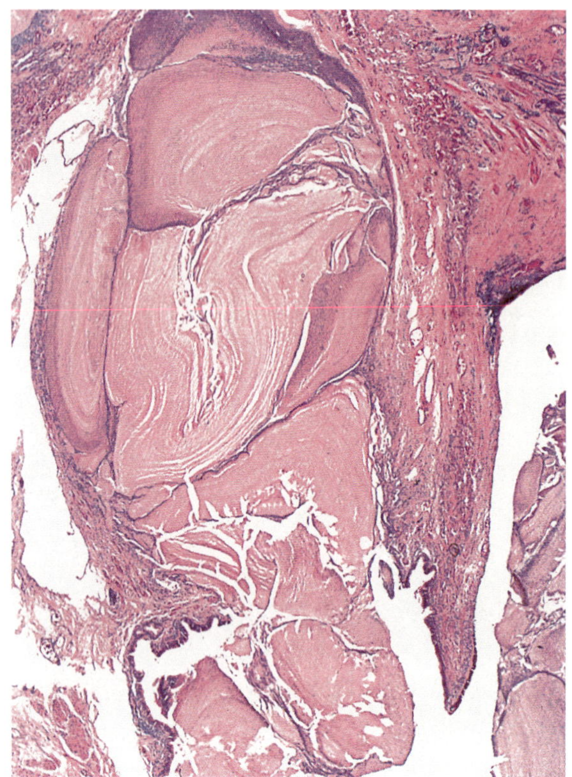

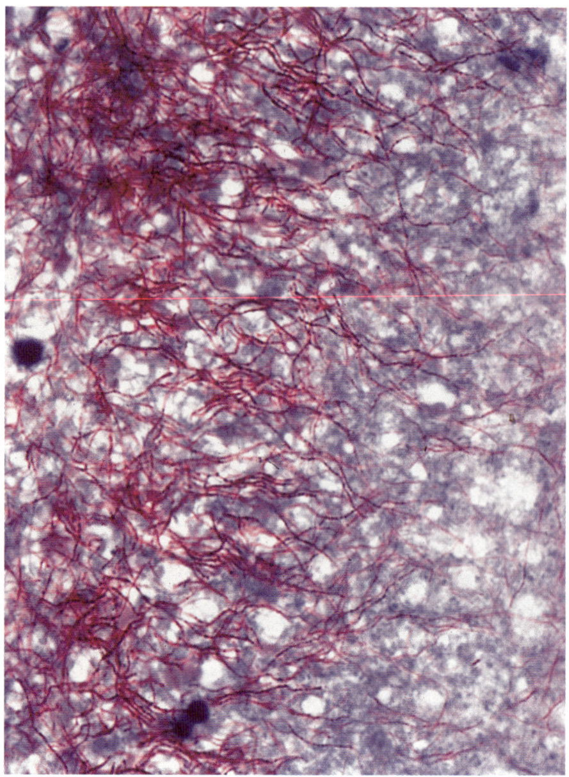

Figure 12-27

NOCARDIA "FUNGUS BALL"

Left: Within this bronchus is a mass or "fungus ball" of *Nocardia* organisms.
Right: The Coates-Fite stain demonstrates a dense mass of acid-fast *Nocardia* organisms.

Nocardia is also weakly acid-fast in contrast to *Actinomyces*. Atypical mycobacteria may sometimes have long, beaded, acid-fast bacilli which conceivably could be confused with *Nocardia* if they are numerous and overlapping. However, mycobacteria are much shorter than *Nocardia,* do not show true branching, and stain with routine acid-fast stains.

Treatment and Prognosis. The optimal treatment for pulmonary nocardiosis is sulfonamide medication. In normal hosts it is usually effective, with less than 5 percent mortality in recent studies (43). Surgery may be necessary to drain empyemas, but antimicrobial therapy is usually effective against lung abscesses (43). Patients with impaired cellular immunity and transplant recipients require more prolonged treatment with similar medication to prevent relapses (43).

Actinomyces Sp

Definition. Actinomycosis is an infection caused by the anaerobic filamentous bacteria, *Actinomyces* sp.

Actinomycosis was at one time a common diagnosis in this country. It still is fairly common in some parts of the world (9). As the numbers of antibiotics and indications for their use have increased, the disease has almost become a medical rarity in the United States. This fact might suggest a paradox in view of the universal presence of *Actinomyces* organisms in every human mouth. Although actinomycetes resemble fungi in appearance, they are actually bacteria. Therefore, it is perhaps not well recognized that the actinomycetes are particularly sensitive to most of the common antibacterials in current usage. These facts have combined to decrease the clinical frequency of the disease as well as effectively reduce the opportunity for securing a satisfactory specimen for laboratory culture in suspected cases. Actinomycosis can manifest in a variety of forms and may mimic other infections or even neoplasms. The clinical pattern of remission and exacerbation of symptoms occurring in parallel sequence with initiation and cessation of antibiotic administration is a phenomenon that should increase suspicion for actinomycosis in any of its manifestations.

Actinomycosis is caused by infection with actinomycetes, and the usual pulmonary organism is *Actinomyces israelii* (27,33,42,55). Less common pathogens include *A. naeslundii, A. viscosus,* and *A. propionica.* The thorax is one of the major sites of infection, which also include the neck, face, abdomen, and pelvis. Thoracic infection typically follows aspiration or extension of cervicofacial infection.

Clinical Features. *Actinomyces,* which normally inhabits the mouth and nose, infects the lung either by aspiration of oropharyngeal contents or by extension from an actinomycotic subdiaphragmatic or liver abscess. Actinomycosis is a chronic granulomatous lesion characterized by suppuration, sulfur granules, abscesses, and sinus tracts. *Actinomyces* may be a component of aspiration pneumonia without causing actinomycosis. Rarely, an endobronchial lesion develops in an HIV-infected patient (15). Disseminated infection with bilateral lung involvement can occur (24). Pulmonary disease manifests insidiously with cough, sputum production, fever, and weight loss. Hemoptysis and pleuritic pain are occasionally present. An elevated WBC count and anemia are common.

Radiologic Findings. The classic chest radiographic appearance of pulmonary actinomycosis is that of peripheral, unilateral, patchy, lower lobe airspace consolidation which may be chronic (fig. 12-28) (80). Mass-like consolidation may be seen and may mimic the radiologic appearance of primary lung cancer (23). Multifocal and nodular opacities have also been described (23). Cross-sectional imaging with CT often demonstrates central low attenuation and cavitation, which may not be visible on radiography (23,80). There may be a peripheral "ring-like" enhancement of parenchymal disease on contrast studies (80). Pleural thickening adjacent to the consolidation is frequently observed, but pleural effusions are less common and usually small (23,80). However, empyema and large pleural effusions have been described. Chronic lung involvement may result in extensive fibrosis. Endobronchial disease may result in atelectasis. Miliary opacities and biapical pulmonary involvement mimicking tuberculosis have also been described (46). Hilar lymphadenopathy is demonstrated on CT in up to 75 percent of patients (80).

Pulmonary actinomycosis may cross anatomic barriers and progress to involve adjacent lobes, the pleura, and the chest wall. These manifestations, while considered classic and characteristic of actinomycosis, are not commonly seen today in the United States. When present, chest wall involvement is characterized by a soft tissue mass or swelling and/or wavy periosteitis or destruction of the affected ribs (fig. 12-28) (27,137). Mediastinal involvement from contiguous spread of adjacent pulmonary disease has been described and primary mediastinal involvement following esophageal perforation may also occur (137). The radiologic differential diagnosis includes primary lung cancer and other infections such as tuberculosis, blastomycosis, and cryptococcosis (27).

Gross Findings. The gross appearance can vary depending on the extent of the infection, the degree of fibrosis, and whether the disease has spread into or through the pleura. The sulfur granules appear as small yellow nodules within abscesses or airways (fig. 12-29). Balls of organisms may grow within cavities, similar to fungus balls (24). A potential complication is rupture of abscesses into the pleura with subsequent empyema or bronchopleural fistulae. Chest wall invasion may also occur. Actinomycosis is frequently suspected to be a malignancy by the clinical presentation, chest radiographs, and gross pathology.

Histologic Findings. The pulmonary reaction to *Actinomyces* infection is an acute suppurative inflammation (figs. 12-30, 12-31, left) (42, 142). Acute bronchopneumonia with abscess formation is the initial reaction and the process typically progresses to fibrosis (fig. 12-30). Around the border of the abscesses there may be a prominent histiocytic reaction. The organisms form sulfur granules that are characterized by the Splendore-Hoeppli phenomenon, which is

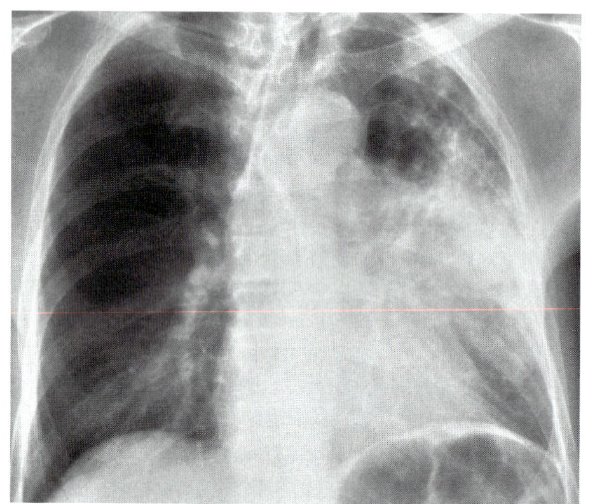
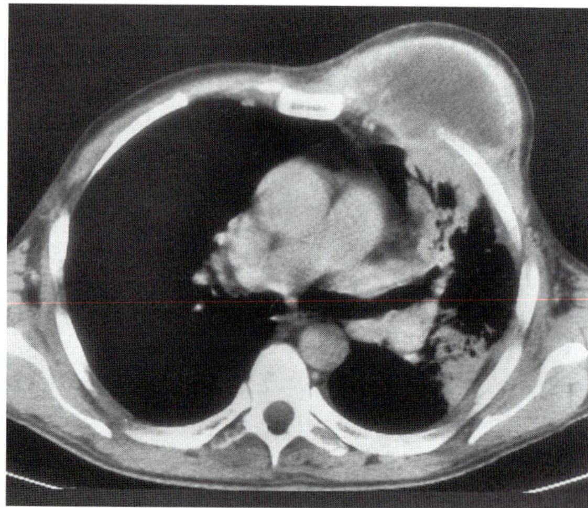

Figure 12-28

ACTINOMYCOSIS

Actinomycosis in a 51-year-old male with a history of gingival swelling, submandibular lymphadenopathy, vomiting, night sweats, and a 15-pound weight loss. The patient also noted a palpable left chest wall mass.

Left: PA chest radiograph demonstrates a left upper lobe parenchymal consolidation.

Right: Contrast-enhanced chest CT (mediastinal window) demonstrates left upper and left lower lobe parenchymal consolidation and contiguous chest wall involvement. Note the left anterior chest wall abscess with peripheral enhancement and central low attenuation.

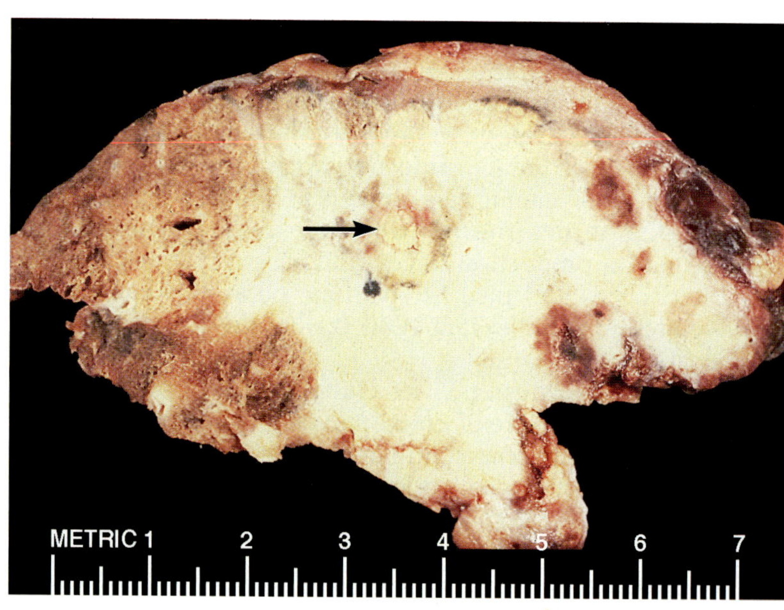

Figure 12-29

ACTINOMYCOSIS: GROSS SPECIMEN

In the center of a large area of dense white-tan consolidation is a small nodular yellow structure within a bronchus that represents a sulfur granule (arrow).

an eosinophilic, amorphous substance around the periphery of a dense mass of organisms (fig. 12-31, left). The organisms are Gram-positive, beaded, branching, filamentous bacteria that are thin, measuring about 1 µm in diameter (fig. 12-31, right). The branching is often at right angles. At the periphery of the granules the filamentous organisms sometimes show a radial orientation, with club-shaped swellings at the periphery. The organisms stain with the GMS and Brown and Brenn Gram stains (fig. 12-31, right).

Differential Diagnosis. The differential diagnosis includes other organisms that can cause the Splendore-Hoeppli phenomenon (18). This can occur with fungal mycetomas as well as botryomycosis. The fungal mycetomas have septate hyphae and chlamydoconidia, and it is rare to see the Splendore-Hoeppli phenomenon in association with fungal pulmonary infections. Botryomycosis consists of clusters of nonfilamentous bacteria that can be either Gram positive or negative. *Nocardia* does not form sulfur granules in the lung and is weakly acid-fast. Negative acid-fast staining is not a reliable way to distinguish *Nocardia* from *Actinomyces* since *Nocardia* is only weakly acid-fast.

Treatment and Prognosis. Penicillin is the drug of choice and results in cure in approximately 90 percent of patients.

UNCOMMON BACTERIAL PNEUMONIAS

Burkholderia Pseudomallei

Definition. Pulmonary melioidosis is an infection caused by the bacteria *Burkholderia pseudomallei*. Synonyms include *Pseudomonas pseudomallei pneumonia* and *false glanders*.

Melioidosis occurs exclusively in tropical regions between the latitudes 20° north and 20° south (94). It is endemic in Southeast Asia. *B. pseudomallei* is an aerobic, bipolar-staining, small, Gram-negative bacterium. Infection is acquired either through a cutaneous route, usually when exposed to contaminated water or

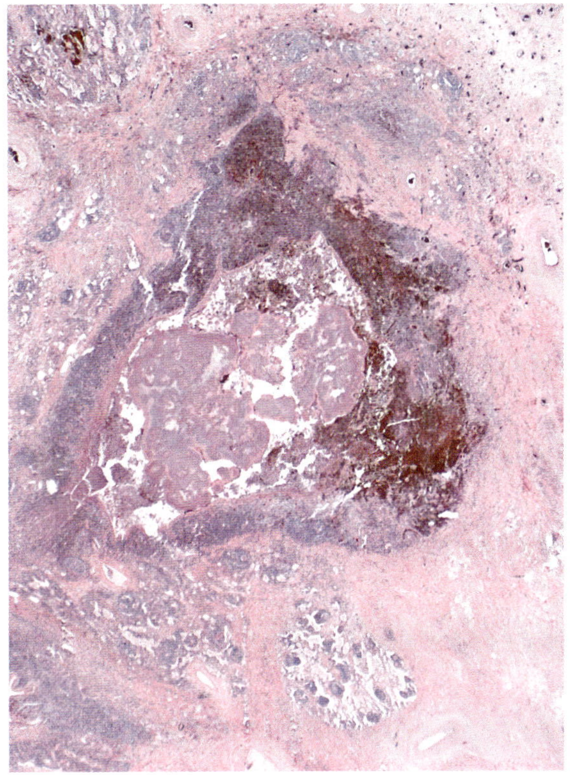

Figure 12-30

ACTINOMYCOSIS: HISTOLOGY

In the center of this bronchus is an actinomycotic sulfur granule. The surrounding lung parenchyma is extensively fibrotic and chronically inflamed.

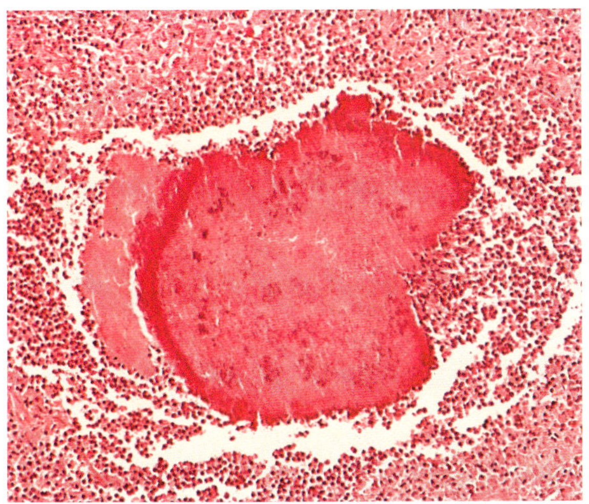

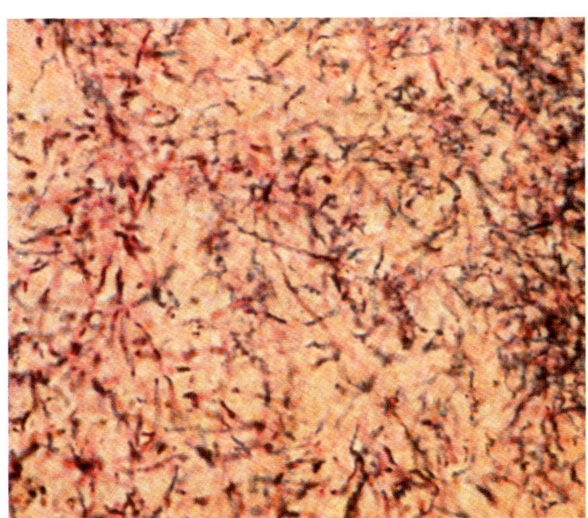

Figure 12-31

ACTINOMYCOSIS: ORGANISMS

Left: A neutrophilic infiltrate surrounds this eosinophilic mass of actinomycetes that form a sulfur granule. At the periphery is the eosinophilic club-like reaction of the Splendore-Hoeppli phenomenon.

Right: With the Brown and Brenn stain, the organisms appear as thin, Gram-positive, beaded, branching, filamentous bacteria.

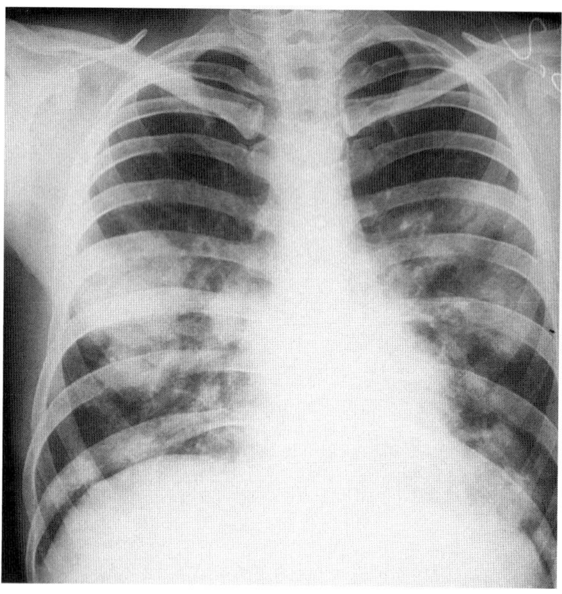

Figure 12-32

PULMONARY MELIOIDOSIS

Melioidosis in a 28-year-old male with multiple skin lesions. PA chest radiograph obtained 1 month later as the patient's clinical status deteriorated demonstrates bilateral, multifocal, confluent mass-like consolidations.

soil, or by inhalation of contaminated aerosolized water or dirt. It is regarded as a "great mimicker" due to the potentially deceptive clinical manifestations, which include skin abscesses, necrotizing pneumonia, and sepsis with abscesses in multiple organs. The major target organ is the lung where it causes a pneumonia that can either be fulminant or indolent.

Clinical Features. Patients with melioidosis present with three clinical syndromes: 1) respiratory, cutaneous; 2) lymphatic, soft tissue, and musculoskeletal; and 3) bacteremic visceral involvement (19,67,70,94). Cellulitis and lymphangitis may be present at the site of the primary skin infection. The latency period may be only 3 days, however, more often it is months to years (19,67,70,94). There is a broad range of clinical severity including an acute, subacute, or chronic pneumonia. Patients with acute pneumonia present with high fever, dyspnea, pleuritic chest pain, prostration, hemoptysis, and purulent sputum. Empyema may be present. Chronic or subacute disease may not cause symptoms and is incidentally found because of an abnormal chest radiograph or because patients present with a chronic disorder resembling pulmonary tuberculosis (19,67,70, 94). Immunosuppressed patients are at risk. Reactivation may occur months or years after initial infection.

Radiologic Findings. Chest radiographs of patients with acute pulmonary melioidosis typically demonstrate multifocal nodular opacities, which may enlarge rapidly, affect the adjacent lung, and demonstrate cavitation (fig. 12-32). The latter develops in 40 to 60 percent of affected patients. Pleural effusion occurs in up to 15 percent of patients and may progress to empyema.

Radiographs of patients with chronic pulmonary melioidosis typically demonstrate peripheral subpleural consolidation, linear opacities, and cavitation. These findings may mimic the radiologic appearance of postprimary tuberculosis. However, melioidosis is reported to spare the subapical lung (35,45,68).

Pathologic Findings. *B. pseudomallei* can cause two histologic patterns of tissue response: acute necrotizing inflammation and poorly formed granulomatous inflammation (fig. 12-33) (57,94). The acute necrotizing lesion consists of numerous neutrophils and macrophages with some giant cells and lymphocytes. The granulomatous pattern is characterized by loose granulomas, which may be associated with necrosis. Some cases may show a mixture of acute and granulomatous inflammation (fig. 12-33, right) (57,94). In cases with the granulomatous reaction, giant cells and macrophages may contain dense clusters of bacilli that are called "globi" (57,94). Most of the organisms are intracellular and much more difficult to identify in specimens showing the acute inflammatory response. In this setting, the organisms may be both intracellular and extracellular (57,94).

Recently, Belchis et al. (8) reported three cases of fatal *B. cepacia* pneumonia in patients without cystic fibrosis. The pathologic findings resembled those of *B. pseudomallei*: necrotizing granulomatous inflammation, which merged with areas of more classic necrotizing acute bronchopneumonia (fig. 12-34).

Recognition of the Gram-negative bacilli in tissue sections can be very helpful, but the diagnosis is best established based on culture (57,94). The organism may take longer than 48

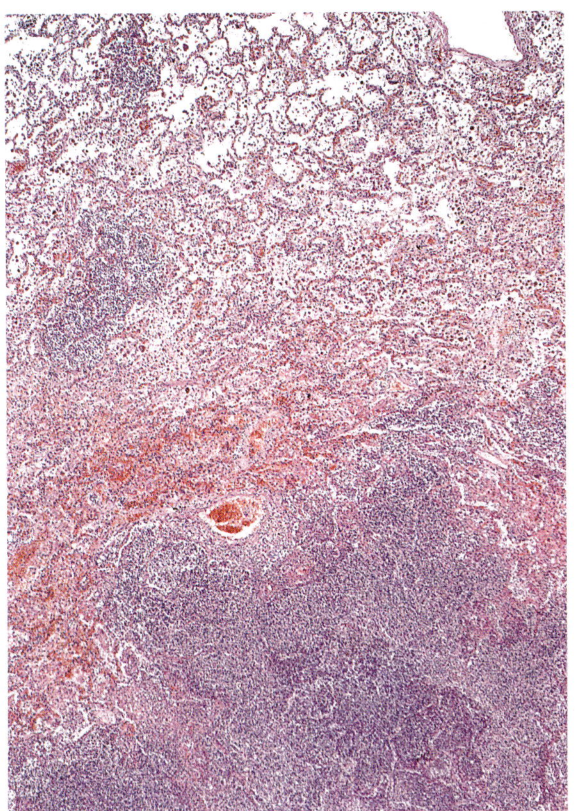

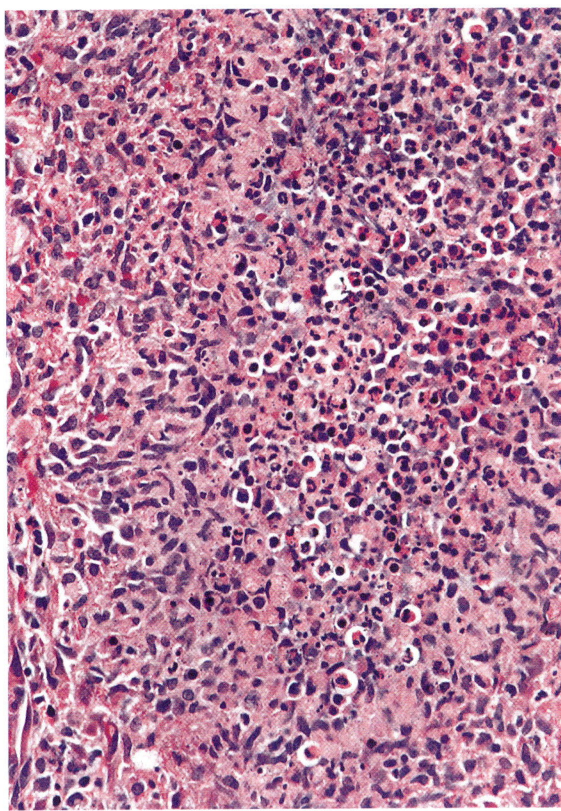

Figure 12-33

PULMONARY MELIOIDOSIS: HISTOLOGY

Left: The lung shows an acute bronchopneumonia (top) with abscess formation (bottom).
Right: A granulomatous reaction consisting of palisading histiocytes is present at the edge of a neutrophilic abscess.

hours to grow in culture. Ashdown's selective medium prevents overgrowth by other contaminants from sputum (57,94).

Differential Diagnosis. Pulmonary melioidosis in the form of a necrotizing pneumonia must be distinguished from necrotizing bacterial pneumonias caused by other organisms such as the Gram-positive *Staphylococcus aureus* and *Streptococcus pyogenes,* and the Gram-negative *Klebsiella pneumoniae* and *Pseudomonas aeruginosa* (67,70,94). Beyond the recognition of Gram-negative bacilli in tissue sections and cultures, knowing whether the patient is from the tropics or traveled to an endemic area can be a valuable clue to the diagnosis (67,70,94).

Treatment and Prognosis. Patients with pulmonary melioidosis tend to respond slowly to treatment if the process remains localized (67, 70,94). Due to the tendency to relapse, prolonged antibiotic therapy is usually required. A variety of medications can be used to treat melioidosis including ceftazidime, tetracyclines, sulfonamides, chloramphenicol, kanamycin, and trimethoprim/sulfamethoxazole. Parenteral therapy with ceftazidime is also effective (67,70,94).

Francisella Tularensis

Definition. Tularemic pneumonia is caused by the small, Gram-negative coccobacillus, *Francisella tularensis* (formerly *Pasteurella tularensis*). Synonyms include *rabbit fever* and *deerfly fever.*

Tularemia is caused by infection with *F. tularensis,* a Gram-negative, pleomorphic coccobacillus that is transmitted through contact with infected animals or a bite by an infected tick or deer fly (39,52). Hunters handling infected rabbits or squirrels are particularly at risk. *F. tularensis* is found in regions of the northern hemisphere between latitudes 30° and 71° north. There are about 150 cases reported in

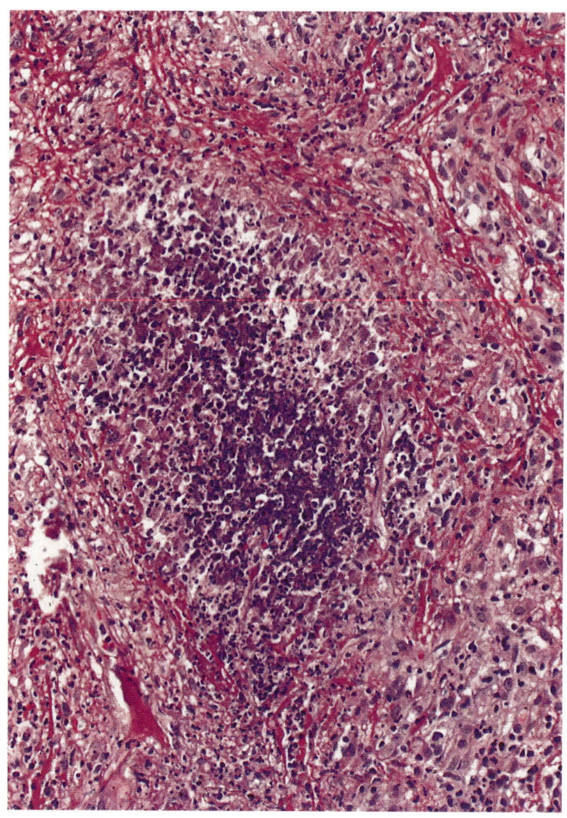

Figure 12-34

BURKHOLDERIA CEPACIA: HISTOLOGY

A dense neutrophilic abscess is surrounded by granulomatous inflammation consisting of palisading histiocytes.

the United States each year. The potential for acquiring the disease from accidental exposure in the laboratory is great.

Clinical Features. Patients with tularemia present with a clinical syndrome initially consisting of abrupt onset of fever, chills, and malaise. This usually develops after a 3- to 5-day incubation period. Subsequently, patients develop a nonproductive cough, dyspnea, and chest pain (39,52,70,96). Symptoms of primary pulmonary tularemia, which result from inhalation of aerosolized contaminated droplets, are rare compared to the other clinical manifestations. Bronchoscopy of patients with primary pulmonary tularemia shows focal to diffuse hemorrhagic erosion of the bronchial mucosa (128). Hilar adenopathy is common.

Tularemia also affects the skin, lymph node, eye, and oropharynx. Patients may have an ulceroglandular infection in which ulceration associated with regional lymphadenopathy occurs at the site of original inoculation (39, 52,70,96). This is the most common form of tularemia, accounting for 70 to 80 percent of all cases (13,52,128).

Tularemia has also been reported to cause pneumonia in a patient with chronic granulomatous disease (88), and to cause a solitary pulmonary nodule after a peripheral blood stem cell transplant for leukemia (104).

Radiologic Findings. Chest radiographic manifestations of pulmonary tularemia are characterized by nonspecific parenchymal consolidation, which may be patchy, segmental, or nonsegmental. Cavitation occurs in up to 20 percent of patients with consolidation. Hilar lymphadenopathy and pleural effusions occur in 50 percent of cases. Miliary disease, isolated intrathoracic lymphadenopathy, and pneumothorax occur less frequently (45,53).

Pathologic Findings. Histologically, tularemia pneumonia is an acute fibrinous and necrotizing pneumonia (fig. 12-35). The alveolar walls undergo necrosis and the airspaces are filled with edema, fibrin, and necrotic neutrophils. Organisms may be seen with immunofluorescent antibody staining. As the lesions resolve they may show fibrosis, calcification, and necrosis (52,96). In one study of patients with primary pulmonary tularemia, bronchoscopic biopsies within the first 45 days showed hemorrhage and edema while a granulomatous reaction was seen in patients 3 to 7 months after onset (128).

Treatment and Prognosis. The optimal therapy is with streptomycin (52,70,96). It is important to initiate treatment early to avoid progression and a fatal outcome. Death occurs in 5 percent of untreated patients.

Yersinia Pestis

Definition. Plague pneumonia is a pulmonary infection caused by *Yersinia pestis* (formerly *Pasteurella pestis,* and also termed *black death, black plague, bubonic plague, septicemic plague, pneumonic plague*).

During the 6th, 14th, 15th–18th, and 19th centuries, millions of deaths occurred due to pandemics of the plague in various parts of the world including Egypt, Europe, Asia Minor, and

China (55,124). The organism is found worldwide but is relatively uncommon today. In the United States, sporadic cases of plague have occurred in rural areas of the southwestern states, especially New Mexico, Arizona, and California. Cases also are reported from parts of Africa, South America, and the Far East (55,124,142). Urban infection can occur in lower socioeconomic environments since rats and fleas carry *Y. pestis*.

Plague is a zoonosis, with the natural hosts being small mammals, mostly rodents such as rats (especially the domestic rat, Rattus rattus), squirrels, rabbits, and prairie dogs (55,124,142). The organism is transmitted to humans through flea bites (especially Xenopsylla cheopis, the rat flea). Aerosol spread occurs by exposure to either infected humans or animals (55,124,142).

The organism is a nonmotile, short, Gram-negative rod. With the Wayson's stain it appears bipolar (55,124,142). It may be encapsulated when it infects tissues.

Clinical Features. Plague causes three major types of disease: bubonic, pneumonic, and septicemic (55,124,142). Pneumonia can occur in the bubonic as well as septicemic forms. The three major forms of plague have different clinical manifestations (55,124,142). The incubation period for *primary pneumonic plague* is usually 2 to 7 days. Patients present initially with high fever and chills. Subsequently, they develop chest pain, cough, dyspnea, and hemoptysis. This form usually occurs following aerosol spread from infected animals or humans (55,124,142).

Patients with pulmonary involvement who have the *bubonic form* of plague also have painful adenopathy (55,124,142). In adults, the inguinal nodes are usually affected while in children the axillary and cervical nodes are typically involved. *Septicemic plague* is the least common form of *Y. pestis* infection, accounting for only 1 percent of cases. Patients have features of Gram-negative septicemic shock such as sudden onset, fever, chills, anxiety, and prostration (55,124,142).

The diagnosis is established with cultures or by utilizing fluorescent antibody stains on sputum or tissue sections (70,124,142). Blood cultures are usually positive. Rapid diagnosis is essential due to the potentially rapid clinical course.

Radiologic Findings. Chest radiographs in patients with pneumonic plague are typically abnormal and demonstrate multiple, bilateral, nodular consolidations which can rapidly progress to diffuse airspace opacity. Pleural effusion may occur as well as hilar or mediastinal lymphadenopathy (fig. 12-36). Initial chest radiographs of patients with bubonic plague may be normal. However, transient focal lower lobe alveolar consolidation may develop. In patients with severe infection and rapidly progressive pulmonary consolidation, parenchymal opacities are secondary to disseminated intravascular coagulation or shock lung (2).

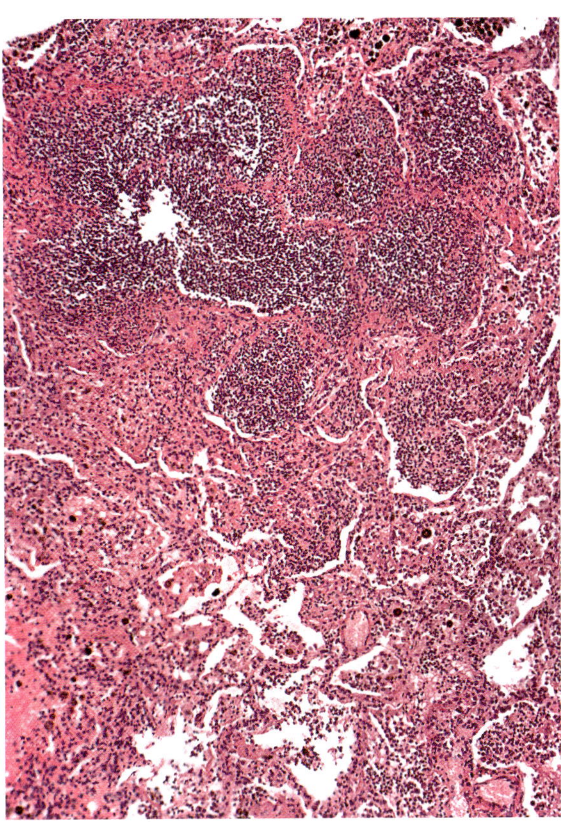

Figure 12-35

TULAREMIC PNEUMONIA: HISTOLOGY

In less affected areas there is intra-alveolar edema (bottom) and neutrophilic infiltration of the alveoli (top).

Pathologic Findings. In primary pneumonic plague, the lungs grossly show nodules of necrosis and hemorrhage (124,142). Histologically, the disease starts as a lobular pneumonia with numerous bacteria and a proteinaceous alveolar exudate (fig. 12-37). This progresses to a necrotic and hemorrhagic pneumonia with

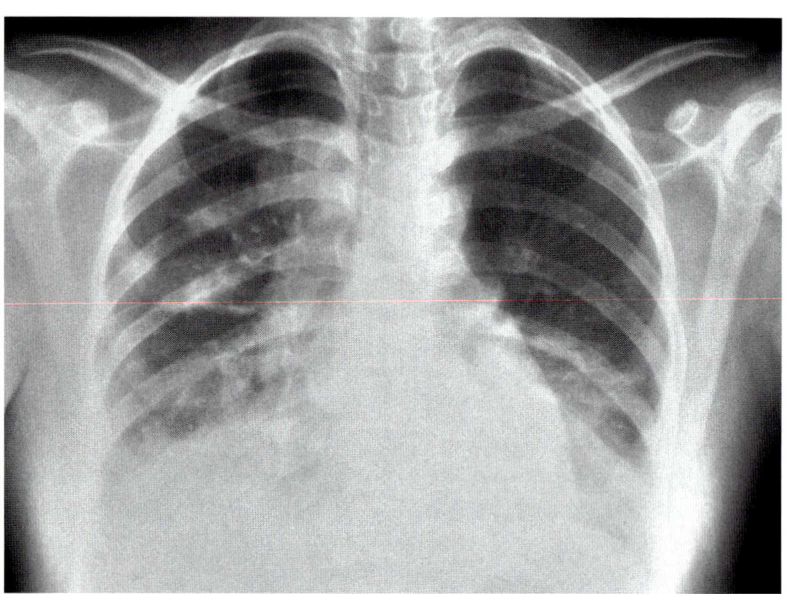

Figure 12-36

YERSINIA PESTIS PULMONARY INFECTION

PA chest radiograph in a 12-year-old female with myalgia, fever, and cough, demonstrates multifocal bilateral parenchymal consolidations. Nodular opacities are noted in the upper lobes and more confluent consolidation in the lower lobes. There are bilateral pleural effusions and marked mediastinal lymphadenopathy.

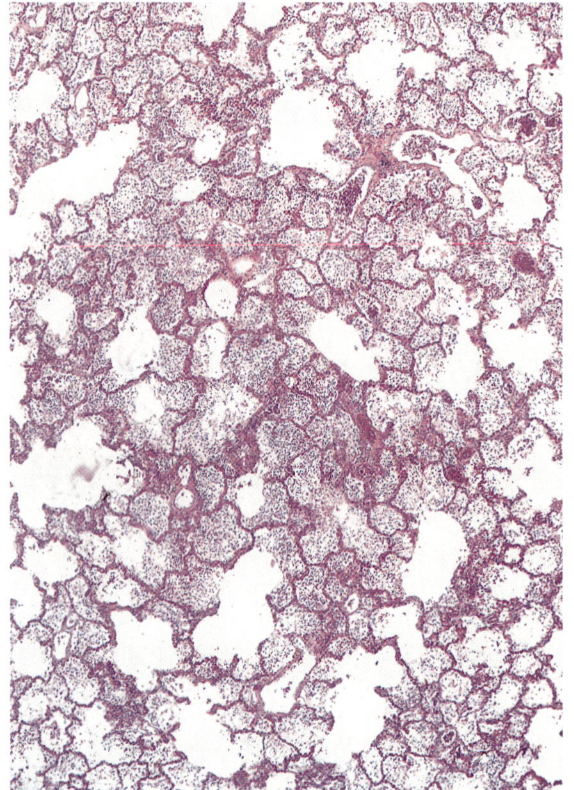

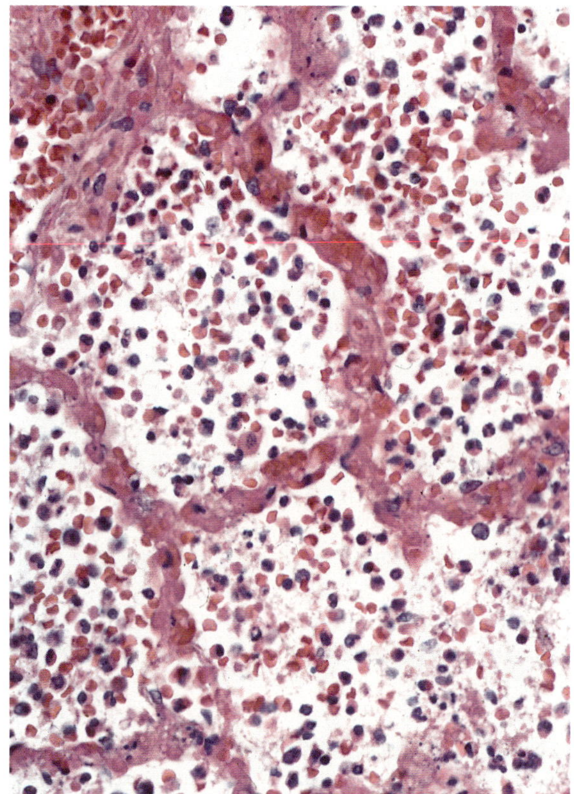

Figure 12-37

YERSINIA PESTIS PNEUMONIA: HISTOLOGY

Left: The lungs show extensive intra-alveolar accumulation of neutrophils and edema. Right: Numerous neutrophils and edema fill the alveolar spaces.

destruction of alveolar walls. There is a paucity of neutrophils relative to the number of organisms. The alveolar exudate lacks fibrin. The overlying pleura may show marked acute pleuritis. Large numbers of organisms are seen in the airways and alveoli. The bacteria are Gram-negative and measure 0.5–1.0 µm to 1.0–2.0 µm (70,124,142). The bacteria are well demonstrated using silver stains (Steiner, Warthin-Starry, or Dieterle) or the Brown and Hopps stain (70,124,142). The bacteria are bipolar and exhibit a "safety-pin" morphology, a feature best seen on touch preparations stained with a Gram or methylene blue stain (55,70,124,142). Direct immunofluorescence can be performed on formalin-fixed, deparaffinized sections to identify the organism (70,124,142).

Treatment and Prognosis. The optimal therapy for serious plague infections is a combination of streptomycin and tetracycline (55, 70,124,142). Due to the risk of aerosol spread, infected patients should be kept in isolation and laboratory workers should handle patient specimens with strict precautions. If untreated, patients with primary pneumonic plague have a high mortality rate of approximately 90 percent within 24 hours; those with bubonic plague have a mortality rate of 60 to 90 percent if untreated; while those with septicemic plague have a mortality of 90 percent within 1 to 2 days (70, 124,142). A vaccine is available for those with potential for exposure.

Rhodococcus Equi and Malakoplakia

Definition. *Rhodococcus* pulmonary infection is caused by *Rhodococcus equi* (formerly *Corynebacterium equi*).

Rhodococcus is a rare cause of pulmonary abscess and pneumonia that usually occurs in immunocompromised patients, especially those with AIDS (1,135,142). *R. equi* is an aerobic, Gram-positive or Gram-variable, pleomorphic coccobacillus (1,79). It is found worldwide in soil and in the feces of some animals. Horses, especially foals, are known to develop *R. equi* pneumonia (1). Human infection is acquired through inhalation of contaminated aerosols. Approximately 30 percent of the reported infected patients have a history of exposure to animals, particularly horses (1). Patients without such an exposure history probably acquired the infection through inhalation of contaminated soil or dust (1).

Pulmonary malakoplakia is a distinctive chronic inflammatory process characterized by a prominent histiocytic component and frequent calcifications in the form of Michaelis-Gutman bodies (see below). It is most commonly associated with *R. equi* infection, but a few cases are reported in association with *E. coli* or *Acinetobacter* sp (25,31,92).

Clinical Features. Patients with *R. equi* pulmonary disease present with a subacute infection characterized by cough, fever, dyspnea, and chest pain. The physical examination is relatively unremarkable. Extrapulmonary infection may be seen in 7 percent of cases and extrapulmonary relapse in 13 percent of cases of pneumonia (135). Extrapulmonary infection can cause brain abscess, endophthalmitis, prostatic abscess, lymph node infection, bacteremia, and pelvic mass due to psoas muscle abscess (1,135). HIV-infected patients usually have CD4 lymphocyte counts of less than 200 cells/mm^3 at the time of *R. equi* pulmonary infection.

The diagnosis is established from sputum, bronchial lavage, or other infected tissue. Blood cultures are often positive. The organism is easily confused with other pleomorphic Gram-positive bacteria so that the clinician should alert the laboratory staff if this organism is suspected.

Most cases of malakoplakia without associated *R. equi* infection involve the urinary tract, especially the urinary bladder (81,92). However, rare cases of pulmonary malakoplakia have been reported in which *R. equi* infection was not found (25,31,59,65). In one case, the patient had a renal mass and multiple bilateral pulmonary nodules resembling metastatic renal cell carcinoma (31). One patient had urinary tract and bone involvement, and bilateral lower lobe masses involving bronchi (59). Another renal transplant patient developed a right lower lobe cavitary mass associated with *E. coli* infection (65). A cardiac transplant patient developed a left upper lobe nodule from which cultures of aspiration specimens grew *Corynebacterium* and *Acinetobacter* sp (25).

Radiologic Findings. Pulmonary infection with *R. equi* manifests radiographically as a dense parenchymal consolidation with a predilection for upper lobe involvement (61,91).

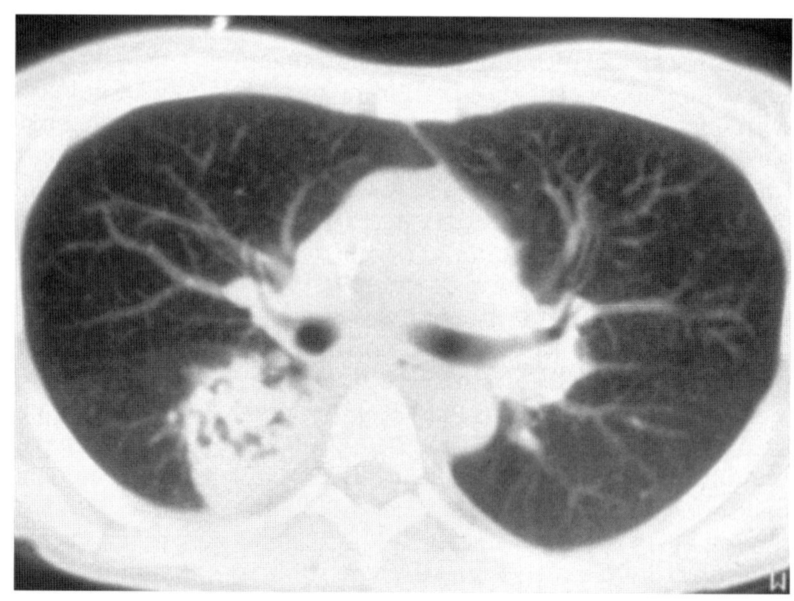

Figure 12-38

RHODOCOCCOSIS

Rhodococcosis in an HIV-positive 36-year-old female with progressive dysphagia, cough, and fever. Chest CT (lung window) demonstrates a large right lower lobe cavitary mass. Other images (not shown) showed multifocal lung nodules.

Cavitation occurs commonly, exhibits thick walls, and may follow initiation of appropriate antibiotic therapy (fig. 12-38) (61,82,91). The above findings may mimic those of postprimary tuberculosis (129). Bilateral pulmonary involvement may occur (82). Multifocal pulmonary opacities involving bronchi and consistent with tracheobronchial dissemination are also described. There may be associated mediastinal lymphadenopathy (61,82,91,129,139).

Pathologic Findings. Gross pulmonary lesions usually consist of large areas of consolidation (fig. 12-39) that may show cavitation. The abscesses measure up to 8 cm in diameter. The histologic reaction to *R. equi* is typically malakoplakia associated with abscesses. The center of the abscess may show numerous neutrophils and necrosis. The surrounding tissue is densely infiltrated by histiocytes with abundant eosinophilic cytoplasm (fig. 12-40A). Organizing pneumonia may be present at the periphery and infiltrates of lymphocytes and plasma cells may be seen. PAS-positive material can be seen in the cytoplasm of the macrophages, but it falls short of the strong positive staining seen in Whipple's disease (see below). By electron microscopy, this PAS-positive material has been shown to consist of large phagolysosomes that contain broken-down organisms of *R. equi*. These may calcify and form Michaelis-Gutmann (MG) bodies, which have a target shape of concentric laminations and measure 2 to 10 µm in diameter (fig. 12-40A) (81,92). The MG bodies are found mostly within macrophages but also in surrounding tissues. They stain pink-red with PAS, dark brown with GMS, green with Grocott, dark blue with Giemsa, brown-red with von Kossa (fig. 12-40B), orange with Alizarin red, dark blue with Prussian blue, and not at all with the S-100 stains (79). The histology of malakoplakia associated with bacteria other than *R. equi* is identical to that associated with that organism (fig. 12-41).

The bacterial organisms are seen easily in tissue sections with tissue Gram stains such as the Brown and Brenn or Brown and Hopps stains (fig. 12-40B,C) (2,79). The organisms appear as small, Gram-positive bacilli that may be pleomorphic in shape, ranging from tiny cocci measuring less than 1 µm in diameter to coccobacilli. The organisms are weakly acid-fast so this feature can only be demonstrated with modified acid-fast stains such as the Coates-Fite, Kinyoun, or Fite-Farraco stain (1,79). *R. equi* does not stain with the Ziehl-Neelsen acid-fast stain.

Differential Diagnosis. The histologic differential diagnosis for *R. equi* infection includes the differential diagnosis for malakoplakia. Pulmonary malakoplakia has been reported in association with other bacterial infections including those caused by *Escherichia coli* and *Acinetobacter* sp (1,79,111). It potentially could also be mistaken for Whipple's disease (see

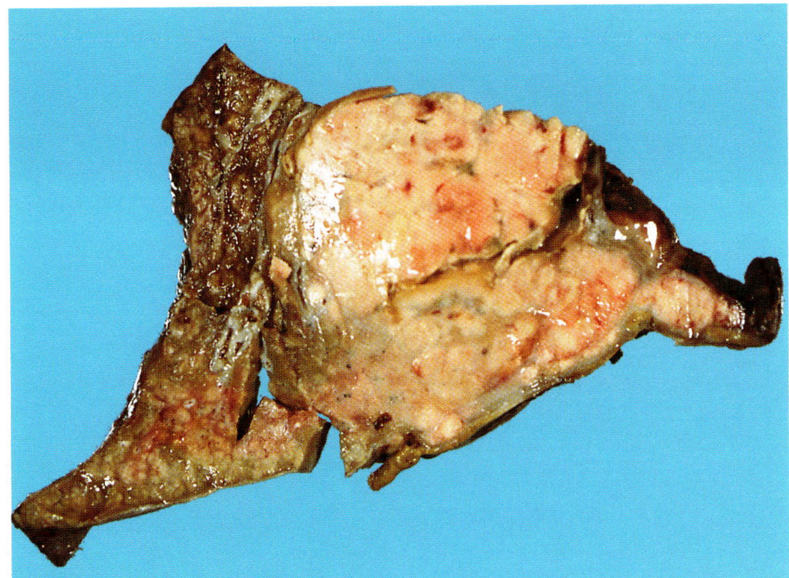

Figure 12-39

RHODOCOCCUS EQUI: GROSS SPECIMEN

The lung shows an extensive area of yellow consolidation, with scattered nodularity.

below) or infection with *Mycobacterium avium-intracellulare* (see Mycobacterial Pneumonias) (60). However, *R. equi* infection can be distinguished by identifying the PAS-positive inclusions in the macrophages, and finding MG bodies, Gram-positive coccobacilli that stain with the GMS stain, and the weakly acid-fast positivity of the organisms (1,60,79,111). Other inflammatory lesions that can have prominent histiocytes include obstructive endogenous lipoid pneumonia, exogenous lipoid pneumonia, or lipid storage disorders such as Gaucher's disease or Nieman-Pick disease (1,79).

Treatment and Prognosis. Multiple antibiotics may be used to treat *R. equi* infection although the organism is frequently resistant to several agents (e.g., penicillins and cephalosporins). Because virulent strains may be resistant to in vitro intracellular killing, it is recommended that *R. equi* infections be treated with antibiotics that can penetrate macrophages. In immunocompetent persons, single agent therapy may be sufficient, probably best provided with an extended-spectrum macrolide or fluoroquinolone. In immunocompromised persons, two or more agents should be initiated, and at least one should have excellent penetration into macrophages.

The treatment is administered for at least 2 months and up to 6 months due to the tendency to relapse without sufficient therapy (1, 70,111). Surgical resection of nodular or cavitary lesions may be required to achieve a cure.

Botryomycosis

Definition. Botryomycosis, also known as *bacterial pseudomycosis,* is an infection caused by nonfilamentous bacteria in which the organisms form eosinophilic granules that have the morphology of sulfur granules resembling actinomycosis.

Botryomycosis is an uncommon, chronic, progressive and localized infection caused by nonfilamentous bacteria. It is found worldwide. In addition to the lung, it can affect most organs including the skin, heart, kidney, central nervous system, prostate, and liver (11,17,33). Infections can be divided into two major clinical forms: skin/soft tissues or visceral (11,17,33). Visceral involvement is rare and usually not associated with cutaneous lesions.

The most common bacterium associated with botryomycosis is *Staphylococcus aureus.* Other organisms that can cause botryomycosis include *Pseudomonas aeruginosa, Escherichia coli, Actinobacillus lignieresii, Neisseria mucosa, Proteus* sp, *Streptococcus* sp, and *Bacteroides* sp (11,17,33). The pathogenesis, including the host and microbial factors that cause the bacterial organisms to form sulfur granules, is poorly understood.

Clinical Features. Pulmonary botryomycosis is rare (11,33,72,108,126). Lung involvement may be primary or secondary (17,108,126).

Pulmonary botryomycosis can take the form of endobronchial infections complicating tuberculous sequelae or bronchiectasis, masses

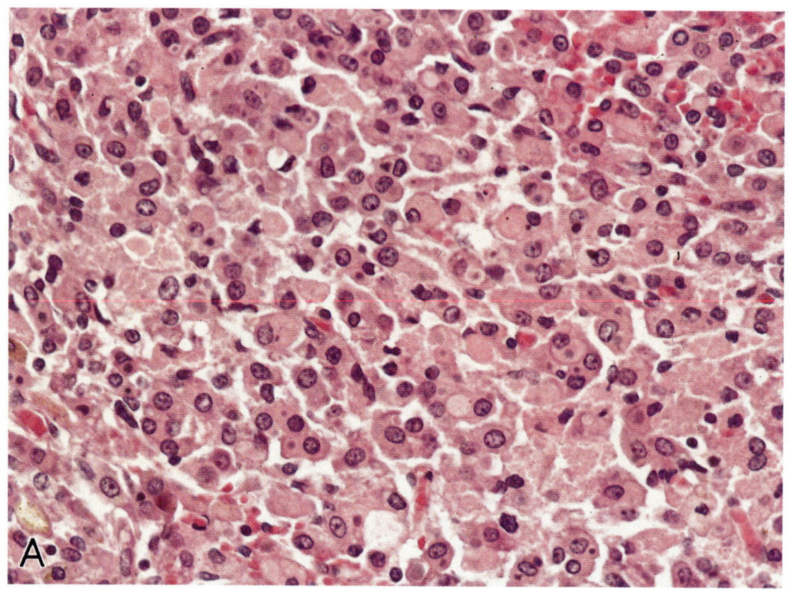

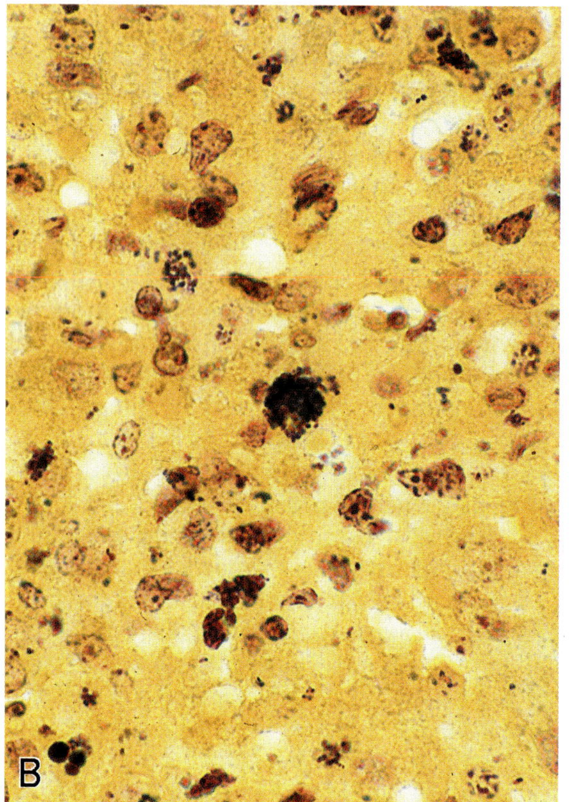

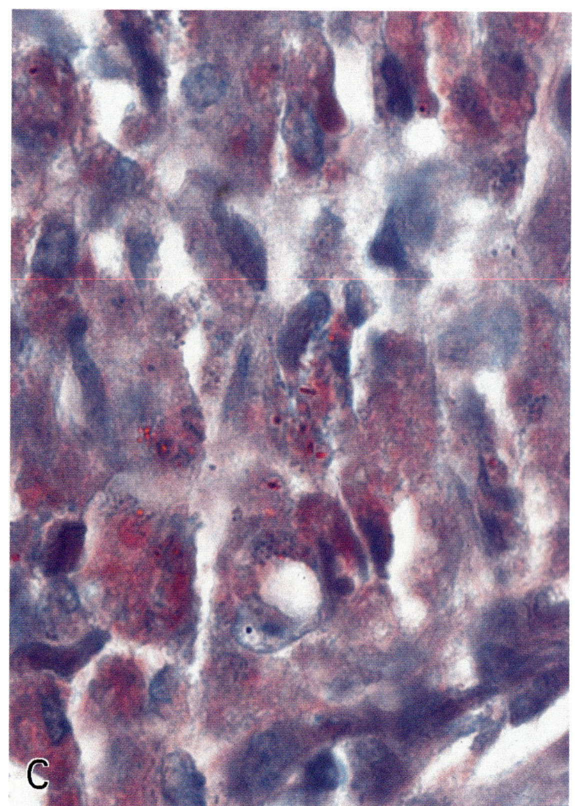

Figure 12-40

MALAKOPLAKIA ASSOCIATED WITH *RHODOCOCCUS EQUI* IN AN HIV-INFECTED PATIENT

A: There is an extensive infiltrate of epithelioid histiocytes.
B: Brown and Brenn stain highlights the small Gram-positive bacilli.
C: The Coates-Fite stain highlights the small bacilli. (Courtesy of Dr. Michael Lewin-Smith, AFIP, Washington, DC.)

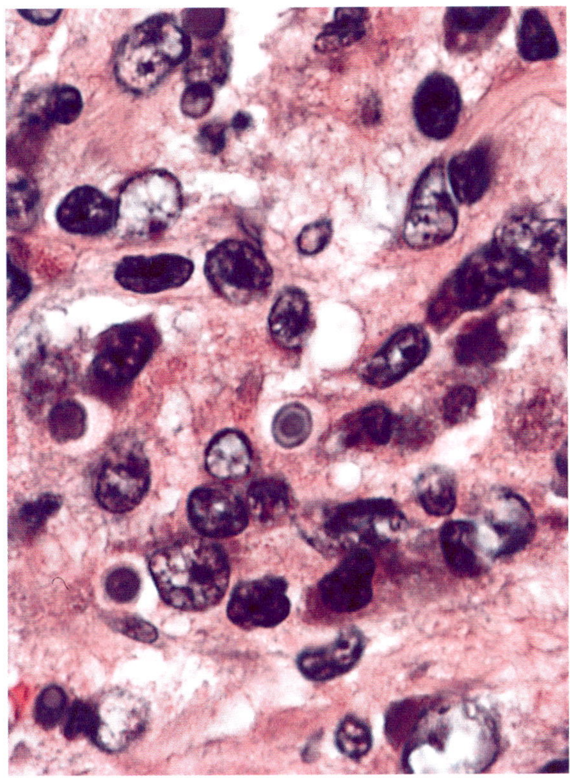
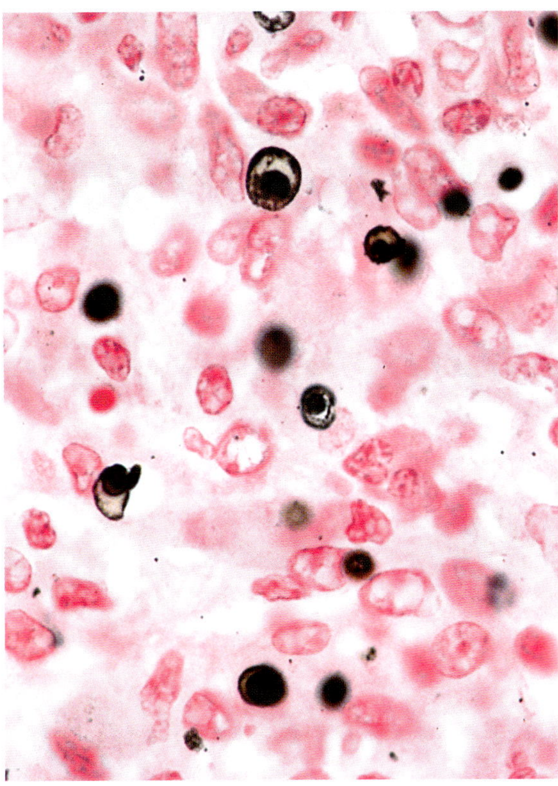

Figure 12-41

MALAKOPLAKIA, NOT ASSOCIATED WITH *RHODOCOCCUS EQUI*

Left: The lung infiltrate consists of histiocytes, lymphocytes, and plasma cells. A few round, concentrically laminated, basophilic Michaelis-Gutmann bodies are present.

Right: This von Kossa stain highlights multiple Michaelis-Gutmann bodies.

or tumor-like lesions, and diffuse pneumonia (11,33). For this reason it can clinically resemble actinomycosis, tuberculosis, or lung malignancy. While most cases occur in immunocompetent individuals, a few cases have been reported in patients with chronic granulomatous disease (108) and AIDS (72). A case of tracheal botryomycosis was reported in a patient with tracheobronchopathia osteoplastica (121).

Radiologic Findings. Atelectasis, multifocal nodules with cavitation, and chest wall involvement have been described in cases of pulmonary botryomycosis (46).

Pathologic Findings. Botryomycosis is diagnosed based on the identification in tissue sections of granules that consist of nonfilamentous bacterial organisms, such as Gram-positive cocci or Gram-negative bacilli, that form sulfur granules (fig. 12-42) (11,17,18,33). The sulfur granules measure up to 2 mm in diameter and are typically situated within areas of suppurative inflammation such as abscesses (17,18). The granules may be seen with careful gross examination and are yellow or white, soft, and friable.

Histologically, the periphery of the abscesses typically shows granulation tissue and fibrosis. Epithelioid histiocytes and giant cells may be seen. The sulfur granule shows the Splendore-Hoeppli phenomenon, with eosinophilic finger-like clubs radiating at the periphery of the bacterial colonies. The organisms may be embedded within a dense matrix that appears amorphous and eosinophilic or amphophilic (17, 18). Organisms are also seen outside the granules, and are Gram-positive cocci or Gram-negative bacilli. They are demonstrated in tissue sections with the Brown and Brenn and Brown and Hopps stains, which best stain

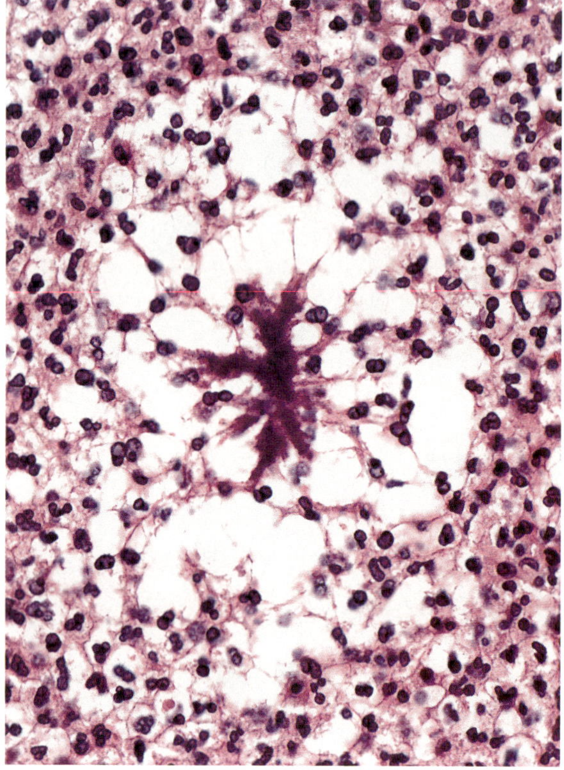

Figure 12-42

PULMONARY BOTRYOMYCOSIS

This cluster of bacterial organisms is growing in a sulfur granule with a peripheral Splendore-Hoeppli effect. The organisms are Gram-positive cocci rather than the branching filamentous bacteria of actinomycosis.

the Gram-positive and Gram-negative bacteria, respectively. The organisms grow in grape-like clusters, hence the name botryomycosis. Rarely, there is a mixture of nonfilamentous bacteria within a single sulfur granule. Culture may be helpful in identifying the specific type of bacterial organism. If the sulfur granules are identified grossly, it is helpful to crush the granules before making the inoculation for culture (17,18).

Differential Diagnosis. The primary differential diagnosis is with actinomycosis but the bacterial organisms do not show the filamentous branching characteristic of that organism. Instead, they consist of Gram-positive cocci or Gram-negative bacilli (17). The organisms may be difficult to see on H&E-stained sections and may require high-power microscopic examination under an oil-immersion objective (17). Degenerated Gram-positive cocci at the periphery of large granules following antibiotic therapy may appear refractile and either Gram-negative or Gram-nonreactive. In such cases, silver stains such as the Dieterle, Steiner, or Warthin-Starry, may highlight the organisms (17).

Treatment and Prognosis. Successful treatment often requires a combination of both surgical resection and long-term antimicrobial therapy. Antibiotic therapy alone is seldom effective.

Bacillary Angiomatosis

Definition. Bacillary angiomatosis is a vascular proliferation that occurs in response to the bacilli of *Bartonella henselae* and *B. quintana*. Synonyms are *epithelioid angiomatosis* and *bacillary ailuronosis*.

Cats are the most common animal host for *B. henselae* and it is thought that transmission to humans occurs by the cat flea, Ctenocephalides felis (83). Infection is acquired by immunocompromised patients who have been scratched, licked, or bitten by cats, particularly kittens. Ticks may also harbor both *B. quintana* and *B. henselae,* but the role of ticks in transmission to humans is not clear. The genus *Bartonella* was previously known as *Rochalimaea*.

Clinical Features. Bacillary angiomatosis most commonly affects the skin, but it has been reported in most organ systems. Several cases of pulmonary bacillary angiomatosis have been reported in AIDS patients who developed a febrile illness with interstitial pneumonitis, lymphadenopathy, and polypoid endobronchial lesions (44,122).

Pathologic Findings. *B. henselae* and *B. quintana* are small coccobacilli measuring 1 to 3 µm in diameter. Ultrastructure demonstrates a trilaminar cell wall. In tissue sections, they grow in clusters in the extracellular spaces.

The vascular lesions consist of proliferating capillaries with plump endothelial cells associated with an infiltrate of macrophages and neutrophils (fig. 12-43). On H&E stains, the masses or colonies of organisms are purple and granular. The organisms are numerous and stain with silver stains such as the Warthin-Starry, Dieterle, and Steiner stains. The Warthin-Starry stain is most effective in demonstrating the bacilli when utilizing a microwave and a pH of 3.2 (83). PAS and acid-fast stains do not demonstrate the organisms very well.

Molecular methods using the polymerase chain reaction (PCR) have been used to confirm the infectious agent. Immunohistochemistry for *B. henselae* is also helpful. However, the diagnosis is usually established by light microscopy with histochemical stains.

Differential Diagnosis. Bacillary angiomatosis must be separated from Kaposi's sarcoma and the prominent granulation tissue associated with ulceration (83). In Kaposi's sarcoma the vascular spaces tend to be slit-like with extravasated erythrocytes, while in bacillary angiomatosis the vessels are more rounded with a frequent neutrophilic infiltrate. Clusters of organisms give a purple appearance that is not seen in Kaposi's sarcoma. In granulation tissue, neutrophils and organisms are found mainly on the ulcerated surface while in bacillary angiomatosis these features are present throughout the lesion (83).

Treatment and Prognosis. Bacillary angiomatosis is usually responsive to antibiotics such as erythromycin and tetracycline (83,122).

Tropheryma Whippelii (Whipple's Disease)

Definition. Whipple's disease is a rare, multiorgan disorder associated with infection by the bacteria, *Tropheryma whippelii*. Patients usually present with diarrhea, weight loss, and malabsorption.

In 1907, Whipple described this disorder and recognized the "rod-shaped organisms" in tissue sections of a mesenteric lymph node (140). Pulmonary involvement is extremely rare (69, 74,113,127,140).

The Whipple bacillus was identified one decade ago using PCR methods which enabled demonstration of a close relationship with the actinomycetes group of Gram-positive bacteria and proposal of the name *Tropheryma whippelii* (98). Although the organism cannot be grown in culture, it has recently been isolated with molecular methods (98).

Clinical and Radiologic Findings. There is a 3 to 1 male predominance and the mean age is 55 years (range, 20 to 82 years) (36,37). The most common manifestations are articular (usually arthralgias), followed by gastrointestinal, general (usually weight loss), and neurologic (usually central nervous system) (36,37). Pleuropulmonary symptoms are reported in 13 to 50 percent of patients and include pleural effusion and chronic cough (21,36–38). Endobronchial lesions in association with pulmonary nodules have been reported (74).

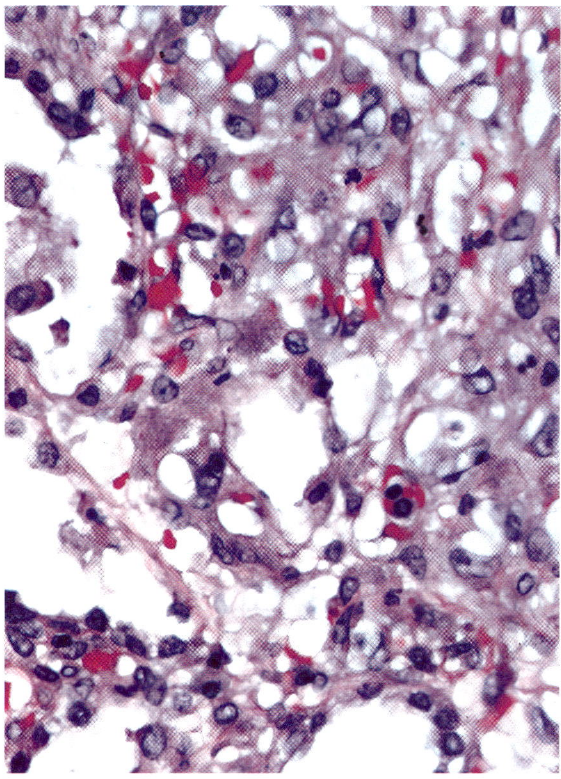

Figure 12-43

BACILLARY ANGIOMATOSIS

There is a prominent vascular proliferation with an associated histiocytic infiltrate.

Patients may have an immunologic defect that predisposes them to this infection, but this has been difficult to prove.

Pathologic Findings. The distinctive histologic finding of Whipple's disease is the accumulation of macrophages with abundant clear cytoplasm that often has a foamy appearance (fig. 12-44A). These macrophages are filled with bacterial organisms and degenerating bacteria that stain with the PAS and silver stains (Warthin-Starry and GMS) (fig. 12-44B). By light microscopy, tiny, thin, sickle-shaped inclusions may be seen (36). By electron microscopy, many bacillary organisms are identified (fig. 12-44C). Prominent peribronchial or peribronchiolar infiltration by macrophages filled with organisms may occur (fig. 12-44D). The histiocytes may also infiltrate the airway submucosa (74).

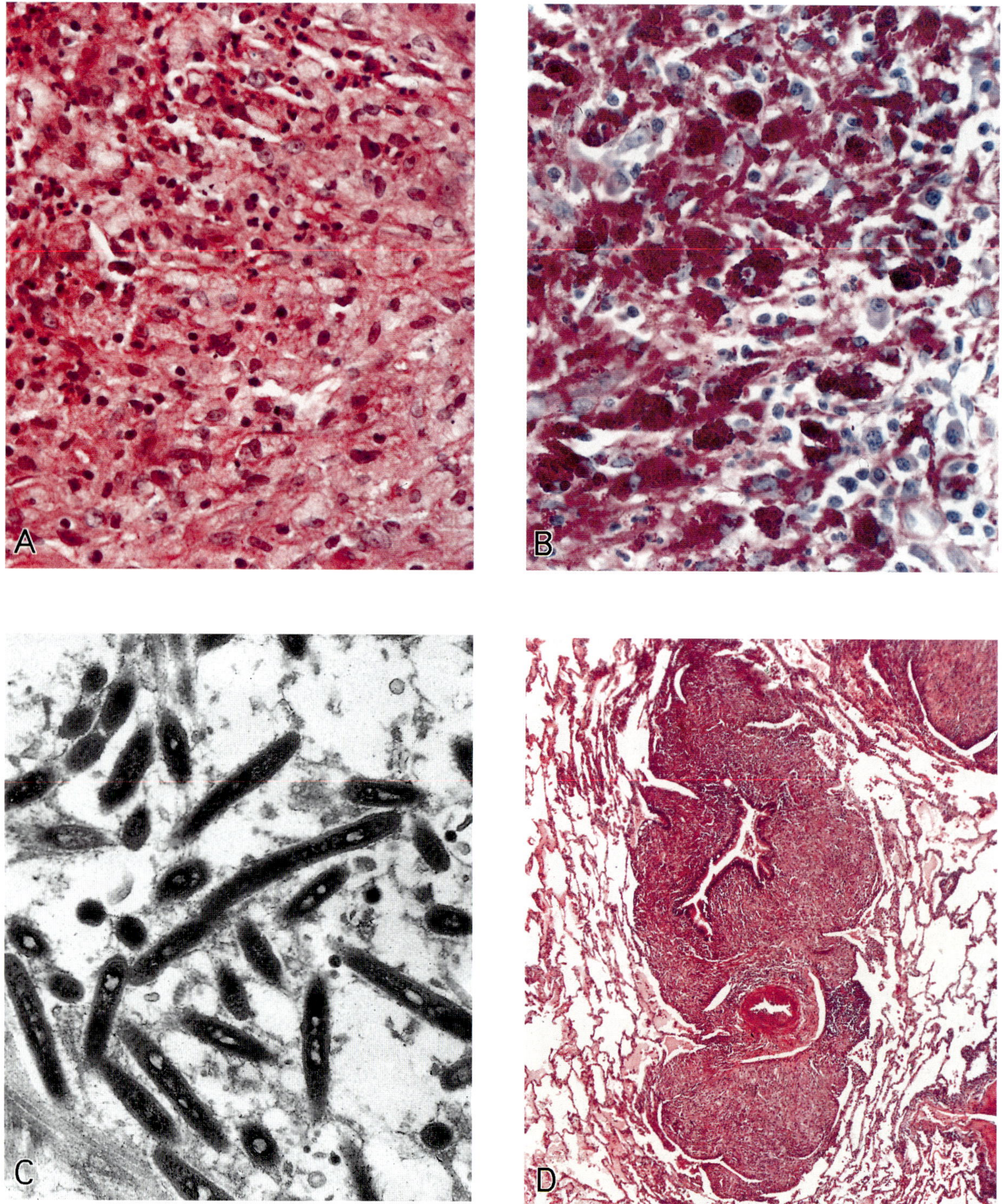

Figure 12-44

WHIPPLE'S DISEASE

A: This lung infiltrate consists of a dense histiocytic infiltrate.
B: The histiocytes stain strongly with the PAS stain.
C: Electron microscopy reveals numerous bacillary organisms.
D: The histiocytic infiltrate is distributed around this bronchiole and its adjacent terminal arteriole.

Granulomatous inflammation is described in 9 percent of liver and lymph node lesions but its frequency in the lung is not known (36). There is little published information about the lung pathology in this disorder (74).

Differential Diagnosis. Pulmonary Whipple's disease must be distinguished from *Mycobacterium avium-intracellulare* (MAI) infection in AIDS patients which can cause pulmonary infiltration by macrophages with abundant cytoplasm filled with bacilli (see Mycobacterial Pneumonias). It also may be confused with diffuse panbronchiolitis (see chapter 8), malakoplakia (see above), and inflammatory pseudotumor (see chapter 17), each of which have distinctive histologic features that differ from Whipple's disease. In addition to morphologic differences, PAS-positive staining of the macrophage cytoplasm and confirmation of the presence of *T. whippelii* using PCR analysis help establish the diagnosis of Whipple's disease (36,98). The Whipple bacilli do not stain strongly with acid-fast stains like the MAI in HIV-infected patients.

Treatment and Prognosis. Patients with Whipple's disease respond to antibiotic therapy. Patients treated with cotrimoxazole appear to have fewer relapses than those treated with tetracycline and penicillin (36,98). Patients with neurologic disease should have parenteral antibiotic therapy to achieve CNS penetration, followed by oral cotrimoxazole (36,98).

Lung Abscess

Definition. Lung abscess is a localized necrotic cavity containing pus. It is most often associated with bacterial pneumonia.

The most common cause of lung abscess is aspiration. Three factors are associated with aspiration: altered consciousness, poor dental hygiene, and immune suppression (32). Most lung abscesses are associated with anaerobic bacteria, which are a common cause of periodontal disease. The most common anaerobes associated with lung abscess are *Fusobacterium nucleatum, Bacteroides melaninogenicus,* and Gram-positive streptococci (32,70). In up to 20 percent of lung abscesses, *Bacteroides fragilis* is present (32). Many abscesses are polymicrobial, with a mixture of bacteria as seen in the oral flora (32,70). Other bacteria that cause lung abscesses include *Klebsiella pneumoniae, Pseudomonas aeruginosa, Staphylococcus aureus, Nocardia,* and *Actinomyces* (32,70). Lung abscess may develop in association with pulmonary infarcts, malignancies (both primary and metastatic), penetrating trauma, necrotizing pneumonias, bronchial obstruction, and necrotic conglomerate lesions of silicosis or coal worker's pneumoconiosis (32,70).

Clinical Features. Patients usually present with low-grade fever, weight loss, and productive cough with copious foul-smelling sputum. If the abscess is not associated with aspiration and anaerobic bacteria, the patients may have a history of acute pneumonia in the setting of hospitalization or immune suppression (32,70). Most lung abscesses occur in men. Chest pain and hemoptysis are less common symptoms. Patients with chronic lung abscess may develop digital clubbing (32,70). Associated conditions that contribute to impaired consciousness and aspiration include alcoholism, drug overdose, neurologic conditions such as epilepsy, and airway obstruction. Most lung abscesses occur in the right lung since the right main bronchus follows the direction of the trachea more closely than the left main bronchus.

The causative organism is best diagnosed by culture, either of blood or pleural fluid, or through invasive methods such as transtracheal aspiration, bronchoscopy with protected brush specimen, and percutaneous lung aspiration. Each of these specimens must be processed in an appropriate manner to enable anaerobic bacteria to grow.

Radiologic Findings. Lung abscesses manifest radiologically as focal or multifocal lung masses that commonly exhibit cavitation. Most cavitary lung abscesses have walls less than 15 mm in thickness, with smooth internal borders (see figs. 12-9, 12-24). Adjacent parenchymal consolidation is common. While thick walls (greater than 15 mm) and irregular internal borders occur, these findings should raise the possibility of a cavitary neoplasm such as bronchogenic carcinoma. Air-fluid levels are commonly encountered. Lung abscess may also manifest as a nonspecific parenchymal consolidation or nodular opacity (47,58). Lung abscesses occur most often in the posterior segment of the right upper lobe and superior segment of the right lower lobe; the next most common location is the posterior segment of the left upper lobe or the superior segment of the left lower lobe (32,70).

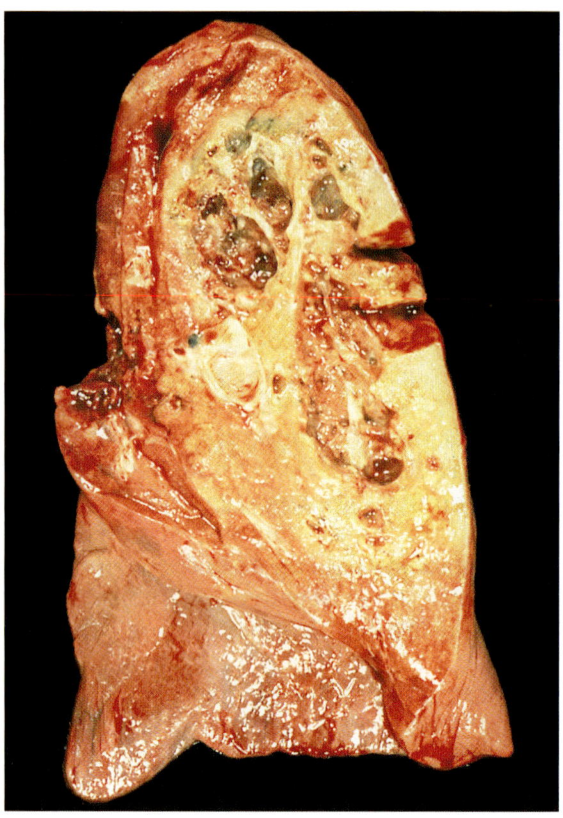

Figure 12-45

ACUTE ABSCESS: GROSS SPECIMEN

This abscess has replaced most of the upper lobe and shows central cavitation and a trabecular cut surface.

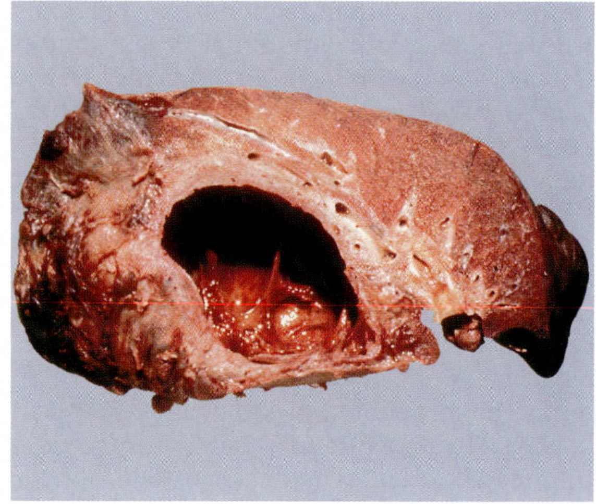

Figure 12-46

CHRONIC ABSCESS: GROSS SPECIMEN

This chronic abscess consists of a cavitary lesion with a thick fibrous wall. (Courtesy of the Gordon Museum, London, England.)

Pathologic Findings. A lung abscess is a localized cavitary lesion that is filled with pus at some point during its evolution (fig. 12-45). Pus is abundant in acute abscesses where necrotic lung tissue and numerous neutrophils are found in the center of the cavity. However, in chronic lesions, the neutrophils become replaced with lymphocytes, plasma cells, and macrophages. The lung abscess is usually 2 to 6 cm in diameter, but may be very large, measuring 10 to 12 cm. The presence of multiple cavities suggests a prior necrotizing pneumonia. If the cavities are evenly distributed throughout both lungs it may suggest hematogenous seeding of an organism from another site such as infective endocarditis or septic thromboemboli. Acute lung abscesses tend to have a thin rim while there is usually a thick wall with chronic abscesses (fig. 12-46). In chronic abscess, granulation tissue develops, and a fibrous wall of varying thickness is seen at the periphery. The wall of a chronic abscess may become lined by ciliated respiratory epithelium that may undergo squamous metaplasia. The lung tissue surrounding the abscess may show prominent organizing pneumonia.

Differential Diagnosis. Lung abscess can be radiologically or clinically mistaken for lung cancer and cavitary tuberculosis. In fact, abscesses are potential complications of both cavitary lung cancers and lesions of tuberculosis.

Pathologists play an important role in the evaluation of a lung abscess by making a careful assessment for infectious agents. This can begin in the frozen section laboratory by performing appropriate cultures using special procedures for anaerobic bacteria if the lesion has a foul smell. Careful evaluation of the gross specimen for sulfur granules may help in recognizing actinomycosis, since the bacteria could be missed if these lesions are not sampled. Some chronic abscesses have an appearance at the periphery that mimics inflammatory pseudotumor by the presence of a prominent lymphoplasmacytic infiltrate. However, recognition of a collection of neutrophils or a prominent neutrophilic infiltrate in the center of the lesion is a helpful clue that the lesion is essentially an acute and organizing abscess.

Cases with lung abscesses were included in the series of inflammatory pseudotumors published by Matsubara et al. (90).

Treatment and Prognosis. Lung abscesses may be complicated by empyema due to rupture into the pleural space, or by severe hemoptysis. Infection may also spread through the airways to the rest of the lung when an abscess ruptures into a bronchus. Chronic cavitary abscesses may become colonized by *Aspergillus,* forming a fungus ball.

Abscesses should be treated with antibiotics that are the most effective against the causative organism. Postural drainage may help in removing pus. If the patient cannot cough, the pus may need to be removed by nasotracheal suction. Bronchoscopy is generally limited only to those patients who do not respond to antibiotics. Some abscesses may be treated via percutaneous drainage.

MYCOBACTERIAL PNEUMONIAS

Tuberculosis is one of the most important infections known to man. It has been identified in the human remains of ancient Egyptians and claimed the lives of many famous historical figures (156,157,163). It was not until 1882 that Robert Koch recognized the tubercle bacillus as the etiologic agent (160). The term tuberculosis commonly refers to disease caused by *Mycobacterium tuberculosis, M. bovis,* or *M. africanum.* Other mycobacteria can cause a similar illness but are less virulent and are not as responsive to treatment.

Following the discovery of antituberculous medications during the 20th century, the incidence of tuberculosis decreased worldwide in most developed countries. However, it remains the most common infectious cause of death in adults worldwide, especially in some developing countries, particularly in Africa and parts of Asia, accounting for approximately 3 million deaths worldwide annually (156,157,163).

In the United States, there was a marked decrease in the incidence of tuberculosis until the mid-1980s when the AIDS epidemic, the increased number of immigrants from Southeast Asia and Haiti, the development of drug-resistant strains, and the growth in numbers of homeless people resulted in a resurgence of this infection (156,157,163). In some developing countries, particularly in Africa and parts of Asia, tuberculosis remains a major public health problem.

In the United States those at particular risk for tuberculosis include the homeless, prisoners, elderly, poor, malnourished, and immunosuppressed, such as those with cancer and AIDS, and transplant recipients. Pneumoconioses, especially silicosis and mixed-dust pneumoconiosis, predispose exposed workers to tuberculosis (156,157,163).

The major defining feature of the *Mycobacteria* sp is the acid-fast staining property, which is very helpful diagnostically in pathologic specimens. The high lipid content of the bacilli helps retain this acid-fast staining even after decolorization with the Ziehl-Neelsen or auramine O stain.

Mycobacterium Tuberculosis

Definition. Pulmonary tuberculosis is a chronic, recurrent infection of the lung that is caused by *Mycobacterium tuberculosis.*

In most cases, tuberculosis is transmitted through inhalation of small, airborne, droplet nuclei measuring 1 to 5 µm that are contaminated with the tubercle bacillus. These particles are small enough that they remain airborne for long periods of time and can reach the alveolar spaces. These droplet nuclei are effectively generated through coughing. In the non-HIV–infected population, the lungs are affected in 80 to 85 percent of patients with tuberculosis, while in HIV-infected patients, pulmonary involvement occurs in 60 to 70 percent of cases (156).

Clinical Features. The clinical manifestations of tuberculosis are quite varied depending on the site of involvement, the host immune status, and whether there are associated diseases. A low-grade fever is the most common finding in patients with primary tuberculosis. Cough (nonproductive or productive of only scant sputum) and chest pain are other common presenting complaints. Rarer symptoms are fatigue, arthralgias, and pharyngitis.

The symptoms of reactivation of tuberculosis are insidious and include cough, weight loss, and fatigue. Many patients have vague or nonspecific symptoms. Fever and night sweats or night sweats alone are present in approximately half of the patients. Often, pulmonary tuberculosis is diagnosed after a hospital admission for unrelated complaints, especially in elderly patients. Dyspnea is uncommon unless there is severe lung involvement. Hemoptysis is usually associated with extensive disease in which there is bronchiectasis from old residual tuberculosis, rupture of a dilated blood vessel in an old tuberculous cavity, infection in an old cavity (especially an *Aspergillus* fungus ball), or broncholithiasis in which calcified lesions erode into the lumen of an airway. Tuberculosis is often associated with other clinical conditions including HIV infection, alcoholism, chronic renal failure, diabetes mellitus, cancer, history of subtotal gastrectomy, or drug abuse (156). Each of these disorders may modify the clinical presentation of tuberculosis. The physical examination is usually normal, although signs of an effusion may be present. Elderly patients may have a more subtle clinical presentation than younger patients (149,168).

Conceptually, tuberculosis is traditionally divided into primary and secondary (or reactivation) forms. A recent statement from the American Thoracic Society (ATS) (146) details the diagnostic strategies for high- and low-risk patient populations based on current knowledge of tuberculosis epidemiology and information on newer technologies, and provides a classification scheme for tuberculosis that is based on pathogenesis. This statement has been prepared as a practical guide and statement of principles for all persons involved in the care of patients with tuberculosis.

Primary Tuberculosis. When droplets contaminated with *M. tuberculosis* deposit in the alveolar spaces, the initial response is a neutrophil reaction followed by macrophages, which phagocytose the organisms. The macrophages either stay in the lung or spread through the lymphatics to regional lymph nodes, which become the site for hematogenous or lymphatic dissemination. The disseminated bacilli often lodge and multiply in the posterior half of the upper lobes of the lungs due to the high oxygen tension and relative lymphostasis; in the upper lobes they are called "Simon foci." The first infection with the tuberculosis bacilli is called a "primary" infection. When primary tuberculosis resolves and forms a parenchymal nodule, it is called a Ghon focus, which often becomes calcified over time. When a Ghon focus is associated with calcified hilar lymph nodes, it is called a Ranke's complex (152).

More than 90 percent of cases of primary tuberculosis heal without progression. Most patients remain asymptomatic and infection is only detected by a positive tuberculin skin test. In 5 to 10 percent of cases, patients develop progressive primary tuberculosis with complications including extension to the pleura with pleural effusion, spread through a pulmonary artery to cause a miliary pattern in the surrounding lung, or spread through an airway to cause either a tuberculous bronchopneumonia or endobronchial tuberculosis. Progressive primary tuberculosis is more likely to occur in individuals with impaired cellular immunity (156).

Secondary Tuberculosis. Secondary tuberculosis occurs when dormant but viable mycobacteria in a previously infected patient become active and cause reinfection or when a previously infected individual acquires a new infection. Secondary tuberculosis usually results in cavitary lesions that affect one or both upper lobes. The apical and posterior segments of the right and left upper lobes are most commonly affected. Immunocompetent patients rarely develop hilar adenopathy. Secondary tuberculosis is the most common form of tuberculosis in adults.

Radiologic Findings. *Primary Tuberculosis.* The most common radiologic manifestations of primary tuberculosis are airspace consolidation and lymph node enlargement. In children, focal airspace consolidation is seen in approximately 70 percent of patients with primary tuberculosis, and hilar or mediastinal lymph node enlargement in 90 to 95 percent (164,165). In adults, lymph node enlargement is less common, seen in 30 to 60 percent of patients (fig. 12-47) (161,172). The airspace consolidation in primary tuberculosis shows no significant predilection for any lung region.

On CT, the enlarged lymph nodes often have low attenuation and demonstrate rim enhancement following intravenous administration of contrast (164). Other radiologic manifestations of primary tuberculosis include tuberculoma, miliary disease, pleural effusion and, rarely, cavitation. The chest radiograph may be normal (152,165).

Follow-up chest radiographs in children with primary tuberculosis demonstrate foci of

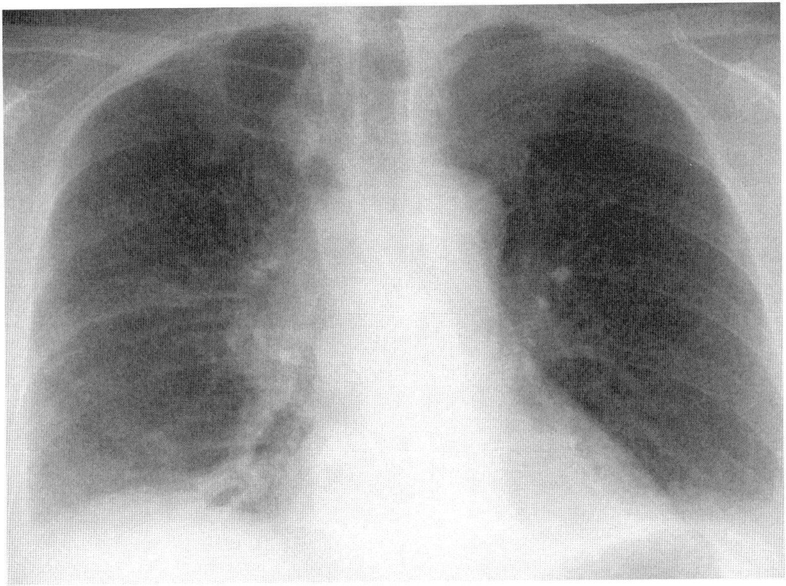

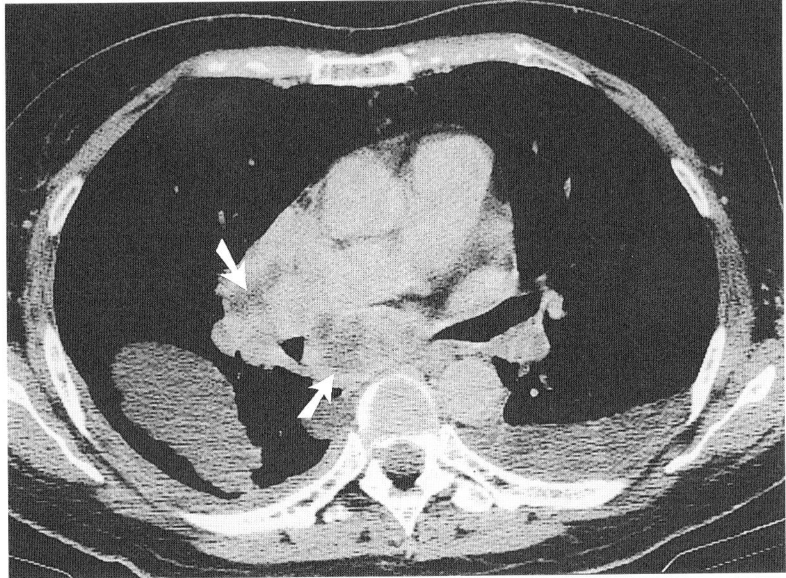

Figure 12-47

PRIMARY TUBERCULOSIS

Top: Chest radiograph in a 57-year-old woman demonstrates an enlarged right hilum and small bilateral pleural effusions.

Bottom: CT scan shows enlarged right hilar and subcarinal lymph nodes (arrows) and bilateral pleural effusions. The enlarged nodes have areas of decreased attenuation, consistent with necrosis.

parenchymal calcification, usually in well-defined tuberculomas, in 10 to 15 percent of cases (152, 165). Lymph node calcification is evident on the radiograph in 5 to 35 percent of cases (152,165).

Secondary Tuberculosis. The characteristic radiologic manifestation of secondary tuberculosis is the presence of focal, heterogeneous areas of consolidation involving the apical and posterior segments of the upper lobes and the superior segments of the lower lobes (fig. 12-48) (152, 165). Cavitation is present in 40 to 45 percent of cases (152,164). The areas of consolidation are often associated with poorly defined nodular opacities. With disease progression, the parenchymal opacities tend to coalesce and there is progressive scarring with development of coarse linear opacities and cephalad retraction of the hilum.

On HRCT, the small nodular opacities seen in secondary tuberculosis have a centrilobular distribution and are often associated with branching linear opacities, giving an appearance that resembles a tree-in-bud (fig. 12-49) (158). This centrilobular distribution reflects a bronchiolocentric process and, in the setting of tuberculosis, is highly suggestive of endobronchial spread. This pattern of spread can be

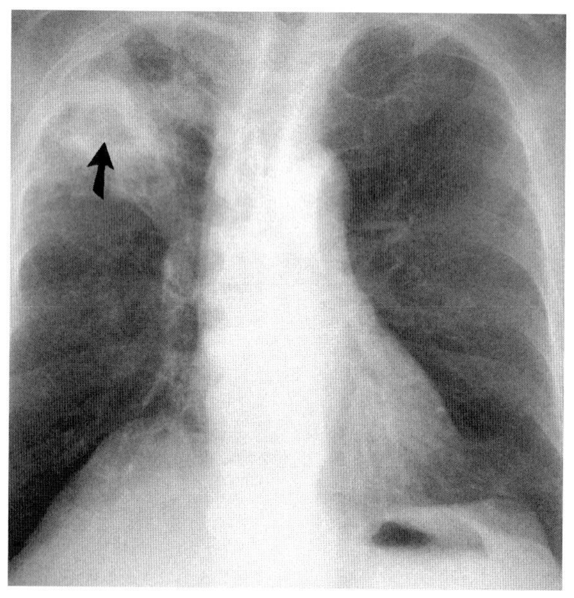

Figure 12-48

SECONDARY TUBERCULOSIS

Chest radiograph in a 71-year-old man demonstrates heterogeneous areas of consolidation and poorly defined nodules in the right upper lobe. Also noted is a cavity (arrow).

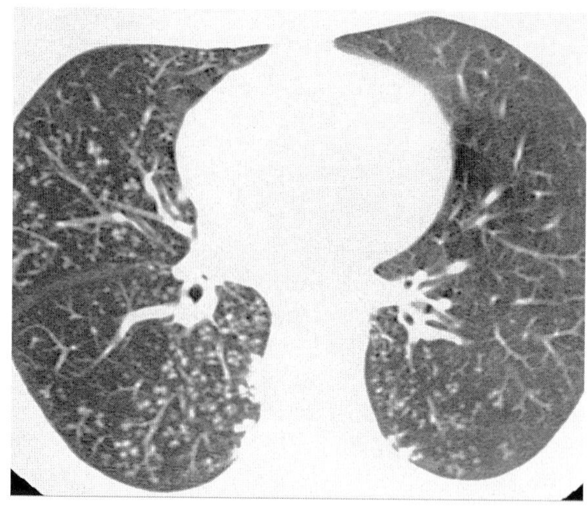

Figure 12-49

ENDOBRONCHIAL SPREAD OF TUBERCULOSIS

CT scan demonstrates centrilobular nodules and small foci of consolidation in the right lung and the left lower lobe. Branching centrilobular linear opacities and nodules give an appearance that resembles a tree-in-bud. (Courtesy of Dr. Jim Barrie, Edmonton, Canada.)

readily distinguished on HRCT from the random distribution of miliary disease.

Hilar or mediastinal lymph node enlargement is present in only 5 to 10 percent of patients with secondary tuberculosis (161,172). Unilateral pleural effusion is seen in 15 to 20 percent (161,172).

The radiologic manifestations of tuberculosis in patients with AIDS are influenced by the level of immunosuppression (152,164). In patients with normal or near-normal cellular immunity, the radiologic findings of reactivation tuberculosis are similar to those seen in the normal host. In severely immunosuppressed patients, the findings tend to resemble those of primary disease and consist predominantly of hilar and mediastinal lymph node enlargement (152,164). The enlarged nodes usually have low attenuation on CT and frequently show rim enhancement after intravenous administration of contrast (152).

Pathologic Findings. Mycobacteria are slender rods measuring approximately 4 µm in length (fig. 12-50). The optimal stain for identifying these organisms is the Ziehl-Neelsen stain, although there are a variety of techniques and stains that can be used in tissue specimens including the auramine-rhodamine fluorescent stain, the Fite stain, and the polymerase chain reaction (PCR) technique for detecting mycobacterial DNA (157,163). It is estimated that 10^6 organisms per millimeter of tissue are required for the Ziehl-Neelsen stain to be positive (157). A positive result with PCR is not regarded as valid diagnostically unless one or more organisms can be identified within tissue specimens with an acid-fast stain.

Culture techniques require 3 to 6 weeks to identify the organism (156,157,163). Rapid identification of *M. tuberculosis* has become possible recently using the BACTEC radiorespiratory detection system, which allows for identification of mycobacteria within 48 hours (156,163).

Skin testing can be performed using the purified protein derivative (PPD) of *M. tuberculosis* (156,157,163). In previously infected individuals with a normal immune system, the skin shows a positive reaction 1 to 3 days following exposure.

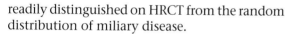

Primary Tuberculosis. The characteristic lesion of primary tuberculosis is the Ghon complex, which consists of a pulmonary parenchymal

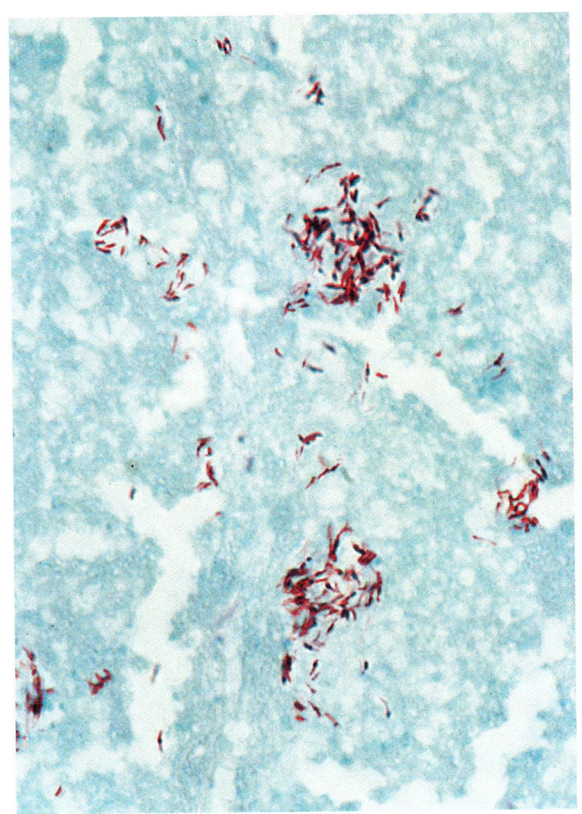

Figure 12-50

MYCOBACTERIAL ACID-FAST BACILLI

Numerous acid-fast bacilli are seen with this Ziehl-Neelsen stain.

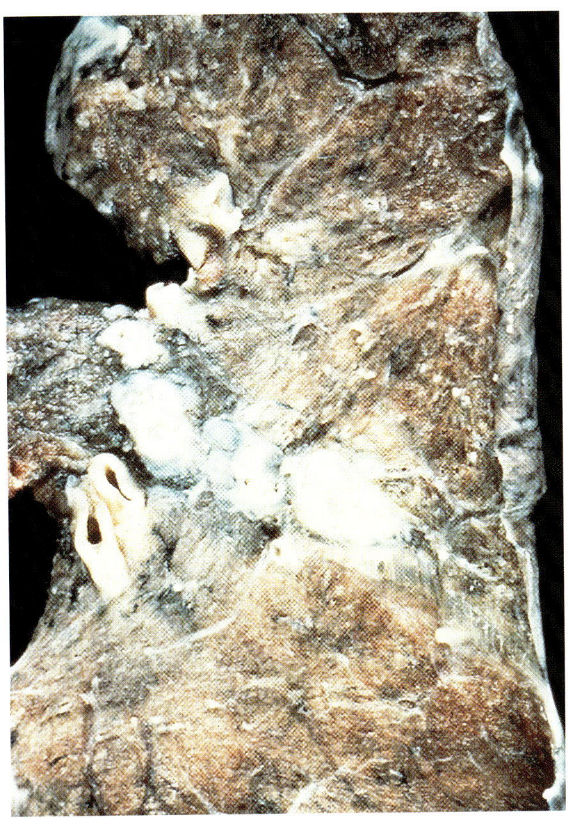

Figure 12-51

RANKE'S COMPLEX: GROSS SPECIMEN

A peripheral, upper lobe necrotizing granuloma, or Ghon focus, is associated with granulomatous involvement of enlarged hilar lymph nodes, forming a Ranke's complex.

nodule usually in the upper lobe. When it is associated with an enlarged hilar lymph node, a Ranke's complex is formed (fig. 12-51). The peripheral lung nodule is round, measures 1 to 2 cm in diameter, and has a necrotic center. Histologically, the lung as well as the mediastinal lymph node show necrotizing granulomas containing mycobacteria (fig. 12-52). The granulomas may have palisading histiocytes, prominent epithelioid cells, and/or Langerhans-type giant cells (fig. 12-52). These necrotizing granulomas can progress to fibrosis and ultimately calcification. The granuloma may heal completely with resolution to normal lung or may progress to a fibrotic and/or calcified nodule. Epithelioid histiocytes are often prominent and fuse to form Langerhans-type giant cells.

Patients with progressive primary tuberculosis develop several pulmonary complications including rupture of the necrotizing granuloma into an artery, the pleura, or a bronchus. The pulmonary necrotizing lesion can enlarge, causing extensive cavitary lesions that extend into the lower lobe. If a necrotizing granuloma invades a pulmonary artery, the bacilli can embolize into the capillary beds of the surrounding lung, resulting in numerous 2 to 3 mm lesions of similar size which mimic the pattern of miliary tuberculosis; if the granuloma invades a vein there may be systemic spread. The pulmonary necrotizing granuloma may also invade the pleura, resulting in a tuberculous empyema (156,157). If a necrotizing granuloma invades into a bronchus, then the organisms spill into the surrounding airways and lung parenchyma causing a tuberculous bronchopneumonia (fig. 12-53) (156,157). Airway spread of tuberculosis can also result in an endobronchial pattern of

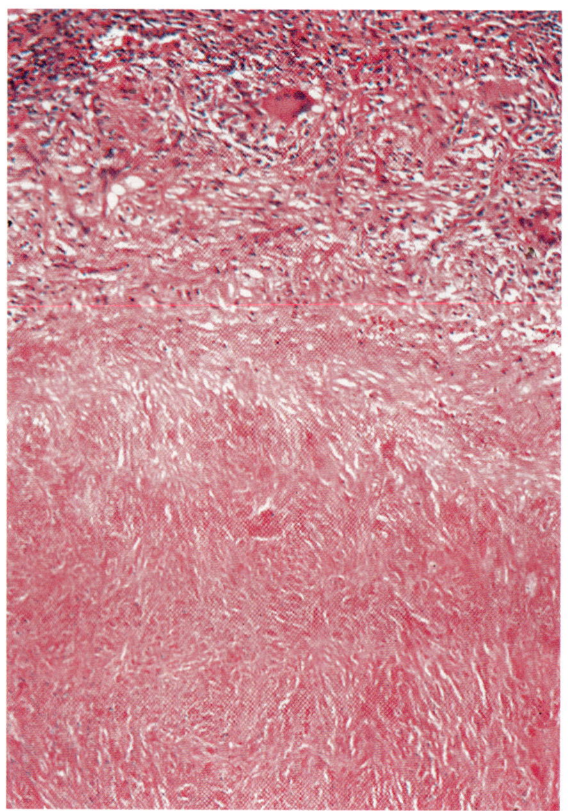

Figure 12-52

NECROTIZING GRANULOMA

A large zone of necrosis is bordered by palisading histiocytes and multinucleated giant cells.

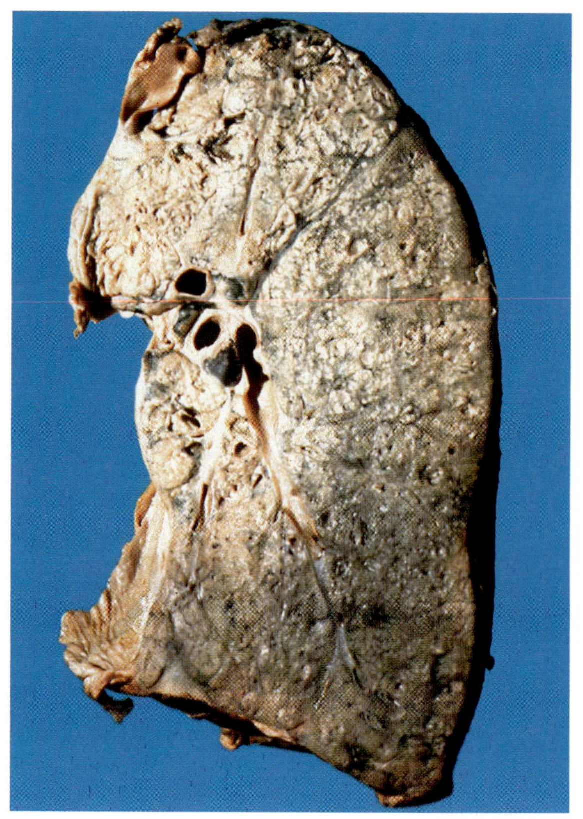

Figure 12-53

PROGRESSIVE PRIMARY TUBERCULOSIS: BRONCHOPNEUMONIA

There is confluent bronchopneumonia causing consolidation of most of the upper lobe and involvement of the lower lobe. (Courtesy of the Gordon Museum, London, England.)

lung involvement. Endobronchial spread occurs through lymphatic spread of bacilli from parenchymal lesions to the bronchial submucosa (156,157). Endobronchial tuberculosis can progress from mucosal ulceration to a hyperplastic inflammatory polyp to healing with bronchostenosis (155,162). Bronchostenosis can resemble bronchogenic carcinoma both grossly and radiographically, and can result in lobar atelectasis (155,162).

The initial lesion enlarges, producing necrotic areas up to 6 cm or more in greatest dimension. Central liquefaction results in cavities (figs. 12-54, 12-55), which may expand to occupy most of the lower lobe. At the same time, the draining lymph nodes display similar histologic changes.

Secondary Tuberculosis. Secondary tuberculosis is also known as *postprimary* or *reactivation tuberculosis* and it consists of those infections that occur in patients who lose their immunity to tuberculosis. The histologic reaction is primarily granulomatous and necrotizing, and cavitation is frequent. These lesions may progress to fibrosis and calcification (fig. 12-56). Cavitary lesions usually range from 3 to 10 cm, typically in the upper lobe apices, but they may be very large and replace an entire lung. Multiple bilateral cavitary lesions may be present (fig. 12-57). The acid-fast bacilli are found within the necrotic material in the cavities.

Pulmonary complications of secondary tuberculosis include miliary tuberculosis resulting from hematogenous dissemination (fig. 12-58), hemoptysis from erosion of pulmonary arteries, bronchopleural fistulae from erosion of cavities

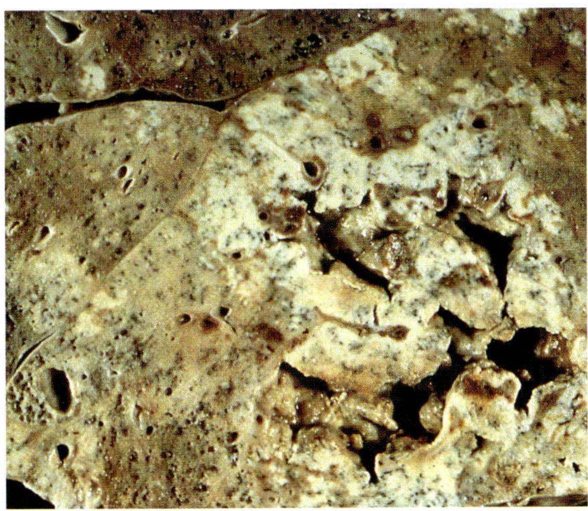

Figure 12-54

PROGRESSIVE PRIMARY TUBERCULOSIS: CAVITARY LESIONS

Multiple cavitary lesions are present within the consolidated areas.

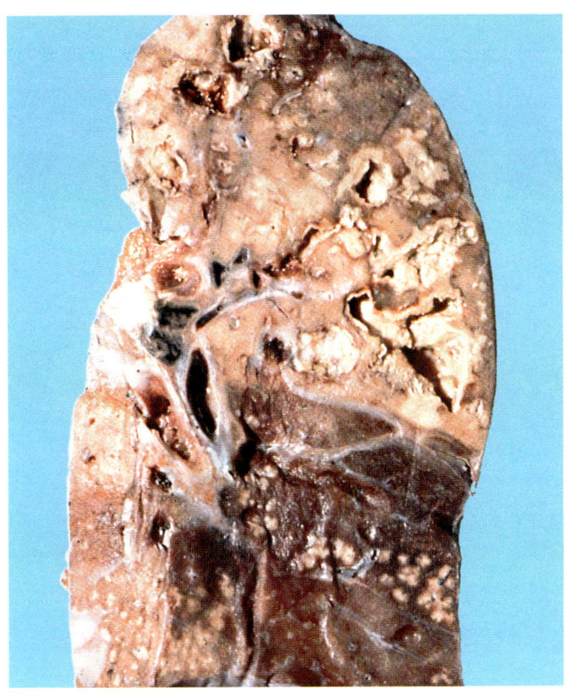

Figure 12-55

PROGRESSIVE PRIMARY TUBERCULOSIS: UPPER LOBE CAVITARY LESIONS

There is upper lobe bronchopneumonia with cavitation and miliary spread to the lower lobe. (Courtesy of the Gordon Museum, London, England.)

into the pleura causing empyema and possibly pneumothorax, and superimposed infections such as aspergillomas (i.e., fungus balls) (156). Carcinomas are also reported to arise in tuberculous scars and cavities (156). Pleural thickening and calcification are complications of prior empyema or spread to the pleural space from the underlying lung (fig. 12-59). Rarely, the entire thoracic cavity undergoes fibrosis and calcification.

Differential Diagnosis. The major entities in the differential diagnosis for the necrotizing granulomatous lesions of *M. tuberculosis* include nontuberculous mycobacterial infection, fungal infection, and Wegener's granulomatosis (WG). The necrotizing granulomas of tuberculosis can be mistaken for WG since a secondary vasculitis may be seen in tuberculous granulomas. Helpful histologic clues to the presence of infection rather than WG include the presence of sarcoidal granulomas, a fibrosing reaction around the granulomas with a relatively thin inflammatory border, and a sharply rounded morphology to the necrotizing granulomas. In addition, the non-necrotizing granulomas of tuberculosis can be mistaken for sarcoidosis (see chapter 3). Careful review of the histology, special stains, and clinicopathologic correlation are needed to separate these entities.

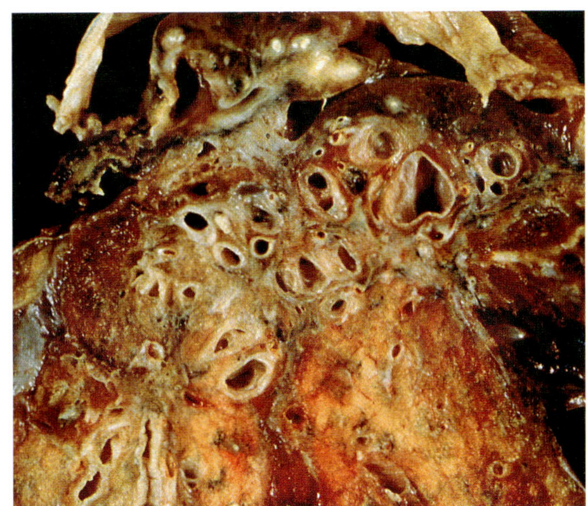

Figure 12-56

SECONDARY TUBERCULOSIS: CAVITARY AND FIBROTIC UPPER LOBE

The lung parenchyma shows consolidation accompanied by fibrosis and cavitary lesions.

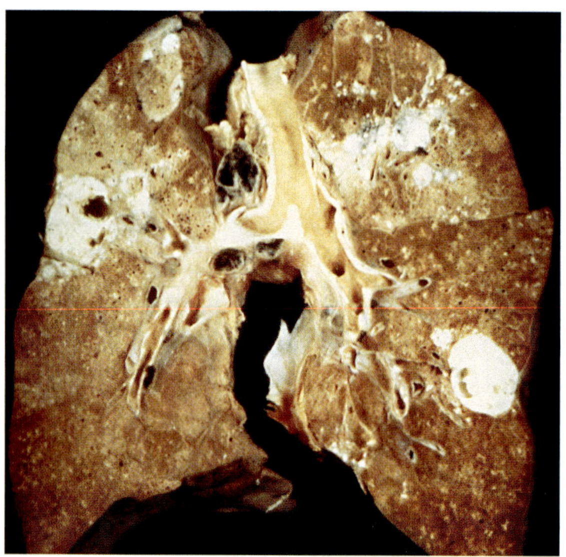

Figure 12-57

SECONDARY TUBERCULOSIS: BILATERAL CAVITARY LESIONS

Multiple bilateral areas of consolidation are present with cavitation.

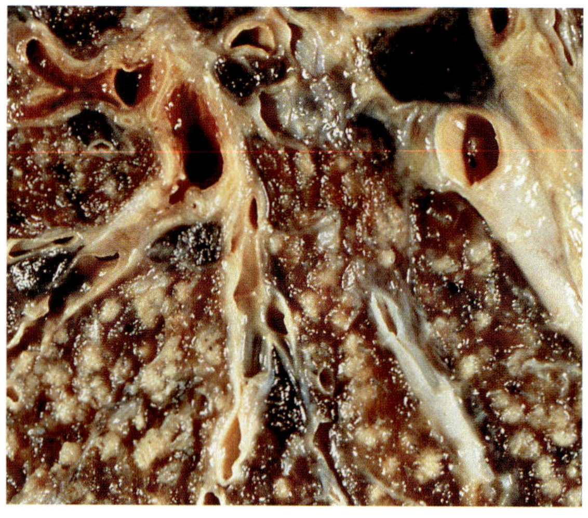

Figure 12-58

SECONDARY MILIARY TUBERCULOSIS

Multiple millimeter-sized granulomas are present throughout this lung.

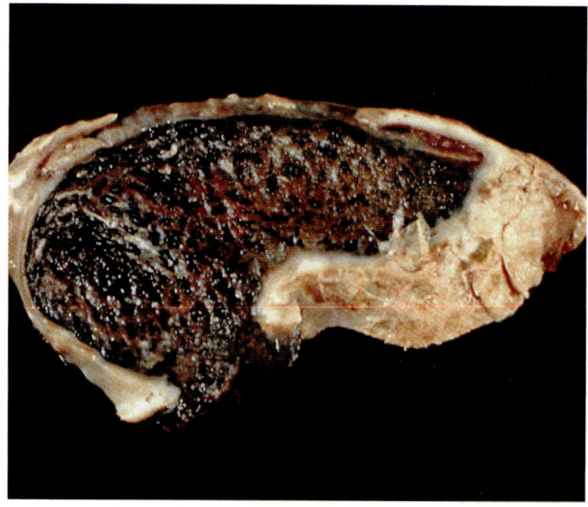

Figure 12-59

SECONDARY TUBERCULOUS PLEURITIS

There is diffuse pleural thickening due to granulomatous pleuritis.

The other major organism that may appear acid fast is *Nocardia* sp whose organisms are long, filamentous, and branching in contrast to the short, nonbranching mycobacteria. However, *Nocardia* is usually only weakly acid fast, requiring the Coates modification of the acid-fast stain. Sometimes mycobacteria lose their acid fastness due to fragmentation and degeneration and they can be detected with the GMS stain. Another pitfall is that extraneous organisms derived from tap water or contaminants that may be floaters from previous specimens can lead to a misdiagnosis of tuberculosis. Noticing that the organisms are not in the same plane of section as the tissue is an important key. In addition, one can sometimes find organisms on the slide away from the tissue section. The unexpected finding of a series of positive stains should also raise concern for such an artifact.

Most of the time the organisms are found within the necrotic centers, not in the surrounding fibroinflammatory reaction. In addition, in most cases, neutrophils are lacking in the center of the granulomas, except in early primary tuberculosis. Therefore, the presence of prominent neutrophils should cause one to consider WG or other infections such as nocardiosis or blastomycosis.

Treatment and Prognosis. The topic of medical therapy for patients with tuberculosis is beyond the scope of this discussion and there are extensive references on this subject (156). The recent statement from the American Thoracic Society (ATS) and the Centers for Disease

Control and Prevention (CDC) on the treatment of tuberculosis includes suggestions relating to monitoring for adequate response to therapy and details of monitoring for drug toxicity (148). Also addressed is the use of the less common antituberculous drugs to minimize the drug toxicity encountered with more common ones, and multidrug-resistant tuberculosis. Successful treatment of tuberculosis requires more than one drug to which the organisms are susceptible, and must be taken regularly, for a sufficient period of time and in appropriate doses. Directly observed therapy (DOT) is the best way to assure the completion of appropriate treatment. The primary medications historically have been isoniazid, para-aminosalicylic acid, streptomycin, rifampin, ethambutol, and pyrazinamide.

The development of drug-resistant strains of *M. tuberculosis* has become a major problem (156). The term drug-resistant tuberculosis refers to cases of tuberculosis caused by an isolate of *M. tuberculosis* which is resistant to one of the first-line antituberculosis drugs: isoniazid, rifampin, pyrazinamide, ethambutol, or streptomycin. Multidrug-resistant tuberculosis (MDR-TB) is caused by an isolate of *M. tuberculosis* which is resistant to two or more of the first-line chemotherapeutic agents, usually isoniazid and rifampin.

Predictors of poor response to therapy include extensive infection with massive numbers of tubercle bacilli, poor compliance, heavy alcohol use, poor nutrition, or serious underlying disease such as cancer or immunodeficiency (156).

Nontuberculous Mycobacteria

Definition. Pulmonary nontuberculous mycobacterial infection is caused by a variety of *Mycobacterium* organisms other than *M. tuberculosis* (MOTT). These organisms are also known as *atypical mycobacteria, anonymous mycobacteria,* and *pseudotubercle bacilli.*

In the lung, the most important nontuberculous mycobacteria are *M. avium-intracellulare, M. kansasii, M. fortuitum,* and *M. chelonei* (153). Nontuberculous mycobacteria were classified by Runyon and Timpe into four groups according to pigmentation, growth rate, catalase activity, morphology, drug susceptibilities, and pathogenicity in animals (157,170,171). According to this classification, photochromogens (group 1, *M. kansasii*) have no color if grown in the dark, but since they can synthesize a carotene pigment, when grown in the light they are yellow to red. The scotochromogens (group 2, *M. scrofulaceum*) are yellow-orange in the dark and red in the light. The nonchromogens (group 3, *M. avium-intracellulare*) have colonies that are small, smooth, circular, and only weakly pigmented. The rapid growers (group 4, *M. fortuitum*) form rough or smooth colonies that typically do not have color.

In one study completed prior to the AIDS epidemic, Good and Snider (153) found that 65 percent of all mycobacteria isolated in 41 states of the United States, were *M. tuberculosis,* 21 percent were *M. avium* complex, 6.5 percent were *M. fortuitum* and *M. cheloni* (rapid growers), 3.5 percent were *M. kansasii,* and 2.3 percent were *M. scrofulaceum.* Since the AIDS epidemic, the incidence of *M. avium-intracellulare* infection has risen since these patients are predisposed to this infection.

The nontuberculous mycobacteria are found in the soil, plants, fresh water, salt water, and animals. Infection is usually acquired from the environment rather than through a person-to-person route. In addition, the majority of patients have underlying lung disease such as COPD, bronchiectasis, interstitial fibrosis, previous tuberculosis, carcinoma of the lung, or mineral oil pneumonia. Other predisposing conditions include AIDS, alcoholism, and diabetes mellitus (156,157).

M. avium and *M. intracellulare* are closely related and often grouped together either as *M. avium* complex or *M. avium-intracellulare* (MAI) (156,157). Prior to the AIDS epidemic, 85 to 90 percent of all isolates of MAI were from the lungs, however, only 30 percent of these individuals were thought to have pulmonary disease (156). For this reason, there is a constant concern to avoid overdiagnosis. Today, there is increasing concern that slowly progressive lung disease can result and patients are carefully followed to make sure that disease progression does not occur.

M. kansasii is not as widespread as MAI since it is found in water rather than in soil or dust. It also tends to be more restricted in geographic distribution. In the United States, it is limited to mid-western states as well as Texas, Louisiana, and Florida.

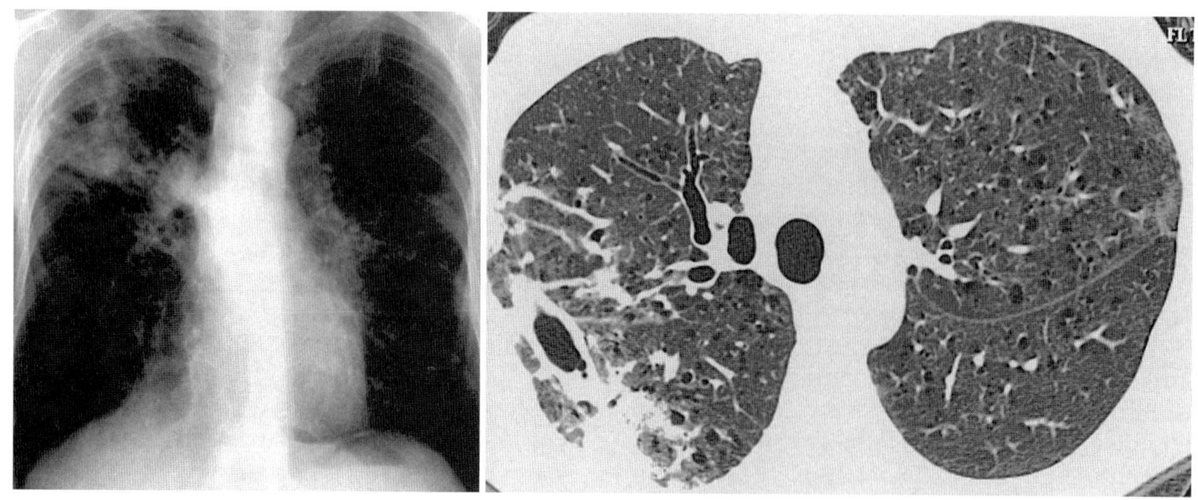

Figure 12-60

MYCOBACTERIUM AVIUM-INTRACELLULARE

Left: Chest radiograph shows right upper lobe consolidation and cavitation.

Right: CT scan in a 62-year-old woman demonstrates foci of consolidation and a cavity in the right upper lobe. Note the centrilobular emphysyema.

Clinical Features. In immunocompetent patients, several criteria must be present to diagnose MAI pneumonia: radiographic signs of cavitary lung disease without another explanation and isolation of the organisms from the sputum on at least three occasions (156). If cavitary lung disease is not present but the organisms is repeatedly isolated from the sputum, the diagnosis is colonization rather than infection. Conversion of the sputum to negative by repeated bronchial hygiene using aerosolized bronchodilators and inhalation of nebulized saline is attempted (145,156). If this approach does not convert the sputum in 2 to 4 months, then the diagnosis of disease by MAI is established. Histologic changes and identification of the organism in tissue by culture or histology are also sufficient to establish the diagnosis (145,156).

Nonimmunosuppressed patients with MAI infection are typically older or middle-aged white men (156). The presenting manifestations are cough, low-grade fever, malaise, and occasionally hemoptysis. Extrapulmonary involvement is uncommon in this clinical setting. While most patients with MAI pulmonary infection have underlying disease, 35 to 40 percent of patients with *M. kansasii* infection have no underlying disease (156). Recently, an association of pulmonary infection with hot-tubs contaminated with MAI has been recognized (150,159).

In HIV-infected individuals, MAI usually causes systemic infection that only seldom involves the lungs (156). In most cases isolation of MAI from the lung is thought to represent colonization. The lung is considered to be the route of initial infection, where the organism remains dormant, until the HIV infection impairs the CD4 counts and dissemination takes place (156). Dissemination can also occur with *M. kansasii* infection in AIDS patients (156).

Radiologic Findings. The most common radiologic manifestations of nontuberculous mycobacterial infection are heterogeneous foci of consolidation and linear and nodular opacities involving the apical and posterior segments of the upper lobes (151,167). Cavitation occurs in 80 to 90 percent of patients (fig. 12-60) (167). These features are indistinguishable from those of reactivation tuberculosis (151,167). Endobronchial spread is common, particularly in patients with cavity formation, and is manifested by unilateral or bilateral, centrilobular nodular opacities. This pattern is seen most commonly in elderly men with underlying lung disease, usually COPD (151).

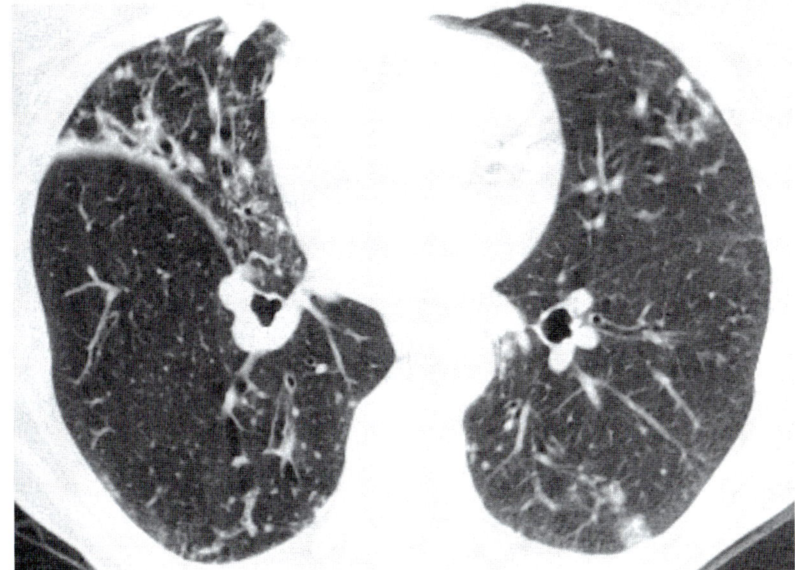

Figure 12-61

MYCOBACTERIUM AVIUM-INTRACELLULARE

HRCT scan in a 77-year-old woman demonstrates cylindrical bronchiectasis in the right middle lobe, right lower lobe, and lingula. There are a few small nodular opacities and small foci of consolidation.

The second most common manifestations are bronchiectasis and multiple, 1- to 5-mm centrilobular nodules (fig. 12-61) (151). The bronchiectasis tends to be most severe in the middle lobe or lingula but often involves all lobes (151, 169). This pattern is seen most commonly in elderly women without underlying disease (151). Less commonly, nontuberculous mycobacterial infection may manifest as single or multiple nodules in asymptomatic patients (151).

AIDS patients with disseminated nontuberculous mycobacterial infection often have normal radiographs. The most common chest radiologic abnormality is hilar or mediastinal lymph node enlargement (151).

Pathologic Findings. MAI usually causes upper lobe cavitary lung lesions (fig. 12-62). The cavities may be thin walled. Histologically, the lungs show granulomatous inflammation with less of a tendency to caseate than with *M. tuberculosis* (157). The necrosis may have serpiginous borders and there may be associated vasculitis resembling Wegener's granulomatosis. Multiple noncaseating granulomas can be seen, sometimes raising the consideration of sarcoidosis. A pattern of bronchocentric granulomatosis can be seen (fig. 12-63). Granulomatous inflammation can involve blood vessels and cause vasculitis, particularly in the setting of extrapulmonary dissemination (fig. 12-64). It can be very difficult to identify organisms in tissue sections. In the hot-tub–associated MAI infections, the granulomas tend to be bronchiolocentric and show a spectrum of relatively small caseating and noncaseating granulomas (fig. 12-65). The granulomas may be within the lumen of the bronchioles (fig. 12-65).

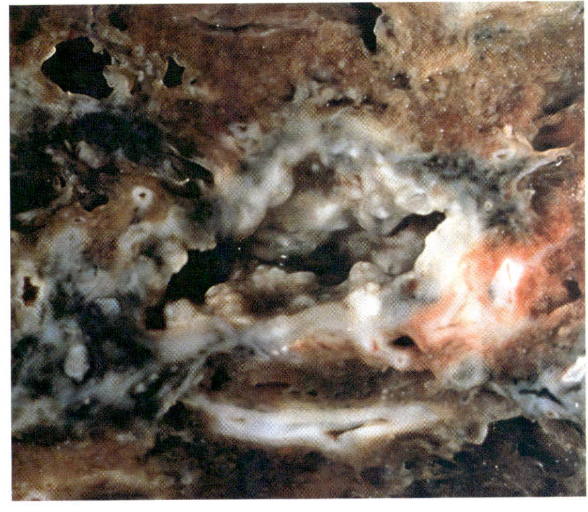

Figure 12-62

CAVITARY *MYCOBACTERIUM AVIUM-INTRA CELLULARE* INFECTION

This localized necrotizing granuloma shows central cavitation.

The morphology of the acid-fast bacilli of most nontuberculous mycobacteria is indistinguishable from that of *M. tuberculosis*. However,

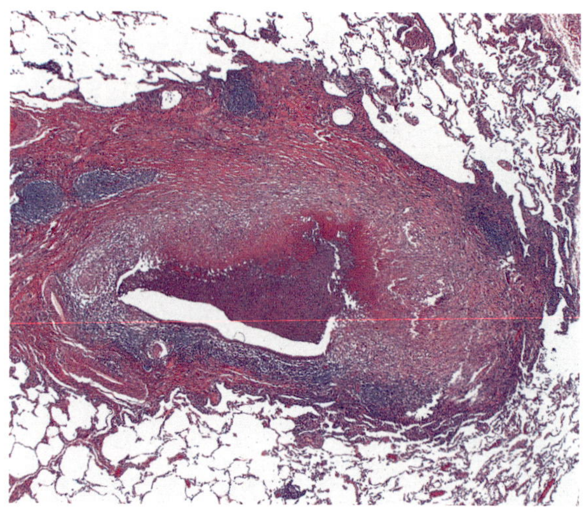

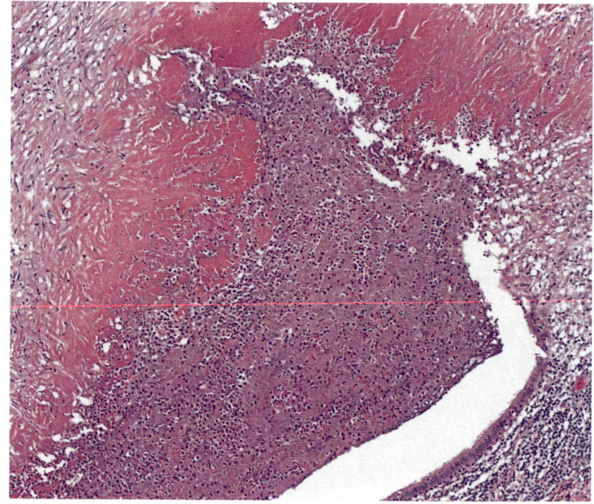

Figure 12-63

BRONCHOCENTRIC GRANULOMATOSIS DUE TO *MYCOBACTERIUM AVIUM-INTRACELLULARE* INFECTION

Left: A large necrotizing granuloma is centered on this bronchiole with the histologic pattern of bronchocentric granulomatosis.

Right: The bronchiolar wall is destroyed by necrotizing granulomatous inflammation. No organisms could be found on review of Ziehl-Neelsen stains, but cultures grew *Mycobacterium avium-intracellulare.*

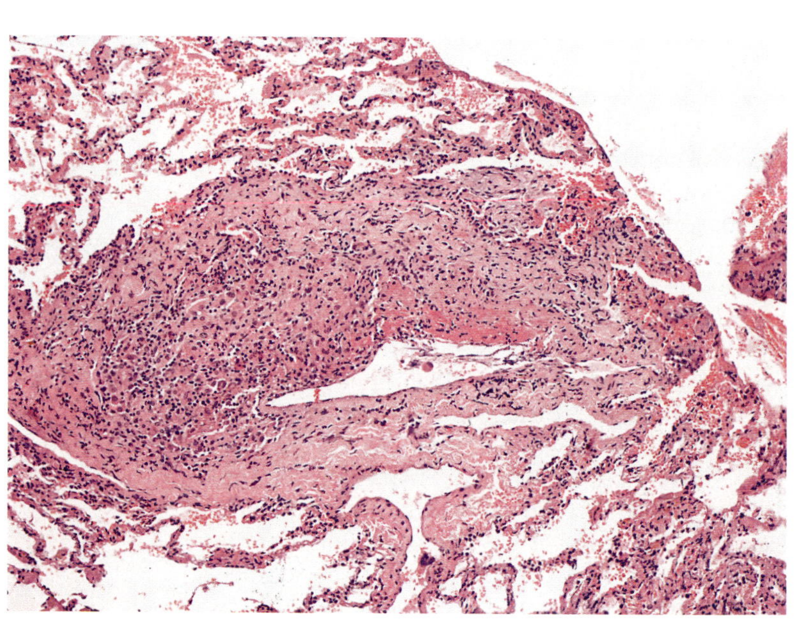

Figure 12-64

MYCOBACTERIUM AVIUM-INTRACELLULARE INFECTION WITH VASCULITIS

Granulomatous vasculitis with extrapulmonary spread.

the acid-fast bacilli of *M. kansasii* tend to be very long and beaded (fig. 12-66).

In AIDS patients, lung involvement typically shows numerous macrophages that contain large numbers of MAI bacilli (157). Well-formed granulomas are usually absent. The histiocytes have a pseudo-Gaucher's appearance due to the massive numbers of bacilli distending the cytoplasm (fig. 12-67) (173). The bacilli can be seen on routine H&E stains as well as the Ziehl-Neelsen stain (173). The organisms can also stain with PAS and GMS (157,173). MAI can cause endobronchial lesions in AIDS patients (166).

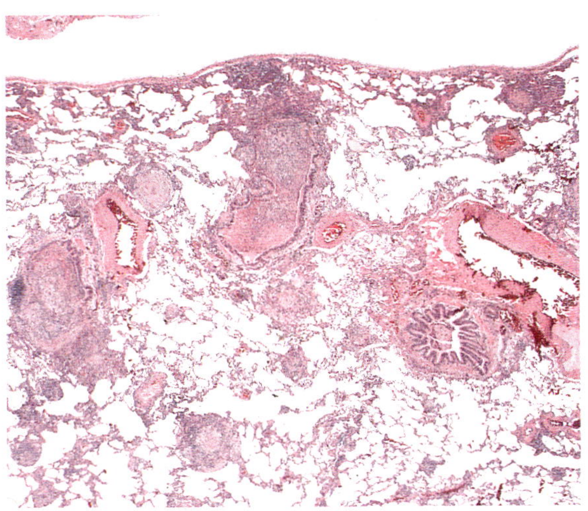

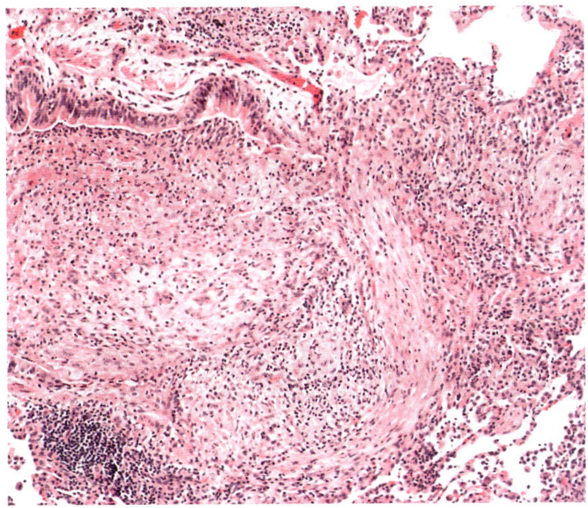

Figure 12-65

MYCOBACTERIUM AVIUM-INTRACELLULARE INFECTION ASSOCIATED WITH CONTAMINATED HOT-TUB

Left: Miliary bronchiolocentric granulomas are present.
Right: The granulomatous inflammation fills the bronchiolar lumen and involves the surrounding tissue.

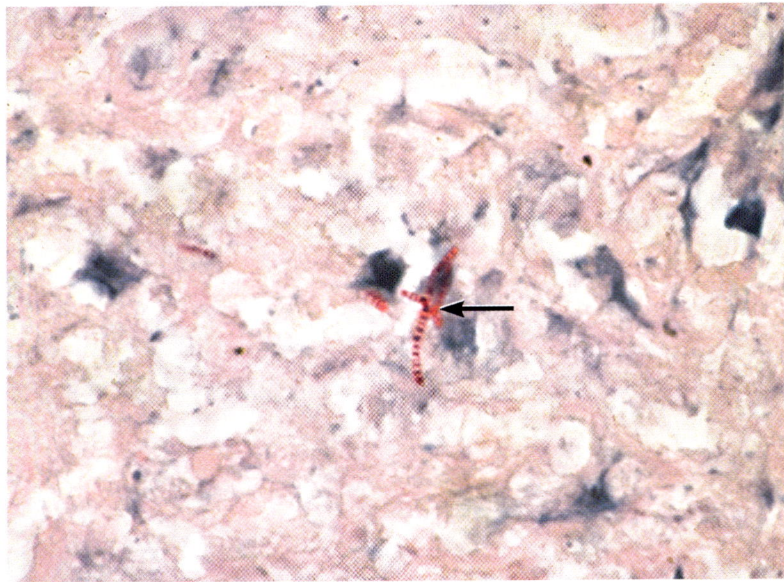

Figure 12-66

MYCOBACTERIUM KANSASII INFECTION

The long, beaded morphology of these acid-fast organisms is characteristic, although not diagnostic, of *M. kansasii* (Ziehl-Neelsen stain).

Differential Diagnosis. The major differential diagnoses for the necrotizing granulomatous lesions of atypical mycobacteria are tuberculosis, fungal infection, and WG. It may be very difficult to identify organisms in tissue sections from patients with nontuberculous mycobacterial infections. In histologic sections, it is impossible to distinguish *M. tuberculosis* from the other nontuberculous mycobacteria.

Just as with tuberculosis, the necrotizing granulomas can be mistaken for WG and the nonnecrotizing granulomas can be mistaken for sarcoidosis. Careful review of the histology, special stains, and clinicopathologic correlation are needed to separate these entities.

In AIDS patients, the extensive histiocytic infiltrates of the MAI pulmonary infection must not be mistaken for a lipoid pneumonia. The

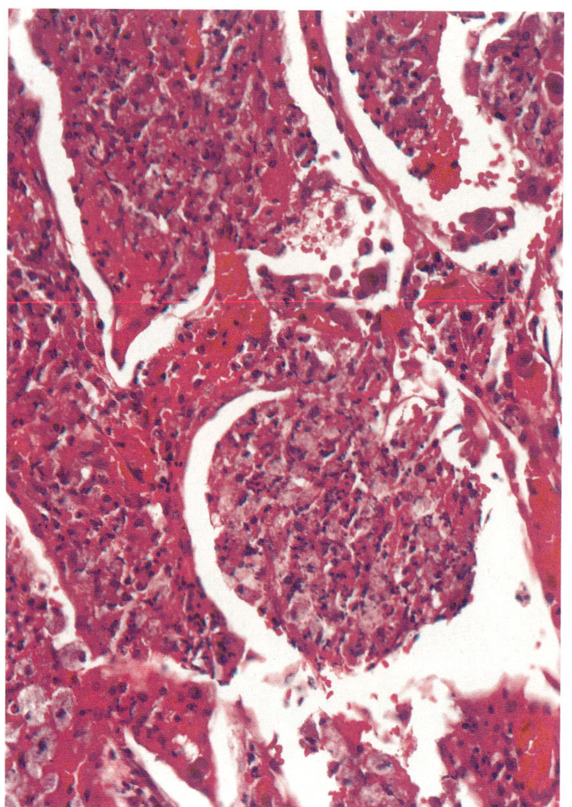

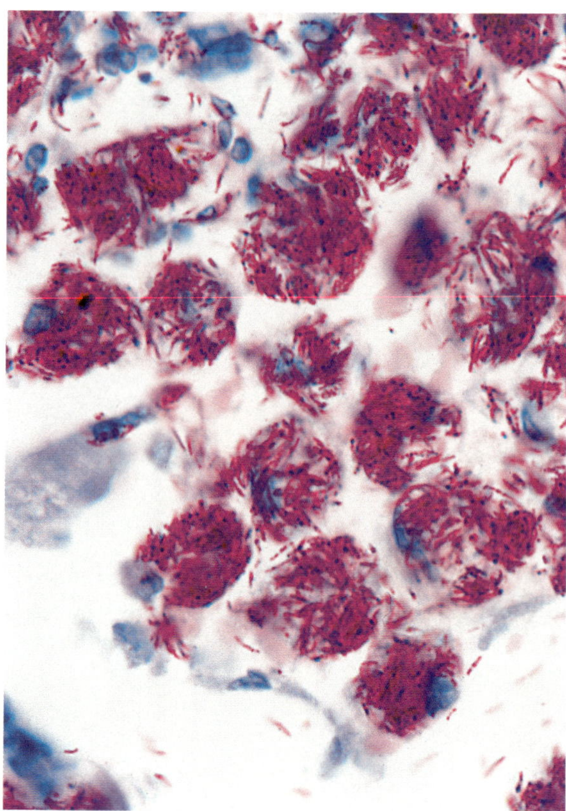

Figure 12-67

MYCOBACTERIUM AVIUM-INTRACELLULARE INFECTION IN AIDS PATIENT

Left: The alveolar spaces are filled with macrophages.
Right: The macrophages are stuffed full of acid-fast bacilli (Ziehl-Neelsen stain).

presence of numerous bacillary rod-shaped organisms gives the histiocytes a very different morphology than the lipid-laden histiocytes of lipoid pneumonia that have many round lipid vacuoles.

Treatment and Prognosis. The most recent recommendations of the ATS in 1997 serve as a useful guide to the diagnosis and treatment of nontuberculous mycobacterial disease in patients with or without HIV co-infection (147). There has been significant improvement in the prognosis of patients with certain nontuberculous pulmonary infections with the use of new drugs including clarithromycin, azithromycin, and rifabutin (154). However, these new medications may have severe toxicities and drug interactions that necessitate careful monitoring of patients. In contrast to MAI infection, *M. kansasii* infection tends to respond well to antituberculous medications.

FUNGAL INFECTIONS

Histoplasma Capsulatum

Definition. Histoplasmosis is a fungal infection caused by the dimorphic fungus *Histoplasma capsulatum.*

This and other fungal infections discussed in this chapter are listed in Table 12-5. Although *Pneumocystis carinii* is now thought to be a fungus, it is discussed separately after the Mycoplasma/Chlamydia section.

H. capsulatum has a natural habitat in the soil where it exists in its mycelial form. It is endemic in the south-central United States, especially in the Mississippi and Ohio valleys. The disease is caused by inhalation of *H. capsulatum* in infected dust, commonly from bird droppings. Exposure to bird droppings can occur in several settings including disturbed chicken

Table 12-5

FUNGAL INFECTIONS

Histoplasmosis (*Histoplasma capsulatum*)
Cryptococcosis (*Cryptococcus neoformans*)
Coccidioidomycosis (*Coccidioides immitis*)
Blastomycosis (*Blastomyces dermatitidis*)
Paracoccidioidomycosis (*Paracoccidioides brasiliensis*)
Aspergillosis (*Aspergillus fumigatus, A. flavus, A. niger*)
Mucormycosis (Zygomycosis, *Rhizopus* sp)
Candidiasis (*Candida* sp)
Sporotrichosis (*Sporothrix schenckii*)
Torulopsosis (*Torulopsis glabrata*)
Fusariosis (*Fusarium* sp)
Pseudoallescheriasis (*Pseudoallescheria boydii*)
Adiaspiromycosis (*Chrysosporium parvum* var *crescens*)
Malasseziasis (*Malassezia furfur*)

Table 12-6

CLINICAL FORMS OF PULMONARY HISTOPLASMOSIS

Benign, self limited
Acute
Acute respiratory distress syndrome
Acute, self limited, upper lobe (in smokers with emphysema)
Chronic
Asymptomatic pulmonary nodules, +/- calcification ("histoplasmoma")
Progressive (chronic cavitary) pulmonary
Progressive disseminated
Mediastinal
Lymphadenopathy with compression of mediastinal structures
Middle lobe syndrome
Fibrosis

coops, bird roosts (pigeons an starlings), or caves and attics where bat guano has accumulated. Infectivity is determined by the ability of the organism to convert from the mycelial to the yeast phase. The stimuli that drive the transformation have not been clearly defined, although temperature appears to be a major factor. The organism is avidly ingested by resident lung phagocytes and then traffics to local lymph nodes. Subsequently, *H. capsulatum* disseminates to many organs that contain a high proportion of mononuclear phagocytes (209).

Clinical Features. In the United States, approximately 500,000 new cases of *H. capsulatum* infection occur annually (207,222,295). The major clinical forms of histoplasmosis are summarized in Table 12-6 (207,222,295). These include benign self-limited, acute, chronic, progressive disseminated, and mediastinal infections.

Primary Pulmonary Histoplasmosis. Most patients are asymptomatic: only 5 to 10 percent of infections cause symptoms. In asymptomatic patients, a patchy pneumonitis may be seen radiographically, which may result in a Ghon-like complex, including a parenchymal granuloma and similar lesions in the draining lymph nodes (207,222,295).

Patients with acute pulmonary infection present clinically with a self-limited disease in the upper lobes that resolves spontaneously with bed rest. Rarely are antifungal agents necessary. When exposed to a very large inoculum, patients can present with a potentially life-threatening illness, with clinical manifestations similar to those of the acute respiratory distress syndrome. Patients usually develop symptoms around 14 days after exposure (207,222,295). The clinical illness is characterized by fever, chills, myalgia, and a nonproductive cough.

Following recovery, the chest radiograph may be normal or show pulmonary nodules with or without calcification, or progressive, chronic cavitary histoplasmosis. Rarely, there are local complications such as extensive fibrosis in the mediastinum that leads to vascular compression and the superior vena cava syndrome. Inflammatory masses may compress the esophagus and cause dysphagia. Calcified nodes may erode into vascular structures and result in hemoptysis.

Progressive Disseminated Histoplasmosis. Progressive dissemination is an extrapulmonary infection that develops in patients who are immunosuppressed due to transplantation, hematologic malignancy, cytotoxic chemotherapy, HIV infection, or old age (203,207,222,295). Such patients develop fever, chills, productive cough, dyspnea, hemoptysis, malaise, headache, weight loss, diarrhea, anemia, purpura, lymphadenopathy, hepatosplenomegaly, and oropharyngeal ulcers. Patients with adrenal involvement may develop Addison's disease. Importantly, up to 50 percent of patients with progressive disseminated histoplasmosis have no symptoms related to the lung. The mortality for patients with disseminated infection is very high, approaching 80 percent in untreated cases. Death occurs within weeks and is usually secondary to respiratory compromise (203).

Chronic Cavitary Histoplasmosis. Chronic infection occurs most commonly in adults (207, 222,295). Chronic infection may progress directly from acute infection or it may develop after a prolonged latency period. The disease resembles reinfection tuberculosis, both in symptoms and radiographic appearance. Chronic infection occurs following resolution of an acute infection in a patient with previously damaged lungs, especially middle-aged men who have smoking-related emphysema. These patients occasionally develop a progressive upper lobe fibrocavitary disease. Treatment is necessary to prevent ongoing pulmonary destruction. Rarely, patients develop mediastinal lymphadenopathy with bronchial obstruction, sclerosing mediastinitis, or pericarditis (207,222,295).

Intradermal skin testing with histoplasmin is not useful in diagnosis. Complement-fixing antibodies to mycelial and yeast phase antigens can be detected 4 to 6 weeks after exposure or 2 to 4 weeks after the onset of symptoms. A titer against the yeast antigen of 1:32 or more suggests histoplasmosis in the proper clinical setting. A four-fold rise of titer is diagnostic of acute histoplasmosis. Unfortunately, a negative test does not rule out histoplasmosis, especially in immunocompromised hosts. The *Histoplasma* polysaccharide antigen test is very useful for diagnosing progressive disseminated histoplasmosis, especially in immunocompromised hosts. Serial measurements of the antigen in urine follow the course of the disease and predict relapses.

Radiologic Findings. The radiologic manifestations of pulmonary histoplasmosis vary according to the type of clinical infection. The majority of patients with acute histoplasmosis have normal chest radiographs. When present, the most common radiographic abnormality is focal or multifocal parenchymal consolidation, which may be associated with ipsilateral hilar lymphadenopathy (250).

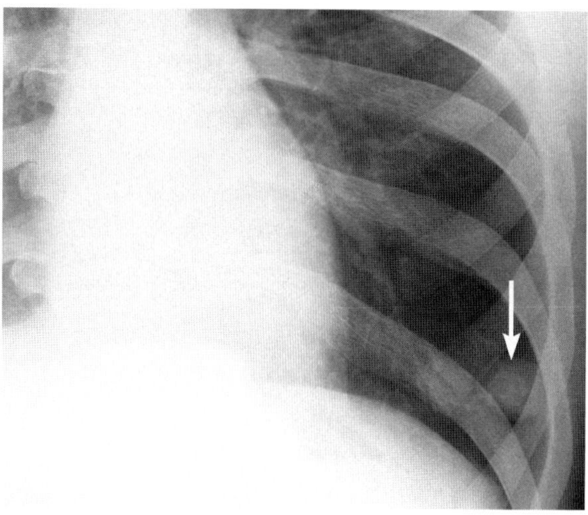

Figure 12-68

HISTOPLASMOMA IN AN ASYMPTOMATIC 20-YEAR-OLD MALE

PA chest radiograph coned-down to the left base demonstrates a 2-cm soft tissue mass with central calcification (arrow). The pattern of calcification is consistent with benignity.

Lymphadenopathy may occur in the absence of radiologically visible parenchymal disease. As parenchymal disease heals, a nodular opacity (histoplasmoma) may develop. While histoplasmomas are usually solitary nodules, satellite nodular lesions are also seen. Calcification may occur and may be central, laminar, or diffuse; in these cases, benignity is confirmed (fig. 12-68). Multifocal histoplasmomas also occur and may calcify and grow over time. Large exposures may result in patchy multifocal airspace disease, large nodular opacities, or small diffuse nodules. In these cases, the nodules may resolve completely or result in multifocal punctate parenchymal calcifications (fig. 12-69) (200,215,224,250).

Chronic pulmonary histoplasmosis typically affects the apical and posterior segments of the upper lobes. Bilateral or unilateral subpleural parenchymal consolidation may surround areas of emphysema or preexisting bullous disease and mimic the radiologic appearance of postprimary tuberculosis. Bullae may develop air-fluid levels and mimic cavitary disease. Adjacent pulmonary linear opacities and pleural thickening may also occur. With therapy and healing there may be resultant upper lobe volume loss (200,215,224,250).

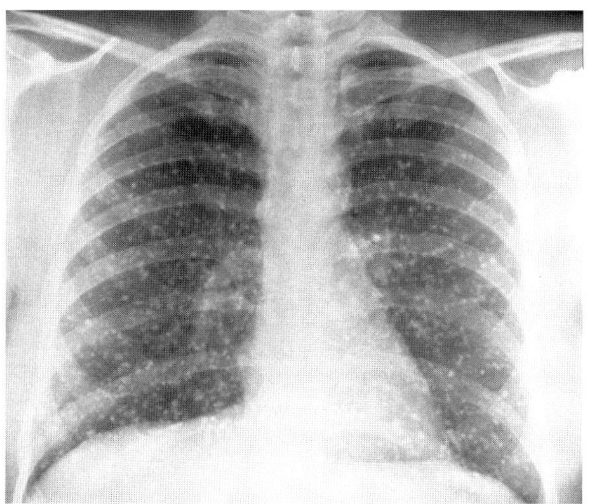

Figure 12-69

HISTOPLASMOSIS IN AN ASYMPTOMATIC 41-YEAR-OLD FEMALE

PA chest radiograph demonstrates multifocal, bilateral, punctate parenchymal calcifications consistent with healed histoplasmosis. (Figure 6 from McAdams HP, Rosado-de-Christenson ML, Lesar M, Templeton PA, Moran CA. Thoracic mycoses from endemic fungi: radiologic-pathologic correlation. Radiographics 1995;15:258.)

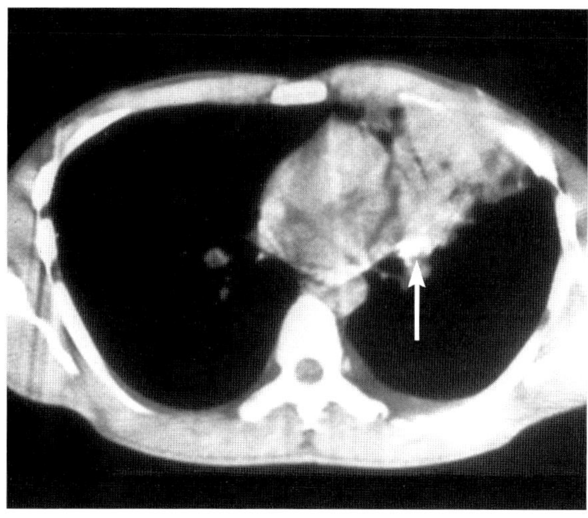

Figure 12-70

BRONCHOLITHIASIS

Broncholithiasis in a 30-year-old male with cough, fever, pleuritic chest pain, and occasional hemoptysis. Unenhanced chest CT (mediastinal window) demonstrates lingular consolidation with associated calcified lymphadenopathy (arrow). Surgery revealed a broncholith and granulation tissue occluding the left upper lobe bronchus.

Parenchymal disease is often associated with hilar or mediastinal lymphadenopathy, which may exhibit calcification on CT imaging. Calcified hilar lymph nodes may erode into the lumen of adjacent bronchi and result in broncholithiasis, which may be complicated by distal obstruction with pneumonia or atelectasis (fig. 12-70). Bronchiectasis and air-trapping may also result from broncholithiasis. In these cases, CT typically demonstrates a densely calcified lymph node, which may appear completely endobronchial or peribronchial, with little evidence of a soft tissue lesion in the bronchus or around it (fig. 12-70) (201).

Immunocompromised patients who are exposed to histoplasmosis may develop disseminated disease, which manifests with bilateral miliary or diffuse reticular and nodular opacities (fig. 12-71). These may progress to diffuse airspace consolidation (200,215).

Mediastinal histoplasmosis may manifest as mediastinal granuloma or fibrosing mediastinitis. Mediastinal granuloma typically appears as a focal, mediastinal, soft tissue mass, which is typically located in the middle mediastinum,

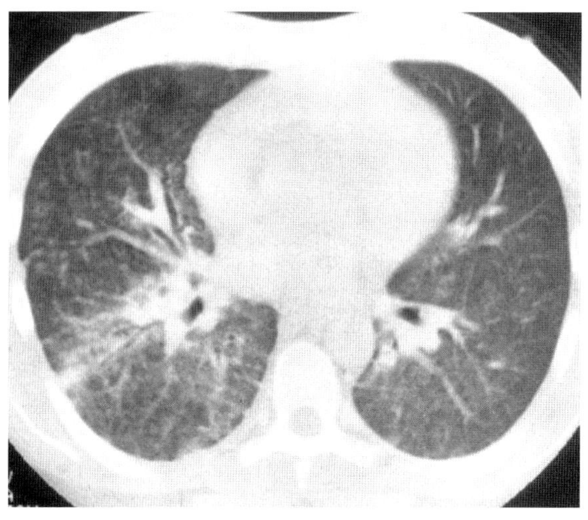

Figure 12-71

DISSEMINATED HISTOPLASMOSIS

Disseminated histoplasmosis in a 36-year-old male with AIDS who presented with dyspnea and fever. Chest CT (lung window) demonstrates consolidation and multifocal miliary parenchymal opacities involving the lungs bilaterally. (Figure 9B from McAdams HP, Rosado-de-Christenson ML, Lesar M, Templeton PA, Moran CA. Thoracic mycoses from endemic fungi: radiologic-pathologic correlation. Radiographics 1995;15:259.)

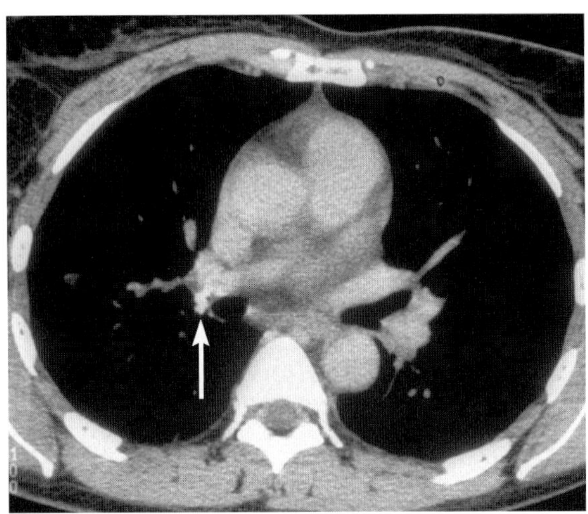

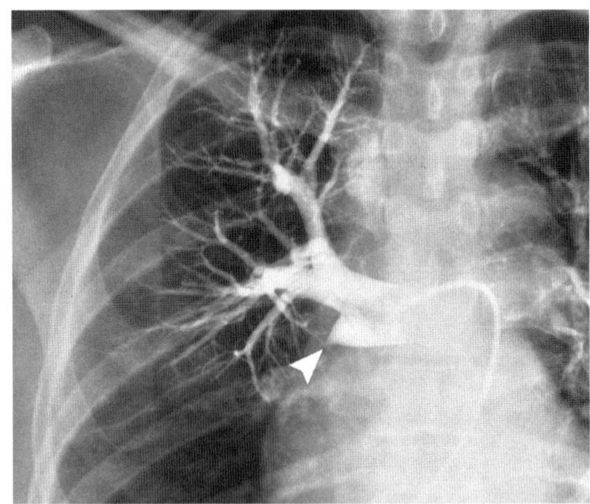

Figure 12-72

FIBROSING MEDIASTINITIS IN A 39-YEAR-OLD FEMALE WITH CHEST PAIN

Left: Unenhanced chest CT (mediastinal window) demonstrates calcification (arrow) in the region of the right pulmonary artery.

Right: Right pulmonary arteriogram demonstrates complete obstruction of the right lower lobe pulmonary artery (arrowhead).

exhibits internal calcification, and may produce mass effect on adjacent structures. Mediastinal granuloma may be associated with hilar lymphadenopathy. The imaging findings may be characteristic, but progressive enlargement of the soft tissue mass and absence of calcification suggest malignant neoplasia, and biopsy is indicated for diagnosis in these cases (200,215,224,250).

Chest radiographs of patients with fibrosing mediastinitis may be normal or demonstrate mediastinal or hilar lymph node enlargement. Airway obstruction may result in atelectasis or pneumonia, and pulmonary vein occlusion may result in interstitial edema. Decreased lung markings may result from pulmonary arterial obstruction. CT demonstrates soft tissue infiltration of the mediastinum, which may encase or obstruct vessels and/or the central aerodigestive tract (fig. 12-72). The presence of calcification within the lesion, which may be stippled or dense, is helpful in suggesting the correct diagnosis and excluding the possibility of metastatic malignancy or lymphoma. Because of its ability to demonstrate calcium, CT is superior to magnetic resonance imaging (MRI) in evaluating these patients. However, in patients with allergy to contrast, MRI may provide useful information regarding vascular involvement by fibrosing mediastinitis (200,215,250).

Pathologic Findings. Morphologic recognition of *H. capsulatum* requires identification of the yeast-like forms in tissue sections (218, 279). They are 2 to 4 µm in diameter, uninucleate, and spherical to oval; have single buds; and are often situated in clusters due to the intracellular growth within histiocytes (fig. 12-73). Budding forms are often difficult to identify although they have a narrow base (fig. 12-73). Rarely, the organisms show "darkly stained foci" similar to those seen in *Pneumocystis carinii* (discussed later in this chapter). A clear space or artifactual "halo" may be apparent on H&E examination due to the retraction of the basophilic fungal cell cytoplasm from the poorly stained cell wall. Hyphal elements are extremely rare in tissue sections except in the setting of intravascular infections (227,279).

It is usually difficult to see the organisms on examination of H&E-stained sections, except in the acute or disseminated forms when organisms are numerous (194). In chronic infection, special stains are usually necessary to identify the organisms and the GMS stain is the best. In chronic infections the organisms stain poorly with the PAS stain, but in acute infections with numerous organisms this stain is useful. Direct immunofluorescence on histologic sections can help establish the diagnosis (195).

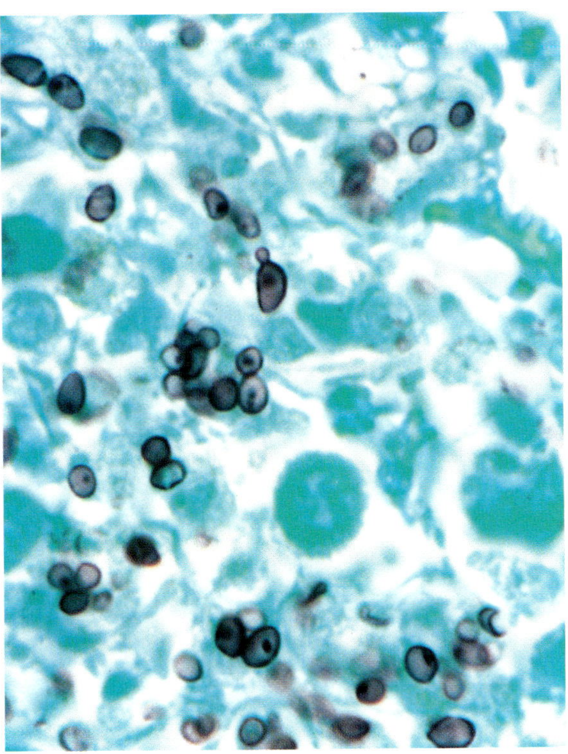

Figure 12-73

HISTOPLASMA CAPSULATUM: YEAST FORMS

Multiple yeast are present with focal narrow-based budding. They are found in clusters. Several yeast forms show darkly stained foci similar to those seen with *Pneumocystis carinii.*

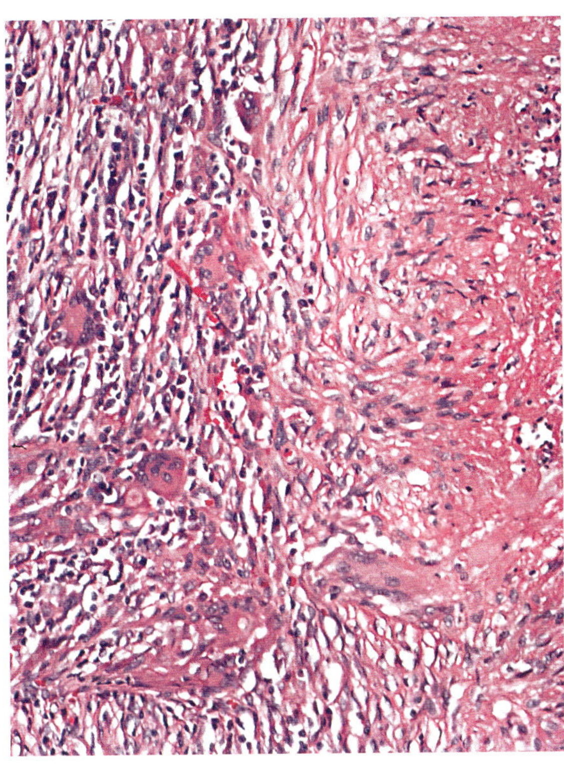

Figure 12-74

HISTOPLASMA CAPSULATUM: NECROTIZING GRANULOMA

The central area of necrosis is surrounded by granulomatous inflammation.

The histologic reaction to *H. capsulatum* varies depending on the pattern of the infection, which in turn is dependent on the severity of the exposure and the host's immune system. The presence of numerous organisms within alveolar spaces and the interstitium characterizes the acute phase. This may manifest as an acute fibrinous pneumonia without granulomatous inflammation. The organisms are typically found within macrophages. This is accompanied by a mononuclear infiltrate, followed by granulomatous inflammation, which may show central areas of necrosis (fig. 12-74). Noncaseating granulomas may also be seen and this may be the only finding on bronchoscopic biopsies, resulting in an appearance similar to that of sarcoidosis.

In chronic infection, the most common reaction is a necrotizing granuloma. These characteristically heal by fibrosis, often with a concentric laminar pattern, which may be appreciated grossly as well as microscopically (fig. 12-75). Fibrosing granulomas are prone to calcify, although central necrotic areas may persist. In such cases, there may be very few organisms and they are found in the necrotic centers of the lesions. The necrotic centers tend to be lost in tissue processing, complicating identification of the organisms.

Chronic fibrosing cases may resemble reactivation tuberculosis. Rarely, the histologic reaction takes the form of bronchocentric granulomatosis (fig. 12-76).

In the disseminated form, as encountered in patients with HIV infection, there is extensive tissue infiltration with many organisms (fig. 12-77). In some cases there is little tissue reaction despite the presence of many organisms (fig. 12-78). The organisms may be intracellular within histiocytes, but they also can freely infiltrate the tissue and resemble "yeast lakes."

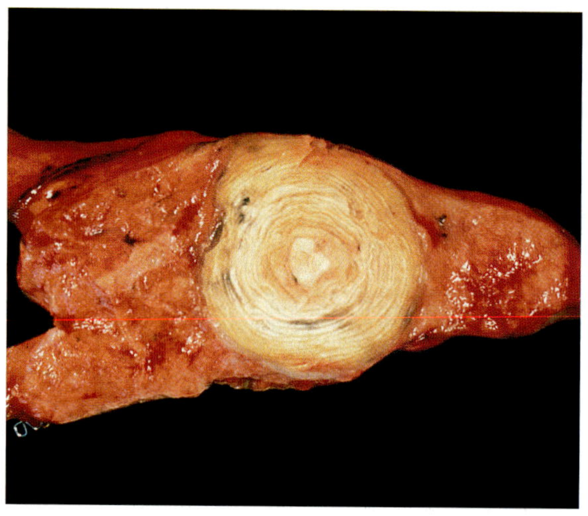

Figure 12-75

HISTOPLASMA CAPSULATUM:
FIBROSING GRANULOMA

This granuloma shows concentric laminating fibrosis.

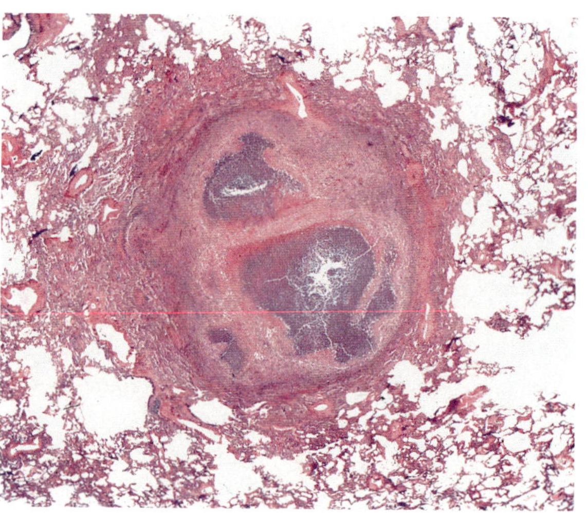

Figure 12-76

HISTOPLASMA CAPSULATUM:
BRONCHOCENTRIC GRANULOMATOSIS

This necrotizing granuloma is centered on a bronchiole. Organisms of *H. capsulatum* were present on a GMS stain (not shown).

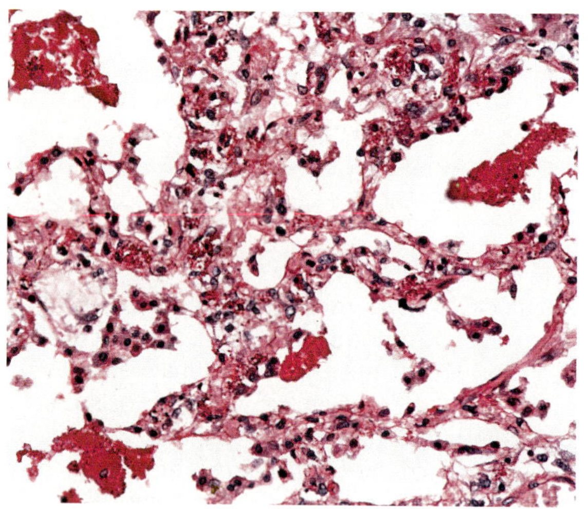

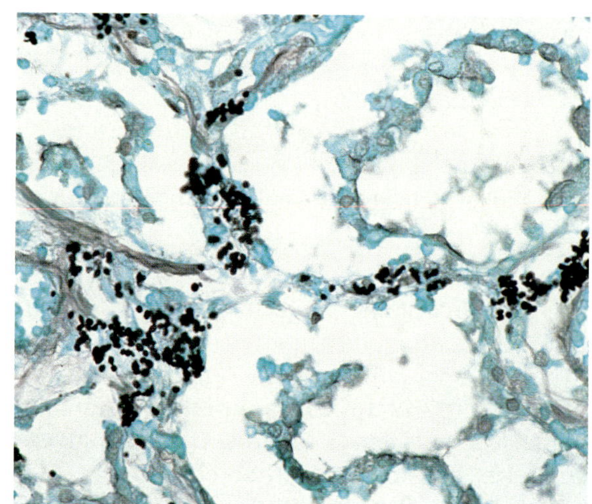

Figure 12-77

HISTOPLASMA CAPSULATUM: PROGRESSIVE DISSEMINATED INFECTION IN HIV-INFECTED PATIENT

Left: The alveolar walls are slightly thickened but no granulomas are seen.
Right: Numerous organisms line the alveolar walls.

Differential Diagnosis. Occasionally, the yeast forms of *H. capsulatum* have dark foci when stained, a staining pattern similar to that of *Pneumocystis carinii;* however, the presence of budding yeast forms as well as the lack of an intra-alveolar location and foamy exudate help diagnose histoplasmosis. The intracellular forms of *Blastomyces dermatitidis* can measure 2 to 4 µm, similar to the yeast forms of *H. capsulatum,* however, the presence of larger sized (8 to 15 µm) yeast forms, broad-based buds, and thick, double-contoured walls aid in the diagnosis of blastomycosis (Table 12-7). Capsule-deficient *Cryptococcus* usually shows a weakly positive reaction with mucicarmine and the size of the organisms is more variable, ranging from 2 to 20 µm. *Torulopsis glabrata* may resemble *H. capsulatum* due to the similar size and propensity for growth within histiocytes. However, *T. glabrata* stains well with the H&E stain, lacks the halo effect seen in *H. capsulatum,* and is usually larger and more variable in size with a broader-based bud than *H. capsulatum.* Rarely, *Candida* sp may be mistaken for *H. capsulatum,* but the presence of pseudohyphae aids in the separation. *Penicillium marneffei* can also be mistaken for *H. capsulatum* since they measure 2.5 to 5.0 µm or larger and are often intracellular. However, no budding is seen and the organisms reproduce by schizogony (fission), forming a conspicuous transverse septum. In addition, they have short hyphal forms, and elongated oval and curved sausage-shaped forms up to 20 µm long with rounded ends and one or more septa.

The cytoplasmic inclusions of cytomegalovirus (CMV) could be mistaken for *H. capsulatum,* however, the presence of intranuclear viral inclusions helps make this distinction. *Toxoplasma gondii* could also be mistaken for *H. capsulatum,* however, they are more often seen in pulmonary epithelial cells rather than histiocytes, are easily seen with the H&E stain, and do not usually stain with the GMS stain.

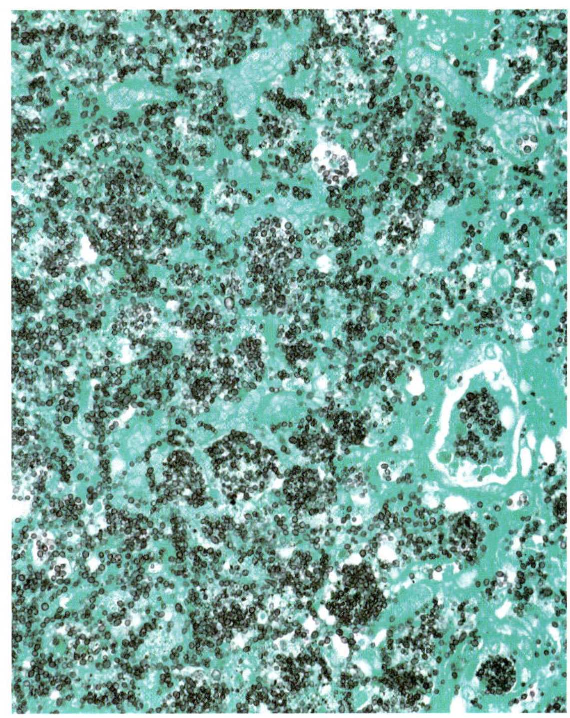

Figure 12-78

HISTOPLASMA CAPSULATUM: PROGRESSIVE DISSEMINATED INFECTION IN HIV PATIENTS

There are sheets of organisms infiltrating the pulmonary interstitium (GMS stain).

Table 12-7

MORPHOLOGIC CHARACTERISTICS OF YEAST-LIKE FUNGI

	Size	Shape	Budding	Cell Wall	Pseudohyphae/ Hyphae	Nuclei	Mucicarmine Staining
Coccidioides immitis	Spherules, 30-100 µm (rarely up to 200 µm), endospores 2-5 µm	Spherical to oval	Endosporulation	Thin	Rare	Single	Negative
Histoplasma capsulatum	2-4 µm	Spherical to oval	Single, narrow based	Thin	Rare	Single	Negative
Cryptococcus neoformans	2-20 µm	Spherical to oval	Single, rarely multiple, narrow based	Thin (thick mucinous capsule)	Rare	Single	Positive
Blastomyces dermatitidis	8-15 µm	Spherical	Single, broad based	Thick	Rare	Multiple	Negative
Candida sp	2-6 µm	Spherical to oval	Single, chains, narrow based	Thin	Pseudohyphae (rare true hyphae)	Single	Negative
Torulopsis galbrata	2-5 µm	Spherical or oval	Single, narrow based	Thin	Absent	Single	Negative

Microcalcification is commonly seen within granulomatous lesions and can be mistaken for the yeast forms of *Histoplasma*. These calcifications appear basophilic on H&E stain and may be positive with the PAS stain. The appearance of budding may occur if calcifications are situated close together. The prominent visibility of microcalcifications with the H&E stain and the lack of reactivity with the GMS stain are important features for diagnosis. Red blood cells may appear reactive with a heavy GMS stain, as can fragments of nuclei of inflammatory cells such as neutrophils that resemble yeast forms.

The diagnosis is most accurately established by culture. In approximately 50 percent of patients with disseminated infection the organisms can be demonstrated in peripheral blood monocytes. Serologic testing of patients with acute and resolving infection is helpful. In deparaffinized sections of formalin-fixed, paraffin-embedded tissue, direct immunofluorescence can confirm the diagnosis (232,233).

Treatment and Prognosis. Most patients do not require antifungal therapy, but it is given to those with progressive chronic cavitary pulmonary and disseminated histoplasmosis (207,222,295). Chronic cavitary infections can be treated with amphotericin B, fluconazole, and ketoconazole. Itraconazole is the agent of choice, especially given the reduced side effects compared to amphotericin B and fluconazole. Disseminated infections in AIDS patients can be treated with itraconazole or fluconazole (in slowly progressive disease), but amphotericin is the mainstay of treatment for disseminated histoplasmosis (207,222,295). Itraconazole can be used as suppressive therapy in HIV-infected patients.

Cryptococcus Sp

Definition. Pulmonary cryptococcosis is caused by inhalation of spores of *Cryptococcus neoformans*.

C. neoformans is a yeast found worldwide in the soil, especially soil contaminated with pigeon droppings (207,211,251). *C. neoformans* var *neoformans* is a more common pathogen than *C. neoformans* var *gatti*.

Clinical Features. Cryptococcal infection has two major clinical forms: pulmonary infection and cerebromeningeal infection due to hematogenous spread from the lung (207,211,251). The time delay between exposure and clinical disease is highly variable, and at one extreme, acute infection shortly after intense exposure has been reported (226). Pulmonary cryptococcal infection can occur in immunocompetent hosts, but immunosuppressed individuals are at greater risk, particularly those with defects in T-cell immunity. Predisposing conditions include hematologic malignancies, particularly Hodgkin's disease, prolonged steroid therapy, diabetes mellitus, HIV infection, and sarcoidosis (207,211,251).

Patients with primary pulmonary cryptococcosis rarely have symptoms. When symptoms are present they include mild fever with nonspecific pulmonary symptoms. One or both lungs may be affected. Most patients with cryptococcal disease have meningitis, with often minor symptoms heralding the onset of the disease (e.g., clouded mental acuity and headaches). Examination of the cerebrospinal fluid shows increased protein, predominant mononuclear pleocytosis, and a reduced glucose level.

Radiologic Findings. There are several radiologic manifestations of pulmonary cryptococcal infection. These include a focal pulmonary nodule or mass with ill-defined or well-defined borders (fig. 12-79), multifocal peripheral pulmonary nodules or masses, and unilateral or bilateral parenchymal consolidation which may contain air bronchograms (fig. 12-80) (215,251,299). An upper lobe predominance has been described (262). Bronchial obstruction with distal atelectasis may occur (215). Cavitation, calcification, and pleural effusion are rare (299). Patients with pulmonary cryptococcosis who develop focal, mass-like lesions and have associated cerebromeningeal infection may exhibit radiologic features that mimic those of primary lung cancer metastatic to the central nervous system (fig. 12-81) (215,251).

Immunocompromised patients with disseminated cryptococcosis may exhibit diffuse, bilateral, reticular or nodular interstitial opacities or diffuse miliary nodules. Parenchymal consolidation may also occur, may be bilateral, and may progress rapidly (299). Cavitation, with associated intrathoracic lymphadenopathy and pleural effusion, is uncommon but occurs more frequently in immunocompromised patients (215,299).

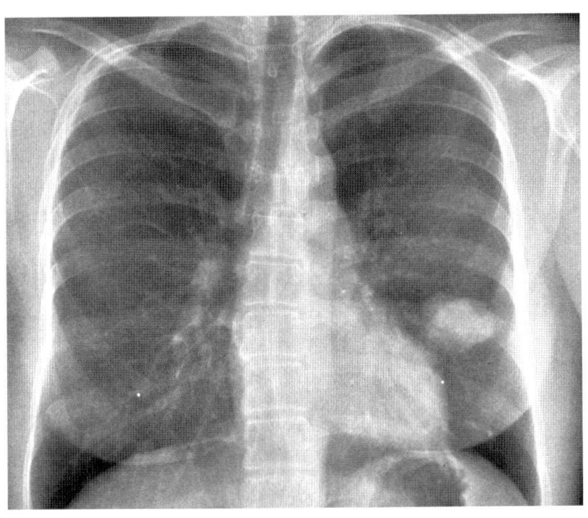

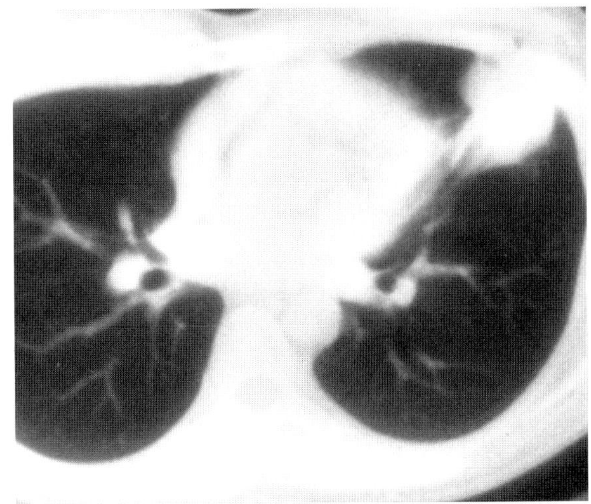

Figure 12-79

PULMONARY CRYPTOCOCCOSIS

Pulmonary cryptococcosis in a 31-year-old female with headache and meningeal signs.
Left: PA chest radiograph demonstrates a well-defined, lobular, 4.5-cm mass located in the lingula.
Right: Chest CT (lung window) demonstrates a well-circumscribed, lobular, peripheral left upper lobe mass.

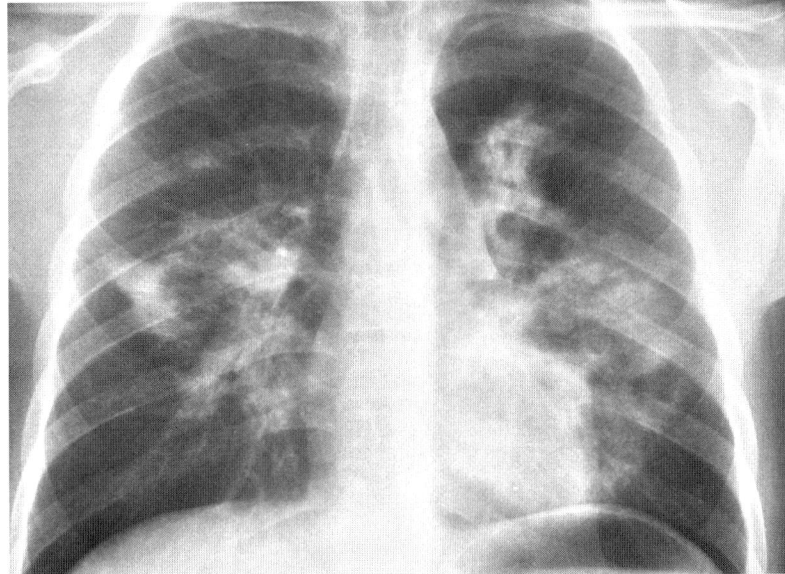

Figure 12-80

PULMONARY CRYPTOCOCCOSIS

Pulmonary cryptococcosis in a 17-year-old male who presented with cough and chest pain and did not respond to antibiotic therapy. PA chest radiograph demonstrates multifocal, bilateral, patchy, parenchymal consolidations. (Figure 4 from McAdams HP, Rosado-de-Christenson ML, Lesar M, Templeton PA, Moran CA. Thoracic mycoses from opportunistic fungi: radiologic-pathologic correlation. Radiographics 1995;15:273.)

Pathologic Findings. In lung tissue, most *C. neoformans* yeast are 4 to 6 µm in diameter although they can range from 2 to 20 µm (figs. 12-82, 12-83) (192,193). The cells are eosinophilic to basophilic, uninucleate, oval to elliptical, and occasionally appear refractile (fig. 12-83). Budding is usually single and narrow based (fig. 12-82). The cells appear to have a halo that actually represents a mucinous capsule (fig. 12-83). This capsule is highlighted with mucin stains such as the mucicarmine (fig. 12-82), DPAS, and Alcian blue. The capsule may measure up to five times the diameter of the fungal cells. Multiple budding and short chains of yeast cells are uncommon. Rarely, germ tubes, pseudohyphae, and branched septate true hyphae can be seen in tissue sections (195).

Capsule-deficient *C. neoformans* is typically found in immunocompetent patients. In the absence of a capsule, the mucicarmine stain is no

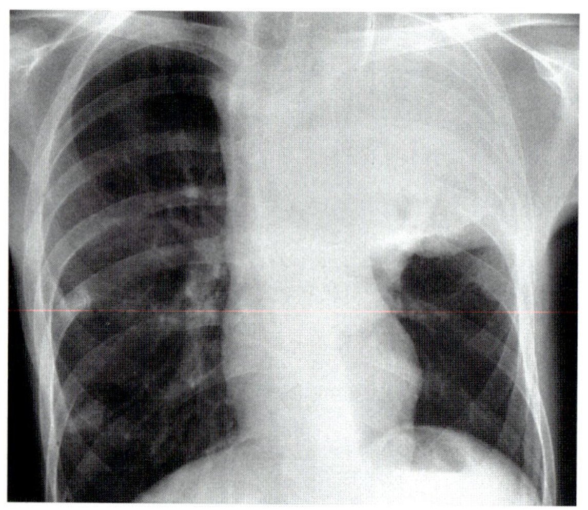

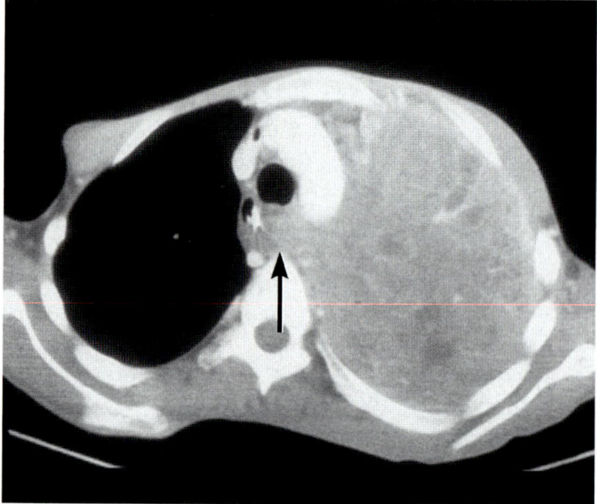

Figure 12-81

PULMONARY CRYPTOCOCCOSIS

Pulmonary cryptococcosis in a 29-year-old male with alcohol abuse and depression.

Left: PA chest radiograph demonstrates a large mass that occupies the left upper lobe.

Right: Chest CT (mediastinal window) demonstrates a heterogeneously enhancing mass in the left upper lobe. Note apparent mediastinal invasion (arrow). Head CT (not shown) demonstrated multifocal enhancing brain lesions. Biopsy was negative for malignancy and diagnostic for cryptococcosis.

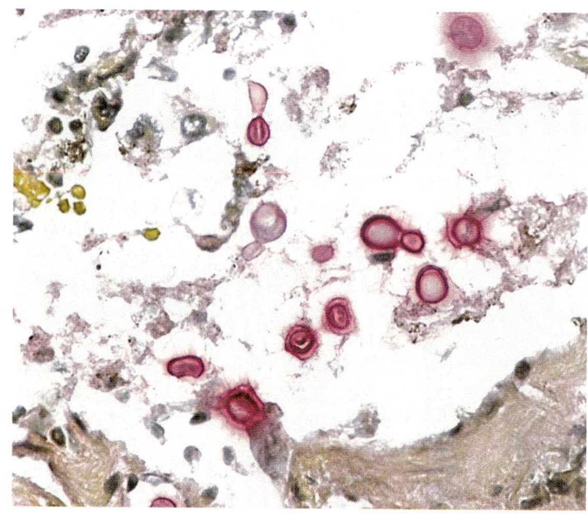

Figure 12-82

CRYPTOCOCCUS: ORGANISM MORPHOLOGY

Multiple organisms stain with the mucicarmine stain. A narrow-based budding yeast is present (center).

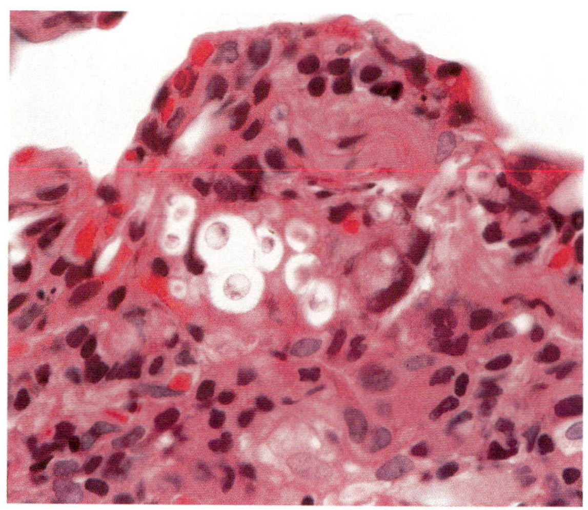

Figure 12-83

CRYPTOCOCCUS: ORGANISM MORPHOLOGY

Several yeast forms appear eosinophilic and are surrounded by a halo.

longer useful in recognizing the organisms. The diagnosis can be established if a few of the organisms retain a recognizable capsule that shows mucicarmine-positive staining. The Fontana-Masson stain is positive in such cases (fig. 12-84) but culture or immunohistochemistry (189) may be necessary to firmly establish the diagnosis.

The histologic response to cryptococcal infection depends on the immune status of the patient and whether the organisms have a

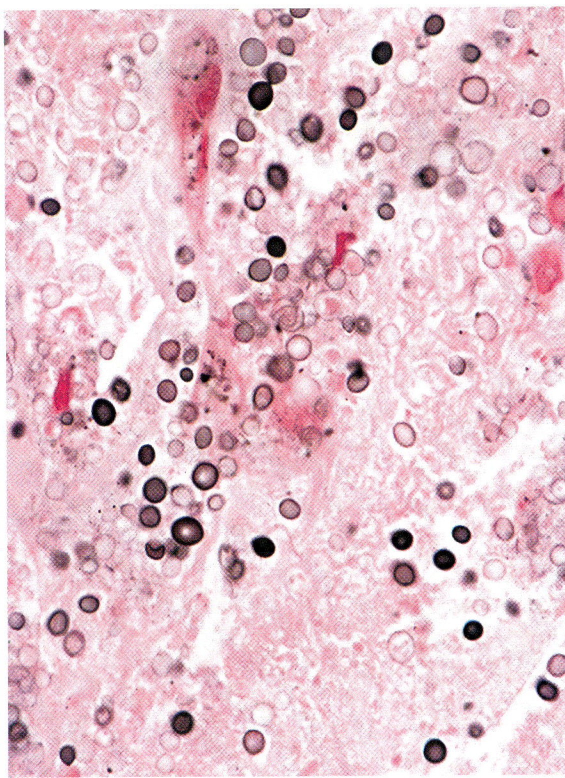

Figure 12-84

CRYPTOCOCCUS: FONTANA-MASSON STAIN

These yeast of *Cryptococcus* stain with the Fontana-Masson stain.

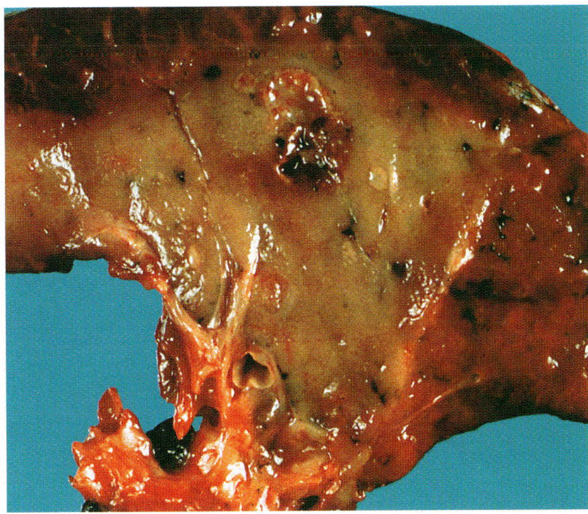

Figure 12-85

CRYPTOCOCCUS: GROSS SPECIMEN

A nodular area of consolidation has a gelatinous cut surface.

capsule. Grossly, lung infiltrates may appear as indistinct areas of consolidation with a gelatinous cut surface (fig. 12-85). When the histologic reaction to the organisms is minimal, the alveolar spaces appear filled with organisms (fig. 12-86). A fibrohistiocytic infiltrate may accompany densely packed organisms (fig. 12-87). This may be mistaken for a lipoid pneumonia. Alternatively, organisms may form nodular granulomas similar to other fungal pulmonary infections. The initial response in patients with an intact immune system may consist of acute necrotizing inflammation. Nodular granulomatous lesions subsequently develop and may progress to fibrocaseous lesions with central necrotic zones and a fibroinflammatory border with granulomatous inflammation (fig. 12-88). Immunosuppressed patients may have extensive tissue infiltration by organisms in a pneumonic fashion, with little tissue response. In some cases cystic lesions develop.

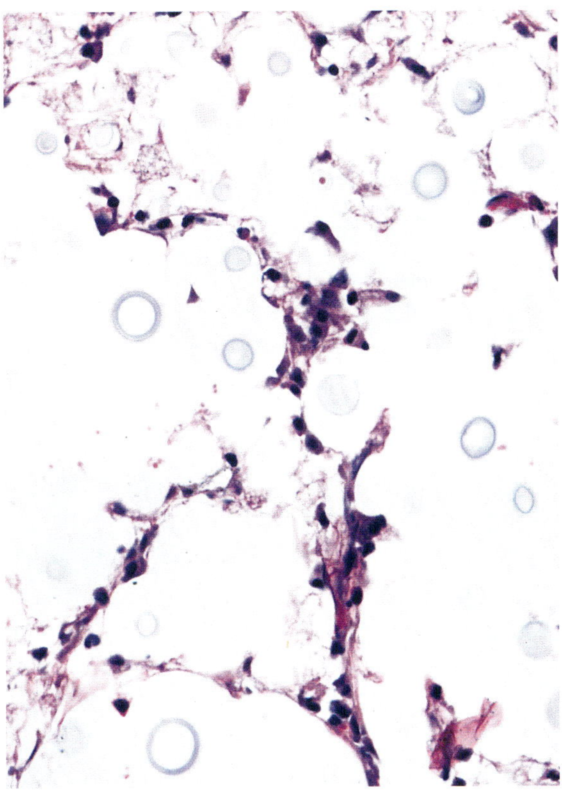

Figure 12-86

CRYPTOCOCCUS: MINIMAL HISTOLOGIC REACTION

Numerous organisms fill the alveolar spaces, with no inflammation in the alveolar walls and no granulomatous

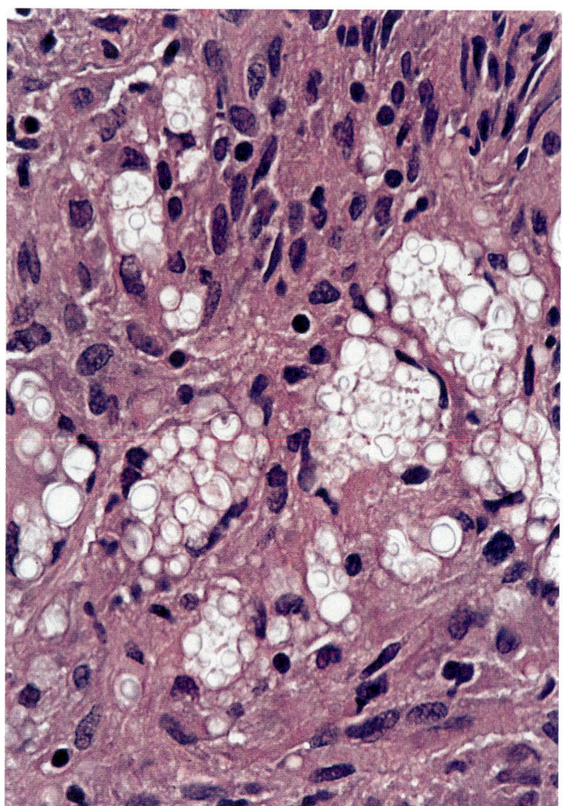

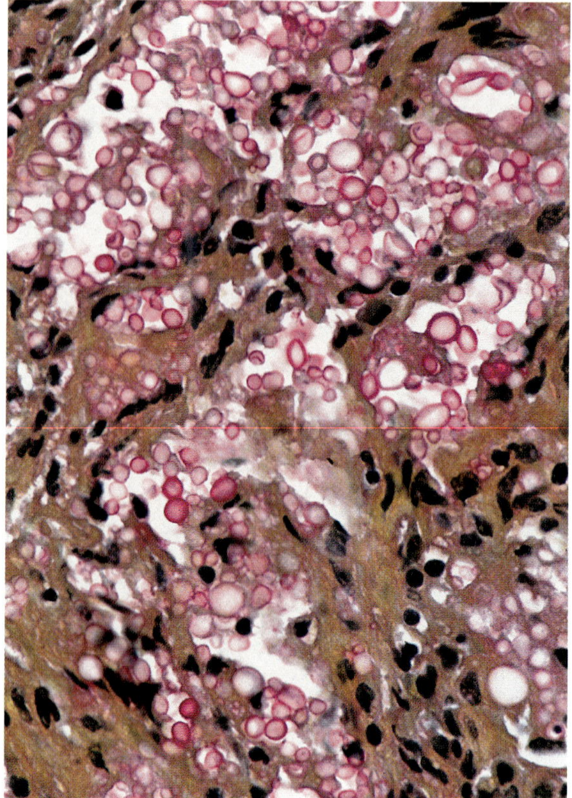

Figure 12-87

CRYPTOCOCCUS: FIBROHISTIOCYTIC RESPONSE

Left: A fibrohistiocytic reaction accompanies numerous organisms. The organisms have a bubbly appearance. Right: The organisms are highlighted by the mucicarmine stain.

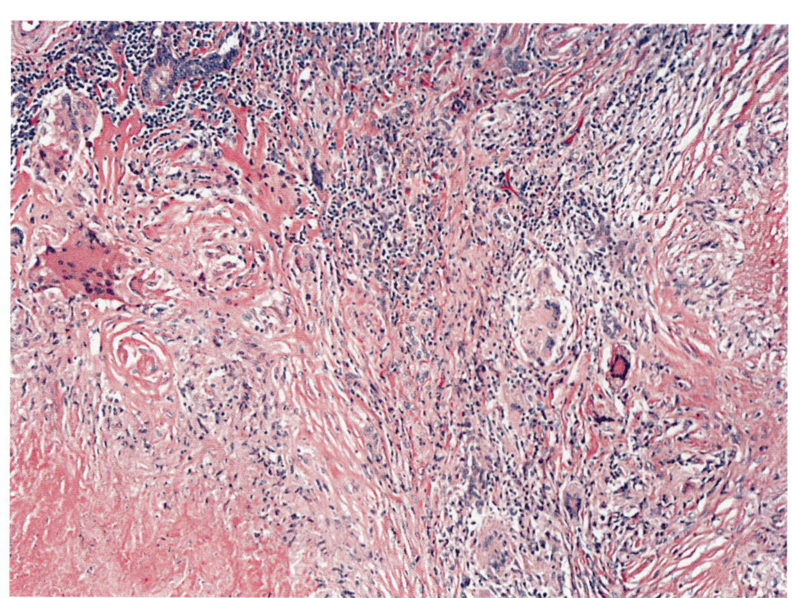

Figure 12-88

CRYPTOCOCCUS: GRANULOMATOUS INFLAMMATION

Granulomatous inflammation and fibrosis surround several areas of necrosis.

Differential Diagnosis. *C. neoformans* can be confused with virtually any yeast-form fungus due to its variable morphology (Table 12-7) (192,195). Recognition of the capsule by its staining with the mucicarmine stain is one of the most helpful ways to distinguish cryptococci from other fungi. The most difficult problems occur with capsule-deficient organisms, although in most of these cases at least a few carminophilic organisms can be identified. Capsule-deficient *C. neoformans* may be confused with *Histoplasma capsulatum, Blastomyces dermatitidis, Sporothrix schenckii, Torulopsis glabrata, Candida* sp, and *Coccidioides immitis.* The Fontana-Masson stain is useful in the differential diagnosis of cryptococcosis (fig. 12-84) since it reacts with the wall and not the capsule, thus staining capsule-deficient organisms (240,273). However, the usefulness of the Fontana-Masson stain in separating *C. neoformans* from other fungi awaits further study in larger numbers of cases. Sporotrichosis and the immature spherules of *C. immitis* also stain with the Fontana-Masson stain. However, *S. schenckii* shows a distinctive cigar-shaped budding yeast morphology. A PAS-positive, eosinophilic, thickened outer layer also surrounds the yeast forms. The broad-based budding in blastomycosis is a morphologic clue that contrasts to the narrow-based buds of *Cryptococcus.* Michaelis-Gutmann bodies may also be mistaken for cryptococci, however, they are laminated and mineralized (192,195).

Treatment and Prognosis. Progressive pulmonary cryptococcosis is best treated with intravenous amphotericin B combined with 5-fluorocytosine. The acute management of cryptococcal meningitis in patients with AIDS requires amphotericin B (with or without 5 fluorocytosine) for the first 2 weeks, and then administration of fluconazole both to complete initial treatment and to provide lifelong suppressive therapy (266). Surgical excision of pulmonary nodules may also be helpful. This course of therapy has led to a considerable reduction in acute mortality (i.e., patients dying in the first 2 weeks). Infection with the *gattii* strain of *C. neoformans* in immunocompetent patients is associated with significant mortality despite conventional treatment, and may lead to blindness in survivors (226).

Table 12-8

PULMONARY MANIFESTATIONS OF COCCIDIOIDOMYCOSIS

Primary Pulmonary Infection
Acute
Persistent
Chronic fibrocavitary
Chronic progressive
Nodules and/or cavities
Mycetoma, rupture into pleural space
Pleural Effusions (eosinophilia)
Chronic Pulmonary Coccidioidomycosis
Disseminated Coccidioidomycosis

Coccidioides Immitis

Definition. Coccidioidomycosis is a pulmonary mycosis caused by the inhalation of fungal spores from the diphasic, multimorphic fungus, *Coccidioides immitis.* Coccidioidomycosis is also known as *San Joaquin Valley fever.*

C. immitis grows optimally in hot, dry climates with sandy, alkaline soil and the mycelial form is present in the desert soil (176,207). The organism is endemic throughout the southwestern United States, northern and central Mexico, and regions of Central and South America (188,195,230,255).

Clinical Features. Most infected patients have no symptoms. Approximately 40 percent have only mild symptoms of a febrile, influenza-like illness that may last 1 to 3 weeks. The usual manifestations are nonproductive cough, myalgias and arthralgias, headaches, and pleuritic chest pain. Erythema multiforme or erythema nodosum occurs in about 20 percent of patients, most often young white women. These manifestations are thought to represent favorable prognostic signs. Most infected patients recover without evidence of persistent disease.

The multiple manifestations of pulmonary coccidioidomycosis are summarized in Table 12-8 (176,207). Primary pulmonary infection may be acute (242), persistent, chronic fibrocavitary, chronic progressive, and nodular with or without cavities (176,207). Mycetomas may occur within cavitary lesions. Pleural complications include rupture into the pleural space (204) and pleural effusions that may be associated with

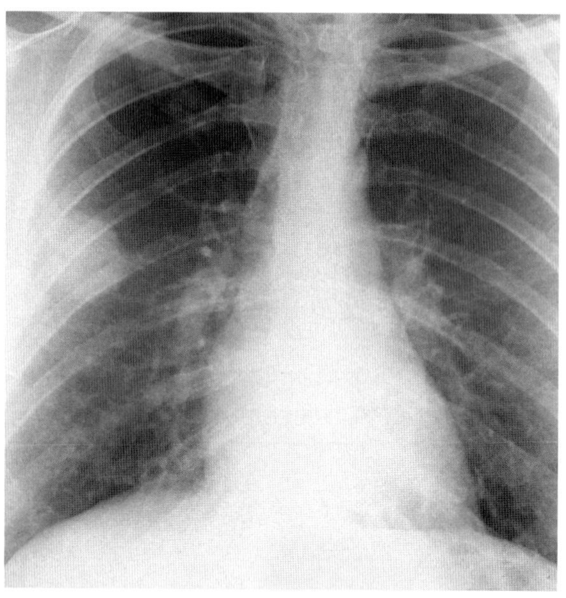

Figure 12-89

COCCIDIOIDOMYCOSIS IN A 34-YEAR-OLD FEMALE WITH CHEST PAIN

PA chest radiograph demonstrates a spherical, cavitary, right upper lobe mass. *Coccidioides immitis* was cultured from the lesion.

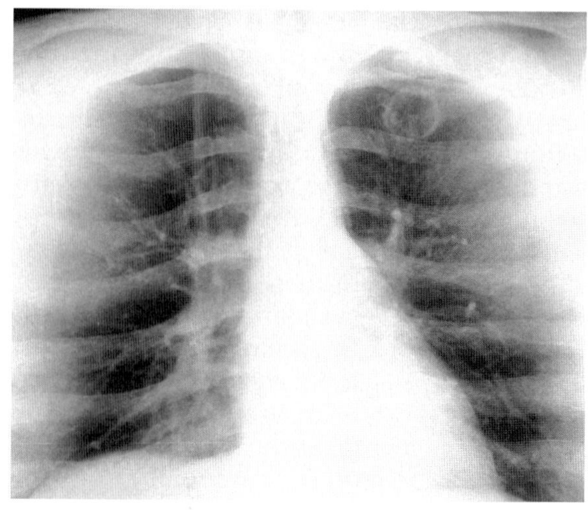

Figure 12-90

COCCIDIOIDOMYCOSIS IN 26-YEAR-OLD MALE WITH COUGH

PA apical lordotic chest radiograph demonstrates a left apical thin-walled cavity. Biopsy demonstrated *Coccidioides immitis.*

eosinophilia (210). Rarely, an endobronchial granuloma causes bronchial obstruction (182).

Disseminated infection is rare (less than 1 percent of patients) and occurs more often in African-Americans, and Filipinos and other Asians compared to Caucasians (176,207). Group B blood type, diabetes mellitus, hematologic neoplasms, HIV infection, transplantation, and the second and third trimesters of pregnancy are additional risk factors for disseminated coccidioidomycosis (176,207,255). Disseminated infection in normal hosts follows local primary infection by several weeks to months. In immunocompromised hosts, there may be a fulminant illness with rapidly diffuse pulmonary opacities, meningitis (headache, change in mental status), and bone and skin lesions. Coccidioidomycosis is being increasingly recognized in HIV-infected patients (CD4+ counts less than 250/mm^3) and may be rapidly progressive and fatal.

Radiologic Findings. Primary pulmonary infection with *C. immitis* results in radiologic manifestations similar to those encountered in patients with acute histoplasmosis. Chest radiographs typically exhibit patchy, unilateral, perihilar or lower lobe parenchymal consolidation. The parenchymal consolidation may resolve in some areas and progress in others, resulting in so-called phantom infiltrates. Multifocal, peripheral, subpleural nodules or masses and peribronchial thickening may also occur. These lesions typically resolve rapidly but in some cases persist for several months (180). Healing may result in a solitary pulmonary nodule or a thin-walled cavity, which may persist for years (figs. 12-89, 12-90). Lymphadenopathy and small pleural effusions occur in approximately 20 percent of cases. Large pleural effusions are rare (180,215,250).

Persistent primary pulmonary coccidioidomycosis (pulmonary disease persisting longer than 6 weeks) manifests radiologically as pulmonary nodules or chronic cavities. Pulmonary nodules are typically single, peripheral, spherical, and well-defined. Calcification is uncommon. CT may demonstrate marked contrast enhancement (180,215). These nodules typically develop in areas of previous consolidation. Single, thin-walled cavities may develop in areas of previous parenchymal consolidation. They occur in up to 15 percent of patients with pulmonary involvement and typically affect the upper lobes (180,215). While thick-walled cavities do occur, thin-walled (grape-skin) cavities, which may change in size over time, are characteristic (fig. 12-90). Cavitary lesions may rupture into the pleural space and produce a pneumothorax or bronchopleural fistula. Chronic parenchymal consolidation and lymphadenopathy may occur as well (180,215,250).

Chronic progressive coccidioidomycosis manifests with persistent unilateral or bilateral apical consolidation, which may cavitate. Multifocal upper lobe cavities, linear and nodular opacities, and volume loss also occur and may mimic the radiologic features of postprimary tuberculosis. Pleural effusion and localized fibrosis may occur (180).

Disseminated pulmonary coccidioidomycosis is a complication of primary disease and usually affects immunocompromised patients. Radiologically, there may be miliary nodules or diffuse reticular and nodular interstitial pulmonary opacities, particularly in patients with AIDS (fig. 12-91). Lymphadenopathy and multiorgan involvement also occur (180).

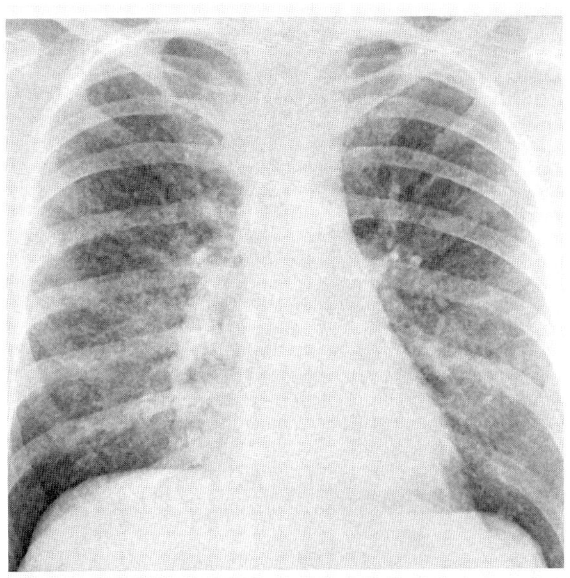

Figure 12-91

COCCIDIOIDOMYCOSIS

Coccidioidomycosis in a 42-year-old HIV-positive male with fever, dyspnea, and hypoxia, which did not respond to treatment for *Pneumocystis carinii* pneumonia. PA chest radiograph demonstrates bilateral, diffuse, miliary nodular interstitial opacities. (Figure 28A from McAdams HP, Rosado-de-Christenson ML, Lesar M, Templeton PA, Moran CA. Thoracic mycoses from endemic fungi: radiologic-pathologic correlation. Radiographics 1995;15:255–70.)

Pathologic Findings. In tissues, *C. immitis* consists of immature spherules, mature spherules, and endospores (195). The morphologic diagnosis of *C. immitis* requires the presence of the endosporulating spherule: a round to oval spherule containing endospores. Most are 30 to 100 µm, but they may measure up to 200 µm (fig. 12-92). The mature spherules have a 1- to 2-µm–thick refractile wall. Immature spherules lack endospores and their walls and granular contents are PAS positive. The uninucleate endospores are 2 to 5 µm in diameter and they have punctate cytoplasmic inclusions that are PAS positive and GMS negative (195). When mature spherules rupture, the endospores spread into the adjacent tissues. In tissues, the endospores stain with both GMS and PAS (fig. 12-93), but the spherule wall stains only with GMS. The spherule walls may become lined with eosinophilic, radiating Splendore-Hoeppli material. When vegetative forms are identified in tissues, they consist of 2- to 4-µm–thick septate hyphae and chains of barrel-shaped arthroconidia (fig. 12-94) (195). Hyphae and arthroconidia are found in 10 to 30 percent of cavitary lesions, particularly if they open into the bronchial tree (255). Fungus balls of *C. immitis* may develop in some pulmonary cavities (fig. 12-95) (255,268,287,297).

The early histologic reaction associated with primary pulmonary coccidioidomycosis consists of an acute suppurative pneumonitis with neutrophilic infiltrates (fig. 12-96). The neutrophilic foci become surrounded by granulomatous inflammation and these lesions can progress to necrotizing granulomas, which can cavitate and become fibrotic (fig. 12-97). Most lung biopsies of *C. immitis* infection show necrotizing granulomatous inflammation. The organisms are typically found within the neutrophilic infiltrates or necrotic zones. It is thought that the spherules induce a granulomatous reaction and the endospores a neutrophilic reaction (255). Eosinophilic pneumonia may be associated with *C. immitis* pulmonary infection (245). In severe pneumonia there may be numerous organisms within alveolar fibrinous exudates (fig. 12-98).

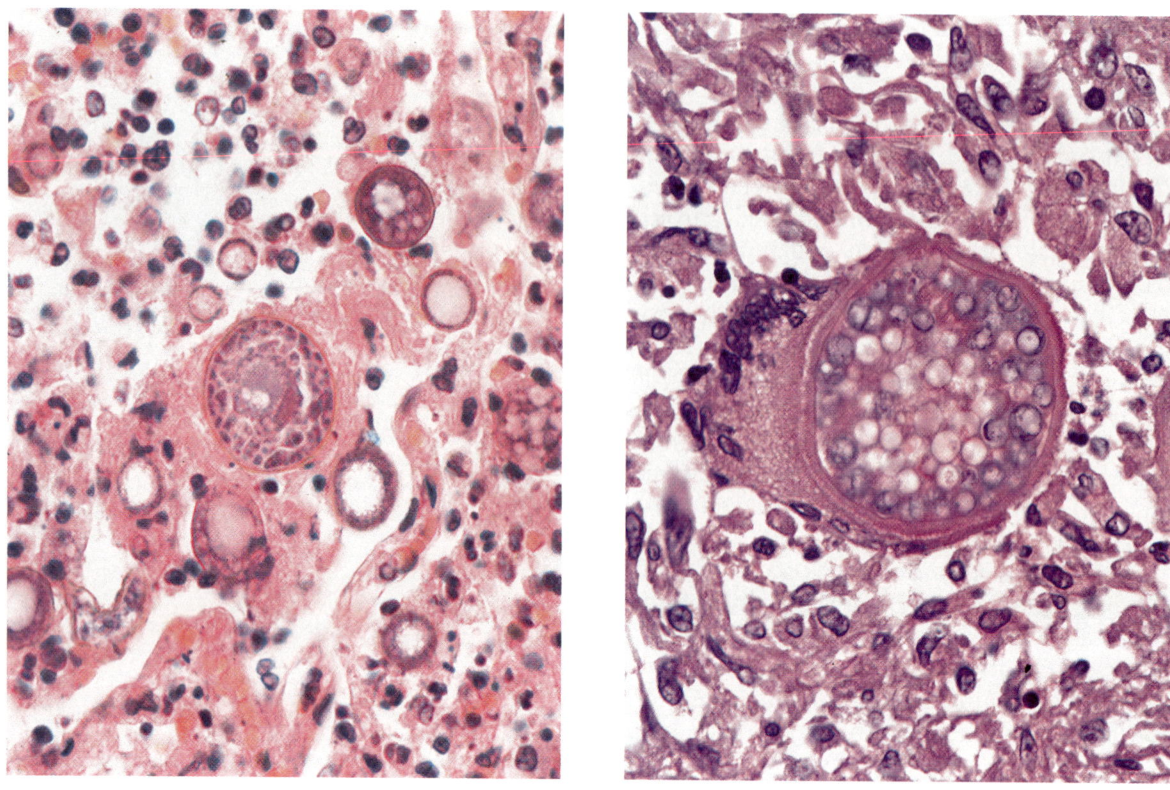

Figure 12-92

COCCIDIOIDOMYCOSIS: ORGANISM MORPHOLOGY

Left: Many immature and mature spherules are present. The mature spherules contain multiple endospores.

Right: This mature spherule is surrounded by a multinucleated giant cell. The spherule wall is thick and refractile. Within the spherule are multiple small endospores.

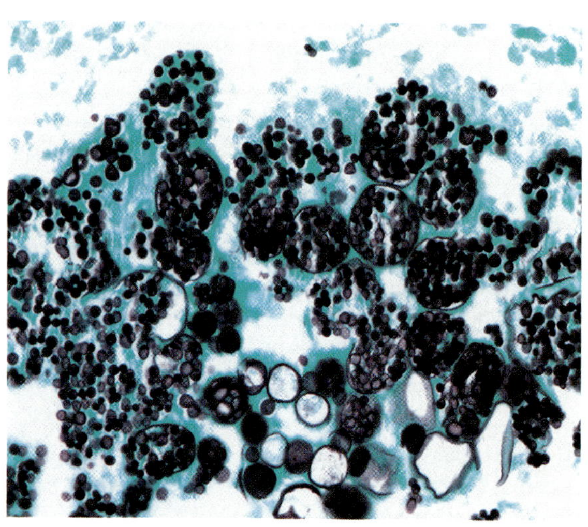

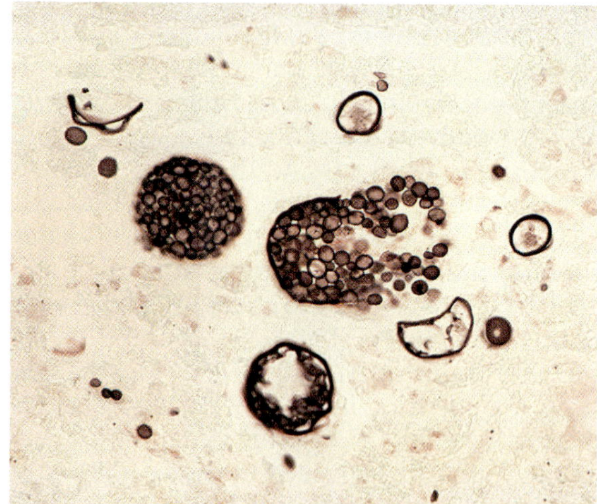

Figure 12-93

COCCIDIOIDOMYCOSIS: ORGANISM MORPHOLOGY

Left: Multiple mature spherules are present and the GMS stain highlights both the spherule wall and the endospores.

Right: Several intact spherules and a rupturing spherule are present.

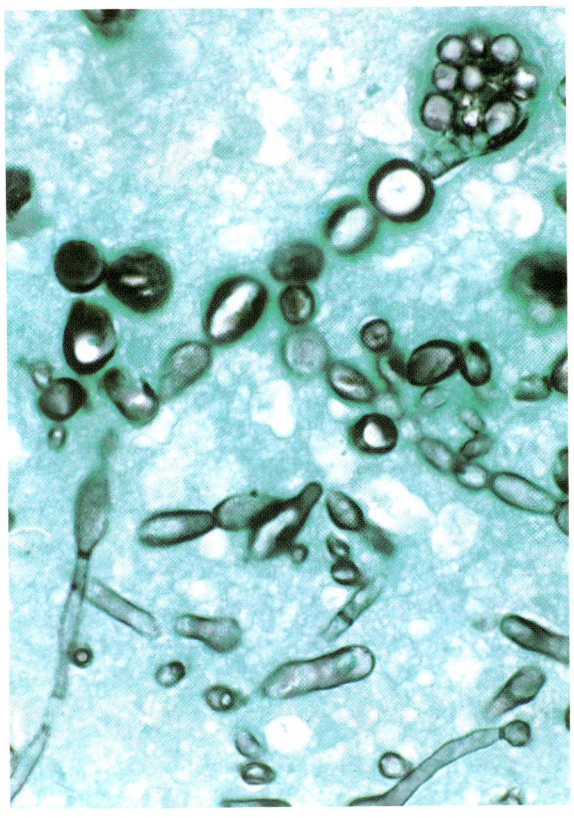

Figure 12-94

COCCIDIOIDOMYCOSIS: VEGETATIVE FORMS

The mycelia (hyphae) produce chains of barrel-shaped arthroconidia.

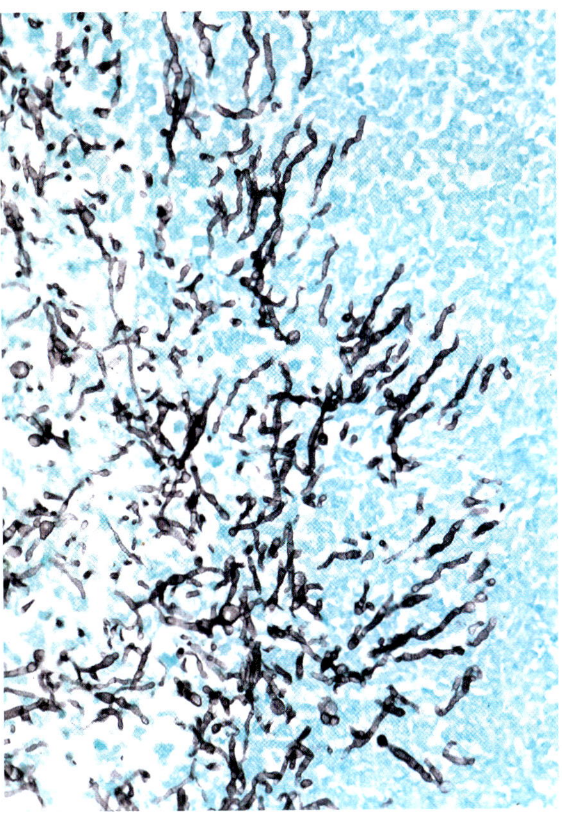

Figure 12-95

COCCIDIOIDOMYCOSIS: MYCELIAL FORMS IN FUNGUS BALL

Mycelial forms consist of septate hyphae.

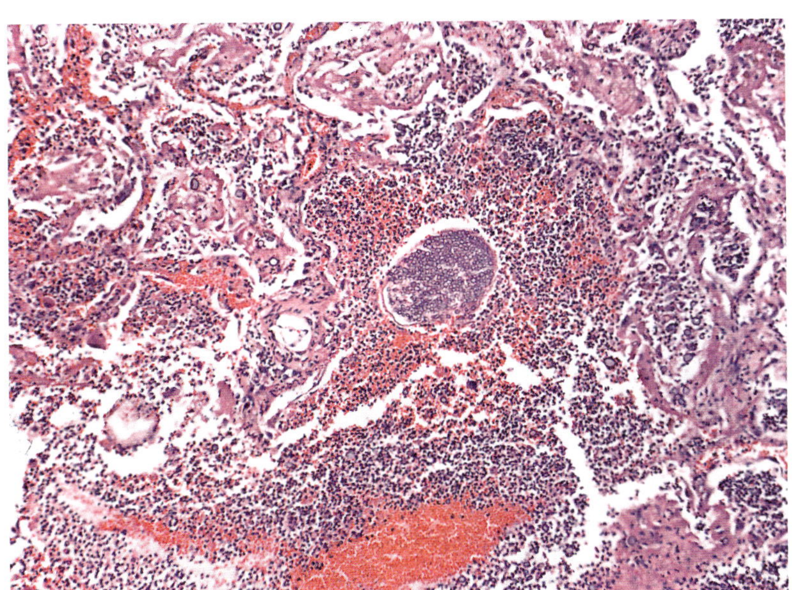

Figure 12-96

COCCIDIOIDOMYCOSIS: ACUTE PNEUMONIA

A marked neutrophilic infiltrate or acute pneumonia is associated with this mature spherule.

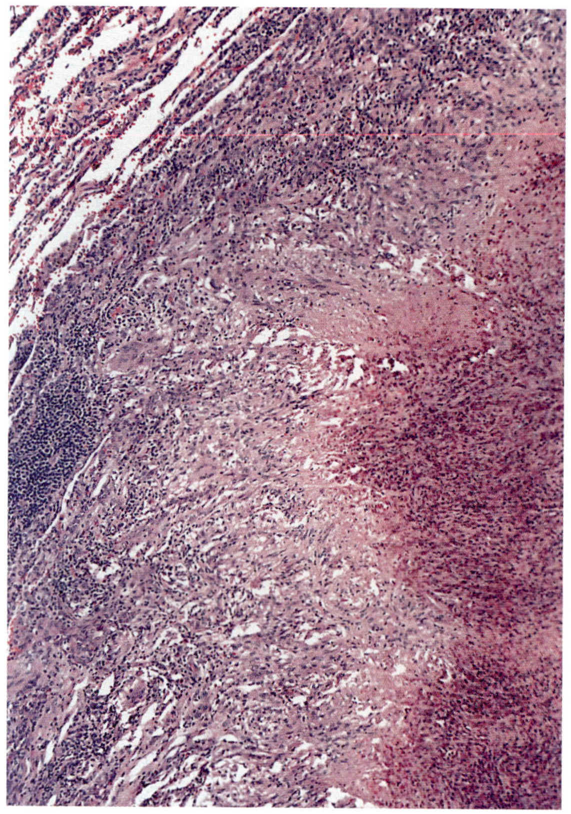

Figure 12-97

COCCIDIOIDOMYCOSIS: NECROTIZING GRANULOMA

The necrotic center is surrounded by granulomatous inflammation.

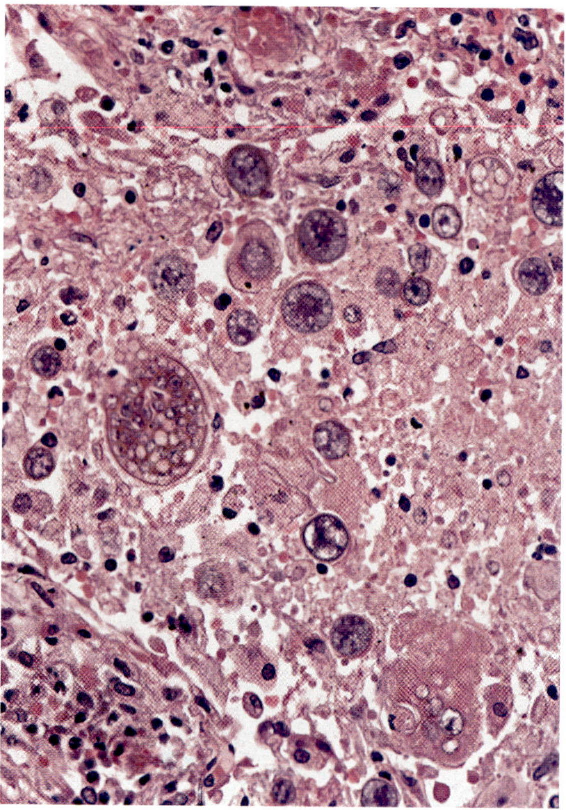

Figure 12-98

COCCIDIOIDOMYCOSIS: DISSEMINATED INFECTION

Numerous organisms, highlighted by the GMS stain, line the alveolar walls and fill the alveolar spaces, which show minimal histologic reaction. No granulomas or neutrophils are seen.

The lung may have diffuse nodular infiltrates affecting areas that measure several millimeters to several centimeters in diameter. These may appear cavitary. Most pulmonary nodules are necrotizing granulomas, with or without fibrosis. Fibrocaseous nodules may be subpleural lesions that manifest as coin lesions on chest radiographs in asymptomatic patients. Histologically, these have a dense collagenous fibrous capsule with a central necrotic zone. Associated with the fibrous capsule are variable numbers of lymphocytes, plasma cells, and giant cells. Within the necrotic zone it may be difficult to identify classic endosporulating spherules. In such cases one may find only occasional immature spherules or distorted fragments of spherule walls. In the appropriate clinical and regional setting, it may be possible to suggest the diagnosis without seeing mature spherules if only atypical forms are identified. Cavitary nodules may contain hyphae and barrel-shaped arthroconidia (255) and these may form fungus balls (274,297). In cases where definite endosporulating spherules cannot be identified, the definitive diagnosis requires culture, serology, or immunofluorescence (231,232).

Differential Diagnosis. In cases where diagnostic mature spherules are absent or difficult to find, the endospores or immature spherules of *C. immitis* may be confused with other fungi (Table 12-7). The endospores of *C. immitis* may be distinguished from yeast forms of *Histoplasma capsulatum* or cryptococci by the presence of buds on the latter two. Immature spherules of *C. immitis* may be difficult to separate from the yeast forms of *Blastomyces dermatitidis* but the presence of broad-based budding would favor the latter.

Serologic testing is helpful in the diagnosis of coccidioidomycosis. Serum IgM antibodies may be detected 2 to 3 weeks after the onset of the infection and can be found in up to 75 percent of patients. They may wane over 4 to 6 months. Serum IgG antibodies are detected later in the illness but are positive in up to 90 percent of patients. High or rising titers should suggest the possibility of disseminating infection. In patients with meningitis, these antibodies may be detected in the cerebrospinal fluid and this finding is diagnostic.

Treatment and Prognosis. Patients with primary pulmonary coccidioidomycosis do not require treatment unless they are immunocompromised or at risk of disseminated disease. Both surgery and medical therapy are useful in pulmonary coccidioidomycosis (207,211,230). Surgery may be beneficial if chronic cavitary infection is associated with hemoptysis or is enlarging and threatening to rupture into the pleural space. Acute pulmonary coccidioidomycosis, disseminated disease, and meningitis require intravenous amphotericin B. Prolonged intrathecal therapy is required for meningeal involvement. Other oral medications such as ketoconazole, fluconazole, or itraconazole may be effective for patients with less severe infections (255). Fluconazole is effective for treatment of meningitis but once started it must be continued because of the high rate of relapse. HIV-infected patients with coccidioidomycosis are difficult to treat and the prognosis is grim.

Blastomyces Dermatitidis

Definition. Pulmonary blastomycosis is an infection caused by inhalation of the dimorphic fungus, *Blastomyces dermatitidis*. Synonyms include *North American blastomycosis* and *Gilchrist's disease*.

B. dermatitidis is a soil fungus (205,207). Inhalation of aerosolized conidia of the mycelial form of *B. dermatitidis* results in pulmonary infection. Blastomycosis occurs primarily in the United States: in the Mississippi, Missouri, and Ohio River valleys; around the Great Lakes; and in the southeast (243). It is also found in southern Manitoba and northwestern Ontario in Canada. Cases have also been reported in Europe, Africa, Central and South America, India, Asia, and the Middle East (205,207).

Clinical Features. The clinical presentation of patients with acute infection is similar to that of an acute bacterial pneumonia: sudden onset of high fever, chills, myalgias, and arthralgias (205,207,260,277,280). Cough is initially nonproductive but becomes productive of mucopurulent sputum. Pleuritic chest pain is usually transient. Chronic infection is more common and patients may have a gradual onset of productive cough, low-grade fever, hemoptysis, weight loss, and pleuritic chest pain (205,207). Extrapulmonary spread can occur to a variety of sites, particularly the skin and bone. Acute deterioration results in the acute respiratory distress syndrome (252,254). This can result from hematogenous or endobronchial spread.

Blastomycosis is not a common infection in immunocompromised patients but it can occur in patients with HIV infection, transplantation, prolonged corticosteroid therapy, and cytotoxic therapy for hematologic and solid malignancies (205,207,256,257,259). Blastomycosis is more aggressive in HIV-infected patients than in normal hosts (221). The former also tend to have more frequent visceral dissemination and central nervous system involvement than other immunocompromised patients (221).

Radiologic Findings. Pulmonary blastomycosis typically manifests radiologically as focal or diffuse parenchymal consolidation, which typically affects the upper lobes of adult patients. Slow radiologic resolution or absence of change helps distinguish blastomycosis from bacterial pneumonia. Solitary or multiple nodules or masses occur in approximately 30 percent of patients. In some cases, focal involvement manifests as a pulmonary mass indistinguishable from primary lung cancer, particularly if there is associated ipsilateral hilar and/or mediastinal lymphadenopathy (fig. 12-99). These focal masses have been described in perihilar and paramediastinal locations (215,239,250). Visualization of air bronchograms and satellite nodules is helpful in suggesting an infectious etiology. Calcification rarely occurs. Cavitation occurs in 15 to 20 percent of cases (215). Cavities may be single or multiple and may exhibit thick or thin walls (239). Miliary and diffuse reticular and nodular opacities are also described but are uncommon features. Peripheral lesions may cross anatomic boundaries to involve the

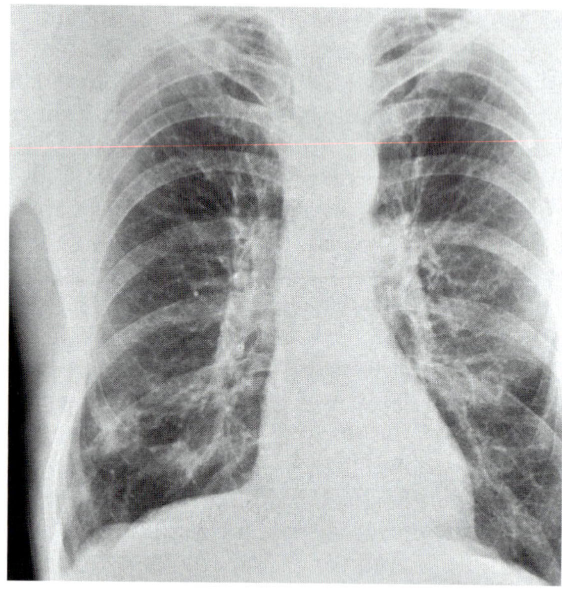

Figure 12-99

BLASTOMYCOSIS

Blastomycosis in a 63-year-old male with productive cough and weight loss. PA chest radiograph demonstrates a spiculated mass in the right lower lung suspicious for lung carcinoma.

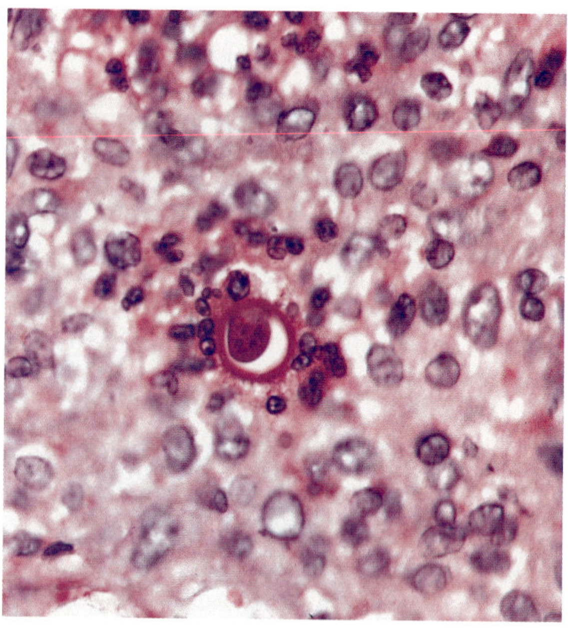

Figure 12-101

BLASTOMYCOSIS: ORGANISM MORPHOLOGY

The PAS stain highlights the thick yeast wall and the nuclei.

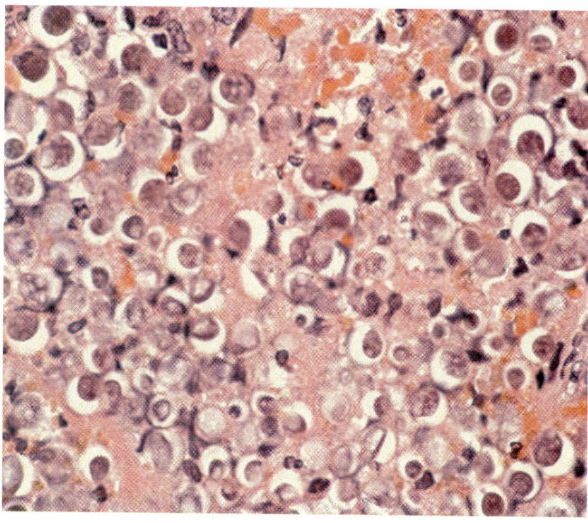

Figure 12-100

BLASTOMYCOSIS: ORGANISM MORPHOLOGY

Multiple yeast forms of blastomycosis have a thick wall.

adjacent pleura, mediastinum, and chest wall, and may mimic the radiologic features of pulmonary infection with actinomycosis or tuberculosis. Pleural effusion is seen in up to 15 percent of cases with parenchymal involvement, but pleural thickening is a more common finding (215).

CT features of blastomycosis include a localized mass and parenchymal consolidation. These masses may reach large sizes and most contain air bronchograms. CT may also demonstrate cavitation within parenchymal disease and hilar and/or mediastinal lymphadenopathy. The enlarged lymph nodes may exhibit calcification (296).

Immunocompromised patients with blastomycosis may exhibit radiologic features similar to those described above. However, diffuse interstitial opacities, cavitation, and progression to acute respiratory distress syndrome are more common (239).

Pathologic Findings. *B. dermatitidis* consists of spherical to oval, yeast-like cells measuring 8 to 15 µm (190,193). The cells are multinucleate (fig. 12-100) and have thick, refractile walls (figs. 12-101, 12-102). Buds are single and broad-based, and represent a useful diagnostic feature (fig. 12-103). The multiple nuclei are best seen on H&E-stained sections and are helpful diagnostically.

Occasionally, the organisms manifest as microforms with numerous, small, yeast-like cells measuring 2 to 4 µm (190,193). In such

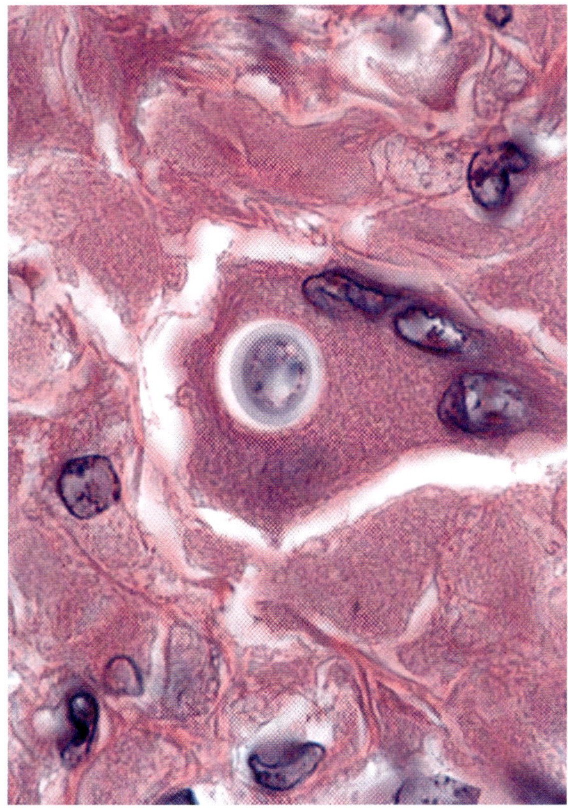

Figure 12-102

BLASTOMYCOSIS: ORGANISM MORPHOLOGY

This yeast form is engulfed by a multinucleated giant cell and has a thick refractile wall.

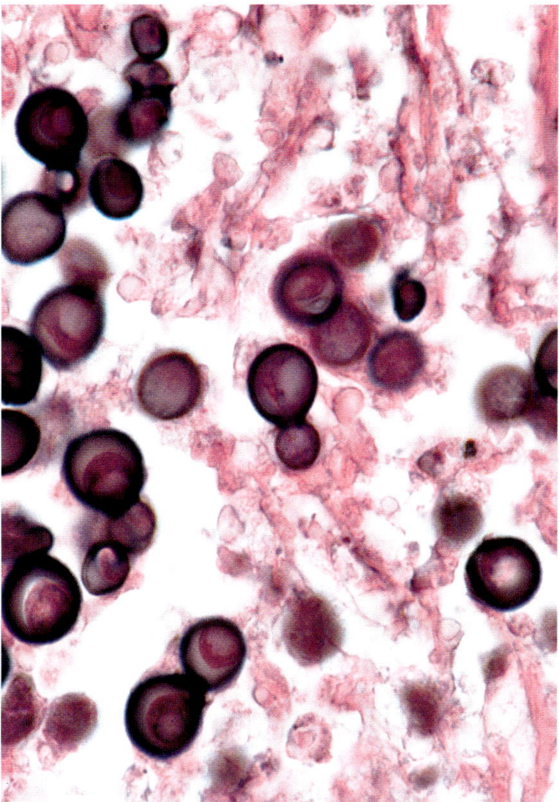

Figure 12-103

BLASTOMYCOSIS: ORGANISM MORPHOLOGY

The GMS stain demonstrates many yeast forms including a broad-based budding yeast (GMS-H&E stain).

cases one must search to identify the larger, more classic forms measuring 8 to 15 µm. Rarely, germ tubes, multiple buds, pseudohyphae, and septate hyphae are seen in tissues. The GMS is the optimal stain to demonstrate the fungal cells, although they stain well with PAS (190,193).

The histologic reaction to *B. dermatitidis* is typically suppurative, with a marked neutrophil response and abscess formation (fig. 12-104) (190, 193). If the process progresses, granulomatous inflammation develops. Even the necrotizing granulomas may show central neutrophilic microabscesses (fig. 12-105). The organisms tend to be more numerous in suppurative than chronic granulomatous lesions. Granulomas may become fibrotic and cavitary, but calcification is uncommon. Rarely, sclerosing mediastinitis occurs (241). In disseminated infection, there is dense infiltration of pulmonary tissues by sheets of organisms forming "yeast lakes." In such cases there may be minimal or no inflammatory reaction and granulomas may be absent (190,195).

Culture is the most definitive way to establish the diagnosis but usually takes up to 3 weeks to be positive. However, direct immunofluorescence on deparaffinized sections and immunohistochemistry are helpful (190,195,231–233). Skin tests are not available. Serologic testing is not a reliable method for making the diagnosis.

Differential Diagnosis. The separation of *B. dermatitidis* from capsule-deficient *Cryptococcus neoformans* may be a challenge if the diagnostic broad-based forms are not present or difficult to find (190,193,195). The mucicarmine stain is usually helpful in this differential diagnosis, but if the organisms are capsule-deficient, the Fontana-Masson stain should be negative in *B. dermatitidis*. Rarely, *B. dermatitidis* may be weakly positive with the mucicarmine

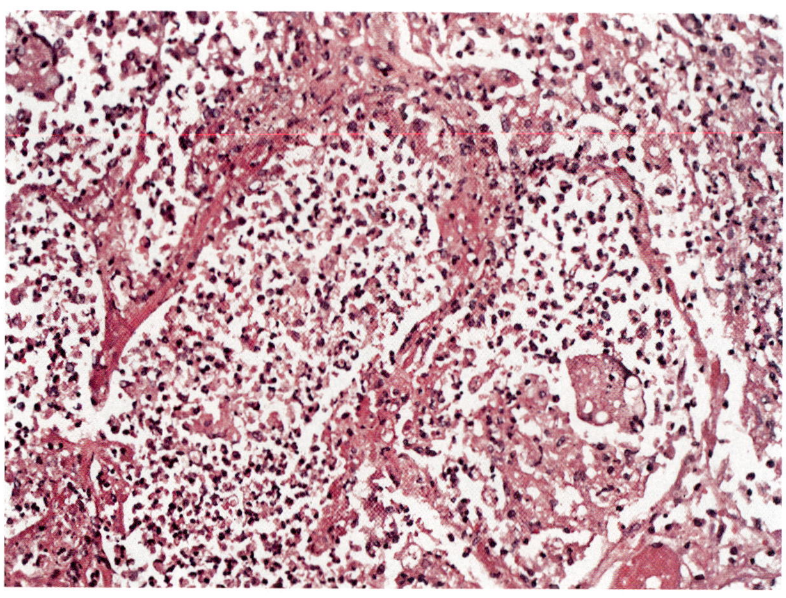

Figure 12-104

BLASTOMYCOSIS: SUPPURATIVE INFLAMMATION

Many neutrophils fill the alveolar spaces, causing an acute pneumonia.

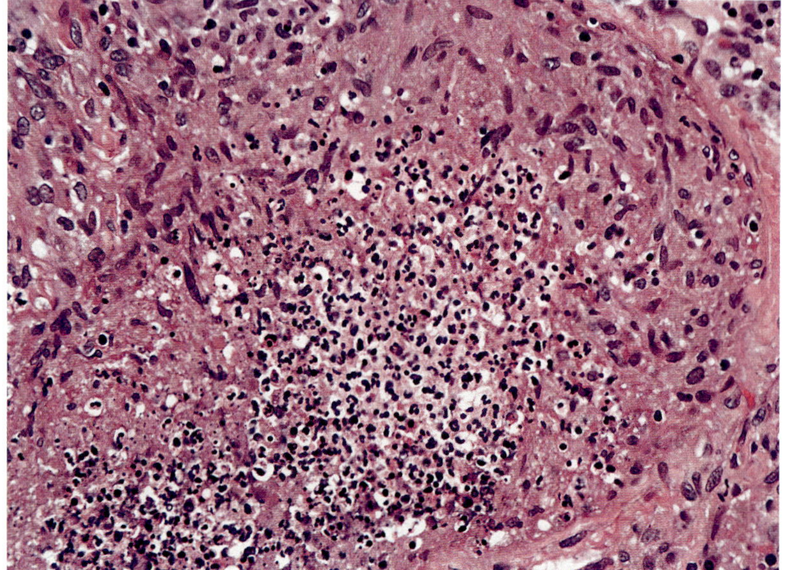

Figure 12-105

BLASTOMYCOSIS: SUPPURATIVE NECROTIZING GRANULOMA

A neutrophilic microabscess is surrounded by palisading histiocytes forming a suppurative necrotizing granuloma.

stain, but other morphologic features usually allow for the distinction from *C. neoformans* (190,193,195). The mucicarmine stain is positive in the cell wall and not the capsule, as seen in cryptococcosis (190,195). *B. dermatitidis* can also be mistaken for *Coccidioides immitis* when large cells without buds are empty or have inner contents that stain poorly. *H. capsulatum* can also be confused with the small, 2- to 4-µm intracellular forms of *B. dermatitidis,* but the latter typically have multiple nuclei, broader-based budding, and cells of larger size (190,193,195).

Treatment. The optimal therapy for patients with severe life-threatening blastomycosis or patients with meningeal involvement is amphotericin B. In patients with mild or moderate disease, ketoconazole or itraconazole are effective (205,207).

Paracoccidioides Brasiliensis

Definition. Pulmonary paracoccidioidomycosis *(South American blastomycosis)* is an infection by the dimorphic fungus, *Paracoccidioides brasiliensis.*

Table 12-9

PULMONARY MANIFESTATIONS OF PARACOCCIDIOIDOMYCOSIS[a]

Asymptomatic or Subclinical Infection
- Primary pulmonary paracoccidioidomycosis

Paracoccidioidomycosis Disease
- Acute or subacute form (juvenile type)
  - Mild
  - Severe
- Chronic form (adult type)
  - Unifocal
    - Chronic pulmonary disease
    - Other locations
  - Multifocal
- Quiescent form or sequelae (latent form)

[a] Table adapted from reference 284.

P. brasiliensis is endemic in the tropical and subtropical regions of Latin America, from Mexico to Argentina. Human infection is thought to be due to inhalation (207,285).

Clinical Features. Paracoccidioidomycosis is seen mostly in adults over 30 years of age (207,285). There is a 15 to 1 male predominance. Alcoholism is a predisposing factor (183, 246,284). The lungs are the primary site of infection, but only about one third of patients have disease limited to the lungs (207,285). The spectrum of clinical manifestations is summarized in Table 12-9.

Asymptomatic subclinical infection can be documented by positive skin tests in 10 percent of the population of Brazil and Colombia (207, 246,285). Pulmonary infection may be acute or chronic (patients present with fever, weight loss, and chronic cough). Immunocompromised patients may have acute respiratory failure and high fever. Disseminated infection often involves the mucous membranes, lymph nodes, liver, central nervous system, and spleen (284).

Radiologic Findings. The radiologic features of paracoccidioidomycosis are indistinguishable from those of other fungal infections and may mimic those of tuberculosis and sarcoidosis. They include transient airspace opacities, focal or multifocal nodular opacities, bilateral linear and reticular opacities, and extensive bilateral airspace consolidation. The radiographic abnormalities have been previously classified as infiltrative, nodular, and fibrotic.

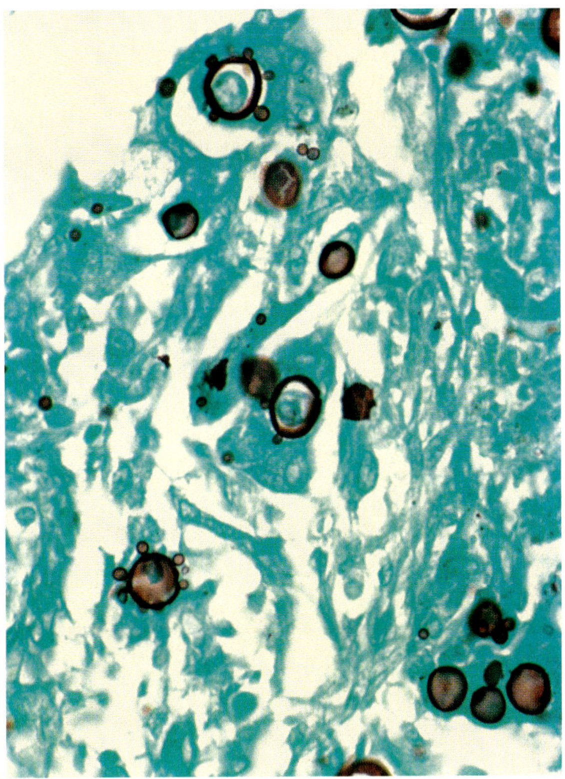

Figure 12-106

PARACOCCIDIOIDOMYCOSIS

Spherical yeast show multiple buds of varying size with a "pilot's wheel" morphology.

Cavitation has been described. Improvement of parenchymal involvement is typically observed after 3 to 6 months of appropriate therapy (215,216).

HRCT features are described as bilateral and symmetric parenchymal opacities affecting all lung zones. These have been characterized as peribronchovascular interstitial thickening with a central predominance and peripheral nodular opacities, often with irregular borders and a tendency to spare the anterior lung. In addition, there may be thickening of the interlobular septa, ground-glass opacities, centrilobular opacities, and evidence of fibrosis (215,216).

Pathologic Findings. The yeast cells of *P. brasiliensis* are spherical, vary markedly in size, and have multiple buds (fig. 12-106) (193,246). Most yeast forms are between 5 and 30 μm, however, the size can range from 4 to 60 μm (193,195, 246,284). The wall of the yeast is thick; doubly contoured walls may appear refractile. Budding blastoconidia have two morphologic appearances: 1) small, oval or tubular shapes or 2) large "teardrop" buds with narrow necks. The multiple buds may have a characteristic "pilot wheel" appearance (fig. 12-106). There may be six or more buds (blastoconidia), which characteristically vary in size. Larger fungal cells tend to break up, forming "soccer ball" or "mosaic" forms (183,246). Occasionally, germ tubes and short hyphal fragments occur; this is more likely in immunosuppressed patients (195,284).

If the infection is active, *P. brasiliensis* can be seen on H&E-stained sections where the multinucleated cytoplasm separates from the cell wall with a clear space or "halo." If the infection is chronic with few organisms, they may not be easily seen with H&E stain. In tissues, the organisms are best demonstrated with the GMS stain.

The histologic features range from an acute suppurative bronchopneumonia to a granulomatous and fibrosing process. Granulomas are poorly or well formed.

Differential Diagnosis. The histologic differential diagnosis includes cryptococcosis, blastomycosis, and sporotrichosis (193,246). *P. brasiliensis* can be separated from *Cryptococcus neoformans* by the presence of characteristic features of budding and lack of staining with mucicarmine. If the organisms are large and empty, they may resemble immature spherules of *Coccidioides immitis* (193,246).

Treatment. Ketoconazole is an effective treatment for active infection. Amphotericin B and itraconazole are also useful. Localized pulmonary nodules may be surgically excised (207,285).

Aspergillus Sp

Definition. Pulmonary aspergillosis is an infection caused by *Aspergillus*, usually *A. fumigatus, A. flavus,* or *A. niger.*

Aspergillus sp are ubiquitous molds found worldwide (207,261). *Aspergillus* spores are inhaled commonly by all individuals. Consequently, colonization of the airways may occur, especially after massive exposure. Although *A. fumigatus, A. flavus,* and *A. niger* are the most common pathogens, there are a wide variety of other species known to cause pulmonary disease (207,261). Pulmonary aspergillosis can take several forms, but the most common is colonization of airways or preexisting cavities, including formation of fungus balls. Other forms of involvement include allergic bronchopulmonary aspergillosis, bronchocentric granulomatosis, noninvasive and invasive infections, and empyema (Table 12-10) (207,261). The clinical, radiologic, and pathologic features of allergic bronchopulmonary aspergillosis are discussed in chapter 9.

Table 12-10

PATTERNS OF PULMONARY ASPERGILLOSIS

Colonization
Fungus ball
Hypersensitivity Reaction
Allergic bronchopulmonary aspergillosis
Eosinophilic pneumonia
Mucoid impaction
Bronchocentric granulomatosis
Hypersensitivity pneumonitis
Invasive
Acute invasive aspergillosis
Necrotizing pseudomembranous tracheobronchitis
Chronic necrotizing aspergillosis
Bronchopleural fistula
Empyema

Clinical Features. There is a broad spectrum of clinical manifestations of pulmonary *Aspergillus* infection (Table 12-10).

Fungus Ball (Aspergilloma). Aspergillus fungus balls result from colonization of preexisting cavities within the lung (207,261). These cavities may be due to a wide variety of causes including tuberculosis, bronchiectasis, sarcoidosis, chronic lung abscess, histoplasmosis, and malignancy. Fungus balls develop in the cavitary infarcts of acute angioinvasive aspergillosis and they are reported in up to 40 percent of cases of chronic necrotizing aspergillosis (193). While most fungus balls are caused by *Aspergillus fumigatus,* they are associated with other *Aspergillus* sp as well as other fungi such as *Coccidioides immitis.*

Fungus balls have a wide variety of clinical manifestations ranging from incidental discovery in an asymptomatic patient to hemoptysis, which can be massive and life-threatening (207,261,270). From 75 to 90 percent of patients have hemoptysis at least once (193). This is thought to be due to erosion of blood vessels adjacent to the cavity. Patients with severe hemoptysis may require surgical resection (206) and 5 percent of patients die from massive hemorrhage (193). The diagnosis is usually based on chest radiographs in conjunction with positive serum precipitins and a history of hemoptysis (193). Serum precipitins against *Aspergillus* are found in 92 to 100 percent of patients with fungus balls (193,206). Bronchopleural fistulas are a potential complication that may result in pleural involvement. Sputum cultures can help identify the *Aspergillus* organisms.

Hypersensitivity Reactions. Two types of pulmonary hypersensitivity reaction occur with *Aspergillus* sp: *allergic bronchopulmonary aspergillosis* (ABPA, chapter 9) and *hypersensitivity pneumonitis* (chapter 3) (181,185,207,261,282,300).

Necrotizing Pseudomembranous Tracheobronchitis. This form accounts for 6 to 9 percent of cases of bronchopulmonary aspergillosis (174, 207,261). It usually occurs in patients with relatively mild impairment of the immune system (199,293): those with hematologic, lymphoreticular, and solid malignancies who have granulocytopenia and a history of prolonged treatment with antibiotics, corticosteroids, and chemotherapy; HIV-infected patients (235); and patients following bone marrow or lung transplantation (238,248). Presenting symptoms include dyspnea, wheezing, and nonproductive cough (193,293).

Acute Invasive Aspergillosis. Acute invasive pulmonary aspergillosis is a life-threatening fulminant infection that is associated with vascular invasion and frequent dissemination (207,261). Patients are typically immunosuppressed and myelosuppressed. Granulocytopenia is the greatest risk factor for this disease. Patients present with clinical features similar to those of an acute bacterial pneumonia (193,206,293): nonproductive cough, high fever, pleuritic pain, and pleural friction rubs. It can be difficult to be certain of the diagnosis since sputum cultures are often negative and a positive result could be from an upper airway contaminant. Open lung biopsy is very helpful in establishing the diagnosis (206).

Chronic Necrotizing Aspergillosis (Semi-Invasive Aspergillosis). This locally invasive and slowly progressive condition typically occurs in patients with severe underlying pulmonary disease (184,193,206,207,214,236,261,289,293, 301). Patients are middle-aged to elderly, and usually have some underlying condition such as chronic obstructive lung disease, diabetes mellitus, a collagen vascular disease, or malnutrition, or are on low-dose corticosteroid therapy. Presenting manifestations include fever, productive cough, and dyspnea. Chest radiographs typically demonstrate upper lobe consolidation, which may cavitate. Fungus balls often form within the cavities. The onset is usually indolent, ranging from months to years. The clinical course, isolation of the fungus from the lung, or identification of the characteristic pathologic features in a surgical specimen help to establish the diagnosis. Patients should also have negative cultures for other pathogens, and there should be no response to antibiotics directed at bacteria and mycobacteria (184,193,206,289,293,301).

Radiologic Findings. *Aspergilloma.* The classic radiologic manifestation of saprophytic aspergillosis (mycetoma) is that of a gravity-dependent, soft tissue nodule or mass within a preexistent pulmonary cavity or bronchiectatic airway (215,217,251). The spherical mass (fungus ball) is usually outlined by a crescent of air along its nondependent surface. This has been termed the Mounod or "air-crescent" sign (215,217, 251). The lesion is typically located in an upper lobe or lung periphery, and the adjacent pleura is thickened. These cavities usually have thin walls and may contain air-fluid levels (215). Occasionally, mycetomas may completely fill the cavity and obscure the air-crescent sign or may adhere to the wall of the cavity and fail to demonstrate mobility within it. Focal thickening of the cavity wall classically precedes the radiologic visualization of an aspergilloma (217,251).

CT helps demonstrate early subtle mycetomas (figs. 12-107, 12-108), and supine and prone chest CT may demonstrate mobility of the mycetoma within the cavity. In addition, CT allows evaluation of early mycetomas, which may only exhibit cavity wall thickening, as well as those that almost completely fill the cavitary lesion (217). Calcification within the fungus ball has been described on chest CT (177). The soft tissue mass may exhibit an irregular shape or heterogeneous attenuation because of

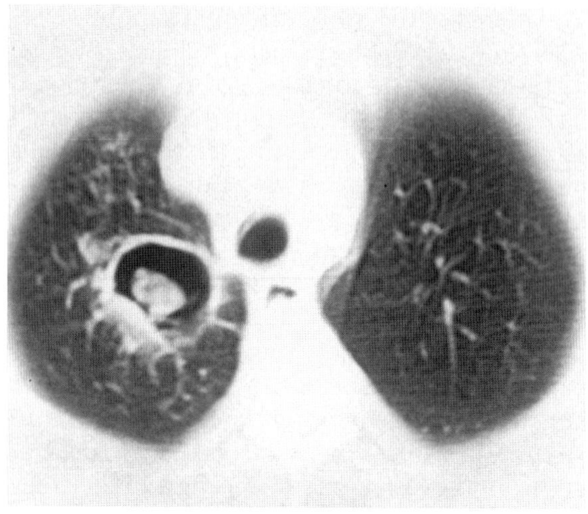

Figure 12-107

ASPERGILLOMA

Aspergilloma in a 59-year-old female with metastatic renal cell carcinoma. Chest CT (lung window) demonstrates a right upper lobe cavity with a dependent heterogeneous soft tissue mass, which represents an aspergilloma. While the cavity was visible on chest radiography, the mycetoma was not.

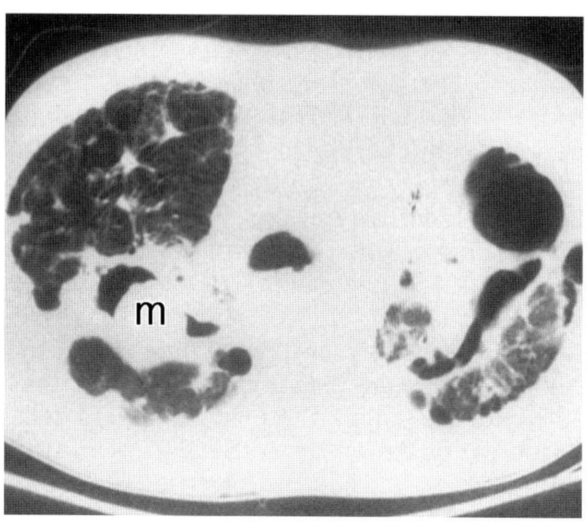

Figure 12-108

ASPERGILLOMA

Aspergilloma in a 38-year-old female with stage IV sarcoidosis and hemoptysis. Supine chest CT (lung window) demonstrates bilateral central pulmonary fibrosis and cystic lung disease. Note the gravity-dependent soft tissue mass (m) in the right cystic space.

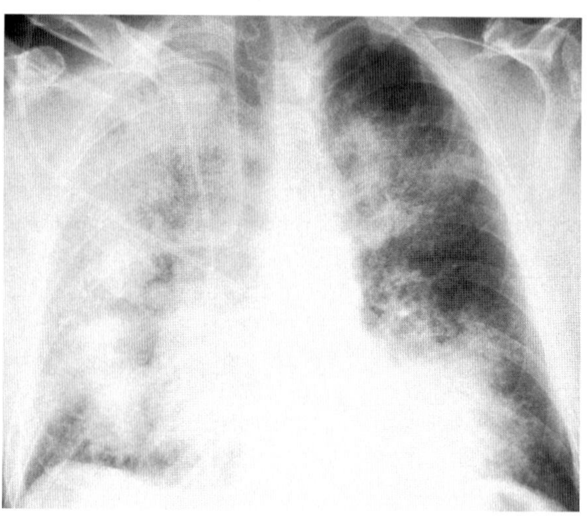

Figure 12-109

INVASIVE ASPERGILLOSIS

Invasive aspergillosis in a 61-year-old male with aplastic anemia, recurrent infections, and abdominal pain. PA chest radiograph demonstrates multifocal, bilateral, confluent consolidation. A central venous catheter is in place.

air trapped in interstices within the fungus ball (fig. 12-107) (217). Multiple mycetomas may be visible within the same cavity or within multiple cavities. The most common etiology of cavitary lung disease complicated by mycetoma formation is tuberculosis, followed by stage IV sarcoidosis, bronchiectasis, and various lung cysts, bullae, and abscesses. The radiologic differential diagnosis includes lung cancer, lung necrosis, parasitic disease, and intracavitary thrombus (215).

Invasive Aspergillosis. Radiographs in patients with invasive aspergillosis demonstrate multifocal pulmonary opacities of ill-defined borders which may rapidly progress to large, bilateral, multifocal consolidations (fig. 12-109). A single large parenchymal consolidation may affect an entire lobe and mimic bacterial pneumonia. The diagnosis is suspected where there is neutropenia and clinical infection. Early in the course of the disease, the chest CT may demonstrate focal or multifocal nodular opacities surrounded by ground-glass attenuation; this has been referred to as the CT "halo sign" (fig. 12-110) (223,251). It correlates with surrounding intra-alveolar hemorrhage, is not diagnostic of angioinvasive fungal infection, and may be seen in other infections, neoplasms, and vasculitides (215,267). A recent study of 11 neutropenic patients described segmental consolidation with surrounding ground-glass attenuation as the most common

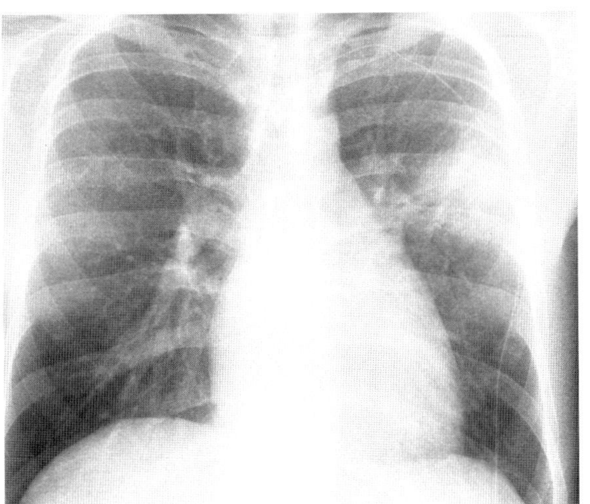

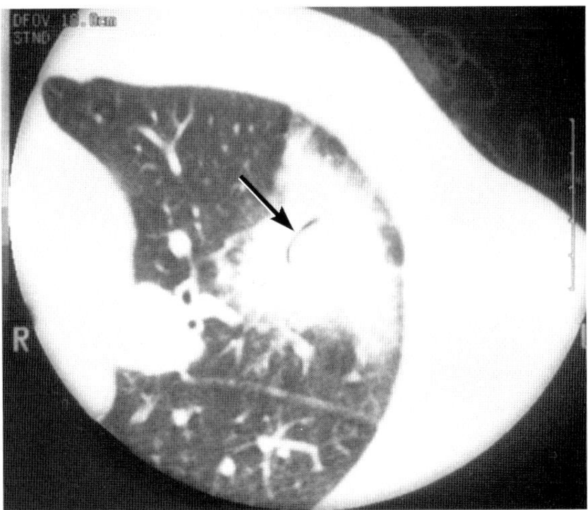

Figure 12-110

INVASIVE ASPERGILLOSIS

A 21-year-old male with acute myelogenous leukemia and chemotherapy-induced neutropenia who developed pleuritic chest pain and dyspnea.

Left: PA chest radiograph demonstrates a left upper lobe consolidation. A central venous catheter is in place.

Right: Thin-section chest CT (lung window) demonstrates a soft tissue mass within the left upper lobe consolidation surrounded by a thin air crescent (arrow). Note the "halo" of ground-glass opacity that surrounds the consolidation.

CT finding of invasive aspergillosis (298). Other radiologic findings include lobar or segmental consolidation, multiple small nodules, reticular opacities, and pleural effusion (251).

The nodular opacities and consolidations of invasive aspergillosis may undergo cavitation during recovery from chemotherapy-induced neutropenia. Characteristically, a spherical mass surrounded by a crescent of air develops within a preexistent nodule or consolidation. The nodular mass represents retracting necrotic lung tissue (fig. 12-110) (177). The radiologic appearance is similar to that of a mycetoma. However, invasive aspergillosis is distinguished from mycetomas by the status of the lung on prior radiographs and the patient's clinical presentation. Mycetomas develop in a preexisting lung cavity (fig. 12-107); in invasive aspergillosis, the air-crescent sign is preceded by a pulmonary nodule, mass, or consolidation without preexistent cavitary disease (fig. 12-109).

Pseudomembranous Tracheobronchitis. Patients with invasive tracheobronchitis secondary to *Aspergillus* infection typically have normal chest radiographs. Atelectasis and patchy peribronchial opacities may be observed (174,215,251).

Chronic Necrotizing Aspergillosis. Chronic necrotizing aspergillosis manifests radiologically with upper lobe parenchymal consolidation, adjacent pleural thickening, and cavitation. An intracavitary mass (aspergilloma) may develop. The course of disease is slow and may span weeks to months. There may be progression to whole lung, mediastinum, chest wall, or blood vessel involvement (177,215,251).

Pathologic Findings. *Morphologic Features of the Organism.* The hyphae of *Aspergillus* sp are septated and branching, and 3 to 6 µm in width (fig. 12-111). The hyphae tend to be uniform and grow in a parallel fashion with septa at regular intervals. The branching is dichotomous, that is, the size of the branches is the same as the parent hyphae. The branching is usually at acute angles, often at 45° (fig. 12-111). The hyphae may show degenerative changes, making them difficult to distinguish from those of other fungi such as in mucormycosis. The degenerative changes may consist of swollen, globose hyphal segments measuring up to 15 µm in diameter (193). The degenerative artifacts also make it difficult to see septation or a branching pattern.

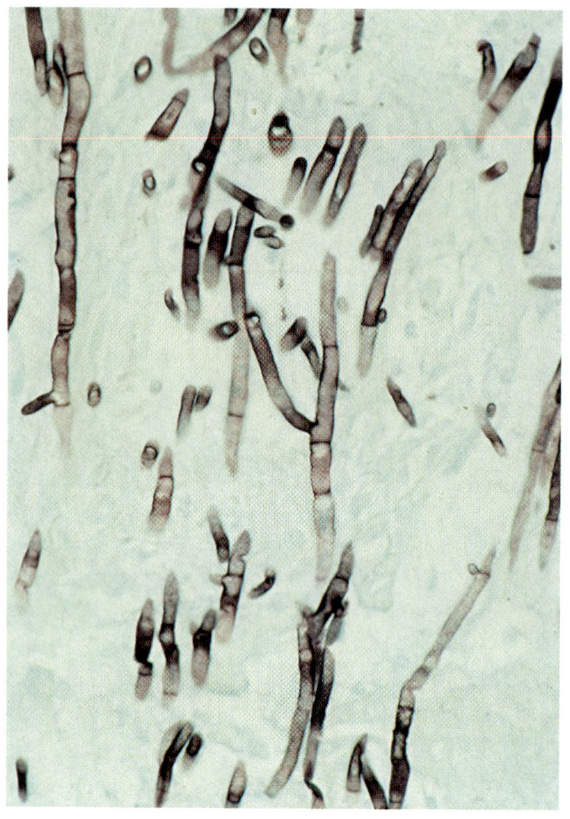

Figure 12-111

ASPERGILLUS: ORGANISM MORPHOLOGY

The hyphae are parallel, uniform, and septate at regular intervals. Branching is at 45° angles.

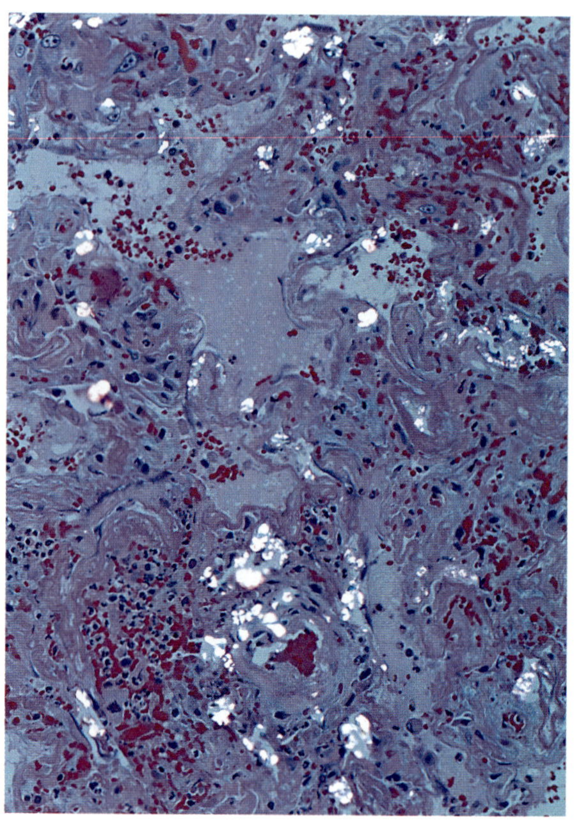

Figure 12-112

ASPERGILLUS: CALCIUM OXALATE CRYSTALS

These birefringent crystals are calcium oxalates.

Aspergillus organisms can be seen with routine H&E stains, but they are better appreciated with a PAS or GMS stain (fig. 12-111). Calcium oxalate crystals are associated with *Aspergillus,* especially *A. niger* (fig. 12-112) (193,293).

Conidial heads of *Aspergillus* organisms (fig. 12-113) occur in lesions where the organism is exposed to air, such as the cavities associated with fungus balls or in pseudomembranous tracheobronchitis. The conidial head is a vesicle with one or two layers of sterigmata and chains of conidia growing from their tips (fig. 12-113). In their conidial form the different types of *Aspergillus* have distinguishing morphologic characteristics that allow their separation, but otherwise the hyphae of most of the species are indistinguishable.

In chronic granulomatous lesions the hyphae may be surrounded by the Splendore-Hoeppli phenomenon. This consists of radiating eosinophilic material (fig. 12-114).

Fungus Balls. The gross appearance of fungus balls vary depending on the type of underlying cavitary disease and the amount of fungal growth. In general, the fungus ball appears as a friable, brown to red mass that is not firmly attached to the cavity wall (fig. 12-115). The cavities range from 1 to 7 cm or larger and typically have a thick fibrous wall measuring up to 0.5 cm. They are usually solitary but may be multiple (193,293).

Fungus balls consist of masses of mycelia that grow in layers within preexisting cavities in the lung (fig. 12-116). They may also develop in the pleural space in areas of scarring such as from adhesions or prior surgical intervention. While other fungi, such as *Mucor,* cause fungus balls as well, most are due to *Aspergillus.* The

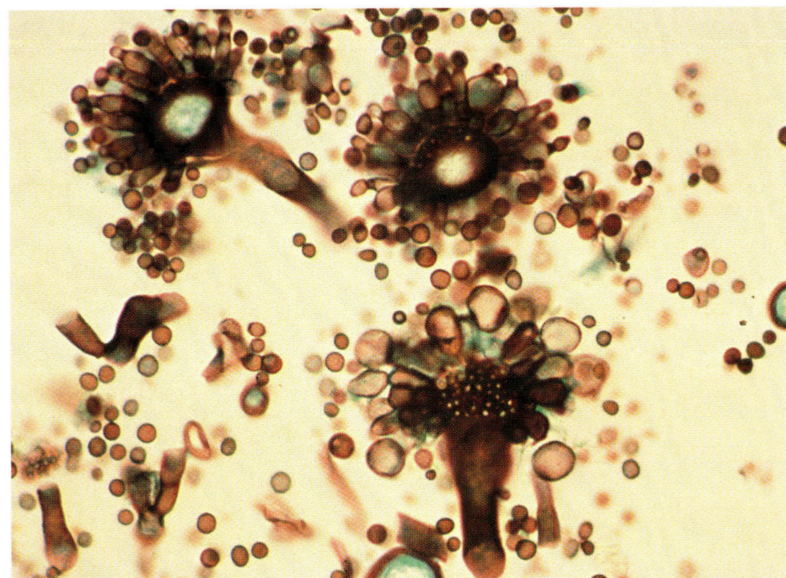

Figure 12-113

ASPERGILLUS: CONIDIAL HEADS

The conidial heads consist of a vesicle with sterigmata and chains of conidia.

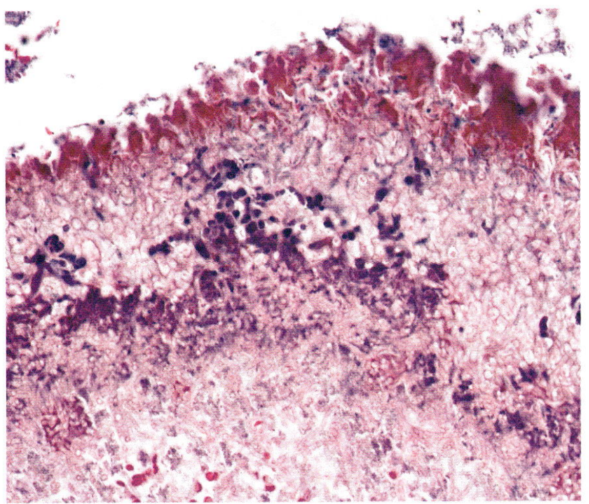

Figure 12-114

ASPERGILLUS: SPLENDORE-HOEPPLI PHENOMENON

At the edge of the mass of fungal hyphae is radiating eosinophilic material.

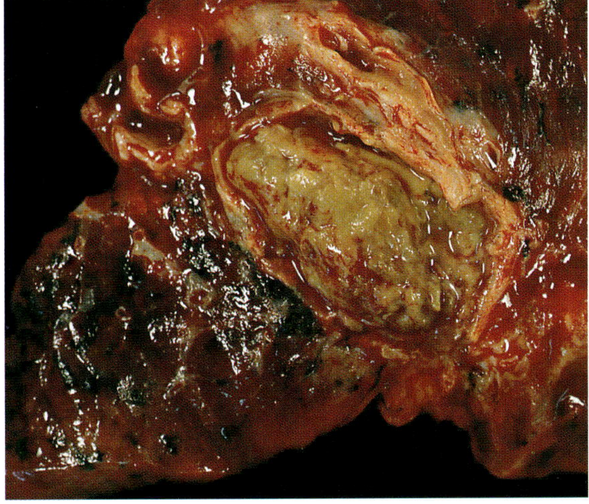

Figure 12-115

ASPERGILLUS: FUNGUS BALL

Within the bronchiectatic cavity is a yellow ball of fungus.

fungi may grow superficially into the cavity walls, but invasive growth and hematogenous spread typically do not occur. In cases where there is high oxygen tension, such as a bronchial stump, fruiting bodies and conidial heads may be seen. The organisms typically consist of concentric layers of hyphae growing in a radial pattern (fig. 12-116, right). In the center of the fungus ball the hyphae tend to be degenerated and can be mistaken for *Mucor* organisms. Rarely, an aspergilloma progresses to a serious invasive infection.

Necrotizing Pseudomembranous Tracheobronchitis. Necrotizing pseudomembranous tracheobronchitis occurs when a pseudomembrane of *Aspergillus* grows along the surface of the tracheal and bronchial mucosa, undermining and eroding the epithelium (fig. 12-117). Histologically, the pseudomembrane consists of an exudate of necrotic tissue, mucus, inflammatory

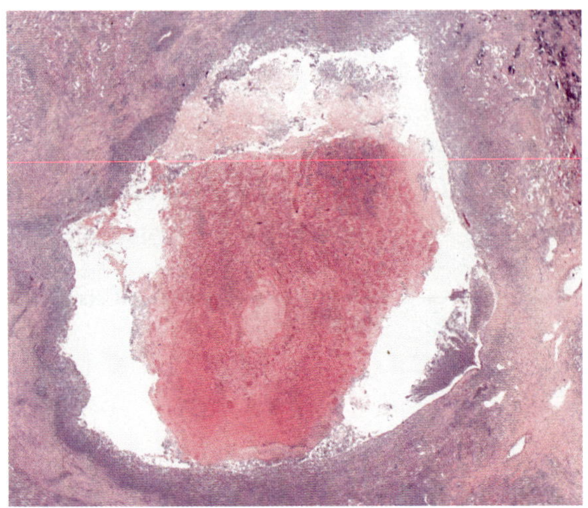

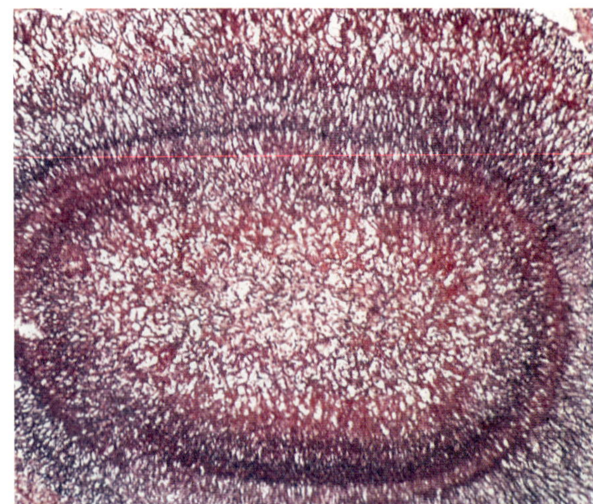

Figure 12-116

ASPERGILLUS: FUNGUS BALL, HISTOLOGY

Left: A mass of fungal hyphae is present within this cavity (PAS stain).
Right: The hyphae are growing in concentric layers in a radial pattern.

Figure 12-117

ASPERGILLUS: PSEUDOMEMBRANOUS TRACHEOBRONCHITIS

A layer of fungus coats the surface of the bronchial wall (GMS stain).

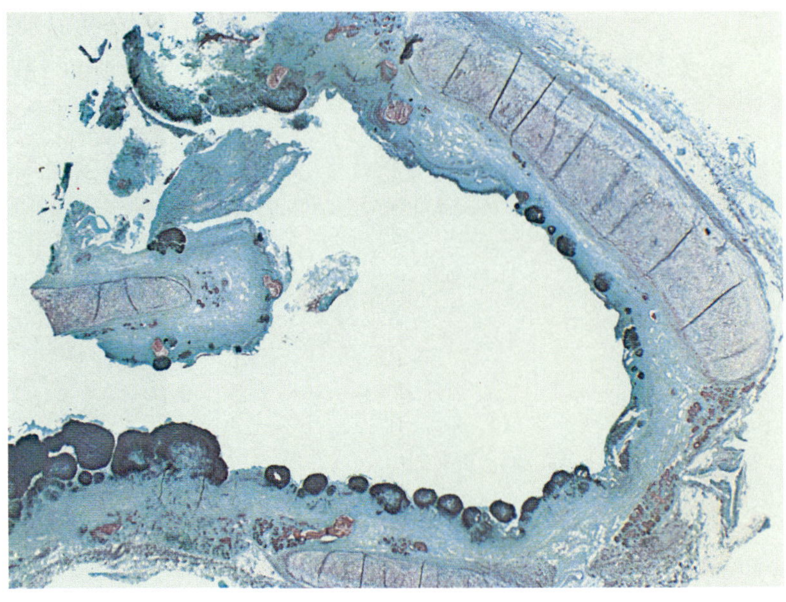

cells, and fungal hyphae that is accompanied by conidial heads in approximately 40 percent of cases (199,235,248,286).

Clarke et al. and others (199,215,251,293) identified two morphologic patterns of necrotizing tracheobronchitis. In some patients the pseudomembrane tends to involve the entire circumference of the bronchial wall and the mucus/fungus plug completely occludes the airway lumen. The second pattern consists of single or multiple discrete plaques on the airway wall and in some cases the fungus invades the adjacent lung parenchyma or pulmonary artery.

Acute Invasive Aspergillosis. The characteristic lesion of acute invasive aspergillosis is the target lesion (fig. 12-118), although it is not specific for *Aspergillus* infection and can occur with other angioinvasive fungi such as *Mucor.* The

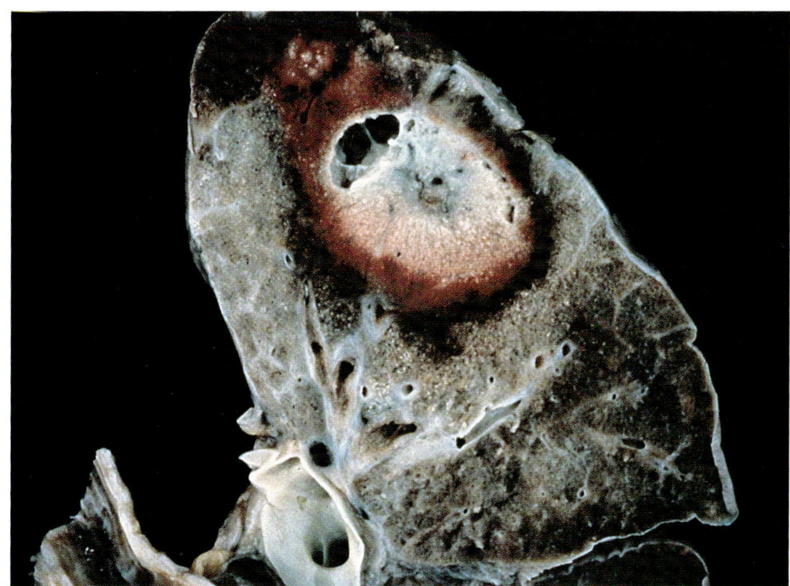

Figure 12-118

ASPERGILLUS: INFARCT

A subpleural nodular infarct consists of a pale yellow necrotic center surrounded by a hemorrhagic rim. At the top is a crescent-shaped space where the necrotic lung has retracted from the surrounding viable tissue.

target lesion is a nodular pulmonary infarct associated with vascular invasion by fungal hyphae. Grossly, these target lesions typically have a central pale necrotic zone surrounded by a hemorrhagic rim (fig. 12-118). There may be a crescent-shaped cavitary space surrounding the central necrotic lung at the periphery. These lesions are usually multiple and peripheral, and range from several millimeters to 3 cm or more in diameter.

Histologically, the lesion consists of infarcts associated with vascular occlusion by fungal hyphae (fig. 12-119). Miliary microabscesses from intrapulmonary dissemination occur in less than 10 percent of cases. If large arteries become occluded by fungus, large wedge-shaped infarcts may be seen (193,293). Cavitation occurs in the infarcts when the patient recovers from the neutropenia (fig. 12-120). In 1 to 6 percent of cases fungus balls develop within necrotic lesions (193,293). The fungi appear to grow radially in waves outward from the center of the lesions (fig. 12-121). In patients who survive due to early diagnosis, aggressive antifungal therapy, or a relatively intact immune system, a granulomatous reaction may develop at the periphery of the infarct. Extrapulmonary hematogenous dissemination occurs in 25 to 35 percent of patients (193,293).

Chronic Necrotizing Aspergillosis (Semi-Invasive Aspergillosis). Chronic necrotizing aspergillosis is characterized pathologically by three major patterns: a necrotizing granulomatous pneumonia (fig. 12-122), granulomatous bronchiectatic cavities, or bronchocentric granulomatosis (fig. 12-123) (193,289,301). In the necrotizing granulomatous pneumonia pattern, there are large areas of parenchymal consolidation by necrotizing granulomas (fig. 12-122). Fungal hyphae are usually seen in the areas of tissue necrosis and parenchymal invasion is present (fig. 12-122). Eosinophilic pneumonia may be present and an organizing pneumonia pattern may be seen at the periphery of the lesions.

When bronchiectatic cavities are present in chronic necrotizing aspergillosis, they contain fungus balls or poorly formed aggregates of fungal hyphae. There is also invasive growth of fungus into surrounding tissue. A clue that the cavities are centered on airways is the presence of respiratory or squamous metaplastic epithelium focally lining the walls. The periphery of the fungus balls may show the Splendore-Hoeppli phenomenon (see fig. 12-114) (193,289,301). Histologically, the lesions appear centered on airways that are grossly distorted by granulomatous inflammation and fibrosis. The surrounding lung parenchyma shows fibrosis and chronic inflammation, which may represent underlying chronic lung disease. A variety of other nonspecific lesions may be seen including lymphoid hyperplasia, acute inflammation, and hemorrhage.

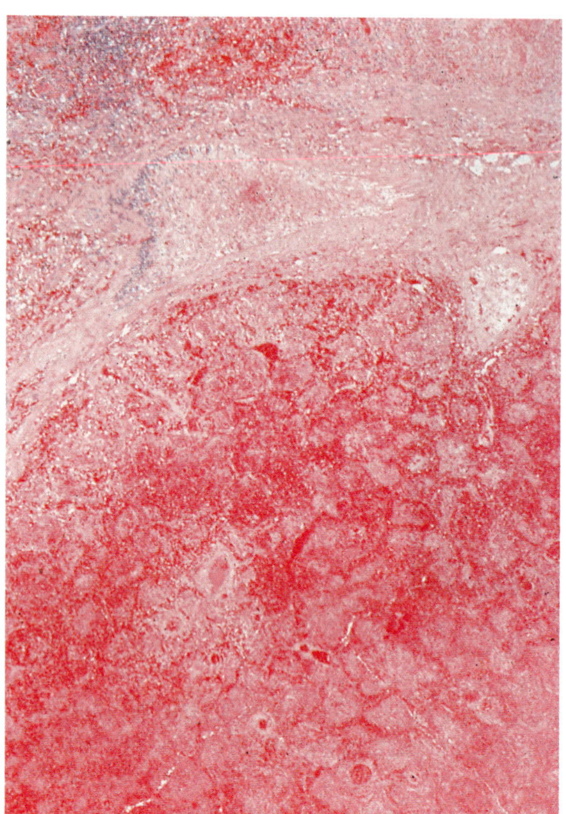

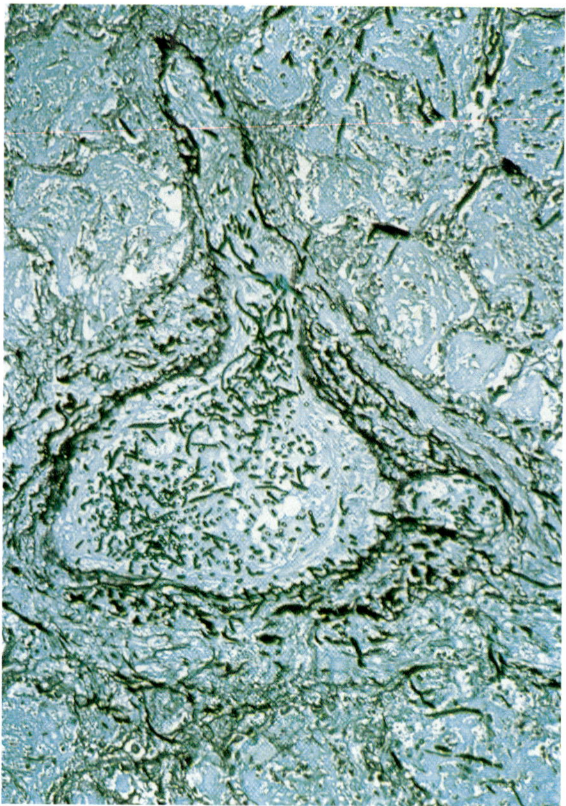

Figure 12-119

ASPERGILLUS: ANGIOINVASIVE WITH INFARCT

Left: This hemorrhagic infarct was associated with angioinvasive aspergillosis.
Right: This blood vessel is occluded by a mass of *Aspergillus* organisms (GMS stain).

Figure 12-120

ASPERGILLUS: CAVITATED INFARCT

This cavitary lesion is from a patient with angioinvasive aspergillosis. Along the surface of the cavity is brown soft material that represents a fungus ball.

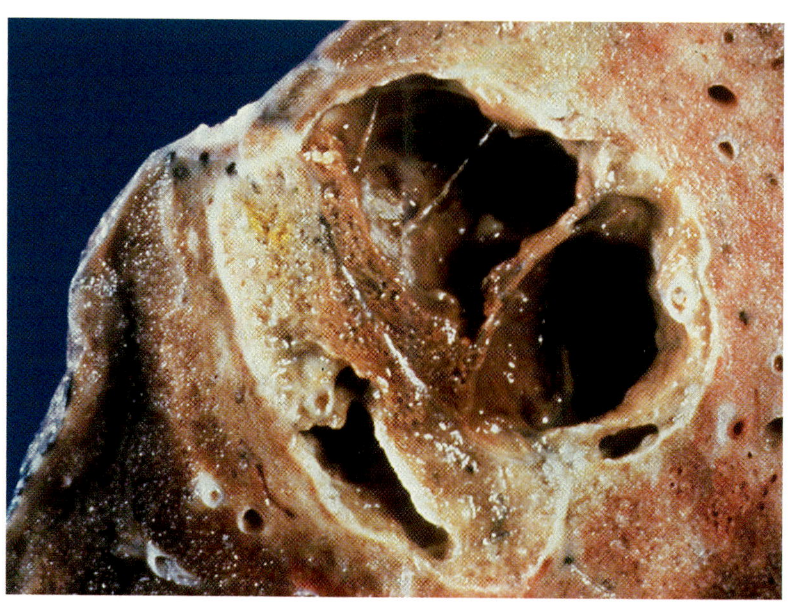

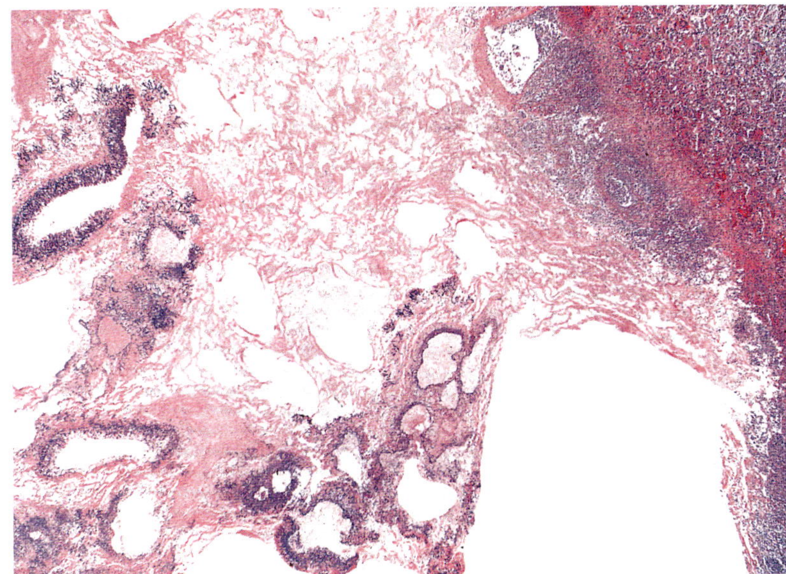

Figure 12-121

ASPERGILLUS: FUNGUS BALL IN CAVITATED INFARCT

Within the center of this necrotic infarct are radial waves of *Aspergillus* hyphae growing outward.

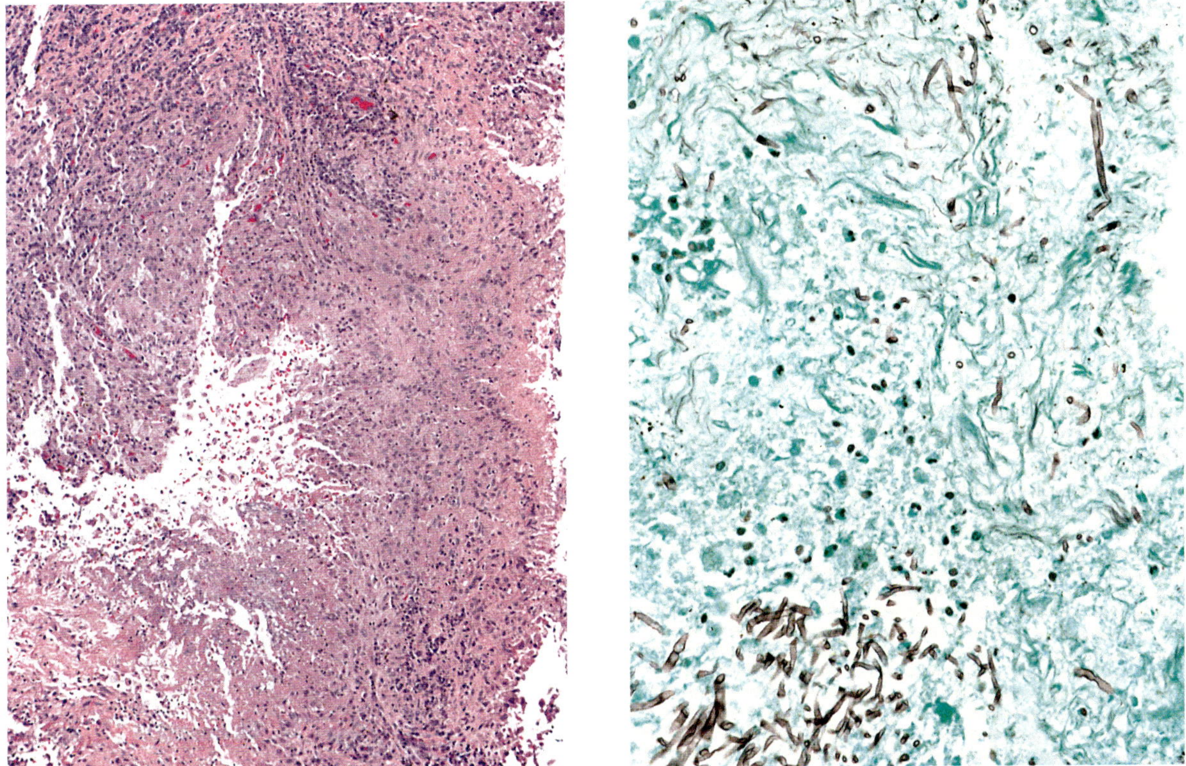

Figure 12-122

ASPERGILLUS: NECROTIZING GRANULOMATOUS PNEUMONIA, HISTOLOGY

Left: This necrotizing granuloma consists of histiocytes and giant cells surrounding a collection of neutrophils. Right: *Aspergillus* hyphae are infiltrating the surrounding tissue.

Table 12-11

MORPHOLOGIC CHARACTERISTICS OF HYPHAL FUNGI[a]

	Width	Contours	Branching Pattern	Orientation	Septation
Aspergillus sp	3-6 µm	Parallel	Dichotomous	Parallel	Frequent
Zygomycetes	5-25 µm	Irregular	Haphazard	Random	Infrequent
Fusarium sp	3-8 µm	Parallel	Right angle	Random	Frequent
Pseudoallescheria boydii	2-5 µm	Parallel	Haphazard	Random	Frequent (Conidiophores)

[a]Modified from Table 10 from reference 195.

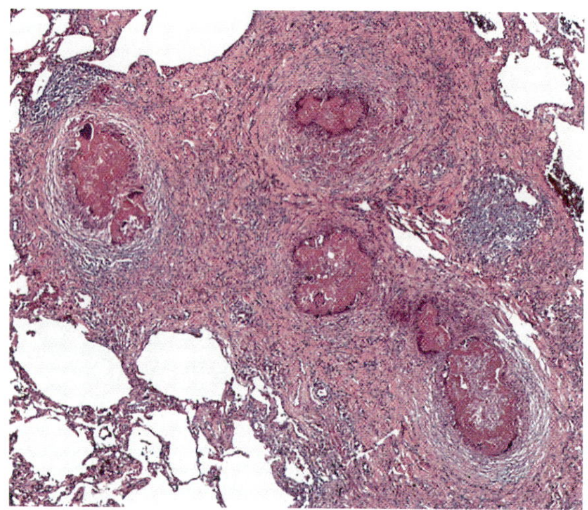

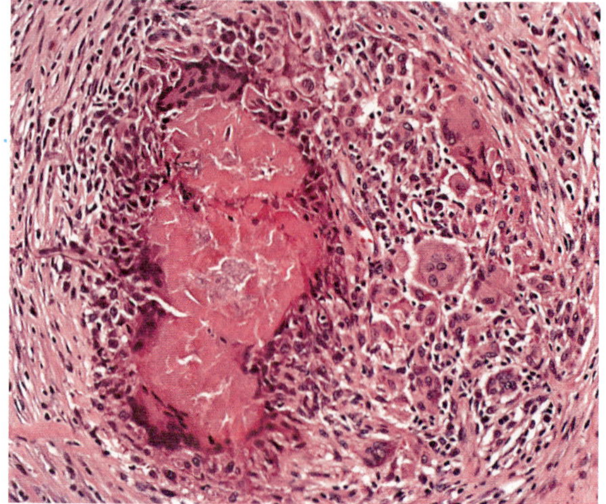

Figure 12-123

ASPERGILLUS: BRONCHOCENTRIC GRANULOMATOSIS IN PATIENT WITHOUT ASTHMA

Left: Necrotizing granulomatous inflammation thickens the wall of this bronchiole.
Right: The lumen is filled with inspisated mucus and fungal hyphae. Eosinophils are absent.

Less commonly, the histologic pattern of bronchocentric granulomatosis is the primary pattern of chronic necrotizing aspergillosis (fig. 12-123) (193,289,301). The lesions primarily affect bronchioles, which are altered by granulomatous inflammation, luminal mucus, necrotic eosinophilic debris, neutrophils, and hyphal fragments of *Aspergillus.* The fungus invades the surrounding parenchyma.

Differential Diagnosis. Due to the degenerative changes that frequently occur in tissue sections, care must be taken in making the diagnosis based on morphology alone unless well-preserved hyphae are present. It can be very difficult to separate *Aspergillus* sp from *Fusarium* sp (Table 12-11) and *Pseudoallescheria boydii,* so absolute confirmation of the diagnosis requires culture or immunologic methods. Separation from zygomycosis is discussed below. *Fusarium* sp has wider hyphae measuring 3 to 8 µm in width and the branching tends to occur at right angles rather than acute angles. The branching also is associated with constrictions at the branch points. *P. boydii* has slightly thinner hyphae, measuring 2 to 5 µm, and a more haphazard branching pattern than *Aspergillus.* Furthermore, *P. boydii* often shows conspicuous vesicles and oval conidia that may be brown, measure 5 to 10 µm, and grow on short conidiophores (195,293). Although it is possible to suggest the diagnosis of *Aspergillosis* sp based on morphology, especially if conidial forms are identified, a definitive diagnosis is established based on culture or immunohistochemistry (195,208,234,264,293).

Treatment and Prognosis. *Fungus Ball.* Most patients with fungus balls require no therapy. Surgical resection may be necessary in patients with severe hemoptysis (270). However, some patients have such severe underlying disease that surgical resection is not possible. Medical therapy is generally not effective. Patients who have associated hemoptysis may benefit from bronchial artery embolization. Percutaneous installation of antifungal agents into the fungus ball has also been successful (207,261).

Necrotizing Pseudomembranous Tracheobronchitis. Kramer et al. (238) reported that oral therapy with itraconazole was successful in five of six patients, with fatal relapse in one. A more recent study described successful therapy using liposomal amphotericin, inhaled amphotericin, gamma interferon, and GM-CSF (186).

Acute Invasive Aspergillosis. Amphotericin B is the therapy of choice for this type of aspergillosis (207,261). Patients who recover from their neutropenia are more likely to improve. Residual nodular lesions and cavities can be surgically excised.

Chronic Necrotizing Aspergillosis. This form of aspergillosis frequently responds to high-dose amphotericin B (207,261).

Zygomycetes

Definition. Zygomycosis is an uncommon but frequently fatal infection that is caused by fungi of the order Mucorales and class *Zygomycetes.* There are two orders of *Zygomycetes*-containing organisms that cause human disease, the Mucorales and the Entomophthorales; the majority of human illness is caused by the Mucorales. While disease is most commonly linked to *Rhizopus* sp, other organisms are also associated with human infection, including *Mucor, Rhizomucor, Absidia, Apophysomyces, Saksenaea, Cunninghamella, Cokeromyces,* and *Syncephalastrum* (271).

Clinical Features. The spores from these molds are transmitted by inhalation, via a variety of percutaneous routes, or by ingestion. Human zygomycosis occurs only rarely in immunocompetent hosts; most cases occur in hosts with one or more of the following risk factors: diabetes mellitus, neutropenia, sustained immunosuppressive therapy, chronic prednisone use, iron chelation therapy, broad-spectrum antibiotic use, severe malnutrition, and primary breakdown in the integrity of the cutaneous barrier such as from trauma, surgical wounds, needle sticks, or burns (271). The disease manifestations reflect the mode of transmission, with rhinocerebral and pulmonary diseases being the most common manifestations. Pulmonary infections are most frequently caused by *Rhizopus arrhizus* (also known as *R. oryzae*) (207,228). Other specific types of Mucorales known to cause pulmonary infection on rare occasion are *Absidia* and *Cunninghamella.* Cutaneous, gastrointestinal, and allergic diseases are also seen (237). There is a strong predilection for vascular invasion and dissemination in immunocompromised patients. Risk factors for respiratory zygomycosis include diabetic ketoacidosis, corticosteroid therapy, granulocytopenia, deferoxamine therapy, burns, and low birth weight or neonatal prematurity (207,228).

Radiologic Findings. Pulmonary zygomycosis typically manifests radiographically as progressive, homogeneous, lobar or multilobar parenchymal consolidation (fig. 12-124). Rounded mass-like consolidation with rapid progression and lobar expansion is also described (215,251). Solitary or multiple pulmonary nodules or masses as well as peripheral wedge-shaped consolidations are seen (229). Nodular opacities may be surrounded by a halo of ground-glass attenuation on CT imaging. Cavitation occurs in up to 40 percent of cases, may exhibit the air-crescent sign, and mimic the radiologic appearance of invasive aspergillosis. CT may demonstrate features of angioinvasive disease which include focal or diffuse low attenuation within consolidations. Lymphadenopathy and pleural effusion occur but are less common features. CT imaging is useful for identifying unsuspected complications such as vascular invasion with resultant pulmonary artery pseudoaneurysms, evidence of hematogenous dissemination, and extrapulmonary invasion (251).

Pathologic Findings. *Zygomycetes* have broad hyphae that range from 5 to 25 µm (193, 197). Due to the thin walls, the hyphae frequently appear twisted or folded (fig. 12-125). The branching pattern is irregular but angles of

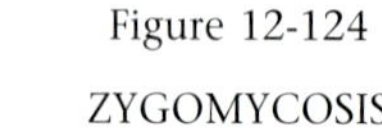

Figure 12-124

ZYGOMYCOSIS

Zygomycosis in a 34-year-old female with endstage renal disease secondary to diabetes mellitus, status postrenal transplant, who became septic. PA chest radiograph demonstrates a right lower lobe consolidation with cavitation (arrow).

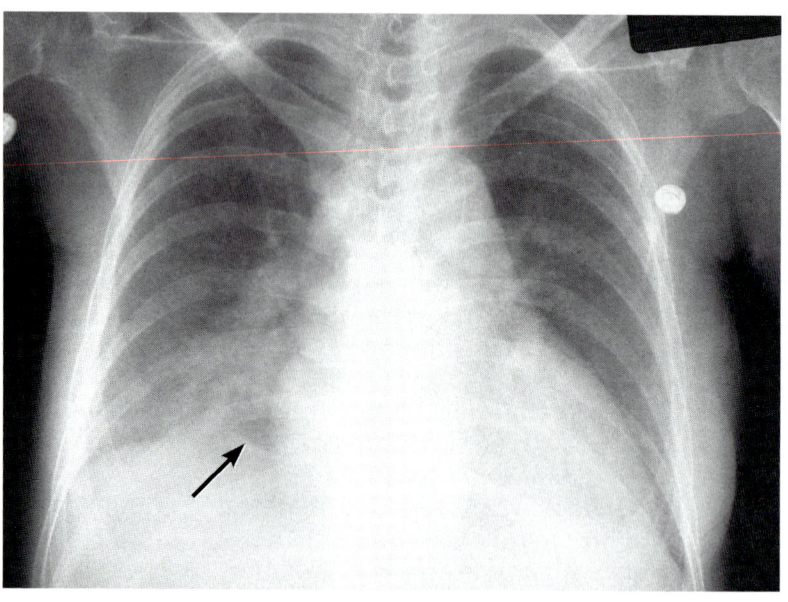

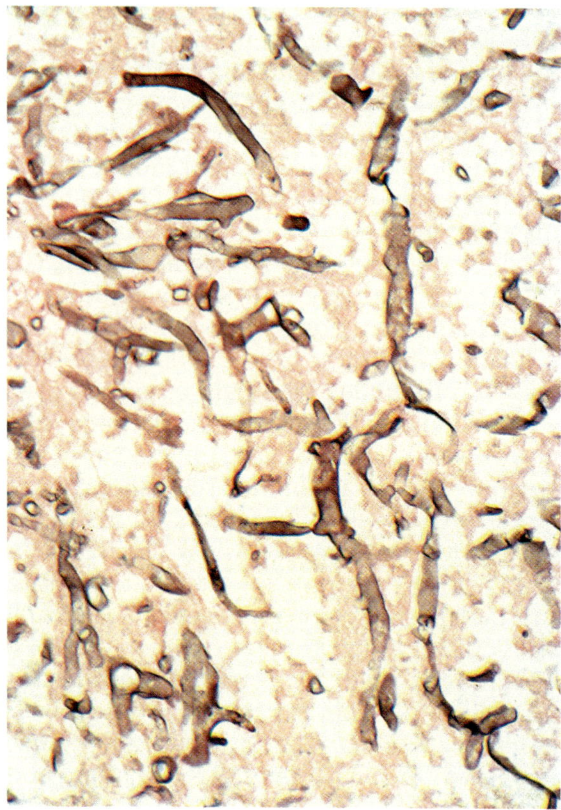

Figure 12-125

ZYGOMYCOSIS: ORGANISM MORPHOLOGY

The hyphae are broad, twisted or folded, and have an irregular branching pattern with some 90° angles.

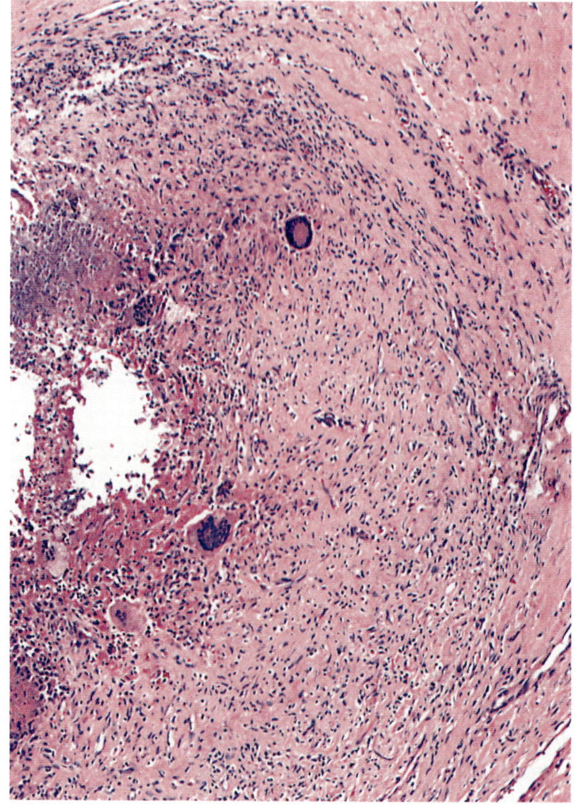

Figure 12-126

ZYGOMYCOSIS: GRANULOMATOUS VASCULITIS IN ANGIOINVASIVE INFECTION

The wall of this artery is thickened by granulomatous inflammation.

90° occur. When cut in cross section, the hyphae often appear round or oval with clear centers. Septation is usually inapparent but is actually inconspicuous. Rarely, chlamydoconidia, which measure 15 to 30 µm, are formed in lesions exposed to ambient air (193,197). These are densely basophilic and PAS positive. They result from local hyperseptation in or at the ends of the hyphae. Following detachment, the thick walled cells form clusters that can appear like yeast-like cells or sporangia. Rarely, sporangia and sporangiospores are seen if the organisms are exposed to ambient air. The separation of the various mucoraceous *Zygomycetes* organisms cannot be achieved in histologic sections and requires cultures (175).

Pulmonary zygomycosis is characterized by invasive growth, especially in blood vessels. This is typically associated with vascular thrombosis and infarcts. Granulomatous vasculitis may be seen (fig. 12-126).

Differential Diagnosis. In most cases it is possible to distinguish between the hyphae of zygomycosis and aspergillosis in tissue sections due to differences in the thickness, uniformity, septation, branching patterns, and orientation of the hyphae (Table 12-11) (193,197). However, it may be difficult, especially if there is crush artifact. The blood vessels within granulation tissue can be mistaken for the hyphae of *Zygomycetes,* however, the vascular walls do not stain with GMS. Culture or immunohistochemical methods are the definitive ways of establishing the diagnosis (175,189,197).

Treatment and Prognosis. Effective therapy of patients with zygomycosis requires a combination of antifungal drugs, surgical intervention, and reversal of the underlying risk factors (237,271).

Candida Sp

Definition. Candidiasis is an infection caused by *Candida* sp.

Candida are common commensal organisms found in the respiratory tract as well as the gastrointestinal and genitourinary tracts. However, they are not pathogens unless the patient becomes immunodeficient and then the organisms invade into the tissues.

There are more than 81 recognized species of *Candida,* but only a small number are pathogenic to humans. The most common is *Candida albicans;* others include *C. tropicalis, C. pseudotropicalis, C. parapsilosis, C. krusei, C. lusitaniae, C. stellatoidea,* and *C. guilliermondii.* There is ongoing debate whether *Torulopsis glabrata* should be classified in the genus *Candida* as *C. glabrata* (191).

Clinical Features. Oropharyngeal candidiasis, or thrush, is a common local infection seen in young infants; patients treated with antibiotics, chemotherapy, or radiation therapy; and those with cellular immune deficiency states, such as AIDS. Patients receiving inhaled corticosteroids for asthma or rhinitis are also subject to this complication. *Candida* esophagitis causes odynophagia or pain on swallowing. Factors that predispose patients to *Candida* pneumonia are summarized in Table 12-12. Pulmonary infection occurs in 50 to 80 percent of patients with disseminated candidiasis (247). The lung may be invaded by hematogenous spread or aspiration from the upper airways.

Table 12-12

FEATURES PREDISPOSING TO *CANDIDA* PNEUMONIA[a]

Hematogenous Pneumonia
Neutropenia
Indwelling intravenous catheter
Extensive abdominal surgery
Intravenous drug use
Intensive adrenocorticosteroid use
Intensive antibiotic therapy
Diabetes mellitus
Total parenteral nutrition
Colonization with *Candida* at multiple sites
Renal Insufficiency
Primary or Aspiration Pneumonia
Debilitation of the newborn
Debilitation of the aged/elderly
Debilitation of chronic disease
Lung transplantation
Congenital Pneumonia
Maternal antibiotic use
Maternal *Candida* vaginitis
Chorioamnionitis
Premature rupture of membranes
Use of cervical sutures

[a]Table 1 from Chu FE, Armstrong D. Candia species pneumonia. In: Sarosi GA, Davies SF, eds. Fungal diseases of the lung, 2nd ed. New York: Raven Press; 1993:1126.

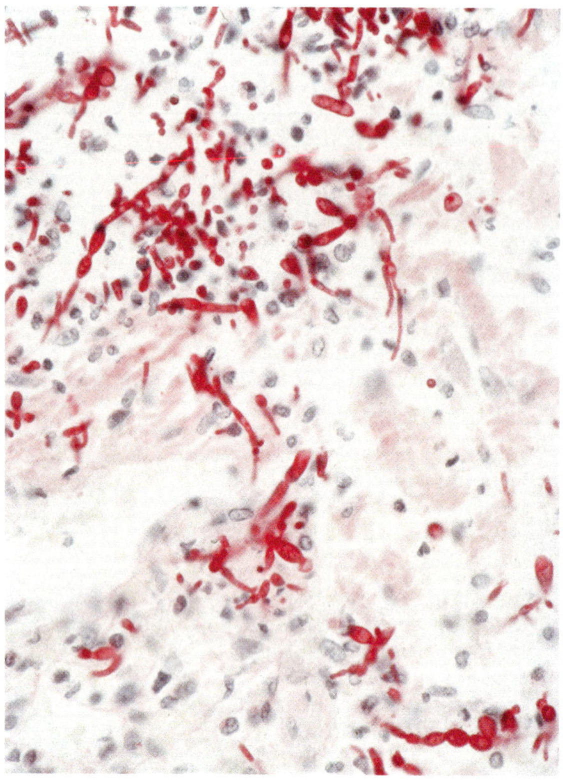

Figure 12-127

CANDIDA: ORGANISM MORPHOLOGY

The organisms consist of pseudohyphae. There are constrictions at the point of attachment between the cells.

Primary candidal pneumonia is unusual but was observed with a frequency of 0.2 and 0.4 percent at autopsy at two major cancer centers (225). Patients usually present with fever and tachypnea (225,249). Immunocompromised hosts and patients in intensive care units are most at risk for the development of nosocomial bloodstream infections (candidemia). *T. glabrata* is typically not a pathogen, but it can cause fulminant fungemia.

Radiologic Findings. Pulmonary candidiasis manifests radiographically with bilateral or unilateral airspace consolidation (215,251). Pulmonary involvement may be lobar, segmental, or patchy. Associated interstitial opacities may occur. Pleural effusion occurs in approximately 25 percent of cases. Cavitation and hilar lymphadenopathy are rarely described. The HRCT features of pulmonary candidiasis include bilateral nodular opacities, bilateral multifocal ground-glass attenuation, and nodules and masses of variable size. The latter may be surrounded by ground-glass attenuation (215,251).

Pathologic Findings. *Candida* sp are oval yeast-like cells that measure 2 to 6 µm in diameter and are accompanied by mycelial forms with pseudohyphae and occasionally true hyphae. The pseudohyphae are elongated yeast-like cells, 3 to 5 µm in width that line up in chains (fig. 12-127); they have constrictions at the attachments between adjacent cells. This differs from the true hyphae that are septate, tubular in shape, 3 to 5 µm in width, and have parallel borders. It is not possible to distinguish the various species of *Candida* by morphology. The organisms stain well with the PAS, GMS, and Gram stains. *T. glabrata* is a spherical to oval yeast measuring 2 to 5 µm. The buds are single and attached by a narrow base to the parent cells. Hyphae and pseudohyphae are not seen.

The tissue response in the lung depends on the route of infection (hematogenous or airway inhalation) and the immune status of the patient. Hematogenous dissemination may result in bilateral, symmetrical, miliary, circumscribed, centrally necrotic nodules that are hemorrhagic at the periphery (figs. 12-128, 12-129). Histologically, these lesions consist of colonies of organisms with associated abscesses oriented around blood vessels (fig. 12-128). Infarcts may occur due to vascular obstruction when organisms grow in the center of the dead tissue (fig. 12-129). Mycotic emboli typically occur in children with indwelling catheters and cause large hemorrhagic infarcts. Patients with massive fungemia may have organisms filling capillaries and spilling over into the surrounding alveolar spaces.

Airway spread of *Candida* from the upper respiratory tract can result in an endobronchial pattern with acute bronchopneumonia (figs. 12-130, 12-131). The small patchy lesions are mostly in the lower lobes. Primary *Candida* pneumonia is characterized histopathologically by bronchopneumonia, hemorrhage, and necrosis (225).

Differential Diagnosis. *Candida* sp are usually readily separated from other fungal yeast forms by the presence of yeast-like cells, pseudohyphae, and true hyphae. They are separated morphologically from *Aspergillus* by the true dichotomous branching in *Aspergillus* at angles of about 45° and the blastoconidia in *Candida* sp (Table 12-11). Cross sections of

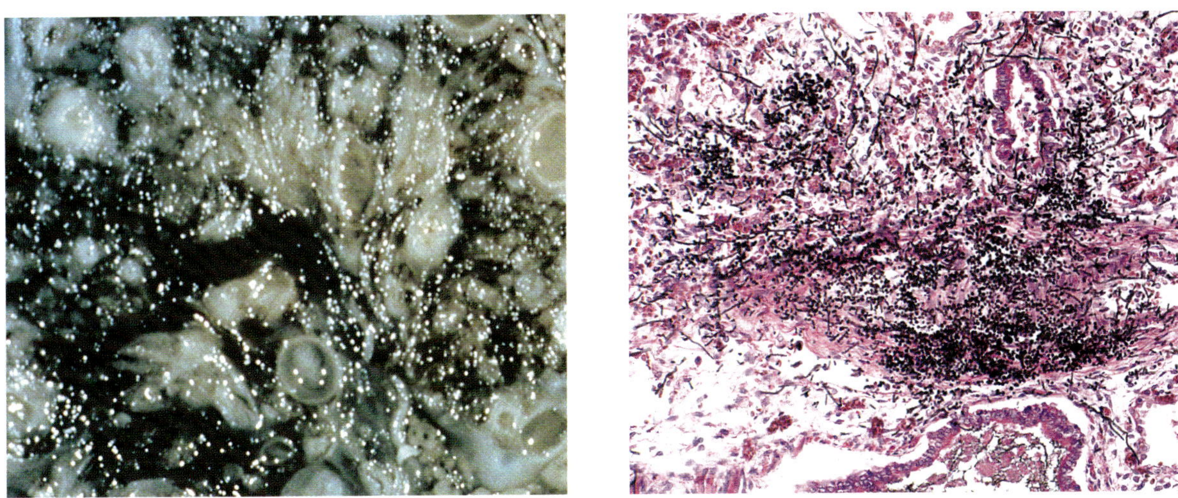

Figure 12-128

CANDIDA: HEMATOGENOUS DISSEMINATION

Left: Gross photograph shows multiple nodular *Candida* abscesses evenly distributed through the lung tissue.

Right: Histology shows colonies of *Candida* centered on blood vessels. There is little inflammatory reaction and no infarction.

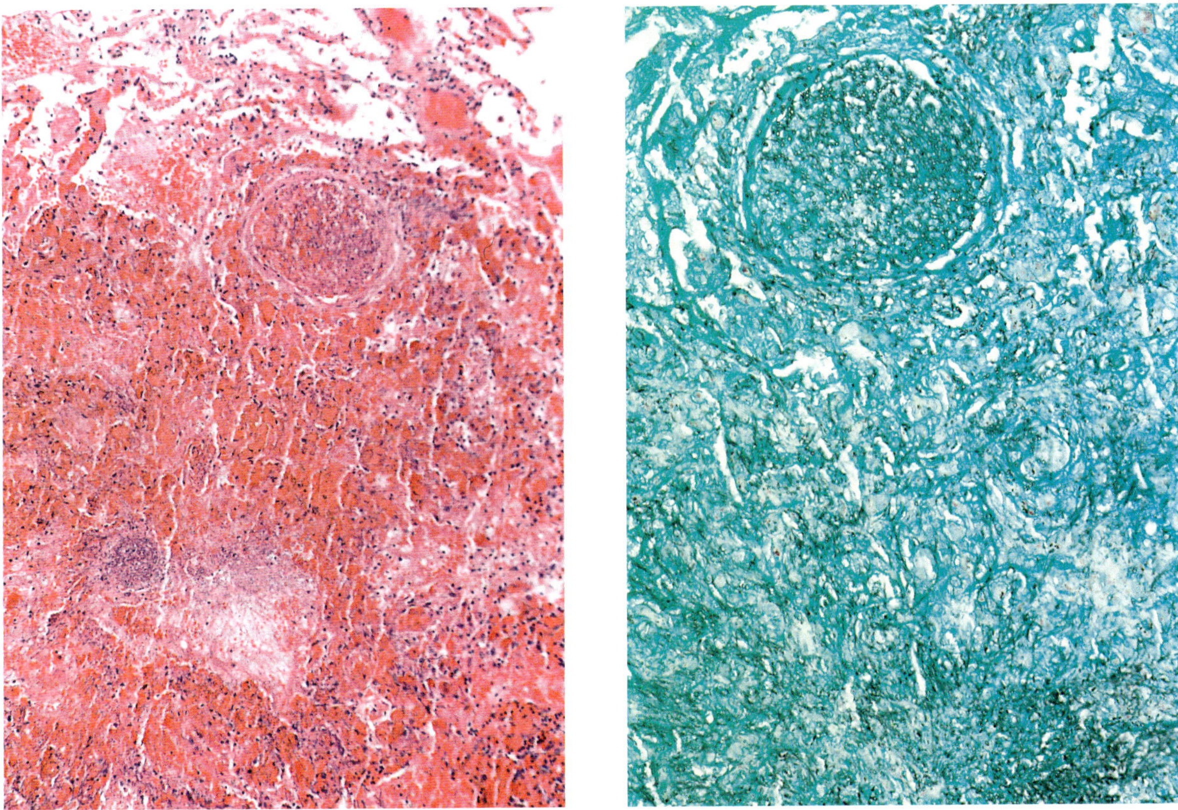

Figure 12-129

CANDIDA: HEMATOGENOUS DISSEMINATION WITH INFARCTION

A hemorrhagic infarct (left) contains fungal pseudohyphae within blood vessels and the infarcted tissue (right, GMS stain).

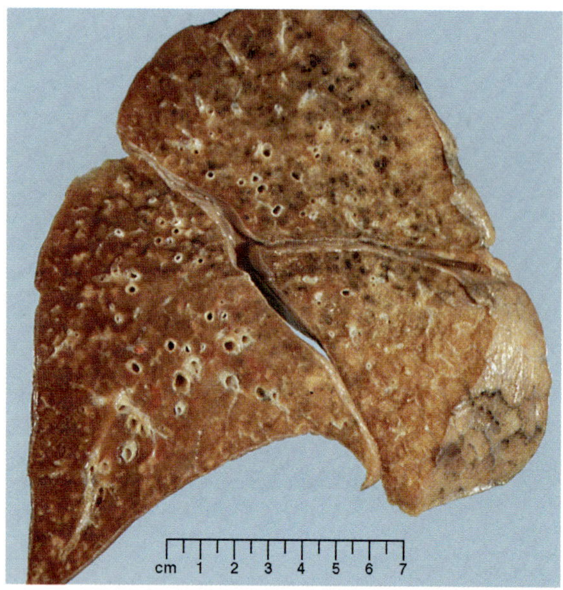

Figure 12-130

CANDIDA: BRONCHOPNEUMONIA

Multiple abscesses are distributed along the airways.

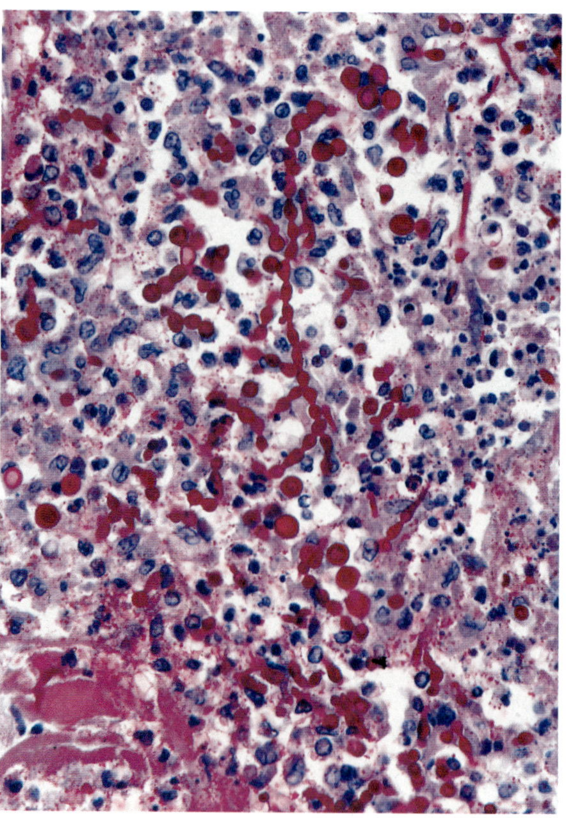

Figure 12-131

CANDIDA: BRONCHOPNEUMONIA, ABSCESS

Candida pseudohyphae stain with the PAS stain and are surrounded by numerous neutrophils within an abscess.

Aspergillus hyphae are hollow and should not be confused with the yeast forms of *Candida* sp.

The most difficult distinction to make is with *Trichosporon* sp, which also consists of yeast-like cells and mycelial elements. However, the average diameter of *Trichosporon* is 5.0 µm rather than 2.5 µm and the yeast form is more pleomorphic. The pseudohyphae of *Trichosporon* are narrow and not as well formed as they are in *Candida*. *Trichosporon* also show radial growth and arthroconidia (247).

Rarely, *Candida* sp show very few pseudohyphae and overlap morphologically with *Histoplasma capsulatum.* If only yeast cells are present and no pseudohyphae, it may be impossible to distinguish the two. However, the yeast forms of *Candida* are much easier to appreciate on H&E-stained sections than the yeast forms of *H. capsulatum* and they stain with tissue Gram stains. Examination of additional sections may be helpful in such cases (247). Another clue is the intracellular location of organisms, which is characteristic of *H. capsulatum* but not *Candida* sp.

Immunohistochemistry can be used to detect *Candida* sp in tissue sections.

Treatment. The treatment of patients with *Candida* sp pulmonary infection requires antifungal agents. In addition to amphotericin B, fluorocytosine and a variety of azole agents have been found to be effective.

Sporothrix Schenckii

Definition. Sporotrichosis is a chronic infection caused by the dimorphic fungus, *Sporothrix schenckii* (219,265).

S. schenckii is found worldwide in climates ranging from temperate to tropical and in a variety of environmental areas including sphagnum moss, decaying wood and other vegetation, hay, and soil. Infection usually occurs as a result of cutaneous injury due to thorns, barbs, straws, or splinters that are contaminated from exposure to soil or plant material. An uncommon risk factor for infection is exposure to animals that are either infected or able to passively transfer the organism from soil through scratching or biting. Most cases are reported from the Americas and Japan. Most outbreaks in the United States have been traced to the Wisconsin sphagnum moss. The disease appears to be endemic in at least one remote area of Peru, with an incidence of 48 to 60 cases/100,000 people and approximately 1 case/1,000 children 7 to 14 years of age (258).

Sporotrichosis most commonly affects the skin, subcutaneous tissues, and lymphatics. However, rarely it disseminates to involve the bones, lungs, meninges, and gastrointestinal tract (193,196,207).

Clinical Features. Inhalation of *S. schenckii* from soil is the presumed method of transmission leading to pulmonary sporotrichosis. Most patients have been involved in an occupation that exposes them to aerosols from soil. Sporotrichosis is associated with alcoholism, diabetes mellitus, chronic obstructive pulmonary disease, and AIDS. The symptoms mimic those of tuberculosis including dyspnea, cough, purulent sputum, hemoptysis, fever, night sweats, weight loss, and fatigue (207,220).

Radiologic Findings. The radiologic manifestations of sporotrichosis are similar to those of postprimary tuberculosis (fig. 12-132) (215): parenchymal nodules or masses, which may undergo cavitation, and diffuse reticular and nodular opacities. Hilar and mediastinal lymphadenopathy may occur in association with pulmonary disease or in isolation. There may be transgression of tissue planes with pleural and chest wall involvement and the formation of sinus tracts (215).

Pathologic Findings. The yeast cells of *S. schenckii* may be very difficult to identify in tissue sections since they tend to be rare and do not stain very well (193,196). They are round, oval, or cigar shaped. Most measure 2 to 6 µm in diameter but they can be up to 10 µm (fig. 12-133). The buds appear elongated or "teardrop" in shape, or they have narrow-based attachments with a "pipe-stem" appearance (fig. 12-133) (193, 196,213). Rarely, asteroid bodies are seen in the lung: the *S. schenckii* cells are surrounded by an eosinophilic Splendore-Hoeppli phenomenon that has a stellate appearance and can measure up to 100 µm. These asteroid bodies are not specific for *S. schenckii* since a similar Splendore-Hoeppli phenomenon can be seen with a variety of other organisms and foreign bodies.

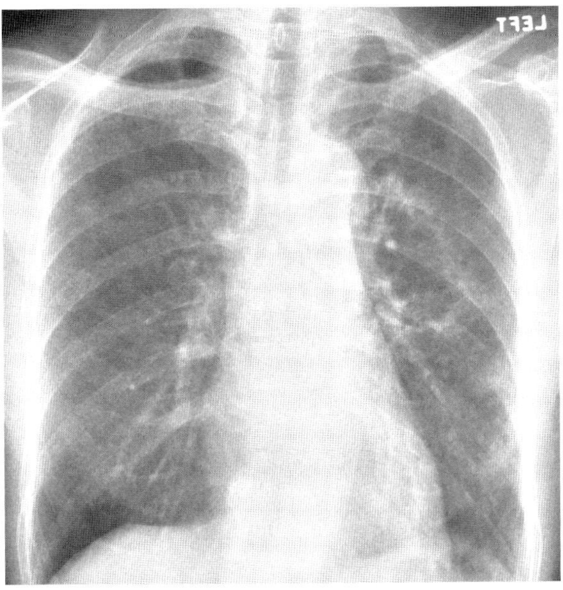

Figure 12-132

SPOROTRICHOSIS IN A 56-YEAR-OLD MALE WITH SPORADIC HEMOPTYSIS

PA chest radiograph demonstrates a large thin-walled cavity in the superior segment of the left lower lobe. Cultures recovered *Sporothrix* and *Candida*.

Differential Diagnosis. The organisms of *S. schenckii* are relatively small and can be confused with those of fungal yeast such as *Histoplasma capsulatum* (193,196,213). However, the elongated, cigar-shaped morphology is not seen in *H. capsulatum*. *S. schenckii* may also be confused with Hamazaki-Wesenberg bodies, which also have an elongated cigar-shaped morphology. These are elliptical bodies seen in the lymph nodes of patients with sarcoidosis. In contrast to *S. schenckii*, they have a yellow-brown pigmentation, lack budding, and usually are smaller (193, 196,213). Grossly, sporotrichosis causes nodular areas of consolidation. The histologic reaction varies from an acute suppurative pneumonia to a necrotizing granulomatous pneumonia.

Treatment and Prognosis. Pulmonary sporotrichosis is difficult to treat due to delayed diagnosis or the underlying illnesses in infected patients. Seriously ill patients require treatment with amphotericin B followed by itraconazole. Surgical resection has proven useful for those patients who have focal lesions and adequate lung function.

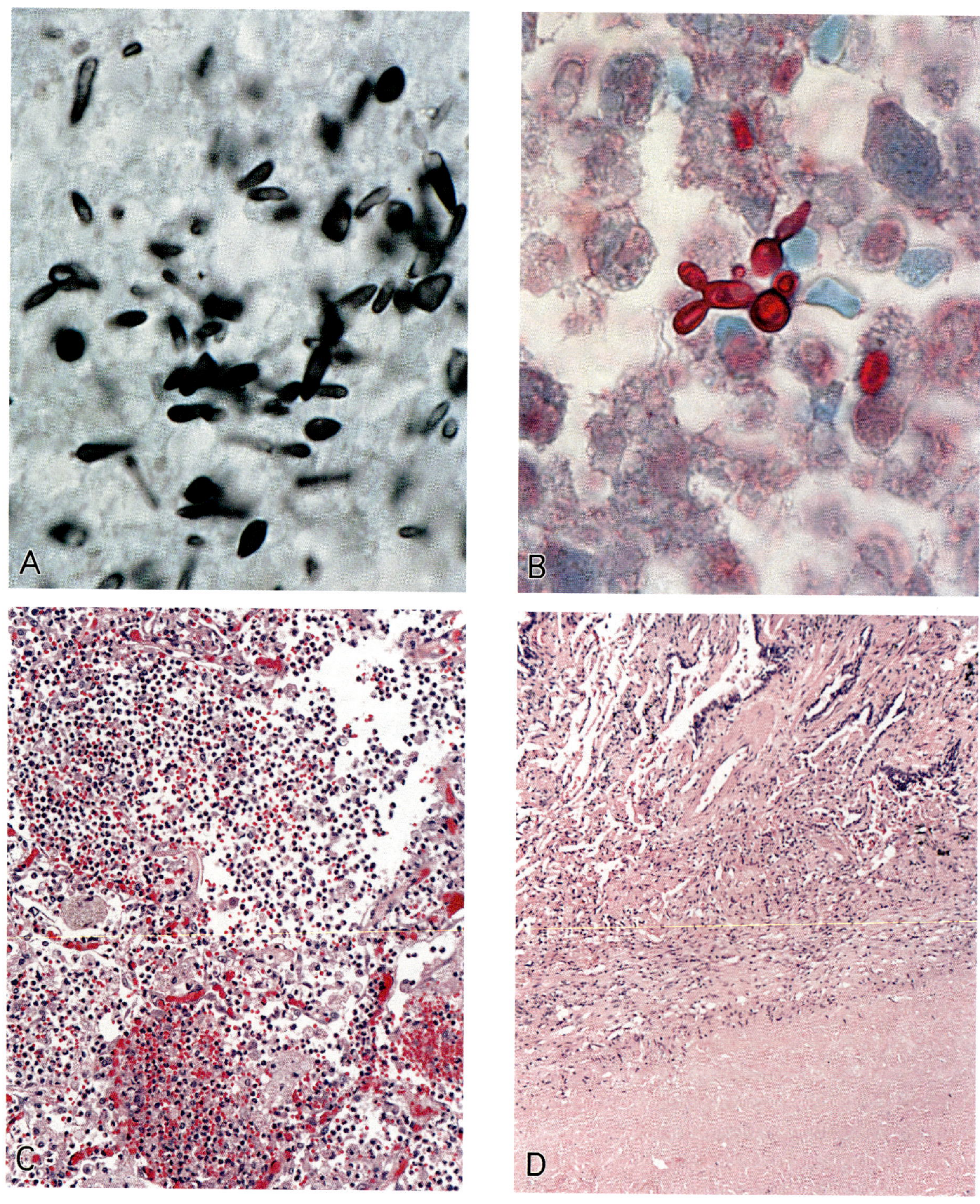

Figure 12-133

SPOROTRICHOSIS

A: The yeast are round, oval, and cigar shaped (GMS stain).
B: The buds appear elongated or "teardrop" in shape (PAS stain).
C: This case consists of a suppurative pneumonia with numerous neutrophils forming microabscesses.
D: Necrotizing granulomatous inflammation characterizes this case.

Fusarium Sp

Definition. Fusariosis is a mycosis caused by *Fusarium* sp, which are ubiquitous soil saprophytes that rarely cause pulmonary infection.

There are three major pathogens including *F. moniliforme, F. oxysporum,* and *F. solani* (294).

Clinical Features. *Fusarium* infection of the lung takes the form of pneumonia, allergic bronchopulmonary fungal disease (179,275), or pulmonary mycotoxicosis (202,263,294). Invasive pulmonary infection usually occurs in immunocompromised patients, particularly in the setting of hematologic malignancies or lung transplantation (178,187,276).

Pathologic Findings. The hyphae of *Fusarium* sp are septate, branched, 3 to 8 µm in diameter, and haphazardly arranged. They typically show 90° angle branching, but may also show the same 45° angle branching as *Aspergillus* sp. Constrictions may be seen at the point of branching from parent hyphae. In invasive infections, the hyphae may appear varicose and terminal (intercalated) chlamydoconidia can be seen.

Differential Diagnosis. A variety of morphologic features may be used to separate *Fusarium* sp and *Aspergillus* sp including hyaline septate hyphae and characteristic reproductive structures known as phialides and phialoconidia (244). However, the degree of morphologic overlap is considerable (193,294). Definitive diagnosis requires cultures or immunohistochemistry (189,234,264,276).

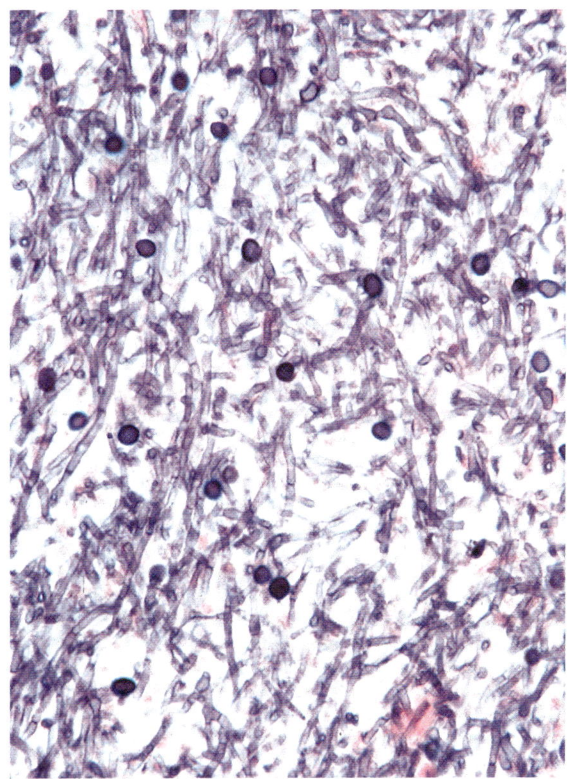

Figure 12-134

PSEUDOALLESCHERIA BOYDII: ORGANISM MORPHOLOGY

The hyphae are septate and have ovoid brown conidia situated terminally or laterally on short conidiophores. (Figure 1 from Travis LB, Roberts GD, Wilson WR. Clinical significance of Pseudoallescheria boydii: a review of 10-years' experience. Mayo Clin Proc 1985;60:531–7.)

Pseudoallescheria Boydii

Definition. Pulmonary pseudoallescheriasis is a pulmonary infection caused by *Pseudoallescheria boydii.*

Clinical Features. *P. boydii* lung infection typically occurs in immunosuppressed patients (207,215,278,288,291). Rarely, it can be associated with allergic bronchopulmonary fungal disease (253).

Radiologic Findings. The radiologic manifestations resemble those of aspergillosis. They include mycetoma, bronchiectasis (in patients with atopy), and nodular opacities, which may exhibit cavitation (215).

Pathologic Findings. *P. boydii* hyphae are septate and branching, however, the pattern is more haphazard than that of *Aspergillus*. The hyphae are narrow, measuring 2 to 5 µm in diameter (fig. 12-134). There may be ovoid, brown conidia of 5 to 10 µm that are present terminally or laterally on short conidiophores. These conidia are seen most often around pulmonary fungus balls.

Differential Diagnosis. In most cases, it is very difficult to distinguish *P. boydii* from *Aspergillus*. However, the presence of conidia is helpful. Otherwise, definitive diagnosis requires culture, immunohistochemistry, or direct immunofluorescence (232,234).

Treatment and Prognosis. *P. boydii* is best treated with miconazole rather than amphotericin B. Ketoconazole and itraconazole are also effective (207).

Chrysosporium Parvum

Definition. Adiaspiromycosis is a pulmonary mycosis caused by *Chrysosporium parvum* var *crescens*.

Adiaspiromycosis is a nonarthropod-transmitted fungal infection that occurs worldwide in lower vertebrates, especially rodents, but usually does not cause infection in humans. Humans may become accidental hosts by inhaling dust-borne spores (conidia) of saprophytic soil fungi. The inhaled fungal spore never germinates in the host but enlarges in size and forms an adiaspore (290).

Clinical Features. Pulmonary adiaspiromycosis can take the form of a solitary granuloma or disseminated infection. Solitary granulomas are usually incidental findings in asymptomatic patients. Disseminated pulmonary adiaspiromycosis is a self-limited infection that can be sparsely or densely nodular. The former is usually asymptomatic and the latter causes progressive dyspnea. Patients with pulmonary involvement complain of cough, dyspnea, and low-grade fever, symptoms that mimic other systemic fungal infections and tuberculosis (290).

Radiologic Findings. Patients with lung disease exhibit diffuse reticular and nodular opacities, which may mimic the appearance of miliary tuberculosis (215).

Pathologic Findings. The lung can show either solitary or multiple nodules, which represent granulomas. The granulomas measure 0.5 to 2.0 mm and are well circumscribed (206,212,292).

C. parvum var *crescens* is a dimorphic fungus in which the small, 2 to 4 µm conidia are inhaled. They progressively enlarge to thick-walled adiaconidia that grow to 200 to 400 µm in diameter (fig. 12-135) (206,212,292). The adiaconidia have refractile walls, 20 to 70 µm in thickness. The outer third of the wall is eosinophilic and refractile (fig. 12-135C). There is a nonstaining fenestrated layer. The inner two thirds of the wall is hyaline and chitinous (fig. 12-135C). The GMS stain decorates the entire wall and highlights the nonstaining fenestrae. The organism does not replicate in human tissues.

The tissue response to *C. parvum* var *crescens* consists of granulomatous inflammation and fibrosis (fig. 12-135) (206,212,292).

Differential Diagnosis. The differential diagnosis includes coccidioidomycosis and lentil pneumonia (206,212,292). *Coccidioides immitis* has a smaller spherule size, which only rarely reaches 200 µm; it has a much thinner wall thickness of 1 to 2 µm; and it has 2 to 5 µm endospores that are lacking in adiaspiromycosis. Lentil pneumonia consists of starch granules of vegetable matter.

Treatment and Prognosis. In non-AIDS patients, lung involvement may regress spontaneously, persist, or progress. Treatment includes azoles or amphotericin B; ketoconazole has also been used with success (290).

Malassezia Furfur

Definition. Malasseziasis is an infection caused by the yeast, *Malassezia furfur. M. furfur* is a dimorphic fungus with hyphal and yeast forms in the skin but in deep organs such as the lung it grows as a yeast.

M. furfur was previously called *Pityrosporum orbicularis* and *P. ovale* (269,283). It is commonly associated with the dermatophytosis pityriasis or tinea versicolor. Rarely, *M. furfur* causes deep infection, particularly in association with intralipid therapy, due to its growth requirement for exogenous lipid (269,283).

Clinical Features. Patients presenting with systemic disseminated *M. furfur* infection are typically totally dependent on parenteral nutrition using Intralipid and have an indwelling central venous catheter (269,283). The central venous catheter becomes colonized and occluded with *M. furfur.* These patients have a variety of associations including avitaminosis, steroid therapy, tropical environment, and possible genetic predisposition (269,283). Infants of low birth weight and adults with severe gastrointestinal disease are affected. Therapy with broad-spectrum antibiotics may render patients susceptible to *M. furfur* by altering normal bacterial flora (269,283).

Radiologic Findings. Chest radiographic features include consolidation that is either within a single lobe or diffuse throughout one lung, localized patchy or streaky opacities, or bilateral consolidation progressing to opacification (269,283).

Pathologic Findings. In deep tissues such as in the lung, the organisms consist of yeast cells that are round to oval and measure 2 to 5 µm in diameter (fig. 12-136). The pattern of budding is distinctive: unipolar with a broad

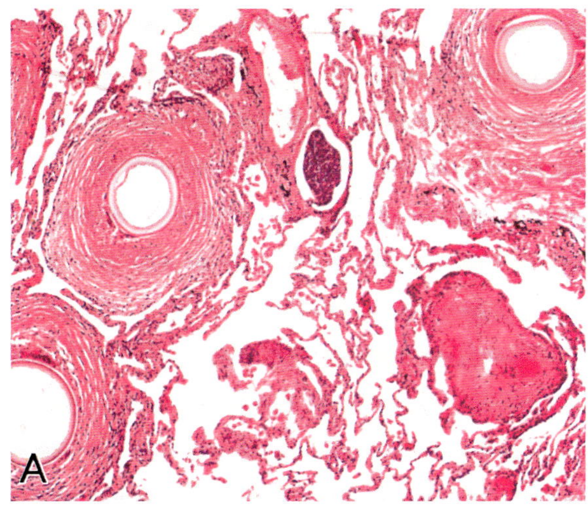

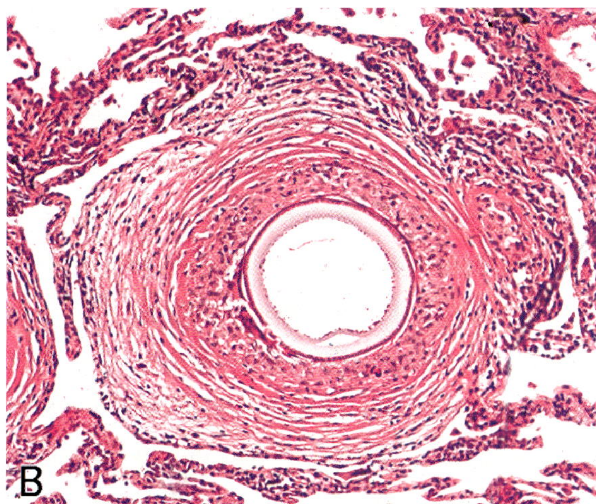

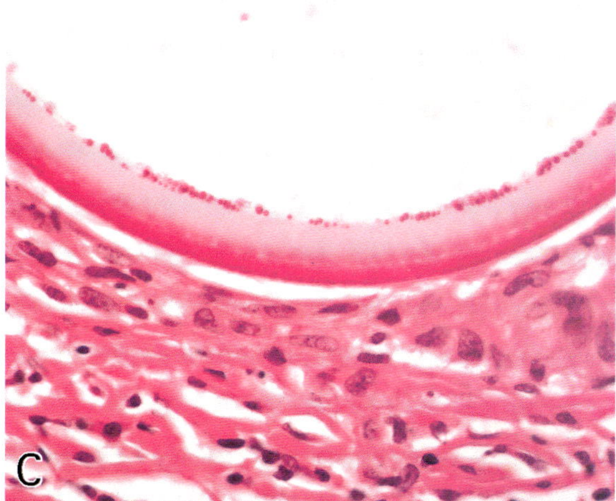

Figure 12-135

ADIASPIROMYCOSIS: ORGANISM MORPHOLOGY

A: The adiaconidia are large, measuring 200 to 400 μm in diameter.

B: They are surrounded by concentric fibrosis.

C: The outer third of the wall is eosinophilic and the inner layer is hyaline and chitinous.

base and extrusion of the daughter bud through a scar collarette at the site of previous budding. The organisms stain with GMS, PAS, Brown and Brenn, and Brown and Hopps stains, but they are only faintly visible with H&E stains. By electron microscopy the organisms have a characteristic thick wall with corrugations along the inner surface and the collarette shows a circumferential thickening of the wall.

Pulmonary infections include mycotic thromboemboli, pneumonia, infarcts, and vasculitis (fig. 12-137) (269,272,283). Target thrombi consist of rings of fungus alternating with layers of thrombus (283). In the lung, the organisms are usually identified within small to medium-sized pulmonary arteries, sometimes in association with lipid that can be confirmed with oil red O stains (269,283). Vasculitis is common (fig. 12-137). The lung may also show features

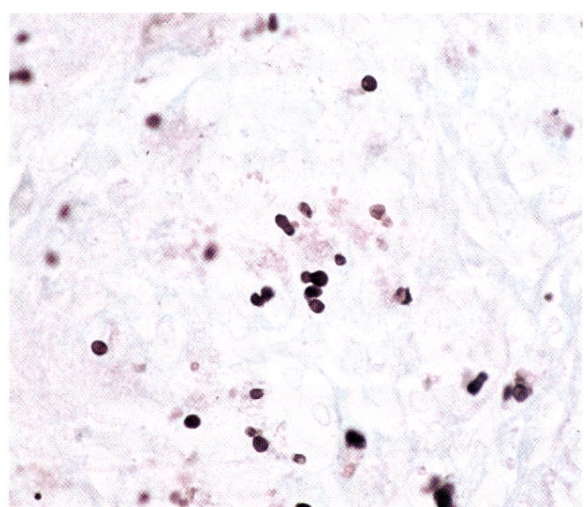

Figure 12-136

MALASSEZIA FURFUR: ORGANISM MORPHOLOGY

The organisms consist of multiple budding yeast.

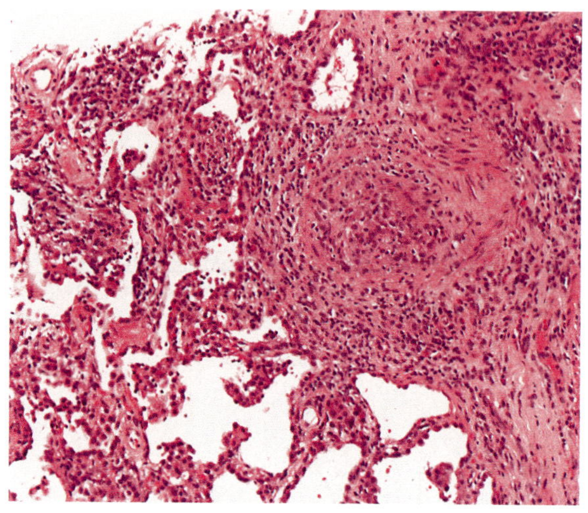

Figure 12-137

MALASSEZIA FURFUR: VASCULITIS

There is marked interstitial inflammation and vasculitis causing severe narrowing of an arteriole (top right).

of underlying disease such as bronchopulmonary dysplasia (269,283).

Disseminated infection occurs rarely. It may cause acute meningitis, necrotizing encephalitis, and interstitial nephritis (281,283).

Differential Diagnosis. The clinical setting and distinctive organism morphology, with frequent intravascular location or mycotic thromboemboli, usually allow for recognition of the diagnosis (283). Morphologically, *M. furfur* must be distinguished from *Histoplasma capsulatum, Cryptococcus neoformans,* and *Candida* sp. While the size is similar to *H. capsulatum,* the latter has much narrower neck budding. *C. neoformans* has a much wider spectrum of yeast size (2 to 10 µm) and also has narrower neck budding. *Candida* sp usually have hyphae, pseudohyphae, and yeast forms and they lack unipolar budding (283).

Treatment and Prognosis. Patients with *M. furfur* are treated with amphotericin B or 5-fluorocytosine. Since this infection is probably underdiagnosed, it should be considered in patients receiving Intralipid therapy when they develop systemic infections (269,283).

VIRAL INFECTIONS

Viral infections are the most common pulmonary infections in man. The viruses discussed in this chapter are listed in Table 12-13.

Table 12-13

VIRAL INFECTIONS IN THE LUNG

Cytomegalovirus
Herpes simplex
Varicella-zoster
Adenovirus
Respiratory syncytial virus
Measles
Parainfluenza virus
Influenza
Hantavirus

The common cold is the most frequent pulmonary infection and viruses such as influenza are a worldwide cause of significant mortality and morbidity (352,434). Although viral respiratory infections are common, they are infrequent problems for the anatomic pathologist since few patients have lung biopsy or autopsy. Nevertheless, the pathologist plays an important role in assessing viral cultures and other special studies performed to establish the diagnosis (352). Only certain viruses cause cytopathic changes that are morphologically distinctive enough to enable the pathologist to recognize a specific diagnosis on routine histologic examination of lung specimens. With the availability of special diagnostic techniques, such as immunohistochemistry, in situ hybridization, and polymerase chain reaction (PCR) testing, many viruses can be detected in formalin-fixed, paraffin-embedded tissue samples even if specific viral inclusions cannot be found in histologic examination of tissue sections. While fresh or frozen tissue samples are optimal for some techniques, recent more sophisticated techniques have allowed for more to be done with formalin-fixed paraffin-embedded tissue samples (352).

Some viruses primarily infect the respiratory tract while others involve the lung while causing a systemic infection (352). The classification of viruses is based on the type of nucleic acid, the properties of the viral structural proteins, and whether or not there is a lipid-containing envelope surrounding the virus particle. The latter issue is important since viruses with an envelope, such as influenza and coronavirus, are prevalent during midwinter periods of relatively low indoor humidity while the viruses lacking an envelope are more common during the spring-summer and autumn when humidity is higher (352).

Cytomegalovirus

Definition. Cytomegalovirus pneumonia is an infection of the lung caused by cytomegalovirus (CMV).

CMV is the most common viral organism causing pneumonia that can be recognized by the anatomic pathologist based on the characteristic cytopathic changes in histologic sections. It is a herpesvirus with a double-stranded DNA and an icosahedral capsid that contains 162 capsomeres. The virus measures 120 to 200 nm and has an envelope that is derived from the nuclear membrane. The DNA of CMV contains the genetic information to approximately 33 structural proteins. CMV replicates in the host cell nucleus.

Clinical Features. CMV causes many types of infection including congenital and perinatal infections, hepatitis, infectious mononucleosis, post-transfusion infection, and opportunistic infection in transplant patients, those receiving immunosuppressive therapy for cancer or immunologic disease, and those with AIDS and other immunodeficiencies (352). Disseminated CMV infection causes fever, leukopenia, thrombocytopenia, pneumonitis, hepatitis, adrenalitis, and encephalitis (434). Clinical manifestations include sustained fever, nonproductive cough, and shortness of breath (352). Physical exam reveals rales. Severe hypoxemia tends to correlate with poor outcome (352).

The diagnosis of CMV pneumonia is based on culture or pathologic evaluation of lung biopsies or bronchoalveolar lavage (BAL) specimens (352). One cannot be sure that CMV is a pulmonary pathogen based on finding it in urine, blood, or respiratory secretions, which only indicates the presence of CMV organisms (352). Serologic signs of CMV infection are inadequate for a diagnosis of CMV pneumonia (352).

Radiologic Findings. The main radiographic manifestation of pulmonary infection by CMV is bilateral nodular or reticular interstitial opacities (fig. 12-138). Ground-glass opacities have also been described. Airspace consolidation and unilateral consolidation occur less frequently (402). Hilar and mediastinal lymphadenopathy are rare. Cavitation and cyst formation have been reported, but rarely occur (402). Pleural effusions occur in 10 to 33 percent of patients and constitute the most common associated finding (401,402).

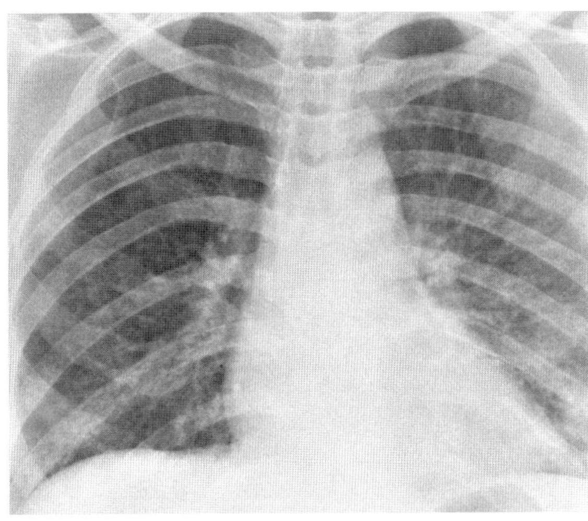

Figure 12-138

CYTOMEGALOVIRUS

CMV infection in a 22-year-old female with systemic lupus erythematosus who developed fever, chills, and myalgias. PA chest radiograph demonstrates diffuse, bilateral, fine reticular and nodular opacities.

In patients with mixed infections there may be additional, and at times confusing, radiologic findings (430). Also, patients with documented infection may have normal radiographs (348).

HRCT studies of transplant recipients who develop CMV pneumonia show micronodules, consolidation, ground-glass opacities, and irregular reticular opacities. Patients with AIDS and CMV infection may exhibit a different pattern of involvement, with nodules and masses that measure between 1 and 3 cm. Bronchiectasis and bronchial wall thickening have also been described in this population (361).

Pathologic Findings. There are four major patterns of CMV infection of the lung (318, 320,370,434): a miliary pattern (fig. 12-39), diffuse interstitial pneumonitis (fig. 12-40), hemorrhagic pneumonia, and CMV inclusions associated with minimal inflammation or lung injury (134). The miliary pattern is thought to

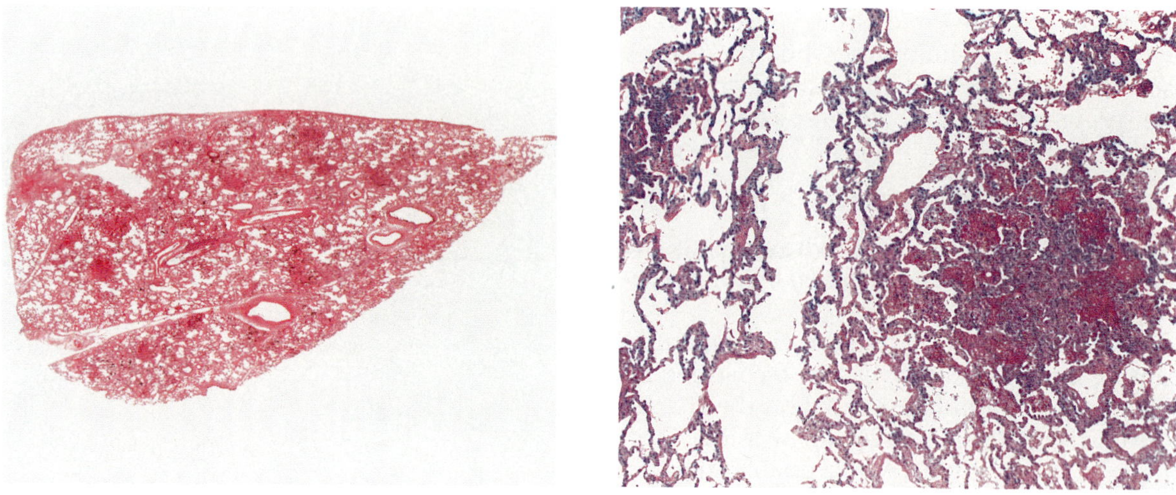

Figure 12-139

CYTOMEGALOVIRUS PNEUMONIA: MILIARY PATTERN

Left: There are multiple nodular inflammatory foci evenly distributed throughout the lung.
Right: This nodule consists of acute and chronic inflammation with alveolar fibrin.

result from hematogenous spread and it shows multicentric lesions that consist of alveolar exudation by fibrin, inflammatory cells, neutrophils, and chronic inflammatory cells (fig. 12-139). Centrally, these lesions may show necrosis, hemorrhage, alveolar fibrin, and inflammatory cells. CMV inclusions are found in these nodular lesions. The diffuse interstitial pneumonitis can range from mild to a pattern of diffuse alveolar damage (fig. 12-140A). The mild interstitial pneumonitis may consist of interstitial chronic inflammation with varying amounts of pneumocyte hyperplasia and alveolar macrophage accumulation. Depending on the phase of diffuse alveolar damage present, one may see a spectrum of interstitial edema, alveolar fibrin, and hyaline membranes, or interstitial fibroblastic proliferation and type 2 pneumocyte hyperplasia. The number of CMV inclusions vary from a few, which may require a careful search for identification, to numerous. In the former, it may be difficult to assess whether the CMV is actually a pulmonary pathogen. If there are isolated CMV viral inclusions, but little or no histologic reaction, one may question whether these findings represent an incidental histologic finding of little clinical significance (318,320,370,434). Rarely, CMV manifests as a single pulmonary nodule (398). CMV infection of pulmonary endothelial cells has been speculated as a possible cause of pulmonary hypertension in an AIDS patient (410).

CMV can infect a wide variety of cell types and in the lung this includes epithelial cells of the airways and alveoli, fibroblasts, macrophages, and endothelial cells (378). The cytopathic effects of CMV include both nuclear and cytoplasmic inclusions. Infected cells show cytomegaly or marked enlargement (fig. 12-140B). The nuclear inclusion is single, measuring up to 20 µm in diameter, while the cytoplasmic inclusions are much smaller, measuring 1 to 3 µm. The nuclear inclusion is usually basophilic but may be eosinophilic. It is round to oval, with a peripheral halo and accentuation of the nuclear membrane. At the edge of the viral inclusion, a rounded clump of peripheral chromatin may be seen extending into the clear region of the halo. The cytoplasmic inclusions are basophilic to amphophilic and indistinct (fig. 12-140B). They may not be present in all cells. These stain with the PAS and GMS stains. The intranuclear inclusions are Feulgen positive and contain viral nuclear, protein, and capsid material (344, 434). The cytoplasmic inclusions are composed of variable amounts of virions or cytoplasmic components such as endoplasmic reticulum, dense bodies, mitochondria, and lysosomes

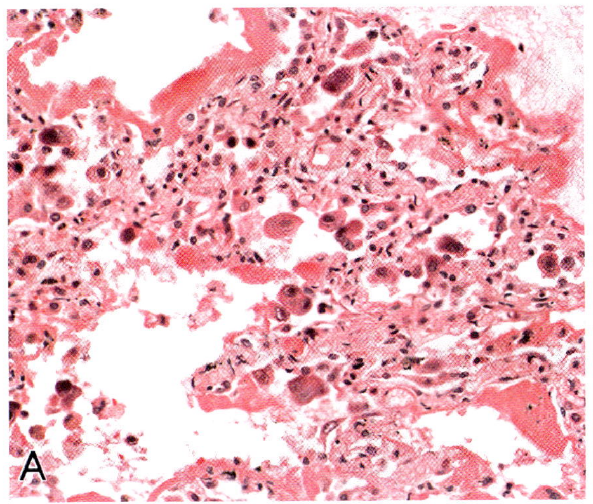

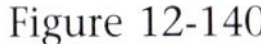

Figure 12-140

CYTOMEGALOVIRUS PNEUMONIA WITH DIFFUSE ALVEOLAR DAMAGE (DAD)

A: The lung shows a DAD pattern in association with numerous basophilic CMV inclusions.

B: Cytopathic changes include cytomegaly, multiple small basophilic cytoplasmic inclusions, and a large nuclear inclusion surrounded by a halo with a thickened nuclear membrane.

C: Immunohistochemistry for CMV shows staining of the nuclear and cytoplasmic inclusions. Immunohistochemistry highlighted many more organisms in this case than were appreciated by examination of the H&E-stained sections.

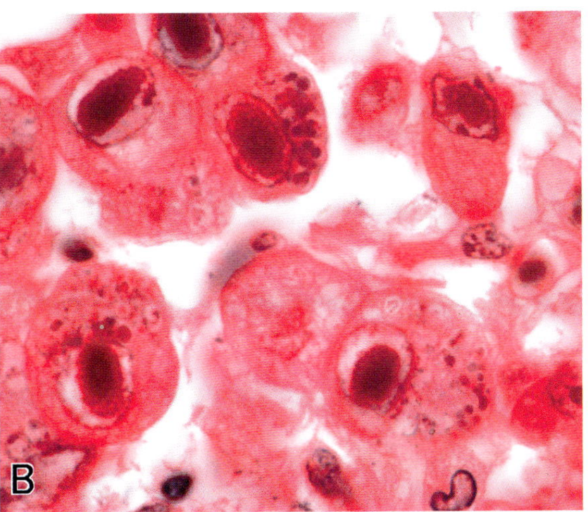

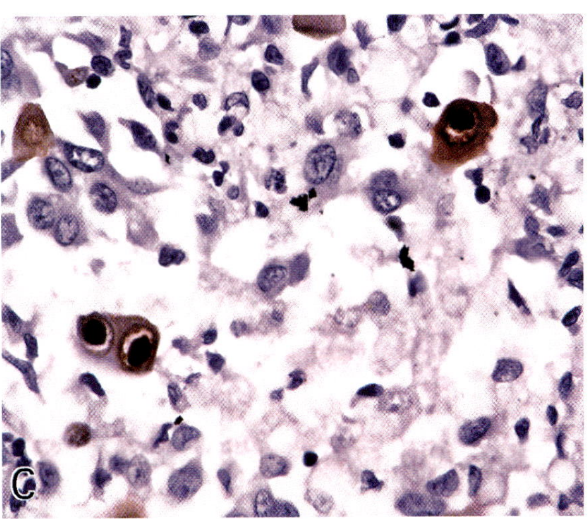

(344,434). Following Ganciclovir therapy, the intranuclear inclusion of CMV has been reported to have a globular and eosinophilic appearance due to loss of viral DNA (356).

If characteristic CMV inclusions are present in the setting of an appropriate histologic reaction, the diagnosis of CMV pneumonia is established with certainty even in the absence of culture or special techniques. However, there are cases in which the inclusions are not easy to recognize or few in number and it is helpful to perform either immunohistochemical staining (fig. 12-140C) or in situ hybridization as a diagnostic aid (305,308,314,315,340, 341,358). Immunohistochemistry (fig. 12-140C) may be easier to interpret than in situ hybridization since it is possible to distinguish the cellular morphology and cytopathic effects as well as the staining results (419,427).

Since CMV pneumonia frequently occurs in immunocompromised patients, one must search for additional infectious agents that might be present. The association with *Pneumocystis carinii* pneumonia is particularly frequent in AIDS patients. Special techniques help to confirm the presence of multiple organisms, especially if more than one virus is present (399,427).

Differential Diagnosis. The differential diagnosis of CMV pneumonia is approached from the histologic reaction to the organism or the morphology of the cytopathic effects. Miliary inflammatory lesions, diffuse alveolar damage, and interstitial pneumonitis can occur with other viruses or infectious agents, but

Table 12-14

HISTOLOGIC AND ULTRASTRUCTURAL FEATURES OF VIRUSES CAUSING PNEUMONIA[a]

Virus	Inclusions (Nuclear/ Cytoplasmic)	Cellular Changes	Tissue Reaction	Ultrastructural Features
Cytomegalovirus	Yes/Yes	Cytomegaly	Interstitial pneumonia, DAD[b]	Particle: 120-200 nm with round core, double membrane
Herpes simplex/ Varicella-zoster	Yes/No	Rare multinucleation	DAD, necrosis	Particle: 150-200 nm with round core, double membrane
Measles	Yes/Yes	Multinucleation	Interstitial pneumonia, DAD	Particle: 120-150 nm, spherical inclusion: 15-20 tubular filaments
Adenovirus	Yes/No	Smudge cells	Necrotizing bronchiolitis, DAD	Particle: 60-90 nm icosahedral particles in crystalline array
Influenza	No/No	None	DAD, necrotizing bronchiolitis, organizing pneumonia	Particle: 80-120 nm, round, oval, or elongated
Respiratory syncytial virus	No/Yes	Occasional multinucleation	Necrotizing bronchiolitis, organizing pneumonia	Particle: 120-300 nm, numerous 12-nm spikes of glycoprotein
Parainfluenza virus	No/Yes	Occasional multinucleation	DAD, interstitial pneumonia	Particle: 150-250 nm, more pleomorphic than influenza
Hantavirus	No/No	None	Edema, early DAD	Particle: 70-120 nm, spherical to oval, granular and filamentous inclusions

[a]From references 362, 364, 370, 433, 441, 442.
[b]DAD = diffuse alveolar damage.

they lack the CMV inclusion cells. Cytologic atypia of pneumocytes in the setting of diffuse alveolar damage can be confused with viral cytopathic changes, including those of CMV. CMV inclusions must be separated from the other types of viral inclusions such as those of herpesvirus, adenovirus, and measles. In most of these cases this separation is fairly straightforward, as summarized in Table 12-14, since none of these viruses have the same collection of changes, including cytomegaly, a single large basophilic nuclear inclusion with a prominent halo, and multiple indistinct cytoplasmic inclusions. CMV inclusions can also be confused with the bradyzoites of toxoplasmosis. However, the cysts of toxoplasmosis lack the large nuclear inclusions seen in CMV. When there is little histologic reaction and rare CMV inclusions one can question whether the organisms are incidental findings. If there is some histologic reaction and the patient has pulmonary symptoms, it is possible they have a very mild CMV pneumonia.

One should also be very cautious about interpreting a positive culture, immunohistochemical stain (fig. 12-140C), PCR result, or in situ hybridization result if the clinical and radiologic findings or a lung biopsy does not show features consistent with a CMV pneumonia.

Treatment and Prognosis. CMV pneumonia may be fatal, especially in immunocompromised patients and in patients with other associated infections. Ganciclovir, foscarnet, and intravenous immunoglobulin may be helpful in patients with transient immunosuppression (352).

Herpes Simplex

Definition. Herpes simplex pneumonia is a lung infection caused by the virus, herpes simplex (HSV).

There are two serotypes of herpes simplex: HSV-1 primarily causes respiratory tract infection and HSV-2 primarily causes genitourinary tract infection (352). HSV has structural characteristics similar to those of the other herpesviruses.

The morphologic and ultrastructural features are summarized in Table 12-14.

Clinical Features. HSV-1 has three major respiratory tract manifestations: 1) acute gingivostomatitis and pharyngitis (342), 2) chronic ulcerative pharyngitis and laryngotracheitis (352, 384,397), and 3) pneumonia (352). Acute gingivostomatitis and pharyngitis are the most common manifestations of HSV-1 infection, seen mostly in children but also in adolescents and young adults (342,352).

Chronic ulcerative pharyngitis and laryngotracheitis occur in immunocompromised patients, including AIDS patients (352,384,397). They can occur as both primary and recurrent HSV infections. Clinically, patients present with 5- to 15-mm, painful ulcers of the oral cavity and upper airway mucous membranes that grow slowly. This clinical syndrome has presenting manifestations of fever, chills, dyspnea, cough, and hypoxemia. Elderly patients, in the absence of immunosuppression or chronic lung disease, may develop a tracheobronchitis that manifests with bronchospasm (352,374,405).

HSV pneumonia is seen in the neonatal period as well as in immunosuppressed patients with malignancy, burns, transplants, or immunodeficiency syndromes such as AIDS (352,384,397). Neonatal HSV-1 pneumonia may be acquired congenitally or in the peripartum period (309,357,376). Patients usually present between the 3rd and 14th day after birth (309, 352,357,376). Mucocutaneous herpes infection precedes herpes pneumonia in most cases. Ramsey et al. (397) studied 20 cases and found that focal HSV pneumonia appears to reach the lungs through contiguous spread from the tracheobronchial tree. However, diffuse HSV pneumonia appears to be associated with hematogenous spread from the upper respiratory or genitourinary tracts.

Radiologic Findings. Chest radiographs of patients with HSV pulmonary infection typically demonstrate segmental and subsegmental, ground-glass opacities and consolidation (fig. 12-141). The findings are typically diffuse and bilateral. CT demonstrates patchy ground-glass opacities with scattered areas of consolidation. These findings are seen in the central, nondependent portions of the lung. Poorly defined nodules with associated ground-glass opacity have also been described (337). In one study (310) the findings were not significantly different in patients concomitantly infected with HSV and other organisms. Thus, coexisting infections cannot be excluded based on radiologic findings alone. In addition, HSV infection may be difficult to detect in patients with acute respiratory distress syndrome in whom ground-glass opacities, consolidations, and reticular opacities also occur. Pleural effusions are common (310). Tracheobronchitis may not be detectable radiographically.

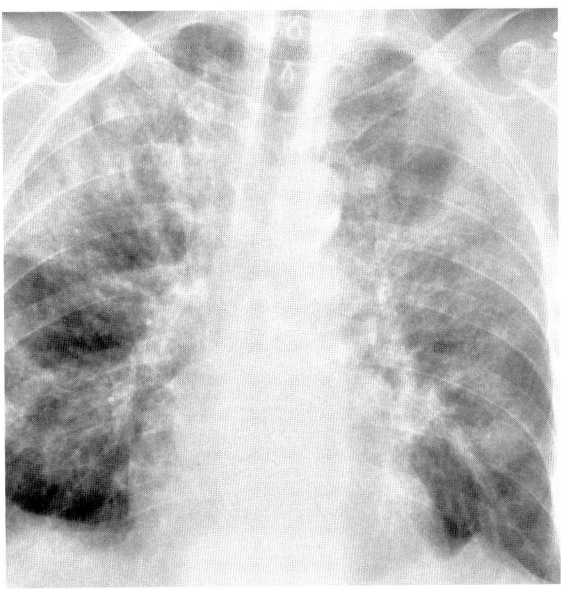

Figure 12-141

HERPES SIMPLEX PULMONARY INFECTION

A 66-year-old male with a history of renal insufficiency, heart failure, recent decreased breath sounds, and nonproductive cough. PA chest radiograph demonstrates multifocal bilateral airspace consolidations and bilateral pleural effusions. The pulmonary abnormalities are most severe in the upper lobes.

Pathologic Findings. HSV can have three primary forms of lung involvement: 1) necrotizing tracheobronchitis, 2) necrotizing pneumonia, and 3) interstitial pneumonitis (345, 384,397). The necrotizing tracheobronchitis is usually ulcerative, resulting in a necrotic and fibrinopurulent exudate along the surface of the airway mucosa (fig. 12-142). In the bronchi this may extend into the submucosal glands. Neutrophils are prominent. A pseudomembrane

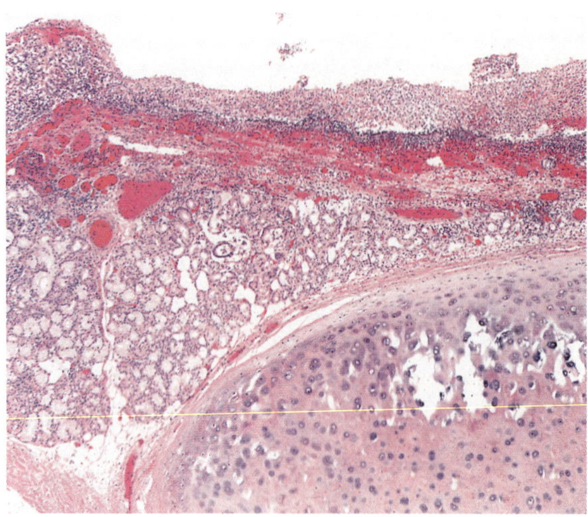

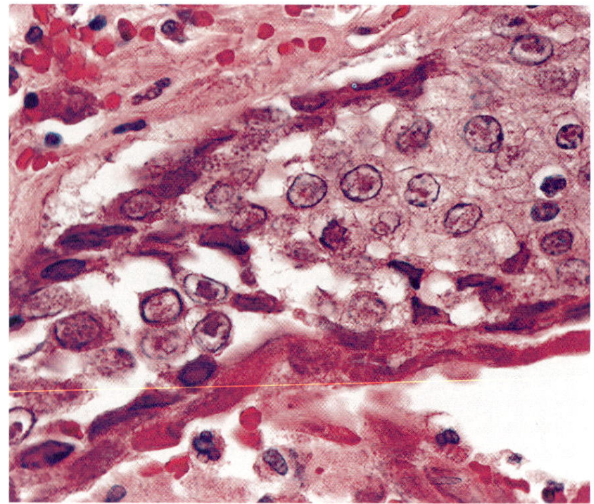

Figure 12-142

HERPES SIMPLEX: NECROTIZING TRACHEOBRONCHITIS

Left: There is diffuse ulceration of the mucosa of the trachea.

Right: Many refractile eosinophilic nuclear inclusions are seen in these squamous metaplastic cells. It consists of a dense, eosinophilic mass surrounded by a clear halo.

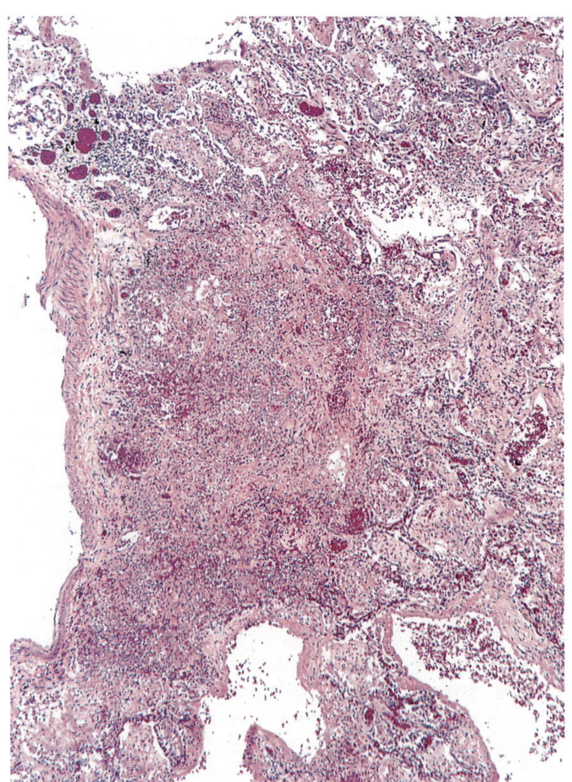

Figure 12-143

HERPES SIMPLEX: NECROTIZING BRONCHIOLITIS

The nodular area of necrosis is centered on a bronchiole.

may result from the extensive necrosis and sloughing of the epithelium (345,384,397,434).

Necrotizing HSV pneumonia is usually airway centered (fig. 12-143). For this reason lesions of necrotizing bronchiolitis are found in the center of the areas of necrotic lung parenchyma unless the entire airway has been destroyed. Within the necrotic areas are abundant fibrin, necrotic debris, and acute inflammation. To identify cells with viral cytopathic effect, one must look at the viable lung parenchyma at the edge of the necrotic zones. Sometimes the viral inclusions are best seen in squamous metaplastic cells in preserved airways (fig. 12-142).

Diffuse interstitial pneumonitis has histologic features that are closest to diffuse alveolar damage (fig. 12-144). Perivascular inflammation may be seen (fig. 12-145). Occasionally, there is a miliary pattern, particularly in cases of hematogenous spread of HSV to the lungs.

The viral inclusions of HSV and varicella-zoster virus are identical. The classic inclusion consists of a dense, eosinophilic mass within the nucleus that is surrounded by a clear halo and peripherally marginated, beaded nuclear chromatin (figs. 12-142, right, 12-146) (305,364, 418,434,439). The inclusions usually are greater than half the nuclear diameter (364), and are sometimes called Cowdry type A inclusions.

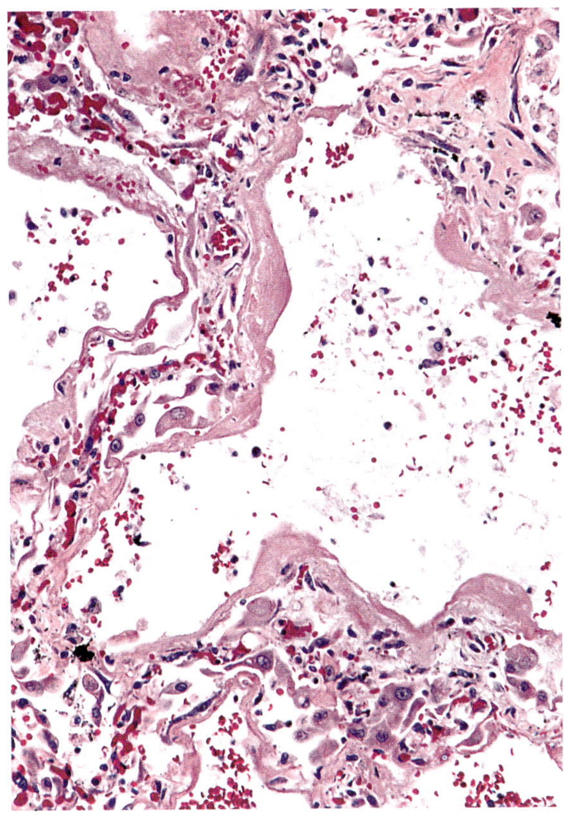

Figure 12-144

HERPES SIMPLEX: DIFFUSE ALVEOLAR DAMAGE

The hyaline membranes, interstitial edema, and pneumocyte hyperplasia are features of diffuse alveolar damage.

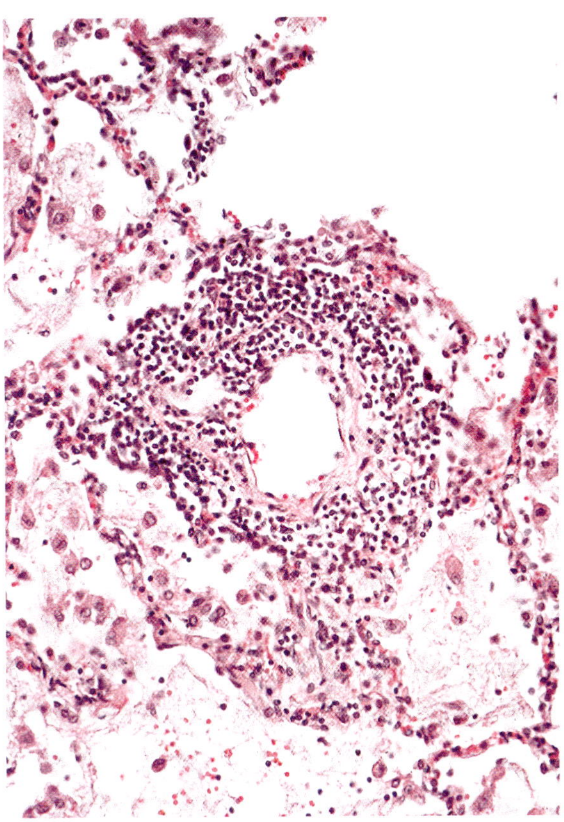

Figure 12-145

HERPES SIMPLEX: PERIVASCULAR INFLAMMATION

This venule is surrounded by a marked chronic inflammatory infiltrate.

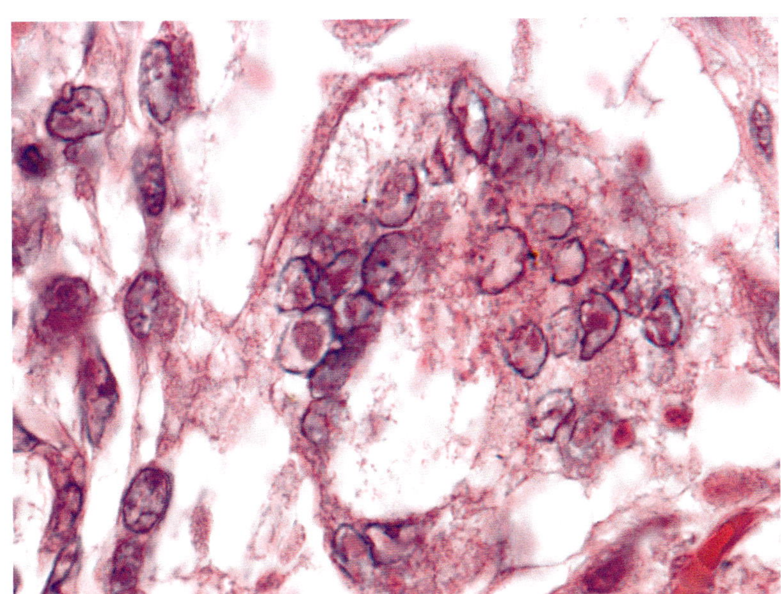

Figure 12-146

HERPES SIMPLEX: MULTINUCLEATED CELL WITH INCLUSIONS

This multinucleated epithelial cell shows multiple nuclei with eosinophilic refractile nuclear inclusions. No cytoplasmic inclusions are seen.

Both HSV and varicella-zoster may form multinucleated cells (fig. 12-146). It may be very difficult to find these viral inclusions, particularly in extensively necrotic samples. Immunohistochemistry or in situ hybridization techniques are helpful (305,419). Electron microscopy shows that the nuclear inclusion consists of viral DNA and nucleocapsids. The encapsulated viral particles with central DNA have a target-like appearance and may be arranged in a lattice-like pattern (364,434,439,440).

Differential Diagnosis. The viral inclusions of HSV must be separated from those of other viruses including adenovirus, cytomegalovirus, and measles (Table 12-14). Separation from adenovirus may be the most difficult since it can produce identical inclusions. Identifying the smudge cells of adenovirus in light microscopic sections makes the distinction. HSV does not produce cytoplasmic inclusions, which should be seen in cytomegalovirus or the multinucleated cells of measles.

Treatment and Prognosis. In immunocompetent patients, primary HSV infection of the upper respiratory tract usually resolves without treatment, although oral acyclovir may reduce symptoms (352). For immunosuppressed patients with chronic pharyngitis and laryngotracheobronchitis, therapy with acyclovir is very important to prevent the infection from disseminating. If the patient recovers, the herpes infection may recur. The effectiveness of acyclovir in HSV pneumonia has not been established, although it is the treatment of choice. Foscarnet is the drug of choice in acyclovir-resistant patients (352).

Varicella-Zoster

Definition. Herpes varicella-zoster pneumonia is a lung infection caused by the herpes varicella-zoster virus (VZV).

VZV is structurally similar to the other herpesviruses. The details of these properties are summarized in the previous section on cytomegalovirus (Table 12-14).

Clinical Features. VZV causes two different clinical syndromes: varicella (chickenpox) and herpes zoster (shingles) (352,428). Varicella is very contagious and causes extensive mucocutaneous lesions. It occurs primarily in children but also in adults. Herpes zoster occurs in adults. It is the result of reactivation of latent infection harbored in the posterior dorsal root ganglia and causes spread along sensory nerves, typically resulting in a unilateral, painful cutaneous eruption in a dermatomal distribution (428). If the patient is immunocompetent the disease is usually limited to a postherpetic neuralgia. However, herpes zoster is more likely to develop in immunosuppressed patients and in up to 50 percent of these patients disseminated infection causes hepatitis, pneumonitis, meningoencephalitis, or uveitis.

Pneumonia is a rare complication of varicella in children, but in adults it is more frequent (335,352,423). In children or adults with impaired cell-mediated immunity, disseminated infection is more likely to cause pneumonia, meningoencephalitis, and hepatitis (328,333,335). Pneumonia develops in up to 45 percent of bone marrow transplant recipients and 33 percent of acute leukemia patients who develop varicella infection. When varicella develops during pregnancy, pneumonia occurs in 10 percent of patients (332,393).

Immunocompetent adults with varicella viral pneumonia present with cough, shortness of breath, pleuritic chest pain, and hemoptysis, 1 to 6 days after presentation with skin lesions (317,323,335,352,423). Pulmonary infarction is an acute complication (335,343).

Radiologic Findings. Chest radiographic abnormalities in patients with VZV pulmonary infection are characterized by multifocal, bilateral, ill-defined nodular opacities that measure 5 to 10 mm in diameter (fig. 12-147, left) (334, 437). Smaller nodules have been described in early infection. These opacities may coalesce to form extensive consolidation. The nodular lesions may mimic metastatic disease. While resolution occurs in 10 days to several months, some patients have persistent parenchymal nodules (fig. 12-147, right). These may densely calcify and uncommonly persist as multifocal, tiny, widespread nodular calcifications of 2 to 3 mm, predominantly in the lower lung zones (334, 337,437). Hilar lymphadenopathy may occur. Pleural effusions are uncommon (334).

Pathologic Findings. VZV pneumonia (both varicella and herpes zoster) causes diffuse multicentric hemorrhage and necrosis. Histologically, the necrotic and hemorrhagic areas may appear centered on airways (fig. 12-148).

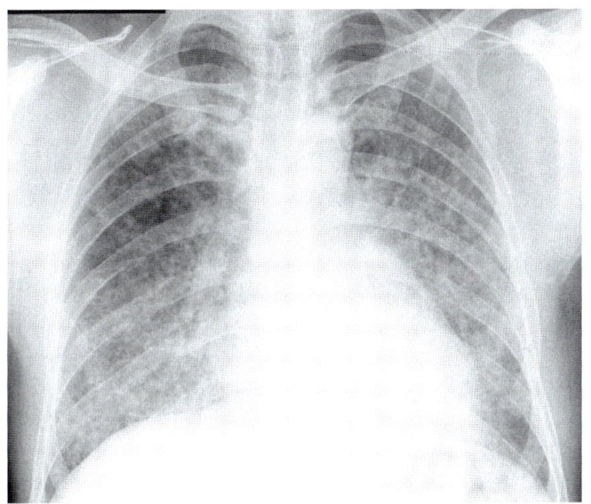

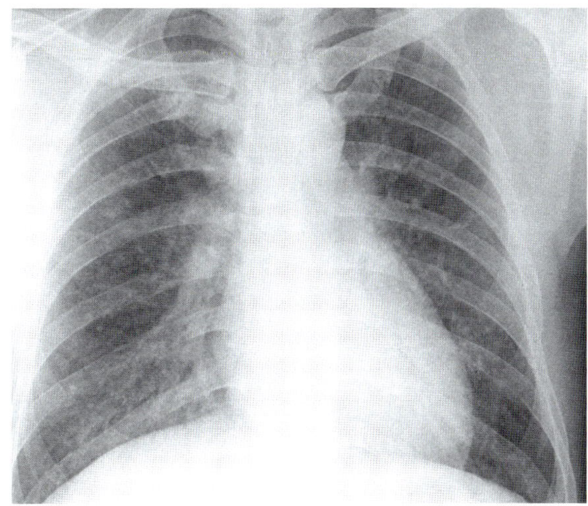

Figure 12-147

VARICELLA-ZOSTER VIRAL PNEUMONIA IN A 35-YEAR-OLD MALE

Left: PA chest radiograph obtained at the time of active pulmonary infection demonstrates bilateral, diffuse nodular opacities with ill-defined borders.

Right: PA chest radiograph obtained 1 month after the acute infection demonstrates residual, small, well-defined, multifocal bilateral pulmonary nodules, some of which exhibit calcification.

A miliary distribution may also occur, consistent with hematogenous spread. An acute lung injury pattern may be present, with interstitial edema, congestion, and inflammation. Alveolar fibrin and hyaline membranes may also be seen (423). Exudates of fibrin and necrotic debris may be seen in the lumens of bronchioles or bronchi. Recurrent pulmonary infarction has been reported (343). Vesicles have been reported on the pleural surface and on the mucosa of the tracheobronchial tree (423). Hypertensive arteriopathy may occur (423).

Viral cytopathic effects can be found in the respiratory epithelium of the trachea, bronchi and bronchioles, alveoli, interstitial connective tissue, and capillary endothelial cells. The viral inclusions are identical to those seen with HSV infection described above, but they are more difficult to find. They are best seen in the viable tissue surrounding the necrotic lesions. One case of giant cell viral pneumonia was reported in a neonate with VZV infection. Resolution of VZV pneumonia can result in calcification (313,396,415) and rare reports of interstitial fibrosis (363). Necrotizing granulomas were described in one adult patient who had persistent pulmonary nodules 1 year after an episode of varicella pneumonia (380).

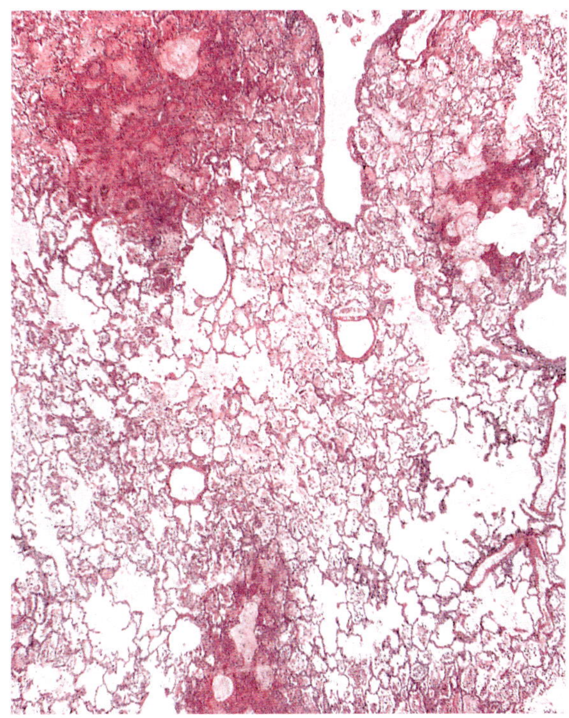

Figure 12-148

VARICELLA-ZOSTER VIRUS NECROTIZING BRONCHIOLITIS

Several hemorrhagic and necrotic foci are centered on bronchioles.

Differential Diagnosis. The differential diagnosis for pulmonary infection due to VZV is similar to that for HSV. Necrotizing tracheobronchitis and interstitial pneumonitis or diffuse alveolar damage are patterns of lung injury that should raise the possibility of a viral agent such as VZV. VZV gives the characteristic viral cytopathic features described above. The viral inclusions of VZV are identical to those of HSV, but they can be distinguished from those of cytomegalovirus, measles, adenovirus, and respiratory syncytial virus (Table 12-14). VZV is difficult to culture, but it can be distinguished from HSV by immunohistochemistry.

Treatment and Prognosis. Treatment for patients with VZV pneumonia is intravenous acyclovir. It is most effective in immunocompetent patients. Infected patients can communicate the virus to other hospital contacts, so isolation procedures should be implemented to prevent the spread of infection.

Adenovirus

Definition. Adenovirus pneumonia is caused by pulmonary infection with adenovirus.

Adenovirus is a linear, double-stranded DNA virus without an envelope that measures approximately 70 to 90 nm in diameter (322, 352,432). It is composed of 240 hexons and 12 pentons or 252 capsomeres arranged in an icosahedral pattern. There are 12 penton capsomeres situated at each vertex from which arises a long projecting fiber that is thought to be the site of host cell attachment. The hexons and fibers are the sites of type-specific antigens to which neutralizing antibody is directed (322,352,432,434). Currently, there are 51 candidate serotypes of adenovirus but all are not pathogenic in humans. The virus infects the nucleus of the host cell and when the cell ruptures the virus spreads to infect new cells.

Adenovirus is thought to spread in a person-to-person fashion. Epidemics are known to occur in military recruits as well as in dense civilian populations such as at colleges and daycare centers (322,352,432,434).

Clinical Features. There are two common clinical presentations of adenovirus infection that primarily affect the upper respiratory tract. Acute respiratory disease was defined initially in military recruits and termed "acute respiratory disease of military recruits" (322,329). A similar condition, called pharyngoconjunctival fever, was recognized in civilians (321). There is considerable overlap in the clinical manifestations, which consist primarily of a moderate to severe pharyngitis; fever, chills, myalgias, and prostration are common (322,352). A severe tracheobronchitis is present more often in acute respiratory disease; conjunctivitis is present more often in pharyngoconjunctival fever. However, the same viral serotypes are associated with both clinical syndromes. Adenovirus is thought to cause approximately 5 percent of the acute respiratory diseases in young children (322,434) and 5 percent of cases of bronchiolitis in the United States (436).

Adenovirus pneumonia also occurs in military recruits as well as civilian adults and children (322,330,352,365). Clinically, patients present with signs and symptoms similar to other pneumonias. The disease can be severe and progress to death in a 2- to 3-week period (322, 352). Adenovirus accounts for 10 percent of neonatal viral pneumonias (394). In this setting it can cause a severe necrotizing bronchiolitis and pneumonitis. For reasons that are not clear, adenovirus is the most aggressive virus to cause neonatal pneumonia (394). Survivors may have chronic complications such as bronchiectasis (352,406), asthma (406), impaired pulmonary function (409), and hyperlucent lung (352,372).

In immunosuppressed patients, adenovirus causes a severe pneumonia that is frequently fatal, particularly in transplant patients and those with immunodeficiency (368,371,375,386, 387,408). The adenovirus serotypes that are frequently involved in this opportunistic pneumonia are 1, 2, 5, 6, 7, 11, 21, 31, and 34 (322,352).

Radiologic Findings. Chest radiographic findings in patients with pulmonary adenovirus infection have classically been described as bilateral hyperaeration, bronchial wall thickening, and diffuse bilateral bronchopneumonia (fig. 12-149). Lobar atelectasis is a frequent complication (337). Radiologic abnormalities typically resolve within 2 weeks. Pleural effusion and lymphadenopathy are rarely described (337,350).

A 1998 review of 32 pediatric patients with pulmonary adenovirus infection described lobar or segmental consolidation in 90 percent and pleural effusion in 62 percent (fig. 12-149)

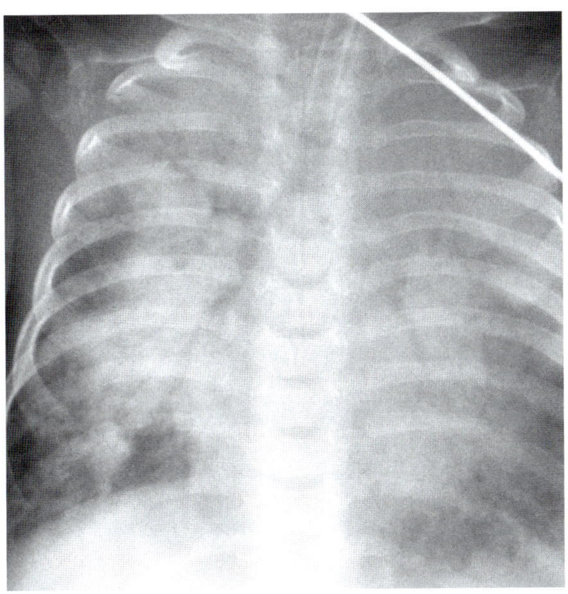

Figure 12-149

ADENOVIRUS INFECTION

Adenovirus infection in a 6-month-old male who developed bronchopneumonia. AP portable chest radiograph demonstrates bilateral, confluent, diffuse, parenchymal consolidations. Note that the patient is intubated. After death, adenovirus type 7 was recovered on culture.

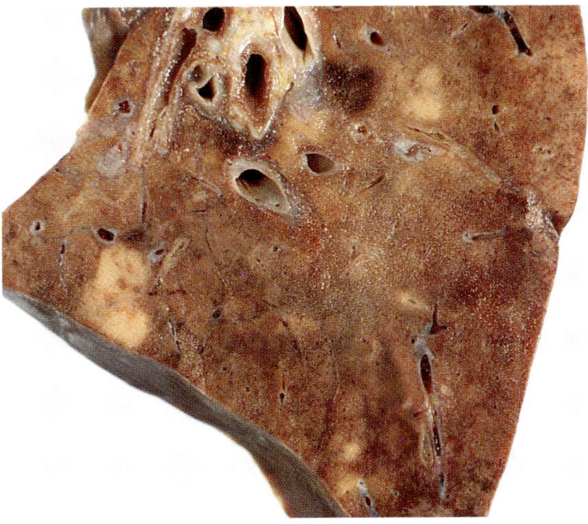

Figure 12-150

ADENOVIRUS PNEUMONIA: GROSS SPECIMEN

Multiple yellow nodules represent a necrotizing bronchopneumonia.

(350). Pneumatoceles were also reported in this study. The above findings are usually described as radiologic features of bacterial pneumonia. The authors suggested that bilateral and multifocal involvement should suggest inclusion of viral pneumonia in the differential diagnosis.

The sequelae of adenovirus infection in children may be serious: chronic lung disease occurs in up to 53 percent of affected patients (337). These patients may develop bronchiectasis, bronchiolitis obliterans, and unilateral hyperlucent lung (337,350).

Pathologic Findings. Adenovirus causes two major patterns of lung injury: a necrotizing bronchitis/bronchiolitis and an interstitial pneumonia that often shows necrosis, hemorrhage, and features of diffuse alveolar damage (346,381,387,394,432,434). In fatal cases, the lungs are heavy and diffusely consolidated with patchy areas of hemorrhage and necrosis (fig. 12-150). Nodular inflammatory and necrotic lesions may be palpable (346,381,387,394,432, 434). The airway mucosa appears congested and hemorrhagic. The bronchiolitis consists of a severe inflammatory infiltrate that causes necrosis of the airway wall. The airway lumens are filled with necrotic eosinophilic granular debris and inflammatory cells. The muscularis of the bronchioles is usually preserved, but the epithelium is frequently destroyed. In the bronchi, the submucosal glands may be involved. In some cases the necrotizing bronchiolitis may be so severe that it is difficult to be certain of the distribution and the lesion may appear to be an extensive necrotizing pneumonia.

The acute alveolitis is frequently associated with lesions of bronchiolitis. Interstitial edema, fibrinous alveolar exudates, and a neutrophilic and mononuclear inflammatory infiltrate are seen (346,381,387,394,432,434). When hyaline membranes are present, the lesion can be recognized as diffuse alveolar damage.

Adenovirus causes two types of nuclear inclusions that are helpful in suggesting the diagnosis (319,418,432,434). The most distinctive is the smudge cell (fig. 12-151), which is a basophilic or amphophilic inclusion that obscures the nuclear membrane, giving a "smudgy" appearance to the nucleus (319,418,432,434). It usually fills the entire nucleus but in some cases it is surrounded by a small halo. The other type of nuclear inclusion is similar to those seen in herpesvirus infections, as it is densely eosinophilic

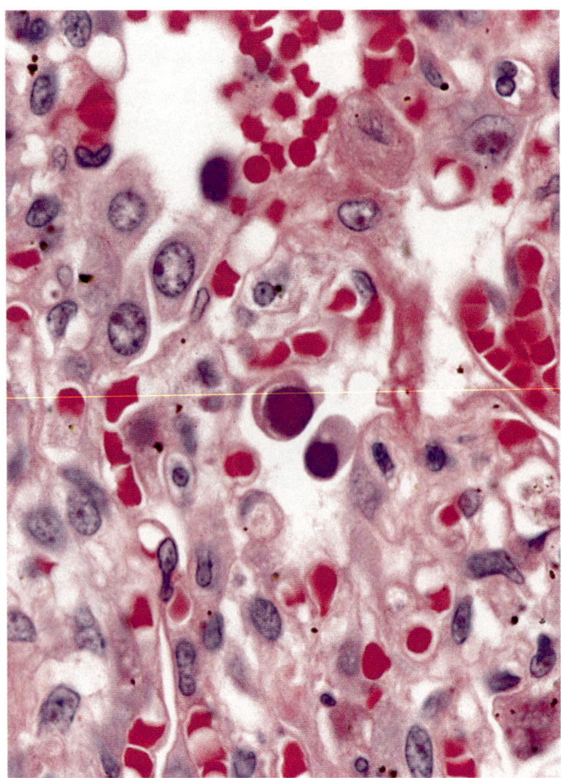

Figure 12-151

ADENOVIRUS: INCLUSION

In the center is an epithelial cell with a basophilic, slightly enlarged nucleus that has a smudgy nuclear membrane.

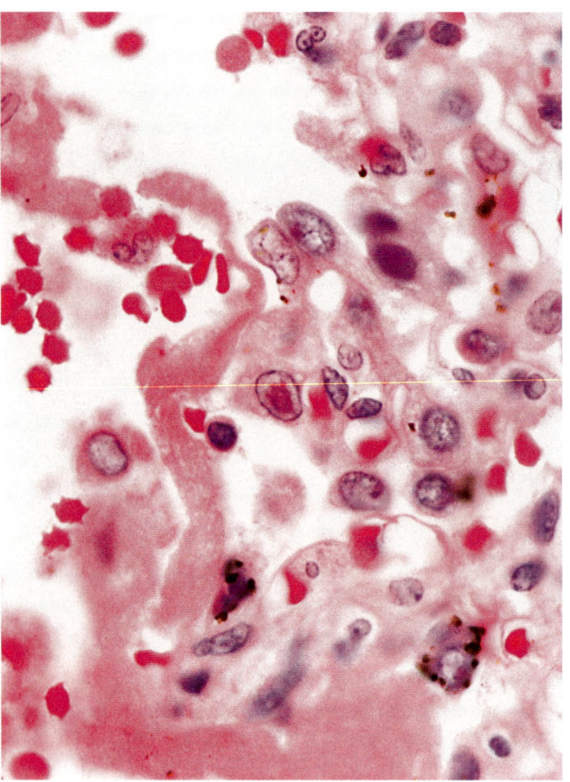

Figure 12-152

ADENOVIRUS: INCLUSION

In the center is a cell with an eosinophilic nuclear inclusion.

and surrounded by a clear halo (fig. 12-152). Inclusions are usually found in the viable tissue at the edges of the necrotic zones. It has been suggested that the eosinophilic inclusions may "mature" to the smudged inclusions through peripheralization of the chromatin and blurring of the nuclear membrane, but some believe the inclusions develop separately (432, 434). By electron microscopy, the nuclear inclusions of adenovirus appear as a lattice-like crystalline array of virions (302,434,439,440).

Chronic pulmonary disease develops in up to 60 percent of infants (436). It may take the form of bronchiectasis, bronchiolitis obliterans, abnormal pulmonary function, and unilateral hyperlucent lung syndrome (312,406, 409,413,434).

Culture is the optimal way to establish the diagnosis of adenovirus infection. This provides the added advantage of serotyping. However, immunohistochemistry (fig. 12-153), in situ hybridization, and other molecular techniques can be applied to formalin-fixed, paraffin-embedded tissue as well as frozen tissue samples. Serology requires the demonstration of an IgM antibody or a four-fold increase in an IgG antibody (432,434). Initially, antihexon genus-reactive serologic tests are performed, followed by type-specific tests if needed.

Differential Diagnosis. The differential diagnosis for pulmonary adenovirus infection includes the other potential causes of necrotizing bronchiolitis and/or diffuse alveolar damage. The inclusions of adenovirus must be distinguished from those of herpes simplex, varicella-zoster, and cytomegalovirus. In herpesvirus infections there are no smudge cells and multinucleation can occur, a feature lacking in adenovirus infections. Adenovirus lacks the combination of nuclear as well as cytoplasmic

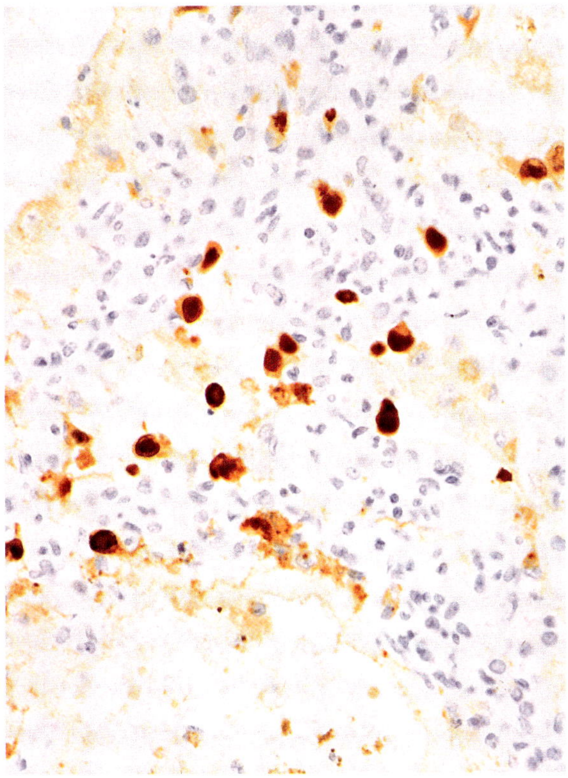

Figure 12-153

ADENOVIRUS: IMMUNOHISTOCHEMISTRY

There are numerous infected cells that stain with an antibody to adenovirus.

inclusions seen in cytomegalovirus, but in some cases this distinction can be difficult (371). Degenerated nuclei may be mistaken for smudge cells of adenovirus. Cultures not only confirm the diagnosis of adenovirus but also type the virus. Search for a characteristic histologic reaction, herpes-like inclusions, and results of cultures, immunohistochemistry (fig. 12-153), PCR, or electron microscopy help to sort out the correct diagnosis (386,387,424).

Treatment and Prognosis. Therapy for adenovirus infections usually consists of management of the patient's clinical manifestations since effective medical therapy is not available. Patients with severe pulmonary infections may be treated with intravenous ribavirin or immunoglobulin (352). Adenovirus pneumonia in immunosuppressed patients is virtually always fatal. Effective vaccines for adenovirus types 4 and 7 are available and used routinely in the military (352).

Respiratory Syncytial Virus

Definition. Respiratory syncytial virus pneumonia is caused by infection due to respiratory syncytial virus (RSV).

RSV is a paramyxovirus with a single-strand RNA genome enclosed within a capsid (352,417,434). It has structural similarities to parainfluenza viruses. Two major antigenic groups exist (group A and B). There is a surface F glycoprotein, which causes fusion of the viral envelope with the host cell membranes and syncytial giant cell formation. In addition, there is a G surface glycoprotein which is involved in the attachment of the virus to host cell receptors (352,417,434). The group A strains appear to be associated with more severe infections (352,417,434).

RSV is found worldwide. It infects up to 50 percent of children in the first year of life and virtually all children by the first few years of life. It is transmitted via person to person through large-particle aerosols or hand contamination of infectious secretions that are subsequently self-inoculated through the eye or nose. Outbreaks are most commonly seen in the late autumn and winter.

Clinical Features. RSV infection presents most commonly as an upper respiratory tract infection, but it can also cause laryngotracheobronchitis and pneumonia, both of which are more serious infections. RSV causes 45 to 90 percent of cases of bronchiolitis and 40 percent of cases of pneumonia in infants and young children (352,417,434). A smaller percentage of cases of croup and bronchitis are caused by RSV. Only about 1 to 2 percent of patients need hospitalization. Predisposing factors for severe infection include cyanotic congenital heart disease, cystic fibrosis, bronchopulmonary dysplasia, and immunosuppression (352,417,425,434).

Patients with bronchiolitis present with tachypnea, wheezing, intercostal and suprasternal retractions, a hyperresonant chest, and inspiratory rales. Hypoxemia may be prolonged, even for several weeks. Apneic episodes occur in up to 20 percent of hospitalized infants (307). Increased risk for these episodes include prematurity and young postnatal age.

In adults, approximately half of recurrent infections are associated with upper respiratory tract disease. Presenting features include coryza,

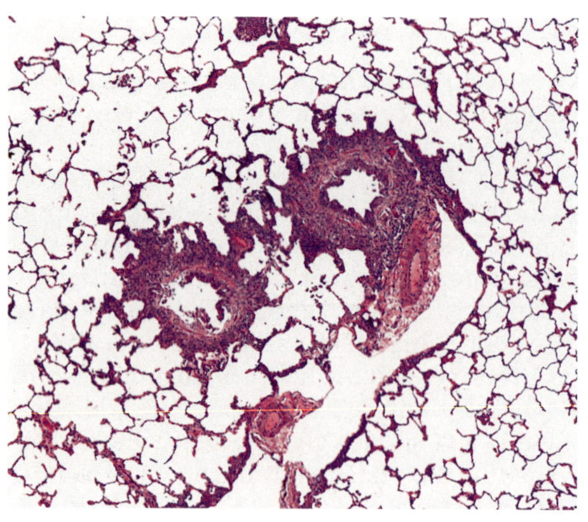

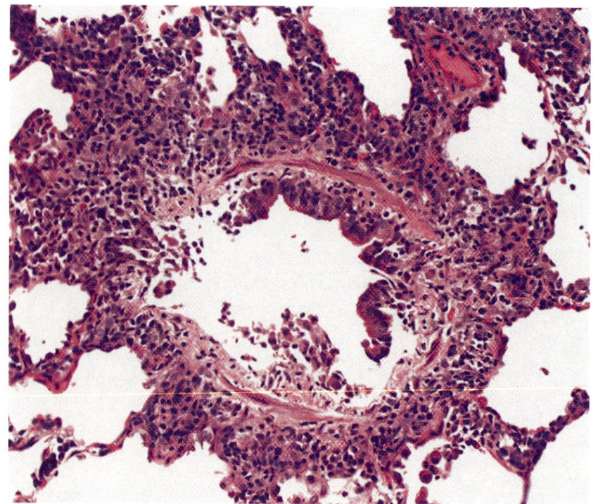

Figure 12-154

RESPIRATORY SYNCYTIAL VIRUS: BRONCHIOLITIS

Left: There is marked bronchiolar and peribronchiolar inflammation.
Right: The inflammation consists primarily of lymphocytes. The bronchiolar epithelium is focally ulcerated.

cough, pharyngitis, and low-grade fever. In elderly patients, it is common to encounter second infections of viral or bacterial bronchopneumonia.

In immunosuppressed children or adults, RSV pneumonia may be very serious. The pneumonia usually follows an upper respiratory tract infection. The diagnosis is made by detecting RSV antigen in BAL specimens. Long-term sequelae of RSV pneumonia include persistent hypoxemia and prolonged pulmonary function abnormalities (353,407).

Radiologic Findings. RSV infections in children typically manifest radiographically with peribronchial thickening and air-trapping, which may be associated with patchy airspace consolidation. Adults typically exhibit bilateral interstitial opacities, patchy consolidation, and rarely, lobar consolidation (337,437).

RSV pneumonia is one of the pulmonary infections seen within the first 10 days after bone marrow transplantation. Radiographs of affected patients may demonstrate localized or diffuse opacities. Bilateral linear or nodular opacities also occur (431).

Pathologic Findings. The pathology of RSV infection includes bronchiolitis (fig. 12-154) and interstitial pneumonia (304,417,434). The lungs typically show changes related to airway inflammation and obstruction. The large and small airways are filled with mucus and necrotic debris. Histologically, the material within the airways consists of mucus, necrotic epithelial cells, and inflammatory cells. The airway epithelium may show ulceration, necrosis (fig. 12-154, right), and regenerative changes such as hyperplasia and squamous metaplasia. Some cases resemble a giant cell viral pneumonia with features of diffuse alveolar damage (fig. 12-155). Syncytial giant cells consist of enlarged epithelial cells that line the bronchi, bronchioles, or alveolar spaces (fig. 12-155).

The characteristic cytopathic effect of RSV is multinucleation and formation of eosinophilic cytoplasmic inclusions (fig. 12-155, right) (326,366). The inclusions may be paranuclear within the cytoplasm, with a clear halo. However, the cytoplasmic inclusions may be difficult to find. The fusion protein that is important for syncytial coalescence of cells facilitates multinucleation. Cellular necrosis of the virally infected cells is common.

Culture and immunofluorescence antibody staining of epithelial cells from the respiratory tract are reliable methods of diagnosis. Enzyme-linked immunosorbent assay (ELISA) or radioimmunoassay (RIA) are used to demonstrate RSV antigen in nasopharyngeal specimens. Serology is less reliable.

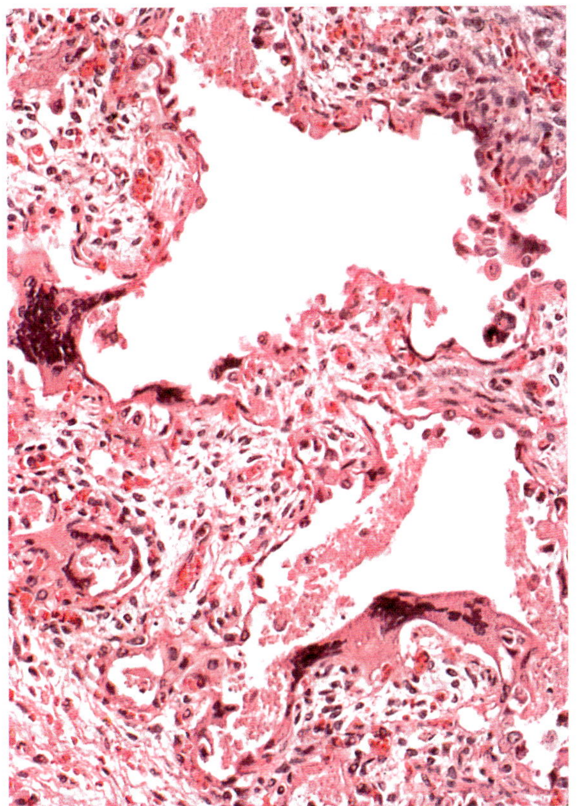
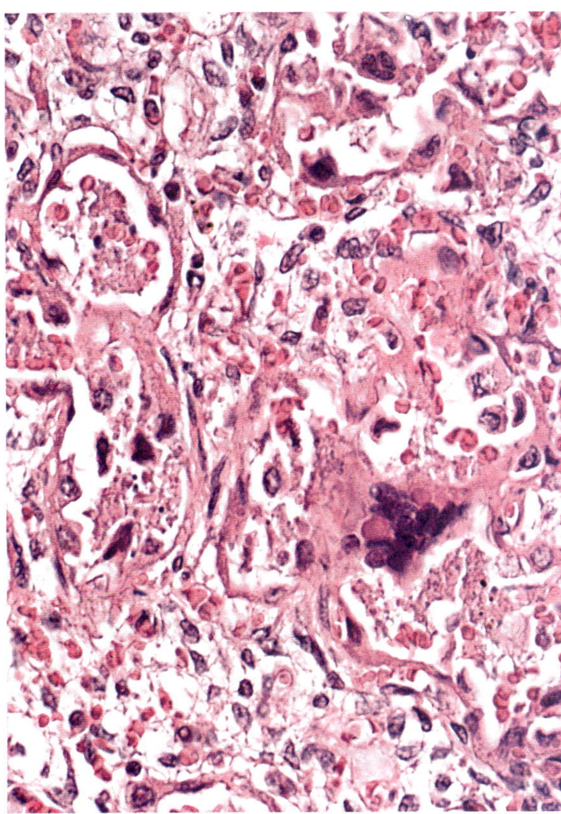

Figure 12-155

RESPIRATORY SYNCYTIAL VIRUS: GIANT CELL VIRAL PNEUMONIA

Left: Diffuse alveolar septal thickening and hyaline membranes form the pattern of diffuse alveolar damage. Syncytial multinucleated cells line the alveolar walls.

Right: There is marked interstitial thickening, alveolar fibrin, as well as a syncytial multinucleated giant cell, which contains an eosinophilic cytoplasmic inclusion. (Both figures courtesy of Dr. Dani Zander, Gainesville, FL.)

Differential Diagnosis. RSV pneumonia must be separated from other forms of giant cell viral pneumonia. The key morphologic features of these other forms are summarized in Table 12-14.

Treatment and Prognosis. For previously healthy infants hospitalized for RSV infection, the mortality is low (0.5 to 1.0 percent), however, it is 15 to 40 percent for immunosuppressed patients or those with underlying disease. If pulmonary hypertension is present, mortality may reach 70 percent.

For patients with RSV pneumonia, it is important to correct the hypoxemia. Aerosolized ribavirin may help by reducing virus titers, severity of disease, and hypoxemia. Careful precautions through hand washing and eye/nose goggles should be taken around infected individuals.

Measles

Definition. Measles pneumonia is a pulmonary infection caused by the measles virus, rubeola.

Measles is a highly contagious, worldwide infection that has been greatly curtailed through the introduction of vaccines, but continues to be significant in underdeveloped countries. In the United States and United Kingdom there was a recrudescence of cases in the past two decades due to the decreased use of the vaccine in children and young adults (352).

Clinical Features. There is an initial incubation period of 1 to 2 weeks, followed by a prodrome in which the patient has fever, rhinorrhea, cough, and conjunctivitis (352). Koplik's spots, consisting of small, irregular spots with a central bluish white speck, appear on the buccal mucosa in 50 to 90 percent of patients. An erythematous maculopapular rash begins on the face 3 to 4 days after the prodrome and spreads to the trunk and extremities. The symptoms slowly resolve and the rash lasts approximately 6 days (352).

Pulmonary complications include a secondary pneumonia, giant cell pneumonia (Hecht's pneumonia) (359,389), and atypical measles pneumonia (352). Secondary pneumonia is caused by bacterial infection and usually develops as the rash fades. It usually responds well to antibiotics. Giant cell pneumonia usually represents an opportunistic infection in a patient immunocompromised due to premature birth, cystic fibrosis (331), malignancy, or immunodeficiency including AIDS (311,359, 383,403,411). It is seen more often in children than adults and is a severe and progressive pneumonia that is usually fatal. A skin rash may be absent in these patients (331,389).

Bronchiolitis obliterans has been reported following measles pneumonia (369,389). In one case an open lung biopsy during active measles infection showed a severe bronchiolitis (369).

Atypical measles pneumonia occurs in patients who were previously vaccinated with an inactivated vaccine and in whom the vaccine failed to induce immunity to the fusion (F) surface glycoprotein that is responsible for the spread of infection (338,349,352). The virus causes segmental or lobar consolidation. Patients have hilar adenopathy and pleural effusions. An atypical rash often starts on the feet and spreads proximally. This type of pneumonia is typically a self-limited illness, and is mainly of historical interest since the use of this type of vaccine has been discontinued (338, 349,352).

Radiologic Findings. Chest radiographs in patients with measles pneumonia demonstrate fine reticular opacities and patchy consolidation throughout the lungs (337,437). Affected children may exhibit bronchial wall thickening, peribronchial opacities, and small nodules. The parenchymal manifestations typically persist throughout the period of time that the skin rash is apparent. Pleural effusion is uncommon (437). Adults with measles pneumonia may exhibit ground-glass opacities, small nodules, and consolidation on CT (337).

Patients with atypical measles pneumonia exhibit diffuse segmental or nodular consolidations. Hilar lymphadenopathy may occur. The radiographic abnormalities can persist for months following clinical resolution (337,437).

Pathologic Findings. In fatal cases, the lungs can be heavy, hemorrhagic, and congested (311). Measles infection of the lung can cause a necrotizing bronchiolitis as well as a giant cell interstitial pneumonitis, which can have features of diffuse alveolar damage. The necrotizing bronchiolitis may be associated with squamous metaplasia and epithelial regenerative changes (311,359). This peribronchiolar distribution can render a nodular appearance to the pulmonary infiltrates (311). Features of the giant cell interstitial pneumonia are interstitial edema, pneumocyte hyperplasia, and hyaline membranes characteristic of diffuse alveolar damage (311). Alveolar macrophages may be prominent. Thromboemboli have been described (311).

Giant cell cytopathic changes affect the tracheal and bronchial mucosa and alveolar epithelial cells (311,331,395). The cytopathic changes consist of very large (100 µm in diameter) multinucleated giant cells which have nuclear and large eosinophilic cytoplasmic inclusions (fig. 12-156) (418,439,442). The giant cells may be numerous or rare and they may have up to 60 nuclei (fig. 12-156) (395). The multinucleated giant cells have viral inclusions in the nuclei as well as the cytoplasm. Inclusions are seen in uninucleate cells as well (359). The nuclear inclusions are homogeneous, eosinophilic, and surrounded by an indistinct clear halo. By electron microscopy, the intranuclear inclusions consist of a worm-like, fibrillar, viral nucleocapsid material (359,395). This material resembles tubules or rod-shaped particles with blunt tips (359). The cytoplasmic inclusions are deeply eosinophilic, granular, and variable in size (fig. 12-156). The ultrastructural nature of the cytoplasmic inclusions is less clear (311, 359). An immunohistochemical study by Sata et al. (403) suggested that the cytoplasmic inclusions originate from the measles virus but differ in the protein content compared to the intranuclear inclusions accounting for variation in the morphologic appearance. In some cases, giant cells may be present, but inclusions are difficult to find (395).

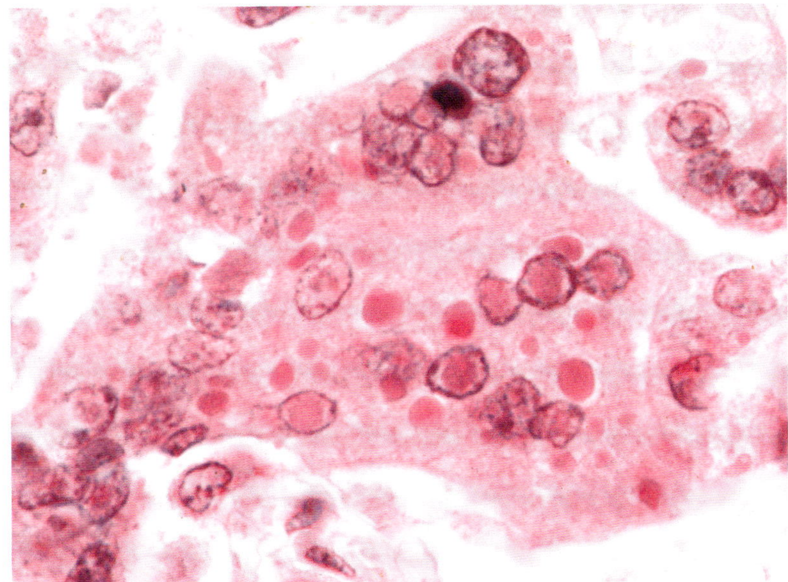

Figure 12-156

MEASLES: GIANT CELL VIRAL PNEUMONIA

This multinucleated giant cell has multiple, irregular cytoplasmic inclusions as well as eosinophilic refractile nuclear inclusions. The histologic background was that of diffuse alveolar damage.

Immunohistochemistry and in situ hybridization can help confirm the measles virus in tissue sections (339,403). Little is known about the lung biopsy findings in patients with atypical measles pneumonia, but the histology typically shows a combination of an Arthus reaction and delayed hypersensitivity (352). The diagnosis of measles pneumonia has been established by BAL (351,382) as well as sputum cytology (303).

Differential Diagnosis. Measles giant cell viral pneumonia is usually not very difficult to recognize due to the distinctive morphologic features of the viral inclusions. More details about the differential diagnosis of giant viral pneumonias are discussed below. However, there is a spectrum of histologic features; in some cases there may be an associated bacterial pneumonia and potentially other viral infections (395,440). When viral inclusions are absent it may be difficult to be certain of the diagnosis without ancillary studies (395).

Giant Cell Viral Pneumonia. Giant cell pneumonia can be caused by measles (331,403), parainfluenza virus (PIV) types 2 and 3 (304,417, 434), respiratory syncytial virus (RSV) (326,434), and varicella-zoster virus (VZV) (400). The light microscopic features may suggest the type of virus causing the infection (418), however, a definitive diagnosis usually requires additional studies such as viral isolation, demonstration of viral antigen by immunofluorescence, serologic testing, or ultrastructural studies. Measles has the most distinctive features, with both nuclear and cytoplasmic inclusions. The giant cells in measles pneumonia need to be distinguished from Warthin-Finkeldey giant cells, which are seen in lymphoid cells rather than epithelial cells (395,440). In contrast, PIV 2 or 3 and RSV have cytoplasmic but not nuclear inclusions. As a result, it may be impossible to distinguish giant cell viral pneumonia caused by PIV 2 or 3 from that caused by RSV by morphology alone. While not seen in every case, in PIV 2 or 3 infection, the multinucleated giant cells can have multiple cytoplasmic inclusions. Occasionally, the syncytial giant cells in RSV contain a few eosinophilic cytoplasmic inclusions. These may be surrounded by a halo, tend to be situated in a paranuclear location, and stain with the Giemsa stain. In RSV, the inclusions tend to be few while in PIV 2 or 3 they may be numerous. In VZV, the viral inclusions are nuclear rather than cytoplasmic.

Giant cell viral pneumonia must be distinguished from giant cell interstitial pneumonia which is usually a manifestation of hard metal pneumoconiosis (324,388,414). The hard metals implicated are tungsten carbide, cobalt, and titanium, which, due to their heat resistance, are used in drill tips, tool edges, and armament components. These metals can be demonstrated in lung tissues by energy dispersive X-ray spectroscopy analysis. In these cases the primary pathologic finding is a combination of chronic interstitial fibrosis, with prominent alveolar macrophages and alveolar multinucleated cells (324,388,414). The multinucleated cells consist of macrophages and alveolar epithelial cells. Although there is some pneumocyte proliferation in giant cell interstitial pneumonia, it is not as exuberant as the marked epithelial proliferation seen in giant cell viral pneumonia, which is reminiscent of that seen in diffuse alveolar damage. In addition, nuclear and cytoplasmic viral inclusions are not seen in giant cell interstitial pneumonia.

Treatment and Prognosis. Although interstitial pneumonia is a well-characterized complication of measles, it is rarely fatal except in immunocompromised patients. Immune globulin can be helpful if given within the first week of exposure. Measles vaccination is helpful if given within 72 hours of exposure (352,395,442).

Parainfluenza

Definition. Parainfluenza pneumonia is a pulmonary infection caused by the parainfluenza virus (PIV).

PIV is a paramyxovirus consisting of a single-strand RNA genome and a protein coat or envelope known as a capsid. The major antigenic subtypes of PIV are types 1, 2, 3, 4A, and 4B. The surface hemagglutinin-neuraminidase (HN) glycoprotein possesses hemagglutinin and neuraminidase activities and is necessary for the attachment of the virus to host cell receptors (352). The F glycoprotein on the surface of the capsid has hemolyzing and membrane-fusing capabilities. It must be cleaved by enzymes in the host cells for the virus to penetrate. In PIV types 2 and 3, the F glycoprotein is involved with the formation of multinucleated syncytial cells.

Clinical Features. Each of the PIV subtypes causes respiratory infection, including upper respiratory infection, laryngotracheobronchitis (croup), bronchitis, bronchiolitis, and interstitial pneumonitis (347). Croup is primarily caused by PIV 1 and 2 in children between 2 and 6 years of age. PIV is associated with approximately 40 percent of cases of croup. PIV 3 causes croup, bronchiolitis, and pneumonia. In children less than 2 years of age, PIV 3 follows respiratory syncytial virus as the second most common cause of bronchiolitis and it is the second most common cause of lower respiratory tract infections that lead to hospitalization in infants. Pneumonia is usually mild and rarely fatal. Transmission is usually via droplet spread by close personal contact. The incubation period is 3 to 6 days.

Patients with PIV types 1 to 3 usually present with a febrile rhinitis, pharyngitis, laryngitis, and bronchitis (352). Fever occurs in up to 80 percent of patients. Lower respiratory tract involvement occurs in up to one third of children (352). PIV may cause severe lower respiratory tract pneumonia in immunosuppressed patients, particularly children with immunodeficiency or leukemia, and transplant patients (325,352,429).

Radiologic Findings. Patients with PIV pulmonary infection exhibit nonspecific radiologic abnormalities. Diffuse interstitial opacities are typically seen. Bronchial wall thickening, peribronchial consolidation, patchy consolidation, and air-trapping have been described (337,437).

Pathologic Findings. Histologically, lung biopsies from patients with PIV infection show bronchiolitis and/or pneumonia (304,417,434). PIV-infected cells are often, but not always, multinucleated (fig. 12-157). Cytoplasmic but not nuclear inclusions may be seen.

Multinucleated giant cells may be numerous in a background of organizing pneumonia and interstitial inflammation (304,417,434). Except for the giant cells, the underlying histologic reaction is often reminiscent of the organizing phase of diffuse alveolar damage. There is exuberant pneumocyte proliferation, alveolar fibrin, small foci of necrosis, organizing interstitial fibrosis, and interstitial inflammation. Many of the giant cells appear to be in continuity with hyperplastic pneumocytes. The giant cells are very large with abundant cytoplasm, which frequently contains numerous small, eosinophilic inclusions. Some nuclei have prominent nucleoli, but distinct nuclear inclusions are not seen.

The histopathology of pulmonary infection by PIV varies with the antigenic subtype and immunologic status of the patient. Giant cell pneumonia is a rare manifestation of PIV infection and can occur with types 2 and 3. The giant cells may contain cytoplasmic inclusions

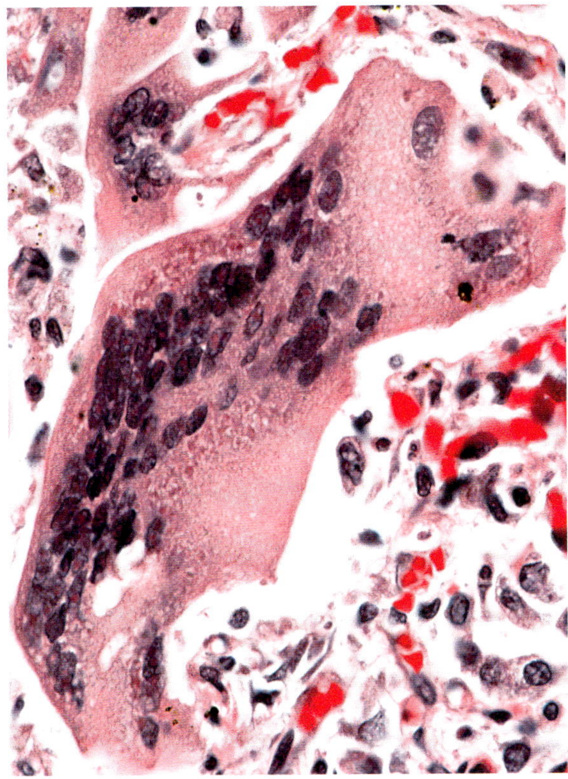

Figure 12-157

PARAINFLUENZA VIRUS:
GIANT CELL VIRAL PNEUMONIA

This multinucleated giant cell has multiple, small cytoplasmic inclusions and many nuclei, which do not show inclusions.

consisting of aggregates of viral nucleocapsids. However, nuclear inclusions are not seen. Extrapulmonary dissemination rarely occurs in patients with PIV 3 giant cell viral pneumonia.

By ultrastructure, it has been shown that most of the multinucleated cells in giant cell viral pneumonia are epithelial cells. Electron microscopy shows that the intracytoplasmic inclusions of PIV 3 consist of material resembling nucleocapsids (306,326).

Differential Diagnosis. The differential diagnosis depends on the histologic reaction. Since PIV does not have a diagnostic viral cytopathic effect, cultures and immunofluorescent techniques are used to firmly establish the diagnosis. Electron microscopy may also be helpful. For cases that have the pattern of giant cell viral pneumonia, the considerations discussed above should be kept in mind (see Giant Cell Viral Pneumonia).

Treatment and Prognosis. There is no proven treatment for PIV infections. For hospitalized patients with croup, supportive care is recommended. A few case reports (422) suggest that aerosolized ribavirin may be helpful for immunosuppressed patients with severe PIV infection. Giant cell viral pneumonia in immunosuppressed children is usually fatal.

Influenza

Definition. Influenza pneumonia is a pulmonary infection caused by the influenza virus.

Influenza belongs to the Myxoviradae family. It is a single-stranded, helical RNA virus measuring 80 to 120 nm (433,434). It reproduces by budding from the cell surface. As it buds through the cell surface, the plasma membrane of the cell becomes the lipid envelope of the virus. The virus has two proteins that protrude through the envelope: hemagglutinin and neuraminidase (433,434). Hemagglutinin is important for attachment to the cell surface and is used most often for diagnosis in cell culture and serology. Neuraminidase is thought to play a role in the destruction of cellular mucins or it may participate in viral budding.

There are three antigenic types of influenza virus, defined by the properties of their genome and proteins. Influenza virus types A and B are the most important causes of respiratory infection while type C causes only mild disease. Influenza viruses A and B both have differences in hemagglutinin and neuraminidase that can be detected serologically.

Influenza viruses are found worldwide and cause annual epidemics. Major worldwide epidemics have occurred in 1890, 1900, 1918, 1957, and 1968. In 1918 to 1919, the influenza epidemic killed 20 to 40 million people and probably accounted for 80 percent of the deaths in the US Army in World War I (432,437).

Clinical Features. Patients with influenza typically have rapid onset of fever, chills, prostration, myalgias, malaise, headache, and anorexia (352,433,434). These systemic manifestations are seen in the initial few days while respiratory symptoms (nasal discharge, sore throat, and dry cough) are more common in the

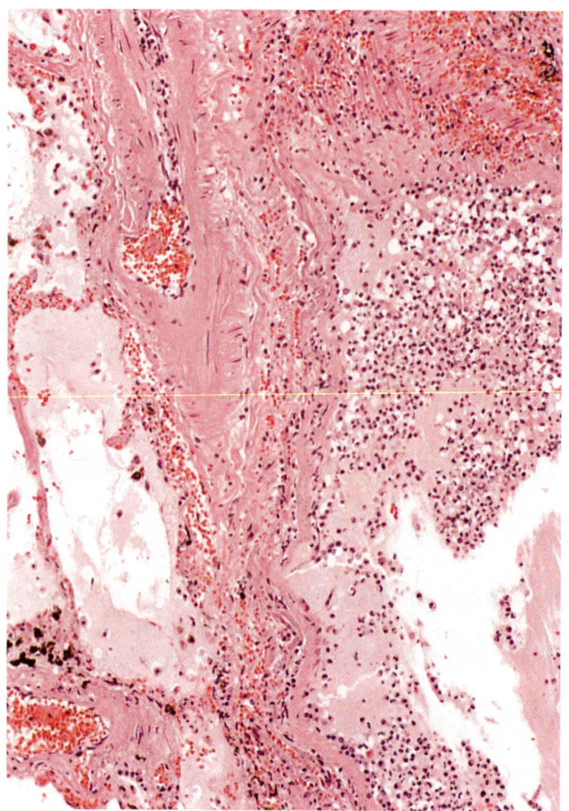

Figure 12-158

INFLUENZA BRONCHIOLITIS

A necrotizing inflammatory infiltrate involves the bronchiolar wall and there is a marked luminal neutrophilic exudate. (Courtesy of Dr. Dani Zander, Gainesville, FL.)

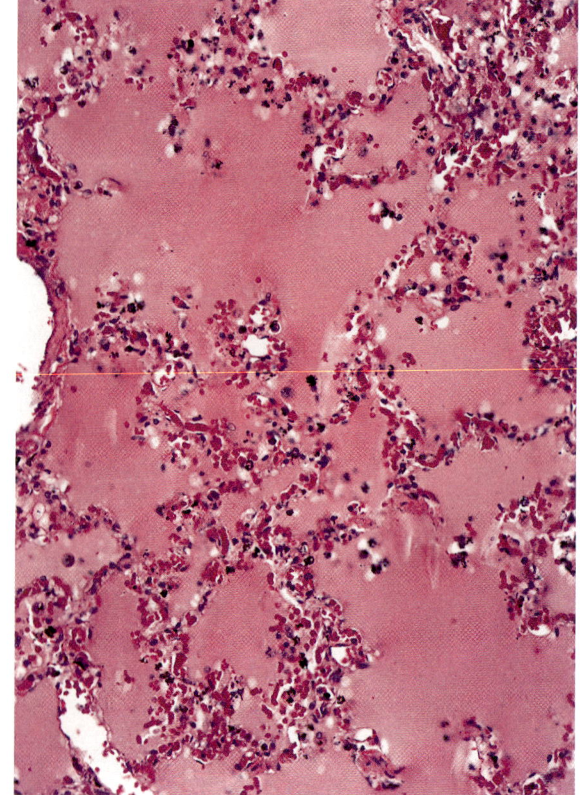

Figure 12-159

INFLUENZA VIRUS: CASE FROM 1918 EPIDEMIC

There is marked pulmonary edema with mild interstitial thickening. (Courtesy of Dr. Jeffrey Taubenberger, AFIP, Washington, DC.)

latter part of the first week of the illness. In the second week patients tend to have nonproductive cough, easy fatigability, and asthenia. Children may have cervical lymphadenopathy, croup, sore throat, and otitis media (352,433,434).

Patients can develop secondary bacterial infection with *Haemophilus influenza, Staphylococcus aureus,* and *Streptococcus pneumoniae.* Herpes simplex can also be a cause of secondary pneumonia. Diffuse pulmonary fibrosis may be a complication. Uncommon systemic complications include myopathy, myocarditis, Guillain-Barre syndrome, toxic shock syndrome, and Reyes' syndrome.

Radiologic Findings. The main radiographic feature of influenza virus pulmonary infection is an ill-defined patchy consolidation, which may progress to confluent lung disease. Pulmonary involvement may be bilateral or unilateral. Pleural effusion is rare (337).

Pathologic Findings. The pulmonary pathologic findings of influenza pneumonia vary depending on the severity of the infection, the stage at which the specimen is obtained, and whether there is an associated infection. Most of the available data come from autopsy specimens, which naturally show advanced stages of infection, often with complications of secondary infection (336,354,355,391,412,435). The pathology ranges from a minimal histologic change to bronchitis, bronchiolitis (fig. 12-158), edema (fig. 12-159), and alveolitis, to severe changes of diffuse alveolar damage (336,355, 360,367,392,416,420,433–435,438).

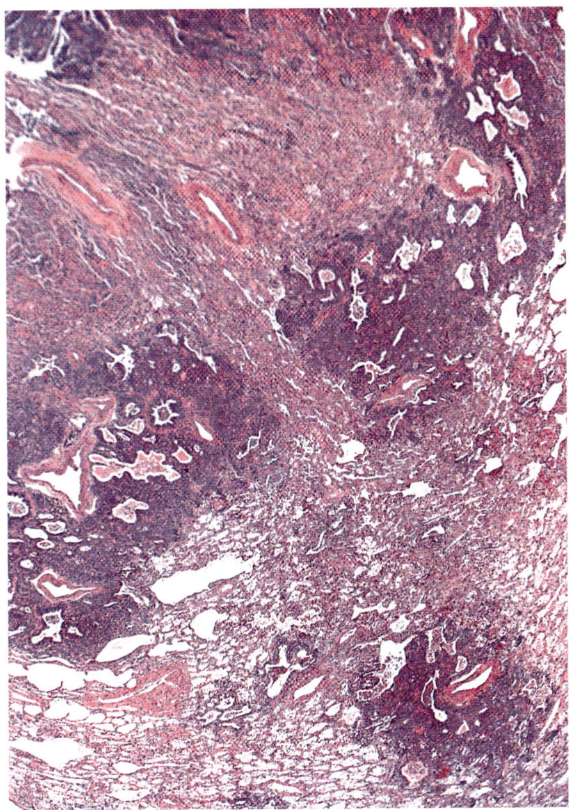

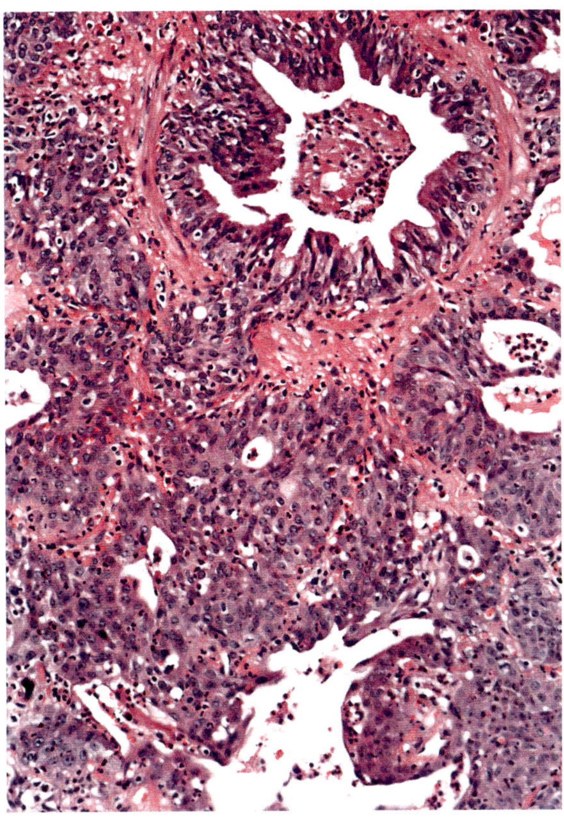

Figure 12-160

INFLUENZA VIRUS: MARKED SQUAMOUS METAPLASIA FOLLOWING INFLUENZA PNEUMONIA

Left: There is a marked epithelial proliferation centered on multiple bronchioles.

Right: The epithelial cells consist of squamous metaplasia extensively replacing the epithelium of the bronchiole and the surrounding airways.

The early pathologic changes of influenza pneumonia consist of a bronchiolitis with necrosis of the ciliated and goblet epithelial cells of the bronchiolar epithelium (355,420,434). A neutrophilic exudate may be present in the bronchiolar lumen. The interstitium may show congestion, edema (fig. 12-159), and a cellular infiltrate. The airspaces may become filled with edema, fibrin, and varying numbers of neutrophils. When hyaline membranes become evident, the process has evolved to frank diffuse alveolar damage (434). These membranes develop as early as the second day or as late as the third week in the course of the disease.

The chronic effects of influenza pneumonia include squamous metaplasia (fig. 12-160) and interstitial fibrosis. Squamous metaplasia may be so severe that the masses of metaplastic epithelia have been referred to as "tumorlets," perhaps because they can be mistaken for carcinoid tumorlets or a malignant neoplasm (fig. 12-160) (336,434). Organizing pneumonia, bronchiolitis, bronchiectasis, and interstitial fibrosis may also develop (373,434,438).

Since influenza pneumonia does not produce characteristic viral cytopathic changes, it is not possible to make the diagnosis based on routine histologic examination of tissue sections. Thus it may be impossible to make the diagnosis without a good clinical history or additional diagnostic methods such as serology, culture, immunohistochemistry (fig. 12-161), in situ hybridization, or PCR for viral nucleic acid (341,377,379,421,433). The presence of neutrophils suggests a bacterial superinfection. When concurrent bacterial pneumonia is present, it

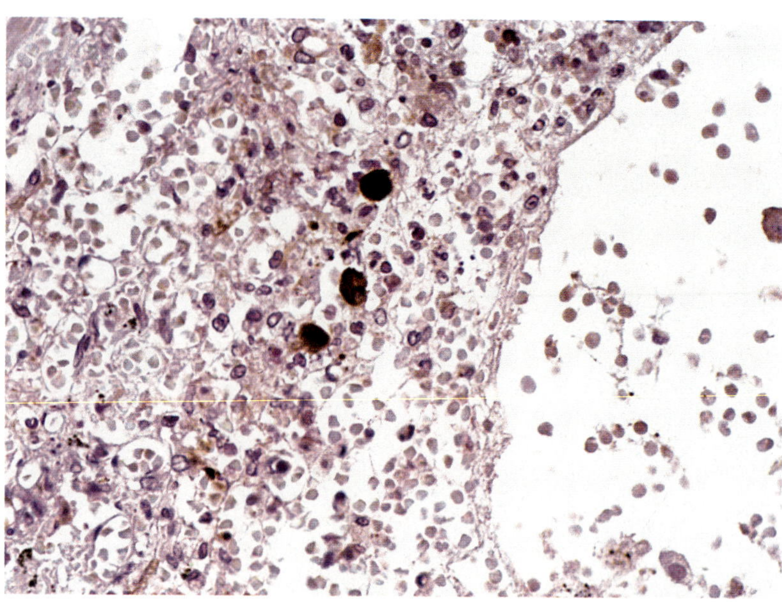

Figure 12-161

INFLUENZA VIRUS: IMMUNOHISTOCHEMISTRY

Several cells stain with an antibody to influenza. (Courtesy of Dr. Dani Zander, Gainesville, FL.)

may be difficult to sort out the pathology of the underlying influenza pneumonia (434,435).

Differential Diagnosis. The lack of distinctive cytopathic effects makes the diagnosis of influenza pneumonia difficult for the anatomic pathologist. Recognition of an acute lung injury pattern, particularly with a necrotizing bronchiolitis, should prompt a viral infectious evaluation including cultures or other special techniques to pursue the cause. One problem in the differential diagnosis of influenza pneumonia is separating the effects of a superimposed bacterial pneumonia, when present, from the underlying viral pneumonia. When severe squamous metaplasia occurs it may mimic a neoplasm, either a carcinoid tumorlet or a well-differentiated squamous cell carcinoma. Recognition of the peribronchiolar orientation of the process as well as correlation with the clinical history and chest radiographs, and confirmation by culture or molecular techniques can help in this distinction.

Clinically, the syndrome associated with influenza pneumonia can be produced by a variety of other viruses including adenovirus, parainfluenza virus, and respiratory syncytial virus, so additional microbiologic methods are necessary to establish a firm diagnosis.

Treatment and Prognosis. Influenza is rarely fatal in the immunocompetent host in developed countries. Management with bed rest, oral hydration, antipyretics, and antitussives is usually sufficient. Antiviral agents may be helpful if given early in the course of disease. In immunosuppressed patients or in underdeveloped countries, patients may not be so fortunate and the infection may be associated with superimposed complications of bacterial pneumonia or a severe life-threatening clinical course (352,367,390,391,433,434).

Hantavirus

Definition. Hantavirus pulmonary syndrome is an infection of the lung caused by one of the hantaviruses.

In May, 1993, an epidemic of a respiratory illness in the southwestern United States led to a massive epidemiologic effort which ultimately implicated hantavirus as the cause (422,426). Hantaviruses are members of the Bunyavirus family and the virus that causes the hantavirus pulmonary syndrome is now called the Sin Nombre virus (SNV) (422). Hantavirus pulmonary syndrome has been seen in other states in association with other hantaviruses including New York (New York virus), Florida (Black Canal virus), and Louisiana (Bayou virus). It has also been seen in other countries such as Argentina, Chile, Paraguay, and Bolivia (422). The viruses are thought to be transmitted by exposure to excreta of rodents such as the deer mouse.

Clinical Features. Patients present with fever, myalgias, headache, and cough, followed by rapid development of respiratory failure.

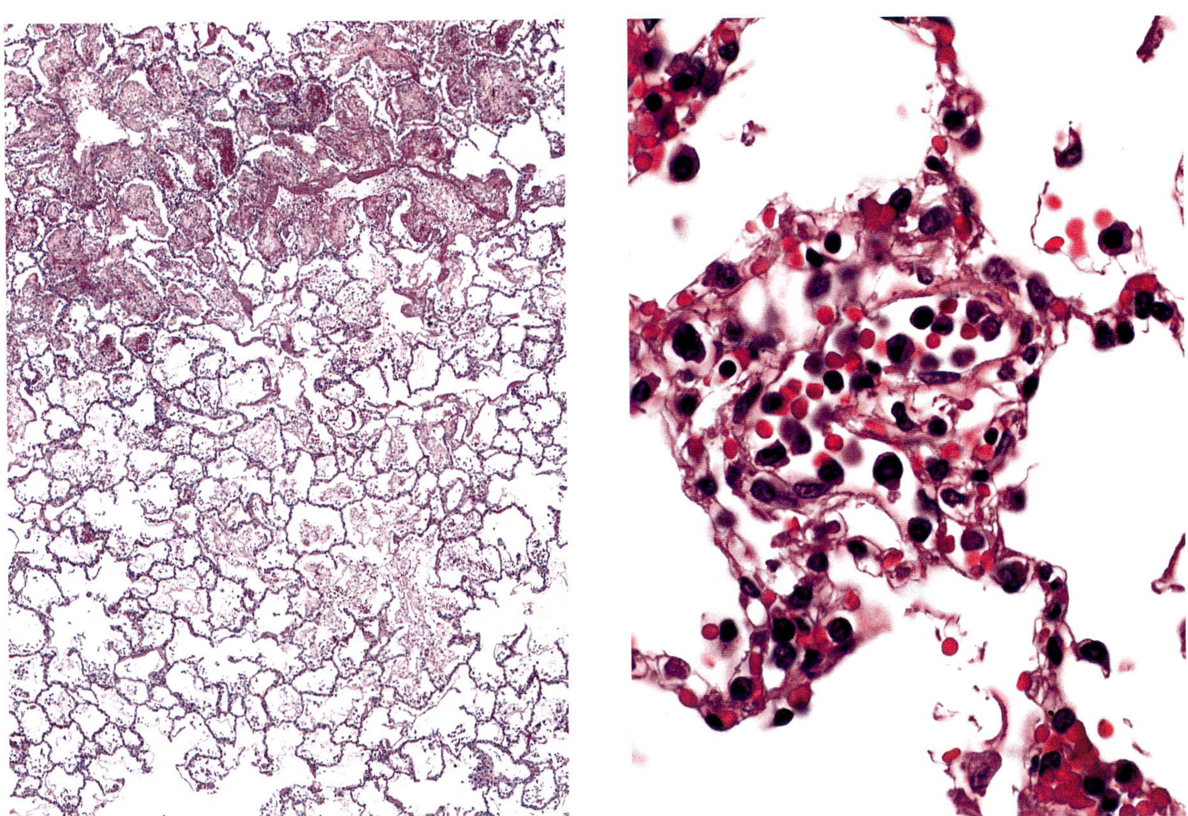

Figure 12-162

HANTAVIRUS PULMONARY SYNDROME

Left: Alveolar edema is the most remarkable histologic feature.
Right: Immature leukocytes are present within alveolar capillaries.

Dizziness and nausea may be present. Laboratory studies reveal thrombocytopenia and left-shifted granulocytes with circulating myeloblasts and immunoblasts. The diagnosis is best established by identifying serum IgM and IgG antibodies with serologic techniques (422).

Radiologic Findings. Chest radiographs show pulmonary edema without consolidation. Pleural effusions are common (337).

Pathologic Findings. The lungs typically show pulmonary edema and mild interstitial thickening with only focal hyaline membranes, resembling early diffuse alveolar damage (fig. 12-162) (316,385,441). Immature leukocytes may be identified within the capillaries (fig. 12-162, right). Pleural effusions may be seen at autopsy. The organisms are identified in lung tissues by immunohistochemistry using monoclonal antibodies (441) and PCR methods (404).

Treatment and Prognosis. The optimal therapy is supportive, with good management of fluid status to avoid worsening pulmonary edema. Ribavirin is being investigated as a potential antimicrobial agent (422). A high mortality (over 50 percent) was seen in early epidemics.

MYCOPLASMAL AND CHLAMYDIAL PNEUMONIAS

Community-acquired pneumonia is a common and serious illness. Bacteria are the most common cause. Community-acquired pneumonias have traditionally been divided into two groups: "typical" (caused by *Streptococcus pneumoniae, Haemophilus influenzae, Staphylococcus aureus*, and other Gram-negative bacteria) and "atypical" (caused by *Legionella* sp, *Mycoplasma pneumoniae, Chlamydia* sp, *Coxiella burnettii*, and a variety of viral agents). *M. pneumoniae, C.*

pneumoniae, or *Legionella* sp cause 7 to 20 percent of community-acquired atypical pneumonias for which a pathogen can be identified. In contrast to patients with more common bacterial pneumonias, those with atypical pneumonia are usually young, otherwise healthy, and tend to be less sick (456). Atypical pneumonia is defined as the association of pneumonitis, fever, and usually a normal peripheral white blood cell count in a patient in whom no bacterial agent can be identified (456). However, recent studies suggest that it is not possible to differentiate the clinical presentation of atypical from typical pneumonia and that co-infections with atypical pathogens and other bacteria are frequent (460). This chapter will focus on the common atypical pneumonias.

Mycoplasma Pneumoniae

Definition. *Mycoplasma* pneumonia is an infection of the lung caused by *Mycoplasma pneumoniae*.

The term "mycoplasma" is widely used to refer to any organism within the class Mollicutes, which is composed of five genera: *Mycoplasma, Ureaplasma, Acholeplasma, Anaeroplasma,* and *Asteroloplasma*. Three species are well-established human pathogens: *Mycoplasma pneumoniae, Mycoplasma hominis,* and *Ureaplasma urealyticum*.

Mycoplasma are bacteria that lack a cell wall and grow in an extracellular location (454,456, 488). They are very small (200 x 10 nm) and are surrounded by a plasma membrane that has three layers (454,456,488). They have a P1 attachment protein that allows the cell to adhere to ciliated respiratory epithelial cells. The organism proliferates outside the cells, producing hydrogen peroxide, superoxides, and cytotoxins, which damage the epithelial cells and interfere with ciliary function.

Clinical Features. The incidence of *M. pneumoniae* infection in the United States is approximately 1/1,000 persons per year (456). It is transmitted person to person through aerosolized droplets (456). Infection occurs most frequently during the fall and winter but may develop year-round. Most patients with pneumonia caused by *M. pneumoniae* infection are children and young adults, however, up to 15 percent of patients are older than 40 years (456, 469). There is an incubation period of 9 to 21 days and patients present with fever, chills, malaise, anorexia, and headache. This is followed by the development of sore throat and dry cough, which may produce mucoid nonpurulent sputum; earache occurs in one third of patients (469). Dyspnea, pleuritic chest pain, and hemoptysis are rare. As the disease progresses, 75 to 100 percent of patients have persistent low-grade fever and an intractable hacking cough. However, only 3 to 10 percent with this intractable, nonproductive cough develop pneumonia. In those with pneumonia, auscultation reveals rhonchi and rales, especially in the lower lobes. Extrapulmonary abnormalities are important and may suggest the diagnosis: hemolysis, cervical lymphadenopathy, joint involvement, pharyngitis, skin rash, conjunctivitis, and symptoms and signs indicative of gastrointestinal tract (nausea, vomiting, diarrhea), central nervous system (aseptic meningitis, meningoencephalitis, peripheral neuropathy, transverse myelitis, cranial nerve palsies, and cerebellar ataxia), and heart (rhythm disturbances, congestive heart failure, chest pain, and conduction abnormalities on the electrocardiogram) involvement (456,469).

The white blood cell count is usually normal although a mild leukocytosis occurs in 25 to 33 percent of patients (469). Cold agglutinins are characteristically present, with a titer greater than 1:32 (456). The diagnosis is often based on the clinical presentation, normal white blood cell count, and elevated titers of cold agglutinins. Cultures require special media. DNA testing can be performed on sputum. A rise of serum titer greater than four-fold using a specific *M. pneumoniae* complement fixation test favors the diagnosis (463).

Rarely, adults or children with *Mycoplasma* pneumonia present with acute respiratory distress syndrome (487). Severe *M. pneumoniae* bronchiolitis can cause a severe restrictive pulmonary function defect in the absence of radiographic findings of pneumonia (447).

Mycoplasma pneumonia may occur in immunocompromised patients with malignancy (leukemia [455] and Ewing's sarcoma [455, 476]), immunodeficiency (443,455), or immunosuppression associated with infectious mononucleosis (451). It is the cause of community-acquired pneumonia in 3 percent of patients with COPD (486).

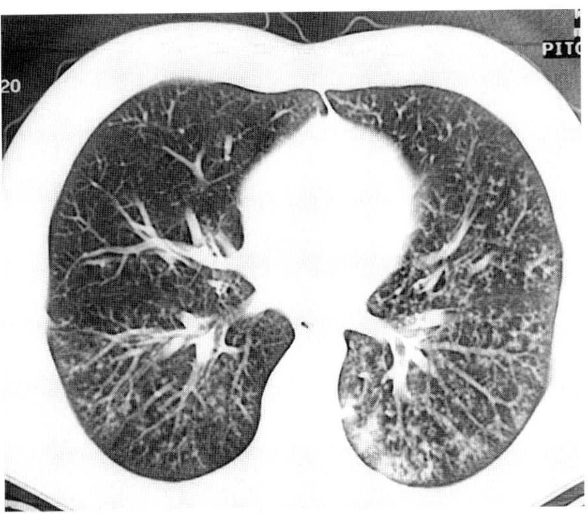

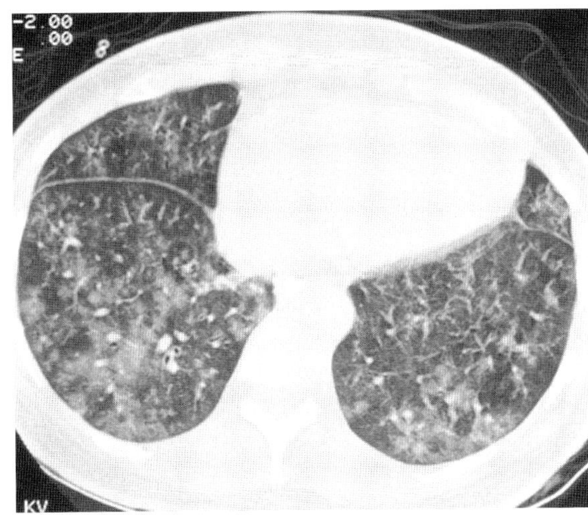

Figure 12-163

MYCOPLASMA PNEUMONIA

Mycoplasma pneumonia in a 60-year-old female with new onset of malaise and dyspnea.

Left: Chest CT demonstrates bilateral centrilobular nodules that are more numerous in the left lung, with focal ground-glass attenuation and consolidation.

Right: Chest CT demonstrates widespread, ill-defined, centrilobular nodules with lobular ground-glass attenuation and consolidation in the lower lobes. (Both figures courtesy of Dr. Rosita M. Shah, Philadelphia, PA.)

Following *M. pneumoniae* infection patients may develop a variety of complications including interstitial fibrosis (487), unilateral hyperlucent lung (Swyer-James syndrome) (482), and impaired pulmonary function (471, 480). *M. pneumoniae* can exacerbate bronchial asthma, however, its role in the initiation of asthma is not clear (491).

Radiologic Findings. Chest radiographs in patients with *Mycoplasma* pneumonia typically demonstrate bilateral airspace consolidations or ground-glass opacities. Consolidations may be segmental or lobar. The lower lobes are more commonly affected. Reticular and nodular opacities, bronchial wall thickening, and small pleural effusions have also been described (478); the latter are reported in up to 30 percent of cases (448).

CT demonstrates poorly defined centrilobular nodules typical of bronchiolitis, lobular patchy airspace consolidation, and ground-glass attenuation (fig. 12-163). These findings are typical of bronchopneumonia. There may be thickening of the peribronchovascular and interlobular septal interstitium (478). Mediastinal lymphadenopathy has also been described (452). Resolution of radiographic abnormalities is relatively rapid and occurs within 4 to 8 weeks in most patients (448). Following *M. pneumoniae* infection the lungs may show mosaic perfusion, bronchiectasis, bronchial wall thickening, decreased vascularity, and air-trapping on expiratory HRCT (465).

Pathologic Findings. Most of the information about the lung pathology of *M. pneumoniae* infection is from autopsy material (464, 466,472,473,484), with only a small number of reports based on surgical lung biopsies (479). The primary histologic finding is a bronchiolitis characterized by a neutrophil-rich luminal exudate and a marked plasma cell–rich chronic inflammatory infiltrate in the bronchiolar wall (fig. 12-164) (479). The epithelium may be ulcerated or show squamous metaplasia. When severe, as seen in autopsy cases, there is necrotizing bronchiolitis and bronchitis. The peribronchiolar alveolar septa may be thickened with prominent type 2 pneumocyte hyperplasia. As this process heals, lesions of bronchiolitis obliterans (461,468,477) and bronchiectasis (459,490) may be seen. Lung abscess has been reported (481).

Diffuse alveolar damage (DAD) and organizing pneumonia are other potential pathologic manifestations (446,479). However, the DAD

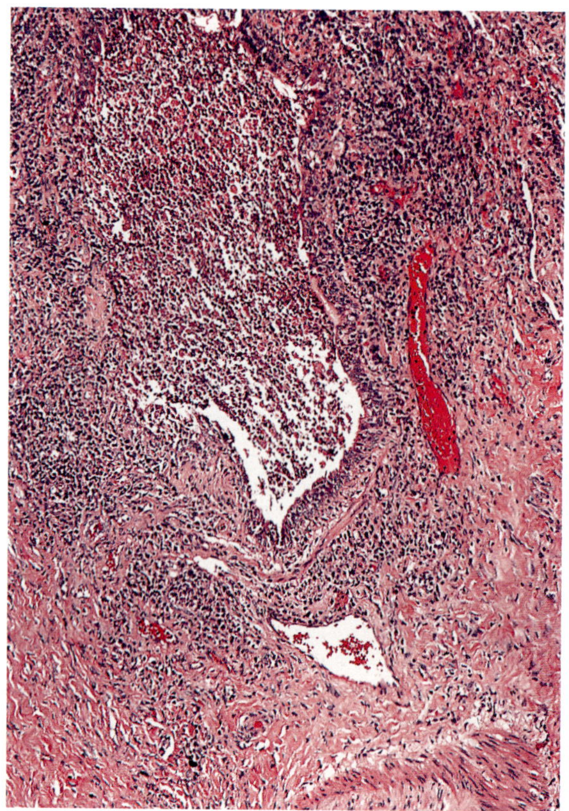

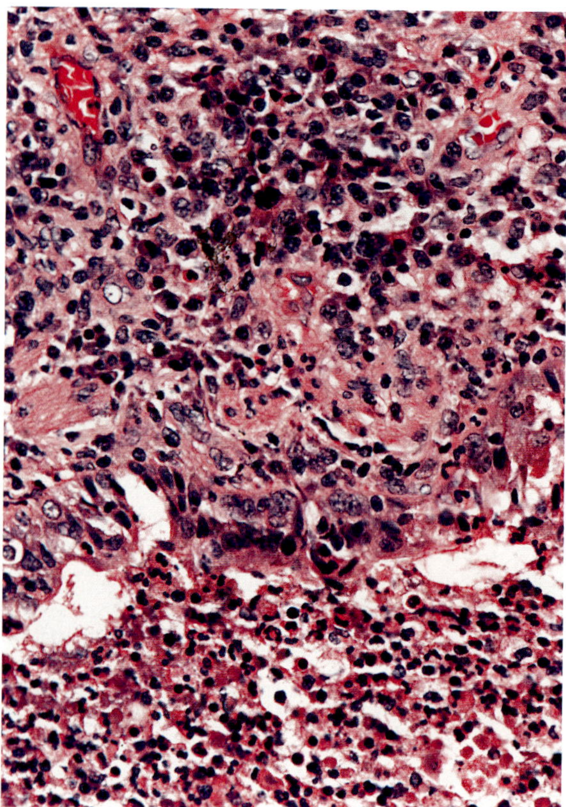

Figure 12-164

MYCOPLASMA PNEUMONIAE: HISTOLOGY

Left: Necrotizing bronchiolitis is characterized by necrosis of the bronchiolar wall accompanied by a prominent chronic inflammatory infiltrate and a neutrophilic exudate in the bronchiolar lumen.

Right: The wall of the bronchiole shows a lymphoplasmacytic infiltrate and numerous neutrophils in the airway lumen.

pattern may show more prominent chronic inflammation and eosinophils than most idiopathic cases (479). Thromboemboli and infarction can be seen (446). Reported cases of diffuse interstitial fibrosis probably represent the fibrosing phase of DAD (464).

None of these histologic features are specific, so when they are recognized they may suggest appropriate clinical tests to confirm the histologic impression. Electron microscopy can show filamentous structures that are suggestive of *M. pneumoniae* organisms, but this is not an optimal way to establish the diagnosis. The diagnosis is usually established by the clinical features in conjunction with serology or culture. However, in some patients the diagnosis is not suspected and only recognition of the characteristic histologic findings on a surgical lung biopsy enables the pathologist to suggest the diagnosis.

Differential Diagnosis. The histologic differential diagnosis for *M. pneumoniae* infection depends on the pattern of lung involvement. The classic differential diagnoses for bronchiolitis or DAD should be considered if that pattern is present. However, a bronchiolitis with a neutrophilic luminal exudate and a prominent plasma cell infiltrate in the bronchiolar wall should raise the possibility of *M. pneumoniae* infection.

Treatment and Prognosis. Patients with *M. pneumoniae* infection usually recover completely. The rare patient who develops the acute respiratory distress syndrome is at higher risk for a fatal outcome (463,489). Sequelae such as bronchiectasis or interstitial fibrosis are potential complications. The main therapy for *M. pneumoniae* infection is doxycycline or erythromycin. Both agents are equally effective and reduce symptom duration (463,489).

Chlamydia Sp

Definition. Chlamydial pneumonias are infections of the lung caused by *Chlamydia trachomatis, C. pneumoniae,* or *C. psittaci.*

Chlamydia are obligate intracellular bacteria that can only grow in host cells and not in artificial media (483,488). They are major causes of genital tract and ocular infections worldwide. Chlamydia replicate by undergoing binary fission (450). The elementary body attaches to the host respiratory epithelial cells, induces phagocytosis, and transforms into the intracellular reticulate body (450). After the metabolically active reticulate body undergoes a set number of cycles of binary fission, infectious elementary bodies are formed and are released, allowing for infection of more epithelial cells (450,483,488). The reticular body is 850 nm in diameter and the elementary body is much smaller, measuring 350 nm (483,488).

C. trachomatis causes pneumonia in infants, *C. pneumoniae* causes a mild pneumonia in children and young adults, and *C. psittaci*, a zoonosis associated with exposure to infected birds, causes a systemic infection primarily affecting the lung (463,483,488).

***Chlamydia psittaci* (Psittacosis, Ornithosis, Parrot Fever).** Psittacosis is acquired most often through exposure to birds that are usually ill due to *C. psittaci* infection. Rarely, it is transmitted person to person through aerosols (463,483,488). Birds usually have an intestinal infection and excrete chlamydial elementary bodies in their feces, which aerosolize and are inhaled by humans. The birds are often pets, most commonly parrots. Psittacosis is an occupational hazard for pet shop employees, veterinarians, zoo personnel, and workers in poultry processing plants (463,483,488).

Patients have a systemic infection characterized by pneumonitis, fever, myalgias, and malaise (463,483,488). The high fever and chills are of sudden or gradual onset. The disease typically follows a 1- to 2-week incubation period. Patients also have headache, arthralgias, and painful myalgias.

The primary pulmonary symptom is severe cough and if there is extensive lung involvement, patients may have chest pain and dyspnea. Extrapulmonary manifestations include splenomegaly, a cutaneous macular rash (also known as Horder's spots), cardiac disease (endocarditis, pericarditis, myocarditis), neurologic disease (altered mental status, encephalitis, meningitis, seizures), glomerulonephritis, pancreatitis, hemolysis, and thyroiditis (463,483,488).

Chest radiographs typically demonstrate homogeneous ground-glass opacities and patchy reticular opacities radiating from the hila. Hilar lymphadenopathy may occur. Radiographic resolution is typically slow (453).

Little is known about the pathologic features of psittacosis since patients are diagnosed clinically and not by lung biopsy. A few reports describe autopsy features. Consolidation can either be lobular or lobar (444,470). Early lesions consist of alveolar exudates of fibrin, neutrophils, and hemorrhage; diffuse alveolar damage (fig. 12-165), which can progress to a mononuclear infiltrate; and interstitial thickening associated with prominent pneumocyte hyperplasia (fig. 12-166) (444,470,483). Bronchiolitis can be severe while lymphocytes and macrophages surround proximal airways. The hyperplastic pneumocytes characteristically contain minute, basophilic, intracytoplasmic coccobacillary inclusions (444,470,483).

The optimal method for establishing the diagnosis is by serology using the complement fixation test, which should demonstrate a fourfold increase in titer (444,470,483). However, a titer of 1:16 or greater is regarded as evidence of infection in a patient with an appropriate history (444,470,483). A microimmunofluorescence method is more sensitive than the complement fixation test (444,470,483). PCR shows promise as a diagnostic tool (485). It is difficult to rely on fluorescent antibody stains of tissue specimens and cultures for inclusion bodies and organisms to establish the diagnosis. The organism can be isolated using tissue culture methods, but the technique is difficult and not widely available (444,470,483).

The clinical course is variable, ranging from a mild illness to a fulminant infection with multisystem involvement. Patients have an excellent prognosis with appropriate therapy, which consists of tetracycline for at least 2 weeks to prevent relapse. Rarely, patients develop complications of encephalitis, hepatitis, renal failure, and disseminated intravascular coagulation. Mortality is 1 percent or less (463).

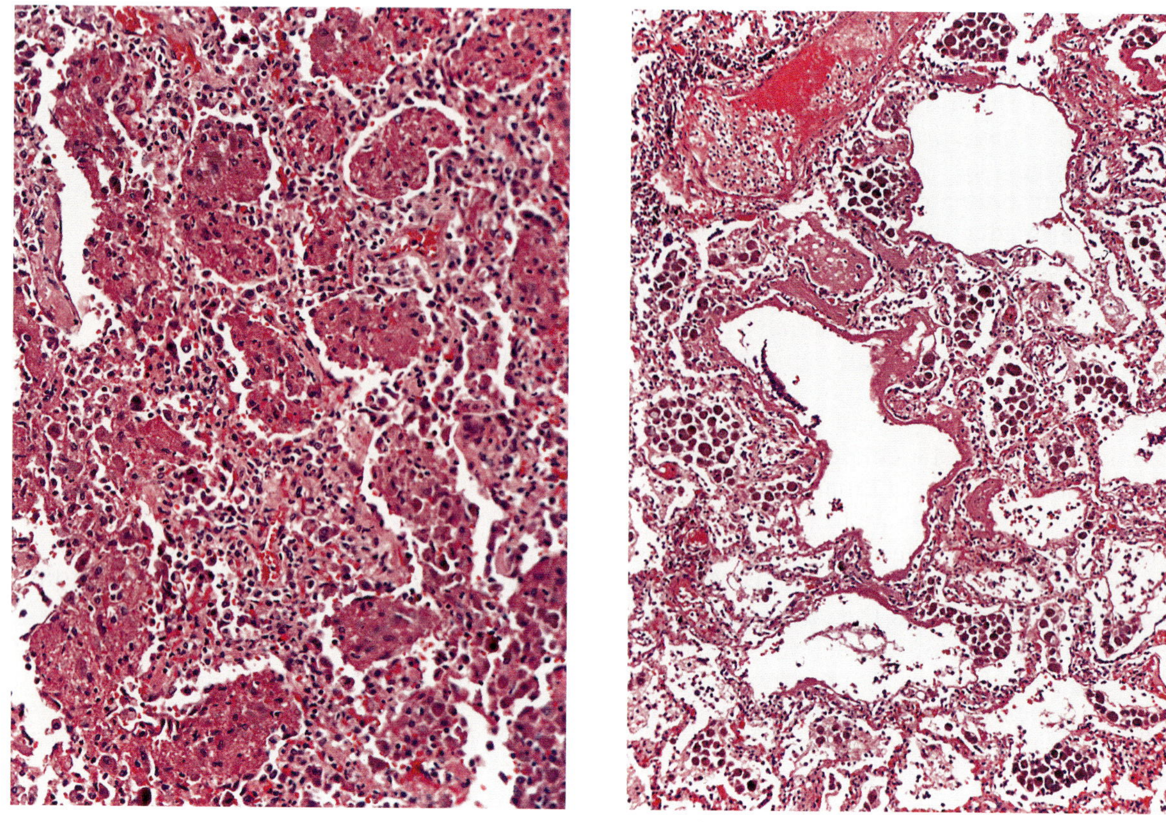

Figure 12-165

CHLAMYDIA PSITTACI PNEUMONIA

Left: The alveoli are filled with edema and fibrin. The alveolar walls are mildly thickened.

Right: Hyaline membranes outline an alveolar duct and there is marked edema and fibrin in the surrounding airspaces. The interstitium is mildly thickened.

Figure 12-166

CHLAMYDIA PSITTACI PNEUMONIA

A chronic inflammatory interstitial infiltrate and hyperplasia of type 2 pneumocytes accompany the alveolar fibrinous exudate.

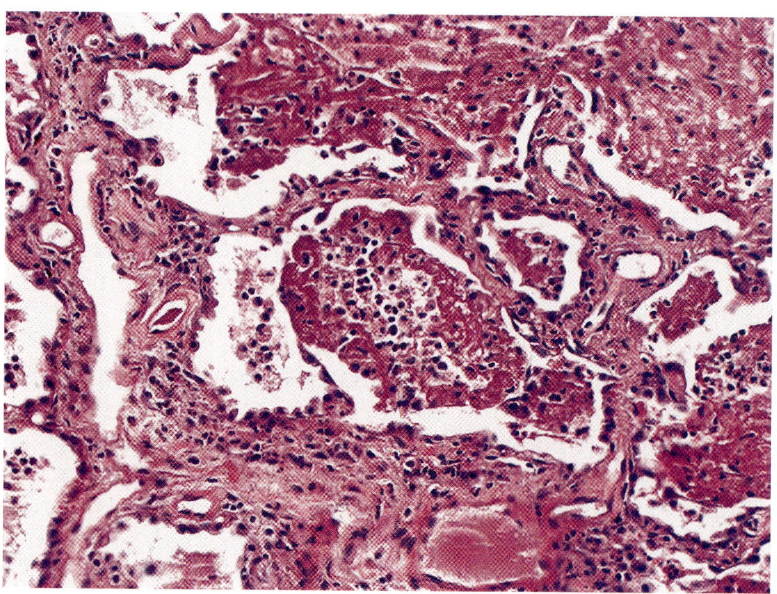

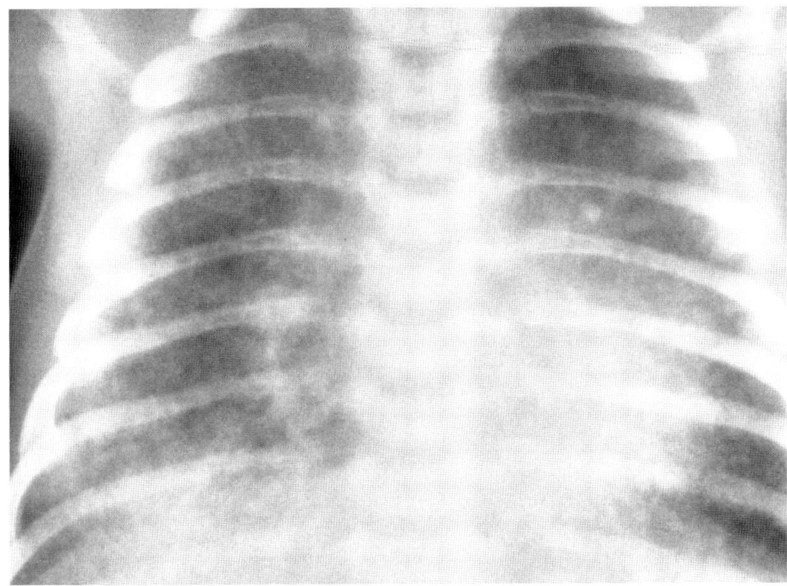

Figure 12-167

CHLAMYDIAL PULMONARY INFECTION IN A 24-DAY-OLD INFANT

AP portable chest radiograph demonstrates bilateral, diffuse, ill-defined parenchymal opacities. Note the normal-to-increased lung volumes.

Chlamydia Trachomatis. *C. trachomatis* causes pneumonia in infants usually between 1 and 6 months of age (463,488). Transmission is during birth from a mother with an endocervical infection (463,488). Patients have gradual tachypnea, staccato coughing, rales, and absence of fever (463,488). Conjunctivitis occurs in approximately 50 percent. The laboratory findings may show peripheral eosinophilia and hyperglobulinemia.

Rarely, *C. trachomatis* is the cause of pneumonia in adults, especially in patients who are immunosuppressed because of bone marrow transplantation, acute leukemia, or HIV infection (462,463,474,488).

The diagnosis is usually established by clinical findings, serology (elevated *Chlamydia* titers in the blood or tears), and isolation of *C. trachomatis* in specimens obtained from the lung. Immunofluorescent antibodies can detect the organism in tissue or cytology specimens (463,488).

Chest radiographs of affected infants demonstrate diffuse bilateral interstitial and airspace opacities with atelectasis and overinflation (fig. 12-167). Pleural effusions and mediastinal lymphadenopathy have also been described (453). There is little known about the histology of *C. trachomatis* pneumonia in infants since virtually all patients survive and do not have surgical lung biopsy (458,474). However, interstitial or alveolar pneumonia and bronchiolitis are reported (458, 488). The inflammatory cells consist of lymphocytes, plasma cells, neutrophils, alveolar macrophages, and eosinophils (458,488).

The lung biopsy in one adult immunosuppressed patient (462) showed multiple bronchiolocentric nodules of alveolar and interstitial inflammation consisting of lymphocytes and histiocytes, with only rare neutrophils, and prominent type 2 pneumocyte hyperplasia. In another study from adult patients who had bone marrow transplants, the most common histologic finding was a diffuse interstitial pneumonia with varying degrees of interstitial fibrosis and pneumocyte hyperplasia (474). Hyaline membranes and acute to subacute organizing pneumonia were also seen (474).

Infants with *C. trachomatis* pneumonia usually recover even without treatment. Optimal therapy includes erythromycin or sulfasoxazole. Ideally, the disease can be prevented by treating infected mothers prior to birth (463,488).

Chlamydia Pneumoniae. *C. pneumoniae* was relatively recently discovered to be a third species of *Chlamydia* that can cause pneumonia and bronchitis (457,467). In 1985, a new strain of *Chlamydia* was recognized based on an epidemic of mild pneumonia in young adults from Finland. It was called the TWAR strain initially due to similarities between the Taiwan (TR-183) and the AR-39 strains, but it was subsequently called *Chlamydia pneumoniae* (463,483,488). It differs from *C. trachomatis* and *C. psittaci* in that it has a pear-shaped elementary body as seen by ultrastructure and less than 10 percent of the DNA shows homology with those species (457,467).

The organism is found worldwide. Serologic studies suggest antibodies are uncommon in children, are found in 40 to 50 percent of the population in their fourth decade of life, and often exceed 80 percent in the elderly (463). The mode of transmission is unknown but thought to be via infected respiratory secretions.

C. pneumoniae infection is most common among children between the ages of 5 and 14 years. Children usually have mild or asymptomatic infections, but adults tend to have disease of greater severity. *C. pneumoniae* is thought to cause approximately 10 percent of cases of pneumonia and 5 percent of cases of bronchitis in the United States (457,467). The most common symptoms are nonproductive cough and fever (457,467). This may be preceded by pharyngitis. Other potential manifestations include bronchitis, sinusitis, and laryngitis. *C. pneumoniae* is a potential cause of respiratory infections in HIV-infected individuals (445,449) and may cause severe acute chest syndrome in children with sickle cell disease. Extrapulmonary manifestations of infection with *C. pneumoniae* include: meningoencephalitis, Guillain-Barré syndrome, reactive arthritis, and myocarditis. *C. pneumoniae* infection may be a trigger for asthma.

Serologic assays using a microimmunofluorescent method are useful in establishing the diagnosis and effective in separating recent from past infections (457,467). The organism can be cultivated in cell culture (457,467). PCR techniques have been shown recently to be valuable for detecting *C. pneumoniae* in respiratory specimens (485).

C. pneumoniae infection manifests radiographically as airspace consolidation, interstitial opacities, or both. Pleural effusions are also reported (453).

Little is known about the histology of *C. pneumoniae* pulmonary infections since these patients have mild disease, usually recover, and do not have surgical lung biopsy or autopsy (488). Presumably the histologic findings consist primarily of an acute and/or chronic bronchiolitis.

Most patients recover completely, although older patients may have a more severe illness. Fatalities are rare and usually associated with other severe underlying diseases. The treatment of choice for *C. pneumoniae* infection is doxycycline. The organism is susceptible to erythromycin and ciprofloxacin in vitro (463). However, few clinical trials have firmly established the optimal therapy. Oral clarithromycin was recently shown to be effective in children (475). Anecdotal data suggest that prolonged therapy (more than 2 weeks up to a month) is need to prevent recurrence (460).

PNEUMOCYSTIS CARINII PNEUMONIA

Definition. *Pneumocystis* pneumonia is an infection of the lung caused by *Pneumocystis carinii*. *P. carinii* pneumonia has been recognized since the early 1900s. In the late 1940s, outbreaks of interstitial plasmacellular pneumonia were seen, especially among premature infants and marasmic orphans (505). Subsequently, *P. carinii* was recognized as an important cause of opportunistic pneumonia in patients with impaired T-cell immunity (519).

P. carinii is a fungus related to the *Saccharomyces* (506). There are two major forms of the organism: trophozoites and cysts. The cysts are thick-walled and have eight internal sporozoites (525,536). The organism is probably acquired through airborne respiratory secretions, but the precise mechanism of transmission is not completely understood (525,536). The epidemiologic pattern of *P. carinii* pneumonia suggests a seasonal periodicity similar to that seen with other upper respiratory tract infections. DNA amplification of induced sputa from healthcare workers exposed to patients with acute *P. carinii* pneumonia shows the presence of *P. carinii*. This finding implies that those in close contact with patients with *P. carinii* pneumonia may develop a carrier state. It is thought that the organism causes subclinical pulmonary infection in most individuals during childhood (65 to 100 percent of children have antibodies to *P. carinii* by the age of 4 years) and then the latent infection develops into an opportunistic pneumonia when the patient becomes immunosuppressed (525,536).

The inability to culture *P. carinii* has inhibited progress in understanding the origin and biologic properties of this organism (532). While lung biopsy was once regarded as the definitive approach to diagnosis, other reliable

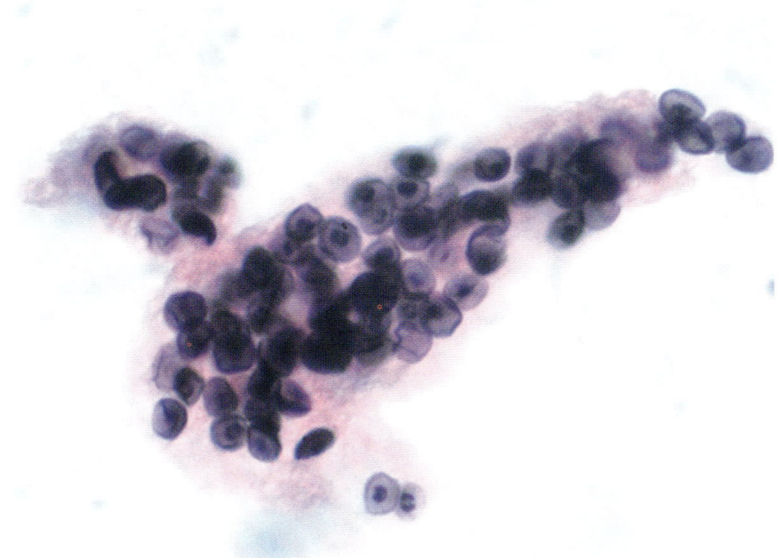

Figure 12-168

PNEUMOCYSTIS CARINII PNEUMONIA

Bronchoalveolar lavage shows multiple cysts of *P. carinii* highlighted with the GMS stain. The cysts are round to oval and have prominent, darkly stained foci.

approaches now include cytologic examination of BAL fluid (diagnostic in 80 to 90 percent of cases) (fig. 12-168) (511), bronchial washings (527), and sputum specimens (495).

Clinical Features. *P. carinii* pneumonia typically develops in patients who are immunocompromised due to a variety of underlying causes including premature birth; malnutrition; receiving chemotherapy for immunologic disease, cancer, or organ transplantation; congenital or acquired disorders affecting cell-mediated immunity; and AIDS. *P. carinii* is the most common cause of pneumonia in AIDs patients, occurring in at least 80 percent at some time during the course of their disease (525,536). However, recent data suggest that this frequency may be decreasing (517).

The clinical presentation of patients with *P. carinii* pneumonia is variable and the spectrum of clinical manifestations has expanded since the onset of the AIDS epidemic (522,534). At one extreme, the symptoms and signs are minimal, whereas at the other, there is rapidly progressive respiratory failure. The typical presentation is with nonproductive cough, dyspnea, and fever. Patients with AIDS have a more indolent presentation with symptoms gradually increasing over weeks to a few months. Tachypnea is present and crackles may be heard on chest examination. In HIV-infected patients, thin-walled cysts may develop and predispose to pneumothorax.

Routine laboratory studies are not helpful in diagnosis. An elevated lactate dehydrogenase level (LDH) is present in 90 percent of HIV-infected patients with *P. carinii* pneumonia and has some prognostic significance, with a rising LDH level despite appropriate treatment portending a poor prognosis. HIV-infected patients with CD4 counts of less than 200 cells/µL are about five times more likely to develop *P. carinii* pneumonia than patients with CD4 counts of over 200 cells/µL. Gas exchange is usually abnormal and 80 to 95 percent of patients have hypoxemia. Lung function testing shows a decrease in the vital capacity, often with an increase residual volume. The diffusing capacity for carbon monoxide (DLCO) is reduced. It is often used as a screening test for the detection of pneumocystosis in AIDS patients with a normal chest radiograph. *P. carinii* pneumonia is highly unlikely if the DLCO is normal.

Patients with *P. carinii* pneumonia are at risk for other infectious processes or neoplasms since they are immunosuppressed. Cytomegalovirus is the most common associated infection (534). Recent data suggest that the presence of cytomegalovirus in bronchoscopy specimens from patients with *P. carinii* pneumonia does not imply a difference in baseline characteristics, long-term survival, acute death rate, or length of stay in the hospital (515). Neoplasms such as Kaposi's sarcoma or malignant

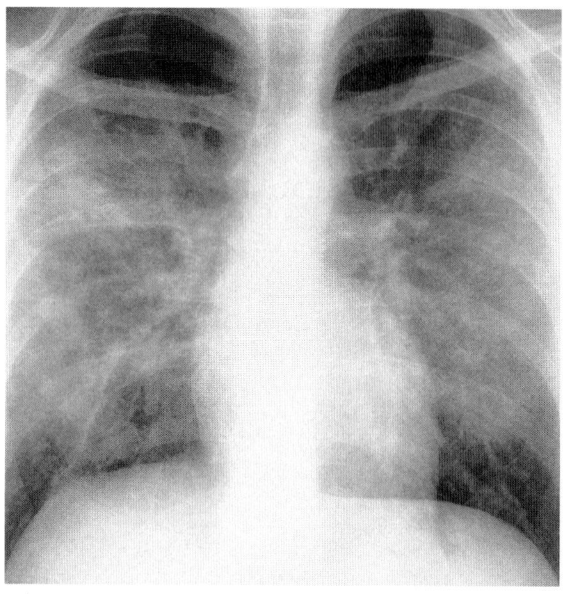

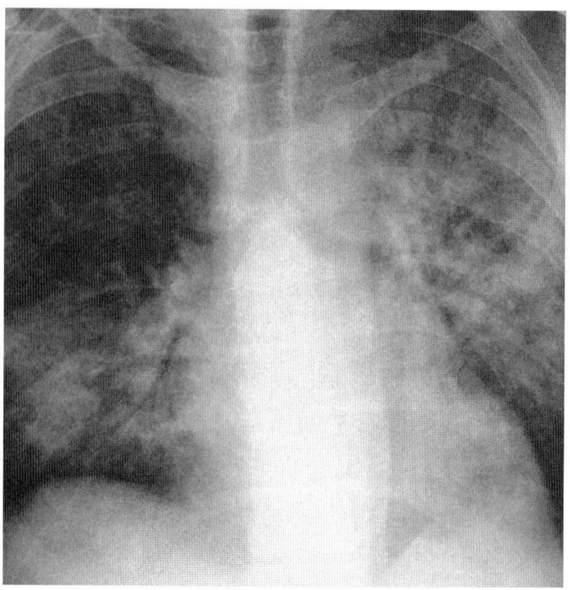

Figure 12-169

PNEUMOCYSTIS CARINII PNEUMONIA

Left: Chest radiograph demonstrates bilateral, hazy, increased opacities (ground-glass pattern) involving mainly the perihilar regions. Airspace consolidation is present in the right upper lobe. The patient was a 32-year-old male with AIDS.

Right: Chest radiograph shows extensive bilateral airspace consolidation. The patient was a 31-year-old male with AIDS.

lymphoma may also be encountered in the lungs of AIDS patients (534).

Radiologic Findings. The earliest manifestation of *P. carinii* pneumonia on the chest radiograph is a fine granular pattern or hazy increased opacity (ground-glass pattern) involving mainly the perihilar regions (fig. 12-169, left) (499,509,510). If untreated, the findings progress to perihilar or diffuse bilateral airspace consolidation (fig. 12-169, right). The consolidation may involve mainly the lower lobes or, less commonly, the upper lobes. The characteristic finding on HRCT is of symmetric, bilateral, ground-glass opacities. These may be diffuse but often have a geographic distribution, with areas of ground-glass attenuation sharply outlined by adjacent normal lung parenchyma (fig. 12-170) (494,509).

AIDS patients with *P. carinii* pneumonia, particularly patients who have received prophylactic aerosolized pentamidine, have a propensity to develop thin-walled cysts (499). Cysts are seen in approximately 10 percent of radiographs and 30 percent of HRCT scans of patients with *P. carinii* pneumonia and AIDS (fig.12-171) (514,530). The cysts usually are bilateral, involve mainly the upper lobes, and often have a predominantly subpleural distribution. Patients with cysts have an increased propensity to develop pneumothorax, sometimes as the presenting manifestation (500).

Although the radiographic and HRCT findings are often suggestive of the diagnosis, atypical manifestations occur in 5 to 10 percent of patients (521). These include single or multiple nodules, thick-walled cavities, focal or asymmetric areas of airspace consolidation, and reticulation (509,521). Approximately 5 percent of patients have normal radiographs (518). In the majority of patients with *P. carinii* pneumonia and normal or equivocal radiographic findings, HRCT scans demonstrate areas of ground-glass attenuation (512,518). Mediastinal lymphadenopathy is uncommon: it is a recognized manifestation in less than 5 percent of AIDS patients due to dissemination of the organism to the lymph nodes (492,499,520).

Pathologic Findings. The cysts of *P. carinii* are round to oval, measure 5 to 7 µm in diameter, and often have very prominent grooves or

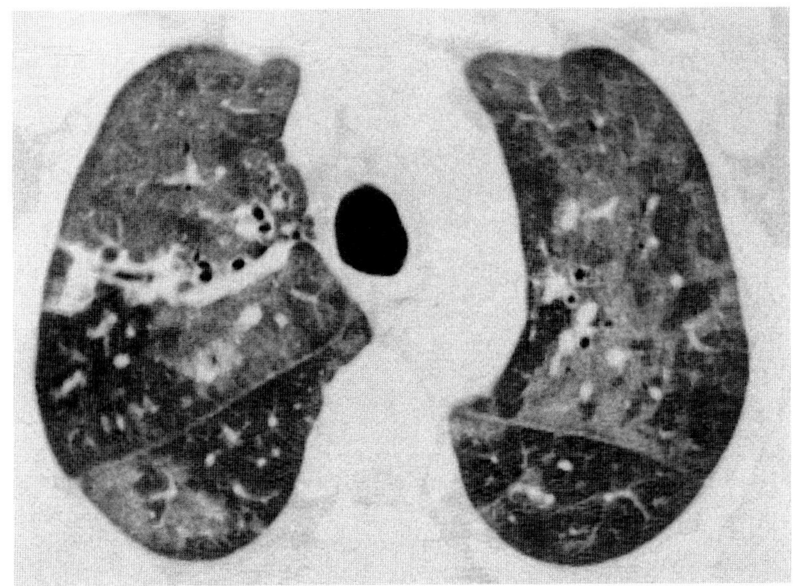

Figure 12-170

PNEUMOCYSTIS CARINII PNEUMONIA

HRCT demonstrates bilateral areas of ground-glass attenuation. Note the geographic distribution with sharp demarcation between normal and abnormal parenchyma. The patient was a 46-year-old male with AIDS.

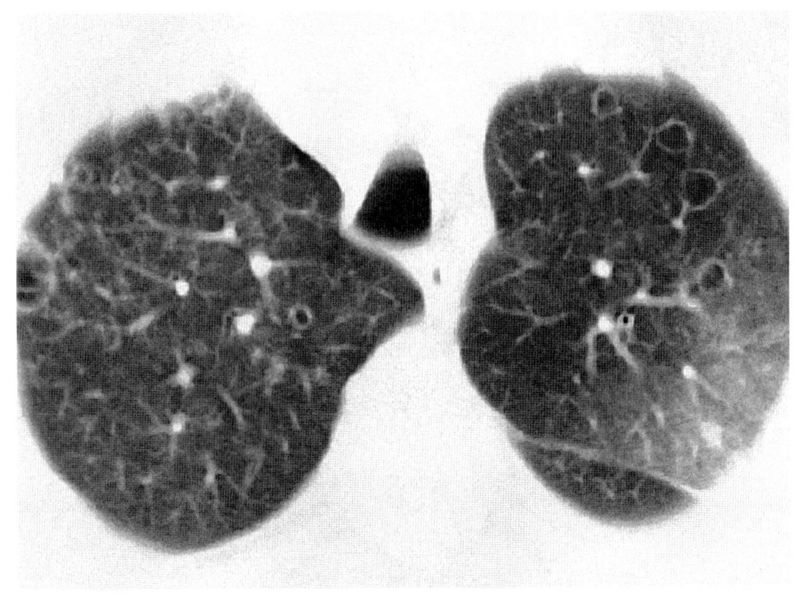

Figure 12-171

PNEUMOCYSTIS CARINII PNEUMONIA

Chest CT demonstrates thin-walled cystic lesions in both upper lobes. Also noted are focal areas of ground-glass attenuation. The patient was a 41-year-old male with AIDS.

folds due to the tendency of the cysts to collapse (fig. 12-172) (493). In addition, darkly stained foci represent discoid thickenings of the cyst capsule. In optimally stained sections, a tiny dot can be identified in the center of many of these small bubbles. Giemsa stains of cytologic preparations can be used to demonstrate the trophozoites, but it is not possible to reliably detect trophozoites by routine light microscopy in histologic sections. The best stain for demonstrating the cysts of *P. carinii* in tissue sections is the GMS stain (534). The toluidine blue stain also highlights the cysts, but it does not stain fungi as well as the GMS stain and is therefore not always as useful in the routine screening of lung biopsies for opportunistic infections.

The classic lesion of *P. carinii* pneumonia consists of an intra-alveolar foamy exudate (fig. 12-173A) in which the organisms appear as small "bubbles" in a background of proteinaceous exudate (fig. 12-173B,C). The alveolar exudate is usually accompanied by a mild interstitial pneumonitis consisting of interstitial chronic inflammation and proliferation of type 2 pneumocytes

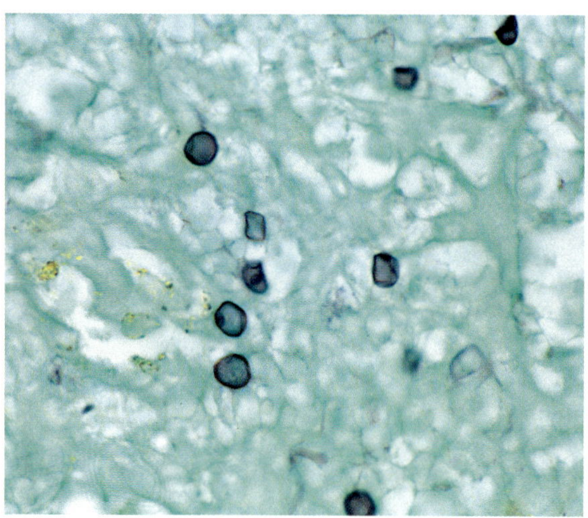

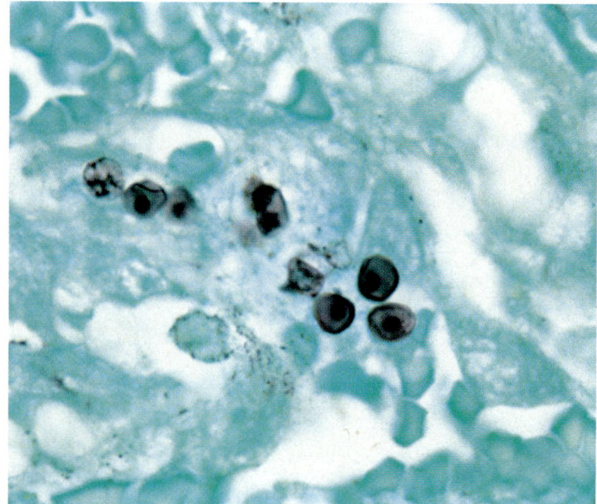

Figure 12-172

PNEUMOCYSTIS CARINII PNEUMONIA

These cysts of *Pneumocystis carinii* are 5 to 7 μm in diameter. The cysts are round to oval and some are folded (left). Several darkly stained foci are present (right) in these cysts.

Figure 12-173

PNEUMOCYSTIS CARINII PNEUMONIA: ALVEOLAR EXUDATE

A: The alveolar spaces are filled with the characteristic foamy eosinophilic exudate. The interstitium is mildly thickened due to inflammation and loose fibrosis, and there is type 2 pneumocyte hyperplasia.

B: The alveolar exudate has a frothy, bubbly appearance due to the many cysts.

C: Within the alveolar exudate are many cysts of *P. carinii*.

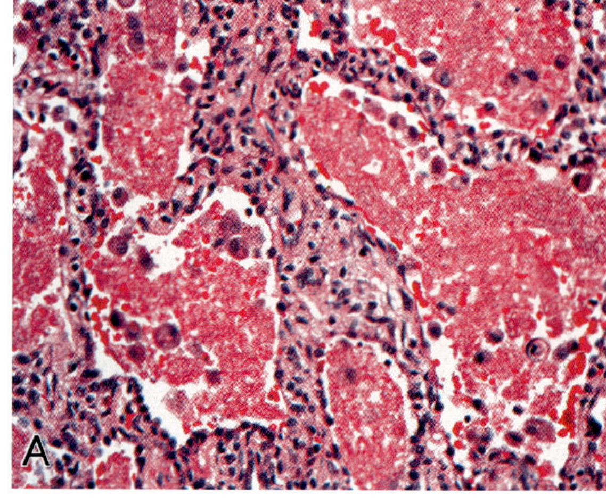

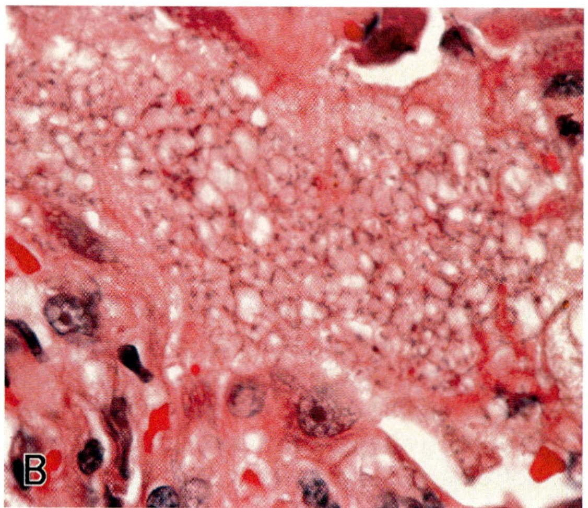

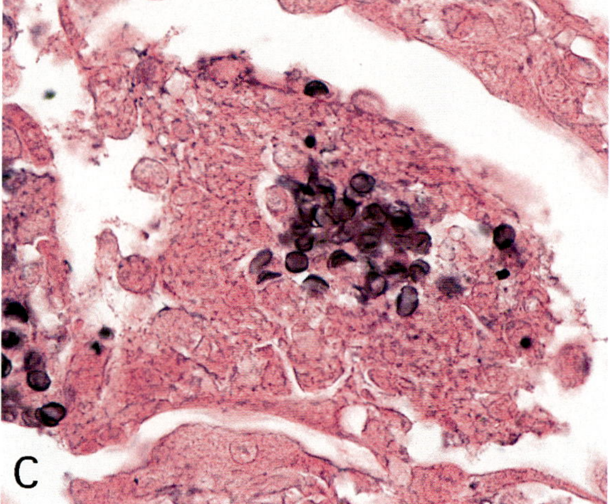

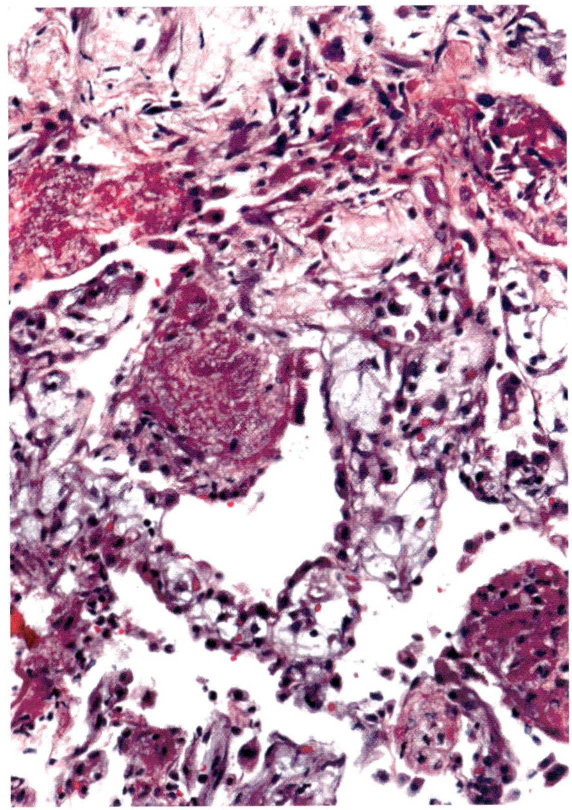

Figure 12-174

PNEUMOCYSTIS CARINII PNEUMONIA: INTERSTITIAL FIBROSIS

The loose organizing interstitial fibrosis is situated primarily in the alveolar walls. Alveolar exudates are being incorporated into the interstitial fibrosis.

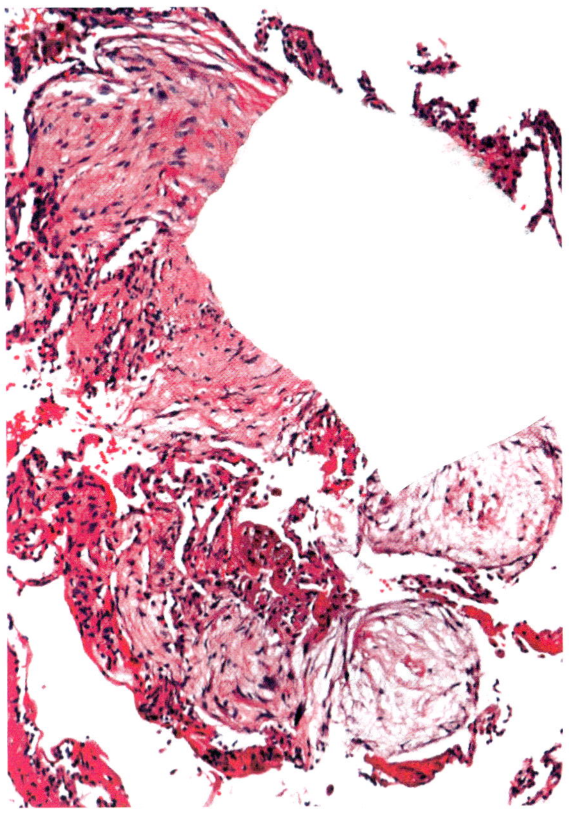

Figure 12-175

PNEUMOCYSTIS CARINII PNEUMONIA: ORGANIZING PNEUMONIA PATTERN

Polypoid plugs of loose connective tissue within these alveolar spaces give the organizing pneumonia pattern in this patient following treatment for *P. carinii* pneumonia.

(fig. 12-173A). Interstitial and intraluminal fibrosis, manifestations of chronic diffuse alveolar damage (fig. 12-174), can be found, respectively, in 63 and 36 percent of lung biopsy specimens from AIDS patients with *P. carinii* pneumonia (534). Biopsies during the resolving phase of the pneumonia may show an organizing pneumonia pattern (fig. 12-175). Severe interstitial fibrosis is seen in patients who die of *P. carinii* pneumonia (529). Less commonly, the acute phase of diffuse alveolar damage with hyaline membranes is seen (fig. 12-176) (534). Hyaline membranes were found in only 4 percent of lung biopsies in one study of AIDS patients with *P. carinii* pneumonia (534).

A variety of unusual pathologic features of *P. carinii* pneumonia have been described in patients with and without AIDS (Table 12-15) (534, 537). Awareness of these unusual manifestations is important since they can result in misleading presenting clinical and/or pathologic features, which can cause diagnostic difficulties.

Absence of the characteristic foamy exudate occurs in up to 47 percent of lung biopsy specimens from non-HIV patients with *P. carinii* pneumonia (537) and up to 19 percent of HIV-infected patients (fig. 12-177; Table 12-15) (534). There are several reasons why the alveolar exudate can be difficult to find, including biopsy artifacts such as intra-alveolar red blood cell accumulation from local hemorrhage or crush artifact causing collapse of alveolar walls. The exudate can also be obscured if the histologic reaction associated with *P. carinii* pneumonia, such as diffuse alveolar damage or lymphocytic interstitial pneumonia, is extensive. In rare cases, the

Figure 12-176

PNEUMOCYSTIS CARINII PNEUMONIA: DIFFUSE ALVEOLAR DAMAGE

Hyaline membranes and prominent interstitial loose fibrosis show the features of acute and organizing diffuse alveolar damage.

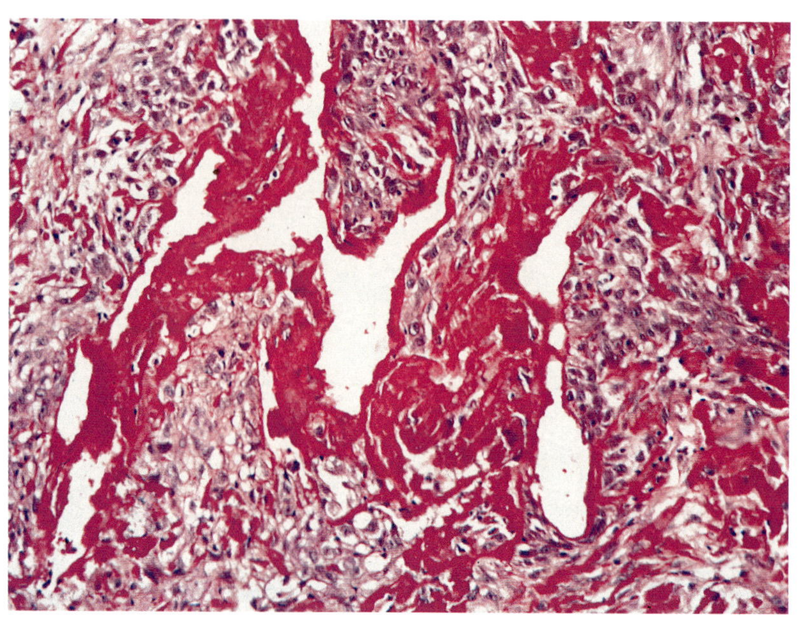

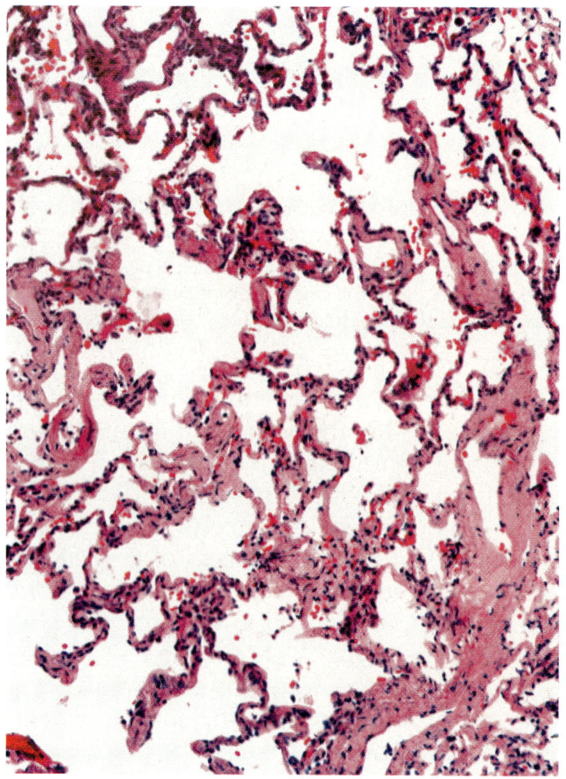

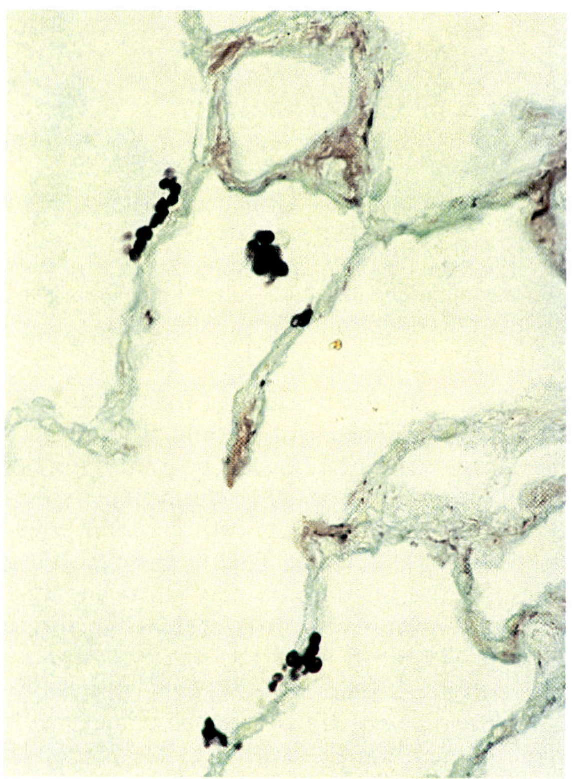

Figure 12-177

PNEUMOCYSTIS CARINII PNEUMONIA: MINIMAL HISTOLOGIC REACTION

Left: There is minimal interstitial reaction of these alveolar walls, without interstitial inflammation and pneumocyte hyperplasia.

Right: The *Pneumocystis* organisms that are lining the alveolar walls stain with the GMS stain.

Table 12-15

LUNG BIOPSY HISTOLOGIC FINDINGS OF *PNEUMOCYSTIS CARINII* PNEUMONIA IN PATIENTS WITH AND WITHOUT HIV INFECTION

	HIV-Infected Patients (% of Lung Biopsies)[a]	Non-HIV-Infected Patients (% of Lung Biopsies)[b]
Interstitial fibrosis	63	NA[c]
Intraluminal fibrosis	36	33
Absent exudate	19	47
Many macrophages	9	9
Granulomas	5	17
Hyaline membranes	4	NA
Lymphocytic interstitial pneumonia	3	8
Cysts	2	NA
Microcalcification	2	3
Minimal histology	2	NA
Vascular invasion	1	NA

[a]From reference 534.
[b]From reference 537.
[c]NA = not available.

cysts of *P. carinii* are found along the alveolar wall and there may be virtually no histologic reaction or alveolar exudate (fig. 12-177, right) (534). Rarely, *P. carinii* may have a miliary pattern of lung involvement (fig. 12-178).

Cavitary pulmonary lesions consist of subpleural bullous emphysematous blebs (fig. 12-179), intraparenchymal cysts (fig. 12-180), infarcts, or necrotizing granulomas (534). The cysts are often situated in the subpleural parenchyma. It is not known why cysts occur in *P. carinii* pneumonia in HIV-infected patients, but several theories have been proposed, including interstitial emphysema, remodeling of the lung parenchyma associated with interstitial fibrosis, infarction, necrotizing granulomas, and necrotizing effects of *P. carinii* pneumonia (534). *P. carinii* organisms may spill into the pleural fluid if a subpleural cavitary lesion ruptures. In such cases, cytologic preparations of pleural fluid using the Diff-Quik stain demonstrate trophozoites (507).

Granulomatous inflammation can be found in 5 percent of lung biopsies from HIV-infected adult patients with *P. carinii* pneumonia (figs. 12-181, 12-182) (534). Granulomatous inflammation consists of clusters of epithelioid histiocytes and/or multinucleated giant cells (fig. 12-181), or rarely, necrotizing granulomas (fig. 12-182). In the latter setting, one must be

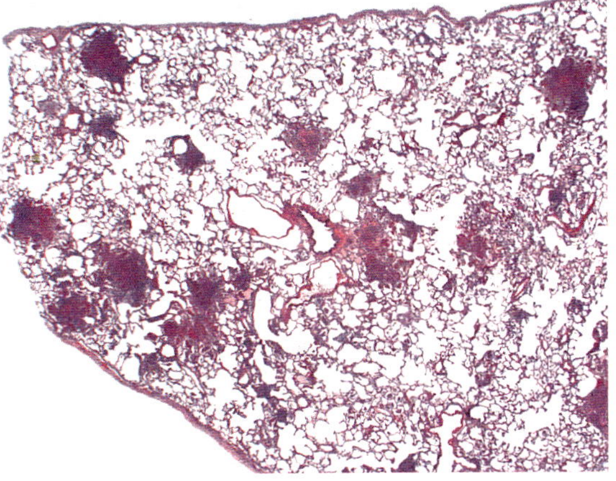

Figure 12-178

PNEUMOCYSTIS CARINII PNEUMONIA: MILIARY PATTERN

Multiple small foci of *P. carinii* are scattered evenly throughout the lung tissue.

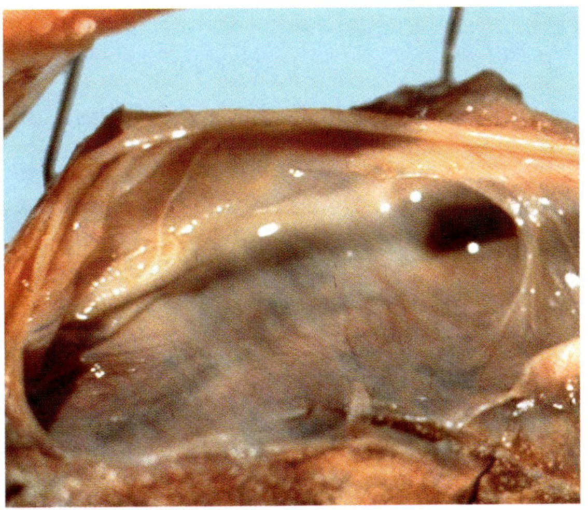

Figure 12-179

PNEUMOCYSTIS CARINII PNEUMONIA: CYSTS

Marked subpleural cystic changes are present in this autopsied lung from an AIDS patient with longstanding recurrent *P. carinii* pneumonia.

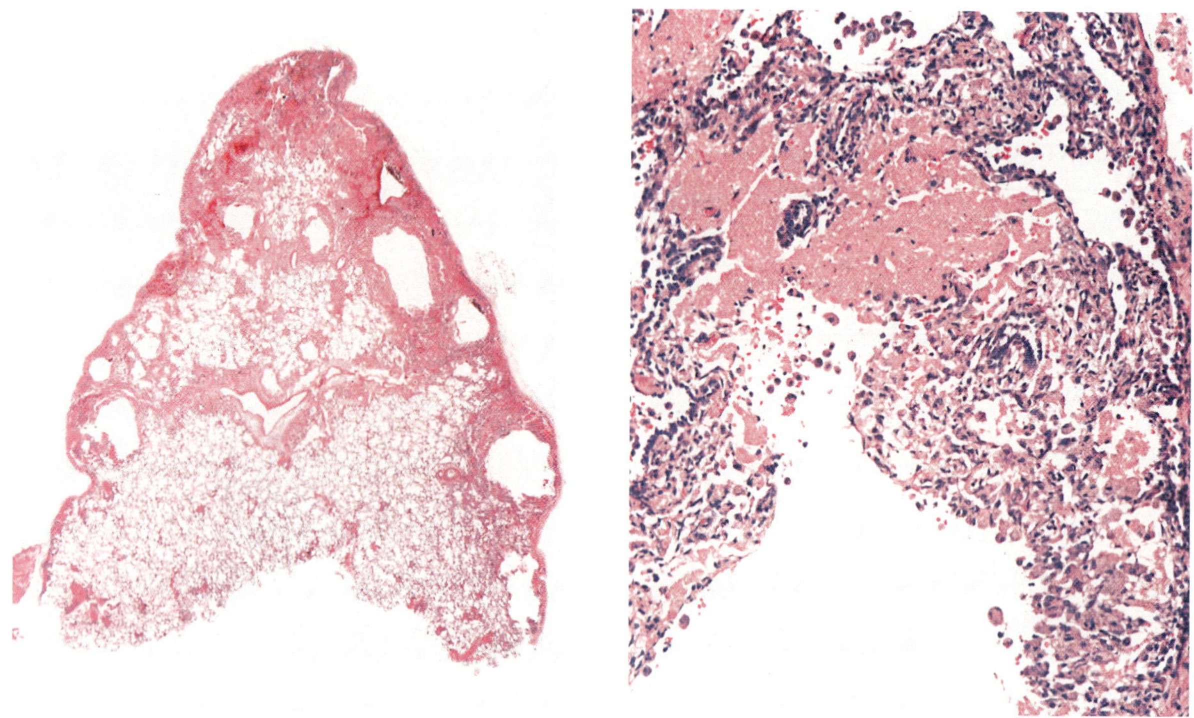

Figure 12-180

PNEUMOCYSTIS CARINII PNEUMONIA: CYSTIC HISTOLOGIC FEATURES

Left: There are multiple cystic spaces, mostly distributed in the subpleural lung parenchyma and accompanied by eosinophilic alveolar exudates.

Right: The wall of this cystic space consists of histiocytes, loose fibrous connective tissue, and alveolar exudates of *P. carinii* pneumonia.

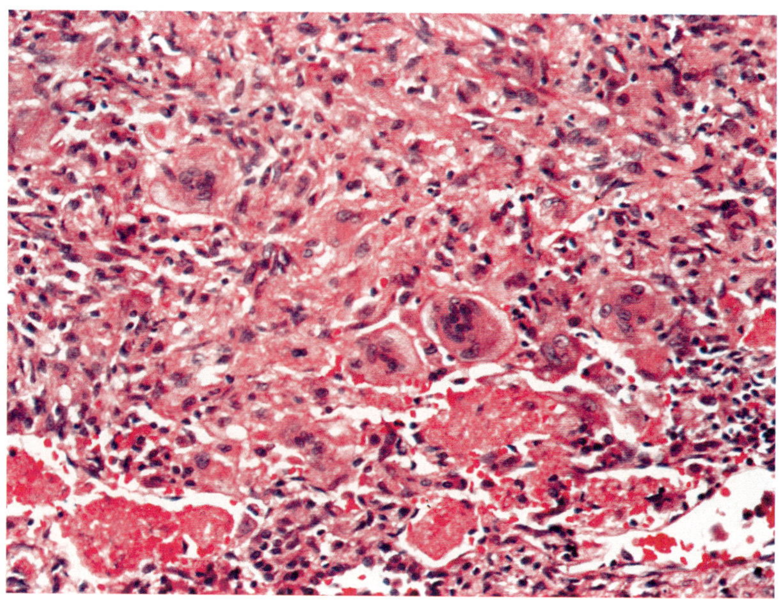

Figure 12-181

PNEUMOCYSTIS CARINII PNEUMONIA: GRANULOMATOUS INFLAMMATION

A cluster of epithelioid histiocytes forms an epithelioid granuloma. A few eosinophilic exudates are present within the granuloma.

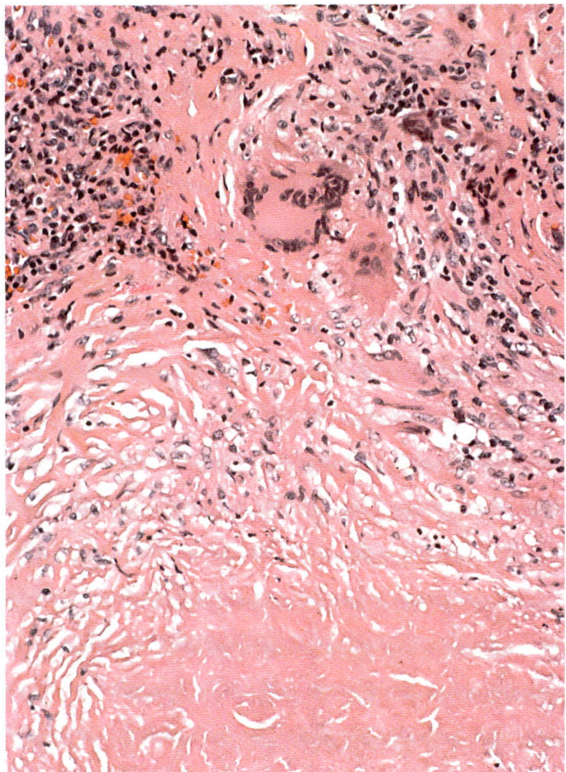

Figure 12-182

PNEUMOCYSTIS CARINII PNEUMONIA: GRANULOMATOUS INFLAMMATION

This granuloma is centrally necrotic and surrounded by multinucleated giant cells, lymphocytes, plasma cells, and fibrosis.

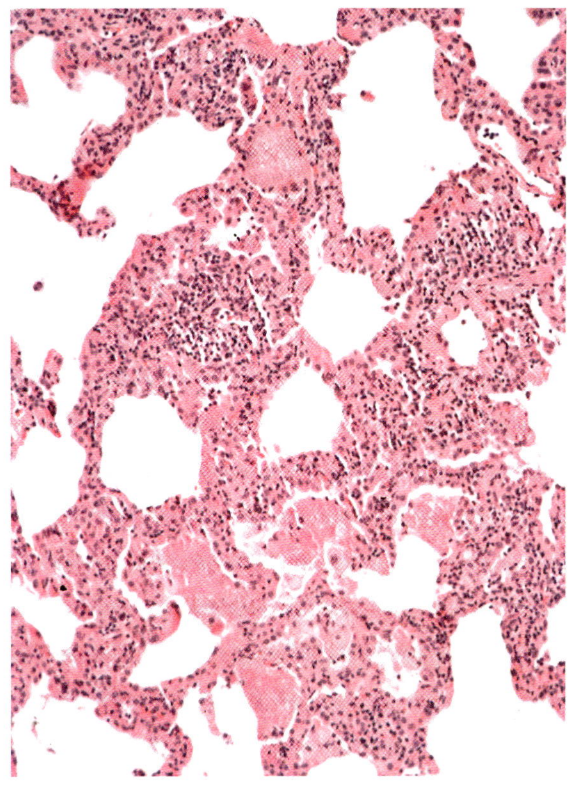

Figure 12-183

PNEUMOCYSTIS CARINII PNEUMONIA: MARKED LYMPHOCYTIC INFILTRATE

The interstitium is involved by a marked lymphocytic infiltrate. The alveolar exudates are obscured by the marked interstitial inflammation. Focal alveolar exudates are present.

cautious about separation from *Histoplasma* infection with darkly stained foci (see *Histoplasma capsulatum* section above). However, the center of the necrotizing granuloma shows the same frothy, bubbly exudate more typically seen in the alveolar spaces in *P. carinii* pneumonia infection, and budding yeasts are not seen. Although one report described granulomas in 17 percent of lung biopsies of patients with *P. carinii* pneumonia prior to the HIV epidemic (537), there were very few papers describing granulomatous *P. carinii* pneumonia in the pre-AIDS literature. However, many examples of granulomatous inflammation have been reported in AIDS patients (496,534).

Prominent lymphoplasmacytic interstitial infiltration is unusual in adult patients with *P. carinii* pneumonia. However, it was a characteristic feature in early descriptions of institutionalized and malnourished infants (505), and in two studies, prominent lymphocytic infiltrates were described in lung biopsy specimens from 8 percent of non-HIV infected patients and 3 percent of AIDS patients (534,537). Rarely, the interstitial infiltrates may be so extensive that they obscure the alveolar exudates and impair morphologic recognition of the diagnosis of *P. carinii* pneumonia (fig. 12-183) (524,534).

Microcalcifications in *P. carinii* pneumonia have been described in 3 percent of lung biopsies from patients without HIV infection (537), and in 2 percent of lung biopsies from HIV-infected patients (fig. 12-184) (516,534). Calcifications can be a helpful histologic clue to the presence of *P. carinii* in lung biopsies where alveolar exudate is absent (516). In addition, identification of calcification in organs such as the

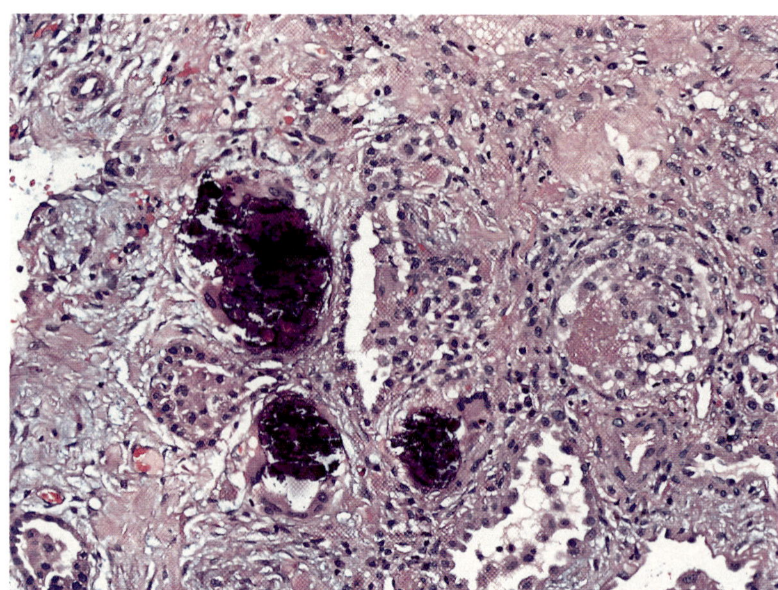

Figure 12-184

PNEUMOCYSTIS CARINII PNEUMONIA: MICROCALCIFICATION AND CYSTIC CHANGE

Microcalcification is present within the interstitium of the lung, which also shows cystic cavitary changes.

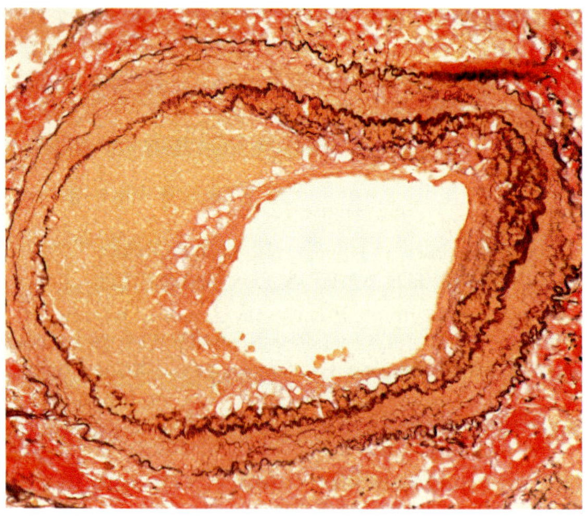

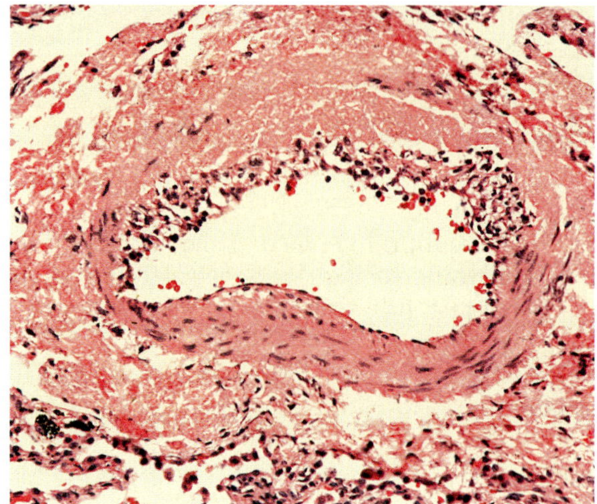

Figure 12-185

PNEUMOCYSTIS CARINII PNEUMONIA: VASCULAR INVASION

Left: The eosinophilic exudate of *Pneumocystis carinii* pneumonia permeates the media of this blood vessel wall (elastic van Gieson stain).

Right: The muscularis on one side of this blood vessel is completely destroyed by alveolar exudates and is associated with intimal chronic inflammation or vasculitis. This patient subsequently developed widespread dissemination.

lymph nodes, liver, spleen, or kidney in an HIV-infected patient suggests the diagnosis of disseminated extrapulmonary *P. carinii* infection (508).

Invasion of pulmonary vessels and vasculitis are seen in 1 percent of lung biopsies from HIV-infected patients with *P. carinii* pneumonia (fig. 12-185) (534). Such invasion has been described in association with necrotizing or cavitary lung lesions (534) and subsequent extrapulmonary dissemination (503,534).

Dissemination of *P. carinii* outside the lung has been described in almost every organ including the thyroid (513,526), pancreas (503), adrenal glands (503), bone marrow (503), spleen (503), liver (503), gastrointestinal tract (504), kidney (503), myocardium (503), thoracic and/

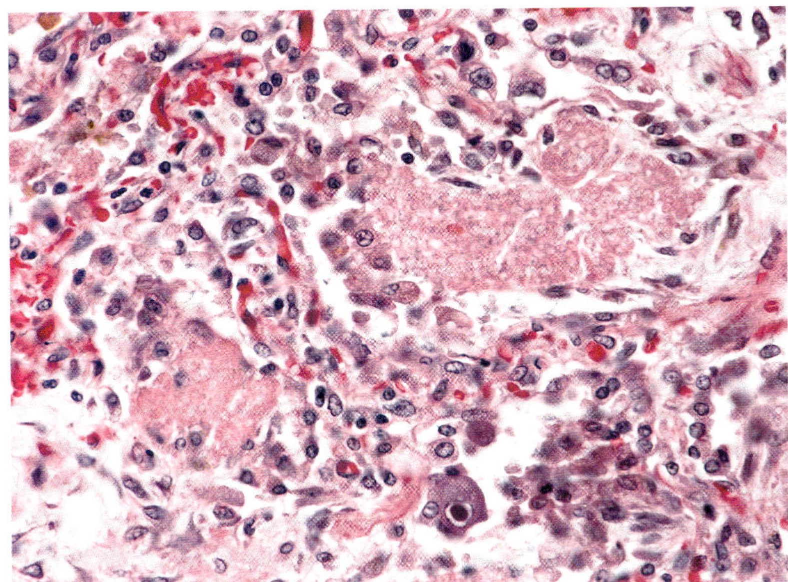

Figure 12-186

PNEUMOCYSTIS CARINII AND CYTOMEGALOVIRUS PNEUMONIA

In addition to the alveolar exudates of *P. carinii* pneumonia there is a pneumocyte showing a CMV inclusion.

or abdominal lymph nodes (508), parathyroid glands (503), skin (503), ear (535), and eye (535). Virtually all of these cases have occurred in AIDS patients. In a substantial number of cases, lung involvement could not be demonstrated at the time of diagnosis of extrapulmonary infection (501). Extrapulmonary dissemination is of clinical importance since *P. carinii* infection can cause hepatic, bone marrow, renal, and thyroid gland dysfunction (523,526,529). Occasionally, radiographs or CT show calcification in organs affected by disseminated *P. carinii* (508).

Other Special Techniques. Immunohistochemistry in formalin-fixed, paraffin-embedded tissue sections plays a limited role in the diagnosis of *P. carinii* infection (502,534). A variety of monoclonal antibodies to *P. carinii* have been described. Monoclonal antibody staining has been shown to be of greater value in the diagnosis of *P. carinii* infection from sputum or BAL specimens (495,497). IgG and IgA antibodies to *P. carinii* detected in BAL fluid have stained organisms in tissue sections from the lung and sites of extrapulmonary infection (498). Immunohistochemical staining of tissue sections is useful for confirming extrapulmonary sites of infection and distinguishing *P. carinii* from *Histoplasma capsulatum*. However, in routine biopsies of the lung, the GMS stain is quicker and cheaper, and enables detection of most fungal organisms.

Detection of *P. carinii* DNA in the serum, sputum, or BAL fluid of AIDS patients has been studied (525,531,536). However, it remains to be established whether a positive result necessarily correlates with clinical disease. After diagnosing *P. carinii* pneumonia, one should make a careful search for additional organisms such as cytomegalovirus (fig. 12-186).

Differential Diagnosis. *P. carinii* pneumonia must be separated from infection by fungi including *Histoplasma capsulatum, Torulopsis glabrata,* and *Cryptococcus neoformans* (536). The presence of budding in the yeast forms of these fungi is a helpful clue since *P. carinii* does not show budding. Separation from *H. capsulatum* is the most common problem since on rare occasion it shows darkly stained foci similar to *P. carinii,* but in such cases the identification of budding helps with the distinction (536). When the cysts rupture, *P. carinii* tends to form cup or helmet shapes, which are not typical of *H. capsulatum.* Also identification of a foamy eosinophilic exudate surrounding the organisms is in favor of *P. carinii,* especially if it is present within alveolar spaces and lacks a granulomatous reaction. Immunohistochemistry may be needed in this differential diagnosis.

Although the intra-alveolar accumulations of *P. carinii* pneumonia and alveolar proteinosis both consist of eosinophilic material, these two disorders should not be confused. The intra-alveolar material in both conditions stain with PAS (see fig. 12-177). Alveolar proteinosis has been reported in a small number of cases of *P. carinii* pneumonia, however, this diagnosis should be made with caution (528,533). In *P. carinii* pneumonia the intra-alveolar material is foamy and vacuolated while in alveolar proteinosis it is finely granular with coarse clumps, and cholesterol clefts are often present. *P. carinii* organisms should be sought rigorously with special stains in cases of suspected alveolar proteinosis, especially in HIV-infected patients. The alveolar material of alveolar proteinosis has been shown to stain with surfactant apoprotein (528,533), and lipoproteinaceous material with myelin-like bodies can be seen by electron microscopy (533).

Treatment and Prognosis. The prognosis for patients with *P. carinii* pneumonia is usually favorable, with a 50 to 95 percent survival rate if appropriately treated. Trimethoprim-sulfamethoxazole and intravenous pentamidine continue to be effective therapy for acute disease (525,536). Early administration of glucocorticoids (within a few hours of beginning chemotherapy) to patients with *P. carinii* pneumonia and severe hypoxemia decrease the risk of respiratory failure and death by over 50 percent. Chemoprevention with oral trimethoprim-sulfamethoxazole continues to be the preferred method of prophylaxis, followed by oral dapsone (525,536). For patients who cannot tolerate these prophylactic regimens, aerosolized pentamidine (AP) is an alternative. Chemoprevention is given to AIDS patients with a prior history of *P. carinii* pneumonia, patients with a CD4 cell count of less than 200 cells/μL, and HIV-infected patients with thrush or persistent fevers (525,536). Patients may have residual pulmonary fibrosis following infection, although it is not clear whether this is caused by the infection or the drugs given therapeutically (525,536). Relapses occur in 50 to 75 percent of AIDS patients unless given further chemotherapy and 10 to 20 percent of other immunosuppressed patients (525, 536). Recent molecular typing of *P. carinii* shows that a few patients who have an apparent relapse after successful therapy actually have new infections with a different strain of *P. carinii* (in contrast to the strain found in the sputum at the original diagnosis).

Table 12-16

PARASITIC INFECTIONS OF THE LUNG

Protozoa
- *Toxoplasma gondii*
- *Entamoeba histolytica*
- *Cryptosporidium*
- *Microsporidium*

Nematoda (roundworms)
- *Dirofilaria immitis*
- *Filaria* sp. (*Wuchereria bancrofti, Brugia malayi,* or *Onchocerca volvulus*)
- *Strongyloides stercoralis*

Trematoda (flukes)
- *Paragonimus westermani*
- *Schistosoma mansoni, S. japonicum, S. haematobium*

Cestoda (tapeworms)
- *Echinococcus granulosus, E. multilocularis*

Pseudoparasitic structures

PARASITIC INFECTIONS

Parasitic disease of the lung is rare in most Western countries, but in parts of the world it may be endemic. The major categories of parasites that cause pulmonary disease are protozoa, nematodes (roundworms), trematodes (flukes), and cestodes (tapeworms) (Table 12-16) (594). This chapter will address some of the better known parasites that affect the lung.

PROTOZOA

Toxoplasmosis

Definition. Pulmonary toxoplasmosis is an infection of the lung caused by the coccidian *Toxoplasma gondii.*

T. gondii is an obligate intracellular protozoan that is found worldwide. There are three forms: tachyzoites (the asexual form), tissue cysts (containing bradyzoites), and oocysts (containing sporozoites) (541,570,575). Only the tachyzoite is capable of invasion, proliferation, and cell destruction. Tissue cysts serve as a reservoir of tachyzoites and are responsible for disease transmission and latent infection. Cats are the definitive host: oocysts are produced in their intestinal epithelium and then shed in the stool.

After sporulation, these oocysts become infectious and may be ingested by humans. Other potential means of exposure include ingestion of raw or undercooked meats, perinatal exposure from infected mother, transfusion of contaminated blood products, and transplantation of infected organs (541,570,575).

Clinical Features. In 80 to 90 percent of immunocompetent hosts, acute pulmonary toxoplasmosis is asymptomatic. Acute toxoplasmosis may cause painless, firm lymphadenopathy confined to one chain of nodes, most commonly cervical. Rarely, the adenopathy is diffuse and associated with a mononucleosis-like syndrome of rash, arthralgias, myalgias, fever, sore throat, and hepatosplenomegaly accompanied by slightly abnormal liver function tests. Although the disease is usually benign and self-limited it can become chronic.

Pulmonary toxoplasmosis occurs in two different clinical settings: in immunocompetent patients and in patients with defective cell-mediated immunity (613). Immunodeficient patients include those undergoing immunosuppressive treatment for cancer (639) and transplantation (561,566,631), and those with AIDS (574). Patients present with shortness of breath and cough, and may have fever and rales.

Disseminated toxoplasmosis manifests most commonly with fever, encephalitis, or brain abscesses, and occasionally by pneumonitis, myocarditis, hepatosplenomegaly, or rash. Up to 33 percent of patients with disseminated toxoplasmosis primarily affecting organs other than the lung have evidence of subclinical pulmonary involvement even though pneumonia had not been diagnosed clinically (613). In disseminated toxoplasmosis organisms are transported to the lung through the bloodstream and/or lymphatics (541,570,575). In the lung, the organisms cause a diffuse, confluent bronchopneumonia that may be fatal. Uncommonly, there is a focal pneumonia and, rarely, cavitation is present. When the lungs are involved in disseminated toxoplasmosis there is also usually extensive brain and heart involvement.

In AIDS patients, the incidence of pulmonary toxoplasmosis is estimated to be 2 to 3 percent and occurs mainly in patients with advanced immunodeficiency (mean CD4+ lymphocyte count, 40/mm^3) (616). Importantly, pulmonary toxoplasmosis must be distinguished from *Pneumocystis carinii* pneumonia in the HIV-infected patient with diffuse pulmonary opacities since the therapy and clinical sequelae are different (574,575,616).

Serology is helpful in the diagnosis, however, acute infection must be distinguished from preexisting infection or passively transferred antibody. The Sabin-Feldman dye test is one of the better serologic tests (titers greater than or equal to 1:1024 are diagnostic) (575,619). Acute and convalescent titers are optimal for demonstrating acute infection (541,570,575). In immunocompromised patients, serology is less reliable since there may be a lower titer of antibodies despite active infection (575). The current recommendation is to perform both the Sabin-Feldman dye test and one of the newer serology methods such as the differential agglutination test (which measures IgG anti-*Toxoplasma* antibodies), IgA ELISA (enzyme-linked immunosorbent assay), IgE ELISA, and the IgE immunosorbent agglutination assay. In equivocal cases, lymph node biopsy may be required for diagnosis of acute toxoplasmosis. Given the very high risk for reactivation of latent toxoplasmosis in HIV-infected patients, the IgG titer should be measured early, before the patient becomes significantly immunocompromised, because a positive serologic finding, regardless of titer, indicates that the patient is at risk and should receive chemoprophylaxis.

Radiologic Findings. Chest radiographs in immunocompetent individuals with pulmonary toxoplasmosis demonstrate focal reticular opacities, airspace consolidation, and/or hilar lymphadenopathy (569). Immunocompromised patients frequently exhibit bilateral, multifocal, coarse pulmonary nodules. However, bilateral, diffuse, fine reticular opacities that mimic the radiologic features of *Pneumocystis carinii* pneumonia also occur. Pleural effusions have been reported (574,578).

Pathologic Findings. In pulmonary toxoplasmosis, the lungs are congested and heavy. Petechial hemorrhages and areas of consolidation and cavitation may be seen. Areas of necrosis and acute fibrinous pneumonia are characteristically present (fig. 12-187, left).

The tachyzoites invade host cells and grow within a vacuole inside the cell cytoplasm to

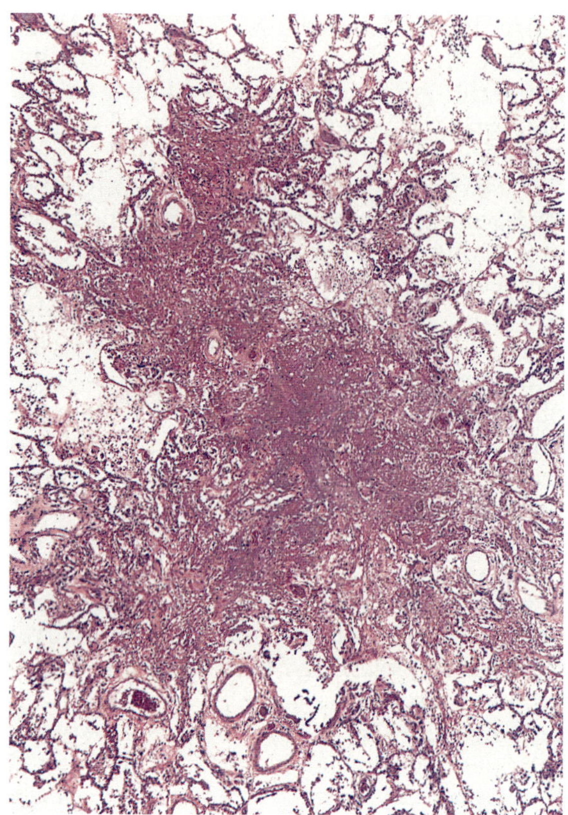

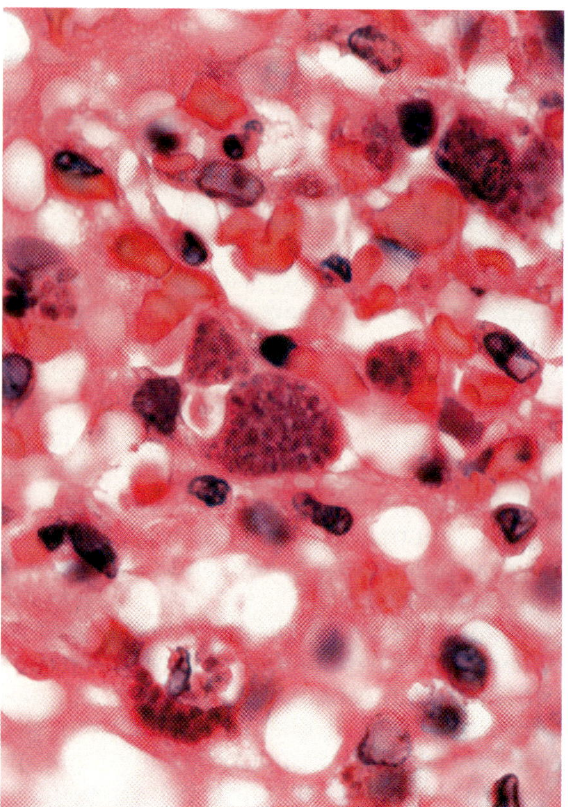

Figure 12-187

TOXOPLASMOSIS: HISTOLOGY

Left: A large area of hemorrhagic necrosis comprises an acute necrotizing pneumonia.
Right: Numerous bradyzoites are contained within the centrally placed cyst.

form tissue pseudocysts (541). Tachyzoites tend to be found within alveolar spaces (fig. 12-187, right). In macrophages, the tachyzoites reside inside phagosomes and inhibit fusion with lysosomes, thus avoiding destruction. If the macrophages become cytokine activated, they are able to destroy the intracellular parasites and when the cell ruptures, tachyzoites are released. Some tachyzoites transform into bradyzoites and grow within a cell, which becomes a true cyst. Bradyzoites grow slowly and are PAS positive because of their amylopectin content (570). True cysts are also PAS positive. Pseudocysts tend to be seen in areas of necrosis or diffusely throughout the lung (541,570). The organisms are seen well on H&E-stained sections.

Immunohistochemistry for *Toxoplasma* antigen using a monoclonal antibody is diagnostically useful (570). PCR for DNA in BAL fluid can be used to make the diagnosis (570,623). *T. gondii* does not grow on artificial media, but it may be cultured by mouse inoculation or in tissue cell culture (559,575). One study by Lavrard et al. (584) suggested that PCR provided little advantage over cell culture in establishing the diagnosis in BAL specimens.

Differential Diagnosis. The diagnosis of pulmonary toxoplasmosis requires identification of tachyzoites in lung tissue or BAL specimens. The primary entity in the differential diagnosis of disseminated toxoplasmosis of the lung is cytomegalovirus with prominent cytoplasmic inclusions. In cytomegalovirus, it is usual to find enlarged cells with large nuclear viral inclusions in addition to the many small basophilic cytoplasmic inclusions.

Treatment and Prognosis. Disseminated toxoplasmosis is usually treated with pyrimethamine and sulfonamides such as sulfadiazine (575). While these drugs will kill the tachyzoites, they do not kill the cysts so patients are susceptible to relapsing infection even following initial therapy. Sulfadiazine and pyrimethamine produce a sequential blockade of folic acid metabolism by acting as enzyme inhibitors at different points along the pathway. Concurrent administration of folic acid attenuates the bone marrow suppression caused by pyrimethamine. There is a high incidence of rash and treatment must be discontinued in up to 50 percent of patients. Seronegative immunodeficient patients should avoid exposure to uncooked meat and eggs, and unpasteurized milk, and avoid cat feces. HIV-infected patients may benefit by prophylaxis against *Pneumocystis carinii* since trimethoprim-sulfamethoxazole or pyrimethamine-sulfamethoxazole also protect against toxoplasmosis (575). HIV patients infected with *T. encephalitis* require suppressive anti-*Toxoplasma* therapy for life.

The mortality among patients with *Toxoplasma* pneumonia is 55 percent (613). However, if the diagnosis is established during life, there is an excellent survival rate for immunocompetent patients and a 40 percent rate for immunosuppressed patients (613).

Amebiasis

Definition. Pulmonary amebiasis is caused by infection of the lung with the protozoan, *Entamoeba histolytica.*

E. histolytica is found worldwide, but most human infections occur in the tropics, particularly in third world countries. Worldwide, approximately 40 to 50 million people are infected annually. In the United States, homosexual men and Mexican Americans have a high rate of infection (575). It is primarily a gastrointestinal infection acquired through ingestion of contaminated food or water. Among homosexual men, it is a sexually transmitted disease.

Clinical Features. Pleuropulmonary complications of amebiasis occur in 7 to 20 percent of patients with hepatic infection and 2 to 3 percent of those with invasive intestinal disease. Four forms of thoracic amebiasis occur: 1) the most common is a "neighborhood reaction" due to the spread of inflammation through the diaphragm with an intact liver abscess; 2) hepatic abscess rupture into the pleural space causing an empyema; 3) hepatic abscess rupture into the lung causing pneumonia, lung abscess, or hepatobronchial fistula; and 4) hematogenous spread (541,548,575). Spread from the liver usually primarily affects the right lung or pleural space.

Patients with thoracopulmonary amebiasis present with cough and dyspnea, or right-sided chest pain, which may be pleuritic. Patients with liver abscesses can appear to have a pulmonary disorder with fever, chills, sweats, cough, and chest pain. Patients with a hepatobronchial fistula may produce copious amounts of "anchovy paste" or "chocolate" sputum (541, 548,575). Some patients with pulmonary involvement also have pericardial amebiasis.

The diagnosis of amebiasis, especially hepatic amebic disease, is confirmed by amebic serologic tests, such as the indirect hemagglutination inhibition or gel diffusion assays. These tests are positive in more than 90 percent of patients.

Radiologic Findings. Patients with amebiasis may exhibit pulmonary or thoracic involvement on chest radiography. Radiographic abnormalities include right diaphragmatic elevation, basilar parenchymal consolidation typically affecting the right lower or middle lobe, and pleural effusion (fig. 12-188) (569, 583). Sonographic evaluation of the liver may demonstrate nonspecific, peripheral hypoechoic lesions. The combination of these findings, with evidence of diaphragmatic disruption, is considered diagnostic (583).

Pathologic Findings. Pulmonary amebiasis forms multiple abscesses ranging from millimeters to up to 10 cm (fig. 12-189) (541). The lung abscesses are usually contiguous with those in the liver. The fluid within the abscess appears yellow-brown. The center of the abscess consists of necrotic debris and inflammatory cells with scattered trophozoites (541). The border of the abscess typically shows marked acute and chronic inflammation accompanied by a fibroblastic proliferation (541).

In tissue sections the trophozoites measure approximately 15 to 25 µm in diameter (fig. 12-190, left) (541,548). They have a sharply defined, thin cell membrane and an amphophilic cytoplasm that contains vacuoles, red blood cells,

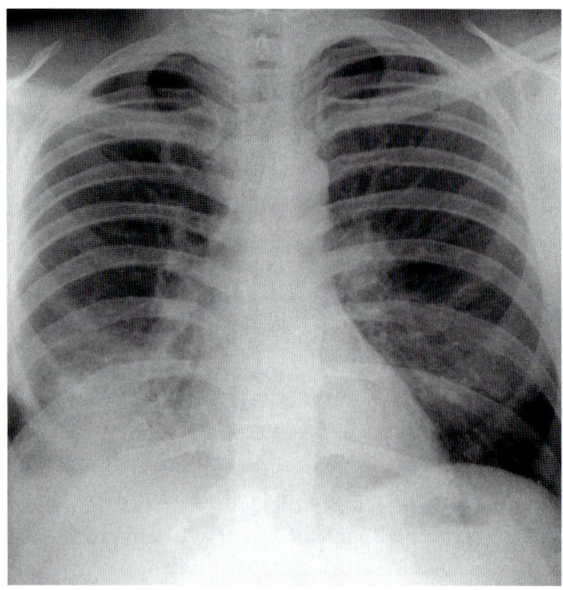

Figure 12-188

AMEBIASIS IN A 33-YEAR-OLD MALE WITH RIGHT CHEST PAIN

PA chest radiograph demonstrates a right lower lobe consolidation. Stool examination demonstrated ova of *Entamoeba histolytica*. The pneumonia responded to treatment with antiamebic agents.

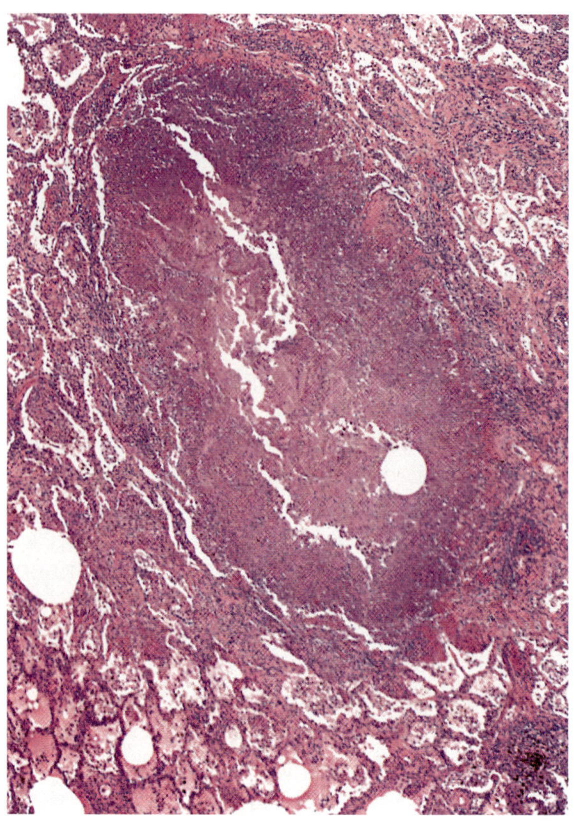

Figure 12-189

AMEBIASIS: PULMONARY ABSCESS

This nodular, cavitated area represents an acute abscess centered on a bronchiole.

nuclear fragments, and other cellular debris (fig. 12-190, left). The trophozoites stain strongly with the PAS stain due to the prominent cytoplasmic glycogen (fig. 12-190, right). The nucleus is small, measuring 2 to 3 µm, with a centrally placed karyosome, and the chromatin is accentuated around the nuclear membrane (541,548). The nucleus appears to be surrounded by a "halo." An iron stain may help demonstrate the cellular organelles of the trophozoites and facilitate the distinction of cells in the surrounding tissue.

Differential Diagnosis. Trophozoites of *E. histolytica* can be confused with histiocytes, particularly if they show erythrophagocytosis. Histiocytes tend to be smaller, the nuclei are larger, and they have coarser chromatin (541,548). One should be cautious about the diagnosis of thoracopulmonary amebiasis unless there is involvement of the gastrointestinal tract or liver, or unless the patient has known predisposing factors.

Treatment and Prognosis. Rupture of a hepatic abscess into the lung or pleura worsens the prognosis of patients with amebiasis. Therapy for pleuropulmonary amebiasis is metronidazole (562). Patients with empyemas require a chest tube. Drainage is sometimes adequate for patients with hepatobiliary fistulas, but medical therapy may also be required (575).

Cryptosporidiosis

Definition. Pulmonary cryptosporidiosis is caused by infection of the lung with *Cryptosporidium parvum*.

Cryptosporidium is an intestinal protozoan that rarely affects the lung (541,636). It is closely related to other coccidian parasites including *Isospora belli* and *Toxoplasma gondii*. *Cryptosporidium* infects the respiratory or gastrointestinal tract of many hosts including fish, birds, reptiles, and mammals. *C. parvum* is easily transmitted by oral ingestion of oocysts and is an important cause of diarrhea in animals

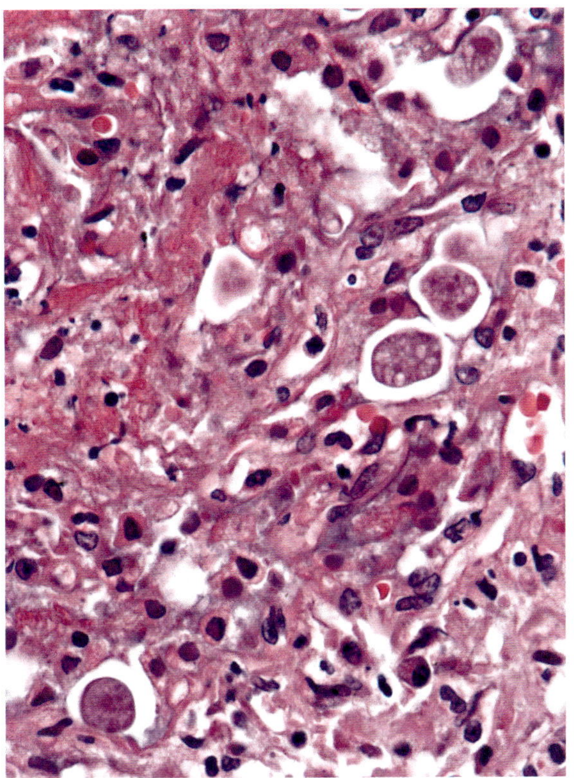

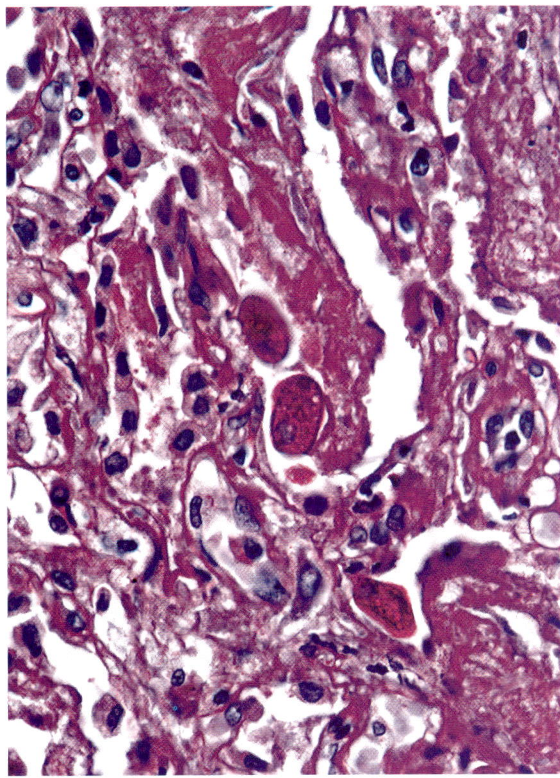

Figure 12-190

AMEBIASIS: ORGANISM MORPHOLOGY

Left: Multiple trophozoites are present in this lung tissue. They have a sharply defined, thin cell membrane and amphophilic cytoplasm that contains vacuoles.

Right: The PAS stain is strongly positive in the trophozoites.

and humans worldwide (602). Animal-to-human transmission can occur, particularly from calves to veterinarians or farmers and from rabbits in the research laboratory to researchers. Person-to-person transmission of *Cryptosporidium* can occur, especially in daycare centers. *Cryptosporidium* has become the most important contaminant of drinking water and is an emerging cause of food-borne disease in domestic settings. Human cryptosporidiosis usually involves the gastrointestinal tract, especially the jejunum, where it causes villous atrophy.

The most likely mode of transmission to the lungs is by aspiration associated with fecal-oral spread or esophageal-oropharyngeal infection (634,636). Other possible routes of transmission include inhalation and hematogenous spread (634,636). Nosocomial transmission of *Cryptosporidium* infection to hospital personnel and to hospitalized patients is a public health concern (550).

Clinical Features. *Cryptosporidium* infection results in a self-limited diarrheal illness that lasts from 4 to 20 days and is associated with abdominal cramping, nausea, vomiting, low-grade fever, and anorexia (602). The presenting features of respiratory cryptosporidiosis include productive cough, dyspnea, fever, and thoracic pain (636). Diarrhea is present in three fourths of the patients with lung involvement (556). Rales may be heard on auscultation of the chest. All patients with respiratory involvement have had gastrointestinal cryptosporidiosis and some type of immunosuppression, most commonly AIDS (541,563,598,610,612, 636,645). An estimated 10 to 15 percent of AIDS patients in the United States develop pulmonary cryptosporidiosis during the course of

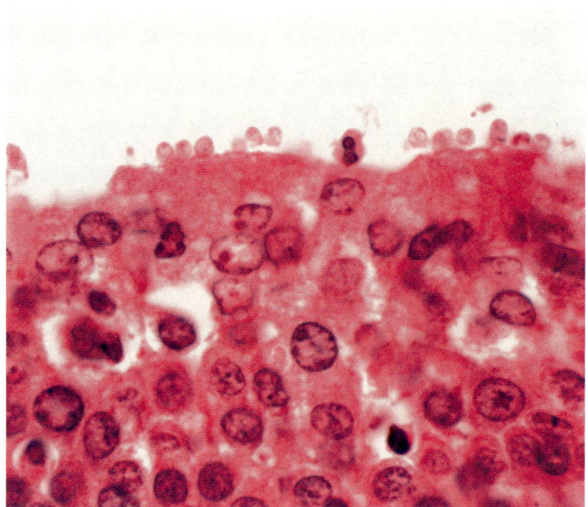

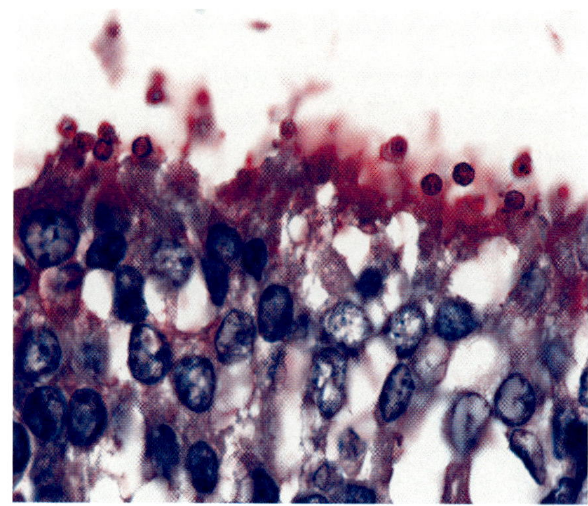

Figure 12-191

CRYPTOSPORIDIOSIS

Left: Multiple 4- to 6-µm, round to oval, basophilic organisms are situated within the apical cytoplasm of the bronchial epithelial cells.

Right: The cryptosporidia are highlighted by the PAS stain.

their disease (634). Most have associated pulmonary processes such as cytomegalovirus, *Pneumocystis carinii, Mycoplasma pneumoniae, Legionella,* or *Aspergillus* pneumonia. The diagnosis is based on the recognition of acid-fast oocysts in sputum or aspirated bronchial material, and in stool specimens (541,563,598,610, 612,634,636,646).

Radiologic Findings. Chest radiographs show diffuse, bilateral interstitial opacities (636). If there are associated lesions, such as invasive *Aspergillus,* there may be other radiographic findings such as bilateral cavitary nodules (636).

Pathologic Findings. Respiratory involvement by cryptosporidiosis typically shows a tracheitis, bronchitis, and bronchiolitis (636). There is a mild to moderate chronic inflammatory infiltrate in the mucosa and submucosa. In most cases, the organisms are seen within the luminal aspect of the mucosa of the trachea, bronchi, and bronchioles (fig. 12-191) (541,563, 598,610,612,636,646). Organisms may extend into the submucosal glands. Rarely, they are seen within an alveolar exudate. The organisms consist of 4- to 6-µm, round to oval, basophilic cryptosporidia. In most cases they are intracellular, within the apical cytoplasm of the epithelial cells, although they appear to lie along the surface. The organisms stain with the Giemsa, PAS, and GMS stains (636). In sputum cytology, the organisms may be weakly acid-fast (636).

Differential Diagnosis. The biggest problem in the diagnosis of respiratory cryptosporidiosis is overlooking the organisms. Since they may not be the only organisms in tissue sections, it is easy to get so distracted by the histopathologic changes in the lung that the cryptosporidia, which typically represent a subtle histologic finding, are not noticed. The differential diagnosis includes infection with *Toxoplasma gondii* and *Pneumocystis carinii,* and cellular debris or nuclear fragments. *T. gondii* and *P. carinii* do not cause the primary lesion of bronchitis and bronchiolitis with limitation of the organisms to the surface of the airway epithelium. Degenerated nuclear debris, situated along the surface of the epithelial cells, could be mistaken for cryptosporidia. However, debris is likely to be irregular in size and shape, and more variable in location compared to the uniform morphology and apical epithelial location of the cryptosporidia.

Treatment and Prognosis. It is not clear how to effectively treat cryptosporidiosis. Paromomycin, a nonabsorbable aminoglycoside, may be efficacious for the treatment of the intestinal disease but it is of limited use in most other cases (579). Inhaled paromomycin has been used for the treatment of symptomatic pulmonary infection (600). In HIV-infected patients, treatment of the underlying retroviral infection with combination antiretroviral therapy that includes a protease inhibitor, restores immunity to *C. parvum* and results in improvement in the clinical manifestations of cryptosporidiosis (552,589).

Microsporidiosis

Definition. Pulmonary microsporidiosis is an infection of the lung caused by the protozoa *Encephalitozoon* sp and *Enterocytozoon bieneusi.*

The protozoa that cause microsporidiosis are obligate, intracellular, spore-forming organisms found in the intestine, liver, kidney, cornea, brain, nerves, and muscles of a variety of wild and domesticated animals. Only six genera of microsporidia are known to infect humans: *Encephalitozoon, Enterocytozoon, Septata, Pleistophora, Nosema*, and *Microsporidium* (608). Prior to the AIDS epidemic, microsporidia caused few human infections, but now in HIV-infected patients they are well-recognized opportunistic pathogens that cause gastrointestinal disease, renal disease, sinusitis, and keratitis (620,625,626,628,644).

Microsporidia are acquired through oral, respiratory, and ocular pathways and are excreted in the stool and urine (608). They can infect a variety of cell types including epithelial, endothelial, and mesenchymal cells as well as macrophages (608). The microsporidial spore injects these host cells with sporoplasm, which undergoes multiple divisions to form many organisms (608). The sporoblasts grow into mature spores, which are composed of an endospore surrounded by an ectospore (608). The spores measure 1 to 6 μm.

Clinical Features. Microsporidia identified in BAL fluid and transbronchial lung biopsies are usually thought to represent colonization. It is not known if microsporidia cause significant clinical pulmonary disease. All of the patients reported to have pulmonary microsporidiosis have underlying AIDS and most have had associated intestinal involvement (576,585,620, 625,628,629,644). The pulmonary disease is usually asymptomatic and patients present with other manifestations of AIDS or other organ involvement by microsporidiosis. When symptomatic, patients may have dyspnea or nonproductive cough (576,585,625).

Disseminated microsporidiosis can involve the central nervous system and respiratory, gastrointestinal, and urinary tracts; it can cause keratoconjuntivitis, sinusitis, myositis, peritonitis, cholangitis, and hepatitis (560,576,620, 625–627,644). Most cases of pulmonary microsporidiosis have been associated with *Encephalitozoon hellem* (576,620,625), although dissemination to the lungs can also occur with *E. cuniculi* and *Enterocytozoon bieneusi* (572).

Radiologic Findings. Chest radiographs may be normal or show multiple bilateral opacities (620,625).

Pathologic Findings. The pathologic diagnosis of pulmonary microsporidiosis is most often established by cytologic examination of BAL fluid (620). The organisms can be highlighted with a fungi-flour fluorescent mycology stain (620). Electron microscopy, cell culture, indirect immunofluorescence assays, protein extraction and immunoblots, and DNA extraction with PCR methods can be used to confirm the presence of *Enterocytozoon* and to identify the specific species (542,576,625,644). PCR techniques utilizing rRNA sequences allow for separation of species with similar electron microscopic features.

The organisms may be identified in sputum, BAL cytology specimens, or lung tissue specimens from biopsies or autopsies. Histologically, the organisms are found mostly within bronchial and bronchiolar epithelial cells (fig. 12-192), although other cells may be infected as mentioned above. *Encephalitozoon* sp grows within vacuoles in the apical aspect of the epithelial cell cytoplasm. The associated histologic findings are tracheitis, bronchitis, and bronchiolitis with superficial erosions and a mixture of neutrophils and mononuclear cells (fig. 12-192) (608). The epithelium may demonstrate alternating areas of hyperplasia and attenuation, and there may be inflammatory cells within the epithelium (608). The spores are very small, 1.0 to 1.5 μm, and they appear slightly basophilic on H&E stain (fig. 12-192B). Although the parasites may be readily recognized on an H&E-stained section, certain special stains may be necessary for definitive diagnosis. The organisms are Gram-positive and can be demonstrated with a Brown and Brenn or Brown and

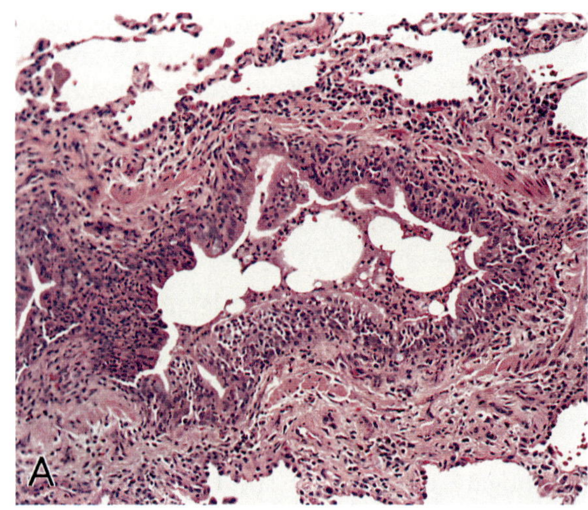

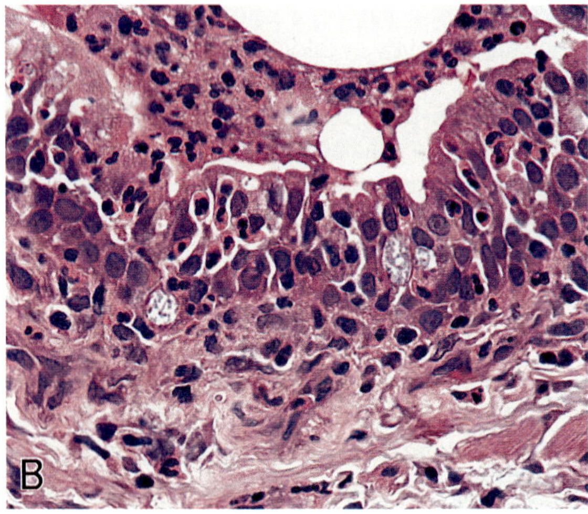

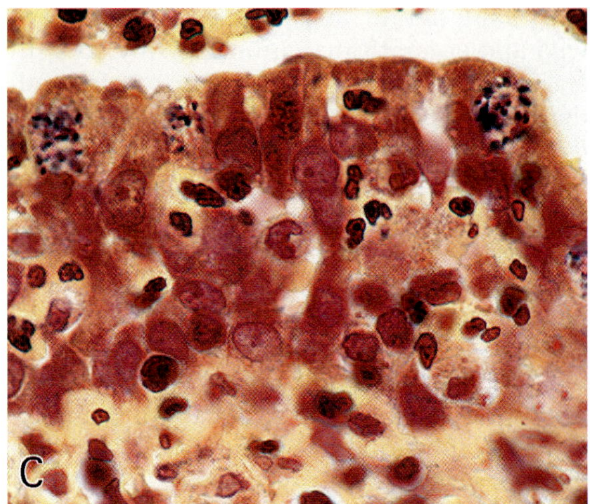

Figure 12-192

MICROSPORIDIOSIS: *ENCEPHALITOZOON CUNICULI*

A: The bronchiole shows mild mucosal and submucosal chronic inflammation and squamous metaplasia.

B: The spores are seen within vacuoles in the apical cytoplasm of the bronchiolar epithelial cells.

C: The organisms within the cytoplasmic vacuoles stain with the Brown and Hopps stain. (Courtesy of Ronald C. Neafie, AFIP, Washington, DC.)

Hopps stain (fig. 12-192C) (608), although with the latter it is easier to visualize the underlying lung tissue. The organisms may also be weakly acid-fast (608). Some organisms are GMS positive. The polar body is PAS positive in some spores (608). A modified Warthin-Starry stain can be helpful in demonstrating microsporidia, especially *E. bieneusi* (608). Parasites are usually birefringent due to the chitin content of the endospores. The birefringence is white with the H&E and Warthin-Starry stains; it appears pink with the Brown and Brenn stain.

There are a variety of morphologic differences between the *Enterocytozoon* and *Encephalitozoon* microsporidia (608). The simplest distinguishing feature is that spores of the *Enterocytozoon* are small (1.0 x 1.5 µm) compared to those of the *Encephalitozoon* (2.0 to 2.5 x 1.0 to 1.5 µm) (608). Other distinguishing features include the type of nuclear division, pleomorphism of the nuclei, and thickness of the ectospore and endospores. In addition, the species and genera of microsporidia are separated depending on whether the development occurs within a membrane derived from the parasite itself (pansporoblastic) or within the host cytoplasm. The *Encephalitozoon* and *Enterocytozoon* grow freely dispersed within the host cytoplasm (pansporoblastic) but the former grow within a vacuole (parasitophorous), while the latter grow in direct contact with the cytoplasm (608).

Differential Diagnosis. The biggest problem in the histologic recognition of microsporidiosis in pulmonary specimens is considering the possibility and then knowing what to look for. Once the diagnosis is suspected on morphologic grounds, appropriate stains and pursuit of other organ involvement confirm the suspicion. The organisms can be confused with *Toxoplasma* (608), *Histoplasma,* and *Coccidiodomyces.* However, *Toxoplasma* does not show tropism for the apical aspect of the cytoplasm of bronchial or bronchiolar epithelial cells and the bradyzoites are not acid-fast. *H. capsulatum* usually demonstrates budding forms that are lacking in microsporidiosis. The yeast of *C. immitis* is usually more spherical and spherules with endospores are diagnostic.

Treatment and Prognosis. The optimal therapy is not clear and no controlled trials for the treatment of microsporidiosis have been published. Albendazole, an inhibitor of tubulin polymerization chemically related to metronidazole, has been effective in some patients. However, it must be continued once improvement occurs because relapse is common in patients who have responded to albendazole when therapy is stopped. Fumagillin and nitazoxanide have promise as effective oral treatments for intestinal microsporidiosis (546,601). Combination antiretroviral therapy is able to greatly modify the course of microsporidiosis in patients infected with HIV (589).

NEMATODA

Dirofilariasis

Definition. Pulmonary dirofilariasis is an infection of the lung caused by the filarial nematode, *Dirofilaria immitis,* the dog heartworm.

Human pulmonary dirofilariasis is thought to be transmitted from dogs to humans by mosquitoes of the genera *Aedes, Culex, Myzorhynchus,* and *Anopheles,* which represent the intermediate host and vector (593,614,622). Dogs are the most common definitive host but cats, foxes, muskrats, wolves, otters, and sea lions may also be infected. Canine dirofilariasis is widespread throughout the United States, but human dirofilariasis is rare, with reports only from 17 states, particularly those along the eastern, southeastern, and southern coasts (555,564). Rare cases are also reported in Europe (549), Asia (540,588, 590,609,622), Australia (605), Central America (549), and South America (595,599,603).

The adult worms reside in the right ventricle of the definitive host (593). Circulating microfilariae are ingested by mosquitoes, where they develop into infective larvae over 2 weeks (614, 622). These larvae are inoculated into a new host by a mosquito bite, where they develop over a 60- to 120-day period into adult worms. Ultimately, the worms reach the right ventricle where they often cause right heart failure. Since humans are unsuitable hosts, the infective larvae usually develop no further and die. In the rare patients who develop pulmonary dirofilariasis, the worm remains immature and reaches the right ventricle, where it dies and then embolizes to pulmonary arteries within the lung parenchyma.

Clinical Features. Pulmonary dirofilariasis is most often detected as an incidental radiographic finding in an asymptomatic patient (567, 593,630). Patients are typically in the fifth or sixth decade of life, with an age range between 28 and 79 years (567,622). There is a 2 to 1 male predominance (555). Approximately 40 percent of patients have various clinical manifestations including cough (23 percent), chest pain (17 percent), hemoptysis (9 percent), and fever (6 percent) (539,622). Eosinophilia may be present in 15 to 20 percent of patients (539,622).

Radiologic Findings. The classic radiologic manifestation of pulmonary dirofilariasis is a solitary, noncalcified, peripheral pulmonary nodule in an asymptomatic adult. The lesion is typically well marginated and measures 1 to 3 cm. Wedge-shaped peripheral lesions have also been described (fig. 12-193). Most lesions occur in the lower lobes. Multifocal nodules, consolidation that resolves as a pulmonary nodule, and pleural effusion have been reported (569,599,642).

Most patients have a solitary subpleural nodule, but up to 10 percent have multiple nodules (555,622). One patient was reported to have three nodules and another had multiple nodules in different lobes of both lungs (622). Approximately 75 percent of nodules measure 2 cm or less, with a range from 1.0 to 4.5 cm (555,622). The nodules can be mistaken for primary or metastatic malignancy (622).

The lesions are typically stable without change in size over time (555,622). However, when detected early, the lesions may initially mimic pneumonia and subsequently evolve into nodules over a period of weeks (622). Calcification is a rare and late complication (555,622).

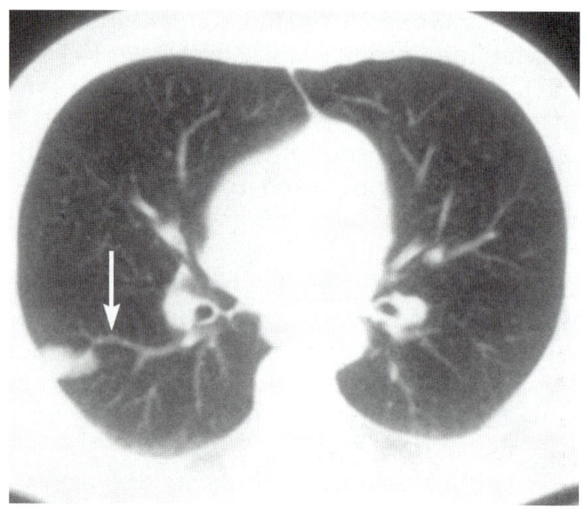

Figure 12-193

DIROFILARIASIS

Dirofilariasis in an asymptomatic 36-year-old male with a 20 pack-year history of smoking. Chest CT (lung window) demonstrates a wedge-shaped peripheral nodule in the right lower lobe. Note the pulmonary artery (arrow) that courses to the lesion, consistent with its embolic nature.

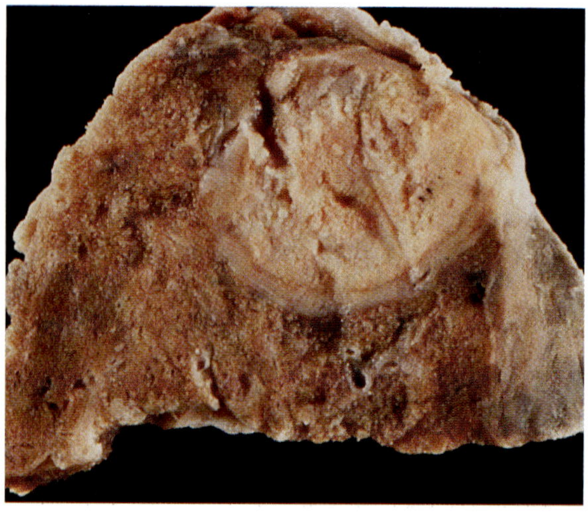

Figure 12-194

DIROFILARIA: GROSS SPECIMEN

This subpleural nodular infarct has a thick fibrous wall.

Pathologic Findings. Grossly, dirofilariasis usually causes a single, circumscribed, rounded, subpleural nodule with a granular, yellow-gray cut surface (fig. 12-194). Multiple nodules are found in 10 percent of patients.

Histologically, the nodule is a rounded infarct surrounded by an inflammatory and fibrotic border (fig. 12-195) (593). In the center of the infarct, the ghosts of alveolar walls can often be seen. There is usually a mild to moderate inflammatory infiltrate at the edge consisting of lymphocytes, plasma cells, and eosinophils. When the eosinophils are numerous, Charcot-Leyden crystals may be present. There may be granulomatous inflammation at the border, with palisading histiocytes and Langhans' giant cells.

The dead immature worm is identified within a small to medium-sized arteriole, within the infarct associated with thrombotic material (fig. 12-196) (593,606,622). The worm often appears fragmented and partly calcified. The blood vessel and worm may be more conspicuous when visualized in sections stained with the Movat pentachrome stain. The worm may appear in multiple cross sections if it is coiled within the arteriole. The infected blood vessel may show vasculitis consisting of chronic inflammation and eosinophils. Vascular occlusion is not caused solely by the presence of the worm but also by the marked intimal fibrosis. The worm measures 125 to 300 µm in diameter. It has a smooth multilayered cuticle, 5 to 25 µm in thickness. There are prominent external transverse striations (606) and internal longitudinal cuticular ridges. There is abundant somatic muscle and a centrally placed intestine (606). The number of reproductive tubes helps determine the sex of the worm since males have one and females have two, but this may be difficult to discern in necrotic worms and is not necessary to establish the diagnosis.

Differential Diagnosis. Most dirofilarial lesions are initially mistaken for infarcts or necrotizing granulomas due to mycobacteria or fungi. Identification of the organism is best appreciated at low-power scanning examination and sometimes requires a search of multiple sections. The eosinophilic staining of the worm makes it difficult to appreciate since the blood vessel and surrounding necrotic tissue are also eosinophilic.

Treatment and Prognosis. The prognosis is excellent since patients are cured by surgical excision.

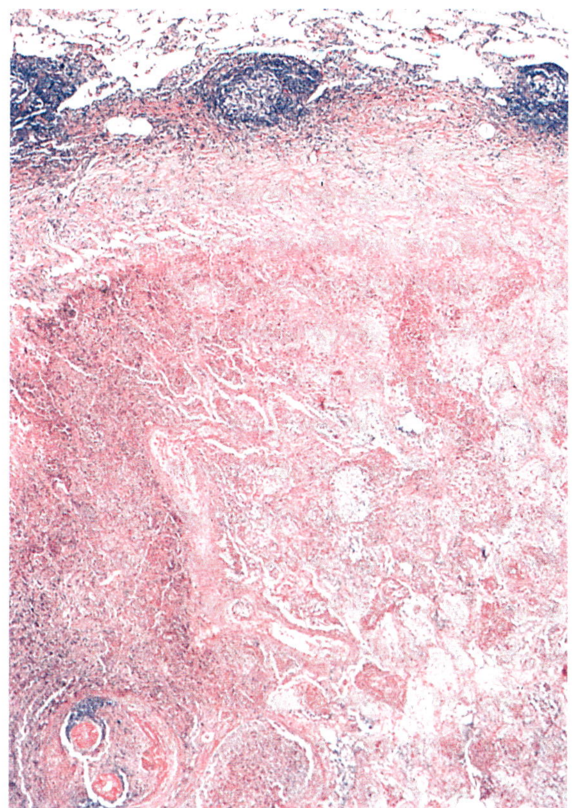

Figure 12-195

DIROFILARIA: HISTOLOGY

This nodular infarct is surrounded by a fibrous wall. Ghosts of the alveolar walls are present within the infarct. Within an arteriole (bottom right) is a *Dirofilaria* worm.

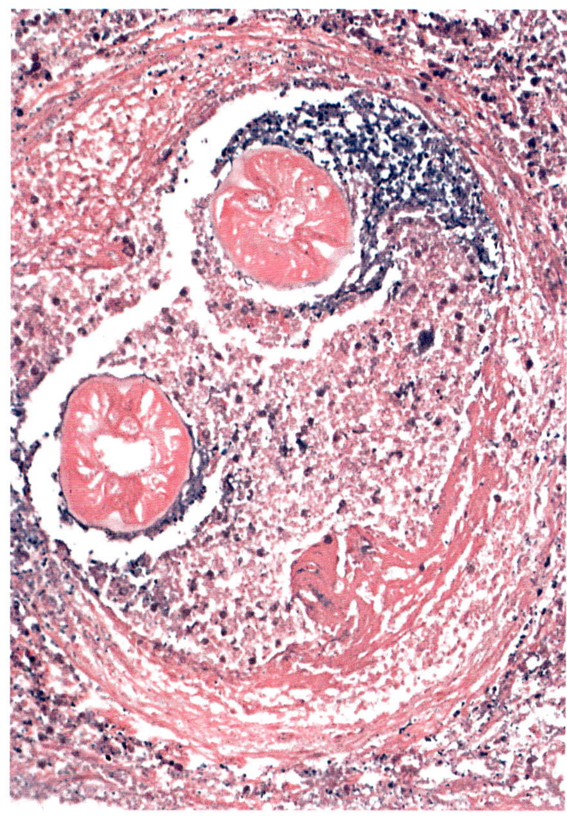

Figure 12-196

DIROFILARIA: HISTOLOGY

This arteriole is filled with a dead worm associated with a thrombus. Two cross sections of the worm are present.

Filariasis

Definition. Pulmonary filariasis is an infection of the lung caused by *Wuchereria bancrofti, Brugia malayi,* or *Onchocerca volvulus.*

Infected mosquitoes are the transmitting agent for bancroftian and brugian filariasis. *B. malayi* infection is found in Southeast and East Asia while *W. bancrofti* infection is encountered in Asia, Africa, and South America (541,597). Blackflies of the genus *Simulium* are the transmitting agent for *O. volvulus.* This infection is encountered in tropical Africa, North Yemen, and Central and South America (541,558).

Clinical Features. The lungs are only secondarily involved in each of these filarial infections. Lymphadenopathy associated with lymphangitis and, rarely, elephantiasis are the primary lesions caused by bancroftian and brugian filariasis. *O. volvulus* typically infects subcutaneous tissues forming a discrete nodule surrounded by a fibrous wall; lymph nodes may be affected. However, microfilariae can be released following therapy with diethylcarbamazine, and they may migrate to internal tissues such as the lungs.

These filarial organisms cause two types of pulmonary disease: tropical pulmonary eosinophilia and pulmonary lesions caused by the adult worms (541). The latter is a very rare phenomenon. The adult worms of *W. bancrofti* and *B. malayi* embolize in small pulmonary arteries and cause an infarct (541). *O. volvulus* has been reported to cause acute respiratory distress and fatal pulmonary edema following therapy with diethylcarbamazine.

Tropical eosinophilia (Weingarten's syndrome) is a hypersensitivity reaction to *W. bancrofti* or *B. malayi* (541,565,575,591). The patients do not have clinical findings of filariasis, although they may have lymphadenopathy and some children have hepatosplenomegaly. The presence of microfilariae within lymph nodes or spleen is called the *Meyers-Kouwenaar syndrome* (541). The peripheral eosinophilia may be striking, with counts above 3,000/mm^3 and sometimes reaching as high as 60,000/mm^3 (575). However, microfilariae are not present in the peripheral blood. Numerous eosinophils may be seen in the BAL fluid or sputum. Patients present with a cough that is worse at night, wheezing, and dyspnea. High titers of antifilarial antibodies are present and there is an increased total serum IgE that is usually above 5,000 ng/mL (575). A favorable response to diethylcarbamazine is supportive of the diagnosis (565,591).

Radiologic Findings. Radiographic abnormalities in patients with tropical eosinophilia consist of reticular and nodular opacities that affect primarily the mid- and lower lung zones. Nodular opacities are typically 2 to 5 mm in diameter. Hilar lymphadenopathy may occur (569).

Pathologic Findings. When the adult worms embolize to the lungs, a nodular infarct ranging from 2 to 8 cm is found (541). The worms are found within pulmonary arteries in adjacent lung tissue associated with thrombi and vasculitis or a perivascular inflammation that may consist of eosinophils, epithelioid cells, and giant cells. Eosinophils may be present around the periphery of the infarct (541).

Within pulmonary arteries the worms of *W. bancrofti* and *B. malayi* show tight coils with multiple cross sections. They are best distinguished by their size and the presence of a thin, finely striated cuticle. *W. bancrofti* are larger (approximately 250 µm for females and 150 µm for males) than *B. malayi* (approximately 100 µm for females and 90 µm for males). It is rare to find microfilariae in the lungs of patients with tropical pulmonary eosinophilia (541,558). The microfilariae of *O. volvulus* have a long cephalic space measuring 7 to 13 µm, with a caudal space measuring 9 to 15 µm, and a finely pointed tail.

In tropical pulmonary eosinophilia, the lung shows a marked eosinophilic pneumonia (541). Similar to eosinophilic pneumonia due to other causes, there may be abscesses associated with a granulomatous reaction.

Differential Diagnosis. The differential diagnosis for tropical pulmonary eosinophilia includes all the various causes of eosinophilic pneumonia such as allergic bronchopulmonary fungal disease, Churg-Strauss syndrome, and Wegener's granulomatosis. This differential is best sorted out based on clinical evidence.

Treatment and Prognosis. The best treatment for filariasis is diethylcarbamazine. Untreated patients with tropical pulmonary eosinophilia may progress to develop pulmonary fibrosis or chronic bronchitis with respiratory failure (558,607). Relapses are treated with another course of diethylcarbamazine (607).

Strongyloidiasis

Definition. Pulmonary strongyloidiasis is an infection of the lung caused by *Strongyloides stercoralis* (threadworm).

S. stercoralis is found worldwide, but human infection is most common in the tropics or subtropics. In the southern United States, the prevalence is estimated as 0.4 to 4.0 percent (541,571,575). At risk are immigrants from developing countries or from southern, eastern, and central Europe; travelers to and natives of eastern states bordering the Appalachian region; military service members from Southeast Asia; and institutionalized individuals (541,571,575).

The skin is penetrated by filariform larvae contracted from soil that is contaminated with larvae-containing feces. The larvae pass through the lungs into the alveolar spaces and cause petechial hemorrhages and an inflammatory reaction of neutrophils and monocytes (541,571). This stage is usually asymptomatic. After molting, the larvae move up the trachea, are swallowed, and pass to the gastrointestinal tract, particularly the small intestine, where they mature into parthenogenic females and produce eggs. Rhabditiform larvae hatch from the eggs, migrate into the lumen of the intestine, and are excreted with feces. A small number of rhabditiform (noninfective) larvae molt to reach the filariform (infective) stage in the wall of the colon and perianal skin. Therefore, in contrast to other helminthic parasites, *S. stercoralis* can complete its life cycle entirely within the human host. This allows for the process of autoinfection, which may persist for decades within the host.

A hyperinfection syndrome occurs when there is accelerated differentiation and endogenous reinfection. In this setting, there is an increased number of filariform larvae in the intestine, and increased invasion of the intestine and migration to the lung. Hyperinfection syndrome occurs when infected patients take steroids or cytotoxic drugs, develop malignancy, or become alcoholics. During this syndrome, hematogenous spread may occur and involve multiple organs including those usually not affected.

Clinical Features. There are three primary sites of clinical disease: the skin, lung, and intestine (571,575). During the initial period following skin penetration there may be a transient urticarial rash. When the first pulmonary migration phase occurs, patients may have transient cough, wheezing, pulmonary infiltration, and eosinophilia. Intestinal manifestations include cramps, diarrhea, malabsorption, and weight loss. When the infection is disseminated, patients have massive larval infection of the lungs, intestines, and occasionally, skin. The brain, liver, and other organs may be involved. Patients have nausea, vomiting, diarrhea, anorexia, and abdominal pain. Pulmonary symptoms of disseminated disease include cough, wheezing, dyspnea, and hemoptysis. Patients may develop the acute respiratory distress syndrome.

Radiologic Findings. Radiographs in patients with pulmonary strongyloidiasis may demonstrate miliary nodules and diffuse reticular opacities during the phase of larval migration through the lung. With heavy infection, multifocal, nonsegmental, patchy airspace consolidation may develop and affect entire lobes (569,647). Reticular and nodular opacities as well as small well-defined nodules that mimic miliary tuberculosis have been described (645). Affected patients may have peripheral eosinophilia in association with the radiographic abnormalities. When there is massive pulmonary larval migration (hyperinfection), diffuse consolidation and pulmonary hemorrhage may occur. Pleural effusions are reported in association with parenchymal disease but also occur as isolated findings (569,645,647). Patients with pulmonary complaints may have normal chest radiographs in spite of documented visualization of the organism on sputum analysis. Cavitation and abscess formation are thought to indicate secondary bacterial infection (569,647).

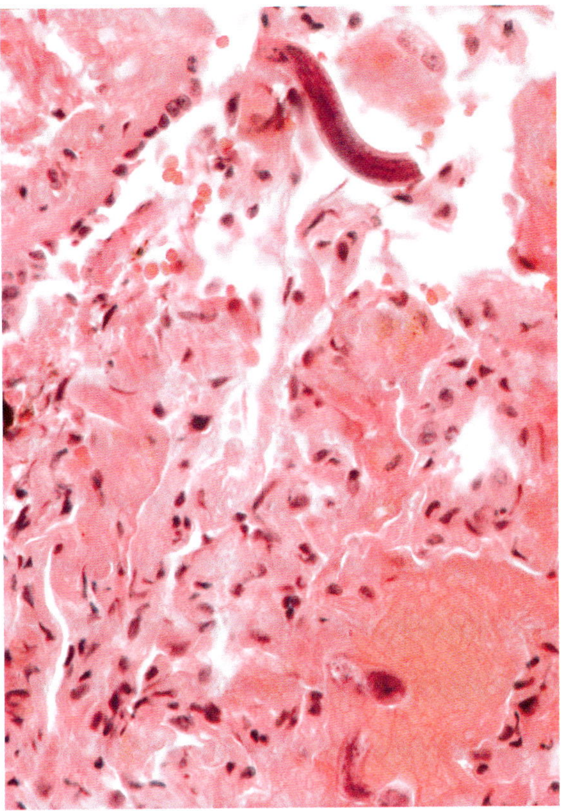

Figure 12-197

STRONGYLOIDES: FILARIFORM LARVA

The lung shows acute hemorrhage and a basophilic curved fragment of a filariform larva (top left).

Pathologic Findings. In the lung, during the initial stages of infection, the filariform larvae invade the alveoli and cause petechial hemorrhages. This results from migration of filariform larvae through the capillaries or small blood vessels. Cavities and abscesses may develop. Adult worms rarely develop in the bronchial mucosa, and probably only during hyperinfection. The finding of filariform larvae in the lung is a sign of hyperinfection (figs. 12-197, 12-198). During this phase, massive pulmonary hemorrhage or diffuse alveolar damage may result.

The filariform larvae are 300 to 600 µm long and 10 to 20 µm wide. They appear basophilic and may be seen within alveolar spaces or bronchioles (figs. 12-197, 12-198). The

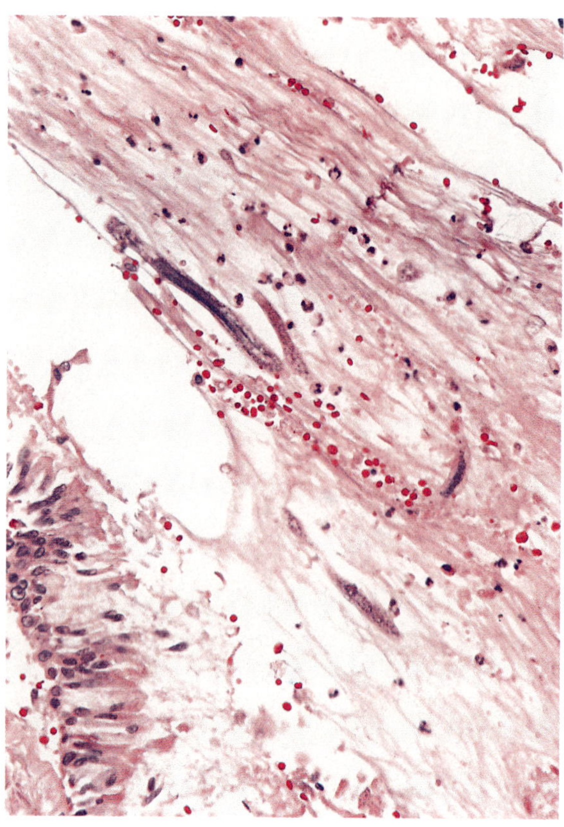

Figure 12-198

STRONGYLOIDES: FILARIFORM LARVAE

rhabditiform larvae are approximately 400 µm long and 10 to 20 µm wide and are rarely found in the lung.

Differential Diagnosis. The classic morphologic features of the parthenogenic females, larvae, and eggs of *Strongyloides* are distinctive (541,571). One has to consider other potential causes of pulmonary hemorrhage and abscesses when these are associated with the larval forms of *Strongyloides*. Although they could be confused with *Strongyloides,* it would be extremely rare to find migrating larvae of *Ascaris lumbricoides* or hookworm in histologic sections from the lung (541,571).

Treatment and Prognosis. It is important to evaluate patients potentially exposed to *Strongyloides* prior to immunosuppressive therapy, especially if they have had any potential manifestations such as a rash, eosinophilia, or diarrhea (575). Treatment of choice is thiabendazole. Recently, ivermectin has been shown to be an effective and better tolerated alternative to thiabendazole (562). Treatment failures and relapses occur with thiabendazole. Only patients with the hyperinfection syndrome have high fatality rates, which increase by the presence of immunosuppression and bacteremia.

TREMATODA

Paragonimiasis

Definition. Pulmonary paragonimiasis is an infection of the lung caused by the trematode *Paragonimus* sp. Other names of this disease are *Oriental lung fluke, Manson hemoptysis, pulmonary distomiasis, parasitic hemoptysis,* and *endemic hemoptysis.*

Approximately 48 species and subspecies of *Paragonimus* are described but only 16 are pathogenic in humans (541,632). The most common species to cause human infection is *P. westermani* and it is found in Asia (541,632). It is estimated that 2.5 million people are infected worldwide (632).

Human infection is acquired through eating raw, pickled, or undercooked freshwater crabs or crayfish that are contaminated with encysted metacercariae (541,575,632).The miracidia reside in the snails of the Pleuroceridae and Thiaridae families. Over a 10- to 12-week period they transform through sporocyst and rediae stages, and eventually become cercariae (541, 632). The cercariae leave the snail and through the water reach the second intermediate host, a crustacean such as a freshwater crab or crayfish (541,632). Here they develop into encysted forms (metacercariae) and human infection results from ingestion of poorly cooked or raw crabs or crayfish contaminated with them. The larvae pass through the human intestine into the peritoneum, through the diaphragm to the chest cavity, and to the lungs where they mature. Five to six weeks later the adult flukes start to lay eggs. The eggs spill into the airways and eventually reach the feces. There are usually very few worms within any individual, but these can survive within humans for more than 20 years.

Clinical Features. The initial illness is characterized by diarrhea, abdominal pain, urticaria, eosinophilia, and malaise that lasts from days to weeks when the immature flukes are migrating. As larvae penetrate the diaphragm and migrate within the pleural cavity, pleuritic chest pain (often bilateral) may develop, occasionally associated with pneumothorax or pleural effusions (an eosinophilic exudative). Pulmonary manifestations include dyspnea, cough, chest pain, night sweats, and hemoptysis (541, 575). Leukocytosis, very prominent blood eosinophilia, and transient pulmonary opacities occur during this time.

In the later chronic stage, when the adult worms inhabit the lungs and produce eggs, patients have chronic cough and bouts of hemoptysis. The sputum may be thick, chocolate brown, and contain eggs. Pleural effusions may be large and cause dyspnea. A bronchopleural fistula is an uncommon complication. The pulmonary manifestations may resolve spontaneously and new lesions appear slowly over months. Extrapulmonary spread is uncommon but can affect the brain, spinal cord, abdominal wall, and skin (541,575,632). Cerebral paragonimiasis occurs in up to 10 percent of patients and can cause masses or seizures.

Radiologic Findings. Chest radiographs in patients with paragonimiasis may be normal. Radiographic abnormalities during larval migration include transient parenchymal consolidations, pleural effusion, and pneumothorax. These findings are typically associated with peripheral eosinophilia (581). Pleural abnormalities are seen in up to 70 percent of affected patients (582).

Chronic paragonimiasis manifests radiographically with ill-defined patchy consolidation (fig. 12-199), cystic changes (worm cysts), and pleural effusion or thickening. Calcified pulmonary lesions may result from worm death and healing. Cystic lesions usually occur in the mid-lungs. They may be associated with linear opacities and intracystic soft tissue. The former is thought to result from worm migration through the lung and is called the "burrow tract" sign; the latter is thought to represent the worm itself (580–582). The worm migration tracks may be air-filled. Fluid-filled cysts may manifest as nodular masses, and those surrounded by consolidation may mimic cavitary disease (580). CT demonstrates mass-like consolidation, air-containing cysts, and linear opacities that course in opposite directions to bronchovascular bundles (580).

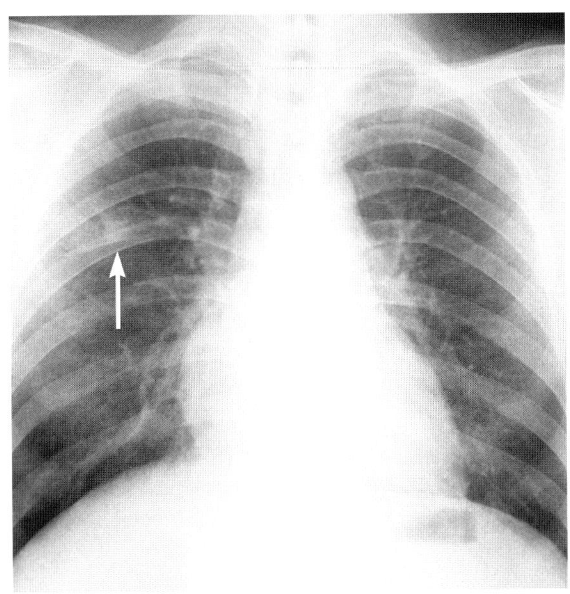

Figure 12-199

PARAGONIMIASIS

Paragonimiasis in a young Korean soldier with hemoptysis and low-grade fever. PA chest radiograph shows a small ill-defined consolidation in the anterior segment of the right upper lobe (arrow), which was initially thought to represent postprimary tuberculosis.

Pleural ultrasound has demonstrated diffuse particulate foci within a pleural effusion in a patient with thoracentesis-proven parasite-containing pleural fluid as well as pleural granulation tissue (638).

Pathologic Findings. In the lung, worms are found adjacent to large bronchioles and are surrounded by an abscess and a fibrous wall forming a small cyst (541,632). The worms are red-brown, yellow, or gray, and measure 1 to 3 mm in diameter. The inflammatory response consists of a mixture of lymphocytes, plasma cells, histiocytes, eosinophils, and giant cells (541,632). The cysts are 1.5 cm in diameter; they may rupture into airways, spilling eggs and debris and leading to hemoptysis. Histologically, a fibrous and granulomatous reaction may be seen in association with the eggs (fig. 12-200). Secondary bronchopneumonia is common. The pleura is frequently also involved. Chronic fibrous pleuritis may be accompanied by an inflammatory reaction to the eggs present in the pleura (fig. 12-201).

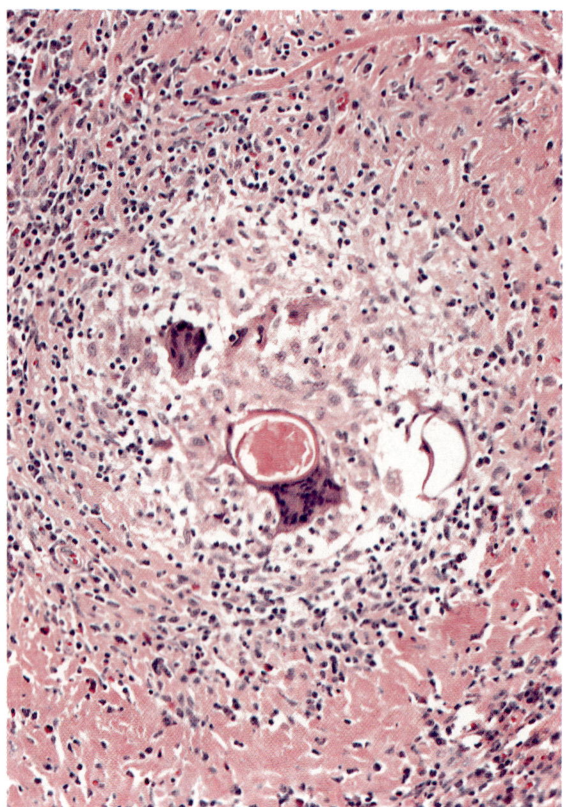
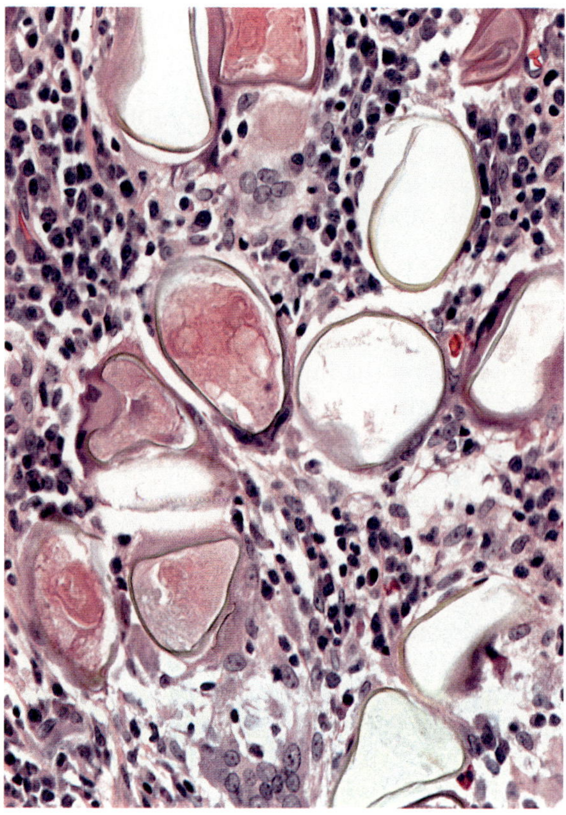

Figure 12-200

PARAGONIMIASIS: HISTOLOGY OF CHRONIC PNEUMONIA

Left: There is a marked granulomatous and fibrous reaction to these eggs of *Paragonimus*.

Right: Multiple eggs are embedded in fibrous tissue and chronic inflammation. The eggs are yellow to brown and oval, and have a thick birefringent shell.

The adult fluke is thick, egg-shaped, red-brown, and has a rounded anterior aspect with a tapered posterior. It measures 7 to 12 mm in length and is 4 to 6 mm thick. In the lung a fibrous capsule forms around the fluke.

The eggs of *P. westermani* are yellow to brown and oval, and have a thick birefringent shell. They measure 75 to 110 μm x 45 to 60 μm and they have a flattened operculum at one end (figs. 12-200, 12-201). The eggs may calcify.

Differential Diagnosis. In pathologic specimens, the eggs of *P. westermani* can be mistaken for *Schistosoma* sp, however, the eggs of the former are generally smaller and have thicker shells than the latter. In addition, *P. westermani* eggs are birefringent whereas those of *Schistosoma* are not (541,632).

Clinically, pulmonary paragonimiasis is frequently mistaken for tuberculosis (541). The diagnosis is usually established by identifying eggs in the sputum or feces. If the organism is in the pleura, the pleural cavity must be aspirated (541).

Treatment and Prognosis. Praziquantel is the medication of choice. There is a very high cure rate of between 90 and 100 percent. Chloroquine phosphate and emetine hydrochloride are less effective (575).

Schistosomiasis

Definition. Pulmonary schistosomiasis is an infection of the lung caused by *Schistosoma mansoni, S. japonicum,* or *S. haematobium.*

Schistosomes are trematodes, or "flukes," found in tropical regions of the world.

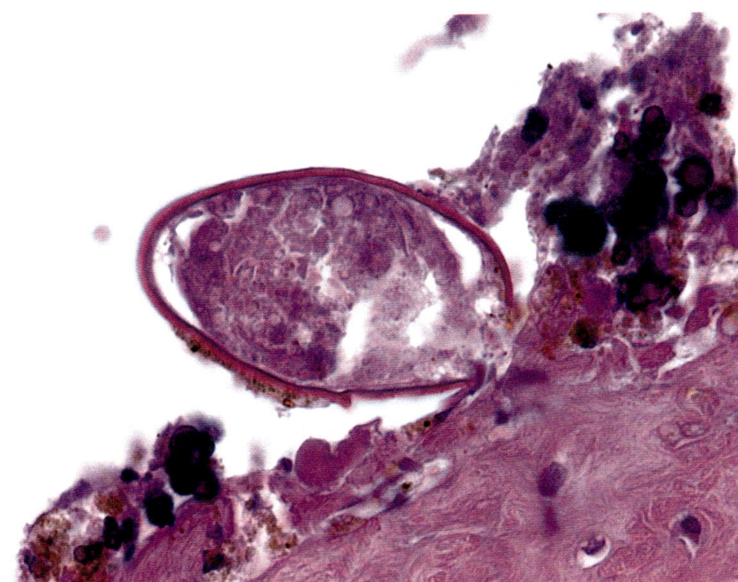

Figure 12-201

PARAGONIMIASIS

The shell of this partly calcified egg is brown and thick. This specimen was from the pleura.

Schistosomiasis is widely found in many parts of Africa including the Nile valley (554). Only *S. mansoni* occurs in the western hemisphere including parts of Brazil, the West Indies, and Puerto Rico. *S. japonicum* is found in the Philippines, China, and Japan (541,640). *S. haematobium,* also called *bilharzia* or *urinary schistosomiasis,* is found throughout Africa, southern Europe, and western Asia (640). The life cycle of the schistosomes alternates between sexual reproduction in the blood vessels of animals and asexual multiplication in snails (640).

Human infection occurs through exposure to water contaminated with infective cercariae (554). The cercariae penetrate the skin and enter the vasculature where they grow into adult worms; the worms reside in copula without causing disease. The adult female worms produce eggs and these migrate to the tissues and cause disease (541,640). The clinical course evolves through several phases, including penetration, prepatent, acute, latent, chronic, and inactive stages (640). The eggs of *S. mansoni* and *S. japonicum* reside mostly in the portal and hepatic venous habitat and they target the gut, liver, and lung. In contrast, the eggs of *S. haematobium* reside mostly in the pelvic region and target the bladder, ureter, and pelvis (640).

Clinical Features. Pulmonary involvement can occur at several stages of infection. A larval pneumonitis occurs during the tissue migration phase following heavy cercarial exposure. A pulmonary component may occur during the acute stage. Late in chronic infection cor pulmonale can develop secondary to the pulmonary hypertension associated with the granulomatous reaction to eggs deposited around pulmonary vessels. In addition, a Loeffler-like syndrome can occur as a response to therapy (575). Occasionally, worms embolize to the lungs and cause a localized pneumonitis or lung mass (541). In endemic areas, schistosome eggs may be an incidental histologic finding in the lung.

Larval pneumonitis may occur days to weeks following heavy cercarial exposure and is characterized by cough, low-grade fever, and peripheral eosinophilia. Patients have transient basilar pulmonary opacities and may have wheezing and basilar crepitant rales.

An acute serum sickness-like syndrome, also known as *Katayama fever,* can develop (575). This fever lasts 2 to 4 weeks and patients have low-grade fever, chills, headache, myalgias, and diarrhea (575,640). Some patients have pulmonary involvement with dry cough and transient pulmonary opacities (575).

Patients who receive antischistosomal therapy for heavy infection may develop an acute Loeffler-like syndrome, with fleeting pulmonary infiltrates associated with peripheral eosinophilia

(541,575). These patients present with cough and wheezing. This is thought to be a hypersensitivity reaction resulting from the release of antigens from dying worms. It resolves more rapidly than larval pneumonitis and the peripheral eosinophilia is less prominent (541,575).

Cor pulmonale typically occurs in patients with chronic infection who have liver disease with portal hypertension, which allows for the eggs to shunt to the lungs (541,575). Eggs deposit in the pulmonary capillaries and elicit a granulomatous and fibrosing response that leads to pulmonary hypertension.

Pulmonary disease occurs in up to 25 percent of patients with hepatosplenomegaly, but no more than 5 percent develop cor pulmonale (575). While cor pulmonale can occur with any of the types of schistosomiasis, it occurs most often in patients with *S. mansoni* infection in Egypt and Brazil (575).

Radiologic Findings. Acute pulmonary schistosomiasis manifests radiologically with patchy parenchymal consolidations associated with peripheral eosinophilia, which develop 2 to 6 weeks after initial infection. Chronic disease manifests with miliary nodular opacities (fig. 12-202). Vascular occlusion by the worms may result in pulmonary arterial hypertension, which manifests with enlarged central pulmonary arteries abruptly tapering towards the lung periphery (fig. 12-202) (569,581).

Pathologic Findings. Little is known about the histologic features of larval pneumonitis or the Loeffler-like syndrome seen in association with schistosomiasis since these patients do not have open lung biopsies. However, the lung probably shows the histologic pattern of an eosinophilic pneumonia.

Histologically in chronic infection, the *Schistosoma* eggs are seen in association with granulomatous inflammation and fibrosis that sometimes has a concentric morphology (fig. 12-203, left) (541). Since these eggs are deposited in a perivascular location, there is typically endarteritis, intimal fibrosis, and medial thickening (fig. 12-204). Pulmonary artery aneurysmal dilatation and angiomatoid and plexiform lesions have been described (541).

The pathologic diagnosis of schistosomiasis is usually established by recognition of the eggs in tissue sections (fig. 12-203, right). The

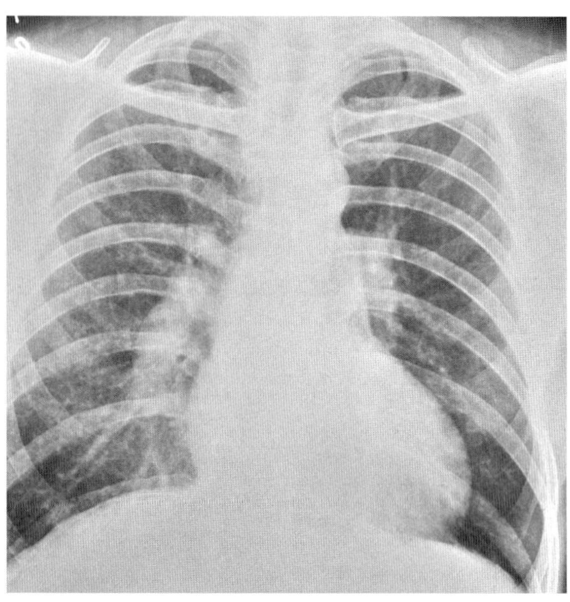

Figure 12-202

SCHISTOSOMIASIS

Schistosomiasis in a 25-year-old male with pulmonary arterial hypertension. PA chest radiograph demonstrates enlarged central pulmonary arteries, particularly on the right. Miliary nodular opacities are also noted in the right lung. The patient had documented pulmonary involvement by *Schistosoma mansoni.*

eggs of the various species have a distinctive morphology: those of *S. haematobium* are terminally spined, those of *S. mansoni* are laterally spined, and those of *S. japonicum* have a small lateral spine (640). These distinguishing features may be difficult to identify in tissue sections. The eggs of *S. haematobium* and *S. mansoni* measure 110-175 x 40-70 µm and those of *S. japonicum* are smaller, measuring 100 µm in greatest dimension (541).

Differential Diagnosis. The primary morphologic differential diagnosis for schistosomiasis is *Paragonimus* infection. *Paragonimus* eggs measure less than 100 µm, which is smaller than most eggs of *Schistosoma;* they have an operculum rather than spines; and they are birefringent (541). Occasionally, it is difficult to resolve these morphologic features in tissue sections.

Treatment and Prognosis. The optimal drug for the treatment of schistosomiasis is praziquantel (541,575). Once hepatosplenic or pulmonary involvement has developed, it is irreversible (541,575).

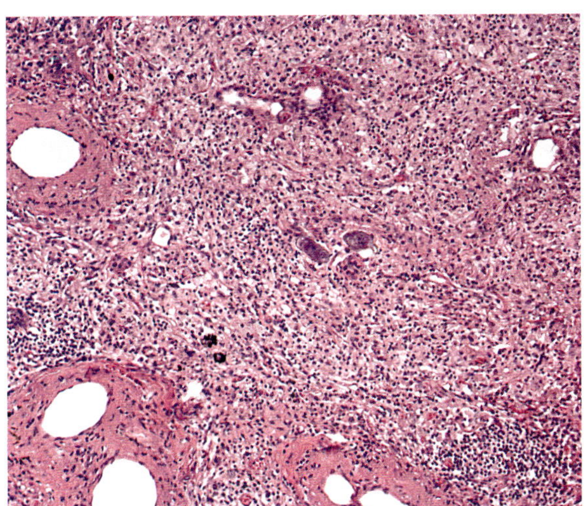

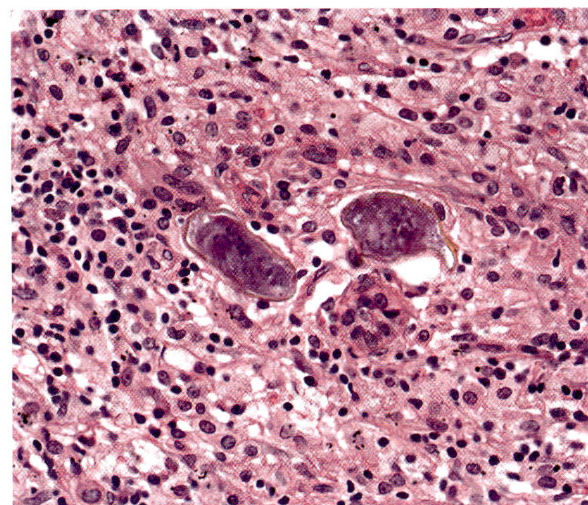

Figure 12-203

SCHISTOSOMIASIS: HISTOLOGY, *S. JAPONICUM*

Left: An inflammatory exudate surrounds the *Schistosoma* eggs.
Right: The eggs have a golden brown refractile wall. (Courtesy of Ronald C. Neafie, AFIP, Washington, DC.)

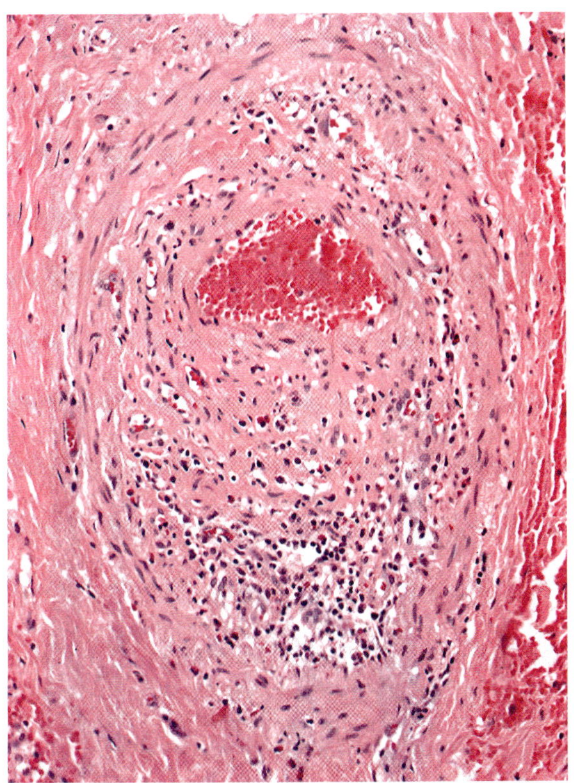

Figure 12-204

SCHISTOSOMIASIS: VASCULAR CHANGES

This artery shows medial thickening and vasculitis with a moderate chronic inflammatory infiltrate in the vessel wall.

CESTODA

Echinococcus is the most important of the cestodes known to cause pulmonary disease. Only rare cases of pulmonary involvement are reported with sparganosis or cysticercosis (541).

Echinococcosis

Definition. Pulmonary echinococcosis (also known as *hydatid disease* and *hydatidosis*) is an infection of the lung caused by the larval tapeworms, *Echinococcus granulosus, E. multilocularis,* and *E. vogeli*.

Echinococcal disease is one of the most important helminthic pulmonary diseases. It is caused by infection with the metacestode stage of the tapeworm *Echinococcus,* which belongs to the family Taeniidae. In its adult stage, the parasite lives in the intestinal tract of carnivores. The head is composed of a double crown of hook-like structures, and the body is formed by three or four rings, the last of which bears the eggs. The four species of *Echinococcus* that are known to cause human disease are *E. granulosus, E. multilocularis, E. oligarthrus,* and *E. vogeli* (541,575,592). The epidemiology and pathology of infections with echinococcal species differ (538).

E. granulosus is found mostly in rural areas where people frequently have contact with carnivores, sheep, cows, and dogs (541,568). There are three strains of *E. granulosus:* 1) the dog/sheep strain is the most widespread, 2) the sylvatic strain found mostly in the arctic regions and affecting moose and wolves, and 3) the Middle Eastern or dog/horse strain (541,568). Echinococcosis is a significant public health problem in South and Central America. It is also prevalent in Australia, New Zealand, northern Canada, cosmopolitan Europe, Asia, South Africa, and the Middle East (541,568). In the United States it is reported in Alaska, Utah, Minnesota, North and South Dakota, Iowa, Nebraska, Montana, Wyoming, and California (541,568). The prevalence of liver and pulmonary echinococcal cysts increases with advancing age, indicating that new infections continue to occur throughout life (557).

E. multilocularis occurs only in the Northern hemisphere, particularly in parts of central Europe, Russia, western China, certain areas of North America, and northern Africa (541,568). The life cycle involves wild foxes as the definitive host and rodents as the natural intermediate host. Domestic dogs or cats may also become infected and can transmit the infection to humans directly or can contaminate food with parasite eggs (541,568). The rate of infection in animals in North America is low and human infection is rare (541,568). The cysts of *E. multilocularis* are slow growing, with an estimated incubation period of 5 to 15 years. The average age at presentation is 55 years.

E. vogeli causes a polycystic form of echinococcosis with clinical features that overlap with those of cystic and alveolar echinococcosis (541,568). It is found most often in Colombia, Ecuador, Venezuela, Panama, Argentina, Brazil, and Costa Rica. It infects wild dogs and paca (541,568), but human infection is rare.

E. oligarthrus causes polycystic echinococcosis. The definitive hosts for the parasite are the wild puma and the jaguar, with intermediate hosts that include rodents and rabbits. The parasite has been reported from northern Mexico to southern Argentina, but only three human cases of *E. oligarthrus* infection have been documented in Venezuela and Brazil (586).

The life cycle of *Echinococcus* begins as an adult tapeworm living within the intestine of a definitive host, which is usually a dog (541,568). A variety of grazing animals, most commonly sheep, serve as the intermediate host after ingesting vegetation contaminated with feces from the dogs that are contaminated with eggs and gravid proglottids of *Echinococcus*. In the intestinal tract of the intermediate host, the eggs hatch and release oncospheres, which pass through the intestinal mucosa into the blood stream to the various organs, where they grow into hydatid cysts (541,568). Humans are accidental hosts and do not play a role in the biological cycle (586).

Clinical Features. The most common site of human *E. granulosus* infection in adults is the liver (60 percent), followed by the lung (20 to 25 percent), and less commonly, the kidney (4 percent), muscle (4 percent), brain (3 percent), and bone (2 percent) (541,568). However, the lungs are the most common site of infection in children (50 percent of cases) (541). Pulmonary involvement can result from extension through the diaphragm from the liver into the right lower lobe or hematogenous dissemination from another cyst. Multiple cysts are common. Approximately 60 percent of pulmonary echinococcosis affects the right lung and 50 to 60 percent involves the lower lobes (544). Approximately 20 to 40 percent of patients with lung cysts also have liver cysts, although the cervid (northern) strain of *E. granulosus* localizes predominantly in the lungs (586).

Most patients with liver or pulmonary lesions are asymptomatic, but pulmonary cysts can cause cough and chest pain (551,575,635). The cysts grow slowly, so the delay of presentation from the time of initial infection may be many years. Dyspnea and hemoptysis can be associated with leakage or rupture of a cyst into a bronchus. Rarely, "grape skin"-like cyst contents may be expectorated (575). Rupture of cysts and leakage of the contents may result in several complications: 1) a hypersensitivity reaction and shock, 2) drowning in aspirated cyst fluid, or 3) dissemination or "metastases" of cysts within the thoracic cavity or lungs. If there is cyst rupture into the pleural cavity it can result in empyema and seeding of the pleura (541,575). Rarely, patients have compressive manifestations such as dysphagia, Horner's syndrome, and superior vena cava syndrome. A life-threatening complication occurs when a hydatid cyst of the right heart ruptures, resulting in pulmonary emboli (541).

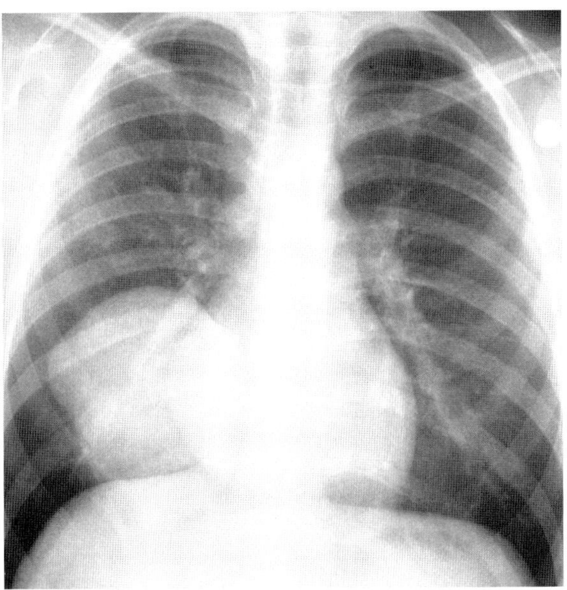

Figure 12-205

ECHINOCOCCOSIS

Echinococcosis in an 11-year-old male who presented with recurrent respiratory infections and bronchospasm. PA chest radiograph demonstrates a well-defined spherical mass in the right lower lobe with lobular contours and adjacent discoid atelectasis.

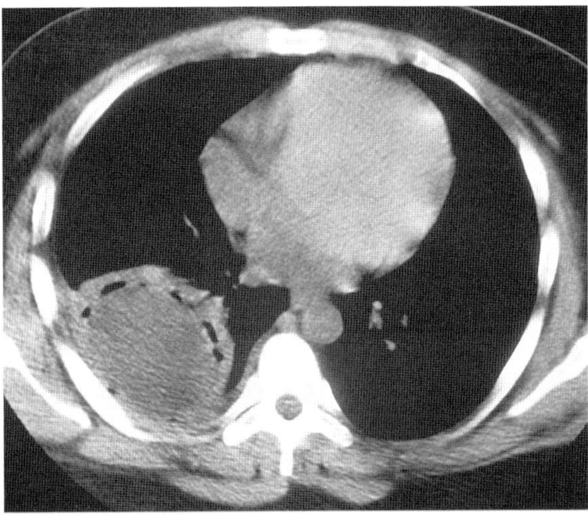

Figure 12-206

ECHINOCOCCOSIS

Echinococcosis in a 21-year-old male with productive cough and fever. Unenhanced chest CT (mediastinal window) demonstrates a right lower lobe mass with a thin linear peripheral air collection surrounding a central area of water attenuation.

E. multilocularis can cause a severe and often fatal infection because the metacestode (hydatid cyst) invades and destroys tissue extending beyond organ borders into adjacent structures, and metastasizes to distant sites (586).The primary infection in humans is located in the liver in almost 100 percent of cases, but spread to other organs, including the lungs and brain, occurs commonly, either by direct extension or hematogenous dissemination. The lung is involved in approximately 15 percent of cases (541,586). The most common presenting complaints include right upper quadrant discomfort due to hepatomegaly, malaise, and weight loss. Cholestatic jaundice, cholangitis, portal hypertension, and the Budd-Chiari syndrome can also occur. Infection is often found incidentally. Rare cases of pulmonary involvement are reported with *E. vogeli* (541).

Routine laboratory tests may be abnormal but are not specific and cannot make the diagnosis. Fewer than 15 percent of patients have eosinophilia and this occurs only if there is leakage of antigenic material (586). Serology using an enzyme-linked immunoelectrotransfer blot assay is a reliable aid in diagnosis since it is positive in 60 to 90 percent of cases (541,545,575).

Radiologic Findings. The typical radiographic appearance of pulmonary echinococcosis in asymptomatic patients is that of a well-marginated, spherical, soft tissue mass of variable size which may mimic a pulmonary neoplasm (fig. 12-205). Closed uncomplicated echinococcal cysts typically affect the lower lobes and may be multiple and bilateral. When multiple, they may mimic metastatic disease. The posterior right lung is most commonly affected. When echinococcal cysts are completely surrounded by lung they exhibit a spherical morphology (fig. 12-205). However, peripheral cysts may conform to the shape of adjacent structures. Large lesions may produce mass effect (543). CT demonstrates a spherical lesion with smooth walls of variable thickness and central water or near-water attenuation (fig. 12-206) (624).

Cysts that rupture result in a variety of radiographic appearances. Communication between the pericyst and bronchi results in a thin crescent of air that surrounds the laminated membrane (exocyst) and mimics the appearance of a

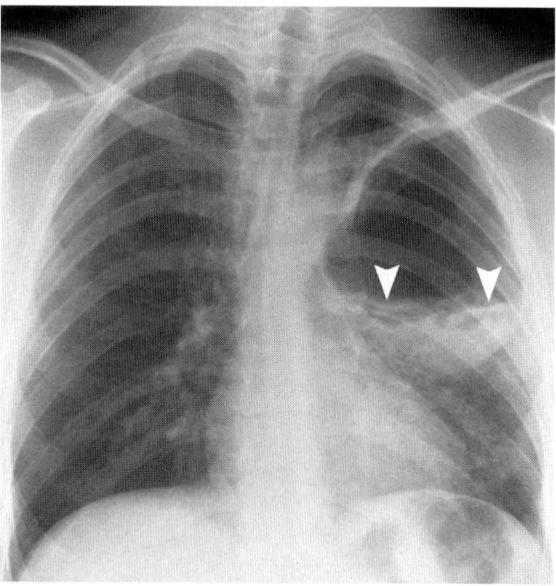

Figure 12-207

ECHINOCOCCOSIS

Echinococcosis in a 15-year-old male with chest pain, cough, fever, and moderate respiratory distress. PA chest radiograph demonstrates a large thin-walled cyst in the left upper lobe. Note the undulating air-fluid level (arrowheads) and dependent debris within the cyst. Adjacent lung parenchymal consolidation is also noted.

mycetoma (fig. 12-206). This is considered a sign of impending cyst rupture (543). CT is helpful in suggesting the diagnosis as the air is visualized around an intact cystic structure of water attenuation. Rupture may result in the sign of the "double arch" where there is an intracystic air-fluid level and a superior air crescent. More characteristically, the cyst membranes collapse within the fluid and produce an undulating air-fluid level referred to as the "water lily" sign or the sign of the "camalote" (fig. 12-207), which is considered a pathognomonic radiologic appearance. Cross-sectional imaging studies may demonstrate daughter cysts. Collapse of the cyst membranes is identified as the "serpent" sign on cross-sectional imaging studies, which refers to visualization of the membranes as linear structures that are roughly parallel to each other within the cyst fluid (641). Collapse of the cyst membranes may also produce a gyrated appearance termed the "spin"or "whirl" sign. Cyst rupture typically leads to superinfection, which may manifest with air bubbles within the cyst fluid. Rim enhancement may be demonstrated because of enhancement of the inflammatory pericyst. A halo sign of parenchymal consolidation or atelectasis surrounding a parenchymal cyst has been described (543). Adjacent consolidation results in irregular lesion margins on radiography and may mimic the appearance of pneumonia or primary lung carcinoma (624). Expectoration of fluid and cyst membranes from a ruptured cyst may result in a thin-walled air-filled parenchymal cystic space (624). Rupture into the pleural space with associated pleural effusion also occurs (641). Confirmatory findings on CT include evidence of hepatic echinococcal disease, which may exhibit peripheral calcification (543).

Pathologic Findings. In the lung, the echinococcal cyst appears as a unilocular (fig. 12-208) or multilocular cyst, depending on whether the infection is due to *E. granulosus* or *E. multilocularis*. The cysts vary in size from several millimeters up to 20 cm.

The cyst wall of *E. granulosus* is thick, measuring 2 to 3 mm, and consists of fibrous tissue from the host. A laminated layer, consisting of an embryonic membrane that measures approximately 1 mm in thickness, lines this wall (fig. 12-209A). A germinal layer that consists of a single cell layer approximately 10 to 25 µm thick covers the embryonic membrane. Clusters of cells bud from the germinal layer, float in the interior, and grow into brood capsules which are attached by stalks to the germinal layer. If brood capsules are present the cyst is fertile, if they are absent the cyst is sterile. When the brood capsule separates from the germinal layer it becomes a daughter cyst. The brood capsule produces several infective protoscolices (fig. 12-209B) (541,568,641). The protoscolices have teeth-like hooklets (fig. 12-209B,C); some of these are acid-fast.

E. multilocularis causes echinococcal cysts that consist of an amorphous mass of sterile proliferative parasitic tissue. The cut surface shows multiple cystic spaces with collapsed membranes. However, in contrast to the cysts of *E. granulosus*, no fluid is seen. The cysts are often surrounded by necrotic debris and they may cavitate.

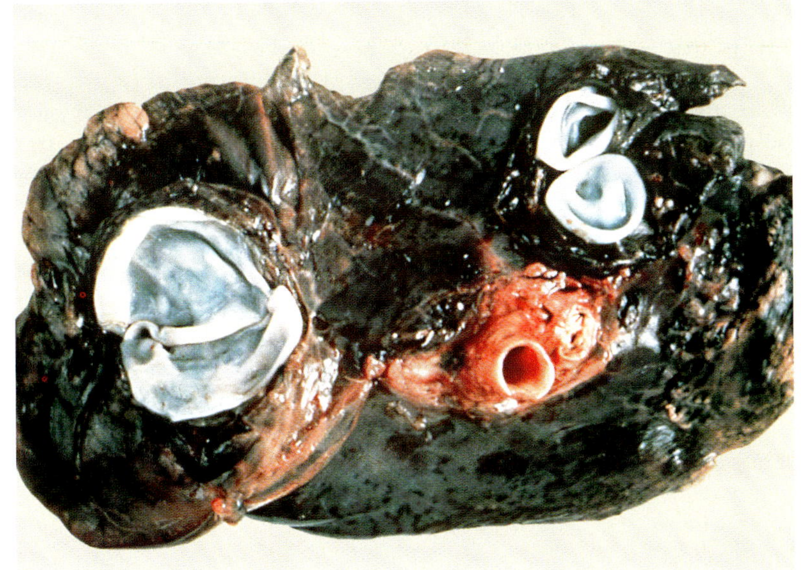

Figure 12-208

ECHINOCOCCUS GRANULOSUS: GROSS SPECIMEN

Two unilocular cysts are present in this lung. The surface of the cyst wall is white and smooth.

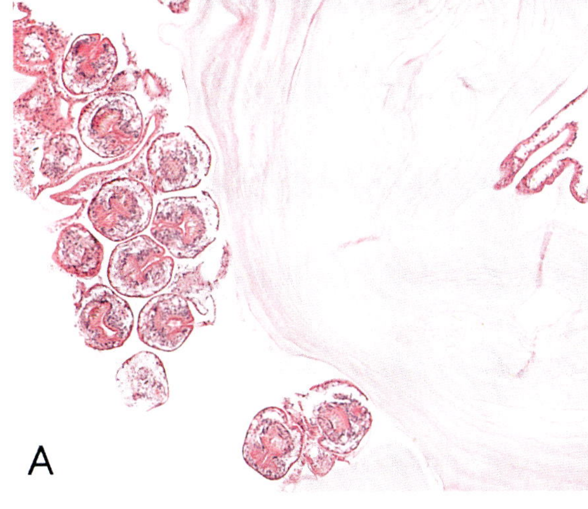

Figure 12-209

ECHINOCOCCUS: ORGANISM MORPHOLOGY

A: A folded, white, laminated membrane is present. Along the surface (right) is a germinal layer that consists of single cells. Several brood capsules (left) with clusters of protoscolices are present.

B: Protoscolices containing teeth-like hooklets are present within the brood capsules.

C: Several hooklets are freely floating adjacent to one protoscolex.

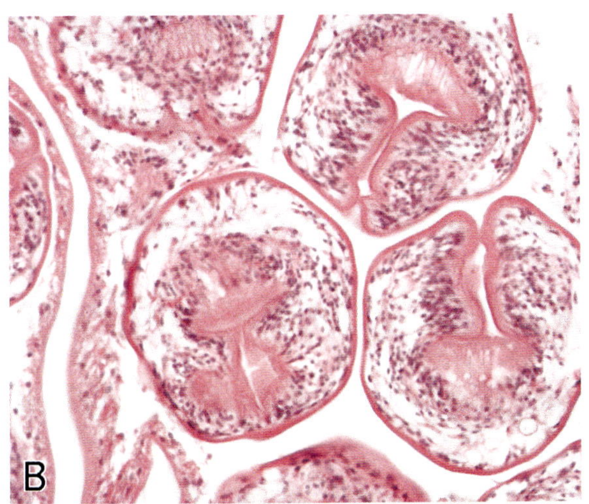

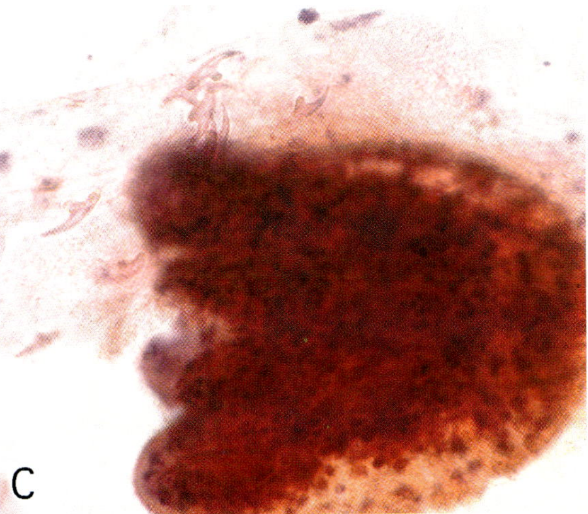

Acute inflammation and abscess formation can occur in cysts that decay or rupture into a bronchus. The cyst wall may elicit a necrotizing granulomatous inflammatory response. Calcification can develop in the cyst wall (541).

Since patients may develop anaphylactic shock or dissemination of infection when the cyst wall is penetrated, needle aspiration is not recommended (541).

Differential Diagnosis. The histologic features are quite distinctive and difficult to confuse with other lesions. The characteristic germinal layer could potentially be overlooked in small biopsy specimens, however, the presence of the protoscolices and hooklets should allow for the diagnosis. If there is extensive necrosis or a suppurative reaction, it might be possible to overlook the characteristic germinal layer.

Treatment and Prognosis. The treatment of choice involves endocystectomy or surgical resection (547,551,553,596,615,617). The surgical options for lung cysts include lobectomy, wedge resection, pericystectomy, intact endocystectomy, and capitonnage. It is important to avoid spilling the cyst contents to avoid anaphylactic shock and dissemination of infection. Simultaneous surgical resection of cysts in the liver and right lower lobe of the lung is sometimes performed. In a large study of 842 patients followed for 3 to 20 years, a recurrence rate of 1.9 percent was noted after intact endocystectomies (615).

The PAIR (percutaneous aspiration, introduction of a protoscolicidal agent, and reaspiration) procedure involves percutaneous puncture of cysts under ultrasound guidance, followed by aspiration of substantial amounts of cyst fluid and injection of a protoscolicidal agent into the cyst cavity (usually hypertonic saline or ethanol). The cyst is then reaspirated after a period of at least 15 minutes. This procedure is used predominantly for liver cysts. Complications have been observed more frequently when PAIR is used for pulmonary cysts. The World Health Organization (WHO) currently recommends PAIR for inoperable patients and for those who refuse surgery. The potential risks of this procedure include anaphylaxis, secondary spillage of hydatid fluid into the peritoneum, hemorrhage, infection, chemical sclerosing cholangitis, and biliary fistulas (586). Adjunctive chemotherapy before and after surgery appears to reduce the risk of recurrence by inactivating protoscolices and lessening the tension of the cysts for easier removal (587).

The optimal drug for medical therapy is albendazole (541,575,620). However, albendazole treatment is not highly successful and prolonged therapy is needed. Also, this agent is teratogenic and hepatotoxic. More recently, mebendazole has been used as an intracavitary agent (573,604,617). If left untreated, more than 90 percent of patients infected with *E. multilocularis* die within 10 years of the onset of clinical symptoms, and virtually 100 percent by 15 years (538). Patients often become infected at an early age and live for 30 to 40 years. Surgical therapy is very difficult and medical therapy is not very effective (541).

PSEUDOPARASITIC STRUCTURES

A variety of structures can be mistaken for parasites in the lung. These include corpora amylacea (see fig. 2-6), lentil pneumonia (see figs. 3-161, 8-16C,D), and other viral or fungal infectious agents. Liesegang rings (577,618,633,637) are peculiar laminated structures observed in cysts in organs such as the kidney and breast, but to date they are not reported in the lung. Rarely, however, similar laminated calcifications occur in areas of mucous stasis in the lung (fig. 12-210).

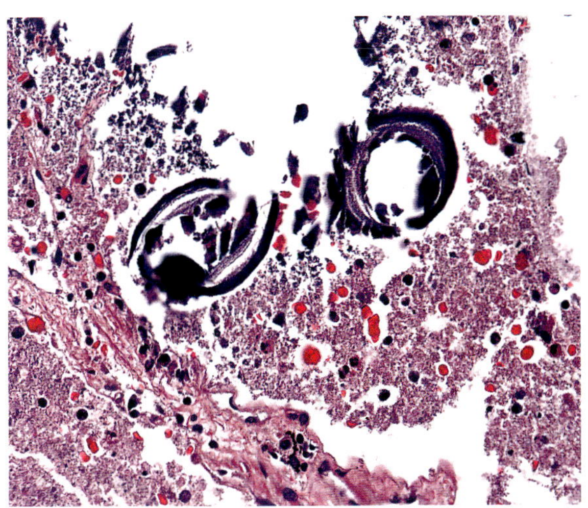

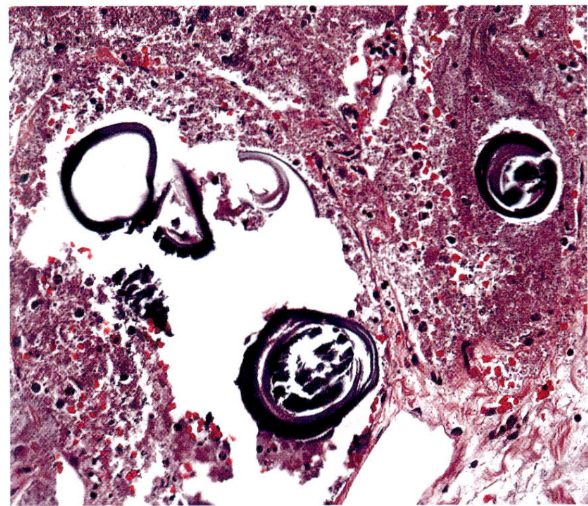

Figure 12-210

LAMINATED MICROCALCIFICATIONS

Left: These laminated, round to oval calcifications were mistaken for possible parasites.
Right: These calcifications were found within areas of mucus stasis.

REFERENCES

Bacterial Pneumonias

1. Allen SD. Rhodococcus equi infections. In: Connor DH, Chandler FW, Manz HJ, et al, eds. Pathology of infectious diseases. Stamford: Appleton & Lange; 1997:781–7.
2. Alsofrom DJ, Mettler FA Jr, Mann JM. Radiographic manifestations of plaque in New Mexico, 1975-1980. A review of 42 proved cases. Radiology 1981;139:561–5.
3. Aronson MD, Komaroff AL, Pasculle W, Myerowitz RL. Legionella micdadei (Pittsburgh pneumonia agent) infection in nonimmunosuppressed patients with pneumonia. Ann Intern Med 1981;94:485–6.
4. Barnett TB, Knowles MR. Diffuse bacterial bronchiolitis with bronchiolar pneumonia in adults. South Med J 1987;80:10–5.
5. Bartlett J. Treatment of community-acquired pneumonia. Chemotherapy 2000;46[Suppl 1]:24–31.
6. Bartlett JG, Dowell SF, Mandell LA, File TM Jr, Musher DM, Fine MJ. Practice guidelines for the management of community-acquired pneumonia in adults. Infectious Diseases Society of America. Clin Infect Dis 2000;31:347–82.
7. Beaman BL, Beaman L. Nocardia species: host-parasite relationships. Clin Microbiol Rev 1994;7:213–64.
8. Belchis DA, Simpson E, Colby T. Histopathologic features of Burkholderia cepacia pneumonia in patients without cystic fibrosis. Mod Pathol 2000;13:369–72.
9. Bennhoff DF. Actinomycosis: diagnostic and therapeutic considerations and a review of 32 cases. Laryngoscope 1984;94:1198–217.
10. Bergqvist G, Trovik M. Neonatal infections with Streptococcus pneumoniae. Scand J Infect Dis 1985;17:33–5.
11. Bersoff-Matcha SJ, Roper CC, Liapis H, Little JR. Primary pulmonary botryomycosis: case report and review. Clin Infect Dis 1998;26:620–4.
12. The British Thoracic Society. Guidelines for the management of community-acquired pneumonia in adults admitted to hospital. Br J Hosp Med 1993;49:346–50.
13. Byrd RP Jr, Vasquez J, Roy TM. Respiratory manifestations of tick-borne diseases in the southeastern United States. South Med J 1997;90:1–4.
14. Carter JB, Wolter RK, Angres G, Saltzman P. Nodular Legionnaire disease. AJR Am J Roentgenol 1981;137:612–3.
15. Cendan I, Klapholz A, Talavera W. Pulmonary actinomycosis. A cause of endobronchial disease in a patient with AIDS. Chest 1993;103: 1886–7.

16. Chandler FW. Nocardiosis. In: Conner DH, Chandler FW, Manz HJ, et al, eds. Pathology of infectious diseases. Stamford: Appleton & Lange; 1997:701–8.
17. Chandler FW, Watts JC. Botryomycosis. In: Connor DH, Chandler FW, Manz HJ, et al, eds. Pathology of infectious diseases. Stamford: Appleton & Lange; 1997:441–5.
18. Chandler FW, Watts JC. Pathologic diagnosis of fungal infections. Chicago: American Society of Clinical Pathologists; 1987.
19. Charoenratanakul S. Tropical infection and the lung. Monaldi Arch Chest Dis 1997;52:376–9.
20. Chastre J, Raghu G, Soler P, Brun P, Basset F, Gibert C. Pulmonary fibrosis following pneumonia due to acute Legionnaires' disease. Clinical, ultrastructural, and immunofluorescent study. Chest 1987;91:57–62.
21. Chears WC, Hargrove MD, Verner JV, Smith AG, Ruffin JM. Whipple's disease: a review of twelve patients from one service. Am J Med 1961;30:226–34.
22. Chenoweth CE, Saint S, Martinez F, Lynch JP, Fendrick AM. Antimicrobial resistance in Streptococcus pneumoniae: implications for patients with community-acquired pneumonia. Mayo Clin Proc 2000;75:1161–8.
23. Cheon JE, Im JG, Kim MY, Lee JS, Choi GM, Yeon KM. Thoracic actinomycosis: CT findings. Radiology 1998;209:229–33.
24. Coelho Filho JC. Pulmonary cavities colonized by actinomycetes: report of six cases. Rev Inst Med Trop Sao Paulo 1990;32:63–6.
25. Colby TV, Hunt S, Pelzmann K, Carrington CB. Malakoplakia of the lung: a report of two cases. Respiration 1980;39:295–9.
26. Coletta FS, Fein AM. Radiological manifestations of Legionella/Legionella-like organisms. Semin Respir Infect 1998;13:109–15.
27. Conant EF, Wechsler RJ. Actinomycosis and nocardiosis of the lung. J Thorac Imaging 1992;7:75–84.
28. Conces DJ Jr. Bacterial pneumonia in immunocompromised patients. J Thorac Imaging 1998;13:261–70.
29. Cordes LG, Myerowitz RL, Pasculle AW, et al. Legionella micdadei (Pittsburgh pneumonia agent): direct flourescent-antibody examination of infected human lung tissue and characterization of clinical isolates. J Clin Microbiol 1981;13:720–2.
30. Corley DE, Winterbauer RH. Infectious diseases that result in slowly resolving and chronic pneumonia. Semin Respir Infect 1993;8:3–13.
31. Crouch E, White V, Wright J, Churg A. Malakoplakia mimicking carcinoma metastatic to lung. Am J Surg Pathol 1984;8:151–6.
32. Dail DH. Bronchial and transbronchial diseases. In: Dail DH, Hammar SP, eds. Pulmonary pathology, 2nd ed. New York: Springer-Verlag; 1994:79–119.
33. de Montpreville VT, Nashashibi N, Dulmet EM. Actinomycosis and other bronchopulmonary infections with bacterial granules. Ann Diagn Pathol 1999;3:67–74.
34. Dedicoat M, Venkatesan P. The treatment of Legionnaires' disease. J Antimicrob Chemother 1999;43:747–52.
35. Dhiensiri T, Puapairoj S, Susaengrat W. Pulmonary melioidosis: clinical-radiologic correlation in 183 cases in northeastern Thailand. Radiology 1988;166:711–5.
36. Dobbins WO III. Whipple's disease. In: Connor DH, Chandler FW, Manz HJ, et al, eds. Pathology of infectious diseases. Stamford: Appleton & Lange; 1997:897–903.
37. Durand DV, Lecomte C, Cathebras P, Rousset H, Godeau P. Whipple disease. Clinical review of 52 cases. The SNFMI Research Group on Whipple Disease. Societe Nationale Francaise de Medecine Interne. Medicine (Baltimore) 1997;76:170–84.
38. Enzinger FM, Helwig EB. Whipple's disease: a review of the literature and report of fifteen patients. Virchows Arch [A] 1963;336:269.
39. Evans ME, Gregory DW, Schaffner W, McGee ZA. Tularemia: a 30-year experience with 88 cases. Medicine (Baltimore) 1985;64:251–69.
40. Farley MM, Stephens DS, Brachman PS Jr, Harvey RC, Smith JD, Wenger JD. Invasive Haemophilus influenzae disease in adults. A prospective, population-based surveillance. CDC Meningitis Surveillance Group. Ann Intern Med 1992;116:806–12.
41. Feigin DS. Nocardiosis of the lung: chest radiographic findings in 21 cases. Radiology 1986;159:9–14.
42. Filice GA. Actinomycosis. In: Sarosi GA, Davies SF, eds. Fungal diseases of the lung, 3rd ed. Philadelphia: Lippincott Williams & Wilkins; 2000:187–96.
43. Filice GA. Nocardiosis. In: Sarosi GA, Davies SF, eds. Fungal diseases of the lung, 3rd ed. Philadelphia: Lippincott Williams & Wilkins; 2000:197–212.
44. Foltzer MA, Guiney WB Jr, Wager GC, Alpern HD. Bronchopulmonary bacillary angiomatosis. Chest 1993;104:973–5.
45. Fraser RS, Müller NL, Colman N, Pare PD. Bacteria other than mycobacteria. In: Fraser RS, Müller NL, Colman N, Pare PD, eds. Fraser and Pare's diagnosis of diseases of the chest, 4th ed. Philadelphia: WB Saunders; 1999:734–97.

46. Fraser RS, Müller NL, Colman N, Pare PD. Fungi and actinomyces. In: Fraser RS, Müller NL, Colman N, Pare PD, eds. Fraser and Pare's diagnosis of diseases of the chest, 4th ed. Philadelphia: WB Saunders; 1999:875–978.
47. Fraser RS, Müller NL, Colman N, Pare PD. General features of pulmonary infection. In: Fraser RS, Müller NL, Colman N, Pare PD, eds. Fraser and Pare's diagnosis of diseases of the chest, 4th ed. Philadelphia: WB Saunders; 1999:697–733.
48. Friedlander C. Uber die Schizomyceten bei der acuten fibrosen Pneumonie. Virchows Arch [Pathol Anat] 1882;87:319.
49. Fujii T, Kadota J, Kawakami K, et al. Long term effect of erythromycin therapy in patients with chronic Pseudomonas aeruginosa infection. Thorax 1995;50:1246–52.
50. Gallivan MV, Davis WA II, Garagusi VF, Paris AL, Lack EE. Fatal-cat transmitted tularemia: demonstration of the organism in tissue. South Med J 1980;73:240–2.
51. Gervaix A, Beghetti M, Rimensberger P, Posfay-Barbe K, Barazzone C. Bullous emphysema after Legionella pneumonia in a two-year-old child. Pediatr Infect Dis J 2000;19:86–7.
52. Geyer SJ, Burkey AR, Chandler FW. Tularemia. In: Connor DH, Chandler FW, Manz HJ, et al, eds. Pathology of infectious diseases. Stamford: Appleton & Lange; 1997:869–73.
53. Gill V, Cunha BA. Tularemia pneumonia. Semin Respir Infect 1997;12:61–7.
54. Gilligan PH, Whittier S. Burkholderia, stenotrophomonas, ralstonia, brevundimonas, comamonas, and acidovorax. In: Murray PR, Baron EJ, Pfaller MA, Tenover FC, Yolken RH, eds. Manual of clinical microbiology, 7th ed. Washington D.C.: ASM Press; 1999:526–38.
55. Goetz MB, Finegold SM. Pyogenic bacterial pneumonia, lung abscess and empyema. In: Murray JF, Nadel JA, Mason RJ, Boushey HA Jr, eds. Textbook of respiratory medicine, 3rd ed. Philadelphia: WB Saunders; 2000:985–1041.
56. Goodman LR, Goren RA, Teplick SK. The radiographic evaluation of pulmonary infection. Med Clin North Am 1980;64:553–74.
57. Greenawald KA, Nash G, Foley FD. Acute systemic melioidosis. Autopsy findings in four patients. Am J Clin Pathol 1969;52:188–98.
58. Groskin SA, Panicek DM, Ewing DK, et al. Bacterial lung abscess: a review of the radiographic and clinical features of 50 cases. J Thorac Imaging 1991;6:62–7.
59. Gupta RK, Schuster RA, Christian WD. Autopsy findings in a unique case of malacoplakia. A cytoimmunohistochemical study of Michaelis-Gutmann bodies. Arch Pathol 1972;93:42–8.
60. Hamrock D, Azmi FH, O'Donnell E, Gunning WT, Philips ER, Zaher A. Infection by Rhodococcus equi in a patient with AIDS: histological appearance mimicking Whipple's disease and Mycobacterium avium-intracellulare infection. J Clin Pathol 1999;52:68–71.
61. Haramati LB, Jenny-Avital ER. Approach to the diagnosis of pulmonary disease in patients infected with the human immunodeficiency virus. J Thorac Imaging 1998;13:247–60.
62. Heath PT, Booy R, Azzopardi HJ, et al. Non-type b Haemophilus influenzae disease: clinical and epidemiologic characteristics in the Haemophilus influenzae type b vaccine era. Pediatr Infect Dis J 2001;20:300–5.
63. Hebert GA, Thomason BM, Harris PP, Hicklin MD, McKinney RM. "Pittsburgh pneumonia agent": a bacterium phenotypically similar to Legionella pneumophila and identical to the TATLOCK bacterium. Ann Intern Med 1980;92:53–4.
64. Henkle JQ, Nair SV. Endobronchial pulmonary nocardiosis. JAMA 1986;256:1331–2.
65. Hodder RV, George-Hyslop P, Chalvardjian A, Bear RA, Thomas P. Pulmonary malakoplakia. Thorax 1984;39:70–1.
66. Hurter T, Rumpelt HJ, Ferlinz R. Fibrosing alveolitis responsive to corticosteroids following Legionnaires' disease pneumonia. Chest 1992;101:281–3.
67. Ip M, Osterberg LG, Chau PY, Raffin TA. Pulmonary melioidosis. Chest 1995;108:1420–4.
68. Iralu JV, Maguire JH. Pulmonary infections in immigrants and refugees. Semin Respir Infect 1991;6:235–46.
69. James TN, Bulkley BH. Whipple bacilli within the tunica media of pulmonary arteries. Chest 1984;86:454–8.
70. Johnson CC, Finegold SM. Pyogenic bacterial pneumonia, lung abscess and empyema. In: Murray JF, Nadel JA, eds. Textbook of respiratory medicine, 2nd ed. Philadelphia: WB Saunders; 1994:1036–93.
71. Kantor HG. The many radiologic facies of pneumococcal pneumonia. AJR Am J Roentgenol 1981;137:1213–20.
72. Katapadi K, Pujol F, Vuletin JC, Katapadi M, Pachter BR. Pulmonary botryomycosis in a patient with AIDS. Chest 1996;109:276–8.
72a. Katzenstein AZ, Davis C, Brande A. Pulmonary changes in neonatal sepsis to group B beta-hemolytic streptococus: relation of hyaline membrane disease. J Infect Dis 1976;133:430–5.
73. Kaufmann AF, McDade JE, Patton CM, et al. Pontiac fever: isolation of the etiologic agent (Legionella pneumophilia) and demonstration of its mode of transmission. Am J Epidemiol 1981;114:337–47.

74. Kelly CA, Egan M, Rawlinson J. Whipple's disease presenting with lung involvement. Thorax 1996;51:343–4.
75. Kissane JM. Staphylococcal Infections. In: Connor DH, Chandler FW, Manz HJ, et al, eds. Pathology of infectious diseases. Stamford: Appleton & Lange; 1997:805–16.
76. Kissane JM. Streptococcal infections and infections by "Streptococcus-like" organisms. In: Connor DH, Chandler FW, Manz HJ, et al, eds. Pathology of infectious diseases. Stamford: Appleton & Lange; 1997:817–32.
77. Kozak AJ, Hall WH, Gerding DN. Cavitary pneumonia associated with tularemia. Chest 1978;73:426–7.
78. Kroboth FJ, Yu VL, Reddy SC, Yu AC. Clinicoradiographic correlation with the extent of Legionnaire disease. AJR Am J Roentgenol 1983;141:263–8.
79. Kwon KY, Colby TV. Rhodococcus equi pneumonia and pulmonary malakoplakia in acquired immunodeficiency syndrome. Pathologic features. Arch Pathol Lab Med 1994;118:744–8.
80. Kwong JS, Müller NL, Godwin JD, Aberle D, Grymaloski MR. Thoracic actinomycosis: CT findings in eight patients. Radiology 1992;183:189–92.
81. Lack EE. Malakoplakia. In: Connor DH, Chandler FW, Manz HJ, et al, eds. Pathology of infectious diseases. Stamford: Appleton & Lange; 1997:1647–54.
82. Lasky JA, Pulkingham N, Powers MA, Durack DT. Rhodococcus equi causing human pulmonary infection: review of 29 cases. South Med J 1991;84:1217–20.
83. LeBoit PE. Bacillary angiomatosis. In: Connor DH, Chandler FW, Manz HJ, et al, eds. Pathology of infectious diseases. Stamford: Appleton & Lange; 1997:407–15.
84. Lerner PI. Nocardiosis. Clin Infect Dis 1996;22: 891–903.
85. Macfarlane J, Holmes W, Gard P, et al. Prospective study of the incidence, aetiology and outcome of adult lower respiratory tract illness in the community. Thorax 2001;56:109–14.
86. Macfarlane J, Rose D. Radiographic features of staphylococcal pneumonia in adults and children. Thorax 1996;51:539–40.
87. Macfarlane JT, Miller AC, Roderick Smith WH, Morris AH, Rose DH. Comparative radiographic features of community acquired Legionnaires' disease, pneumococcal pneumonia, mycoplasma pneumonia, and psittacosis. Thorax 1984;39:28–33.
88. Maranan MC, Schiff D, Johnson DC, Abrahams C, Wylam M, Gerber SI. Pneumonic tularemia in a patient with chronic granulomatous disease. Clin Infect Dis 1997;25:630–3.
89. Marley EF, Campos JM. Haemophilus influenzae infection. In: Connor DH, Chandler FW, Manz HJ, et al, eds. Pathology of infectious diseases. Stamford, CT: Appleton & Lange; 1997:579–82.
90. Matsubara O, Tan-Liu NS, Kenney RM, Mark EJ. Inflammatory pseudotumors of the lung: progression from organizing pneumonia to fibrous histiocytoma or to plasma cell granuloma in 32 cases. Hum Pathol 1988;19:807–14.
91. Mayor B, Jolidon RM, Wicky S, Giron J, Schnyder P. Radiologic findings in two AIDS patients with Rhodococcus equi pneumonia. J Thorac Imaging 1995;10:121–5.
92. McClure J. Malakoplakia. J Pathol 1983;140: 275–330.
93. McNeil MM, Brown JM, Georghiou PR, Allworth AM, Blacklock ZM. Infections due to Nocardia transvalensis: clinical spectrum and antimicrobial therapy. Clin Infect Dis 1992;15:453–63.
94. Meier FA. Melioidosis. In: Connor DH, Chandler FW, Manz HJ, et al, eds. Pathology of infectious diseases. Stamford: Appleton & Lange; 1997:647–56.
95. Meier FA. Pseudomonas aeruginosa. In: Connor DH, Chandler FW, Manz HJ, et al, eds. Pathology of infectious diseases. Stamford: Appleton & Lange; 1997:739–57.
96. Miller RP, Bates JH. Pleuropulmonary tularemia. A review of 29 patients. Am Rev Respir Dis 1969;99:31–41.
97. Miron D, Dennehy PH, Josephson SL, Forman EN. Catheter-associated bacteremia with Nocardia nova with secondary pulmonary involvement. Pediatr Infect Dis J 1994;13:416–7.
98. Misbah SA, Mapstone NP. Whipple's disease revisited. J Clin Pathol 2000;53:750–5.
99. Monteforte JS, Wood CA. Pneumonia caused by Nocardia nova and Aspergillus fumigatus after cardiac transplantation. Eur J Clin Microbiol Infect Dis 1993;12:112–4.
100. Moon WK, Im JG, Yeon KM, Han MC. Complications of Klebsiella pneumonia: CT evaluation. J Comput Assist Tomogr 1995;19:176–81.
101. Moore EH, Webb WR, Gamsu G, Golden JA. Legionnaires' disease in the renal transplant patient: clinical presentation and radiographic progression. Radiology 1984;153:589–93.
102. Muder RR, Reddy SC, Yu VL, Kroboth FJ. Pneumonia caused by Pittsburgh pneumonia agent: radiologic manifestations. Radiology 1984; 150:633–7.

103. Mwandumba HC, Beeching NJ. Pyogenic lung infections. Curr Opin Pulm Med 1999;5:151–6.
104. Naughton M, Brown R, Adkins D, DiPersio J. Tularemia—an unusual cause of a solitary pulmonary nodule in the post-transplant setting. Bone Marrow Transplant 1999;24:197–9.
105. Niederman MS, Bass JB, Campbell GD, et al. Guidelines for the initial management of adults with community-acquired pneumonia: diagnosis, assessment of severity, and initial antimicrobial therapy. American Thoracic Society. Medical Section of the American Lung Association. Am Rev Respir Dis 1993;148:1418–26.
106. Osoagbaka OU, Njoku-Obi AN. Presumptive diagnosis of pulmonary nocardiosis: value of sputum microscopy. J Appl Bacteriol 1987;63:27–38.
107. Pascual J, Gomez Aguinaga MA, Vidal R, et al. Alveolar proteinosis and nocardiosis: a patient treated by bronchopulmonary lavage. Postgrad Med J 1989;65:674–7.
108. Paz HL, Little BJ, Ball WC Jr, Winkelstein JA. Primary pulmonary botryomycosis: a manifestation of chronic granulomatous disease. Chest 1992;101:1160–2.
109. Pearlberg J, Haggar AM, Saravolatz L, Beute GH, Popovich J. Hemophilus influenzae pneumonia in the adult. Radiographic appearance with clinical correlation. Radiology 1984;151:23–6.
110. Peltola H. Worldwide Haemophilus influenzae type b disease at the beginning of the 21st century: global analysis of the disease burden 25 years after the use of the polysaccharide vaccine and a decade after the advent of conjugates. Clin Microbiol Rev 2000;13:302–17.
111. Peralta-Venturina MN, Clubb FJ, Kielhofner MA. Pulmonary malacoplakia associated with Rhodococcus equi infection in a patient with acquired immunodeficiency syndrome. Am J Clin Pathol 1994;102:459–63.
112. Pitchenik AE, Zaunbrecher F. Superior vena cava syndrome caused by Nocardia asteroides. Am Rev Respir Dis 1978;117:795–8.
113. Pollock JJ. Pleuropulmonary Whipple's disease. South Med J 1985;78:216–7.
114. Pope TL Jr, Armstrong P, Thompson R, Donowitz GR. Pittsburgh pneumonia agent: chest film manifestations. AJR Am J Roentgenol 1982;138:237–41.
115. Quigley MJ, Fraser RS. Pulmonary pneumatocele: pathology and pathogenesis. AJR 1988;150:1275–7.
116. Raby N, Forbes G, Williams R. Nocardia infection in patients with liver transplants or chronic liver disease: radiologic findings. Radiology 1990;174:713–6.
117. Ruiz M, Ewig S, Marcos MA, et al. Etiology of community-acquired pneumonia: impact of age, comorbidity, and severity. Am J Respir Crit Care Med 1999;160:397–405.
118. Salh B, Fegan C, Hussain A, Jaulim A, Whale K, Webb A. Pulmonary infection with Nocardia caviae in a patient with diabetes mellitus and liver cirrhosis. Thorax 1988;43:933–4.
119. Schwartz DA, Geyer SJ. Klebsiella and rhinoscleroma. In: Connor DH, Chandler FW, Manz HJ, et al, eds. Pathology of infectious diseases. Stamford: Appleton & Lange; 1997:589–95.
120. Sethi S. Infectious exacerbations of chronic bronchitis: diagnosis and management. J Antimicrob Chemother 1999;43[Suppl A]:97–105.
121. Shih JY, Hsueh PR, Chang YL, et al. Tracheal botryomycosis in a patient with tracheopathia osteochondroplastica. Thorax 1998;53:73–5.
122. Slater LN, Min KW. Polypoid endobronchial lesions. A manifestation of bacillary angiomatosis. Chest 1992;102:972–4.
123. Smego RA Jr, Gallis HA. The clinical spectrum of Nocardia brasiliensis infection in the United States. Rev Infect Dis 1984;6:164–80.
124. Smith JH, Reisner BS. Plague. In: Connor DH, Chandler FW, Manz HJ, et al, eds. Pathology of infectious diseases. Stamford: Appleton & Lange; 1997:729–38.
125. Soave R, Murray HW, Litrenta MM. Bacterial invasion of pulmonary vessels. Pseudomonas bacteremia mimicking pulmonary thromboembolism with infarction. Am J Med 1978;65:864–7.
126. Speir WA Jr, Mitchener JW, Galloway RF. Primary pulmonary botryomycosis. Chest 1971;60:92–3.
127. Symmons DP, Shepherd AN, Boardman PL, Bacon PA. Pulmonary manifestations of Whipple's disease. Q J Med 1985;56:497–504.
128. Syrjala H, Sutinen S, Jokinen K, Nieminen P, Tuuponen T, Salminen A. Bronchial changes in airborne tularemia. J Laryngol Otol 1986;100:1169–76.
129. Takasugi JE, Godwin JD. Lung abscess caused by Rhodococcus equi. J Thorac Imaging 1991;6:72–4.
130. Teplitz C. Pathogenesis of Pseudomonas vasculitis and septic lesions. Arch Pathol Lab Med 1965;80:297–307.
131. Tillotson JR, Lerner AM. Characteristics of nonbacteremic Pseudomonas pneumonia. Ann Intern Med 1968;68:295–307.
132. Tomashefski JF, Thomassen MJ, Bruce MC, Goldberg HI, Konstan MW, Stern RC. Pseudomonas cepacia-associated pneumonia in cystic fibrosis. Relation of clinical features to histopathologic patterns of pneumonia. Arch Pathol Lab Med 1988;112:166–72.

133. Tsukamura M, Shimoide H, Kaneda K, Sakai R, Seino A. A case of lung infection caused by an unusual strain of Nocardia farcinica. Microbiol Immunol 1988;32:541–6.
134. Vergis EN, Indorf A, File TM, et al. Azithromycin vs cefuroxime plus erythromycin for empirical treatment of community-acquired pneumonia in hospitalized patients: a prospective, randomized, multicenter trial. Arch Intern Med 2000;160:1294–300.
135. Verville TD, Huycke MM, Greenfield RA, Fine DP, Kuhls TL, Slater LN. Rhodococcus equi infections of humans. 12 cases and a review of the literature. Medicine (Baltimore) 1994;73:119–32.
136. Vezza PR, Lack EE, Chandler FW. Legionellosis. In: Connor DH, Chandler FW, Manz HJ, et al, eds. Pathology of infectious diseases. Stamford: Appleton & Lange; 1997:597–604.
137. Webb WR, Sagel SS. Actinomycosis involving the chest wall: CT findings. AJR Am J Roentgenol 1982;139:1007–9.
138. Weisenburger DD, Helms CM, Renner ED. Sporadic Legionnaires' disease. A pathologic study of 23 fatal cases. Arch Pathol Lab Med 1981;105:130–7.
139. Wicky S, Cartei F, Mayor B, et al. Radiological findings in nine AIDS patients with Rhodococcus equi pneumonia. Eur Radiol 1996;6: 826–30.
140. Winberg CD, Rose ME, Rappaport H. Whipple's disease of the lung. Am J Med 1978;65:873-80.
141. Winer-Muram HT, Jennings SG, Wunderink RG, Jones CB, Leeper KV Jr. Ventilator-associated Pseudomonas aeruginosa pneumonia: radiographic findings. Radiology 1995;195:247–52.
142. Winn WC Jr, Chandler FW. Bacterial infections. In: Dail DH, Hammar SP, eds. Pulmonary pathology, 2nd ed. New York: Springer-Verlag; 1994:255–330.
143. Winn WC Jr, Myerowitz RL. The pathology of the Legionella pneumonias. A review of 74 cases and the literature. Hum Pathol 1981;12:401–22.
144. Yoon HK, Im JG, Ahn JM, Han MC. Pulmonary nocardiosis: CT findings. J Comput Assist Tomogr 1995;19:52–5.

Mycobacterial Pneumonias

145. Ahn CH, McLarty JW, Ahn SS, Ahn SI, Hurst GA. Diagnostic criteria for pulmonary disease caused by Mycobacterium kansasii and Mycobacterium intracellulare. Am Rev Respir Dis 1982;125:388–91.
146. American Thoracic Society. Diagnosis and treatment of disease caused by nontuberculous mycobacteria. Am J Respir Crit Care Med 1997;156:S1–25.
147. American Thoracic Society and the Centers for Disease Control and Prevention. Diagnostic standards and classification of tuberculosis in adults and children. Am J Respir Crit Care Med 2000;161:1376–95.
148. Bass JB, Farer LS, Hopewell PC, et al. Treatment of tuberculosis and tuberculosis infection in adults and children. American Thoracic Society and The Centers for Disease Control and Prevention. Am J Respir Crit Care Med 1994;149:1359–74.
149. Dutt AK, Stead WW. Tuberculosis in the elderly. Med Clin North Am 1993;77:1353–68.
150. Embil J, Warren P, Yakrus M, et al. Pulmonary illness associated with exposure to Mycobacterium-avium complex in hot tub water. Hypersensitivity pneumonitis or infection? Chest 1997;111:813–6.
151. Erasmus JJ, McAdams HP, Farrell MA, Patz EF Jr. Pulmonary nontuberculous mycobacterial infection: radiologic manifestations. Radiographics 1999;19:1487–505.
152. Fraser RS, Müller NL, Colman N, Pare PD. Mycobacteria. In: Fraser RS, Müller NL, Colman N, Pare PD, eds. Fraser and Pare's diagnosis of diseases of the chest, 4th ed. Philadelphia: WB Saunders; 1999:798–873.
153. Good RC, Snider DE Jr. Isolation of nontuberculous mycobacteria in the United States, 1980. J Infect Dis 1982;146:829–33.
154. Griffith DE. Nontuberculous mycobacteria. Curr Opin Pulm Med 1997;3:139–45.
155. Han JK, Im JG, Park JH, Han MC, Kim YW, Shim YS. Bronchial stenosis due to endobronchial tuberculosis: successful treatment with self-expanding metallic stent. AJR Am J Roentgenol 1992;159:971–2.
156. Hopewell PC, Bloom BR. Tuberculosis and other mycobacterial diseases. In: Murray JF, Nadel JA, Mason RJ, Boushey HA Jr, eds. Textbook of respiratory medicine, 3rd ed. Philadelphia: WB Saunders; 2000:1043–105.
157. Hruban RH, Hutchins GM. Mycobacterial infections. In: Dail DH, Hammar SP, eds. Pulmonary pathology, 2nd ed. New York: Springer-Verlag; 1994:331–50.
158. Im JG, Itoh H, Shim YS, et al. Pulmonary tuberculosis: CT findings–early active disease and sequential change with antituberculous therapy. Radiology 1993;186:653–60.
159. Kahana LM, Kay JM, Yakrus MA, Waserman S. Mycobacterium avium complex infection in an immunocompetent young adult related to hot tub exposure. Chest 1997;111:242–5.
160. Koch R. Die Aetiologie der Tuberculose. Berlin Klin Wochenschr 1882;19:221–30.

161. Krysl J, Korzeniewska-Kosela M, Müller NL, FitzGerald JM. Radiologic features of pulmonary tuberculosis: an assessment of 188 cases. Can Assoc Radiol J 1994;45:101–7.
162. Kurasawa T, Kuze F, Kawai M, et al. Diagnosis and management of endobronchial tuberculosis. Intern Med 1992;31:593–8.
163. Lack EE, Connor DH. Tuberculosis. In: Connor DH, Chandler FW, Manz HJ, et al, eds. Pathology of infectious diseases. Stamford: Appleton & Lange; 1997:857–68.
164. Leung AN. Pulmonary tuberculosis: the essentials. Radiology 1999;210:307–22.
165. Leung AN, Müller NL, Pineda PR, FitzGerald JM. Primary tuberculosis in childhood: radiographic manifestations. Radiology 1992;182:87–91.
166. Mehle ME, Adamo JP, Mehta AC, Wiedemann HP, Keys T, Longworth DL. Endobronchial mycobacterium avium-intracellulare infection in a patient with AIDS. Chest 1989;96:199–201.
167. Miller WT Jr. Spectrum of pulmonary nontuberculous mycobacterial infection. Radiology 1994;191:343–50.
168. Morris CD. Pulmonary tuberculosis in the elderly: a different disease? Thorax 1990;45:912–3.
169. Primack SL, Logan PM, Hartman TE, Lee KS, Müller NL. Pulmonary tuberculosis and mycobacterium avium-intracellulare: a comparison of CT findings. Radiology 1995;194:413–7.
170. Runyon EH. Anonymous bacteria in pulmonary disease. Med Clin North Am 1959;43:273–90.
171. Timpe A, Runyon EH. The relationship of "atypical" acid-fast bacteria to human disease. J Lab Clin Med 1954;44:202–9.
172. Woodring JH, Vandiviere HM, Fried AM, Dillon ML, Williams TD, Melvin IG. Update: the radiographic features of pulmonary tuberculosis. AJR Am J Roentgenol 1986;146:497–506.
173. Zakowski P, Fligiel S, Berlin GW, Johnson L Jr. Disseminated mycobacterium avium-intracellulare infection in homosexual men dying of acquired immunodeficiency. JAMA 1982;248: 2980–2.

Fungal Infections

174. Ahn MI, Park SH, Kim JA, Kwon MS, Park YH. Pseudomembranous necrotizing bronchial aspergillosis. Br J Radiol 2000;73:73–5.
175. American Lung Association. Laboratory diagnosis of mycotic and specific fungal infections. Am Rev Respir Dis 1985;132:1373–9.
176. Ampel NM. Coccidioidomycosis. In: Sarosi GA, Davies SF, eds. Fungal disease of the lung, 3rd ed. Philadelphia: Lippincott Williams & Wilkins; 2000:59–78.
177. Aquino SL, Kee ST, Warnock ML, Gamsu G. Pulmonary aspergillosis: imaging findings with pathologic correlation. AJR Am J Roentgenol 1994;163:811–5.
178. Arney KL, Tiernan R, Judson MA. Primary pulmonary involvement of Fusarium solani in a lung transplant recipient. Chest 1997;112: 1128–30.
179. Backman KS, Roberts M, Patterson R. Allergic bronchopulmonary mycosis caused by Fusarium vasinfectum. Am J Respir Crit Care Med 1995;152:1379–81.
180. Batra P. Pulmonary coccidioidomycosis. J Thorac Imaging 1992;7:29–38.
181. Baur X, Richter G, Pethran A, Czuppon AB, Schwaiblmair M. Increased prevalence of IgG-induced sensitization and hypersensitivity pneumonitis (humidifier lung) in nonsmokers exposed to aerosols of a contaminated air conditioner. Respiration 1992;59:211–4.
182. Beller TA, Mitchell DM, Sobonya RE, Barbee RA. Large airway obstruction secondary to endobronchial coccidioidomycosis. Am Rev Respir Dis 1979;120:939–42.
183. Bethlem EP, Capone D, Maranhao B, Carvalho CR, Wanke B. Paracoccidioidomycosis. Curr Opin Pulm Med 1999;5:319–25.
184. Binder RE, Faling LJ, Pugatch RD, Mahasaen C, Snider GL. Chronic necrotizing pulmonary aspergillosis: a discrete clinical entity. Medicine (Baltimore) 1982;61:109–24.
185. Blyth W, Grant IW, Blackadder ES, Greenberg M. Fungal antigens as a source of sensitization and respiratory disease in Scottish maltworkers. Clin Allergy 1977;7:549–62.
186. Boots RJ, Paterson DL, Allworth AM, Faoagali JL. Successful treatment of post-influenza pseudomembranous necrotizing bronchial aspergillosis with liposomal amphotericin, inhaled amphotericin B, gamma interferon and GM-CSF. Thorax 1999;54:1047–9.
187. Boutati EI, Anaissie EJ. Fusarium, a significant emerging pathogen in patients with hematologic malignancy: ten years' experience at a cancer center and implications for management. Blood 1997;90:999–1008.
188. Cantanzaro A. Coccidioidomycosis. In: Sarosi GA, Davies SF, eds. Fungal diseases of the lung, 2nd ed. New York: Raven Press; 1993:65–83.
189. Cartun RW. Use of immunohistochemistry in the surgical pathology laboratory for the diagnosis of infectious diseases. Pathology Case Reviews 1999;4:260–5.
190. Chandler FW. Blastomycosis. In: Connor DH, Chandler FW, Manz HJ, et al, eds. Pathology of infectious disease. Stamford: Appleton & Lange; 1997:943–51.

191. Chandler FW, Ajello L. Torulopsis. In: Connor DH, Chandler FW, Manz HJ, et al, eds. Pathology of infectious diseases. Stamford: Appleton & Lange; 1997:1105–8.
192. Chandler FW, Watts JC. Cryptococcus. In: Connor DH, Chandler FW, Manz HJ, et al, eds. Pathology of infectious disease. Stamford: Appleton & Lange; 1997:989–97.
193. Chandler FW, Watts JC. Fungal Infections. In: Dail DH, Hammar SP, eds. Pulmonary pathology, 2nd ed. New York: Springer-Verlag; 1994:351–427.
194. Chandler FW, Watts JC. Histoplasmosis capsulati. In: Conner DH, Chandler FW, Manz HJ, et al, eds. Pathology of infectious diseases. Stamford, Connecticut: Appleton & Lange; 1997:1007–15.
195. Chandler FW, Watts JC. Pathologic diagnosis of fungal infections. Chicago: American Society of Clinical Pathologists; 1987.
196. Chandler FW, Watts JC. Sporotrichosis. In: Connor DH, Chandler FW, Manz HJ, et al, eds. Pathology of infectious disease. Stamford: Appleton & Lange; 1997:1089–96.
197. Chandler FW, Watts JC. Zygomycosis. In: Connor DH, Chandler FW, Manz HJ, et al, eds. Pathology of infectious diseases. Stamford: Appleton & Lange; 1997:1113–9.
198. Chu FE, Armstrong D. Candia species pneumonia. In: Sarosi GA, Davies SF, eds. Fungal diseases of the lung, 2nd ed. New York: Raven Press; 1993:125–31.
199. Clarke A, Skelton J, Fraser RS. Fungal tracheobronchitis. Report of 9 cases and review of the literature. Medicine (Baltimore) 1991;70:1–14.
200. Conces DJ Jr. Histoplasmosis. Semin Roentgenol 1996;31:14–27.
201. Conces DJ Jr, Tarver RD, Vix VA. Broncholithiasis: CT features in 15 patients. AJR Am J Roentgenol 1991;157:249–53.
202. Connolly JE Jr, McAdams HP, Erasmus JJ, Rosado de Christenson ML. Opportunistic fungal pneumonia. J Thorac Imaging 1999;14:51–62.
203. Corti ME, Cendoya CA, Soto I, et al. Disseminated histoplasmosis and AIDS: clinical aspects and diagnostic methods for early detection. AIDS Patient Care STDS 2000;14:149–54.
204. Cunningham RT, Einstein H. Coccidioidal pulmonary cavities with rupture. J Thorac Cardiovasc Surg 1982;84:172–7.
205. Davies SF, Sarosi GA. Blastomycosis. In: Sarosi GA, Davies SF, eds. Fungal diseases of the lung, 3rd ed. Philadelphia: Lippincott Williams & Wilkins; 2000:47–59.
206. Davies SF, Sarosi GA. Fungal infections. In: Murray JF, Nadel JA, eds. Textbook of respiratory medicine, 2nd ed. Philadelphia: WB Saunders; 1994:1161–200.
207. Davies SF, Sarosi GA. Fungal infections. In: Murray JF, Nadel JA, Mason RJ, Boushey HA Jr, eds. Textbook of respiratory medicine, 3rd ed. Philadelphia: WB Saunders, 2000:1107–41.
208. De Repentigny L, Kaufman L, Cole GT, Kruse D, Latge JP, Matthews RC. Immunodiagnosis of invasive fungal infections. J Med Vet Mycol 1994;32[Suppl 1]:239–52.
209. Deepe GS. Immune response to early and late Histoplasma capsulatum infections. Curr Opin Microbiol 2000;3:359–62.
210. Dolan MJ, Lattuada CP, Melcher GP, Zellmer R, Allendoerfer R, Rinaldi MG. Coccidioides immitis presenting as a mycelial pathogen with empyema and hydropneumothorax. J Med Vet Mycol 1992;30:249–55.
211. Ehrensing ER, Saag MS. Cryptococcosis. In: Sarosi GA, Davies SF, eds. Fungal diseases of the lung, 3rd ed. Philadelphia: Lippincott Williams & Wilkins; 2000:91–104.
212. England DM, Hochholzer L. Adiaspiromycosis: an unusual fungal infection of the lung. Report of 11 cases. Am J Surg Pathol 1993;17:876–86.
213. England DM, Hochholzer L. Sporothrix infection of the lung without cutaneous disease. Primary pulmonary sporotrichosis. Arch Pathol Lab Med 1987;111:298–300.
214. Franquet T, Müller NL, Gimenez A, Domingo P, Plaza V, Bordes R. Semiinvasive pulmonary aspergillosis in chronic obstructive pulmonary disease: radiologic and pathologic findings in nine patients. AJR Am J Roentgenol 2000;174:51–6.
215. Fraser RS, Müller NL, Colman N, Pare PD. Fungi and actinomyces. In: Fraser RS, Müller NL, Colman N, Pare PD, eds. Fraser and Pare's diagnosis of diseases of the chest, 4th ed. Philadelphia: WB Saunders; 1999:875–978.
216. Funari M, Kavakama J, Shikanai-Yasuda MA, et al. Chronic pulmonary paracoccidioidomycosis (South American blastomycosis): high-resolution CT findings in 41 patients. AJR Am J Roentgenol 1999;173:59–64.
217. Gefter WB. The spectrum of pulmonary aspergillosis. J Thorac Imaging 1992;7:56–74.
218. George RB, Penn RL. Histoplasmosis. In: Sarosi GA, Davies SF, eds. Fungal diseases of the lung, 2nd ed. New York: Raven Press; 1993:39–50.
219. Gerding DN. Sporotrichosis. In: Sarosi GA, Davies SF, eds. Fungal disease of the lung, 2nd ed. New York: Raven Press; 1993:113–23.
220. Gerding DN. Sporotrichosis. In: Sarosi GA, Davies SF, eds. Fungal diseases of the lung, 3rd ed. Philadelphia: Lippincott Williams & Wilkins; 2000:105–14.

221. Glassroth J. Fungal infections complicating HIV infection. In: Sarosi GA, Davies SF, eds. Fungal diseases of the lung, 3rd ed. Philadelphia: Lippincott Williams & Wilkins, 2000:213–8.
222. Goldman M, Johnson PC, Sarosi GA. Fungal pneumonias. The endemic mycoses. Clin Chest Med 1999;20:507–19.
223. Goyal R, White CS, Templeton PA, Britt EJ, Rubin LJ. High attenuation mucous plugs in allergic bronchopulmonary aspergillosis: CT appearance. J Comput Assist Tomogr 1992;16: 649–50.
224. Gurney JW, Conces DJ. Pulmonary histoplasmosis. Radiology 1996;199:297–306.
225. Haron E, Vartivarian S, Anaissie E, Dekmezian R, Bodey GP. Primary Candida pneumonia. Experience at a large cancer center and review of the literature. Medicine (Baltimore) 1993;72:137-42.
226. Harrison TS. Cryptococcus neoformans and cryptococcosis. J Infect 2000;41:12–7.
227. Hutton JP, Durham JB, Miller DP, Everett ED. Hyphal forms of Histoplasma capsulatum. A common manifestation of intravascular infections. Arch Pathol Lab Med 1985;109:330–2.
228. Irwin RG, Rinaldi MG, Walsh TJ. Zygomycosis of the respiratory tract. In: Sarosi GA, Davies SF, eds. Fungal diseases of the lung, 3rd ed. Philadelphia: Lippincott Williams & Wilkins; 2000:163–86.
229. Jamadar DA, Kazerooni EA, Daly BD, White CS, Gross BH. Pulmonary zygomycosis: CT appearance. J Comput Assist Tomogr 1995;19:733–8.
230. Johnson PC, Davies SF, Sarosi GA. Fungal diseases of the lung. In: Niederman MS, Sarosi GA, Glassroth J, eds. Respiratory infections. A scientific basis for management. Philadelphia: WB Saunders; 1994:387–415.
231. Kaplan W, Kraft DE. Demonstration of pathogenic fungi in formalin-fixed tissues by immunofluorescence. Am J Clin Pathol 1969;52:420–32.
232. Kaufman L. Immunohistologic diagnosis of systemic mycoses: an update. Eur J Epidemiol 1992;8:377–82.
233. Kaufman L. Laboratory methods for the diagnosis and confirmation of systemic mycoses. Clin Infect Dis 1992;14[Suppl 1]:S23–9
234. Kaufman L, Standard PG, Jalbert M, Kraft DE. Immunohistologic identification of Aspergillus spp. and other hyaline fungi by using polyclonal fluorescent antibodies. J Clin Microbiol 1997;35:2206–9.
235. Kemper CA, Hostetler JS, Follansbee SE, et al. Ulcerative and plaque-like tracheobronchitis due to infection with Aspergillus in patients with AIDS. Clin Infect Dis 1993;17:344–52.
236. Kim SY, Lee KS, Han J, et al. Semiinvasive pulmonary aspergillosis: CT and pathologic findings in six patients. AJR Am J Roentgenol 2000;174:795–8.
237. Kontoyiannis DP, Wessel VC, Bodey GP, Rolston KV. Zygomycosis in the 1990s in a tertiary-care cancer center. Clin Infect Dis 2000;30:851–6.
238. Kramer MR, Denning DW, Marshall SE, et al. Ulcerative tracheobronchitis after lung transplantation. A new form of invasive aspergillosis. Am Rev Respir Dis 1991;144:552–6.
239. Kuzo RS, Goodman LR. Blastomycosis. Semin Roentgenol 1996;31:45–51.
240. Kwon-Chung KJ, Hill WB, Bennett JE. New, special stain for histopathological diagnosis of cryptococcosis. J Clin Microbiol 1981;13:383–7.
241. Lagerstrom CF, Mitchell HG, Graham BS, Hammon JW Jr. Chronic fibrosing mediastinitis and superior vena caval obstruction from blastomycosis. Ann Thorac Surg 1992;54:764–5.
242. Larsen RA, Jacobson JA, Morris AH, Benowitz BA. Acute respiratory failure caused by primary pulmonary coccidioidomycosis. Two case reports and a review of the literature. Am Rev Respir Dis 1985;131:797–9.
243. Lemos LB, Baliga M, Guo M. Acute respiratory distress syndrome and blastomycosis: presentation of nine cases and review of the literature. Ann Diagn Pathol 2001;5:1–9.
244. Liu K, Howell DN, Perfect JR, Schell WA. Morphologic criteria for the preliminary identification of Fusarium, Paecilomyces, and Acremonium species by histopathology. Am J Clin Pathol 1998;109:45–54.
245. Lombard CM, Tazelaar HD, Krasne DL. Pulmonary eosinophilia in coccidioidal infections. Chest 1987;91:734–6.
246. Londero AT, Chandler FW. Paracoccidioidomycosis. In: Connor DH, Chandler FW, Manz HJ, et al, eds. Pathology of infectious disease. Stamford: Appleton & Lange; 1997:1045–53.
247. Luna MA. Candidiasis. In: Connor DH, Chandler FW, Schwartz DA, et al, eds. Pathology of infectious diseases. Stamford: Appleton & Lange; 1997:953–64.
248. Machida U, Kami M, Kanda Y, et al. Aspergillus tracheobronchitis after allogeneic bone marrow transplantation. Bone Marrow Transplant 1999;24:1145–9.
249. Masur H, Rosen PP, Armstrong D. Pulmonary disease caused by Candida species. Am J Med 1977;63:914–25.
250. McAdams HP, Rosado-de-Christenson ML, Lesar M, Templeton PA, Moran CA. Thoracic mycoses from endemic fungi: radiologic-pathologic correlation. Radiographics 1995;15:255–70.

251. McAdams HP, Rosado-de-Christenson ML, Templeton PA, Lesar M, Moran CA. Thoracic mycoses from opportunistic fungi: radiologic-pathologic correlation. Radiographics 1995;15:271–86.
252. Meyer KC, McManus EJ, Maki DG. Overwhelming pulmonary blastomycosis associated with the adult respiratory distress syndrome. N Engl J Med 1993;329:1231–6.
253. Miller MA, Greenberger PA, Amerian R, et al. Allergic bronchopulmonary mycosis caused by Pseudoallescheria boydii. Am Rev Respir Dis 1993;148:810–2.
254. Mukkamala R, Mehta JB, Myers JW, Cole CP. Pulmonary blastomycosis with acute respiratory failure as predominant clinical feature. South Med J 1997;90:847–50.
255. Pappagianis D, Chandler FW. Coccidioidomycosis. In: Connor DH, Chandler FW, Manz HJ, et al, eds. Pathology of infectious disease. Stamford: Appleton & Lange; 1997:977–87.
256. Pappas PG. Blastomycosis in the immunocompromised patient. Semin Respir Infect 1997;12:243–51.
257. Pappas PG, Pottage JC, Powderly WG, et al. Blastomycosis in patients with the acquired immunodeficiency syndrome. Ann Intern Med 1992;116:847–53.
258. Pappas PG, Tellez I, Deep AE, Nolasco D, Holgado W, Bustamante B. Sporotrichosis in Peru: description of an area of hyperendemicity. Clin Infect Dis 2000;30:65–70.
259. Pappas PG, Threlkeld MG, Bedsole GD, Cleveland KO, Gelfand MS, Dismukes WE. Blastomycosis in immunocompromised patients. Medicine (Baltimore) 1993;72:311–25.
260. Patel RG, Patel B, Petrini MF, Carter RR, III, Griffith J. Clinical presentation, radiographic findings, and diagnostic methods of pulmonary blastomycosis: a review of 100 consecutive cases. South Med J 1999;92:289–95.
261. Paterson DL, Boots RJ. Aspergillus. In: Sarosi GA, Davies SF, eds. Fungal diseases of the lung, 3rd ed. Philadelphia: Lippincott Williams & Wilkins; 2000:123–62.
262. Patz EF Jr, Goodman PC. Pulmonary cryptococcosis. J Thorac Imaging 1992;7:51–5.
263. Perry LP, Iwata M, Tazelaar HD, Colby TV, Yousem SA. Pulmonary mycotoxicosis: a clinicopathologic study of three cases. Mod Pathol 1998;11:432–6.
264. Phillips P, Weiner MH. Invasive aspergillosis diagnosed by immunohistochemistry with monoclonal and polyclonal reagents. Hum Pathol 1987;18:1015–24.
265. Pluss JL, Opal SM. Pulmonary sporotrichosis: review of treatment and outcome. Medicine (Baltimore) 1986;65:143–53.
266. Powderly WG. Current approach to the acute management of cryptococcal infections. J Infect 2000;41:18–22.
267. Primack SL, Hartman TE, Lee KS, Müller NL. Pulmonary nodules and the CT halo sign. Radiology 1994;190:513–5.
268. Putnam JS, Harper WK, Greene JF Jr, Nelson KG, Zurek RC. Coccidioides immitis. A rare cause of pulmonary mycetoma. Am Rev Respir Dis 1975;112:733–8.
269. Redline RW, Redline SS, Boxerbaum B, Dahms BB. Systemic Malassezia furfur infections in patients receiving intralipid therapy. Hum Pathol 1985;16:815–22.
270. Regnard JF, Icard P, Nicolosi M, et al. Aspergilloma: a series of 89 surgical cases. Ann Thorac Surg 2000;69:898–903.
271. Ribes JA, Vanover-Sams CL, Baker DJ. Zygomycetes in human disease. Clin Microbiol Rev 2000;13:236–301.
272. Richet HM, McNeil MM, Edwards MC, Jarvis WR. Cluster of Malassezia furfur pulmonary infections in infants in a neonatal intensive-care unit. J Clin Microbiol 1989;27:1197–200.
273. Ro JY, Lee SS, Ayala AG. Advantage of Fontana-Masson stain in capsule-deficient cryptococcal infection. Arch Pathol Lab Med 1987;111:53–7.
274. Rohatgi PK, Schmitt RG. Pulmonary coccidioidal mycetoma. Am J Med Sci 1984;287:27–30.
275. Saini SK, Boas SR, Jerath A, Roberts M, Greenberger PA. Allergic bronchopulmonary mycosis to Fusarium vasinfectum in a child. Ann Allergy Asthma Immunol 1998;80:377–80.
276. Saito T, Imaizumi M, Kudo K, et al. Disseminated Fusarium infection identified by the immunohistochemical staining in a patient with a refractory leukemia. Tohoku J Exp Med 1999;187:71–7.
277. Sarosi GA, Davies SF. Blastomycosis. Am Rev Respir Dis 1979;120:911–38.
278. Sawada M, Isogai S, Miyake S, Kubota T, Yoshizawa Y. Pulmonary pseudoallescherioma associated with systemic lupus erythematosus. Intern Med 1998;37:1046–9.
279. Schwarz J. Pathology of histoplasmosis. Pathol Annu 1968;3:335–66.
280. Schwarz J, Salfelder K. Blastomycosis. A review of 152 cases. Curr Top Pathol 1977;65:165–200.
281. Shek YH, Tucker MC, Viciana AL, Manz HJ, Connor DH. Malassezia furfur–disseminated infection in premature infants. Am J Clin Pathol 1989;92:595–603.

282. Storms WW. Occupational hypersensitivity lung disease. J Occup Med 1978;20:823–4.
283. Stöppler MC. Malasseziasis. In: Connor DH, Chandler FW, Manz HJ, et al, eds. Pathology of infectious diseases. Stamford: Appleton & Lange; 1997:1029–33.
284. Taborda AB, Arechavala AI. Paracoccidioidomycosis. In: Sarosi GA, Davies SF, eds. Fungal diseases of the lung, 2nd ed. New York: Raven Press; 1993:85–94.
285. Taborda AB, Arechavala AI. Paracoccidioidomycosis. In: Sarosi GA, Davies SF, eds. Fungal diseases of the lung, 3rd ed. Philadelphia: Lippincott Williams & Wilkins; 2000:79–90.
286. Tasci S, Schafer H, Ewig S, Luderitz B, Zhou H. Pseudomembraneous Aspergillus fumigatus tracheobronchitis causing life-threatening tracheobronchial obstruction in a mechanically ventilated patient [Letter]. Intensive Care Med 2000;26:143–4.
287. Thadepalli H, Salem FA, Mandal AK, Rambhatla K, Einstein HE. Pulmonary mycetoma due to Coccidioides immitis. Chest 1977;71:429–30.
288. Travis LB, Roberts GD, Wilson WR. Clinical significance of Pseudoallescheria boydii: a review of 10 years' experience. Mayo Clin Proc 1985;60:531–7.
289. Tron V, Churg A. Chronic necrotizing pulmonary aspergillosis mimicking bronchocentric granulomatosis. Pathol Res Pract 1986;181: 621–6.
290. Turner D, Burke M, Bashe E, Blinder S, Yust I. Pulmonary adiaspiromycosis in a patient with acquired immunodeficiency syndrome. Eur J Clin Microbiol Infect Dis 1999;18:893–5.
291. Walsh M, White L, Atkinson K, Enno A. Fungal Pseudoallescheria boydii lung infiltrates unresponsive to amphotericin B in leukaemic patients. Aust N Z J Med 1992;22:265–8.
292. Watts JC, Chandler FW. Adiaspiromycosis. In: Connor DH, Chandler FW, Manz HJ, et al, eds. Pathology of infectious diseases. Stamford: Appleton & Lange; 1997:929–32.
293. Watts JC, Chandler FW. Aspergillosis. In: Connor DH, Chandler FW, Manz HJ, et al, eds. Pathology of infectious diseases. Stamford: Appleton & Lange; 1997:933–41.
294. Watts JC, Chandler FW. Fusariosis. In: Conner DH, Chandler FW, Schwartz DA, et al, eds. Pathology of infectious diseases. Stamford: Appleton & Lange; 1997:999–1001.
295. Wheat LJ. Histoplasmosis. In: Sarosi GA, Davies SF, eds. Fungal diseases of the lung, 3rd ed. Philadelphia: Lippincott Williams & Wilkins; 2000:31–46.
296. Winer-Muram HT, Rubin SA. Pulmonary blastomycosis. J Thorac Imaging 1992;7:23–8.
297. Winn RE, Johnson R, Galgiani JN, Butler C, Pluss J. Cavitary coccidioidomycosis with fungus ball formation. Diagnosis by fiberoptic bronchoscopy with coexistence of hyphae and spherules. Chest 1994;105:412–6.
298. Won HJ, Lee KS, Cheon JE, et al. Invasive pulmonary aspergillosis: prediction at thin-section CT in patients with neutropenia—a prospective study. Radiology 1998;208:777–82.
299. Woodring JH, Ciporkin G, Lee C, Worm B, Woolley S. Pulmonary cryptococcosis. Semin Roentgenol 1996;31:67–75.
300. Yoshida K, Ueda A, Yamasaki H, Sato K, Uchida K, Ando M. Hypersensitivity pneumonitis resulting from Aspergillus fumigatus in a greenhouse. Arch Environ Health 1993;48:260–2.
301. Yousem SA. The histological spectrum of chronic necrotizing forms of pulmonary aspergillosis. Hum Pathol 1997;28:650–6.

Viral Infections

302. Abbondanzo SL, English CK, Kagan E, McPherson RA. Fatal adenovirus pneumonia in a newborn identified by electron microscopy and in situ hybridization. Arch Pathol Lab Med 1989;113:1349–53.
303. Abreo F, Bagby J. Sputum cytology in measles infection. A case report. Acta Cytol 1991;35:719–21.
304. Adams JM. Primary virus infection with cytoplasmic inclusion bodies. Study of an epidemic involving thirty-two infants, with nine deaths. JAMA 1947;116:1037–9.
305. Akhtar N, Ni J, Langston C, Demmler GJ, Towbin JA. PCR diagnosis of viral pneumonitis from fixed-lung tissue in children. Biochem Mol Med 1996;58:66–76.
306. Akizuki S, Nasu N, Setoguchi M, Yoshida S, Higuchi Y, Yamamoto S. Parainfluenza virus pneumonitis in an adult. Arch Pathol Lab Med 1991;115:824–6.
307. Anas N, Boettrich C, Hall CB, Brooks JG. The association of apnea and respiratory syncytial virus infection in infants. J Pediatr 1982;101:65–8.
308. Andersen CB. Detection of cytomegalovirus-infected cells in autopsy material by in situ hybridization. APMIS 1990;98:363–8.
309. Andersen RD. Herpes simplex virus infection of the neonatal respiratory tract. Am J Dis Child 1987;141:274–6.
310. Aquino SL, Dunagan DP, Chiles C, Haponik EF. Herpes simplex virus 1 pneumonia: patterns on CT scans and conventional chest radiographs. J Comput Assist Tomogr 1998;22:795–800.

311. Archibald RW, Weller RO, Meadow SR. Measles pneumonia and the nature of the inclusion-bearing giant cells: a light- and electron-microscope study. J Pathol 1971;103:27–34.
312. Becroft DM. Bronchiolitis obliterans, bronchiectasis, and other sequelae of adenovirus type 21 infection in young children. J Clin Pathol 1971;24:72–82.
313. Brunton FJ, Moore ME. A survey of pulmonary calcification following adult chicken-pox. Br J Radiol 1969;42:256–9.
314. Buffone GJ, Frost A, Samo T, Demmler GJ, Cagle PT, Lawrence EC. The diagnosis of CMV pneumonitis in lung and heart/lung transplant patients by PCR compared with traditional laboratory criteria. Transplantation 1993;56:342–7.
315. Cenacchi G, Musiani M, Gentilomi G, et al. In situ hybridization at the ultrastructural level: localization of cytomegalovirus DNA using digoxigenin labelled probes. J Submicrosc Cytol Pathol 1993;25:341–5.
316. Colby TV, Zaki SR, Feddersen RM, Nolte KB. Hantavirus pulmonary syndrome is distinguishable from acute interstitial pneumonia. Arch Pathol Lab Med 2000;124:1463–6.
317. Conti JA, Karetzky MS. Varicella pneumonia in the adult. N J Med 1989;86:475–8.
318. Craighead JE. Cytomegalovirus pulmonary disease. Pathobiol Annu 1975;5:197–220.
319. Craighead JE. Cytopathology of adenoviruses types 7 and 12 in human respiratory epithelium. Lab Invest 1970;22:553–7.
320. Craighead JE. Pulmonary cytomegalovirus infection in the adult. Am J Pathol 1971;63:487–504.
321. D'Angelo LJ, Hierholzer JC, Keenlyside RA, Anderson LJ, Martone WJ. Pharyngoconjunctival fever caused by adenovirus type 4: report of a swimming pool-related outbreak with recovery of virus from pool water. J Infect Dis 1979;140:42–7.
322. Dascomb HE, Hilleman MR. Clinical and laboratory studies in patients with respiratory disease caused by adenoviruses. Am J Med 1956; 21:161–74.
323. Davidson RN, Lynn W, Savage P, Wansbrough-Jones MH. Chickenpox pneumonia: experience with antiviral treatment. Thorax 1988;43:627–30.
324. Davison AG, Haslam PL, Corrin B, et al. Interstitial lung disease and asthma in hard-metal workers: bronchoalveolar lavage, ultrastructural, and analytical findings and results of bronchial provocation tests. Thorax 1983;38:119–28.
325. Delage G, Brochu P, Pelletier M, Jasmin G, Lapointe N. Giant-cell pneumonia caused by parainfluenza virus. J Pediatr 1979;94:426–9.
326. Delage G, Brochu P, Robillard L, Jasmin G, Joncas JH, Lapointe N. Giant cell pneumonia due to respiratory syncytial virus. Occurrence in severe combined immunodeficiency syndrome. Arch Pathol Lab Med 1984;108:623–5.
327. Demos TC. Mediastinal lymphadenopathy in mycoplasmal pneumonia. AJR Am J Roentgenol 1994;162:1499–500.
328. Dolin R, Reichman RC, Mazur MH, Whitley RJ. NIH conference. Herpes zoster-varicella infections in immunosuppressed patients. Ann Intern Med 1978;89:375–88.
329. Dudding BA, Top FH Jr, Winter PE, Buescher EL, Lamson TH, Leibovitz A. Acute respiratory disease in military trainees: the adenovirus surveillance program, 1966-1971. Am J Epidemiol 1973;97:187–98.
330. Dudding BA, Wagner SC, Zeller JA, Gmelich JT, French GR, Top FH Jr. Fatal pneumonia associated with adenovirus type 7 in three military trainees. N Engl J Med 1972;286:1289–92.
331. Enders JF, McCarthy K, Mitus A, Cheatham WJ. Isolation of measles virus at autopsy in cases of giant cell pneumonia without rash. N Eng J Med 1959;261:875.
332. Esmonde TF, Herdman G, Anderson G. Chickenpox pneumonia: an association with pregnancy. Thorax 1989;44:812–5.
333. Feldman S. Varicella zoster infections of the fetus, neonate, and immunocompromised child. Adv Pediatr Infect Dis 1986;1:99–115.
334. Feldman S. Varicella-zoster virus pneumonitis. Chest 1994;106:22S–7S.
335. Feldman S, Stokes DC. Varicella zoster and herpes simplex virus pneumonias. Semin Respir Infect 1987;2:84–94.
336. Finckh ES, Bader L. Pulmonary damage from Hong Kong influenza. Aust N Z J Med 1974;4: 16–22.
337. Fraser RS, Müller NL, Colman N, Pare PD. Viruses, mycoplasmas, chlamydiae, and rickettsiae. In: Fraser RS, Müller NL, Colman N, Pare PD, eds. Fraser and Pare's diagnosis of diseases of the chest, 4th ed. Philadelphia: WB Saunders; 1999:979–1032.
338. Frey HM, Krugman S. Atypical measles syndrome: unusual hepatic, pulmonary, and immunologic aspects. Am J Med Sci 1981;281:51–5.
339. Gendelman HE, Moench TR, Narayan O, Griffin DE, Clements JE. A double labeling technique for performing immunocytochemistry and in situ hybridization in virus infected cell cultures and tissues. J Virol Methods 1985;11:93–103.

340. Gleaves CA, Myerson D, Bowden RA, Hackman RC, Meyers JD. Direct detection of cytomegalovirus from bronchoalveolar lavage samples by using a rapid in situ DNA hybridization assay. J Clin Microbiol 1989;27:2429–32.
341. Gleaves CA, Smith TF, Wold AD, Wilson WR. Detection of viral and chlamydial antigens in open-lung biopsy specimens. Am J Clin Pathol 1985;83:371–4.
342. Glezen WP, Fernald GW, Lohr JA. Acute respiratory disease of university students with special reference to the etiologic role of Herpesvirus hominis. Am J Epidemiol 1975;101:111–21.
343. Glick N, Levin S, Nelson K. Recurrent pulmonary infarction in adult chickenpox pneumonia. JAMA 1972;222:173–7.
344. Gorelkin L, Chandler FW, Ewing EP Jr. Staining qualities of cytomegalovirus inclusions in the lungs of patients with the acquired immunodeficiency syndrome: a potential source of diagnostic misinterpretation. Hum Pathol 1986;17:926–9.
345. Graham BS, Snell JD Jr. Herpes simplex virus infection of the adult lower respiratory tract. Medicine (Baltimore) 1983;62:384–93.
346. Green WR, Williams AW. Neonatal adenovirus pneumonia. Arch Pathol Lab Med 1989; 113:190–1.
347. Greenberg SB. Viral pneumonia. Infect Dis Clin North Am 1991;5:603–21.
348. Gulati M, Kaur R, Jha V, Venkataramu NK, Gupta D, Suri S. High-resolution CT in renal transplant patients with suspected pulmonary infections. Acta Radiol 2000;41:237–41.
349. Hall WJ, Hall CB. Atypical measles in adolescents: evaluation of clinical and pulmonary function. Ann Intern Med 1979;90:882–6.
350. Han BK, Son JA, Yoon HK, Lee SI. Epidemic adenoviral lower respiratory tract infection in pediatric patients: radiographic and clinical characteristics. AJR Am J Roentgenol 1998; 170:1077–80.
351. Harboldt SL, Dugan JM, Tronic BS. Cytologic diagnosis of measles pneumonia in a bronchoalveolar lavage specimen. A case report. Acta Cytol 1994;38:403–6.
352. Hayden FG, Gwaltney JM. Viral infections. In: Murray JF, Nadel JA, eds. Textbook of respiratory medicine, 2nd ed. Philadelphia: WB Saunders; 1994:977–1035.
353. Henry RL, Milner AD, Stokes GM, Hodges IG, Groggins RC. Lung function after acute bronchiolitis. Arch Dis Child 1983;58:60–3.
354. Hers JF, Masurel N, Mulder J. Bacteriology and histopathology of the respiratory tract and lungs in fatal Asian influenza. Lancet 1958;2:1141–3.
355. Hers JF, Mulder J. Changes in the respiratory mucosa resulting from infection with influenza virus B. B J Pathol Bacteriol 1957;73:565–8.
356. Hruban Z, Kuzo R, Heimann P, Weisenberg E, Hruban RH. Globular changes in cytomegaloviral inclusions after Ganciclovir treatment. Arch Virol 1989;108:287–93.
357. Hubbell C, Dominguez R, Kohl S. Neonatal herpes simplex pneumonitis. Rev Infect Dis 1988;10:431–8.
358. Jiwa NM, Raap AK, van de Rijke FM, et al. Detection of cytomegalovirus antigens and DNA in tissues fixed in formaldehyde. J Clin Pathol 1989;42:749–54.
359. Joliat G, Abetel G, Schindler AM, Kapanci Y. Measles giant cell pneumonia without rash in a case of lymphocytic lymphosarcoma. An electron microscopic study. Virchows Arch [A] 1973;358:215–24.
360. Joshi VV, Escobar MR, Stewart L, Bates RD. Fatal influenza A2 viral pneumonia in a newborn infant. Am J Dis Child 1973;126:839–40.
361. Kang EY, Patz EF Jr, Müller NL. Cytomegalovirus pneumonia in transplant patients: CT findings. J Comput Assist Tomogr 1996;20:295–9.
362. Katzenstein AL, Askin FB. Surgical pathology of non-neoplastic lung disease. Philadelphia: WB Saunders; 1997.
363. Keane J, Gochuico B, Kasznica JM, Kornfeld H. Usual interstitial pneumonitis responsive to corticosteroids following varicella pneumonia. Chest 1998;113:249–51.
364. Khalifa MA, Lack EE. Herpes simplex viral infection. In: Connor DH, Chandler FW, Manz HJ, et al, eds. Pathology of infectious diseases. Stamford: Appleton & Lange; 1997:147–52.
365. Kim JS, Han HS, Park SH, Chun YK, Lee HJ, Chi JG. Neonatal adenoviral pneumonia—report of three autopsy cases. J Korean Med Sci 1997;12:146–50.
366. King JC Jr, Burke AR, Clemens JD, et al. Respiratory syncytial virus illnesses in human immunodeficiency virus- and noninfected children. Pediatr Infect Dis J 1993;12:733–9.
367. Klimek JJ, Lindenberg LB, Cole S, Ellison LH, Quintiliani R. Fatal case of influenza pneumonia with suprainfection by multiple bacteria and herpes simplex virus. Am Rev Respir Dis 1976;113:683–8.
368. Kramer MR, Marshall SE, Starnes VA, Gamberg P, Amitai Z, Theodore J. Infectious complications in heart-lung transplantation. Analysis of 200 episodes. Arch Intern Med 1993;153:2010–6.
369. Kumar L, Singh M, Mandal AK, Singhi PD, Bushnurmath SR. Bronchiolitis obliterans following measles. Indian Pediatr 1988;25:1201–5.

370. Lack EE, Chandler FW, Pearson GR. Cytomegalovirus infection. In: Connor DH, Chandler FW, Manz HJ, et al, eds. Pathology of infectious diseases. Stamford: Appleton & Lange; 1997:91–9.
371. Landry ML, Fong CK, Neddermann K, Solomon L, Hsiung GD. Disseminated adenovirus infection in an immunocompromised host. Pitfalls in diagnosis. Am J Med 1987;83:555–9.
372. Lanning P, Simila S, Linna O. Late pulmonary sequelae after type 7 adenovirus pneumonia. Ann Radiol (Paris) 1980;23:132–6.
373. Laraya-Cuasay LR, DeForest A, Huff D, Lischner H, Huang NN. Chronic pulmonary complications of early influenza virus infection in children. Am Rev Respir Dis 1977;116:617–25.
374. Legge RH, Thompson AB, Linder J, et al. Acyclovir-responsive herpetic tracheobronchitis. Am J Med 1988;85:561–3.
375. Levy J, Wodell RA, August CS, Bayever E. Adenovirus-related hemophagocytic syndrome after bone marrow transplantation. Bone Marrow Transplant 1990;6:349–52.
376. Lissauer TJ, Shaw PJ, Underhill G. Neonatal herpes simplex pneumonia. Arch Dis Child 1984;59:668–70.
377. McIntosh K, Halonen P, Ruuskanen O. Report of a workshop on respiratory viral infections: epidemiology, diagnosis, treatment, and prevention. Clin Infect Dis 1993;16:151–64.
378. McKenzie R, Travis WD, Dolan SA, et al. The causes of death in patients with human immunodeficiency virus infection: a clinical and pathologic study with emphasis on the role of pulmonary diseases. Medicine (Baltimore) 1991;70:326–43.
379. McQuillin J, Madeley CR, Kendal AP. Monoclonal antibodies for the rapid diagnosis of influenza A and B virus infections by immunofluorescence. Lancet 1985;2:911–4.
380. Meyer B, Stalder H, Wegmann W. Persistent pulmonary granulomas after recovery from varicella pneumonia. Chest 1986;89:457–9.
381. Myerowitz RL, Stalder H, Oxman MN, et al. Fatal disseminated adenovirus infection in a renal transplant recipient. Am J Med 1975;59:591–8.
382. Myou S, Fujimura M, Yasui M, Ueno T, Matsuda T. Bronchoalveolar lavage cell analysis in measles viral pneumonia. Eur Respir J 1993; 6:1437–42.
383. Nadel S, McGann K, Hodinka RL, Rutstein R, Chatten J. Measles giant cell pneumonia in a child with human immunodeficiency virus infection. Pediatr Infect Dis J 1991;10:542–4.
384. Nash G, Foley FD. Herpetic infection of the middle and lower respiratory tract. Am J Clin Pathol 1970;54:857–63.
385. Nolte KB, Feddersen RM, Foucar K, et al. Hantavirus pulmonary syndrome in the United States: a pathological description of a disease caused by a new agent. Hum Pathol 1995;26: 110–20.
386. Nuovo MA, Nuovo GJ, Becker J, Gallery F, Delvenne P, Kane PB. Correlation of viral infection, histology, and mortality in immunocompromised patients with pneumonia. Analysis by in situ hybridization and the polymerase chain reaction. Diagn Mol Pathol 1993;2:200–9.
387. Ohori NP, Michaels MG, Jaffe R, Williams P, Yousem SA. Adenovirus pneumonia in lung transplant recipients. Hum Pathol 1995;26:1073–9.
388. Ohori NP, Sciurba FC, Owens GR, Hodgson MJ, Yousem SA. Giant-cell interstitial pneumonia and hard-metal pneumoconiosis. A clinicopathologic study of four cases and review of the literature. Am J Surg Pathol 1989;13:581–7.
389. Omar AH, Manan A. Bronchiolitis obliterans in children—a report of six cases. Med J Malaysia 1989;44:204–9.
390. Oppenheim IA, Shields DF. Fatal interstitial pneumonitis and English (London) influenza. Three case reports which illustrate the typical bacteria-free course of infection. Clin Pediatr (Phila) 1973;12:681–3.
391. Oseasohn R, Adelson L, Kaji M. Clinicopathologic study of thirty-three fatal cases of Asian influenza. N Engl J Med 1959;260:509–18.
392. Parker RG. The pathology of uncomplicated influenza. Postgrad Med J 1963;39:564–6.
393. Paryani SG, Arvin AM. Intrauterine infection with varicella-zoster virus after maternal varicella. N Engl J Med 1986;314:1542–6.
394. Pinto A, Beck R, Jadavji T. Fatal neonatal pneumonia caused by adenovirus type 35. Report of one case and review of the literature. Arch Pathol Lab Med 1992;116:95–9.
395. Radoycich GE, Zuppan CW, Weeks DA, Krous HF, Langston C. Patterns of measles pneumonitis. Pediatr Pathol 1992;12:773–86.
396. Raider L. Calcification in chickenpox pneumonia. Chest 1971;60:504–7.
397. Ramsey PG, Fife KH, Hackman RC, Meyers JD, Corey L. Herpes simplex virus pneumonia: clinical, virologic, and pathologic features in 20 patients. Ann Intern Med 1982;97:813–20.
398. Ravin CE, Smith GW, Ahern MJ, McLoud T, Putman C, Milchgrub S. Cytomegaloviral infection presenting as a solitary pulmonary nodule. Chest 1977;71:220–2.

399. Reed JA, Slater LN, Hemann BA, Brigati DJ. Dual organism infection in biopsy specimens from immunocompromised patients: two cases demonstrated by immunocytochemistry. J Clin Lab Anal 1993;7:168–73.
400. Saito F, Yutani C, Imakita M, Ishibashi-Ueda H, Kanzaki T, Chiba Y. Giant cell pneumonia caused by varicella zoster virus in a neonate. Arch Pathol Lab Med 1989;113:201–3.
401. Salomon N, Gomez T, Perlman DC, Laya L, Eber C, Mildvan D. Clinical features and outcomes of HIV-related cytomegalovirus pneumonia. AIDS 1997;11:319–24.
402. Salomon N, Perlman DC. Cytomegalovirus pneumonia. Semin Respir Infect 1999;14:353–8.
403. Sata T, Kurata T, Aoyama Y, Sakaguchi M, Yamanouchi K, Takeda K. Analysis of viral antigens in giant cells of measles pneumonia by immunoperoxidase method. Virchows Arch [A] 1986;410:133–8.
404. Schwarz TF, Zaki SR, Morzunov S, Peters CJ, Nichol ST. Detection and sequence confirmation of Sin Nombre virus RNA in paraffin-embedded human tissues using one-step RT-PCR. J Virol Methods 1995;51:349–56.
405. Sherry MK, Klainer AS, Wolff M, Gerhard H. Herpetic tracheobronchitis. Ann Intern Med 1988;109:229–33.
406. Simila S, Linna O, Lanning P, Heikkinen E, Ala-Houhala M. Chronic lung damage caused by adenovirus type 7: a ten-year follow-up study. Chest 1981;80:127–31.
407. Sims DG, Downham MA, Gardner PS, Webb JK, Weightman D. Study of 8-year-old children with a history of respiratory syncytial virus bronchiolitis in infancy. Br Med J 1978;1:11–4.
408. Simsir A, Greenebaum E, Nuovo G, Schulman LL. Late fatal adenovirus pneumonitis in a lung transplant recipient. Transplantation 1998;65: 592–4.
409. Sly PD, Soto-Quiros ME, Landau LI, Hudson I, Newton-John H. Factors predisposing to abnormal pulmonary function after adenovirus type 7 pneumonia. Arch Dis Child 1984;59:935–9.
410. Smith FB, Arias JH, Elmquist TH, Mazzara JT. Microvascular cytomegalovirus endothelialitis of the lung: a possible cause of secondary pulmonary hypertension in a patient with AIDS. Chest 1998;114:337–40.
411. Sobonya RE, Hiller FC, Pingleton W, Watanabe I. Fatal measles (rubeola) pneumonia in adults. Arch Pathol Lab Med 1978;102:366–71.
412. Soto PJ, Broun GO, Wyatt JP. Asian influenzal pneumonitis. A structural and virologic analysis. Am J Med 1959;27:18–25.
413. Spigelblatt L, Rosenfeld R. Hyperlucent lung: long-term complication of adenovirus type 7 pneumonia. Can Med Assoc J 1983;128:47–9.
414. Stettler LE, Groth DH, Platek SF. Automated characterization of particles extracted from human lungs: three cases of tungsten carbide exposure. Scan Electron Microsc 1983;[Pt. 1]:439–48.
415. Stevens W, Vermeire P, Van De SR. Pulmonary calcifications and varicella. Acta Clin Belg 1977;32:264–70.
416. Stinson SF, Ryan DP, Hertweck S, Hardy JD, Hwang-Kow SY, Loosli CG. Epithelial and surfactant changes in influenzal pulmonary lesions. Arch Pathol Lab Med 1976;100:147–53.
417. Stocker JT, Conran RM, Fishback N. Respiratory syncytial virus. In: Connor DH, Chandler FW, Manz HJ, et al, eds. Pathology of infectious diseases. Stamford: Appleton & Lange; 1997:287–95.
418. Strano AJ. Light microscopy of selected viral diseases (morphology of viral inclusion bodies). Pathol Annu 1976;11:53–75.
419. Strickler JG, Manivel JC, Copenhaver CM, Kubic VL. Comparison of in situ hybridization and immunohistochemistry for detection of cytomegalovirus and herpes simplex virus. Hum Pathol 1990;21:443–8.
420. Sung RY, Chan RC, Tam JS, Cheng AF, Murray HG. Epidemiology and aetiology of acute bronchiolitis in Hong Kong infants. Epidemiol Infect 1992;108:147–54.
421. Taubenberger JK, Reid AH, Krafft AE, Bijwaard KE, Fanning TG. Initial genetic characterization of the 1918 "Spanish" influenza virus. Science 1997;275:1793–6.
422. Treanor JJ, Hayden FG. Viral infections. In: Murray JF, Nadel JA, Mason RJ, Boushey HA Jr, eds. Textbook of respiratory medicine, 3rd ed. Philadelphia: WB Saunders; 2000:929–84.
423. Triebwasser JH, Harris RE, Bryant RE, Rhoades ER. Varicella pneumonia in adults. Report of seven cases and a review of literature. Medicine (Baltimore) 1967;46:409–23.
424. Turner PC, Bailey AS, Cooper RJ, Morris DJ. The polymerase chain reaction for detecting adenovirus DNA in formalin-fixed, paraffin-embedded tissue obtained post mortem. J Infect 1993;27:43–6.
425. van Dissel JT, Zijlmans JM, Kroes AC, Fibbe WE. Respiratory syncytial virus, a rare cause of severe pneumonia following bone marrow transplantation. Ann Hematol 1995;71:253–5.

426. Warner GS. Hantavirus illness in humans: review and update. South Med J 1996;89:264–71.
427. Weiss RL, Colby TV, Spruance SL, Salmon VC, Hammond ME. Simultaneous cytomegalovirus and herpes simplex virus pneumonia. Arch Pathol Lab Med 1987;111:242–5.
428. Weller TH. Varicella and herpes zoster. Changing concepts of the natural history, control, and importance of a not-so-benign virus. N Engl J Med 1983;309:1362–8; 1434–40.
429. Whimbey E, Bodey GP. Viral pneumonia in the immunocompromised adult with neoplastic disease: the role of common community respiratory viruses. Semin Respir Infect 1992;7:122–31.
430. Wilczek B, Wilczek HE, Heurlin N, Tyden G, Aspelin P. Prognostic significance of pathological chest radiography in transplant patients affected by cytomegalovirus and/or Pneumocystis carinii. Acta Radiol 1996;37:727–31.
431. Winer-Muram HT, Gurney JW, Bozeman PM, Krance RA. Pulmonary complications after bone marrow transplantation. Radiol Clin North Am 1996;34:97–117.
432. Winn WC. Adenovirus. In: Connor DH, Chandler FW, Manz HJ, et al, eds. Pathology of infectious diseases. Stamford: Appleton & Lange; 1997:63–9.
433. Winn WC. Influenza and parainfluenza viruses. In: Connor DH, Chandler FW, Manz HJ, et al, eds. Pathology of infectious diseases. Stamford: Appleton & Lange; 1997:221–7.
434. Winn WC, Walker DH. Viral infections. In: Dail DH, Hammar SP, eds. Pulmonary pathology, 2nd ed. New York: Springer-Verlag; 1994:429–64.
435. Winternitz MG, Watson IM, McNamara FP. The pathology of influenza. New Haven: Yale University Press; 1920.
436. Wohl ME, Chernick V. State of the art: bronchiolitis. Am Rev Respir Dis 1978;118:759–81.
437. Yang E, Rubin BK. "Childhood" viruses as a cause of pneumonia in adults. Semin Respir Infect 1995;10:232–43.
438. Yeldandi AV, Colby TV. Pathologic features of lung biopsy specimens from influenza pneumonia cases. Hum Pathol 1994;25:47–3.
439. Yunis EJ, Agostini RM Jr, Atchison RW. An atlas of viral particles from human specimens. Perspect Pediatr Pathol 1978;4:387–429.
440. Yunis EJ, Hashida Y, Haas JE. The role of electron microscopy in the identification of viruses in human disease. Pathol Annu 1977;12[Pt. 1]:311–30.
441. Zaki SR. Hantavirus-associated diseases. In: Connor DH, Chandler FW, Manz HJ, et al, eds. Pathology of infectious diseases. Stamford: Appleton & Lange; 1997:125–36.
442. Zaki SR, Bellini WJ. Measles. In: Connor DH, Chandler FW, Manz HJ, et al, eds. Pathology of infectious diseases. Stamford: Appleton & Lange; 1997:233–44.

Mycoplasmal and Chlamydial Pneumonias

443. Andersen RD, Larson LA, Smith TF. Mycoplasma pneumoniae and Nocardia asteroides in lung biopsy tissue of an immunodeficient infant. Diagn Microbiol Infect Dis 1985;3:175–7.
444. Binford CH, Hauser GH. An epidemic of a severe pneumonitis in the bayou region of Louisiana. III. Report of autopsy on two cases. Pub Health Rep 1944;59:1363–74.
445. Blasi F, Boschini A, Cosentini R, et al. Outbreak of Chlamydia pneumoniae infection in former injection-drug users. Chest 1994;105:812–5.
446. Case records of the Massachusetts General Hospital. Weekly clinicopathological exercises. Case 5-1992. A 20-year-old man with diffuse pulmonary infiltrates and disseminated intravascular coagulation. N Engl J Med 1992;326:324–36.
447. Chan ED, Kalayanamit T, Lynch DA, et al. Mycoplasma pneumoniae-associated bronchiolitis causing severe restrictive lung disease in adults: report of three cases and literature review. Chest 1999;115:1188–94.
448. Corley DE, Winterbauer RH. Infectious diseases that result in slowly resolving and chronic pneumonia. Semin Respir Infect 1993;8:3–13.
449. Cosentini R, Esposito S, Blasi F, et al. Incidence of Chlamydia pneumoniae infection in vertically HIV-1 infected children. Eur J Clin Microbiol Infect Dis 1998;17:720–3.
450. Dean D. Chlamydial infections, Chlamydia trachomatis. In: Connor DH, Chandler FW, Manz HJ, et al, eds. Pathology of infectious diseases. Stamford: Appleton & Lange; 1997: 473–90.
451. Dearth JC, Rhodes KH. Infectious mononucleosis complicated by severe Mycoplasma pneumoniae infection. Am J Dis Child 1980;134:744–6.
452. Demos TC. Mediastinal lymphadenopathy in mycoplasmal pneumonia. AJR Am J Roentgenol 1994;162:1499–500.
453. Fraser RS, Müller NL, Colman N, Pare PD. Viruses, mycoplasmas, chlamydiae, and rickettsiae. In: Fraser RS, Müller NL, Colman N, Pare PD, eds. Fraser and Pare's diagnosis of diseases of the chest, 4th ed. Philadelphia: WB Saunders; 1999:979–1032.
454. Gal AA. Mycoplasma pneumoniae infections. In: Connor DH, Chandler FW, Manz HJ, et al, eds. Pathology of infectious diseases. Stamford: Appleton & Lange; 1997:675–80.

455. Ganick DJ, Wolfson J, Gilbert EF, Joo P. Mycoplasma infection in the immunosuppressed leukemic patient. Arch Pathol Lab Med 1980;104:535-6.
456. Goetz MB, Finegold SM. Pyogenic bacterial pneumonia, lung abscess and empyema. In: Murray JF, Nadel JA, Mason RJ, Boushey HA Jr, eds. Textbook of respiratory medicine, 3rd ed. Philadelphia: WB Saunders; 2000:985–1041.
457. Grayston JT. Chlamydia pneumoniae, strain TWAR. Chest 1989;95:664-9.
458. Griffin M, Pushpanathan C, Andrews W. Chlamydia trachomatis pneumonitis: a case study and literature review. Pediatr Pathol 1990;10:843–52.
459. Halal F, Brochu P, Delage G, Lamarre A, Rivard G. Severe disseminated lung disease and bronchiectasis probably due to Mycoplasma pneumoniae. Can Med Assoc J 1977;117:1055–6.
460. Hammerschlag MR. Chlamydia pneumoniae and the lung. Eur Respir J 2000;16:1001–7.
461. Isles AF, Masel J, O'Duffy J. Obliterative bronchiolitis due to Mycoplasma pneumoniae infection in a child. Pediatr Radiol 1987;17:109–11.
462. Ito JI Jr, Comess KA, Alexander ER, et al. Pneumonia due to Chlamydia trachomatis in an immunocompromised adult. N Engl J Med 1982;307:95–8.
463. Johnson CC, Finegold SM. Pyogenic bacterial pneumonia, lung abscess and empyema. In: Murray JF, Nadel JA, eds. Textbook of respiratory medicine, 2nd ed. Philadelphia: WB Saunders; 1994:1036–93.
464. Kaufman JM, Cuvelier CA, Van der Straeten M. Mycoplasma pneumonia with fulminant evolution into diffuse interstitial fibrosis. Thorax 1980;35:140–4.
465. Kim CK, Chung CY, Kim JS, Kim WS, Park Y, Koh YY. Late abnormal findings on high-resolution computed tomography after Mycoplasma pneumonia. Pediatrics 2000;105:372–8.
466. Koletsky RJ, Weinstein AJ. Fulminant Mycoplasma pneumoniae infection. Report of a fatal case, and a review of the literature. Am Rev Respir Dis 1980;122:491–6.
467. Kuo CC, Jackson LA, Campbell LA, Grayston JT. Chlamydia pneumoniae (TWAR). Clin Microbiol Rev 1995;8:451–61.
468. Leong MA, Nachajon R, Ruchelli E, Allen JL. Bronchitis obliterans due to Mycoplasma pneumonia. Pediatr Pulmonol 1997;23:375–81.
469. Levine DP, Lerner AM. The clinical spectrum of Mycoplasma pneumoniae infections. Med Clin North Am 1978;62:961–78.
470. Lillie RD. Pathology of psittacosis in man. NIH Bull 1933;161:1.
471. Macfarlane JT, Morris MJ. Abnormalities in lung function following clinical recovery from Mycoplasma pneumoniae pneumonia. Eur J Respir Dis 1982;63:337–41.
472. Maisel JC, Babbitt LH, John TJ. Fatal Mycoplasma pneumoniae infection with isolation of organisms from lung. JAMA 1967;202:287–90.
473. Meyers BR, Hirschman SZ. Fatal infections associated with Mycoplasma pneumoniae: discussion of three cases with necropsy findings. Mt Sinai J Med 1972;39:258–64.
474. Meyers JD, Hackman RC, Stamm WE. Chlamydia trachomatis infection as a cause of pneumonia after human marrow transplantation. Transplantation 1983;36:130–4.
475. Numazaki K, Sakamoto Y, Umetsu M, et al. Therapeutic effect of clarithromycin for respiratory-tract infections in children caused by Chlamydia pneumoniae. Research Group of Sapporo for Pediatric Chlamydial Infections. Int J Antimicrob Agents 2000;13:219–22.
476. Perez CR, Leigh MW. Mycoplasma pneumoniae as the causative agent for pneumonia in the immunocompromised host. Chest 1991;100: 860–1.
477. Prabhu MB, Barber D, Cockcroft DW. Bronchiolitis obliterans and Mycoplasma pneumonia. Respir Med 1991;85:535–7.
478. Reittner P, Müller NL, Heyneman L, et al. Mycoplasma pneumoniae pneumonia: radiographic and high-resolution CT features in 28 patients. AJR Am J Roentgenol 2000;174:37-41.
479. Rollins S, Colby T, Clayton F. Open lung biopsy in Mycoplasma pneumoniae pneumonia. Arch Pathol Lab Med 1986;110:34–41.
480. Sabato AR, Martin AJ, Marmion BP, Kok TW, Cooper DM. Mycoplasma pneumoniae: acute illness, antibiotics, and subsequent pulmonary function. Arch Dis Child 1984;59:1034-7.
481. Siegler DI. Lung abscess associated with Mycoplasma pneumoniae infection. Br J Dis Chest 1973;67:123–7.
482. Stokes D, Sigler A, Khouri NF, Talamo RC. Unilateral hyperlucent lung (Swyer-James syndrome) after severe Mycoplasma pneumoniae infection. Am Rev Respir Dis 1978;117:145–52.
483. Strano AJ. Ornithosis (psittacosis). In: Connor DH, Chandler FW, Manz HJ, et al, eds. Pathology of infectious diseases. Stamford: Appleton & Lange; 1997:713–5.
484. Talkington DF, Thacker WL, Keller DW, Jensen JS. Diagnosis of Mycoplasma pneumoniae infection in autopsy and open-lung biopsy tissues by nested PCR. J Clin Microbiol 1998;36: 1151–3.

485. Tong CY, Donnelly C, Harvey G, Sillis M. Multiplex polymerase chain reaction for the simultaneous detection of Mycoplasma pneumoniae, Chlamydia pneumoniae, and Chlamydia psittaci in respiratory samples. J Clin Pathol 1999;52:257–63.
486. Torres A, Dorca J, Zalacain R, et al. Community-acquired pneumonia in chronic obstructive pulmonary disease: a Spanish multicenter study. Am J Respir Crit Care Med 1996;154:1456-61.
487. Van Bever HP, Van Doorn JW, Demey HE. Adult respiratory distress syndrome associated with Mycoplasma pneumoniae infection. Eur J Pediatr 1992;151:227–8.
488. Walker DH. Mycoplasmal, chlamydial, and rickettsial pneumonias. In: Dail DH, Hammar SP, eds. Pulmonary pathology, 2nd ed. New York: Springer-Verlag; 1994:465–74.
489. Waris ME, Toikka P, Saarinen T, et al. Diagnosis of Mycoplasma pneumoniae pneumonia in children. J Clin Microbiol 1998;36:3155–9.
490. Whyte KF, Williams GR. Bronchiectasis after mycoplasma pneumonia. Thorax 1984;39:390-1.
491. Yano T, Ichikawa Y, Komatu S, Arai S, Oizumi K. Association of Mycoplasma pneumoniae antigen with initial onset of bronchial asthma. Am J Respir Crit Care Med 1994;149:1348–53.

Pneumocystis Pneumonia

492. Afessa B, Green WR, Williams WA, et al. Pneumocystis carinii pneumonia complicated by lymphadenopathy and pneumothorax. Arch Intern Med 1988;148:2651–4.
493. Bedrossian CW. Ultrastructure of Pneumocystis carinii: a review of internal and surface characteristics. Semin Diagn Pathol 1989;6:212–37.
494. Bergin CJ, Wirth RL, Berry GJ, Castellino RA. Pneumocystis carinii pneumonia: CT and HRCT observations. J Comput Assist Tomogr 1990;14:756–9.
495. Bigby TD, Margolskee D, Curtis JL, et al. The usefulness of induced sputum in the diagnosis of Pneumocystis carinii pneumonia in patients with the acquired immunodeficiency syndrome. Am Rev Respir Dis 1986;133:515–8.
496. Bleiweiss IJ, Jagirdar JS, Klein MJ, et al. Granulomatous Pneumocystis carinii pneumonia in three patients with the acquired immune deficiency syndrome. Chest 1988;94:580–3.
497. Blumenfeld W, Kovacs JA. Use of a monoclonal antibody to detect Pneumocystis carinii in induced sputum and bronchoalveolar lavage fluid by immunoperoxidase staining. Arch Pathol Lab Med 1988;112:1233–6.
498. Blumenfeld W, McCook O, Griffiss JM. Detection of antibodies to Pneumocystis carinii in bronchoalveolar lavage fluid by immunoreactivity to Pneumocystis carinii within alveoli, granulomas, and disseminated sites. Mod Pathol 1992;5:107–13.
499. Boiselle PM, Crans CA Jr, Kaplan MA. The changing face of Pneumocystis carinii pneumonia in AIDS patients. AJR Am J Roentgenol 1999;172:1301–9.
500. Chow C, Templeton PA, White CS. Lung cysts associated with Pneumocystis carinii pneumonia: radiographic characteristics, natural history, and complications. AJR Am J Roentgenol 1993;161:527–31.
501. Cohen OJ, Stoeckle MY. Extrapulmonary Pneumocystis carinii infections in the acquired immunodeficiency syndrome. Arch Intern Med 1991;151:1205–14.
502. Cote RJ, Rosenblum M, Telzak EE, May M, Unger PD, Cartun RW. Disseminated Pneumocystis carinii infection causing extrapulmonary organ failure: clinical, pathologic, and immunohistochemical analysis. Mod Pathol 1990;3:25–30.
503. Davey RT Jr, Margolis D, Kleiner D, Deyton L, Travis W. Digital necrosis and disseminated Pneumocystis carinii infection after aerosolized pentamidine prophylaxis. Ann Intern Med 1989;111:681–2.
504. Dieterich DT, Lew EA, Bacon DJ, Pearlman KI, Scholes JV. Gastrointestinal pneumocystosis in HIV-infected patients on aerosolized pentamidine: report of five cases and literature review. Am J Gastroenterol 1992;87:1763–70.
505. Dutz W. Pneumocystis carinii pneumonia. Pathol Annu 1970;5:309–41.
506. Edman JC, Kovacs JA, Masur H, Santi DV, Elwood HJ, Sogin ML. Ribosomal RNA sequence shows Pneumocystis carinii to be a member of the fungi. Nature 1988;334:519–22.
507. Elwood LJ, Dobrzanski D, Feuerstein IM, Solomon D. Pneumocystis carinii in pleural fluid. The cytologic appearance. Acta Cytol 1991;35:761–4.
508. Feuerstein IM, Francis P, Raffeld M, Pluda J. Widespread visceral calcifications in disseminated Pneumocystis carinii infection: CT characteristics. J Comput Assist Tomogr 1990;14: 149-51.
509. Fraser RS, Müller NL, Colman N, Pare PD. Pneumocystis carinii pneumonia. In: Fraser RS, Müller NL, Colman N, Pare PD, eds. Fraser and Pare's diagnosis of diseases of the chest, 4th ed. Philadelphia: WB Saunders; 1999:1660–7.
510. Goodman PC. Pneumocystis carinii pneumonia. J Thorac Imaging 1991;6:16–21.

511. Griffiths MH, Kocjan G, Miller RF, Godfrey-Faussett P. Diagnosis of pulmonary disease in human immunodeficiency virus infection: role of transbronchial biopsy and bronchoalveolar lavage. Thorax 1989;44:554–8.
512. Gruden JF, Huang L, Turner J, et al. High-resolution CT in the evaluation of clinically suspected Pneumocystis carinii pneumonia in AIDS patients with normal, equivocal, or nonspecific radiographic findings. AJR Am J Roentgenol 1997;169:967–75.
513. Guttler R, Singer PA, Axline SG, Greaves TS, McGill JJ. Pneumocystis carinii thyroiditis. Report of three cases and review of the literature. Arch Intern Med 1993;153:393–6.
514. Hartman TE, Primack SL, Müller NL, Staples CA. Diagnosis of thoracic complications in AIDS: accuracy of CT. AJR Am J Roentgenol 1994;162:547–53.
515. Jacobson MA, Mills J, Rush J, et al. Morbidity and mortality of patients with AIDS and first-episode Pneumocystis carinii pneumonia unaffected by concomitant pulmonary cytomegalovirus infection. Am Rev Respir Dis 1991;144:6–9.
516. Lee MM, Schinella RA. Pulmonary calcification caused by Pneumocystis carinii pneumonia. A clinicopathological study of 13 cases in acquired immune deficiency syndrome patients. Am J Surg Pathol 1991;15:376–80.
517. Masliah E, DeTeresa RM, Mallory ME, Hansen LA. Changes in pathological findings at autopsy in AIDS cases for the last 15 years. AIDS 2000;14:69–74.
518. Mason AC, Müller NL. The role of computed tomography in the diagnosis and management of human immunodeficiency virus (HIV)-related pulmonary diseases. Semin Ultrasound CT MR 1998;19:154–66.
519. Masur H, Lane HC, Kovacs JA, Allegra CJ, Edman JC. NIH conference. Pneumocystis pneumonia: from bench to clinic. Ann Intern Med 1989;111:813–26.
520. Mayor B, Schnyder P, Giron J, Landry M, Duvoisin B, Fournier D. Mediastinal and hilar lymphadenopathy due to Pneumocystis carinii infection in AIDS patients: CT features. J Comput Assist Tomogr 1994;18:408–11.
521. McGuinness G. Changing trends in the pulmonary manifestations of AIDS. Radiol Clin North Am 1997;35:1029–82.
522. McKenzie R, Travis WD, Dolan SA, et al. The causes of death in patients with human immunodeficiency virus infection: a clinical and pathologic study with emphasis on the role of pulmonary diseases. Medicine (Baltimore) 1991;70:326–43.
523. Merkel IS, Good CB, Nalesnik M, Roseman SR. Chronic Pneumocystis carinii infection of the liver. A case report and review of the literature. J Clin Gastroenterol 1992;15:55–8.
524. Murphy PM, Fox C, Travis WD, Koenig S, Fauci AS. Acquired immunodeficiency syndrome may present as severe restrictive lung disease. Am J Med 1989;86:237-40.
525. Petersen C, Mills J. Parasitic infections. In: Murray JE, Nadel JA, eds. Respiratory medicine, 2nd ed. Philadelphia: WB Saunders; 1994:1201–43.
526. Ragni MV, Dekker A, DeRubertis FR, et al. Pneumocystis carinii infection presenting as necrotizing thyroiditis and hypothyroidism. Am J Clin Pathol 1991;95:489–93.
527. Rorat E, Garcia RL, Skolom J. Diagnosis of Pneumocystis carinii pneumonia by cytologic examination of bronchial washings. JAMA 1985;254:1950–1.
528. Ruben FL, Talamo TS. Secondary pulmonary alveolar proteinosis occurring in two patients with acquired immune deficiency syndrome. Am J Med 1986;80:1187–90.
529. Saldana MJ, Mones JM, Martinez GR. The pathology of treated Pneumocystis carinii pneumonia. Semin Diagn Pathol 1989;6:300–12.
530. Sandhu JS, Goodman PC. Pulmonary cysts associated with Pneumocystis carinii pneumonia in patients with AIDS. Radiology 1989;173:33–5.
531. Schluger N, Godwin T, Sepkowitz K, et al. Application of DNA amplification to pneumocystosis: presence of serum Pneumocystis carinii DNA during human and experimentally induced Pneumocystis carinii pneumonia. J Exp Med 1992;176:1327–33.
532. Sloand E, Laughon B, Armstrong M, et al. The challenge of Pneumocystis carinii culture. J Eukaryot Microbiol 1993;40:188–95.
533. Tran Van Nhieu J, Vojtek AM, Bernaudin JF, Escudier E, Fleury-Feith J. Pulmonary alveolar proteinosis associated with Pneumocystis carinii. Ultrastructural identification in bronchoalveolar lavage in AIDS and immunocompromised non-AIDS patients. Chest 1990;98:801–5.
534. Travis WD, Pittaluga S, Lipschik GY, et al. Atypical pathologic manifestations of Pneumocystis carinii pneumonia in the acquired immune deficiency syndrome. Review of 123 lung biopsies from 76 patients with emphasis on cysts, vascular invasion, vasculitis, and granulomas. Am J Surg Pathol 1990;14:615–25.

535. Wasserman L, Haghighi P. Otic and ophthalmic pneumocystosis in acquired immunodeficiency syndrome. Report of a case and review of the literature. Arch Pathol Lab Med 1992;116:500–3.
536. Watts JC, Chandler FW. Pneumocystosis. In: Connor DH, Chandler FW, Manz HJ, et al, eds. Pathology of infectious diseases. Stamford: Appleton & Lange; 1997:1241–51.
537. Weber WR, Askin FB, Dehner LP. Lung biopsy in Pneumocystis carinii pneumonia: a histopathologic study of typical and atypical features. Am J Clin Pathol 1977;67:11–9.

Parasitic Infections

538. Ammann RW, Eckert J. Cestodes. Echinococcus. Gastroenterol Clin North Am 1996;25: 655–89.
539. Asimacopoulos PJ, Katras A, Christie B. Pulmonary dirofilariasis. The largest single-hospital experience. Chest 1992;102:851-5.
540. Badhe BP, Sane SY. Human pulmonary dirofilariasis in India: a case report. J Trop Med Hyg 1989;92:425–6.
541. Baird JK, Neafie RC, Marty AM. Parasitic infections. In: Dail DH, Hammar SP, eds. Pulmonary pathology, 2nd ed. New York: Springer-Verlag; 1994:491–536.
542. Beckers PJ, Derks GJ, Gool T, Rietveld FJ, Sauerwein RW. Encephalocytozoon intestinalis-specific monoclonal antibodies for laboratory diagnosis of microsporidiosis. J Clin Microbiol 1996;34:282–5.
543. Beggs I. The radiology of hydatid disease. AJR Am J Roentgenol 1985;145:639–48.
544. Bhatia G. Echinococcus. Semin Respir Infect 1997;12:171–86.
545. Biava MF, Dao A, Fortier B. Laboratory diagnosis of cystic hydatic disease. World J Surg 2001;25:10–4.
546. Bicart-See A, Massip P, Linas MD, Datry A. Successful treatment with nitazoxanide of Enterocytozoon bieneusi microsporidiosis in a patient with AIDS. Antimicrob Agents Chemother 2000;44:167–8.
547. Bosanac ZB, Lisanin L. Percutaneous drainage of hydatid cyst in the liver as a primary treatment: review of 52 consecutive cases with long-term follow-up. Clin Radiol 2000;55:839–48.
548. Braunstein H, Connor DH. Amebiasis-infection by Entamoeba histolytica. In: Connor DH, Chandler FW, Manz HJ, et al, eds. Pathology of infectious diseases. Stamford: Appleton & Lange; 1997:1127–33.
549. Brenes R, Beaver PC, Monge E, Zamora L. Pulmonary dirofilariasis in a Costa Rican man. Am J Trop Med Hyg 1985;34:1142–3.
550. Bruce BB, Blass MA, Blumberg HM, Lennox JL, del Rio C, Horsburgh CR. Risk of Cryptosporidium parvum transmission between hospital roommates. Clin Infect Dis 2000;31:947–50.
551. Burgos R, Varela A, Castedo E, et al. Pulmonary hydatidosis: surgical treatment and follow-up of 240 cases. Eur J Cardiothorac Surg 1999;16:628–34.
552. Carr A, Marriott D, Field A, Vasak E, Cooper DA. Treatment of HIV-1-associated microsporidiosis and cryptosporidiosis with combination antiretroviral therapy. Lancet 1998;351: 256–61.
553. Celik M, Senol C, Keles M, et al. Surgical treatment of pulmonary hydatid disease in children: report of 122 cases. J Pediatr Surg 2000; 35:1710–3.
554. Cheever AW, Neafie RC. Schistosomiasis. In: Meyers WM, Neafie RC, Marty AM, Wear DJ, eds. Pathology of infectious diseases. Washington, D.C.: Armed Forces Institute of Pathology; 2000:23–48.
555. Ciferri F. Human pulmonary dirofilariasis in the United States: a critical review. Am J Trop Med Hyg 1982;31:302–8.
556. Clavel A, Arnal AC, Sanchez EC, et al. Respiratory cryptosporidiosis: case series and review of the literature. Infection 1996;24:341–6.
557. Cohen H, Paolillo E, Bonifacino R, et al. Human cystic echinococcosis in a Uruguayan community: a sonographic, serologic, and epidemiologic study. Am J Trop Med Hyg 1998;59:620–7.
558. Connor DH, Neafie RC. Onchocerciasis. In: Binford CH, Connor DH, eds. Pathology of tropical and extraordinary diseases, 2nd ed. Washington, D.C.: Armed Forces Institute of Pathology; 1976:360–72.
559. Contini C, Romani R, Magno S, Delia S. Diagnosis of Toxoplasma gondii infection in AIDS patients by a tissue-culture technique. Eur J Clin Microbiol Infect Dis 1995;14:434–40.
560. Cowley GP, Miller RF, Papadaki L, Canning EU, Lucas SB. Disseminated microsporidiosis in a patient with acquired immunodeficiency syndrome. Histopathology 1997;30:386–9.
561. Derouin F, Devergie A, Auber P, et al. Toxoplasmosis in bone marrow-transplant recipients: report of seven cases and review. Clin Infect Dis 1992;15:267–70.
562. Drugs for parasitic infections. Med Lett Drugs Ther 1998;40:1–12.
563. Dupont C, Bougnoux ME, Turner L, Rouveix E, Dorra M. Microbiological findings about pulmonary cryptosporidiosis in two AIDS patients. J Clin Microbiol 1996;34:227–9.

564. Echeverri A, Long RF, Check W, Burnett CM. Pulmonary dirofilariasis. Ann Thorac Surg 1999;67:201–2.
565. Enzenauer RJ, Underwood GH Jr, Ribbing J. Tropical pulmonary eosinophilia. South Med J 1990;83:69–72.
566. Evans TG, Schwartzman JD. Pulmonary toxoplasmosis. Semin Respir Infect 1991;6:51–7.
567. Flieder DB, Moran CA. Pulmonary dirofilariasis: a clinicopathologic study of 41 lesions in 39 patients. Hum Pathol 1999;30:251–6.
568. Fraiji EK Jr, Connor DH. Echinococcosis. In: Connor DH, Chandler FW, Manz HJ, et al, eds. Pathology of infectious diseases. Stamford: Appleton & Lange; 1997:1405–13.
569. Fraser RS, Müller NL, Colman N, Pare PD. Protozoa, helminths, arthropods, and leeches. In: Fraser RS, Müller NL, Colman N, Pare PD, eds. Fraser and Pare's diagnosis of diseases of the chest, 4th ed. Philadelphia: WB Saunders; 1999:1033–66.
570. Frenkel JK. Toxoplasmosis. In: Connor DH, Chandler FW, Manz HJ, et al, eds. Pathology of infectious diseases. Stamford: Appleton & Lange; 1997:1261–78.
571. Genta RM, Haque AK. Strongyloidiasis. In: Connor DH, Chandler FW, Manz HJ, et al, eds. Pathology of infectious diseases. Stamford: Appleton & Lange; 1997:1567–76.
572. Georges E, Rabaud C, Amiel C, et al. Enterocytozoon bieneusi multiorgan microsporidiosis in a HIV-infected patient. J Infect 1998;36:223–5.
573. Gil-Grande LA, Rodriguez-Caabeiro F, Prieto JG, et al. Randomized controlled trial of efficacy of albendazole in intra-abdominal hydatid disease. Lancet 1993;342:1269–72.
574. Goodman PC, Schnapp LM. Pulmonary toxoplasmosis in AIDS. Radiology 1992;184:791–3.
575. Gopinath R, Nutman TB. Parasitic diseases. In: Murray JF, Nadel JA, Mason RJ, Boushey HA Jr, eds. Textbook of respiratory medicine, 3rd ed. Philadelphia: WB Saunders; 2000:1143–71.
576. Gunnarsson G, Hurlbut D, DeGirolami PC, Federman M, Wanke C. Multiorgan microsporidiosis: report of five cases and review. Clin Infect Dis 1995;21:37–44.
577. Gupta RK, McHutchison AG, Fauck R. Liesegang rings in a needle aspirate from a breast cyst. Acta Cytol 1991;35:700–2.
578. Haramati LB, Jenny-Avital ER. Approach to the diagnosis of pulmonary disease in patients infected with the human immunodeficiency virus. J Thorac Imaging 1998;13:247–60.
579. Hewitt RG, Yiannoutsos CT, Higgs ES, et al. Paromomycin: no more effective than placebo for treatment of cryptosporidiosis in patients with advanced human immunodeficiency virus infection. AIDS Clinical Trial Group. Clin Infect Dis 2000;31:1084–92.
580. Im JG, Whang HY, Kim WS, Han MC, Shim YS, Cho SY. Pleuropulmonary paragonimiasis: radiologic findings in 71 patients. AJR Am J Roentgenol 1992;159:39–43.
581. Iralu JV, Maguire JH. Pulmonary infections in immigrants and refugees. Semin Respir Infect 1991;6:235–46.
582. Kagawa FT. Pulmonary paragonimiasis. Semin Respir Infect 1997;12:149–58.
583. Landay MJ, Setiawan H, Hirsch G, Christensen EE, Conrad MR. Hepatic and thoracic amaebiasis. AJR Am J Roentgenol 1980;135: 449–54.
584. Lavrard I, Chouaid C, Roux P, et al. Pulmonary toxoplasmosis in HIV-infected patients: usefulness of polymerase chain reaction and cell culture. Eur Respir J 1995;8:697–700.
585. Leder K, Ryan N, Spelman D, Crowe SM. Microsporidial disease in HIV-infected patients: a report of 42 patients and review of the literature. Scand J Infect Dis 1998;30:331–8.
586. Leder K, Weller PF. Life cycle and epidemiology of echinococcal species. In: Rose BD, ed. Uptodate in medicine. Wellesley: BDR-Uptodate; 2001.
587. Leder K, Weller PF. Treatment and prevention of echinococcosis. In: Rose BD, ed. Uptodate in medicine. Wellesley: BDR-Uptodate; 2001.
588. Lee KJ, Park GM, Yong TS, et al. The first Korean case of human pulmonary dirofilariasis. Yonsei Med J 2000;41:285–8.
589. Maggi P, Larocca AM, Quarto M, et al. Effect of antiretroviral therapy on cryptosporidiosis and microsporidiosis in patients infected with human immunodeficiency virus type 1. Eur J Clin Microbiol Infect Dis 2000;19:213–7.
590. Makiya K. Recent increase of human infections with dog heart worm Dirofilaria immitis in Japan. Parassitologia 1997;39:387–8.
591. Marshall BG, Wilkinson RJ, Davidson RN. Pathogenesis of tropical pulmonary eosinophilia: parasitic alveolitis and parallels with asthma. Respir Med 1998;92:1–3.
592. Marty AM, Johnson LK, Neafie RC. Hydatidosis (echinococcosis). In: Meyers WM, Neafie RC, Marty AM, Wear DJ, eds. Pathology of infectious diseases. Washington, D.C.: Armed Forces Institute of Pathology; 2000:145–64.
593. Marty AM, Neafie RC. Dirofilariasis. In: Meyers WM, Neafie RC, Marty AM, Wear DJ, eds. Pathology of infectious diseases. Washington, D.C.: Armed Forces Institute of Pathology; 2000:275–85.

594. Marty AM, Neafie RC. Overview of the pathogenic helminths with discussion of nonpathogenic worms, arthropods, and other structures. In: Meyers WM, Neafie RC, Marty AM, Wear DJ, eds. Pathology of infectious diseases, vol. I. Washington, D.C.: Armed Forces Institute of Pathology; 2000:1–21.
595. Marty P. Human dirofilariasis due to Dirofilaria repens in France. A review of reported cases. Parassitologia 1997;39:383–6.
596. Mawhorter S, Temeck B, Chang R, Pass H, Nash T. Nonsurgical therapy for pulmonary hydatid cyst disease. Chest 1997;112:1432–6.
597. Meyers WM, Neafie RC, Connor DH. Bancroftian and Malayan filariasis. In: Binford CH, Connor DH, eds. Pathology of tropical and extraordinary diseases, 2nd ed. Washington, D.C.: Armed Forces Institute of Pathology; 1976:340–55.
598. Meynard JL, Meyohas MC, Binet D, Chouaid C, Frottier J. Pulmonary cryptosporidiosis in the acquired immunodeficiency syndrome. Infection 1996;24:328–31.
599. Milanez de Campos Jr, Barbas CS, Filomeno LT, et al. Human pulmonary dirofilariasis: analysis of 24 cases from Sao Paulo, Brazil. Chest 1997;112:729–33.
600. Mohri H, Fujita H, Asakura Y, et al. Case report: inhalation therapy of paromomycin is effective for respiratory infection and hypoxia by cryptosporidium with AIDS. Am J Med Sci 1995;309:60–2.
601. Molina JM, Goguel J, Sarfati C, et al. Trial of oral fumagillin for the treatment of intestinal microsporidiosis in patients with HIV infection. ANRS 054 Study Group. Agence Nationale de Recherche sur le SIDA. AIDS 2000;14:1341–8.
602. Mosier DA, Oberst RD. Cryptosporidiosis. A global challenge. Ann N Y Acad Sci 2000;916:102–11.
603. Muro A, Genchi C, Cordero M, Simon F. Human dirofilariasis in the European Union. Parasitol Today 1999;15:386–9.
604. Nahmias J, Goldsmith R, Soibelman M, el On J. Three- to 7-year follow-up after albendazole treatment of 68 patients with cystic echinococcosis (hydatid disease). Ann Trop Med Parasitol 1994;88:295–304.
605. Narine K, Brennan B, Gilfillan I, Hodge A. Pulmonary presentation of Dirofilaria immitis (canine heartworm) in man. Eur J Cardiothorac Surg 1999;16:475–7.
606. Neafie RC, Piggott J. Human pulmonary dirofilariasis. Arch Pathol 1971;92:342–9.
607. Ong RK, Doyle RL. Tropical pulmonary eosinophilia. Chest 1998;113:1673–9.
608. Orenstein JM. Microsporidiosis. In: Connor DH, Chandler FW, Manz HJ, et al, eds. Pathology of infectious diseases. Stamford: Appleton & Lange; 1997:1223–39.
609. Pampiglione S, Rivasi F, Canestri Trotti G. Human pulmonary dirofilariasis in Italy [Letter]. Lancet 1984;1:333.
610. Pellicelli AM, Palmieri F, Spinazzola F, et al. Pulmonary cryptosporidiosis in patients with acquired immunodeficiency syndrome. Minerva Med 1998;89:173–5.
611. Pickup CM, Nee PA, Randall PE. Radiographic features in 1016 adults admitted to hospital with acute asthma. J Accid Emerg Med 1994;11:234–7.
612. Poirot JL, Deluol AM, Antoine M, et al. Broncho-pulmonary cryptosporidiosis in four HIV-infected patients. J Eukaryot Microbiol 1996;43:78S–9S.
613. Pomeroy C, Filice GA. Pulmonary toxoplasmosis: a review. Clin Infect Dis 1992;14:863–70.
614. Portnoy LG. Dirofilariasis. In: Connor DH, Chandler FW, Manz HJ, et al, eds. Pathology of infectious diseases. Stamford: Appleton & Lange; 1997:1391–6.
615. Qian, ZX. Thoracic hydatid cysts: a report of 842 cases treated over a thirty-year period. Ann Thorac Surg 1988;46:342–46.
616. Rabaud C, May T, Lucet JC, Leport C, Ambroise-Thomas P, Canton P. Pulmonary toxoplasmosis in patients infected with human immunodeficiency virus: a French national survey. Clin Infect Dis 1996;23:1249–54.
617. Ramos G, Orduna A, Garcia-Yuste M. Hydatid cyst of the lung: diagnosis and treatment. World J Surg 2001;25:46–57.
618. Raso DS, Greene WB, Finley JL, Silverman JF. Morphology and pathogenesis of Liesegang rings in cyst aspirates: report of two cases with ancillary studies. Diagn Cytopathol 1998;19:116–9.
619. Reiter-Owona I, Petersen E, Joynson D, et al. The past and present role of the Sabin-Feldman dye test in the serodiagnosis of toxoplasmosis. Bull World Health Organ 1999;77:929–35.
620. Remadi S, Dumais J, Wafa K, MacGee W. Pulmonary microsporidiosis in a patient with the acquired immunodeficiency syndrome. A case report. Acta Cytol 1995;39:1112–6.
621. Reuter S, Jensen B, Buttenschoen K, Kratzer W, Kern P. Benzimidazoles in the treatment of alveolar echinococcosis: a comparative study and review of the literature. J Antimicrob Chemother 2000;46:451–6.

622. Ro JY, Tsakalakis PJ, White VA, et al. Pulmonary dirofilariasis: the great imitator of primary or metastatic lung tumor. A clinicopathologic analysis of seven cases and a review of the literature. Hum Pathol 1989;20:69–76.
623. Roth A, Roth B, Höffken G, Steuber S, Khalifa KI, Janitschke K. Application of the polymerase chain reaction in the diagnosis of pulmonary toxoplasmosis in immunocompromised patients. Eur J Clin Microbiol Infect Dis 1992;11: 1177–81.
624. Saksouk FA, Fahl MH, Rizk GK. Computed tomography of pulmonary hydatid disease. J Comput Assist Tomogr 1986;10:226–32.
625. Scaglia M, Gatti S, Sacchi L, et al. Asymptomatic respiratory tract microsporidiosis due to Encephalitozoon hellem in three patients with AIDS. Clin Infect Dis 1998;26:174–6.
626. Scaglia M, Sacchi L, Croppo GP, et al. Pulmonary microsporidiosis due to Encephalitozoon hellem in a patient with AIDS. J Infect 1997;34:119–26.
627. Schwartz DA, Bryan RT, Hewan-Lowe KO, et al. Disseminated microsporidiosis (Encephalitozoon hellem) and acquired immunodeficiency syndrome. Autopsy evidence for respiratory acquisition. Arch Pathol Lab Med 1992;116:660–8.
628. Schwartz DA, Sobottka I, Leitch GJ, Cali A, Visvesvara GS. Pathology of microsporidiosis: emerging parasitic infections in patients with acquired immunodeficiency syndrome. Arch Pathol Lab Med 1996;120:173–88.
629. Schwartz DA, Visvesvara GS, Leitch GJ, et al. Pathology of symptomatic microsporidial (Encephalitozoon hellem) bronchiolitis in the acquired immunodeficiency syndrome: a new respiratory pathogen diagnosed from lung biopsy, bronchoalveolar lavage, sputum, and tissue culture. Hum Pathol 1993;24:937–43.
630. Shah MK. Human pulmonary dirofilariasis: review of the literature. South Med J 1999;92:276-9.
631. Sing A, Leitritz L, Roggenkamp A, et al. Pulmonary toxoplasmosis in bone marrow transplant recipients: report of two cases and review. Clin Infect Dis 1999;29:429–33.
632. Sinniah B. Paragonimiasis. In: Connor DH, Chandler FW, Manz HJ, et al, eds. Pathology of infectious diseases. Stamford: Appleton & Lange; 1997:1527–30.
633. Sneige N, Dekmezian RH, Silva EG, Cartwright J, Ayala AG. Pseudoparasitic Liesegang structures in perirenal hemorrhagic cysts. Am J Clin Pathol 1988;89:148–53.
634. Soave R, Johnson WD. Cryptosporidium and Isospora belli infections. J Infect Dis 1988; 157:225–9.
635. Tor M, Ozvaran K, Ersoy Y, et al. Pitfalls in the diagnosis of complicated pulmonary hydatid disease. Respir Med 2001;95:237–9.
636. Travis WD, Schmidt K, MacLowry JD, Masur H, Condron KS, Fojo AT. Respiratory cryptosporidiosis in a patient with malignant lymphoma. Report of a case and review of the literature. Arch Pathol Lab Med 1990;114:519–22.
637. Tuur SM, Nelson AM, Gibson DW, et al. Liesegang rings in tissue. How to distinguish Liesegang rings from the giant kidney worm, Dioctophyma renale. Am J Surg Pathol 1987;11:598–605.
638. Uchida K, Sekiguchi S, Doi Y, Yamazaki H. Pulmonary paragonimiasis with pleural effusion containing paragonimus ova: sonographical appearance of pleural effusion. Intern Med 1995;34:1178–80.
639. Vietzke WM, Gelderman AH, Grimley PM, Valsamis MP. Toxoplasmosis complicating malignancy. Experience at the National Cancer Institute. Cancer 1968;21:816–27.
640. von Lichtenberg F. Schistosomiasis. In: Connor DH, Chandler FW, Manz HJ, et al, eds. Pathology of infectious diseases. Stamford: Appleton & Lange; 1997:1537–51.
641. von Sinner W, te Strake L, Clark D, Sharif H. MR imaging in hydatid disease. AJR Am J Roentgenol 1991;157:741–5.
642. von Sinner WN. New diagnostic signs in hydatid disease: radiography, ultrasound, CT and MRI correlated to pathology. Eur J Radiol 1991;12:150–9.
643. Wand A, Kasirajan LP, Sridhar S. Solitary pulmonary nodule due to dirofilariasis. J Thorac Imaging 2000;15:198–200.
644. Weber R, Kuster H, Keller R, et al. Pulmonary and intestinal microsporidiosis in a patient with the acquired immunodeficiency syndrome. Am Rev Respir Dis 1992;146:1603–5.
645. Wehner JH, Kirsch CM. Pulmonary manifestations of strongyloidiasis. Semin Respir Infect 1997;12:122–9.
646. Wells GM, Gajjar A, Pearson TA, Hale KL, Shenep JL. Brief report. Pulmonary cryptosporidiosis and Cryptococcus albidus fungemia in a child with acute lymphocytic leukemia. Med Pediatr Oncol 1998;31:544–6.
647. Woodring JH, Halfhill H 2nd, Reed JC. Pulmonary strongyloidiasis: clinical and imaging features. AJR Am J Roentgenol 1994;162:537–42.

13
INTERPRETATION OF LUNG BIOPSIES FROM IMMUNOCOMPROMISED PATIENTS AND PATIENTS WITH ACQUIRED IMMUNODEFICIENCY SYNDROME

There has been a dramatic increase in the number of lung biopsies performed to assess pulmonary complications in immunocompromised patients. Three major events have fueled this increase: the use of ablative chemotherapy regimens in cancer patients, the rise of solid organ and bone marrow transplantation, and the impact of the epidemic of infections by the human immunodeficiency virus (HIV) (27,47, 59). These patients are particularly susceptible to infections, often resulting in new syndromes due to agents that were thought to be relatively benign organisms (such as *Microsporida, Cryptosporidia,* and *Rhodococcus equi*) or with a degree of severity out of proportion to the native virulence of the offending organism (such as cavitary *Pneumocystis carinii* pneumonia). Furthermore, pathologists now recognize that there is a much broader spectrum of histopathologic findings in this setting, leading to new concepts concerning the pathogenesis of many patterns of lung injury and repair.

The surgical pathologist plays a critical role, with the clinician and radiologist, in the diagnosis of pulmonary disease in the immunocompromised patient. Given the wide array of potential pathogens, the frequency of atypical and multiple infections, and the urgency of the diagnosis of infection in the immunocompromised host, a systematic approach to diagnosis of lung disease in these patients is imperative. Often, immunocompromised patients with pulmonary complications do not present with the expected signs and symptoms. Thus, the clinician and pathologist must continue to look for new pathogens or unusual presentations of known pathogens in these patients. The goal of this chapter is to provide an overview of the general principles that guide the evaluation of lung biopsies in the immunocompromised patient, with special emphasis on patients with the acquired immunodeficiency syndrome (AIDS).

The clinical history as well as the radiologic pattern of the pulmonary lesions are important to the pathologist interpreting a biopsy from an immunocompromised patient. They may provide clues to the type of pathologic lesion or organism to look for when examining the specimen, or help determine that a biopsy has not sampled the lesion in question.

DIAGNOSIS OF PULMONARY COMPLICATIONS IN IMMUNOCOMPROMISED PATIENTS

The clinical evaluation of an immunocompromised patient requires that a series of steps be taken to ensure that a rapid and accurate diagnosis is obtained (see chapter 12). Infection must be considered first; a discussion of the specific categories of pulmonary infection is found in chapter 12. Many processes that mimic infection must be ruled out including cytotoxic and noncytotoxic drug reactions, interstitial lung diseases, and neoplasms.

The chest radiograph is an important first step for identifying the presence of lung disease and monitoring response to treatment. It seldom allows a confident specific diagnosis; this can come only from microbiologic or histologic information. The chest radiograph may be normal in up to 10 percent of immunocompromised patients with pulmonary complications (52,87). High-resolution computerized tomography (HRCT) is superior to the chest radiograph for demonstrating the pattern, distribution, and extent of lung disease (37,52,79). HRCT can help determine if the pneumonia is necrotizing, if the consolidation is associated with bronchial obstruction (from a tumor), if there is an associated pleural effusion, if a circumscribed lesion is a fungus ball within a cavity, or if bronchiectasis is present.

Assessment of the radiologic pattern, combined with clinical and epidemiologic information, can narrow the diagnostic possibilities while other tests are being obtained. Review of these imaging studies should include careful inspection of both lungs for comparison of the bronchovascular markings, and overall density of right and left lung from the apices to the diaphragm. The analysis also should include careful examination of the hila, mediastinum, heart, and pleura in order to detect associated findings such as lymph node enlargement and pleural effusion. Comparison with previous chest imaging studies is crucial for the detection of subtle parenchymal opacities and for defining the pattern of progression of these opacities.

LUNG BIOPSY INTERPRETATION IN IMMUNOCOMPROMISED PATIENTS

Interpretation of lung biopsy specimens from immunocompromised patients is a difficult challenge (see chapter 2) (103). Accurate interpretation of these biopsies is essential since these patients are often critically ill and the pathologic diagnosis often determines whether the patient is given antimicrobial therapy or continues to receive immunosuppressive medication.

A number of important principles must be applied when interpreting lung biopsies from immunocompromised patients. Infection is the most common pulmonary complication in immunocompromised patients, so lung biopsies must be carefully evaluated for infectious agents. Underlying disease, such as neoplastic infiltrates, collagen vascular disease, or vasculitis, may account for new lung lesions. For this reason it is important for pathologists to have some clinical and radiologic history so they know what to look for, especially when lesions are subtle or when it is necessary to sort out the pathologic effects of drugs or radiation (see chapter 7). Transplant-related lung injury may cause a spectrum of lesions including bronchiolitis obliterans (graft versus host disease in bone marrow transplant patients or chronic rejection in heart-lung transplant patients) or Epstein-Barr virus–associated lymphoproliferative disorders (see chapter 14).

Immunocompromised patients may develop new lung disorders such as pulmonary emboli or aspiration sequelae. In addition, these patients often have more than one lesion or more than one infectious agent at the same time, so one must continue to search for additional pathology or organisms after an initial positive finding.

Lung biopsy specimens must be routinely processed with a complete battery of special stains to search for infectious organisms. Immunocompromised patients may not be able to mount an appropriate inflammatory response, making it difficult for a pathologist to suspect the correct organism. In some cases there is no histologic response and the lung may appear normal.

When interpreting special stains for organisms, one must be critical about whether the criteria for finding an organism are actually met. If the morphologic features are not clear-cut one should be cautious about making a definitive diagnosis. There are a variety of steps that can be used to help assess such a situation. Some organisms can be recognized without special stains, but if the organism does not stain appropriately, there may be a problem with the stains, or the structures identified may be something other than an organism. Control slides should be evaluated to make sure the stain worked properly; if the control slides did not work, then the stains should be repeated until they stain appropriately. Things that get confused with organisms range from aspirated or inhaled vegetable material (see chapter 3), Hamazaki-Wesenberg bodies (see chapter 3), calcification (see chapter 17), atypical reactive pneumocytes, and contaminants in the reagents used for preparing histologic slides and special stains. In some cases special techniques such as immunohistochemistry may help to confirm the presence of organisms such as cytomegalovirus. Unusual organisms must be considered in the search for infectious agents, particularly in patients with HIV infection.

Only certain organisms can be seen in histologic sections; to diagnose infections due to other agents, cultures, immunohistochemistry, or serologic or skin tests are used. A number of nucleic acid amplification tests (polymerase chain reactions [PCR]) are available or in development that allow more rapid and direct detection of pulmonary pathogens. A substantial percentage of lung biopsies from immunocompromised patients show a negative result and this information is often valuable.

RADIOLOGIC PATTERNS IN IMMUNOCOMPROMISED PATIENTS

Radiographic and HRCT assessments of pulmonary complications are based on the pattern and distribution of the parenchymal abnormalities, the presence of associated findings such as hilar or mediastinal lymph node enlargement, and the clinical history. The main patterns of

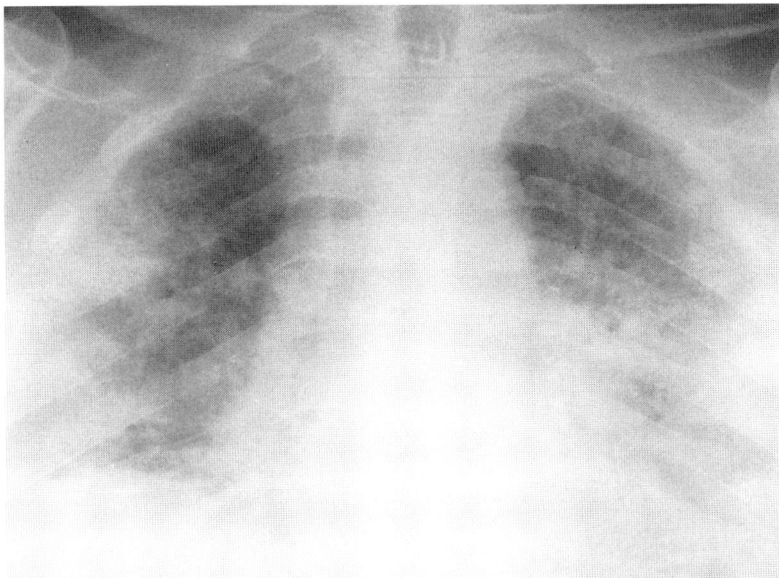

Figure 13-1

DRUG REACTION

Chest radiograph demonstrates extensive bilateral airspace consolidation involving mainly the peripheral lung regions. The consolidation was shown to represent acute respiratory distress syndrome (ARDS) caused by an adverse drug reaction to bleomycin.

abnormality seen in immunocompromised patients are airspace consolidation, hazy increase in opacity (ground-glass pattern), and nodules.

Airspace or Alveolar Opacities. Lobar, segmental, or focal consolidation is usually due to bacterial infection (4,63). In immunocompromised non-AIDS patients, diffuse consolidation is a relatively nonspecific finding that may result from severe pneumonia, drug reaction, or hemorrhage (fig. 13-1) (79, 87,111). In patients with AIDS, diffuse consolidation is most commonly due to pneumonia caused by *Pneumocystis carinii.*

A hazy increase in opacity (ground-glass pattern) is often difficult to recognize on the radiograph but can be readily seen on HRCT. This pattern usually reflects the presence of relatively mild interstitial or airspace disease. In patients with AIDS, it is most suggestive of *P. carinii* pneumonia (42,63). In immunocompromised non-AIDS patients, the ground-glass pattern is nonspecific, being seen in opportunistic infections, drug reactions, pulmonary hemorrhage, and pulmonary edema (63,87,111).

Interstitial Opacities. A reticular or peribronchovascular pattern of opacities may occur in some atypical, mycoplasma, and viral pneumonias. These opacities may progress to produce patchy airspace consolidation. Noninfectious causes of such a pattern include drug reaction (e.g., bleomycin), early radiation pneumonitis, and pulmonary edema.

Nodular Opacities. A nodular pattern is most suggestive of pulmonary infection or neoplasm (fig. 13-2). Nodules less than 1 cm in diameter are most commonly due to viral or bacterial pneumonia, or tuberculosis (29,63,87). The nodules seen in pulmonary infections usually have a centrilobular distribution on HRCT (29). Nodules measuring more than 1 cm in diameter are most common in invasive aspergillosis, septic embolism, Kaposi's sarcoma, lymphoma, and post-transplant lymphoproliferative disorders (29,63,87). The nodules in Kaposi's sarcoma typically have irregular margins and a peribronchovascular distribution while the nodules in lymphoma and post-transplant lymphoproliferative disorders tend to have smooth margins and a random distribution (42,87).

Lymphadenopathy. Hilar and/or mediastinal lymph node enlargement is most suggestive of mycobacterial infection or a neoplastic process, most commonly lymphoma. The enlarged nodes in lymphoma, post-transplant lymphoproliferative disorders, and Kaposi's sarcoma usually have homogeneous attenuation on CT while the enlarged nodes in *Mycobacterium tuberculosis* and *M. avium-intracellulare* infection tend to have heterogeneous attenuation (58,81). HIV-seropositive patients with tuberculosis, particularly those who have fewer than 200 CD4 cells/μL, have a significantly higher prevalence of enlarged hilar and mediastinal nodes than HIV-seronegative patients (49,58). En-

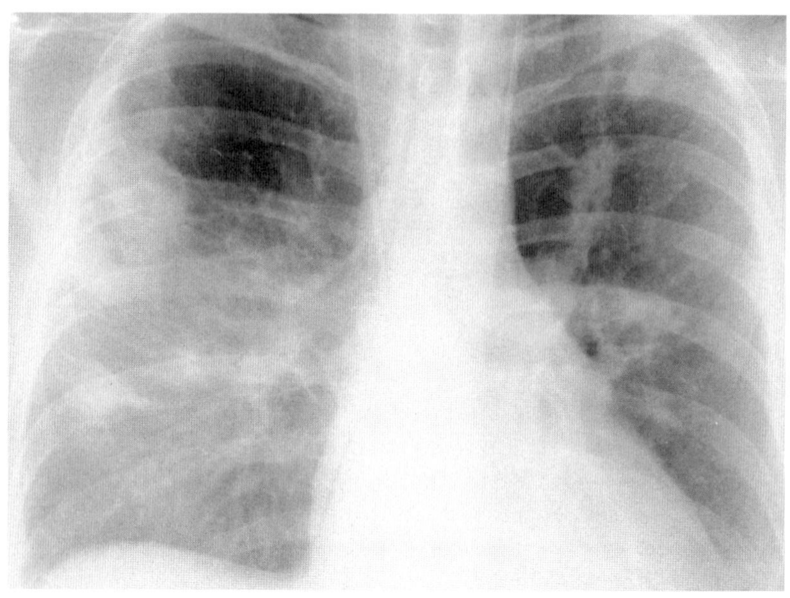

Figure 13-2

SEPTIC EMBOLISM

Chest radiograph shows poorly defined nodules ranging from 0.5 to 2.0 cm in diameter. There are small focal areas of consolidation. The patient was a 36-year-old intravenous drug abuser. Blood cultures grew *Staphylococcus aureus*.

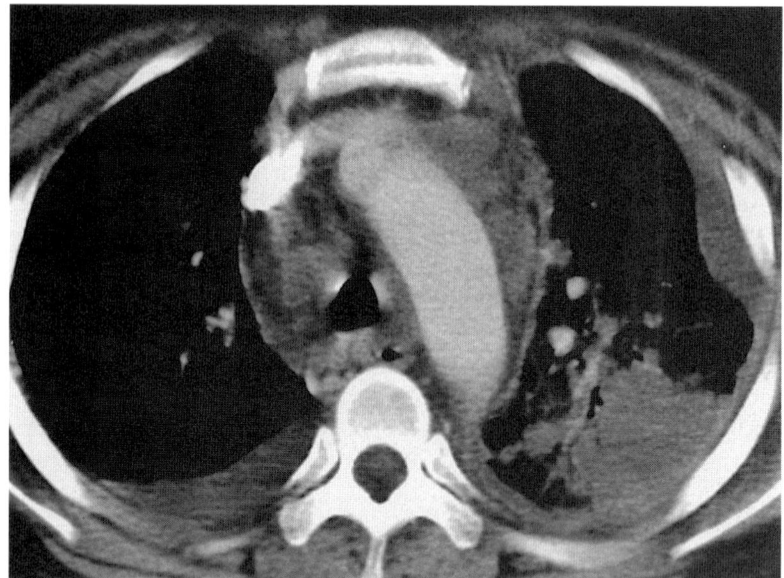

Figure 13-3

TUBERCULOSIS

Contrast-enhanced chest CT demonstrates enlarged mediastinal lymph nodes. The nodes have low attenuation centers and show slight rim enhancement. Also noted are bilateral pleural effusions and a focal area of consolidation in the left upper lobe. The patient was a 43-year-old woman with AIDS.

larged nodes in patients with tuberculosis frequently show low attenuation centers and rim enhancement following intravenous administration of contrast material (fig. 13-3) (58,81).

PATHOLOGIC PATTERNS IN LUNG BIOPSIES FROM IMMUNOCOMPROMISED PATIENTS

A key principle in the approach to interpreting lung biopsies from immunocompromised patients is to recognize the morphologic pattern of lung injury. Infectious agents tend to produce a distinctive set of histologic patterns of lung injury. Familiarity with these patterns can provide helpful clues to the diagnosis of pulmonary infections. Since each of the major organisms are discussed elsewhere in this textbook, this section primarily addresses the general principle of using these morphologic patterns as an aid in the diagnosis of lung biopsies from immunocompromised hosts. If an infectious etiology is excluded, careful clinical and radiologic correlation may be necessary to determine whether an underlying condition or a new pulmonary process caused the lung injury.

Diffuse alveolar damage (DAD) is a very common histologic reaction to infection. As discussed in chapter 3, it can occur in a variety of clinical settings, but the most common is pulmonary infection. Whenever DAD is encountered, the presence of foci of necrosis or microabscesses is strong evidence of infection. Secondary bacterial pneumonia is a common complication of DAD, so it can sometimes be difficult to sort out whether a bacterial pneumonia or a superimposed infection was the underlying cause of the DAD. Once a DAD pattern has been recognized, one should look for infectious agents that can be recognized morphologically in lung biopsy specimens such as viral inclusions (especially herpes, cytomegalovirus, measles), fungi, or *Pneumocystis carinii*. The recently described *hantavirus pulmonary syndrome* typically causes marked pulmonary edema, alveolar fibrin deposits, and an interstitial mononuclear infiltrate which may resemble the early stages of DAD but does not usually produce a classic picture of DAD with hyaline membranes (60,74).

Pulmonary infections frequently manifest as multiple or single nodules. *Nodular necrotizing granulomas,* often with cavitation, are frequently seen with mycobacterial and fungal infections such as histoplasmosis, coccidioidomycosis, blastomycosis, and cryptococcosis. *Dirofilaria* infection usually manifests as a solitary coin lesion which has the appearance of an infarct with a worm in a central artery. Rarely, *P. carinii* infection causes cavitary granulomatous inflammation. Nodular infiltrates with cavitation may also be seen with certain bacteria that cause pneumonias such as *Staphylococcus aureus,* due to their tendency to undergo necrosis and form abscesses.

Poorly formed granulomas can be seen with mycobacterial (particularly with atypical mycobacteria) infections, histoplasmosis, coccidioidomycosis, cryptococcosis, chronic necrotizing aspergillosis, and *P. carinii* pneumonia. Neutrophil microabscesses are likely to be present with blastomycosis, actinomycosis, nocardiosis, botryomycosis, melioidosis (*Burkholderia pseudomallei*), and sporotrichosis.

Granulomas, necrosis, and microabscesses can cause *diffuse micronodular infiltrates* associated with infectious organisms. If the infection is acquired by the airways, the nodules may be centered on bronchioles, but if it reaches the lungs through a hematogenous route, it may be centered either on blood vessels or alveolar walls. These millimeter-sized nodules consist of neutrophils, fibrinous exudates, histiocytes, granulomas, and foci of necrosis. This pattern of diffuse micronodular inflammatory infiltration can occur in a variety of infections including viral infection (including herpes, varicella, and cytomegalovirus), fungal infection (especially from *Candida*), miliary tuberculosis, nocardiosis, histoplasmosis, toxoplasmosis, and *Pneumocystis* and *Strongyloides* pneumonia.

Bronchiolitis may occur in a variety of settings but is characteristically observed in collagen-vascular disease, bone marrow and heart-lung transplantation, AIDS, and with certain infections by viruses such as adenovirus, influenza, parainfluenza, herpes simplex, and respiratory syncytial; *Mycoplasma pneumoniae;* and *Chlamydia* (19,65). *Necrotizing bronchiolitis* is characteristically seen with herpesvirus, respiratory syncytial virus, and adenoviral pneumonitis. Bronchiolitis may also encountered in bronchocentric fungal infections (especially with *Aspergillus*). Bronchiolitis may also be due to bacterial infection and represents an early form of bronchopneumonia.

Organizing pneumonia is a nonspecific pattern that has been called the bronchiolitis obliterans organizing pneumonia (BOOP) pattern. As discussed in chapter 8, it is best known for its association with the idiopathic condition described by Epler et al. (31). However, it is commonly seen in association with infection. Numerous reports have documented an organizing pneumonia histologic pattern due to infectious agents, including *P. carinii* (106), mycoplasma, *Nocardia asteroides* (15), *Legionella* (93), and the viruses influenza, parainfluenza, adenovirus, and herpes. In the setting of infection, there are often histologic clues to the underlying cause, such as the presence of neutrophils, microabscesses, foci of bronchopneumonia or necrosis, and granulomatous inflammation. Patients with cancer may develop organizing pneumonia associated with medications such as bleomycin or as an idiopathic problem (cryptogenic organizing pneumonia [COP]). The clinical and radiologic picture may mimic metastatic cancer to the lungs.

Perivascular chronic inflammation is a nonspecific lesion that may be seen in association with infection, lung transplant rejection, graft versus host disease, lymphoid hyperplasia, malignant lymphomas, and post-transplant lymphoproliferative disorders. This pattern of inflammation can be seen with cytomegalovirus pneumonia, *P. carinii* pneumonia, or as a systemic reaction to viruses such as Coxsackie virus, echovirus, and Epstein-Barr virus.

Cystic parenchymal changes occur in necrotizing granulomas, abscesses, or infarcts; in AIDS patients they are a frequent complication of *P. carinii* pneumonia (62,106). The cysts are often subpleural and may be associated with spontaneous pneumothorax.

The presence of foci of *acute inflammation* or *acute pneumonia* in a lung biopsy should raise the possibility of an infectious pneumonia, especially in an immunocompromised patient. The pathologic patterns of pneumonia in immunocompromised patients may be similar to those seen in normal hosts: bronchopneumonia, lobar pneumonia, and pneumonia associated with septicemia. In open lung biopsy specimens it is sometimes possible to recognize a septicemic pneumonia if the inflammation and organisms are concentrated around vessels, or if infarction is present. However, the pathologic response to a given infectious agent may be altered if the patient is leukopenic, and in some cases of neutropenia one may only see consolidation with alveolar edema and fibrin exudate with the pattern of acute fibrinous pneumonia. Airspace accumulations of neutrophils are often an indication of bacterial infection but may also be seen with many other organisms, particularly in immunocompromised patients. Neutrophilic microabscesses associated with granulomatous inflammation may be a prominent histologic lesion in other underlying diseases such as Wegener's granulomatosis and chronic granulomatous disease of childhood.

Necrotizing pneumonia is associated with extensive parenchymal necrosis. Identification of necrosis in a lung biopsy specimen should suggest an infectious process, and the pattern of necrosis can sometimes provide a clue to the underlying cause. Small foci of necrosis can be seen with viral agents, fungi, *P. carinii,* and *Toxoplasma.* Suppurative necrosis with numerous neutrophils and microabscesses can be seen with bacterial, fungal, and mycobacterial pneumonias. Large areas of infarct-like necrosis are characteristically seen with angioinvasive fungal organisms (*Aspergillus* and *Zygomyces*). Miliary foci of necrosis can occur with viruses such as cytomegalovirus and herpesvirus, especially if they spread in a hematogenous fashion.

Histologically, *lung abscesses* are walled-off collections of acute inflammatory cells (41) that may be acute or chronic. They may arise within cavitary lesions or necrotizing neoplasms. Lung abscesses may also arise in the setting of aspiration pneumonia, septic infarction, and necrotizing pneumonia. Abscesses are discussed in more detail in chapter 12.

Giant cell viral pneumonia can be caused by measles (30), parainfluenza (61), herpes varicella-zoster (92), or respiratory syncytial virus (23). In these cases, the cells exhibiting a giant cell morphology are primarily epithelial cells that demonstrate cytopathic changes (see chapter 12).

Vasculitis is a common secondary reaction to pulmonary infection. Bacterial pneumonia, most notably due to *Pseudomonas aeruginosa* (98,101) or *Legionella* species, is known to cause vasculitis. Granulomatous vasculitis can be seen with mycobacteria, granulomatous fungi such as *Histoplasma capsulatum,* and angioinvasive fungi, especially *Aspergillus* and *Mucor.* Angioinvasive fungal infections cause multiple bilateral pulmonary nodules with extensive hemorrhagic infarcts. Cytomegalovirus can cause an endothelialitis and, rarely, a necrotizing vasculitis. Noninfectious causes of pulmonary vasculitis include drug toxicity (busulfan, chlorophentermine, cromoglycate, intravenous drugs, and sulfonamides) and underlying diseases such as severe pulmonary hypertension, Wegener's granulomatosis, allergic angiitis and granulomatosis, or collagen vascular disease.

PULMONARY COMPLICATIONS OF HIV INFECTION AND AIDS

HIV is a chronic viral infection and progressive decline in immune function that predisposes to opportunistic infection or neoplasm. AIDS is the syndrome caused by infection with HIV; it is characterized by immune deficiency and one or more associated opportunistic infections,

Table 13-1

CD4 LYMPHOCYTE COUNT AND TYPE OF PULMONARY DISEASE IN HIV-INFECTED PATIENTS

Any CD4 count: upper respiratory tract illness (sinusitis, pharyngitis), acute bronchitis, bacterial pneumonia, tuberculosis, non-Hodgkin's lymphoma, pulmonary embolism, bronchogenic carcinoma

Less than 500 cells/mm^3: bacterial pneumonia, mycobacterial pneumonia (nontuberculous)

Less than 200 cells/mm^3: *Pneumocystis carinii* pneumonia, *Cryptococcus neoformans,* disseminated or extrapulmonary tuberculosis

Below 100 cells/mm^3: bacterial pneumonia, especially Gram-negative bacilli and *Staphylococcus aureus,* toxoplasmosis, cytomegalovirus, disseminated *Mycobacterium avium-intracellulare* complex, nontuberculous mycobacteria, *Histoplasma capsulatum, Coccidioides immitis,* nonendemic fungi (*Aspergillus* and *Candida* species), Kaposi's sarcoma, lymphoma

neoplasms, or conditions consistent with an acquired defect in cell-mediated immunity.

A complete discussion of HIV infection is beyond the scope of this chapter. However, several general comments about this infection are important to review. HIV infection is divided into several stages: 1) viral transmission; 2) primary HIV infection (acute HIV infection or acute seroconversion syndrome); 3) seroconversion; (4) clinical latent period with or without persistent generalized lymphadenopathy; (5) early symptomatic HIV infection; (6) AIDS; and (7) advanced HIV infection characterized by a CD4 cell count below 50/mm^3.

The rate of progression from HIV infection to AIDS depends on several factors (9): the mode of transmission (about 7 years for transfusion recipients, 10 years for hemophiliacs, 10 years for intravenous drug users, and 8 to 12 years for gay men); age at the time of seroconversion, with shorter conversion time for those 35 years or older compared to younger individuals (median, 6 years for those 35 years or older versus 15 years for patients aged 16 to 24 years); characteristics of the virus itself which influence the rate of progression, with some strains having a long latent period; and the characteristics of the CD4 count, with a worse prognosis for patients with a lower CD4 count, a steeper CD4 decline, and a higher viral burden. The rank order of first AIDS-defining conditions in the Center for Disease Control (CDC) Adult/Adolescent Spectrum of HIV Disease Sentinel Surveillance Project is as follows: *P. carinii* pneumonia, 42.6 percent; esophageal candidiasis, 15.0 percent; wasting, 10.7 percent; Kaposi's sarcoma, 10.7 percent; disseminated *M. avium* infection, 4.8 percent; tuberculosis, 4.5 percent; cytomegalovirus disease, 3.7 percent; HIV-associated dementia, 3.6 percent; recurrent bacterial pneumonia, 3.0 percent; toxoplasmosis, 2.6 percent; immunoblastic lymphoma, 1.9 percent; chronic cryptosporidiosis, 1.5 percent; Burkitt's lymphoma, 1.5 percent; disseminated histoplasmosis, 1.0 percent; invasive cervical cancer, 0.9 percent; and chronic herpes simplex, 0.5 percent.

The diagnosis of pulmonary disease in HIV-positive patients requires the multistep approach discussed in the preceding section of this chapter. Certain epidemiologic factors may predict specific disease patterns, which may be helpful when formulating a differential diagnosis in HIV-infected patients (99). For example, homosexual men have a higher incidence of Kaposi's sarcoma than other groups with AIDS and intravenous drug abusers are at increased risk for bacterial pneumonia and tuberculosis. Environmental exposures are important sources of opportunistic pathogens, e.g., homeless shelters are potential areas for transmitting tuberculosis while travel to, or living in, areas endemic for histoplasmosis and coccidioidomycosis, such as the Mississippi River Valley and the southwest, can increase the risk of these infections. Exposure to some pets is a risk factor for acquiring *Cryptosporidium, Toxoplasma,* and bacterial organisms such as *Pasteurella multocida.* Knowledge of the CD4 lymphocyte count (and possibly the viral load) can give a clue regarding the type of pulmonary disease to which the patient is susceptible (Table 13-1) (99).

There have been substantial improvements in the treatment of patients with HIV infection in the last decade. Four treatment strategies have resulted in prolonged survival in these individuals: antiretroviral therapy, *P. carinii* prophylaxis, *M. avium* prophylaxis, and improved care by physicians expert in the management of HIV-infected patients (9). As a result, hospitalization rates have fallen 45 to 50 percent and the rate of AIDS deaths has fallen dramatically since mid-1990. Only non-Hodgkin's lymphoma increased as an AIDS-defining condition since 1995 (9,67).

Highly active antiretroviral therapy (HAART) suppresses viral replication and improves immune function (110). The introduction of HAART during therapy for tuberculosis may be followed by a systemic inflammatory response within 1 to 2 weeks (14,17,35,48,55,73,82). Fishman et al. (33) reported transient worsening on radiography in 14 (45 percent) of 31 AIDS patients receiving HAART, including 7 patients (23 percent) who showed severe worsening. Worsening was first noted between 1 and 5 weeks after initiation of HAART, with improvement occurring 2 weeks to 3 months later. Four patients with severe worsening converted their tuberculin PPD (purified protein derivative) responses from anergic to positive. Organizing pneumonia with multiple necrotizing granulomas without acid-fast bacilli can be found on lung biopsy, and cultures are negative for *M. tuberculosis* or other pathogens. Continued treatment with HAART and directly observed antituberculosis therapy result in clinical improvement. After initiating HAART, clinicians should be aware of the possibility of an immunorestitution syndrome (an acute symptomatic or paradoxical deterioration) of a (presumably) preexisting infection, subacute hypersensitivity pneumonitis, or sarcoid-like granulomatous reaction that is temporally related to the recovery of the immune system (16,72).

Noninfectious Pulmonary Complications of HIV Infection

Infection is the most common pulmonary complication in patients with HIV and AIDS. In recent years the frequency of pneumonia from *Pneumocystis carinii*, cytomegalovirus, and *Mycobacterium avium-intracellulare* has decreased and there has been a rise in the incidence of bacterial pneumonias (44,67). The pathology of pulmonary infections in HIV-infected patients has some general differences compared to that of patients with an intact immune system, and most of these are described in chapter 12 where each organism is specifically discussed. However, there is a group of noninfectious pulmonary complications of HIV that are the subject of this discussion (38,51,54,83,104).

The most common of these complications are the lymphoid proliferations, including lymphocytic interstitial pneumonia (LIP), pulmonary lymphoid hyperplasia (PLH), and chronic interstitial pneumonia (CIP); the latter is the most common lung biopsy finding in HIV-positive patients with nonspecific interstitial pneumonia (NSIP/HIV) (12,105,107). Other pulmonary inflammatory complications of HIV infection include bronchiectasis (5,11,43), organizing pneumonia (BOOP, see chapter 8) (50,57), eosinophilic pneumonia (28,69), sarcoidosis, pulmonary hypertension, and alveolar proteinosis (Table 13-2) (20,36,64). The definitions and histologic features of these lesions are essentially the same as in non-HIV infected patients, so in this chapter, with the exception of LIP and CIP, the pathologic features are only briefly described, with emphasis on differences in HIV-infected patients and reference to the chapter in the text where the pathologic features are reported in more detail.

Pulmonary Lymphoid Lesions

In HIV-infected patients there is a histologic spectrum of non-neoplastic pulmonary lymphoid lesions including LIP (discussed in chapter 5), lymphoid hyperplasia, and mild cellular interstitial pneumonia (12,44,104). In addition, bronchoalveolar lavage (BAL) studies have demonstrated a lymphocytic alveolitis in HIV-infected patients (1,8,40). A diffuse infiltrative lymphocytosis syndrome that resembles Sjögren's syndrome develops in some HIV-infected patients with LIP (45,46). Each of these lymphoid proliferations can be viewed as part of a continuum, but they can usually be separated into distinct clinicopathologic syndromes which are summarized in Table 13-3.

Chronic Interstitial Pneumonia Associated with Nonspecific Interstitial Pneumonia

Definition. Chronic interstitial pneumonia (CIP) is a histologic lesion which consists of mild or moderate interstitial lymphoid infiltrates without alveolar septal infiltration that fall short of LIP.

Table 13-2

PULMONARY COMPLICATIONS OF HIV INFECTION

Infection	Interstitial and Inflammatory Lesions
Pneumocystis carinii	Lymphoid lesions
Fungi	Lymphocytic interstitial pneumonia
Bacteria	Lymphoid hyperplasia (follicular bronchiolitis)
Viruses	Chronic interstitial pneumonia (clinically known as nonspecific interstitial pneumonia)
Mycobacteria	Lymphocytic alveolitis
Parasites	Diffuse infiltrative lymphocytosis syndrome
Neoplasms	Diffuse alveolar damage
Kaposi's sarcoma	Organizing pneumonia (bronchiolitis obliterans organizing pneumonia)
Lymphoproliferative disorders	Bronchiectasis
Lung carcinoma	Eosinophilic pneumonia
	Sarcoidosis
	Alveolar proteinosis

Table 13-3

FEATURES THAT DISTINGUISH CHRONIC INTERSTITIAL PNEUMONIA FROM LYMPHOCYTIC INTERSTITIAL PNEUMONIA IN HIV-INFECTED PATIENTS[a]

Distinguishing Feature	CIP/NSIP[b]	LIP
Clinical		
Age	Common in adults; can occur in up to 33% of symptomatic patients; frequency in children is unknown	Rare in adults; common in children
Severity of symptoms	Mild; can occur in up to 48% of asymptomatic adults	Moderate to severe respiratory symptoms
Extrapulmonary involvement	Uncommon	Common both in children and adults; generalized lymphadenopathy in up to 94%; intrathoracic adenopathy in up to 25%; parotid enlargement; lymphocytic infiltration of kidney, liver, nasopharynx, bone marrow, and GI tract
Peripheral CD8 lymphocytosis	Not known	Common
Radiologic		
Normal chest radiograph	Common (up to 44%)	Uncharacteristic
Subtle increased perihilar markings	Common (up to 36%)	Uncharacteristic
Prominent nodular, interstitial or alveolar infiltrates	Uncharacteristic (up to 6%)	Characteristic
Pleural effusion	Uncommon (up to 11%)	Common (up to 31%)
Pathologic		
Severity of lymphoid infiltrate	Mild/moderate	Marked
Distribution along lymphatic routes: peribronchiolar, perivascular, pleural, interlobular septal	Characteristic	Characteristic
Alveolar septal infiltration	Uncharacteristic	Characteristic
Lymphoid aggregates (with or without germinal cancers)	Common	Common

[a]Table 1 from Travis WD, Fox CH, Devaney KO, et al. Lymphoid pneumonitis in 50 adult patients infected with the human immunodeficiency virus: lymphocytic interstitial pneumonitis versus nonspecific interstitial pneumonitis. Hum Pathol 1992;23:538.

[b]CIP/NSIP = chronic interstitial pneumonia/nonspecific interstitial pneumonia; LIP = lymphocytic interstitial pneumonia.

CIP is the most common histologic finding in lung biopsies from HIV-infected patients with the clinicopathologic syndrome described as NSIP (77,97,100). For the purposes of distinguishing NSIP in HIV patients from idiopathic NSIP, we will refer to the former as NSIP/HIV. Suffredini et al. (100) proposed the concept of NSIP to describe a group of HIV-infected adults who had clinical evidence of pneumonia in the absence of a detectable infectious agent based on lung biopsy or BAL findings. As such, NSIP is not a pathologic term but rather a clinical term. Suffredini et al. found NSIP in 38 percent of patients with AIDS and pulmonary symptoms. While some of these patients had Kaposi's sarcoma, prior *Pneumocystis carinii* pneumonia, or previous drug therapy, in some there was no other explanation for the pulmonary disease except HIV infection. In a follow-up study, Ognibene et al. (77) found CIP in 48 percent of asymptomatic HIV-infected adults. At autopsy, CIP/NSIP was found in 13 percent of AIDS patients, but it was not the primary cause of death in any patient (70). NSIP is not well characterized in children, although the term has been used without a good pathologic description (13). Thus CIP can be a histologic finding in lung biopsies from patients with mild respiratory symptoms or in asymptomatic HIV-infected patients.

Clinical Features. Patients usually present with mild symptoms of dyspnea, nonproductive cough, and fever (77,94,100). The clinical features may be impossible to separate from those of *Pneumocystis carinii* pneumonia (77,94,100).

Radiologic Findings. The radiologic features of chronic interstitial pneumonitis mimic those of other infectious and noninfectious conditions, particularly *P. carinii* pneumonia. The most common abnormality is a fine reticular or reticulonodular pattern which may be diffuse or involve predominately or exclusively the perihilar regions (39,97). A small percentage of patients have associated pleural effusion or hilar lymphadenopathy (39,97). Up to 44 percent of patients have a normal chest radiograph (97).

Pathologic Findings. The pathologic term, CIP, has been applied to these cases (104). This is the most common histologic pattern found in patients with the clinical syndrome of HIV-associated NSIP (104).

The typical histologic finding in CIP associated with NSIP/HIV is mild to moderate, interstitial, chronic inflammation, frequently in a peribronchiolar and/or perivascular location (fig. 13-4). The lymphoid infiltrate lacks the extensive alveolar septal infiltration seen in LIP. Mild hyperplasia of type 2 pneumocytes can be present (fig. 13-4).

Lymphoid hyperplasia can occur in association with the CIP of NSIP/HIV as well as LIP. A case reported as lymphocytic bronchiolitis by Ettensohn et al. (32), probably fits best into this group of lesions. Follicular bronchiolitis or bronchus-associated lymphoid tissue (BALT) hyperplasia also may occur by itself as the primary pulmonary lesion. It is characterized by enlarged or hyperplastic lymphoid aggregates situated adjacent to bronchioles (fig. 13-5) (51,104,112).

Differential Diagnosis. CIP is a diagnosis of exclusion after the presence of an opportunistic infection has been ruled out by BAL analysis or review of special stains for organisms on lung biopsies. It is distinguished from LIP in that the interstitial lymphoid infiltrates are mild, without extensive infiltration of alveolar septa.

Treatment and Prognosis. Patients with the clinical syndrome of NSIP who have a CIP pattern on lung biopsy usually have a mild clinical course (44,77,94,100). Most patients experience spontaneous resolution without treatment. If patients deteriorate, repeat bronchoscopy with biopsy should be considered to pursue a different clinical problem, especially an infection (44,100). Patients with NSIP/HIV usually do not die from this condition (95): in one study, long-term survival was less than 3 years but death was due to infections or neoplasms (39).

Pathogenesis of Lymphoid Lesions in HIV-Infected Patients

Both host genetic and immune factors are thought to play a role in the pathogenesis of pulmonary lymphoid lesions in HIV infection, although the pathogenesis is not completely understood (45,46,68). HIV itself as well as other viruses, such as Epstein-Barr virus or cytomegalovirus, have been considered potential causative agents (68). HIV was initially demonstrated in pulmonary specimens from HIV-infected patients by Ziza et al. (113), and subsequently by many other investigators (18,85,89). HIV has

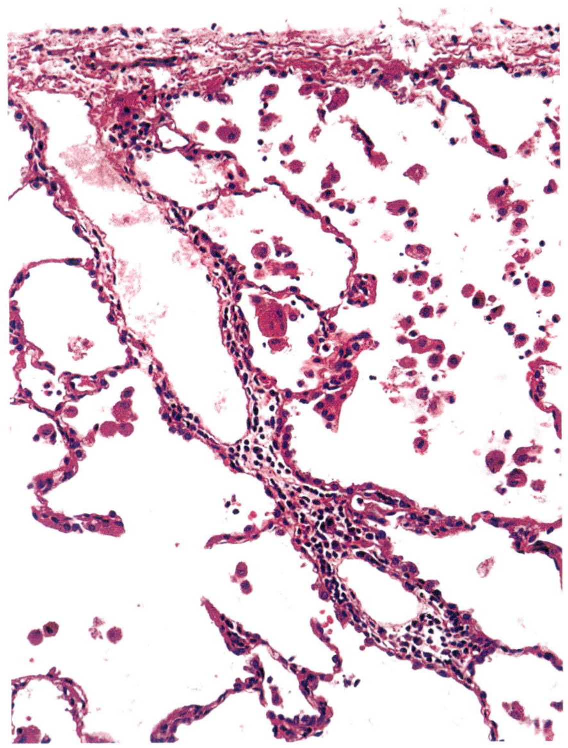

Figure 13-4

NONSPECIFIC INTERSTITIAL PNEUMONIA/ CHRONIC INTERSTITIAL PNEUMONIA IN HIV-INFECTED ADULT

Alveolar septa are infiltrated by mild interstitial chronic inflammation.

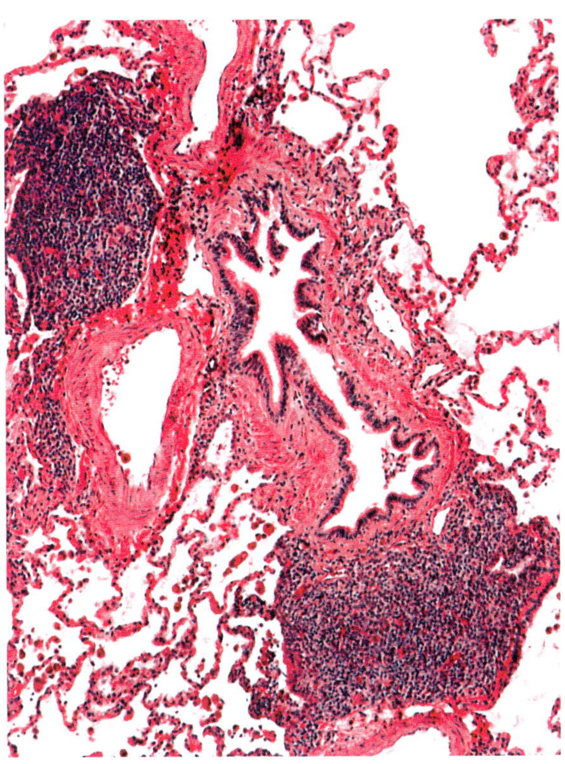

Figure 13-5

FOLLICULAR BRONCHIOLITIS OR HYPERPLASIA OF THE BALT IN HIV-INFECTED ADULT

There are hyperplastic lymphoid follicles adjacent to a bronchiole.

been shown to infect alveolar macrophages, CD4 lymphocytes, fibroblasts, and dendritic cells both in vivo and in vitro (68,85). Few studies have demonstrated HIV directly in lung biopsy tissue. Using in situ hybridization, HIV was shown to be concentrated in the germinal centers in a patient with LIP (104). This correlates with data from lymphoid tissue, which shows that lymphoid germinal centers are reservoirs of HIV (34). A variety of cytokines are abnormally expressed in vitro by HIV-infected cells including IL-1, IL-2, IL-6, IL-8, IL-10, tumor necrosis factor (TNF)-alpha, and granulocyte-macrophage colony-stimulating factor (GM-CSF) (24,25,56,68). The cytokines may be mediators that influence lung injury, inflammatory cell recruitment, or HIV replication (68). In addition, immune complexes have been seen in the BAL fluid of HIV-infected children (75) and adults. The absence of other infectious agents combined with the presence of HIV suggest that HIV plays an important causative role in pulmonary lymphoid lesions (96,113).

Epstein-Barr virus has also been proposed to play a role in LIP associated with HIV infection. In several studies, it has been recovered from some lung biopsies from HIV-infected patients with LIP (6,66,91,104).

Lymphocytic Alveolitis

Lymphocytic alveolitis is commonly found by BAL fluid analysis in HIV-infected patients (7,8,22,40,80,86,108,109). BAL lymphocytosis was seen by Guillon (40) in 78 percent of 154 HIV-infected patients with lung infections or tumors and in 72 percent of 122 patients without lung infections or tumors. The immunophenotypes of the majority of the BAL lymphocytes were CD8+ and CD44+ (40). Studies by Autran et al. (7) and Plata et al. (84) showed

Table 13-4

DIFFUSE INFILTRATIVE LYMPHOCYTOSIS SYNDROME (DILS) IN HIV INFECTION VERSUS SJÖGREN'S SYNDROME[a]

	Sjögren's Syndrome	DILS
Glandular manifestations	Moderate parotid enlargement	Massive parotid enlargement
Extraglandular manifestations	Infrequent; may have pulmonary, gastrointestinal, renal, and neurologic involvement	Prominent; pulmonary, gastrointestinal, renal, and neurologic involvement
Infiltrative lymphocytic phenotype	CD4 predominant	CD8 predominant
Autoantibodies	High frequency rheumatoid factor, ANA[b], anti-Ro/SSA, anti LA/SSB	Low frequency rheumatoid factor, ANA, anti-Ro/SSA, anti LA/SSB
HLA association	B8, DR2, DR3, DR4 (rheumatoid arthritis)	DR5, DR6 (blacks), DR6 (whites)

[a]Table 1 from Itescu S. Diffuse infiltrative lymphocytosis syndrome in children and adults infected with HIV-1: a model of rheumatic illness caused by acquired viral infection. Am J Reprod Immunol 1992;28:248.
[b]ANA = antinuclear antibody; HLA = human leukocyte antigen.

that the BAL cytotoxic T lymphocytes have cytolytic activity against HIV-infected alveolar macrophages and that this activity is restricted by class I human leukocyte antigen (HLA) transplantation antigens. The open lung biopsy findings in four patients with BAL lymphocytic alveolitis reported by Guillon et al. showed CIP consisting of CD8+ lymphocytes. This observation combined with the finding that CIP/NSIP and lymphocytic alveolitis are found in a similar percentage of asymptomatic HIV-infected patients (48 percent [77] and 59 percent [40], respectively) suggests that they represent the same pulmonary inflammatory lesion detected by different methods.

Diffuse Infiltrative Lymphocytosis Syndrome

The diffuse infiltrative lymphocytosis syndrome (DILS) was described by Itescu et al. (46) in HIV-infected patients who develop a Sjögren's syndrome–like disorder. There is a bimodal age pattern, with a peak at 14 years of age and between 22 to 62 years of age (45). Bilateral parotid gland enlargement and xerostomia or xerophthalmia are common. Generalized lymphadenopathy and LIP are frequent. Less often, patients have neurologic involvement or lymphocytic infiltration of the gastrointestinal tract (46). Most patients have a polyclonal hypergammaglobulinemia (46). The infiltrating lymphocytes are CD8+ T cells that have a memory phenotype (45). DILS and Sjögren's syndrome are compared in Table 13-4.

Immunologic and genetic factors are important in DILS (45,46), as shown by data that susceptibility in blacks is associated with HLA-DR5 and HLA-DR6 while in whites it is only associated with HLA-DR6 (46).

Diffuse Alveolar Damage

When the histologic pattern of diffuse alveolar damage (DAD) is found in the lungs of an HIV-infected patient, it is usually associated with infection. Rarely, however, it occurs in the absence of a detectable etiology (88,100). Ramaswamy et al. (88) described 12 AIDS patients with lung biopsies showing DAD without detectable infection. Studies from the National Institutes of Health (NIH) of 46 HIV-infected adults with NSIP revealed a DAD pattern in 6.5 percent (77,100,104). The histologic features of DAD in HIV-infected patients are similar to those seen in patients without HIV infection (53,78).

Organizing Pneumonia (Cryptogenic Organizing Pneumonia/Bronchiolitis Obliterans Organizing Pneumonia)

Rare HIV-infected patients have been reported to develop cryptogenic organizing pneumonia (COP)/bronchiolitis obliterans organizing pneumonia (BOOP) (3,50,57) The clinical and histologic features are similar to the organizing

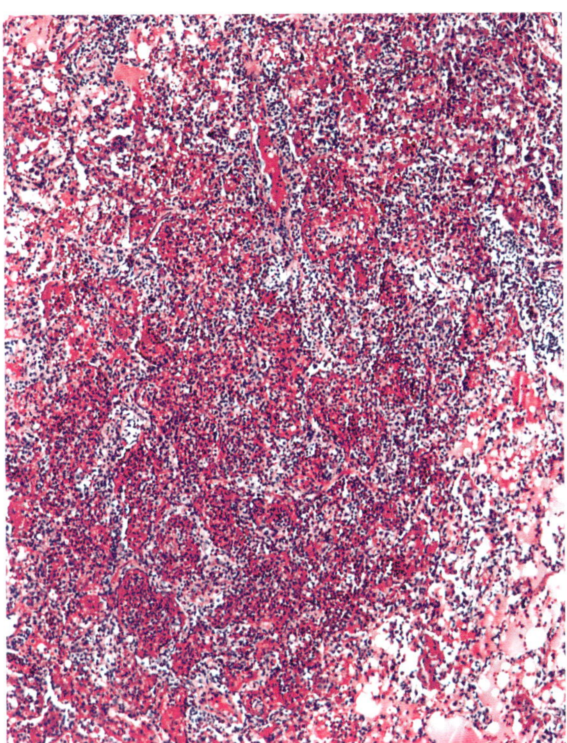
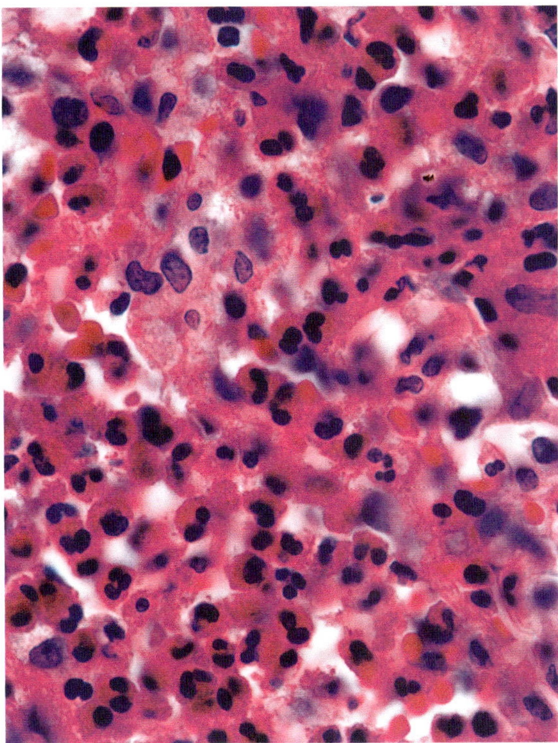

Figure 13-6

EOSINOPHILIC PNEUMONIA

Eosinophilic pneumonia in a pediatric HIV-infected patient with associated *Bipolaris* sp fungal infection from an intravenous line.

Left: The lung shows an extensive intra-alveolar cellular infiltrate.

Right: There are numerous eosinophils indicating eosinophilic pneumonia. No fungus was found in the lung.

pneumonia pattern seen in patients without HIV infection (21,31) (see chapter 3). In HIV-infected patients it is particularly important for pathologists to exclude an infectious etiology, especially *Pneumocystis carinii* pneumonia (106).

Obstructive Lung Disease and Bronchiectasis

Obstructive lung disease is commonly found in HIV-infected patients (44,76). O'Donnell et al. (76) found decreased forced expiratory flow rates in up to one third of HIV-infected patients; two thirds of these patients responded to bronchodilators (44). Diaz et al. (26) recently found evidence of early emphysema in HIV-infected patients by demonstrating decreased diffusing capacity with abnormal HRCT scans. A history of asthma is reported in 21 percent of patients prior to developing HIV infection (44). Up to 17 percent of HIV-infected patients have asthma, which progresses in 60 percent in these patients (44).

A few cases of bronchiectasis have been reported HIV-infected patients, mostly in children (5,11,43). Amorosa et al. (5) found bronchiectasis in 4 of 32 patients with LIP. Holmes et al. (43) reported bronchiectasis in seven patients without lymphocytic interstitial pneumonitis, six of whom had recurrent episodes of infection. Bronchiectasis tends to occur in HIV-infected patients after many years.

Eosinophilic Pneumonia

A few cases of eosinophilic pneumonia have been reported in HIV-infected patients (28,69). These included several cases of acute eosinophilic pneumonia (2,69). The clinical features were similar to those described in chapter 8 (2, 69), however, associations with drugs such as maloprim (10) or pentamidine (28) were reported. Eosinophilic pneumonia may also occur in association with fungal infections (fig. 13-6).

Sarcoidosis

Rarely, HIV-infected patients develop sarcoidosis (20,36,64). Patients present with fever, weight loss, fatigue, and pulmonary symptoms as well as cutaneous anergy and elevated serum polyclonal gammaglobulin levels (64). BAL analysis shows a lymphocytic alveolitis characterized by a CD4 predominance in contrast to the CD8 predominance typically seen in most HIV-infected patients. The clinical features, diagnostic criteria, and histologic features are similar to those in patients without HIV-infection (see chapter 3). It is very important to exclude infection since granulomas are also found in HIV-infected patients with fungal, mycobacterial, or *Pneumocystis carinii* infection. Patients may respond to corticosteroid therapy (64).

Alveolar Proteinosis

Rare cases of alveolar proteinosis are reported in AIDS patients (90,102). For pathologists, the major concern in the diagnosis of alveolar proteinosis is distinction from *Pneumocystis carinii* pneumonia, which has a similar eosinophilic alveolar exudate. This differential diagnosis is discussed in chapter 3. The distinction may be difficult, especially if the pneumonia has been treated and the organisms have either been reduced markedly in number or eliminated entirely.

Pulmonary Hypertension

Pulmonary hypertension is a well recognized but relatively uncommon pulmonary complication of HIV infection (71). Mesa et al. (71) recently reviewed 88 patients with pulmonary hypertension and HIV infection. There was a male predominance (61 percent) and a mean age of 32 years (range, 2 to 56 years). Patients typically presented with dyspnea. Of the 33 patients with histologic evaluation of lung tissue, a plexogenic pattern was seen in 28 (85 percent), followed by 3 with thrombotic pulmonary arteriopathy, and 2 with veno-occlusive disease. Mesa et al. could not find any correlation between onset of pulmonary hypertension and CD4 counts or previous pulmonary infections. It is thought that in most cases the pulmonary hypertension is associated with chronic HIV infection. The 1-year survival rate was 51 percent and in most cases death was thought to be due to pulmonary hypertension.

REFERENCES

1. Agostini C, Zambello R, Trentin L, et al. Prognostic significance of the evaluation of bronchoalveolar lavage cell populations in patients with HIV-1 infection and pulmonary involvement. Chest 1991;100:1601–6.
2. Allen JN, Pacht ER, Gadek JE, Davis WB. Acute eosinophilic pneumonia as a reversible cause of noninfectious respiratory failure. N Engl J Med 1989;321:569–74.
3. Allen JN, Wewers MD. HIV-associated bronchiolitis obliterans organizing pneumonia. Chest 1989;96:197–8.
4. Amin Z, Miller RF, Shaw PJ. Lobar or segmental consolidation on chest radiographs of patients with HIV infection. Clin Radiol 1997;52:541–5.
5. Amorosa JK, Miller RW, Laraya-Cuasay L, et al. Bronchiectasis in children with lymphocytic interstitial pneumonia and acquired immune deficiency syndrome. Plain film and CT observations. Pediatr Radiol 1992;22:603–6.
6. Andiman WA, Eastman R, Martin K, et al. Opportunistic lymphoproliferations associated with Epstein-Barr viral DNA in infants and children with AIDS. Lancet 1985;2:1390–3.
7. Autran B, Mayaud CM, Raphael M, et al. Evidence for a cytotoxic T-lymphocyte alveolitis in human immunodeficiency virus-infected patients. AIDS 1988;2:179–83.
8. Autran B, Sadat-Sowti B, Hadida F, et al. HIV-specific cytotoxic T lymphocytes against alveolar macrophages: specificities and downregulation. Res Virol 1991;142:113–8.
9. Bartlett JG. Natural history and classification of HIV-1 infection. In: Rose BD, ed. Uptodate in medicine 2000. Wellesley: BDR-Uptodate; 2000.

10. Begbie S, Burgess KR. Maloprim-induced pulmonary eosinophilia. Chest 1993;103:305–6.
11. Berdon WE, Mellins RB, Abramson SJ, Ruzal-Shapiro C. Pediatric HIV infection in its second decade–the changing pattern of lung involvement. Clinical, plain film, and computed tomographic findings. Radiol Clin North Am 1993;31:453–63.
12. Brodie SJ, de la Rosa C, Howe JG, Crouch J, Travis WD, Diem K. Pediatric AIDS-associated lymphocytic interstitial pneumonia and pulmonary arterio-occlusive disease: role of VCAM-1/VLA-4 adhesion pathway and human herpesviruses. Am J Pathol 1999;154:1453–64.
13. Bye MR, Bernstein L, Shah K, Ellaurie M, Rubinstein A. Diagnostic bronchoalveolar lavage in children with AIDS. Pediatr Pulmonol 1987;3:425–8.
14. Cabie A, Abel S, Brebion A, Desbois N, Sobesky G. Mycobacterial lymphadenitis after initiation of highly active antiretroviral therapy. Eur J Clin Microbiol Infect Dis 1998;17:812–3.
15. Camp M, Mehta JB, Whitson M. Bronchiolitis obliterans and Nocardia asteroides infection of the lung. Chest 1987;92:1107–8.
16. Cheng VC, Yuen K, Chan WM, Wong SS, Ma ES, Chan RM. Immunorestitution disease involving the innate and adaptive response. Clin Infect Dis 2000;30:882–92.
17. Chien JW, Johnson JL. Paradoxical reactions in HIV and pulmonary TB. Chest 1998;114:933–6.
18. Clarke JR, Mitchell D. Evidence for human immunodeficiency virus infection of the lung. Monaldi Arch Chest Dis 1993;48:360–5.
19. Colby TV, Myers JL. Clinical and histologic spectrum of bronchiolitis obliterans, including bronchiolitis obliterans organizing pneumonia. Semin Respir Med 1992;13:119–33.
20. Coots LE, Lazarus AA. Bronchoalveolar lavage in sarcoidosis and HIV infection [Letter]. Chest 1990;98:517–8.
21. Davison AG, Heard BE, McAllister WA, Turner-Warwick ME. Cryptogenic organizing pneumonitis. Q J Med 1983;207:382–94.
22. de Blic J, Blanche S, Danel C, Le Bourgeois M, Caniglia M, Scheinmann P. Bronchoalveolar lavage in HIV infected patients with interstitial pneumonitis. Arch Dis Child 1989;64:1246–50.
23. Delage G, Brochu P, Robillard L, Jasmin G, Joncas JH, Lapointe N. Giant cell pneumonia due to respiratory syncytial virus. Occurrence in severe combined immunodeficiency syndrome. Arch Pathol Lab Med 984;108:623–5.
24. Denis M, Ghadirian E. Alveolar macrophages from subjects infected with HIV-1 express macrophage inflammatory protein-1 alpha (MIP-1 alpha): contribution to the CD8+ alveolitis. Clin Exp Immunol 1994;96:187–92.
25. Denis M, Ghadirian E. Dysregulation of interleukin 8, interleukin 10, and interleukin 12 release by alveolar macrophages from HIV type 1-infected subjects. AIDS Res Hum Retroviruses 1994;10:1619–27.
26. Diaz PT, King MA, Pacht ER, et al. The pathophysiology of pulmonary diffusion impairment in human immunodeficiency virus infection. Am J Respir Crit Care Med 1999;160:272–7.
27. Dichter JR, Levine SJ, Shelhamer JH. Approach to the immunocompromised host with pulmonary symptoms. Hematol Oncol Clin North Am 1993;7:887–912.
28. Dupon M, Malou M, Rogues AM, Lacut JY. Acute eosinophilic pneumonia induced by inhaled pentamidine isethionate. BMJ 1993;306:109.
29. Edinburgh KJ, Jasmer RM, Huang L, et al. Multiple pulmonary nodules in AIDS: usefulness of CT in distinguishing among potential causes. Radiology 2000;214:427–32.
30. Enders JF, McCarthy K, Mitus A, Cheatham WJ. Isolation of measles virus at autopsy in cases of giant-cell pneumonia without rash. N Eng J Med 1959;261:875–81.
31. Epler GR, Colby TV, McLoud TC, Carrington CB, Gaensler EA. Bronchiolitis obliterans organizing pneumonia. N Engl J Med 1985;312:152–8.
32. Ettensohn DB, Mayer KH, Kessimian N, Smith PS. Lymphocytic bronchiolitis associated with HIV infection. Chest 1988;93:201–2.
33. Fishman JE, Saraf-Lavi E, Narita M, Hollender ES, Ramsinghani R, Ashkin D. Pulmonary tuberculosis in AIDS patients: transient chest radiographic worsening after initiation of antiretroviral therapy. AJR Am J Roentgenol 2000;174:43–9.
34. Fox CH, Tenner-Racz K, Racz P, Firpo A, Pizzo PA, Fauci AS. Lymphoid germinal centers are reservoirs of human immunodeficiency virus type 1 RNA. J Infect Dis 1991;164:1051–7.
35. Furrer H, Malinverni R. Systemic inflammatory reaction after starting highly active antiretroviral therapy in AIDS patients treated for extrapulmonary tuberculosis. Am J Med 1999;106:371–2.
36. Gowda KS, Mayers I, Shafran SD. Concomitant sarcoidosis and HIV infection. Can Med Assoc J 1990;142:136–7.
37. Graham NJ, Müller NL, Miller RR, Shepherd JD. Intrathoracic complications following allogeneic bone marrow transplantation: CT findings. Radiology 1991;181:153–6.

38. Grieco MH, Chinoy-Acharya P. Lymphocytic interstitial pneumonia associated with the acquired immune deficiency syndrome. Am Rev Respir Dis 1985;131:952–5.
39. Griffiths MH, Miller RF, Semple SJ. Interstitial pneumonitis in patients infected with the human immunodeficiency virus. Thorax 1995;50:1141–6.
40. Guillon JM, Autran B, Denis M, et al. Human immunodeficiency virus-related lymphocytic alveolitis. Chest 1988;94:1264–70.
41. Hagan JL, Hardy JD. Lung abscess revisited. A survey of 184 cases. Ann Surg 1983;197:755–62.
42. Hartman TE, Primack SL, Müller NL, Staples CA. Diagnosis of thoracic complications in AIDS: accuracy of CT. AJR Am J Roentgenol 1994;162:547–53.
43. Holmes AH, Trotman-Dickenson B, Edwards A, Peto T, Luzzi GA. Bronchiectasis in HIV disease. Q J Med 1992;85:875–82.
44. Huang L, Stansell JD. Pulmonary complications of human immunodeficiency virus infection. In: Murray JF, Nadel JA, Mason RJ, Boushey HA Jr, eds. Textbook of respiratory medicine, 3rd ed. Philadelphia: WB Saunders; 2000:2171–221.
45. Itescu S. Diffuse infiltrative lymphocytosis syndrome in children and adults infected with HIV-1: a model of rheumatic illness caused by acquired viral infection. Am J Reprod Immunol 1992;28:247–50.
46. Itescu S, Brancato LJ, Buxbaum J, et al. A diffuse infiltrative CD8 lymphocytosis syndrome in human immunodeficiency virus (HIV) infection: a host immune response associated with HLA-DR5. Ann Intern Med 1990;112:3–10.
47. Janzen DL, Adler BD, Padley SP, Müller NL. Diagnostic success of bronchoscopic biopsy in immunocompromised patients with acute pulmonary disease: predictive value of disease distribution as shown on CT. AJR Am J Roentgenol 1993;160:21–4.
48. John M, French MA. Exacerbation of the inflammatory response to Mycobacterium tuberculosis after antiretroviral therapy. Med J Aust 1998;169:473–4.
49. Jones BE, Young SM, Antoniskis D, Davidson PT, Kramer F, Barnes PF. Relationship of the manifestations of tuberculosis to CD4 cell counts in patients with human immunodeficiency virus infection. Am Rev Respir Dis 1993;148:1292–7.
50. Joseph J, Harley RA, Frye MD. Bronchiolitis obliterans with organizing pneumonia in AIDS [Letter]. N Engl J Med 1995;332:273.
51. Joshi VV, Oleske JM, Minnefor AB, et al. Pathologic pulmonary findings in children with the acquired immunodeficiency syndrome: a study of ten cases. Hum Pathol 1985;16:241–6.
52. Kang EY, Staples CA, McGuinness G, Primack SL, Müller NL. Detection and differential diagnosis of pulmonary infections and tumors in patients with AIDS: value of chest radiography versus CT. AJR Am J Roentgenol 1996;166:15–9.
53. Katzenstein AL, Bloor CM, Leibow AA. Diffuse alveolar damage—the role of oxygen, shock, and related factors. A review. Am J Pathol 1976;85: 209–28.
54. Kornstein MJ, Pietra GG, Hoxie JA, Conley ME. The pathology and treatment of interstitial pneumonitis in two infants with AIDS. Am Rev Respir Dis 1986;133:1196–8.
55. Kunimoto DY, Chui L, Nobert E, Houston S. Immune mediated 'HAART' attack during treatment for tuberculosis. Highly active antiretroviral therapy. Int J Tuberc Lung Dis 1999;3:944–7.
56. Lairmore MD, Butera ST, Callahan GN, DeMartini JC. Spontaneous interferon production by pulmonary leukocytes is associated with lentivirus-induced lymphoid interstitial pneumonia. J Immunol 1988;140:779–85.
57. Leo YS, Pitchon HE, Messler G, Meyer RD. Bronchiolitis obliterans organizing pneumonia in a patient with AIDS. Clin Infect Dis 1994;18:921–4.
58. Leung AN, Brauner MW, Gamsu G, et al. Pulmonary tuberculosis: comparison of CT findings in HIV-seropositive and HIV-seronegative patients. Radiology 1996;198:687–91.
59. Levine SJ. An approach to the diagnosis of pulmonary infections in immunosuppressed patients. Semin Respir Infect 1992;7:81–95.
60. Levy H, Simpson SQ. Hantavirus pulmonary syndrome. Am J Respir Crit Care Med 1994;149:1710–3.
61. Little BW, Tihen WS, Dickerman JD, Craighead JE. Giant cell pneumonia associated with parainfluenza virus type 3 infection. Hum Pathol 1981;12:478–81.
62. Liu YC, Tomashefski JF Jr, Tomford JW, Green H. Necrotizing Pneumocystis carinii vasculitis associated with lung necrosis and cavitation in a patient with aquired immunodeficiency syndrome. Arch Pathol Lab Med 1989;113:494–7.
63. Logan PM, Primack SL, Staples C, Miller RR, Müller NL. Acute lung disease in the immunocompromised host. Diagnostic accuracy of the chest radiograph. Chest 1995;108:1283–7.
64. Lowery WS, Whitlock WL, Dietrich RA, Fine JM. Sarcoidosis complicated by HIV infection: three case reports and a review of the literature. Am Rev Respir Dis 1990;142:887–9.
65. Lugo RA, Nahata MC. Pathogenesis and treatment of bronchiolitis. Clin Pharm 1993;12:95–116.

66. Malamou-Mitsi V, Tsai MM, Gal AA, Koss MN, O'Leary TJ. Lymphoid interstitial pneumonia not associated with HIV infection: role of Epstein-Barr virus. Mod Pathol 1992;5:487–91.
67. Masliah E, DeTeresa RM, Mallory ME, Hansen LA. Changes in pathological findings at autopsy in AIDS cases for the last 15 years. AIDS 2000;14:69–74.
68. Mayaud CM, Cadranel J. HIV in the lung: guilty or not guilty? Thorax 1993;48:1191–5.
69. Mayo J, Collazos J, Martinez E, Diaz F. Acute eosinophilic pneumonia in a patient infected with the human immunodeficiency virus. Tuber Lung Dis 1995;76:77–9.
70. McKenzie R, Travis WD, Dolan SA, et al. The causes of death in patients with human immunodeficiency virus infection: a clinical and pathologic study with emphasis on the role of pulmonary diseases. Medicine (Baltimore) 1991;70:326–43.
71. Mesa RA, Edell ES, Dunn WF, Edwards WD. Human immunodeficiency virus infection and pulmonary hypertension: two new cases and a review of 86 reported cases. Mayo Clin Proc 1998;73:37–45.
72. Morris AM, Nishimura S, Huang L. Subacute hypersensitivity pneumonitis in an HIV infected patient receiving antiretroviral therapy. Thorax 2000;55:625–7.
73. Narita M, Ashkin D, Hollender ES, Pitchenik AE. Paradoxical worsening of tuberculosis following antiretroviral therapy in patients with AIDS. Am J Respir Crit Care Med 1998; 158:157–61.
74. Nolte KB, Feddersen RM, Foucar K, et al. Hantavirus pulmonary syndrome in the United States: a pathological description of a disease caused by a new agent. Hum Pathol 1995; 26:110–20.
75. Nowakowski M, Clarke LM, Amaro R, Pellegrino MG, Sierra MF, Steiner P. Characterization of cells, immunoglobulins, and immune complexes present in the bronchoalveolar lavage of pediatric AIDS patients. Reg Immunol 1992;4:34–40.
76. O'Donnell CR, Bader MB, Zibrak JD, Jensen WA, Rose RM. Abnormal airway function in individuals with the acquired immunodeficiency syndrome. Chest 1988;94:945–8.
77. Ognibene FP, Masur H, Rogers P, et al. Nonspecific interstitial pneumonitis without evidence of Pneumocystis carinii in asymptomatic patients infected with human immunodeficiency virus (HIV). Ann Intern Med 1988;109:874–9.
78. Olson J, Colby TV, Elliott CG. Hamman-Rich syndrome revisited. Mayo Clin Proc 1990;65:1538–48.
79. Padley SP, Adler B, Hansell DM, Müller NL. High-resolution computed tomography of drug-induced lung disease. Clin Radiol 1992;46:232–6.
80. Palange P, Carlone S, Venditti M, et al. Alveolar cell population in HIV infected patients. Eur Respir J 1991;4:639–42.
81. Pastores SM, Naidich DP, Aranda CP, McGuinnes G, Rom WN. Intrathoracic adenopathy associated with pulmonary tuberculosis in patients with human immunodeficiency virus infection. Chest 1993;103:1433–7.
82. Phillips P, Kwiatkowski MB, Copland M, Craib K, Montaner J. Mycobacterial lymphadenitis associated with the initiation of combination antiretroviral therapy. J Acquir Immune Defic Syndr Hum Retrovirol 1999;20:122–8.
83. Pitt J. Lymphocytic interstitial pneumonia. Pediatr Clin North Am 1991;38:89-95.
84. Plata F, Autran B, Martins LP, et al. AIDS virus-specific cytotoxic T lymphocytes in lung disorders. Nature 1987;328:348–51.
85. Plata F, Garcia-Pons F, Ryter A, et al. HIV-1 infection of lung alveolar fibroblasts and macrophages in humans. AIDS Res Hum Retroviruses 1990;6:979–86.
86. Plaza V, Jimenez P, Xaubet A, et al. Bronchoalveolar lavage cell analysis in patients with human immunodeficiency virus related diseases. Thorax 1989;44:289–91.
87. Primack SL, Müller NL. High-resolution computed tomography in acute diffuse lung disease in the immunocompromised patient. Radiol Clin North Am 1994;32:731–44.
88. Ramaswamy G, Jagadha V, Tchertkoff V. Diffuse alveolar damage and interstitial fibrosis in acquired immunodeficiency syndrome patients without concurrent pulmonary infection. Arch Pathol Lab Med 1985;109:408–12.
89. Resnick L, Pitchenik AE, Fisher E, Croney R. Detection of HTLV-III/LAV-specific IgG and antigen in bronchoalveolar lavage fluid from two patients with lymphocytic interstitial pneumonitis associated with AIDS-related complex. Am J Med 1987;82:553–6.
90. Ruben FL, Talamo TS. Secondary pulmonary alveolar proteinosis occurring in two patients with acquired immune deficiency syndrome. Am J Med 1986;80:1187–90.
91. Rubinstein A, Morecki R, Silverman B, et al. Pulmonary disease in children with acquired immune deficiency syndrome and AIDS-related complex. J Pediatr 1986;108:498–503.
92. Saito F, Yutani C, Imakita M, Ishibashi-Ueda H, Kanzaki T, Chiba Y. Giant cell pneumonia caused by varicella zoster virus in a neonate. Arch Pathol Lab Med 1989;113:201–3.

93. Sato P, Madtes DK, Thorning D, Albert RK. Bronchiolitis obliterans caused by Legionella pneumophila. Chest 1985;87:840–2.
94. Sattler F, Nichols L, Hirano L, et al. Nonspecific interstitial pneumonitis mimicking Pneumocystis carinii pneumonia. Am J Respir Crit Care Med 1997;156:912–7.
95. Schneider RF. Lymphocytic interstitial pneumonitis and nonspecific interstitial pneumonitis. Clin Chest Med 1996;17:763–6.
96. Setoguchi Y, Takahashi S, Nukiwa T, Kira S. Detection of human T-cell lymphotropic virus type I-related antibodies in patients with lymphocytic interstitial pneumonia. Am Rev Respir Dis 1991;144:1361–5.
97. Simmons JT, Suffredini AF, Lack EE, et al. Nonspecific interstitial pneumonitis in patients with AIDS: radiologic features. AJR Am J Roentgenol 1987;149:265–8.
98. Soave R, Murray HW, Litrenta MM. Bacterial invasion of pulmonary vessels. Pseudomonas bacteremia mimicking pulmonary thromboembolism with infarction. Am J Med 1978;65:864–7.
99. Stover DE. Approach to the HIV-infected patient with pulmonary symptoms. In: Rose BD, ed. Uptodate in medicine 2000. Wellesley: BDR-Uptodate; 2000.
100. Suffredini AF, Ognibene FP, Lack EE, et al. Nonspecific interstitial pneumonitis: a common cause of pulmonary disease in the acquired immunodeficiency syndrome. Ann Intern Med 1987;107:7–13.
101. Teplitz C. Pathogenesis of Pseudomonas vasculitis and septic lesions. Arch Pathol Lab Med 1965;80:297–307.
102. Tran Van Nhieu J, Vojtek AM, Bernaudin JF, Escudier E, Fleury-Feith J. Pulmonary alveolar proteinosis associated with Pneumocystis carinii. Ultrastructural identification in bronchoalveolar lavage in AIDS and immunocompromised non-AIDS patients. Chest 1990;98:801–5.
103. Travis WD. Surgical pathology of pulmonary infections. Semin Thorac Cardiovasc Surg 1995;7:62–9.
104. Travis WD, Fox CH, Devaney KO, et al. Lymphoid pneumonitis in 50 adult patients infected with the human immunodeficiency virus: lymphocytic interstitial pneumonitis versus nonspecific interstitial pneumonitis. Hum Pathol 1992;23:529–41.
105. Travis WD, Lack EE, Ognibene FP, Suffredini AF, Shelhamer J. Lung biopsy interpretation in the acquired immunodeficiency syndrome: experience of the National Institutes of Health with literature review. Prog AIDS Pathol 1989;1:51–84.
106. Travis WD, Pittaluga S, Lipschik GY, et al. Atypical pathologic manifestations of Pneumocystis carinii pneumonia in the acquired immune deficiency syndrome. Review of 123 lung biopsies from 76 patients with emphasis on cysts, vascular invasion, vasculitis, and granulomas. Am J Surg Pathol 1990;14:615–25.
107. Travis WD, Roth DB. Histopathologic evaluation of lung biopsy specimens. In: Shelhamer J, Pizzo PA, Parrillo JE, Masur H, eds. Respiratory disease in the immunosuppressed host. Philadelphia: JB Lippincott; 1991:182–217.
108. Venet A, Clavel F, Israel-Biet D, et al. Lung in acquired immune deficiency syndrome: infectious and immunological status assessed by bronchoalveolar lavage. Bull Eur Physiopathol Respir 1985;21:535–43.
109. Wallace JM, Barbers RG, Oishi JS, Prince H. Cellular and T-lymphocyte subpopulation profiles in bronchoalveolar lavage fluid from patients with acquired immunodeficiency syndrome and pneumonitis. Am Rev Respir Dis 1984;130:786–90.
110. Wendland T, Furrer H, Vernazza PL, et al. HAART in HIV-infected patients: restoration of antigen-specific CD4 T-cell responses in vitro is correlated with CD4 memory T-cell reconstitution, whereas improvement in delayed type hypersensitivity is related to a decrease in viraemia. AIDS 1999;13:1857–62.
111. Worthy SA, Flint JD, Müller NL. Pulmonary complications after bone marrow transplantation: high-resolution CT and pathologic findings. Radiographics 1997;17:1359–71.
112. Yousem SA, Colby TV, Carrington CB. Follicular bronchitis/bronchiolitis. Hum Pathol 1985;16:700–6.
113. Ziza JM, Brun-Vezinet F, Venet A, et al. Lymphadenopathy-associated virus isolated from bronchoalveolar lavage fluid in AIDS-related complex with lymphoid interstitial pneumonitis [Letter]. N Engl J Med 1985;313:183.

14
TRANSPLANTATION PATHOLOGY

Among the many complications that follow organ transplantation, pulmonary complications are more common than those in any other organ. Given the marked immunosuppression induced by modern regimens to prevent organ rejection, it is not surprising that these patients are at risk for almost the entire range of respiratory tract pathogens. Discussion of these infections is beyond the scope of this chapter and can be found in chapters 12 and 13. In addition to infections, many other types of pulmonary injury can occur in the immunosuppressed patient, and these are reviewed in chapter 13. This chapter focuses on the types of pulmonary injury unique to the transplant recipient: reperfusion injury, including acute and chronic rejection, and post-transplant lymphoproliferative disorders.

GENERAL PRINCIPLES IN DIAGNOSIS OF PULMONARY COMPLICATIONS IN TRANSPLANT RECIPIENTS

Diagnosis of Pulmonary Complications

Transplant recipients are at such tremendous risk from pulmonary complications that clinicians must maintain a very low threshold for early, aggressive and definitive approaches to making a correct diagnosis. Unfortunately, the usual clinical and radiologic manifestations are unreliable in this setting; tissue examination is commonly required and immediate help is sought from the pathologist.

Some pulmonary complications are more often encountered with certain types of organ transplant; however, most are nonspecific and occur in any organ recipient. Perhaps the most useful approach to the initial assessment of pulmonary complications in these patients is to recognize that certain distinct problems occur at different time intervals following the transplant. The general timetable is remarkably similar among the many different solid organ and bone marrow transplantation procedures: early (occurring within 100 days following transplantation) and late (occurring 100 or more days after transplantation). Knowledge of the relative likelihood of a potential problem allows the clinician to use a stepwise diagnostic approach and to implement appropriate empirical therapy while awaiting test results.

Early Complications. Bacterial infections are overwhelmingly the most common cause of pulmonary infection in the first month after transplantation. The rate of early pneumonia tends to be lower among bone marrow and renal transplant recipients and highest among liver, heart-lung, and heart transplant recipients. Other pulmonary complications in this setting include: pulmonary edema (due to fluid overload, myocardial injury, drug toxicity, sepsis), acute respiratory distress syndrome, diffuse alveolar hemorrhage, interstitial pneumonitis, and veno-occlusive disease.

Late Complications. Opportunistic infectious complications increase in importance with ongoing immunosuppression. Bronchiolitis obliterans, nonspecific interstitial pneumonitis, and lymphocytic interstitial pneumonia are important entities to consider. Also, a number of diseases have been reported to recur in the lung allograft including sarcoidosis, lymphangioleiomyomatosis, giant cell interstitial pneumonitis, diffuse panbronchiolitis, pulmonary alveolar proteinosis, desquamative interstitial pneumonia, pulmonary Langerhans' cell histiocytosis, bronchioloalveolar carcinoma, and idiopathic pulmonary hemorrhage.

Evaluation of Transbronchial Lung Biopsies

Fiberoptic bronchoscopy, with bronchoalveolar lavage (BAL) and transbronchial lung biopsies, is the method of choice for diagnosing pulmonary complications in transplant recipients. The lavage specimens and lung biopsies should be processed and read as emergent procedures, with same day turnaround, if possible. Transbronchial biopsy has a high overall rate of positivity (63 to 83 percent) when performed for assessment of a clinical problem. Periodic transbronchial biopsy for surveillance in asymptomatic, clinically and physiologically stable recipients remains controversial and is less sensitive.

Table 14-1

THE INTERNATIONAL SOCIETY FOR HEART AND LUNG TRANSPLANTATION WORKING FORMULATION FOR THE GRADING OF PULMONARY ALLOGRAFT REJECTION[a]

Grade of Rejection	Histologic Findings
Acute rejection	
Grade A0 (no rejection)	No perivascular lymphoid infiltrates
Grade A1 (minimal rejection)	Rare perivascular lymphoid infiltrates, found with difficulty at low magnification
Grade A2 (mild rejection)	Frequent perivascular lymphoid infiltrates, readily seen at low magnification; eosinophils and plasma cells may be admixed
Grade A3 (moderate rejection)	Infiltrates extend into alveolar septal interstitium
Grade A4 (severe rejection)	Diffuse interstitial lymphoid infiltrates with diffuse alveolar damage, hemorrhage, and/or parenchymal necrosis
With bronchial/bronchiolar inflammation	
Grade B0	No inflammation
Grade B1	Rare lymphocytes in airways submucosa
Grade B2	Circumferential band of lymphocytes, without epithelial inflammation or necrosis
Grade B3	Circumferential band of lymphocytes, with epithelial inflammation or necrosis
Grade B4	Circumferential band of lymphocytes, with epithelial inflammation, and ulceration and necrosis
Grade Bx	Not gradable
Chronic rejection (obliterative bronchiolitis)	
Grade Ca (active)	Fibrosis with mononuclear infiltrates
Grade Cb (inactive)	Fibrosis with minimal inflammation
Chronic vascular rejection (graft vasculopathy)	
Grade D	

[a]Adapted from references 8 and 14.

The bronchoscopist should obtain 3 to 5 fragments of alveolated tissue (5) (preferably containing at least 100 alveoli and one bronchiole in each fragment), which reduces to less than 5 percent the possibility of missing rejection (14). Biopsies of the bronchial anastomotic site may also be done to evaluate whether there is colonization by fungi.

As a routine, the pathologist should obtain at least three hematoxylin and eosin (H&E)–stained tissue levels of the biopsy, a methenamine silver stain for fungi and *Pneumocystis,* and a Gram stain for bacteria (8). Biopsy sections are usually combined with cytospins and/or cell blocks of BAL fluid stained with H&E, Gomori methenamine silver (GMS), and Gram stains to evaluate for viral inclusions, fungi, *Pneumocystis,* and bacteria. BAL fluid is also typically cultured for viruses, fungi, and bacteria. When lung rejection is a major consideration, elastic and trichrome stains of the biopsy tissue are of value to highlight the perivascular location of lymphoid cells in acute rejection and to better assess the lung architecture in chronic rejection.

Acute allograft rejection (described below) remains a significant problem in lung transplantation. The specificity and sensitivity of transbronchial lung biopsy for detecting acute rejection is 93 percent and 77 percent, respectively (assuming an adequate specimen) (10). The diagnosis should be accompanied by a rejection grade, presuming the biopsy is adequate (Table 14-1) (8). It is important to compare the current biopsy to any previous biopsies to determine whether it shows ongoing rejection or evidence of resolution (8). The sensitivity of transbronchial biopsy falls considerably when

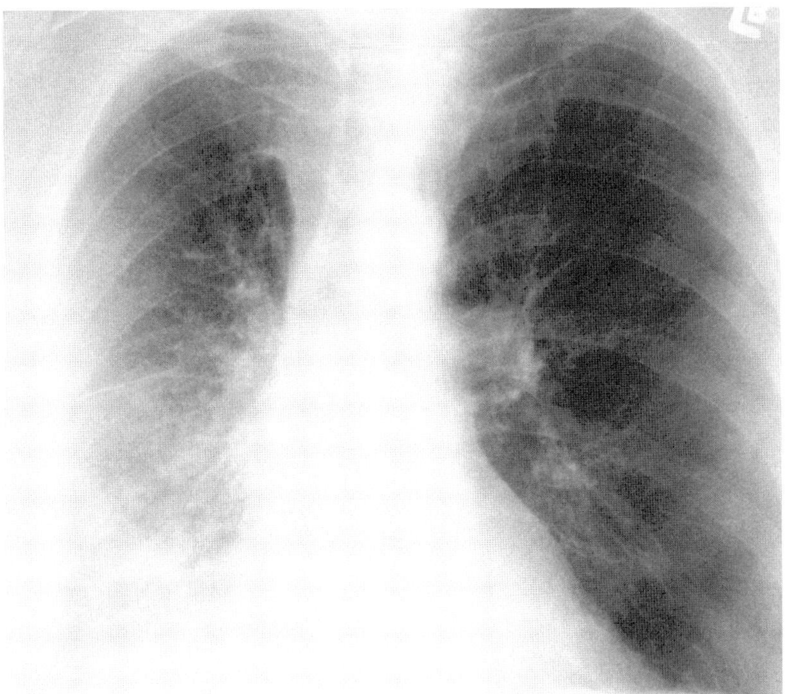

Figure 14-1

ACUTE REJECTION OF LUNG TRANSPLANT

A 62-year-old woman underwent right lung transplantation for emphysema. Chest radiograph performed 6 days later demonstrates prominent interstitial markings in the right lung, ground-glass opacities in the right middle and lower lung zones, and a small right pleural effusion. The diagnosis was confirmed by transbronchial biopsy. The left lung is overinflated and has decreased vascularity due to panacinar emphysema.

the diagnosis of bronchiolitis obliterans, the histologic counterpart of chronic allograft rejection, is considered. Surgical lung biopsy has a role in the evaluation of obliterative bronchiolitis and lymphoproliferative disorders. Increasingly, the diagnosis of bronchiolitis obliterans is usually based on clinical findings.

EARLY COMPLICATIONS

Reperfusion Injury

Definition. Reperfusion injury refers to noncardiogenic pulmonary edema resulting from capillary injury. The injury is produced by the lung ischemia that results from the lung or heart-lung transplantation procedure itself, but is manifested when the circulation to the lung is re-established. A synonymous term is *reimplantation response.*

Clinical Features. Reperfusion injury occurs in up to 80 percent of patients who undergo lung transplantation (2). Clinically, the manifestations typically occur within 3 to 4 days after transplantation and are associated with reduced lung compliance and an increased alveolar-arterial oxygen gradient.

Radiologic Findings. The radiologic abnormalities range from subtle, perihilar, hazy opacities to confluent airspace consolidation involving mainly the perihilar regions and lower lobes (fig. 14-1) (4). Radiologic manifestations are usually present within 24 hours of transplantation and reach a peak by day 3 or 4 (7).

Gross Findings. The cut section of the lung is tan to red, rubbery or firm to palpation, with a slimy or slippery surface.

Histologic Findings. The principal histologic finding is diffuse alveolar damage (DAD) (see chapter 3) (3). In the acute phase, there are hyaline membranes, congestion, interstitial edema, intra-alveolar macrophages, and type 2 cell hyperplasia (fig. 14-2). Small numbers of neutrophils may be present in the interstitium, a rather common finding in DAD and one not to be misconstrued with early acute pneumonia. The reparative phase is characterized by organization of the alveolar exudate, with intra-alveolar tufts of fibrous connective tissue (Masson bodies) and interstitial fibrosis (fig. 14-3).

Differential Diagnosis. DAD occurring after the early post-transplantation period (more than 2 weeks after transplantation)

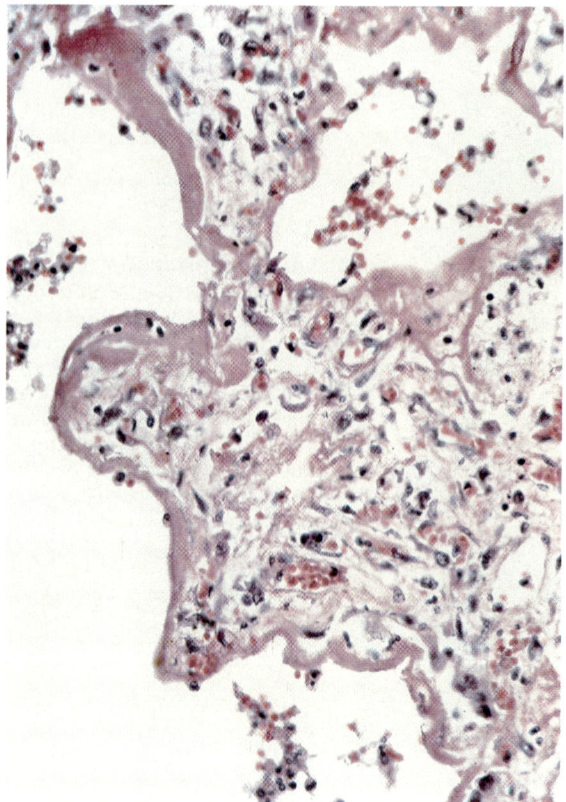

Figure 14-2

LUNG TRANSPLANTATION: REPERFUSION INJURY, ACUTE PHASE

The initial microscopic appearance of reperfusion injury shows hyaline membranes; hence, it represents a form of diffuse alveolar damage.

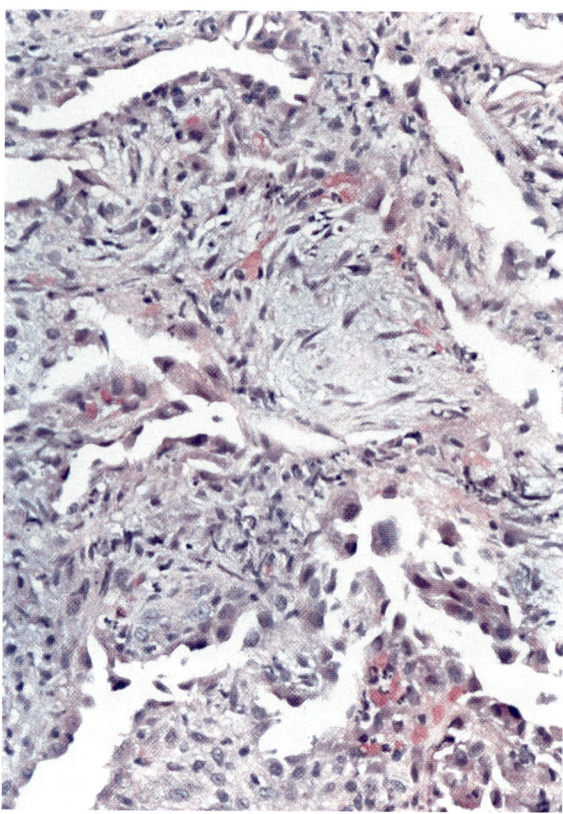

Figure 14-3

LUNG TRANSPLANTATION: REPERFUSION INJURY, HEALING PHASE

Reperfusion injury heals by the organization of the hyaline membranes as alveolar plugs of fibrous tissue. Note the young, pale, myxoid fibrous connective tissue plug, the replicating alveolar lining cells, and the thickened alveolar septa.

should raise the possibility of etiologies other than reperfusion injury, such as severe acute rejection, aspiration, drug toxicity, and cytomegalovirus pneumonia (8). Thus, chronologic information is very important in evaluating the transplant biopsy.

The presence of reperfusion injury does not exclude a second process, particularly acute cellular rejection. In particular, more than a scattering of interstitial lymphocytes is unusual in reperfusion injury, and the finding of perivascular lymphoid infiltrates more than seven cell layers in diameter, particularly when they contain eosinophils, supports acute rejection. Another potential problem involves separating combined mild acute rejection and reperfusion injury from severe acute rejection (grade A4, Table 14-1), which typically has a component of DAD. When the biopsy is taken in the early post-transplant course (first week), when it shows DAD, and when lymphoid infiltrates are restricted to around the vessels without extension into the interstitium, the best diagnosis is combined reperfusion injury and mild (grade A2) rejection. When the DAD occurs in conjunction with perivascular lymphoid infiltrates that extend widely into the interstitium, then severe acute rejection (grade A4) is the better diagnosis. This is particularly the case if the biopsy is done after the first 2 post-transplant weeks, when one would not expect to see the hyaline membranes of reperfusion injury.

Treatment and Prognosis. Early postoperative care focuses on ventilatory support and weaning, fluid and hemodynamic management, immunosuppression, detection of early rejection, and prevention or treatment of infection. Inhaled nitric oxide has been proposed as a method to ameliorate ischemia-reperfusion injury because it can mediate pulmonary vasodilatation. Future use of this therapy may improve perioperative pulmonary function and reduce ventilatory requirements.

Acute Cellular Rejection

Definition. Acute cellular rejection refers to cell-mediated (lymphocyte-mediated) rejection of the allograft.

Clinical Features. Acute rejection is common in the first 3 to 6 months after transplantation. Over 80 percent of lung transplant patients and two thirds of heart-lung transplant patients have at least one episode (6). The first episode can occur as early as 5 to 7 days post-transplantation; recurrence is not unusual (1), but episodes after the first year are less frequent. Clinically, acute rejection often produces shortness of breath, cough, and low-grade fever, but patients can be asymptomatic. It is often difficult to distinguish acute rejection from infection. The most sensitive clinical indicator is reduced forced expiratory volume flow rates (FEV1), but other diseases may produce similar reductions. A decline of 10 percent in spirometric values that persists for more than 2 days indicates either rejection or infection. Severe rejection is very rare, except in patients who are noncompliant in taking their immunosuppressive medications.

Radiologic Findings. The radiographic abnormalities are nonspecific and resemble those of interstitial pulmonary edema (7). The most common findings consist of a reticular interstitial pattern, septal (Kerley B) lines, perihilar haze, and new or increasing pleural effusions (7). Severe rejection may lead to ground-glass opacities or confluent areas of airspace consolidation involving mainly the perihilar regions and lower lung zones. It should be noted, however, that in approximately 50 percent of patients with acute rejection the chest radiograph is normal (12).

Histologic Findings. Histologically, the earliest manifestation of acute cellular rejection is perivascular (and in particular, perivenular) lymphoid cuffing. The cells are small lymphocytes, immunoblasts, and monocytes. The density of the lymphoid cells ought to be at least seven cell layers thick, but the infiltrates are often difficult to see at low magnification because of the few vessels involved (minimal acute cellular rejection, grade A1; Table 14-1; figs. 14-4, 14-5). As the rejection increases in intensity, the lymphoid infiltrate spreads to small arteries and increasing numbers of vessels overall, and the perivascular lymphoid infiltrates become more readily visible at low magnification (mild acute rejection, grade A2; figs. 14-6, 14-7). At this point, the lymphoid cells may be associated with small numbers of eosinophils and plasma cells, but neutrophils are not seen. In more severe grades of acute rejection, infiltrates extend

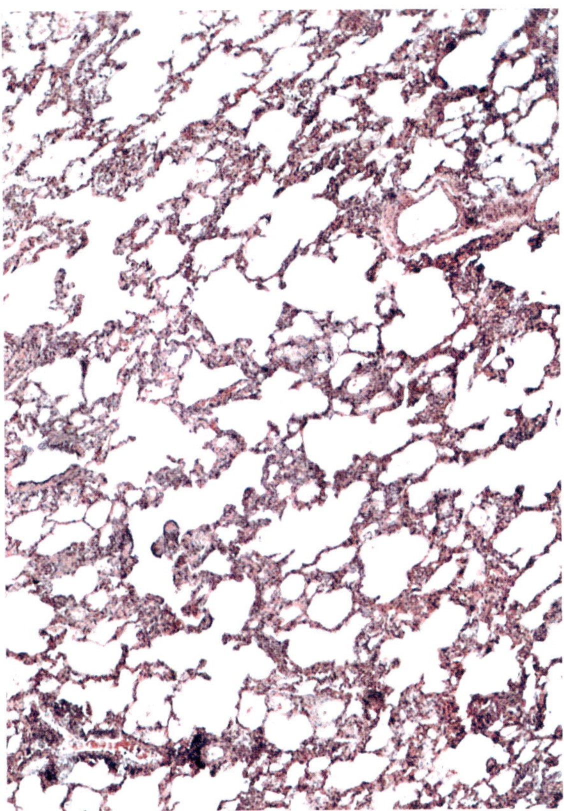

Figure 14-4

LUNG TRANSPLANTATION: ACUTE CELLULAR REJECTION, GRADE A1

The hallmark of acute rejection is perivascular lymphoid aggregates, but in grade A1 disease, at low magnification, they are typically hard to demonstrate. (Courtesy of Dr. Charles Marboe, New York, NY.)

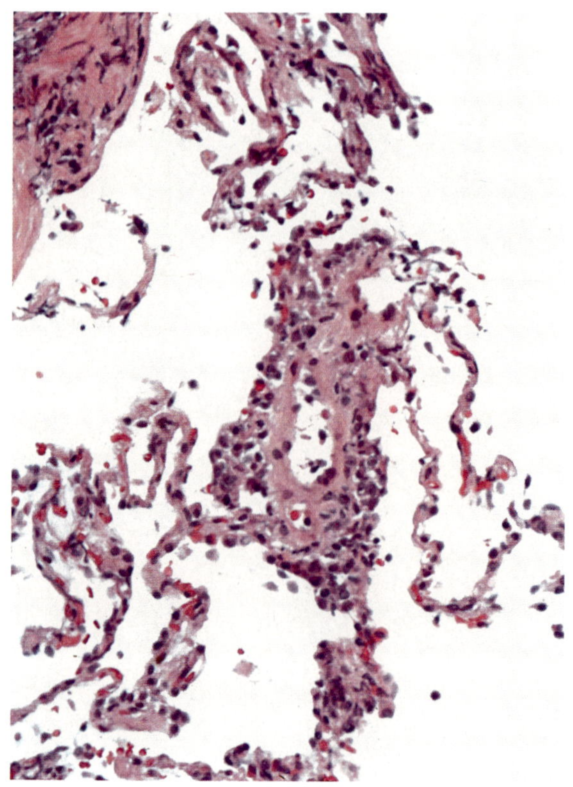

Figure 14-5

LUNG TRANSPLANTATION: ACUTE CELLULAR REJECTION, GRADE A1

At high magnification, and after search, small perivascular lymphoid aggregates can be found.

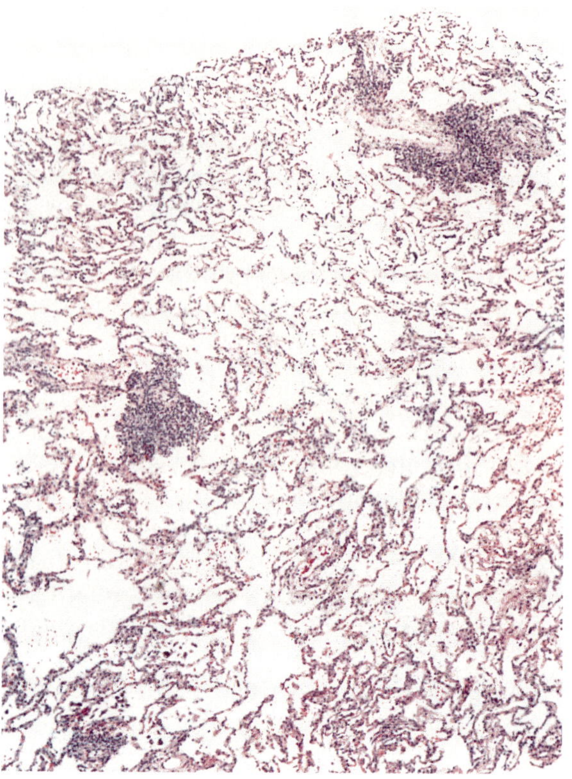

Figure 14-6

LUNG TRANSPLANTATION: ACUTE CELLULAR REJECTION, GRADE A2

At low magnification, perivascular lymphoid aggregates at least seven cell layers thick are easily seen, but the lymphoid cells do not substantially extend into the alveolar interstitium.

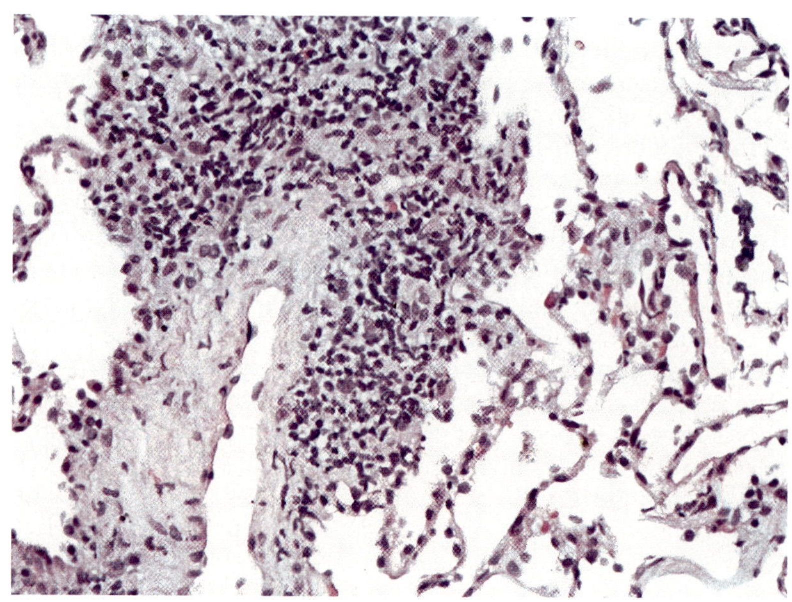

Figure 14-7

LUNG TRANSPLANTATION: ACUTE CELLULAR REJECTION, GRADE A2

High magnification shows a thick cuff of lymphoid cells, including small lymphocytes and lymphoblasts, surrounding a portion of the circumference of the vessel wall. Note the minimal extension into alveolar septa.

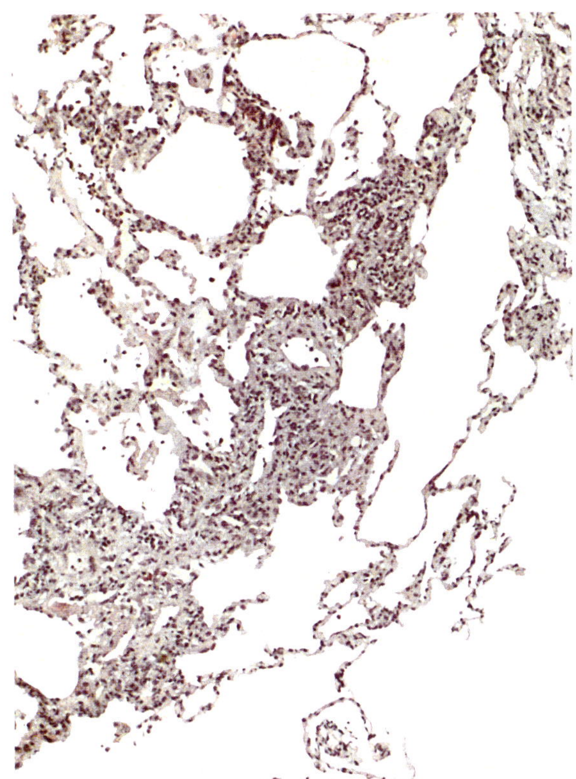

Figure 14-8

LUNG TRANSPLANTATION:
ACUTE CELLULAR REJECTION, GRADE A3

The lymphoid infiltrate extends from the perivascular area to involve the alveolar interstitium. (Courtesy of Dr. Charles Marboe, New York, NY.)

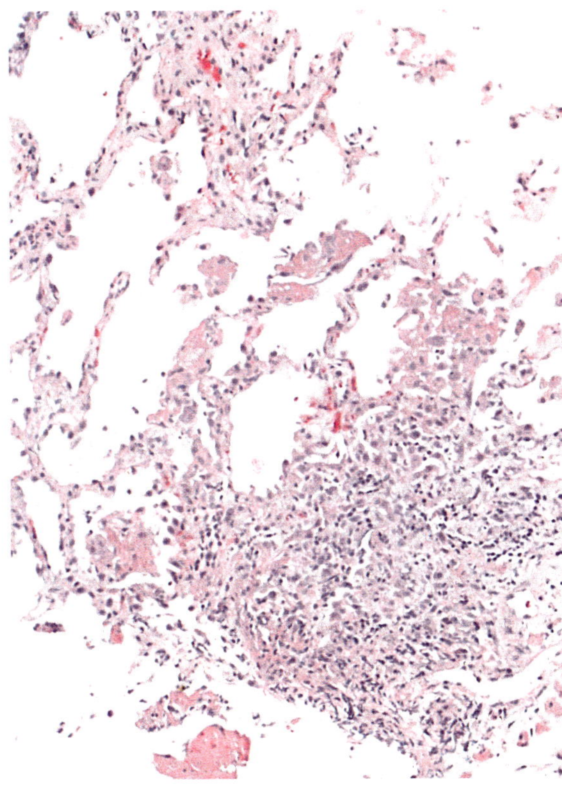

Figure 14-9

LUNG TRANSPLANTATION:
ACUTE CELLULAR REJECTION, GRADE A3-4

The lymphoid infiltrate extends from the perivascular zone to involve the pulmonary interstitium, and there is an early fibrinous exudate within the alveolar lumens.

into the perivascular and peribronchiolar alveolar interstitium (moderate rejection, grade A3; fig. 14-8), eventually provoking DAD, hemorrhage, and parenchymal necrosis or infarction (severe rejection, grade A4; figs. 14-9, 14-10). Neutrophils in small numbers may be present along with the other inflammatory cells in more severe grades of acute rejection (grades A3 and A4). Also, patients with higher grades of acute rejection may show endothelialitis, but this is not a prominent feature.

Lymphoid infiltration of airways often accompanies acute rejection, but it can also occur in the absence of parenchymal rejection, apparently independent of it (Table 14-1). It varies from scant lymphocytic inflammation of the submucosa of bronchioles and bronchi (grade B1) to band-like, circumferential lymphoid infiltrates (grade B2; fig. 14-11). More severe forms of airway inflammation produce epithelial infiltration and necrosis (grade B3) and, eventually, extensive airway epithelial ulceration (grade B4). Still, the clinical meaning of lymphocytic bronchitis/bronchiolitis in the absence of parenchymal acute rejection is unclear; it has been suggested that lymphocytic bronchitis/bronchiolitis may be a precedent event for obliterative bronchiolitis (9,13).

Differential Diagnosis. Acute cellular rejection is diagnosed only after infection is excluded (8). Perivascular lymphoid infiltrates can be seen in cytomegalovirus infection and *Pneumocystis* pneumonia, which may be difficult to distinguish from acute rejection without a careful examination for inclusions or organisms and performance of special stains (11). On the other hand, neutrophils may be seen in severe acute rejection and may incorrectly

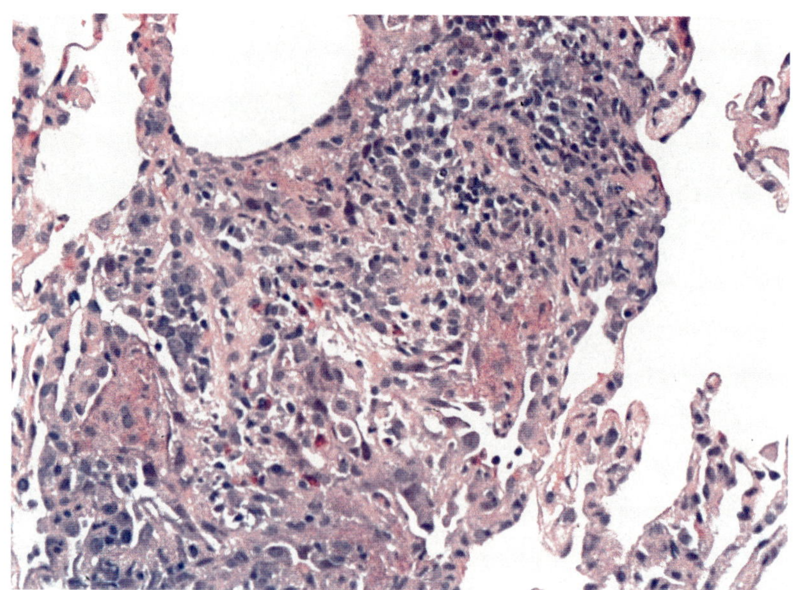

Figure 14-10

LUNG TRANSPLANTATION: ACUTE CELLULAR REJECTION, GRADE A3-4

There is not only involvement of the alveolar interstitium, but there is a fibrinous exudate within the alveolar lumens.

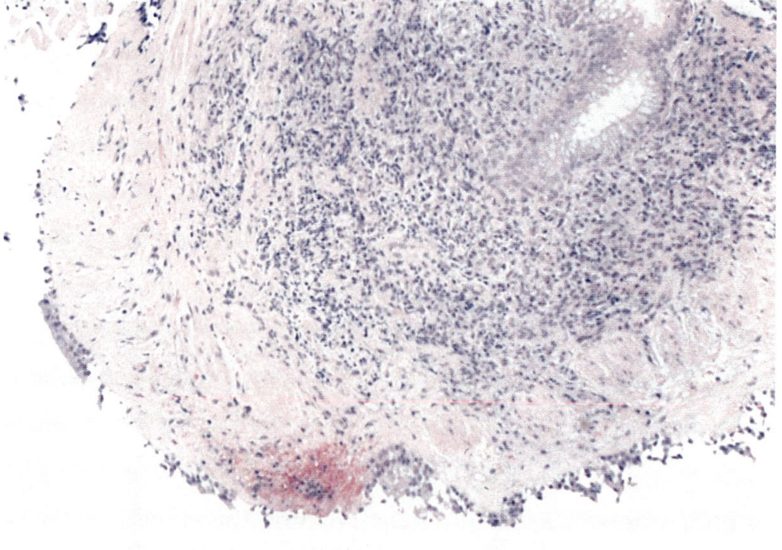

Figure 14-11

LUNG TRANSPLANTATION: ACUTE REJECTION WITH BRONCHIAL WALL INVOLVEMENT (B2)

A band-like infiltrate of lymphocytes is present deep within the bronchial wall. The loss of the epithelium is artefactual.

suggest the diagnosis of acute pneumonia. The severity of the perivascular and interstitial lymphoid infiltrates favors severe acute rejection.

The problem of distinguishing reperfusion injury from mild acute rejection (grade A2) from severe acute rejection (grade 4) has already been discussed (see differential diagnosis of reperfusion injury, above).

Treatment and Prognosis. A 3-day course of high-dose corticosteroids followed by tapering is typical treatment (1). In refractory cases, antilymphocyte antibodies, cytotoxic drugs (such as methotrexate or cyclophosphamide), tacrolimus, or aerosolized cyclosporine can be used.

Diffuse Alveolar Hemorrhage

Definition and Clinical Features. Bone marrow transplantation can be complicated by extensive pulmonary alveolar hemorrhage, without a microscopically discernible source. It usually occurs relatively soon after transplantation, within 7 to 45 days (19), in 5 to 35 percent of patients with bone marrow transplants, particularly in those with autologous transplants,

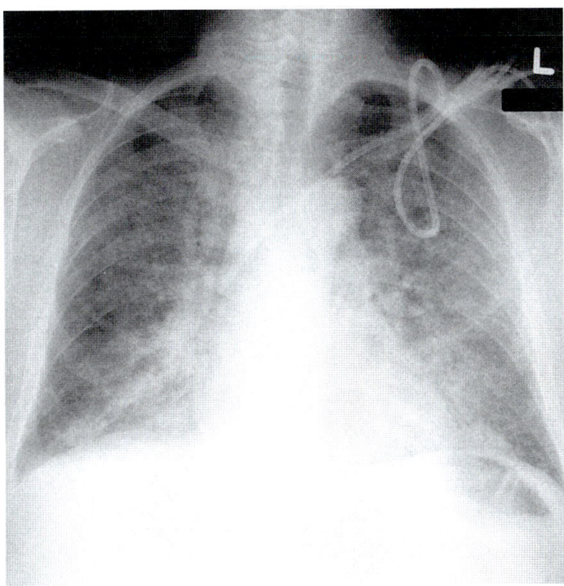

Figure 14-12

DIFFUSE PULMONARY HEMORRHAGE AFTER BONE MARROW TRANSPLANTATION

Chest radiograph demonstrates diffuse, bilateral, ground-glass opacities and airspace consolidation. There is relative sparing of the peripheral lung regions. The diagnosis was confirmed by diagnostic bronchoalveolar lavage.

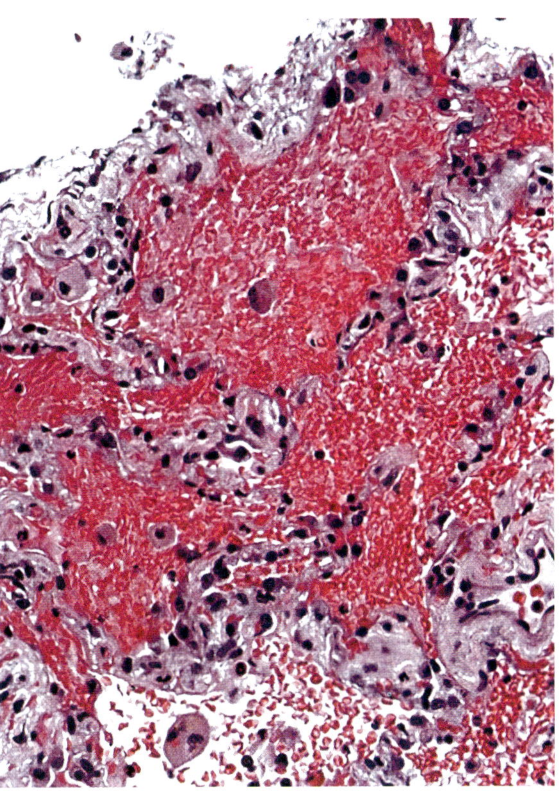

Figure 14-13

ACUTE PULMONARY HEMORRHAGE FOLLOWING BONE MARROW TRANSPLANTATION

Numerous red blood cells fill alveolar lumens.

but occasionally in those with allogeneic transplants (17,19).

The symptoms are usually of sudden onset. They include dyspnea, fever, cough, and sometimes hemoptysis. This dangerous complication occurs particularly in older patients (those more than 40 years old) and in those who have renal insufficiency, a history of total body irradiation, or an underlying malignancy (20).

Radiologic Findings. The typical radiologic manifestation of pulmonary hemorrhage is the presence of areas of airspace consolidation (21). These areas may be patchy or confluent, but they are usually bilateral, although they can be asymmetric (fig. 14-12).

Histologic Findings. Transbronchial lung biopsy and BAL show hemosiderin-laden macrophages and red blood cells (fig. 14-13). In biopsy material, these cells lie within alveoli, without observable capillaritis, vasculitis, or other distinct pathologic findings.

Etiology and Pathogenesis. The pathogenesis is uncertain, although radiation effects, drug toxicity, and possibly infection may play a role (15). An immunologic pathogenesis is suggested by the timing of the onset of disease, which correlates with an influx of neutrophils from the bone marrow transplant into the lung (16).

Treatment and Prognosis. Treatment is reduction of the immunosuppressive state, although one recent study suggested a role for corticosteroid therapy (18). Nevertheless, the mortality rate is high, ranging from 50 to 100 percent (17,19).

LATE COMPLICATIONS

Obliterative (Constrictive) Bronchiolitis

Definition. Obliterative (constrictive) bronchiolitis refers to progressive airflow limitation caused by fibrosis, with or without minimal chronic inflammation, in the walls and contiguous tissues of membranous and respiratory

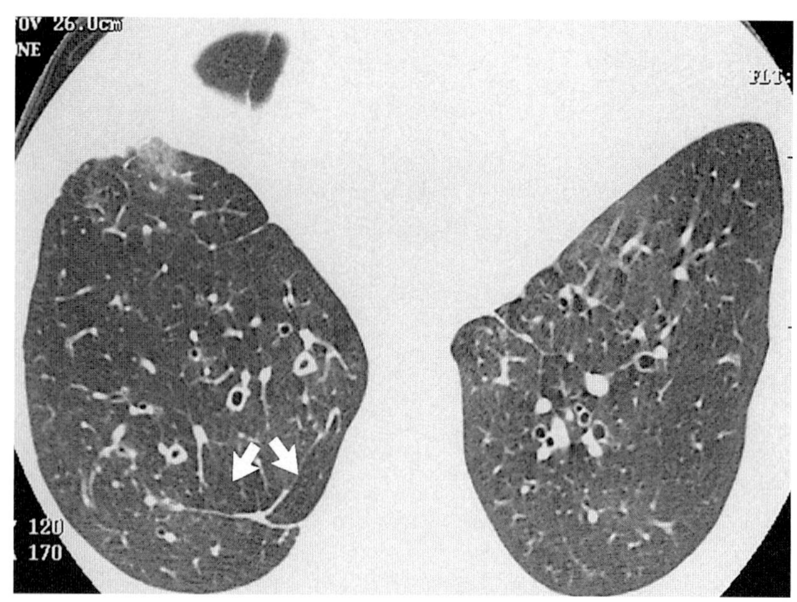

Figure 14-14

OBLITERATIVE BRONCHIOLITIS FOLLOWING LUNG TRANSPLANTATION

HRCT through the lower lobes demonstrates dilated bronchi, some of which have thick walls. Also noted are localized areas of decreased attenuation and vascularity (arrows). The diagnosis was confirmed by transbronchial biopsy.

bronchioles, leading to narrowing or obliteration of their lumens. It most often represents a form of chronic rejection in lung, heart-lung, and bone marrow transplantations. Constrictive bronchiolitis is a term preferred by some because obliterative bronchiolitis can lead to confusion with bronchiolitis obliterans organizing pneumonia (BOOP), a morphologically and etiologically different pattern of injury (see chapter 3) (44). However, because obliterative bronchiolitis (OB) is a term that is frequently used in the clinical transplantation literature, we will continue to use it here.

Clinical Features. The incidence of OB in lung and heart-lung transplant patients ranges from 15 to 25 percent. In this setting, it is viewed most often as an indicator of chronic rejection (23,45). It typically occurs more than 6 months after lung or heart-lung transplantation. It also develops in 2 to 13 percent of allogeneic bone marrow transplant patients who survive more than 3 months (48). Symptoms include cough, dyspnea, and wheezing, either gradual or rapid in onset (23). Physiologically, there is a progressive reduction in FEV1, eventually accompanied by diffusion impairment and ultimately, respiratory failure. A decrease in FEV1 can be used to support the clinical impression of OB in the transplant patient, even when there is no histologic proof of it (26). The term *bronchiolitis obliterans syndrome (BOS)* is used to denote this clinical dysfunction, which likely corresponds to OB.

Radiologic Findings. The chest radiograph is often normal but it may show decreased peripheral lung markings, overinflation with flattening of the diaphragm, and increase in the retrosternal airspace. High-resolution computed tomography (HRCT) is the imaging modality of choice in the assessment of patients with suspected OB. The characteristic findings consist of bronchial dilatation and areas of decreased attenuation and vascularity (fig. 14-14) (52). HRCT performed at end-expiration shows air-trapping (35).

Histologic Findings. Biopsy is the gold standard for the diagnosis of OB, even though clinical criteria are increasingly being used to suggest it (see bronchiolitis obliterans syndrome, above). Because of the importance of OB, the pathologist, in assessing the adequacy of transplant biopsies, must report whether bronchioles are present in the specimen. Even so, the diagnosis is infrequent in transbronchial biopsies for the reasons noted below (36). In one series, the sensitivity of transbronchial lung biopsy for the diagnosis of OB was only 28 percent, while the specificity was 75 percent (43).

In the normal bronchiole, the epithelium lies contiguous to the underlying elastica. OB is

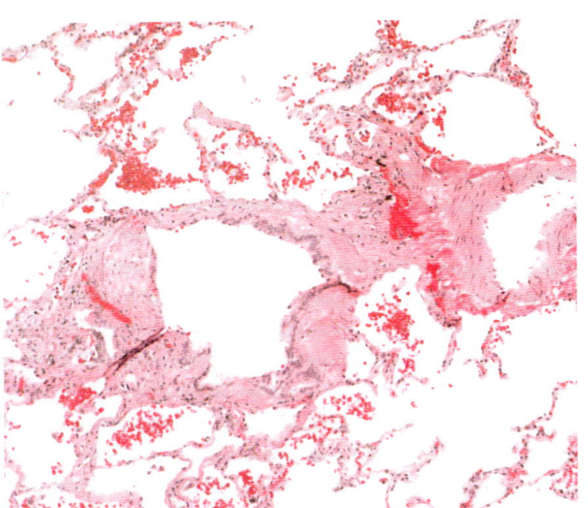

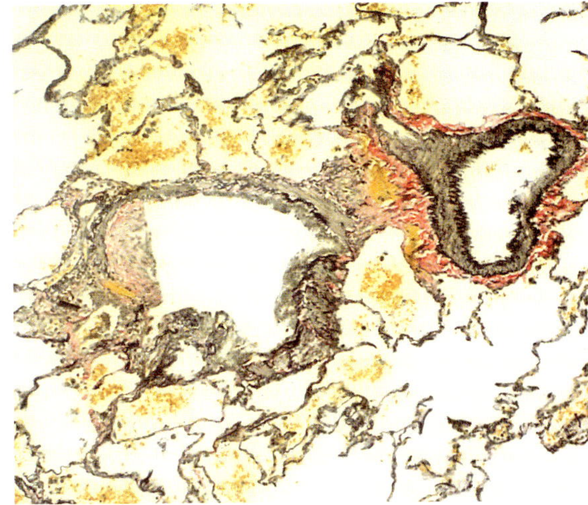

Figure 14-15

LUNG TRANSPLANTATION: OBLITERATIVE BRONCHIOLITIS

Left: Hematoxylin and eosin (H&E) stain shows very subtle fibrosis of the wall of the bronchiole, affecting a segment of its circumference between the 3 and 5 o'clock positions.

Right: The same bronchiole stained for elastic tissue readily demonstrates the eccentric submucosal fibrosis and luminal narrowing, illustrating the advantage of this stain for diagnosing obliterative bronchiolitis. (Left and right are figure 3, top and bottom, from Schlesinger C, Meyer CA, Veeraraghavan S, Koss MN. Constrictive (obliterative) bronchiolitis: diagnosis, etiology, and a critical review of the literature. Ann Diagn Pathol 1998;2:326.)

characterized by either concentric or eccentric deposition of fibrous tissue within the submucosa of the bronchioles, so that the epithelium appears lifted from the underlying elastica and the lumens of the airways are narrowed (hence the value of the descriptive term constrictive bronchiolitis) (fig. 14-15). OB is most easily diagnosed in elastic-stained sections (fig. 14-15, right). There is likely an initial stage of inflammation, with resulting epithelial necrosis and fibrosis, but in practice epithelial necrosis or a purely inflammatory bronchiolitis is rarely recognized. OB with a mixed fibrotic and inflammatory component is referred to as "active" in the 1995 Revised Working Formulation for the Classification of Pulmonary Allograft Rejection (Table 14-1; fig. 14-16) (36,54). However, by light microscopy most cases of OB show only bland fibrosis with minimal or no chronic inflammation (fig. 14-17). This is referred to as "inactive" OB in the Working Formulation for the classification of pulmonary allograft rejection. Ectasia of bronchioles proximal to the obstructed airway can also occur.

In severe cases of inactive OB with complete cicatricial destruction of bronchioles, the fibrosing process can obliterate the bronchiole, producing one or more nondescript scars in the

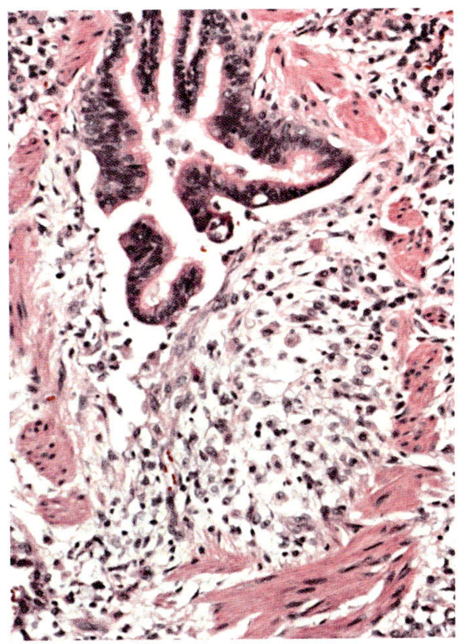

Figure 14-16

LUNG TRANSPLANTATION: OBLITERATIVE BRONCHIOLITIS, ACTIVE

There is a mixture of chronic inflammatory cells, fibrous tissue, and edema in the submucosa, and narrowing of the bronchiolar lumen. (Courtesy of Dr. Corey Schlesinger, Columbus, OH.)

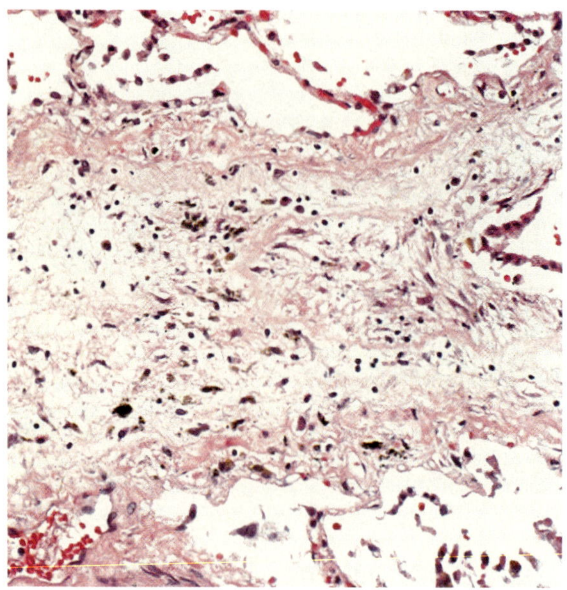

Figure 14-17

LUNG TRANSPLANTATION: OBLITERATIVE BRONCHIOLITIS, INACTIVE

The bronchiole lumen is completely obliterated by bland fibrous connective tissue with a scant admixture of pigmented macrophages and lymphocytes. (Figure 4 from Schlesinger C, Meyer CA, Veeraraghavan S, Koss MN. Constrictive (obliterative) bronchiolitis: diagnosis, etiology, and a critical review of the literature. Ann Diagn Pathol 1998;2:327.)

parenchyma whose significance is easily overlooked in H&E-stained sections (fig. 14-18, left) (36,42,44,54). The histologic clue is the absence of the distal bronchial tree, which in the normal lung should lie adjacent to the pulmonary arteries. In this setting, staining for elastica is of great value, since it often shows residual elastic fibers of a bronchiole within the scarred area (fig. 14-18, right). For this reason, elastic stains should be performed on all tissue blocks of allograft lungs. Also, since OB can be patchy in its involvement of airways, the finding of a normal bronchiole does not exclude the diagnosis. In sum, the lack of bronchioles in many transbronchial biopsies, the focal involvement of airways, and the subtlety of airway involvement are confounding factors leading to the relatively poor diagnostic sensitivity of transbronchial biopsy in OB. The histologic grading of OB is shown in Table 14-1.

Etiology and Pathogenesis. Possible causes of OB in lung transplant patients include repeated or late episodes of acute rejection, cytomegalovirus infection and, in both pulmonary and bone marrow transplantation, autoimmunity to the bronchial tree (44). Acute lung

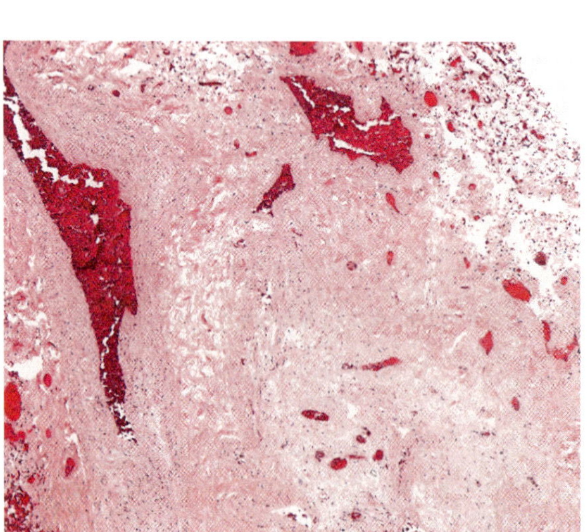

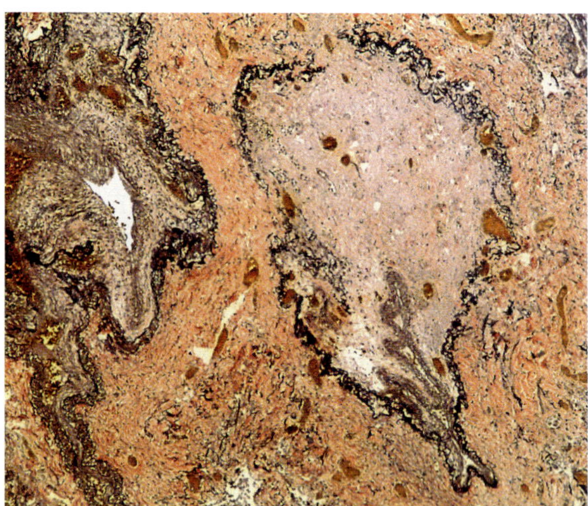

Figure 14-18

LUNG TRANSPLANTATION: OBLITERATIVE BRONCHIOLITIS, INACTIVE

Left: A supposedly nondescript scar in the lung parenchyma, whose significance could easily be overlooked, is noted with H&E stain.

Right: The nondescript scar, when stained for elastic tissue, shows residual elastic fibers of a bronchiole, in keeping with late stage obliterative bronchiolitis and illustrating the importance of the elastic stain in diagnosing obliterative bronchiolitis. (Left and right, figure 6 from Schlesinger C, Meyer CA, Veeraraghavan S, Koss MN. Constrictive (obliterative) bronchiolitis: diagnosis, etiology, and a critical review of the literature. Ann Diagn Pathol 1998;2:328.)

rejection, either as recurrent episodes of significant rejection or as late acute rejection, is a risk factor for OB (25,27,33,50). Also, in a rat model, delay in treatment of acute rejection is correlated with subsequent development of OB (28).

An important role for human leukocyte antigen (HLA) class I mismatches has been postulated in the development of OB (27,30,44,47). OB may be mediated not only by individual episodes of acute rejection but also by continuous subclinical immunologic injury, which may occur even when there is adequate immunosuppression (39,51).

Cytomegalovirus infection may be another risk factor for OB (25,31,33,34). In particular, it appears that cytomegalovirus pneumonitis produces a significantly increased relative risk for the development of OB in the transplant patient (33). In this situation, it may be that CD8+ T cells are the mediators of bronchiolar epithelial damage that results in OB (29,37). Platelet-derived growth factors alpha and beta, and endothelin (a vasoconstrictive peptide) may be potential mediators for the production of airway fibrosis in OB (32,49).

Large and small airway inflammation, both acute and chronic, may lead to OB (27,41, 53). In one study, nearly half of the patients with isolated lymphocytic bronchitis/bronchiolitis either had OB or developed it (24). It is for this reason that the Revised Working Formulation for the classification of pulmonary allograft rejection includes a separate category "B" to grade the degree of airway inflammation, even though the exact significance of this finding is still unclear (Table 14-1) (54).

After inflammation of the small airways, the development of small airway fibrosis may be mediated by transforming growth factor-beta (TGF-beta), CD44-bearing inflammatory cells, and bronchial fibroblasts (27,56).

Differential Diagnosis. OB should be distinguished from BOOP, also termed cryptogenic organizing pneumonia (see chapter 3). In this pattern of disease, polyps of fibrous connective tissue occur within the lumens of bronchioles, alveolar ducts, and alveoli (fig. 14-19). In lung allografts, a BOOP pattern can be seen in the first 6 months after transplantation. It is caused by factors such as intercurrent infection, aspiration, or more proximal airway involvement (22,36). It is unclear whether a BOOP pattern of disease leads to OB. Several studies have examined this relationship, but due to different methods and conflicting results, no definitive conclusions can be drawn (38,46,55).

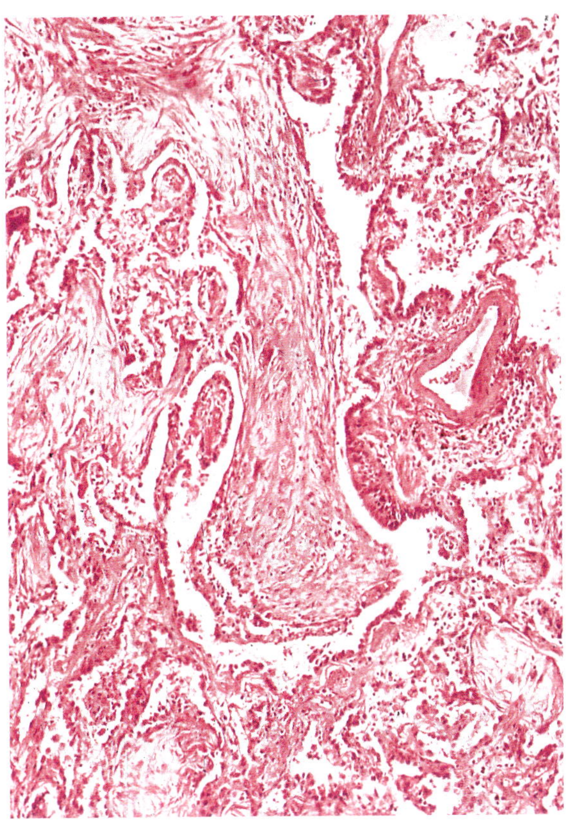

Figure 14-19

DIFFERENTIAL DIAGNOSIS OF OBLITERATIVE BRONCHIOLITIS: BRONCHIOLITIS OBLITERANS ORGANIZING PNEUMONIA (BOOP) PATTERN

Note the plugs of fibrous tissue (Masson bodies) within a bronchiole (center) and adjacent alveoli. BOOP pattern can be seen in the transplanted lung after intercurrent infection, aspiration, or more proximal airway involvement.

Treatment and Prognosis. The clinical course of patients with OB varies. There may be: 1) rapid onset with a relentlessly progressive course; 2) rapid onset and initial progression followed by clinical and physiologic stabilization; or 3) insidious onset with a subtle but progressive course (40). Treatment has included high doses of corticosteroids, azathioprine, plasmapheresis, cyclosporine, anti-OKT-3 antibody, and methotrexate (44). Unfortunately, the results of treatment, whether in the setting of lung, heart-lung, or bone marrow transplantation, are poor. OB is the leading cause of death among long-term lung transplant patients. Among bone marrow allograft patients with OB, there is a 3-year mortality rate of 65 percent (48).

Post-Transplant Lymphoproliferative Disorders

Definition. Post-transplant lymphoproliferative disorder (PTLD) is an abnormal proliferation of lymphoid cells, typically associated with the presence of Epstein-Barr virus, and occurring in the setting of the chronic immunosuppression required for organ transplantation. The lymphoid proliferations show a broad histologic, immunophenotypic, genotypic, and clinical spectrum of disease. Most are B-cell lesions; rarely, T-cell proliferations can occur.

Clinical Features. The incidence of PTLD in patients who survive more than 1 month after solid organ transplantation varies depending on the organ transplanted (59). In patients who undergo lung and heart-lung transplants, and who generally require high levels of immunosuppression, the incidence ranges from 3.8 to nearly 10 percent (65,66). The disease usually occurs in the first year after transplantation. The major risk factor is primary infection with Epstein-Barr virus. Other potential risks are nonrenal transplantation, history of cytomegalovirus sero-mismatch (positive donor, negative recipient), and the type and intensity of immunosuppression (in particular, the use of cyclosporine and antilymphocyte antibodies) (57). The lung is involved in up to 60 percent of pulmonary transplant recipients, whereas heart or lung involvement is present in only 18 percent of cardiac transplant patients. Patients present with either infectious mononucleosis-like symptoms, gastrointestinal symptoms, or single or multiple pulmonary nodules or infiltrates. Open lung biopsy is often necessary for diagnosis.

Radiologic Findings. The main radiologic manifestation of PTLD is the presence of single or multiple pulmonary nodules. Nodules are seen on CT examination in approximately 90 percent of patients with PTLD (60). Hilar and/or mediastinal lymph node enlargement is evident in 30 percent of patients (60). Less common findings include ground-glass opacities and interlobular septal thickening (60).

Table 14-2

SELECTED CLASSIFICATIONS OF POST-TRANSPLANT LYMPHOPROLIFERATIVE DISEASES

Frizzera et al. (modified by Shapiro et al.) (61,67,68)
- Plasmacytic hyperplasia (atypical lymphoid hyperplasia)
- Polymorphic diffuse B-cell hyperplasia
- Polymorphic diffuse B-cell lymphoma
- Monomorphic lymphoma/immunoblastic sarcoma of B cells

Third Annual Workshop of Society for Hematopathology (62)
- Early lesions
  - reactive plasmacytic hyperplasia
  - infectious mononucleosis-like
- Post-transplant lymphoproliferative disorder
  - polymorphic polyclonal (rare)
  - monoclonal
- Post-transplant lymphoproliferative disorder-monomorphic B-cell lymphoma
  - diffuse large B-cell (immunoblastic)
  - Burkitt's/Burkitt's-like
- T-cell lymphoma
  - peripheral T-cell lymphoma (unspecified)
  - anaplastic large cell lymphoma (T or null)
  - other (eg., T-NK [natural killer])
- Other
  - T-cell–rich/Hodgkin's disease-like large B-cell lymphoma
  - plasmacytoma-like
  - myeloma

Knowles et al. (63,68)
- Plasmacytic hyperplasia
- Polymorphic lymphoproliferative disorder
- Malignant lymphoma/multiple myeloma

Histologic Findings. Histologically, PTLD in the lung usually manifests as infiltrates of lymphoid cells occurring in a lymphangitic pattern, that is, around bronchi, arteries, and veins, and beneath pleura, or as nodules that obliterate the underlying alveolar parenchyma. Several classification schemes have been proposed (Table 14-2; fig. 14-20). All recognize that the disease encompasses lesions that appear histologically benign as well as those that microscopically resemble traditional lymphomas. There is now an increasing move towards combining molecular and phenotypic features in the classification of PTLD. The classification of Knowles et al. (58,63,68) is discussed in more detail below as an example of the categorizing efforts that have been made.

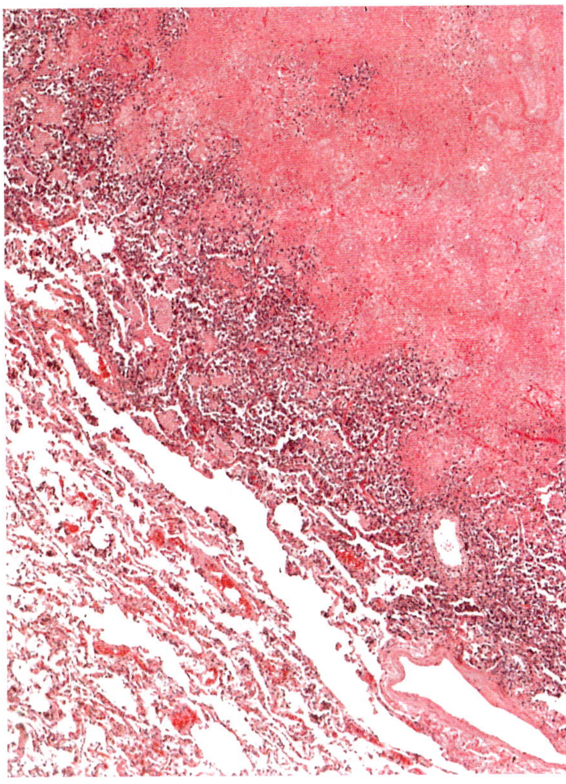

Figure 14-20

POST-TRANSPLANT LYMPHOPROLIFERATIVE DISEASE

A lymphoid nodule with central necrosis obliterates the underlying lung architecture. This is one of the possible histologic presenting manifestations of this disease in lung. Not infrequently, the disease also manifests as infiltrates of lymphoid cells occurring in a lymphangitic pattern around blood vessels and airways.

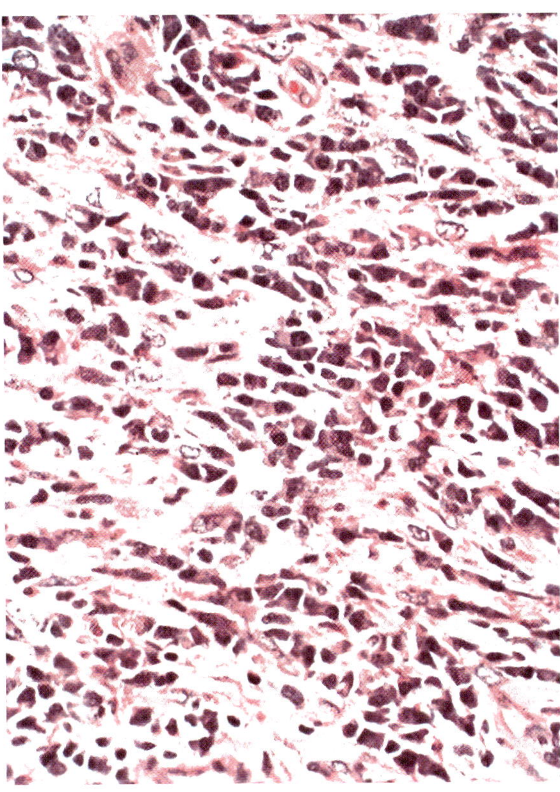

Figure 14-21

POST-TRANSPLANT LYMPHOPROLIFERATIVE DISEASE: PLASMACYTIC HYPERPLASIA

Plasmacytic hyperplasia consists of a mixture of small lymphocytes, often numerous plasma cells, and scattered immunoblasts. In this case, numerous mature plasma cells are present in addition to fibrous connective tissue. (Courtesy of Dr. Glauco Frizzera, New York, NY.)

Plasmacytic hyperplasia represents a benign reactive process (58). There is retention of the underlying lung architecture and a mixture of small lymphocytes, often numerous plasma cells, and scattered immunoblasts (fig. 14-21). In general, the lymphocytes are both B and T cells that are polyclonal (64). Epstein-Barr nucleic acid, which may be polyclonal or monoclonal, is present in most cases. There is no evidence of clonality in either immunoglobulin light or heavy chain genes or T-cell receptor genes, and oncogenes are not present (Table 14-3). Plasmacytic hyperplasia is seen most often in children and young adults after transplantation.

Polymorphic lymphoproliferative disorder is characterized by a lymphoid infiltrate that obliterates the underlying alveolar architecture. There is a spectrum of lesions, varying from those composed predominantly of plasmacytoid cells and immunoblasts to lesions composed of lymphocytes with atypical lymphoblasts (fig. 14-22). There can be admixed "swiggle" cells (T cells with angulated cytoplasm) (61). The atypical immunoblasts may even resemble Reed-Sternberg cells. Almost all cases show necrosis, ranging from small foci to large zones (58,63). The lymphoid infiltrate typically expresses B-cell antigens, which may be monoclonal or polyclonal with respect to immunoglobulin light chain expression on cell surfaces. The lymphoid cells always show clonal rearrangement of the immunoglobulin light chain gene and Epstein-Barr virus; no oncogenes are expressed (Table 14-3).

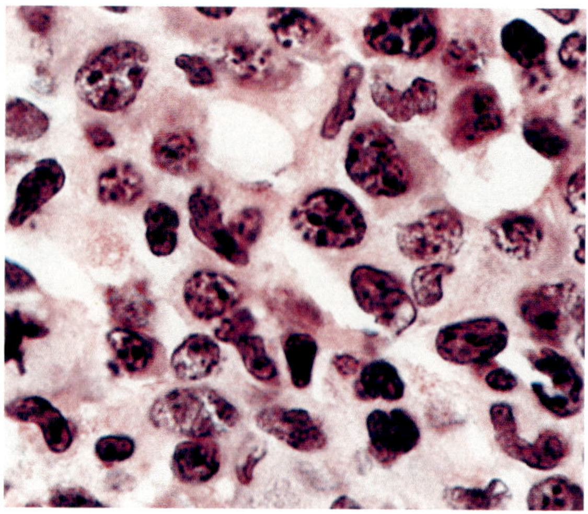

Figure 14-22

POST-TRANSPLANT LYMPHOPROLIFERATIVE DISEASE: POLYMORPHIC LYMPHOPROLIFERATIVE DISORDER

There is an admixture of lymphocytes, plasmacytoid cells, and occasional immunoblasts. (Courtesy of Dr. Glauco Frizzera, New York, NY.)

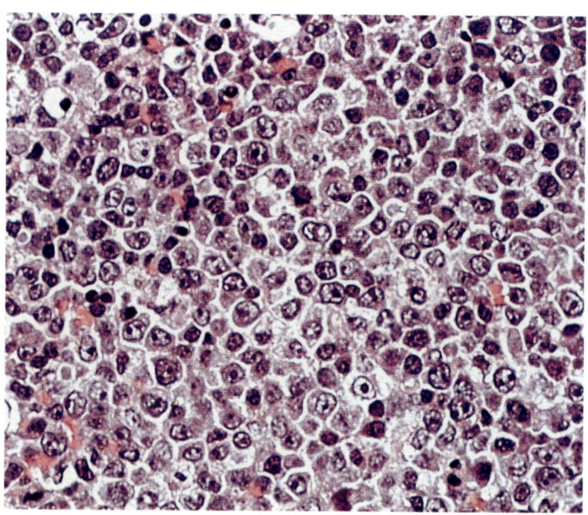

Figure 14-23

POST-TRANSPLANT LYMPHOPROLIFERATIVE DISEASE: MALIGNANT LYMPHOMA

There is a sheet-like growth of monotonous cells with immunoblastic differentiation. (Courtesy of Dr. Glauco Frizzera, New York, NY.)

Table 14-3

MOLECULAR ANALYSIS OF 28 CASES OF POST-TRANSPLANT LYMPHOPROLIFERATIVE DISEASE[a]

Type	Ig[b] Gene Rearrangement (%)	EBV Present (%)	*c-myc* Present (%)	p53/*ras* Present (%)	Died of Disease (%)
Plasmacytic hyperplasia	9	45	0	0/0	13
Polymorphic lymphoproliferative disorder	100	94	0	0/0	0
Malignant lymphoma	100	100	33	25/75	75

[a]Modified from Table 2 from reference 58.

[b]Ig = immunoglobulin; EBV = Epstein-Barr virus.

Malignant lymphoma/multiple myeloma refers to a tumor that histologically resembles malignant lymphoma or multiple myeloma (58). The cells are generally monotonous in appearance and show plasmacytoid or immunoblastic differentiation (fig. 14-23). Most of these tumors are diffuse large B-cell lymphomas; there are occasional small noncleaved cell lymphomas as well (fig. 14-24). Immunophenotypically, the tumors are either B cell or null cell, but they always show clonal immunoglobulin and Epstein-Barr viral gene rearrangements. Of interest and potential diagnostic importance, they can show p53 overexpression and *c-myc* and *ras* expression (Table 14-3).

Treatment and Prognosis. The clinical course depends on a complex of findings, including histologic subtype, clonality, and oncogene expression (Table 14-3). In general, plasmacytic hyperplasia regresses after reduction of immunosuppression and therapy with antiviral agents. Polymorphic lymphoproliferative disorder has a variable clinical course, and progression to lymphoma in a given case cannot be predicted. Treatment is usually a short period of reduced immunosuppression, which, if there is no clinical improvement, is followed by chemotherapy. Patients who have malignant lymphomas typically show widespread (stage III or IV) disease and have a poor outcome (58).

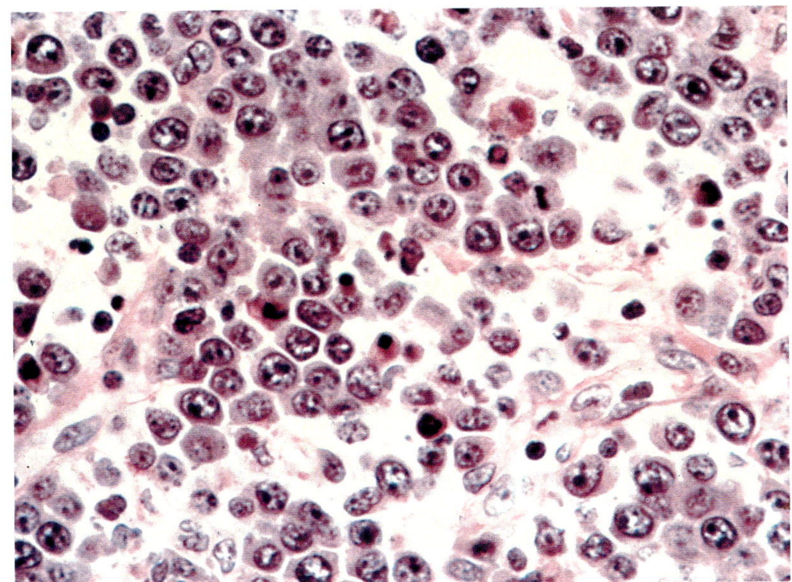

Figure 14-24

POST-TRANSPLANT LYMPHOPROLIFERATIVE DISEASE: MALIGNANT LYMPHOMA

This case shows a monotonous infiltrate of neoplastic cells with distinctly plasmacytoid differentiation. (Courtesy of Dr. Glauco Frizzera, New York, NY.)

REFERENCES

Reperfusion Injury and Acute Rejection

1. Alam S, Chan KM. Noninfectious pulmonary complications after organ transplantation. Curr Opinion Pulmon Med 1996;2:412–8.
2. Bierman MI, Stein KL, Stuart RS, Dauber J. Critical care management of lung transplant recipients. J Intens Care Med 1991;6:135–42.
3. Chaparro C, Chamberlain DW, Maurer J, et al. Acute lung injury in human allografts. J Heart Lung Transplant 1995;14:267–73.
4. Garg K, Zamora MR, Tuder R, Armstrong JD II, Lynch DA. Lung transplantation: indications, donor and recipient selection, and imaging of complications. Radiographics 1996;16:355–67.
5. Higenbottam T, Stewart S, Penketh A, Wallwork J. Transbronchial lung biopsy for the diagnosis of rejection in heart-lung transplant patients. Transplantation 1988;46:532–9.
6. Keenan RJ, Bruzzone P, Paradis IL, et al. Similarity of rejection patterns among heart-lung and double lung transplant recipients. Transplantation 1991;51:176–80.
7. Kundu S, Herman SJ, Larhs A, et al. Correlation of chest radiographic findings with biopsy-proven acute lung rejection. J Thorac Imaging 1999;14:178–84.
8. Marboe C. Pathology of lung transplantation. In: Marchevsky A, Koss M, eds. Pathology: state of the art review. Philadelphia: Hanley & Belfus; 1996:73–101.
9. Ohori NP, Iacono AT, Grgurich WF, Yousem SA. Significance of acute bronchitis/bronchiolitis in the lung transplant recipient. Am J Surg Pathol 1994;18:1192–204.
10. Pomerance A, Madden B, Burke MM, Yacoub MH. Transbronchial biopsy in heart and lung transplantation: clinicopathologic correlations. J Heart Lung Transplant 1995;14:761–73.
11. Tazelaar HD. Perivascular inflammation in pulmonary infections: implications for the diagnosis of lung rejection. J Heart Lung Transplant 1991;10:437–41.
12. Ward S, Müller NL. Pulmonary complications following lung transplantation. Clin Radiol 2000;55:332–9.
13. Yousem SA. Lymphocytic bronchitis/bronchiolitis in lung allograft recipients. Am J Surg Pathol 1993;17:491–6.
14. Yousem SA, Berry G, Cagle PT, et al. Revision of the 1990 working formulation for the classification of pulmonary allograft rejection: Lung Rejection Study Group. J Heart Lung Transplant 1996;15:1–15.

Diffuse Alveolar Hemorrhage

15. Alam S, Chan KM. Noninfectious pulmonary complications after organ transplantation. Curr Opinion Pulmon Med 1996;2:412–8.
16. Duncan SR. Pulmonary complications of transplantation. In: Tierney DF, ed. Current pulmonology. St. Louis: Mosby; 1993:199–241.

17. Jules-Elysee K, Stover DE, Yahalom J, White DA, Gulati SC. Pulmonary complications in lymphoma patients treated with high-dose therapy autologous bone-marrow transplantation. Am Rev Resp Dis 1992;146:485–91.
18. Metcalf JP, Rennard SI, Reed EC, et al. Corticosteroids as adjunctive therapy for diffuse alveolar hemorrhage associated with bone marrow transplantation. University of Nebraska Medical Center Bone Marrow Transplant Group. Am J Med 1994;96:327–34.
19. Robbins RA, Linder J, Stahl MG, et al. Diffuse alveolar hemorrhage in autologous bone marrow transplant recipients. Am J Med 1989;87:511–8.
20. Soubani AO, Miller KB, Hassoun PM. Pulmonary complications of bone marrow transplantation. Chest 1996;109:1006–77.
21. Worthy SA, Flint JD, Müller NL. Pulmonary complications after bone marrow transplantation: high-resolution CT and pathologic findings. Radiographics 1997;17:1359–71.

Obliterative (Constrictive) Bronchiolitis

22. Abernathy EC, Hruban RH, Baumgartner WA, Reitz BA, Hutchins GM. The two forms of bronchiolitis obliterans in heart-lung transplant patients. Hum Pathol 1991;22:1102–10.
23. Alam S, Chan KM. Noninfectious pulmonary complications after organ transplantation. Curr Opinion Pulmon Med 1996;2:412–8.
24. Badizadegan K, Perez-Atayde AR. Pathology of lung allografts in children and young adults. Hum Pathol 1997;28:704–13.
25. Bando K, Paradis IL, Similo S, et al. Obliterative bronchiolitis after lung and heart-lung transplantation: an analysis of risk factors and management. J Thorac Cardiovasc Surg 1995;110:4–14.
26. Cooper JD, Billingham M, Egan T, et al. A working formulation for the standardization of nomenclature and for clinical staging of chronic dysfunction in lung allografts. J Heart Lung Transplant 1993;12:713–6.
27. El-Gamel A, Sim E, Hasleton P, et al. Transforming growth factor beta (TGF-beta) and obliterative bronchiolitis following pulmonary transplantation. J Heart Lung Transplant 1999;18:828–37.
28. Hirt SW, You XM, Moller F, et al. Development of obliterative bronchiolitis after allogeneic rat lung transplantation: implication of acute rejection and the time point of treatment. J Heart Lung Transplant 1999;18:542–8.
29. Holland VA, Cagle PT, Windsor NT, et al. Lymphocyte subset populations in bronchiolitis obliterans after heart-lung transplantation. Transplantation 1990;50:955–9.
30. Jaramillo A, Smith MA, Phelan D, et al. Development of ELISA-detected anti-HLA antibodies precedes the development of bronchiolitis obliterans syndrome and correlates with progressive decline in pulmonary function after lung transplantation. Transplantation 1999;67:1155–61.
31. Keenan RJ, Lega ME, Dummer JS, et al. Cytomegalovirus serologic status and postoperative infection correlated with risk of developing chronic rejection after pulmonary transplantation. Transplantation 1991;51:433–8.
32. Koskinen PK, Kallio EA, Bruggeman CA, Lemstorm KB. Cytomegalovirus infection enhances experimental obliterative bronchiolitis in rat allografts. Am J Respir Crit Care Med 1997;155:2078–88.
33. Kroshus TJ, Kshettry VR, Savik K, John R, Hertz MI, Bolman RM. Risk factors for the development of bronchiolitis obliterans syndrome after lung transplantation. J Thorac Cardiovasc Surg 1997;114:195–202.
34. Kshettry VR, Kroshus TJ, Savik K, Hertz MI, Bolman RM. Primary pulmonary hypertension as a risk factor for the development of obliterative bronchiolitis in lung allograft recipients. Chest 1996;110:704–9.
35. Leung AN, Fisher K, Valentine V, et al. Bronchiolitis obliterans after lung transplantation: detection using expiratory HRCT. Chest 1998;113:365–70.
36. Marboe C. Pathology of lung transplantation. In: Marchevsky A, Koss M, eds. Pathology: state of the art review. Philadelphia: Hanley & Belfus; 1996:73–101.
37. Milne DS, Gascoigne A, Wilkes J, et al. The immunohistopathology of obliterative bronchiolitis following lung transplantation. Transplantation 1992;54:748–50.
38. Milne DS, Gascoigne AD, Ashcroft T, et al. Organizing pneumonia following pulmonary transplantation and the development of obliterative bronchiolitis. Transplantation 1994;57:1757–62.
39. Nagano H, Tilney NL. Chronic allograft failure: the clinical problem. Am J Med Sci 1997;313:305–9.
40. Nathan SD, Ross DJ, Belman MJ, et al. Bronchiolitis obliterans in single-lung transplant recipients. Chest 1995;107:967–72.
41. Ohori NP, Iacono AT, Grgurich WF, Yousem SA. Significance of acute bronchitis/bronchiolitis in the lung transplant recipient. Am J Surg Pathol 1994;18:1192–204.

42. Paradis I, Yousem SA, Griffith B. Airway obstruction and bronchiolitis obliterans after lung transplantation. Clin Chest Med 1993;14:751–63.
43. Pomerance A, Madden B, Burke MM, Yacoub MH. Transbronchial biopsy in heart and lung transplantation: clinicopathologic correlations. J Heart Lung Tranplant 1995;14:761–73.
44. Schlesinger C, Veeraraghavan S, Koss MN. Constrictive (obliterative) bronchiolitis. 1998;4: 288–93.
45. Scott JP, Sharples L, Mullins P, et al. Further studies on the natural history of obliterative bronchiolitis following heart-lung transplantation. Transplant Proc 1991;23:1201–2.
46. Siddiqui MT, Garrity ER, Husain AN. Bronchiolitis obliterans organizing pneumonia-like reaction: a nonspecific response or an atypical form of rejection or infection in lung allograft recipients? Hum Pathol 1996;27:714–9.
47. SivaSai KS, Smith MA, Poindexter NJ, et al. Indirect recognition of donor HLA class I peptides in lung transplant recipients with bronchiolitis obliterans syndrome. Transplantation 1999;67:1094–8.
48. Soubani AO, Miller KB, Hassoun PM. Pulmonary complications of bone marrow transplantation. Chest 1996;109:1006–77.
49. Takeda SI, Sawa Y, Minami M, et al. Experimental bronchiolitis obliterans induced by in vivo HVJ-liposome-mediated endothelin-1 gene transfer. Ann Thorac Surg 1997;63:1562–7.
50. Theodore J, Starnes VA, Lewiston NJ. Obliterative bronchiolitis. Clin Chest Med 1990;11:309–21.
51. Tullius SG, Tilney NL. Both alloantigen-dependent and -independent factors influence chronic allograft rejection. Transplantation 1995;59:313–8.
52. Worthy SA, Park CS, Kim JS, Müller NL. Bronchiolitis obliterans after lung transplantation: high-resolution CT findings in 15 patients. AJR Am J Roentgenol 1997;169:673–7.
53. Yousem SA. Lymphocytic bronchitis/bronchiolitis in lung allograft recipients. Am J Surg Pathol 1993;17:491–6.
54. Yousem SA, Berry G, Cagle PT, et al. Revision of the 1990 working formulation for the classification of pulmonary allograft rejection: Lung Rejection Study Group. J Heart Lung Transplant 1996;15:1–15.
55. Yousem SA, Duncan SR, Griffith BP. Interstitial and airspace granulation tissue reactions in lung transplant recipients. Am J Surg Pathol 1992;16:877–84.
56. Zander DS, Baz MA, Massey JK. Patterns and significance of CD44 expression in lung allografts. J Heart Lung Transplant 1999;18:646–53.

Post-Transplant Lymphoproliferative Disorders

57. Alam S, Chan KM. Noninfectious pulmonary complications after organ transplantation. Curr Opinion Pulmon Med 1996;2:412–8.
58. Chadburn A, Cesarman E, Knowles DM. Molecular pathology of posttransplantation lymphoproliferative disorders. Semin Diagn Pathol 1997;14:15–26.
59. Chen JM, Barr ML, Chadburn A, et al. Management of lymphoproliferative disorders after cardiac transplantation. Ann Thorac Surg 1993;56:527–38.
60. Collins J, Müller NL, Leung AN, et al. Epstein-Barr-Virus-associated lymphoproliferative disease of the lung: CT and histologic findings. Radiology 1998;208:749–59.
61. Frizzera G, Hanto DW, Gajl-Peczalska KJ, et al. Polymorphic diffuse B-cell hyperplasias and lymphomas in renal transplant recipients. Cancer Res 1981;41:4262–79.
62. Harris NL, Ferry JA, Swerdlow SH. Posttransplant lymphoproliferative disorders: summary of Society of Hematopathology Workshop. Semin Diagn Pathol 1997;14:8–14.
63. Knowles DM, Cesarman E, Chadburn A, et al. Correlative morphologic and molecular genetic analysis demonstrates three distinct categories of posttransplantation lymphoproliferative disorders. Blood 1995;85:552–65.
64. Nalesnik MA, Jaffe R, Starz TE, et al. The pathology of posttransplantation lymphoproliferative disorders occurring in the setting of cyclosporine A-prednisone immunosuppression. Am J Pathol 1988;133:173–92.
65. Nalesnik MA, Locker J, Jaffe R, et al. Experience with posttransplant lymphoproliferative disorders in solid organ transplant recipients. Clin Transplant 1992;6:249–58.
66. Randhawa PS, Yousem SA, Paradis IL, et al. The clinical spectrum, pathology and clonal analysis of Epstein-Barr virus-associated lymphoproliferative disorders in heart-lung transplant recipients. Am J Clin Pathol 1989;92:177–85.
67. Shapiro RS, McClain K, Frizzera G, et al. Epstein-Barr virus associated B cell lymphoproliferative disorders following bone marrow transplantation. Blood 1988;71:1234–43.
68. Swerdlow SH. Classification of the posttransplant lymphoproliferative disorders: from the past to the present. Semin Diagn Pathol 1997;14:2–7.

15
PULMONARY HYPERTENSION AND OTHER VASCULAR DISORDERS

Pulmonary vascular disorders constitute a large and diverse group of illnesses that primarily affect the blood vessels in the lung (e.g., primary pulmonary hypertension) or affect the blood vessels as a consequence of processes that originate in sites outside the lungs (e.g., pulmonary thromboembolism). Pulmonary hypertension can be defined as an elevated mean resting arterial pressure greater than 25 mm Hg (88), however, it is not a single entity but includes a spectrum of lesions with a broad range of clinical and morphologic features as well as many potential etiologies. This chapter will focus on several major vascular disorders leading to pulmonary hypertension: pulmonary arterial hypertension; pulmonary venous hypertension; and pulmonary hypertension associated with disorders of the respiratory system and/or hypoxemia, those due to chronic thrombotic and/or embolic disease, and those due to disorders directly affecting the pulmonary vasculature. Details of many of the specific conditions that may involve the pulmonary circulation are found elsewhere in this book. Pulmonary vasculitis is discussed in chapter 4.

NORMAL PULMONARY CIRCULATION

Knowledge of the normal vascular anatomy of the lung is critical to the understanding of pathologic lesions. The blood supply to the lung is derived from two different sources: the pulmonary circulation and the bronchial circulation. The general anatomic organization of the two circulations and their histologic components are described in chapter 1. The pulmonary circulation extends from the pulmonary valve (the vascular exit from the right heart) to the orifices of the pulmonary veins in the wall of the left atrium (the entrance into the left heart) (49). The normal pulmonary circulation is a low-pressure, high-flow vascular bed that accommodates the entire cardiac output with each heartbeat (62). The normal low pulmonary arterial pressure in the lungs, while at rest, depends on a pulmonary circulation with a large cross-sectional area and a low resistance to blood flow (49). Pulmonary artery pressure increases with increases in cardiac output and left atrial pressure (62). Given the remarkable capacity of the pulmonary circulation to sustain these increases in flow and venous pressure, pulmonary hypertension does not occur in the healthy subject. However, pulmonary hypertension, an elevated mean resting arterial pressure greater than 25 mm Hg, can occur if there is an increase in pulmonary vascular resistance caused by a decrease in the cross-sectional area of the vascular bed. Thus, sufficient narrowing of any segment of the pulmonary circulation will cause hypertension by vasoconstriction or by structural changes (e.g., obstruction or obliteration) of blood vessels, or by both (49,62,88). More detail about this subject can be found in several sources (75,76).

The pulmonary arterial vasculature consists of elastic arteries, muscular arteries, and arterioles; the pulmonary venous vessels consist of veins and venules; and the bronchial vessels consist of bronchial arteries and veins (75,76,88).

Elastic pulmonary arteries include the pulmonary trunk, main pulmonary arteries, and intrapulmonary arteries. The elastic laminae are well developed, and parallel. These arteries usually measure at least 1.0 mm in diameter or 0.5 mm if the arteries are not injected. There is a gradual transition to muscular arteries as the elastic arteries become smaller. As this occurs the elastic laminae become less complete and more disorderly. The muscular pulmonary arteries have a media consisting primarily of a muscular layer lined by an outer and an inner elastic lamina. Most arteries less than 500 µm are muscular in type. Most of the arterioles track with the bronchioles although there are also supernumerary arteries that do not. As the muscular arteries extend to smaller and smaller branches they eventually lose their muscular coat and become arterioles. These vessels are usually smaller than 100 µm. They empty into capillaries in the alveolar walls that consist of a single layer of endothelial cells resting on a basement membrane (75,76,88).

The pulmonary venules have a media consisting of collagen and elastic fibers (75,76,88). These can closely resemble arterioles and the distinction may require serial sections to track the

Table 15-1

WHO NOMENCLATURE AND CLASSIFICATION OF PULMONARY HYPERTENSION[a]

1. Pulmonary Arterial Hypertension
   - 1.1 Primary pulmonary hypertension
     - a. Sporadic
     - b. Familial
   - 1.2 Related to:
     - a. Collagen vascular disease
     - b. Congenital systemic to pulmonary shunts
     - c. Portal hypertension
     - d. Human immunodeficiency virus (HIV) infection
     - e. Drugs/toxins
       - 1) Anorexigens
       - 2) Other
     - f. Persistent pulmonary hypertension of the newborn
     - g. Other
2. Pulmonary Venous Hypertension
   - 2.1 Left-sided atrial or ventricular heart disease
   - 2.2 Left-sided valvular heart disease
   - 2.3 Extrinsic compression of central pulmonary veins
     - a. Fibrosing mediastinitis
     - b. Adenopathy/tumors
   - 2.4 Pulmonary veno-occlusive disease
   - 2.5 Other
3. Pulmonary Hypertension Associated with Disorders of the Respiratory System and/or Hypoxemia
   - 3.1 Chronic obstructive pulmonary disease
   - 3.2 Interstitial lung disease
   - 3.3 Sleep disordered breathing
   - 3.4 Alveolar hypoventilation disorders
   - 3.5 Chronic exposure to high altitude
   - 3.6 Neonatal lung disease
   - 3.7 Alveolar-capillary dysplasia
   - 3.8 Other
4. Pulmonary Hypertension due to Chronic Thrombotic and/or Embolic Disease
   - 4.1 Thromboembolic obstruction of proximal pulmonary arteries
   - 4.2 Obstruction of distal pulmonary arteries
     - a. Pulmonary embolism (thrombus, tumor, ova and/or parasites, foreign material)
     - b. In situ thrombosis
     - c. Sickle cell disease
5. Pulmonary Hypertension due to Disorders Directly Affecting the Pulmonary Vasculature
   - 5.1 Inflammatory
     - a. Schistosomiasis
     - b. Sarcoidosis
     - c. Other
   - 5.2 Pulmonary capillary hemangiomatosis

[a]Modified from reference 53.

connection to larger vessels with more distinguishing characteristics. Larger veins have more medial collagen and elastic fibers as well as smooth muscle cells. The veins have an internal elastic lamina that may be discontinuous in smaller veins but continuous in larger veins.

Bronchial arteries are associated with the cartilage-bearing bronchi. Smaller nonmuscular branches can be followed to the level of the bronchioles; however, these are very difficult to recognize without serial sections (75,76,88). They have a thicker media than pulmonary arteries although their caliber is smaller than that of pulmonary arteries associated with the same bronchus. There is a prominent internal elastic lamina but the outer elastic lamina is less distinct or absent. The bronchial veins are closely associated with the bronchial arteries. They are thin-walled and contain valves. Through anastomoses they communicate extensively with pulmonary veins (75,76,88).

WORLD HEALTH ORGANIZATION CLASSIFICATION OF PULMONARY HYPERTENSION

The World Health Organization (WHO) has recently proposed a new classification of pulmonary hypertension (Table 15-1) (53). The previous WHO classification from 1975 was primarily based on pathology and included: 1) plexogenic pulmonary arteriopathy, 2) pulmonary veno-occlusive disease, and 3) recurrent pulmonary thromboembolism (28). The new WHO proposal recommends that the previous pathologic classification be dropped and a combined clinical, epidemiologic, and pathologic classification be used to classify pulmonary hypertension.

Previously, several schemes were proposed for grading the severity of the vascular changes in pulmonary hypertension associated with congenital heart disease (29,55,60,85,87). The one proposed by Heath and Edwards in 1958 (29) is particularly well known (Table 15-2). In patients with congenital heart disease, the presence of plexiform lesions, concentric laminar fibrosis, or arteritis suggests that the disease is irreversible even with surgical intervention. Unfortunately, these grading schemes are not reliable for assessing the severity of morphologic changes of primary pulmonary arterial hypertension in patients without congenital heart

Table 15-2

HEATH AND EDWARDS GRADING SCHEME FOR HYPERTENSIVE PULMONARY VASCULAR DISEASE

Grade 1:	Distal extension of muscle into distal arterioles and medial thickening of muscular arteries
Grade 2:	Cellular intimal proliferation limited to small muscular arteries, usually mostly cellular endothelial reaction
Grade 3:	Medial hypertrophy and concentric laminar intimal fibrosis
Grade 4:	Progressive generalized arterial dilatation with plexiform lesions
Grade 5:	Chronic dilatation with medial as well as intimal fibrosis; prominent plexiform lesions, vein-like branches and angiomatoid lesions; pulmonary hemosiderosis
Grade 6:	Necrotizing arteritis

[a]Modified from reference 29.

disease (4,7,76). Therefore, the WHO committee also recommended that the previous grading schemes be abandoned since they do not consistently correlate with clinical and hemodynamic findings outside of the setting of congenital heart disease (53).

Role of Histologic Assessment in Diagnosis of Pulmonary Vascular Diseases

Lung biopsy can play a helpful role in the diagnosis of primary pulmonary arterial hypertension, pulmonary arterial hypertension associated with congenital systemic to pulmonary shunts, pulmonary veno-occlusive disease, chronic thrombotic pulmonary hypertension due to obstruction of distal pulmonary arteries, and pulmonary capillary hemangiomatosis. However, pulmonary vascular disease is frequently overlooked histologically due to the subtlety of the vascular changes and the frequent "normal" appearance of the rest of the lung biopsy. Part of the challenge in accurate assessment of lung biopsies for pulmonary hypertension is the need for systematic evaluation of all types of blood vessels and their individual components as well as the surrounding lung tissue. The approach recommended by the 1998 WHO Symposium on Primary Pulmonary Hypertension is shown in Table 15-3 (53).

Although isolated blood vessels may show individual lesions, the vascular changes should be generalized before classifying a specific histologic pattern of pulmonary hypertension. Elastic stains are essential for evaluating lung biopsies for pulmonary hypertension. The most useful stain is the Movat pentachrome stain, which highlights both the elastic fibers and the intimal fibrosis. Inflation of the specimen through the largest artery or directly into the lung tissue can also be helpful. Despite the value of lung biopsy in classifying the type of pulmonary hypertension, in up to one fourth of cases, the histologic findings are indeterminate (73).

Certain artifacts can cause problems in the histologic assessment of the pulmonary vasculature. Traction artifact, also known as a pedunculated nodule, can result from the invagination of the elastic artery wall into the vessel lumen (fig. 15-1). This can resemble a thrombus, embolus, or a pulmonary hypertensive change. Tangential sections can also give the impression of intimal thickening or fibrosis.

PULMONARY ARTERIAL HYPERTENSION

Definition. Pulmonary arterial hypertension is a clinical syndrome characterized by elevated pulmonary arterial pressures. The WHO definition of pulmonary hypertension is a systolic pulmonary artery pressure of more than 40 mm Hg, which corresponds to a tricuspid regurgitant velocity on Doppler echocardiography of 3.0 to 3.5 m/sec (53). Histologically, the pulmonary arteries can show a spectrum of findings, including medial hypertrophy, concentric laminar intimal fibrosis, plexiform lesions, dilatation lesions, and vasculitis. Synonyms include *primary plexiform arteriopathy, plexogenic pulmonary arteriopathy, primary pulmonary arteriopathy,* and *arterial pulmonary hypertension, plexiform type.* Primary pulmonary arterial hypertension can occur as a primary sporadic disorder of unknown cause, as a familial condition, or in the

Table 15-3

PROTOCOL FOR EVALUATION OF LUNG BIOPSIES FOR PULMONARY HYPERTENSION[a]

I. Vasculature
- A. Vessels
  Elastic preacinar and intra-acinar arteries, microvessels, postacinar and intra-acinar veins, capillaries, lymphatics, and bronchial vessels. The vessel lumen should be commented on with respect to thrombi (recent or old) and abnormal cellular and matrix components.
- B. Components
  1. Endothelium/intima
     a. Cellular components (endothelial cells and smooth muscle cells)
     b. Matrix (elastin, collagen, mucopolysaccharides)
  2. Media
     a. Pattern (eccentric or concentric)
     b. Cellular components (smooth muscle and/or other cells)
     c. Matrix
  3. Adventitia
     a. Cellular components (fibroblasts)
     b. Matrix
  4. Complex vascular lesions: dilatation complexes, plexiform lesions, fibrinoid necrosis, arteritis, hemosiderosis, granulomas
  5. Inflammatory cells
     a. Types (neutrophils and mononuclear cells)
     b. Sites (perivascular or vascular wall)
- C. Quantification
  Identify arteries by type of accompanying airways. An assessment of the number of affected vessels in proportion to total vessels at a given airway level should be given. The number of vessels in relation to the alveoli should be determined.

II. Lung Tissue
Components: Preacinar and intra-acinar airways, alveoli, interstitium, and pleura
The description should include:
1. Source of tissue (postmortem, explant, or open lung biopsy) with a comment on size
2. Sample site: lobe, central, or peripheral (avoid the lingula)
3. Preparation of tissue (fixation in inflation either via airways or by needle injection of unclamped biopsy is preferred)
4. Stains: hematoxylin and eosin (H&E), pentachrome, alpha-actin, factor VIII, and iron.

Comments: Description of state of inflation and adequacy of sample size, airway, and parenchyma including evidence of associated parenchymal disease. Any other abnormalities or hemorrhage.

[a]Modified from reference 53.

context of a variety of associated exposures or underlying diseases (Table 15-1) (51,53).

Clinical Features. *Sporadic Primary Pulmonary Hypertension (PPH).* Sporadic PPH is a rare condition diagnosed when pulmonary arterial hypertension is present in patients without other defined risk factors. PPH is most commonly found in young women, but it can occur at any age.

Familial PPH. Familial PPH is an extremely rare condition that has been found in families worldwide. The prevalence of genetic or familial PPH is uncertain but is at least 6 percent of all PPH cases (53). The disease appears to be genetically transmitted as an autosomal dominant trait with incomplete penetrance. The locus of a gene linked to familial PPH has been identified on chromosome 2q31-32 and an association with mutations in the bone morphogenetic protein receptor-II gene has been demonstrated (18,19). Vertical transmission has been demonstrated in as many as five generations in one family and is highly indicative of a single dominant gene for PPH (53).

Secondary Pulmonary Arterial Hypertension. Pulmonary arterial hypertension can also be associated with a wide variety of conditions (Table 15-1), including collagen vascular disease (27, 40,89), congenital systemic to pulmonary shunts (29,54,86), portal hypertension, human

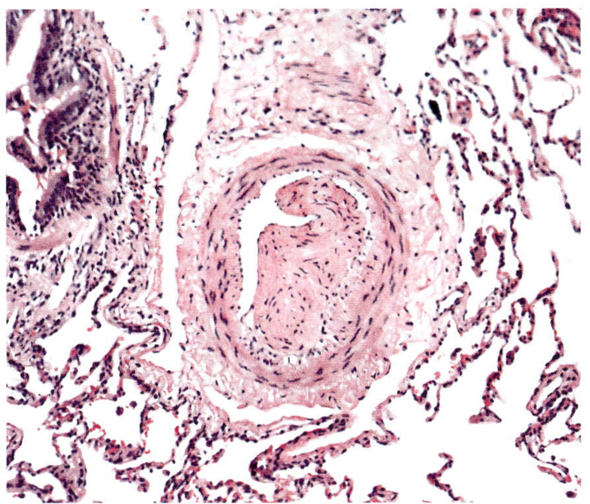
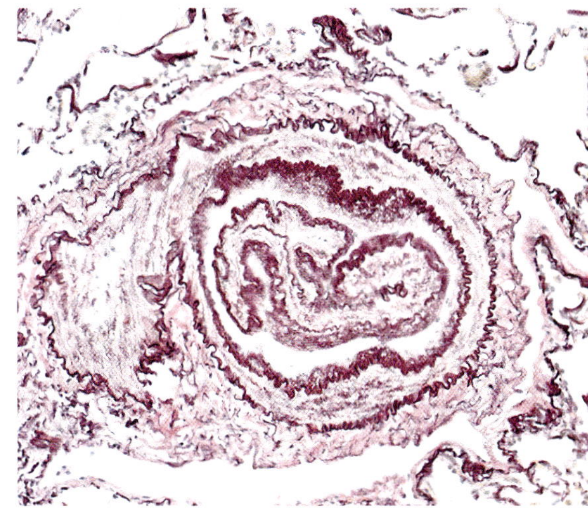

Figure 15-1

TELESCOPED ARTERIOLE

Left: The initial review of this vessel gave the impression of marked medial thickening.
Right: The elastic stain highlights how the vessel has invaginated into its own lumen, causing a telescopic artifact.

immunodeficiency virus (HIV) infection (10,15) drugs/toxins (17,38), and persistent pulmonary hypertension of the newborn (12). Risk factors for primary pulmonary arterial hypertension are summarized in Table 15-4.

Most patients with PPH present late in their clinical course with exertional dyspnea. As the disease progresses, patients develop exertional chest pain, syncope, and edema because of severe pulmonary hypertension and impaired right heart function. Physical examination is usually unremarkable until signs of cor pulmonale develop. Patients invariably progress to a fatal outcome. Serum uric acid, the final product of purine degradation, has been proposed as a marker for impaired oxidative metabolism and a possible predictor of mortality in patients with chronic heart failure. Hyperuricemia occurs commonly in patients with severe pulmonary hypertension (72), and the serum uric acid increases in proportion to the clinical severity of PPH and has an independent association with long-term mortality of patients with PPH (50).

The diagnosis of PPH rarely requires histopathologic confirmation and is made on clinical grounds, based on a comprehensive evaluation which includes pulmonary function testing, connective tissue serology, echocardiography, complete cardiac catheterization, ventilation-perfusion lung scanning, and pulmonary angiography.

Table 15-4

RISK FACTORS FOR PRIMARY PULMONARY HYPERTENSION[a]

I. Drugs and Toxins
- A. Definite: aminorex, fenfluramine, dexfenfluramine, toxic rapeseed oil
- B. Very likely: amphetamines, L-tryptophan
- C. Possible: meta-amphetamines, cocaine, chemotherapeutic agents
- D. Unlikely: antidepressants, oral contraceptives, estrogen therapy, cigarette smoking

II. Demographics and Medical Conditions
- A. Definite: gender
- B. Possible: pregnancy, systemic hypertension
- C. Unlikely: obesity

III. Diseases
- A. Definite: HIV infection
- B. Very likely: portal hypertension/liver disease, collagen vascular diseases, congenital systemic-pulmonary cardiac shunts
- C. Possible: thyroid disorders

[a]Modified from reference 53.

Radiologic Findings. The radiologic manifestations of pulmonary arterial hypertension are similar, regardless of the specific etiology. The findings consist of enlargement of the

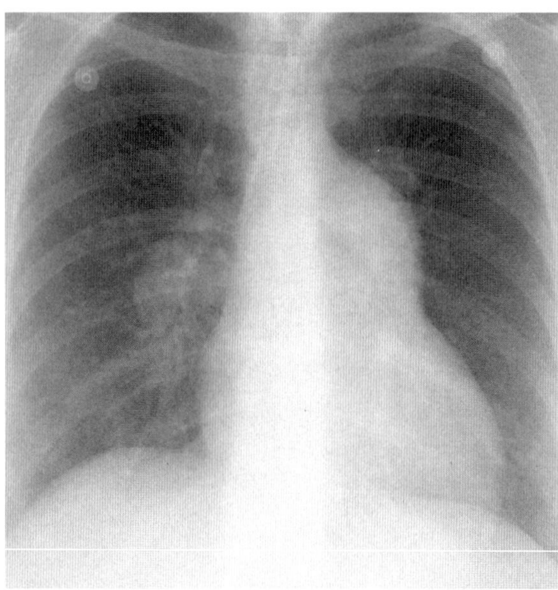

Figure 15-2

PULMONARY ARTERIAL HYPERTENSION

The chest radiograph shows marked dilatation of the main pulmonary artery, resulting in a focal convexity between the level of the aortic arch and left main bronchus. The right interlobar pulmonary artery is enlarged and measures approximately 2 cm in diameter. The patient was a 36-year-old woman with primary pulmonary arterial hypertension.

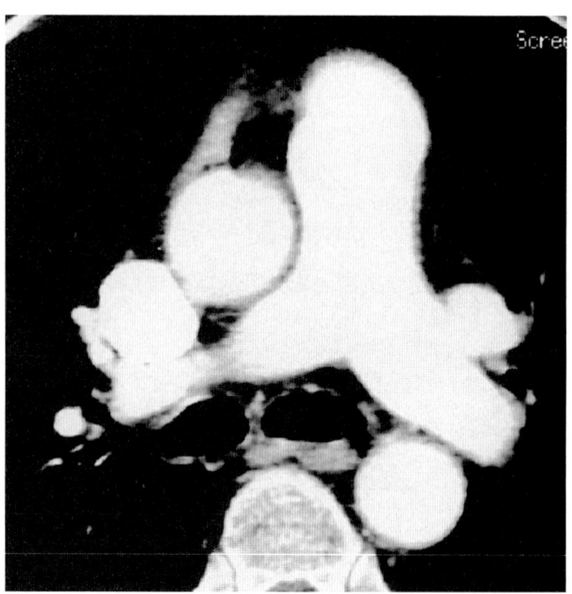

Figure 15-3

PULMONARY ARTERIAL HYPERTENSION

Contrast-enhanced chest CT demonstrates enlargement of the main pulmonary artery, which has a diameter of 31 mm, slightly greater than the diameter of the aorta. The patient was a 68-year-old man with acute pulmonary arterial hypertension due to pulmonary embolism.

central pulmonary arteries, rapid decrease in size (tapering) of the pulmonary arteries as they course distally, and peripheral oligemia (fig. 15-2) (24). The assessment of rapid tapering and peripheral oligemia is subjective and often difficult. The chest radiograph only allows reliable measurement of the right interlobar pulmonary artery, which is considered enlarged if it measures more than 16 mm in diameter (8,24). Computed tomography (CT) and magnetic resonance imaging (MRI) allow assessment of the main pulmonary artery. The main pulmonary artery is considered enlarged when its diameter is greater than 29 mm (fig. 15-3) (24,39,70).

Enlargement of the central pulmonary arteries can be seen in other conditions, particularly increased blood flow due to left-to-right shunts. Furthermore, there is often poor correlation between the diameter of the central pulmonary arteries and the severity of pulmonary arterial hypertension. The chest radiograph, CT, and MRI, therefore, play a limited role in the diagnosis of pulmonary arterial hypertension. Their main value lies in the diagnosis of possible underlying causes such as interstitial lung disease, pulmonary venous hypertension, and chronic thromboembolic disease (see below). The most accurate noninvasive method to diagnose pulmonary arterial hypertension is echocardiography (24).

Pathologic Findings. The pathology of pulmonary hypertension includes changes to the vascular endothelium, smooth muscle cells, and extracellular matrix. The major morphologic features include a spectrum of lesions, although in the appropriate setting, concentric laminar fibrosis, plexiform lesions, and vasculitis with fibrinoid necrosis are the only ones that are strongly suggestive of this type of pulmonary hypertension (Table 15-5). Generalized and uniform dilatation of muscular pulmonary arteries is typically associated with systemic to pulmonary shunts, especially atrial septal defects. If all the pulmonary arteries are wider than the caliber of the adjacent bronchi then the dilatation is probably generalized (76).

Medial hypertrophy due to thickening of the arteriolar muscular layer is the earliest and

Table 15-5

CHARACTERISTIC MORPHOLOGIC CHANGES IN PRIMARY PULMONARY ARTERIAL HYPERTENSION[a]

Medial hypertrophy and muscularization of arterioles
Cellular proliferation of intima
Concentric laminar intimal fibrosis
Dilatation lesions (angiomatoid lesions)
Fibrinoid necrosis
Plexiform lesions
Occasional additional lesions include:
Tortuosity
General dilatation
Intimal longitudinal smooth muscle

[a]Adapted from reference 76.

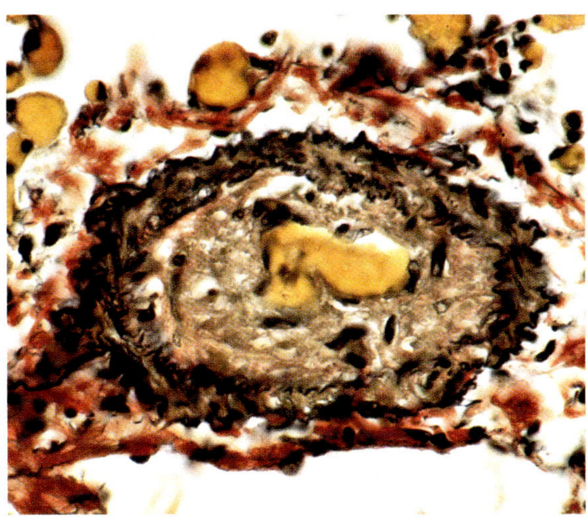

Figure 15-5

PULMONARY ARTERIAL HYPERTENSION: CELLULAR INTIMAL PROLIFERATION

A cellular proliferation of the intima of this small arteriole has caused narrowing of the lumen.

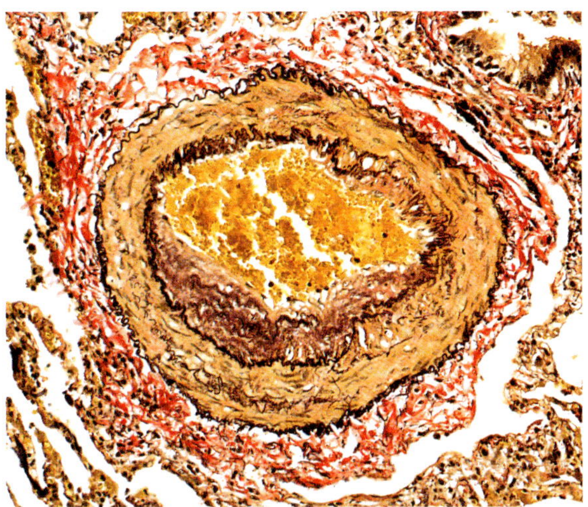

Figure 15-4

PULMONARY ARTERIAL HYPERTENSION: MEDIAL THICKENING

The elastic stain highlights the mild thickening of the media of this arteriole.

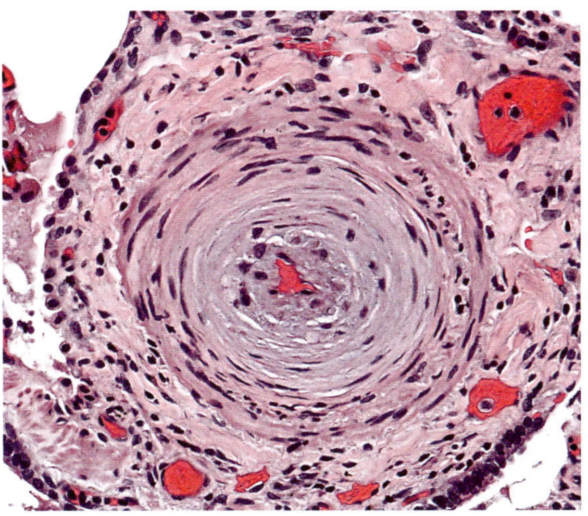

Figure 15-6

PULMONARY ARTERIAL HYPERTENSION: CONCENTRIC LAMINAR INTIMAL FIBROSIS

The concentric laminar fibrosis of this arteriole has caused severe narrowing of the vessel lumen.

most common alteration (fig. 15-4). In general, there is a correlation between the degree of medial hypertrophy and the pulmonary arterial pressure (76). The average, normal arteriolar medial thickness in adults is 3 to 7 percent of the external vascular diameter. Mild, moderate, and marked medial thicknesses range from 7 to 9 percent, 10 to 14 percent, and greater than 15 percent, respectively (76). However, there is a continuum of severity and it is difficult to make a sharp distinction between categories.

There are two forms of intimal thickening in primary pulmonary arterial hypertension: cellular intimal proliferation and concentric laminar intimal fibrosis (figs. 15-5, 15-6). They often occur together and when severe can cause marked narrowing or obliteration of the arteriolar lumen. Unlike medial hypertrophy, which results from an increase in the thickness of an existing vascular component, thickening of the

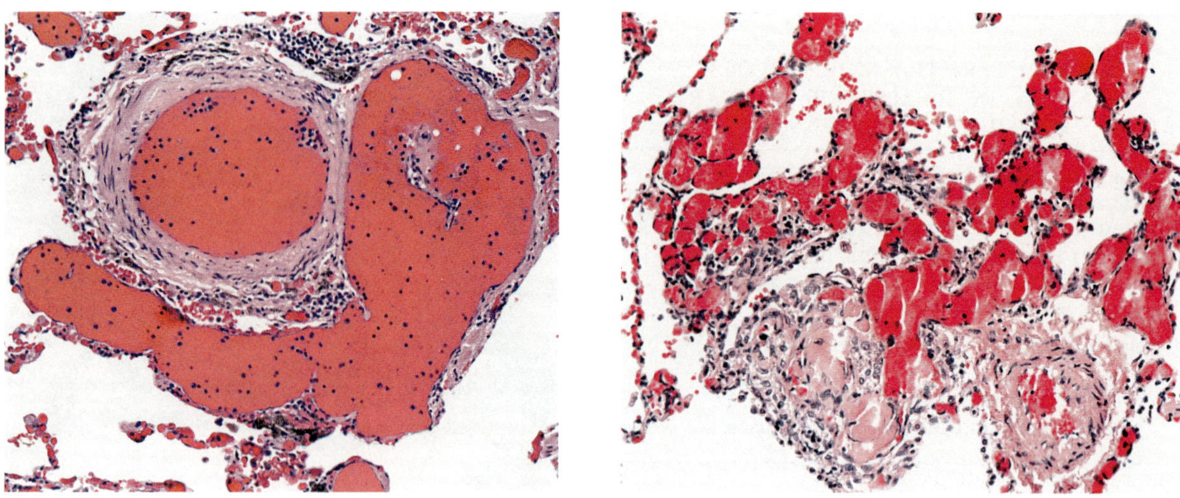

Figure 15-7

PULMONARY ARTERIAL HYPERTENSION: DILATATION LESION

Left: A dilated, vein-like, thin-walled arterial branch surrounds the parent arteriole which shows medial hypertrophy.
Right: Dilatation lesion with angiomatoid features. Adjacent to this parent artery is a large collection of dilated, thin-walled branches forming an angiomatoid lesion.

intima is caused by a cellular proliferation within a normally noncellular region between the endothelium and internal elastic lamina. The matrix of the cellular intimal proliferation may be mucopolysaccharide rich, but usually there is no increased deposition of collagen. Concentric laminar intimal fibrosis is associated with collagen or elastin deposition within the matrix of a cellular intimal proliferation. As these lesions progress, they become more fibrotic and demonstrate a concentric laminar morphology, usually with central placement of the arteriolar lumen. This lesion is distinctive for primary pulmonary arterial hypertension, especially if present in multiple arteries (76).

Localized dilatation of pulmonary arteries occurs in the setting of sustained pulmonary hypertension resulting in widening of the lumen and thinning of the arterial wall. This can result in "vein-like branches of arteries" that contrast markedly to the thickened parent artery (fig. 15-7). The vein-like arteries form clusters around the thickened artery and are sometimes complex enough to form "angiomatoid lesions" due to the resemblance to a small angioma (fig. 15-8) (76). These lesions have sometimes been grouped together with plexiform lesions (29).

Plexiform lesions are seen in severe pulmonary hypertension (20,52,76,78). They typically affect arteries measuring 80 to 150 µm in diameter and are situated close to the branch point from the parent artery. They consist of areas of dilatation due to arterial wall destruction by thinning of the media, loss of smooth muscle cells, and rupture or complete loss of the elastic lamina (fig. 15-9). Within the dilated lumen a glomeruloid plexus of narrow slit-like channels develops. In the early stages, a fibrin clot develops that becomes organized and recanalized, forming the plexus of vessels (fig. 15-10). Plexiform lesions may be difficult to find and require examination of multiple tissue sections, or they may be prominent. The pathogenesis of the plexiform lesion is not known, however, it is speculated that it develops in areas of fibrinoid necrosis in association with spastic vasoconstriction (76).

Fibrinoid necrosis and arteritis are advanced lesions found in patients with severe pulmonary hypertension and portend a poor prognosis (figs. 15-11, 15-12) (20,52,76,78). Fibrinoid necrosis usually affects arteries smaller than 100 µm in diameter and results from necrosis and fibrin deposition in the vascular wall, particularly the medial smooth muscle. Necrotizing arteritis tends

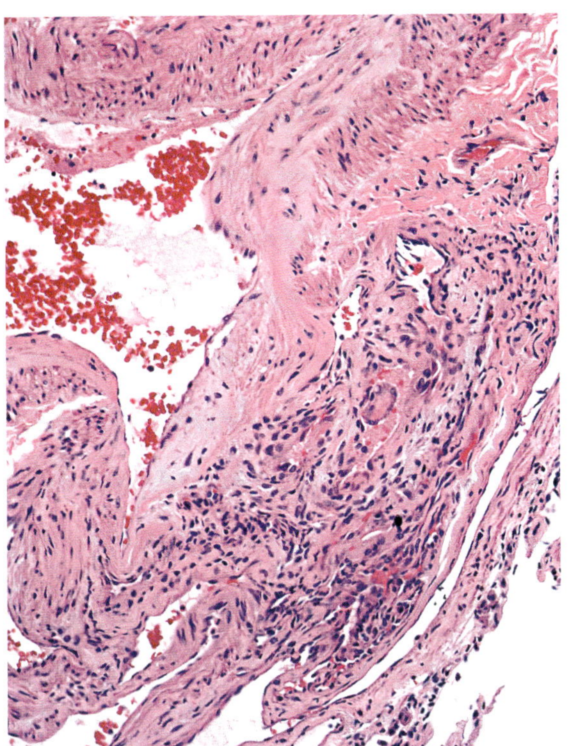

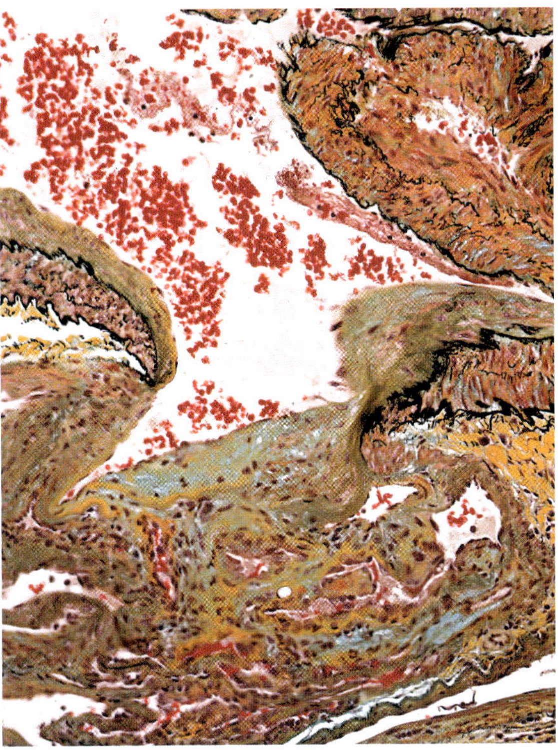

Figure 15-8

PULMONARY ARTERIAL HYPERTENSION: PLEXIFORM LESION

Left: A glomeruloid plexus of slit-like vascular channels is present adjacent to an arteriole.

Right: The plexiform lesion (bottom) highlighted by the Movat stain protrudes through the wall of the arteriole. The elastic laminae of the arteriole are lost at the base of the lesion.

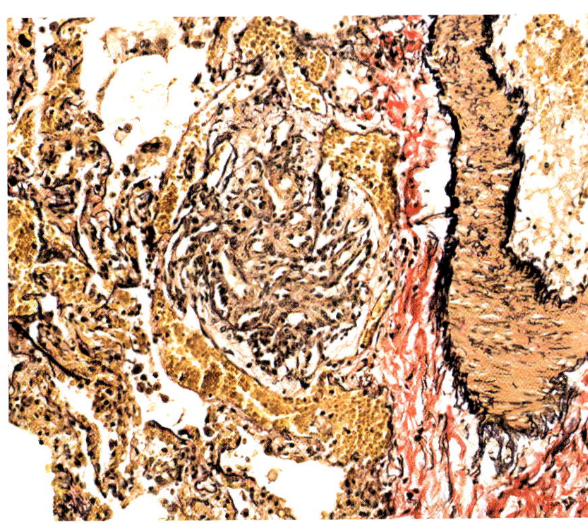

Figure 15-9

PULMONARY ARTERIAL HYPERTENSION: PLEXIFORM LESION

An elastic stain demonstrates a plexiform lesion adjacent to an arteriole.

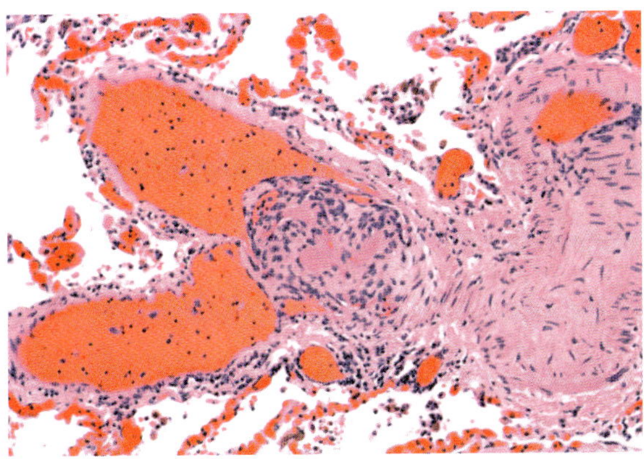

Figure 15-10

PULMONARY ARTERIAL HYPERTENSION: EARLY PLEXIFORM LESION

An early plexiform lesion is developing as the fibrin clot (center) becomes recanalized. The lesion is situated adjacent to the parent artery (right) and within a dilatation lesion consisting of vein-like arteriolar branches (left).

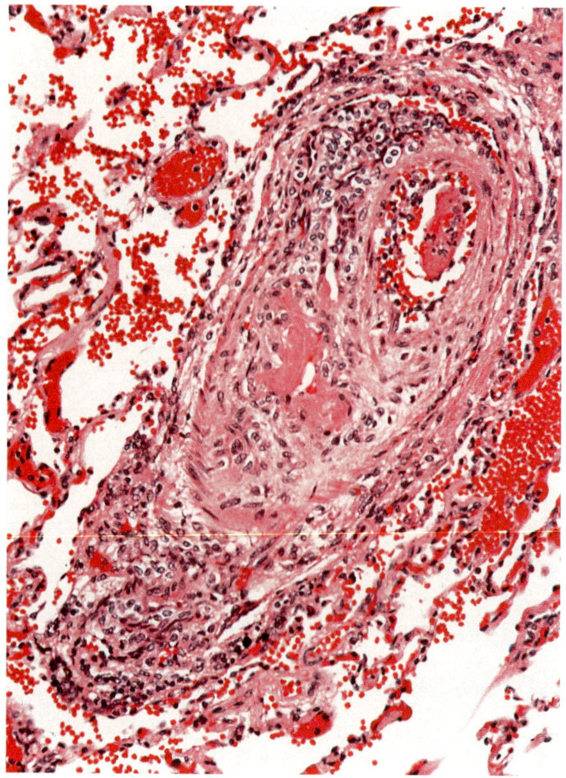

Figure 15-11

PULMONARY ARTERIAL HYPERTENSION: FIBRINOID NECROSIS

The wall of this arteriole shows fibrinoid necrosis. At the lower pole of the vessel is an early plexiform lesion with a plexus of slit-like vascular channels.

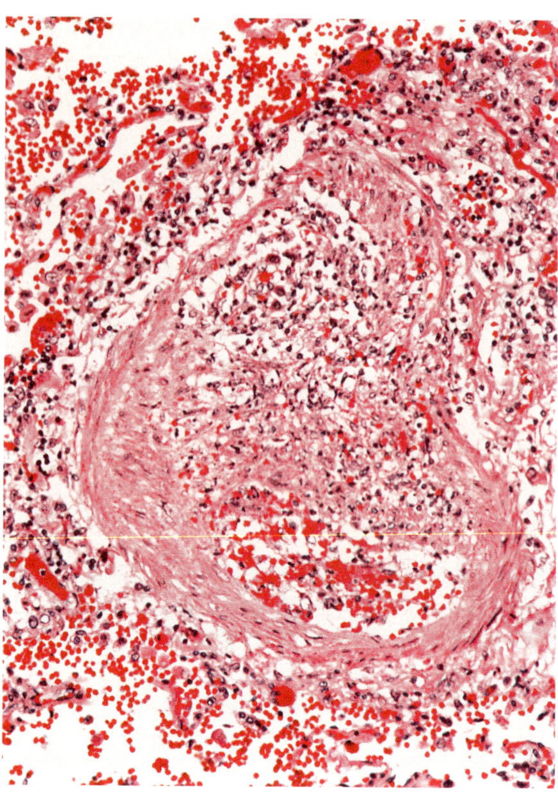

Figure 15-12

PULMONARY ARTERIAL HYPERTENSION: VASCULITIS

This arteriole shows a severe necrotizing vasculitis with a marked inflammatory infiltrate permeating the media.

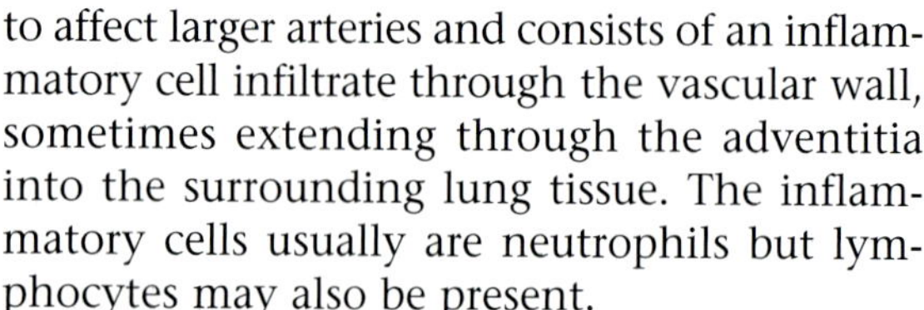

to affect larger arteries and consists of an inflammatory cell infiltrate through the vascular wall, sometimes extending through the adventitia into the surrounding lung tissue. The inflammatory cells usually are neutrophils but lymphocytes may also be present.

In patients with congenital heart disease, concentric laminar fibrosis, plexiform lesions, and arteritis are regarded as irreversible changes.

Pathogenesis. The pathogenesis of PPH is not known. It probably involves a variety of factors: intense spastic vasoconstriction with an apparent imbalance in the vasoconstricting and vasodilating mediators or substances involved in the control of pulmonary vascular tone; the influence of local hemodynamics and sheer stress on vascular remodeling; alterations in matrix protein synthesis; endothelial damage and alteration of the endothelial cell phenotype (loss of expression of prostacyclin synthase enzyme and gene in the lung, reduced expression of nitric oxide synthase); alterations in vascular smooth muscle; and platelet reactivity and thrombosis in situ (9,53). The plexiform lesion is a distinctive lesion, the pathogenesis of which is poorly understood. Angiogenesis and/or various growth factors are probably involved (9).

Treatment and Prognosis. Chronic oxygen therapy is important since patients with PPH may experience hypoxemia at rest or during activity. Diuretics can be used cautiously for control of edema. Patients with PPH require life-long anticoagulation because they are at increased risk for intrapulmonary thrombosis and thromboembolism. The risk factors responsible for these problems include sluggish pulmonary blood flow, dilated right heart chambers, venous stasis, and sedentary lifestyle (63). Anticoagulants appear to improve survival. The anticoagulant of choice is warfarin, with the goal of therapy to achieve a prothrombin time with an International Normalized Ratio (INR) of approximately of 1.5 to 2.0; however, different clinical circumstances may require adjustment of this range (53,63).

Vasoconstriction plays a role in the pathogenesis of PPH. Consequently, there has been increasing interest in vasodilator therapy for these patients. Between 25 and 35 percent of patients with this disorder are "responders" to the acute administration of nitric oxide, epoprostenol, or other vasodilators (calcium channel blockers) (63). The usefulness of calcium channel blockers in patients with PPH is believed to be based on the ability to cause vasodilatation of pulmonary vascular smooth muscle (53).

The creation of an atrial septostomy in PPH patients has been suggested as a bridge to transplantation if deterioration occurs despite maximum medical therapy (53,61,63). The rationale is based on experimental and clinical observations suggesting that an intra-atrial defect allowing right to left shunting in the setting of severe pulmonary hypertension leads to improvement in pulmonary artery pressures and the patient's hemodynamic status. Heart-lung and single and bilateral lung transplantation have been performed successfully in patients with PPH (32,83). The major decision is when to refer the patient for transplantation since most run the risk of dying while waiting, given that suitable organs for transplantation are limited. Patients who fall into New York Heart Association functional class III or IV and have hemodynamic parameters predicting poor survival should be evaluated for transplantation. The operative mortality ranges from 16 to 29 percent and is affected by the primary diagnosis (53). The 5-year survival rate is between 40 and 45 percent (53). Recurrence of PPH after transplantation has not been reported. Patients with PPH of unknown cause usually die within 1 to 3 years, although there are rare long-term survivors (6). The natural history of precapillary pulmonary hypertension shows that the most important measure of severity and predictor of poor survival is cardiac output (31). Patients who have a cardiac output in excess of 2.5 L/min and have a capacity to vasodilate have the best survival rates in response to oral treatment with vasodilators and anticoagulants. Patients with severe pulmonary hypertension are the ones most likely to respond to long-term treatment with intravenous epoprostenol or iloprost (an analogue of prostacyclin) (31). In the United States the mortality of patients with PPH has increased notably since 1979. Some portion of this increase is likely do to improvements in diagnostic recognition, however, it has been suggested the increase may be related to the introduction of anorexigens during this time period (41,58).

PULMONARY VENOUS HYPERTENSION

Definition. Pulmonary venous hypertension results from obstruction of pulmonary venous outflow. Obstruction of pulmonary venous outflow causes a variety of changes including medial hypertrophy and muscularization of arterioles, medial hypertrophy and arterialization of veins, dilatation of lymphatics, hemosiderosis, interstitial edema, and fibrosis. Pulmonary venous hypertension is usually cardiac in origin, most often due to mitral valve disease or left ventricular failure. In addition to cardiac causes, pulmonary venous hypertension can be due to external compression of large pulmonary veins by mediastinal fibrosis (11), adenopathy, or neoplasms (5). Pulmonary veno-occlusive disease is another rare cause (see below) (1,79,80).

Clinical Features. Common causes of pulmonary venous hypertension are summarized in Table 15-1 (76,82). Left-sided ventricular failure is the most common cause and it may be due to coronary heart disease, myocarditis, or hypertension. Left mitral valve dysfunction due to congenital stenosis, atresia, or rheumatic disease is associated with severe venous hypertension and substantial pulmonary artery hypertension. Rare congenital causes include pulmonary vein abnormalities such as congenital stenosis of major pulmonary veins and total anomalous pulmonary venous connection. Left atrial disorders include cor triatriatum and myxoma (76). Pulmonary venous hypertension is also caused by disorders of the aortic valve such as congenital stenosis or atresia, acquired stenosis or incompetence, and aortic coarctation (76).

Radiologic Findings. Normally, in the upright individual, the upper lobe vessels are smaller than the lower lobe vessels due to the

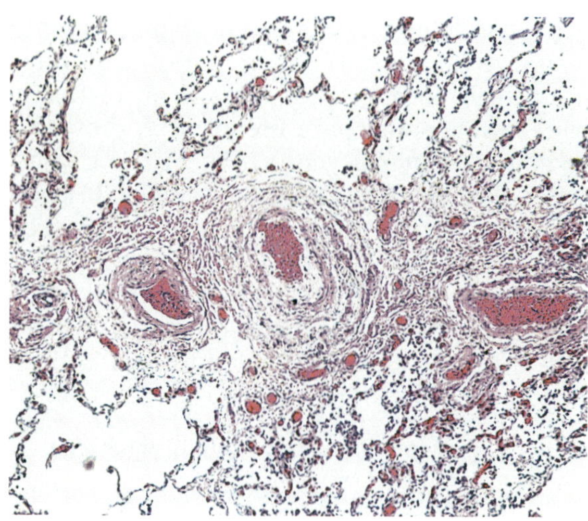

Figure 15-13

PULMONARY VENOUS HYPERTENSION: ATERIOLAR INTIMAL FIBROSIS

The intimal fibrosis is eccentric, unlike the concentric laminar changes in primary pulmonary ateriopathy.

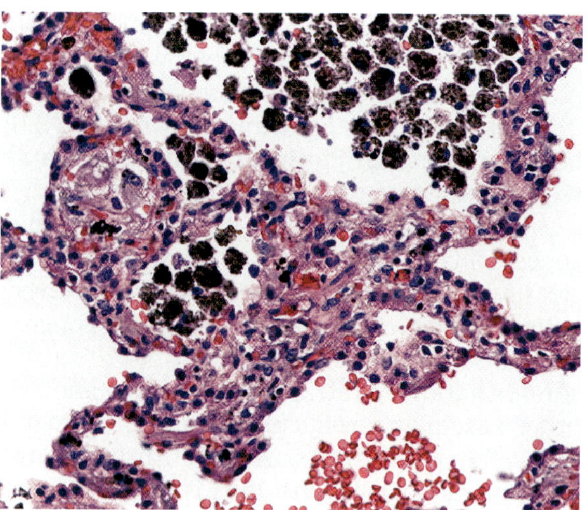

Figure 15-14

PULMONARY VENOUS HYPERTENSION: HEMOSIDEROSIS

Many hemosiderin-laden macrophages are present in these alveolar spaces and there is mild thickening of the alveolar walls.

Table 15-6

CHARACTERISTIC MORPHOLOGIC CHANGES IN CONGESTIVE VASCULOPATHY[a]

Pulmonary Arteries
Prominent medial hypertrophy and muscularization of arterioles
Prominent eccentric, nonlaminar, nonobstructive intimal fibrosis over long distances
Pulmonary Veins
Medial hypertrophy and arterialization
Moderate intimal fibrosis
Lymphatics
Dilatation
Lung Tissue
Interstitial edema, interstitial fibrosis, hemosiderosis

[a]Adapted from reference 76.

effect of gravity on pulmonary blood flow. The earliest radiographic manifestation of pulmonary venous hypertension is blood flow redistribution to the upper lobes. This results in upper lobe vessels of similar or larger size than lower lobe vessels (24,56). Pulmonary venous hypertension secondary to left ventricular failure is commonly associated with cardiomegaly. Findings of pulmonary edema, such as indistinct margins of the lower lobe vessels, perihilar haze, thickening of the interlobular septa (septal or Kerley B lines), and small pleural effusions are often present (24,56). Pulmonary venous hypertension secondary to mitral valve disease is associated with prominence of the left atrial appendage, which can be readily recognized as a focal prominence of the left heart border immediately below the level of the left main bronchus.

Pathologic Findings. In congestive vasculopathy, the elastic pulmonary arteries commonly show intimal fibrosis (fig. 15-13), which is often extensive and severe (Table 15-6). It is usually eccentric and lacks the concentric onion-skin pattern of primary pulmonary arteriopathy (see fig. 15-7). In addition, muscular arteries can appear normal or show medial hypertrophy. Congestive vasculopathy differs from thrombotic arteriopathy in that the intimal fibrosis of the muscular pulmonary arteries extends over longer distances. The veins and venules show medial hypertrophy and arterialization, with moderate intimal fibrosis. The arterialization results from changes in the elastic tissue, with condensation of the fibers to form internal and external elastic laminae. Lymphatics are dilated. The surrounding lung tissue shows hemosiderosis (fig. 15-14), interstitial fibrosis, chronic congestion, and interstitial edema of the vessel walls, pleura, interlobular septa, and parenchyma.

Treatment and Prognosis. The most effective treatment for patients with pulmonary venous hypertension is an aggressive approach to establishing the underlying cause. Surgical correction of an atrial septal defect or mitral stenosis will lead to improvement in the pulmonary venous hypertension. Data from autopsies of several patients showed marked regression of the severe arterial medial hypertrophy and intimal fibrosis as well as venous medial hypertrophy and arterialization that was seen in lung biopsies at the time of mitral valve surgery (76). Many patients do well following mitral valve replacement despite the severe vascular changes seen on lung biopsies at the time of valve surgery (76). For this reason, lung biopsies are rarely used to evaluate the reversibility of pulmonary venous hypertension.

PULMONARY VENO-OCCLUSIVE DISEASE

Definition. Pulmonary veno-occlusive disease (PVOD) is a rare cause of pulmonary hypertension in which small pulmonary veins and venules are occluded by intimal fibrosis.

Clinical Features. PVOD accounts for 10 percent of cases of pulmonary hypertension of unknown etiology (62). In children, there is no sex predilection but in adults there is a 2 to 1 male to female ratio. More than half of the cases are encountered in the first three decades of life. Patients present with symptoms similar to those of other types of pulmonary hypertension including dyspnea on exertion and fatigue in the early stages, and cyanosis, hemoptysis, and syncope in the late stages. Bibasilar crackles may occasionally be heard on chest examination. PVOD may be difficult to distinguish from congestive heart failure and PPH. The disease has been reported to follow viral infections, exposure to toxic agents, and chemotherapy (67).

Radiologic Findings. The radiologic manifestations of PVOD include enlargement of the central pulmonary arteries due to arterial hypertension and findings of interstitial pulmonary edema (indistinct margins of the lower lobe vessels and thickening of the interlobular septa) (24). The left atrium is not enlarged and there is no redistribution of blood flow to the upper lobes. These findings are helpful in distinguishing PVOD from left ventricular failure and mitral valve disease. High-resolution (HR) CT demonstrates normal-sized pulmonary veins, extensive interlobular septal thickening, and areas of ground-glass attenuation due to interstitial pulmonary edema (69). Another common finding on the radiograph and HRCT is the presence of small bilateral pleural effusions.

Table 15-7

CHARACTERISTIC MORPHOLOGIC CHANGES IN PULMONARY VENO-OCCLUSIVE DISEASE[a]

Pulmonary Veins and Venules
Obstructive intimal fibrosis, initially of a loose texture
Recanalization and septa formation
Recent thrombi scarce
Medial hypertrophy and arterialization
Pulmonary Arteries
Sometimes similar intimal changes, often with recent thrombi
Sometimes medial hypertrophy
Lung Tissue
Prominent hemosiderosis, focal congestion, and interstitial fibrosis

[a]Adapted from reference 76.

Pathologic Findings. Histologically, the veins and venules show an obstructive intimal fibrosis (Table 15-7; figs. 15-15, 15-16) (30,76, 79). The fibrosis is often loose and edematous initially and becomes denser with time. Recanalization of the intimal fibrosis with formation of intravascular fibrous septa is common (30,76,79). The media of the veins may show hypertrophy and arterialization.

In up to 50 percent of cases, muscular pulmonary arteries show loose intimal fibrosis similar to that seen in the veins (fig. 15-17) (76,80). Hypertensive arterial changes and recent thrombi are also often seen. This can cause obliteration of the arterial lumen and recanalization; formation of intravascular septa is common. Veins may become arterialized and develop a double elastic layer, making it very difficult to separate veins from arteries (13).

Fibrous thickening of the interlobular septa is characteristic (fig. 15-18). Sclerotic veins may be seen within the septa and in some cases,

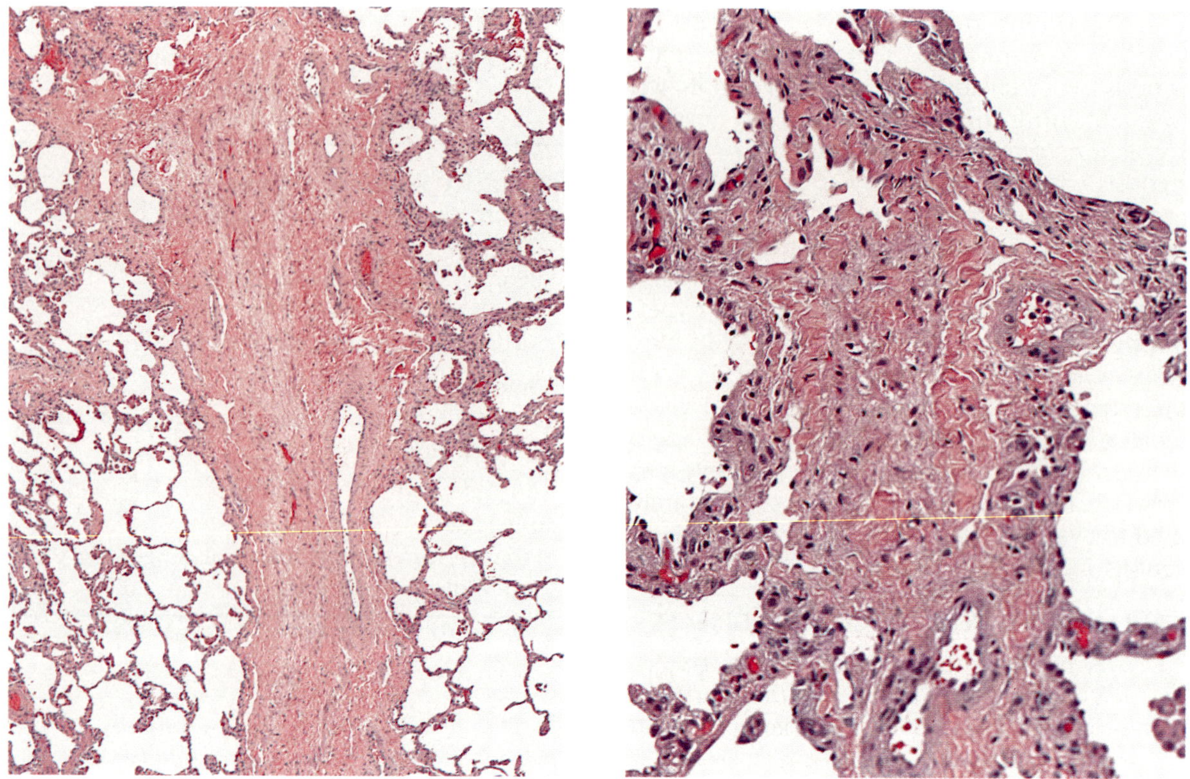

Figure 15-15

PULMONARY VENO-OCCLUSIVE DISEASE

Left: The interstitium appears fibrotically thickened, however, these lesions are actually scarred veins. Right: This is a small vein that is completely obliterated by occlusive fibrosis.

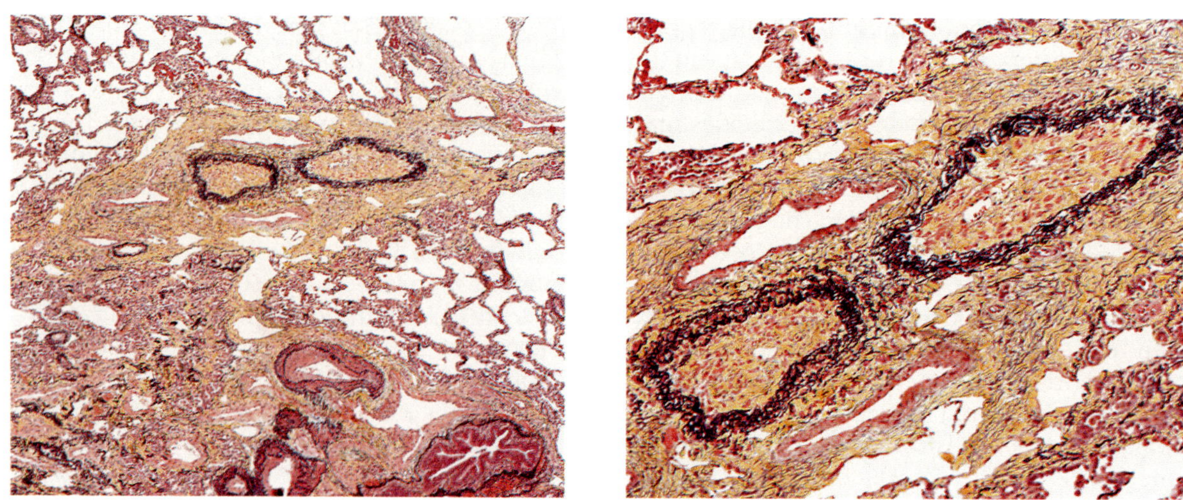

Figure 15-16

PULMONARY VENO-OCCLUSIVE DISEASE

Left: This Movat stain highlights the venous occlusion and interstitial thickening around the vein. Right: This vein is completely obliterated by occlusive fibrosis.

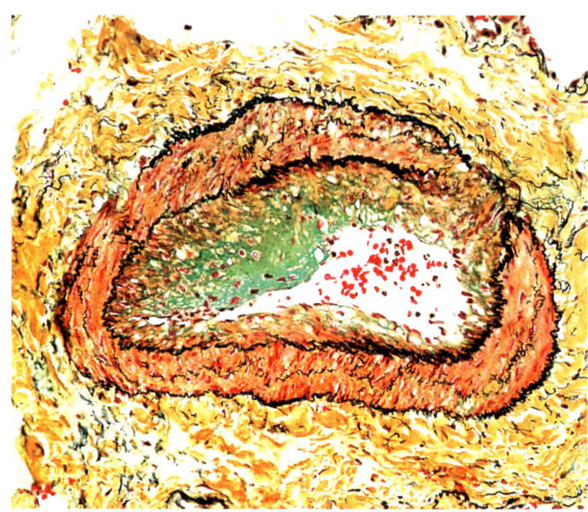

Figure 15-17

PULMONARY VENO-OCCLUSIVE DISEASE: ARTERIAL INTIMAL FIBROSIS

The Movat stain highlights the loose intimal fibrosis in this arteriole.

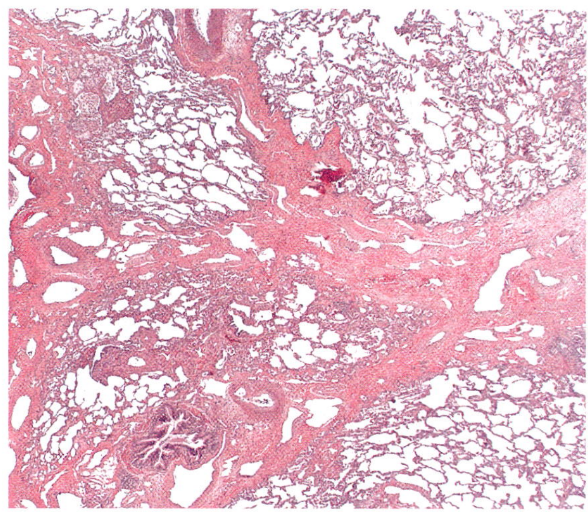

Figure 15-18

PULMONARY VENO-OCCLUSIVE DISEASE: SEPTAL THICKENING

The interlobular septa show marked fibrous thickening.

lymphatic spaces become dilated, raising the possibility of lymphangiomatosis. Areas of alveolar capillary proliferation may give the appearance of capillary hemangiomatosis (see below).

The lungs can show foci of severe congestion or interstitial fibrosis. Hemosiderosis is common. When prominent it may be associated with iron encrustation of blood vessel walls (also known as endogenous pneumoconiosis; see fig. 2-9) (13). Interstitial inflammation and hyaline membranes are rarely seen.

Pathogenesis. The cause of PVOD is not known. Thrombosis is thought to play a role, with a variety of potential initiating events. PVOD is associated with respiratory infections (especially viral infections), toxic exposures (chemotherapy), malignancies (65), bone marrow transplantation (65), scleroderma (46), and renal transplantation (76,80). Genetic factors may be involved, as there are several reports of siblings with PVOD (80).

Differential Diagnosis. Concentric laminar intimal fibrosis and plexiform lesions are characteristic of pulmonary arterial hypertension and are not seen in PVOD disease even when the intimal fibrosis is circumferential. The presence of interstitial fibrosis, hemosiderosis, and congestion can result in confusion with interstitial fibrotic disorders, idiopathic pulmonary hemorrhage, and chronic passive congestion. Whenever these lesions are suspected, PVOD should be considered and the veins carefully examined with elastic stains (76,79). Capillary hemangiomatosis may be present.

Treatment and Prognosis. Patients with PVOD tend to have a more fulminant clinical course than those with PPH. Median survival in one series was 84 days with 71 percent mortality in the first 6 months (52). No effective therapy exists except for heart-lung transplantation.

PULMONARY HYPERTENSION ASSOCIATED WITH DISORDERS OF THE RESPIRATORY SYSTEM AND/OR HYPOXEMIA

Definition. Lung diseases are the most common causes of pulmonary hypertension. This type of pulmonary hypertension usually is not evident until the underlying lung disease is severe, often endstage.

Clinical Features. Pulmonary hypertension can be caused by any condition that causes hypoxemia. Some of the many potential causes are summarized in Table 15-8. Recently, it was shown that pulmonary hypertension can develop following lung reduction surgery in patients with emphysema (81). The underlying pathogenesis of this type of pulmonary hypertension is vasoconstriction of small pulmonary arteries.

Table 15-8

CAUSES OF HYPOXIC PULMONARY ARTERIOPATHY[a]

Upper Airway Obstruction
Hyperplastic adenoids
Facioskeletal malformations
Chronic Obstructive Lung Disease
Chronic bronchitis
Emphysema
Bronchial asthma
Interstitial fibrosis
Alveolar Hypoventilation on Central Basis
Central nervous system disorders
Pickwickian syndrome
Sleep apnea syndrome
Neuromuscular Disorders
Progressive muscular dystrophy
Poliomyelitis
Thoracic Skeletal Disorders
Kyphoscoliosis
Thoracic ankylosing spondylitis
Pediatric Disorders
Neonatal lung disease
Alveolar-capillary dysplasia
High Altitude

[a]Information from references 76 and 82.

Table 15-9

CHARACTERISTIC MORPHOLOGIC CHANGES IN HYPOXIC ARTERIOPATHY[a]

Increased muscularity of small arterial branches (medial hypertrophy and peripheral extension of smooth muscle); large arteries are normal or have mild medial hypertrophy
Longitudinal smooth muscle bundles or layers in intima of small arterial branches
Similar changes to a lesser extent in small pulmonary veins

[a]Data from reference 76.

Radiologic Findings. The radiologic findings of pulmonary hypertension caused by underlying lung disease consist of enlargement of the central pulmonary arteries, rapid decrease in size (tapering) of the pulmonary arteries as they course distally, and peripheral oligemia (24). In patients with pulmonary arterial hypertension due to chronic obstructive or interstitial lung disease, the chest radiograph and HRCT are helpful in assessing the severity and extent of the underlying lung disease.

Pathologic Findings. The vascular changes in hypoxia are often overlooked since the changes primarily affect small arterioles while larger muscular arterioles greater than 100 µm are often normal or only show mild medial hypertrophy (Table 15-9). Small arteries typically have increased muscularity due to medial hypertrophy and peripheral extension of smooth muscle. The longitudinal smooth muscle that appears in small arterioles tends to be in the intima within a reduplicated internal elastic lamina. In some cases, the smooth muscle may involve the media or adventitia. In the setting of interstitial fibrosis, the arterioles often show medial as well as intimal thickening (see fig. 3-12). In patients with chronic obstructive lung disease, post-thrombotic lesions are common and result in eccentric intimal fibrosis.

Treatment and Prognosis. The prognosis is determined by the underlying illness. In general, the presence of pulmonary hypertension is a poor prognostic sign. The treatment plan should focus on the underlying disease. Supplemental oxygen can correct the arterial hypoxemia and may reduce the pulmonary arterial hypertension. Long-term supplemental oxygen therapy may improve prognosis and survival.

PULMONARY HYPERTENSION DUE TO CHRONIC THROMBOTIC AND/OR EMBOLIC DISEASE

Definition. Thrombotic arteriopathy is a form of pulmonary hypertension due to thromboembolic disease, which causes obstruction of proximal or distal pulmonary arteries.

Clinical Features. Distal pulmonary artery obstruction can occur due to pulmonary embolism by thrombi, tumor (16,22,53), ova and/or parasites, and foreign material. It can also be caused by in situ thrombosis (4) or sickle cell disease. Sickle cell disease is characterized by both acute and chronic pulmonary complications which are the most common cause of death in adults with the disease. Recurrent microvascular obstruction appears to be the mechanism that results in the development of pulmonary hypertension in these patients. Bone marrow infarction resulting from microvascular occlusion is the probable pathogenic mechanism common to the initiation of both fat and bone

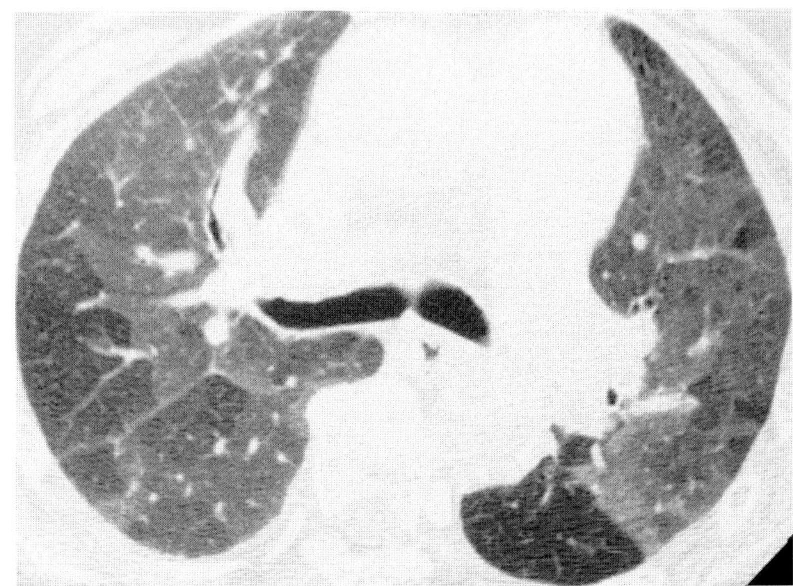

Figure 15-19

PULMONARY ARTERIAL HYPERTENSION

HRCT demonstrates patchy areas of decreased vascularity and attenuation, and blood flow redistribution to other areas of the lung. The overall appearance is known as mosaic perfusion. The patient was a 73-year-old woman with pulmonary arterial hypertension secondary to chronic pulmonary thromboembolism.

marrow emboli. Autopsy data of the lungs of patients with sickle cell disease reveal fibrin thromboembolism in larger arteries, with or without infarction, and extensive thrombosis in smaller arteries (in situ thrombosis).

Acute pulmonary thromboembolism rarely causes significant pulmonary hypertension, unless it is a submassive or massive embolism obstructing more than half of the pulmonary vascular bed (62). However, about 2 percent of patients with pulmonary thromboembolism have recurrent emboli and can develop progressive and sustained pulmonary hypertension. The clinical presentation of these patients is often nonspecific and the diagnosis is delayed or missed. The diagnosis is confirmed by ventilation-perfusion lung scanning, spiral CT scanning, or pulmonary angiography (see below). Lung biopsy, when obtained, usually confirms the primary diagnosis but does not diagnose the cause of the pulmonary hypertension.

Radiologic Findings. The radiologic manifestations of pulmonary arterial hypertension secondary to chronic pulmonary thromboembolism consist of enlargement of the central pulmonary arteries, cardiomegaly with right-sided enlargement, and patchy areas of decreased vascularity (mosaic oligemia) (84). The areas of decreased vascularity are clearer on HRCT and ventilation-perfusion scintigraphy than on the radiograph (fig. 15-19) (3,24,36).

Ventilation-perfusion scintigraphy is a highly sensitive test for diagnosing thromboembolic pulmonary arterial hypertension. However, it has a relatively low specificity and does not provide information about the morphology of the pulmonary vasculature and occluding thromboemboli (64,68). Contrast-enhanced spiral CT is currently the method of choice for the assessment of patients with suspected chronic pulmonary thromboembolism (24,36,59,66). The diagnosis of chronic thromboembolism on spiral CT is based on the presence of at least two of the following findings: eccentric filling defect contiguous to the vessel wall, evidence of recanalization within the intraluminal filling defect, arterial stenosis or web, abrupt narrowing of a pulmonary artery with a greater than 50 percent reduction of the arterial diameter, and complete occlusion at the level of the stenosed arteries (fig. 15-20) (57).

Pathologic Findings. Wagenvoort et al. (67) used the term *thrombotic arteriopathy* and argued that it is not important whether the thrombi are formed within the pulmonary arteries or if they migrate to the pulmonary circulation as emboli (76). Involvement of proximal large elastic arteries favors an embolic origin. Thrombosis of peripheral deep veins is a risk factor for pulmonary emboli. The histologic lesions of thrombotic arteriopathy are summarized in Table 15-10.

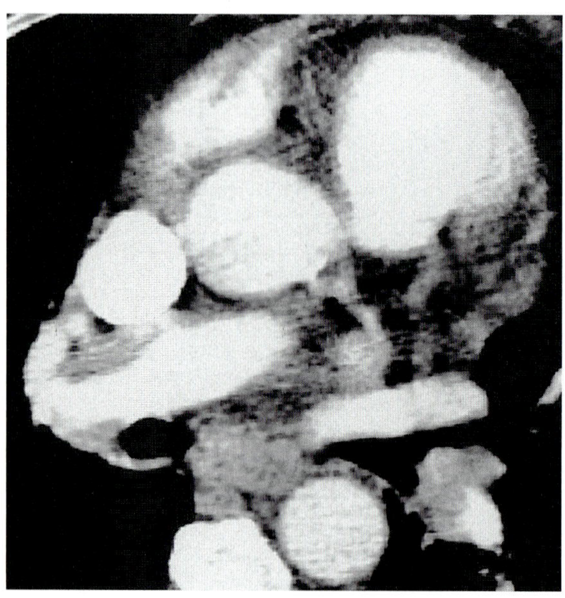

Figure 15-20

CHRONIC PULMONARY THROMBOEMBOLISM

Contrast-enhanced spiral CT demonstrates eccentric filling defects adjacent to the walls of the right interlobar and left lower lobe pulmonary arteries. Note irregular narrowing of the lumen of the involved arteries. The patient was a 56-year-old woman with chronic pulmonary thromboembolism.

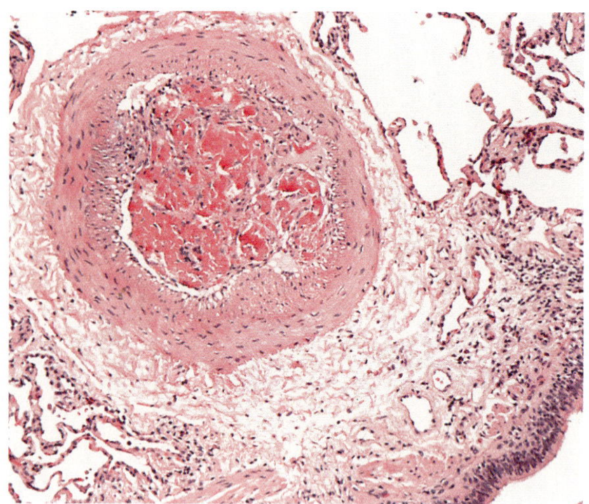

Figure 15-21

THROMBOTIC ARTERIOPATHY

A recent organizing thrombus is present in this arteriole.

Table 15-10

CHARACTERISTIC MORPHOLOGIC CHANGES IN THROMBOTIC ARTERIOPATHY

Medial hypertrophy: mild or absent
Recent thrombi: scarce
Eccentric intimal fibrosis (nonlaminar, often obliterating)
Recanalization

In thrombotic arteriopathy, the medial hypertrophy is usually mild or absent (47,76). Recent or organizing thrombi may be seen (figs. 15-21, 15-22). Eccentric intimal fibrosis often obliterates the arteriolar lumen, but it does not have a concentric laminar appearance. Recanalization of thrombi is common (fig. 15-23). Recent thrombi show capillary-like recanalization channels; however, as the thrombi become more organized the intimal fibrosis may show large recanalization channels. Large elastic arteries show

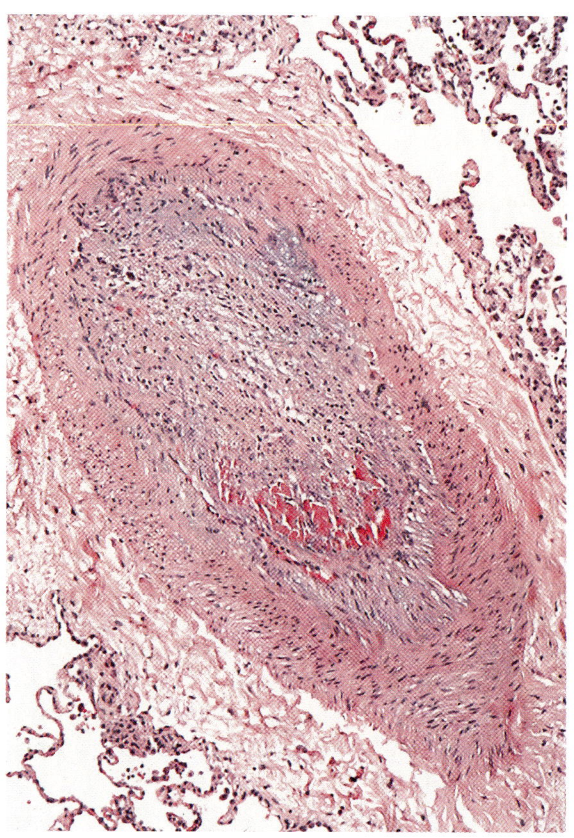

Figure 15-22

THROMBOTIC ARTERIOPATHY

This mostly organized thrombus eccentrically occludes virtually the entire lumen of this arteriole.

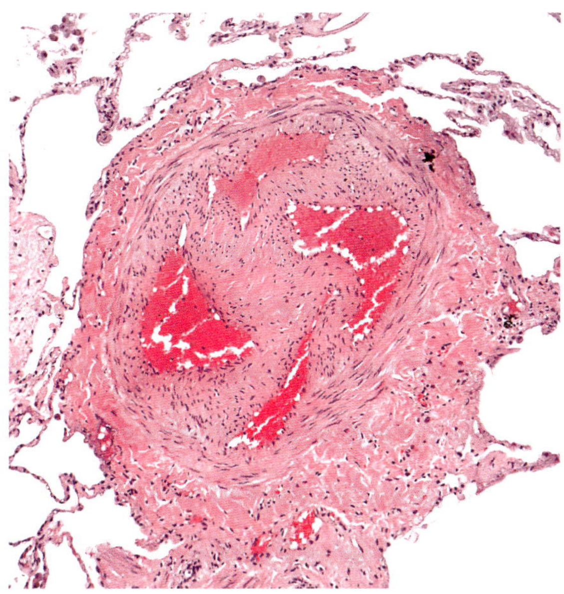

Figure 15-23

THROMBOTIC ARTERIOPATHY

This arteriole shows muscularized webs traversing the lumen of an arteriole.

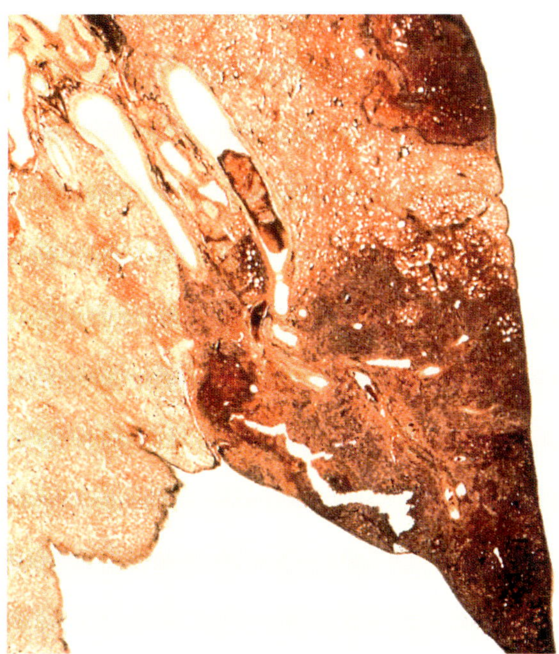

Figure 15-24

INFARCT: GOUGH MOUNTED SECTION

This wedge-shaped brown area represents dead lung tissue situated just beneath the pleura. A thrombus is present in a proximal artery. (Courtesy of the Gordon Museum, London, England.)

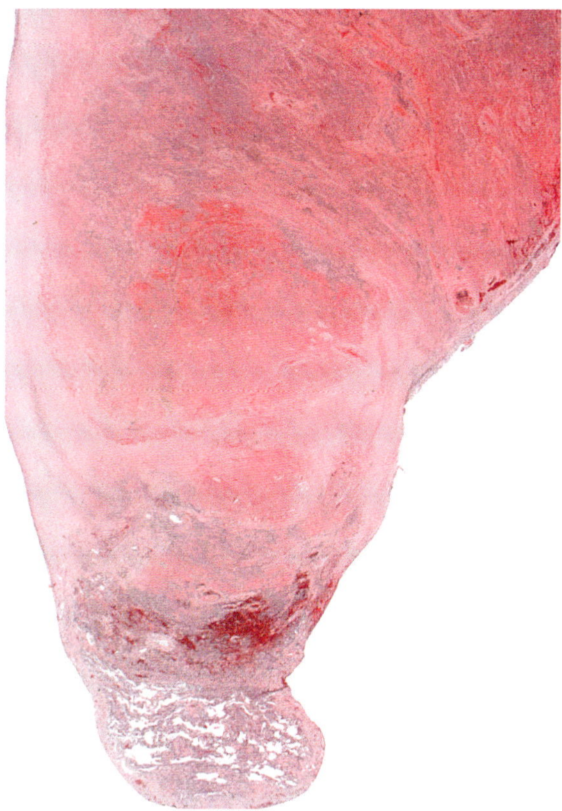

Figure 15-25

INFARCT: HISTOLOGY

This hemorrhagic, subpleural, wedge-shaped lesion represents the dead lung tissue of an infarct.

intravascular fibrous septa or webs (fig. 15-23). A spectrum of recent and organized thrombi is often seen. Thrombotic arteriopathy typically lacks plexiform lesions, the veins and venules are normal, and the media of arterioles is normal or only mildly thickened.

Large emboli have a tendency to locate within the right lung and lower lobes. This differs from primary thrombosis of the pulmonary arteries which tends to affect the upper lobes (76). Large emboli are often associated with infarcts that are usually situated in the periphery of the lung, often giving a subpleural wedge-shaped appearance (figs. 15-24, 15-25). Acute infarcts typically show extensive hemorrhage with dead alveolar walls (fig. 15-25). As infarcts organize they can show a spectrum of changes including organizing pneumonia, squamous metaplasia (fig. 15-26), and hemosiderin or hematoidin (fig. 15-27).

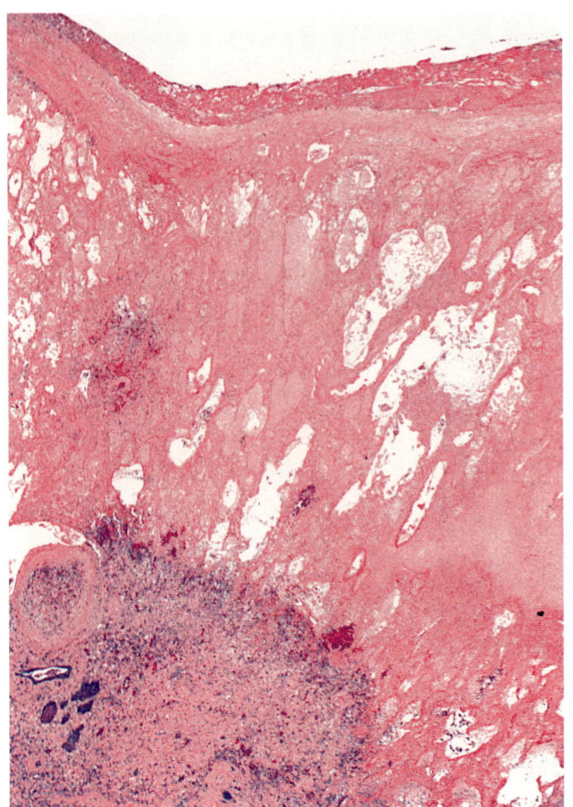

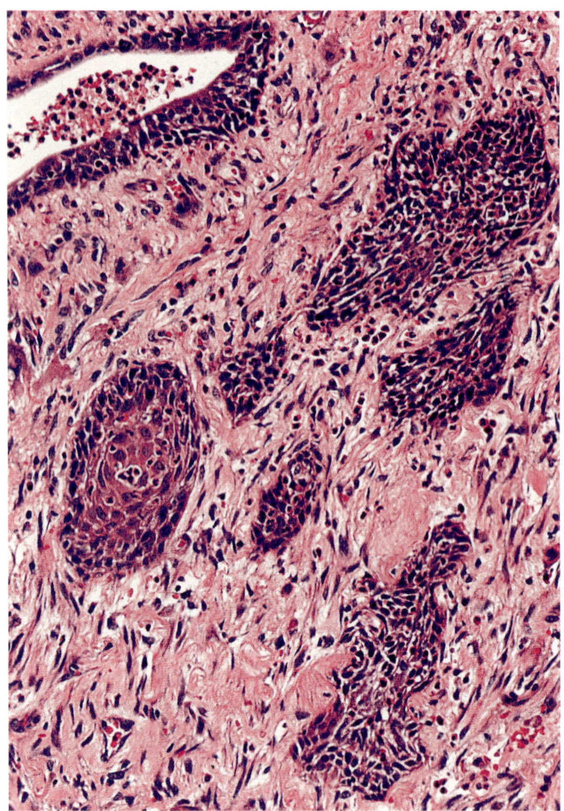

Figure 15-26

INFARCT: SQUAMOUS METAPLASIA

Left: The lung beneath this infarct shows squamous metaplasia (bottom left).
Right: Squamous metaplasia consists of evenly spaced nests of squamous cells within a fibrous stroma.

Figure 15-27

INFARCT: HEMATOIDIN PIGMENT

The orange-yellow hematoidin pigment was found in the wall of an organizing infarct.

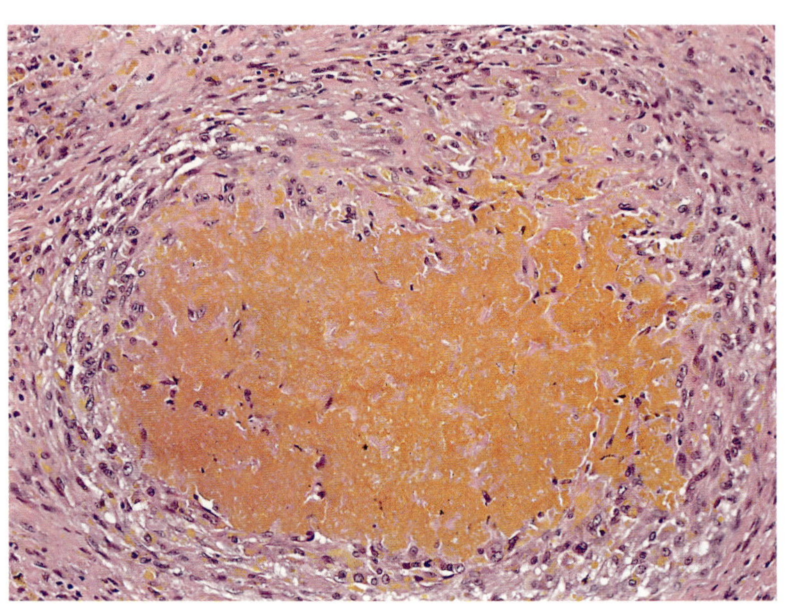

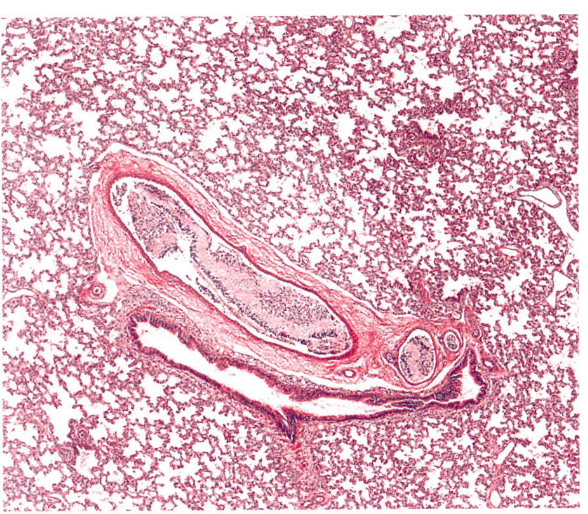

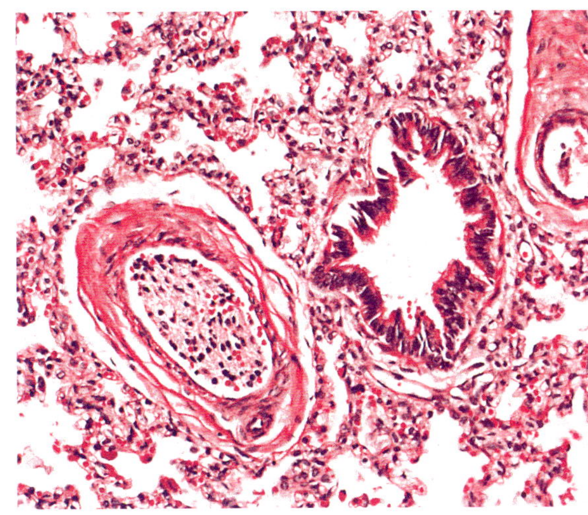

Figure 15-28

BRAIN EMBOLI

These pulmonary arteries are occluded by glial tissue.

Treatment and Prognosis. All patients require appropriate anticoagulant therapy. Patients with chronic thromboembolism may benefit from pulmonary thromboendarterectomy, sometimes with dramatic improvement. Unfortunately, postoperative complications are common and operative mortality is high, about 10 percent.

PULMONARY HYPERTENSION DUE TO DISORDERS DIRECTLY AFFECTING THE PULMONARY VASCULATURE

Definition. Pulmonary hypertension can occur in association with conditions that directly affect the vasculature including intravenous drug abuse, schistosomiasis, and sarcoidosis.

Clinical Features. Schistosomiasis is a common cause of pulmonary hypertension and cor pulmonale in endemic areas and among immigrant populations in the United States. Pulmonary granulomatosis associated with intravenous drug abuse is an increasingly recognized cause of pulmonary hypertension worldwide. Drug users commonly pulverize tablets intended for oral use, dissolve them in water, and inject them intravenously. Pulmonary hypertension, emphysema, and interstitial fibrosis can occur if the granulomatosis is severe (35). Drugs with sympathomimetic properties (e.g., cocaine, methamphetamine) may produce transient pulmonary vasoconstriction. Chronic use of these drugs can lead to irreversible injury and production of a syndrome indistinguishable from primary pulmonary hypertension (35). Patients who are HIV positive may develop pulmonary arterial hypertension with plexiform lesions and medial hypertrophy (35).

There are a variety of nonthrombotic pulmonary emboli including fat, bone, skin and hairs, liver, brain (fig. 15-28), trophoblasts, decidua, and amniotic fluid (fig. 15-29) (77). Most of these are incidental findings except for amniotic fluid embolism and massive fat embolism. Amniotic fluid embolism occurs during labor. When it is massive, it can be rapidly fatal by causing dyspnea, cyanosis, and shock. Histologically, material from amniotic fluid including squamous epithelial cells, lanugo hairs, fat, mucus, and bile from the meconium is found within pulmonary vessels (fig. 15-28) (2,14,26). Mucin stains may help demonstrate the amniotic fluid. Kobayashi et al. (37) found immunohistochemical staining for TKH-2, which is an antibody directed against sialyl Tn, NeuAc alpha 2-6GalNAc and reacts with meconium- and amniotic fluid-derived mucin-type glycoprotein. Disseminated intravascular coagulation is a possible complication.

Fat embolism occurs in a variety of settings including trauma to bone or subcutaneous adipose tissue as well as various diseases such as diabetes, pancreatitis, and sickle cell anemia (43,

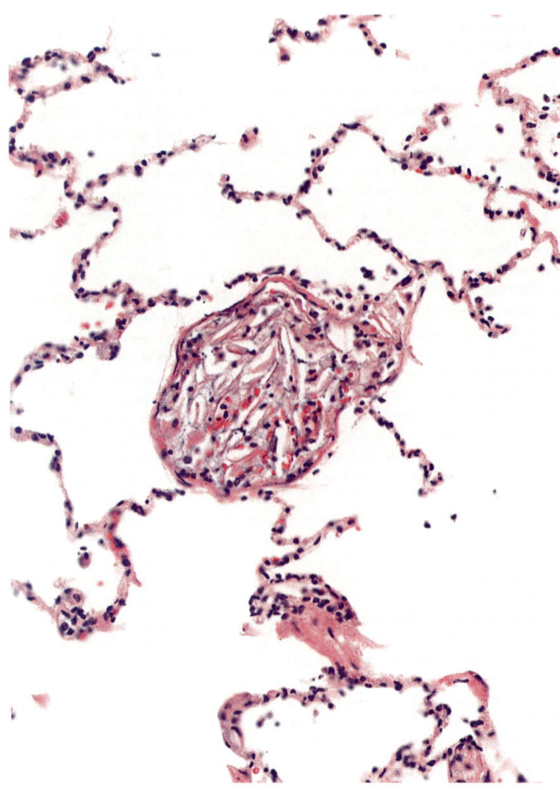

Figure 15-29

AMNIOTIC FLUID EMBOLISM

Squamous epithelial cells and a mucinous matrix occlude this small pulmonary vein.

45,48). Grossly, the lung may show an oily cut surface (77). Histologically, embolic fat droplets are found within alveolar capillaries (77). Intracellular fat deposits may be seen in macrophages obtained by bronchoalveolar lavage (BAL) (25,71). Fat stains such as oil red O can be used to stain the emboli (77). In the minority of patients, fat emboli cause acute respiratory distress syndrome, which is associated with the histologic features of diffuse alveolar damage.

Radiologic Findings. The manifestations are similar to those described above for PPH. Intravenous drug users have an increased prevalence of bullous lung damage and emphysema, predominantly in the upper lobes and lung periphery, with sparing of the central portions of the lungs. It is unclear whether this finding is a marker for the presence or development of pulmonary vascular disease in this setting.

Pathologic Findings. The ova of schistosomiasis, particularly *Schistosoma mansoni* and *S. haematobium,* embolize to small muscular arteries where they infiltrate through the walls. They elicit a foreign body reaction causing vasculitis and/or thrombosis (see fig. 12-204) (77).

In intravenous drug abusers, the talc, starch, cotton, and cellulose used as filler agents in tablets may be carried by the bloodstream until they lodge in the pulmonary capillary bed. Perivascular deposits of birefringent crystalline material, such as talc, are associated with a foreign body granulomatous reaction as well as fibrosis and narrowing of the arterioles (see chapter 7).

PULMONARY CAPILLARY HEMANGIOMATOSIS

Definition. Pulmonary capillary hemangiomatosis is a rare manifestation of pulmonary hypertension that is characterized by a proliferation of capillaries within the alveolar septa (23,34,44,53,74).

Clinical Features. This lesion occurs in patients 12 to 71 years of age. There is no sex predilection (21,23,34,44,74).

Radiologic Findings. Chest radiographs typically show a diffuse, bilateral, reticulonodular pattern with enlarged central pulmonary arteries (42). CT shows enlarged pulmonary arteries and multiple, bilateral, small, poorly defined nodular opacities (42). Ventilation perfusion scans may show matched defects.

Pathologic Findings. Histologically, the lung shows a multifocal, widespread, dense proliferation of capillary-like endothelial-lined vessels within the alveolar walls, interlobular septa, peribronchial and perivascular connective tissue, and pleura (fig. 15-30) (21,23,34,44,74). The alveolar septal capillaries appear engorged and may extend around and into both arteries and veins. Pulmonary veins or venules may show narrowing or obliteration, with features similar to PVOD. Hemosiderosis and interstitial fibrosis may be seen. Muscular pulmonary arteries may show medial hypertrophy.

Differential Diagnosis. The differential diagnosis of capillary hemangiomatosis includes PVOD, acute congestion, and atelectasis artifact. In some cases of PVOD, one may see foci of capillary hemangiomatosis. In capillary hemangiomatosis, there may be some venous occlusion,

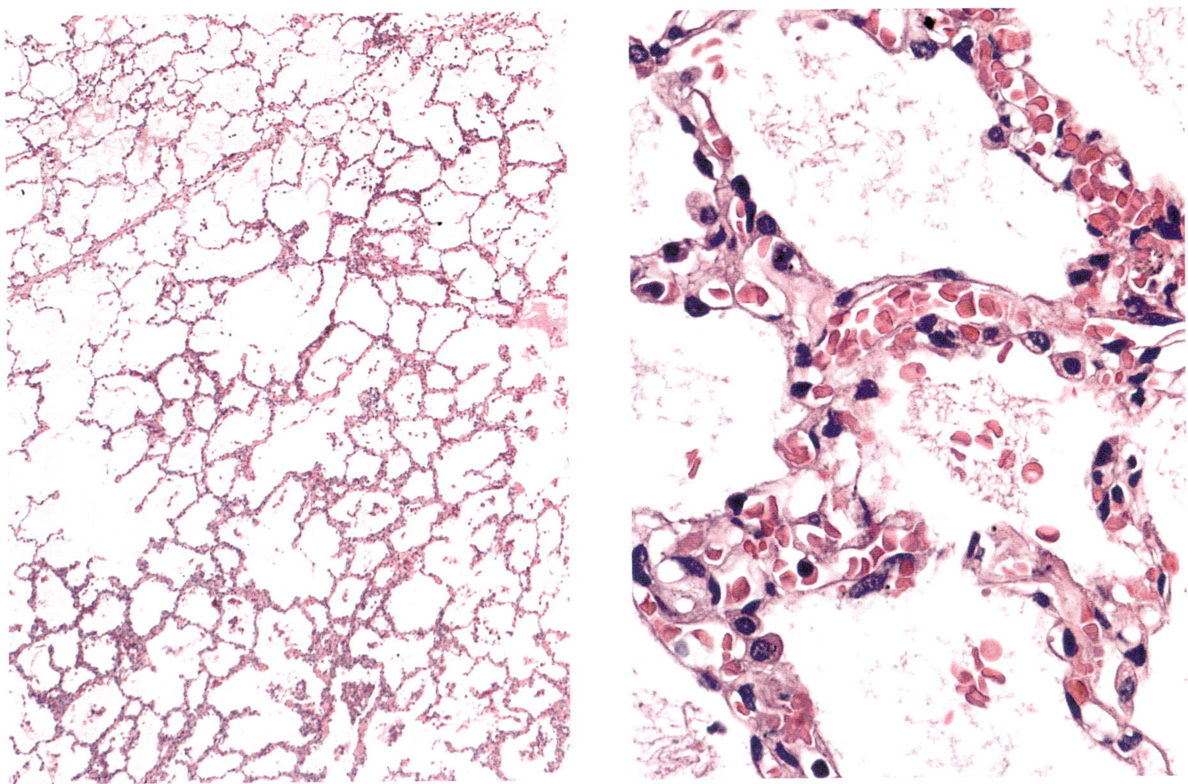

Figure 15-30

PULMONARY CAPILLARY HEMANGIOMATOSIS

Left: The abnormal area shows slightly thicker alveolar walls than the normal lung (lower right).
Right: The alveolar walls show a dense proliferation of capillary-like endothelial-lined vessels.

but it is not widespread. In fact, some regard the distinction between PVOD and capillary hemangiomatosis to be arbitrary (13). Congestion can cause engorgement of alveolar capillaries and give the impression of capillary hemangiomatosis, however, there is no increased density with proliferation of capillaries. Atelectasis only shows collapse of alveolar walls, which are normal, without capillary proliferation.

Treatment and Prognosis. No optimal therapy for capillary hemangiomatosis is established due to its rarity. Humbert et al. (33) recently reported that prostacyclin therapy was complicated by pulmonary edema. Other potential therapies include lung transplantation, inhaled nitrous oxide, and angiogenesis inhibitors such as interferon (33).

REFERENCES

1. Arnett EN, Bacos JM, Macher AM, et al. Fibrosing mediastinitis causing pulmonary arterial hypertension without pulmonary venous hypertension. Clinical and necropsy observations. Am J Med 1977;63:634–43.
2. Attwood HD, Delprado WJ. Amniotic fluid embolism: fatal case confirmed at autopsy five weeks after delivery. Pathology 1988;20:381–2.
3. Bergin CJ, Rios G, King MA, Belezzuoli E, Luna J, Auger WR. Accuracy of high-resolution CT in identifying chronic pulmonary thromboembolic disease. AJR Am J Roentgenol 1996;166:1371–7.
4. Bjornsson J, Edwards WD. Primary pulmonary hypertension: a histopathologic study of 80 cases. Mayo Clin Proc 1985;60:16–25.

5. Bloch KE, Marincek B, Amann FW, Russi EW. Pulmonary hypertension five years after left pneumonectomy for adenoid cystic carcinoma. Chest 1991;99:1018–9.
6. Brenot F. Primary pulmonary hypertension. Case series from France. Chest 1994;105:33S–6S.
7. Burke AP, Farb A, Virmani R. The pathology of primary pulmonary hypertension. Mod Pathol 1991;4:269–82.
8. Chang CH. The normal roentgenographic measurement of the right descending pulmonary artery in 1085 cases. AJR Am J Roentgenol 1962;87:929–35.
9. Cool CD, Kennedy D, Voelkel NF, Tuder RM. Pathogenesis and evolution of plexiform lesions in pulmonary hypertension associated with scleroderma and human immunodeficiency virus infection. Hum Pathol 1997;28: 434–42.
10. Coplan NL, Shimony RY, Ioachim HL, et al. Primary pulmonary hypertension associated with human immunodeficiency viral infection. Am J Med 1990;89:96–9.
11. Cordasco EM Jr, Ahmad M, Mehta A, Rubio F. The effects of steroid therapy on pulmonary hypertension secondary to fibrosing mediastinitis. Cleve Clin J Med 1990;57:647–52.
12. Cullinane C, Cox PN, Silver MM. Persistent pulmonary hypertension of the newborn due to alveolar capillary dysplasia. Pediatr Pathol 1992;12:499–514.
13. Dail DH. Uncommon tumors. In: Dail DH, Hammar SP, eds. Pulmonary pathology, 2nd ed. New York: Springer-Verlag; 1994:1279–461.
14. Davies S. Amniotic fluid embolus: a review of the literature. Can J Anaesth 2001;48:88–98.
15. de Chadarevian JP, Lischner HW, Karmazin N, Pawel BR, Schultz TE. Pulmonary hypertension and HIV infection: new observations and review of the syndrome. Mod Pathol 1994;7:685–9.
16. de Luis DA, Darriba J, San Miguel P, Rull SG, Cuesta C, Fogue I. A case of secondary pulmonary hypertension due to microscopic pulmonary tumor cell embolism from gallbladder carcinoma. Respiration 1997;64:244–6.
17. Delcroix M, Kurz X, Walckiers D, Demedts M, Naeije R. High incidence of primary pulmonary hypertension associated with appetite suppressants in Belgium. Eur Respir J 1998;12:271–6.
18. Deng Z, Haghighi F, Helleby L, et al. Fine mapping of PPH1, a gene for familial primary pulmonary hypertension, to a 3-cM region on chromosome 2q33. Am J Respir Crit Care Med 2000;161:1055–9.
19. Deng Z, Morse JH, Slager SL, et al. Familial primary pulmonary hypertension (gene PPH1) is caused by mutations in the bone morphogenetic protein receptor-II gene. Am J Hum Genet 2000;67:737–44.
20. Edwards WD. Pathology of pulmonary hypertension. Cardiovasc Clin 1988;18:321–59.
21. Eltorky MA, Headley AS, Winer-Muram H, Garrett HE Jr, Griffin JP. Pulmonary capillary hemangiomatosis: a clinicopathologic review. Ann Thorac Surg 1994;57:772–6.
22. Feller HA, Janis JF. Pulmonary hypertension, resulting from tumor emboli to pulmonary arteries. Dis Chest 1968;54:68–70.
23. Fernandez-Alonso J, Zulueta T, Reyes-Ramirez JR, Castillo-Palma MJ, Sanchez-Roman J. Pulmonary capillary hemangiomatosis as cause of pulmonary hypertension in a young woman with systemic lupus erythematosus [Letter]. J Rheumatol 1999;26:231–3.
24. Fraser RS, Müller NL, Pare PD. Pulmonary hypertension. In: Fraser and Pare's diagnosis of diseases of the chest. Philadelphia: WB Saunders; 1999:1879–945.
25. Godeau B, Schaeffer A, Bachir D, et al. Bronchoalveolar lavage in adult sickle cell patients with acute chest syndrome: value for diagnostic assessment of fat embolism. Am J Respir Crit Care Med 1996;153:1691–6.
26. Green BT, Umana E. Amniotic fluid embolism. South Med J 2000;93:721–3.
27. Gurubhagavatula I, Palevsky HI. Pulmonary hypertension in systemic autoimmune disease. Rheum Dis Clin North Am 1997;23:365–94.
28. Hatano S, Strasser T. Primary pulmonary hypertension: report on a WHO meeting, Geneva, 15-17, October 1973. Geneva: World Health Organization, 1975.
29. Heath D, Edwards JE. The pathology of hypertensive pulmonary vascular disease. A description of six grades of structural changes in the pulmonary arteries with special reference to congenital cardiac septal defects. Circulation 1958;18:533–47.
30. Heath D, Scott O, Lynch J. Pulmonary venoocclusive disease. Thorax 1971;26:663–74.
31. Higenbottam T, Stenmark K, Simonneau G. Treatments for severe pulmonary hypertension. Lancet 1999;353:338–40.
32. Huerd SS, Hodges TN, Grover FL, et al. Secondary pulmonary hypertension does not adversely affect outcome after single lung transplantation. J Thorac Cardiovasc Surg 2000;119:458–65.
33. Humbert M, Maitre S, Capron F, Rain B, Musset D, Simonneau G. Pulmonary edema complicating continuous intravenous prostacyclin in pulmonary capillary hemangiomatosis. Am J Respir Crit Care Med 1998;157:1681–5.

34. Ishii H, Iwabuchi K, Kameya T, Koshino H. Pulmonary capillary haemangiomatosis. Histopathology 1996;29:275–8.
35. Karpel JP. Overview of pulmonary disease in intravenous drug abusers. In: Rose BD, ed. Uptodate in medicine. Wellesley: BDR-Uptodate; 2001.
36. King MA, Ysrael M, Bergin CJ. Chronic thromboembolic pulmonary hypertension: CT findings. AJR Am J Roentgenol 1998;170:955–60.
37. Kobayashi H, Ooi H, Hayakawa H, et al. Histological diagnosis of amniotic fluid embolism by monoclonal antibody TKH-2 that recognizes NeuAc alpha 2-6GalNAc epitope. Hum Pathol 1997;28:428–33.
38. Kramer MS, Lane DA. Aminorex, dexfenfluramine, and primary pulmonary hypertension. J Clin Epidemiol 1998;51:361–4.
39. Kuriyama K, Gamsu G, Stern RG, Cann CE, Herfkens RJ, Brundage BH. CT-determined pulmonary artery diameters in predicting pulmonary hypertension. Invest Radiol 1984;19:16–22.
40. Li EK, Tam LS. Pulmonary hypertension in systemic lupus erythematosus: clinical association and survival in 18 patients. J Rheumatol 1999;26:1923–9.
41. Lilienfeld DE, Rubin LJ. Mortality from primary pulmonary hypertension in the United States, 1979-1996. Chest 2000;117:796–800.
42. Lippert JL, White CS, Cameron EW, Sun CC, Liang X, Rubin LJ. Pulmonary capillary hemangiomatosis: radiographic appearance. J Thorac Imaging 1998;13:49–51.
43. Maitre B, Habibi A, Roudot-Thoraval F, et al. Acute chest syndrome in adults with sickle cell disease. Chest 2000;117:1386–92.
44. Masur Y, Remberger K, Hoefer M. Pulmonary capillary hemangiomatosis as a rare cause of pulmonary hypertension. Pathol Res Pract 1996;192:290–5.
45. Mellor A, Soni N. Fat embolism. Anaesthesia 2001;56:145–54.
46. Morassut PA, Walley VM, Smith CD. Pulmonary veno-occlusive disease and the CREST variant of scleroderma. Can J Cardiol 1992;8:1055–8.
47. Moser KM, Bloor CM. Pulmonary vascular lesions occurring in patients with chronic major vessel thromboembolic pulmonary hypertension. Chest 1993;103:685–92.
48. Mudd KL, Hunt A, Matherly RC, et al. Analysis of pulmonary fat embolism in blunt force fatalities. J Trauma 2000;48:711–5.
49. Murray JF. Disorders of the pulmonary circulation. General principles and diagnostic approach. In: Murray JF, Nadel JA, Mason RJ, Boushey HA, eds. Textbook of respiratory medicine, 3rd ed. Philadelphia: WB Saunders; 2000:1485–502.
50. Nagaya N, Uematsu M, Satoh T, et al. Serum uric acid levels correlate with the severity and the mortality of primary pulmonary hypertension. Am J Respir Crit Care Med 1999;160:487–92.
51. Peacock AJ. Primary pulmonary hypertension. Thorax 1999;54:1107–18.
52. Pietra GG, Edwards WD, Kay JM, et al. Histopathology of primary pulmonary hypertension. A qualitative and quantitative study of pulmonary blood vessels from 58 patients in the National Heart, Lung, and Blood Institute, Primary Pulmonary Hypertension Registry. Circulation 1989;80:1198–206.
53. Primary pulmonary hypertension. Executive summary from the world symposium—primary pulmonary hypertension 1998. Evian, France: World Health Organization (www.who.int/ncd/cvd/pph.html), 1999.
54. Rabinovitch M. Problems of pulmonary hypertension in children with congenital cardiac defects. Chest 1988;93:119S–26S.
55. Rabinovitch M, Haworth SG, Vance Z, et al. Early pulmonary vascular changes in congenital heart disease studied in biopsy tissue. Hum Pathol 1980;11:499–509.
56. Ravin CE. Pulmonary vascularity: radiographic considerations. J Thorac Imaging 1988;3:1–13.
57. Remy-Jardin M, Louvegny S, Remy J, et al. Acute central thromboembolic disease: posttherapeutic follow-up with spiral CT angiography. Radiology 1997;203:173–80.
58. Rich S, Rubin L, Walker AM, Schneeweiss S, Abenhaim L. Anorexigens and pulmonary hypertension in the United States: results from the surveillance of North American pulmonary hypertension. Chest 2000;117:870–4.
59. Roberts HC, Kauczor HU, Schweden F, Thelen M. Spiral CT of pulmonary hypertension and chronic thromboembolism. J Thorac Imaging 1997;12:118–27.
60. Roberts WC. A simple histologic classification of pulmonary arterial hypertension. Am J Cardiol 1986;58:385–6.
61. Rothman A, Sklansky MS, Lucas VW, et al. Atrial septostomy as a bridge to lung transplantation in patients with severe pulmonary hypertension. Am J Cardiol 1999;84:682–6.
62. Rounds S, Cutaia MV. Pulmonary hypertension: pathophysiology and clinical disorders. In: Baum GL, Crapo JD, Celli BR, Karlinsky JB, eds. Textbook of pulmonary diseases. Philadelphia: Lippincott-Raven; 1998:1273–95.
63. Rubin LJ. Treatment of primary pulmonary hypertension. In: Rose BD, ed. Uptodate in medicine. Wellesley: BDR-Uptodate; 2000.

64. Ryan KL, Fedullo PF, Davis GB, Vasquez TE, Moser KM. Perfusion scan findings understate the severity of angiographic and hemodynamic compromise in chronic thromboembolic pulmonary hypertension. Chest 1988;93:1180–5.
65. Salzman D, Adkins DR, Craig F, Freytes C, LeMaistre CF. Malignancy-associated pulmonary veno-occlusive disease: report of a case following autologous bone marrow transplantation and review. Bone Marrow Transplant 1996;18:755–60.
66. Schwickert HC, Schweden F, Schild HH, et al. Pulmonary arteries and lung parenchyma in chronic pulmonary embolism: preoperative and postoperative CT findings. Radiology 1994;191:351–7.
67. Seguchi M, Hirabayashi N, Fujii Y, et al. Pulmonary hypertension associated with pulmonary occlusive vasculopathy after allogeneic bone marrow transplantation. Transplantation 2000;69:177–9.
68. Spies WG, Burstein SP, Dillehay GL, Vogelzang RL, Spies SM. Ventilation-perfusion scintigraphy in suspected pulmonary embolism: correlation with pulmonary angiography and refinement of criteria for interpretation. Radiology 1986;159:383–90.
69. Swensen SJ, Tashjian JH, Myers JL, et al. Pulmonary venoocclusive disease: CT findings in eight patients. AJR Am J Roentgenol 1996;167:937–40.
70. Tan RT, Kuzo R, Goodman LR, Siegel R, Haasler GB, Presberg KW. Utility of CT scan evaluation for predicting pulmonary hypertension in patients with parenchymal lung disease. Medical College of Wisconsin Lung Transplant Group. Chest 1998;113:1250–6.
71. Vedrinne JM, Guillaume C, Gagnieu MC, Gratadour P, Fleuret C, Motin J. Bronchoalveolar lavage in trauma patients for diagnosis of fat embolism syndrome. Chest 1992;102:1323–7.
72. Voelkel MA, Wynne KM, Badesch DB, Groves BM, Voelkel NF. Hyperuricemia in severe pulmonary hypertension. Chest 2000;117:19–24.
73. Wagenvoort CA. Lung biopsy specimens in the evaluation of pulmonary vascular disease. Chest 1980;77:614–25.
74. Wagenvoort CA, Beetstra A, Spijker J. Capillary haemangiomatosis of the lungs. Histopathology 1978;2:401–6.
75. Wagenvoort CA, Denolin H. Pulmonary circulation. New York: Elsevier; 1989.
76. Wagenvoort CA, Mooi WJ. Biopsy pathology of the pulmonary vasculature. London: Chapman and Hall; 1989.
77. Wagenvoort CA, Mooi WJ. Vascular diseases. In: Dail DH, Hammar SP, eds. Pulmonary pathology, 2nd ed. New York: Springer-Verlag; 1994:985–1025.
78. Wagenvoort CA, Wagenvoort N. Primary pulmonary hypertension: a pathologic study of the lung vessels in 156 clinically diagnosed cases. Circulation 1970;42:1163–84.
79. Wagenvoort CA, Wagenvoort N. The pathology of pulmonary veno-occlusive disease. Virchows Arch [A] 1974;364:69–79.
80. Wagenvoort CA, Wagenvoort N, Takahashi T. Pulmonary veno-occlusive disease: involvement of pulmonary arteries and review of the literature. Hum Pathol 1985;16:1033–41.
81. Weg IL, Rossoff L, McKeon K, Michael GL, Scharf SM. Development of pulmonary hypertension after lung volume reduction surgery. Am J Respir Crit Care Med 1999;159:552–6.
82. White CS, Romney BM, Mason AC, Austin JH, Miller BH, Protopapas Z. Primary carcinoma of the lung overlooked at CT: analysis of findings in 14 patients. Radiology 1996;199:109–15.
83. Whyte RI, Robbins RC, Altinger J, et al. Heart-lung transplantation for primary pulmonary hypertension. Ann Thorac Surg 1999;67:937–41.
84. Woodruff WW III, Hoeck BE, Chitwood WR Jr, Lyerly HK, Sabiston DC Jr, Chen JT. Radiographic findings in pulmonary hypertension from unresolved embolism. AJR Am J Roentgenol 1985;144:681–6.
85. Yamaki S, Wagenvoort CA. Comparison of primary plexogenic arteriopathy in adults and children. A morphometric study in 40 patients. Br Heart J 1985;54:428–34.
86. Yamaki S, Wagenvoort CA. Medial thickness of intrarenal arteries in congenital heart disease. Arch Pathol Lab Med 1980;104:483–6.
87. Yamaki S, Wagenvoort CA. Plexogenic pulmonary arteriopathy: significance of medial thickness with respect to advanced pulmonary vascular lesions. Am J Pathol 1981;105:70–5.
88. Yi ES, Rich S, Giaid A. Chronic pulmonary hypertension: pathobiology, diagnosis, and treatment. In: Wardlaw A, Hamid Q, eds. Textbook of respiratory cell and molecular biology. United Kingdom: Harwood Academic Publisher; 2002.
89. Young ID, Ford SE, Ford PM. The association of pulmonary hypertension with rheumatoid arthritis. J Rheumatol 1989;16:1266–9.

16
OCCUPATIONAL LUNG DISEASES AND PNEUMOCONIOSES

INTRODUCTION AND GENERAL PRINCIPLES

Occupational lung disease includes many disorders, some of which are covered in other chapters of this monograph. Occupational lung disease is not entirely synonymous with pneumoconiosis. Pneumoconiosis refers to the retention of, and the pathologic effects from, the inhalation of dust particulates. Many of the conditions comprising occupational lung disease do not fit this definition.

Clinical Evaluation. In most cases, the diagnosis of occupational lung disease is made without tissue examination. The diagnosis is based on a combination of clinical, epidemiologic, and radiologic findings related to a history of exposure to occupational and environmental sources. When making the diagnosis, several issues are important: 1) is there clear evidence of exposure to a known agent that is associated with the findings identified; 2) how strong is the association and the relative risk of developing the disease; 3) what is the temporal sequence of the exposure with the onset of illness; and 4) is exposure linked to a single disease.

Radiographic assessment of the presence, type, and severity of parenchymal and pleural abnormalities is made by comparison with a set of standard radiographs provided by the International Labor Office (ILO) (29). The ILO classification provides a means of recording the chest radiographic findings semiquantitatively in a uniform and reproducible manner. Parenchymal and pleural abnormalities are evaluated for size and shape as well as extent (profusion) (11).

Occupational lung diseases are inextricably intertwined with medicolegal issues, many of which do not directly apply to the diagnosis and management in individual cases. The medicolegal aspects are often contentious; in this section we concentrate only on the medical aspects of these conditions. The literature on this topic is voluminous and there are many excellent texts; for this chapter we have primarily relied on the works of Churg and Green (11), and Parkes (57).

Physical Properties of Dust Particles. Particle size, chemical composition, and mineralogic aspects all affect the potency of a specific dust to cause lung injury. In order for dust particles to reach the lung parenchyma, they generally have to be less than 10 μm and often less than 5 μm in diameter (11). Fibers are an exception, particularly asbestos, and these may reach the alveoli when considerably larger than 10 μm, with the width appearing to be the critical factor.

Latency of Exposure. There is generally a latency period between the onset of exposure and the development of clinically apparent disease (11). During the latent period, which may be years or even decades, there is ongoing clearance of dust which varies with the dust itself, the intensity and persistence of the exposure, and the adequacy of clearance methods. The lung burden of a given dust thus depends on its total cumulative deposition (be it from continuous or intermittent exposure) minus the dust that has been cleared, primarily via the mucociliary escalator and the lymphatics. Mucociliary clearance may be affected by many factors, particularly cigarette smoking; thus smoking may be an indirect factor in the pathologic findings related to some dust exposures.

Pathologic Reaction Patterns to Dusts. Among the classic pneumoconioses, it is conceptually useful to categorize the general pathologic reactions as follows: 1) nonfibrogenic dusts (e.g., carbon, and many others) and 2) fibrogenic dusts (e.g., silica, asbestos). Patterns of fibrosis include diffuse interstitial fibrosis (e.g., asbestosis) and nodular fibrosis (e.g., silicosis). While conceptually useful, these divisions frequently are blurred since mixed dust exposures are common (i.e., mixed dust pneumoconioses).

Pathologic changes in the pneumoconioses can often be correlated with the physiology of dust inhalation and clearance: early deposition along airways and clearance along lymphatic routes. This is well seen in silica and silicate exposures. Such a scheme is not so readily applicable in cases of diffuse interstitial fibrosis and massive fibrosis.

For the most part, pathologic lesions of the classic pneumoconioses fall into the groups shown in Table 16-1. *Centriacinar emphysema* is similar to that associated with cigarette smoking.

Table 16-1

PLEUROPULMONARY PATHOLOGIC LESIONS IN CLASSIC PNEUMOCONIOSES[a]

Centriacinar emphysema
Centriacinar dust macules
Mineral dust airway disease
Dust-laden macrophages along lymphatic routes of clearance
Nodular fibrosis
Massive fibrosis
Diffuse interstitial fibrosis
Miscellaneous other reactions
Pleuritis and pleural fibrosis
Hyaline pleural plaques

[a]Summarized from reference 11.

It is sufficiently characteristic in some exposures that it has become part of the definition (e.g., coal worker's pneumoconiosis). In this circumstance, it may be referred to as *focal emphysema.*

Dust macules are accumulations of dust-filled macrophages in the walls of respiratory bronchioles and alveolar ducts. There is little associated fibrosis and not surprisingly, macules are one of the most prominent features of nonfibrogenic dusts.

Mineral dust airway disease is related to the dust macule, although there is more scarring of the respiratory bronchioles and alveolar ducts, probably as a result of increased fibrogenicity of the dusts involved (fig. 16-1).

Lymphatic clearance of dust leads to accumulations of dust-laden macrophages along the lymphatic routes (around bronchovascular bundles, in interlobular septa, and in the pleura). This is best seen in silica and silicate exposures.

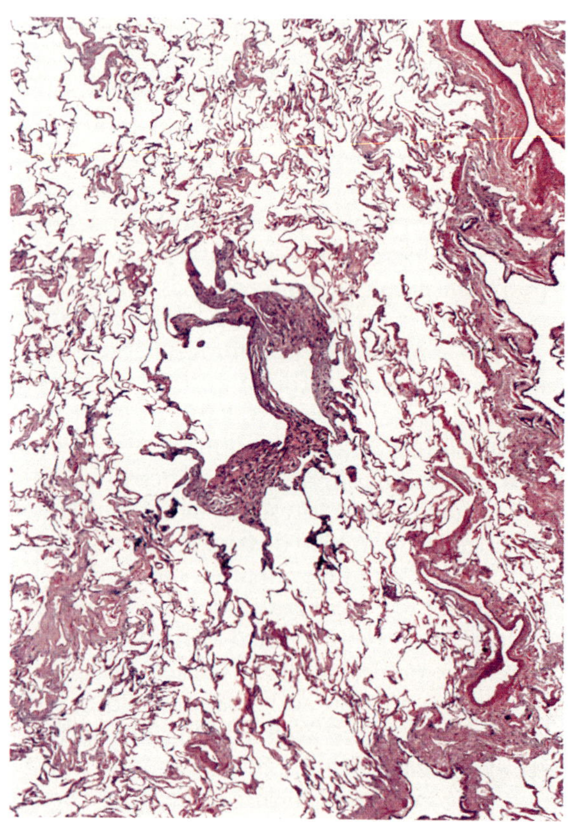

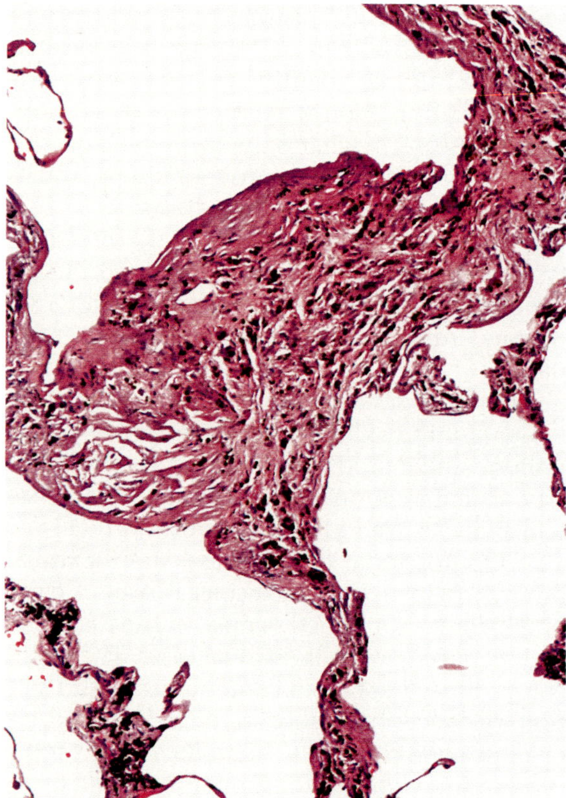

Figure 16-1

MINERAL DUST AIRWAY DISEASE

The lesion centers on a respiratory bronchiole and there is associated interstitial thickening, fibrosis, and prominent dust-laden macrophages.

Nodules are firm to palpation, usually round, and often arise in a background of sheets of dust-laden macrophages. Nodules may be identified in centrilobular regions and along sites of lymphatic clearance (along bronchovascular bundles, in septa, and adjacent to the pleura), and occasionally scattered in the parenchyma. Nodules can be broadly divided into silicotic, mixed dust, and giant cell/granulomatous types.

Diffuse interstitial fibrosis, in the context of the pneumoconioses, refers to the fibrosis and architectural remodeling of lung tissue that is more diffuse and widespread than seen with discrete nodular fibrosis. There is typically abundant dust associated with the fibrosis. This pattern has been likened to usual interstitial pneumonia, but with the relatively strict definition of usual interstitial pneumonia used in this monograph (see chapter 3), most cases of diffuse interstitial fibrosis in the pneumoconioses would not fit perfectly in this category.

Massive fibrosis (progressive massive fibrosis or *complicated pneumoconiosis)* typically occurs in a background of dust macules and nodules, and is defined as zones of fibrosis greater than 1.0 cm in diameter. Massive fibrosis may be identified as large amorphous zones of fibrosis with abundant dust-filled macrophages or as a coalescence of smaller fibrotic nodules. Degenerative changes with cavity formation may be found centrally in zones of massive fibrosis.

COAL WORKER'S PNEUMOCONIOSIS

Definition. Coal worker's pneumoconiosis (CWP) is the parenchymal lung disease that results from the inhalation of, retention of, and host response to coal dust (11,38,57).

Mineralogy and Exposure. The four major types of coal are anthracite, bituminous, subbituminous, and lignite (11). Coal dust typically has variable amounts of other minerals including silicates, sulfides, carbonates, silica, and feldspars, but coal may contain any element found in the earth's crust. Sufficient silica is frequently present to produce pathologic effects (see below).

The burning of coal produces ash, some particles of which are small enough to escape into the smoke; these are termed "fly ash" (57). For the most part, fly ash consists of aluminosilicate spheres which are respirable, but deleterious health effects are not adequately characterized (11).

The most significant factor in the development of CWP is the cumulative exposure to coal dust (11). Among coal miners, exposure is higher among those who work in underground mines than those who work in surface mines. The composition of the dust is a factor in determining the type of histologic lesion identified (see below) (15). Coal miners have an increased risk for developing simple and complicated CWP even at the current permissible exposure limits of the Mine Safety and Health Administration (11).

Clinical Features. The prevalence rate of CWP is influenced by the dust level, worksite, and length of exposure. The prevalence of CWP among exposed workers varies from 4 percent in Britain to 10 percent in the United States. Less than 0.5 percent of workers with CWP develop complicated CWP. Importantly, all exposed workers are at risk for the development of coal dust–related illnesses: "industrial bronchitis," silicosis, bronchogenic carcinoma, and tuberculosis. The diagnosis of CWP is based on a history of exposure and appropriate radiographic abnormalities.

CWP is divided into simple CWP and complicated CWP (progressive massive fibrosis [PMF]) (11,38,57). These are defined radiologically and pathologically (see below). Patients with *simple CWP* are generally asymptomatic although there may be chronic productive cough and sputum that is tinged black. Routine pulmonary function tests may be normal or show mild obstruction and decreased diffusing capacity. The severity of simple CWP is generally defined radiologically (see below).

Complicated CWP (or PMF) develops in a background of simple CWP. It is usually associated with dyspnea, cough, and sputum production and, in severe cases, congestive heart failure may supervene. Significant functional deficits may be present: usually a restrictive ventilatory defect and abnormalities in gas exchange (57). PMF may progress even in the absence of continued exposure to dust.

Rheumatoid pneumoconiosis (Caplan's syndrome) is a severe form of CWP in which the affected individuals have rheumatoid arthritis or a circulating rheumatoid factor with the attendant radiologic and pathologic findings described below. Rheumatoid pneumoconiosis is

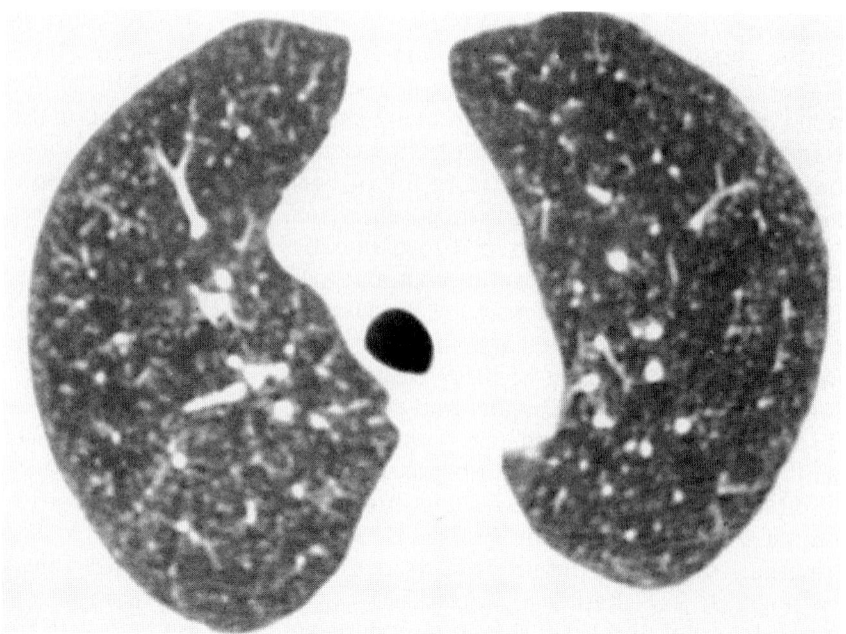

Figure 16-2

COAL WORKER'S PNEUMOCONIOSIS

HRCT through the upper lobes demonstrates numerous bilateral nodules. The nodules measure approximately 2 to 3 mm in diameter and have sharply circumscribed margins. The patient was a 56-year-old coal worker.

Table 16-2

PATHOLOGIC LESIONS IN COAL WORKER'S PNEUMOCONIOSIS[a]

Coal dust macules and focal emphysema (simple CWP)[b]
Progressive massive fibrosis (complicated CWP)
Coal nodules
Diffuse interstitial fibrosis
Rheumatoid pneumoconiosis (Caplan's syndrome)
Lymphatic and lymph node deposits of coal dust
Silicotic nodules

[a]Modified from references 11 and 58.
[b]CWP = coal worker's pneumoconiosis.

relatively rare, particularly in North America. In Great Britain, the incidence in miners with identifiable CWP is between 2 and 6 percent (57).

Radiologic Findings. Radiographically, CWP consists of multiple small nodules. The nodules may be diffuse throughout both lungs but tend to involve mainly the upper lobes (71). Increased severity of lung involvement correlates with an increase in the number and size of the nodules (62). Computed tomography (CT) is superior to chest radiography in demonstrating the presence and distribution of nodules (62). On CT, the nodules usually have a random distribution, although a centrilobular predominance may be seen in some cases (fig. 16-2).

PMF is characterized by the presence of opacities of greater than 1 cm in diameter. The large opacities are usually bilateral and symmetric, and involve the upper lobes. In the majority of patients, the opacities have irregular borders and are associated with adjacent emphysema and cephalad retraction of the hila; less commonly, they have regular borders and are not associated with emphysema. The latter form appears to result not from conglomeration of nodules and fibrosis but from enlargement of single nodules in lungs with a high carbon content (62).

The radiographic manifestations of rheumatoid pneumoconiosis consist of single or multiple well-defined nodules measuring 0.3 to 5.0 cm in diameter (62). The radiograph usually shows little if any evidence of concomitant pneumoconiosis (62).

Pathologic Findings. Inhaled coal dust is identified histologically as black particulates in macrophages, although free dust may be admixed with fibrous tissue. Some of the particles may be ferruginated and superficially resemble an asbestos body (so-called coal bodies) (57), although a dark core is present in contrast to the

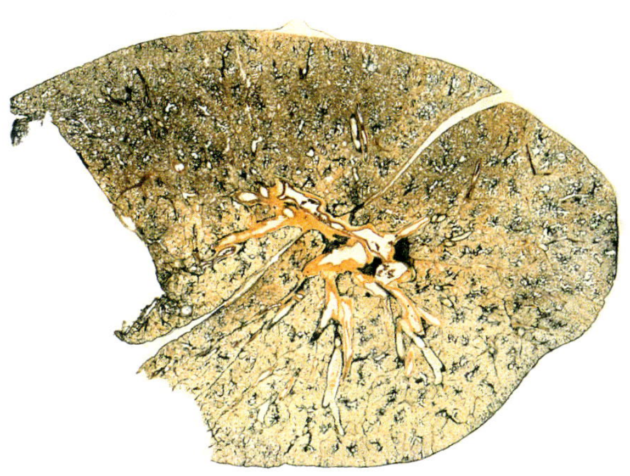
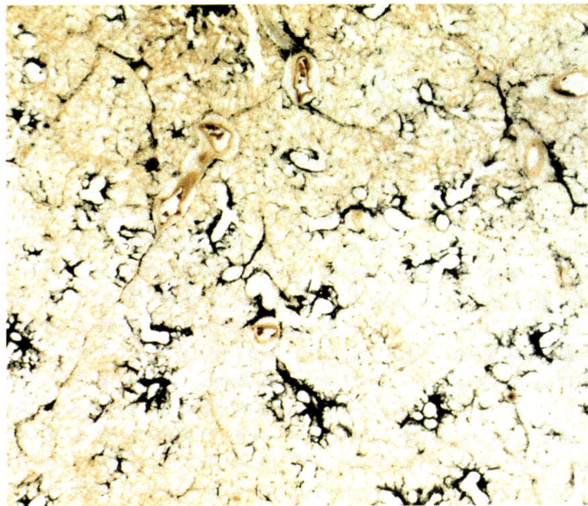

Figure 16-3

COAL WORKER'S PNEUMOCONIOSIS

This Gough section shows anthracotic dust macules involving respiratory bronchioles with associated centriacinar emphysema.

lucent core of an asbestos body. The pathologic lesions of CWP are summarized in Table 16-2.

The pathologic features of *simple CWP* include the presence of dust macules and focal emphysema, and both are required for pathologic diagnosis (11,57,58). Grossly, coal dust macules are discrete regions of black pigmentation that are more prominent in the upper lobes and upper portions of the lower lobes (fig. 16-3). Macules vary from 0.5 to 6.0 mm in diameter and correspond to the accumulation of pigmented macrophages in the walls of respiratory bronchioles and their immediately adjacent alveoli (fig. 16-4). A mild increase in interstitial connective tissue may be present. The amount of coal dust present (anthracotic pigmentation) is much more than typically associated with cigarette smoking or urban dwelling, although there is an overlap (21). Focal emphysema refers to the airspace enlargement immediately around the coal dust macule; it represents a form of centriacinar emphysema.

Patients with *complicated CWP* show features of PMF, identified grossly as zones of pigmented fibrosis that tend to be bilateral and distributed in the upper lobes posteriorly (figs. 16-5–16-7) (11,57,58). Some patients have massive uniform zones of fibrosis whereas others develop coalescence of coal nodules (see below). PMF is well demarcated from the surrounding tissue. It violates normal anatomic structures such as fissures, bronchi, and vessels, all of which may become engulfed and destroyed within larger fibrous lesions. There is replacement of lung tissue by fibrosis, with interspersed, abundant, pigmented coal dust. Central liquefactive necrosis may develop. A giant cell reaction to degenerating tissue may be identified, although its presence should raise the possibility of infection, particularly tuberculosis. Vessels are typically destroyed or show endarteritis obliterans. Lung tissue away from the zones of PMF shows simple CWP.

Coal nodules are nodular lesions occurring in a background of CWP (fig. 16-7) (11,21,57,58). Coal nodules are considered a form of mixed dust pneumoconiosis in which coal has been contaminated by fibrogenic dusts, particularly silica, leading to the formation of pigmented fibrous nodules. Some authors require the presence of coal nodules for a histologic diagnosis of CWP (21). Coal nodules are more numerous in the upper zones, and in addition to involving respiratory bronchioles, may also be found in subpleural and peribronchial connective tissue. When nodules form conglomerates greater than 1 cm in diameter, the designation of PMF is appropriate. Coal nodules may show degenerative changes similar to those seen in PMF, including calcification and liquefactive necrosis with cholesterol clefts.

Figure 16-4

COAL WORKER'S PNEUMOCONIOSIS

There are centriacinar dust macules with associated centrilobular emphysema (A,B). The macules are composed of numerous anthracotic dust-filled macrophages with little associated fibrosis (C).

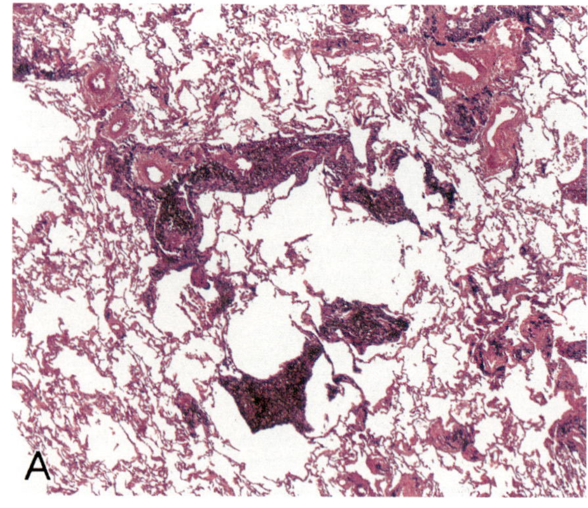

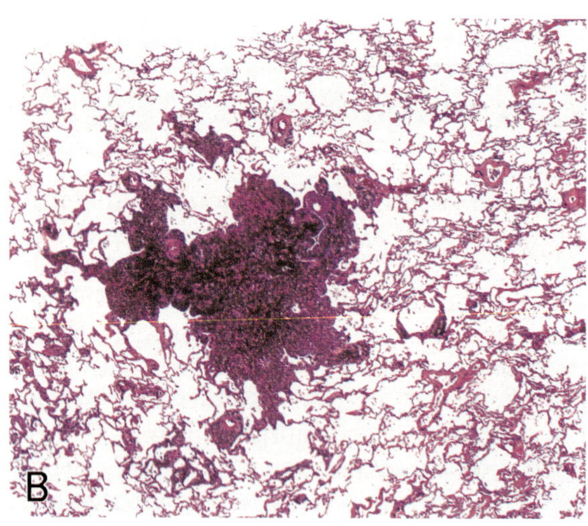

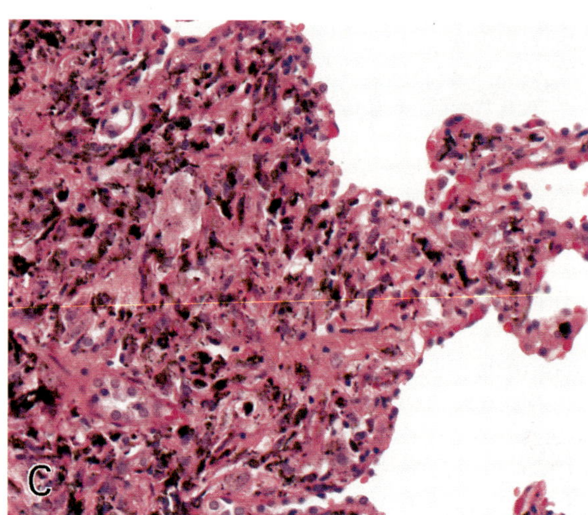

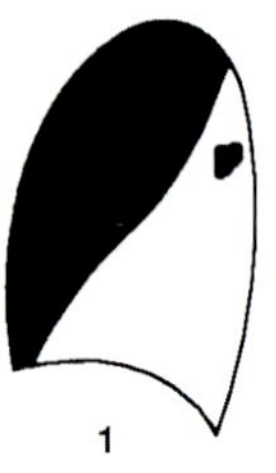

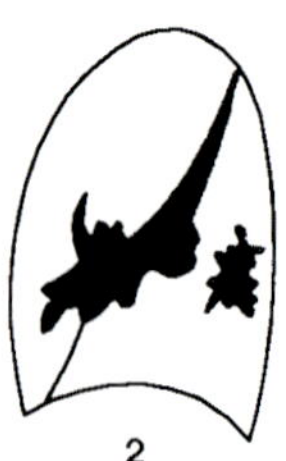

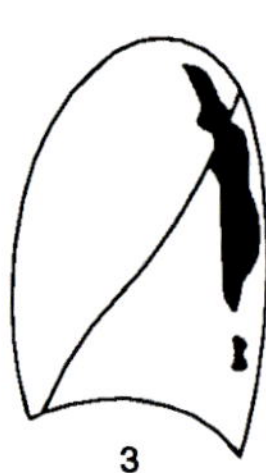

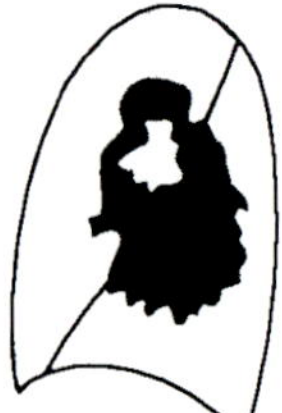

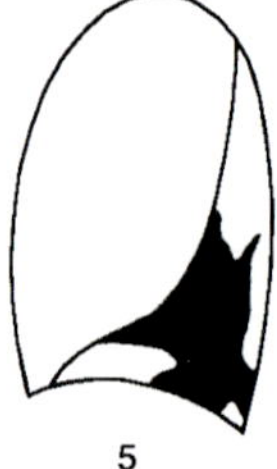

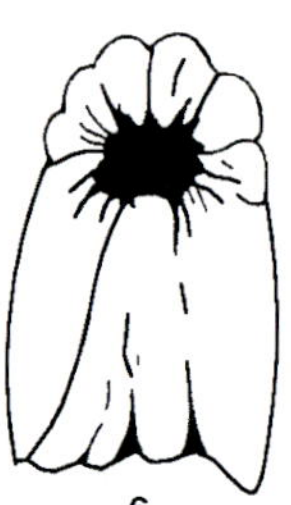

Figure 16-5

COAL WORKER'S PNEUMOCONIOSIS WITH PROGRESSIVE MASSIVE FIBROSIS

These diagrams illustrate various gross and radiologic appearances of progressive massive fibrosis in coal worker's pneumoconiosis. (Figure 13.15 from Parkes WR. Occupational lung disorders, 3rd ed. Oxford: Butterworth Heinemann; 1994:361.)

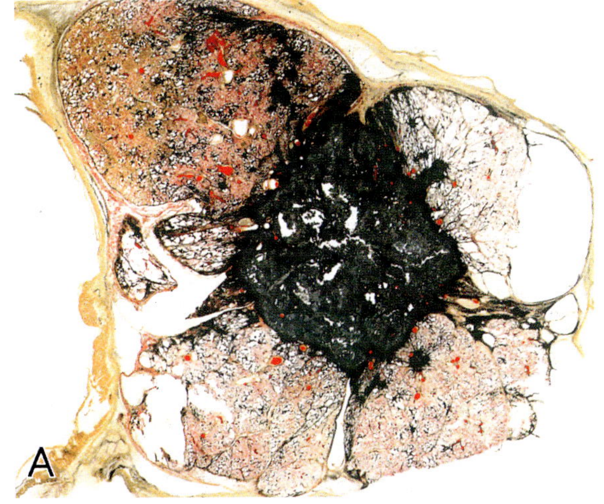

Figure 16-6

COAL WORKER'S PNEUMOCONIOSIS WITH PROGRESSIVE MASSIVE FIBROSIS

The Gough section shows a large zone of scarring and anthracosis involving both upper and lower lobes (A). Histologic sections show dense fibrosis with numerous anthracotic dust-laden macrophages (B,C).

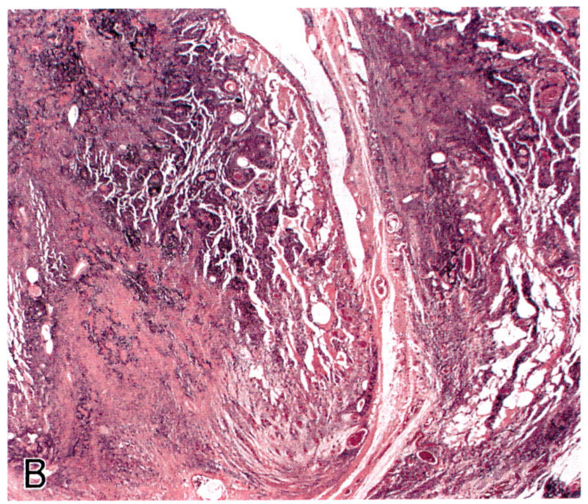

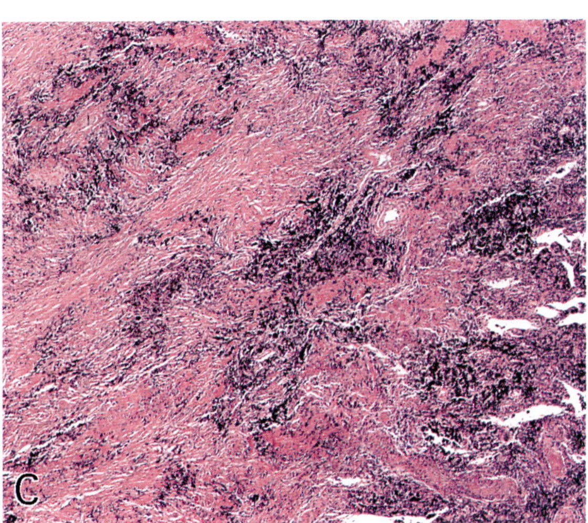

Dust-filled macrophages may be identified along lymphatic regions in the septa and pleura, along bronchovascular bundles, and in hilar lymph nodes. Coal nodules may show a similar lymphatic distribution. Pigmentation of pleural lymphatics by coal dust is one of the distinctive gross features of CWP.

Diffuse interstitial pulmonary fibrosis has been identified in up to one fifth of autopsied coal miners in some studies (11,57). Grossly, the findings are similar to those of other forms of diffuse fibrosis with architectural remodeling. Histologically, there are varying degrees of interstitial fibrosis with honeycomb change. The fibrous tissue may show prominent coal dust pigmentation as in other lesions of CWP, but this is not true of all cases. According to Churg and Green (11) "it seems reasonable to consider the pigmented type of interstitial fibrosis to be caused by exposure to coal mine dust."

In *rheumatoid pneumoconiosis* there are scattered nodules that measure up to 5 cm or more in diameter (fig. 16-8) (11,57). They are situated mostly in the subpleural parenchyma. They tend to undergo cavitation and may be secondarily calcified. The nodules have concentric, pale pigmented bands around the center. Histologically, they resemble subcutaneous rheumatoid nodules with central eosinophilic necrotic debris that is abruptly demarcated from a surrounding layer of fibroblasts, and macrophages with occasional giant cells. The distinction from an infectious granuloma may be difficult. Plasma cells and palisaded fibroblasts are more characteristic of rheumatoid pneumoconiosis and rare in tuberculosis and other infections.

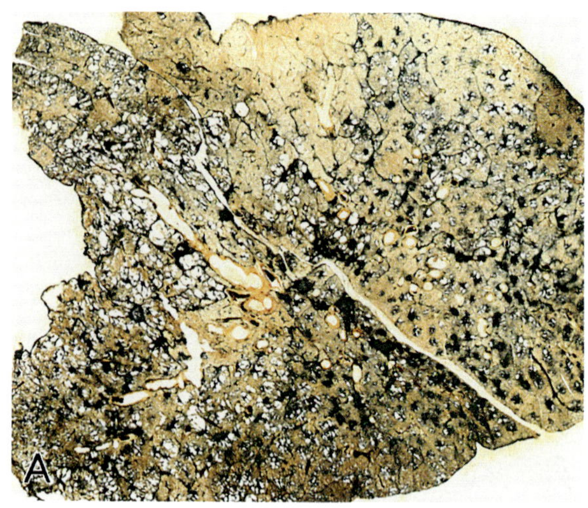

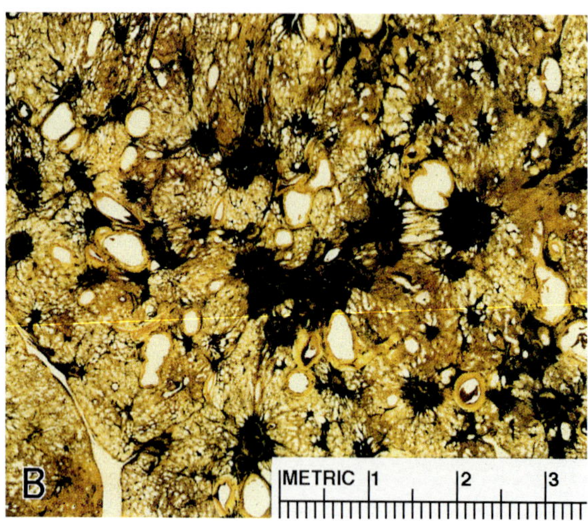

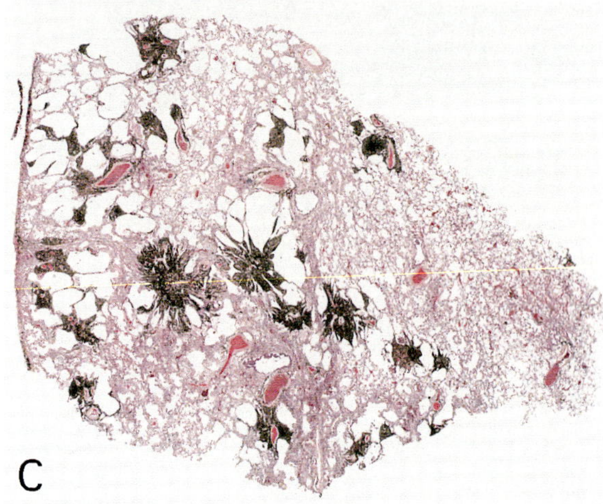

Figure 16-7

COAL NODULES

Anthracotic pigmented nodules with background coal worker's pneumoconiosis are seen in Gough sections (A,B). Histologic section shows a 3-mm nodular accumulation of dust-laden macrophages (C).

Dust rings are more pronounced in rheumatoid pneumoconiosis than in infection. From a practical point of view, the designation of rheumatoid pneumoconiosis should not be applied unless the characteristic clinical or serologic and histologic features are present and an infection has been rigorously excluded.

Silicotic nodules may be identified in cases of CWP (fig. 16-9) (11,15). They should have relatively little pigment and be densely collagenized and rounded, in contrast to the irregular ("Medusa head") contour of the mixed dust coal nodules. The occurrence of silicotic nodules in CWP is not surprising given the frequency with which silica may contaminate coal dust. With individual lesions, the distinction between a silicotic nodule and a mixed dust pneumoconiotic coal nodule may be arbitrary.

Pathogenesis. Since no coal dust is "pure" and since dust composition varies from mine to mine, a straightforward pathogenesis may not be possible. Carbon by itself is considered nonfibrogenic, although it may produce macules (57). Coal contaminated with quartz (silica) probably is involved in the development of nodular and fibrotic lesions in CWP (57). The factors responsible for the development of complicated CWP in the setting of simple CWP are not well understood; probably the most important factor is cumulative dust exposure (11). Once coal dust reaches the lungs it is thought to interact with macrophages, leading to a variety of macrophage products that are associated with the development and progression of CWP (38).

Diagnosis. The presence of marked pigmentation of hilar or mediastinal lymph nodes (with

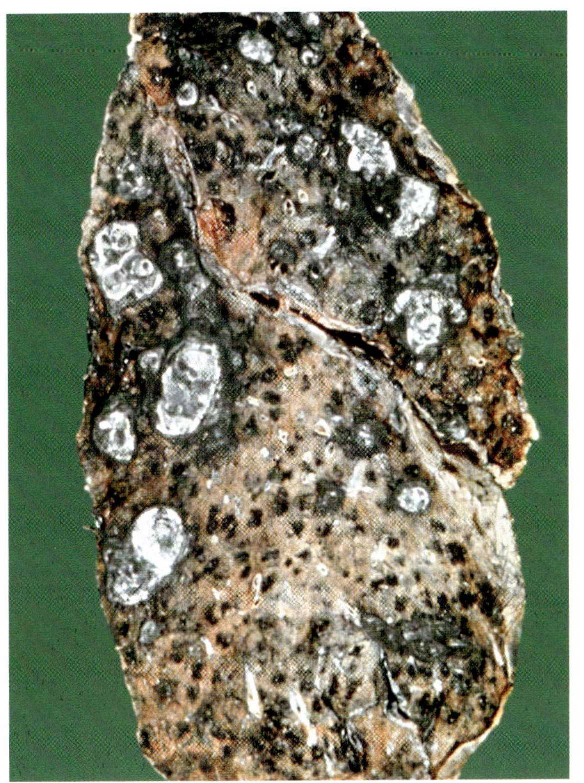

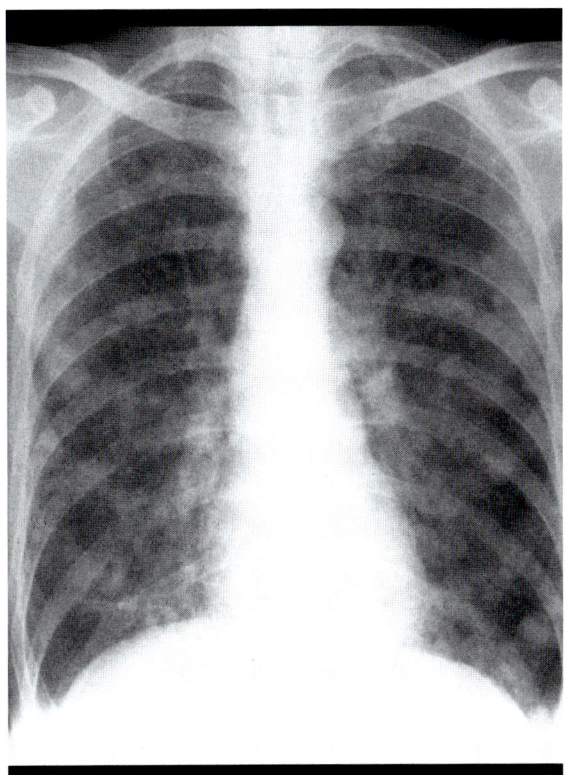

Figure 16-8

RHEUMATOID PNEUMOCONIOSIS

Left: Grossly, rheumatoid pneumoconiosis shows discrete nodules with central necrosis and peripheral layering. (Courtesy of Dr. Alan R. Gibbs, Wales, United Kingdom.)

Right: Radiologically, multiple nodules are apparent. (Courtesy of Dr. Sujal Desai, United Kingdom.)

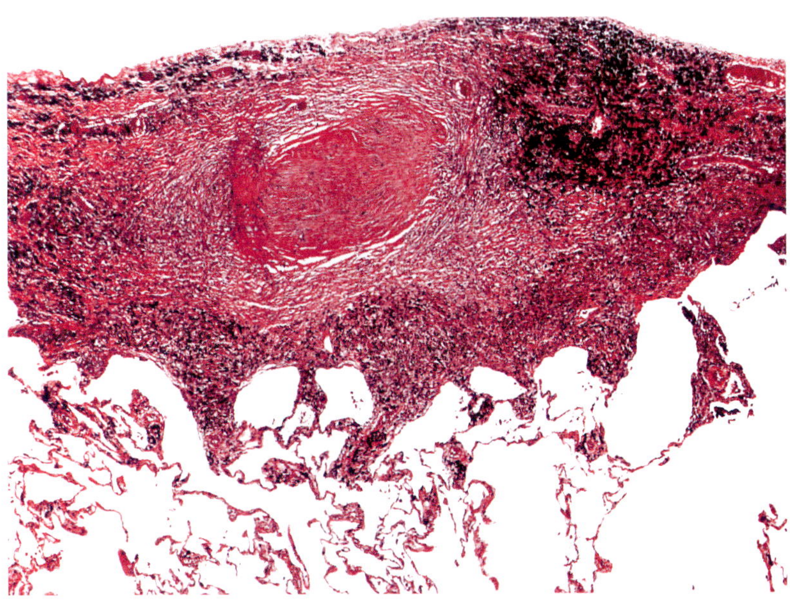

Figure 16-9

SILICOTIC NODULE IN COAL WORKER'S PNEUMOCONIOSIS

A nonpigmented, dusty, collagenized silicotic nodule (upper center) is surrounded by anthracotic pigment-laden macrophages.

Figure 16-10

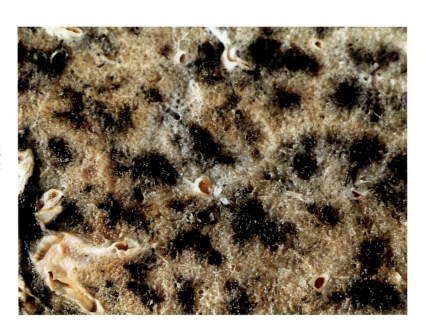

GRAPHITE PNEUMOCONIOSIS

This gross photograph shows numerous centriacinar anthracotic dust macules.

or without an associated fibrotic reaction) is insufficient for a diagnosis of CWP. The diagnosis requires pathologic or radiologic recognition of the characteristic parenchymal lung changes.

In most cases, the diagnosis of CWP, whether simple or complicated, is made on the basis of radiologic findings in an individual with the appropriate exposure history: rounded opacities at the apices for the former and confluence of opacities or large opacities in the latter (11). Pathologically, the diagnosis can be made on the basis of finding simple CWP (coal dust macules and focal emphysema) in a patient with the appropriate history. In cases of PMF, the diagnosis is based on pathologic findings and the background presence of simple CWP.

Treatment and Prognosis. No specific treatment for CWP exists. Prevention is possible and depends upon adequate ventilation and improved work practices at each step in the extraction and processing of the coal. Importantly, cigarette smoke is responsible for more of the ventilatory impairment in these workers than is coal dust.

The most important factor in the development, progression, and prognosis of CWP is cumulative exposure to respirable dust. Progression appears to be greater in individuals who have been exposed to dust with relatively high levels of silica and in younger workers with radiologically identifiable disease (57). The development of isolated simple pneumoconiosis does not require cessation of mining and leaving the work environment. However, the more severe the profusion of the opacities, the more likely is the development of PMF. Consequently, workers with simple pneumoconiosis should be monitored regularly for disease progression. Documented worsening of simple CWP should exclude a worker from further coal dust exposure. Unfortunately, complicated CWP may progress despite stopping coal dust exposure. Rheumatoid pneumoconiosis leads to more rapid progression of both simple and complicated CWP (57). Currently, approximately 4 percent of coal miners die of causes directly attributable to CWP (11).

PNEUMOCONIOSIS FROM OTHER CARBONACEOUS MATERIALS

Forms of pneumoconiosis that are essentially identical to CWP may be associated with exposure to activated carbon, graphite (fig. 16-10), lamp black, carbon black, and the dust and fumes generated in carbon electrode manufacturing (11,57). As with CWP, those dusts that contain relatively little silica produce primarily macules whereas those with appreciable amounts of silica are associated with the development of nodules.

Anthracosis of the airways has been described in individuals chronically exposed to indoor smoke (7). Domestic woodburning has been implicated in causing interstitial lung disease, and iron-coated wood fibers are demonstrated in addition to interstitial inflammatory changes (60).

SILICOSIS

Definition. Silicosis is a chronic lung disease characterized by the development of progressive parenchymal nodules and pulmonary fibrosis after the inhalation of crystalline free silica (11,57,67).

Mineralogy and Exposure. When silicon combines with oxygen it forms tetrahedral silicon tetroxide (SiO_4) (57). Silica is a three-dimensional network of these tetrahedra in which two of the oxygen atoms are shared, resulting in giant molecules that have an average stoicheiometric formula of SiO_2. Uncombined silica is referred to as free silica; when silica combines with various cations, silicates are formed. The most common cations are magnesium, calcium, and aluminum (11). Fibrous silicates are included under the term asbestos and separated from other silicates, as discussed below.

Free silica occurs naturally in amorphous and crystalline forms. Quartz is the most abundant form of crystalline silica and is found in most types of rock. It is the most abundant mineral in the earth's crust and most cases of silicosis are related to exposure to quartz.

Silicosis is the oldest recognized occupational lung disease, having been identified in Egyptian mummies. Although recognized for decades, cases continue to occur, as shown in recent surveillance studies (64). Exposure occurs in: rock mining, quarrying, tunneling through rock, stone cutting, engraving, polishing rock, manufacture and use of silica-containing fillers and abrasives, foundries, ceramics and refractories industries, and sandblasting and grinding.

Clinical Features. Silica-induced lung disease may be chronic, accelerated, or acute, depending upon the intensity and duration of the silica dust exposure. *Acute silicoproteinosis* is similar to pulmonary alveolar proteinosis (see chapter 3). There is very heavy exposure to finely particulate silica, as may occur in sandblasting, among silica flour workers, and in some of the ceramic industries. The patients are generally symptomatic within 3 years of exposure and most reported cases have been fatal (11,57,67).

Chronic (classic or *nodular) silicosis* is the most common form and usually occurs decades after the onset of exposure to relatively low levels of dust. Typically, classic silicosis requires a latency period of at least 20 years after onset of exposure. When the disease manifests within 3 to 10 years of exposure, the term *accelerated silicosis* has been suggested. Among cases of classic silicosis, *simple silicosis* applies to cases with nodules 10 mm or less in diameter and *complicated silicosis (PMF)* when nodules are greater than 1 cm in diameter.

Clinical findings in patients with simple silicosis are generally lacking. In the more advanced stages of disease, dyspnea develops. Cough and sputum production may also occur but are frequently due to chronic bronchitis in smokers or to concurrent infections. Fever and weight loss suggest the development of infection, especially mycobacterial lung disease, a known complicating illness in silicotics. Signs of cor pulmonale may develop in individuals with severe, longstanding, silica-induced lung disease and interstitial fibrosis. Crackles on auscultation and clubbing are uncommon and suggest another diagnosis, such as bronchogenic carcinoma or infection. The laboratory findings are nonspecific and may include the presence of rheumatoid factor, antinuclear antibodies, and serum immune complexes, and a polyclonal increase in immunoglobulins.

Connective tissue diseases, especially scleroderma, rheumatoid arthritis, and systemic lupus erythematosus, have been identified in individuals with a history of exposure to silica (6,35). In such cases, the signs and symptoms are those of the connective tissue disease; silicosis is not always evident radiologically.

Radiologic Findings. The characteristic radiographic manifestation of silicosis is multiple nodules that mainly or exclusively involve the upper lobes (fig. 16-11) (71). The nodules are well-circumscribed, of fairly uniform size, and usually less than 5 mm in diameter. They tend to coalesce over time and form conglomerate masses measuring greater than 1 cm in diameter (PMF). PMF is usually bilateral and associated with marked volume loss of the upper lobes, cephalad retraction of the hila, and compensatory hyperinflation of the lower lobes. CT is superior to chest radiography in demonstrating the presence and distribution of silicotic nodules (9).

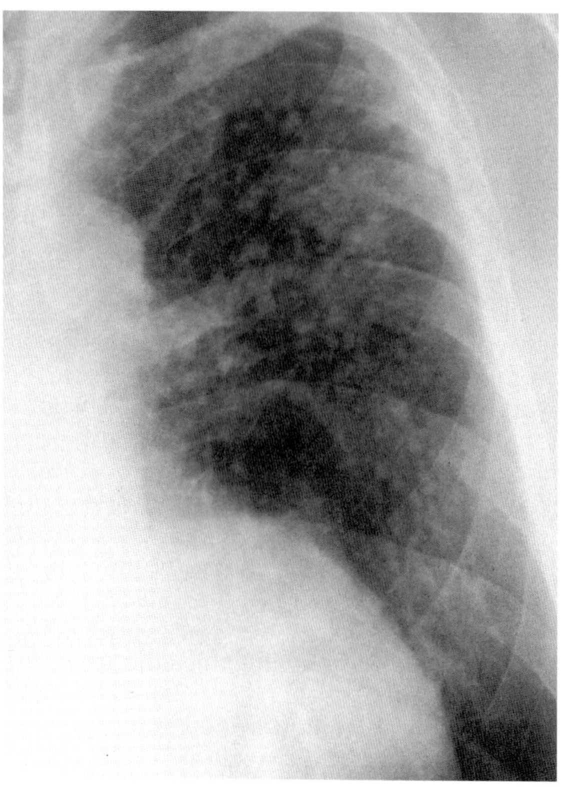

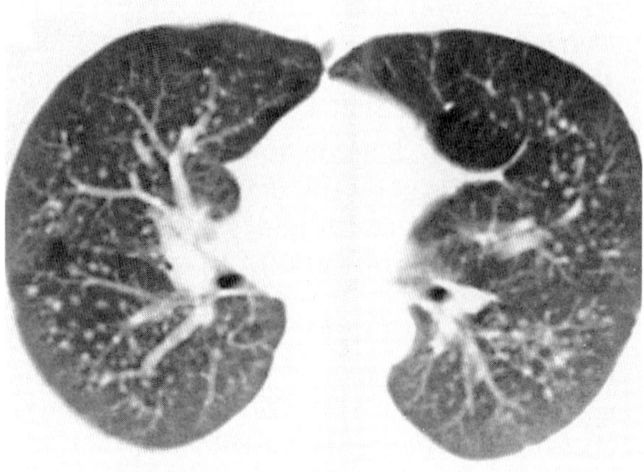

Figure 16-11

SILICOSIS

Left: View of the left lung from a PA chest radiograph shows small nodules involving mainly the upper and middle lung zones.

Above: Conventional 10-mm collimation CT demonstrates bilateral nodules. The nodules have sharply circumscribed margins and measure 2 to 4 mm in diameter. The patient was a 55-year-old man with longstanding silicosis.

Table 16-3

PATHOLOGIC LESIONS ASSOCIATED WITH SILICA EXPOSURE[a]

Acute silicoproteinosis
Nodular silicosis
Simple silicosis
Complicated silicosis/progressive massive fibrosis
Silicotuberculosis
Rheumatoid pneumoconiosis (Caplan's syndrome)
Mixed dust fibrosis
Diffuse interstitial fibrosis
Pleural fibrosis

[a]Modified from references 11 and 67.

Pathologic Findings. The pathologic lesions associated with silica exposure are shown in Table 16-3 (11,67).

Silicoproteinosis resembles pulmonary alveolar proteinosis (fig. 16-12). Grossly, the lung tissue is characterized by irregular zones of consolidation. Histologically, there is granular, eosinophilic, lipoproteinaceous material filling airspaces. Some poorly formed silicotic nodules and granulomas may also be present. The eosinophilic material is periodic acid–Schiff (PAS) positive (diastase resistant) and lipid rich; it may contain cholesterol clefts and nodular or amorphous eosinophilic cell debris. Mild interstitial inflammation and collagenization may be present. Polarization may or may not reveal weakly birefringent silica particles, depending on the size of the particles; some are too small to be seen with the light microscope.

Nodular silicosis is characterized grossly by discrete fibrous nodules 3 to 6 mm in diameter (figs. 16-13, 16-14) which are firm, rounded, and well demarcated on cut section; these may appear somewhat flattened and are often surrounded by a cuff of pigmentation when on the pleural surface. Hilar lymph nodes are typically involved by silicotic nodules and secondary calcification may be present. The nodules may be pigmented depending on the amount of concomitant coal dust exposure; when the nodules lose their rounded shape, a designation of mixed dust fibrosis may be appropriate (see below).

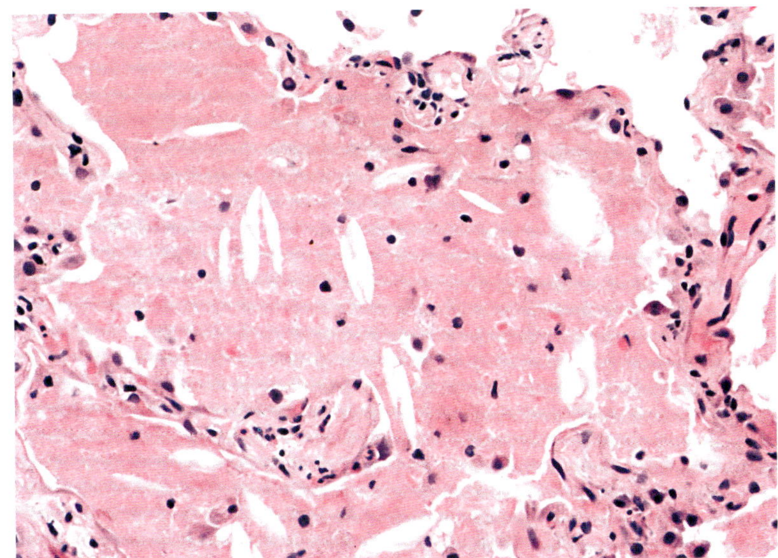

Figure 16-12

SILICOPROTEINOSIS

The alveolar spaces are filled with granular eosinophilic debris including fragments of cells and prominent cholesterol clefts.

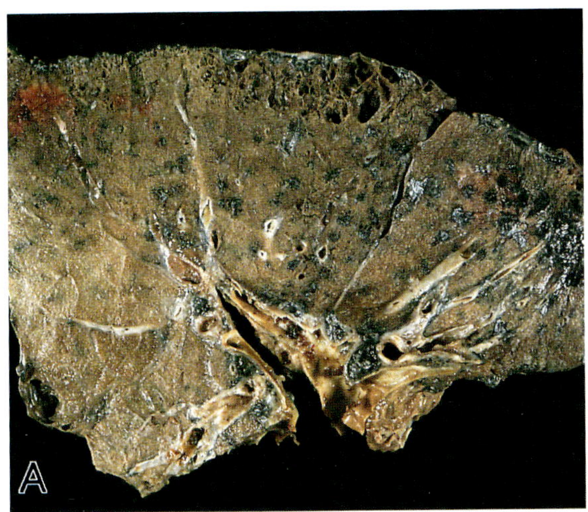

Figure 16-13

SILICOSIS

Three cases of silicosis are grossly illustrated. The first patient was asymptomatic and had only radiologic changes; a few gray-black silicotic nodules are noted in the upper lobe with some emphysema (A). More dramatic changes are noted in the other cases with PMF and confluent nodules (B,C). Some cavitation is present in C. (Courtesy of Dr. Andrew Churg, Vancouver, Canada.)

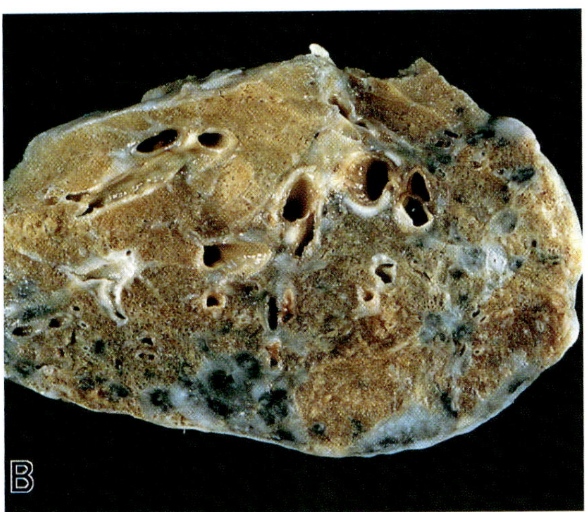

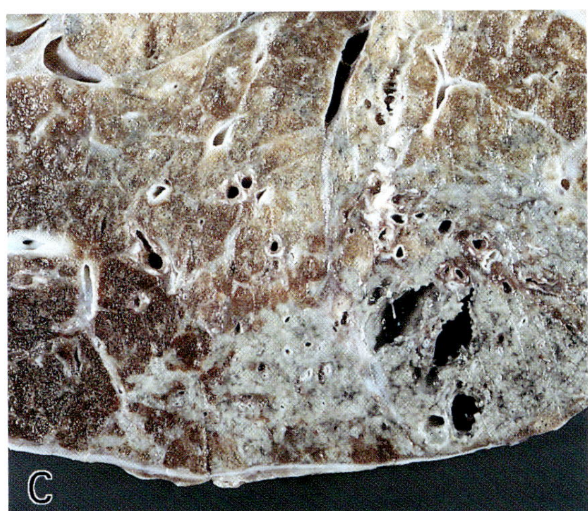

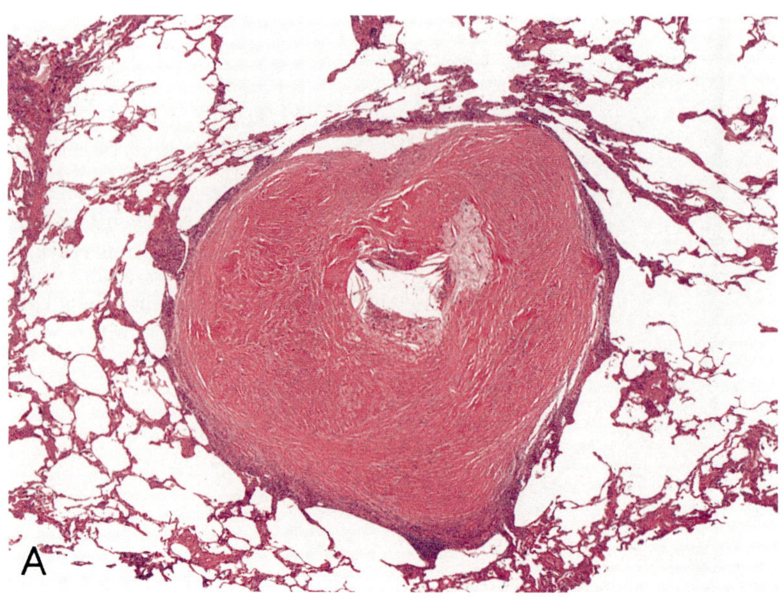

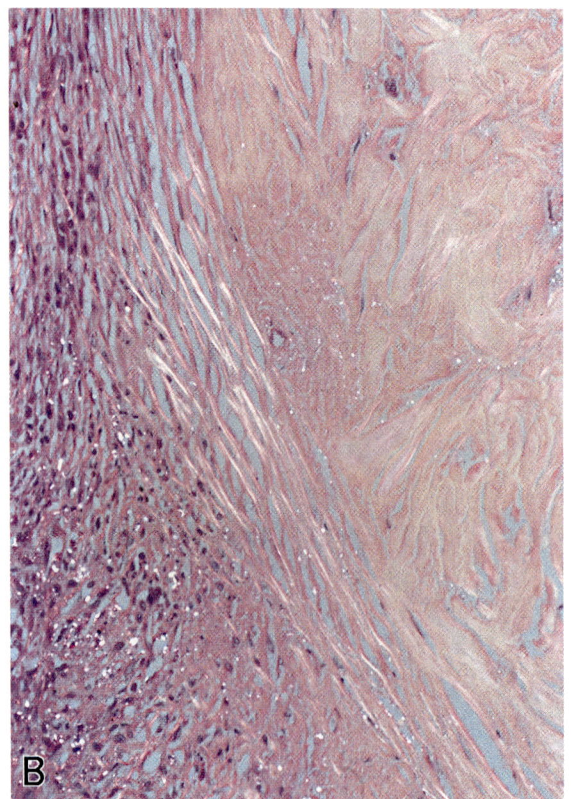

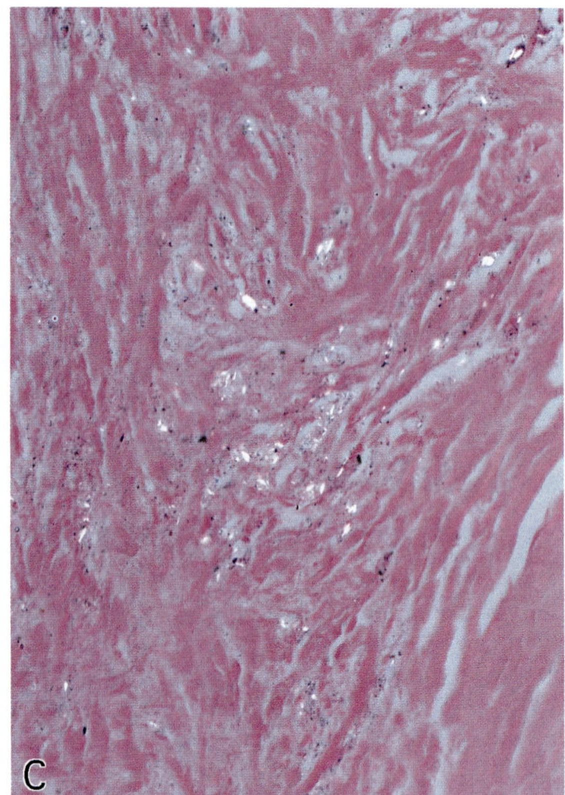

Figure 16-14

SILICOSIS

In chronic nodular silicosis there is dense lamellar fibrosis with little surrounding infiltrate (A). The collagen is dense, lamellar, and birefringent (B). Weakly birefringent silica particles and more strongly birefringent silicate particles are seen both within the fibrosis and in the surrounding infiltrate (B,C).

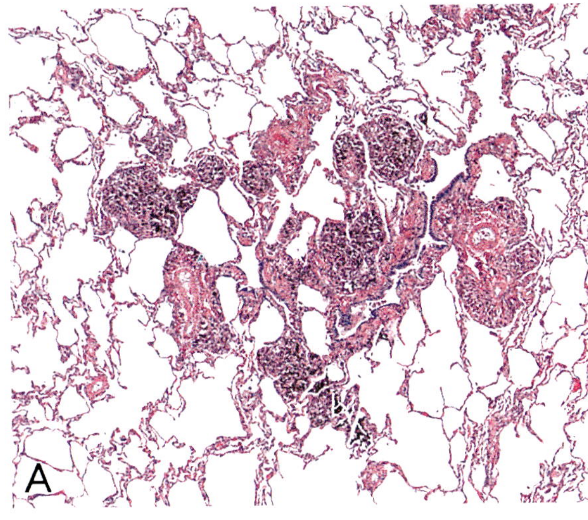

Figure 16-15

SILICOSIS

This case shows early/cellular silicosis with infiltrates of dust-laden macrophages producing a centriacinar dust macule (A). There is nodular accumulation of dust-filled macrophages along perivenular lymphatic routes adjacent to veins and in the pleura (B,C).

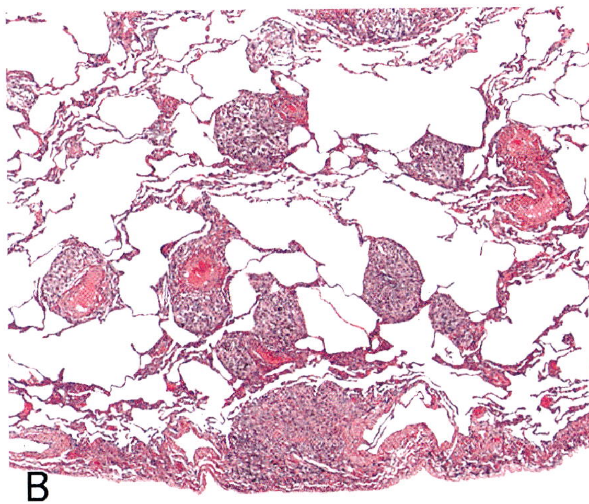

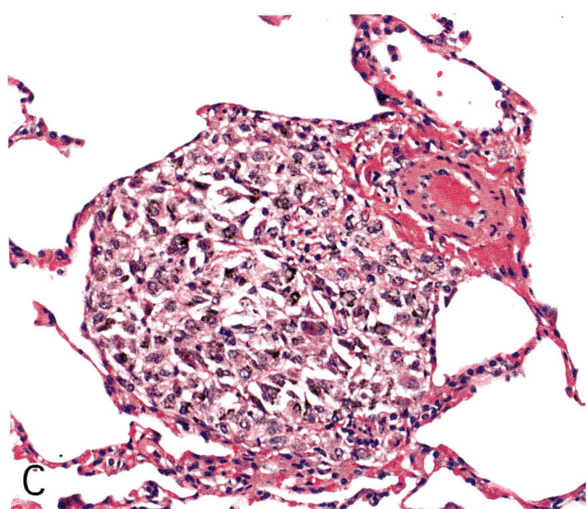

Silicotic nodules arise in a background of dust-filled macrophages distributed along lymphatic routes, around bronchovascular bundles, and in the pleura and septa (figs. 16-15–16-17). In early ("cellular") cases only macrophages may be present. Sarcoid-like granulomas are not seen. Developing silicotic nodules can be identified as foci of increased reticulin and fibrosis in the sheets of dust-laden macrophages; micronodules enlarge to form the discrete rounded nodules, of classic silicosis. Late in the course of the disease and after exposure has stopped, the predominant pattern may be that of fibrous nodules with few surrounding histiocytes. Some surrounding emphysematous change is common. Early in the course of silicosis, particularly in accelerated silicosis, dust-filled macrophages may be the most prominent finding, with only scattered silicotic nodules.

Silicotic nodules are composed of dense lamellar collagen. They may become calcified, hyalinized, or undergo secondary central degenerative changes. Polarized light reveals weakly birefringent silica (and commonly, more strongly birefringent silicates [42]), both within the nodules and in the surrounding cuff of dust-filled macrophages.

Individual lesions and conglomerates of lesions greater than 1 cm in diameter are defined as *PMF* (figs. 16-13, 16-18). Lesions this large may develop cavitation and necrosis. When these occur, infection, particularly tuberculosis, should be carefully excluded.

Silicotuberculosis is suggested when silicotic nodules show central necrosis with a histocytic and recognizable epithelioid granulomatous reaction. Silicosis by itself is not associated with a sarcoid-like granulomatous reaction (fig. 16-19).

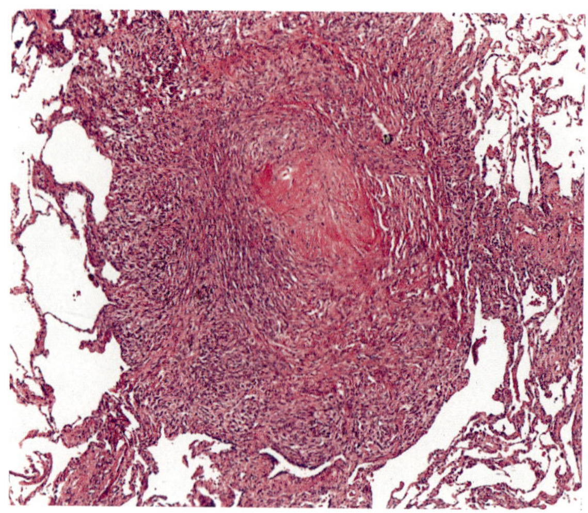

Figure 16-16

SILICOSIS

Silicotic nodules arise in a background of infiltrates of dust-laden macrophages, here seen in an intralobular septum. The silicotic nodules are seen as zones of dense eosinophilic collagen arising in this background.

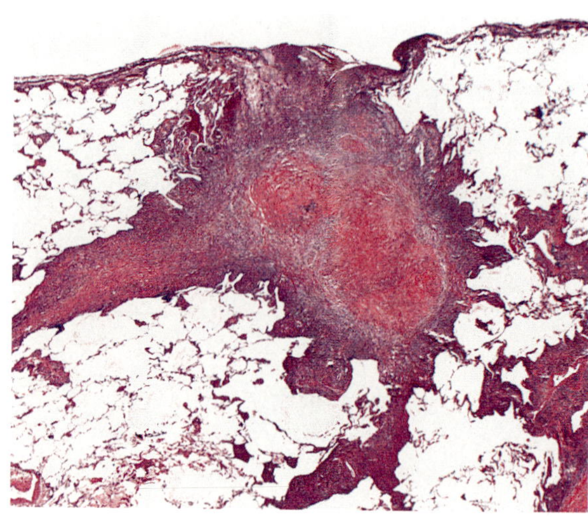

Figure 16-17

SILICOSIS

Silicotic nodule formation is apparent in an intralobular septum.

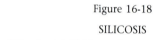

Figure 16-18

SILICOSIS

Silicosis with PMF may show conglomerates of silicotic nodules (A) or more widespread fibrosis with increased associated dust-laden macrophages (B,C).

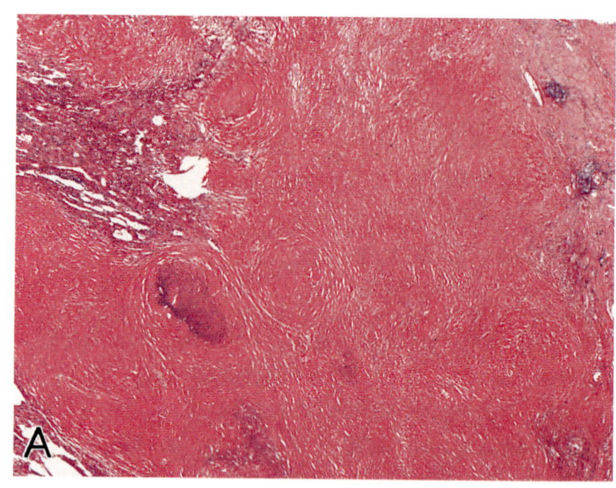

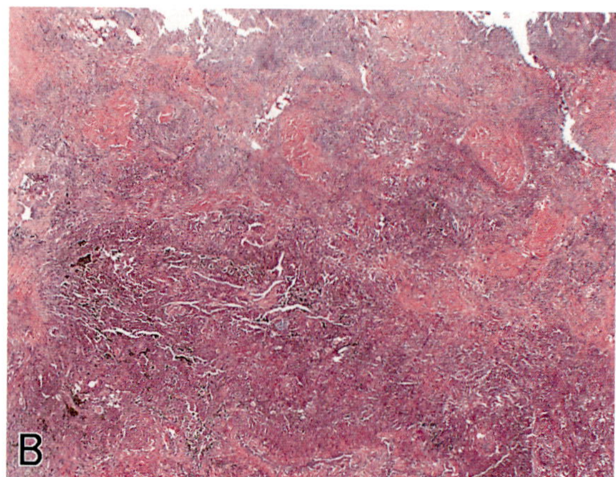

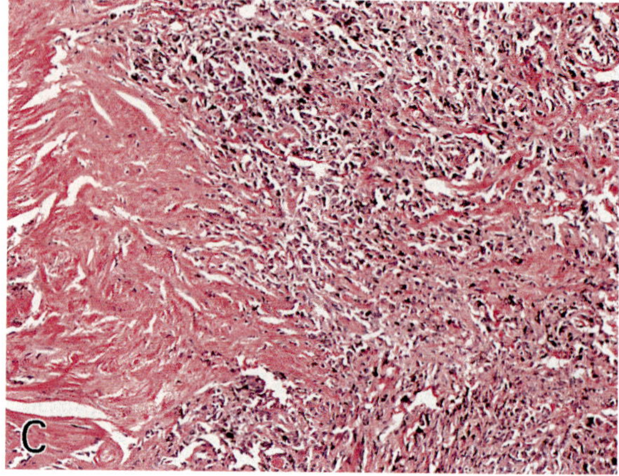

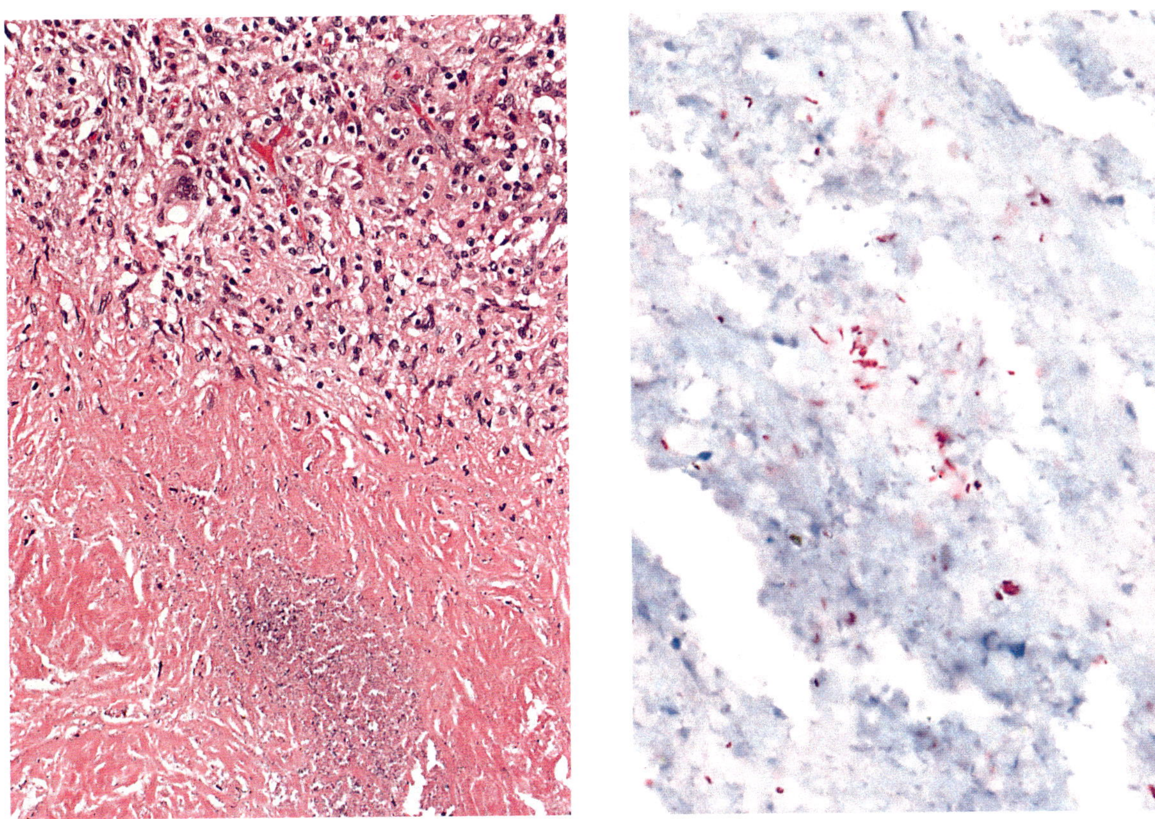

Figure 16-19

SILICOTUBERCULOSIS

Left: There is necrosis with adjacent granulomatous inflammation including giant cells. Right: Numerous acid-fast organisms are identified with the Ziel-Nielsen stain.

From a practical point of view, any necrosis in silicotic nodules and any granulomatous inflammation (epithelioid histiocytes and giant cells) should be considered tuberculosis until that possibility has been rigorously excluded.

In *rheumatoid pneumoconiosis,* nodules classically have necrotic centers and laminations of light and dark tissue around the periphery. They measure 5 cm or more in diameter. Histologically, there is central necrosis surrounded by rings of variably pigmented tissue. Around the necrosis are palisaded histiocytes, neutrophils, fibroblasts, and collagen. Some cases closely resemble infectious granulomas (fig. 16-20). The distinction from tuberculosis may be very difficult and knowledge of the clinical history and serologic findings is helpful.

Silica is so frequently associated with other (less fibrogenic) dusts that the recognition of *mixed dust fibrosis* (i.e., *mixed dust pneumoconiosis*) as one of the patterns of silicosis is expedient (figs. 16-21, 16-22). The nodular lesions in mixed dust fibrosis are pigmented and have a "Medusa head" appearance in contrast to the pale round nodules of classic silicosis. Typically, there is whorled fibrosis in the center with variable amounts of pigmentation (depending on the exposure). A cuff of surrounding histiocytes tapers off into the surrounding interstitium rather than being rounded and sharply demarcated as in the classic silicotic nodule.

Diffuse interstitial fibrosis is recognized in a significant portion of lungs from individuals who have been exposed to silica (sometimes in conjunction with other fibrogenic dusts) (fig. 16-23). In a study of slate workers from north Wales, it was found that more than 20 percent had severe interstitial fibrosis, sometimes with

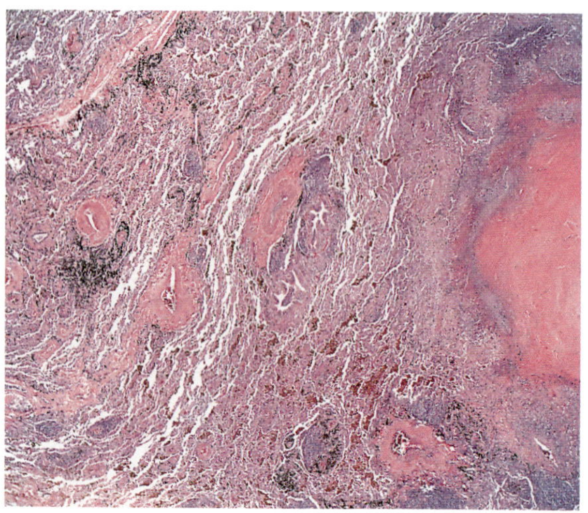

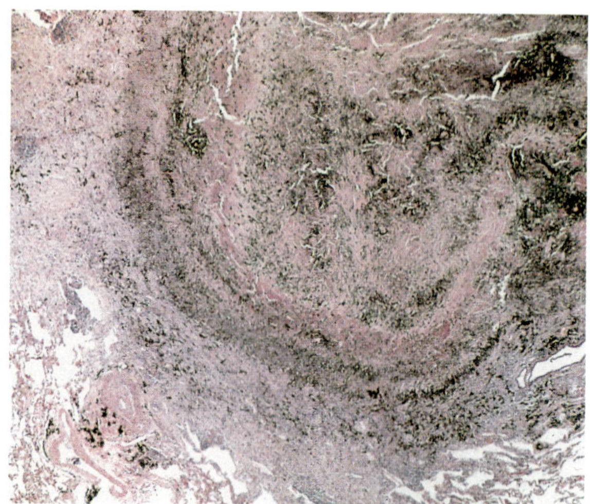

Figure 16-20

RHEUMATOID PNEUMOCONIOSIS

Left: There are extensive carbon dust deposits surrounding a nodule with central fibrinoid necrosis.

Right: A palisaded histiocytic reaction is present around the zone of necrosis. Extensive carbon dust deposits are present within and surrounding the rheumatoid nodule. Although the lesion resembles an infectious granuloma, there is an absence of non-necrotizing sarcoid-like granulomas. (Courtesy of Dr. Alan R. Gibbs, Wales, United Kindgom.)

associated honeycombing (11). By description, the fibrosis does not show the heterogeneity seen in usual interstitial pneumonia as currently defined (see chapter 3). Patients with silicosis and extensive fibrosis of any type may show the changes of pulmonary hypertension and secondary cor pulmonale.

Pleural fibrosis is commonly a component of parenchymal silicosis. Isolated pleural involvement mimicking a malignant mesothelioma has been described (fig. 16-24) (81). In established silicosis, silicotic nodules may protrude as "pleural pearls" (61).

Peritoneal silicotic nodules have also been described in patients with established silicosis (44). Slavin et al. (68) described more widespread dissemination of silica, with lesions identified in liver, spleen, bone marrow, and extrathoracic lymph nodes.

Silicotic fibrous pseudotumors may occur in the mediastinum and peribronchial lymph nodes. These are recognized as expansile masses even in the absence of established silicosis in the lungs (fig. 16-25). They may mimic sarcomas and show infiltrative and destructive growth (8).

Pathogenesis. Silicosis is caused by the inhalation of particles less than 10 µm in diameter. Those approximately 1 µm in diameter are thought to be the most pathogenic (11,57).

The most important factors in the pathogenesis of silicosis are the intensity and duration of the exposure to silica. Once silica particles are deposited in the lung, damage occurs, either by direct cytotoxicity or via the production of oxidants and other mediators (11,47). The exact sequence of events in the development of lung injury and fibrosis has not been worked out. Toxic effects of silica on alveolar lining cells have been implicated in the development of silicoproteinosis (67).

Diagnosis. The diagnosis of silicosis should be reserved for individuals who show the lung parenchymal abnormalities described above. These may be identified radiologically or pathologically, and in most cases, the history of exposure can be readily elicited. According to Parkes, criteria for the diagnosis are as follows: 1) an appropriate exposure history; 2) radiologic findings consistent with silicosis; and 3) absence of other diseases to explain the radiologic findings (57). The finding of silica, silicates, silicotic nodules, and increased dust in hilar and mediastinal lymph nodes alone is not sufficient for a diagnosis of silicosis. Virtually

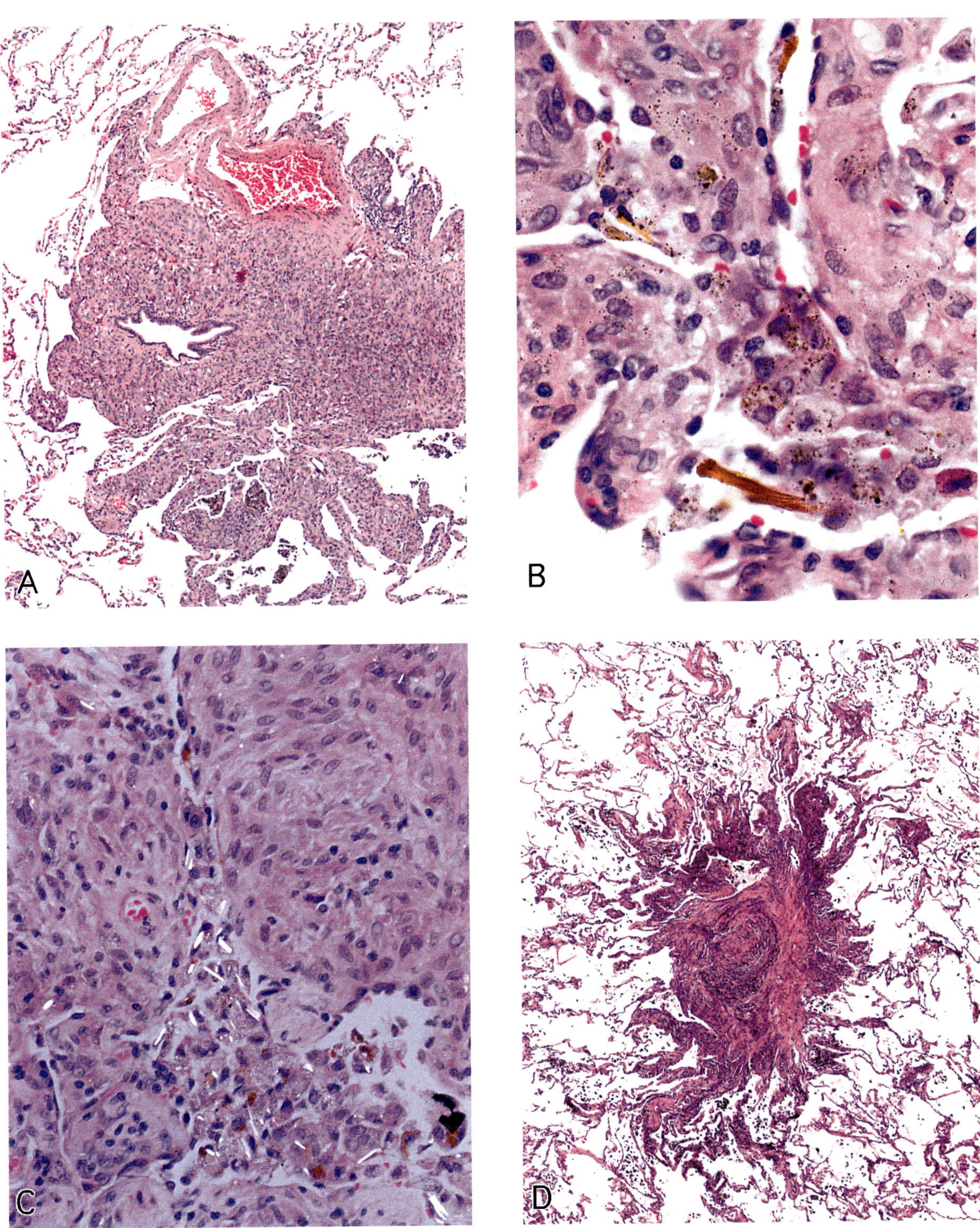

Figure 16-21

MIXED DUST PNEUMOCONIOSIS

Early cellular lesions are identified in centriacinar regions along bronchioles (A). In this case there was both asbestos exposure with asbestos bodies (B) and silicates seen with birefringence (C). In another case, a typical mixed dust nodule with its "Medusa head" appearance is illustrated (D).

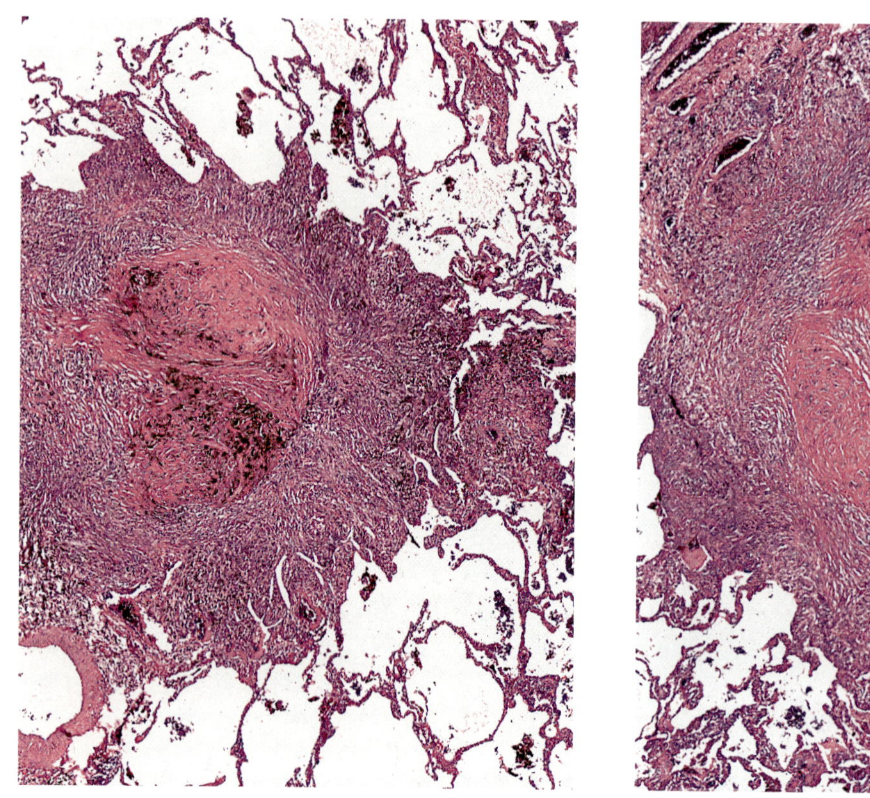
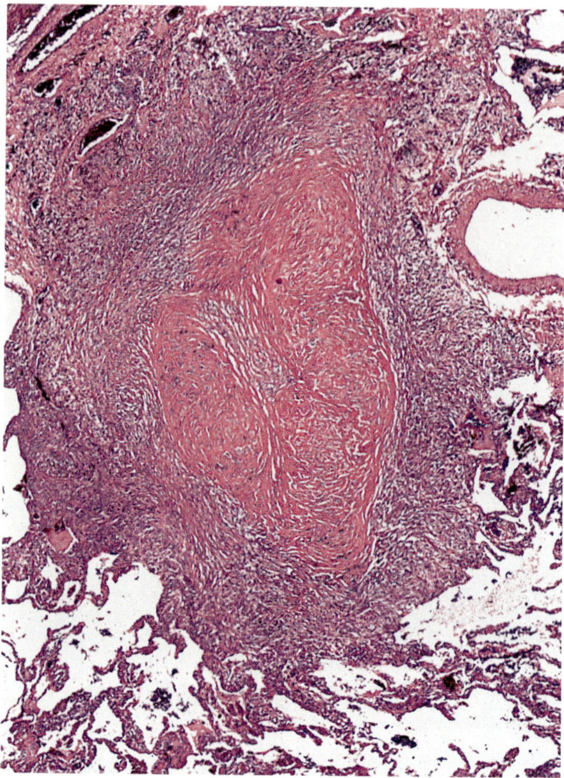

Figure 16-22

MIXED DUST PNEUMOCONIOSIS

Left: Some nodules show central pigmentation.
Right: Other nodules are typical of eosinophilic, densely fibrotic, silicotic-type nodules.

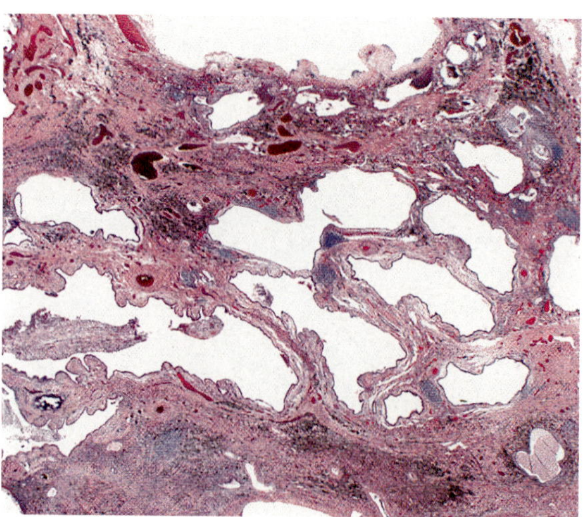
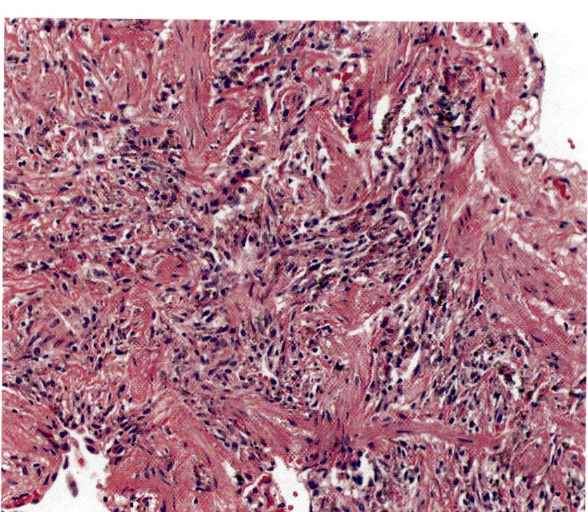

Figure 16-23

SILICOSIS WITH DIFFUSE INTERSTITIAL FIBROSIS

Left: There is diffuse fibrosis with architectural destruction and honeycomb formation.
Right: Within the fibrosis are numerous dust-laden macrophages.

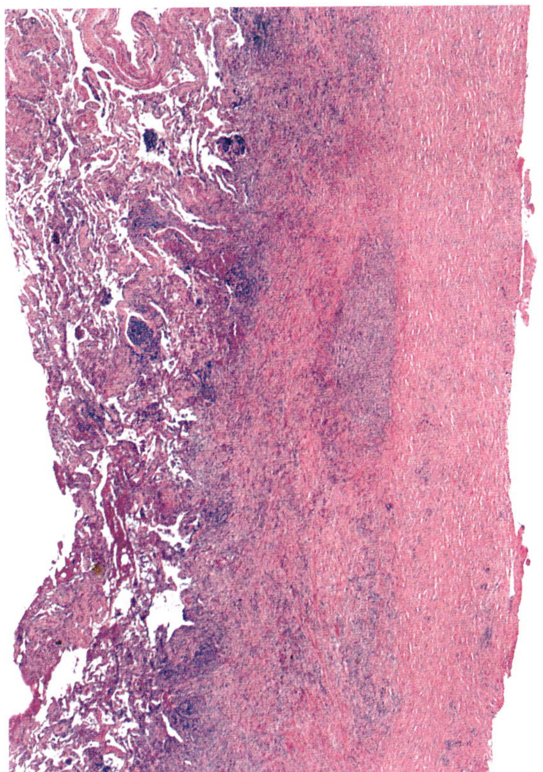

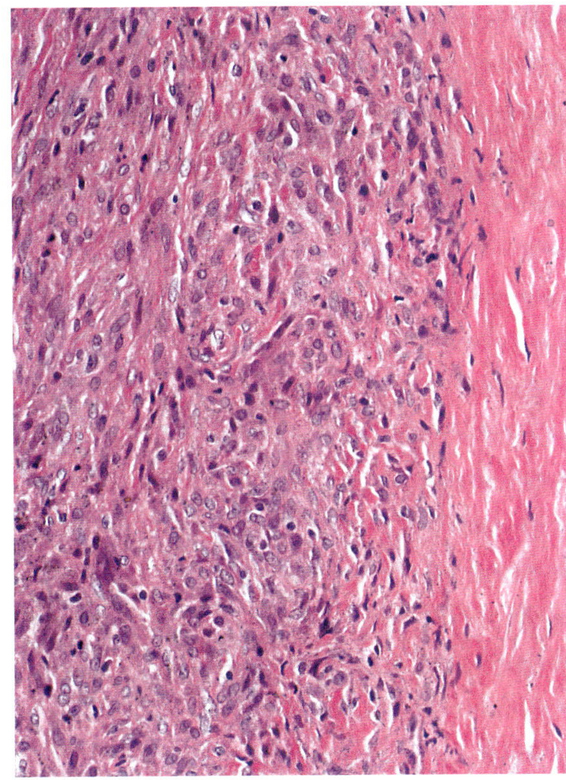

Figure 16-24

PLEURAL SILICOSIS

There is marked pleural thickening (left) with associated dust-laden macrophages (right); there was no evidence of parenchymal silicosis. Clinically, the process mimicked malignant mesothelioma.

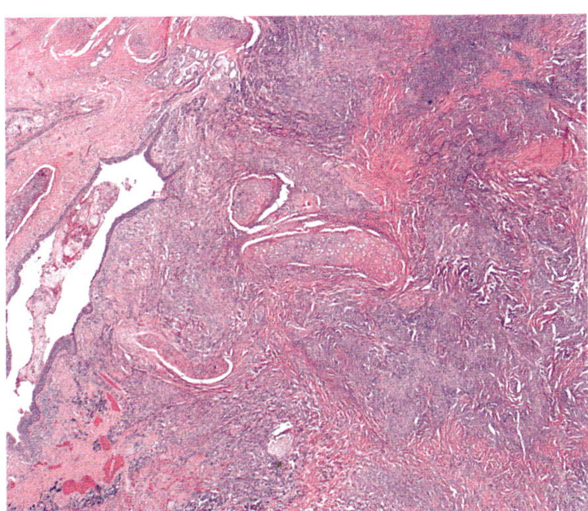

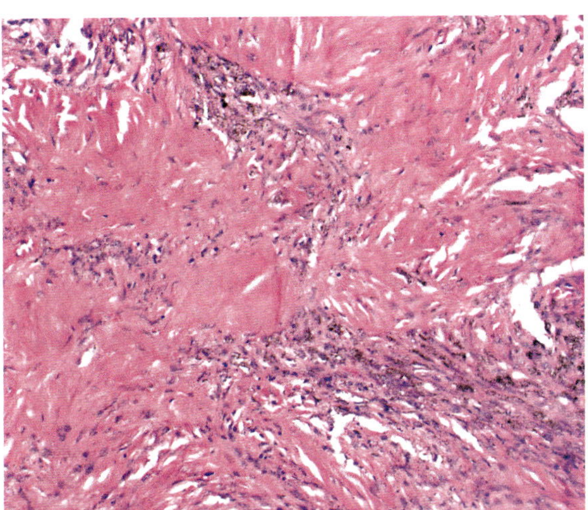

Figure 16-25

SILICOTIC FIBROUS PSEUDOTUMOR

Dust-laden macrophages and proliferative fibrosis destroy a bronchus. This was associated with distal obstructive pneumonia.

Table 16-4

METHODS OF QUANTIFYING ASBESTOS BURDEN IN HUMAN LUNG TISSUE[a]

Identifying and quantifying asbestos bodies in routine tissue sections of lung tissue (may be highlighted with Prussian blue staining)
Counting asbestos bodies in lung tissue digest preparations with the light microscope
Counting uncoated asbestos fibers in lung tissue digest preparations with a phase microscope
Counting and identifying uncoated asbestos fibers with an appropriately equipped electron microscope

[a]Summarized from reference 11.

all adults have a small amount of silica and silicates associated with anthracotic pigment along lymphatic routes in their lungs and in hilar and mediastinal lymph nodes.

Treatment and Prognosis. Most affected patients remain symptom free and have a normal lifespan (57). A small percentage do have progressive respiratory disability. There is no known effective therapy to prevent or ameliorate the course of silicosis after the inhalation of silica dust. Therefore, efforts have been directed at preventing the disease. The development of tuberculosis is associated with increased morbidity. The presence of rheumatoid pneumoconiosis or silicotuberculosis complicating PMF portends an unfavorable prognosis. The prognosis of patients with established silicoproteinosis is poor.

ASBESTOSIS AND OTHER NON-NEOPLASTIC DISEASES CAUSED BY ASBESTOS

Background, Mineralogy, and Exposure

Asbestos refers to a group of fibrous silicates that are useful in industry because of their strength, resistance to heat and chemical degradation, and ability to be woven (11,12,57,63). Six types of asbestos are recognized: chrysotile, amosite, crocidolite, anthophyllite, tremolite, and actinolite (11). These are generally divided into the chrysotiles (the first) and the amphiboles (the remaining five types). Chrysotile asbestos tends to be relatively fragile and not chemically stable under biologic conditions, whereas amphiboles are more stable and resistant. Inhaled chrysotile is more easily cleared from the lung than amphibole asbestos, and chrysotile is also thought to be a weaker human mesothelial carcinogen. The ability of asbestos fibers to reach the deep lung parenchyma is a reflection more of their diameter (usually less than 3 µm) than their length; fibers up to several hundred microns may be found in the alveoli.

The toxic effects of asbestos have been recognized for decades and exposure to asbestos is regulated in virtually all industrialized nations (11,57). Asbestos is sufficiently common in ambient air that nearly everyone is exposed to a minor degree. Occupations associated with high levels of exposure to asbestos include work in mining and milling of asbestos and production and use of asbestos cement products, asbestos insulation products, asbestos friction products, asbestos textiles, asbestos floor tiles, asbestos paper products, and others.

For many asbestos-related lung disorders there is a correlation between the level of exposure and the severity of the disease, and quantitative evaluation of the lung burden of asbestos may be of importance. Asbestos in the lung is found either as uncoated fibers or as asbestos bodies. One theory is that the outer golden brown coat of iron particles is due to reduction of the oxide to hemosiderin (occurring from the outside in), and not due to ferrugination. Another view is that asbestos bodies are asbestos fibers that are "ferruginated" with an iron protein coat by macrophages. Some believe that true ferrugination only occurs on fibrous particulates approximately 20 µm or greater in length. Asbestos bodies are visible with the light microscope and can be distinguished from other ferruginous bodies by their segmented appearance: clubbed ends and a thin, straight, lucent central core (figs. 16-26, 16-27) (11,13,63). Asbestos fibers are not visible with the light microscope and require electron microscopy to be identified. In general, there are many more asbestos fibers in the lung tissue than asbestos bodies. There are a number of methods of quantifying asbestos in the lung and these are summarized in Table 16-4.

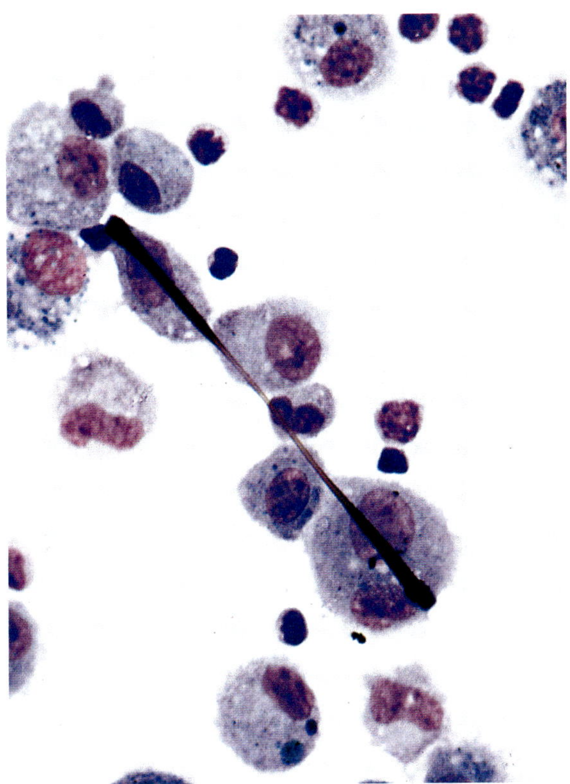
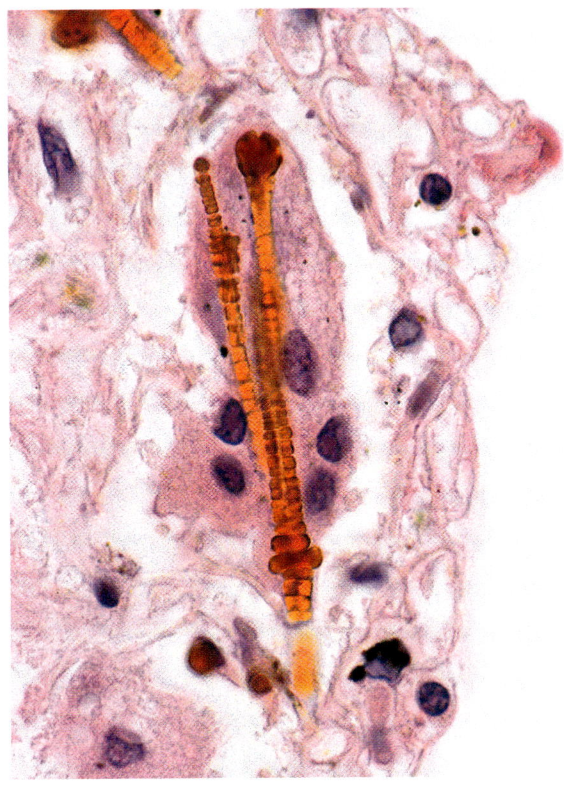

Figure 16-26

ASBESTOS BODIES

Left: Asbestos bodies in BAL fluid. Note the beaded character with clubbing at either end and faintly visible central lucent core. The latter feature is diagnositc of an asbestos body.

Right: Asbestos bodies in tissue section.

Asbestos bodies are most commonly encountered in the lung or hilar lymph nodes. Asbestos fibers may be distributed more widely in the body and may be identified in sites of the development of mesothelioma, including pleura, omentum, and mesentery (19). Special techniques, including filtrations of digested tissue and analytical transmission electron microscopy, are required to identify asbestos in these sites (19).

In general, the identification of asbestos bodies in routine histologic sections of lung tissue with the light microscope is simple but insensitive; the number of uncoated asbestos fibers cannot be assessed. In routine sections, the presence of asbestos bodies is indicative of a heavy lung burden (63). Conversely, the counting and identification of uncoated asbestos fibers with an appropriately equipped electron microscope is expensive and time consuming, but a very sensitive method of quantification. Details of these methods are discussed elsewhere (11,63).

The thoracic diseases associated with asbestos exposure can be divided into neoplastic and non-neoplastic diseases (Table 16-5). Neoplasms are not within the scope of this monograph.

Asbestosis

Definition. Asbestosis is bilateral diffuse interstitial fibrosis of the lungs caused by the inhalation of asbestos fibers (11,12,63). Asbestosis generally requires heavy exposure to asbestos; the severity and rate of progression of asbestosis parallel the exposure level. The heavier the exposure, the shorter the latency from exposure to the appearance of clinical manifestations.

Clinical Features. The clinical findings in asbestosis are those of diffuse interstitial fibrosis: cough and shortness of breath. Physical

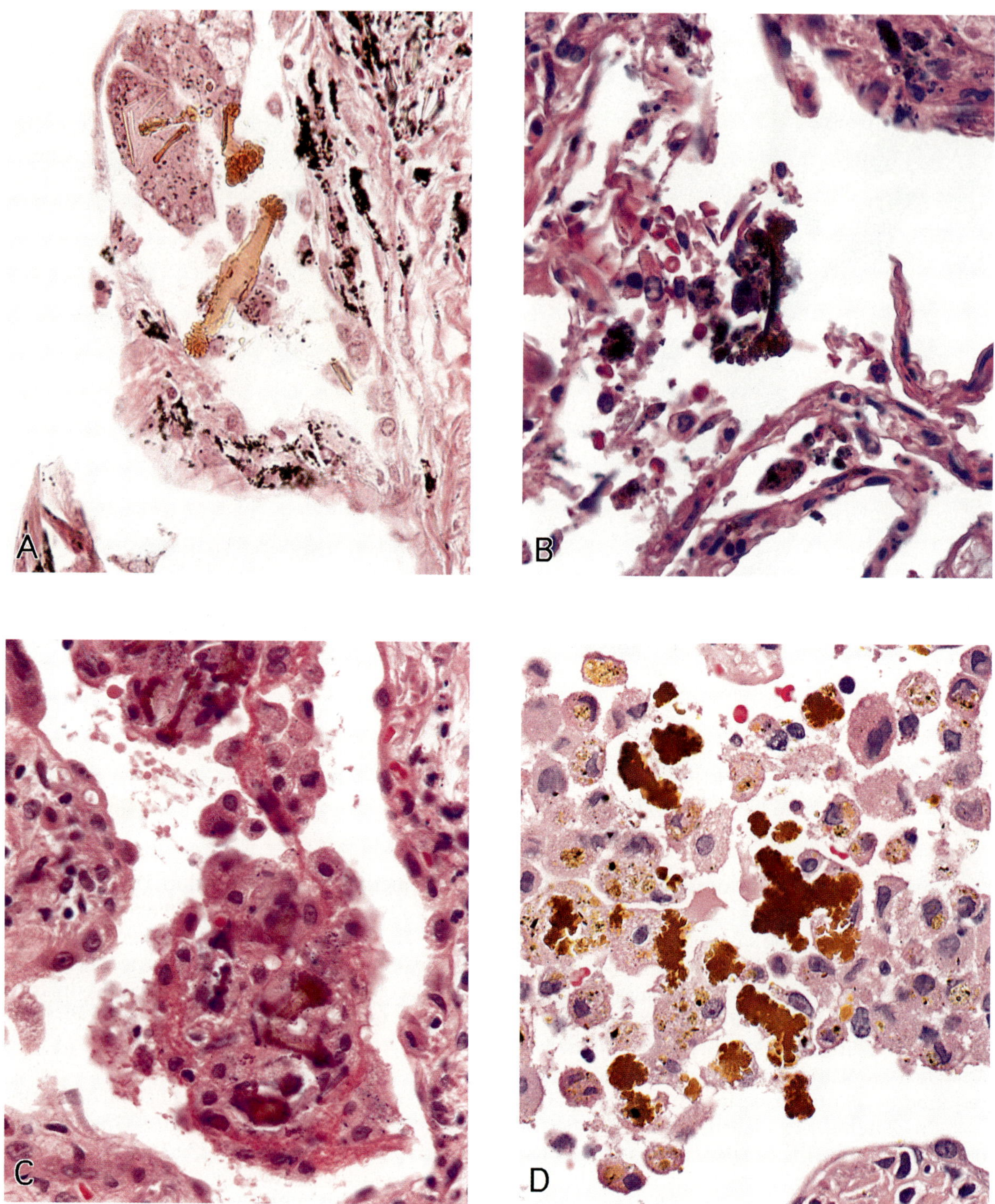

Figure 16-27

FERRUGINOUS BODIES

A variety of foreign materials may become ferruginated when retained in the alveolar space. Asbestos bodies are the best known, but ferruginous bodies may also be seen with mica (A), in foundry workers where the core appears to be carbon particles (B), and in inhalational talcosis (C). In some instances the material is so heavily ferruginated that it is difficult to determine the core material without specific analysis, as in this case of mixed dust pneumoconiosis (D).

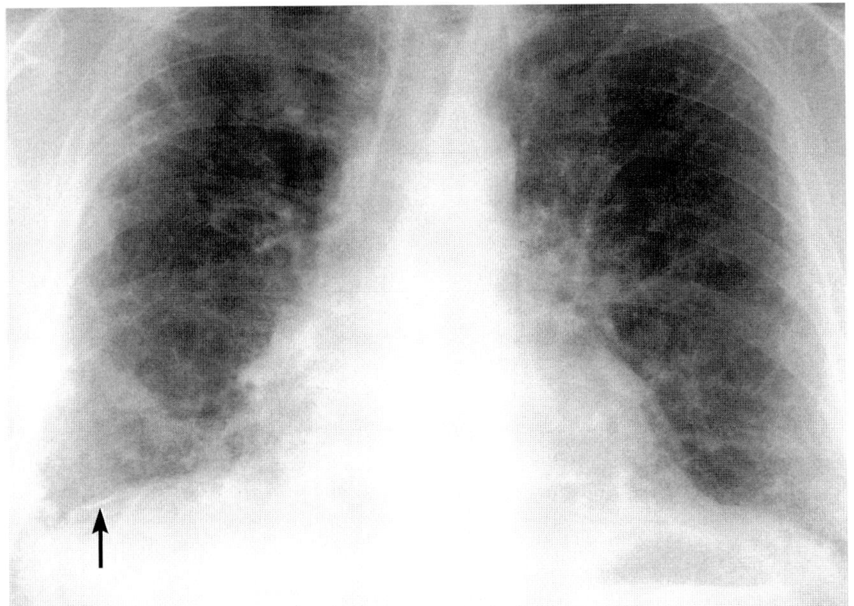

Figure 16-28

ASBESTOSIS

PA chest radiograph demonstrates a reticular pattern involving mainly the subpleural regions and the lower lobes. Also seen are bilateral pleural plaques. A right diaphragmatic pleural plaque is calcified (arrow). The patient was a 58-year-old man with asbestosis.

examination shows dry inspiratory rales at the lung bases on auscultation and possibly clubbing. Pulmonary function studies reflect a restrictive pattern, with low lung volumes and decreased diffusing capacity. Airflow limitation in some patients is due to large airway inflammation caused by asbestos deposition along the respiratory bronchioles and at the bifurcation of the alveolar ducts. Arterial blood gases often demonstrate hypoxemia with exercise early in the course of asbestosis and at rest with advanced disease. Asbestos bodies are frequently encountered in bronchoalveolar lavage (BAL) specimens but their presence is indicative of exposure and not necessarily of disease (57).

Radiologic Findings. The typical radiographic findings of asbestosis are bilateral, symmetrical, irregular linear opacities that result in a reticular pattern, which mainly involves the lower lobes (fig. 16-28). Pleural involvement is a hallmark of asbestos exposure that differentiates asbestos-induced pulmonary disease from many other interstitial lung disorders. CT, particularly high-resolution (HR) CT, allows detection of parenchymal abnormalities not evident on the radiograph (70). The most common HRCT manifestations of asbestosis are intralobular linear opacities, irregular thickening of interlobular septa, subpleural curvilinear opacities, parenchymal bands, and honeycombing (fig. 16-29). The abnormalities involve mainly the subpleural lung regions of the lower lobes. Parenchymal bands consist of linear opacities measuring 2 to 5 cm in length coursing through the lung, usually to an area of pleural thickening. Pathologic correlation has shown that these bands reflect the presence of fibrosis along the bronchovascular sheath or interlobular septa (3). In most cases, HRCT demonstrates concomitant pleural plaques or diffuse pleural thickening (70).

Table 16-5

DISEASES ASSOCIATED WITH ASBESTOS EXPOSURE[a]

Asbestosis
Asbestos airway disease
Non-neoplastic pleural disorders
Benign asbestos effusion
Visceral pleural fibrosis
Hyaline pleural plaque
Rounded atelectasis
Carcinoma of the lung
Malignant mesothelioma

[a]Summarized from references 11, 13, and 63.

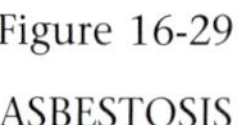

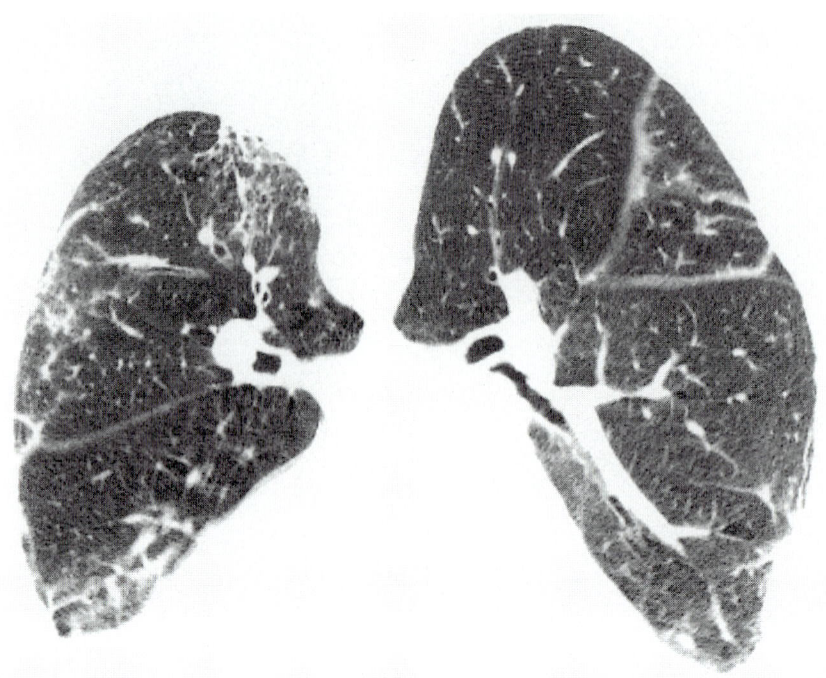

Figure 16-29

ASBESTOSIS

HRCT performed with the patient prone shows intralobular linear opacities and irregular thickening of the interlobular septa, causing a reticular pattern. Also noted are focal areas of ground-glass attenuation. The abnormalities have a patchy distribution and involve mainly the subpleural lung regions. The patient was a 70-year-old man with asbestosis.

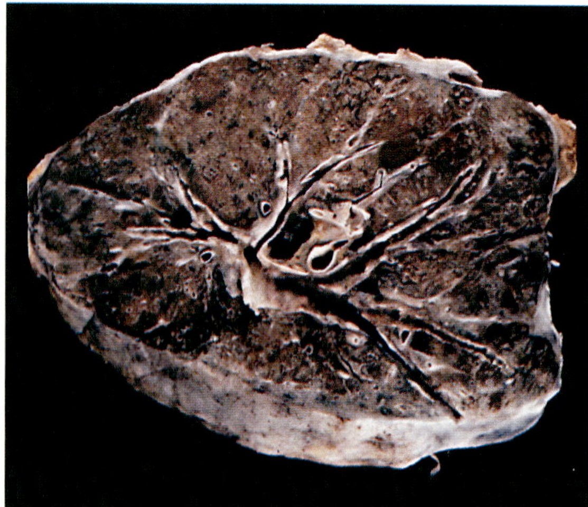

Figure 16-30

ASBESTOSIS

There is patchy gray-white fibrosis which is more severe in the lower zones and associated with visceral pleural fibrosis.

Pathologic Findings. Grossly, there is often pleural as well as parenchymal fibrosis (fig. 16-30) (11,12,57,63). The parenchymal fibrosis is typically worse in the lower lung zones and subpleural regions, and may include honeycomb change. The gross extent of the fibrosis should be documented by the pathologist.

The histologic findings are those of interstitial fibrosis, with or without associated visceral pleural fibrosis (figs. 16-31–16-34) (11,12, 63). The interstitial fibrosis is patchy and accentuated in the subpleural regions. It resembles usual interstitial pneumonia, although the fibroblastic foci characteristic of the latter are not prominent. According to Craighead et al. (12), the minimal feature that allows a diagnosis of asbestosis is "discrete foci of fibrosis in the walls of respiratory bronchioles associated with accumulations of asbestos bodies." As mentioned below, some might consider this asbestos airway disease and as such, separate from asbestosis. For the histologic diagnosis of asbestosis one must find asbestos bodies in routine histologic sections in association with interstitial fibrosis. In most cases these are easily identified, but the presence of even a single asbestos body in a case of interstitial fibrosis in an individual with an appropriate exposure history is sufficient for a diagnosis of asbestosis (12). For cases clinically suspected of being asbestosis in which no asbestos bodies are identified, one can quantitate asbestos fibers (Table 16-4): there are rare cases of asbestosis that have heavy fiber burdens but an absence of identifiable asbestos bodies (11).

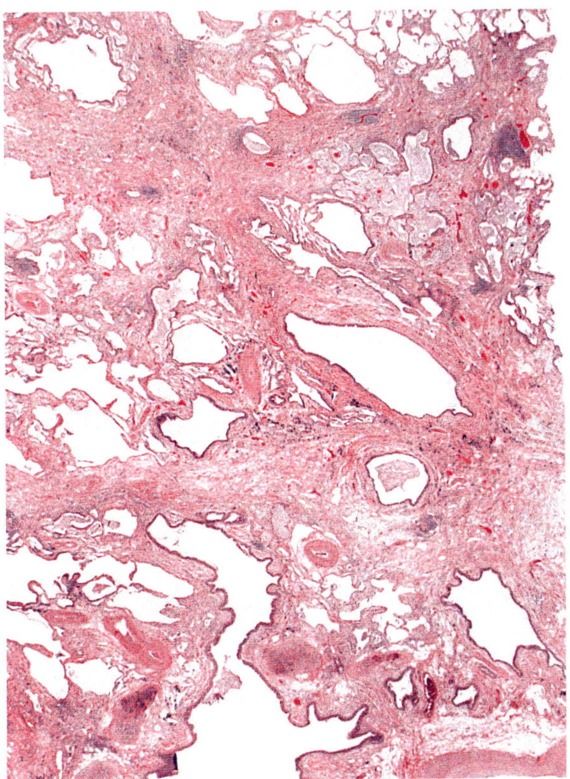
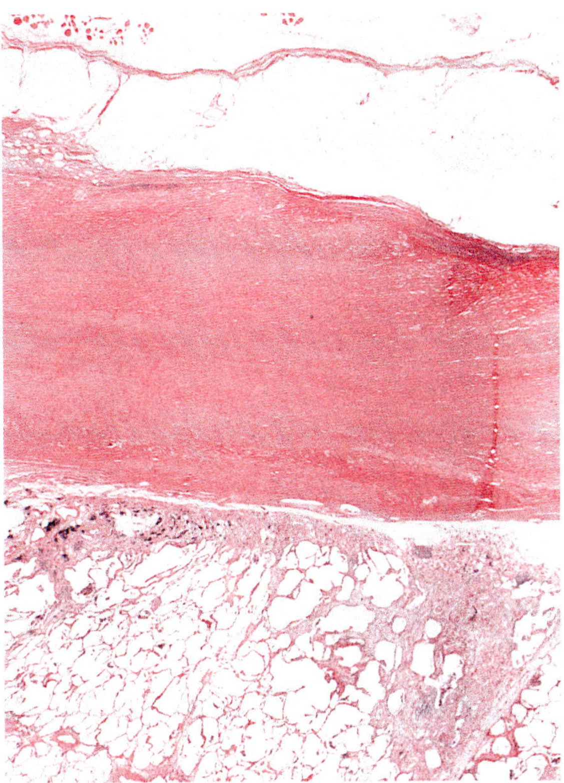

Figure 16-31

ASBESTOSIS

Left: There is fibrosis, honeycomb change, and architectural revision involving the lung tissue.
Right: In this case there is also marked visceral pleural fibrosis.

Changes associated with the fibrosis include metaplastic epithelium, mild chronic inflammatory infiltrate in the interstitium, and stasis of secretions in airspaces. The following are unusual in asbestosis: large honeycomb cysts, smooth muscle proliferation, lymphoid hyperplasia, large zones of increased alveolar macrophages, and sarcoid-like granulomas (57).

Asbestosis can be graded according to the scheme of Craighead et al. (12), shown in Table 16-6. The grading is designed for examination of autopsy material with extensive sampling. In practice, there is rarely sufficient tissue for full grading, and a designation of mild, moderate, or severe histologic asbestosis is practically expedient. The modifier "histologic" is added here since a full knowledge of the clinical, functional, and radiologic findings is not always available, and not all histologically identified changes translate into clinical or radiologic findings. For practical purposes, the simplified grading scheme suggested by Roggli (63) is useful and shown in Table 16-7.

Pathogenesis. The pathogenesis of asbestosis is not established. Current evidence suggests that lung injury is related to the physical properties of the asbestos fibers and mediated by reactive oxygen species, macrophage-derived cytokines, and growth factors (32).

Diagnosis. The histologic criteria for the identification of asbestosis are outlined above. While interstitial pneumonias unrelated to asbestos may occur in individuals with prior asbestos exposure (24), the finding of asbestos bodies in histologic sections of lung tissue in cases of diffuse interstitial fibrosis is sufficient for the pathologic diagnosis. In the absence of tissue evaluation, clinical and radiologic criteria have been suggested. According to the American Thoracic Society, the finding of an ILO category greater than 1/1 on chest radiographs, a decrease in diffusing capacity less than

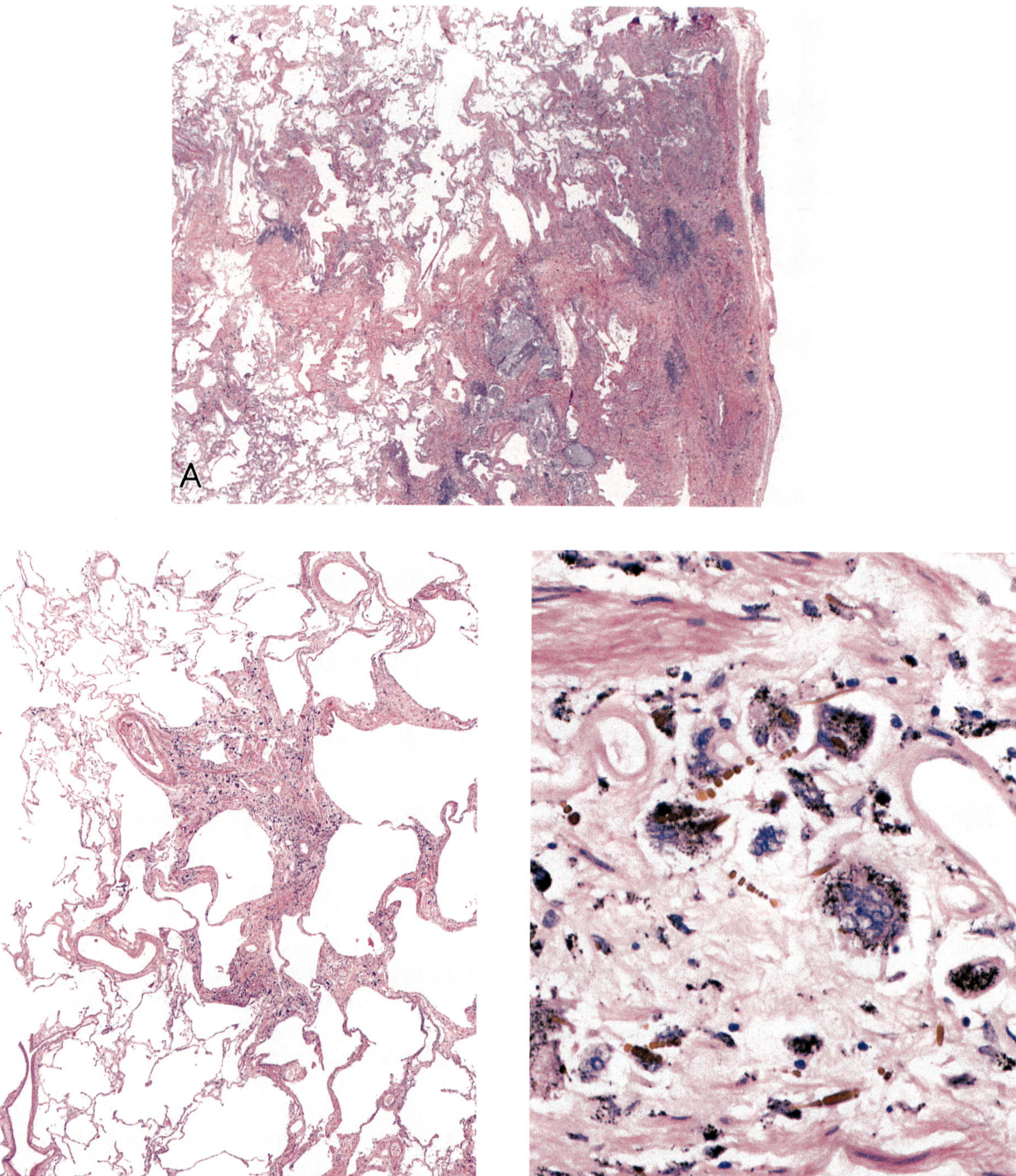

Figure 16-32

ASBESTOSIS

A: There is patchy fibrosis that is more severe in the subpleural zones.

B: In other regions there is fibrous thickening along respiratory bronchioles and alveolar ducts consistent with so-called asbestos airway disease.

C: Asbestos bodies are easily demonstrated.

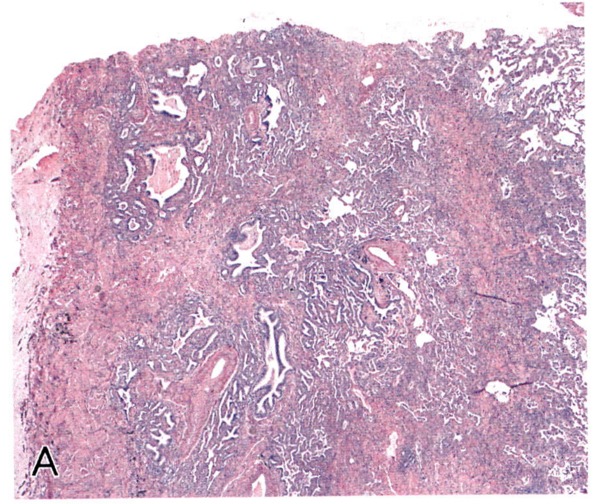

Figure 16-33

ASBESTOSIS

This case shows prominent associated visceral pleural fibrosis and fibrinous pleuritis (A). The underlying lung tissue shows interstitial inflammation and fibrosis (B), with asbestos bodies in the airspaces (C).

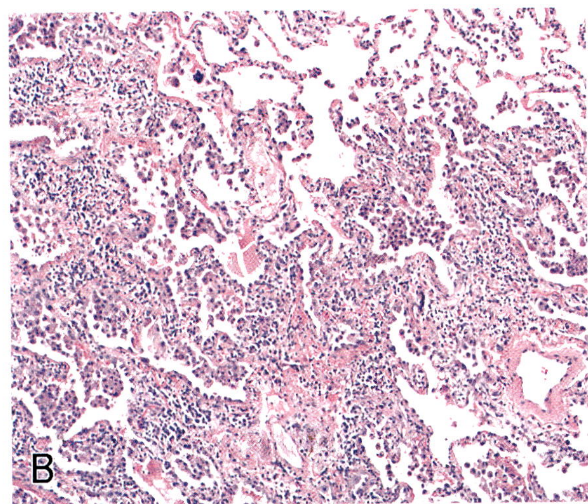

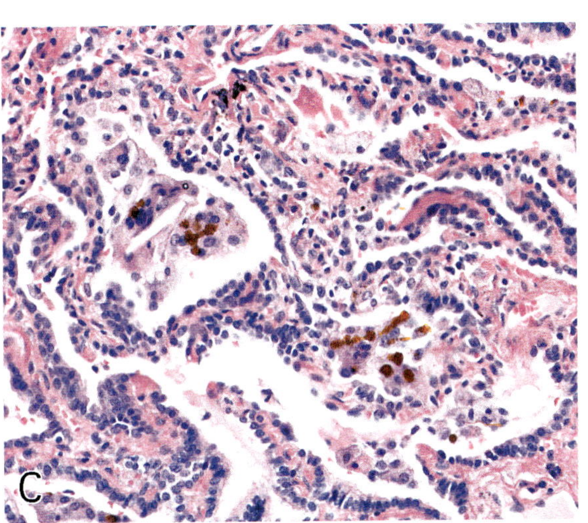

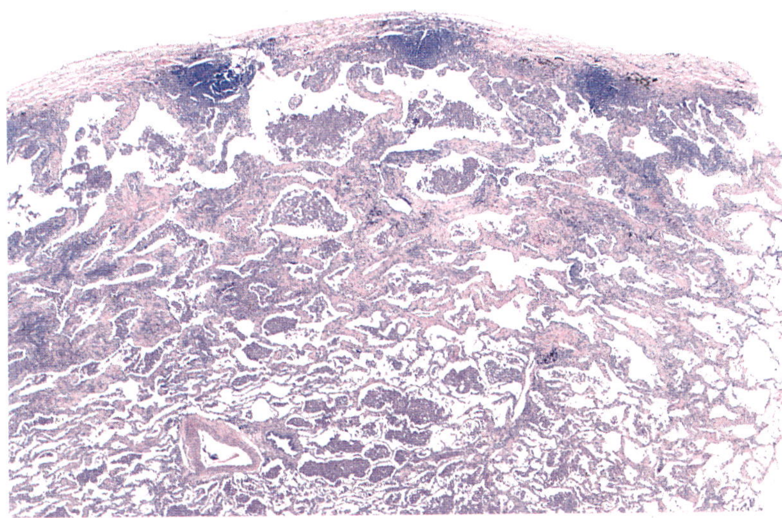

Figure 16-34

ASBESTOSIS

There is interstitial widening and prominent alveolar macrophages in the subpleural zones, resembling desquamative interstitial pneumonia.

Table 16-6

CRAIGHEAD'S HISTOLOGIC GRADING OF ASBESTOSIS[a]

Severity		Extent	
Grade 0:	No fibrosis	Grade A (1):	Only occasional bronchioles involved
Grade 1:	Fibrosis involving the wall of at least one respiratory bronchiole	Grade B (2):	More than occasional involvement present but less than half the bronchioles involved
Grade 2:	Fibrosis as in grade 1 plus involvement of alveolar ducts or two or more layers of adjacent alveoli	Grade C (3):	More than half of all bronchioles involved
Grade 3:	Fibrosis as in grade 2 but with coalescence of fibrosis such that all the alveoli between two adjacent bronchioles are involved		
Grade 4:	Fibrosis as in grade 3 but with the formation of abnormal airspaces (i.e., honeycombing)		

Explanation of scoring: The severity is multiplied by the extent for each slide, an average of the slides for each lobe is calculated, the total scores for all the lobes are added and divided by the number of lobes involved to reach a final grade of asbestosis.

[a]Modified from reference 12.

Table 16-7

ROGGLI'S HISTOLOGIC GRADING OF ASBESTOSIS[a]

Grade 0:	No appreciable peribronchiolar fibrosis or less than half of the bronchioles affected
Grade 1:	Fibrosis is confined to the walls of respiratory bronchioles with minimal alveolar involvement and involvement of more than half the bronchioles on the slide
Grade 2:	Extension of fibrosis to alveolar ducts and/or two or more tiers of adjacent alveoli, with some sparing of alveoli between bronchioles
Grade 3:	Fibrotic thickening of the walls of all the alveoli between at least two adjacent respiratory bronchioles
Grade 4:	Honeycomb change (includes microscopic honeycombing)

[a]Modified from reference 63.

the lower limit of normal, and a history of exposure are sufficient for a clinical diagnosis (5). In disputed cases or cases in which the diagnosis is in doubt, quantitative tissue analysis may be helpful and the reader is referred to the large amount of literature on this topic (11,63).

Treatment and Prognosis. There is no specific treatment for asbestosis. The disease may progress more slowly with early withdrawal from exposure, but it may still progress even though exposure has ceased (76). Risk factors for progression of asbestos-induced fibrosis include cumulative asbestos exposure, duration of exposure, and fiber type (crocidolite exposure is associated with the most frequent progression). Progression, as determined by changes in the chest roentgenogram or pulmonary function studies, occurs in up to 30 percent of individuals with asbestosis and about one fifth die as a result of it (32).

Asbestos Airway Disease

Definition. Asbestos airway disease is the fibrosis and thickening of bronchioles and alveolar ducts associated with asbestos inhalation (11,80). Although the concept of asbestos airway disease has not been universally accepted, the histologic findings are similar to those seen with a variety of inhaled dusts and the concept is appealing. Whether or not asbestos-induced

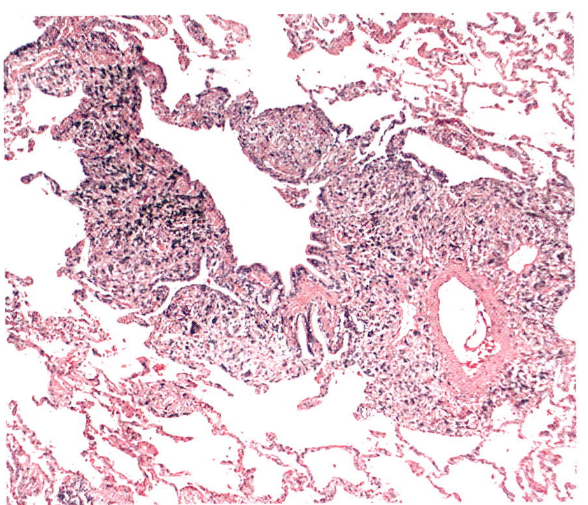

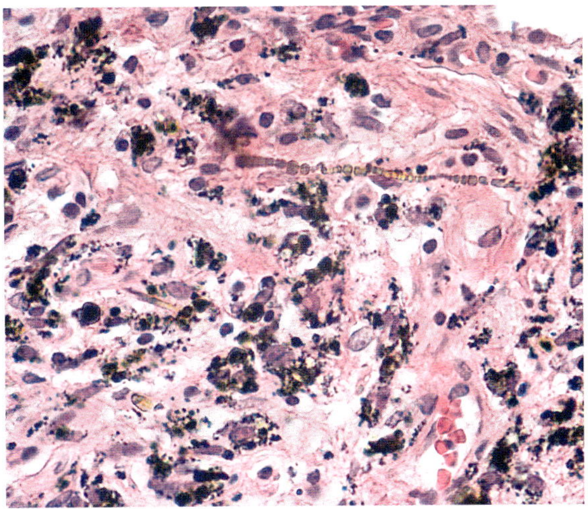

Figure 16-35

ASBESTOS AIRWAY DISEASE

Left: Asbestos airway disease with dust-laden macrophages along a distal bronchiole.
Right: Asbestos bodies are readily identified within the dust-laden macrophages (upper center).

airway fibrosis is a precursor to asbestosis (63), as described above, is controversial and not universally agreed upon.

Clinical Features. Clinical findings are not well documented. Minor abnormalities in the functioning of the small airways (e.g., obstruction) may be noted.

Radiologic Findings. Peribronchiolar fibrosis results in subpleural, dot-like or small, branching linear opacities that are evident on HRCT (4). These opacities are present in patients with normal radiographs (4). Serial HRCT scans have shown these opacities to progress to subpleural fibrosis (4).

Pathologic Findings. Respiratory bronchioles and alveolar ducts show mural thickening, fibrosis with a scant inflammatory infiltrate, and scattered to numerous asbestos bodies (fig. 16-35) (11,80). The fibrosis tends to be mature and well collagenized, and is associated with dust-filled macrophages in addition to asbestos bodies. Evidence of other dust exposures may be apparent (fig. 16-36). There is some resemblance to the changes associated with cigarette smoking (and affected individuals may also be cigarette smokers) but the amount of fibrosis is more than that seen with cigarette smoking alone. Furthermore, the fibrosis with cigarette smoking is more prominent in membranous and respiratory bronchioles, whereas the fibrosis associated with asbestos airway disease preferentially involves alveolar ducts and respiratory bronchioles, particularly the former.

Benign Asbestos Pleural Effusion (Benign Asbestos Pleurisy)

Definition. Benign asbestos pleural effusion is defined by four criteria (11,27,63): a history of asbestos exposure, radiologic or thoracentesis confirmation of pleural effusion, absence of another disease that could cause the pleural effusion, and no malignant tumor developing within 3 years.

Clinical Features. Benign asbestos effusions are rare (less than 3 percent of workers followed serially) and usually encountered within 10 years of the first exposure to asbestos (11,57). However, in one review (27), the mean latency period was 30 years, with a range of 1 to 58 years. Most patients are asymptomatic. Some have pleuritic chest pain, fever, cough, or dyspnea. The effusions are hemorrhagic in about half the cases; eosinophils are prominent in one fourth of cases. Biochemically, the exudate is fluid with a normal glucose level.

Radiologic Findings. There is a pleural effusion that is usually unilateral.

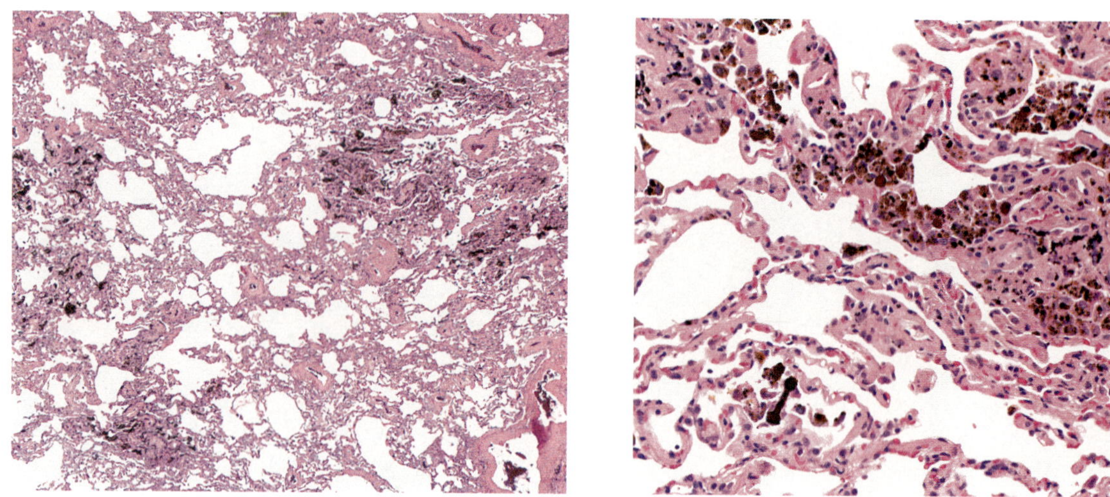

Figure 16-36

ASBESTOS AIRWAY DISEASE WITH SIDEROSIS IN A WELDER

Left: There is dust deposition and mural fibrosis involving alveolar ducts.

Right: Dust-laden macrophages are apparent and a few asbestos bodies are identified (lower left). Much of the hemosiderosis represents welder's siderosis.

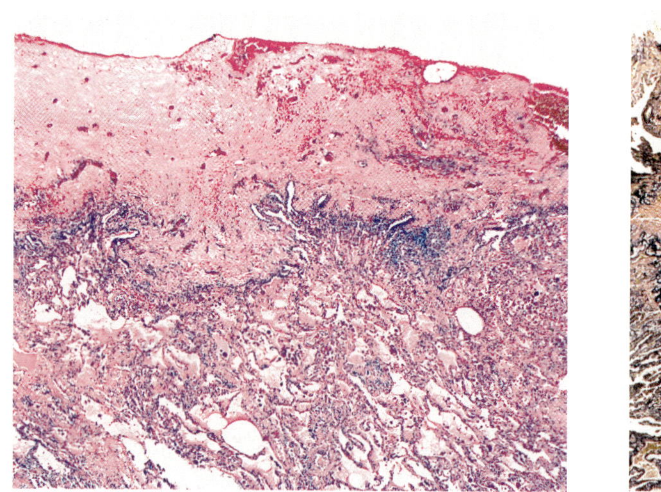

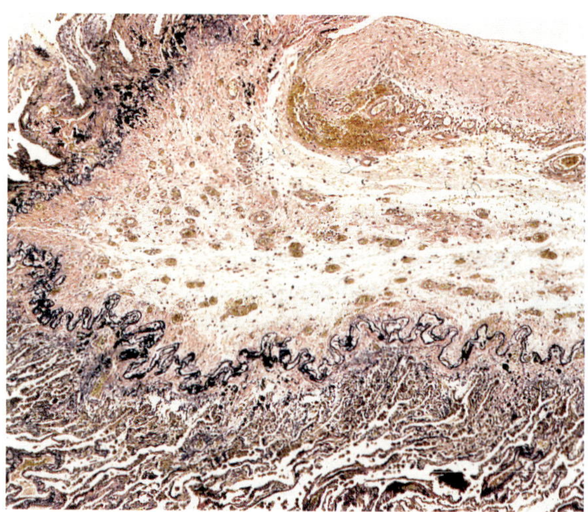

Figure 16-37

PLEURA IN BENIGN ASBESTOS EFFUSION

Left: There is visceral pleural fibrosis with an overlying hemorrhagic organizing pleuritis.

Right: A more chronic case shows some pleural scarring and retraction highlighted by elastic tissue staining.

Pathologic Findings. The pathologic findings are nonspecific (11,63). There is an organizing fibrinous or hemorrhagic pleuritis associated with varying degrees of pleural fibrosis (fig. 16-37). Coexisting hyaline plaques, visceral pleural fibrosis, or rounded atelectasis may be found.

Pathogenesis. The pathogenesis of asbestos pleural disease is unknown. Benign asbestos effusion may be seen after lower levels of exposure than typically associated with asbestosis.

Treatment and Prognosis. Most effusions resolve spontaneously over weeks to months.

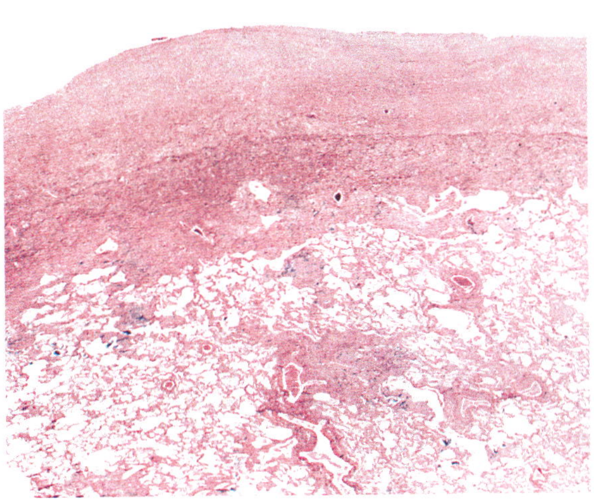

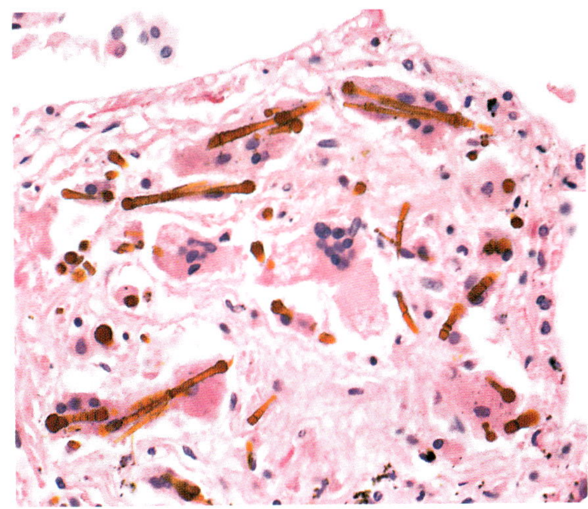

Figure 16-38

VISCERAL PLEURAL FIBROSIS ASSOCIATED WITH ASBESTOS EXPOSURE

Left: There is marked visceral pleural fibrosis.

Right: The underlying parenchyma shows patchy interstitial fibrosis and numerous asbestos bodies, indicative of associated asbestosis.

Recurrences develop in up to one third of patients (27). They may leave a residue of visceral pleural fibrosis (see below). Follow-up is recommended to rule out mesothelioma.

Visceral Pleural Fibrosis

Definition. Visceral pleural fibrosis, usually diffuse and bilateral, results from asbestos exposure (11,57,63,72).

Clinical Features. In individuals heavily exposed to asbestos who have been followed for more than 15 years, approximately 20 percent have diffuse visceral pleural fibrosis (57). The clinical findings in asbestos-induced pleural fibrosis depend on the extent and severity of scarring (11,72). Most patients are asymptomatic. Those with severe visceral pleural fibrosis may have signs and symptoms of restrictive lung disease. Some patients have a history of prior benign asbestos effusion or pleurisy (65).

Radiologic Findings. The radiologic findings depend on the severity of the process. In mild cases, chest radiolographic abnormalities may not be apparent. In severe cases, visceral pleural thickening may be identifiable and associated with small lung volumes. The fibrosis may be unilateral or bilateral. CT scanning usually shows visceral pleural thickening and associated parietal pleural plaques.

Pathologic Findings. The pathologic findings are nonspecific. There are varying degrees of visceral pleural thickening by fibrous tissue with relatively little inflammatory infiltrate (fig. 16-38). Some overlying remnants of pleural fibrinous pleuritis may be apparent. The fibrosis may extend a short distance into the lung as interstitial tendrils. Parenchymal changes of asbestosis may or may not be present. In some cases, the dense basket-weave collagenization typical of hyaline pleural plaques (see below) is seen. Surface adhesions may be present.

Pathogenesis. The pathogenesis of visceral pleural fibrosis is unknown (11,72).

Diagnosis. The diagnosis is based on clinical and radiologic findings as well as the histologic features described in patients with well-documented asbestos exposure. In contrast to desmoplastic malignant mesothelioma, visceral pleural fibrosis tends to be relatively acellular and to lack a storiform pattern (11). When active pleuritis is present, there is zonation from the cellular zones of active pleuritis to the underlying acellular fibrotic zones. Unlike desmoplastic mesothelioma, visceral pleural fibrosis does not invade the underlying parenchyma and lacks independent expansile cellular nodules. This issue is also addressed in chapter 18.

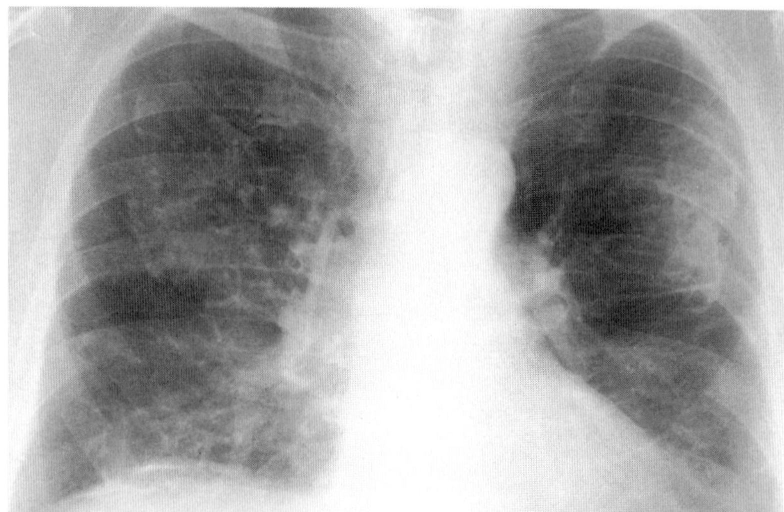

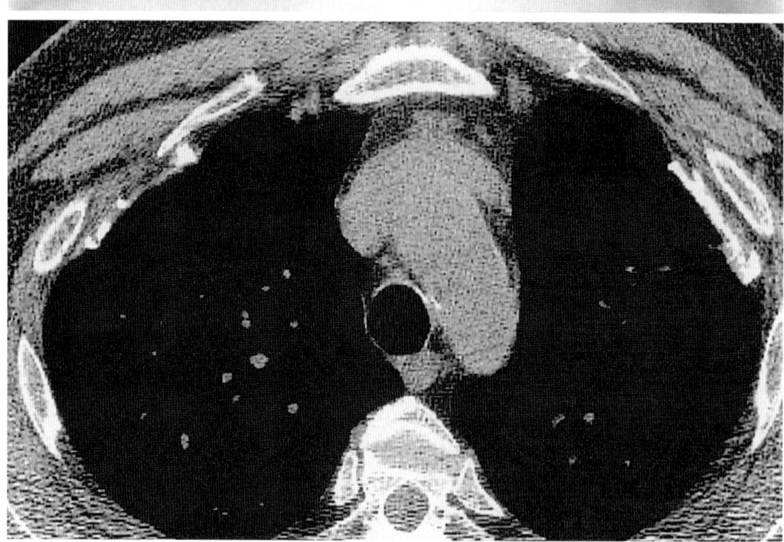

Figure 16-39

ASBESTOS-RELATED PLEURAL PLAQUES

Top: PA chest radiograph shows bilateral calcified pleural plaques.

Bottom: HRCT demonstrates calcified pleural plaques in the anterolateral aspect of the right and left chest. The patient was a 72-year-old man who had worked for several years in a shipyard.

Prognosis. The process may be slowly progressive. Morbidity is related to the extent of pleural scarring.

Hyaline Parietal Pleural Plaques

Definition. Hyaline pleural plaques are localized plaques of dense fibrous tissue that tend to occur on the posterior inferior parietal pleura and surface of the diaphragm (11,12,57,63). They are usually bilateral, though not necessarily symmetrical.

While characteristic and distinctive, hyaline parietal pleural plaques are not unique to individuals with asbestos exposure and may be the result of other exposures or the residue of healed inflammatory processes (11,57). However, when bilateral and symmetrical, they are virtually always related to exposure to fibrous minerals, most often asbestos.

Clinical Features. Plaques by themselves are asymptomatic and most cases are incidental findings at the time of radiologic studies, surgery, or autopsy (11,57).

Radiologic Findings. Hyaline pleural plaques are identified radiologically as focal areas of pleural thickening in the lower half of the thorax. They may be smooth or nodular and are seen most commonly on the posterolateral chest wall between the seventh and tenth ribs, and on the domes of the diaphragm. Calcification may be apparent (fig. 16-39). It should be noted that the chest radiograph has a low sensitivity for the detection of pleural plaques: plaques are evident on the radiograph

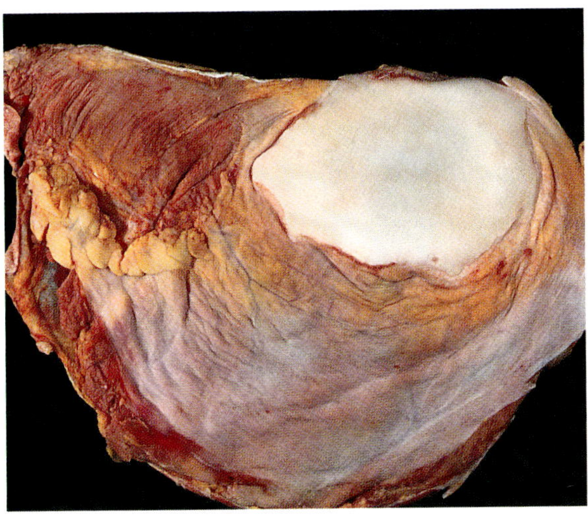

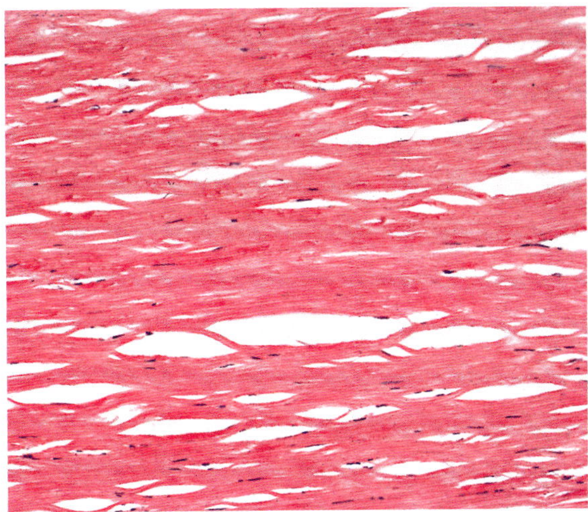

Figure 16-40

HYALINE PLEURAL PLAQUE

Left: This diaphragmatic plaque is well circumscribed, densely fibrous, and covered by a shiny mesothelial surface. Right: Histology shows dense, relatively acellular, "basket weave" collagen.

in fewer than 50 percent of cases in which they are demonstrable at autopsy (22). HRCT has a greater sensitivity and specificity than chest radiography for their detection (70).

Pathologic Findings. Hyaline pleural plaques are very firm, discrete elevations of the pleura that have a shiny surface (fig. 16-40); some are associated with adhesions to the adjacent lung (11,12,57,63). Plaques are irregular in shape and may attain diameters of 12 to 15 cm. Calcification may be apparent grossly. Small lesions have been likened to drippings of candle wax (63). The pericardium or peritoneum may be affected (63).

Histologically, plaques are composed of dense acellular collagen with a basket-weave pattern (fig. 16-40). There may be some fibroblastic proliferation and chronic inflammation around the edges of the plaque, but the center is paucicellular.

Pathogenesis. The pathogenesis of asbestos-related hyaline pleural plaques is unknown. Plaques are induced by much lower levels of exposure to asbestos than is asbestosis (11).

Diagnosis. The radiologic and gross features are diagnostic.

Prognosis. Hyaline pleural plaques by themselves are asymptomatic and in and of themselves are associated with little morbidity. Another asbestos-related disease may eventually develop (65).

Rounded Atelectasis

Definition. Rounded atelectasis is a focal, pleural-based lesion that is the result of pleural and subpleural scarring and atelectasis of the adjacent lung tissue (fig. 16-41) (11,28,63).

Clinical Features. Most patients with rounded atelectasis are asymptomatic and the lesion is an incidental radiologic finding. There may be other asbestos-related pleural changes. Rarely, the lesions are multiple and bilateral (28). Rounded atelectasis may be resected to exclude the possibility of a neoplasm.

Radiologic Findings. The characteristic radiologic manifestation of rounded atelectasis is a round or oval, pleural-based nodule or mass-like opacity, with pulmonary vessels and bronchi curving into it, giving an appearance that resembles a comet tail (43). The nodule or mass-like opacity typically abuts an area of pleural thickening or pleural effusion and is associated with volume loss. Rounded atelectasis may occur anywhere in the lungs but is found most commonly in the dorsal surface of the lower lobes. In a review of 174 cases, Hillerdal (28) found that rounded atelectasis was distributed as follows: upper lobes, 6 percent; middle lobe/lingula, 39 percent; and lower lobes, 55 percent.

Pathologic Findings. Rounded atelectasis is a pleural-based mass, 2 to 7 cm in diameter

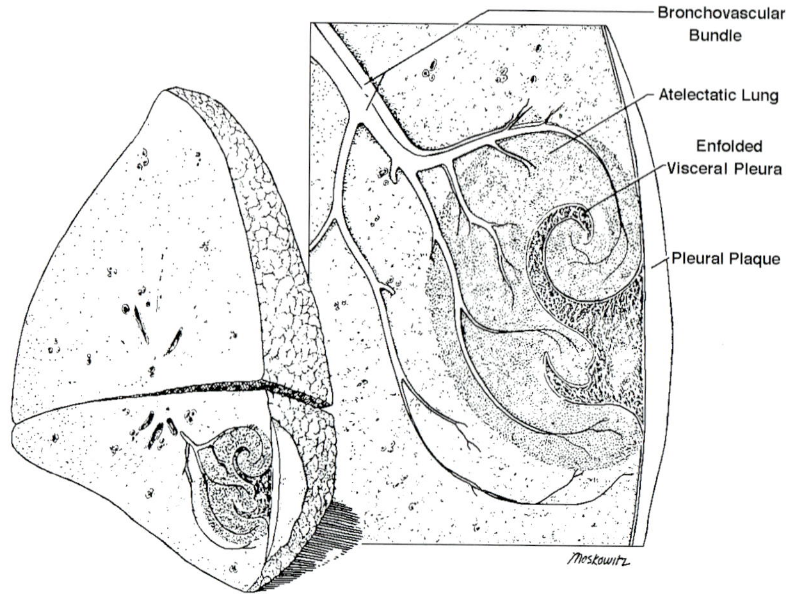

Figure 16-41

ROUNDED ATELECTASIS

Schematic drawing showing proposed pathogenesis of the lesion. The fibrotic pleura of a lower lobe enfolds in a spiral manner, entrapping and collapsing subjacent lung. The folding of the lung gives a curvilinear configuration to bronchovascular structures feeding the entrapped parenchyma ("comet's tail sign"). (Fig. 4 from Mark EJ. Case records of the Massachusetts General Hospital. Case 24-1983. N Eng J Med 1983;308:1469.)

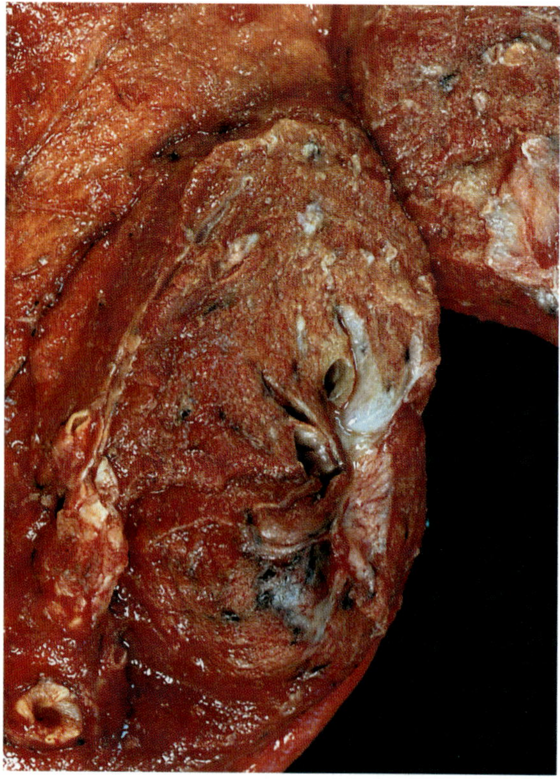

Figure 16-42

ROUNDED ATELECTASIS

Grossly, there is a zone of pleural scarring and retraction associated with atelectasis of the underlying lung tissue, producing a mass-like lesion.

(fig. 16-42) (63). In some cases bands of fibrosis can be seen emanating from the pleura along septa. Typically, when a lesion is resected and dissected by the pathologist, the "mass" seems to disappear. Histologically, there is marked pleural and septal fibrosis, with associated atelectasis of the adjacent lung tissue (fig. 16-43) (11,63). Lymphoid follicles and chronic inflammation may be present. Overlying active pleuritis may be identified.

Pathogenesis. Rounded atelectasis may be the residue of a healed pleural effusion with relatively localized pleural scarring that contracts and produces the radiologically apparent lesion. While it is known to occur in association with asbestos, it can occur with pleural fibrosis due to any cause.

Diagnosis and Prognosis. Cases diagnosed on the basis of typical radiologic findings (and negative bronchoscopy) may be followed prospectively without surgery (28). Most lesions recognized pathologically are entirely resected (to exclude a neoplasm) and recurrences are not a problem, or they are incidental findings in resection or autopsy material. For the most part, rounded atelectasis shows little change at follow-up; some increase in fibrosis may be noted, as well as other pleural or parenchymal asbestos-related lesions (28).

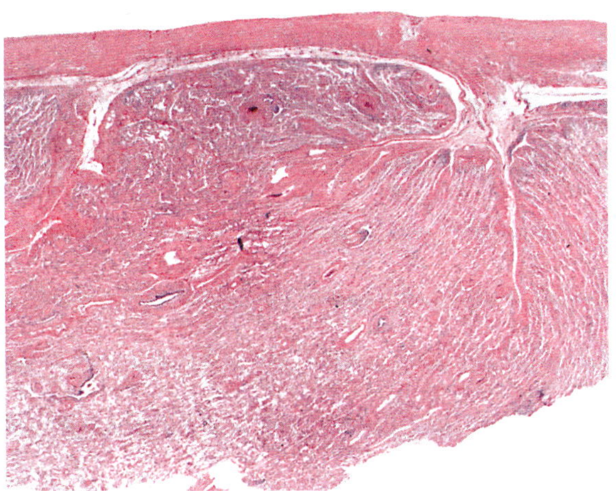

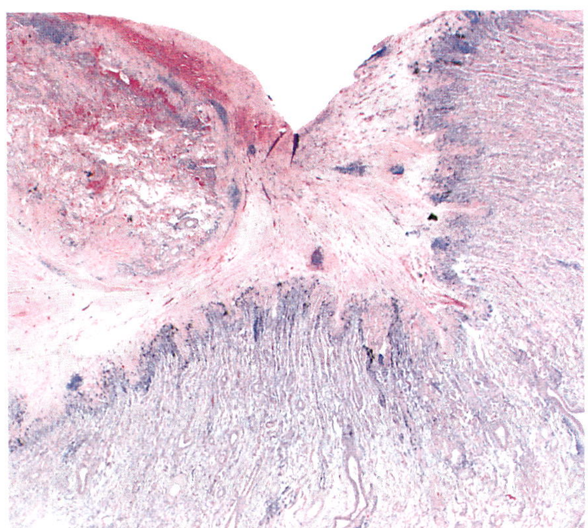

Figure 16-43

ROUNDED ATELECTASIS

Pleural fibrosis is associated with traction on the underlying lung parenchyma and associated atelectasis.

Overlap Among Non-Neoplastic Asbestos-Related Diseases of the Lung and Pleura

The above categories of non-neoplastic disorders caused by asbestos are conceptually convenient but in practice there is considerable overlap among them (63). For example, patients with severe visceral pleural fibrosis may have concomitant parietal pleural fibrosis that resembles hyaline pleural plaque (72). Patients with benign asbestos effusion may have coexisting recognizable or developing rounded atelectasis. Patients with asbestosis typically have a variable degree of pleural thickening, and accompanying hyaline pleural plaques are common. In established asbestosis, there may be zones of less affected lung tissue that show features of asbestos airways disease.

The benign asbestos-related pleural diseases are the most common clinically and pathologically recognized abnormalities associated with asbestos exposure.

SILICATOSES

Definition. The silicatoses are pneumoconioses associated with the inhalation of nonasbestos silicates (11).

Mineralogy and Exposure. Silicates are minerals formed when silicon dioxide combines with one or more cations, usually magnesium, calcium, and aluminum (11). Silicates make up about one third of all the minerals and a substantial portion of the earth's crust. They comprise the most common mineral species identified in human lung tissue. The nonasbestos silicates are grouped together because they share common clinical and pathologic features, and are divided into the following groups (11): sheet silicates: talc, mica, vermiculite, kaolin, fuller's earth, sepiolite, attapulgite; framework silicates: feldspars, zeolites; chain silicates: wollastonite; and orthosilicates: mullite.

The sheet silicates are usually implicated in pulmonary disease (11). As a group, the nonasbestos silicates are strongly birefringent particulates, recognized as plate-like in the case of sheet silicates; their birefringence is much brighter than that of silica. Particles that reach the alveoli and are deposited in lung tissue are usually between 1 and 5 µm in diameter. A few silicate particles are common incidental findings associated with anthracotic pigment in otherwise normal adult lungs. Silicates may become ferruginated, resulting in ferruginous bodies that differ from asbestos bodies by having a different central core and shape. Asbestos bodies have a straight, thin, lucent core in contrast to ferruginous bodies with cores of nonasbestos silicates, which are broad, plate-like, shorter, and more irregular in shape (see fig. 16-26).

Table 16-8

SILICATES MOST COMMONLY IMPLICATED AS CAUSES OF DISEASE[a]

Kaolin:	Used in the manufacture of pharmaceuticals, ceramics, plastic, rubber, and paper
Talc:	Used in the production of ceramics, paper, paints, refractories, building materials, rubber, insecticides, plastics, cosmetics, pharmaceuticals, and confectionery
Mica:	Used primarily in thermal and electrical insulation; building products; as a filler in adhesives, cements, textured paints, mastics, enamels, and asphalts; in oil-well drilling; and in lubrication of molds
Fuller's Earth:	Used in industries because of its absorbent properties

[a]Data from reference 11.

Recognizing diseases caused by nonasbestos silicates has been controversial since exposure usually includes variable amounts of silica and asbestos (57). Nevertheless, there are well-documented cases and the existence of pneumoconioses caused by nonasbestos silicates is accepted (11,14,25,26,37,46,57,75,77). For the most part, these are clinically mild disorders that are the result of exposure to high concentrations of dust over long periods of time, with only a small percentage of exposed individuals developing significant disease. The silicates most commonly implicated as causes of disease are shown in Table 16-8.

Clinical Features. The majority of patients with silicatosis are asymptomatic but have abnormal radiographs (see below) (11,14,25,26,37, 46,57,75,77). Those with more severe disease have signs and symptoms of interstitial lung disease. The latency period between exposure and development of disease may be many years; with heavy exposures this period is shorter. Pulmonary function may be normal despite extensive nodular opacities radiologically (e.g., talcosis).

Radiologic Findings. The radiographic findings of talc and mica pneumoconiosis are usually similar to those of asbestos exposure (22). The most common radiographic abnormality is the presence of pleural plaques. The parenchymal abnormalities usually consist of a reticular pattern of fibrosis involving mainly the lower lung zones. The radiologic manifestations of Fuller's earth and kaolin exposure resemble those of silicosis and consist of numerous small nodular opacities that can occasionally conglomerate into large opacities (progressive massive fibrosis) (22).

Pathologic Findings. The pathologic findings in the silicatoses can be grouped as follows (11). *Macules* with dust and dust-laden macrophages and relatively little associated fibrosis involve the respiratory bronchioles and alveolar ducts. *Mineral dust airway disease* is similar to macules, but with a greater degree of fibrosis involving the walls of membranous respiratory bronchioles and alveolar ducts; distortion of the airway lumen is often present. *Granulomatous reaction,* a feature that separates patients with the nonasbestos silicates from those with most other pneumoconioses, has been described with exposure to talc (fig. 16-44), mullite, kaolin, and feldspars.

Nodules are the most common lesion described in silicate pneumoconioses. They measure from 2 to 10 mm in diameter and are gray, brown, blue, or black depending on the dust that is present. The nodules show a predilection for the upper and middle lung zones. Some nodules have a disorganized collagenous center and a stellate periphery similar to the "Medusa head" nodules of mixed dust pneumoconiosis. The degree of hyalinization in the center correlates with the amount of silica present. Other nodules consist of masses of dust particles with associated fibrosis and intermingled giant cells (granulomatous nodules). These are distinct and separable from nodules associated with mixed dust pneumoconiosis and they lack the well-hyalinized center of a silicotic nodule.

Progressive massive fibrosis (complicated silicate pneumoconiosis) has been reported with exposures to talc, kaolin, mica, feldspars, and other silicates (fig. 16-45). Progressive massive fibrosis is due to the coalescence of multiple small and large nodules; the fibrosis tends to be sharply defined, bilateral, and may replace an entire lobe. Mid- or upper lung zones are preferentially involved. Histologically, there are innumerable refractory particles and macrophages with intermixed collagen.

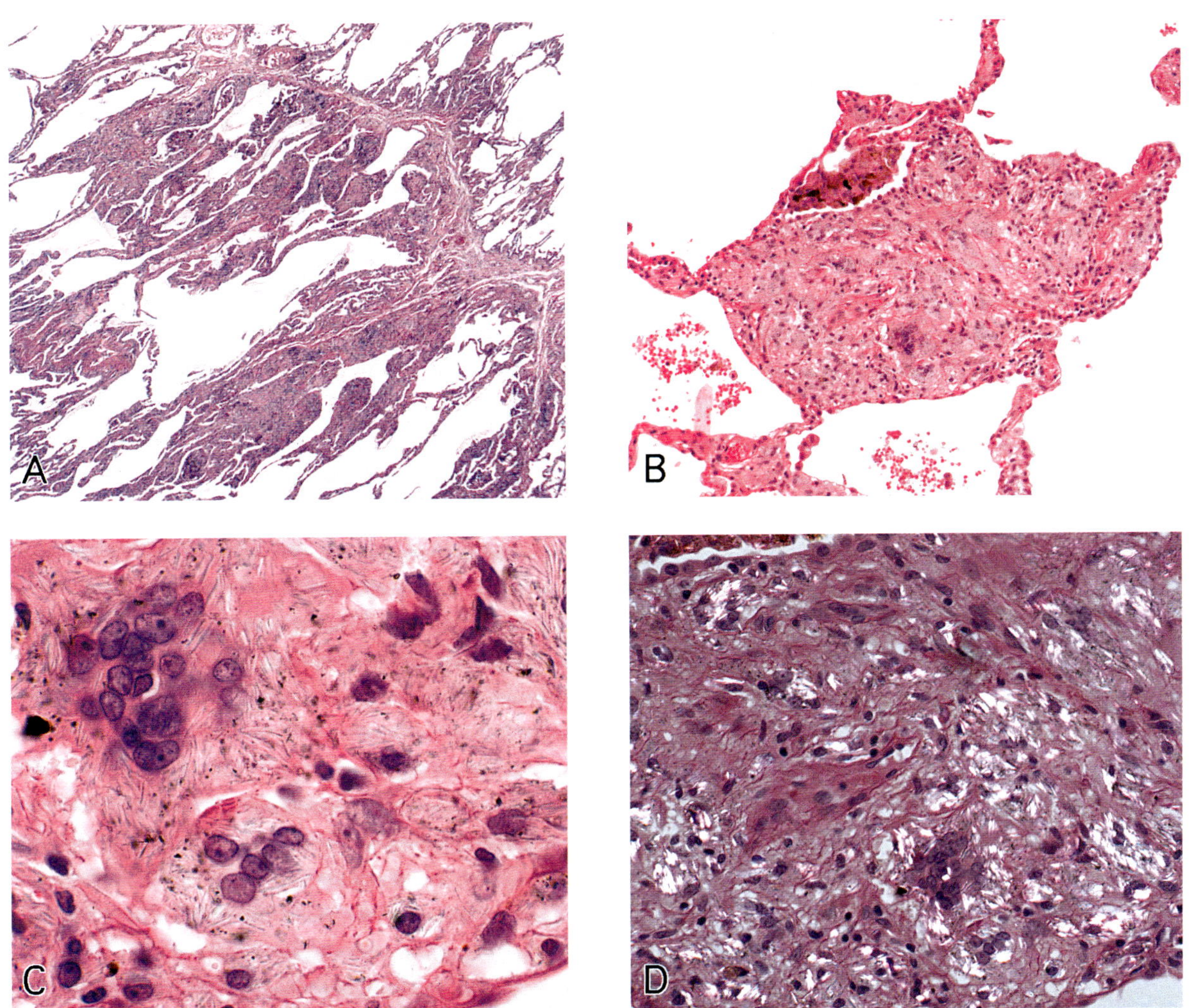

Figure 16-44

INHALATION TALCOSIS

There are nodular aggregates of histiocytes (A,B), with giant cells that resemble granulomas (B,C). Polarization shows large amounts of brightly birefringent plate-like talc (D).

Diffuse interstitial fibrosis has been reported with exposure to most of the nonasbestos silicates. Two forms can be identified: in one, nodules are linked with fibrosis, and in the other, nodules are scanty or absent and the process bears some resemblance to usual interstitial pneumonia with lower zonal fibrosis and honeycombing. Microscopically, there are numerous refractile particles and occasional giant cells in addition to the widespread fibrosis. In one series, a subset of patients with presumed idiopathic pulmonary fibrosis was found to have unrecognized exposure to silicates which were implicated as causative (45).

Pleural fibrosis and thickening have been described in a number of patients exposed to silicates.

Pathogenesis. In many of the silicatoses, contamination of dust with asbestos or silica has been implicated as a cause of the fibrosis (57). Talc causes a foreign body reaction. While most of the nonasbestos silicates are relatively nonfibrogenic, high levels of exposure may be associated with disease, either on the basis of the density of the infiltrates of dust-laden macrophages, the low level of associated fibrosis, or both.

Diagnosis. An appropriate exposure and compatible radiologic or pathologic findings

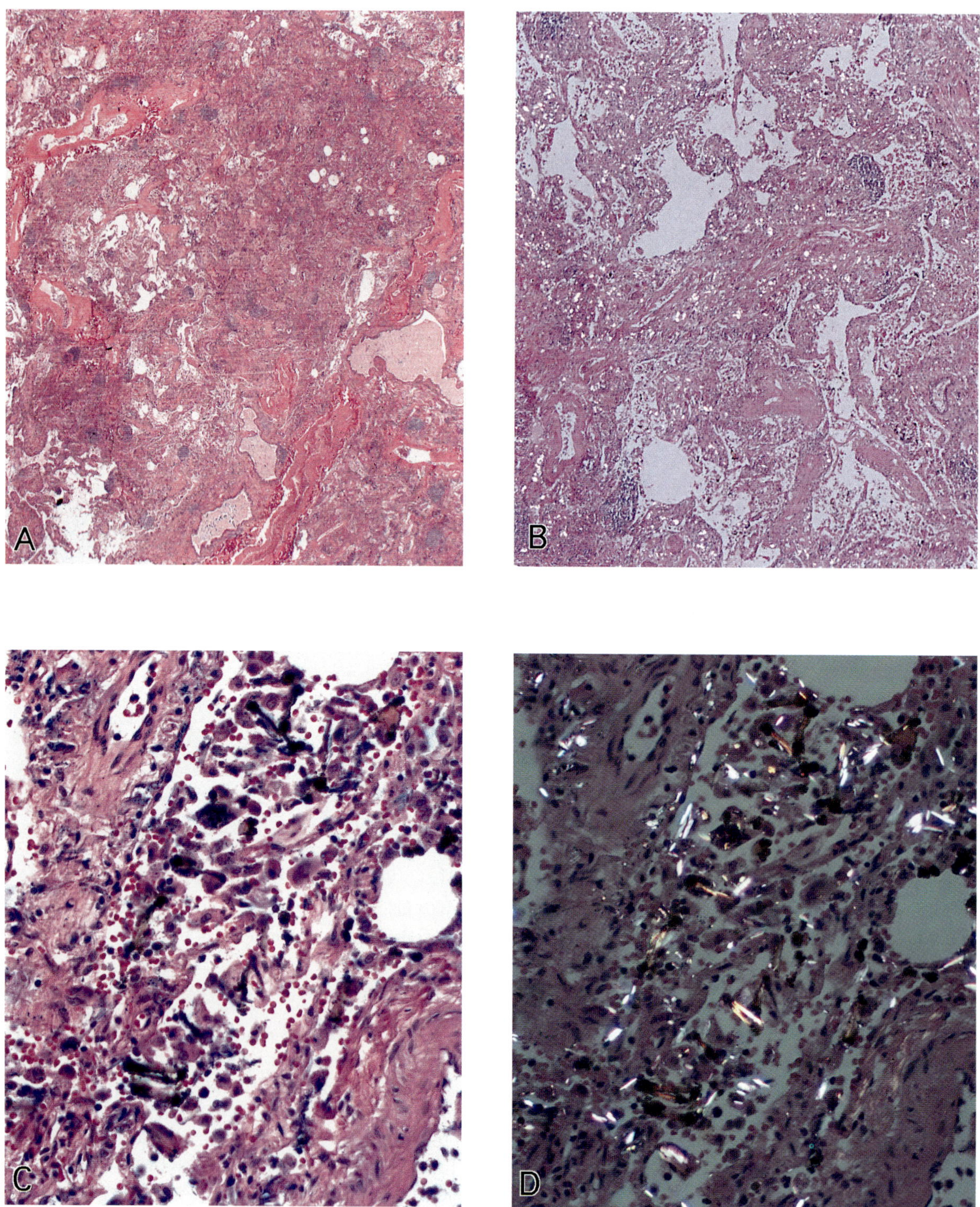

Figure 16-45

PROGRESSIVE MASSIVE FIBROSIS FROM INHALED TALC

There is marked fibrosis and destruction of lung architecture (A,B). Polarization of the field in B shows large amounts of brightly birefringent talc (C). Detail shows an increase in alveolar macrophages as well as irregular ferruginous bodies that lack features of asbestos bodies (D). Polarization of the field in D shows large amounts of bright birefringent talc.

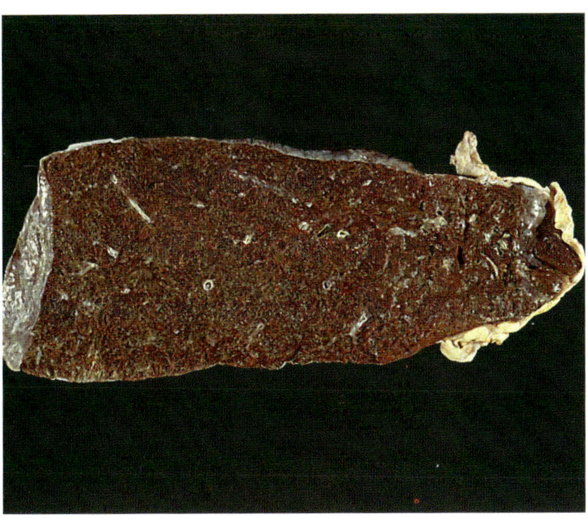

Figure 16-46

PULMONARY SIDEROSIS

This gross photograph of the lung of a hematite miner shows deep brown pigmentation.

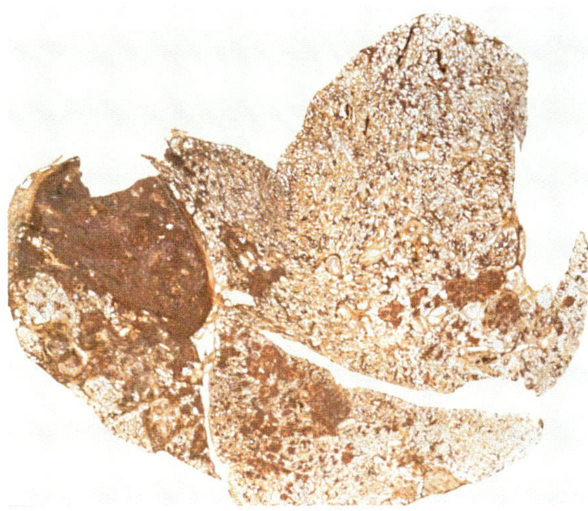

Figure 16-47

PULMONARY SIDEROSIS

This Gough section of lung from a hematite miner shows large zones of brownish consolidation. (Courtesy of the Gordon Museum in London, England.)

allow a diagnosis of silicatosis. The relative frequency of mixed dust exposure leads to a frequent incidence of mixed dust pneumoconiosis. In such cases one should look for the predominant pathologic pattern: macules and dust-filled macrophages along lymphatic routesare seen in relatively pure silicatoses, fibrous nodule formation (including classic silicotic nodules) in cases with appreciable amounts of silica exposure, and more diffuse fibrosis similar to that seen in asbestosis when appreciable amounts of asbestos fibers are present.

Treatment and Prognosis. In most cases the disease progresses slowly and many patients enjoy a normal lifespan (57). Morbidity and mortality are increased in the small percentage of cases that are associated with progressive massive fibrosis. There is no known treatment although the foreign body granulomas of talc exposure may show some response to steroids.

PULMONARY SIDEROSIS

Definition. Pulmonary siderosis is the deposition of iron or iron oxides in the lung following inhalation exposure. The iron is recognized in its ferruginated state (see below).

Mineralogy and Exposure. Among occupational exposures in general, exposure to iron is very common. It occurs in mining (hematite, magnetite, limonite, siderite, and emery), steel mills, foundries, boiler scaling, welding, and in the grinding, polishing, and refining of metal alloys (11,57,66). In many of these situations, there is also exposure to other particulates, especially silica. Siderosis in the background of a mixed dust pneumoconiosis is relatively common.

Clinical Features. Pure exposure to iron is rarely associated with clinically significant disease unless other (more fibrogenic) dusts are also present, such as silica. Individuals with very high levels of inhaled iron may show some abnormalities in small airway function and evidence of emphysema.

Radiologic Findings. The radiologic manifestations of siderosis consist of diffuse or predominantly upper lobe micronodules and a reticulonodular pattern (22).

Pathologic Findings. Grossly, macular lesions are red, reddish brown, gray, or black, and centrilobular (figs. 16-46, 16-47) (11,57). Histologically there is: 1) the presence of macules with iron-filled macrophages involving respiratory bronchioles and alveolar ducts; 2) mineral dust airways disease with dust and macrophages associated with fibrosis of alveolar ducts; or 3) nodular fibrosis (fig. 16-48) (11). Focal emphysema may be identified. Siderosis shows a strong

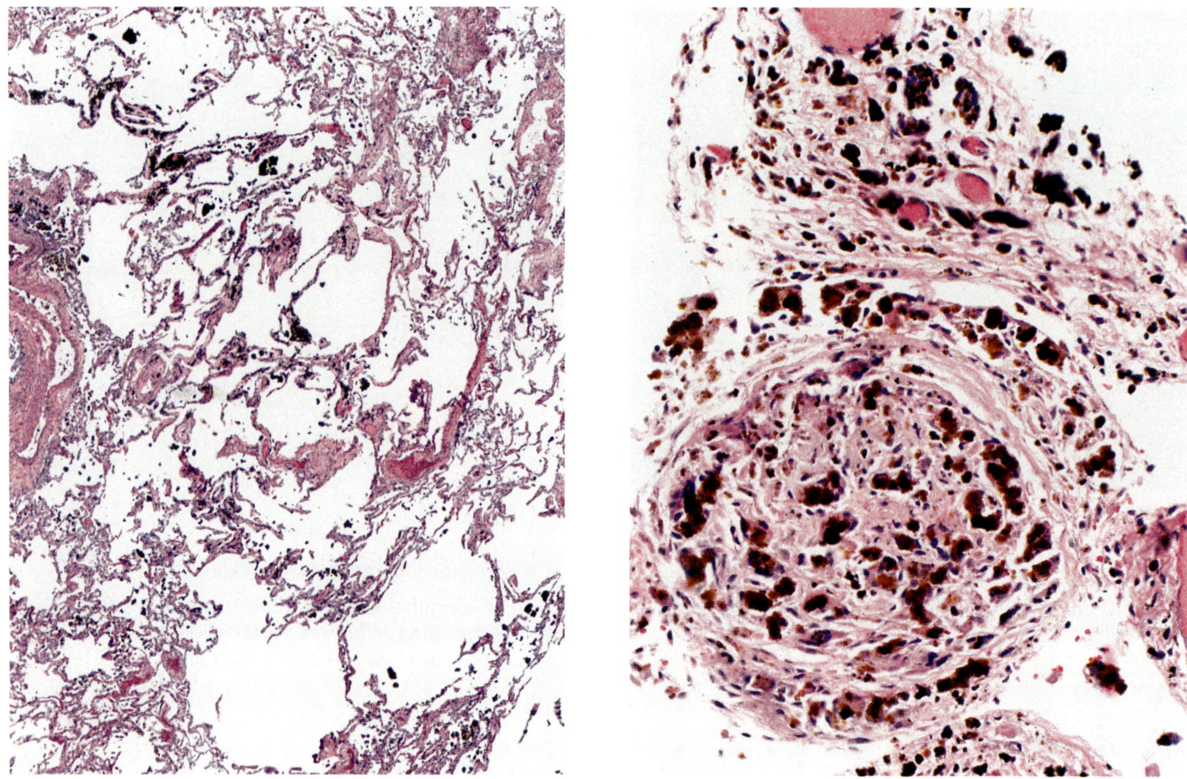

Figure 16-48

PULMONARY SIDEROSIS DUE TO WELDING

Left: There is a centrilobular infiltrate of dust-filled macrophages associated with centriacinar emphysema (dust macule). Right: Detail shows numerous macrophages with iron oxides/welder's pigment.

reaction to the Prussian blue stain. The presence of other particulates, such as silica or asbestos, modifies the pathologic changes accordingly.

Pathogenesis. Iron inhalation produces primarily dust macules with hemosiderin-filled macrophages.

Diagnosis. Pulmonary siderosis is diagnosed on the basis of documented exposure and the radiologic or pathologic findings described above. Contamination with other particulates is common and results in a mixed dust pneumoconiosis.

Treatment and Prognosis. There is no specific treatment. Cessation of exposure may be associated with some radiologic improvement as the dust is cleared from the lungs (11,57).

MIXED DUST REACTIONS

Exposures to mixtures of dust are frequent. In fact, most industrial exposures are mixed, leading to a relatively high frequency of mixed dust reactions in the lung (figs. 16-8, 16-9, 16-20–16-22, 16-36). This explains, for example, the frequency of anthracosilicosis, the common finding of asbestos bodies in welders with siderosis, and the presence of classic silicotic nodules in many of the patients with silicatoses. The nodules of mixed dust fibrosis have classically been described as "Medusa head" in configuration, with less collagen, less developed collagen bundles, and pigmented macrophages around the periphery extending as tentacles into the surrounding lung tissue in contrast to the discrete rounded character of a silicotic nodule. Needless to say, the nodules found in a given case may show a broad spectrum of appearances, and precise characterization as a silicotic nodule, coal nodule, mixed dust nodule, etc., may be impossible. When appreciable amounts of sheet silicates (particularly talc) are present, giant cells may be an additional finding.

When asbestos bodies are identified in a mixed dust reaction, they may be incidental (fig. 16-36) or they may be significant. Their significance is determined by whether or not fibrosis of the type found in asbestosis is present.

BERYLLIOSIS

Definition. Berylliosis is caused by exposure to beryllium or compounds containing it. Acute and chronic forms are recognized and in chronic beryllium disease the clinical manifestations are part of a systemic disease process (11,36,50,52–54,57).

Mineralogy and Exposure. Beryllium is a metal that is useful because of its light weight, thermal and electrical conductivity, modulus of elasticity, sound conductivity, high rate of fusion, ability to be a moderator and reflector of neutrons, and because it is nonmagnetic and translucent to X rays (11,57). It is primarily mined in the form of beryl from which beryllium hydroxide, beryllium oxide (beryllia), beryllium silicates, and beryllium metal alloys are produced. Beryllium and all compounds containing it are potentially toxic to humans (11,57).

Exposure to beryllium may occur in the following settings: extraction of beryllium from beryl, fluorescent lamp manufacturing (mostly of historical interest), metal working, ceramic manufacturing, electronics and computer industry, rocket and space industry, dental labs using beryllium alloys, and nuclear weapons industry research with beryllium, as well as among individuals who work in beryllium processing plants but are not directly exposed to beryllium, live in the vicinity of factories using beryllium, or handle the clothing of beryllium workers (11, 36,57). The latter three settings represent bystander exposures. Currently, 2 percent of exposed individuals develop chronic beryllium disease even though beryllium levels in manufacturing are strictly regulated (50).

Clinical Features. Beryllium lung disease is divided into acute and chronic forms (11,57). Acute beryllium disease is primarily of historical interest except for massive accidental exposures. Direct acute exposure can cause conjunctivitis, periorbital edema, nasopharyngitis, tracheobronchitis, and pneumonitis. The acute chemical pneumonitis is characterized by dyspnea, cough, sputum production, chest pain, tachycardia, crackles, and cyanosis. Patients may develop a fulminant disease with acute respiratory distress syndrome (ARDS).

Chronic beryllium disease is a multisystem disease caused by hypersensitivity to beryllium (11,36,50,52–54,57). It has clinical, radiologic, and pathologic similarities to sarcoidosis. Chronic beryllium disease may develop while the individual is still exposed to beryllium, up to 40 years or more after the onset of exposure, or long after exposure has ceased. The long latency period reemphasizes the importance of a careful occupational history (49).

Patients with chronic beryllium disease may be asymptomatic or have signs and symptoms of interstitial lung disease with progressive dyspnea and cough (11,57). Physical examination may be normal but occasionally reveals bibasilar crackles on chest examination, lymphadenopathy, and hepatosplenomegaly. Clubbing of the digits may occur. Manifestations of the involvement of some other organ system (such as skin granulomas) may occur before the lung disease is identified. As disease severity increases, the clinical findings resemble those of progressive fibrosing interstitial pneumonia.

Patients with chronic beryllium disease have a number of nonspecific abnormalities in laboratory tests: hyperuricemia, hypercalcemia, hypercalciuria, elevations in hepatocellular injury tests, elevated serum angiotensin converting enzyme, and elevation in serum immunoglobulins. The physiologic changes in chronic disease are quite variable. In early disease the lung function may be normal. Obstructive changes, independent of cigarette smoking, are found in approximately one third of patients. A restrictive or mixed pattern is found in most patients, especially those with advanced disease. Gas exchange abnormalities are common.

Radiologic Findings. The radiologic features of acute beryllium disease are those of acute chemical pneumonitis. The chest radiograph initially shows a diffuse, bilateral, hazy increase in opacity (ground-glass pattern), which progresses to patchy areas of consolidation (22).

Chronic beryllium disease resembles sarcoidosis (22). The most common radiologic finding is the presence of ill-defined nodules throughout both lungs, sometimes associated with hilar and mediastinal lymph node enlargement.

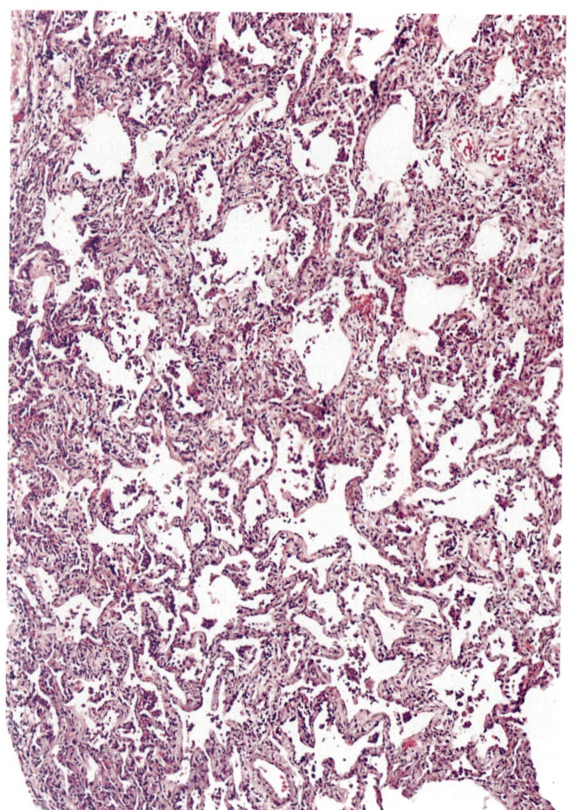

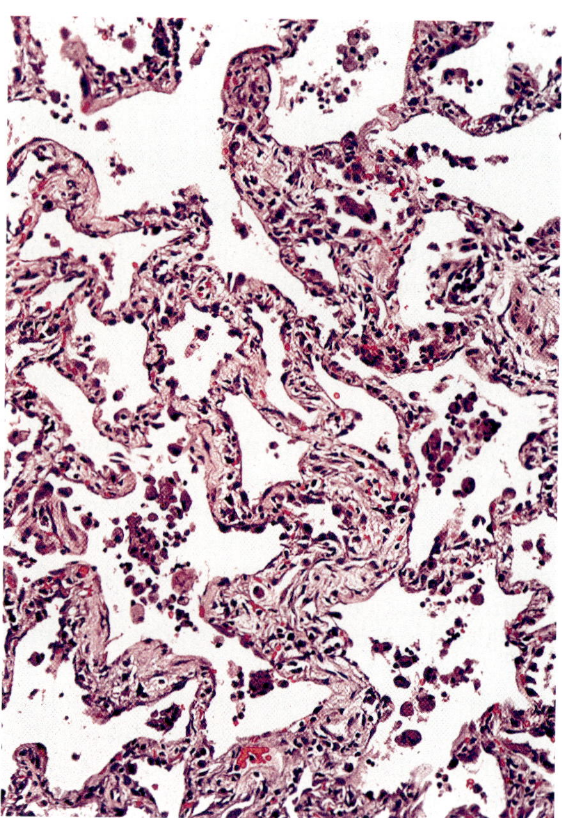

Figure 16-49

ACUTE BERYLLIOSIS

Acute berylliosis with organizing acute lung injury manifesting as edematous alveolar septal widening and type 2 cell metaplasia.

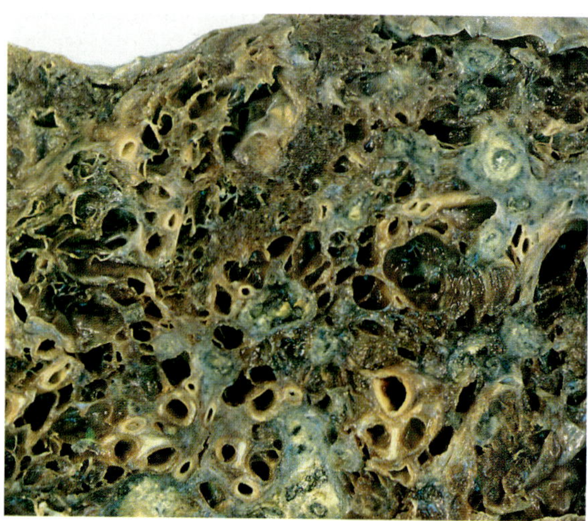

Figure 16-50

CHRONIC BERYLLIOSIS

Grossly, these fibrotic nodules are associated with emphysematous change.

The chest radiograph has limited sensitivity in demonstrating the parenchymal abnormalities in beryllium disease: in one investigation of 28 patients with biopsy-proven disease, abnormalities were detected by radiograph in 15 (54 percent) patients and by HRCT in 25 (89 percent) (51). The most common abnormalities on HRCT were small nodules and thickening of the interlobular septa.

Pathologic Findings. The histologic features of acute beryllium disease are those of nonspecific acute lung injury (fig. 16-49); in severe cases the features of diffuse alveolar damage are present (11). In milder cases there is interstitial edema, a mild interstitial inflammatory infiltrate, and prominent reactive type 2 cells.

The gross findings of chronic beryllium disease are primarily nodules representing coalesced granulomas (fig. 16-50) and associated fibrosis (11,23,31). The nodules may be 2 cm or

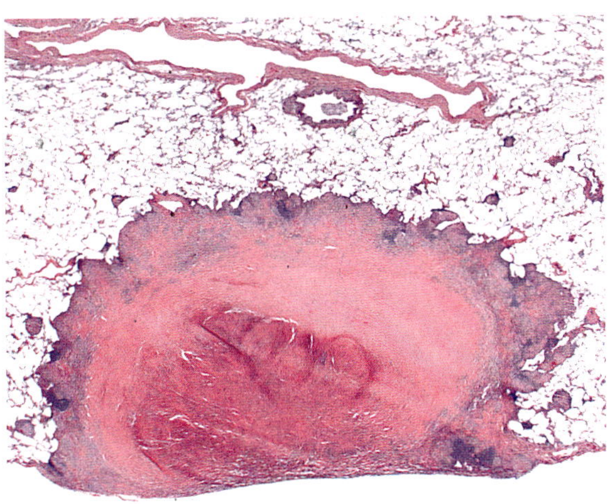

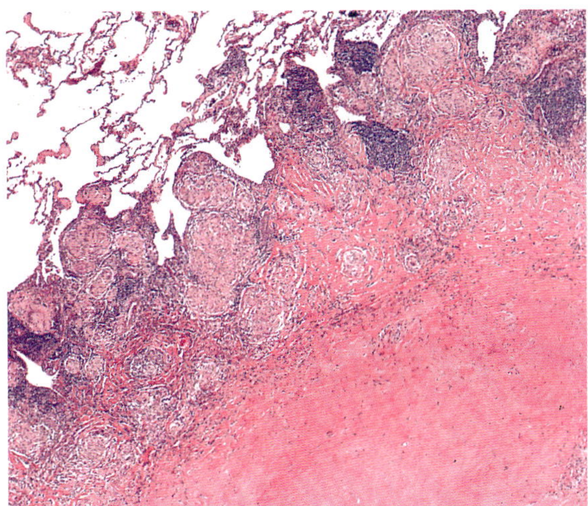

Figure 16-51

CHRONIC BERYLLIOSIS

There is a chronic granulomatous nodule with central fibrosis and degenerative change, and a rim of non-necrotizing granulomas.

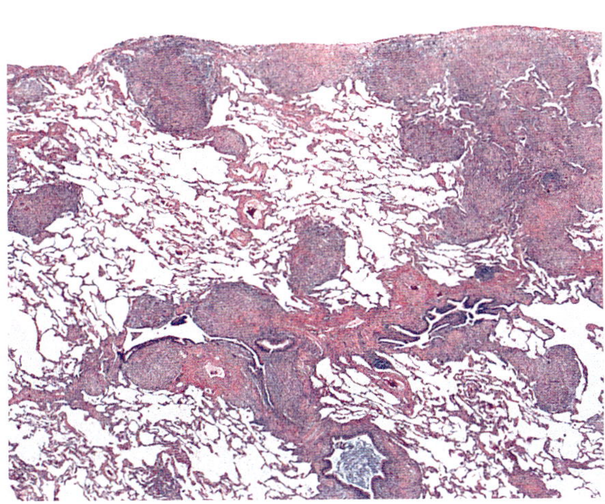

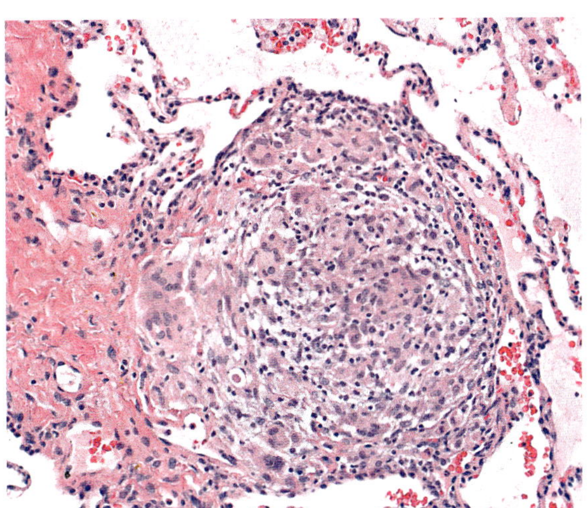

Figure 16-52

CHRONIC BERYLLIOSIS

Left: This case is similar to sarcoidosis, with non-necrotizing granulomas distributed along lymphatic routes in the pleura and bronchovascular bundles.

Right: The granulomas are indistinguishable from those of sarcoidosis.

greater in diameter. Interstitial fibrosis and honeycomb change are occasionally found.

The histologic changes of chronic disease are identical to those of sarcoidosis: confluent granulomas distributed along lymphatic routes (figs. 16-51–16-53); in other cases there are scattered small granulomas associated with interstitial inflammation and varying degrees of interstitial fibrosis (11,23,31,53,57). As the disease progresses, honeycomb change can develop and the granulomas may disappear over time. The granulomas typically coalesce to form large hyalinized nodules which can show degenerative changes, including necrosis (fig. 16-51).

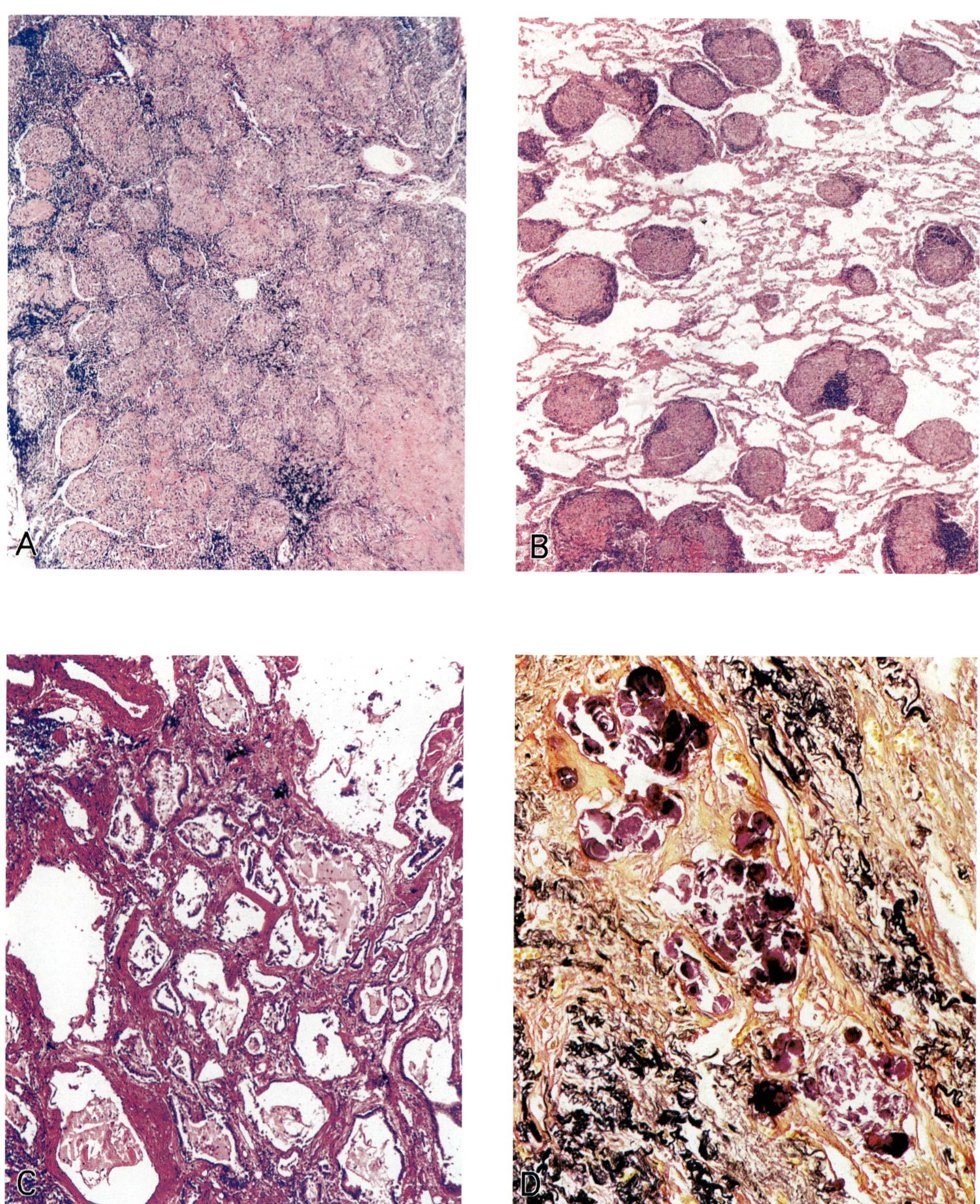

Figure 16-53

CHRONIC BERYLLIOSIS

Biopsies of a hilar lymph node (A) and lung (B) show numerous non-necrotizing granulomas. At autopsy over two decades later, this patient's lungs showed only diffuse interstitial fibrosis without active granulomas (C), but numerous residual Schaumann bodies (D).

Distinction from infection is important and special stains should be performed. Schaumann bodies are particularly prominent in berylliosis (fig. 16-53). Extrapulmonary lesions in chronic beryllium disease may be identical to those of sarcoidosis.

Although the pathology of berylliosis is not specific, the presence of non-necrotizing granulomas, with or without an interstitial infiltrate, the tendency of granulomas to form large hyalinized nodules in the lung and/or lymph nodes, and the presence of large numbers of Schaumann bodies in the connective tissue of a fibrotic lung are clues to the diagnosis. Obviously, none of these findings are specific but since the latency period for the development of chronic beryllium disease may be extremely long, pathologic examination of tissues may provide the initial clue which ultimately leads to recognition of a case. Practically speaking, whenever sarcoidosis is considered, chronic beryllium disease should be included in the differential diagnosis (49,52).

Pathogenesis. Acute beryllium pneumonitis is a toxic chemical pneumonitis. Chronic berylliosis is a chronic hypersensitivity reaction to beryllium. Human leukocyte antigen (HLA)-DP is a marker for susceptibility to chronic beryllium disease among exposed individuals, but not all individuals with a HLA-DP genotype develop disease if exposed (50). Patients with chronic disease show beryllium-stimulated release of inflammatory cytokines from cells in the BAL specimen (73).

Diagnosis. Documentation of beryllium in urine or tissue was formerly used in assessing individuals suspected of having chronic beryllium disease (11). These tests are expensive, require relatively large amounts of material for analysis in order to be reliable, and may be falsely negative due to sampling and the fact that only low levels of beryllium may persist in individuals who have the disease. Other methods can be used to document the presence of beryllium in tissue, such as laser microprobe mass spectrometry (79). However, the finding of beryllium with these methods reflects only exposure and not necessarily disease.

Any person suspected of having beryllium disease should undergo an evaluation that includes fiberoptic bronchoscopy with BAL to obtain cells for lymphocyte transformation testing, and lymph node or lung biopsy to confirm histopathologic alterations. Documentation of a beryllium-specific immune response is now possible with beryllium lymphocyte proliferation testing (BLPT), which can be performed on lymphocytes from peripheral blood or BAL (36, 50,53). While BLPT on BAL lymphocytes may be more sensitive, the use of peripheral blood lymphocytes is accurate in over 90 percent of cases.

Table 16-9

PROPOSED CRITERIA FOR THE DIAGNOSIS OF CHRONIC BERYLLIUM DISEASE[a]

1. History of exposure to beryllium
2. Beryllium-specific immune response; positive blood or BAL BLPT[b]
3. Lung biopsy histopathology consistent with chronic beryllium disease (granulomas and/ or mononuclear cell infiltrates)
4. Clinical manifestations that include any of the following:
   - respiratory signs or symptoms
   - reticulonodular infiltrates on chest imaging
   - altered pulmonary physiology with restrictive and/or obstructive changes
   - decreased diffusing capacity, ventilatory impairment, or altered gas exchange on exercise testing

[a]Modified from reference 53.
[b]BAL BLPT = Bronchoalveolar lavage beryllium lymphocyte proliferation testing.

Proposed criteria for the diagnosis of chronic beryllium disease, subclinical beryllium disease, and beryllium sensitization are shown in Table 16-9. A definitive diagnosis of chronic beryllium disease requires all four criteria, the diagnosis of subclinical beryllium disease requires criteria 1 to 3, and the diagnosis of beryllium sensitization requires 1 and 2 (53).

Treatment and Prognosis. Acute beryllium disease is now rare (11); in historical series there was about a 10 percent mortality. Patients generally recovered in 1 to 6 months, and approximately 10 percent developed chronic beryllium disease.

Patients with chronic beryllium disease should be removed from exposure. Resolutions and long-term remissions of chronic disease have been documented, with or without steroid therapy (11). No controlled study of corticosteroid therapy has been reported. However, many patients improve clinically and radiographically after such treatment. Often, the disease recurs when treatment is discontinued, necessitating prolonged therapy. In older series, primarily derived from cases identified in the 1940s and 1950s, the mortality rate was 30 percent.

More recently, it has been documented that stringent control of levels of exposure may be associated with fewer cases of disease and radiologic improvement in those with disease (11,54). In one study, patients with only a granulomatous reaction fared the best, whereas those with a marked mononuclear cell reaction and no or poorly formed granulomas fared the worst (23). A cohort mortality study of beryllium-exposed workers has shown an excess mortality from lung cancer and from nonmalignant beryllium disease (11).

HARD METAL (COBALT) LUNG DISEASE

Definition. Hard metal (cobalt) lung disease is caused by exposure to cobalt, usually as a component of hard metal or in association with diamond dust (2,11,16,39,40,55,57).

Mineralogy and Exposure. Hard metal is a synthetic compound that combines tungsten carbide with cobalt as well as a number of other metals. It has a hardness nearly that of diamond which makes it useful in the cutting and grinding of metal tools, and most documented cases have occurred in this setting. An identical disease has been documented in diamond polishers who are not exposed to hard metal. Cobalt is now implicated in both. Prior to the identification of cobalt as central to the disease, most biopsied cases had been morphologically categorized as giant cell interstitial pneumonia according to the classification of Liebow (16).

Clinical Features. Hard metal lung disease manifests in three ways: interstitial lung disease, immunoglobulin (Ig)E-mediated asthma, and a syndrome resembling extrinsic allergic alveolitis (11). The clinical and radiologic findings are nonspecific, and correspond to the syndromes described. Many workers exposed to cobalt develop rhinitis, conjunctival irritation, and contact dermatitis. Asthma is a much more common manifestation than interstitial lung disease (10.9 percent versus 0.7 percent) (2), and these patients have a history of chest tightness, dyspnea, and wheezing. There is a strong relationship between the asthmatic symptoms and obstructive airflow, and the cobalt exposure. These patients do not have evidence of diffuse parenchymal lung disease. Patients with interstitial disease have clinical manifestations common to interstitial lung disease in general, i.e., breathlessness with exertion and nonproductive cough. Patients with cobalt-related interstitial lung disease may have a latency period ranging from 2 to 25 years (57).

There are no specific abnormalities detected in the routine laboratory tests among exposed or diseased workers. Several methods for monitoring exposure to cobalt utilize blood or urine analyses. Urinary levels of cobalt have been shown to reflect exposure. Blood cobalt concentration appears to have a linear relationship with exposure when levels are greater than 0.1 mg/m^3. The usefulness of monitoring blood levels is not known. Serum IgE antibodies to cobalt have been demonstrated. In addition, the transformation of blood lymphocytes by cobalt has been shown in patients with cobalt asthma and cobalt-induced dermatitis. BAL analysis shows an increase in neutrophils and lymphocytes, and may also demonstrate giant cells.

Radiologic Findings. There are no distinctive radiographic features of cobalt-associated occupational asthma. However, in a cross-sectional study of hard metal workers, slight radiographic abnormalities (0/1, 1/1 according to the ILO classification) were more frequent in exposed workers compared to controls. In hard metal–associated interstitial lung disease, the chest radiograph usually shows small irregular opacities, predominately in the lower lung zones. With progression of the disease, more widespread and coarser opacities can be seen and endstage honeycombing may develop. A normal chest radiograph does not preclude the presence of significant clinical and physiologic impairment. Therefore, in symptomatic patients, the diagnosis of hard metal disease should not be delayed until radiographic abnormalities are present since these may lag behind other evidence of disease.

Pathologic Findings. The most distinctive histologic finding is multinucleated giant cells of histiocytic origin within airspaces, hence, the

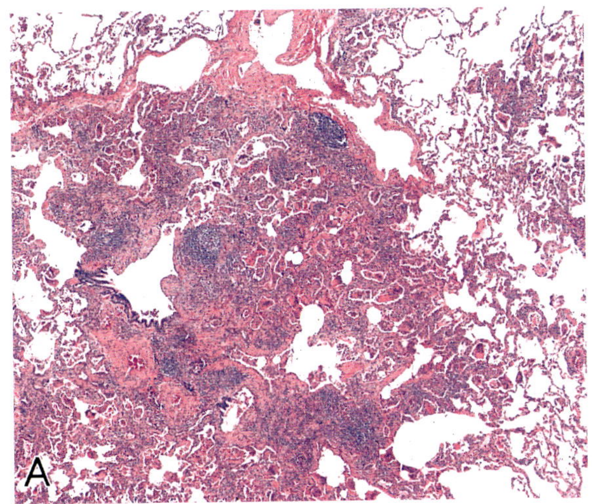

Figure 16-54

HARD METAL LUNG DISEASE

In this case the centrilobular distribution of the nodule is not so apparent (A), although the characteristic intra-alveolar giant cells, some of which contain phagocytosed histiocytes, are very prominent (B,C).

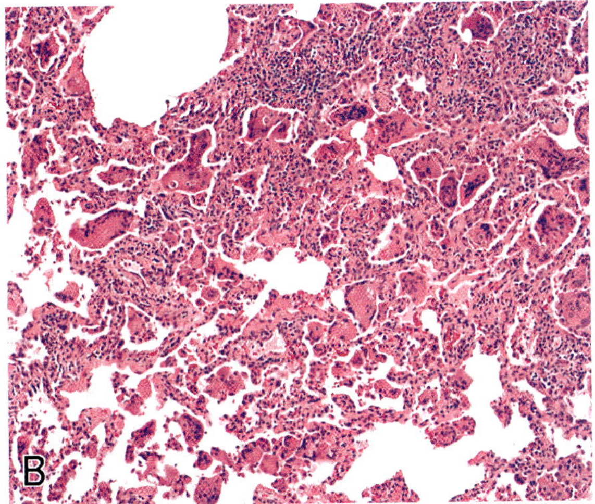

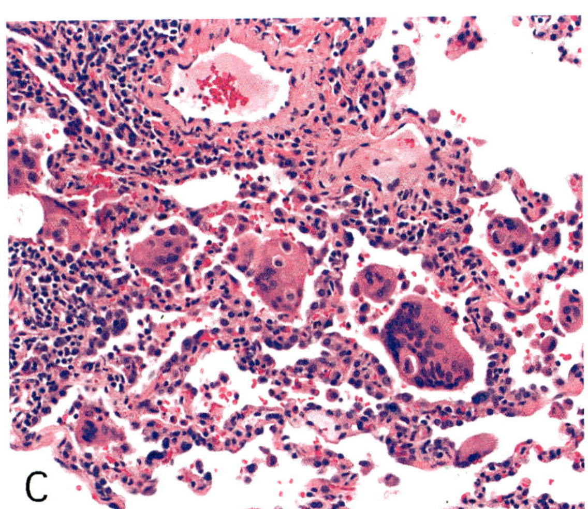

previous classification of most cases as giant cell interstitial pneumonia (fig. 16-54) (11,16,39,40, 52). The giant cells often contain macrophages in their cytoplasm. Multinucleated alveolar lining cells may also be identified. The presence of a centrilobular inflammatory process that produces vague nodules centering on membranous bronchioles is at least as useful diagnostically as the giant cells (fig. 16-55). A lymphoid reaction that includes germinal centers is common. Other cases are indistinguishable from desquamative interstitial pneumonia, and a few resemble usual interstitial pneumonia. Particulate black material, which may be birefringent, may be found in macrophages and giant cells. Cobalt, tungsten, tantalum, and other metals have been identified with energy dispersive X-ray spectroscopy, but their presence suggests exposure and not necessarily disease. Their absence does not exclude the diagnosis since cobalt is soluble in the lung and may not persist.

Pathogenesis. Hard metal lung disease is presumably immunologically mediated but the specifics are not well worked out (57). The classic histologic lesion (described above) is nearly unique and does not resemble any of the well-characterized immunologic reactions in the lung.

Diagnosis. Asthma associated with hard metal exposure is unlikely to lead to tissue evaluation by the pathologist. In patients with interstitial lung disease, the possibility of hard metal disease should be considered in those with known exposure and compatible histologic findings. Giant cell interstitial pneumonia with centrilobular nodular accentuation alone should suggest reevaluation of the exposure

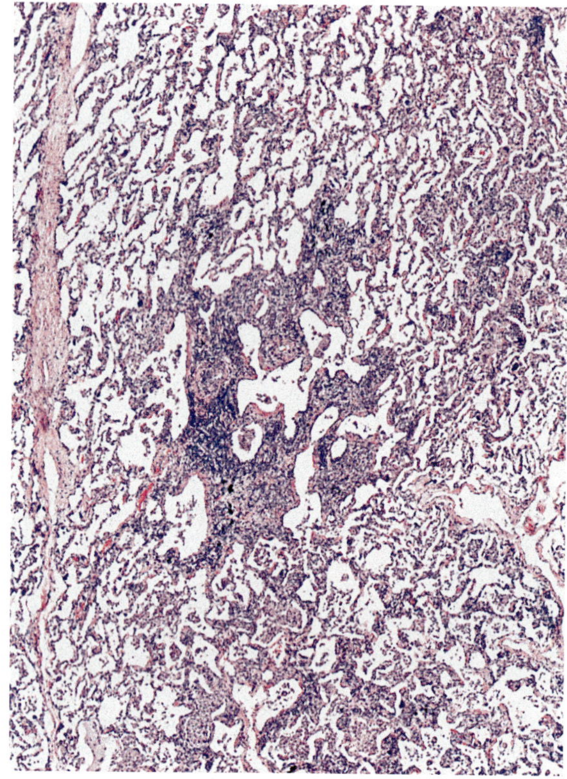

Figure 16-55

HARD METAL LUNG DISEASE

Scanning power microscopy high-lights the centrilobular inflammatory and fibrotic nodular lesions that are the result of peribronchiolar alveolar septal widening.

history. The presence of components of hard metal in the lung tissue may be further confirmatory evidence but is not always required.

Treatment and Prognosis. Patients with established occupational asthma and interstitial lung disease should be removed from further exposure. Although no control studies exist, patients with cobalt pneumoconiosis often require corticosteroid therapy to speed recovery and (hopefully) prevent disease progression (11,57). Recurrences may occur in patients who return to the work environment after being successfully treated by removal from exposure and corticosteroid therapy. A few patients have required cytotoxic treatment with cyclophosphamide or azathioprine when they did not improve with corticosteroid therapy alone. Fatal cases have been documented (48). Lung transplantation has been used as a last resort and there are reports of recurrence of the disease in the allograft (74).

PULMONARY DISEASE AND EXPOSURE TO OTHER METALS

In addition to the metals already mentioned, other metals and related compounds have been implicated in human disease: aluminum, aluminum oxide, antimony, antimony trichloride, pentachloride, arsenic, barium, cadmium, chromium, copper, lanthanum and rare earths, nickel and its salts, silicon carbide, tin, titanium, zinc oxide, chloride, and zirconium (11).

Exposure to tin, barium, and antimony; chromium; or zirconium and titanium produces "benign pneumoconioses" characterized by relatively dramatic radiologic findings and comparatively few clinical findings (11). Pathologic descriptions are few but macules appear to be the dominant histologic finding. The implicated agent is readily identified from the exposure history.

Exposure to aluminum and alumina ($AL_2 0_3$), primarily in the aluminum smelting industry, is implicated in potroom asthma, chronic obstructive lung disease, lung cancer, and pulmonary fibrosis (11). The fumes from aluminum smelting contain approximately 29 to 44 percent silica and 41 to 62 percent alumina. Aluminum welders and smelters exposed to aluminum fumes in poorly ventilated areas can develop *metal fume fever* (see below). A potentially severe and fatal mixed dust pneumoconiosis (*Shaver's disease*) can result from exposure to these fumes, particularly in furnace feeders or crane operators. Other rare pulmonary diseases have been reported including a granulomatous lung reaction, pulmonary alveolar proteinosis, and desquamative interstitial pneumonia (17). Grossly, the lungs have a slate gray color. There are a few cases that show a nodular fibrosing process whereas others have a more diffuse fibrosis resembling usual interstitial pneumonia (figs. 16-56, 16-57) (11,30). Early lesions are seen as centrilobular macules with histiocytes showing grayish tan pigmentation (fig. 16-58). Often, dense accumulations of macrophages containing a granular, gray-brown, metallic material are present in both the nodular masses and the interstitium of the fibrotic tissue. The

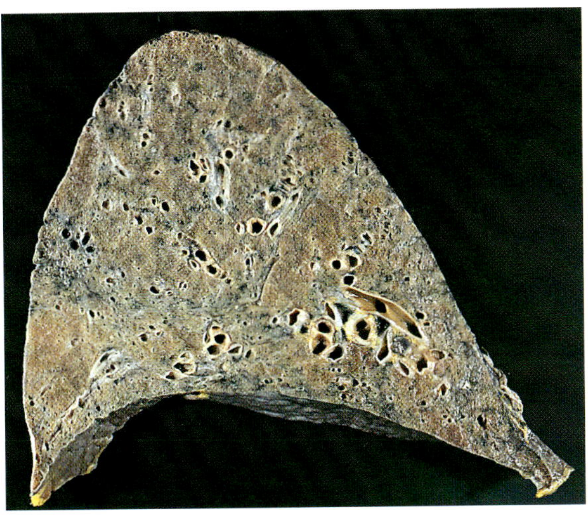

Figure 16-56

ALUMINUM FIBROSIS

This gross photograph shows grayish fibrosis with focal peripheral honeycomb change. (Courtesy of Dr. Andrew Churg, Vancouver, Canada.)

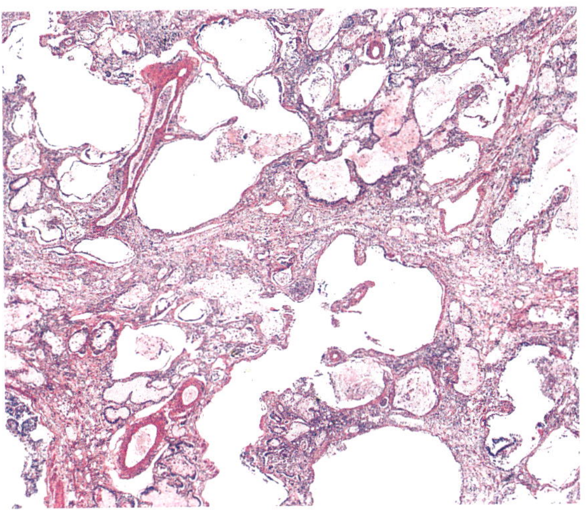

Figure 16-57

ALUMINUM FIBROSIS

This case of aluminum pneumoconiosis shows diffuse interstitial fibrosis and architectural loss.

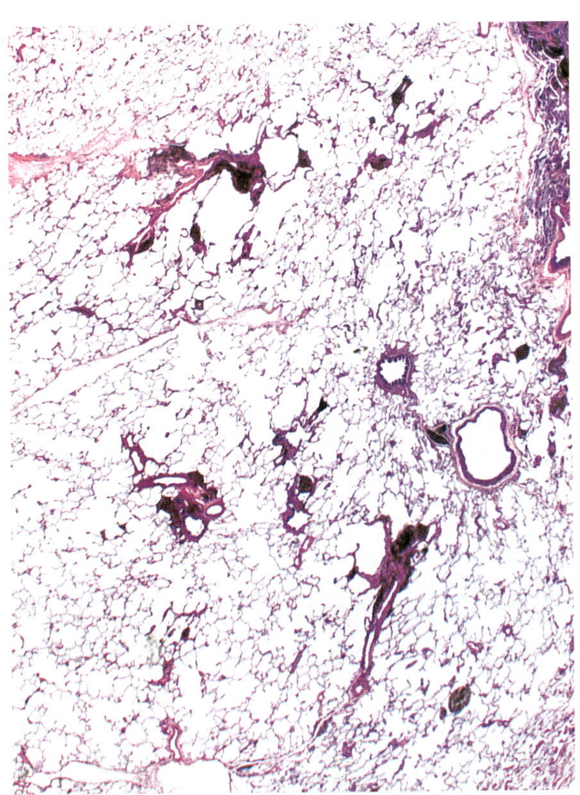

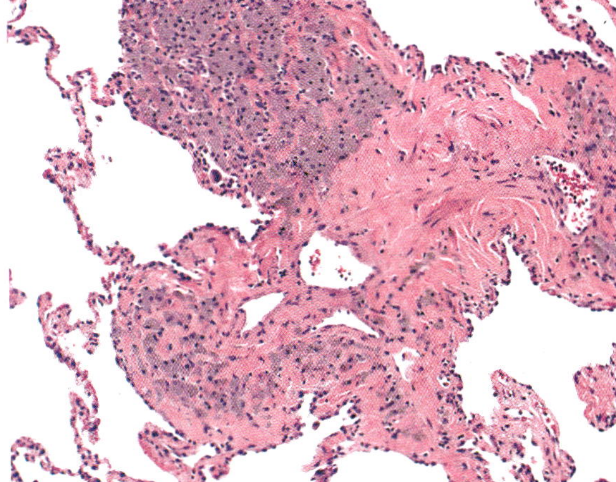

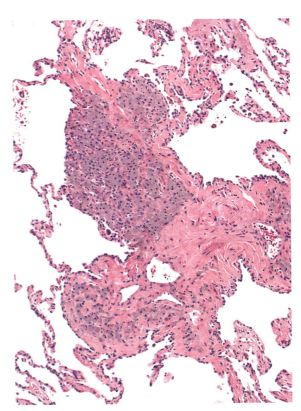

Figure 16-58

ALUMINUM MACULES

The centriacinar macules (left) are composed of macrophages laden with grayish tan dust (right). The patient was asymptomatic.

fibrogenic potential of alumina dust appears to be much less than that of other inorganic dusts, especially asbestos, silica, or coal. As in other exposures, the presence of excessive quantities of aluminum (often 1,000 times higher than controls) in the tissue or cells does not correlate directly with the development of disease.

Silicon carbide (carborundum) is an abrasive formed by heating silica and carbon at high temperatures (11,41). Nodular and reticulonodular disease have been reported in workers exposed to silicon carbide. Histologically, both nodular fibrosis and diffuse interstitial fibrosis have been described, and given the presence of silica these likely represent silicosis or mixed dust pneumoconiosis (11,41,57).

Table 16-10

PULMONARY DISEASES CAUSED BY GASES AND FUMES[a]

Acute respiratory distress syndrome
Necrotizing bronchitis or bronchiolitis
Organizing pneumonia
Constrictive bronchiolitis
Bronchiectasis
Asthma
Chronic bronchitis
Chronic airflow obstruction
Metal fume fever

[a]Data from reference 11.

Acute inhalation of cadmium oxide fumes (for example, from smelting or welding) may cause a delayed toxic fume type reaction with upper airway irritation, dyspnea, chest pain, and cough followed by pulmonary edema. Metal fume fever may also develop (see below). These symptoms usually resolve over days and only rarely does this condition progress to pulmonary fibrosis or cause death. Both chronic bronchitis and emphysema may be found with increased incidence in cadmium workers (11,57). Chronic cadmium poisoning primarily causes kidney problems. Urinary cadmium may be a useful guide to cadmium exposure but is not used to make the diagnosis of cadmium-related disease.

PULMONARY DISEASE ASSOCIATED WITH INHALATION OF GASES AND FUMES

A large number of gases and fumes may be encountered in the workplace and they cause a variety of pulmonary diseases (Table 16-10) (11). Agents that have been documented to produce ARDS (the usual histologic correlate of which is diffuse alveolar damage) are shown in Table 16-11.

Noxious gases and fumes may produce acute necrotizing bronchitis and bronchiolitis, and diffuse alveolar damage (see above) in the distal parenchyma. As the process heals, organizing pneumonia (bronchiolitis obliterans with intraluminal polyps) may be encountered.

Table 16-11

INHALED AGENTS ASSOCIATED WITH ACUTE RESPIRATORY DISTRESS SYNDROME[a]

Acetaldehyde	Hydrogen bromide	Ozone
Acrolein	Hydrogen chloride	Perchloroethylene
Ammonia	Hydrogen selenide	Phosgene
Antimony trichloride or pentachloride	Hydrogen sulfide	Phosphorus tribromide
Beryllium	Mercury	Sulfur dioxide
Boranes	Methyl bromide	Sulfuric acid
Cadmium and cadmium salts	Methylene chloride (paint remover)	Thionyl chloride
Chlorine	Nickel (fume)	Titanium tetrachloride
Cobalt metal	Nickel carbonyl	Zinc oxide and chloride
Fire smoke	Nitrogen oxides	Zirconium chloride

[a] Modified from reference 11.

Table 16-12

INHALED AGENTS ASSOCIATED WITH CONSTRICTIVE BRONCHIOLITIS[a]

Ammonia	Hydrogen selenide
Chlorine	Oxides of nitrogen
Fire smoke	Sulfur dioxide
Hydrogen bromide	Thionyl chloride

[a] Modified from reference 11.

Table 16-13

INHALED AGENTS ASSOCIATED WITH BRONCHIECTASIS[a]

Ammonia
Fire Smoke
Kerosene
Nickel carbonyl
Phosgene

[a] Modified from reference 11.

In the late stages, constrictive bronchiolitis or bronchiectasis, with airflow obstruction, may occur. Agents known to produce constrictive bronchiolitis and bronchiectasis are shown in Tables 16-12 and 16-13, respectively.

Metal fume fever is generally encountered in shipyard welders exposed to oxides of zinc, copper, magnesium, and occasionally, cadmium (11,57,66). Clinically, affected individuals complain of excessive thirst and a metallic taste in the mouth 4 to 8 hours after beginning work. These are followed by flu-like symptoms with fever and myalgia. The symptoms subside in 1 to 2 days. Tolerance may develop and the symptoms decrease over the course of the work week; they are worse at the beginning of the week, hence the name "Monday morning fever" (11). The pathologic findings are not known.

Exposure to the oxides of nitrogen produces one of the best known clinical syndromes. *Silo-filler's disease* results from exposure to high concentrations of nitrogen dioxide (NO_2) that develop in the space above the silage as a yellow-red-orange vapor (11). Acute high exposure results in death from asphyxiation (*silo suffocation*). Individuals with less severe exposures may develop necrotizing bronchiolitis or ARDS with diffuse alveolar damage. Constrictive bronchiolitis is an occasional late effect of the small airway injury that occurs during the acute phase (see chapter 8).

Firefighters are exposed to a wide variety of gases and fumes (11). Inhalation injuries resulting in acute necrotizing bronchitis/bronchiolitis and diffuse alveolar damage may be encountered. Late effects of constrictive bronchiolitis are also recognized (chapter 8).

EFFECTS OF INHALATION OF SYNTHETIC FIBERS ON THE LUNG

Synthetic fibers, which are made of polymers that do not occur naturally, may be divided into inorganic (usually called man-made vitreous fibers [MMVF)] and organic fibers including carbon, aramids, and polyolefin fibers (11). The size and shape of the synthetic fibers are such that there is a potential for them to be inhaled into the lower respiratory tract and to cause diseases analogous to those caused by naturally occurring fibers such as asbestos. Despite the potential for respiratory tract disease, the pathogenicity of synthetic fibers has not been well documented (11,18). Recently, a distinctive form of lung disease has been associated with the inhalation of nylon flock (see below).

Man-made vitreous fibers are amorphous glassy silicates that can be divided into four main groups (11,18): slag wools, rock wools, glass wools, and filaments. Industrially, they are used in textiles and insulation. Organic fibers including polyvinyl alcohol, polyacrylonitrile, polyolefins, aramid fibers, graphite, and other types of carbon fibers are, for the most part, too big to be respirable (11).

Nylon Flock Worker's Lung

Definition. Pulmonary disease caused by the inhalation of nylon flock (10,20,33,34).

Exposure and Pathogenesis. Nylon is a generic term for a group of synthetic polyamide fibers used in the textile industry (55). Nylon flock is used to make the plush surface of upholstery. While the actual fibers themselves may not be respirable, the ends sheared off during the production are, and these are implicated pathogenetically (34).

Clinical Features. The following case definition has been used for patients with flock worker's lung: persistent respiratory symptoms, current/previous work in the flocking industry, and histologic evidence of interstitial lung disease without better explanation.

Symptoms of flock worker's lung are chronic dyspnea and dry cough, with or without chest pain. Crackles are rarely heard. Pulmonary function studies show restriction and impaired diffusion. Symptoms may be present for months or years before clinical diagnosis.

Radiologic Findings. The chest radiograph may be normal or show reticulonodular opacities or, occasionally, patchy areas of consolidation (33). HRCT demonstrates patchy hazy areas of increased density (ground-glass opacities), areas of consolidation, or, occasionally, a micronodular pattern or peripheral honeycombing (33).

Pathologic Findings. The most characteristic pathologic finding in flock worker's lung is a lymphocytic bronchiolitis and peribronchiolitis; scanning power microscopy reveals an inflammatory process centered on bronchioles and alveolar ducts (fig. 16-59). Lymphoid follicles with germinal centers are common. Some cases have more diffuse interstitial lymphocytic infiltrates with germinal centers. Less commonly, bronchiolitis obliterans organizing pneumonia, desquamative interstitial pneumonia, and usual interstitial pneumonia patterns have been noted. Granulomas and birefringent material are lacking.

Diagnosis and Prognosis. Most affected workers have histories of heavy exposure and avoidance of exposure has been associated with clinical improvement. To date, no patients have died of this condition.

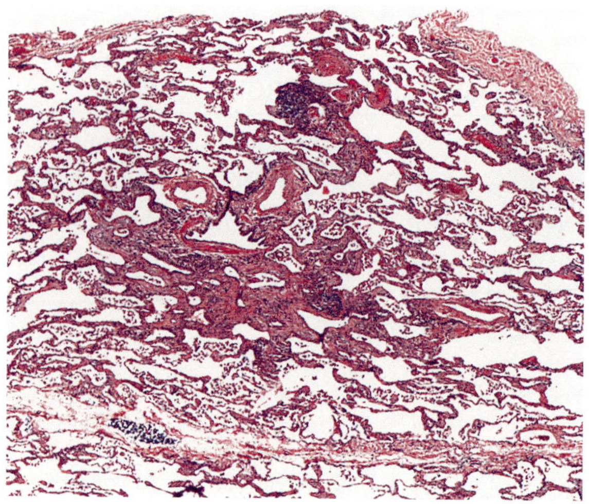

Figure 16-59

FLOCK WORKER'S LUNG

There is a centrilobular inflammatory nodule reminiscent of those seen in hard metal disease. Lymphoid follicles are present. Descriptively, this lesion has been termed "lymphocytic bronchiolitis and peribronchiolitis."

OCCUPATIONAL ASTHMA AND REACTIVE AIRWAYS DYSFUNCTION SYNDROME

Occupational asthma is defined as "variable airflow limitation and/or airway hyperresponsiveness due to causes and conditions attributable to a particular occupational environment and not to stimuli encountered outside the workplace" (11).

Two types of occupational asthma are recognized (11): occupational asthma with prior sensitization, and reactive airways dysfunction syndrome (RADS) which shows no latency or prior sensitization and is initiated by a single exposure to high concentrations of an irritant.

Occupational asthma with prior sensitization is similar in its clinical, functional, and radiologic appearances to nonoccupational asthma (11). Patients develop symptoms acutely upon entering the workplace, the symptoms may be delayed by several hours, or the response may be delayed until the early hours of the next morning. Workers with occupational asthma have a progressive decline in pulmonary function if they remain in the workplace (11). Removal from exposure and the use of inhaled steroids are associated with improvement but a minority of individuals have persistent asthma or longstanding bronchial hyperreactivity.

Occupational asthma represents over one third of the cases of occupational lung disease reported to the National Institute of Occupational Safety and Health (NIOSH) (11). The causes are numerous and major categories are summarized in Table 16-14. In the United States, 3 to 10 percent of the general population have asthma and it is estimated that 2 to 15 percent of these have occupational asthma

Table 16-14

CAUSES OF OCCUPATIONAL ASTHMA[a]

High Molecular Weight Sensitizing Agents
Animal-derived products
Insects
Plants
Biologic enzymes
Vegetable gums
Low Molecular Weight Sensitizing Agents
Aliphatic amines
Fluxes
Wood dust
Diisocycanates
Anhydrides
Metals
Drugs
Chemicals

[a]Modified from reference 11.

Table 16-15

AGENTS REPORTED TO CAUSE REACTIVE AIRWAY DYSFUNCTION SYNDROME[a]

Hydrogen sulfide	Sulfuric acid
Nitrogen dioxide	Hydrochloric acid
Sulphur dioxide (bleach)	Sodium hypochlorite
Ammonia	Acetic acid
Chlorine	Formaldehyde
Ethylene oxide	Phosphoric acid
Phosgene	Tear gas
Ether	Spray paint
Butadiene	Welding fumes
Toluene diisocyanate	Smoke inhalation
Metam sodium (pesticide)	

[a] Modified from reference 11.

(11). The prevalence of occupational asthma in the workplace depends on the asthmagenicity of the agents to which individuals are exposed, and varies from 3 to over 50 percent. In general, high molecular weight antigens are more asthmagenic than low molecular weight sensitizing agents. The pathologic findings of occupational asthma are identical to those of nonoccupational asthma.

For the diagnosis of RADS, the following should be present (11): 1) confirmed exposure to high concentrations of an irritant with symptoms developing within hours thereafter; 2) symptoms persisting for at least 3 months although most persist for several years. An exacerbation of previously diagnosed asthma does not qualify as RADS; 3) persistence of asthma-like symptoms and documented evidence of bronchial hyperreactivity by the histamine or methacholine challenge study; and 4) no symptoms caused by low level exposures to the inciting irritant. If specific IgE or IgG antibodies can be demonstrated, the diagnosis of RADS is excluded. Approximately 10 percent of workers who carry a diagnosis of occupational asthma probably fulfill the above criteria (11).

The pathogenesis of RADS is unknown; causes are shown in Table 16-15. The pathologic findings of RADS are not well characterized (11). There appears to be a mild chronic bronchiolitis with epithelial metaplasia in the airways, mild lymphocytic infiltrates in the airway mucosa and wall, and goblet cell metaplasia. Basement membrane thickening and smooth muscle hypertrophy may be present. Eosinophils may or may not be seen.

OCCUPATIONAL EXTRINSIC ALLERGIC ALVEOLITIS

Extrinsic allergic alveolitis (hypersensitivity pneumonitis) may be caused by exposure in the workplace to organic antigens as well as some simple inorganic chemical compounds. In many cases, the exposure is obvious (for example, farmer's lung disease or malt worker's lung), whereas in others the exposure is much more difficult to identify, such as to contamination in a ventilation system. The clinical, radiologic, and pathologic features of extrinsic allergic alveolitis are covered in chapter 3.

BYSSINOSIS

Byssinosis refers to respiratory complaints (mill fever, chronic bronchitis, airway hyperresponsiveness) associated with exposure to cotton dust, flax, and soft hemp (11,57). *Mill fever,* for which the term byssinosis is usually used, is most likely a form of organic dust toxic syndrome (see below). It is associated with cough, wheezing, chest tightness, and shortness of breath, developing within 4 hours of starting work on a Monday morning.

Table 16-16

CLINICAL FEATURES OF ORGANIC DUST TOXIC SYNDROME (ODTS) COMPARED TO ACUTE FARMER'S LUNG DISEASE (FLD)[a]

	ODTS	FLD
Exposure	Massive organic dust (moldy silage, haylage, grain, etc.; silo cleaning)	Variety of antigens (classically, thermophilic actinomycetes); exposure need not be massive
Occurrence	Nearly all heavily exposed individuals, occasionally in clusters	Susceptible individuals only
Season	Summer (July-September)	Winter-early spring (Jan.-Mar.)
Latent interval from exposure to symptoms	4–8 hours	4–8 hours
Duration of illness	Hours to a few weeks	Hours to a few weeks
Symptoms	Fever, chills, cough, dyspnea, myalgias, headache, and irritation of the eyes and nose	Fever, chills, cough, dyspnea
Chest radiography	Normal or mild diffuse infiltrates	Bilateral interstitial infiltrate
Peripheral white blood cell counts	Leukocytosis with increased neutrophils	Leukocytosis with increased neutrophils
Serum precipitins to causative antigens	Negative	Positive
BAL fluid	Neutrophils increased	Lymphocytes increased
Recurrence	None except for re-exposure to massive dust	Yes, with re-exposure
Chronicity	No	Possible

[a]Summarized from reference 59 and personal communication from M. Iwata, M.D. (1993).

There are few distinctive histologic features (11). Changes of chronic bronchitis with mucous gland hypertrophy and goblet cell metaplasia may be found, as well as some increase in bronchial smooth muscle. A small proportion of cases may show birefringent cotton fibers and structures termed byssinosis bodies, which represent iron-encrusted cotton fibers. Byssinosis bodies are spherical, range up to 10 µm in diameter, and have a central black nidus surrounded by a clear halo. They are a marker of exposure and not necessarily of disease.

ORGANIC DUST TOXIC SYNDROME

Organic dust toxic syndrome (ODTS) is a systemic syndrome that follows massive exposure to organic dusts containing toxic quantities of microorganisms or their products (especially endotoxin) (11,59). ODTS is most commonly found in farmers who are exposed to grains or moldy hay contaminated with spores of fungi and actinomyces, or to endotoxins, or other workers exposed to textile materials contaminated with *Fusarium,* an aflatoxin-producing fungus.

ODTS produces an acute and systemic illness characterized by fever, malaise, aches and pains, and occasionally, vomiting (11,59). Respiratory symptoms may be present and these include dry cough and bibasilar rales. Symptoms typically develop within 4 to 8 hours of exposure; the course is benign with full recovery within 3 days. Leukocytosis, diffuse opacities on chest radiography, restrictive ventilatory defects, and reduced diffusing capacity for carbon monoxide (DLCO) are common laboratory abnormalities. The clinical features of patients with ODTS, as compared to those with acute farmer's lung disease (extrinsic allergic alveolitis), with which it is often confused, are shown in Table 16-16. These cases are thought not to represent true hypersensitivity reactions because no prior sensitization is required and there is a lack of serologic response to common fungal antigens.

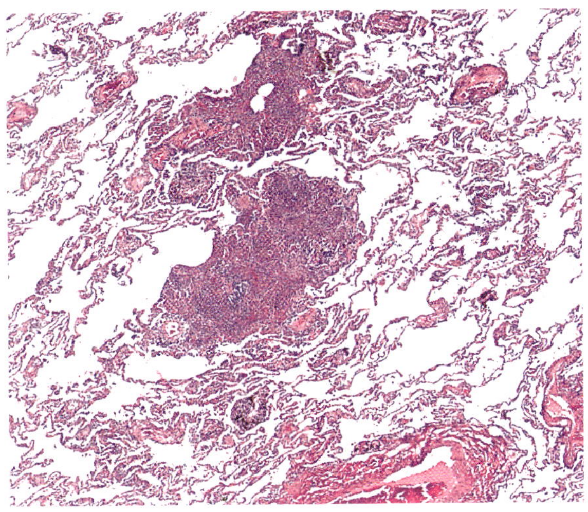

Figure 16-60

PULMONARY MYXOTOXICOSIS

There is an acute bronchiolitis manifested by inflammatory cells filling the lumen of a small bronchiole. Multiple fungal organisms were identified by culture. (Courtesy of Dr. Samuel Yousem, Pittsburgh, PA.)

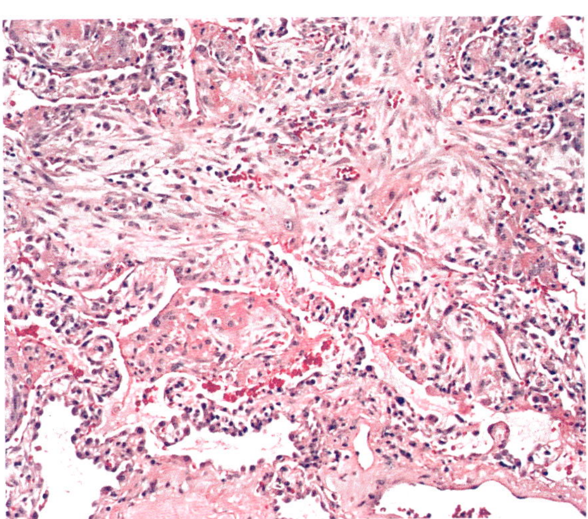

Figure 16-61

PULMONARY MYXOTOXICOSIS

There is nonspecific, organizing, diffuse alveolar damage, with airspace exudate and organization.

Table 16-17

HISTOLOGIC FEATURES OF ORGANIC DUST TOXIC SYNDROME (ODTS) COMPARED TO FARMER'S LUNG DISEASE (FLD)[a]

	ODTS	FLD
Main region	Intra-alveolar space	Interstitium
Cellular infiltrates	Neutrophils, histiocytes	Lymphocytes, plasma cells, histiocytes
Granulomas	Absent	Present
Bronchiolitis	Acute (neutrophils)	Chronic (lymphocytes)
Organisms	Fungal spores and hyphae	None[b]

[a]Summarized from reference 59 and personal communication from M. Iwata, M.D. (1993).
[b]*Cryptostroma corticale* in maple bark stripper's disease is a rare exception.

Pathologic studies of ODTS are few (59). Some patients have an acute bronchiolitis. Large numbers of organisms are found on culture or identified with special stains (fig. 16-60). Other patients have features of diffuse alveolar damage (fig. 16-61). A histologic comparison of ODTS with extrinsic allergic alveolitis is shown in Table 16-17.

ODTS appears to be the direct effect of inhalation of large amounts of toxins that mobilize nonimmune defense systems.

PULMONARY DISEASE ASSOCIATED WITH INTRAVENOUS DRUG EXPOSURE

The many pulmonary complications associated with intravenous drug abuse are shown in Table 16-18. Some of these conditions are related to infections that result from intravenous drug use and others are due to the materials that are injected which become lodged in the lung. The distinctive pathologic changes in the lung are due to the fillers used in the manufacture of pills that are intended for oral use but are

Table 16-18

PULMONARY COMPLICATIONS OF INTRAVENOUS DRUG EXPOSURE[a]

Infections (including HIV)	Pulmonary edema	Bullous lung disease and emphysema
Pneumonia	Acute respiratory distress syndrome	Foreign body granuloma
Abscesses	Pulmonary hypertension	Pulmonary alveolar hemorrhage
Mycotic aneurysms	Interstitial fibrosis	Pneumothorax
Septic emboli	Massive fibrosis	Asthma

[a]Summarized from reference 11.

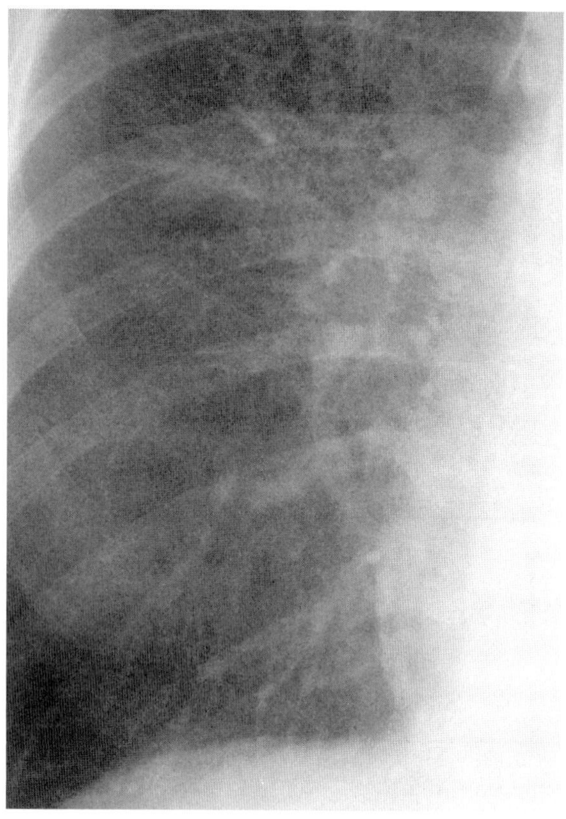

Figure 16-62

INTRAVENOUS TALCOSIS

View of the right lung from a PA chest radiograph shows diffuse, pinpoint, fine nodularity. The patient was a 27-year-old intravenous drug abuser.

crushed and injected intravenously. The most commonly used fillers are talc, microcrystalline cellulose, and cornstarch (11). Cornstarch is recognizable by its round shape and Maltese cross pattern of birefringence. Talc is identified as large, irregular, plate-like crystals that are strongly birefringent and may be pale yellow on routine H&E–stained sections. Microcrystalline cellulose particles are elongated crystalline structures that are positive with the digested PAS, methenamine silver, and Congo red stains. In general, many of these particles are larger than 10 µm. Their relatively large size and perivascular distribution are helpful in excluding an origin from an inhalational route. Additional clues to an intravenous origin are absence of ferruginated material and absence of particles in the alveolar spaces.

The most common radiologic manifestation of talcosis from intravenous drug abuse is a diffuse, pinpoint micronodular pattern in the lung (fig. 16-62) (56). Long-term follow-up often shows conglomeration of the micronodules into upper lobe masses, cephalad retraction of the hila, and lower lobe emphysema (56). HRCT often demonstrates increased attenuation of the conglomerate masses due to accumulation of talc (78). Patients developing talcosis secondary to methylphenidate abuse often develop characteristic findings of predominantly lower lobe panacinar emphysema on HRCT (78).

The pathologic lesions associated with intravenous drug exposure and their clinical correlates are shown in Table 16-19. The most distinctive histologic feature of intravenous drug abuse is an interstitial and perivascular granulomatous and giant cell reaction to birefringent particulate material, so-called talc granulomatosis (figs. 16-63–16-65). The granulomatous reaction is seen in parallel with the vascular thrombotic lesions. Pulmonary hypertension may develop. Acutely, the foreign material is intravascular (fig. 16-66).

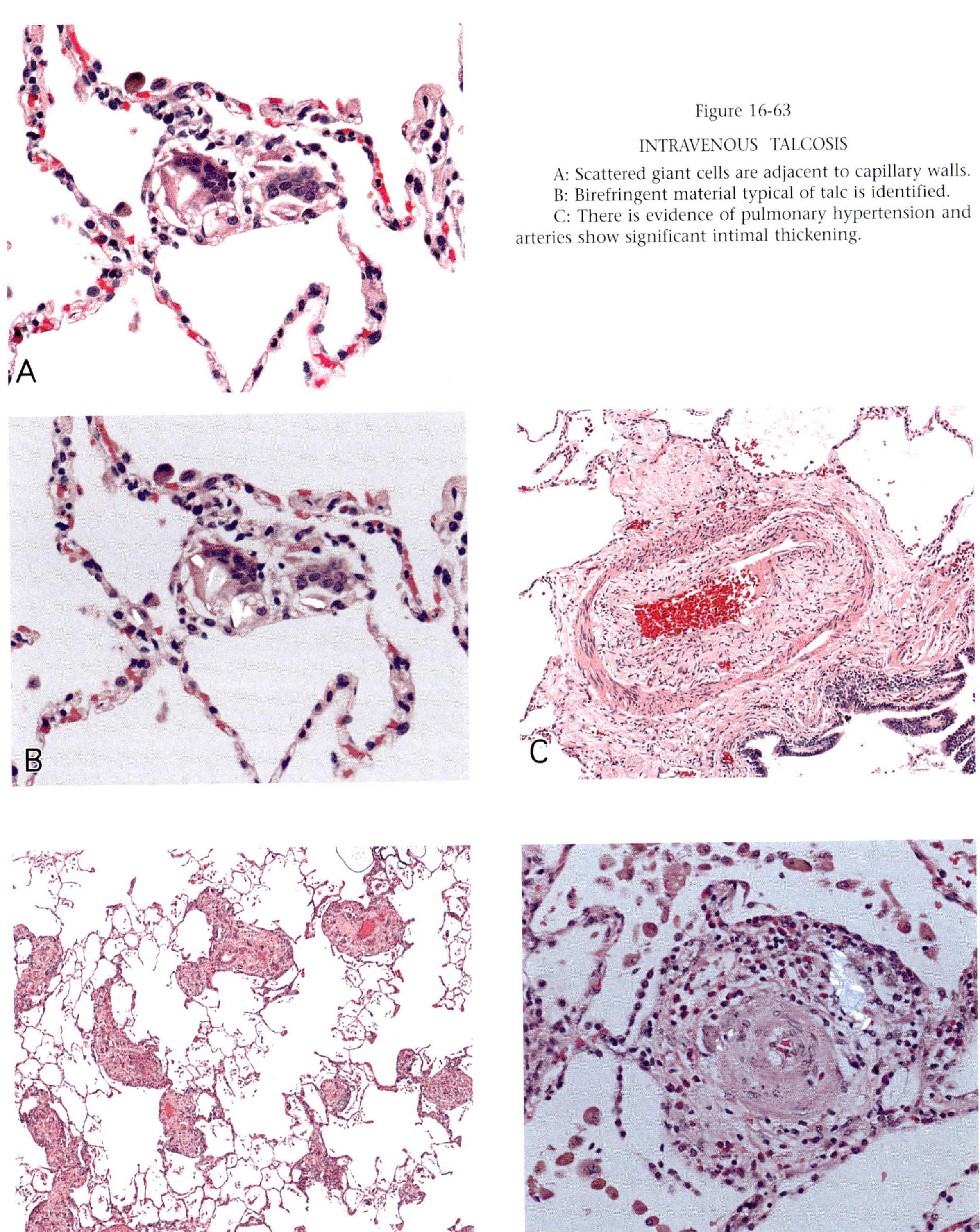

Figure 16-63

INTRAVENOUS TALCOSIS

A: Scattered giant cells are adjacent to capillary walls.
B: Birefringent material typical of talc is identified.
C: There is evidence of pulmonary hypertension and arteries show significant intimal thickening.

Figure 16-64

INTRAVENOUS TALCOSIS

Left: There is a prominent perivascular and granulomatous fibrotic reaction.
Right: Arterioles show mural thickening typical of pulmonary hypertension, with adjacent birefringent material.

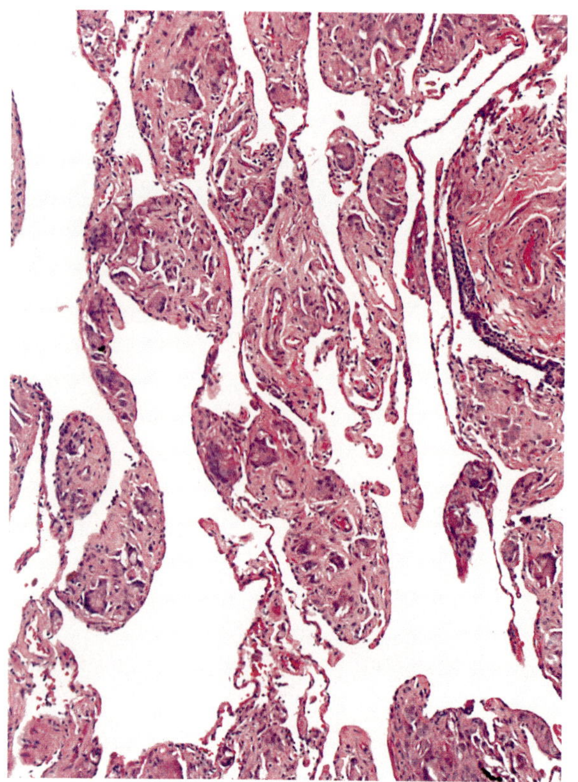
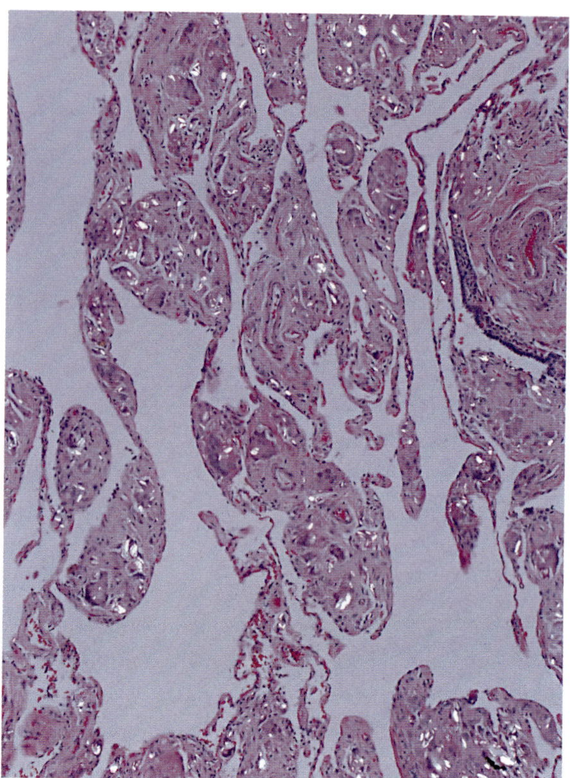

Figure 16-65

INTRAVENOUS TALCOSIS

Left: This case shows moderate perivascular and interstitial pulmonary fibrosis with a granulomatous reaction. Right: Prominent birefringent material is seen.

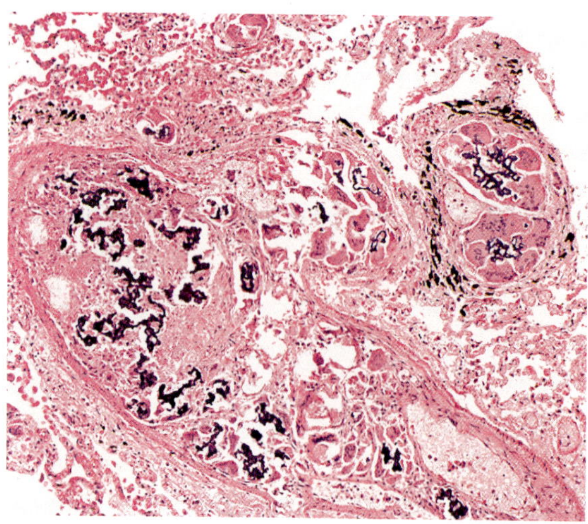
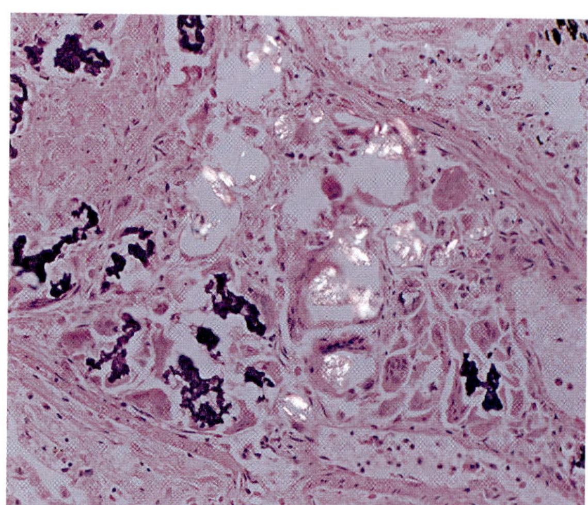

Figure 16-66

INTRAVENOUS TALCOSIS ASSOCIATED WITH TOTAL PARENTERAL NUTRITION

This patient had been injecting crushed drugs via a total parenteral nutrition (TPN) line and there is both birefringent as well as nonbirefringent material stuffing vessels.

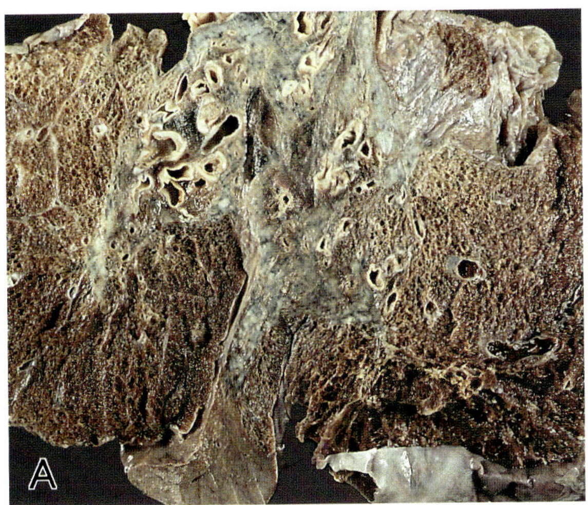

Figure 16-67

INTRAVENOUS TALCOSIS WITH PROGRESSIVE MASSIVE FIBROSIS

Grossly, there is a large zone of fibrosis that extends across the major fissure (A). Histologically, there is dense fibrosis with scattered lymphoid follicles (B) in which large amounts of birefringent talc are seen (C). (Courtesy of Dr. Andrew Churg, Vancouver, Canada.)

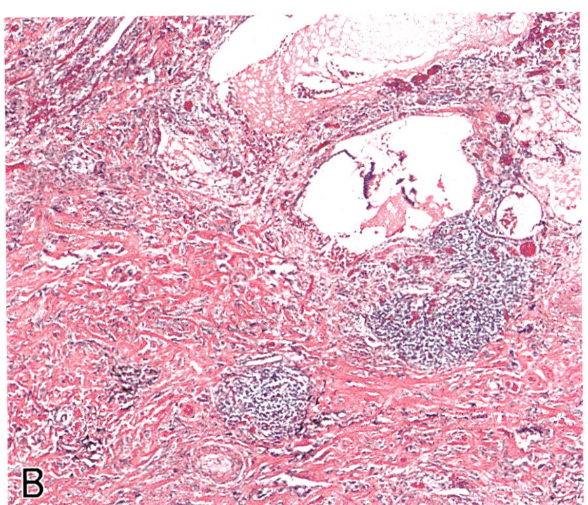

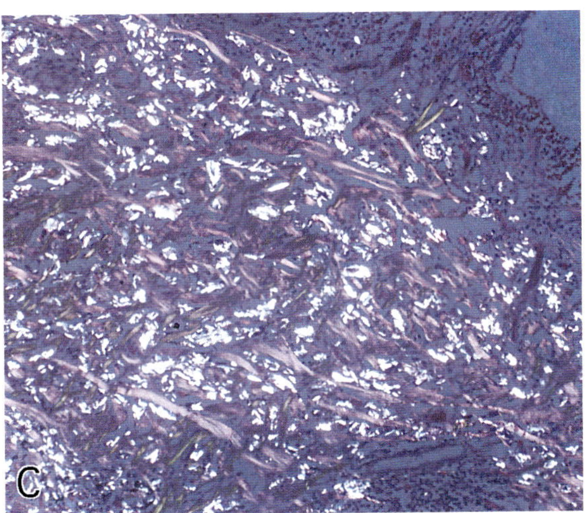

Table 16-19

PULMONARY LESIONS ASSOCIATED WITH INTRAVENOUS INJECTION OF DRUGS INTENDED FOR ORAL USE[a]

Pathologic Lesions	Clinical Syndrome
Vascular, perivascular, and interstitial foreign body granulomas to injected particles	Pulmonary hypertension (may cause sudden death)
Progressive massive fibrosis	Emphysema
Emphysema	Mixture of these
Mixture of these	

[a] Summarized from reference 11.

Less commonly, there is extensive interstitial fibrosis associated with the foreign body reaction. Rarely, progressive massive fibrosis is encountered (fig. 16-67). Emphysema has been classically associated with intravenous abuse of methylphenidate. The pathologic lesions may progress even after discontinuation of all drug abuse (56).

REFERENCES

1. Aberle DR, Gamsu G, Ray CS. High-resolution CT of benign asbestos-related diseases: clinical and radiographic correlation. AJR Am J Roentgenol 1988;151:883–91.
2. Abraham JL. The spectrum of pulmonary pathologic reaction and lung dust burden in 30 cases of cobalt pneumonitis (hard metal lung; giant cell interstitial pneumonia) [Abstract]. Am Rev Respir Dis 1990;141:A28.
3. Akira M, Yamamoto S, Yokoyama K, et al. Asbestosis: high-resolution CT-pathologic correlation. Radiology 1990;176:389–94.
4. Akira M, Yokoyama K. Yamamoto S, et al. Early asbestosis: evaluation with high-resolution CT. Radiology 1991;178:409–16.
5. American Thoracic Society. Diagnosis of nonmalignant diseases related to asbestos. Am Rev Respir Dis 1986;134:363–68.
6. American Thoracic Society Committee of the Scientific Assembly on Environmental and Occupational Health. Adverse effects of crystalline silica exposure. Am J Respir Crit Care Med 1997;155:761–65.
7. Amoli K. Bronchopulmonary disease in Iranian housewives chronically exposed to indoor smoke. Eur Respir J 1998;11:659–63.
8. Argani P, Ghossein R, Rosai J. Anthracotic and anthracosilicotic spindle cell pseudotumors of mediastinal lymph nodes: report of 5 cases of a reactive lesion that simulates malignancy. Hum Pathol 1998;29:851–5.
9. Begin R, Ostiguy G, Fillion R, Colman N. Computed tomography scan in the early detection of silicosis. Am Rev Respir Dis 1991;144:697–705.
10. Boag AH, Colby TV, Fraire AE, et al. The pathology of interstitial lung disease in nylon flock worker's. Am J Surg Pathol 1999;23:1539–45.
11. Churg A, Green FH. Pathology of occupation lung disease, 2nd ed. Baltimore: Williams & Wilkins; 1998.
12. Craighead JE, Abraham JL, Churg A, et al. The pathology of asbestos-associated diseases of the lungs and pleural cavities: diagnostic criteria and proposed grading schema. Arch Pathol Lab Med 1982;106:544–96.
13. Crouch E, Churg A. Ferruginous bodies and the histologic evaluation of dust exposure. Am J Surg Pathol 1984;8:109–16.
14. Crouch E, Churg A. Progressive massive fibrosis of the lung secondary to intravenous injection of talc. A pathologic and mineralogic analysis. Am J Clin Pathol 1983;80:520–6.
15. Davis JM, Chapman J, Collings P, et al. Variations in the histological patterns of the lesions of coal worker's pneumoconiosis in Britain and their relationship to lung dust content. Am Rev Respir Dis 1983;128:118–24.
16. Demedts M, Gheysens B, Nagels J, et al. Cobalt lung in diamond polishers. Am Rev Respir Dis 1984;130:130–5.
17. De Vuyst P, Dumortier P, Schandene L, Estenne M, Verhest A, Yernault JC. Sarcoidlike lung granulomatosis induced by aluminum dusts. Am Rev Respir Dis 1987;135:493–7.
18. De Vuyst P, Dumortier P, Swaen GM, Pairon JC, Brochard P. Respiratory health effects of man-made vitreous (mineral) fibres. Eur Respir J 1995;8:2149–73.
19. Dodson RF, O'Sullivan MF, Huang J, Holiday DB, Hammar SP. Asbestos in extrapulmonary sites: omentum and mesentery. Chest 2000;117:486–93.
20. Eschenbacher WL, Kreiss K, Lougheed MD, Pransky GS, Day B, Castellan RM. Nylon flock-associated interstitial lung disease. Am J Respir Crit Care Med 1999;159:2003–8.
21. Fisher ER, Watkins G, Lam NV, et al. Objective pathological diagnosis of coal workers' pneumoconiosis. JAMA 1981;245:1829.
22. Fraser RS, Müller NL, Colman N, Pare PD, eds. Inhalation of inorganic dust (pneumoconiosis). In: Fraser RS, Müller NL, Colman N, Pare PD, eds. Fraser and Pare's diagnosis of diseases of the chest. Philadelphia: WB Saunders; 1999:2386–484.
23. Freiman DG, Hardy HL. Beryllium disease: the relation of pulmonary pathology to clinical course and prognosis based on a study of 130 cases from the U.S. Beryllium Case Registry. Hum Pathol 1970;1:25–44.
24. Gaensler EA, Jederlinic PJ, Churg A. Idiopathic pulmonary fibrosis in asbestos-exposed workers. Am Rev Respir Dis 1991;144:689–96.
25. Gibbs AE, Pooley FD, Griffiths DM, Mitha R, Craighead JE, Ruttner JR. Talc pneumoconiosis: a pathologic and mineralogic study. Hum Pathol 1992;23:1344–54.
26. Gysbrechts C, Michiels E, Verbeken E, et al. Interstitial lung disease more than 40 years after a 5 year occupational exposure to talc. Eur Respir J 1998;11:1412–5.
27. Hillerdal G. Asbestos-related pleural disease. Sem Respir Med 1987;9:65–74.
28. Hillerdal G. Rounded atelectasis. Clinical experience with 74 patients. Chest 1989;95:836–41.
29. International Labour Office. Guidelines for the use of ILO international classification of radiographs for pneumoconiosis. Occup Safety Health Services 1980;22:1–48.

30. Jederlinic PJ, Abraham JL, Churg A, Himmelstein JS, Epler GR, Gaensler EA. Pulmonary fibrosis in aluminum oxide workers. Investigation of nine workers, with pathologic examination and microanalysis in three of them. Am Rev Respir Dis 1990;142:1179–84.
31. Jones Williams W. A histological study of the lungs in 52 cases of chronic beryllium disease. Br J Ind Med 1958;15:84–91.
32. Kamp DW, Weitzman SA. Asbestosis: clinical spectrum and pathogenic mechanisms. Proc Society Exp Biol Med 1997;214:12–26.
33. Kern DG, Crausman RS, Durand KT, Nayer A, Kuhn C III. Flock worker's lung: chronic interstitial lung disease in the nylon flocking industry. Ann Intern Med 1998;129:261–72.
34. Kern DG, Kuhn C, Ely EW, et al. Flock worker's lung: broadening the spectrum of clinicopathology, narrowing the spectrum of suspected etiologies. Chest 2000;117:251–9.
35. Koeger AC, Lan T, Alcaix D, et al. Silica-associated connective tissue disease. Medicine 1995;74:221–37.
36. Kreiss K, Mroz MM, Zhen B, et al. Epidemiology of beryllium sensitization and disease in nuclear workers. Am Rev Respir Dis 1993;148:985–91.
37. Lapenas D, Gale P, Kennedy T, Rawlings W Jr, Dietrich P. Kaolin pneumoconiosis. Radiologic, pathologic, and mineralogic findings. Am Rev Respir Dis 1984;130:282–8.
38. Lapp NL, Parker JE. Coal workers' pneumoconiosis. Clin Chest Med 1992;13:243–52.
39. Lauwerys R, Lison D. Health risks associated with cobalt exposure—an overview. Sci Total Environ 1994;150:1–6.
40. Lison D, Lauwerys R, Demedts M, Nemery B. Experimental research into the pathogenesis of cobalt/hard metal lung disease. Eur Respir J 1996;9:1024–8.
41. Masse S, Begin R, Cantin A. Pathology of silicon carbide pneumoconiosis. Mod Pathol 1988;1:104–8.
42. McDonald JW, Roggli VL. Detection of silica particles in lung tissue by polarizing light microscopy. Arch Pathol Lab Med 1995;119:242–6.
43. McHugh K, Blaquiere RM. CT features of rounded atelectasis. AJR Am J Roentgenol 1989;153:257–60.
44. Miranda RN, McMillan PN, Pricolo VE, Finkelstein SD. Peritoneal silicosis. Arch Pathol Lab Med 1996;120:300–2.
45. Monso E, Tura JM, Marsal M, Morell F, Pujadas J, Morera J. Mineralogic microanalysis of idiopathic pulmonary fibrosis. Arch Environ Health 1990;45:185–8.
46. Morgan WK, Donner A, Higgins IT, Pearson MG, Rawlings W. The effects of kaolin on the lung. Am Rev Respir Dis 1988;138:813–20.
47. Mossman BT, Churg A. Mechanisms in the pathogenesis of asbestosis and silicosis. Am J Respir Crit Care Med 1998;157:1666–80.
48. Nemery B, Nagels J, Verbeken E, Dinsdale D, Demedts M. Rapidly fatal progression of cobalt lung in a diamond polisher. Am Rev Respir Dis 1990:141:1373–8.
49. Newman LS. Beryllium disease and sarcoidosis: clinical and laboratory links. Sarcoidosis 1995;12:7–19.
50. Newman LS. Immunology, genetics, and epidemiology of beryllium disease. Chest 1996;109:40s–3s.
51. Newman LS, Buschman DL, Newell JD Jr, Lynch DA. Beryllium disease: assessment with CT. Radiology 1994;190:835–40.
52. Newman LS, Kreiss K. Nonoccupational beryllium disease masquerading as sarcoidosis: identification of blood lymphocyte proliferative response to beryllium. Am Rev Respir Dis 1992;145:1212–4.
53. Newman LS, Kreiss K, King TE Jr, Seay S, Campbell PA. Pathologic and immunologic alterations in early stages of beryllium disease. Am Rev Respir Dis 1989;139:1479–86.
54. Newman LS, Lloyd J, Daniloff E. The natural history of beryllium sensitization and chronic beryllium disease. Environ Health Perspect 1997;104[Suppl 5]:937–43.
55. Nordberg G. Assessment of risks in occupational cobalt exposures. Sci Total Environ 1994;150:201–7.
56. Pare JP, Cote G, Fraser RS. Long-term follow-up of drug abusers with intravenous talcosis. Am Rev Respir Dis 1989;139:233–41.
57. Parkes WR. Occupational lung disorders, 3rd ed. Oxford: Butterworth-Heinemann; 1994.
58. Pathology standards for coal workers' pneumoconiosis. Report of the Pneumoconiosis Committee of the College of American Pathologists to the National Institute for Occupational Safety and Health. Arch Pathol Lab Med 1979;103:375–432.
59. Perry LP, Iwata M, Tazelaar HD, Colby TV, Yousem SA. Pulmonary mycotoxicosis: a clinicopathologic study of 3 cases. Mod Pathol 1998;11:432–6.
60. Ramage JE Jr, Roggli VL, Bell DY, Piantadosi CA. Interstitial lung disease and domestic wood burning. Am Rev Respir Dis 1988;137:1229–32.
61. Rashid AM, Green FH. Pleural pearls following silicosis: a histological and electron microscopic study. Histopathology 1995;26:84–7.

62. Remy-Jardin M, Remy J, Farre I, Marquette CH. Computed tomographic evaluation of silicosis and coal worker's pneumoconiosis. Radiol Clin North Am 1992:30:1155–76.
63. Roggli VL, Greenberg SD, Pratt PC, eds. Pathology of asbestos-associated disease. Boston: Little Brown; 1992.
64. Rosenman KD, Reilly MJ, Kalinowski DJ, Watt FC. Silicosis in the 1990s. Chest 1997;111:779–86.
65. Rudd RM. New developments in asbestos-related pleural disease. Thorax 1996;51:210–6.
66. Sferlazza SJ, Beckett WS. The respiratory health of welders. Am Rev Respir Dis 1991;143:1134–48.
67. Silicosis and Silicate Disease Committee. Disease associated with exposure to silica and nonfibrous silicate minerals. Arch Pathol Lab Med 1988;112:673–720.
68. Slavin RE, Swedo JL, Brandes D, Gonzalez-Vitale JC, Osornio-Vargas A. Extrapulmonary silicosis: a clinical, morphologic, and ultrastructural study. Hum Pathol 1985;6:393–412.
69. Sprince NL, Oliver LC, Eisen EA, Greene RE, Chamberlin RI. Cobalt exposure and lung disease in tungsten carbide production. A cross-sectional study of current workers. Am Rev Respir Dis 1988;138:1220–6.
70. Staples CA. Computed tomography in the evaluation of benign asbestos-related disorders. Radiol Clin North Am 1992;30:1191–207.
71. Stark P, Jacobson F, Shaffer K. Standard imaging in silicosis and coal worker's pneumoconiosis. Radiol Clin North Am 1992;30:1147–54.
72. Stephens M, Gibbs AR, Pooley FD, Wagner JC. Asbestos induced diffuse pleural fibrosis: pathology and mineralogy. Thorax 1987;42:583–8.
73. Tinkle S, Kittle L, Schwitters PW, Addison JR, Newman LS. Beryllium stimulates release of T helper 1 cytokines interleukin-2 and interferon gamma from BAL cells in chronic beryllium disease. Chest 1996;109:5S–6S.
74. Trulock EP. Lung transplantation. Am J Respir Crit Care Med 1997;155:789–818.
75. Vallyathan NV, Craighead JE. Pulmonary pathology in workers exposed to nonasbestiform talc. Hum Pathol 1981;12:28–35.
76. Wagner GR. Asbestosis and silicosis. Lancet 1997;349:1311–5.
77. Wagner JC, Pooley FD, Gibbs A, Lyons J, Sheers G, Moncrieff CB. Inhalation of china stone and china clay dusts: relationship between the mineralogy of dust retained in the lungs and pathological changes. Thorax 1986;41:190–6.
78. Ward S, Heyneman LE, Reittner P, Kazerooni EA, Godwin JD, Müller NL. Talcosis associated with IV abuse of oral medications: CT findings. AJR Am J Roentgenol 2000;174:789–93.
79. Williams WJ, Wallach ER. Laser microprobe mass spectrometry (LAMMS) analysis of beryllium, sarcoidosis, and other granulomatous diseases. Sarcoidosis 1989;6:111–7.
80. Wright JL, Churg A. Morphology of small-airway lesions in patients with asbestos exposure. Hum Pathol 1984;15:68–74.
81. Zeren EH, Colby TV, Roggli VL. Silica-induced pleural disease: an unusual case mimicking malignant mesothelioma. Chest 1997;112:1436–8.

17
MISCELLANEOUS DISEASES OF UNCERTAIN ETIOLOGY

INTRODUCTION

A variety of miscellaneous non-neoplastic lesions occur in the lung. In this chaper we review inflammatory pseudotumor, hyalinizing granuloma, amyloidosis, light chain disease, metastatic calcification, dystrophic pulmonary ossification, tracheobronchopathia osteochondroplastica, endometriosis, bronchial inflammatory polyp, and inborn errors of metabolism (Gaucher's disease, Niemann-Pick disease, Fabry's disease, Hermansky-Pudlak syndrome, Marfan's syndrome, and Ehlers-Danlos syndrome).

INFLAMMATORY PSEUDOTUMOR (INFLAMMATORY MYOFIBROBLASTIC TUMOR)

Definition. Inflammatory pseudotumor of lung consists of a spectrum of fibroblastic and myofibroblastic cellular proliferations that contain a varying infiltrate of chronic inflammatory cells, including plasma cells, lymphocytes, macrophages with or without giant cells, and foamy macrophages (167). The lesions are typically well demarcated, usually solitary, and destroy and replace the underlying lung tissue. They range from a primarily myofibroblastic or fibroxanthomatous appearance to one that has a heavy infiltrate of plasma cells (167). Sclerosed or predominantly fibrotic pseudotumors are also seen.

There have been many synonyms for this lesion, reflecting the evolving knowledge of the component cell types and theories of pathogenesis. Among them are *postinflammatory tumor, histiocytoma, xanthofibroma, xanthoma* and *xanthogranuloma, sclerosing hemangioma* (a misnomer), *plasma cell granuloma,* and *mast cell granuloma.* The term *inflammatory myofibroblastic tumor* has recently become popular (32,33,136), since it reflects the latest ultrastructural and immunohistochemical evidence of the principal cell type in these lesions. We will therefore use this as an equivalent term in this text. The histologic overlap of inflammatory pseudotumors (IPT)/inflammatory myofibroblastic tumors (IMT) led Spencer (154) to suggest the term *plasma cell granuloma-histiocytoma complex,* but this is not frequently used, probably because plasma cell granuloma is a misleading term.

Clinical Features. IPT is found most frequently in the lung, but histologically similar lesions occur in virtually all major organs as well as the retroperitoneum, mesentery, mediastinum, dura, and abdominal cavity (33,74). Patients with pulmonary lesions vary greatly in age, ranging from 1 to 77 years; however, about 60 percent are under 40 years of age and the average age is about 30 years (15,115,136). In fact, IPT is reported to account for the majority of benign lung "tumors" in children (34). There is no sex predilection (115).

Most patients are asymptomatic, and the lesion is discovered incidentally on chest radiography; however, they can present with cough, fever, chest pain, or hemoptysis. Sputum and biopsy cultures usually fail to show organisms. In most instances, the lesion is diagnosed by resection, but in 30 percent of cases the diagnosis is made by bronchoscopic biopsy (124).

Radiologic Findings. IPT typically manifests radiographically as a solitary peripheral pulmonary nodule or mass (fig. 17-1, top). Most lesions have well-defined lobular borders, but the borders can be irregular or ill-defined (fig. 17-1). Endoluminal airway involvement occurs in 10 percent of cases (2,9). Involvement of mediastinal or hilar structures and multifocal lesions have been described (2,22,28). Intralesional calcification occurs in about 15 percent of cases (fig. 17-2). Computed tomography (CT) typically demonstrates a well-circumscribed, lobulated, solitary nodule or mass (fig. 17-1, bottom). The lesion may be homogeneous or heterogeneous (fig. 17-2). It is usually of heterogeneous attenuation or enhancement after contrast administration (fig. 17-3). Calcification is best demonstrated on CT and is characterized as punctate, dense, curvilinear, or flocculent (fig. 17-2). Magnetic resonance imaging (MRI) shows a heterogeneous lesion of intermediate signal intensity on T1-weighted images and of high signal intensity on T2-weighted images. The most important differential diagnostic consideration

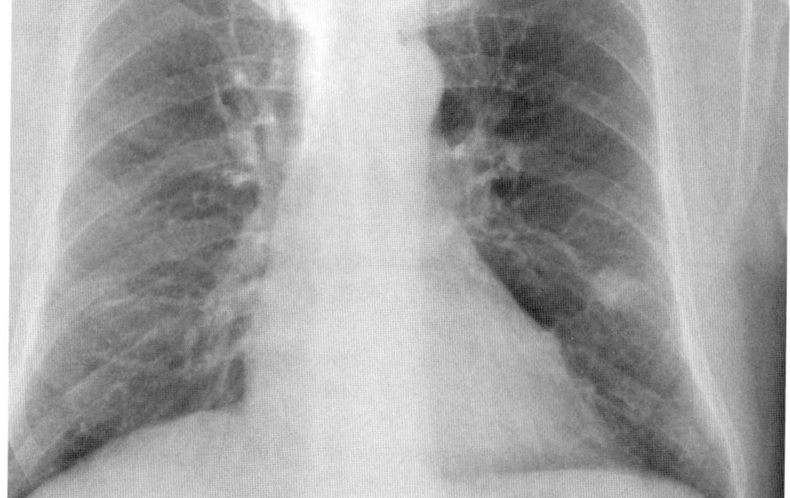

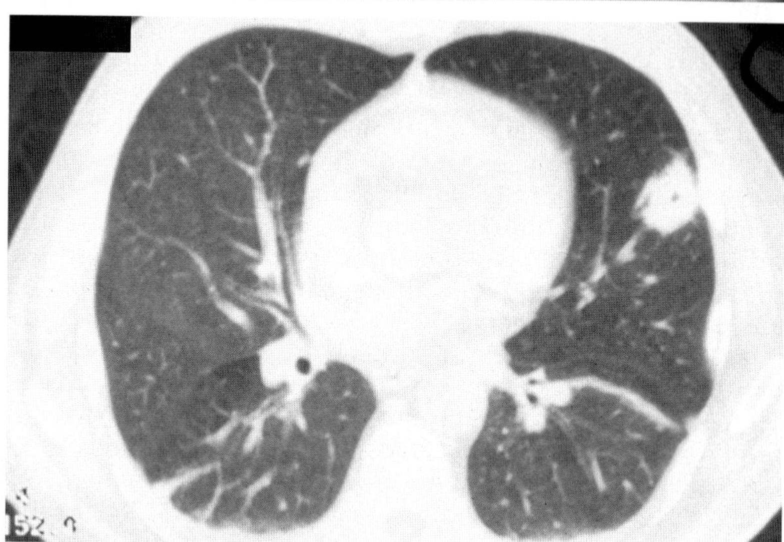

Figure 17-1

INFLAMMATORY PSEUDOTUMOR

The patient was an asymptomatic 64-year-old man with a 75 pack/year history of smoking and a history of prior melanoma and prostatic carcinoma.

Top: Posteroanterior (PA) chest radiograph demonstrates a 2.4-cm left upper lobe mass with irregular borders.

Bottom: Chest CT (lung window) demonstrates a lobular left upper lobe mass with a central focus of cavitation.

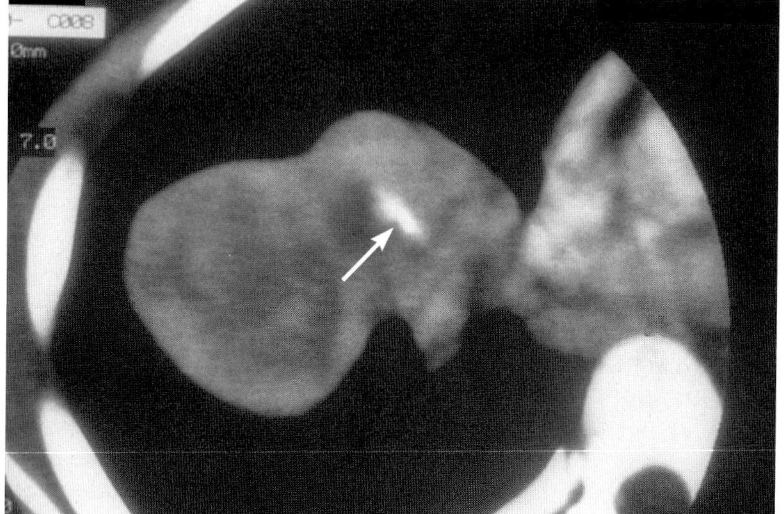

Figure 17-2

INFLAMMATORY PSEUDOTUMOR

The patient was a 14-year-old boy with a history of repeated respiratory infection. Contrast-enhanced chest CT demonstrates a lobular mass of heterogeneous enhancement with central low attenuation and focal linear calcification (arrow).

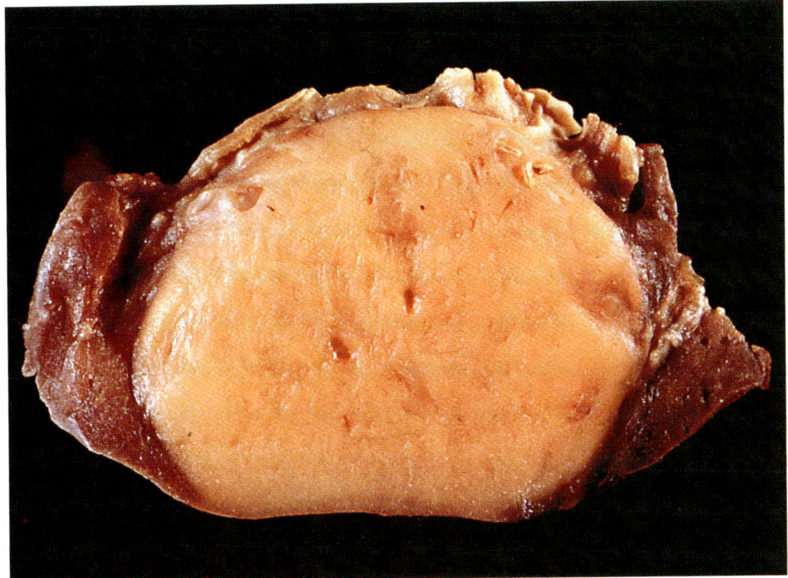

Figure 17-3

INFLAMMATORY PSEUDOTUMOR: GROSS SPECIMEN

This lesion is a fibroxanthoma that is rich in lipid, imparting a distinctly yellow color. Note the sharp demarcation from the surrounding lung.

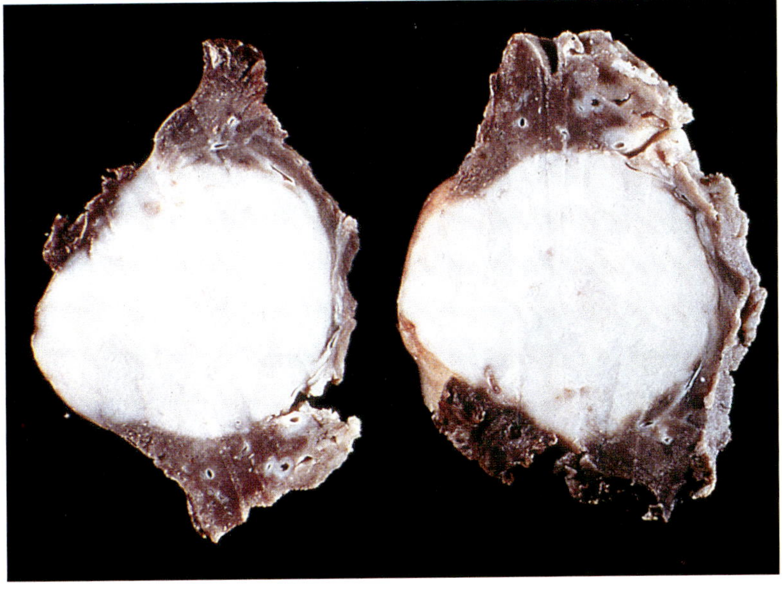

Figure 17-4

INFLAMMATORY PSEUDOTUMOR: GROSS SPECIMEN

The lesion showed abundant fibrous tissue, which is responsible for the white color. Note the sharp circumscription.

in adults who present with IPT is primary lung cancer (2,9).

Gross Findings. The lesions are typically well-circumscribed, solitary, round or ovoid intrapulmonary masses measuring 1 to 6 cm in diameter (136), but they can be as large as 36 cm (15). In about 12 percent of cases, they occur as polypoid endobronchial lesions (115). Grossly, they penetrate the pleura; 6 percent of cases extend into adjacent mediastinal structures.

The color of these lesions varies with their histologic composition: yellow is associated with abundant lipid and numerous xanthoma cells (fig. 17-3), tan with large numbers of plasma cells and lymphocytes, and white with abundant fibrous connective tissue (fig. 17-4). There may be red or brown foci, indicating recent or old hemorrhage (115). Up to 10 percent of cases show calcification and minute foci of necrosis.

Histologic Findings. Microscopically, IPT manifests as a mass consisting of a mixture of chronic inflammatory cells, particularly plasma cells, lymphocytes, macrophages, a few eosinophils, and fibroblasts, as well as fibrous connective

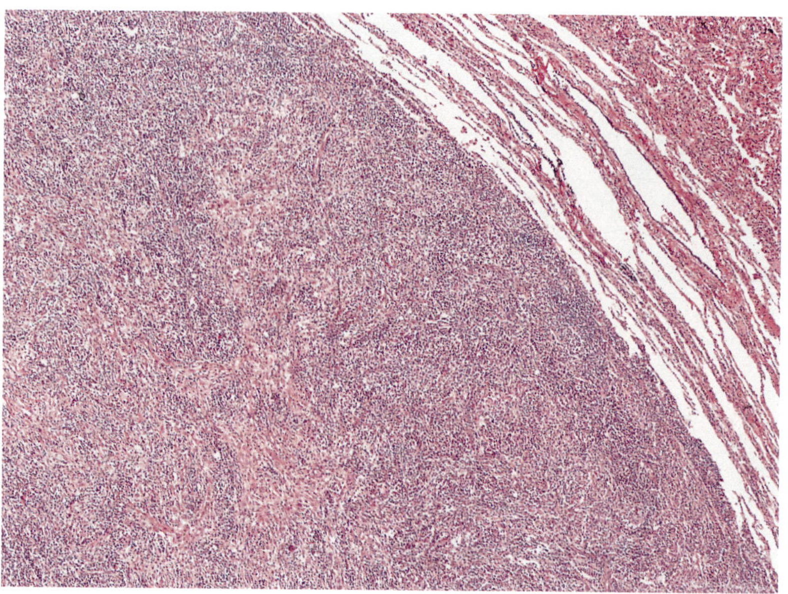

Figure 17-5

INFLAMMATORY PSEUDOTUMOR

The alveolar architecture within the lesion is obliterated, a characteristic finding in these lesions. Note the sharp circumscription from the surrounding lung.

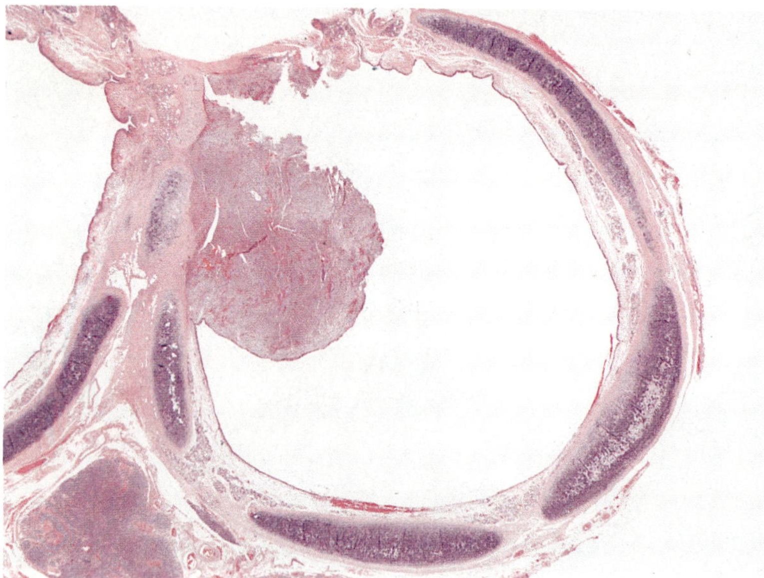

Figure 17-6

ENDOBRONCHIAL INFLAMMATORY PSEUDOTUMOR

The lesion protrudes into the lumen of a bronchus as a broad-based polyp. (Courtesy of Drs. Nancy Warner and Yan-Ling Ma, Los Angeles, CA.)

tissue (fig. 17-5) (15,115,154,167). While there may be preservation of the alveolar architecture, with organizing pneumonia at the margin of the lesion, within the lesion itself there is destruction of the normal alveolar parenchyma and replacement by the inflammatory tissue (fig. 17-5) (115). When endobronchial lesions occur, they are typically polypoid and may or may not extend beyond the bronchial wall (fig.17-6).

As noted above, IPT can show a fibrohistiocytic pattern, which consists of spindled cells (myofibroblasts and fibroblasts) arrayed in a storiform pattern, admixed macrophages, foamy macrophages, multinucleated Touton-type giant cells, lymphocytes, and plasma cells (figs. 17-7–17-9) (115,165). There may be osseous metaplasia and calcification. Mitoses are infrequent. A myxoid stroma may be prominent (28). The lipid found in the fibroxanthomatous lesions contains ethanolamine and N-acetyl neuraminic acid, which is endogenous in origin (fig. 17-9) (107,177).

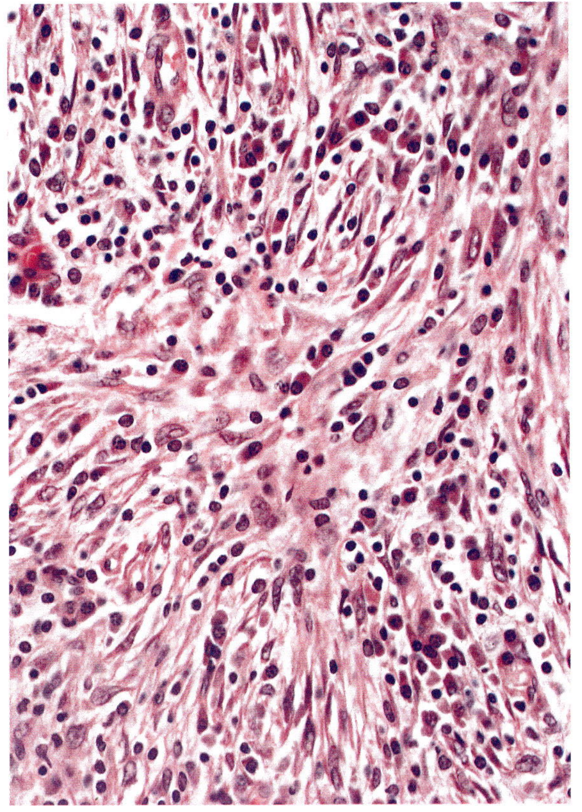

Figure 17-7

INFLAMMATORY PSEUDOTUMOR, FIBROHISTIOCYTIC TYPE

The lesion consists of benign spindle cells (predominantly myofibroblasts) with a storiform (pinwheel) pattern of growth and admixed lymphocytes and plasma cells.

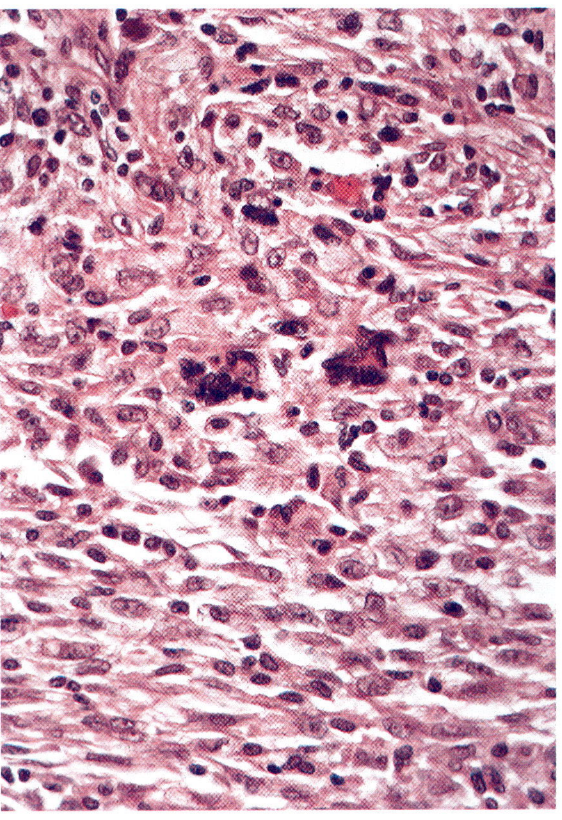

Figure 17-8

INFLAMMATORY PSEUDOTUMOR, FIBROHISTIOCYTIC TYPE

The benign spindle cells (myofibroblasts) are admixed with multinucleated giant cells and lymphocytes.

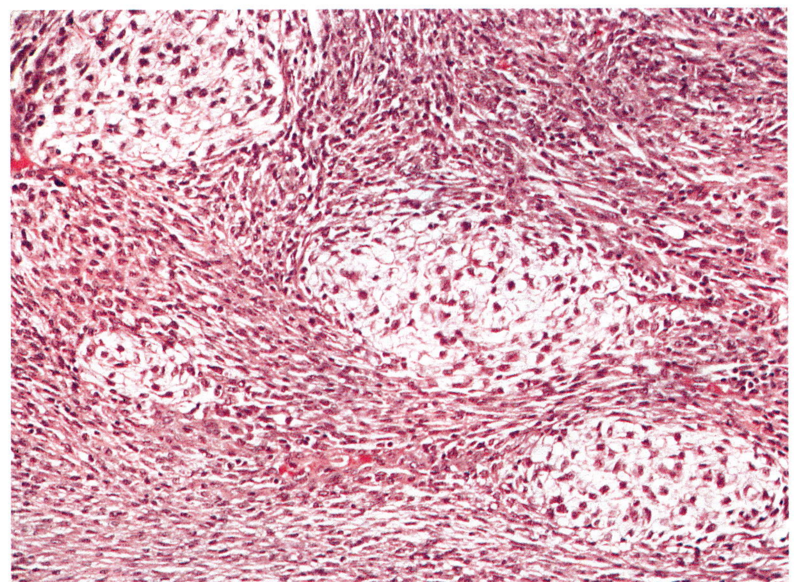

Figure 17-9

INFLAMMATORY PSEUDOTUMOR, FIBROHISTIOCYTIC TYPE

Multiple foci of xanthoma cells are present in addition to the distinctive spindled myofibroblastic cell population of this lesion.

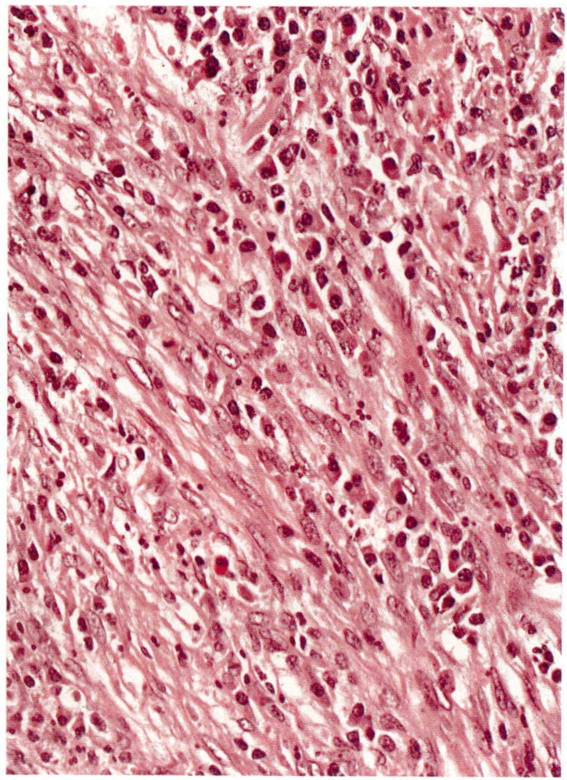

Figure 17-10

INFLAMMATORY PSEUDOTUMOR

There are numerous plasma cells interspersed among fascicles of spindled myofibroblastic cells, a feature that led to the use of the term "plasma cell granuloma" to describe such a lesion.

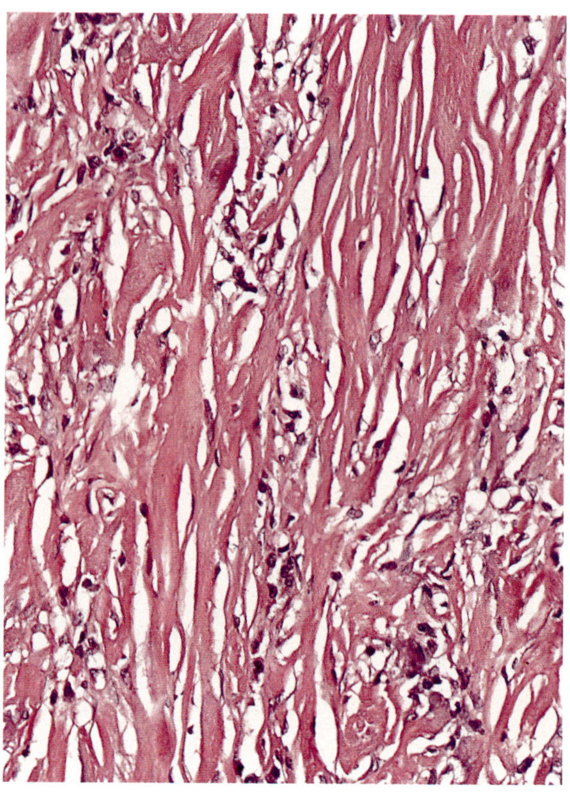

Figure 17-11

INFLAMMATORY PSEUDOTUMOR WITH EXTENSIVE FIBROSIS

The lesion shows extensive fibrosis. It may have demonstrated fibrohistiocytic or "plasma cell granuloma" features earlier in the clinical course. (Figure 19-10 from Fascicle 13, 3rd Series, Atlas of Tumor Pathology.)

IPT can also show spindled fibroblasts and myofibroblasts arranged in fascicles or files, rather than in a pinwheel or cartwheel pattern, and there may be abundant plasma cells. The latter feature led to the term, plasma cell granuloma (fig. 17-10). This term is to be avoided because of the incorrect inferences that may be drawn from the word "granuloma." A mixture of inflammatory cells, including numerous lymphocytes, foamy macrophages, eosinophils, and significant numbers of mast cells can be found. Granulomas and neutrophils are usually inconspicuous or absent (115).

While fibrous connective tissue is a component of most IPTs, largely sclerotic or fibrosed lesions do occur (fig. 17-11). Matsubara and colleagues (115) introduced the concept of an organizing pneumonia type of IPT. It is true that on occasion focal organizing pneumonias show central destruction of alveolar architecture, simulating pseudotumor (115). However, these pneumonias characteristically have numerous intra-alveolar plugs of fibrous connective tissue (Masson bodies). Destruction of alveoli is particularly likely to follow a pneumonia that is complicated by a postpneumonic abscess with consequent scarring. Thus, if the bulk of the lesion shows preservation of alveoli or if a central abscess is present, it is probably best viewed as organizing pneumonia. Still, these pneumonias with central fibrosis provide evidence that pneumonias might evolve to IPT.

Coffin and associates (33) have used somewhat different terms to describe the microscopic patterns of IPT (Table 17-1). These include a

Table 17-1

HISTOLOGIC SUBTYPES OF INFLAMMATORY PSEUDOTUMOR[a]

Fibrohistiocytic: spindled cells (myofibroblasts and fibroblasts) arrayed in a storiform pattern with admixed macrophages, xanthoma cells, Touton giant cells, lymphocytes, and plasma cells	**Compact spindle cell pattern:** spindle cells arrayed in either storiform or fascicular arrays with admixed plasma cells, eosinophils, and lymphoid cells; includes fibrohistiocytic and plasma granuloma subtypes
Plasma cell granuloma: spindled cells arrayed in a fascicular pattern with abundant plasma cells and lymphocytes	**Hypocellular fibrous type:** dense collagen with sparse spindle cells and a mixture of chronic inflammatory cells and eosinophils
Largely sclerosed or fibrosed: collagenized stroma	**Myxoid/vascular pattern:** spindle, polygonal, or stellate myofibroblasts arrayed in an abundant myxoid edematous stroma

[a]Data from reference 32.

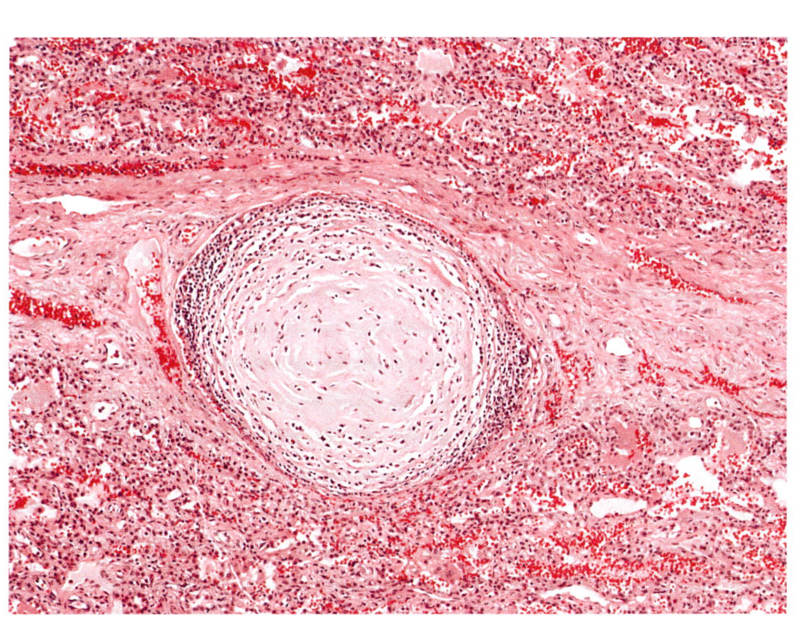

Figure 17-12

INFLAMMATORY PSEUDOTUMOR SHOWING VASCULAR INVASION

Invasion of pulmonary vessels distant from the main mass, as in this example, is relatively infrequent, and should raise the possibility of low-grade fibrosarcoma.

compact spindle cell pattern (akin to the fibrohistiocytic and plasma cell–rich patterns described above), in which spindle cells are arrayed in either storiform or fascicular arrays with admixed plasma cells, eosinophils, and lymphoid cells. There is also a hypocellular fibrous pattern, characterized by dense collagen with sparse spindle cells and a mixture of chronic inflammatory cells and eosinophils. Finally, they report a myxoid/vascular pattern, in which there are spindle, polygonal, or stellate myofibroblasts arrayed in an abundant myxoid edematous stroma.

Small foci of coagulative necrosis have been found in up to 15 percent of cases of IPT (115). Eosinophils may be present in the tissue adjacent to these areas, but neutrophils or abscess-like necrosis argues against IPT and for a postpneumonic abscess, as noted above.

IPT can invade incorporated or contiguous small vessels, particularly veins (fig. 17-12). Invasion of pulmonary vessels distant from the main mass also occurs, but this is rare. In one case, extension of a purported IPT into large pulmonary veins and pericardium led to the patient's death (174).

IPT can also invade pleura (110), chest wall (128), hilum, spine (71), and mediastinum (31). In these cases, the lesions may show cellularity or cytologic atypia, raising the possibility of a low-grade fibrosarcoma. Still, there is no single histologic feature that accurately predicts prognosis.

The spindle cells of IPT are decorated by antibodies to vimentin and often muscle-specific actin. Some cases show focal desmin staining. This pattern of reactivity is in keeping with a myofibroblastic immunophenotype (136). Cytokeratin may be present, but it is probably due to staining of residual entrapped pneumocytes. Lysozyme and alpha-1-antichymotrypsin are observed in macrophages. They can be prominent when xanthoma cells are abundant. The plasma cells are typically polyclonal (12,136,174).

A consistent electron microscopic finding is the presence of numerous myofibroblasts, fibroblasts, and cells intermediate between the two, as well as admixed lymphocytes, plasma cells, macrophages, and entrapped pneumocytes (22, 28,98,147). There are also small vessels containing endothelial cells and pericytes (22).

Cytologic studies of IPT are few, and preoperative diagnosis is rare. One lesion, apparently of fibrohistiocytic subtype, was reached with a bronchial brush. The resulting smears showed short, spindle cells with basophilic cytoplasm and enlarged, mildly atypical, oval nuclei (170). These cells were initially interpreted as epithelioid histiocytes, but in retrospect they appeared to have a storiform pattern.

Fine-needle aspiration biopsies show a mixture of histiocytes, fibroblasts, lymphocytes, and plasma cells (10,108). These findings are not specific; they can be seen in many types of inflammatory lesions. Also, they do not exclude a malignant neoplasm. In this situation, immunohistochemical staining may help in the differential diagnosis (10). In general, fine-needle aspiration is more useful for diagnosing malignant neoplasms than benign lesions, and surgical biopsy remains the most accurate method of diagnosing IPT.

Etiology and Pathogenesis. From the first discovery of IPT, its etiology has been a subject of contention. The initial presumption was that these lesions were reactive processes of inflammatory origin. Certainly, the finding of morphologically compatible cases in extrapulmonary and respiratory tract locations, associated with infectious agents such as *Campylobacter jejuni, Actinomyces,* mycobacteria, and even *Histoplasma* (in patients with acquired immunodeficiency syndrome [AIDS]) lends support to an infectious etiology (30). Further, many adults and some children have a history of respiratory infection, which is of interest in view of the argument that these lesions are reparative processes responding to an initial insult.

Two studies, using immunohistochemistry and reverse transcriptase–polymerase chain reaction, have shown local production of the interleukins (IL)-1ß, IL-6, and IL-8 (a neutrophil attractant) and monocyte chemoattractant protein-1 (a monocyte attractant) within IPTs (139,146). These results confirm the local production of cytokines and raise the possibility that a problem in cytokine regulation produces the disease.

DNA flow cytometry and cytogenetic studies provide intriguing results about the histogenesis of IPT (32). In one report, flow cytometry was done on nine pediatric patients with pseudotumors (17). Four lesions had aneuploid (hyperdiploid) indices, in keeping with a possible neoplastic process. Of these four patients, one had local recurrence and two had distant metastases, and both of the latter died. No definite histologic features separated these cases from the others. In a more recent study, cytogenetic analysis of an inflammatory myoblastic tumor of lung showed the abnormal karyotype 47, XX+r(ring) (157). Finally, clonal abnormalities in t(1:2)(q21; p23) and del(4)(q27) were found in another pseudotumor (153). While these studies suggest that at least some IPTs are actually low-grade mesenchymal neoplasms, the number of cases studied is small. Further, these cases may be more indicative of the difficulty of separating IPTs histologically from low-grade malignant neoplasms, particularly inflammatory fibrosarcoma, which can mimic them (see Differential Diagnosis). Additional clonality and cytogenetic studies on histologically typical IPTs are needed.

Differential Diagnosis. The microscopic resemblance of lesions with a storiform histologic pattern to fibrous histiocytoma of the soft tissues, as well as occasional instances of recurrence, raises the possibility that some of these lesions are tumors, either benign or malignant. This problem is highlighted by Spencer's report of two cases of "inflammatory pseudotumor" that had foci suggestive of malignant fibrous histiocytoma (154). From our own experience (59) and that of others (41,147), there appears to be a small group of fibrohistiocytic lesions (given such names as atypical fibrohistiocytic proliferations, "borderline" lesions, or fibrous histiocytomas) whose precise histogenesis and biologic potential are difficult to judge. Unlike classic IPT, they lack intermixed lymphocytes and plasma cells, they show focal increased cellularity or poor histologic circumscription, and they have focal necrosis, demonstrate increased mitoses (up to 2 per 50 high-power fields), or invade blood vessels (41,59,147). The small number of patients reported to date have had a benign course, but additional experience is necessary to determine their ultimate prognosis. We view these lesions as fibrohistiocytic lesions of uncertain prognosis.

If a fibrohistiocytic lesion has a storiform pattern of growth, nuclear hyperchromatism and pleomorphism, bizarre multinucleated cells, necrosis of greater than 15 percent of the tumor, and frequent mitoses (more than 3 per 50 high-power fields), it is best termed malignant fibrous histiocytoma (MFH) (59,183). MFH usually metastasizes to lung from sites in the soft tissues, but on rare occasion, it arises as a primary tumor in the lung (160,183). It typically manifests as a solitary large mass. Immunohistochemical staining for p53 may be of value in separating sarcomas, including MFH, from IPT. In one small study, 4 of 6 pulmonary sarcomas showed nuclear staining for p53, while 0 of 8 IPTs stained (100).

Wick and associates (145,178) reported 3 cases of "inflammatory sarcomatoid carcinoma of lung" and compared them to 10 IPTs. The carcinomas occurred in smokers 44 to 64 years of age, and they appeared as peripheral upper lobe masses in the lung. Histologically, these sarcomatoid carcinomas were relatively bland spindle cell proliferations with storiform and fascicular arrays, admixed plasma cells and lymphocytes, and foci of keloid-like fibrous connective tissue, suggesting pseudotumor. Still, they often had at least a partially myxoid stroma, lacked xanthoma cells, had small foci of epithelioid cells (in 2 of the 3 cases), showed intrabronchial or extravascular spread, had occasional foci of necrosis, and had at least some mitoses (2 or fewer per 10 high-power fields). Importantly, they stained uniformly with antibodies to keratin or epithelial membrane antigen, and this appears to be the best way to distinguish the two lesions (126,134,178).

An important tumor to consider is inflammatory fibrosarcoma (117,118). This neoplasm was originally described in the mesentery or retroperitoneum of children and young adults. It can affect the lung, extend into the parenchyma of adjacent organs, and lead to the death of the patient. Histologically, it is a low-grade sarcoma composed of fascicles or whorls of fibroblastic and myofibroblastic cells, with admixed plasma cells and variable amounts of collagen (figs. 17-13, 17-14). Mitoses are rare, but the spindle cells show significant nuclear atypia. We have now encountered a few cases in the lung and mediastinum. They can be very difficult to distinguish histologically from IPT. A cellular, fascicular growth pattern, nuclear atypia, or invasive growth into larger vessels and through pleura should alert one to this tumor. We suspect that a number of IPTs that show aggressive behavior, as well as some of those demonstrating flow and cytogenetic abnormalities, are actually inflammatory fibrosarcomas.

The term "invasive fibrous tumor of the tracheobronchial tree" describes a spindle cell fibroblastic tumor that involves the major bronchi and trachea (161). Histologically, this tumor consists of fibroblast-like cells growing in fascicles with a focal storiform pattern, slight or moderate nuclear atypia, enlarged nucleoli, occasional multinucleated cells, and mitotic counts of less than 2 per 10 high-power fields. Reportedly, it differs from IPT in the absence of an inflammatory component, i.e., xanthoma cells or an intimately admixed lymphoplasmacytic infiltrate.

Extramedullary plasmacytomas are neoplastic proliferations of plasma cells occurring outside of bone. They are exceedingly rare in lung, and more commonly involve the head and neck (94). Still, they may enter into the differential diagnosis, particularly when only small biopsy fragments or fine needle aspirates are available (80). Microscopically, extramedullary plasmacytomas consist largely of plasma cells

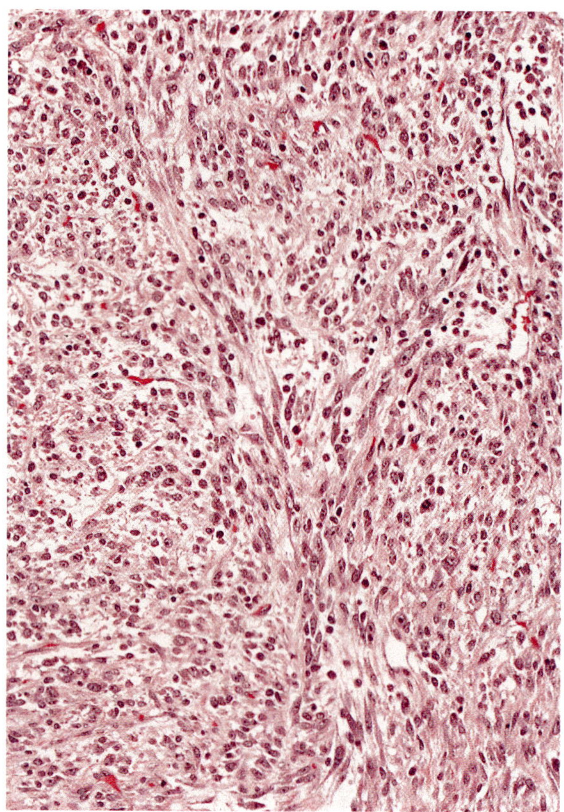

Figure 17-13

DIFFERENTIAL DIAGNOSIS OF INFLAMMATORY PSEUDOTUMOR: INFLAMMATORY FIBROSARCOMA

The low-power appearance of this lesion mimics inflammatory pseudotumor, with short fascicles of spindle cells and a sprinkling of admixed lymphocytes.

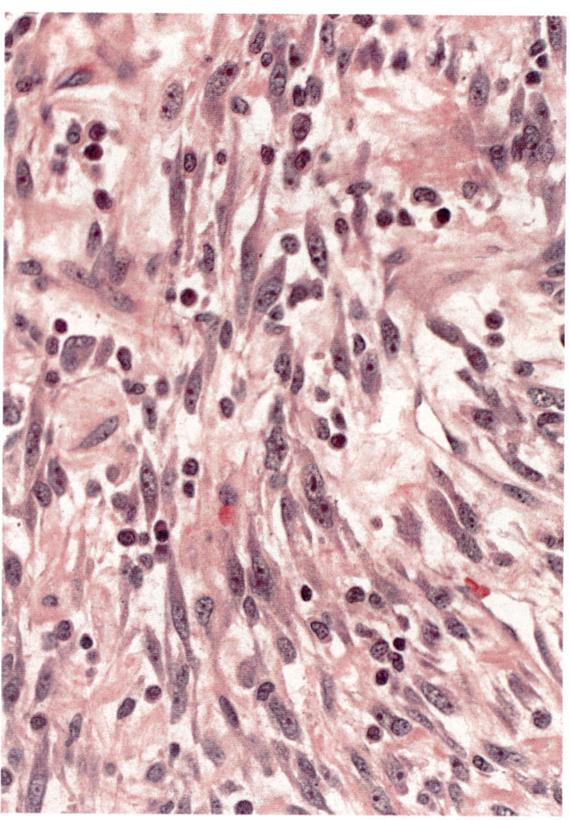

Figure 17-14

DIFFERENTIAL DIAGNOSIS OF INFLAMMATORY PSEUDOTUMOR: INFLAMMATORY FIBROSARCOMA

At higher magnification, the spindled fibroblastic cells show greater nuclear atypia than is seen in inflammatory pseudotumor.

that show nuclear pleomorphism, abundant mitoses, scant fibrous stroma, and a monoclonal pattern of staining for immunoglobulin light chains, features not seen in IPT (94).

On the reactive side, a spindle cell and storiform appearance can, rarely, occur with infections. The problem of distinguishing organizing pneumonias from IPT has been discussed above. In immunosuppressed patients, infection by the mycobacteria *Campylobacter, Actinomyces,* and *Histoplasma* can sometimes produce one or more nodules composed of spindle cells with foamy macrophages. Special bacterial or fungal stains usually demonstrate numerous organisms within macrophages (30,151,169). In nonimmunosuppressed patients, Q fever can produce a pulmonary mass composed of a mixture of monocytic cells, simulating IPT (105).

Treatment and Prognosis. Most cases of IPT are both diagnosed and cured by surgical resection. There remains argument about the extent of surgery. Conservative surgery in the form of segmental resection of peripheral lesions or sleeve resection of endobronchial nodules is favored by some (119). There are even reports of biopsy followed by spontaneous and long-term disappearance of the lesion (111,115). Still, Warter and associates (174), based on their experience of regional spread of IPT in some of their cases, suggested "radical and precocious" surgical resection. In our view, the best approach is one in which there is complete excision, with a reasonably wide margin of uninvolved tissue. Corticosteroids can be tried and may be effective in some cases in which, because of location, residual lesion is left after initial treatment (48).

The prognosis of patients with completely resected lesions is excellent: between 78 and 100 percent are alive and well after average follow-up of 3.3 years (9,15,174). Most IPTs remain constant in size or shrink, but 10 percent grow slowly over years (9,15), or even enlarge rapidly (56). Intrathoracic recurrence is seen in 5 percent of cases (9,15). As noted above, this usually occurs when a wide margin of excision is not obtained, as when a lesion is shelled out or when an endobronchial lesion is resected with a narrow margin of normal tissue. Aggressive lesions that extend into parietal pleura, chest wall, or mediastinum, or that invade pulmonary veins may become unresectable or recur months to years later, leading to the death of the patient (25,27,56,79,83,109,128,154,174). There are reports of metachronous development of "pseudotumors" in extrapulmonary sites, such as brain, ipsilateral pleural cavity, and contralateral lung, but these probably represent low-grade inflammatory fibrosarcomas that have metastasized (27).

One other point raised by Copin et al. (37) is that an initial small biopsy may show IPT, but that on rare occasion other lesions, such as carcinoma, can be present in association, so that complete resection is necessary for a final diagnosis.

PULMONARY HYALINIZING GRANULOMA

Definition. Pulmonary hyalinizing granulomas are nodules consisting of lamellar hyaline collagen (167). The nodules may be solitary or multiple; their etiology is unknown. The term granuloma is a misnomer, since epithelioid cells and giant cells are not intrinsic components.

Clinical Features. In one series of solitary necrotizing granulomas of lung, about 2 percent were termed hyalinizing granuloma (168), but the disease is probably less frequent. In fact, by 1991, only 62 cases had been reported (52, 75,102,184).

The patients average 45 years of age. They usually have symptoms, such as cough, dyspnea, chest pain, or hemoptysis, but 25 percent are asymptomatic (52,184).

Hyalinizing granuloma can occur in association with other sclerosing diseases. Sclerosing mediastinitis occurs in about 20 percent of cases, while retroperitoneal fibrosis is found in 8 percent (26,184). One patient had a combination of constrictive pericarditis, retroperitoneal fibrosis, mediastinal fibrosis, fibrosis of peritoneal and pleural surfaces, fibrosis of the soft tissues, and fibrosis of the hilus of the liver (97). Riedel's thyroiditis can occur (167). These diseases may precede, occur at the same time, or occasionally follow the onset of pulmonary lesions (167). Individual cases have also been reported in association with multiple sclerosis (77) and Castleman's disease (8).

Radiologic Findings. Pulmonary hyalinizing granuloma manifests radiographically as multiple or solitary pulmonary nodules with well-defined borders, ranging in size from 2 to 4 cm (fig. 17-15, left). Calcification and cavitation have been described (fig. 17-15, right) (58). When multifocal nodules are present, the differential diagnostic considerations include primary or metastatic neoplasia, granulomatous disease, vasculitis, and infection (75,135).

Gross Findings. The lung contains intrapulmonary, often subpleural, firm, well-circumscribed nodules measuring 0.2 to 9.0 cm (fig. 17-16). They are white or gray and are infrequently cystic (75). Rare hyalinizing lesions are reported in unusual sites, such as the kidney and tonsil (26,184).

Histologic Findings. Microscopically, the lesions are reasonably well circumscribed (fig. 17-17). They consist of thick, lamellar bands of collagen (fig. 17-18). The collagen is arranged in a whorled or concentric pattern around small blood vessels (fig. 17-19). Large blood vessels within the nodule may be completely obliterated (fig. 17-20). Scattered plasma cells and lymphocytes are present, more so at the margin of the nodules (fig. 17-21). There may also be scattered macrophages and a few multinucleated giant cells, neutrophils, or eosinophils, but no epithelioid granulomas are seen. Broad areas of necrosis are rare; they suggest fungal or bacterial infection (150,184). Factitious staining with Congo red can occur. Electron microscopic studies show that the stained material in these lesions is electron-dense, homogeneous, and amorphous, amid swollen collagen fibrils rather than amyloid (46,52,67,150).

Etiology and Pathogenesis. Neither the etiology nor the pathogenesis of hyalinizing granuloma is known. Possibly, a chronic immune reaction to endogenous or exogenous antigens or

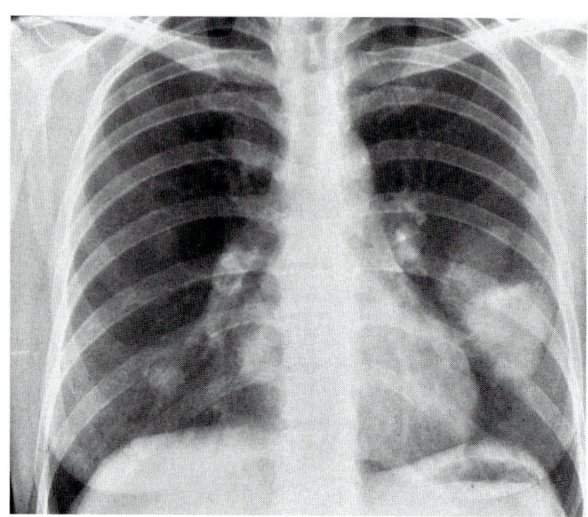
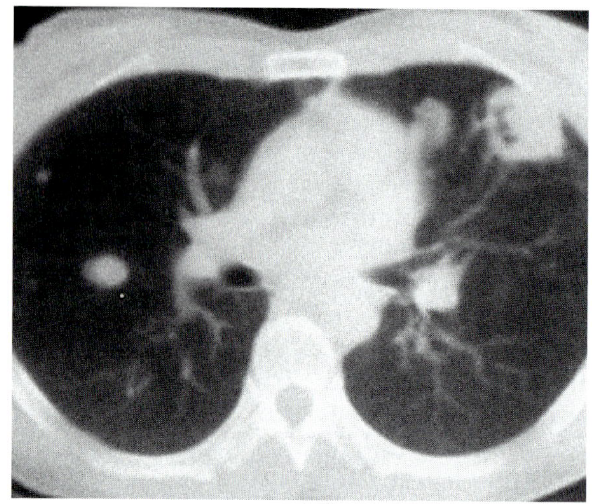

Figure 17-15

PULMONARY HYALINIZING GRANULOMA IN AN ASYMPTOMATIC 40-YEAR-OLD WOMAN

Left: PA chest radiograph demonstrates multiple pulmonary masses of spherical and lobular contours, located predominantly in the lower lung zones.

Right: Chest CT (lung window) demonstrates bilateral, multifocal, spherical and lobular nodules and masses. Note the presence of cavitation in one of the lesions in the left upper lobe.

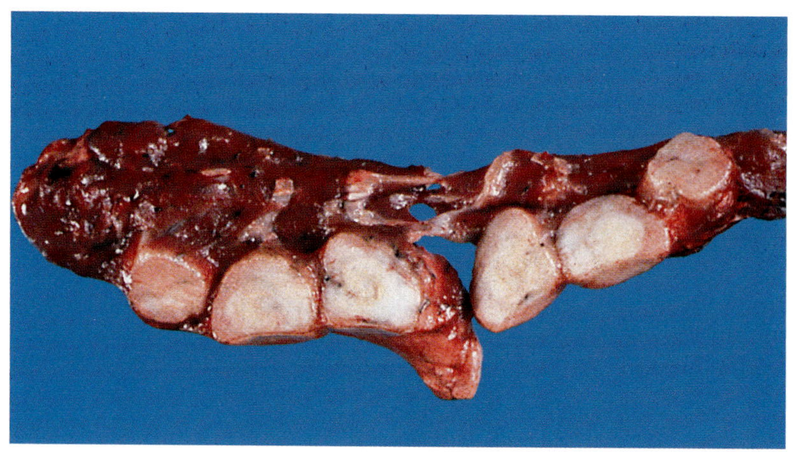

Figure 17-16

PULMONARY HYALINIZING GRANULOMA

The typical gross appearance of this lesion is in the form of multiple, subpleural, white nodules.

infectious agents (such as *Histoplasma capsulatum* or mycobacteria) occurs in an individual predisposed to marked scar formation (112,184). Pulmonary hyalinizing granuloma is not only histologically similar to sclerosing mediastinitis, but the two diseases can even occur together. They may, therefore, have a common pathogenesis (112). Sclerosing mediastinitis can occur in association with histoplasmosis or tuberculosis and may result from an exaggerated immunologic response to these organisms. The same may be true for pulmonary hyalinizing granuloma. Rarely, patients with hyalinizing granuloma show healed histoplasmosis prior to the development of hyalinizing granuloma (26), and we have also seen rare cases in which *Histoplasma* granulomas and hyalinizing granulomas occur synchronously. However, documented exposure or lesions of fungi or tuberculosis are present in only a subset of patients (52,135,184).

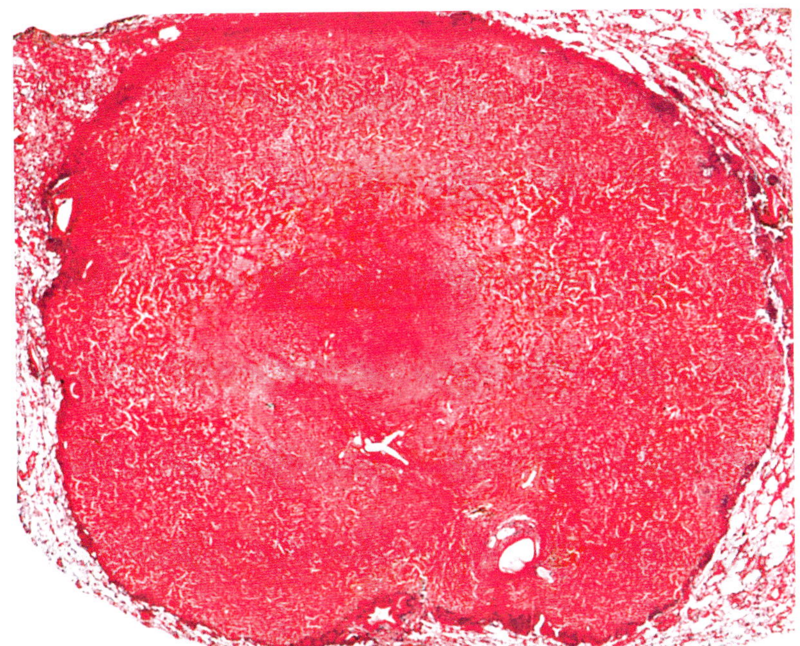

Figure 17-17

PULMONARY HYALINIZING GRANULOMA

In this low magnification view, the lesion obliterates the underlying lung architecture and appears well circumscribed. Small lymphoid aggregates are present at the edge of the lesion.

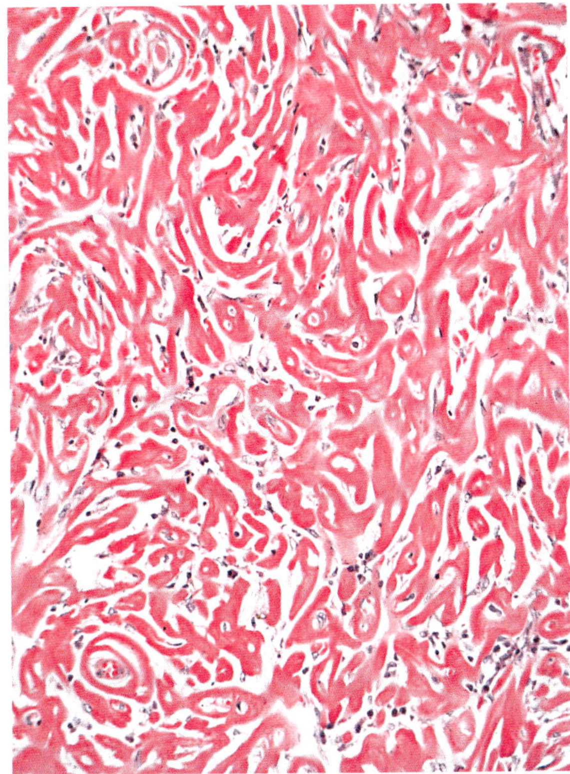

Figure 17-18

PULMONARY HYALINIZING GRANULOMA

The characteristic ropy or lamellar hyaline collagen is arrayed in a whorled or storiform fashion.

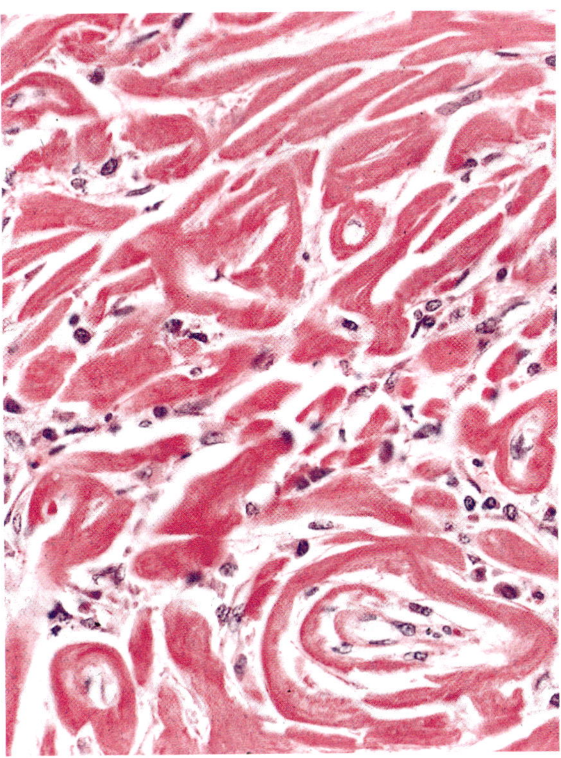

Figure 17-19

PULMONARY HYALINIZING GRANULOMA

Higher magnification shows the thick collagen bundles that are concentrically layered around small blood vessels, along with a scattering of interspersed mononuclear cells (principally lymphocytes and plasma cells).

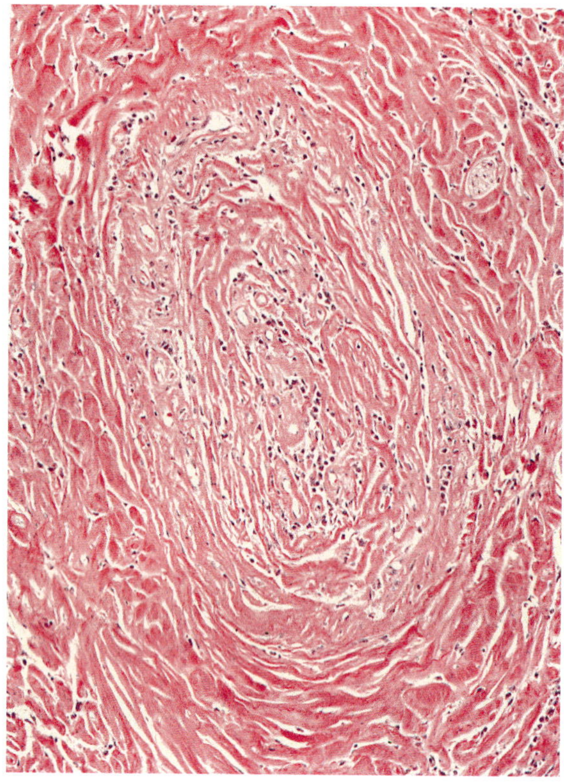

Figure 17-20

LARGE BLOOD VESSEL IN PULMONARY HYALINIZING GRANULOMA

The vascular lumen is obliterated by concentrically arrayed fibrous tissue.

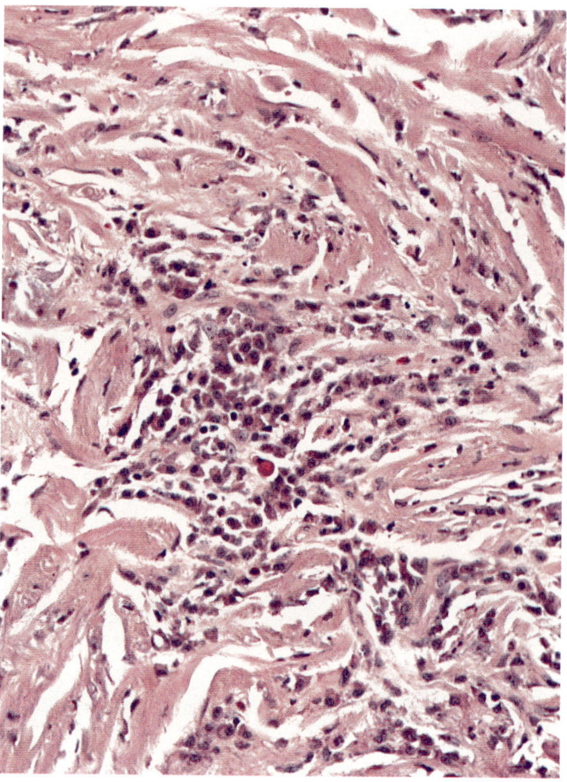

Figure 17-21

PULMONARY HYALINIZING GRANULOMA

Chronic inflammatory cell infiltrates are usually scant in these lesions, but they may be more prominent toward the periphery of the lesion, as seen here.

There is evidence of autoimmunity in the form of elevated titers to antinuclear, anti-smooth muscle, antimicrosomal, and antithyroglobulin antibodies and increased levels of rheumatoid factor in 60 percent of patients (46, 97,150,184). Whether autoimmunity is a preexisting or predisposing factor or occurs subsequent to the onset of the disease is unclear. One patient had hypergammaglobulinemia, with markedly elevated immunoglobulin E (82), while a second had antineutrophil cytoplasmic antibody (63).

Differential Diagnosis. It has been suggested that some cases of hyalinizing granuloma may be fibrotic IPTs (see fig. 17-11) (184). There are some differences. IPTs, unlike hyalinizing granulomas, are usually solitary. They also show a more diffuse infiltrate of plasma cells and lymphocytes, and they usually lack the lamellar collagen typical of hyalinizing granuloma.

Intrapulmonary fibrous tumors are the intrapulmonary analogues of localized fibrous tumors of the pleura. They are solitary rather than multiple, and subpleural rather than of diverse location. Further, intrapulmonary fibrous tumors are more cellular, lack a lymphoid infiltrate, show a variety of histologic patterns including storiform or hemangiopericytoma-like, and stain diffusely with CD34 and bcl-2, as opposed to hyalinizing granuloma.

Nodular amyloidosis has a smudgier appearance microscopically, does not show the extensive lamellar collagenous bands of hyalinizing granuloma, and has more foreign body giant cells (see Amyloidosis, this chapter). As noted above, on occasion, hyalinizing granulomas may be overstained with Congo red, leading to a false diagnosis of amyloidosis, but electron microscopy shows that hyalinizing granuloma lacks the typical fibrillar substructure of amyloid.

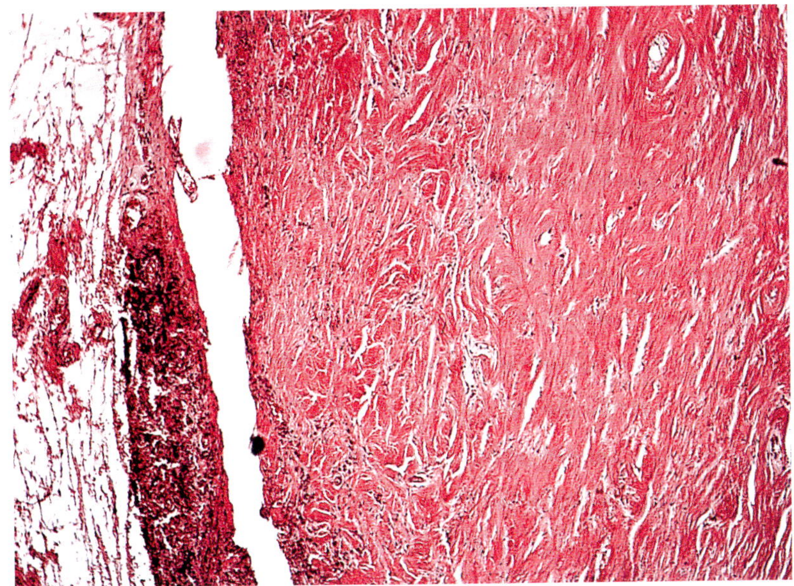

Figure 17-22

SCLEROSING MEDIASTINITIS

A mass composed of dense eosinophilic collagen is external to the lung (left).

Infectious granulomas, especially those of histoplasmosis, may show hyaline fibrosis, but the collagen bundles are generally arrayed in parallel around areas of central necrosis rather than distributed in a haphazard manner as in hyalinizing granuloma. The presence of necrotizing granulomatous inflammation favors infection, as does the finding of calcified hilar lymph nodes. Nevertheless, distinguishing between the two diseases may be difficult and, as noted above, we have seen examples of hyalinizing granuloma in which a small satellite focus of necrotizing granuloma is present, suggesting that *Histoplasma* or some other infectious agent may initiate hyalinizing granulomas (135).

Pulmonary hyalinizing granuloma can be histologically similar to sclerosing mediastinitis (figs. 17-22, 17-23). Hyalinizing granuloma is intrapulmonary, while sclerosing mediastinitis affects the mediastinum or hilus and only secondarily invades lung.

Treatment and Prognosis. There is no effective therapy, but prognosis is still quite good. Patients have been followed up to 28 years with stable or slowly enlarging nodules. Radiologic progression may sometimes be accompanied by increasing dyspnea. Rarely, coalescent nodules lead to respiratory insufficiency. When mediastinal or retroperitoneal sclerosis occurs concurrently with hyalinizing granuloma, there can be entrapment of vessels and airways, with resultant ischemic and obstructive findings (26,52).

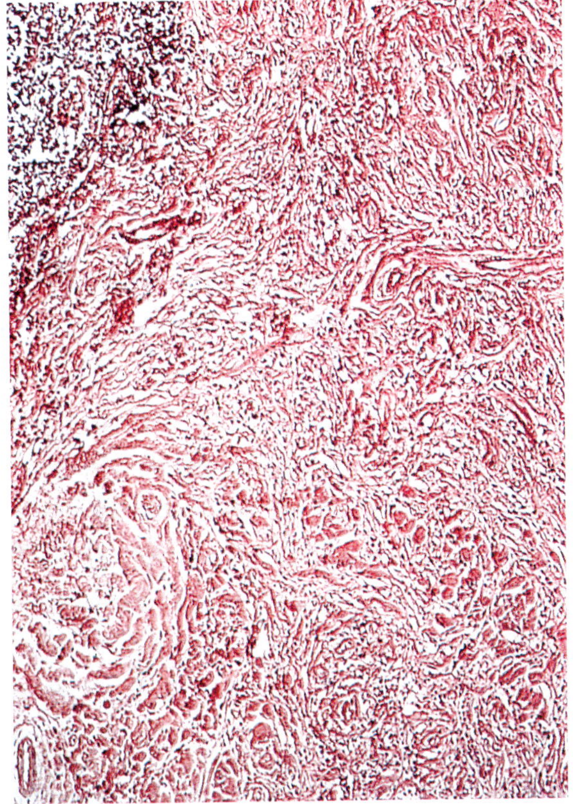

Figure 17-23

SCLEROSING MEDIASTINITIS

This lesion is composed of ropy collagen, similar to that seen in pulmonary hyalinizing granuloma.

Table 17-2

AMYLOIDOSIS OF THE LOWER RESPIRATORY TRACT[a]

Clinical Type	Biochemical Type
Generalized Amyloidosis	
Idiopathic (primary) amyloidosis, associated with myeloma or macroglobulinemia	AL
Reactive (secondary) amyloidosis	AA
Familial Mediterranean fever	AA
Systemic senile amyloidosis	ATTR (transthyretin)
Associated with chronic dialysis	beta-2-microglobulin
Limited Amyloidosis	
Nodular: solitary, multinodular, and miliary	Mostly AL
Tracheobronchial	Mostly AL
Diffuse Alveolar Septal	Mostly AL[b]
Pleural[c]	Mostly AL

[a]Data from references 29, 53, and 90.
[b]Alveolar septal amyloidosis also occurs in the setting of systemic senile amyloidosis (137), and reactive (secondary) amyloidosis.
[c]From references 84 and 90.

PULMONARY AMYLOIDOSIS

Definition. Pulmonary amyloidosis is the accumulation of various insoluble fibrillar proteins (amyloid) in the lung. Amyloid is composed of chemically diverse protein fibrils that have in common their ability to form a twisted, beta-pleated sheet (53,61). Recent classifications have tended to link classic terms such as primary and secondary amyloidosis to their chemical make-up (Table 17-2) (53,61).

Amyloidosis can affect the lung either as a local manifestation of systemic amyloidosis or as a disease strictly localized to lung or manifesting primarily there. There are three major types of amyloid: 1) AL protein, which has an N-terminal sequence that is homologous to a portion of the variable region of an immunoglobulin light chain and occurs in primary amyloidosis and in amyloidosis associated with multiple myeloma; 2) AA protein, which has a unique N-terminal sequence of a nonimmunoglobulin protein and occurs in patients with secondary amyloidosis; and 3) transthyretin, a prealbumin molecule that has a single amino acid substitution and is associated with familial amyloid polyneuropathy.

Several types of systemic or generalized amyloidosis can affect the lung. They include secondary (AA or protein A-derived), familial, systemic senile, and beta-2-microglobulin–derived amyloidoses, but the most frequent form of systemic amyloidosis to involve lung is AL, or light chain-derived amyloid, which is the biochemical type in both myeloma-associated and primary amyloidosis.

Primary amyloidosis can be a systemic disease or localized to a specific organ such as the lung. Primary amyloidosis involves the lung in 30 to 90 percent of cases, depending on the method of analysis, with most cases discovered at autopsy. In one study, 35 of 55 patients with pulmonary amyloidosis had primary systemic amyloidosis (171). Primary amyloidosis usually produces few pulmonary symptoms, although radiologic abnormalities are common (38,53,61,88, 171). Occasionally, the pulmonary involvement is marked enough to lead to dyspnea; more often, it merely produces physiologic impairment of gas exchange. Monoclonal proteins are found in the serum or urine of 10 percent of patients with limited pulmonary amyloidosis (73).

Secondary amyloidosis can manifest in the lung as well. It does so as diffuse interstitial or multinodular disease in patients with rheumatoid arthritis, Crohn's disease, ankylosing spondylitis, tuberculosis, bronchiectasis, and familial Mediterranean fever (14,18,53,61,78,106,158). AL, or light chain–derived amyloid, can deposit in the lung in monoclonal gammopathies accompanying systemic lymphoid proliferations, for example, with IgG gammopathy (53,61,159) and Waldenstrom's macroglobulinemia with IgM gammopathy (53,60,61). In the latter disease, about 10 percent of patients develop amyloid in the lung (53,60,61).

Pulmonary hypertension is a rare manifestation of pulmonary amyloidosis associated with multiple myeloma (AL amyloidosis), visceral beta-2-microglobulin, and secondary (AA) amyloidosis associated with familial Mediterranean fever (38,53,60,61). *Senile systemic amyloidosis* is typically an incidental finding in elderly patients at autopsy (38,171).

There are three main types of limited amyloidosis that manifest primarily in the lower respiratory tract: *nodular parenchymal, tracheobronchial,* and *diffuse parenchymal* (also termed *alveolar septal*) *amyloidoses.* Rare cases of *pleural amyloidosis* manifesting either as solitary nodules or in the setting of pleural effusion have been reported, but they are too few to merit further attention here (53,61,84,90).

Clinical Features. Patients who have amyloidosis manifesting within or limited to the lung range from 27 to 82 years of age, but most are in the sixth and seventh decades of life. In one large series, the mean ages of patients with nodular parenchymal, tracheobronchial, and diffuse parenchymal amyloidosis were 54, 64, and 55 years of age, respectively (73). There is no sex predilection and no known relation to smoking.

Nodular parenchymal amyloidosis refers to a mass or tumor-like lesion consisting of amyloid deposits, generally associated with a lymphoplasmacytic infiltrate and multinucleated foreign body giant cells. Patients with nodular parenchymal amyloidosis usually present with an asymptomatic incidental finding on radiographs obtained for other reasons (16,19,45,53,61,70). Often, infection or malignancy must be excluded. About one third have a single, rounded "coin" lesion (amyloidoma). When multiple nodules are present, symptoms such as cough, hemoptysis, or pleuritic chest pain due to pleural effusion occur (29,53,61,73,179). A variety of lymphoproliferative processes, both benign and malignant, occur in lung in association with nodular parenchymal amyloidosis. The diagnosis is usually established by transthoracic needle biopsy.

In tracheobronchial amyloidosis, amyloid deposits are located primarily in the submucosa of the trachea or large bronchi, but they may extend to the level of segmental bronchi, constricting the airways (89). Tracheobronchial amyloidosis most frequently produces dyspnea, wheezing (often misdiagnosed as asthma), recurrent pneumonia, and atelectasis, which are sequelae of the narrowed airways (6,53,61,64,73,83,89,171). Stridor or hemoptysis can occur (162). The disease can also be asymptomatic. Pulmonary function tests usually show fixed obstruction (89).

Diffuse parenchymal amyloidosis occurs with either primary or secondary amyloidosis and shows diffuse or multifocal deposits in the pulmonary interstitium. Dyspnea and cough are the most common symptoms (73). Cardiac involvement (amyloid cardiomyopathy) and pulmonary vascular involvement are common.

Monoclonal proteins occur in the serum or urine of 10 percent of patients with limited pulmonary amyloidosis (16,73). In fact, a variety of lymphoproliferative processes, both benign and malignant, can also occur in the lung in association with nodular parenchymal amyloidosis. These include nodular lymphoid hyperplasia, lymphoid interstitial pneumonia, marginal zone B-cell lymphoma (MALToma), and plasmacytoma.

In many cases of pulmonary amyloidosis, the diagnosis is made at thoracotomy or autopsy. Increasingly, transbronchial biopsy is used, which one Mayo Clinic study concluded was a safe and effective technique in this setting (171). Percutaneous fine-needle aspiration biopsy may be a helpful initial procedure for diagnosis with the potential of avoiding thoracotomy, but in this situation one must maintain vigilance for the presence of an associated neoplasm with an amyloid-rich stroma (49,53,61,68,103).

Radiologic Findings. Nodular parenchymal amyloidosis of the lung typically manifests as solitary or multiple pulmonary nodules of well-defined smooth or lobular borders located in the lung periphery and lower lung zones (fig. 17-24) (171). Lesion size is variable and calcification is rarely evident radiographically (fig. 17-25). However, CT demonstrates calcification within nodules in 20 to 50 percent of cases (figs. 17-25, 17-26) (88). Cavitation is rare. The radiologic differential diagnosis includes primary and secondary neoplasia, metastatic disease, and granulomatous disease (103). Slow growth over many years has been documented (53,54,61,113,137).

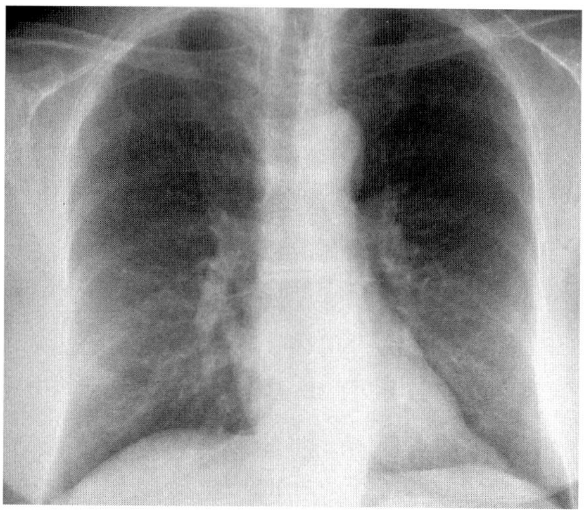

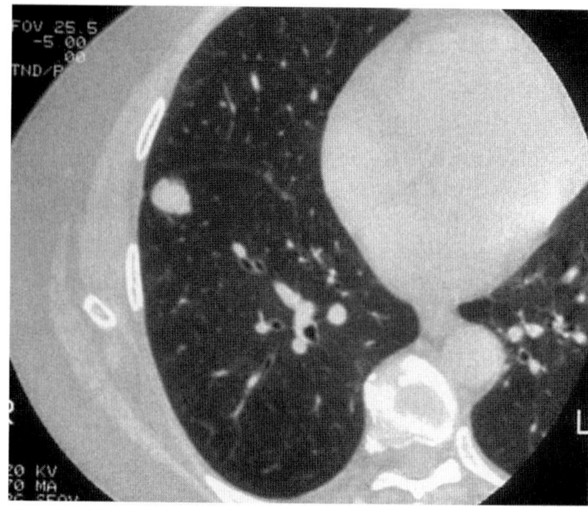

Figure 17-24

NODULAR PARENCHYMAL AMYLOIDOSIS

The patient was a 63-year-old woman with sicca syndrome, rheumatoid arthritis, and a growing right lower lobe nodule.

Left: PA chest radiograph demonstrates an ill-defined nodular opacity in the right lower lung.

Right: Chest CT (lung window) demonstrates a right lower lobe nodule of ill-defined borders. At thoracotomy, additional nodules were found, excised, and diagnosed as nodular amyloidosis.

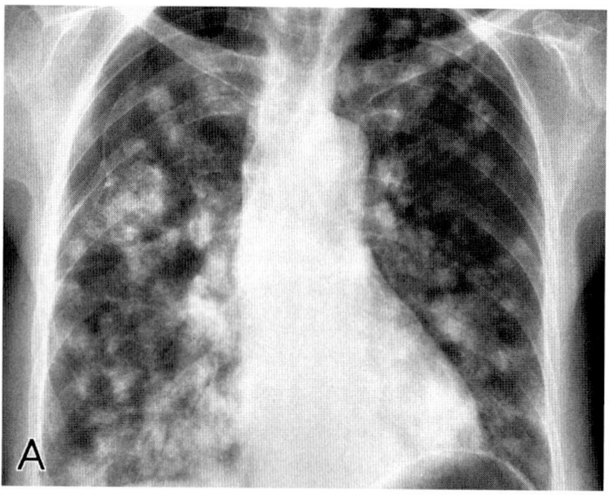

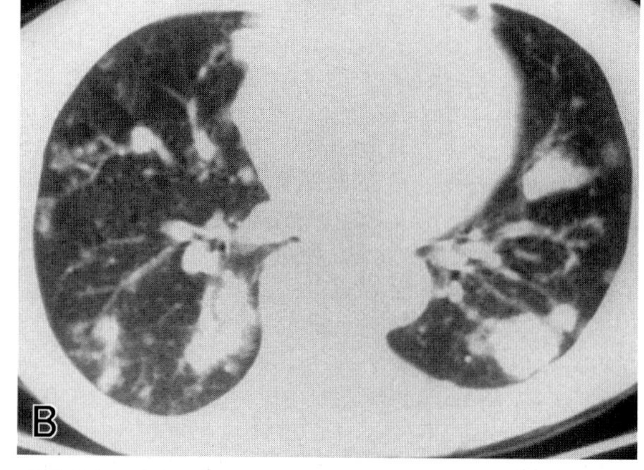

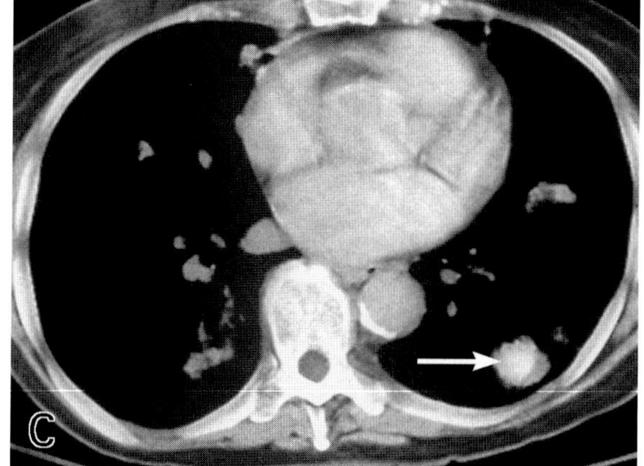

Figure 17-25

NODULAR PARENCHYMAL AMYLOIDOSIS

The patient was a 74-year-old woman evaluated for hypothyroidism.

A: PA chest radiograph demonstrates bilateral multifocal pulmonary nodules and masses.

B,C: Chest CT (lung and mediastinal window) demonstrates multifocal parenchymal masses and nodules of varying sizes. The mediastinal window (image C) shows calcification in one of the lung nodules (arrow).

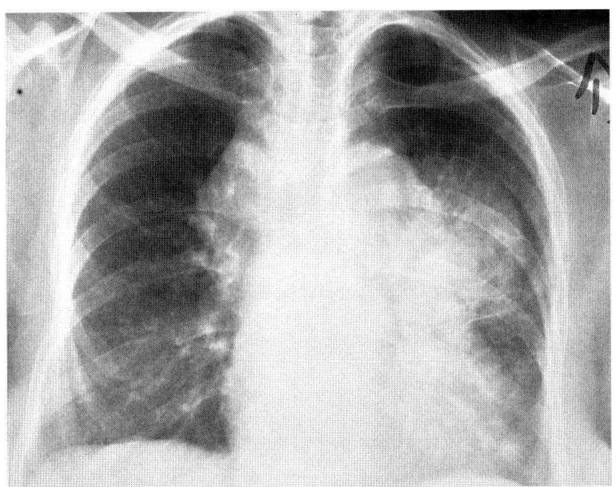

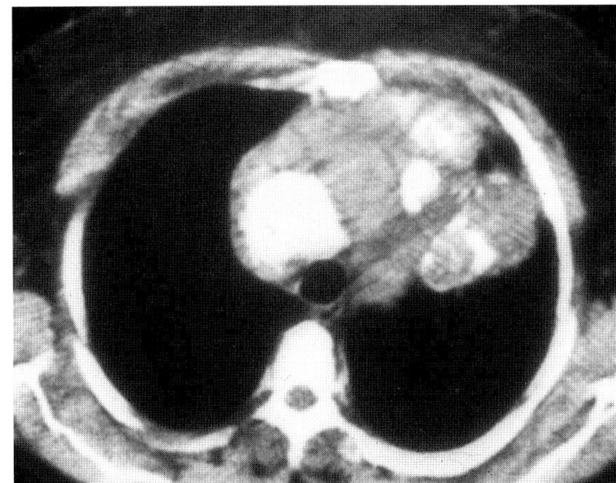

Figure 17-26

AMYLOIDOSIS

The patient was a 68-year-old woman with increasing dyspnea and a palpable neck mass.

Left: PA chest radiograph demonstrates large, lobular, mediastinal masses that extend to both sides of the midline and prominent interstitial lung markings.

Right: Unenhanced chest CT (mediastinal window) demonstrates large prevascular and paratracheal lymphadenopathy with dense calcification.

Patients with primary pulmonary amyloidosis may exhibit diffuse interstitial lung disease. This typically manifests as interstitial linear or nodular subpleural opacities that may be calcified (101,137,171).

Patients with systemic amyloidosis and lung involvement typically have both lymphadenopathy and parenchymal disease. The lymphadenopathy can be widespread and can affect hilar and mediastinal lymph nodes in the thorax (43). The enlarged lymph nodes may exhibit calcification (fig. 17-26). Parenchymal lung disease is characterized by small (less than 1.5 cm) nodules, honeycomb lung, or patchy ground-glass opacities. Thickening of the interlobular septa and irregular linear opacities also occur. These findings may be peripheral and basilar in distribution (fig. 17-27). Punctate calcification may be present within parenchymal linear and nodular opacities. Cystic changes may be demonstrated by CT in patients with associated lymphocytic infiltration

The radiologic manifestations of tracheobronchial amyloidosis include focal or diffuse thickening of the airway wall, a localized nodule within the airway lumen, and the sequelae of airway obstruction (atelectasis, postobstructive pneumonia, and overinflation of the distal lung) (89,162).

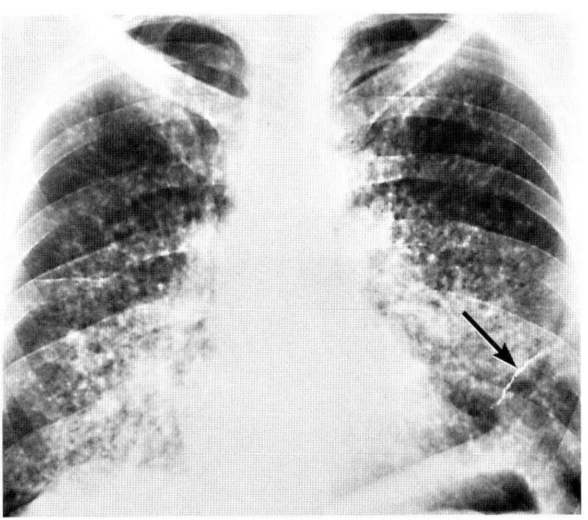

Figure 17-27

DIFFUSE PARENCHYMAL AMYLOIDOSIS

The patient was a 51-year-old man with slowly progressive dyspnea. PA chest radiograph demonstrates profuse, bilateral, nodular and reticular interstitial opacities, most numerous in the lung bases. Note evidence of prior open lung biopsy (arrow).

Gross Findings. Amyloid nodules or masses are irregular in outline and vary from 0.6 to 15.0 cm in diameter (figs. 17-28, 17-29) (73,99). They can be waxy, firm, or gritty (when calcified) in consistency, and yellow, gray, tan, or white (fig.

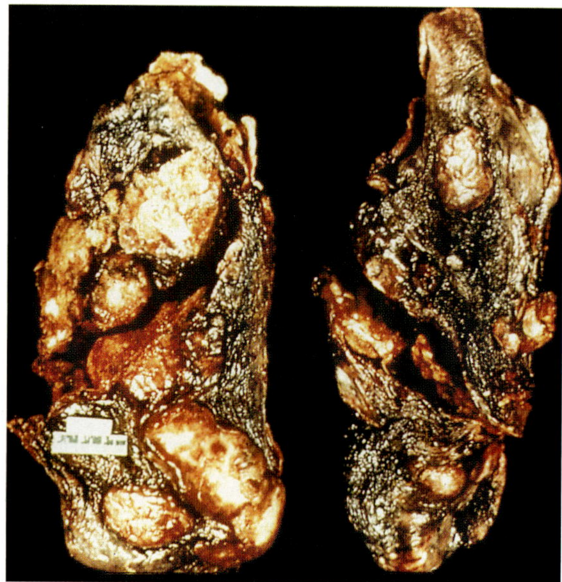

Figure 17-28

NODULAR PARENCHYMAL AMYLOIDOSIS: GROSS SPECIMEN

Bilateral, well-defined masses are present in these lungs at autopsy. (Figure 2 from Fenoglio C, Pascal RR. Nodular amyloidosis of the lungs. An unusual case associated with chronic lung disease and carcinoma of the bladder. Arch Pathol 1970;90:578.)

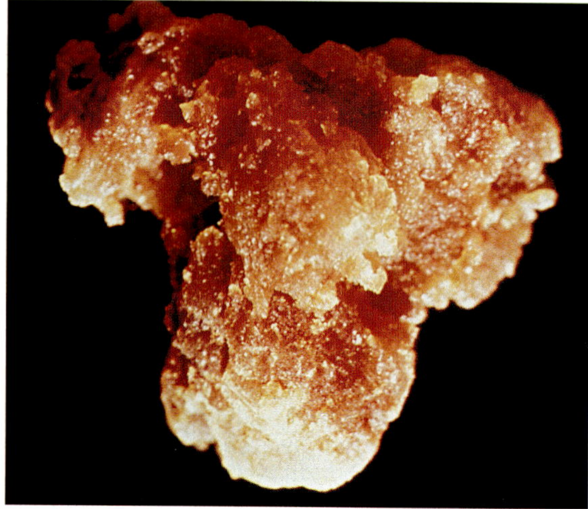

Figure 17-29

NODULAR PARENCHYMAL AMYLOIDOSIS: GROSS SPECIMEN

This nodule of amyloid was shelled out from the lung as an irregular, tan, waxy mass.

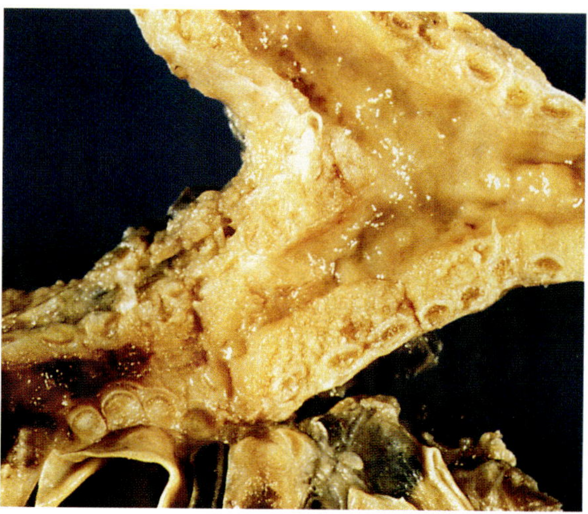

Figure 17-30

TRACHEOBRONCHIAL AMYLOIDOSIS: GROSS SPECIMEN

The cut surfaces of the tracheal and bronchial walls appear tan and thickened, while the mucosal surface of the airway shows a cobblestone appearance.

17-29) (17,18,36). In tracheobronchial amyloid, the airway wall appears thickened and irregular (fig. 17-30). The degree of involvement can be so marked as to cause nearly complete obstruction.

Histologic Findings. The usual histologic appearance of primary systemic (AL) amyloidosis involving lung is that of diffuse parenchymal disease, in which fine interstitial or vascular, amorphous, eosinophilic deposits occur (fig. 17-31). The pleura can also be involved. This appearance may be readily mistaken for interstitial fibrosis, but the interstitial chronic inflammation seen in most interstitial pneumonitides is absent. Congo red staining is very helpful in making the diagnosis.

In secondary amyloidosis involving lung, the amyloid deposits are most often restricted to blood vessels and bronchial glands; alveolar walls are infrequently involved, although there are a few reports to the contrary (140). There are also mild deposits of amyloid in senile cardiac amyloidosis, primarily in small vessels of the lung.

In limited amyloidosis of nodular parenchymal type, the normal lung is replaced by a mass of amorphous, eosinophilic, extracellular material (figs. 17-32, 17-33). The amyloid concentrically wraps around blood vessels within the deposits (figs. 17-33, 17-34). It also often involves

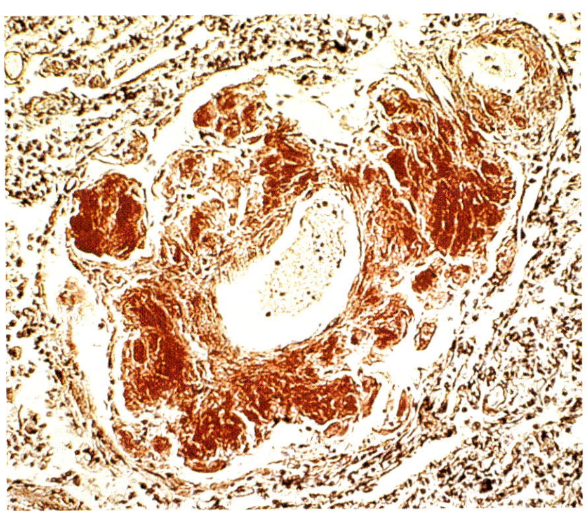

Figure 17-31

PULMONARY AMYLOIDOSIS

This view shows amorphous Congo red–positive deposits in vessel walls (Congo red stain).

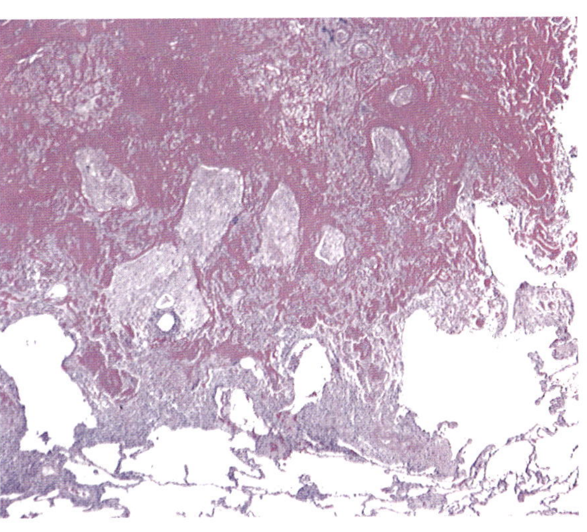

Figure 17-32

NODULAR PARENCHYMAL AMYLOIDOSIS

Low-power view shows obliteration of the pulmonary parenchyma by a solid mass that sends short tendrils into the contiguous lung.

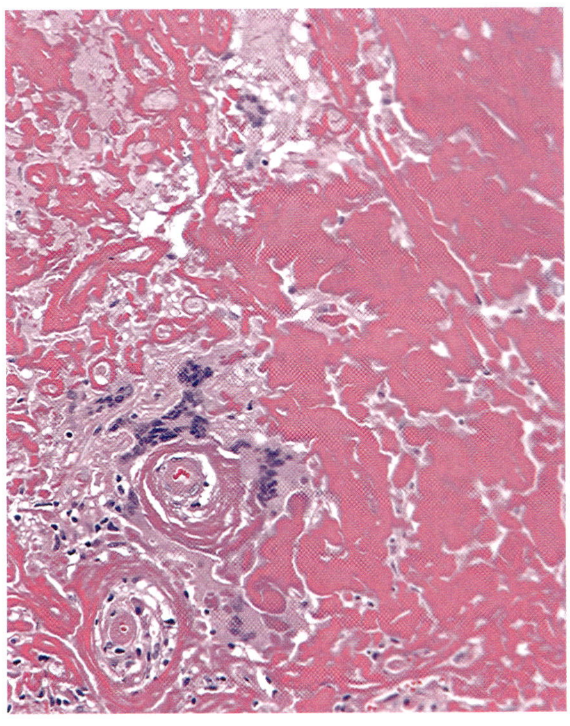

Figure 17-33

NODULAR PARENCHYMAL AMYLOIDOSIS

The amyloid consists of a solid mass of amorphous, eosinophilic, extracellular material. A multinucleated giant cell reaction is present, a typical finding in pulmonary amyloidosis. There is concentric involvement of blood vessels.

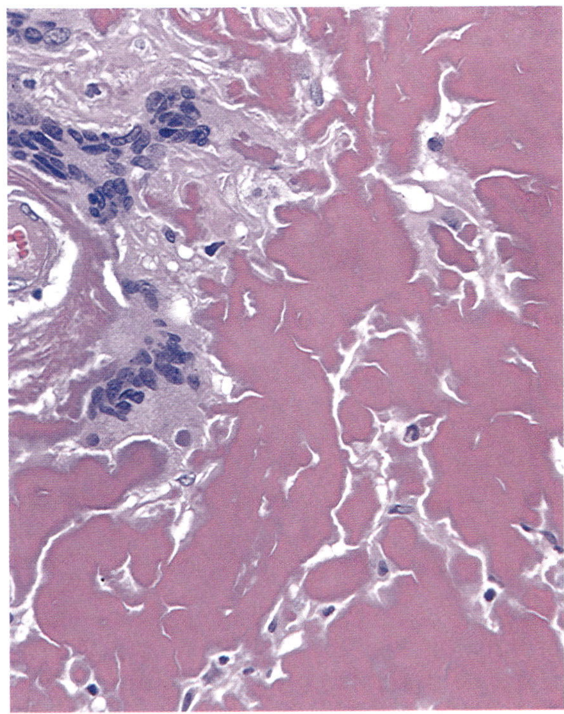

Figure 17-34

NODULAR PARENCHYMAL AMYLOIDOSIS WITH SMALL VESSEL INVOLVEMENT

In this view, the amyloid forms amorphous eosinophilic masses. Multinucleated giant cells are also seen.

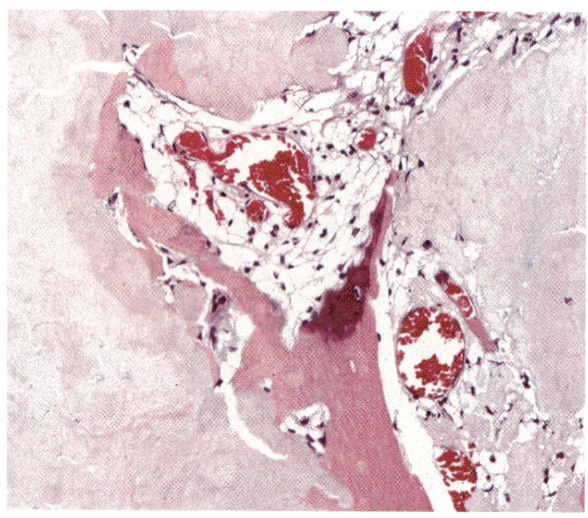

Figure 17-35

NODULAR PARENCHYMAL AMYLOIDOSIS SHOWING OSSIFICATION

Spicules of bone are adjacent to deposits of amyloidosis.

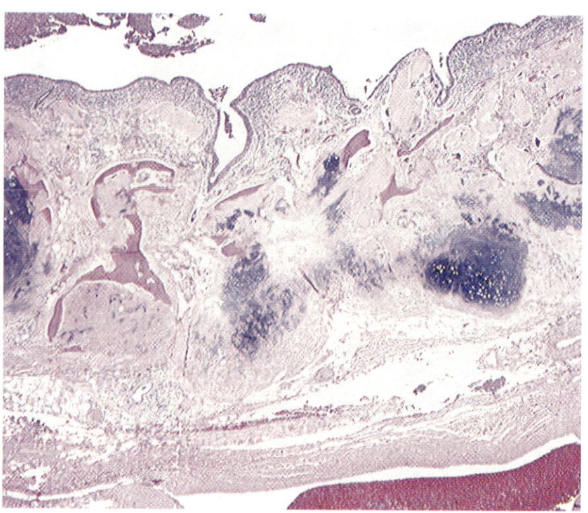

Figure 17-36

TRACHEOBRONCHIAL AMYLOIDOSIS: MICROSCOPIC VIEW

There is a diffuse sheet of eosinophilic, extracellular amorphous material, compatible with amyloid, in the bronchial submucosa. Ossification is also present.

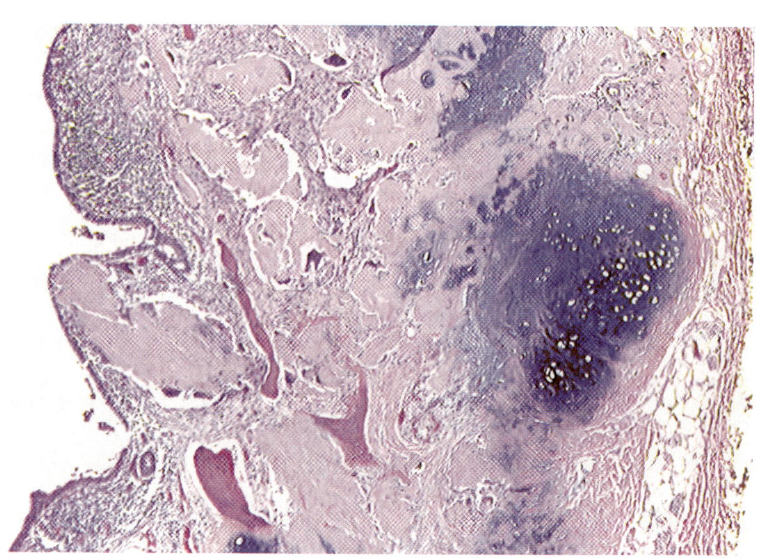

Figure 17-37

TRACHEOBRONCHIAL AMYLOIDOSIS

The amyloid appears as eosinophilic, nodular and sheet-like material involving the submucosa and small submucosal vessels. The bronchial epithelium and lumen appear to the left. Spicules of bone are also present.

the walls of small arteries and veins adjacent to the nodular deposits. Small numbers of lymphocytes, plasma cells, and multinucleated giant cells are found throughout the deposits (figs. 17-33, 17-34), but they are usually most abundant at the edge of the nodules. Calcification or ossification often occurs (figs. 17-35–17-37).

In tracheobronchial amyloidosis, the amyloid is deposited in irregular nodular masses or diffuse sheets in the tracheal or bronchial wall (figs. 17-36, 17-37) (78,166). Small submucosal vessels frequently show amyloid in their walls. Osseous metaplasia, giant cells, macrophages, and plasma cells can be present (fig. 17-38) (73,166).

Diffuse parenchymal amyloidosis manifests as diffuse, uniform, interstitial deposits; multiple small interstitial or perivascular nodules; or confluent larger nodules (fig. 17-39). Most cases show only a scant infiltrate of plasma cells

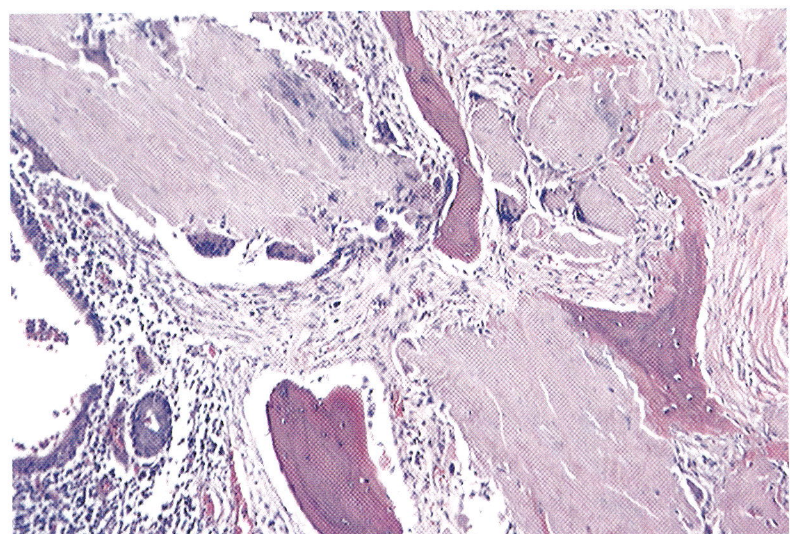

Figure 17-38

TRACHEOBRONCHIAL AMYLOIDOSIS

Amyloid appears as nodular masses surrounded by a chronic inflammatory infiltrate and multinucleated giant cells. Spicules of bone are present. The bronchial mucosa and lumen are on the left.

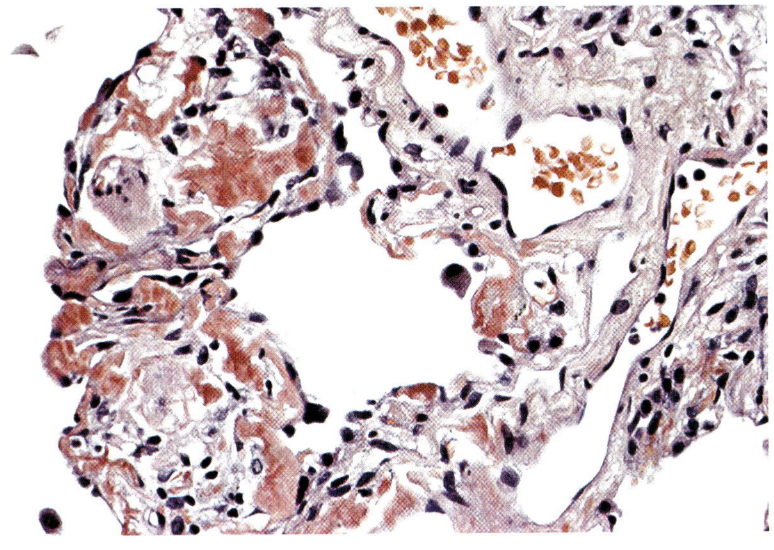

Figure 17-39

DIFFUSE PARENCHYMAL AMYLOIDOSIS

The interstitium is widened by deposition of eosinophilic, amorphous amyloid.

or giant cells, but more ample cellular infiltrates accompany the larger nodular deposits (73).

Combinations of these patterns, particularly tracheobronchial and nodular parenchymal, but even all three, occur (73,123).

When the lung is stained with Congo red and examined by polarizing microscopy, the amyloid deposits show an apple-green birefringence in most, but not all, cases (fig. 17-40). When the amyloid deposits lack or show weak birefringence, thick (12 to 15 μm) histologic sections may be needed to demonstrate them better. Antibodies to amyloid A are usually, but not always, negative. Studies with potassium permanganate oxidation usually indicate that the amyloid is of non-AA type (19,45,73,99). Electron microscopy shows nonbranching, hollow-core, 7.5 to 12.0 nm in diameter fibrils of indeterminate length arrayed in a disorderly fashion (fig. 17-41).

Etiology and Pathogenesis. The cause of amyloid production and its deposition in tissues remains unknown. Most nodular parenchymal and tracheobronchial deposits in lung appear to be light chain–derived (AL) amyloid. A light chain origin has been suggested by the finding of serum monoclonal immunoglobulins, and by biochemical evaluation, potassium permanganate oxidation, and immunohistochemical methods (39,45,53,73,121,133,166). Possibly, a localized intrapulmonary clonal proliferation of

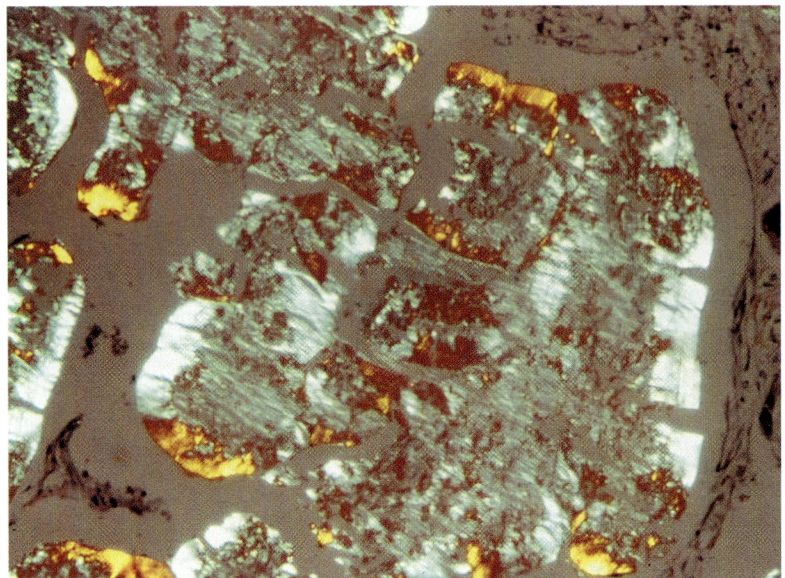

Figure 17-40

NODULAR PARENCHYMAL AMYLOIDOSIS

A Congo red–stained section viewed under polarizing microscopy demonstrates classic apple-green birefringence. This staining is sometimes hard to elicit in standard histologic sections; it may require thicker (12 to 15 μm) sections.

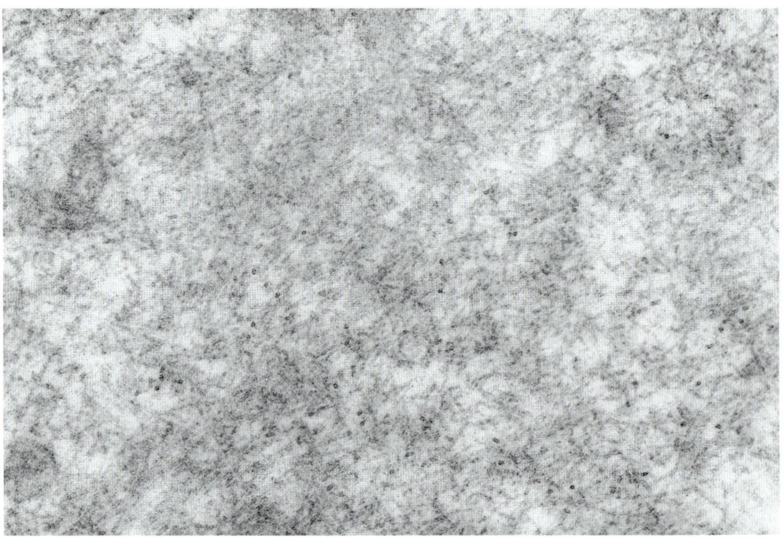

Figure 17-41

AMYLOIDOSIS

Electron micrograph shows the typical mesh of linear nonbranching fibrils measuring 8 to 10 nm in diameter. (Figure 24-9 from Fascicle 13, 3rd Series, Atlas of Tumor Pathology.)

lymphoid cells produces the amyloid deposits (133). While the plasma cells adjacent to these localized forms of amyloid are most often polytypic (53,166), there have been reports of clonally imbalanced or even monoclonal plasma cell or small lymphocytic proliferations (45,53,73,91). For example, a recent study of a patient with localized nodular parenchymal amyloidosis showed a predominance of kappa-bearing plasma cells adjacent to the amyloid nodule and a discrete, amplified, monoclonal band by polymerase chain reaction, supporting local accumulation of monoclonal plasma cells and their secreted immunoglobulin product (122). There has also been a case report of multinodular amyloidosis associated with primary pulmonary lymphoma, apparently of lymphoplasmacytic type, in which both the amyloid and the lymphoma showed a predominance of kappa light chains (89). Nodular AA amyloidosis can also be seen in patients with chronic diseases, such as Sjögren's syndrome and Crohn's disease, or even in those without an identifiable systemic disease (14,180). One interesting study found immunohistochemical staining for transthyretin, but not for amyloid AA, AL, or beta-2-microglobulin, in 6 of 11 patients with tracheobronchial amyloidosis (134).

Differential Diagnosis. Light chain deposition disease can manifest as amyloid-like pulmonary nodules (25,87,155). Light microscopy shows interstitial deposits of amorphous eosinophilic material that resembles amyloid (fig. 17-42A,B), however, these deposits do not show apple-green birefringence with the Congo-red stain. Also, rather than a fibrillar ultrastructure, the deposits of light chain disease are composed of extracellular, finely granular, electron-dense angulated (crystalloid-like) material or sinuous arrays of rounded or globular deposits (fig. 17-42C,D). Pulmonary light chain deposit disease may be nodular or diffuse, similar to amyloidosis (16,87). Light chain deposition disease is usually associated with kappa light chain deposits (16,137). Amyloid-like masses have also been reported in a pulmonary plasmacytoma, but the deposits failed to show either the histochemical or ultrastructural features of amyloidosis and consisted rather of immunoglobin (Ig)G kappa (125). Finally, light chain deposition in lung may produce in the same specimen both amyloid-like fibrillar material and finely granular material having a greater resemblance to that seen in kappa light chain disease, indicating the close relationship of these manifestations of light chain disease (155). A major differential diagnosis for tracheobronchial amyloid is tracheobroncheopathia osteoplastica which lacks amyloid deposits (see below).

Lymphoproliferative disorders as well as primary and metastatic solid neoplasms in lung can show amyloid deposits, but they are microscopic, not macroscopic, in amount. Up to 10 percent of cases of diffuse lymphoid hyperplasia (lymphocytic interstitial pneumonitis), about 3 percent of lymphoplasmacytic lymphomas, and rare cases of multiple myeloma or extramedullary plasmacytoma show amyloid deposits (93, 95,156). Typically, the amyloid is overshadowed by the lymphoid proliferation, but rarely, a full-fledged amyloidoma is present in association with a low-grade B-cell lymphoma (45).

Rarely, nonlymphoid tumors in lung show microscopic amyloid deposits. Neuroendocrine tumors, particularly carcinoids and small cell carcinomas, are the most frequent neoplasms in this group (1,4,47,50,62,144). One carcinoid tumor showed calcitonin gene-related peptide antigen in both tumor cells and amyloid stroma (1). One renal cell carcinoma metastatic to bronchus showed stromal amyloid (47), an interesting finding because of the known association of this tumor with stromal deposits of AA amyloid.

Hyalinized fibrous connective tissue in lung can produce factitious staining with Congo red in overstained sections. This is a problem that can occur in localized scars of diverse etiology and in lesions such as pulmonary hyalinizing granuloma. Usually, the stained material is green or blue with the trichrome stain and does not show convincing birefringence by polarization.

Treatment and Prognosis. Other than surgical excision of localized disease, no proven therapy exists for amyloidosis. There have been anecdotal reports of successful treatment of pulmonary amyloidosis using dimethylsulfoxide (DMSO) (76). Patients with nodular pulmonary amyloidosis generally have a benign prognosis (171). In particular, for solitary amyloid nodules, resection is both diagnostic and curative. There are exceptional reports of numerous and confluent nodules leading to respiratory insufficiency over a 10-year period (17). Lung transplantation has recently been used to treat advanced pulmonary amyloidosis (173).

Although the overall survival rate of patients with tracheobronchial amyloidosis in several series is only 31 to 43 percent at 4 to 6 years (8,173), patients with localized tracheobronchial amyloidosis may benefit from laser therapy or bronchoscopic methods for removal of deposits (162,171).

The prognosis of patients with diffuse parenchymal amyloidosis presenting with clinical symptoms is poor. In one series, the median survival period of patients with primary systemic amyloidosis affecting the lung was 16 months (171). Most patients progress to respiratory failure within 2 years, irrespective of whether disease is limited to lung or affects other organs as well (73).

METASTATIC CALCIFICATION

Definition. Metastatic calcification is the deposition of calcium salts in tissues of the lung, usually as a result of abnormalities of calcium or phosphorus metabolism.

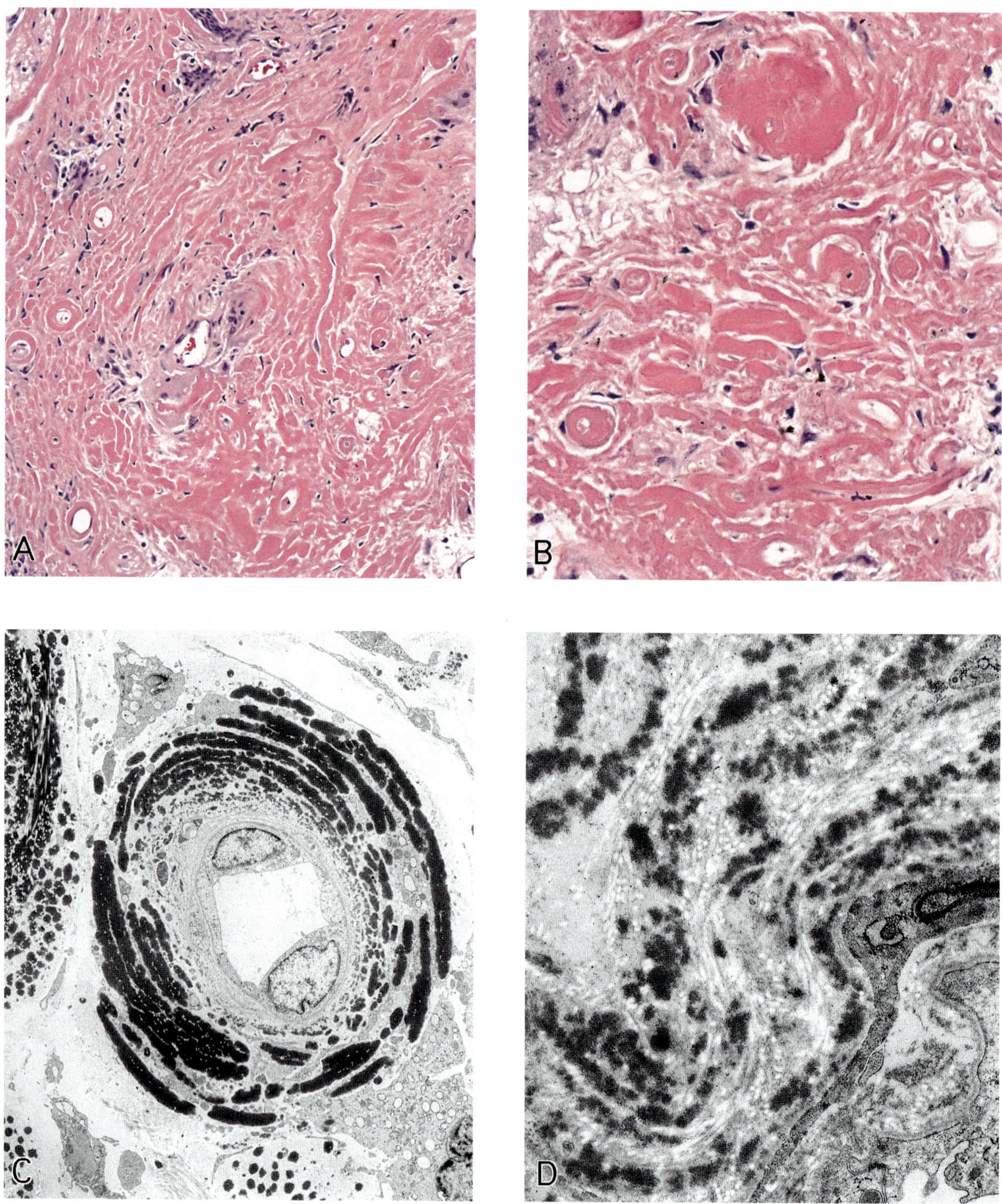

Figure 17-42

LIGHT CHAIN DEPOSITION DISEASE

A: Dense eosinophilic deposits expand the interstitium.

B: The deposits are amorphous, similar to those of amyloidosis.

C: Pulmonary capillary shows granular electron-dense deposits in the wall, in adventitia, and around myointimal cells.

D: In a wall of a small capillary are coarse granular electron-dense deposits. The capillary lumen is at the top left. (Courtesy of Dr. Sharda G. Sabnis, Armed Forces Institute of Pathology.)

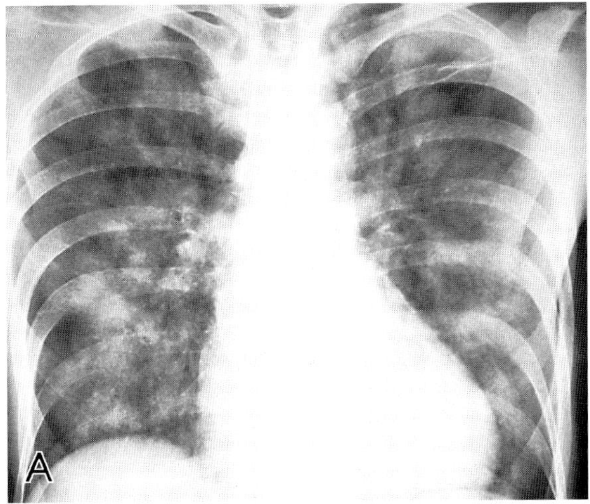

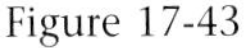

Figure 17-43

METASTATIC CALCIFICATION

The patient was a 53-year-old woman on hemodialysis for renal failure who had progressive respiratory insufficiency.

A: PA chest radiograph demonstrates bilateral, multifocal, patchy nodular airspace opacities.

B: Chest CT (lung window) demonstrates bilateral multifocal areas of ground-glass opacity.

C: CT (soft tissue window) demonstrates extensive calcification of abdominal vascular structures (arrowheads).

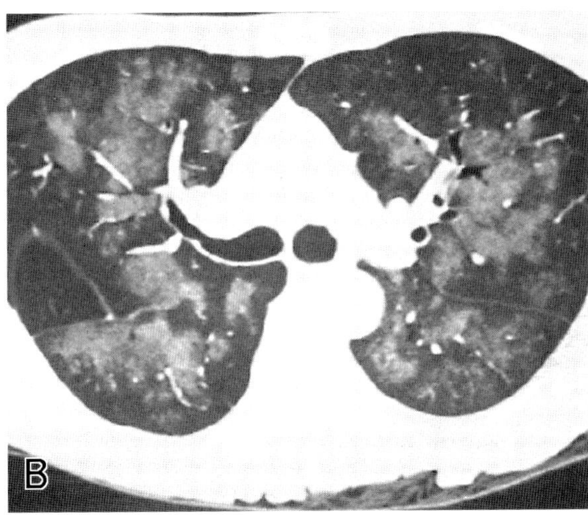

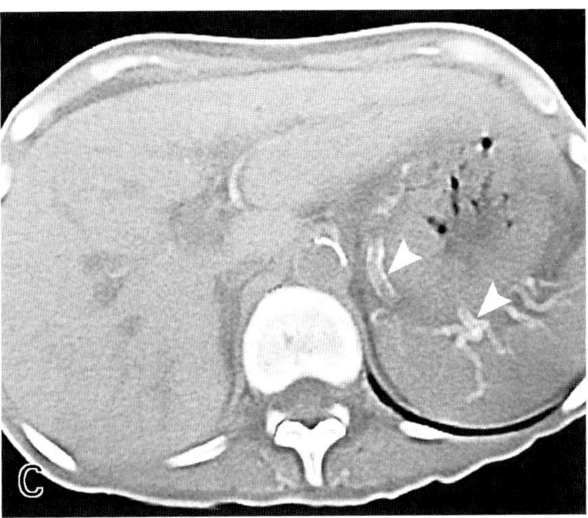

Clinical Features. Metastatic calcification usually occurs in patients with chronic renal insufficiency, especially in those undergoing chronic hemodialysis (36). It also occurs in systemic sclerosis, following orthotopic liver transplantation, and in a variety of skeletal disorders (36). The latter include osteitis fibrosa due to hyperparathyroidism, hypervitaminosis D, hypervitaminosis A (24), sarcoidosis, and tumors extensively involving bone (multiple myeloma and leukemia) and neoplastic parathormone-like activity (40,86). Metastatic calcification also occurs in patients with human T-cell lymphotrophic virus (HTLV)-1–associated malignant lymphoma (42,96). Rarely, it occurs following pyloric stenosis (associated with alkalosis).

Metastatic calcification affects patients from infancy to 70 years of age. The calcium deposits often involve not only the lung but other organs, such as the kidneys, cardia of the stomach, and myocardium and intima of blood vessels (40). Pulmonary calcification usually does not produce symptoms; rather, it is most often found at autopsy. Still, significant edema can develop as progressive calcification of the alveolar walls destroys the alveolar capillary barrier. Metastatic calcification can cause acute respiratory failure and death (42,116).

Radiologic Findings. Metastatic calcification in the lung typically manifests radiologically as multifocal, calcified, nodular opacities or as ill-defined opacities that mimic airspace disease (fig. 17-43). When extensive, the latter may mimic consolidation or edema, as calcification may not be evident on radiography. CT may demonstrate calcification in the lesions as well as associated findings, such as extensive vascular, cardiac, or skin calcification (fig. 17-43) (57).

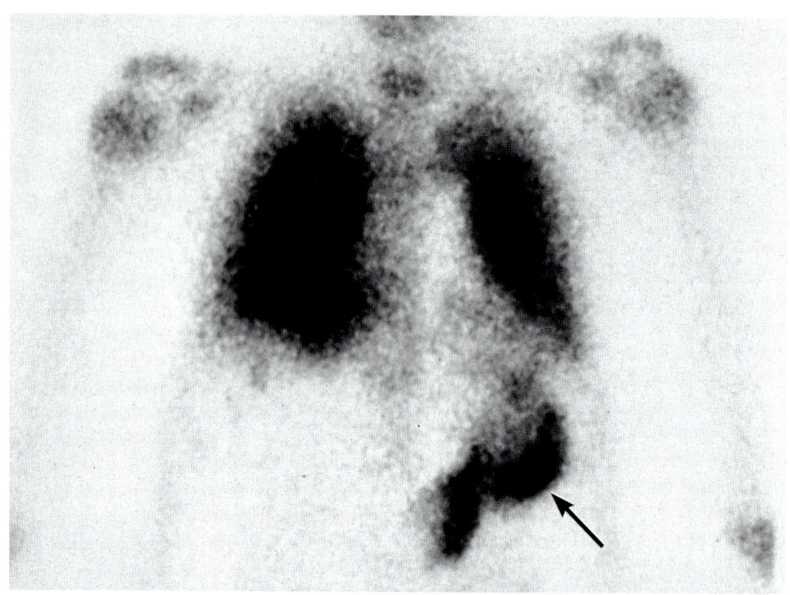

Figure 17-44

METASTATIC CALCIFICATION

The patient was a 60-year-old man on hemodialysis for chronic renal failure who had increasing dyspnea. This 99m technetium-methylene diphosphonate (99m Tc-MDP) bone scan demonstrates marked abnormal uptake in the lung parenchyma and throughout the stomach (arrow). Chest radiography (not shown) had demonstrated bilateral, diffuse, fine reticular opacities.

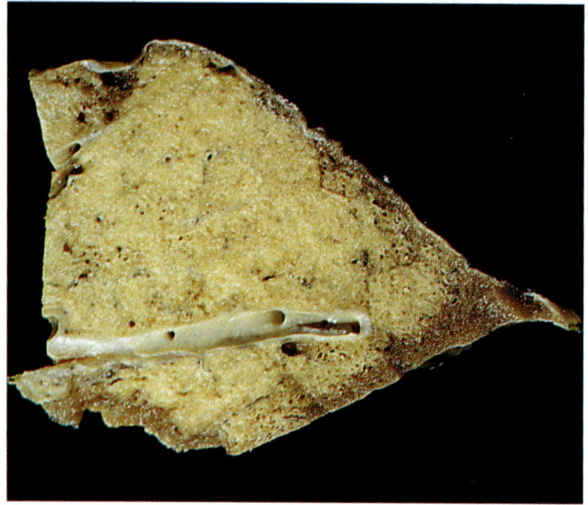

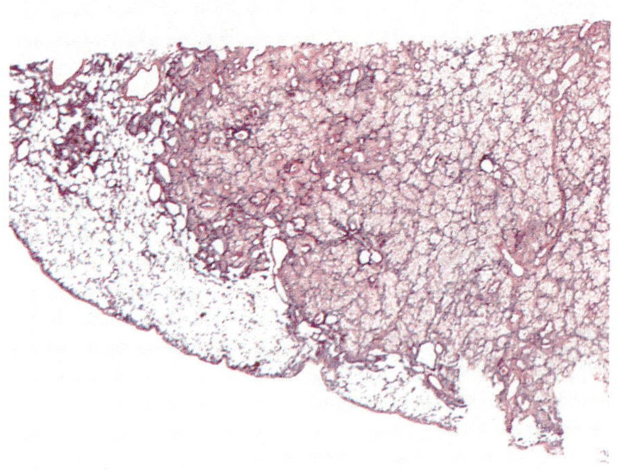

Figure 17-45

METASTATIC CALCIFICATION

Left: The lung parenchyma has a cream-colored gross appearance. It had a gritty feel on palpation.
Right: Low-power microscopic view shows extensive parenchymal involvement by calcification, with associated alveolar fibrosis.

In some cases, radionuclide bone scanning demonstrates diffuse uptake in the lungs because the radionuclide concentrates in areas of active calcium deposition. In fact, radionuclide imaging may detect metastatic calcification not evident with other imaging modalities (fig. 17-44) (132).

Pathologic Findings. Grossly, the lungs have an unusual resistance to palpation and a slightly gritty feel (fig. 17-45, left). Microscopically, metastatic calcium deposits in the lung appear as a layer of hematoxyphilic material in alveolar walls, vessel walls, and basement membranes of small airways (figs. 17-45, right, 17-46, 17-47) (38,40). A von Kossa stain can be used to prove that there are calcium deposits (38,40). Fibrosis can occur within the alveolar lumens, perhaps due to organization of exudate released in response to the calcium salts (figs. 17-46, 17-47).

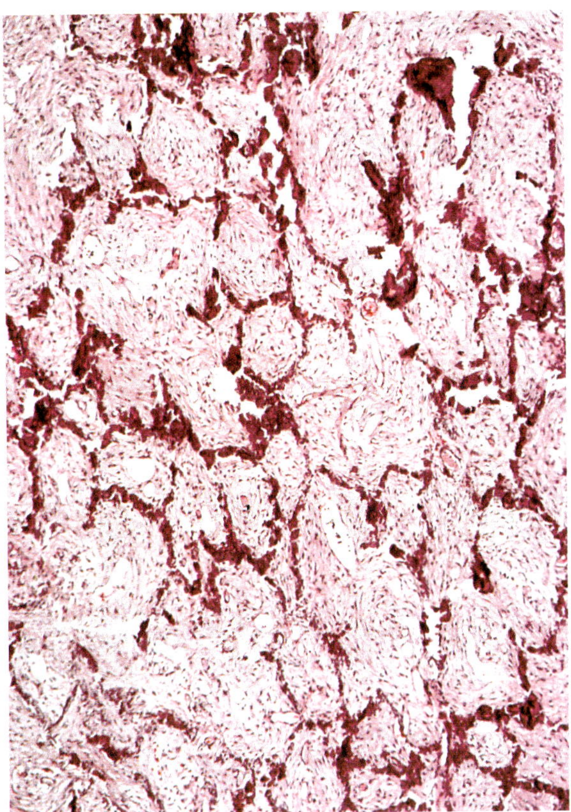

Figure 17-46

METASTATIC CALCIFICATION

The calcium appears as a layer of hematoxyphilic material in alveolar and vessel walls. Note the fibrous tissue within the alveolar lumens, perhaps due to organization of exudate released in response to the calcium salts.

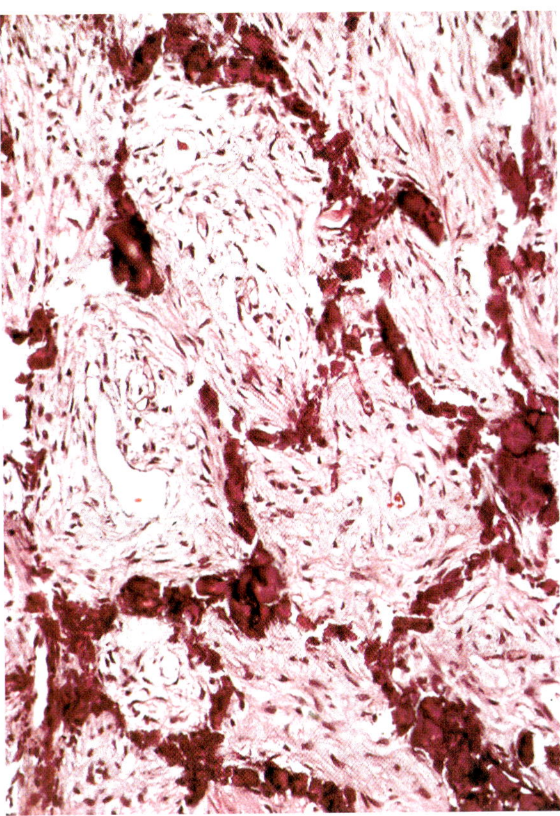

Figure 17-47

METASTATIC CALCIFICATION

The alveolar walls are decorated by basophilic spicules of calcium. Note the fibrous tissue within the alveolar lumens, perhaps due to organization of exudate released in response to the calcium salts.

Treatment and Prognosis. The management of patients with metastatic calcification remains poorly understood. In patients with endstage renal disease, progressive metastatic calcification is often associated with hyperphosphatemia that is refractory to oral phosphate binders. In this setting, parathyroid hormone (PTH)-induced release of phosphate from bone contributes to the persistent elevation in the plasma phosphate concentration. Parathyroidectomy tends to minimize further deposition by lowering the plasma calcium and phosphate concentrations. In patients with chronic hemodialysis, long-term duration of dialysis (over 6 years) and high serum aluminum levels are the two factors that favor metastatic calcification.

DYSTROPHIC PULMONARY OSSIFICATION

Definition. Dystrophic pulmonary ossification is the formation of branching bone in the lung. There are two types of ossification, localized and diffuse.

Localized deposits of bone are common. They are due to bone that is laid down in foci of dystrophic calcification, such as scars and healing granulomas; in tracheobronchopathia osteochondroplastica; in nodular amyloid deposits; and in the bronchial cartilage of aging individuals (38,40). As far as the last is concerned, the necrotic cartilage plates first undergo calcification, then they are invaded by vessels, and finally are transformed into bone, replete with bone marrow and fat, within the bony trabeculae.

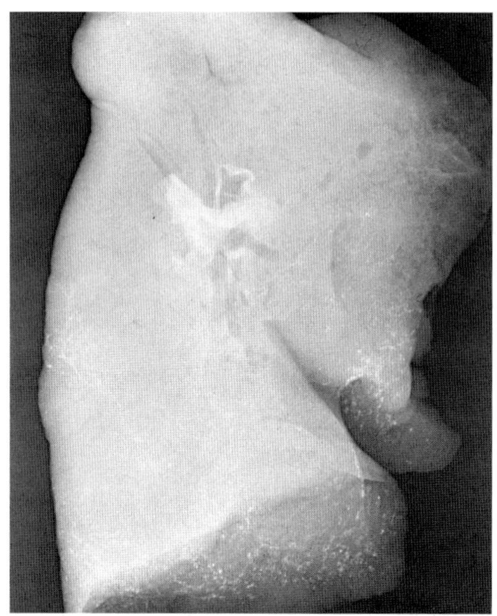
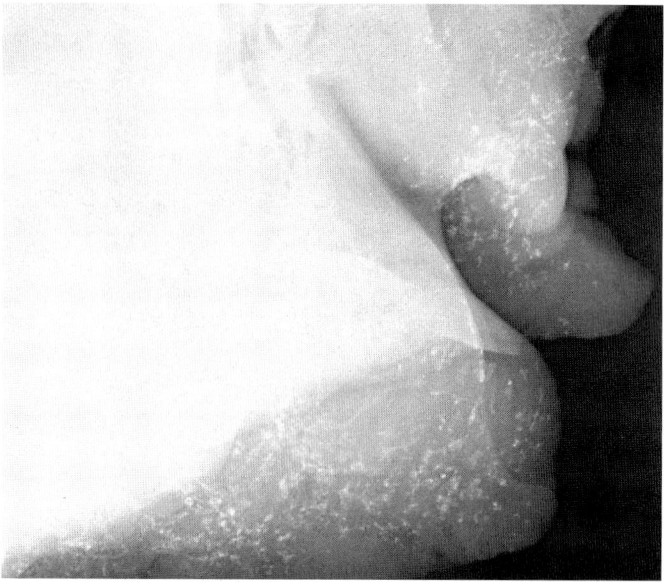

Figure 17-48

RACEMOSE OR DENDRIFORM OSSIFICATION

Lung specimen radiography from a 76-year-old man who died with metastatic colon carcinoma and opportunistic infection.

Left: Postmortem digital radiograph of the left lung demonstrates diffuse branching ossification in the inferior lower and upper lobes.

Right: Coned-down view of the left base shows branching calcified opacities.

Disseminated pulmonary ossification is rare. There are two types. *Racemose, dendriform,* or *branching ossification* is associated with chronic lung disease (79,127,131). It is characterized by bone spicules laid down in a diffuse, branching manner (79,127,131). Other synonyms include *bony metaplasia of the lung, pulmonary osteopathia, ossifying pneumonitis,* and *disseminated pulmonary ossification* (65). The second type is *nodular circumscribed ossification* which is associated with mitral stenosis (141, 176). In this form, bone occurs as scattered, small (less than 0.5 cm) nodules in lung (176).

Clinical Features. Racemose (or dendriform) pulmonary ossification usually occurs in men who are 40 to 60 years old (40,79,127,131). The ossification itself does not cause symptoms and is infrequently diagnosed during life. Rather, symptoms are typically due to underlying chronic pulmonary disease, including interstitial fibrosis, chronic inflammation, bronchiectasis, and amyloid deposits.

Nodular circumscribed ossification occurs in relatively young individuals who average about 35 years of age. Men outnumber women by a ratio of 4 to 1 (44). This form of ossification occurs almost exclusively in association with longstanding mitral stenosis and prolonged chronic congestion, although there are a few reports of it in chronic left ventricular failure, idiopathic hypertrophic subaortic stenosis, and nephrosclerosis (23,44). Radiographs show lungs that contain finely stippled densities to scattered nodules. The lesions are most common in the lung bases and central zones (23,44,66). They can persist radiographically; in one case they were present for 8 years.

Pathologic Findings. The hallmark of racemose ossification is the presence of racemose or branching bone within the lung, which can be well visualized by radiography or lung digestion techniques (fig. 17-48). There is often a background of interstitial fibrosis, organized pneumonia, or zones of fibrosis.

Histologically, there are irregular, branching, slender tubules of woven bone, often with associated marrow elements. While these spicules of bone may be surrounded by fibrosis within interstitium and alveoli, they are not embedded within dense fibrotic scars like the

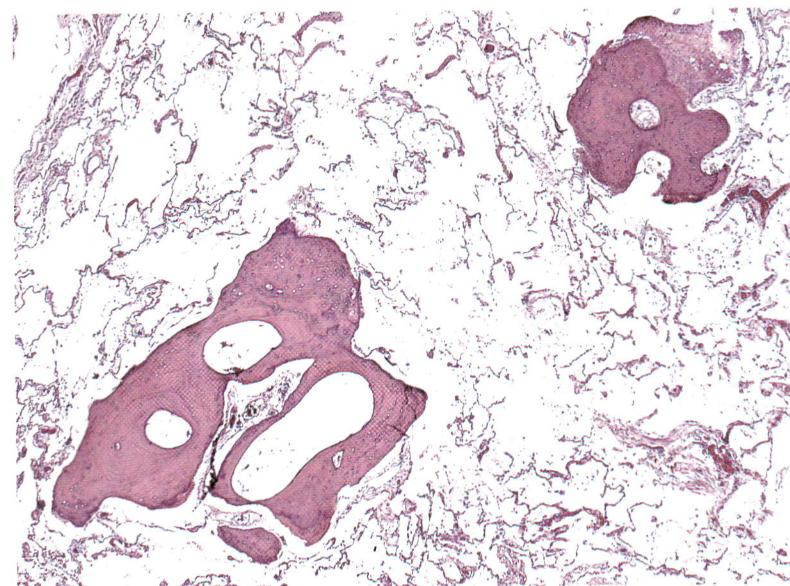

Figure 17-49

RACEMOSE OR DENDRIFORM OSSIFICATION

Microscopically, there is branching bone within the alveolar lumens.

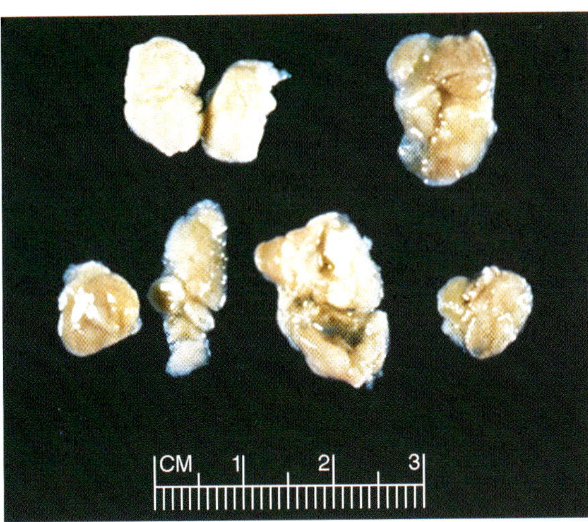

Figure 17-50

NODULAR OSSIFICATION: GROSS SPECIMEN

These numerous, discrete, gray-white stones were removed from the lung parenchyma.

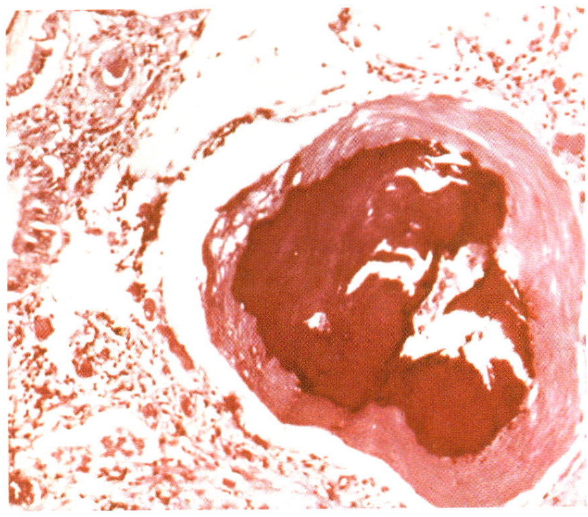

Figure 17-51

NODULAR OSSIFICATION

Oval nodule of bone fills the lumens of a single alveolus or a cluster of alveoli.

metaplastic bone seen in interstitial fibrotic disorders (fig. 17-49). The gross appearance is the key to the diagnosis, but in microscopic sections, the finding of branch points in the bone spicules is suggestive (fig. 17-49) (79,127,131).

The lungs in nodular ossification are brown and indurated, reflecting the underlying chronic passive congestion. There are usually numerous nodules that are gray-white (fig. 17-50). They are commonly less than 0.5 cm in diameter and discrete, and most often occur in the lower lobes. They are frequently found near the pleura.

The bone in nodular ossification occurs in the form of thin plaques or round to irregular nodular masses that contain small regular osteocytes (44,51). The nodules fill the lumens of a single alveolus or a cluster of alveoli (figs. 17-51, 17-52). The bone is of woven type, and marrow is usually absent. Osteoid deposits may be present at the margin of the bony trabeculae (44,51,176).

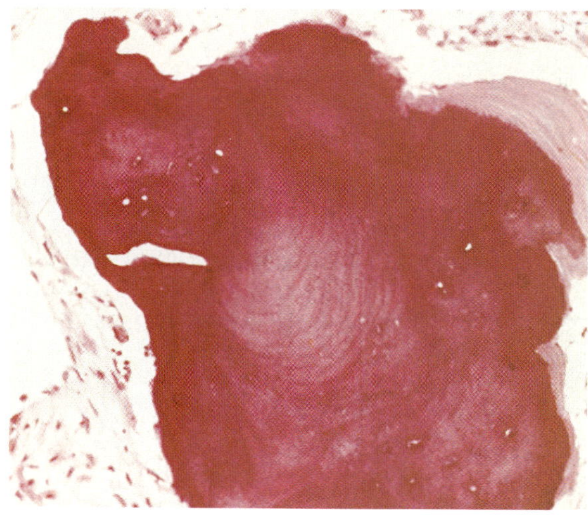

Figure 17-52

NODULAR OSSIFICATION

An irregular nodule of bone is present within an alveolus. Note the small, regular osteocytes.

Intra-alveolar hemorrhage and alveolar capillary engorgement are due to chronic passive congestion, and intra-alveolar hemosiderin-laden macrophages are often present (44,65).

TRACHEOBRONCHOPATHIA OSTEOCHONDROPLASTICA

Definition. Tracheobronchopathia osteochondroplastica (TBO) is an uncommon condition in which multiple submucosal nodules of metaplastic bone and cartilage protrude into the lumen of the trachea and bronchi (3,7,13,120, 142,172,175,182).

Clinical Features. The incidence of TBO identified at bronchoscopy varies from 0.02 to 0.7 percent (142,172,175,182). TBO typically is found in adults over the age of 50 years, although children can have the disease. It is more common in men than women. Patients are generally asymptomatic and the TBO is an incidental finding at the time of radiologic examination, bronchoscopy, or intubation. The minority of patients who have symptoms report cough, sputum production, wheezing, dyspnea, or hemoptysis. Pulmonary function testing rarely shows significant airflow obstruction. Some patients develop obstructive pneumonias and secondary *Mycobacterium avium-intracellulare* infection (13). The diagnosis of TBO is based on radiologic evaluation of the large airways (especially by CT and MRI), bronchoscopic evaluation, and histologic confirmation of the nature of the nodular lesions identified (114). Follow-up data are unremarkable in most cases. Some patients have persistent obstructive or infectious complications.

Radiologic Findings. Radiologic studies may suggest the diagnosis. There are often scalloped nodular opacities on the anterior and lateral walls of the trachea; calcification is also apparent. The lesions are best demonstrated by CT imaging; MRI studies are also useful (114).

Pathologic Findings. Grossly and at bronchoscopy, multiple, hard, submucosal nodules, 2 to 3 mm in diameter are identified (fig. 17-53). The lower trachea tends to be most severely affected and the nodules may be attached to the perichondrium of the cartilaginous plates. The overlying mucosa is intact.

Histologically, metaplastic cartilage and bone (with or without bone marrow) are found in the submucosa (fig. 17-54). The nodules may have a rim of fibrous tissue that is continuous with the perichondrium of the cartilage. The overlying mucosa may appear normal or show metaplastic changes.

Differential Diagnosis. Tracheobronchial amyloidosis is the primary condition in the differential diagnosis. TBO and tracheobronchial amyloidosis are separated histologically by the finding of submucosal amyloid deposits in the latter. The amyloid may show secondary ossification (see figs. 17-36–17-38). Other conditions that may be associated with mucosal and submucosal nodular lesions in the large airways include endobronchial sarcoidosis, endobronchial granulomatous infection (particularly tuberculosis), papillomatosis, and tracheobronchial calcinosis (172).

ENDOMETRIOSIS

Endometriosis may affect the pleura (see chapter 18) or the lung (56,72). Pulmonary endometriosis occurs mostly in women of child-bearing age, but it can also occur in postmenopausal women taking exogenous hormones (56,72). The most common manifestation is catamenial hemoptysis (56,72). Presenting manifestation as an endobronchial lesion has been reported

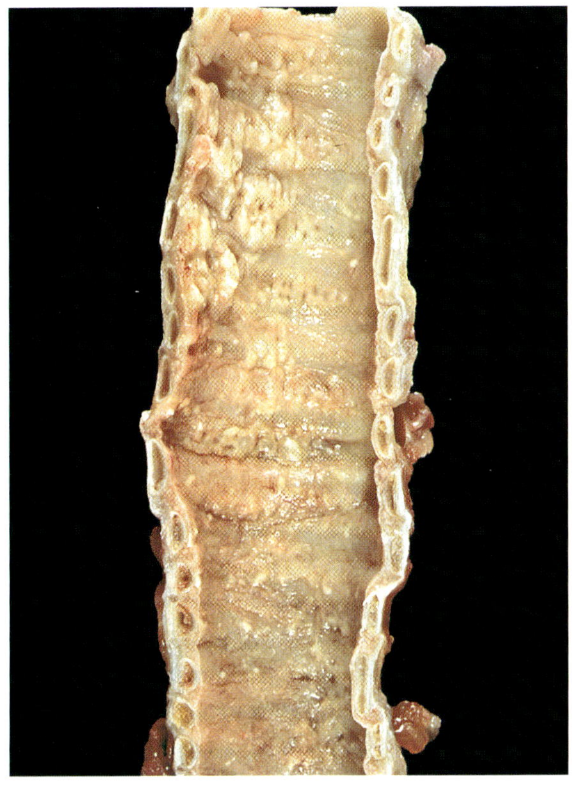

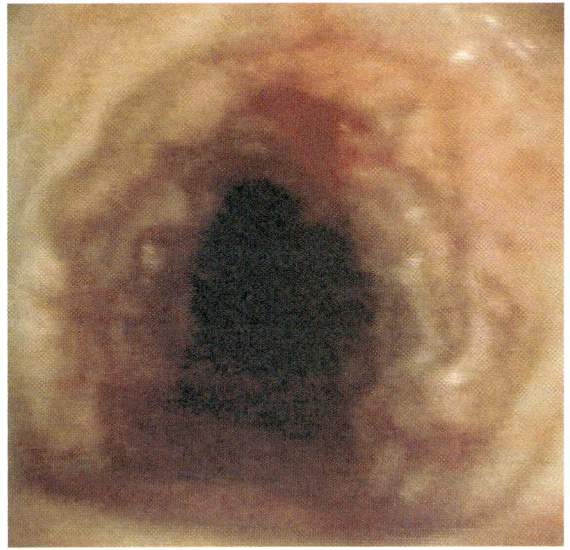

Figure 17-53

TRACHEOBRONCHOPATHIA OSTEOCHONDROPLASTICA

Left: Gross view of the trachea shows multiple submucosal nodules, 2 to 3 mm in diameter.

Above: Endoscopic view shows multiple submucosal nodules. (Courtesy of Dr. Robert Knapp, Lansing, MI.)

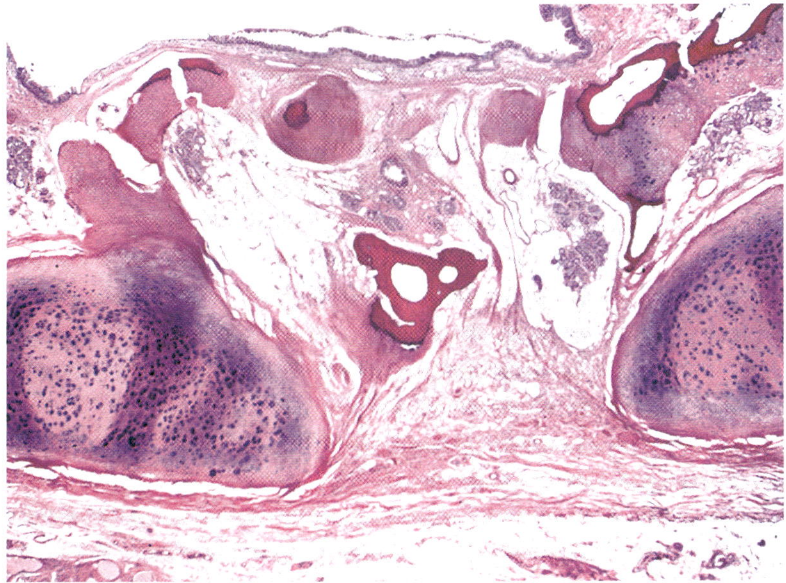

Figure 17-54

TRACHEOBRONCHOPATHIA OSTEOCHONDROPLASTICA

Several nodules of metaplastic bone are present in the submucosa of the trachea.

(163). Chest radiographs show several patterns: discrete 1- to 3-cm nodules that are usually solitary; opacities that can be mistaken for infarcts; or airspace consolidation (56,72,152). Thoracic endometriosis manifests as lung nodules in 6 percent of cases (81). Grossly, the lesions appear as nodules or areas of hemorrhagic lung parenchyma. Histologically, the lesions consist of a circumscribed, but unencapsulated proliferation of endometrial glands and stroma, frequently associated with hemorrhage (fig. 17-55) (56). The biphasic appearance can be confused with

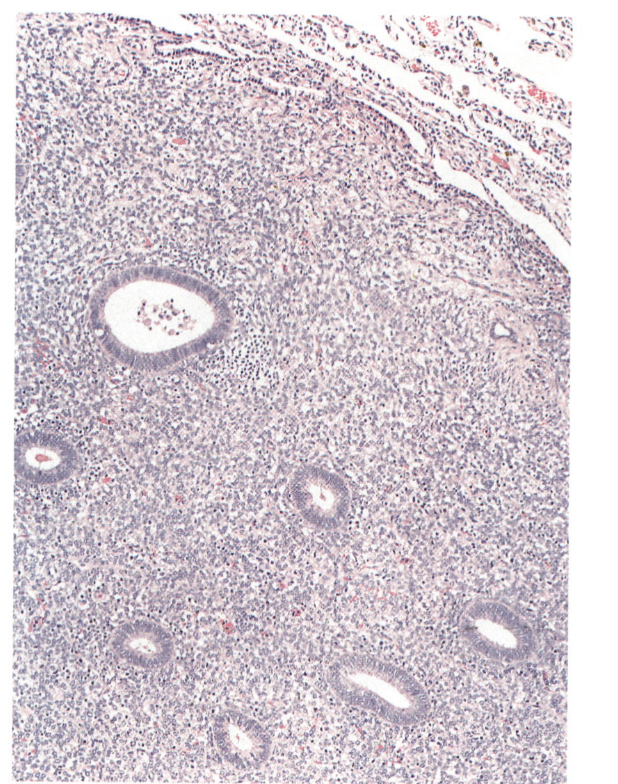

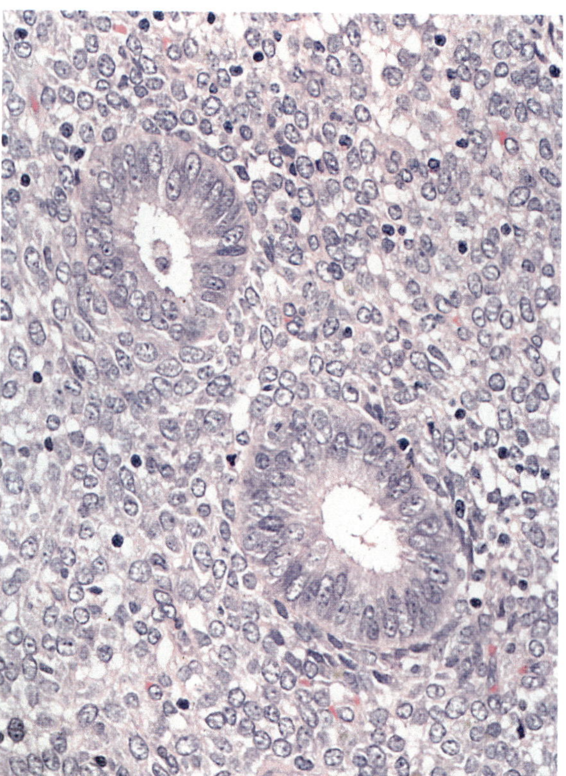

Figure 17-55

INTRAPULMONARY ENDOMETRIOSIS

Left: This nodule of endometrial tissue is circumscribed, but not encapsulated.
Right: The nodule consists of endometrial stroma and glands.

a variety of lesions including well-differentiated fetal adenocarcinoma (56). Pulmonary deciduosis is a related lesion that consists of stromal nodules in a lymphangitic pattern; the nodules are composed of cells with abundant eosinophilic, granular cytoplasm, and distinct cell borders but lack endometrial stroma or glands (56).

Surgical resection is usually effective in treating patients with solitary pulmonary nodules of endometriosis. One case of endobronchial endometriosis was treated by subsegmentectomy (163). Hormonal therapy has also been used (92,126).

BRONCHIAL INFLAMMATORY POLYPS

Inflammatory polyps are rare intraluminal bronchial lesions that can manifest in young children or in adults. In adults, the lesions have a more chronic appearance, with respiratory epithelium overlying a fibrovascular and chronic inflammatory stroma (fig. 17-56). In young children, there may be a history of intubation and the polyps may resemble granulation tissue (fig. 17-57). A papillary growth pattern may raise consideration of a papilloma. However, the lesion consists mostly of a polypoid expansion of submucosal stroma rather than squamous or glandular epithelium. There may be varying amounts of chronic inflammation including lymphoid aggregates. The overlying mucosa consists mostly of ciliated pseudostratified respiratory epithelium, but squamous metaplasia may be present.

PULMONARY INVOLVEMENT IN INBORN ERRORS OF METABOLISM

The lung is involved by many inborn errors of metabolism, and in a number of these clinically significant pulmonary disease may occur (35).

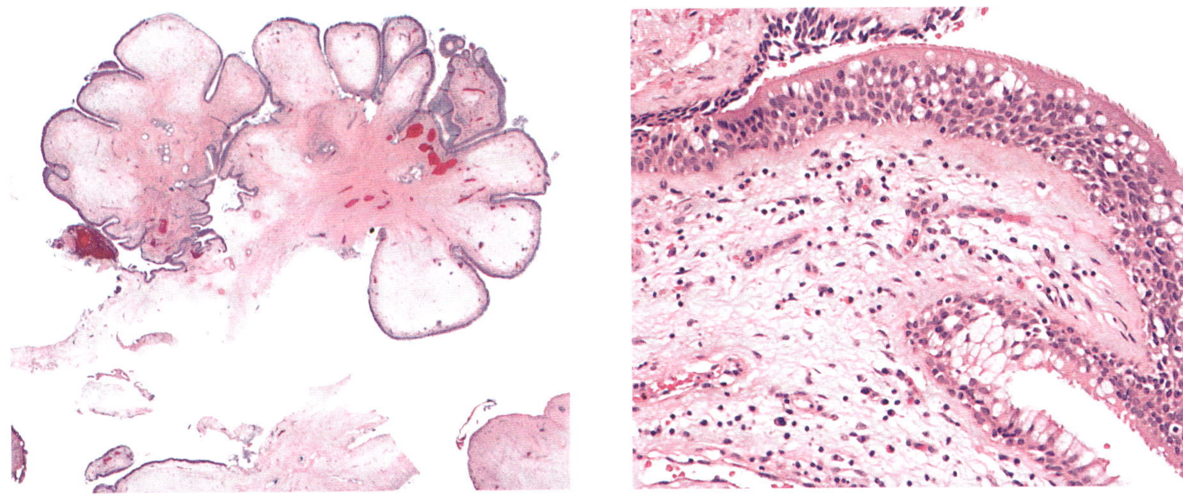

Figure 17-56

INFLAMMATORY POLYP

Left: This polypoid lesion consists of edematous and fibroinflammatory expansion of the submucosa.
Right: The submucosa shows chronic inflammation and loose fibrous tissue.

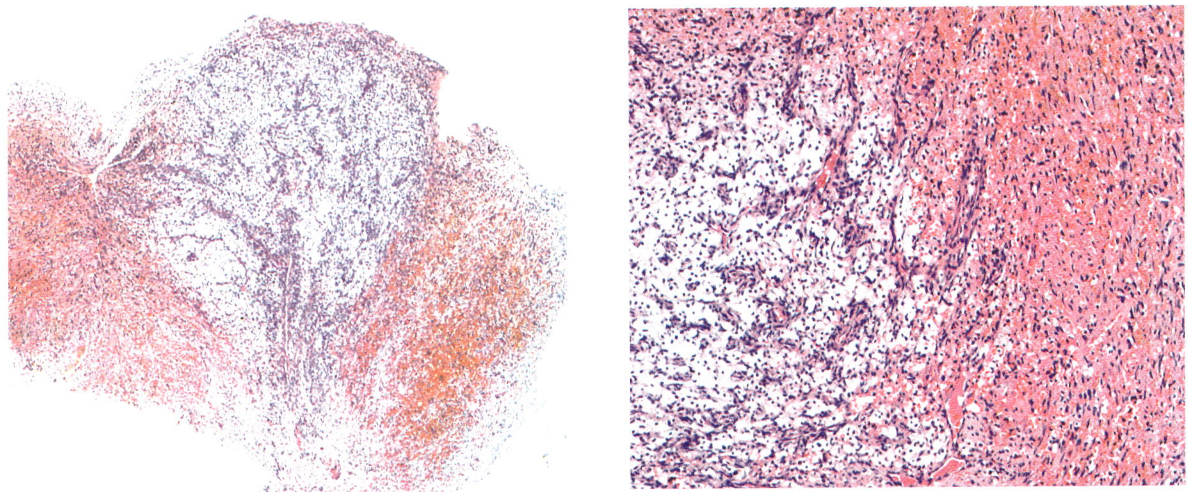

Figure 17-57

INFLAMMATORY POLYP IN CHILD FOLLOWING INTUBATION

Left: Polypoid granulation tissue protrudes from the mucosal surface.
Right: The surface of the lesion shows hemorrhage and numerous capillaries with loose intervening stroma. (Courtesy of Dr. Andrew Nicholson, London.)

Gaucher's Disease

Pulmonary involvement occurs in both infantile and adult forms of Gaucher's disease (11, 85). In clinically significant cases, the signs and symptoms may be those of interstitial lung disease. Abnormal pulmonary function (abnormal diffusion, small airways obstruction, reduced expiratory flow, reduction in lung volume) is more frequently identified than radiologic abnormalities (85).

Histologically, Gaucher cells show the following four patterns: intracapillary, patchy interstitial infiltrates along a lymphatic distribution, massive thickening of alveolar septa, and

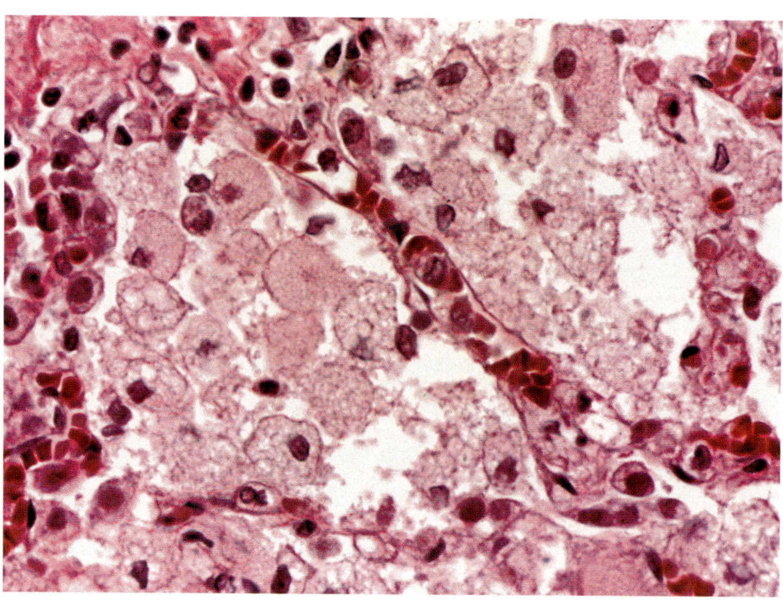

Figure 17-58

GAUCHER'S DISEASE

There is an accumulation of cells with foamy cytoplasm within the alveoli.

intra-alveolar collections of foam cells (figs. 17-58, 17-59) (5). Involvement of the pulmonary capillaries was universal in one autopsy series (5). Gaucher's disease has also been associated with pulmonary hypertension when Gaucher cells occlude the pulmonary capillary network (69,164). L444P homozygotes appear to be the individuals at major risk for developing pulmonary disease (148). Improvement of lung pathology with ceredase treatment has been documented in some patients (11). The differential diagnosis includes mycobacterial infection which can cause pseudo-Gaucher cells with numerous mycobacteria (usually *Mycobacterium avium-intracellulare*) within macrophages (104), and crystal-storing histiocytosis with accumulation of immunoglobulin light chains (usually kappa) associated with low-grade lymphoplasmacytic lymphomas (149).

Niemann-Pick Disease

Pulmonary involvement is relatively common in infantile forms of the disease; it is less common in adults with Niemann-Pick disease (35,55). The clinical and radiologic findings are those of interstitial lung disease (35,55). Histologically, the alveoli are stuffed by foamy Niemann-Pick cells that may also infiltrate the alveolar septa, pleura, and lymphatics. Fibrosis is a late finding. BAL is useful for retrieving cells for biochemical analysis (138).

Fabry's Disease (Angiokeratoma Corporus Diffusinum Universali)

Fabry's disease has been associated with evidence of airflow obstruction. In one large series, 9 of 25 patients (36 percent) had airflow obstruction on spirometry (21).

Hermansky-Pudlak Syndrome

Hermansky-Pudlak syndrome is an autosomal recessive condition that includes defects in platelet aggregation, oculocutaneous albinism, and the accumulation of ceroid-filled histiocytes in many tissues (20,130,143). Pulmonary involvement manifests as interstitial lung disease clinically, radiologically, and functionally. Histologically, the interstitial fibrosis has been likened to usual interstitial pneumonia. In some cases the pattern of interstitial fibrosis is closer to that of nonspecific interstitial pneumonia, cellular and fibrosing patterns (fig. 17-60A,B). In addition to the interstitial fibrosis, there are increased numbers of ceroid-filled histiocytes in the airspaces and interstitium. These histiocytes may be identified in BAL fluid. Nakatani et al. (130) recently described giant lamellar body degeneration of type 2 pneumocytes, visible by light microscopy, as markedly vacuolated pneumocytes (fig. 17-60C) in five patients with the Hermansky-Pudlak syndrome, interstitial fibrosis, bronchiolar fibrosis, and constrictive bronchiolitis.

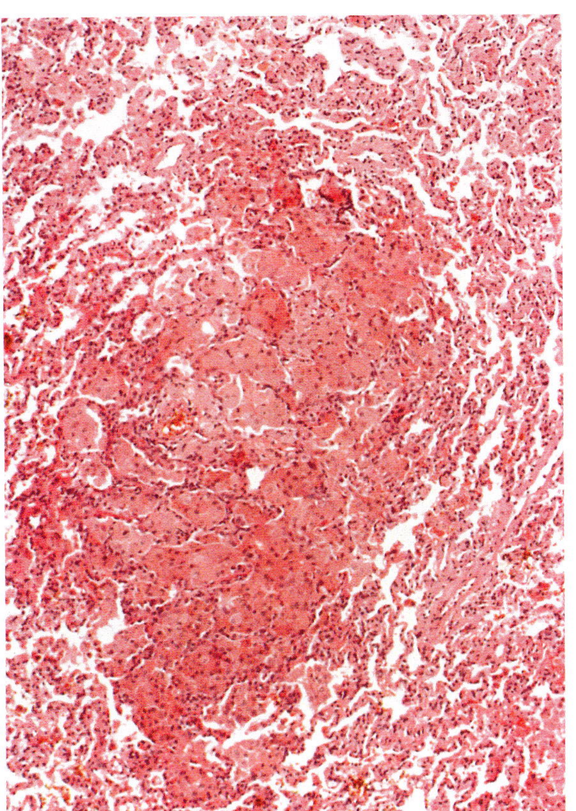

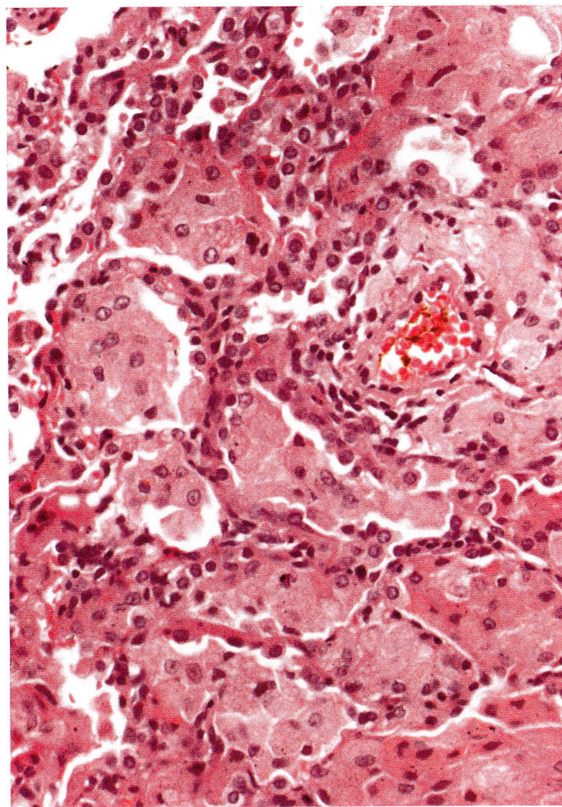

Figure 17-59

GAUCHER'S DISEASE

Left: Nodular lesions are present in this case.
Right: Higher magnification of the nodule reveals alveolar lipid-bearing cells.

Marfan's Syndrome

The pulmonary changes that have been described in Marfan's syndrome include interstitial lung disease with honeycombing, bullous emphysema, congenital malformations of the airways, diffuse cystic changes of the lung, increased respiratory tract infections, bronchiectasis, and spontaneous pneumothoraces (35).

Ehlers-Danlos Syndrome

The reported pulmonary complications of Ehlers-Danlos syndrome include spontaneous pneumothoraces, bronchial dilation, arteriovenous anastomoses, pulmonary cyst formation, and fibrous nodules thought to be secondary to an abnormal reparative reaction (35,129). Fatal hemoptysis has been described (181).

Miscellaneous Diseases

Other rare inborn errors of metabolism have been associated with pulmonary disease. *Infantile GM1 gangliosidosis* shows accumulations of foamy cells in the lung. *Krabbe's disease (globoid leukodystrophy)* has infiltrates of distinctive macrophages with dense eosinophilic cytoplasm and amber brown inclusions. *Pompe's disease (type II glycogenosis/acid maltase deficiency)* shows increased glycogenation of alveolar macrophages. Finally, *Farber's disease (disseminated lipogranulomatosis)* manifests as sheets of histiocytes associated with a background of lymphocytes and plasma cells (181).

Figure 17-60

HERMANSKY-PUDLAK SYNDROME

A: Interstitial fibrosis and chronic inflammation show a pattern similar to that of nonspecific interstitial pneumonia, fibrosing pattern.

B: The interstitium is expanded by dense collagen and a moderate chronic inflammatory infiltrate.

C: These type 2 pneumocytes show marked cytoplasmic vacuolization.

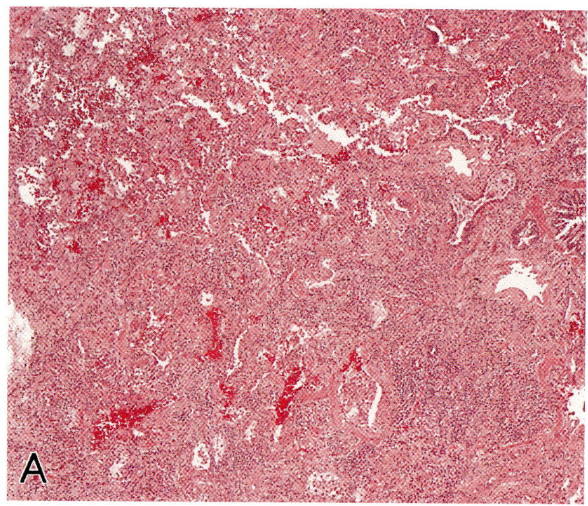

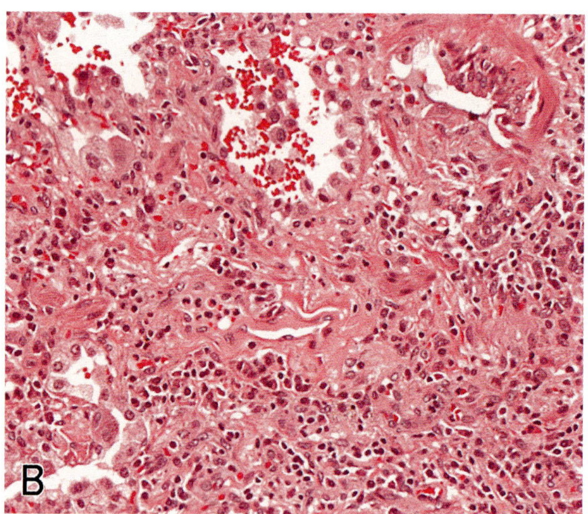

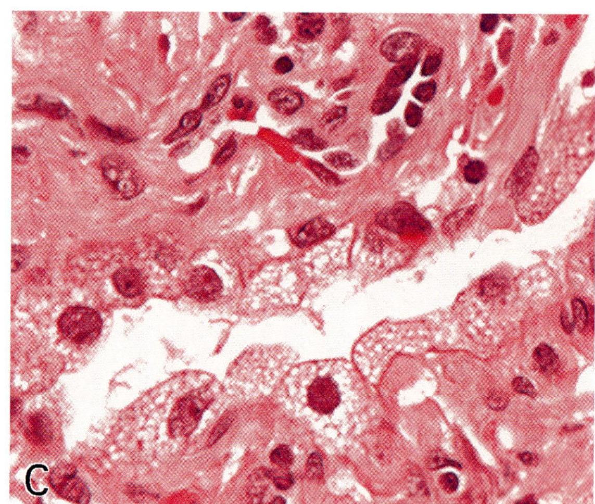

REFERENCES

1. Abe Y, Utsunomiya H, Tsutsumi Y. Atypical carcinoid tumor of the lung with amyloid stroma. Acta Pathol Jpn 1992;42:286–92.
2. Agrons GA, Rosado-de-Christenson ML, Kirejczyk WM, Conran RM, Stocker JT. Pulmonary inflammatory pseudotumor: radiologic features. Radiology 1998;206:511–8.
3. Akyol MU, Martin AA, Dhurandhar N, Miller RH. Tracheobronchopathia osteochondroplastica: a case report and a review of the literature. Ear Nose Throat J 1993;72:347–50.
4. Al-Kaisi N, Abdul-Karim FW, Mendelsohn G, Jacobs G. Bronchial carcinoid tumor with amyloid stroma. Arch Pathol Lab Med 1988;112:211–4.
5. Amir G, Ron N. Pulmonary pathology in Gaucher's disease. Hum Pathol 1999;30:666–70.
6. Antunes ML, Vieira da Luz JM. Primary diffuse tracheo-bronchial amyloidosis. Thorax 1969;24:307–11.
7. Ashley DJ. Bony metaplasia in trachea and bronchi. J Pathol 1970;102:186–8.
8. Atagi S, Sakatani M, Akira M, Yamamoto S, Ueda E. Pulmonary hyalinizing granuloma with Castleman's disease. Intern Med 1994;33:689–91.
9. Bahadori M, Liebow AA. Plasma cell granulomas of the lung. Cancer 1973;31:191–208.
10. Bakhos R, Wojcik EM, Olson MC. Transthoracic fine-needle aspiration cytology of inflammatory pseudotumor, fibrohistiocytic type: a case report with immunohistochemical studies. Diagn Cytopathol 1998;19:216–20.

11. Banjar H. Pulmonary involvement of Gaucher's disease in children: a common presentation in Saudi Arabia. Ann Trop Paediatr 1998;18:55–9.
12. Barbareschi M, Ferrero S, Aldovini D, et al. Inflammatory pseudotumour of the lung. Immunohistochemical analysis of four new cases. Histol Histopathol 1990;5:205-11.
13. Baugnee PE, Delaunois LM. Mycobacterium avium-intracellulare associated with tracheobronchopathia osteochondroplastica. Eur Respir J 1995;8:180–2.
14. Beer TW, Edwards CW. Pulmonary nodules due to reactive systemic amyloidosis (AA) in Crohn's disease. Thorax 1993;48:1287–8.
15. Berardi RS, Lee SS, Chen HP, Stines GJ. Inflammatory pseudotumors of the lung. Surg Gynecol Obstet 1983;156:89–96.
16. Bignold LP, Martyn M, Basten A. Nodular pulmonary amyloidosis associated with benign hypergammaglobulinemic purpura. Chest 1980;78:334–6.
17. Biselli R, Ferlini C, Fattorossi A, Boldrini R, Bosman C. Inflammatory myofibroblastic tumor (inflammatory pseudotumor): DNA flow cytometric analysis of nine pediatric cases. Cancer 1996;77:778–84.
18. Blavia R, Toda MR, Vidal F, Benet A, Razquin S, Richart C. Pulmonary diffuse amyloidosis and ankylosing spondylitis. A rare association. Chest 1992;102:1608–10.
19. Bonner H Jr, Ennis RS, Geelhoed GW, Tarpley TM Jr. Lymphoid infiltration and amyloidosis of lung in Sjögren's syndrome. Arch Pathol 1973;95:42–4.
20. Brantly M, Avila NA, Shotelersuk V, Lucero C, Huizing M, Gahl WA. Pulmonary function and high-resolution CT findings in patients with an inherited form of pulmonary fibrosis, Hermansky-Pudlak syndrome, due to mutations in HPS-1. Chest 2000;117:129–36.
21. Brown LK, Miller A, Bhuptani A, et al. Pulmonary involvement in Fabry disease. Am J Respir Crit Care Med. 1997;155:1004–10.
22. Buell R, Wang NS, Seemayer TA, Ahmed MN. Endobronchial plasma cell granuloma (xanthomatous pseudotumor); a light and electron microscopic study. Hum Pathol 1976;7:411–26.
23. Buja LM, Roberts WC. Pulmonary parenchymal ossific nodules in idiopathic hypertrophic subaortic stenosis. Am J Cardiol 1970;25:710–5.
24. Bush ME, Dahms BB. Fatal hypervitaminosis A in a neonate. Arch Pathol Lab Med 1984; 108:838–42.
25. Buxbaum J, Gallo G. Nonamyloidotic monoclonal immunoglobulin deposition disease. Light-chain, heavy-chain, and light- and heavy-chain deposition diseases. Hematol Oncol Clin North Am 1999;13:1235–48.
26. Chalaoui J, Grégoire P, Sylvestre J, Lefebvre R, Amyot R. Pulmonary hyalinizing granuloma: a cause of pulmonary nodules. Radiology 1984;152:23–6.
27. Chan YF, White J, Brash H. Metachronous pulmonary and cerebral inflammatory pseudotumor in a child. Pediatr Pathol 1994;14:805–15.
28. Chen HP, Lee SS, Berardi RS. Inflammatory pseudotumor of the lung. Ultrastructural and light microscopic study of a myxomatous variant. Cancer 1984;54:861–5.
29. Chen KT. Amyloidosis presenting in the respiratory tract. Pathol Annu 1989;24[Pt 1]:253–73.
30. Chen KT. Mycobacterial spindle cell pseudotumor of lymph nodes. Am J Surg Pathol 1992; 16:276–81.
31. Childress W, Adie G. Plasma cell tumors of the mediastinum and lung: report of two cases. J Thorac Surg 1950;19:794–9.
32. Coffin CM, Humphrey PA, Dehner LP. Extrapulmonary inflammatory myofibroblastic tumor: a clinical and pathological survey. Semin Diagn Pathol 1998;15:85–101.
33. Coffin CM, Watterson J, Priest JR, Dehner LP. Extrapulmonary inflammatory myofibroblastic tumor (inflammatory pseudotumor). A clinicopathologic and immunohistochemical study of 84 cases. Am J Surg Pathol 1995;19:859–72.
34. Cohen MC, Kaschula RO. Primary pulmonary tumors in childhood: a review of 31 years' experience and the literature. Pediatr Pulmonol 1992;14:222–32.
35. Colby TV, Carrington CB. Interstitial lung disease. In: Thurlbeck WM, Churg AM, eds. Pathology of the lung, 2nd ed. New York: Thieme Medical Publishers; 1995:589–737.
36. Conger JD, Hammond WS, Alfrey AC, Contiguglia SR, Stanford RE, Huffer WE. Pulmonary calcification in chronic dialysis patients. Clinical and pathologic studies. Ann Intern Med 1975;83:330–6.
37. Copin MC, Gosselin BH, Ribet ME. Plasma cell granuloma of the lung: difficulties in diagnosis and prognosis. Ann Thorac Surg 1996;61: 1477–82.
38. Corrin B. Pulmonary manifestations of systemic disease. In: Corrin B, ed. Pathology of the lungs. London: Churchill Livingstone; 2000: 423–46.
39. Crestani B, Monnier A, Kambouchner M, Battesti JP, Reynaud P, Valeyre D. Tracheobronchial amyloidosis with hilar lymphadenopathy associated with a serum monoclonal immunoglobulin. Eur Respir J 1993;6:1569–71.

40. Dail DH. Metabolic and other diseases. In: Dail DH, Hammar SP, eds. Pulmonary pathology, 2nd ed. New York: Springer Verlag; 1994:707–77.
41. Dail DH. Uncommon tumors. In: Dail DH, Hammar SP, eds. Pulmonary pathology, 2nd ed. New York: Springer-Verlag; 1994:1279–461.
42. Daisley H, Charles WP. Fatal metastatic calcification in a patient with HTLV-1-associated lymphoma. West Indian Med J 1993;42:37–9.
43. Dalton HR, Featherstone T, Athanasou N. Organ limited amyloidosis with lymphadenopathy. Postgrad Med J 1992;68:47–50.
44. Daugavietis HE, Mautner LS. Disseminated nodular pulmonary ossification with mitral stenosis. Arch Pathol 1957;63:7–12.
45. Davis CJ, Butchart EG, Gibbs AR. Nodular pulmonary amyloidosis occurring in association with pulmonary lymphoma. Thorax 1991;46: 217–8.
46. Dent RG, Godden DJ, Stovin PG, Stark JE. Pulmonary hyalinizing granuloma in association with retroperitoneal fibrosis. Thorax 1983;38: 955–6.
47. Dictor M, Hasserius R. Systemic amyloidosis and non-hematologic malignancy in a large autopsy series. Acta Pathol Microbiol Scand [A] 1981;89:411–6.
48. Doski JJ, Priebe CJ Jr, Driessnack M, Smith T, Kane P, Romero J. Corticosteroids in the management of unresected plasma cell granuloma (inflammatory pseudotumor) of the lung. J Pediatr Surg 1991;26:1064–6.
49. Dundore PA, Aisner SC, Templeton PA, Krasna MJ, White CS, Seidman JD. Nodular pulmonary amyloidosis: diagnosis by fine-needle aspiration cytology and a review of the literature. Diagn Cytopathol 1993;9:562–4.
50. el-Gatit A, Al-Kaisi N, Moftah S, et al. Atypical bronchial carcinoid tumour with amyloid deposition. Eur J Surg Oncol 1994;20:586–7.
51. Elkeles A, Glynn LE. Disseminated parenchymatous ossification in the lungs in association with mitral stenosis. J Pathol Bacteriol 1946;58:517–22.
52. Engleman P, Liebow AA, Gmelich J, Friedman PJ. Pulmonary hyalinizing granuloma. Am Rev Respir Dis 1977;115:997–1008.
53. Falk RH, Skinner M. The systemic amyloidoses: an overview. Adv Intern Med 2000;45:107–37.
54. Fenoglio C, Pascal RR. Nodular amyloidosis of the lungs. An unusual case associated with chronic lung disease and carcinoma of the bladder. Arch Pathol 1970;90:577–82.
55. Ferretti GR, Lantuejoul S, Brambilla E, Coulomb M. Case report. Pulmonary involvement in Niemann-Pick disease subtype B: CT findings. J Comput Assist Tomogr 1996;20:990–2.
56. Flieder DB, Moran CA, Travis WD, Koss MN, Mark EJ. Pleuro-pulmonary endometriosis and pulmonary ectopic deciduosis: a clinicopathologic and immunohistochemical study of 10 cases with emphasis on diagnostic pitfalls. Hum Pathol 1998;29:1495–503.
57. Fraser RS, Müller NL, Colman N, Pare PD. Metabolic pulmonary disease. In: Fraser RS, Müller NL, Colman N, Pare PD, eds. Fraser and Pare's diagnosis of diseases of the chest, 4th ed. Philadelphia: WB Saunders; 1999:2699–736.
58. Fraser RS, Müller NL, Colman N, Pare PD. Neoplasms of uncertain histogenesis and non-neoplastic tumors. In: Fraser RS, Müller NL, Colman N, Pare PD, eds. Fraser and Pare's diagnosis of diseases of the chest, Philadelphia: WB Saunders; 1999:1363–80.
59. Gal AA, Koss MN, McCarthy WF, Hochholzer L. Prognostic factors in pulmonary fibrohistiocytic lesions. Cancer 1994;73:1817–24.
60. Gertz MA, Kyle RA, Noel P. Primary systemic amyloidosis: a rare complication of immunoglobulin M monoclonal gammopathies and Waldenstrom's macroglobulinemia. J Clin Oncol 1993;11:914–20.
61. Gertz MA, Lacy MQ, Dispenzieri A. Amyloidosis. Hematol Oncol Clin North Am 1999;13: 1211–33.
62. Gordon HW, Miller R Jr, Mittman C. Medullary carcinoma of the lung with amyloid stroma: a counterpart of medullary carcinoma of the thyroid. Hum Pathol 1973;4:431-6.
63. Gorini M, Forloni F, Pezzoli A, Pezzica E. Pulmonary hyalinizing granuloma. A limited form of Wegener's granulomatosis? Ann Ital Med Int 1998;13:176–9.
64. Gottlieb LS, Gold WM. Primary tracheobronchial amyloidosis. Am Rev Respir Dis 1972;105:425–9.
65. Green JD, Harle TS, Greenberg SD, Weg JG, Nevin H, Jenkins DE. Disseminated pulmonary ossification. A case report with demonstration of electron-microscopic features. Am Rev Respir Dis 1970;101:293–8.
66. Grishman A, Kane IJ. Disseminated calcified and bony nodules in the lungs associated with mitral disease. AJR Am J Roentgenol 1945;53: 575–81.
67. Guccion JG, Rohatgi PK, Saini N. Pulmonary hyalinizing granuloma. Electron microscopic and immunologic studies. Chest 1984;85:571–3.
68. Halliday BE, Silverman JF, Finley JL. Fine-needle aspiration cytology of amyloid associated with nonneoplastic and malignant lesions. Diagn Cytopathol 1998;18:270–5.

69. Harats D, Pauzner R, Elstein D, et al. Pulmonary hypertension in two patients with type I Gaucher disease while on alglucerase therapy. Acta Haematol 1997;98:47–50.
70. Holmes S, Desai JB, Sapsford RN. Nodular pulmonary amyloidosis: a case report and review of literature. Br J Dis Chest 1988;82:414–7.
71. Hong HY, Castelli MJ, Walloch JL. Pulmonary plasma cell granuloma (inflammatory pseudotumor) with invasion of thoracic vertebra. Mt Sinai J Med 1990;57:117–21.
72. Hong YJ, Paik HC, Kim HJ, et al. A case of parenchymal pulmonary endometriosis. Yonsei Med J 1999;40:514–7.
73. Hui AN, Koss MN, Hochholzer L, Wehunt WD. Amyloidosis presenting in the lower respiratory tract. Clinicopathologic, radiologic, immunohistochemical, and histochemical studies on 48 cases. Arch Pathol Lab Med 1986;110:212–8.
74. Hurt MA, Santa Cruz DJ. Cutaneous inflammatory pseudotumor. Lesions resembling "inflammatory pseudotumors" or "plasma cell granulomas" of extracutaneous sites. Am J Surg Pathol 1990;14:764–73.
75. Ikard RW. Pulmonary hyalinizing granuloma Chest 1988;93:871–2.
76. Iwasaki T, Hamano T, Aizawa K, Kobayashi K, Kakishita E. A case of pulmonary amyloidosis associated with multiple myeloma successfully treated with dimethyl sulfoxide. Acta Haematol 1994;91:91–4.
77. John PG, Rahman J, Payne CB. Pulmonary hyalinizing granuloma: an unusual association with multiple sclerosis. South Med J 1995;88:1076–7.
78. Johnson WJ, Lie JT. Pulmonary hypertension and familial Mediterranean fever: a previously unrecognized association. Mayo Clin Proc 1991;66:919–25.
79. Joines RW, Roggli VL. Dendriform pulmonary ossification. Report of two cases with unique findings. Am J Clin Pathol 1989;91:398–402.
80. Joseph G, Pandit M, Korfhage L. Primary pulmonary plasmacytoma. Cancer 1993;71:721–4.
81. Joseph J, Sahn SA. Thoracic endometriosis syndrome: new observations from an analysis of 110 cases. Am J Med 1996;100:164–70.
82. Kadoyama C, Yokosuka T, Otsuji M, Suzuki M. [Pulmonary hyalinizing granuloma diagnosed by thoracoscopy]. Nihon Kokyuki Gakkai Zasshi 1999;37:481–4.
83. Kamberg S, Loitman BS, Holtz S. Amyloidosis of the tracheobronchial tree. N Engl J Med 1962;266:587–91.
84. Kaw YT, Esparza AR. Solitary pleural amyloid nodules occurring as coin lesions diagnosed by fine-needle aspiration biopsy. Diagn Cytopathol 1991;7:304–7.
85. Kerem E, Elstein D, Abrahamov A, et al. Pulmonary function abnormalities in type I Gaucher disease. Eur Respir J 1996;9:340–5.
86. Khafif RA, DeLima C, Silverberg A, Frankel R. Calciphylaxis and systemic calcinosis. Collective review. Arch Intern Med 1990;150:956–9.
87. Kijner CH, Yousem SA. Systemic light chain deposition disease presenting as multiple pulmonary nodules. A case report and review of the literature. Am J Surg Pathol 1988;12:405–13.
88. Kim HY, Im JG, Song KS, et al. Localized amyloidosis of the respiratory system: CT features. J Comput Assist Tomogr 1999;23:627–31.
89. Kirchner J, Jacobi V, Kardos P, Kollath J. CT findings in extensive tracheobronchial amyloidosis. Eur Radiol 1998;8:352–4.
90. Knapp MJ, Roggli VL, Kim J, Moore JO, Shelburne JD. Pleural amyloidosis. Arch Pathol Lab Med 1988;112:57–60.
91. Kobayashi H, Matsuoka R, Kitamura S, Tsunoda N, Saito K. Sjögren's syndrome with multiple bullae and pulmonary nodular amyloidosis. Chest 1988;94:438–40.
92. Koizumi T, Inagaki H, Takabayashi Y, Kubo K. Successful use of gonadotropin-releasing hormone agonist in a patient with pulmonary endometriosis. Respiration 1999;66:544–6.
93. Koss MN, Hochholzer L, Langloss JM, Lazarus AA, Wehunt WD. Lymphoid interstitial pneumonitis: clinicopathologic and immunopathologic findings in 18 patients. Pathology 1987;19:178–85.
94. Koss MN, Hochholzer L, Moran CA, Frizzera G. Pulmonary plasmacytomas: a clinicopathologic and immunohistochemical study of five cases. Ann Diagn Pathol 1998;2:1–11.
95. Kradin RL, Mark EJ. Benign lymphoid disorders of the lung, with a theory regarding their development. Hum Pathol 1983;14:857–67.
96. Kumamoto H, Ichinohasama R, Sawai T, et al. Multiple organ failure associated with extensive metastatic calcification in a patient with an intermediate state of human T lymphotropic virus type I (HTLV-I) infection: report of an autopsy case. Pathol Int 1998;48:313–8.
97. Kuramochi S, Kawai T, Yakumaru K, et al. Multiple pulmonary hyalinizing granulomas associated with systemic idiopathic fibrosis. Acta Pathol Jpn 1991;41:375–82.
98. Kuzela DC. Ultrastructural study of a postinflammatory "tumor" of the lung. Cancer 1975;36:149–56.
99. Laden SA, Cohen ML, Harley RA. Nodular pulmonary amyloidosis with extrapulmonary involvement. Hum Pathol 1984;15:594–7.

100. Ledet SC, Brown RW, Cagle PT. p53 immunostaining in the differentiation of inflammatory pseudotumor from sarcoma involving the lung. Mod Pathol 1995;8:282–6.
101. Lee KS, Kim TS, Han J, et al. Diffuse micronodular lung disease: HRCT and pathologic findings. J Comput Assist Tomogr 1999;23:99–106.
102. Lhote F, Chapelon C, Piette JC, Andrien JM, Chomette G, Godeau P. Pulmonary hyalinizing granuloma. Apropos of 2 new cases. Rev Mal Respir 1991;8:246–8.
103. Liaw YS, Kuo SH, Yang PC, Chen CL, Luh KT. Nodular amyloidosis of the lung and the breast mimicking breast carcinoma with pulmonary metastasis. Eur Respir J 1995;8:871–3.
104. Links TP, Karrenbeld A, Steensma JT, Weits J, van der Jagt EJ, Postmus PE. Fatal respiratory failure caused by pulmonary infiltration by pseudo-Gaucher cells. Chest 1992;101:265–6.
105. Lipton JH, Fong TC, Gill MJ, Burgess K, Elliott PD. Q fever inflammatory pseudotumor of the lung. Chest 1987;92:756–7.
106. Livneh A, Langevitz P, Pras M. Pulmonary associations in familial Mediterranean fever. Curr Opin Pulm Med 1999;5:326–31.
107. Long FL, Nott DB, MacArthur EB. Xanthomatous tumour of the lung with identification of lipid content. Australas Ann Med 1970;19: 362–5.
108. Machicao CN, Sorensen K, Abdul-Karim FW, Somrak TM. Transthoracic needle aspiration biopsy in inflammatory pseudotumors of the lung. Diagn Cytopathol 1989;5:400–3.
109. Maier HC, Sommers SC. Recurrent and metastatic pulmonary fibrous histiocytoma/plasma cell granuloma in a child. Cancer 1987;60: 1073–6.
110. Makela V, Mattila S, Makinen J. Plasma cell granuloma (histiocytoma) of the lung and pleura. Report on three cases. Acta Pathol Microbiol Scand [A] 1972;80:634–40.
111. Mandelbaum I, Brashear RE, Hull MT. Surgical treatment and course of pulmonary pseudotumor (plasma cell granuloma). J Thorac Cardiovasc Surg 1981;82:77–82.
112. Massachusetts General Hospital, Case Records. Weekly clinicopathological exercises. Case 6-1989. A 57-year-old man with increasing dyspnea and a mediastinal mass. N Engl J Med 1989;320:380–9.
113. Mata JM, Caceres J, Senac JP, Giron J, Alegret X. General case of the day. Nodular amyloidosis of the lung. Radiographics 1991;11:716–8.
114. Mathlouthi A, Ben Rehouma C, Ben M'Rad S, et al. [Tracheobronchopathia osteochondroplastica. Personal observation and review of the literature]. Rev Pneumol Clin 1993;49:156–62.
115. Matsubara O, Tan-Liu NS, Kenney RM, Mark EJ. Inflammatory pseudotumors of the lung: progression from organizing pneumonia to fibrous histiocytoma or to plasma cell granuloma in 32 cases. Hum Pathol 1988;19:807–14.
116. Matsuo T, Tsukamoto Y, Tamura M, et al. Acute respiratory failure due to "pulmonary calciphylaxis" in a maintenance haemodialysis patient. Nephron 2001;87:75–9.
117. Meis JM, Enzinger FM. Inflammatory fibrosarcoma of the mesentery and retroperitoneum. A tumor closely simulating inflammatory pseudotumor. Am J Surg Pathol 1991;15:1146–56.
118. Meis-Kindblom JM, Kjellstrom C, Kindblom LG. Inflammatory fibrosarcoma: update, reappraisal, and perspective on its place in the spectrum of inflammatory myofibroblastic tumors. Semin Diagn Pathol 1998;15:133–43.
119. Messineo A, Mognato G, D'Amore ES, Antoniello L, Guglielmi M, Cecchetto G. Inflammatory pseudotumors of the lung in children: conservative or aggressive approach? Med Pediatr Oncol 1998;31:100–4.
120. Meyer CN, Dossing M, Broholm H. Tracheobronchopathia osteochondroplastica. Respir Med 1997;91:499–502.
121. Miura K, Shirasawa H. Lambda III subgroup immunoglobulin light chains are precursor proteins of nodular pulmonary amyloidosis. Am J Clin Pathol 1993;100:561–6.
122. Miyamoto T, Kobayashi T, Makiyama M, et al. Monoclonality of infiltrating plasma cells in primary pulmonary nodular amyloidosis: detection with polymerase chain reaction. J Clin Pathol 1999;52:464–7.
123. Monreal FA. Pulmonary amyloidosis: ultrastructural study of early alveolar septal deposits. Hum Pathol 1984;15:388–90.
124. Monzon CM, Gilchrist GS, Burgert EO Jr, et al. Plasma cell granuloma of the lung in children. Pediatrics 1982;70:268–74.
125. Morinaga S, Watanabe H, Gemma A, et al. Plasmacytoma of the lung associated with nodular deposits of immunoglobulin. Am J Surg Pathol 1987;11:989–95.
126. Morita Y, Tsutsumi O, Taketani Y. Successful hormonal treatment of pulmonary parenchymal endometriosis. Int J Gynaecol Obstet 1997;59:61–3.
127. Muller KM, Friemann J, Stichnoth E. Dendriform pulmonary ossification. Pathol Res Pract 1980;168:163–72.
128. Muraoka S, Sato T, Takahashi T, Ando M, Shimoda A. Plasma cell granuloma of the lung with extrapulmonal extension. Immunohistochemical and electron microscopic studies. Acta Pathol Jpn 1985;35:933–44.

129. Murray RA, Poulton TB, Saltarelli MG, et al. Rare pulmonary manifestation of Ehlers-Danlos syndrome. J Thorac Imaging 1995;10:138–41.
130. Nakatani Y, Nakamura N, Sano J, et al. Interstitial pneumonia in Hermansky-Pudlak syndrome: significance of florid foamy swelling/degeneration (giant lamellar body degeneration) of type-2 pneumocytes. Virchows Arch [A] 2000;437:304–13.
131. Ndimbie OK, Williams CR, Lee MW. Dendriform pulmonary ossification. Arch Pathol Lab Med 1987;111:1062–4.
132. Nizami MA, Gerntholtz T, Swanepoel CR. The role of bone scanning in the detection of metastatic calcification: a case report. Clin Nucl Med 2000;25:407–9.
133. Page DL, Isersky C, Harada M, Glenner GG. Immunoglobulin origin of localized nodular pulmonary amyloidosis. Res Exp Med (Berl) 1972;159:75–86.
134. Papla B, Dubiel-Bigaj M. Tracheobronchial amyloidosis. Pol J Pathol 1998;49:27–34.
135. Patel Y, Ishikawa S, MacDonnell KF. Pulmonary hyalinizing granuloma presenting as multiple cavitary calcified nodules. Chest 1991; 100:1720–1.
136. Pettinato G, Manivel JC, De Rosa N, Dehner LP. Inflammatory myofibroblastic tumor (plasma cell granuloma). Clinicopathologic study of 20 cases with immunohistochemical and ultrastructural observations. Am J Clin Pathol 1990;94:538–46.
137. Pickford HA, Swensen SJ, Utz JP. Thoracic cross-sectional imaging of amyloidosis. AJR Am J Roentgenol 1997;168:351–5.
138. Piercecchi MD, Sault MC, Cailleres S, Blanc AP, Sudan N. [Interstitial pneumopathy revealing type B Niemann Pick disease in an adult]. Rev Med Interne 1999;20:597–601.
139. Pilozzi E, Stoppacciaro A, Rendina E, Ruco LP. Monocyte chemotactic protein-1 in the inflammatory pseudotumour of the lung. Mol Pathol 1998;51:50–2.
140. Planes C, Kleinknecht D, Brauner M, Battesti JP, Kemeny JL, Valeyre D. Diffuse interstitial lung disease due to AA amyloidosis. Thorax 1992;47:323–4.
141. Popelka CG, Kleinerman J. Diffuse pulmonary ossification. Arch Intern Med 1977;137:523–5.
142. Pounder DJ, Pieterse AS. Tracheopathia osteoplastica: a study of the minimal lesion. J Pathol 1982;138:235–9.
143. Reynolds SP, Davies BH, Gibbs AR. Diffuse pulmonary fibrosis and the Hermansky-Pudlak syndrome: clinical course and postmortem findings. Thorax 1994;49:617–8.
144. Richmond I, Hasleton PS, Samadian S. Systemic amyloid associated with carcinoma of the bronchus. Thorax 1990;45:156–7.
145. Ritter JH, Humphrey PA, Wick MR. Malignant neoplasms capable of simulating inflammatory (myofibroblastic) pseudotumors and tumefactive fibroinflammatory lesions: pseudopseudotumors. Semin Diagn Pathol 1998;15:111–32.
146. Rohrlich P, Peuchmaur M, Cocci SN, et al. Interleukin-6 and interleukin-1 beta production in a pediatric plasma cell granuloma of the lung. Am J Surg Pathol 1995;19:590–5.
147. Sajjad SM, Begin LR, Dail DH, Lukeman JM. Fibrous histiocytoma of lung—a clinicopathological study of two cases. Histopathology 1981;5:325–34.
148. Santamaria F, Parenti G, Guidi G, et al. Pulmonary manifestations of Gaucher disease: an increased risk for L444P homozygotes? Am J Respir Crit Care Med 1998;157:985–9.
149. Schaefer HE. Gammopathy-related crystal-storing histiocytosis, pseudo- and pseudo-pseudo-Gaucher cells. Critical commentary and mini-review. Pathol Res Pract 1996;192:1152–62.
150. Schlosnagle DC, Check IJ, Sewell CW, Plummer A, York RM, Hunter RL. Immunologic abnormalities in two patients with pulmonary hyalinizing granuloma. Am J Clin Pathol 1982;78:231–5.
151. Sekosan M, Cleto M, Senseng C, Farolan M, Sekosan J. Spindle cell pseudotumors in the lungs due to Mycobacterium tuberculosis in a transplant patient. Am J Surg Pathol 1994;18:1065–8.
152. Shimizu I, Nakanishi R, Yoshino I, Yasumoto K. An endometrial nodule in the lung without pelvic endometriosis. J Cardiovasc Surg (Torino) 1998;39:867–8.
153. Snyder CS, Dell'Aquila MD, Haghighi P, Baergen RN, Suh YK, Yi ES. Clonal changes in inflammatory pseudotumor of the lung. A case report. Cancer 1995;76:1545–9.
154. Spencer H. The pulmonary plasma cell/histiocytoma complex. Histopathology 1984;8:903–16.
155. Stokes MB, Jagirdar J, Burchstin O, Kornacki S, Kumar A, Gallo G. Nodular pulmonary immunoglobulin light chain deposits with coexistent amyloid and nonamyloid features in an HIV-infected patient. Mod Pathol 1997;10:1059–65.
156. Strimlan CV, Rosenow EC, Weiland LH, Brown LR. Lymphocytic interstitial pneumonitis. Review of 13 cases. Ann Intern Med 1978;88:616–21.
157. Su LD, Atayde-Perez A, Sheldon S, Fletcher JA, Weiss SW. Inflammatory myofibroblastic tumor: cytogenetic evidence supporting clonal origin. Mod Pathol 1998;11:364–8.

158. Sumiya M, Ohya N, Shinoura H, et al. Diffuse interstitial pulmonary amyloidosis in rheumatoid arthritis. J Rheumatol 1996;23:933–6.
159. Takashi S, Koizumi T, Yamazaki Y, et al. Diffuse pulmonary amyloidosis with monoclonal IgG-kappa gammopathy. Intern Med 1997;36:357–9.
160. Tanino M, Odashima S, Sugiura H, Matsue T, Kajikawa M, Maeda S. Malignant fibrous histiocytoma of the lung. Acta Pathol Jpn 1985;35: 945–50.
161. Tan-Liu NS, Matsubara O, Grillo HC, Mark EJ. Invasive fibrous tumor of the tracheobronchial tree: clinical and pathologic study of seven cases. Hum Pathol 1989;20:180–4.
162. Tariq SM, Morrison D, McConnochie K. Solitary bronchial amyloid presenting with haemoptysis. Eur Respir J 1990;3:1230–1.
163. Terada Y, Chen F, Shoji T, Itoh H, Wada H, Hitomi S. A case of endobronchial endometriosis treated by subsegmentectomy. Chest 1999;115:1475–8.
164. Theise ND, Ursell PC. Pulmonary hypertension and Gaucher's disease: logical association or mere coincidence? Am J Pediatr Hematol Oncol 1990;12:74–6.
165. Titus JL, Harrison EG, Clagett OT, Anderson MW, Knaff LJ. Xanthomatous and inflammatory pseudotumors of the lung. Cancer 1962;15:522–38.
166. Toyoda M, Ebihara Y, Kato H, Kita S. Tracheobronchial AL amyloidosis: histologic, immunohistochemical, ultrastructural, and immunoelectron microscopic observations. Hum Pathol 1993;24:970–6.
167. Travis WD, Colby TV, Corrin B, Shimosato Y, Brambilla E, in collaboration with L. H. Sobin and pathologists from 14 countries. Histological typing of lung and pleural tumors, 3rd ed. Berlin: Springer; 1999.
168. Ulbright TM, Katzenstein AL. Solitary necrotizing granulomas of the lung: differentiating features and etiology. Am J Surg Pathol 1980;4:13–28.
169. Umlas J, Federman M, Crawford C, O'Hara CJ, Fitzgibbon JS, Modeste A. Spindle cell pseudotumor due to Mycobacterium avium-intracellulare in patients with acquired immunodeficiency syndrome (AIDS). Positive staining of mycobacteria for cytoskeleton filaments. Am J Surg Pathol 1991;15:1181–7.
170. Usuda K, Saito Y, Imai T, et al. Inflammatory pseudotumor of the lung diagnosed as granulomatous lesion by preoperative brushing cytology. A case report. Acta Cytol 1990;34:685–9.
171. Utz JP, Swensen SJ, Gertz MA. Pulmonary amyloidosis. The Mayo Clinic experience from 1980 to 1993. Ann Intern Med 1996;124:407–13.
172. Vilkman S, Keistinen T. Tracheobronchopathia osteochondroplastica. Report of a young man with severe disease and retrospective review of 18 cases. Respiration 1995;62:151–4.
173. Ware LB, Keith FM, Gordon RL, et al. Lung transplantation for pulmonary amyloidosis: a case report. J Heart Lung Transplant 1998;17: 1129–32.
174. Warter A, Satge D, Roeslin N. Angioinvasive plasma cell granulomas of the lung. Cancer 1987;59:435–43.
175. Weber AL. Radiologic evaluation of the trachea. Chest Surg Clin N Am 1996;6:637–73.
176. Wells HG, Dunlap CE. Disseminated ossification of the lungs. Arch Pathol 1943;35:420–6.
177. Wentworth P, Lynch MJ, Fallis JC, Turner JA, Lowden JA, Conen PE. Xanthomatous pseudotumor of lung. A case report with electron microscope and lipid studies. Cancer 1968;22:345–55.
178. Wick MR, Ritter JH, Nappi O. Inflammatory sarcomatoid carcinoma of the lung: report of three cases and clinicopathologic comparison with inflammatory pseudotumors in adult patients. Hum Pathol 1995;26:1014–21.
179. Wilson SR, Sanders DE, Delarue NC. Intrathoracic manifestations of amyloid disease. Radiology 1976;120:283–9.
180. Wong BC, Wong KL, Ip MS, Wang EP, Chan KW, Cheng LC. Sjögren's syndrome with amyloid A presenting as multiple pulmonary nodules. J Rheumatol 1994;21:165–7.
181. Yost BA, Vogelsang JP, Lie JT. Fatal hemoptysis in Ehlers-Danlos syndrome. Old malady with a new curse. Chest 1995;107:1465–7.
182. Young RH, Sandstrom RE, Mark GJ. Tracheopathia osteoplastica: clinical, radiologic, and pathological correlations. J Thorac Cardiovasc Surg 1980;79:537–41.
183. Yousem SA, Hochholzer L. Malignant fibrous histiocytoma of the lung. Cancer 1987;60: 2532–41.
184. Yousem SA, Hochholzer L. Pulmonary hyalinizing granuloma. Am J Clin Pathol 1987;87:1–6.

18
PLEURAL DISORDERS

The pleura is a serous membrane consisting of a visceral component that lines the lung parenchyma and a parietal component that covers the mediastinum, diaphragm, and rib cage (22,30). The visceral and parietal pleurae merge at the root of the lung at the pulmonary hilus. The pulmonary ligament consists of a thin double fold of pleura posterior to the lung root (30). A thin layer of pleural fluid lubricates the surfaces of the visceral and parietal pleurae, allowing them move easily during respiration. The right and left pleural spaces are separated by the mediastinum (22,30).

Histologically, the visceral pleura consists of five layers: a single layer of mesothelial cells; a submesothelial layer of connective tissue; an inner thin elastic fiber layer; an outer layer of interstitial connective tissue; and a thick elastic fiber layer (22). The normal pleura may be very thin, making it difficult to appreciate each of these layers; in the parietal pleura these layers are not as distinct. The pleura is rich in blood vessels that consist of arteries, veins, and capillaries, as well as many lymphatics. The diaphragmatic and costal parietal pleura, contains sensory nerves, which are supplied by branches of the intercostal nerves in the costal and part of the diaphragmatic pleura and by the phrenic nerve for the central diaphragm.

The mesothelial cells are normally only about 1 µm thick. They have numerous long surface microvilli that can be seen by electron microscopy. Stomata or openings between the mesothelial cells on the parietal pleura are thought to communicate directly with underlying lymphatics. The mesothelial cells are very sensitive to injury and often show a reactive mesothelial hyperplasia.

Since the pleura is so sensitive to injury, there are a variety of subtle, nonspecific changes that can occur. These include inflammation, fibrosis, and mesothelial hyperplasia. In a scanning electron microscopic study, Peng et al. (44) demonstrated subclinical surface alterations of the pleura in patients with pulmonary or cardiac disease. They found that damage to the pleura results in exposure of the basal lamina or the underlying connective tissue matrix of collagen bundles and wavy elastic fibers; repair occurs by the proliferation of reactive mesothelial cells.

PNEUMOTHORAX

Definition. Pneumothorax is the presence of air or gas within the pleural space, between the visceral and parietal pleurae.

Pneumothoraces can be spontaneous or traumatic, and a subset of the latter is iatrogenic. *Spontaneous pneumothorax* may be primary or secondary. Primary spontaneous pneumothorax occurs in patients without preexisting lung disease or when there is no apparent provoking factor. Secondary spontaneous pneumothorax occurs in individuals with known lung disease (Table 18-1) (16,21,30).

Most cases result from rupture of subpleural emphysematous blebs in the lung apices. This often occurs in patients with emphysema when associated blebs rupture (see chapter 10). Bronchial anomalies, found on bronchoscopy, increase the risk of spontaneous pneumothorax more than 200-fold (3).

Iatrogenic pneumothorax is a recognized complication of invasive procedures that penetrate the pleura such as diagnostic interventions: transthoracic needle aspiration, placement of a catheter in the subclavian vein, thoracentesis, pleural biopsy, and barotrauma. *Traumatic pneumothorax* is the result of penetrating or blunt trauma to the chest, with air entering the pleural space directly through the chest wall; visceral pleural penetration; or alveolar rupture due to sudden compression of the chest (47). *Tension pneumothorax* is present when the intrapleural pressure exceeds the atmospheric pressure throughout expiration and often during inspiration as well. This is a medical emergency seen most often in patients receiving mechanical ventilation and is characterized by sudden deterioration in cardiopulmonary status. *Catamenial pneumothorax* is pneumothorax associated with menstruation and is typically recurrent (30). It is very rare and occurs most often on the right. The pathogenesis of catamenial pneumothorax

Table 18-1

CAUSES OF SECONDARY SPONTANEOUS PNEUMOTHORAX[a]

Airway Disease
- Emphysema
- Cystic fibrosis
- Status asthmaticus

Infectious Lung Disease
- *Pneumocystis carinii* pneumonia
- Tuberculosis
- Necrotizing pneumonias

Interstitial Lung Disease
- Sarcoidosis
- Idiopathic pulmonary fibrosis
- Langerhans' cell histiocytosis
- Lymphangioleiomyomatosis
- Tuberous sclerosis
- Connective tissue disease
- Marfan's syndrome
- Ehlers-Danlos syndrome

Miscellaneous
- Malignancy
- Infarction
- Pneumonitis (chemical, radiation)
- Toxic drug effect (e.g., oxygen, pentamidine)
- Drug abuse (e.g., cocaine, marijuana)
- Pneumoperitoneum (via diaphragm defects)
- Esophageal rupture
- Thoracic endometriosis

[a]Information from references 3, 16, and 34.

is unknown, but some cases are shown to be associated with pleural endometriosis. Diaphragmatic defects allowing air to enter the pleural cavity from the peritoneum have been proposed. Another potential cause of pneumothorax is bronchopleural fistula, which is a fistula between a bronchus and the pleural cavity. Such fistulas occur following lung surgery or as a complication of underlying pulmonary disease; they occur in 1 to 4 percent of patients following lobectomy or pneumonectomy.

Clinical Features. The age-adjusted incidence of spontaneous pneumothorax in Olmstead County, Minnesota (between 1950 and 1974) was 7.9/100,000 person-years (36). Primary and secondary pneumothoraces occur more frequently in men: the male to female ratio was 6 to 1 for primary pneumothorax compared to 3 to 1 for secondary pneumothorax (36). A recent review from England described incidences of 16.8/100,000 for outpatients and 11.1/100,000 for emergency admissions (20). A bimodal age distribution has been described, with the first peak between 20 and 24 years and the second between 80 and 84 years for men; women have an early peak at 30 to 34 years. Young healthy patients tend to have primary pneumothoraces due to subpleural apical blebs or a congenital abnormality of the pleura (5,27). Older patients are more likely to have pneumothoraces associated with emphysema or lung fibrosis (43,57,59,60). Pneumothoraces are rare in children. Cigarette smoking dramatically increases the risk of spontaneous pneumothorax: 22 times for men and 8 times for women (4). The risk is dose related.

Most patients have onset of symptoms between 5 and 8 am, during a period of inactivity or low activity (6). Most patients (80 to 90 percent) experience a sudden onset of chest pain and shortness of breath (21 to 64 percent) (48). Less common symptoms include cough and generalized malaise (48,59,60). A small number of patients (6 to 30 percent) are asymptomatic or have minor, nonspecific complaints; the pneumothorax is found incidentally on radiographic evaluation (48,60). The chest pain usually lateralizes to the side of the pneumothorax, since it is rare for spontaneous pneumothoraces to be bilateral (about 5 percent of cases) (36). The pain may be pleuritic, increasing with respiration. Most patients are able to define a specific time of onset of chest pain, with the duration typically less than 24 hours (usually 1 to 2 hours). Typically, symptoms are more severe in those with secondary pneumothorax, given the limited pulmonary reserve in patients with underlying lung disease. Splinting provides partial pain relief.

Patients with pneumothorax are usually taller and thinner than control subjects (37,61). Specifically, thin tall males are thought to be the prototypic patient for pneumothorax. However, a series of Japanese patients demonstrated that the association is more with low body weight/obesity indices and lung height, rather than body height (25). Tachypnea and tachycardia are common. Inspection may reveal decreased chest wall movement on the side of the pneumothorax. Auscultation demonstrates diminished or absent breath sounds and hyperresonance on

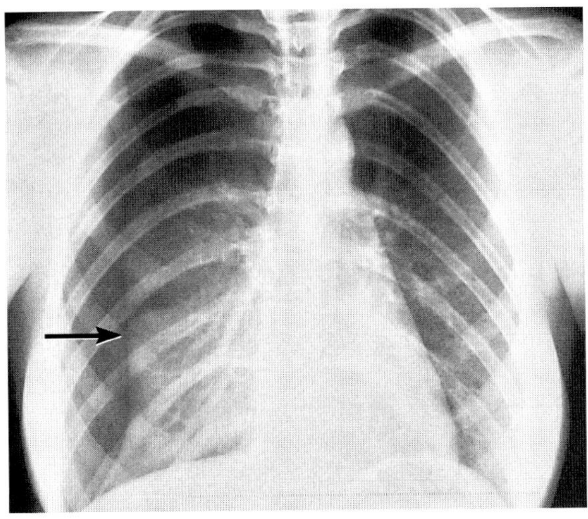

Figure 18-1

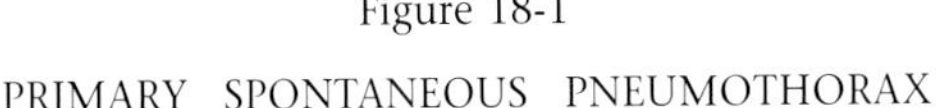

PRIMARY SPONTANEOUS PNEUMOTHORAX

Primary spontaneous pneumothorax in a 19-year-old female with recurrent right-sided pneumothoraces. Expiratory posteroanterior (PA) chest radiograph demonstrates a large pneumothorax. The white pleural line facilitates visualization (arrow). Distal pulmonary markings are absent. The underlying lung has a low volume but is otherwise unremarkable. At surgery, subpleural blebs and fibrous pleuritis were identified.

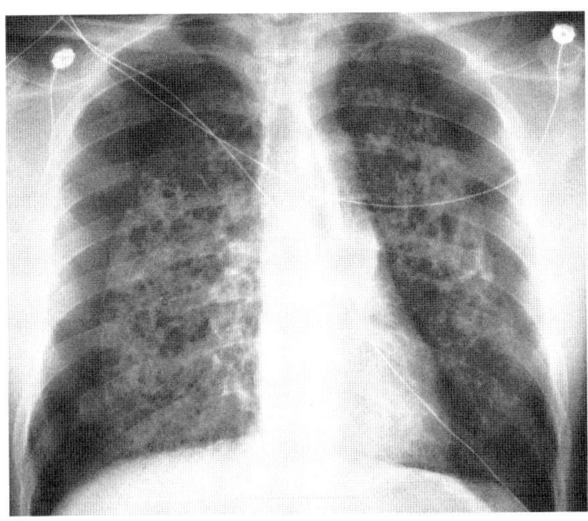

Figure 18-2

SECONDARY SPONTANEOUS PNEUMOTHORAX

Secondary spontaneous pneumothorax in a 26-year-old male smoker who presented to the emergency room with acute progressive dyspnea. PA chest radiograph demonstrates moderate to large, bilateral pneumothoraces. Note the bilateral diffuse cystic lung disease. The biopsy revealed Langerhans' cell histiocytosis.

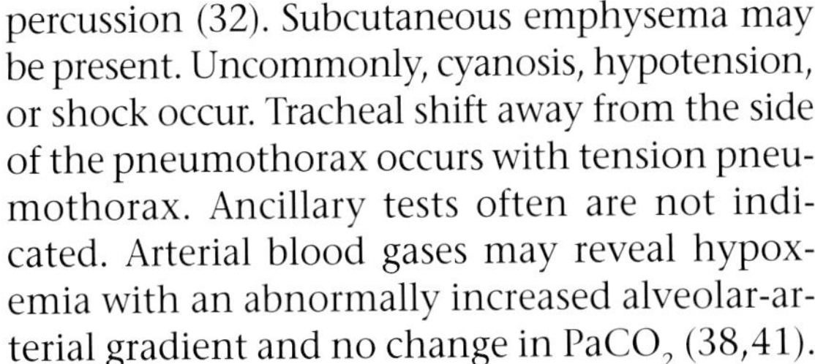

percussion (32). Subcutaneous emphysema may be present. Uncommonly, cyanosis, hypotension, or shock occur. Tracheal shift away from the side of the pneumothorax occurs with tension pneumothorax. Ancillary tests often are not indicated. Arterial blood gases may reveal hypoxemia with an abnormally increased alveolar-arterial gradient and no change in $PaCO_2$ (38,41).

Radiologic Findings. The chest radiograph is an excellent method for diagnosing pneumothorax. The pneumothorax is identified when a thin white pleural line with a radiolucent space along its periphery is noted (19). The absence of normal pulmonary markings beyond the pleural line is confirmatory evidence (fig. 18-1). Pleural air typically accumulates in the nondependent aspect of the pleural space. Thus, visualization of a pneumothorax may depend on the position of the patient during radiography. Upright expiratory radiography is optimal for diagnosis. Expiration decreases the volume of the lung, increases its radiographic opacity, and enhances the conspicuity of a pneumothorax. Decubitus radiography may also be helpful (19). In patients with underlying bullous disease the distinction between bullae and pneumothoraces may be difficult (58). In this instance, computed tomography (CT) of the chest is the most sensitive diagnostic tool (60).

Primary spontaneous pneumothorax typically occurs in the absence of radiographically visible pulmonary disease (fig. 18-1). However, the majority of affected patients have evidence of emphysema on CT, typically located in the apical lung periphery. Secondary spontaneous pneumothorax occurs in association with underlying pulmonary disease, such as cavitary conditions, emphysema, chronic obstructive pulmonary disease, chronic infiltrative lung disease (fig. 18-2), or malignant neoplasia (19). The chest radiograph or CT scan may also show evidence of trauma or iatrogenic etiologies through visualization of rib fractures, pulmonary contusions, evidence of prior invasive procedures such as thoracentesis or lung biopsy, or evidence of mechanical ventilation, invasive monitoring, and life support devices (52,53). Large cysts or emphysematous bullae, skin folds, the inner border of the scapula, chest bandages, and a large diaphragmatic hernia with a herniated air-

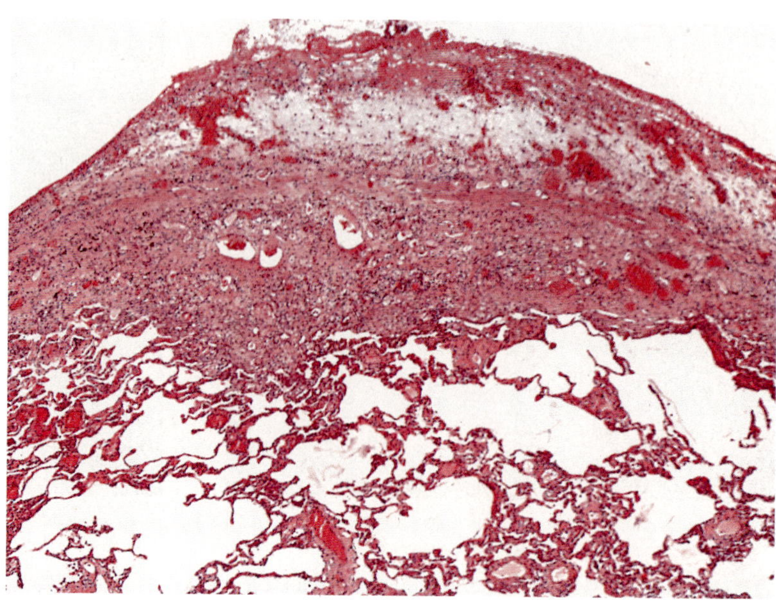

Figure 18-3

FIBROSING PLEURITIS

Fibrosing pleuritis in a pleural biopsy from a patient with spontaneous pneumothorax.

filled viscus may simulate a pneumothorax on chest radiography (60).

Pathologic Findings. Jordan et al. (24) described the pathologic findings of a large series of patients with spontaneous pneumothorax. These authors found emphysema with bullae formation in 80 percent of patients. Irregular emphysema was the most common pattern identified, followed by distal acinar (paraseptal), mixed irregular and distal acinar, mixed irregular and centrilobular, and unclassifiable emphysema (see chapter 10) (24). When biopsies of the parietal pleura were available, either a nonspecific reactive pleuritis or normal pleura was seen.

Idiopathic spontaneous pneumothorax is frequently associated with pleural fibrosis (fig. 18-3) as well as a variety of vascular changes such as medial hypertrophy and intimal fibrosis, which can be misinterpreted as pulmonary hypertension (12). Cottin et al. (11) observed arteriolar intimal fibrosis in 39 percent of 79 patients with idiopathic spontaneous pneumothorax. Lichter and Gwynne (28) found arteriolar endarteritis in 45 percent of 20 cases of idiopathic spontaneous pneumothorax.

Tomashefski et al. (54) studied the pleural tissues following spontaneous pneumothorax in patients with and without cystic fibrosis (CF). They found distorted elastic fibers in areas of pleural fibrosis, adhesions, and air "cysts" in both groups. Following idiopathic spontaneous pneumothorax, they found chronic inflammation, granulation tissue, fibrosis, mesothelial hyperplasia, and reactive eosinophilic pleuritis. Although the pleura seemed more inflamed in CF patients, the main difference was the presence of myxoid connective tissue and vascular proliferation. Columnar, vacuolated mesothelial cells, also known as the Dunnill lesion, were focally observed only in patients with CF. They concluded that extensive degenerative pleural changes might be a nonspecific response to inflammation and predispose to pneumothorax in patients with CF.

Pleural biopsies from patients with catamenial pneumothorax often show the nonspecific histologic findings of pleuritis. In some cases the biopsy specimen may show pleural endometriosis (fig. 18-4), which is characterized by deposits of endometrial stroma, glands often associated with chronic hemorrhage, pleural inflammation, and fibrosis (17). Endometriosis may also involve the lung parenchyma, causing nodular masses (see chapter 17) (17).

Differential Diagnosis. The clinical differential diagnosis of pneumothorax includes pulmonary embolism or infarction, pericarditis, tracheal/esophageal perforation, pleural effusion, and pneumonia. Pulmonary embolism can produce symptoms and signs similar to those of pneumothorax, although clinical examination does not usually reveal asymmetry of breath sounds or hyperresonance. Pericarditis may produce sudden pleuritic pain, usually substernal

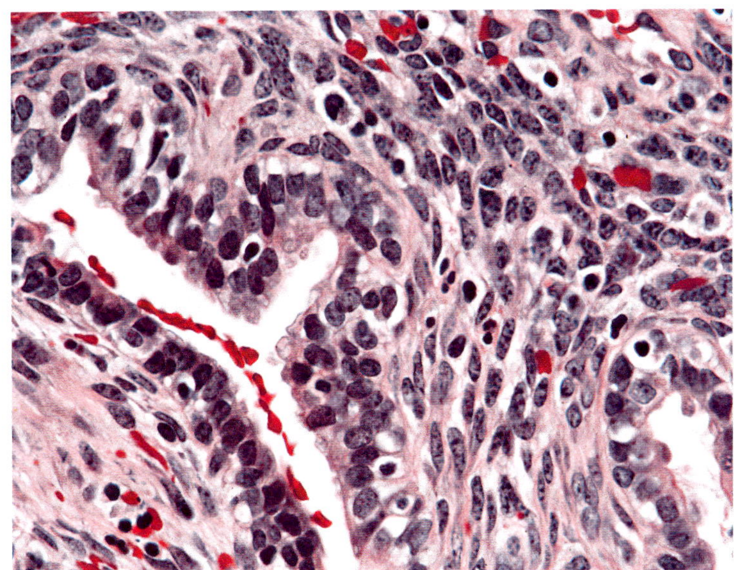

Figure 18-4

PLEURAL ENDOMETRIOSIS

Cleft-like spaces are lined by cuboidal to columnar epithelial cells overlying a cellular stroma. The stroma has an endometrial appearance consisting of bland spindle-shaped cells sprinkled with lymphocytes.

and not unilateral. Esophageal or tracheal disruption may be associated with a pneumothorax or pneumomediastinum. Pleural effusions and pneumonia may produce unilateral pleuritic chest pain, although this is usually slow to evolve.

Treatment and Prognosis. The goals of therapy in any patient with pneumothorax are to remove air from the pleural space to restore normal lung function as quickly as possible, and to prevent recurrence and mortality (12,29, 47). Important considerations include the stability of the patient, the size of the pneumothorax, the presence (and persistence of) an air leak, the number of prior pneumothoraces, and the predicted risk of recurrence (and patient's reserve to tolerate such a recurrence). Recurrences are common (approximately 50 percent of patients). Most recurrences occur within the first 6 months of the initial pneumothorax (31). Of the patients with a second spontaneous pneumothorax, the rate of recurrence is 60 percent and is 80 percent for those with a third pneumothorax. Death from spontaneous pneumothorax is rare and usually due to tension pneumothorax.

In a stable patient with a small pneumothorax (less than 20 percent), the most conservative approach is observation alone. Without intervention, air absorption occurs at a rate of 1.25 percent of the volume of the hemithorax per day (42). Supplemental oxygen therapy accelerates the rate of pleural air absorption by at least four times (14,29,42). Additional intervention is recommended for patients with pneumothoraces of greater than 20 percent (given the prolonged time for resolution) despite successful management of stable patients with larger pneumothoraces (42). Additional therapeutic options include: simple aspiration of air (thoracentesis with a small needle, about 16 gauge); drainage by a tube placed in the pleural space; pleurodesis (tube thoracostomy with the instillation of sclerosant, for example, talc slurry); thoracoscopy (with/without pleurodesis); and parietal pleurectomy. Pleurodesis reduces the rate of recurrence (31,43,48). The presence of a bronchopleural fistula (persistent air leak) necessitates surgical management. There is insufficient evidence on the effects of surgical pleurodesis compared to chemical pleurodesis. Unilateral pulmonary edema (reexpansion pulmonary edema) may occur following rapid expansion of a lung that has been collapsed for several days (60).

PLEURAL EFFUSION

Definition. Pleural effusion is an accumulation of fluid within the pleural cavity.

Pleural fluid normally flows from the capillaries on the parietal pleural surface through the pleural space and into the visceral pleura, where it is resorbed. The formation and movement of pleural fluid can result from an increase in hydrostatic pressure or a decrease in the oncotic pressure in the microvascular circulation, a decrease

Table 18-2

PLEURAL EFFUSIONS: DIFFERENTIAL DIAGNOSIS OF TRANSUDATES AND EXUDATES[a]

	Transudative Effusions	
Congestive heart failure	Peritoneal dialysis	Pulmonary embolism
Cirrhosis	Atelectasis	Urinothorax
Nephrotic syndrome	Myxedema	
	Exudative Effusions	
Malignancy	Other inflammatory	Drug-induced
Lung	Pulmonary embolism	Drug-induced lupus
Lymphoma	Dressler's syndrome	Nitrofurantoin
Mesothelioma	Asbestos	Dantrolene
Metastatic	Uremia	Amiodarone
	Trapped lung	Methysergide
Infectious	Radiation therapy	Procarbazine
Parapneumonic	Meig's syndrome	Practolol
Tuberculosis		Bromocriptine
Fungal	Lymphatic disease	Minoxidil
Viral	Chylothorax	Bleomycin
Parasitic	Lymphangioleiomyomatosis	Methotrexate
Abdominal abscess	Yellow nail syndrome	Mitomycin
Hepatitis		
Noninfectious gastrointestinal	Collagen vascular disease	Trauma
Pancreatitis	Lupus erythematosus	
Esophageal rupture	Rheumatoid arthritis	Vasculitis
Abdominal surgery	Sjögren's syndrome	Wegner's granulomatosis
Variceal sclerotherapy		Churg-Strauss syndrome
	Diseases That Can Present with Transudative or Exudative Effusions	
	Pulmonary embolism (usually exudate)	Diuresed transudate

[a]Table 1 from Bartter T, Santarelli R, Akers SM, Bratter MR. The evaluation of pleural effusion. Chest 1994;106:1210.

in pressure in the pleural space, increased permeability of the microvascular circulation, impaired lymphatic drainage from the pleural space, and migration of fluid from the peritoneal space (22).

There are a wide variety of causes of pleural effusion, ranging from infection to neoplasms (Table 18-2) (46,55). Pleural effusions are often divided into exudates and transudates (46). Exudative pleural effusions meet at least one of the following criteria, whereas transudative pleural effusions meet none of them: pleural fluid protein/serum protein ratio greater than 0.5; pleural fluid lactic acid dehydrogenase (LDH)/serum LDH ratio greater than 0.6; pleural fluid LDH ratio greater than two thirds of the normal serum LDH. Transudates are clear, straw-colored, have a low protein concentration, and have few cells. Whether a pleural effusion is a transudate or an exudate is helpful in the differential diagnosis since each pattern is associated with a group of characteristic disorders. In addition, there are a variety of other features such as pH and glucose levels that are helpful in sorting out the underlying cause.

Clinical Features. The clinical presentation of pleural effusion varies depending on the cause of the effusion and the rapidity of accumulation of the fluid. Some patients develop pleuritic chest pain, dyspnea, and cough. Others are asymptomatic and the effusion is found on a chest radiograph.

Table 18-3

EXUDATIVE PLEURAL FLUID: DIFFERENTIAL DIAGNOSIS[a]

Decreased Glucose (<60mg/dL)	Increased Red Blood Cells (>100,000/mm^3)
Complicated parapneumonic	Trauma
Rheumatoid	Malignancy
Malignant	Pulmonary embolism
Tuberculous	Hematocrit >50 percent of systemic level (hemothorax)
Paragonimiasis	Increased Lymphocytes (>50%)
Decreased pH (<7.2)	Lymphoma
Empyema	Other malignancy
Complicated parapneumonic	Chronic infection
Rheumatoid	Tuberculosis
Esophageal rupture	Fungi
Tuberculosis	Postpericardiotomy syndrome
Malignancy	Sarcoidosis
Paragonimiasis	Increased Eosinophils
Hemothorax	Air in pleural space
Systemic acidosis	Blood in pleural space
Increased Amylase (> upper limit of normal for serum)	Drug-induced
	Nitrofurantoin
Esophageal rupture	Dantrolene
Pancreatitis	Asbestos
Malignancy	Malignancy
	Paragonimiasis

[a]Modified from reference 2a.

Ferrer et al. (15) found *idiopathic pleural effusions* in 13.5 percent of patients with pleural effusions. They reported clinical details in 40 patients (30 men and 10 women). The mean age was 54 years; presenting manifestations were chest pain (77.5 percent), dyspnea (52.5 percent), weight loss (14.6 percent), fever (12.2 percent), and pericardial effusion (5 percent). Approximately half of the patients had a positive tuberculin test. The pleural effusion was left (60 percent), right (32.5 percent), bilateral (7.5 percent), massive (7.5 percent), and higher than half the hemithorax (22.5 percent).

Small effusions are usually not detected on physical examination. Larger effusions produce diminished vesicular breath sounds, dullness to percussion, and decreased tactile fremitus. Egophony and bronchial sounds may be appreciated at the superior aspect of an effusion. A pleural friction rub, caused by irritation of the pleural surfaces, is sometimes audible.

Once pleural effusion is suspected, thoracentesis can be performed for diagnostic and therapeutic reasons. To avoid reexpansion pulmonary edema in the underlying lung, no more than 1,000 to 1,500 mL of pleural fluid is removed at one time. Pleural fluid obtained should be sent to the laboratory for analysis. Serum and pleural protein levels as well as serum and pleural LDH levels are used to distinguish between transudative and exudative effusions. If a transudate is confirmed, further diagnostic tests of the pleural fluid are usually not necessary.

If an exudate is present, however, further tests guided by the clinical situation help establish the etiology (Table 18-3). Rheumatoid pleural effusions are characteristically associated with pleural fluid glucose levels below 30 mg/dL. Small amounts of erythrocytes in the pleural fluid are seen with a traumatic thoracentesis. If the hematocrit of the pleural fluid is more than 50 percent of the serum hematocrit, hemothorax is present and thoracostomy tube drainage is usually required. The differential cell count of the pleural fluid is of more clinical use than the absolute cell count. If the pleural fluid contains predominantly polymorphonuclear leukocytes, it is due to an acute disease process such as pneumonia, pulmonary embolism, pancreatitis, intra-abdominal abscess, or early tuberculosis. If more than 50 percent of the leukocytes in an exudative pleural effusion are lymphocytes, a diagnosis of malignancy or tuberculosis should be strongly considered. If cytology and tuberculosis cultures are negative, pleural biopsy should be considered to establish a diagnosis. If the pleural fluid is turbid or milky, cholesterol and triglyceride levels should be obtained. Immunologic studies of the pleural fluid are helpful in selected cases. Patients with lupus pleuritis frequently have antinuclear antibody titers greater than 1:160 in the pleural fluid. Similarly, patients with rheumatoid pleuritis often have pleural fluid rheumatoid factor titers of 1:320 or higher. Pleural fluid from patients with undiagnosed exudative pleural effusions should be cultured for bacteria, mycobacteria, and fungi; Gram stain, acid-fast bacillus smear, and fungal stain are useful.

In most cases, the cause of the pleural effusion is apparent after the initial clinical assessment and a diagnostic thoracentesis. A needle biopsy of the pleura is useful mainly for establishing the diagnosis of tuberculous pleural effusions. In patients with tuberculous pleuritis, the initial biopsy is positive for granulomas in 60 to 80 percent of cases. When tuberculous pleuritis is suspected, a portion of the pleural biopsy specimen should be cultured for mycobacteria because this increases the overall diagnostic yield.

Hepatic Hydrothorax. Pleural effusions occur in about 5 percent of patients with cirrhosis and ascites. The effusion results from the direct movement of peritoneal fluid into the pleural space through small holes in the diaphragm. In addition, the hypoalbuminemia accompanying the cirrhosis may contribute to the formation of the pleural effusion. The effusions are typically right-sided and frequently are large enough to produce severe dyspnea.

Parapneumonic Effusions. A parapneumonic effusion is any pleural effusion associated with underlying pneumonia, lung abscess, or bronchiectasis. Parapneumonic effusion is the most common cause of exudative pleural effusion. It occurs because of inflammation and increased permeability of the pleura adjacent to an area of parenchymal infection. A complicated parapneumonic effusion is one that has become loculated or filled with proteinaceous fibrinous debris. An *empyema* refers to frank pus in the pleural space. Organisms are present in Gram-stained pleural fluid of patients with an empyema. Gram-negative anaerobic organisms are responsible for most culture-positive parapneumonic effusions in adults.

Hemothorax. Hemothorax is blood within the pleural space. It is a recognized complication of infection, malignancy involving the pleura, or rarely, rupture of the aorta.

Malignant Pleural Effusion. This occurs secondary to cancerous involvement of the pleura and is the second most common type of exudative pleural effusion. Pleural effusion in malignancy occurs because of tumor obstruction of pleural lymphatic drainage, obstructive pneumonia, or direct metastatic spread to the pleural surface. Malignant pleural effusions are most commonly seen in patients with lung cancer, breast cancer, stomach cancer, or lymphoma.

Chylothorax. Chylothorax is the accumulation of lymphatic fluid within the pleural space (30). It occurs when the thoracic duct is disrupted and chyle leaks into the pleural cavity. The effusion has a high concentration of emulsified fats: chylothorax is associated with pleural fluid triglyceride levels over 110 mg/dL (49). If triglyceride levels are between 50 and 100 mg/dL, lipoprotein analysis should be performed to identify chylomicrons and confirm the diagnosis of chylothorax (49). With *pseudochylothorax,* the pleural fluid cholesterol level is elevated, but the triglyceride level is normal.

Chylothorax is associated with thoracic malignancies, lymphangioleiomyomatosis, lymphangiomatosis, traumatic rupture of the thoracic duct, and superior vena cava thrombosis (30). In over 50 percent of malignancies the tumor is a malignant lymphoma (30). Rare cases of congenital chylothorax occur and there is a mortality rate of 30 percent (30). Chylothorax occurs in 17 percent of patients with Gorham's syndrome, which is an intraosseous proliferation of vascular or lymphatic channels that results in the disappearance of bones (51).

Radiologic Findings. The typical radiographic manifestation of pleural effusion is

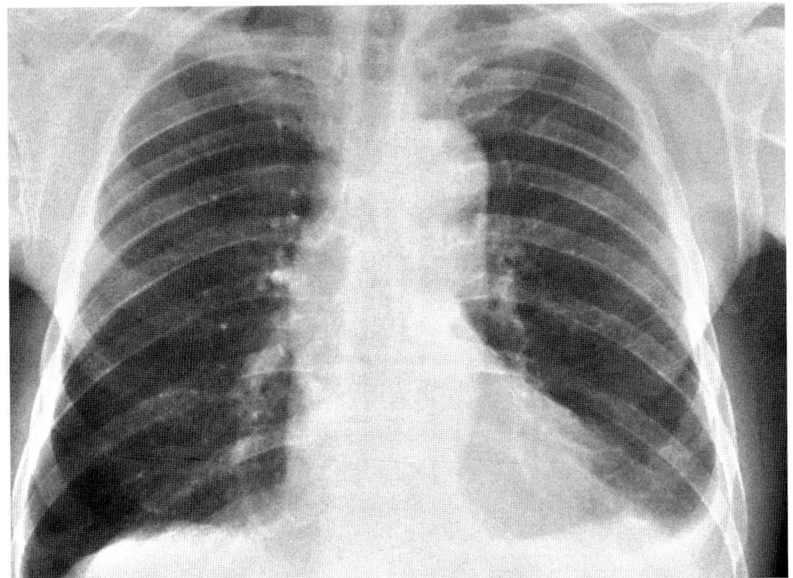

Figure 18-5

PLEURAL EFFUSION

Pleural effusion in a 66-year-old male with a history of rheumatoid arthritis and occupational exposure to asbestos. PA chest radiograph demonstrates blunting of the left costophrenic angle by the pleural fluid. It can be estimated that there is at least 200 mL of fluid in the pleural space.

blunting of a posterior or lateral costophrenic angle on upright radiography (fig. 18-5). The earliest visualization of pleural effusion is accomplished on lateral radiographs because blunting of the posterior costophrenic angle occurs with as little as 25 mL of pleural fluid. By the time costophrenic angle blunting is visualized on a frontal radiograph, the amount of pleural fluid is usually at least 200 mL (7). As most effusions are freely mobile in the pleural space, decubitus radiography can markedly increase the sensitivity for fluid visualization, detecting as little as 5 mL of fluid (40). Cross-sectional imaging studies such as CT, ultrasound, and MRI are also highly sensitive for detecting pleural fluid. Pleural fluid may become loculated and appear as a fixed, nonmobile pleural "mass." In these patients, the clinical features of infection point to a pleural abscess or empyema.

Histologic Findings. Pleural fluid cytology is diagnostic in 40 to 90 percent of patients with malignant pleural effusion, depending on the tumor type, the amount of fluid submitted, and the skill of the cytologist. Immunohistochemical tests using monoclonal antibodies can facilitate the differentiation of adenocarcinoma cells, benign mesothelial cells, and malignant mesothelial cells. In patients in whom malignancy is suspected, if the initial thoracentesis is negative, a second thoracentesis should be performed because this has a higher yield for malignant cells than a closed pleural biopsy.

Pleural biopsies from patients with idiopathic pleural effusion show varying degrees of chronic inflammation and fibrosis. The main role of pleural biopsy is to exclude underlying causes such as infection, granulomatous inflammation, or tumor. Pleural tissue from patients with hemothorax is likely to show acute or chronic hemorrhage. Careful examination should be made for tumor cells. Pleural specimens from patients with chylothorax should be examined for lesions of lymphangioleiomyomatosis as well as malignancy.

Treatment and Prognosis. In most patients, the pleural effusion spontaneously resolves within months, but in about 10 percent relapses occur. The initial step in the management of a patient with a malignant pleural effusion is to identify the site of the primary tumor so that a decision concerning chemotherapy and radiotherapy can be made. The treatment of complicated parapneumonic effusions and empyemas requires antibiotic therapy and usually requires thoracostomy tube drainage or surgical decortication. Chest tube drainage is indicated if there is gross pus in the pleural space, if microorganisms are visible on Gram stain of the pleural fluid, if the pleural fluid pH is less than 7.0, or if the pleural fluid glucose is less than 50 mg/dL. Successful chest tube drainage of a complicated parapneumonic effusion is associated with improvement in the clinical and radiologic status of the patient within 24 to 48 hours. Lack of improvement indicates that either the pleural drainage is unsatisfactory or the antibiotic coverage is inadequate. In such situations, ultrasound or CT examination of the chest should be performed to assess the adequacy of the pleural drainage. Another chest tube should be inserted or the patient should be taken to surgery if the pleural space has been inadequately drained. This decision should be based on the clinical status of the patient and not solely on radiologic data.

If medical management of the underlying disease fails to control the pleural effusion or there is recurrent malignant pleural effusions, it may be necessary to perform a tube thoracostomy followed by chemical pleurodesis. Pleurodesis is accomplished by injecting an agent into the pleural space that creates an intense inflammatory response, resulting in fusion of the visceral and parietal pleurae and obliteration of the pleural space.

PLEURITIS

Definition. Pleuritis is an inflammation of the pleura. Pleurisy or pleuritic chest pain is the most common symptom of patients with pleuritis. A spectrum of histologic patterns of pleuritis can occur ranging from acute, to chronic, fibrosing, eosinophilic, granulomatous, and xanthomatous, as well as fat necrosis.

Pleuritis occurs in patients of any age or gender and in a variety of clinical situations (Tables 18-2 and 18-4). In young patients (less than 40 years old), the most common etiologies are idiopathic (presumably viral infection in 53 percent of the cases), infectious pneumonitis (18 percent), and pulmonary embolism (21 percent) (8). Immunologic causes of pleurisy are also common. Pleural involvement in patients with connective tissue diseases may occur in previously diagnosed patients or may be a presenting manifestation that does not correlate with other signs of systemic disease activity. In the postcardiac injury syndrome, the pleurisy usually begins approximately 3 weeks following cardiac injury (50); the pain may be recurrent over several months. Drug-induced pleural disease is relatively uncommon compared to drug-induced parenchymal lung disease (39). Many drugs have been associated with the development of pleuritis (especially chemotherapeutic agents or drugs associated with a lupus-like syndrome) (39). Radiation therapy can produce pleurisy (with and without associated effusions), usually occurring within 6 months of treatment. Other events or illnesses that cause pleurisy include asbestos-related pleural disease, uremia, yellow nail syndrome, and lymphangioleiomyomatosis.

Table 18-4

CAUSES OF PLEURITIS

Infection
Collagen vascular disease
Neoplastic infiltration
Drug-induced
Pneumoconiosis
Iatrogenic causes
Pleurodesis: talc or tetracycline
Trauma
Gastrointestinal disorders
Pancreatitis

Clinical Features. The onset of pleuritic chest pain is usually sudden. Pleuritic pain arises from the inflammation involving the parietal pleura (as the visceral pleura lacks innervation) and is localized directly over the affected area. If the central diaphragmatic surface is affected, the pain may be referred to the shoulder or neck via the phrenic nerve. Irritation of the posterior and peripheral portions of the diaphragmatic pleura (supplied by the lower six intercostal nerves) results in pain referred to the epigastric region of the lower chest wall and may simulate intra-abdominal disease. The pain varies from vague discomfort to intense, sharp, burning or stabbing pain. Characteristically, the pain varies with the respiratory cycle. In fact it is the intensification of the pain with inspiration that is the hallmark of pleuritic pain. Similarly, coughing, yawning, laughing, or any other movement of the chest wall may exacerbate the discomfort. Given the variety of inciting factors for pleurisy, the associated symptoms may also be quite variable. Dyspnea and cough may be present.

Physical examination may reveal rapid shallow (often grunting) respirations with decreased diaphragmatic excursion because deep breathing induces pain. A pleural friction rub (squeaky rubbing sound) may be auscultated,

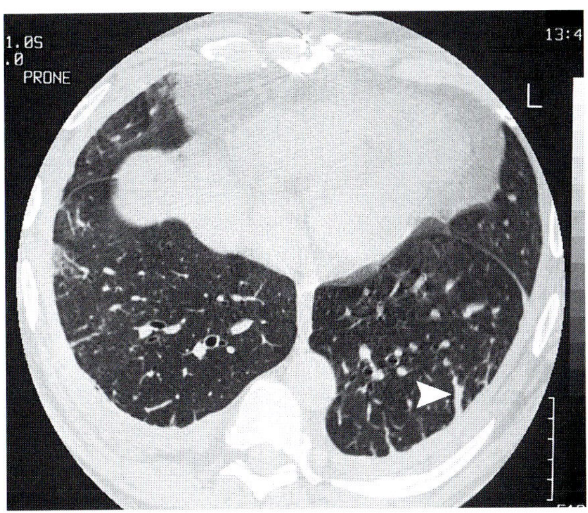

Figure 18-6

DIFFUSE PLEURAL FIBROSIS IN AN ELDERLY MALE WITH DYSPNEA

Prone chest CT (lung window) demonstrates diffuse, relatively smooth pleural thickening and loss of volume in the lower lobes. There is prominent thickening of the interlobular septa (arrowhead).

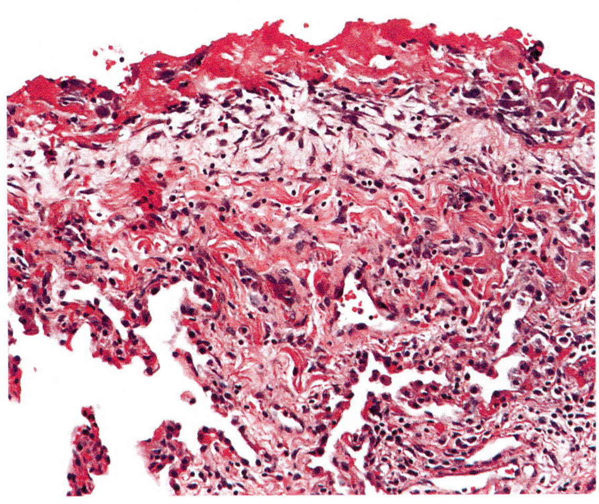

Figure 18-7

ACUTE FIBRINOUS PLEURITIS IN A PATIENT WITH RHEUMATOID ARTHRITIS

The pleural surface is coated with a layer of fibrin and the underlying connective tissue shows edema.

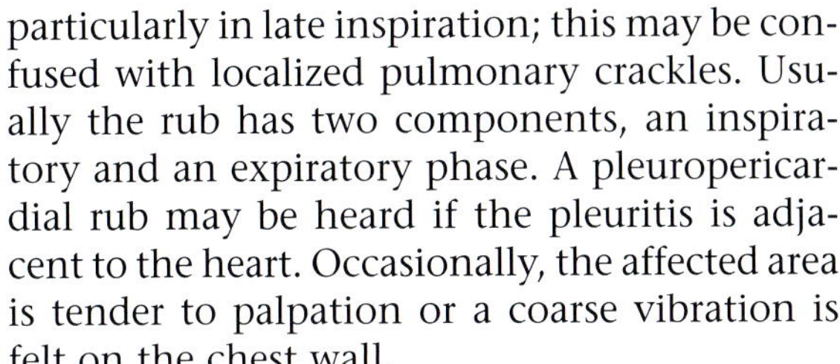

particularly in late inspiration; this may be confused with localized pulmonary crackles. Usually the rub has two components, an inspiratory and an expiratory phase. A pleuropericardial rub may be heard if the pleuritis is adjacent to the heart. Occasionally, the affected area is tender to palpation or a coarse vibration is felt on the chest wall.

Radiologic Findings. Radiographic evaluation includes chest radiographs in the upright and decubitus positions. The main importance of chest radiographs is to reveal the presence of parenchymal lung inflammation or pleural effusion. The earliest detection of pleural fluid may be in the posterior costophrenic sulcus on the lateral view (45). The typical manifestation of pleural fibrosis is pleural thickening which can be detected by chest radiography or earlier by cross-sectional imaging (18). Diffuse pleural fibrosis manifests radiographically as smooth, continuous pleural thickening over at least one fourth of the chest wall. The process may involve the entire pleural surface and may be confused with diffuse malignant mesothelioma (fig. 18-6) (18).

Histologic Findings. There are multiple histologic types of pleuritis (Table 18-5).

Acute Pleuritis. Bacterial pneumonia is one of the more common causes of acute pleuritis. This occurs by extension of acute inflammation from the lung parenchyma to the pleura. If severe, the process can invade through the pleura, causing an exudative pleural effusion and empyema. Acute fibrinous pleuritis is relatively common and may be noninfectious, as in collagen vascular disease (fig. 18-7). Acute pleuritis may also occur as multiple nodular neutrophilic abscesses (fig. 18-8).

Granulation tissue may be prominent in acute or chronic pleuritis (figs. 18-9, 18-10). It may appear as the granulation tissue seen in fibrous adhesions (fig. 18-9). Occasionally, the vascular proliferation may be so extensive that it raises concern for malignancy (fig. 18-10). However, the orderly arrangement of the vessels and the zonation effect, with maturation of the connective tissue and blood vessels toward the lung or chest wall (or lack of invasion), are helpful in recognizing the reactive nature of the lesion.

Chronic Pleuritis. Chronic pleuritis usually is characterized by mild to moderate infiltration by lymphocytes and plasma cells. Rarely, chronic pleuritis consists of extensive lymphocytic

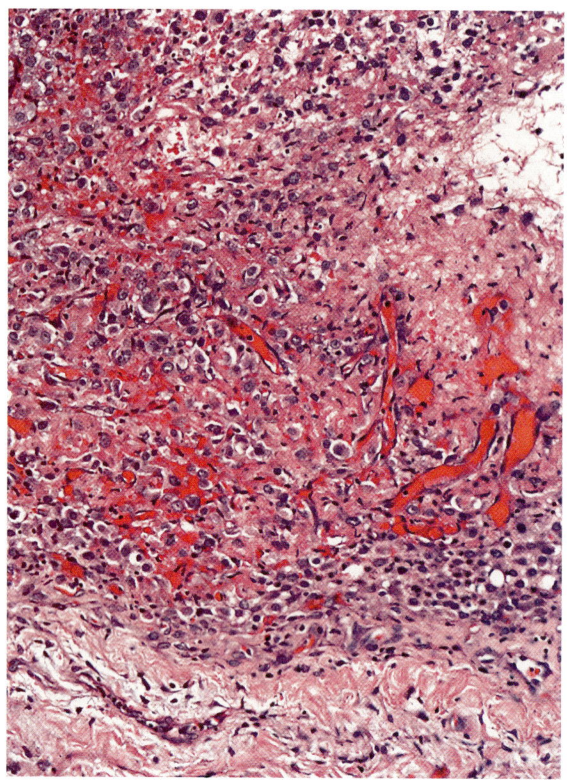

Figure 18-8

ACUTE SUPPURATIVE PLEURITIS

The pleura was studded with multiple, nodular, suppurative abscesses consisting of pockets of neutrophils.

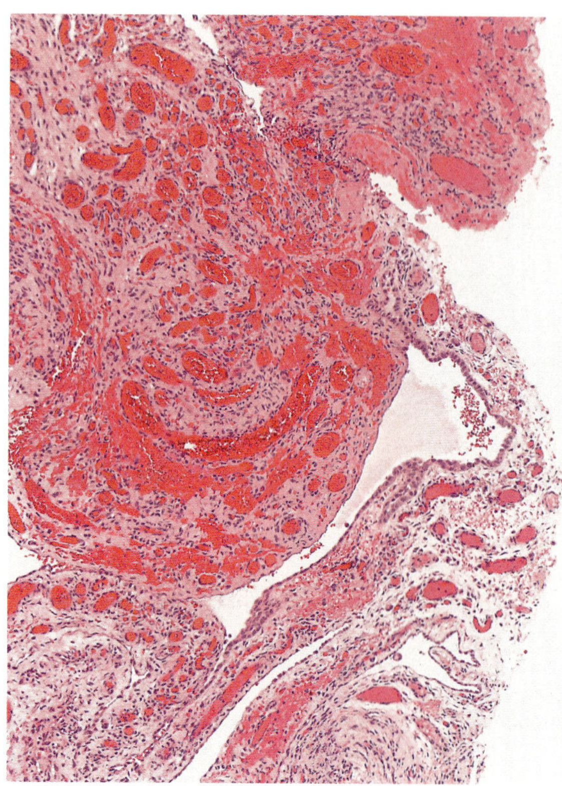

Figure 18-9

GRANULATION TISSUE IN PLEURAL ADHESION

Prominent blood vessel proliferation within this fibrous adhesion gives a granulation tissue–like appearance.

Table 18-5

HISTOLOGIC TYPES OF PLEURITIS

Acute
Suppurative
Fibrinous
Granulation tissue-like
Chronic
Lymphocytic/follicular
Fibrous
Plaque-like
Loculated
(Mesothelial hyperplasia)
Granulomatous
Non-necrotizing
Necrotizing
Foreign body reaction
Eosinophilic
Xanthomatous/xanthogranulomatous
Fat necrosis
Mixed patterns

infiltrates, with or without lymphoid follicles (fig. 18-11). This may raise concern for a malignant lymphoma.

Fibrosing Pleuritis. Fibrosing pleuritis is the fibrous thickening of the pleura (fig. 18-12). It consists of acellular dense fibrosis that may be associated with varying degrees of chronic inflammation. Most often, it is associated with another pathologic lesion, such as a tumor or an underlying condition such as a collagen vascular disease. Rare cases of severe cryptogenic fibrosing pleuritis with diffuse, sometimes bilateral, pleural thickening occur (9). Familial cryptogenic fibrosing pleuritis has been described in patients with Fanconi's syndrome (23). Another familial syndrome of fibrosing serositis was reported in two sisters with infantile contractures of fingers and toes in whom pleuritis, pericarditis, and synovitis were present (56). Plaque-like features can be seen focally (fig. 18-13) as can

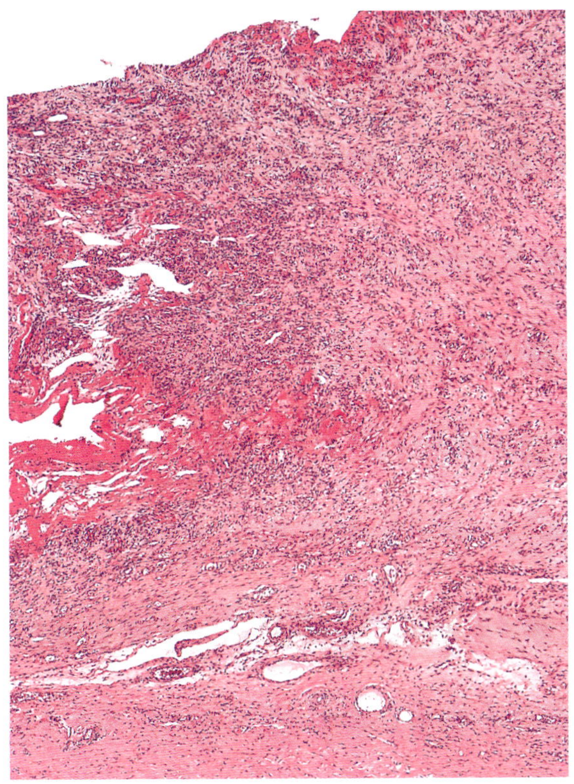

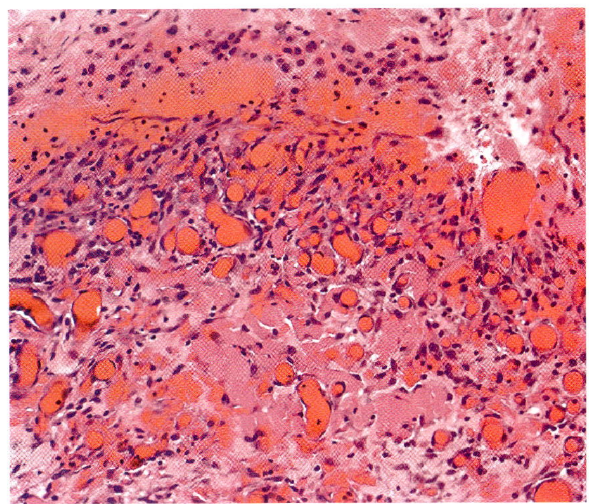

Figure 18-10

GRANULATION TISSUE: SEVERE

The vascular proliferation in this granulation tissue is so severe it raised concern for a vascular malignancy.

Left: The underlying chronic pleural fibrosis (bottom) sharply separated the vascular proliferation (top) from the underlying parietal pleura, so the granulation tissue was on the pleural surface associated with the inflammatory process.

Above: Numerous capillary-sized blood vessels formed

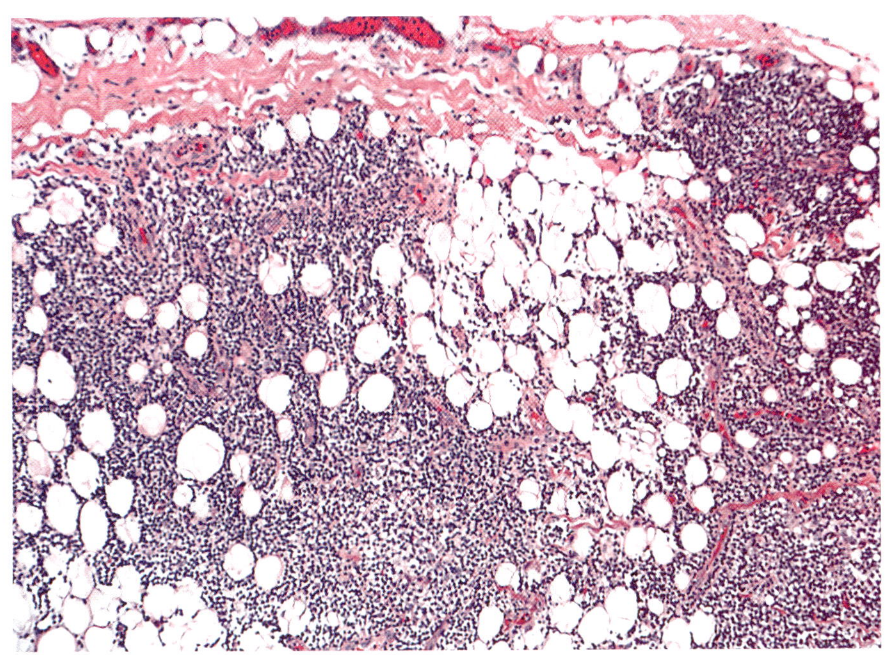

Figure 18-11

CHRONIC LYMPHOCYTIC PLEURITIS

The pleura is extensively infiltrated by lymphocytes and plasma cells.

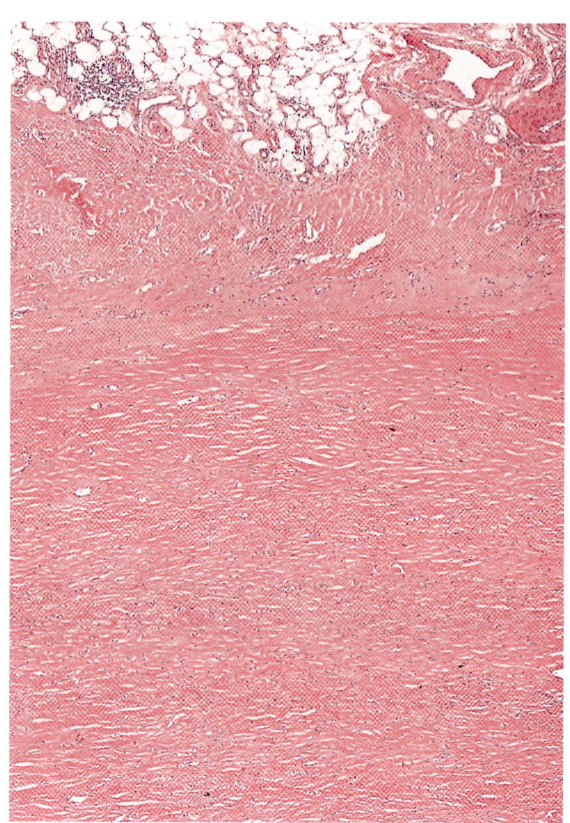

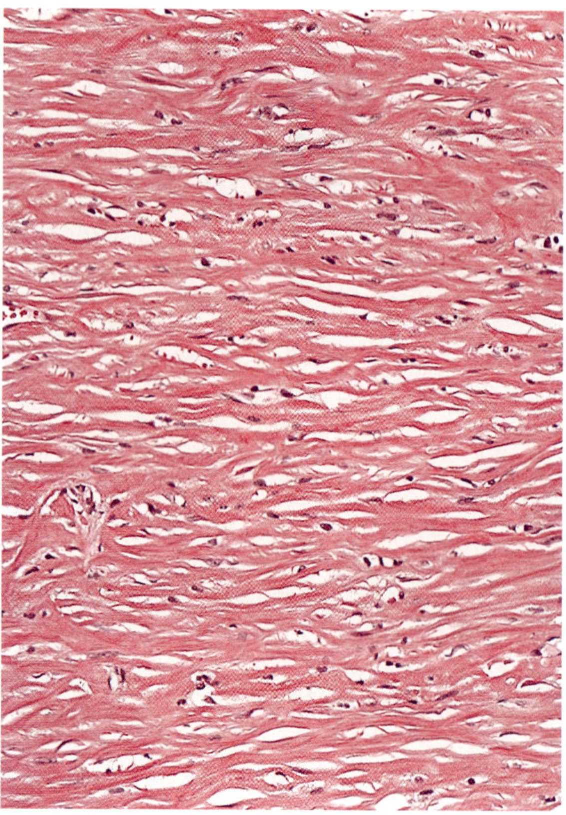

Figure 18-12

CHRONIC FIBROSING PLEURITIS

Left: The pleura is markedly thickened by dense fibrosis.
Right: The connective tissue is very dense, with only rare lymphocytes.

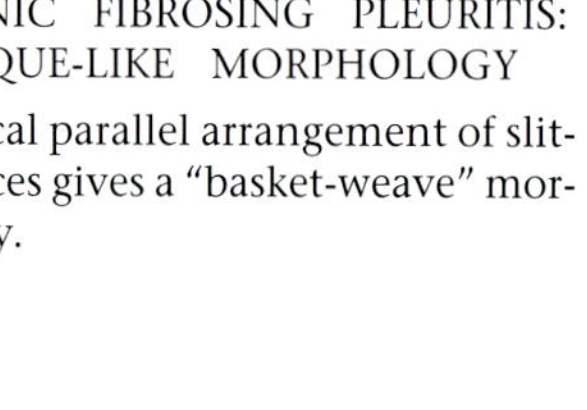

Figure 18-13

CHRONIC FIBROSING PLEURITIS: PLAQUE-LIKE MORPHOLOGY

Focal parallel arrangement of slit-like spaces gives a "basket-weave" morphology.

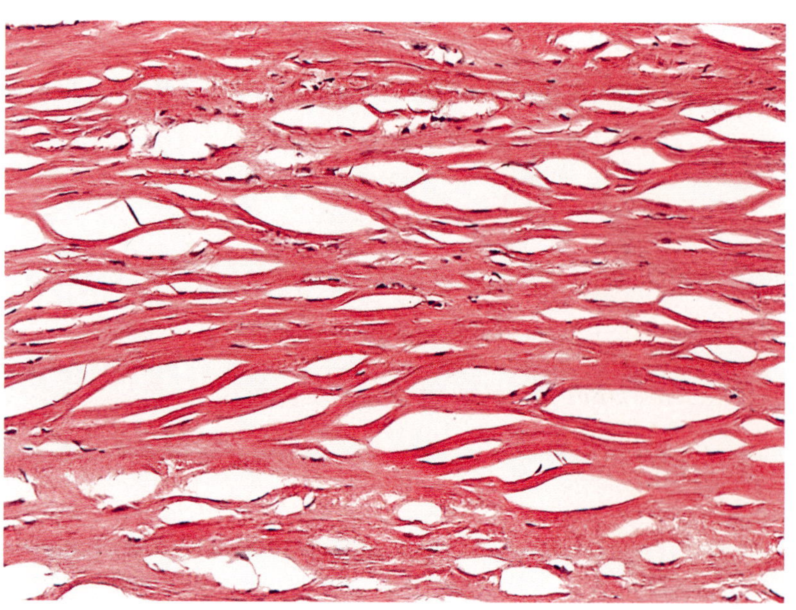

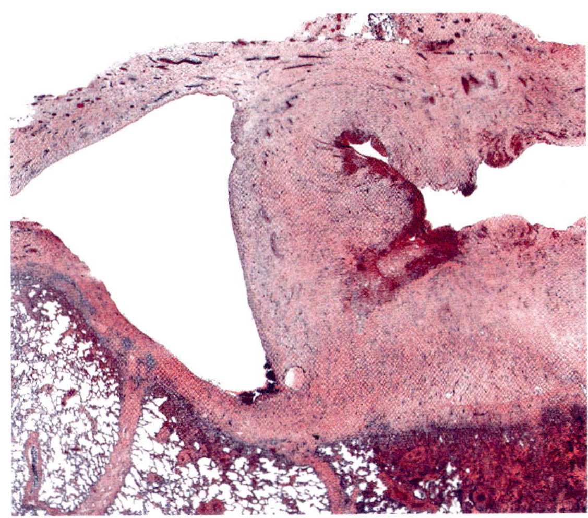

Figure 18-14

MULTILOCULAR CHRONIC FIBROSING PLEURITIS

The fibrosing pleuritis is forming two large cystic locular spaces.

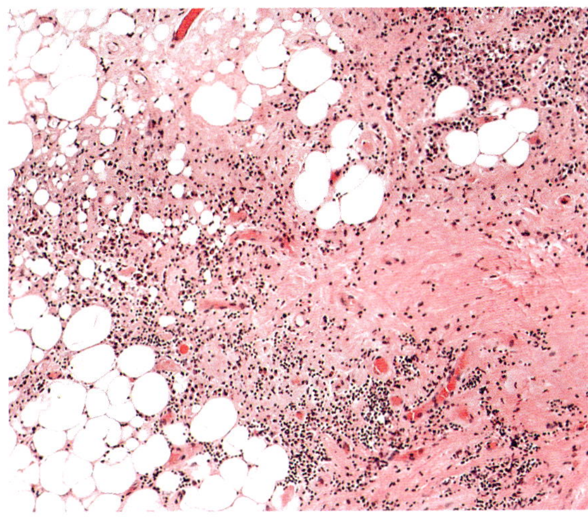

Figure 18-15

CHRONIC FIBROSING PLEURITIS INVOLVING FAT

Tongues of bland fibrous tissue extend into the fat of the parietal pleura. However, these areas consist purely of dense fibrous tissue without atypia or increased cellularity.

multilocular cystic spaces (fig. 18-14). In the presence of inflammation there may be distortion of cleft-like spaces; this appearance focally mimics that of desmoplastic malignant mesothelioma. However, the lack of invasion, necrosis, sarcomatous foci, and cytologic atypia allows for distinction (34).

The fibrous connective tissue may extend into the fat of the parietal pleura, mimicking invasive growth (fig. 18-15). However, these areas consist purely of dense fibrous tissue without atypia or increased cellularity. The presence of blood vessels running parallel to each other but perpendicular to the pleural surface in an orderly fashion is a feature that favors a benign process (fig. 18-16).

Hyperplasia of mesothelial cells is frequently seen in association with pleuritis. In most cases it is mild and inconspicuous, but in some cases it may be worrisome for malignancy (figs. 18-17, 18-18) (10). The lack of invasive growth and the presence of inflammation are two of the major criteria that point to a reactive process (10).

Reactive Eosinophilic Pleuritis. This is an incidental histologic finding associated with pneumothorax due to virtually any cause (2,35). It is characterized by fibrous thickening of the pleura associated with mesothelial cell hyperplasia and an inflammatory infiltrate that consists of histiocytes, eosinophils, and lymphocytes (fig. 18-

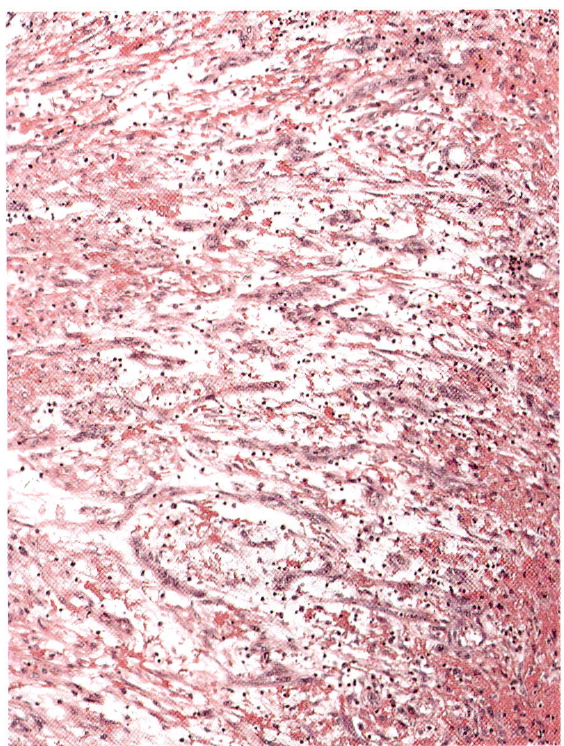

Figure 18-16

CHRONIC PLEURITIS WITH ORDERLY PARALLEL VASCULAR ORIENTATION

These blood vessels run parallel to each other but perpendicular to the pleural surface.

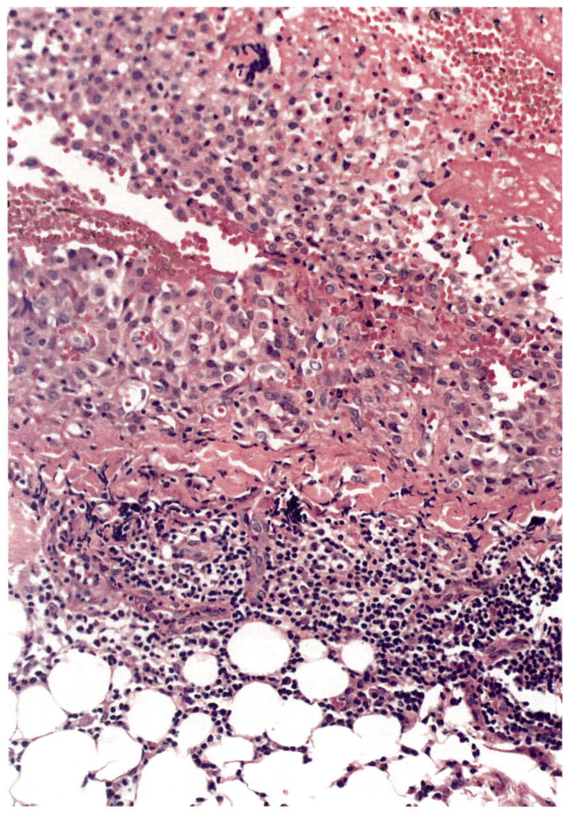

Figure 18-17

CHRONIC PLEURITIS WITH REACTIVE MESOTHELIAL HYPERPLASIA

In addition to chronic pleuritis (bottom) with inflammation in the underlying pleura, there is mesothelial hyperplasia along the surface, with no invasion.

19). Occasionally, the histiocytes are multinucleated and a few have grooved nuclei, resembling Langerhans' cell histiocytosis (fig. 18-19) (2,35). However, the cells do not express CD1a and are typically positive for KP1 (CD68), indicating they are histiocytes. In contrast to Langerhans' cell histiocytosis, which is primarily an interstitial nodular lesion within the lung parenchyma, reactive eosinophilic pleuritis is exclusively situated in the pleura. Rarely, eosinophilic vasculitis may be seen in the underlying lung parenchyma (33).

Granulomatous Pleuritis. Granulomatous pleuritis is necrotizing or non-necrotizing. The main differential diagnosis includes infection, especially tuberculous or fungal, sarcoidosis, and rare disorders such as Wegener's granulomatosis. In patients with rheumatoid arthritis, the possibility of rheumatoid nodules should be considered. In most cases, the presence of necrotizing granulomas strongly suggests infection. A foreign body reaction to material such as talc is another form of granulomatous pleuritis (fig. 18-20).

Xanthomatous Pleuritis. Occasionally, chronic pleuritis may be associated with a prominent accumulation of foamy macrophages (fig. 18-21). This can be mistaken for malignancies such as renal cell carcinoma, mesothelioma, or malignant melanoma, especially in a patient with a prior history of malignancy. Immunohistochemical positivity for KP1 confirms the histiocytic nature of the cells.

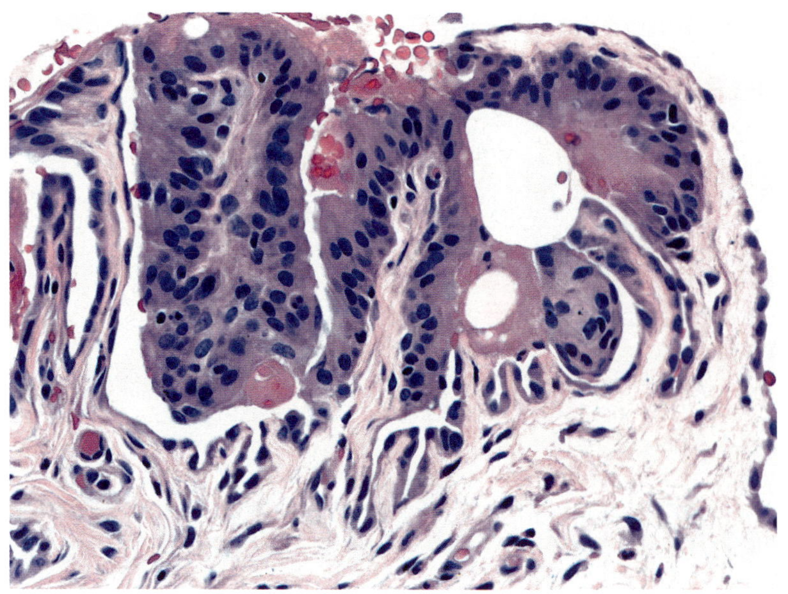

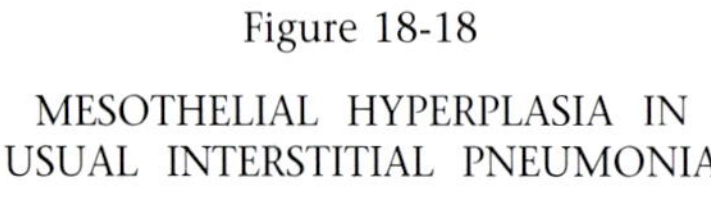

Figure 18-18

MESOTHELIAL HYPERPLASIA IN USUAL INTERSTITIAL PNEUMONIA

This prominent papillary mesothelial proliferation was an incidental finding in a case of usual interstitial pneumonia.

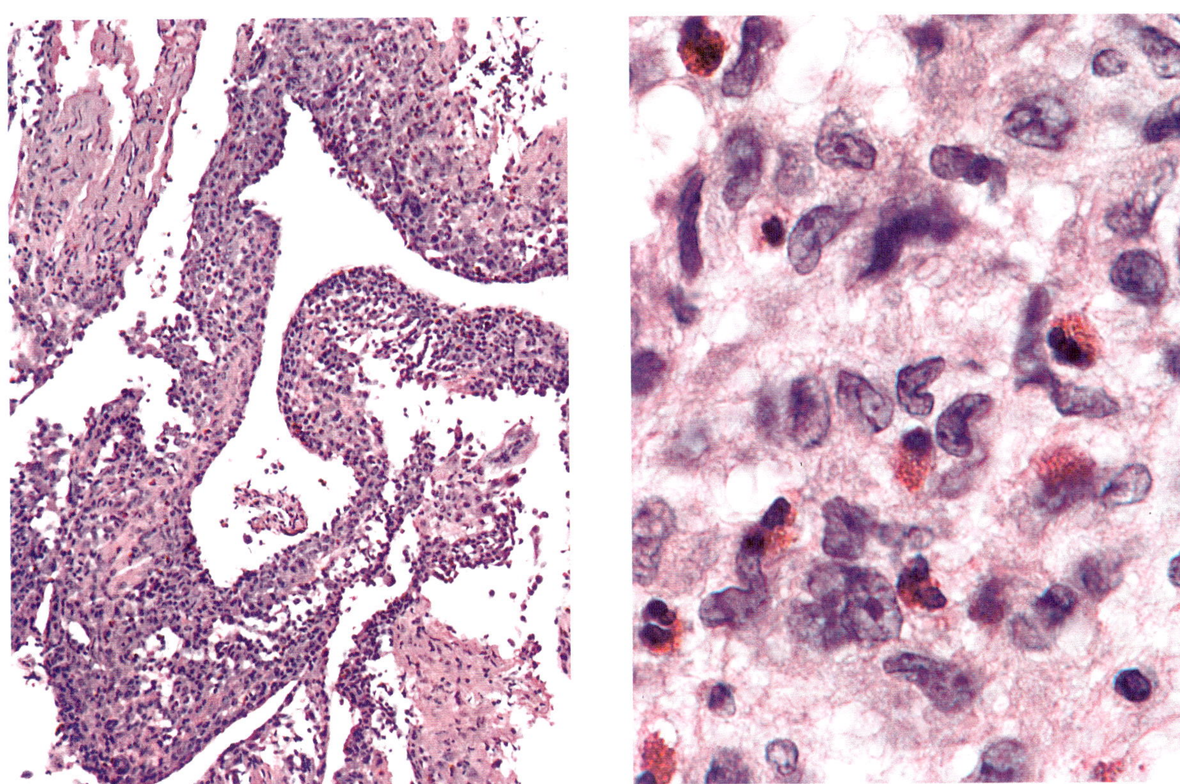

Figure 18-19

REACTIVE EOSINOPHILIC PLEURITIS

Left: The pleura is thickened by a chronic inflammatory infiltrate with mesothelial hyperplasia. Strips of the pleura are detached from the underlying lung in a somewhat papillary fashion.

Right: The infiltrate consists of histiocytes and eosinophils.

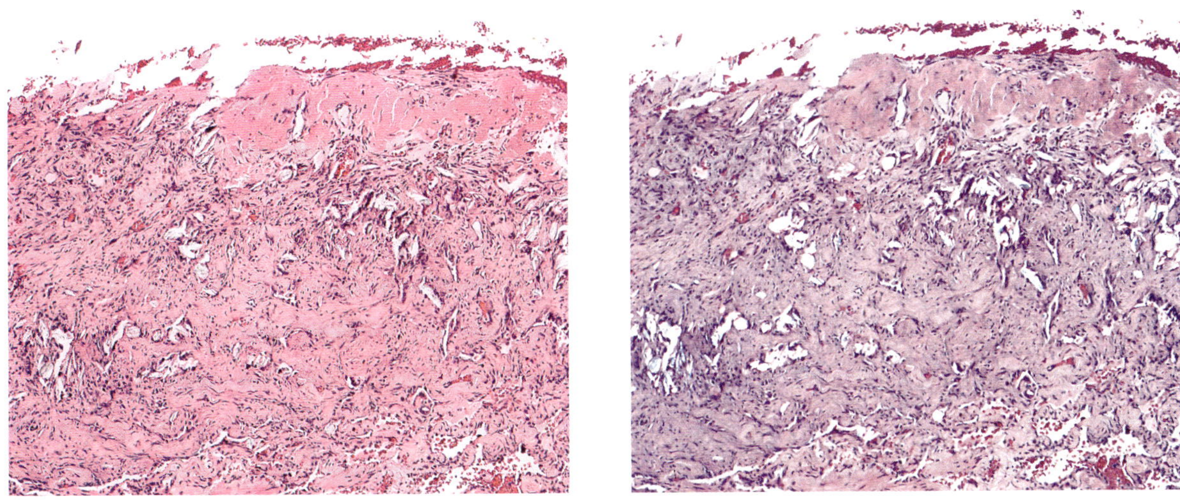

Figure 18-20

TALC PLEURITIS IN PATIENT FOLLOWING TALC PLEURODESIS

Left: Multiple foreign body giant cells are associated with crystalline particles of talc.

Right: These particles are birefringent with polarized light.

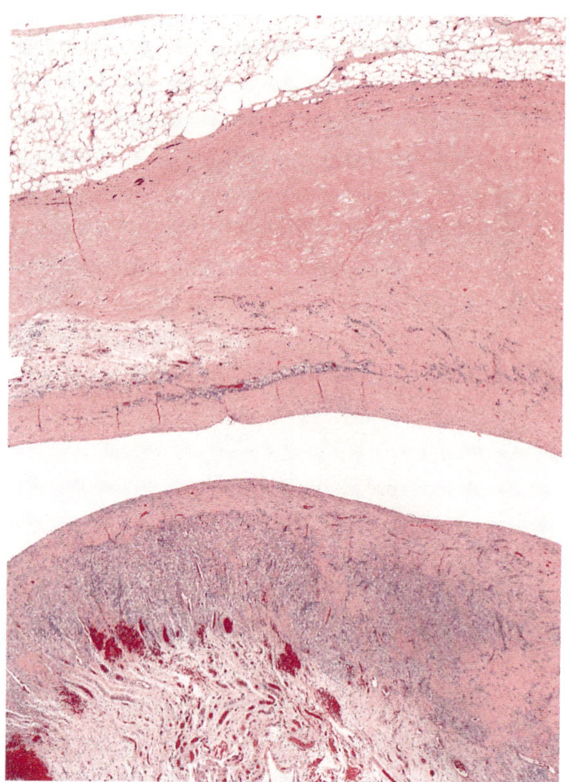

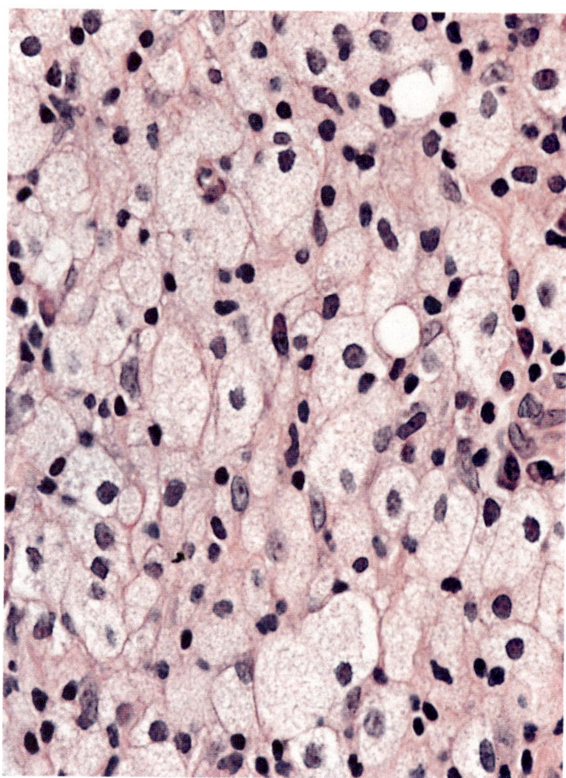

Figure 18-21

XANTHOMATOUS PLEURITIS

Left: There is fibrous thickening of the pleura associated with a prominent infiltrate of foamy macrophages.
Right: The infiltrate consists of foamy macrophages.

Fat Necrosis. Fat necrosis in parietal pleural soft tissues is a rare condition. It can be associated with trauma or as a complication of pancreatitis (1,13,26). It appears like fat necrosis in other locations, showing cavitation, a marked histiocytic reaction, acute and chronic inflammation, and fibrosis (fig. 18-22).

Differential Diagnosis. The clinical differential diagnosis of pleurisy involves distinction of the various precipitating causes noted in Table 18-2. In addition, the chest pain must be distinguished from that of other processes such as pneumothorax, pneumomediastinum, chest wall inflammation (myositis, neuritis, rib pathology, pleurodynia), and pericardial inflammation. Epidemic pleurodynia (Bornholm's disease [the devil's grip]) is severe pain in the side, generally associated with the Coxsackie B viral infection. It occurs at any age but is seen most commonly in children and young adults, usually as part of an epidemic. Pleurodynia is a disease of skeletal muscle.

Treatment and Prognosis. The treatment depends on the underlying cause of the pleuritis (for example, antibiotics for infection). Anti-inflammatory agents for pain relief may be of benefit while awaiting resolution of the primary disease process. Indomethacin has been shown to be effective in treating the pleurisy associated with infectious, embolic, and traumatically induced disease. Corticosteroids can produce dramatic improvement in patients with postmyocardial infarction syndrome. Codeine or other narcotics may be required but should be avoided because suppression of the cough reflex and hypoventilation may increase the risk of pneumonia. In patients with severe pain, intradermal lidocaine around the site of pain may provide dramatic relief. Rarely, intercostal nerve blocks are given with local anesthesia. General management of the associated pleural effusion is discussed above.

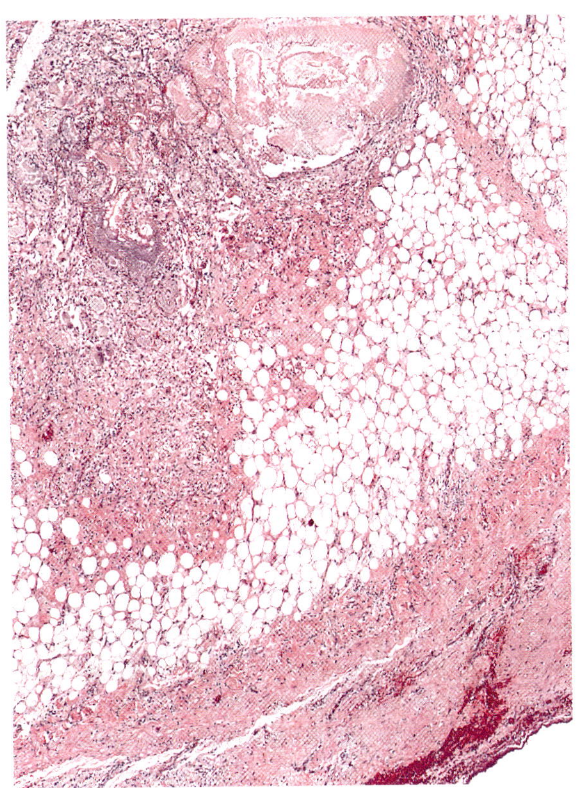

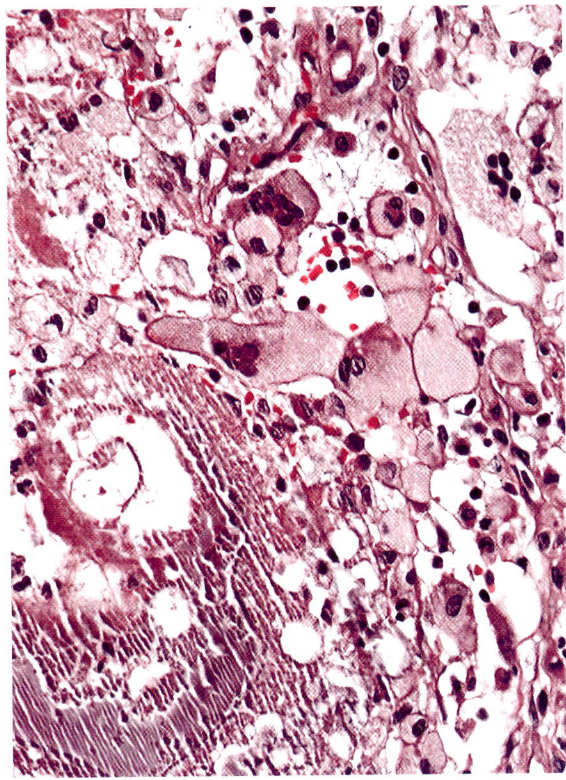

Figure 18-22

PLEURAL FAT NECROSIS IN PATIENT WITH PANCREATITIS

Left: The fat of the parietal pleura shows focal cavitary necrosis (left, top) and an extensive histiocytic infiltrate. Right: The necrosis (left) is surrounded by acute inflammation and multinucleated foamy histiocytes.

REFERENCES

1. Adams DB. Peripheral fat necrosis after penetrating pancreatic trauma: a case report. Am Surg 1993;59:769–71.
2. Askin FB, McCann BG, Kuhn C. Reactive eosinophilic pleuritis: a lesion to be distinguished from pulmonary eosinophilic granuloma. Arch Pathol Lab Med 1977;101:187–91.

2a. Bartter T, Santarelli R, Akers SM, Bratter MR. The evaluation of pleural effusion. Chest 1994;106: 1209–14.

3. Bense L, Eklund G, Wiman LG. Bilateral bronchial anomaly. A pathogenetic factor in spontaneous pneumothorax. Am Rev Respir Dis 1992;146:513–6.
4. Bense L, Eklund G, Wiman LG. Smoking and the increased risk of contracting spontaneous pneumothorax. Chest 1987;92:1009–12.
5. Bense L, Lewander R, Eklund G, Hedenstierna G, Wiman LG. Nonsmoking, non-alpha 1-antitrypsin deficiency-induced emphysema in nonsmokers with healed spontaneous pneumothorax, identified by computed tomography of the lungs. Chest 1993;103:433–8.
6. Bense L, Wiman LG, Hedenstierna G. Onset of symptoms in spontaneous pneumothorax: correlations to physical activity. Eur J Respir Dis 1987;71:181–6.
7. Blackmore CC, Black WC, Dallas RV, Crow HC. Pleural fluid volume estimation: a chest radiograph prediction rule. Acad Radiol 1996;3:103–9.
8. Branch WT, McNeil BJ. Analysis of the differential diagnosis and assessment of pleuritic chest pain in young adults. Am J Med 1983;75:671–9.
9. Buchanan DR, Johnston ID, Kerr IH, Hetzel MR, Corrin B, Turner-Warwick M. Cryptogenic bilateral fibrosing pleuritis. Br J Dis Chest 1988;82:186–93.

10. Churg A, Colby TV, Cagle P, et al. The separation of benign and malignant mesothelial proliferation. Am J Surg Pathol 2000;24:1183–200.
11. Cottin V, Streichenberger N, Gamondes JP, Thevenet F, Loire R, Cordier JF. Respiratory bronchiolitis in smokers with spontaneous pneumothorax. Eur Respir J 1998;12:702–4.
12. Cyr PV, Vincic L, Kay JM. Pulmonary vasculopathy in idiopathic spontaneous pneumothorax in young subjects. Arch Pathol Lab Med 2000;124:717–20.
13. Dahl PR, Su WP, Cullimore KC, Dicken CH. Pancreatic panniculitis. J Am Acad Dermatol 1995;33:413–7.
14. England GJ, Hill RC, Timberlake GA, et al. Resolution of experimental pneumothorax in rabbits by graded oxygen therapy. J Trauma 1998;45:333–4.
15. Ferrer JS, Munoz XG, Orriols RM, Light RW, Morell FB. Evolution of idiopathic pleural effusion: a prospective, long-term follow-up study. Chest 1996;109:1508–13.
16. Feuerstein IM, Archer A, Pluda JM, et al. Thin-walled cavities, cysts, and pneumothorax in Pneumocystis carinii pneumonia: further observations with histopathologic correlation. Radiology 1990;174:697–702.
17. Flieder DB, Moran CA, Travis WD, Koss MN, Mark EJ. Pleuro-pulmonary endometriosis and pulmonary ectopic deciduosis: a clinicopathologic and immunohistochemical study of 10 cases with emphasis on diagnostic pitfalls. Hum Pathol 1998;29:1495–503.
18. Fraser RS, Müller NL, Colman N, Pare PD. Pleural fibrosis. In: Fraser RS, Müller NL, Colman N, Pare PD, eds. Fraser and Pare's diagnosis of diseases of the chest, 4th ed. Philadelphia: WB Saunders; 1999:2795–806.
19. Fraser RS, Müller NL, Colman N, Pare PD. Pneumothorax. In: Fraser RS, Müller NL, Colman N, Pare PD, eds. Fraser and Par's diagnosis of diseases of the chest, 4th ed. Philadelphia: WB Saunders; 1999:2781–94.
20. Gupta D, Hansell A, Nichols T, Duong T, Ayres JG, Strachan D. Epidemiology of pneumothorax in England. Thorax 2000;55:666–71.
21. Hall JR, Pyeritz RE, Dudgeon DL, Haller JA Jr. Pneumothorax in the Marfan syndrome: prevalence and therapy. Ann Thorac Surg 1984;37:500–4.
22. Hammar SP. Pleural diseases. In: Dail DH, Hammar SP, eds. Pulmonary pathology, 2nd ed. New York: Springer-Verlag; 1994:1463–579.
23. Hayes JP, Wiggins J, Ward K, Muldowney F, FitzGerald MX. Familial cryptogenic fibrosing pleuritis with Fanconi's syndrome (renal tubular acidosis). A new syndrome. Chest 1995;107:576–8.
24. Jordan KG, Kwong JS, Flint J, Muller NL. Surgically treated pneumothorax. Radiologic and pathologic findings. Chest 1997;111:280–5.
25. Kawakami Y, Irie T, Kamishima K. Stature, lung height, and spontaneous pneumothorax. Respiration 1982;43:35–40.
26. Lee MS, Lowe PM, Nevell DF, Fryer J, Le Guay J. Subcutaneous fat necrosis following traumatic pancreatitis. Australas J Dermatol 1995;36:196–8.
27. Lesur O, Delorme N, Fromaget JM, Bernadac P, Polu JM. Computed tomography in the etiologic assessment of idiopathic spontaneous pneumothorax. Chest 1990;98:341–7.
28. Lichter I, Gwynne JF. Spontaneous pneumothorax in young subjects. A clinical and pathological study. Thorax 1971;26:409–17.
29. Light RW. Management of spontaneous pneumothorax. Am Rev Respir Dis 1993;148:245–8.
30. Light RW. Pleural diseases, 3rd ed. Baltimore: Williams & Wilkins; 1995.
31. Light RW, O'Hara VS, Moritz TE, et al. Intrapleural tetracycline for the prevention of recurrent spontaneous pneumothorax. Results of a Department of Veterans Affairs cooperative study. JAMA 1990;264:2224–30.
32. Lippert HL, Lund O, Blegvad S, Larsen HV. Independent risk factors for cumulative recurrence rate after first spontaneous pneumothorax. Eur Respir J 1991;4:324–31.
33. Luna E, Tomashefski JF Jr, Brown D, Clarke RE, Kleinerman J. Reactive eosinophilic pulmonary vascular infiltration in patients with spontaneous pneumothorax. Am J Surg Pathol 1994;18:195–9.
34. Mangano WE, Cagle PT, Churg A, Vollmer RT, Roggli VL. The diagnosis of desmoplastic malignant mesothelioma and its distinction from fibrous pleurisy: a histologic and immunohistochemical analysis of 31 cases including p53 immunostaining. Am J Clin Pathol 1998;110:191–9.
35. McDonnell TJ, Crouch EC, Gonzalez JG. Reactive eosinophilic pleuritis. A sequela of pneumothorax in pulmonary eosinophilic granuloma. Am J Clin Pathol 1989;91:107–11.
36. Melton LJ III, Hepper NG, Offord KP. Incidence of spontaneous pneumothorax in Olmsted County, Minnesota: 1950 to 1974. Am Rev Respir Dis 1979;120:1379–82.
37. Melton LJ III, Hepper NG, Offord KP. Influence of height on the risk of spontaneous pneumothorax. Mayo Clin Proc 1981;56:678–82.
38. Moran JF, Jones RH, Wolfe WG. Regional pulmonary function during experimental unilateral pneumothorax in the awake state. J Thorac Cardiovasc Surg 1977;74:396–402.

39. Morelock SY, Sahn SA. Drugs and the pleura. Chest 1999;116:212–21.
40. Moskowitz H, Platt RT, Schachar R, Mellins H. Roentgen visualization of minute pleural effusion. An experimental study to determine the minimum amount of pleural fluid visible on a radiograph. Radiology 1973;109:33–5.
41. Norris RM, Jones JG, Bishop JM. Respiratory gas exchange in patients with spontaneous pneumothorax. Thorax 1968;23:427–33.
42. Northfield TC. Oxygen therapy for spontaneous pneumothorax. Br Med J 1971;4:86–8.
43. O'Rourke JP, Yee ES. Civilian spontaneous pneumothorax. Treatment options and long-term results. Chest 1989;96:1302–6.
44. Peng MJ, Wang NS, Vargas FS, Light RW. Subclinical surface alterations of human pleura. A scanning electron microscopic study. Chest 1994;106:351–3.
45. Rudikoff JC. Early detection of pleural fluid. Chest 1980;77:109–11.
46. Sahn SA. The pathophysiology of pleural effusions. Annu Rev Med 1990;41:7–13.
47. Sahn SA, Heffner JE. Spontaneous pneumothorax. N Engl J Med 2000;342:868–74.
48. Seremetis MG. The management of spontaneous pneumothorax. Chest 1970;57:65–8.
49. Staats BA, Ellefson RD, Budahn LL, Dines DE, Prakash UB, Offord K. The lipoprotein profile of chylous and nonchylous pleural effusions. Mayo Clin Proc 1980;55:700–4.
50. Stelzner TJ, King TE, Antony VB, Sahn SA. The pleuropulmonary manifestations of the postcardiac injury syndrome. Chest 1983;84: 383–7.
51. Tie ML, Poland GA, Rosenow EC III. Chylothorax in Gorham's syndrome. A common complication of a rare disease. Chest 1994;105:208–13.
52. Tocino IM, Miller MH, Fairfax WR. Distribution of pneumothorax in the supine and semirecumbent critically ill adult. AJR Am J Roentgenol 1985;144:901–5.
53. Tocino IM, Westcott JL. Barotrauma. Radiol Clin North Am 1996;34:59–81.
54. Tomashefski JF Jr, Dahms B, Bruce M. Pleura in pneumothorax. Comparison of patients with cystic fibrosis and idiopathic spontaneous pneumothorax. Arch Pathol Lab Med 1985;109:910–6.
55. Valdes L, Alvarez D, Valle JM, Pose A, San Jose E. The etiology of pleural effusions in an area with high incidence of tuberculosis. Chest 1996; 109:158–62.
56. Verma UN, Misra R, Radhakrisnan S, Maitra SC, Agarwal SS, Singh RR. A syndrome of fibrosing pleuritis, pericarditis, and synovitis with infantile contractures of fingers and toes in 2 sisters: "familial fibrosing serositis." J Rheumatol 1995;22:2349–55.
57. Wait MA, Estrera A. Changing clinical spectrum of spontaneous pneumothorax. Am J Surg 1992;164:528–31.
58. Waitches GM, Stern EJ, Dubinsky TJ. Usefulness of the double-wall sign in detecting pneumothorax in patients with giant bullous emphysema. AJR Am J Roentgenol 2000;174:1765–8.
59. Watt AG. Spontaneous pneumothorax. A review of 210 consecutive admissions to Royal Perth Hospital. Med J Aust 1978;1:186–8.
60. Weissberg D, Refaely Y. Pneumothorax. Chest 2000;117:1279–85.
61. Withers JN, Fishback ME, Kiehl PV, Hannon JL. Spontaneous pneumothorax. Am J Surg 2000;108:772–6.

Index*

*Numbers in boldface indicate table and figure pages.